CLINICAL TEXTBOOK
FOR VETERINARY TECHNICIANS

CLINICAL TEXTBOOK
FOR VETERINARY TECHNICIANS

Fifth Edition

DENNIS M. McCURNIN, DVM, MS, DIPL ACVS

Professor, Department of Veterinary Clinical Sciences
Hospital Director, Veterinary Teaching Hospital and Clinics
School of Veterinary Medicine
Louisiana State University
Baton Rouge, Louisiana

JOANNA M. BASSERT, VMD

Professor and Director
Program of Veterinary Technology
Manor College
Jenkintown, Pennsylvania

W.B. SAUNDERS COMPANY
A Division of Harcourt Brace and Company
Philadelphia   London   New York   St. Louis   Sydney   Tokyo

W.B. SAUNDERS COMPANY

A Division of Harcourt Brace & Company

The Curtis Center
Independence Square West
Philadelphia, Pennsylvania 19106

Editor-in-Chief: *John A. Schrefer*
Editorial Manager: *Linda L. Duncan*
Senior Developmental Editor: *Teri Merchant*
Project Manager: *John Rogers*
Project Specialist: *Beth Hayes*
Interior/Cover Design: *Kathi Gosche*
Cover Art and Chapter Opener Art: *Breaking the Silence,* oil, © Anne Embree

Library of Congress Cataloging in Publication Data
Clinical textbook for veterinary technicians / [edited by] Dennis M. McCurnin, Joanna M. Bassert.—5th ed.
    p. ; cm.
    Includes bibliographical references and index.
    ISBN 0-7216-9164-1
      1. Veterinary medicine. I. McCurnin, Dennis M. II. Bassert, Joanna M.
    [DNLM: 1. Veterinary Medicine. 2. Animal Technicians. SF 745 C641 2002]
    SF745 .C625 2002
    636.089—dc21

                              2001020898

CLINICAL TEXTBOOK FOR VETERINARY TECHNICIANS   ISBN 0-7216-9164-1

FIFTH EDITION

Printed in the United States of America

Last digit is the print number: 9 8 7 6 5 4 3 2 1

DEDICATION

We dedicate the fifth edition to the thousands of practicing Veterinary Technicians who provide the technical support needed in high-quality veterinary medical practices worldwide.

We also dedicate this volume to our best teachers:

To my grandson, Evan M. McCurnin—DMM

To my mother, Lauretta H. Bassert—JMB

CONTRIBUTOR LIST

Marvene Augustus, PharmD
Pharmacy Manager
Veterinary Teaching Hospital and Clinics
School of Veterinary Medicine
Louisiana State University
Baton Rouge, Louisiana

Joanna M. Bassert, VMD
Professor and Director
Program of Veterinary Technology
Manor College
Jenkintown, Pennsylvania

Susan A. Berryhill, BS, RVT
Technician Affairs Manager
Hill's Pet Nutrition, Inc.
Topeka, Kansas

Sandra S. Brackenridge, MSW, BCD, LCSW
Associate Professor of Social Work
Idaho State University
Pocatello, Idaho

Daniel J. Burba, DVM, Dipl ACVS
Associate Professor
Equine Surgery
Department of Veterinary Clinical Sciences
School of Veterinary Medicine
Louisiana State University
Baton Rouge, Louisiana

Chistopher K. Cebra, VMD, MA, MS, Dipl ACVIM
Assistant Professor
Large Animal Medicine
College of Veterinary Medicine
Oregon State University
Corvallis, Oregon

Margaret L. Cebra, VMD, MS, Dipl ACVIM
Corvallis, Oregon

Sharee A. Chavis, RHIA
Health Information Supervisor
Veterinary Teaching Hospital and Clinics
School of Veterinary Medicine
Louisiana State University
Baton Rouge, Louisiana

Janyce L. Cornick-Seahorn, DVM, MS, Dipl ACVA, ACVIM
Medical Director
Vet-scans.com
Lexington, Kentucky

Lais R.R. Costa, MV, MS, Dipl ACVIM
Clinical Fellow
Equine Medicine
Department of Veterinary Clinical Sciences
School of Veterinary Medicine
Louisiana State University
Baton Rouge, Louisiana

Jacqueline R. Davidson, DVM, MS, Dipl ACVS
Associate Professor
Companion Animal Surgery
School of Veterinary Medicine
Louisiana State University
Baton Rouge, Louisiana

Jorge De la Calle, DVM, MS
Resident
Equine Surgery
Veterinary Teaching Hospital and Clinics
School of Veterinary Medicine
Louisiana State University
Baton Rouge, Louisiana

Susan C. Eades, DVM, PhD, Dipl ACVIM
Associate Professor of Equine Medicine
Department of Veterinary Clinical Sciences
School of Veterinary Medicine
Louisiana State University
Baton Rouge, Louisiana

Lee Ann Eddleman, CVT, VTS (Emergency and Critical Care)
Head Nurse
Small Animal Intensive Care Unit
Veterinary Teaching Hospital and Clinic
Louisiana State University
Baton Rouge, Louisiana

Erick L. Egger, DVM, Dipl ACVS
Veterinary Orthopedic Consultant
Veterinary Specialists of Northern Colorado
Loveland, Colorado

Bruce E. Eilts, DVM, MS, Dipl ACT
Professor of Theriogenology
Department of Veterinary Clinical Sciences
School of Veterinary Medicine
Louisiana State University
Baton Rouge, Louisiana

Dennis D. French, DVM, Dipl ABVP
Professor of Clinical Sciences
Department of Veterinary Clinical Sciences
School of Veterinary Medicine
Louisiana State University
Baton Rouge, Louisiana

Marjorie S. Gill, DVM, MS, Dipl ABVP
Associate Professor
Food Animal Medicine and Surgery
School of Veterinary Medicine
Louisiana State University
Baton Rouge, Louisiana

Michael G. Groves, DVM, MPH, PhD, Dipl ACVM, ACVPM
Dean
School of Veterinary Medicine
Louisiana State University
Baton Rouge, Louisiana

Perry L. Habecker, VMD, Dipl ACVP
Pathology Service
New Bolton Center
School of Veterinary Medicine
University of Pennsylvania
Kennett Square, Pennsylvania

Kathleen Story Harrington, MS
Instructor
Department of Pathobiological Sciences
School of Veterinary Medicine
Louisiana State University
Baton Rouge, Louisiana

Suzanne Hetts, PhD
Certified Applied Animal Behaviorist
Animal Behavior Associates, Inc.
Littleton, Colorado

Giselle Hosgood, BVSc, MS, FACVSc, Dipl ACVS
Professor of Veterinary Surgery
Department of Veterinary Clinical Sciences
School of Veterinary Medicine
Louisiana State University
Baton Rouge, Louisiana

Johnny D. Hoskins, DVM, PhD, Dipl ACVIM
DocuTech Services, Inc.
Professor Emeritus
Veterinary Clinical Medicine
School of Veterinary Medicine
Louisiana State University
Baton Rouge, Louisiana

Judith L. Hutton, RHIT
Health Information Coding Specialist
Veterinary Teaching Hospital and Clinics
School of Veterinary Medicine
Louisiana State University
Baton Rouge, Louisiana

Tracy J. Jaffe, DVM
Detroit Metro Veterinary Services
Senior Year Guest Lecturer
Veterinary Technology Program
Wayne County Community College
Wayne State University
Detroit, Michigan

Stephanie W. Johnson, BA, MSW
Counselor II, Adjunct Faculty
Department of Veterinary Clinical Sciences
School of Veterinary Medicine
Louisiana State University
Baton Rouge, Louisiana

Robert L. Jones, DVM, PhD, Dipl ACVM
Professor, Department of Microbiology
College of Veterinary Medicine and Biomedical Sciences
Colorado State University
Fort Collins, Colorado

Susan Kretzmer, CAHT
Head Surgery Technician
Veterinary Specialists of Northern Colorado
Loveland, Colorado

Roger L. Lukens, DVM
Professor and Director of Veterinary Technology
School of Veterinary Medicine
Purdue University
West Lafayette, Indiana

Steven L. Marks, BVSc, MS, MRCVS, Dipl ACVIM
Assistant Professor of Internal Medicine
Head, Small Animal Intensive Care Unit
Department of Veterinary Clinical Sciences
School of Veterinary Medicine
Louisiana State University
Baton Rouge, Louisiana

G. Neil Mauldin, DVM, Dipl ACVIM (Internal Medicine and Oncology), ACVR (Radiation Oncology)
Assistant Professor of Veterinary Oncology
Department of Veterinary Clinical Sciences
School of Veterinary Medicine
Louisiana State University
Baton Rouge, Louisiana

Glenna E. Mauldin, DVM, MS, Dipl ACVIM (Oncology)
Assistant Professor of Veterinary Oncology
Department of Veterinary Clinical Sciences
School of Veterinary Medicine
Louisiana State University
Baton Rouge, Louisiana

Dennis M. McCurnin, DVM, MS, Dipl ACVS
Professor of Clinical Sciences
Department of Veterinary Clinical Sciences
Hospital Director
Veterinary Teaching Hospital and Clinics
School of Veterinary Medicine
Louisiana State University
Baton Rouge, Louisiana

Diane McKelvey, BSc, DVM
Kamloops Veterinary Clinic
Kamloops, British Columbia, Canada

Ellen Miller, DVM, Dipl ACVIM
Veterinary Specialist
Animal Emergency Services of Northern Colorado
Loveland, Colorado

Rustin M. Moore, DVM, PhD, Dipl ACVS
Associate Professor
Equine Surgery
Director
Equine Health Studies Program
Department of Veterinary Clinical Sciences
School of Veterinary Medicine
Louisiana State University
Baton Rouge, Louisiana

T. Mark Neer, DVM, Dipl ACVIM
Professor
Small Animal Internal Medicine
Department of Veterinary Clinical Sciences
School of Veterinary Medicine
Louisiana State University
Baton Rouge, Louisiana

Ashley B. Oakes, DVM, Dipl AVDC
Veterinary Dentist
Tampa Bay Veterinary Dentistry
Tampa Bay Veterinary Specialists, Inc.
Largo, Florida

Matt G. Oakes, DVM, Dipl ACVS
Veterinary Surgeon
Tampa Bay Veterinary Surgery
Tampa Bay Veterinary Specialists, Inc.
Largo, Florida

Dale L. Paccamonti, DVM, MS, Dipl ACT
Professor
Theriogenology
Department of Veterinary Clinical Sciences
School of Veterinary Medicine
Louisiana State University
Baton Rouge, Louisiana

Beth Paugh Partington, DVM, MS, Dipl ACVR
Associate Professor of Veterinary Radiology
Department of Veterinary Clinical Sciences
School of Veterinary Medicine
Louisiana State University
Baton Rouge, Louisiana

Carlos R.F. Pinto, MedVet, Dipl ACT
Clinical Fellow
Theriogenology
Department of Veterinary Clinical Sciences
School of Veterinary Medicine
Louisiana State University
Baton Rouge, Louisiana

Philip Roudebush, DVM
Veterinary Fellow
Hill's Science and Technology Center
Topeka, Kansas
Adjunct Professor
College of Veterinary Medicine
Kansas State University
Manhattan, Kansas

Ray L. Russell, DVM, MAM, CPBA
President, ExecuTrends, Executive Education
Management Advisor, State of Arizona
Executive Coach and Professional Speaker/Leadership
    Consultant
Graduate Management Faculty
University of Arizona
Phoenix, Arizona

Jill E. Sackman, DVM, PhD, Dipl ACVS
Director
Surgical Research and Development
Ethicon Endo Surgery, Inc.
Cincinnati, Ohio

William D. Schoenherr, PhD
Principal Nutritionist
Hill's Science and Technology Center
Topeka, Kansas

E. David Stearns, RVT
Practice Technology Consultant
Informatics Consultant
Altoona, Wisconsin

Joseph Taboada, DVM, Dipl ACVIM
Professor and Director of Professional Instruction and
    Curriculum
School of Veterinary Medicine
Louisiana State University
Baton Rouge, Louisiana

Thomas N. Tully, Jr., DVM, MS, Dipl ABVP (Avian)
Associate Professor
Bird Zoo, Exotic Animal Service
Department of Veterinary Clinical Sciences
School of Veterinary Medicine
Louisiana State University
Baton Rouge, Louisiana

Katie M. Underwood, BS
Intern and Graduate Student
Clinical Social Work
Louisiana State University
Baton Rouge, Louisiana

Jan L. VanSteenhouse, DVM, PhD, Dipl ACVP
Clinical Pathologist
Antech Diagnostics
Smyrna, Georgia

Thomas J. Van Winkle, VMD, Dipl ACVP
Associate Professor
Laboratory of Pathology and Toxicology
School of Veterinary Medicine
University of Pennsylvania
Philadelphia, Pennsylvania

PREFACE

The fifth edition of *Clinical Textbook for Veterinary Technicians* continues to grow in scope and purpose to meet the needs of the professional veterinary technician in the twenty-first century. The book has begun to receive a high level of trust and acceptance in the profession and presents information ranging from basic procedures to clinical sciences to management of small, large, and exotic species.

The text continues to focus on the clinical needs of the technical student and practicing technician. A single reference text cannot possibly provide all needed information; however, this book has been adopted by many training programs and practices worldwide. The first edition in 1985 used 30 contributors to produce just over 500 pages contained in 24 chapters. The fifth edition uses over 50 contributors for over 900 pages divided into 37 chapters.

The organization of the book has been revised and divided into six major parts for easier referencing: Part One, Clinical Procedures; Part Two, Clinical Sciences; Part Three, Patient Management and Nutrition; Part Four, Anesthesia and Pharmacology; Part Five, Surgical and Medical Nursing; and Part Six, Practice Management and Self Management.

Numerous chapters have been completely rewritten as new chapters and include Restraint and Handling, Basic Necropsy Procedures, Animal Behavior, and Dentistry. Several chapters have been heavily revised and updated: Clinical Pathology; Emergency Nursing; Birds, Reptiles, and Small Mammals; Veterinary Oncology; Medical Records; Computer Applications; and Veterinary Practice Management. The remaining chapters have been updated to reflect the rapid increase of new knowledge: Diagnostic Imaging, Preventive Health Programs, Companion Animal Nutrition, Veterinary Anesthesia, Pain Management, and Pharmacology and Pharmacy.

We have included numerous features to aid readers in using this text. Technician Notes boxes are integrated throughout the text and summarize and highlight key concepts discussed in the text. Recommended Readings lists feature other reading, organizations, and Internet sources appropriate for veterinary technicians. The book also contains hundreds of tables and boxes summarizing important assessment and treatment protocols. Learning is often promoted by strong visual aids; the book is lavishly illustrated with hundreds of photographs and line drawings, including a color insert. Finally, a helpful appendix of common abbreviations is included.

As a result of feedback from users of the textbook, we are also pleased to offer with the fifth edition an Instructor's Manual containing more than 1600 test questions in a variety of formats. The Manual is free to instructors using the text in their programs.

This fifth edition continues to be dedicated to the many users in the technical and veterinary medical professions. We must all continue to work in teams to achieve levels of excellence in clinical medicine. To this end, I would especially like to welcome my new co-editor, Dr. Joanna Bassert, to our team.

Dennis M. McCurnin, DVM, MS
Diplomate, ACVS

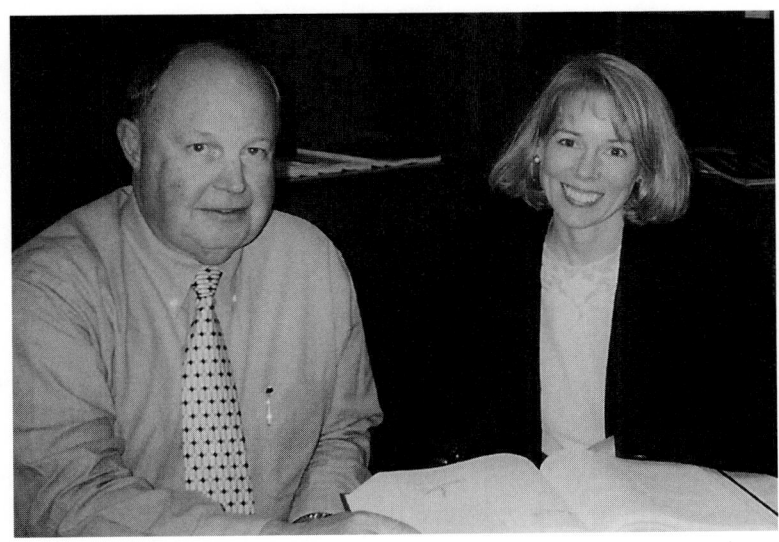

CONTENTS

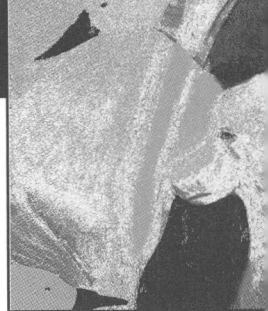

An Introduction to the Profession of Veterinary Technology

Joanna M. Bassert

I solemnly dedicate myself to aiding animals and society by providing excellent care and services for animals, by alleviating animal suffering, and by promoting public health.

I accept my obligations to practice my profession conscientiously and with sensitivity, adhering to the profession's Code of Ethics, and furthering my knowledge and competence through a commitment to lifelong learning.

Veterinary Technician Oath

The veterinary technician has emerged as a critical component of the veterinary health care team. Like the registered nurse in the human health care field, the veterinary technician supports the clinical activities of the supervising doctor. However, unlike registered nurses, veterinary technicians are expected to perform the duties of a radiology and laboratory technician as well as those of a medical and surgical nurse. In addition, veterinary technicians must be prepared to work with multiple species rather than just one. Thus the veterinary technician has a surprisingly broad range of clinical responsibilities.

Over the past 40 years, veterinary medicine has become highly sophisticated. Many veterinarians find they can no longer meet their practice goals, in terms of both providing a high level of medical care and attaining acceptable profit margins, without the skilled assistance of veterinary technicians. In addition, the development of veterinary-centered television programs has given the public a look into the inner workings of the animal hospital. For the first time, the public is able to see the important role veterinary technicians play in the real-life drama of saving animal lives. Thus there is heightened awareness of veterinary technology and an increased expectation, for both the practitioner and the pet owner, that animal patients will receive excellent veterinary nursing care. This introduction presents an overview of the profession of veterinary technology. It discusses the profession's history, laws, and ethics and presents job-related opportunities, duties, salaries, and professional organizations.

HISTORY OF VETERINARY TECHNOLOGY

Historically, many veterinarians practiced independently and performed many of the laboratory and nursing duties themselves. Often spouses and other lay persons served as the veterinary assistant, receptionist, and office manager. Today, many practices employ multiple veterinarians and require a staff of veterinary technicians, assistants, receptionists, and kennel workers to carry out the many duties required in running a successful practice. This team approach is a fundamental part of veterinary practice management today, and the veterinary technician often serves as an important link between the veterinarian and support personnel.

The profession of veterinary technology began to take form in the early 1960s with the establishment of the first organization of veterinary assistants and the first veterinary technician training program. The period that followed 1960 is rich with the accomplishments of dedicated veterinarians and veterinary technicians whose professional developments are listed in Box 1. Today, there are approximately 90 American Veterinary Medical Association (AVMA)-accredited programs of veterinary technology, and thousands of individuals have graduated from these programs. The number of veterinary technology programs continues to grow as the demand for educated, skilled personnel increases.

1

| Box 1 | SOME IMPORTANT EVENTS IN THE HISTORY OF VETERINARY TECHNOLOGY |

1960 The Alameda-Contra Costa Veterinary Medical Assistants Association, based in California, is established. The American Association of Laboratory Animal Science (AALAS) certifies three levels of on-the-job trained animal technicians employed in research institutions.

1961 The first animal technician training program is established at the State University of New York (SUNY) Agricultural and Technical College at Delhi.

1963 Eight pioneering students make up the first graduating class from Delhi.

1967 The American Veterinary Medical Association (AVMA) is charged with establishing criteria for acceptable animal technician training programs. Maryland's Veterinary Medical Association becomes the first organization of veterinarians to test and register veterinary assistants.

1968 and **1969** Seven new veterinary technician programs are established in seven different states.

1969 Nebraska becomes the first state to certify animal technicians.

1970s An unprecedented number of new veterinary technology programs form during this decade.

1972 Michigan State University and University of Nebraska, School of Technical Agriculture, become the first programs of veterinary technology to receive AVMA accreditation. The first national continuing education meeting for animal technicians is held at the Western States Veterinary Conference in Las Vegas.

1973 The Association of Veterinary Technician Educators (AVTE) is formed.

1976 The first professional journal for veterinary technicians, *Methods: The Journal for Animal Health Technicians*, is published.

1980 *The Compendium on Continuing Education for the Animal Health Technician* (later called *Veterinary Technician*) is first published.

1981 The North American Veterinary Technician Association (NAVTA) is organized.

1984 NAVTA develops and adopts the code of ethics for veterinary technicians.

1985 The AVMA forms the Animal Technician Testing Committee, which in turn validates the Animal Technician National Examination (ATNE).

1989 The AVMA approves changing the terminology from Animal Technician to Veterinary Technician. The ATNE becomes the VTNE (Veterinary Technician National Examination).

The Canadian Association of Animal Health Technologists and Technicians (CAAHTT) is funded.

1994 The Committee on Veterinary Technician Specialties (CVTS) is formed by NAVTA.

1995 The American Association of Veterinary State Boards (AASVB) replaces the AVMA in its oversight of the VTNE.

1996 The first meeting of the Pennsylvania Association of Veterinary Technician Educators (PAVTE) is held.

1997 PAVTE expands to include educators from neighboring states and is incorporated as the Northeast Veterinary Technician Educators Association (NEVTEA).

1999 Eighty programs of veterinary technology are accredited by the AVMA. The AVMA incorporates language recommended by NAVTA in the AVMA's model practice act, which delineates the roles of the veterinary technician and the veterinary assistant.

2000 Eighty-six programs are accredited by the AVMA, including two distance learning programs.

Modified from the 1999 AVTE Symposium Proceeding notes by Roger L. Lukens, AVTE historian.

THE VETERINARY TECHNICIAN TODAY

Veterinary technicians work in a wide range of facilities, perform many different kinds of tasks, and may encounter all manner of animal species. For example, veterinary technicians may work in private veterinary practices, such as companion animal, equine, food animal, or mixed practices. (A mixed practice is one that treats both farm and companion animals.) Veterinary technicians may also work in zoos, aquariums, wildlife rehabilitation centers, and research facilities. In addition, they may work for pharmaceutical companies as sales representatives of veterinary products, or they may become entrepreneurs by establishing their own kennel facility or pet-sitting business. Qualified veterinary technicians may also become instructors in veterinary technology programs or other academic programs. The range of job opportunities for the veterinary technician today is broader than ever before. (Table 1 shows the distribution of career paths selected by recent graduates of AVMA-accredited programs.)

Within this diverse array of opportunities, veterinary technicians may also narrow their field of work and concentrate on specific areas. For example, a technician working in a practice that treats exotic species, such as birds and reptiles, will develop skills and knowledge particular to that aspect of veterinary medicine. In addition, some veterinary practices are called "specialty" or "referral" practices because they employ veterinarians who have completed special training in a particular aspect of veterinary medicine, such as dermatology, surgery, internal medicine, radiology, or ophthalmology. The veterinary hospitals associated with schools of veterinary medicine are examples of very large specialty practices. They are also the hospitals where most veterinary specialists complete their specialty training. Veterinarians who are general practitioners and not specialists may refer particularly challenging or difficult cases to specialty practices. Veterinary technicians who work in specialty practices see unusual cases and become skilled in addressing the particular needs of these critically ill patients. It is not uncommon for specialty practices to share their facility with an emergency and trauma practice. Some veterinary technicians prefer the challenge and excitement of emergency practice, rather than general practice, and have dedicated their careers to this aspect of veterinary technology.

Recently, veterinary technicians have also been given the opportunity to become specialists. In February 1994, the North American Veterinary Technician Association (NAVTA) formed the Committee on Veterinary Technician Specialties (CVTS) to address a growing interest among veterinary technicians to be recognized for a higher level of skill, knowledge, and interest in a particular aspect of veterinary technology. For this reason, CVTS established a process and a list of criteria for the formation of academies in specialized fields of veterinary technology.

The first step in this process is for a group of veterinary technicians who share an interest in a particular field of veterinary technology to establish a professional society or association. After the society has grown in size, it may then petition CVTS for recognition as an academy. The organizing committee of the proposed academy, together with CVTS, establishes the advanced requirements and examination process for becoming a veterinary technician specialist. As of this printing, NAVTA has recognized two academies in veterinary technology: the Academy of Veterinary Emergency and Critical Care Technicians and the Academy of Veterinary Technician Anesthetists. Veterinary technicians who have achieved specialty status are signified

TABLE 1	DISTRIBUTION OF EMPLOYMENT AND SALARIES FOR RECENT VETERINARY TECHNICIAN GRADUATES		
Employment Setting or Field	**Percentage (%) of Recent Graduates Working in this Field**	**Salary Range ($)**	**Average Starting Salary ($)**
Companion animal practice	73	10,717-40,000	18,755
Food animal practice	2	14,560-24,000	15,968
Equine practice	2	15,000-30,000	20,906
Mixed animal practice	12	10,717-27,560	17,238
Specialty practice	4	15,000-30,000	20,256
Industry/sales	1	20,000-28,000	21,000
Veterinary technician education	0.2	N/A	N/A
Government	0.4	20,000-28,000	23,625
Diagnostic/research laboratories	2	10,717-30,000	22,807
Other	3	12,480-25,000	20,896
Overall average salary			20,161

From the 1999 AVMA survey results of accredited programs in veterinary technology at www.avma.org.
N/A, Not applicable.

by the initials *VTS* (and their field of specialty in parentheses) after their names.

JOB PROSPECTS, SALARIES, AND ATTRITION

Presently there are widespread shortages of veterinary technicians nationwide, and graduates of veterinary technology programs are therefore finding ample job opportunities. Although job opportunities are bright, salaries vary depending on the field of interest and the level of experience. For example, in 1999 the AVMA reported that the average salary for new graduates in companion animal practice was $18,755, and for experienced graduates in the same field, the average salary was $21,860. Similarly, the average salary in diagnostic and research laboratories was $22,807 for recent graduates and $26,635 for experienced graduates. The salaries within a particular field can vary greatly. For example, salaries for experienced technicians in industry/sales ranged from $13,000 to $81,000, and in mixed animal practice they ranged from $11,000 to $32,000.

In addition to salary compensation, many employers offer a range of benefits, including health care coverage, retirement plans, and payment of continuing education and professional membership fees. Large companies or practices are generally better equipped to provide more complete benefit packages than small private businesses.

The profession of veterinary technology has a high rate of attrition, estimated to be about 65% after only 4 years of employment. Graduate technicians report leaving the profession because of lack of appreciation and underutilization by their employer, low pay, and lack of advancement opportunities. Attrition from the profession is a critical part of the current shortage problem. Many states have shortages of veterinarians and veterinary assistants as well as technicians.

EDUCATION

Like nursing schools in the human health care field, programs of veterinary technology may include 2, 3, or 4 years of undergraduate study and may result in either an associate of science degree (2 or 3 years) or a bachelor of science degree (4 years). Programs in the United States are accredited by the Committee on Veterinary Technician Education and Activities (CVTEA), which is under the auspices of the AVMA. For accreditation a program must meet 11 essential criteria for curricula, faculty, facility, and

Box 2	TYPES OF COURSES REQUIRED IN VETERINARY TECHNOLOGY PROGRAMS

BASIC MATH AND SCIENCE COURSES
Technical math
Biology
Chemistry
Microbiology
Comparative anatomy and physiology
Medical terminology
Computer science

VETERINARY TECHNOLOGY COURSES
Introduction to veterinary technology
Veterinary practice management
Animal management and nutrition
Farm animal clinical procedures
Companion animal clinical procedures
Laboratory animal science
Animal medicine
Veterinary radiology
Animal parasitology
Veterinary hematology
Veterinary clinical chemistry and urinalysis
Veterinary surgical assisting
Veterinary pharmacology and anesthesiology

admissions requirements. Each program must submit reports to CVTEA for review semiannually, annually, or biannually depending on the age and stability of the program. In addition, the CVTEA carries out on-site visits of each program. Based on the on-site evaluation, recommendations by CVTEA are classified into three categories: critical, major, and minor recommendations. Programs must document in reports to the CVTEA progress made in addressing the deficits cited by the on-site committee.

The curriculum of veterinary technology programs includes general college-level courses, such as biology and chemistry, as well as courses specific to clinical practice, such as veterinary parasitology, medicine, and clinical chemistry. In addition, there are approximately 200 "essential" and 84 "recommended" tasks listed in the Accreditation Policies and Procedures Handbook of the CVTEA, which constitutes the foundation of the hands-on curriculum for laboratories and practical training. Refer to Box 2 for a list of courses typically offered in veterinary technology programs.

Distance Education

Although most veterinary technology programs are offered to students in the traditional on-campus fashion, some programs have begun to offer an exciting new type of veterinary technology course using the Internet and teleconferencing. A handful of institutions have made an entire program available to distance-education students.

Continuing Education

Most states require veterinary technicians to attend continuing education lectures and workshops to maintain licensure, certification, or registration. These lectures are available at various national, regional, and local professional conferences and workshops throughout the United States and through AVMA-accredited programs of veterinary technology. As veterinary medicine progresses at a surprisingly rapid rate, it is particularly important for veterinary technicians to commit themselves to a career of life-long learning.

RESPONSIBILITIES OF THE VETERINARY TECHNICIAN

Veterinary technicians perform a myriad of animal care-related duties, but they may also be involved in nonclinical tasks, such as office management, client education, and inventory control. Veterinary practices are organized into distinct working areas. A veterinary technician, depending on his or her job description and the size of the practice, may work in all, a few, or only one of the areas discussed below.

Reception Area

Although many practices hire receptionists, and not veterinary technicians, to work in the reception area, it is important for the clinical staff to be cross-trained in this aspect of the practice so that important information can be accessed easily when the receptionist is not available. The veterinary technician should be familiar with the computer network system and practice management software used by the practice. This will facilitate obtaining existing records, creating new patient records, and accessing medical histories and billing information during emergencies that may occur after hours.

Examination Rooms and Out-patients

The veterinary technician ensures that office visits are handled in an efficient and professional manner. This involves directing clients to the appropriate examination room or treatment area, getting a brief history, weighing the patient, and acquiring the necessary vaccines, instruments, and materials needed for the visit. The veterinary technician may also draw blood at this time and obtain skin scrapings and fecal, urine, and cytology samples for laboratory testing. In addition, the veterinary technician provides important information to clients regarding preventive care, diet, behavior modification, medication, discharge instructions, and spay and neutering procedures for their animal.

Because pet owners often feel more at ease talking to the veterinary technician than to the doctor, the technician can be a valuable support person for bereaved or worried pet owners. In addition, the veterinary technician answers clients' questions both in person and over the telephone and occasionally must address difficult or angry pet owners.

Laboratory and Pharmacy

The veterinary technician has the skills to perform all the routine laboratory tests used in practice. How many of the laboratory tests are actually performed on site varies from practice to practice. In veterinary hospitals that make full use of these skills, veterinary technicians perform complete blood counts, differentials, and morphologic examinations of blood. They perform urinalysis, including examination of urine sediment, and fecal analysis for evidence of parasites. Veterinary technicians are skilled in the use of enzyme-linked immunosorbent assay (ELISA) test kits, dextrometers, refractometers, and dry chemistry analyzers. In addition, veterinary technicians are familiar with interpreting common cytologic preparations, such as ear swabs and vaginal smears.

Technician Note

Being able to take initiative and think quickly during unexpected events is an important quality of the veterinary technician.

Once a diagnosis is made, the veterinarian prescribes, either in writing or verbally, a treatment for the animal patient. The veterinary technician then interprets the prescription language and fills and dispenses the medication to the pet owner with instructions for its use. In addition, veterinary technicians are often responsible for ensuring that the pharmacy is well stocked, that expired drugs are discarded, and that controlled substances are handled appropriately.

Radiology

The x-ray (also known as a radiograph) is an important diagnostic tool for veterinarians. Veterinary technicians are skilled in radiographic techniques, including positioning of the patient, making the proper settings, and taking exposures at the appropriate times. In addition, veterinary technicians are skilled in both manual and automatic development techniques and in problem shooting technical errors. If an x-ray service is not employed by the practice, veterinary technicians may be responsible for maintaining the development and fixative solutions and for keeping the x-ray screens and other equipment clean and in good working order. In addition, the technician ensures that the hospital staff protects itself from harmful radiation by wearing appropriate protective clothing, such as lead aprons, gloves, and thyroid shields, and that dosimeters are used routinely to monitor x-ray exposure. Often the technician is responsible for managing the ordering and mailing of the dosimeters. Finally, veterinary technicians may also assist with special imaging and contrast studies, such as ultrasound studies and those that employ gas, barium sulfate, or other contrast agents.

Treatment Room

Most veterinary hospitals have a treatment room where patients are brought for various procedures and where animals are prepped for surgery. In more contemporary hospital designs, the treatment area is a large central room that may include a bank of cages for the postoperative and critical care patients. This arrangement facilitates the monitoring of in-house patients and enables the technical staff to be more efficient in completing important treatment duties. Dental operatories and procedure sinks may also be part of the main treatment room where dentistries and minor surgical procedures are completed.

Veterinary technicians are responsible for carrying out treatment orders given by the supervising veterinarian. This involves giving medications by all routes (e.g., orally, intramuscularly, intravenously). It may also involve setting up and monitoring intravenous fluids. Collection of small amounts of blood may be performed every few hours, and the animal might be routinely checked for alertness, temperature, pulse, respiration, urination, and defecation. For critical cases, treatments might include changing bandages, lavaging open wounds, placing and monitoring nasal oxygen, and maintaining chest, tracheal, urethral, or abdominal tubes. Veterinary technicians are responsible for recording all treatments, data, and physical findings in the patient's record. The patient record is an important legal document as well as a means of ensuring that errors in treatment are not made.

The veterinary technician prepares the patient before it enters the operating room. This involves ensuring that the animal has not had anything to eat or drink and that the animal urinates before surgery. The technician is responsible for weighing the animal and calculating and administering preoperative anesthetic agents. In many veterinary practices, the veterinary technician is responsible for induction and maintenance of anesthesia. Although there are many ways to anesthetize an animal, this usually involves placing an intravenous catheter, setting up fluids, placing an endotracheal tube, and administering intravenous and/or gas anesthetic agents. Monitoring equipment, such as a pulse oximeter, esophageal stethoscope, Dynamap, Doppler ultrasound, or oscilloscope, may be used by the technician to assist in monitoring the anesthetized patient. Before moving the patient to the operating room, the technician clips hair from the region of the animal that will undergo surgery and performs an initial cleansing of the area.

Often technicians are responsible for performing routine dental prophylaxis procedures, which must be done while the animal is anesthetized. In this situation, the technician must perform two important jobs at once, namely, monitor the patient under anesthesia and clean and polish the animal's teeth. The veterinary technician must be prepared for an anesthetic emergency and should be familiar with the emergency drugs and procedures needed to resuscitate animals that are in crisis.

Technician Note

NAVTA has designated the third week in October as National Veterinary Technician Week! Mark your calendars!

Operating Room

The operating room technician or circulating nurse positions the animal patient on the operating table and completes the final surgical scrub. Instruments, equipment, and materials needed by the surgeon are made available. In addition, the technician acts to retrieve additional materials requested during the procedure. In some practices, the technician acts simultaneously as anesthetist and as circulating nurse. Occasionally, technicians are asked to assist during a particularly challenging operation and must be skilled in proper sterile techniques, including gloving and gowning. After the procedure, the technician washes and dries the surgical instruments and reorganizes them into surgical packs for sterilization.

Wards

Veterinary technicians can play an important role on the wards, not only in ensuring that treatments are given correctly and in a timely manner, but also in providing animals with compassion and a gentle touch. Nurturing animals when they are sick is an important part of their recovery. Even healthy animals that are being boarded can benefit from some special care and reassurance from the technical staff.

Hospital Management

Veterinary technicians, particularly those with a background in business, may act as hospital managers. They may oversee the veterinary staff and assist with scheduling, hiring, bookkeeping, and inventory control. Increasingly, veterinary technicians, particularly in large practices, are drawn into some management duties, such as personnel management and ordering supplies.

TERMINOLOGY AND THE VETERINARY HEALTH CARE TEAM

A productive and efficiently managed veterinary practice depends on the dedication of a team of veterinary professionals and support personnel (Box 3). As described below, each member of the team plays a collaborative role in helping to provide quality health care for the animal patient.

Veterinarian

A veterinarian typically completes 4 years of study at an AVMA-accredited school of veterinary medicine. Graduates are distinguished by the initials *DVM* after their name, unless they have graduated from the University of Pennsylvania, in which case they will have the initials *VMD* after their name. In order to practice, veterinarians are required to be licensed by the state in which they work. Typically, this requires successful completion of national and state

---

Box 3	AVMA NOMENCLATURE

The American Veterinary Medical Association (AVMA) has published the following definitions:

"Veterinary Technology" is the science and art of providing professional support service to veterinarians in the practice of their profession.

A "Veterinary Technician" is a person who has graduated from a two- or three-year, AVMA-accredited program in veterinary technology.

A "Veterinary Technologist" is a graduate of a four-year, AVMA-accredited program who holds a baccalaureate degree from such study.

"Veterinary Assistants": The adjectives "animal," "veterinary," "ward," or "hospital" combined with the nouns "attendant," "caretaker," or "assistant" are titles sometimes used for individuals where training, knowledge, and skills are less than that required for identification as a veterinary technician, veterinary technologist, or laboratory animal technician. The basic tasks performed by veterinary assistants include feeding, watering, bathing, restraining, moving and exercising animals; and cleaning, and clerical/office duties, and other, similar entry-level activities.

From the November 2000 accreditation policies and procedures of the Committee on Veterinary Technician Education and Activities (CVTEA) blue book.

examinations and the payment of a licensing fee. In addition, graduates of foreign veterinary medical colleges that are not accredited by the AVMA are eligible to apply for licensure in most states following certification by the Educational Commission of Foreign Veterinary Graduates (ECFVG).

Veterinary Technician Specialist

The veterinary technician specialist is a veterinary technician who has reached a higher level of skill and understanding in a particular field of veterinary technology. The veterinary specialist must meet the following criteria:

- Be a graduate of an AVMA-accredited program of veterinary technology and/or be legally credentialed to practice veterinary technology in his or her respective state, province, or country,
- Successfully complete the education, training, and experience requirements established by the respective academy of specialists
- Be reviewed and approved for specialist status by the academy

As already mentioned, veterinary technician specialists are distinguished by the initials *VTS* and the field of specialty in parentheses after their name. For additional information about veterinary technician specialists, refer to the section titled The Veterinary Technician Today.

Veterinary Technologist

The veterinary technologist holds a bachelor of science degree (B.S.) in veterinary technology from a 4-year, AVMA-accredited program. The veterinary technologist works in positions that may require a greater level of education than the veterinary technician, such as project leader, practice supervisor, or teacher in a veterinary technology program. Some veterinary technologists, particularly those employed in teaching hospitals of veterinary medical schools, may become highly skilled in a particular aspect of veterinary technology. Some institutions and practices use the term *veterinary technologist* to refer to a veterinary technician who holds a B.S. degree in any field.

Veterinary Technician

A veterinary technician is a person who has earned an associate of science (A.S.) degree in veterinary technology from a 2- or 3-year, AVMA-accredited program of veterinary technology. In many states, veterinary technicians are required to complete national and state examinations before they can be licensed, registered, or certified. Frequently, veterinary technicians are required to pay a fee to the state or state veterinary association in order to receive a license, certification, or registration.

Technician Note

Veterinary technicians must take responsibility for their own safety. The first step involves having personal health care coverage and always staying up-to-date with rabies and tetanus immunizations.

Veterinary Assistant

The term *veterinary assistant* is used to describe those individuals involved in the care of animals, but who are not veterinary technicians, laboratory animal technicians, or veterinarians. Typically, veterinary assistants are responsible for assisting the veterinary technician and the veterinarian by restraining animals, setting up equipment and supplies, cleaning and maintaining clinic and laboratory facilities, and feeding and exercising patients. Most veterinary assistants are trained on the job by a supervising veterinary technician or veterinarian, but some assistants complete 4 to 6 months of training in a formal course of study.

The profession of veterinary technology started to take form in the early 1960s. Before this time, veterinary technicians, as defined today, did not exist and veterinary practices depended exclusively on the skill of on-the-job–trained veterinary assistants. Today, veterinary assistants continue to constitute a large and important portion of the work force in veterinary practices nationwide. Veterinary technicians and veterinary assistants work together in many veterinary practices, and although the AVMA and NAVTA make clear distinctions between the two groups, some states have confused these distinctions.

As the number of traditional and distance AVMA-accredited programs grow, education in the field of veterinary technology becomes increasingly more accessible to veterinary support staff members who wish to become veterinary technicians.

Veterinary Nurse

The term *veterinary nurse* rather than veterinary technician is used in European countries.

CERTIFICATION, REGISTRATION, AND LICENSURE

The requirements for certification, registration, or licensure vary from state to state. Some states, for example, require successful completion of the Veterinary Technician National Examination (VTNE), whereas other states require their own state examination. Still others may require completion of both national and state examinations.

The Veterinary Technician National Examination

The VTNE is developed under a contractual agreement between the American Association of Veterinary State Boards (AAVSB) and the Professional Examination Service (PES). The AAVSB is represented by the Veterinary Technician Testing Committee (VTTC), which is composed of veterinarians and veterinary technicians who are engaged in clinical practice or academia. Members of the committee are appointed by the executive boards of AVMA, NAVTA, AVTE, and the Canadian Association of Animal Health Technologists and Technicians (CAAHTT). PES provides the committee with two draft examinations for their review and validation. These drafts are developed from a computerized bank of questions, originally written by veterinarians and veterinary technicians from all aspects of the veterinary medical profession. The questions are reviewed independently for accuracy, relevance to the field of veterinary technology, and level of difficulty. In addition, the questions are further screened for grammar, style, and conformity to psychometric principles. Each state licensing board is responsible for the administration of the examination and establishes the location and date and times when it is offered. Although PES provides test-scoring services, the state boards are responsible for reporting the scores to the veterinary technician candidates.

The examination is offered in many states and Canadian provinces on the second Friday in June and January of every year. It is composed of 200 multiple-choice questions that cover the following seven primary areas or domains within the profession of veterinary technology:

- Pharmacy and pharmacology
- Surgical preparation and assisting
- Laboratory procedures
- Animal nursing
- Radiology, ultrasound, and other electronic imaging
- Anesthesia
- Office and hospital procedures

On a scale from 200 to 800, the VTNE Standard Setting Committee has established the passing score at 425. A total score and a locally derived scale score may also accompany the test-results report that is sent to each candidate. Candidates who need to have their VTNE scores sent to multiple state boards must register with the Interstate Reporting Service (IRS). There is a fee for registration with the IRS and a second fee for each transfer.

Technician Note

Candidates have 4 hours to complete the VTNE. Because candidates receive no additional penalties for incorrect responses, test takers are encouraged to answer all the questions even if it means guessing.

Laboratory Animal Science

The American Association for Laboratory Animal Science (AALAS) has established a certification program that certifies the following three levels of animal technicians:

- Assistant laboratory animal technician (ALAT)
- Laboratory animal technician (LAT)
- Laboratory animal technologist (LATG)

AALAS-certified animal technicians care for the laboratory animals used in research facilities and teaching institutions. These facilities are registered by the U.S. Department of Agriculture (USDA) and may be located in pharmaceutical companies, universities, and colleges. A technician does not need to be a graduate of an AVMA-accredited program of veterinary technology to be eligible for AALAS certification; however, many are. Graduates of AVMA-accredited programs must complete 6months of additional training in a USDA-registered facility before they are eligible for the level one ALAT examination.

Like the VTNE, AALAS-certification examinations are developed and administered by the Professional Examination Service (PES), but they fall under the auspices of AALAS rather than the AAVSB. All three levels of examinations are multiple choice, but each level becomes more rigorous and asks more questions. For example, the ALAT is composed of 100 questions, the LAT 125, and the LATG 150. Candidates must complete a specified amount of on-the-job experience to qualify for the next level of AALAS certification.

LAWS GOVERNING VETERINARY TECHNOLOGY

As the sophistication of veterinary medicine increases, the responsibilities of the veterinary technician in clinical practice have broadened. Slowly veterinarians are moving away from doing the nursing and laboratory tasks themselves and are delegating these tasks to the veterinary technician. However, there is much variability among veterinary practices in the way in which veterinary technicians are used. In a well-managed practice, veterinary technicians perform all the duties associated with the care and treatment of animal patients except those tasks that by law can only be performed by the veterinarian. Although the state laws that define veterinary medicine differ, it is widely accepted that veterinary technicians may **not** do the following: prescribe, diagnose, or perform surgery.

Additional restrictions vary from state to state. For example, some states may prohibit a veterinary technician from extracting teeth (because it is considered surgery), whereas other states may not. It is amazing that there are still some states that do not recognize veterinary technicians in the law. Because these states have no laws to guide the profession in the use of veterinary technicians, there is much left to the interpretation and judgment of the supervising veterinarian.

The law that governs the practice of veterinary medicine is called a *practice act*. Each state writes its own practice act. In an effort to standardize technician utilization from state to state and to help eliminate confusion between the roles of the veterinary technician and the veterinary assistant, AVMA has developed a model practice act (Box 4). The practice act and any changes to it must be approved by the state house and senate of each state and later signed into law by the governor. Based on the laws outlined in the practice act, more specific laws, called rules and regulations, are written by the state veterinary board. Refer to Box 5 for the AVMA's model of rules and regulations. The board may be formally known as the board of veterinary medical examiners, the board of veterinary governors, or the licensing board of veterinary medicine depending on the state. Typically, there is a state board for every profession that requires licensure. However, unlike the human nursing field, which has its own state boards, there are currently no state boards of veterinary technology. Veterinary technology falls under the governance of the state board of veterinary medicine if the veterinary technicians are licensed in that state.

In veterinary medicine, state boards are responsible for distributing licenses, collecting renewal fees, and evaluating complaints of malpractice or unethical conduct by veterinarians (and by veterinary technicians if they are licensed in the state). With adequate evidence of wrongdoing, a board can revoke the license of a veterinarian (or veterinary technician). Members of a state board are typically appointed by the governor and generally include members of the veterinary profession (usually veterinarians), one government official, and one or two members of the general public. In addition, each board is given legal counsel by the state to ensure that the laws (both in the practice act and in the rules and regulations) are interpreted and upheld correctly. The state's legal counsel also assists the board in writing the rules and regulations. Although the rules and regulations do not need approval by the state house or senate, as does the practice act, they must be reviewed and approved by the state's independent regulatory commission.

The rules and regulations must support the practice act and cannot overrule it. They tend to be more specific laws than those of the practice act and often list the tasks that may or may not be carried out by the veterinary technician. They may also define the level of supervision that is required by the employing veterinarian. Because of the variability of laws among states, it is important for veterinary technicians to be aware of the particular laws in their state that govern what they can and cannot do in practice.

Box 4   MODEL PRACTICE ACT FOR VETERINARY TECHNICIANS

SECTION I. TITLE
This act shall be known and may be cited as the "Model Practice Act."

SECTION II. LEGISLATIVE INTENT AND PURPOSE
The practice of veterinary technology is privilege granted by legislative authority to maintain public health, safety and welfare and to protect the public from being misled by unauthorized individuals.

SECTION III. DEFINITIONS
When used in the text that follows, except where otherwise indicated by context the words and phrases below shall have the following meanings:

1. Animal—Any mammalian animal other than man, and any avian, amphibian, fish or reptile, wild or domestic.
2. Board—The _____ State Board of Veterinary Medical Examiners or Board of Governors.
3. Veterinary Technology—The science and art of providing all aspects of professional medical care and treatment for animals with the exception of diagnosis, prognosis, surgery and prescription.
4. Emergency—When an animal has been placed in a life-threatening condition and immediate treatment is necessary to sustain life; or where death is imminent and action is necessary to relieve pain or suffering.
5. Licensed Veterinarian—An individual who is validly and currently licensed by the Board to practice veterinary medicine in _____ .
6. Veterinary Technician (Licensed, Registered or Certified) —An individual who has graduated from a veterinary technology program that is accredited according to the standards adopted by the American Veterinary Medical Association's Committee on Veterinary Technician Education and Activities and who has passed the examination requirements as prescribed by the Board in _____ shall be known as a licensed, registered or certified veterinary technician.

SECTION IV. TASKS
Certain tasks may be performed ONLY by a licensed veterinarian OR licensed, registered or certified veterinary technician under the direction, supervision and control of a veterinarian licensed to practice in the state of _____ .
    See the Rules and Regulations Document for a list of tasks.

SECTION V. EXAMINATION FOR LICENSURE, REGISTRATION OR CERTIFICATION
Veterinary technicians applying for licensure, registration or certification shall be required to pass the Veterinary Technician National Examination, with scores as set by the Board prior to licensure, registration or certification.
    See the Rules and Regulations Document for a list of tasks.

SECTION VI. CONTINUING EDUCATION
All licensed, registered or certified veterinary technicians shall be required to continue their professional education as a condition of maintenance of his/her status in the state of _____ .
    See the Rules and Regulations Document for a list of tasks.

SECTION VII. DENIAL, SUSPENSION, OR REVOCATION OF VETERINARY TECHNICIAN LICENSES, REGISTRATIONS OR CERTIFICATIONS
The Board may suspend, revoke or deny the issuance or renewal of license, registration or certification of any veterinary technician if after a hearing by his/her peers, has been found guilty of any of the following:

1. Fraud or misrepresentation in applying for license, registration, or certification.
2. Criminal offense relating to veterinary medicine.
3. Any violation of the Uniform Controlled Substances Act or the Legend Drug Act.
4. Convicted of cruelty to animals.
5. Violation of any of the rules or regulations stated in the Rules and Regulations Document.

From the American Veterinary Medical Association (AVMA) membership directory.

MALPRACTICE AND COMMON LAW

The society in which we live today is litigious. The workplace for the veterinary technician is no different and includes legal risks. Because veterinary technicians are becoming increasingly skilled and are taking on greater levels of responsibility in clinical practice, they become increasingly more vulnerable to the possibility of litigation against them. Although veterinarians typically bear the brunt of legal action, veterinary technicians can be and are sued. It is important therefore for veterinary technicians to understand what constitutes malpractice.

As already mentioned, much of the legal framework of our society is defined by laws that are written, approved, and enforced by governmental bodies. These rules constitute what is called *legislative law*, because the laws are written down. The veterinary practice act, professional rules and regulations, and local ordinances are examples of legislative laws. They define the profession of veterinary medicine and provide clear guidelines for the management of veterinary practices. In contrast, however, *common law* is not written down. Rather, it is a series of laws that have

evolved over time based on established professional conduct, customs, and practices. Common law is also derived from and enforced by the decisions of judges made during civil suits when someone has been injured. Thus common law is not enforced by governmental bodies, but by judges in a court of law.

Common law dictates many things to veterinary practices. For example, it dictates that practice owners must provide a reasonably safe environment for their employees and clients. Failure to provide this constitutes *ordinary negligence*. In addition, common law dictates that veterinary practitioners must provide a level of medical care to their patients that is in keeping with a reasonably prudent veterinary practitioner of similar training under similar circumstances. Failure to comply with common law under these circumstances constitutes *professional negligence* or *malpractice*.

Malpractice may be subject to litigation if the plaintiff can prove three things:

- The veterinarian or veterinary technician agreed to treat and *did* treat that particular patient.

Box 5 MODEL RULES AND REGULATIONS FOR VETERINARY TECHNICIANS

I. LICENSED, REGISTERED OR CERTIFIED VETERINARY TECHNICIAN ACTIVITIES

A. Tasks
1. Levels of supervision defined
   a. Immediate supervision—A licensed veterinarian is within direct eyesight and hearing range
   b. Direct supervision—A licensed veterinarian is on the premises, and is readily available
   c. Indirect supervision—A licensed veterinarian is not on the premises, but is able to perform the duties of a licensed veterinarian by maintaining direct communication
2. The following tasks may be performed ONLY by a licensed, registered or certified veterinary technician (or licensed veterinarian) under the direction, supervision and control of a veterinarian licensed to practice in _____ provided said veterinarian makes a daily physical examination of the patient treated:
   a. Immediate supervision
      (1) Induction of anesthesia
      (2) Dental extraction not requiring sectioning of the tooth or the resectioning of bone
      (3) Surgical assistant to a licensed veterinarian within the rules and regulations issued by the _____ Board of Veterinary Medical Examiners and the laws of the state of _____
   b. Direct supervision
      (1) Euthanasia
      (2) Blood or blood component collection, preparation and administration
      (3) Application of splints and slings
      (4) Dental procedures including, but not limited to the removal of calculus, soft deposits, plaque and stains; the smoothing, filing and polishing of teeth; or the flotation or dressing of equine teeth
   c. Indirect supervision
      (1) Administration and application of treatments, drugs, medications and immunological agents by parenteral and injectable routes (subcutaneous, intramuscular, intraperitoneal and intravenous) except when in conflict with government regulations
      (2) Initiation of parenteral fluid administration
      (3) Intravenous catheterizations
      (4) Radiography including settings, positioning, processing and safety procedures
      (5) Collection of blood; collection of urine by expression, cystocentesis or catheterization; collection and preparation of tissue, cellular or microbiological samples by skin scrapings, impressions or other non-surgical methods except when in conflict with government regulations
      (6) Routine laboratory test procedures
      (7) Supervision of the handling of biohazardous waste materials
   d. Other
      (1) Services which a licensed, registered or certified veterinary technician is competent to perform under the appropriate degree of supervision
3. Under conditions of emergency, a licensed, registered or certified veterinary technician may render the following life-saving aid and treatment:
   a. Application of tourniquets and/or pressure bandages to control hemorrhage
   b. Administration of pharmacological agents and parenteral fluids shall only be performed after direct communication with a veterinarian authorized to practice in _____ and such veterinarian is either present or en route to the location of the distressed animals
   c. Resuscitative procedures
   d. Application of temporary splints or bandages to prevent further injury to bones or soft tissue
   e. Application of appropriate wound dressings and external supportive treatment in severe wound and burn cases
   f. External supportive treatment in heat prostration cases
4. HOWEVER, nothing shall be construed to permit a licensed, registered or certified veterinary technician to do the following:
   a. Make any diagnosis or prognosis
   b. Prescribe any treatments, drugs, medications or appliances
   c. Perform surgery

II. EXAMINATIONS

A. Examinations of applicants for licensure, registration or certification as a veterinary technician in _____ shall be held at least annually at a time, place and date set by the Board no later than ninety (90) days prior to the scheduled examination.
B. An applicant shall be required to pass the Veterinary Technician National Examination (VTNE) with scores as set by the Board prior to licensure, registration or certification.

III. CONTINUING EDUCATION REQUIREMENTS FOR LICENSED, REGISTERED OR CERTIFIED VETERINARY TECHNICIANS

A. All licensed, registered or certified veterinary technicians shall be required to continue their professional education as a condition of maintaining his/her license of veterinary technology in the state of _____ with _____ hours of continuing education required annually.

IV. REMOVAL OF VETERINARY TECHNICIAN LICENSES, REGISTRATIONS OR CERTIFICATIONS

A. All licenses, registrations or certifications issued to veterinary technicians in the state of _____ shall expire on _____ of every year unless renewed.
B. All license, registration or certification holders shall submit renewal fees and a current mailing address by the dates determined by the Board on a renewal form that shall be provided by the Board and mailed to all license, registration or certification holders.
C. All license, registration or certification holders will be required to submit evidence of the necessary amount of continuing education in the fields of veterinary medicine to the Board as required by the Board for license, registration or certification renewal.
D. Failure to submit the appropriate license, registration or certification renewal fee by the dates determined by the Board shall result in forfeiture of all privileges and rights extended by the license, registration or certification and the license, registration or certification holder must immediately cease and desist in engaging further in the performance of veterinary technician activities under the _____ veterinary practice act until payment of delinquency fee in addition to the license, registration or certification renewal fee had been received by the Board.

From the American Veterinary Medical Association (AVMA) membership directory.

- The veterinarian or veterinary technician failed to provide a reasonable level of medical care to the patient and in this way was professionally negligent.
- The patient was injured as a result of the negligence.

Although veterinary technicians can be and are sued for malpractice, it is still relatively rare. Legal responsibility for the clinical actions of veterinary technicians generally falls on the supervising veterinarian. Under the common law doctrine of *respondeat superior*, veterinarians may be found negligent for the injurious actions of veterinary technicians. For example, if a veterinary technician gives a cat 6 ml of insulin instead of 0.06 ml, as directed by the veterinarian, and the cat dies as a result of the overdose, the veterinarian may be found negligent and not the veterinary technician. On the other hand, in rare circumstances, veterinary technicians may be found negligent for carrying out the injurious instructions of the supervising veterinarian.

ETHICS AND THE WORKPLACE

Working and living within their respective communities, people are faced with ethical issues, which may be divided into three classifications: societal, personal, and professional.

Societal Ethics

The ethics that are established by society are generally written into law. The laws may include federal legislation against major offenses such as committing murder, rape, embezzlement, and arson, or they may be local ordinances that require people to walk their dogs on leashes or that prohibit loitering. Individuals may not be aware of all the ordinances, rules, and regulations that govern what they should and should not do, but most people are taught from an early age about the most important laws, such as those that prohibit stealing.

Personal Ethics

In addition to the laws of society, each person is guided by an array of personal principles that give him or her a sense of what is right and wrong and what is fair and unfair. For example, issues concerning sexuality, gender roles, dress, family structure, religious choice, and political beliefs are left to the individual to consider. For Americans, the right to make personal choices regarding family, religion, and politics is a fundamental right, but this is not the case in all cultures. In some countries, these issues are controlled by legislative laws and thus become societal rather than personal ethics.

Professional Ethics

As with all citizens, the individuals that make up a profession are bound by societal laws and ethics. In addition, a code of ethics is established by members of the profession to help define and encourage conduct specific to that profession. This code is important and helps to provide additional guidelines by which people carry out their jobs. In veterinary technology, the professional code of ethics has been established by NAVTA. Box 6 outlines NAVTA's nine-point code of ethics.

Professional Ideals

In addition, to the profession's code of ethics, NAVTA has established a list of ideals and recommended behaviors. These encourage veterinary technicians to take pride in their work, dress, and overall presentation; to participate

---

Box 6	THE PROFESSION'S CODE OF ETHICS

Veterinary technicians shall:

1. Aid society and animals through providing excellent care and services for animals.
2. Prevent and relieve the suffering of animals.
3. Promote public health by assisting with the control of zoonotic diseases and informing the public about these diseases.
4. Assume accountability for individual professional actions and judgments.
5. Protect confidential information provided by clients.
6. Safeguard the public and the profession against individuals deficient in professional competence or ethics.
7. Assist with efforts to ensure conditions of employment consistent with the excellent care for animals.
8. Remain competent in veterinary technology through commitment to lifelong learning.
9. Collaborate with members of the veterinary medical profession in efforts to ensure quality health care services for all animals.

From the *2000 Resource Guide of the North American Veterinary Technician Association (NAVTA)*.

---

in professional organizations; and to promote veterinary technology by participating in career days and by giving talks to community groups. As already mentioned, it is important for veterinary technicians to continue their education by attending professional conferences and by being receptive to new ideas and suggestions at work. In addition, veterinary technicians should be respectful of confidential information, should avoid gossip, and should be honest when dealing with co-workers and clients. Finally, veterinary technicians should strive to improve the standards of their profession by contributing to the profession's body of knowledge and by supporting legislation that defines and strengthens the role of the veterinary technician.

PROFESSIONAL AND RELATED ORGANIZATIONS

Many associations and professional societies support the education, professional interests, and activities of the veterinary technician. NAVTA, which represents the profession of veterinary technology in North America, has been a particular leader in shaping and supporting the profession. NAVTA, for example, has written the code of ethics, the veterinary technician oath, and the veterinary technician portion of the model practice act and has brought about important changes in the profession's terminology. In Canada, the Canadian Association of Animal Health Technologists and Technicians (CAAHTT) represents seven provencial associations and is dedicated to promoting the profession of veterinary technology within the animal community and the public in general. Continued growth of veterinary technology therefore depends heavily on the efforts of individuals within this and other professionally related organizations. Graduate veterinary technicians can assist in advancing their profession by joining and being active members of national, state (or provencial), and regional veterinary technician associations, some of which are listed below.

AVMA's Listing of Veterinary Technician Associations

Web site: http://www.avma.org/care4pets/vtassns.htm

Academy of Veterinary Emergency and Critical Care Technicians (Acad. VECCT)
Organizing Committee, c/o VECCS
15729 San Pedro, San Antonio, TX 78232
Phone: (210) 826-1488
Web site: http://veccs.org/technicians

American Society of Veterinary Dental Technicians (ASVDT)
PO Box 1636, Venice, FL 34284-1636

Association of Zoo Veterinary Technicians (AZVT)
Virginia Crossett, Executive Director, Louisville Zoo
PO Box 37250, Louisville, KY 40233
Phone: (502) 451-0440, ext. 345; fax: (502) 459-2196
E-mail: jtutnage@sandiegozoo.org
Web site: http://www.worldzoo.org/AZVT

Canadian Association of Animal Health Technologists and Technicians (CAAHTT)
c/o Sandy Hass
Box 91, Grandora, SK S0K 1V0 Canada
Phone: (306) 329-8660; fax: (306) 329-4700
E-mail: s.vettech@sk.Sympatico.ca
Web site: www.caahtt-acttsa.com

International Veterinary Nurses and Technicians Association (IVNTA)
Web site: http://www.vetweb.co.uk/sites/ivna/index.htm

North American Veterinary Technician Association (NAVTA)
Battleground, IN 47920
Phone or fax: (765) 742-2216
E-mail: NAVTA@compuserv.com

Veterinary Technician Anesthetist Society (VTAS)
Stephanie Plattner, Purdue University
1249 Lynn Hall, West Lafayette, IN 47907

Related Organizations

American Animal Hospital Association (AAHA)
PO Box 150899, Denver, CO 80215-0899
Phone: (303) 986-2800; fax: (303) 986-1700

American Association for Laboratory Animal Science (AALAS)
Michael Sonday, Executive Director
9190 Crestwyn Hills Dr, Memphis, TN 38125
Phone: (901) 754-8620
Web site: http://www.aalas.org

American Association of Veterinary State Boards (AAVSB)
3100 Main St, Suite 208, Kansas City, MO 64111
Phone: (816) 931-1504, fax: (816) 931-1604

American Veterinary Medical Association (AVMA)
Suite 100, 1931 North Meacham Rd
Schaumburg, IL 60173
Phone: (847) 925-8070; fax: (847) 925-1329
Web site: http://www.avma.org

Association of Veterinary Technician Educators (AVTE)
Terry Teeple, DVM, Pierce College
9401 Farwest Dr SW, Tacoma, WA 98498
Phone: (253) 964-6668; fax: (253) 964-6599
Web site: http://www.br.cc.va.us/avte/

Committee on Veterinary Technician Education and Activities (CVTEA)
AVMA
Suite 100, 1931 North Meacham Rd
Schaumburg, IL 60173
Phone: (847) 925-8070; fax: (847) 925-1329

Northeast Veterinary Technician Educators Association (NEVTEA)
Wendy Curtis-Uhle, CVT,
Veterinary Hospital, University of Pennsylvania
38th and Spruce St, Philadelphia, PA 19104

Professional Examination Service (PES)
475 Riverside Dr, New York, NY 10115-0089 (for information regarding the Veterinary Technician National Examination or the AALAS Animal Technician Certification Program)

Veterinary Emergency and Critical Care Society (VECCS)
8015 Broadway, Suite 201, San Antonio, TX 78209

RECOMMENDED READING

The Veterinary Technician Professional journal by Veterinary Learning Systems
Jennifer Schori-Deery, Editor-in-Chief
425 Phillips Blvd., Trenton, NJ 08618

NAVTA Newsletter
Monthly publication by NAVTA
PO Box 224, Battleground, IN 47920
Phone or fax: (765) 742-2216
E-mail: NAVTA@compuserv.com

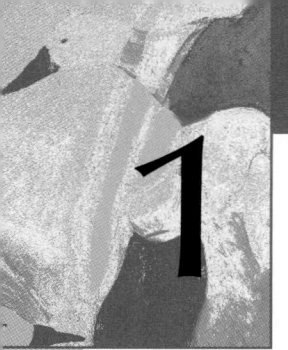

Restraint and Handling of Animals

Dennis D. French • *Thomas N. Tully*

Most people entering the field of veterinary medicine have had experience with some animals, but few have had the experience necessary to deal with all species that may be encountered. To assume all animals respond in the same manner is not correct and can be quite dangerous. Restraint techniques differ markedly among species, and the response of different animals to restraint also is highly variable. The wise individual is able to ascertain what the body language of a particular animal means and respond to the actions of that animal appropriately. Animals that are herd oriented present unique problems for the uninitiated.

This chapter is intended to be a guide to the behavior, handling, and restraint of animals commonly encountered in veterinary practice. It is not intended to be an exhaustive text, but rather to provide a range of techniques to build confidence and competence.

INDICATIONS FOR RESTRAINT

The most obvious reason for restraint of an animal is to control it for an examination or a procedure. The reaction of the animal to unpleasant experiences, sometimes simply avoiding the people trying to restrain it, can be disastrous. Environmental factors must be considered when developing a plan for restraint. Veterinary personnel should be aware from the time that they accept the animal from the owner that situations may develop that are potentially dangerous for the animals. Two dogs passing in the reception area may decide that they are mortal enemies, and a fight may ensue. Dogs and cats are generally examined on tables, and scrambling off the table may result in a damaging fall. Large animals are often held in extremely hazardous environments. Fences constructed of barbed wire can cause massive cuts to equine skin, an unacceptable outcome for all when attempting to catch a horse for a routine examination. Buildings with tin walls that do not extend completely underground will cause heel bulb lacerations

when the horse wheels away from a would-be handler and catches the foot under the bottom of the tin. Protruding nails in a stall may cause skin lacerations or a puncture of the cornea as the horse spins away from the handler trying to halter it. Low sheds can result in severe damage to the head in both horses and cattle. Veterinary personnel must try to make the reception and examination areas as safe as possible. The unfortunate truth is that clients will blame the veterinary practice and the people involved if their animals are injured during an examination.

Restraint for the purpose of physical examination, diagnostic, or therapeutic procedures commonly performed on animals may be unpleasant for them, and most animals will attempt to escape or at least resist. To avoid excessive discomfort for the animal the application of restraint should be to the minimum effective level. The procedure and the animal's response will determine the level of restraint. For example, the examination of a cat's mouth can usually be performed with a minimal hold on the animal, whereas the examination of a cow's mouth will require significant restraint.

Another reason for proper restraint and handling is to prevent the animal from harming itself during the procedure. Venipuncture may result in torn vessels, hematomas, and free-flowing blood if the animal is not properly restrained for the procedure. In pigs, bleeding from the anterior vena cava without proper restraint may result in laceration of the vessel, or phrenic nerve, and subsequent death of the animal. Rectal palpation of a struggling horse may result in a rectal tear for the horse or serious musculoskeletal injury of the veterinary staff. Surgical procedures performed on inadequately restrained animals are doomed to failure. Restraining devices (Elizabethan collars, neck cradles) are used in many aspects of veterinary practice to protect the animal from self-mutilation following procedures.

Probably the most important reason for restraint is to protect the personnel involved in the procedure. All veterinary personnel rely on their own functioning body parts to perform their job and make a living. Slight injuries may result in significant loss of income or efficiency. Bruised and swollen hands from bites and scratches cannot assist in surgery. The use of crutches or wheelchairs severely limits mobility and restraint capabilities around large animals. Severe injuries, including disfigurement or septicemia, may occur from bites. Kicks and body slams from large animals may also result in significant damage to personnel, with subsequent loss of time and income. The veterinarian and associated personnel are legally responsible for any injuries to the client while performing a veterinary procedure. This liability begins when the client enters the practice facility or the truck stops in the driveway. The liability includes injuries occurring during the initial capture of the animal.

Technician Note

Protection of personnel involved in veterinary procedures may be the most important reason for the use of restraint.

Effective restraint is paramount to success of a veterinary practice. Quality practice begins with the physical examination, and this can only be accomplished with the animal properly restrained. The health and safety of the animals and people involved must be identified as the primary goal. Human perception of animal behavior can be used to better control and maneuver animals. This involves interspecies communication that is usually silent. The popularity of behavioral science and the "horse whisperers" is simply a study in animal-to-animal behavior into which humans have been interjected. The unspoken language of gestures, touches, and actions is all a part of animal communication to which humans have become responsive.

We all possess innate abilities to control and manipulate animals that can be consciously developed according to interest or occupation. The perceptive student of animal communication may acquire these techniques quickly, and the use of these techniques will greatly facilitate handling of any animal. Caution and analysis of each situation are warranted, however, because animals that have disease do not react in the same manner as healthy animals. A normal feedlot steer does not usually challenge pen riders, but a bad case of "foot rot" may make him charge the horse and rider in an effort to convince the threat to go away. Another consideration that will affect behavior, especially in herd situations, is the mixing of males and females. A normally docile stallion placed into a brood-mare band will protect his band of mares against intruders. The presence of young, unweaned animals still under the watchful eye of their dam may totally change the expected reactions of a mare, cow, or sow.

Thoughtful assessment of the situation, careful application of the knowledge of species behavior, and the use of appropriate equipment will facilitate restraint of all animals.

ANIMAL PERCEPTION AND BEHAVIOR

All animals are aware of their environment and the changes occurring around them. They use their five senses just as we do, particularly those of sight, smell, and hearing. The question of how an animal senses your encroachment into its environment must be a primary consideration in approaching that animal.

Smell

The sense of smell is well developed in all domestic mammals. The rabbit and cat have improved olfaction because of olfactory epithelium that is nearly 14 times more developed than in humans.

Horses will snort when faced with a smell with which they are unfamiliar. Bulls may react by pawing and blowing when they are faced with a different smell. It is sometimes said that animals can smell fear. Behaviorists point out that body language is more likely to convey lack of confidence, and this may be misconstrued as the smell of fear. However, the language of smell undoubtedly has a more extensive vocabulary in animals than in humans.

Hearing

All domestic mammals have well-developed methods for collecting sound waves into the external ear. Domestic animals are able to move the pinnae, the skin-covered cartilaginous sound collectors of the ear, with muscles, which enables them to focus on the source of the sound. This is advantageous to the handler as an approach is made to a new animal. Slight sounds will elicit movement of the ears and allow the animal to become aware of the presence of someone new. Low, smooth, confidant tones will allow the animal to become comfortable with your presence. The response of the ear is important to assess the animal's attitude. The ears-back position in a horse or llama signals that the animal is upset or aggressive. A dog pricks its ears forward when dominant or actively aggressive, whereas a submissive dog wrinkles and flattens its ears. Cats with their ears pinned back should be considered dangerous.

Vision

Domestic animals, with the exception of pigs, have a special layer behind the lens called the *tapetum* that permits them better vision in low light.

Herbivorous animals have wide fields of vision enabling them to detect the encroachment of predators from various angles. This is particularly evident in the horse and rabbit, both of which enjoy nearly circumferential vision without moving the head.

Technician Note

With the exception of pigs, domestic animals have a special layer behind the lens called the *tapetum*, which permits them better vision in low light.

The eyes of domestic animals focus by means of muscles controlling the shape of the lens. Most animals accommodate the eye on near objects much less readily than do humans. The horse has a particularly sluggish accommodation. What some handlers may perceive as fractious and spooky may in fact be nothing more than the horse attempting to visually accommodate. This is particularly noticeable when an already nervous human makes fast movements near a horse. The horse moves about in a rapid manner trying to ascertain what the human wants. Horses apparently have very acute vision at middle and far distances, which is not surprising for a prey species. Many of the behavioral displays of horses are visual in nature, and subtle movements by handlers at seemingly great distances will generate responses from horses.

The dog's ability to discriminate form and pattern is thought to be poor when compared to human abilities. This is particularly important when dealing with those dogs that are noted to be "fear biters."

Cats have excellent night vision, which is consistent with their nocturnal habits. They are also acutely aware of a small movement, which facilitates the precision of their rush after stalking their prey. Unfortunately, this also enhances the ability of a fearful or vengeful feline patient to strike out against those humans who move too suddenly or come too close.

Touch

The sense of touch is becoming more important in the handling of animals. Numerous behaviorists and trainers are now proponents of contact on different body parts to enhance communication between animals and among animals and humans. Contact behaviors that appear to result from or resolve conflict are the ones most described in handling. Dominant animals use biting, scratching, kicking, or striking to teach youngsters proper behavior. Dogs have been observed to bite or hold the scruff of puppies' necks, hold their muzzles, or force them prone by the application of weight over the withers as a show of dominance if their behavior is unacceptable. This is why hanging dogs or shaking them by the scruff or collar is often a potent punishment. Horses kick or slam a shoulder into other horses to demonstrate dominance and make a point of their supremacy. Mares training youngsters in a herd will actually keep a particularly hardheaded yearling out of the herd by biting and kicking at it. Some people will use blows to correct unacceptable equine behavior. However, when using these techniques the target must be carefully selected, and the individual must possess the physical strength to make the procedure effective. As a general rule, humans will end up hurting themselves much more than the horse they were trying to correct.

The actual method of how to touch animals is a manner of skill. Tentative, light touches or repeated patting makes many species nervous and apprehensive. Steady, firm strokes are reassuring to most species. Watching animals in a natural setting provides the insight into how to most effectively touch them when they are nervous. You will never observe one animal slapping another to calm it down in a natural setting. Clever individuals learn to read the animals that they are asked to restrain and develop the touch necessary to keep them calm.

Agonistic Behaviors

Agonistic behaviors are those associated with conflict. Many animals have to be maneuvered into a position in which restraint is possible, or they must be restrained from the outset as a safety measure. Such maneuvering is perceived by the animal as conflict, and to understand the principles of maneuvering each species, it is wise to become familiar with the predominant forms of agonistic behavior in the different species. Agonistic behaviors cover the range of response to conflict from passive avoidance through the assertion of dominance to the extreme of aggression and fighting. In nature, overt aggressive attacks that lead to fights with other animals of the same or different species are not common outside sexual or predatory behavior. Dominance and submissive behaviors represent the more common method of resolving disagreement over things such as territory and favors. Chapter 13 gives additional information on animal behavior.

Fight or Flight

When a stranger approaches an animal the same basic principles apply whether it is a domestic or wild animal. Each species in a given environment has its own degree of response, but the factors or cues giving rise to the response are common to all animals in varying degrees. Each animal has a fight-or-flight distance. When that space is invaded the animal goes into a state of alert. The sympathetic nervous system releases epinephrine from the adrenal gland. This hormone causes increased heart rate and subsequent increase in blood flow to the skeletal muscles, lungs, and brain. Further encroachment into the animal's space will lead to action that may take the form of avoidance (the cow or horse crash through a fence, the dog runs off down the road) or aggression (the dog bites, the cow runs over the stranger). This action is aptly termed the *fight-or-flight response*. The response will vary from animal to animal of the same species and may vary from time to time for the same animal. When this happens it is very difficult to come up with a good restraint plan.

Aggressive Behavior

Aggressive behavior is the form of agonistic or conflict behavior that leads to and includes fighting. Aggression is not the result of a single cause. The different forms of aggression are classified according to the stimuli or circumstances giving rise to the ferocity.

Irritable or Pain-Induced Aggression

Inevitably, pain-induced aggression is a common problem in the veterinary hospital and in field situations. Herd animals that have become incapacitated and are incapable of keeping up with the herd must resort to aggression to stay alive. Injections and certain manipulations, such as treatment of wounds, cause pain and discomfort that animals may resent. Even the initial injection of a local anesthetic can be most uncomfortable no matter how skilled the anesthetist. The state of mind of the patient has a lot to do with an aggressive outcome. If the animal is initially apprehensive and nervous, the probability for aggression is high. This is the reason that calming and familiarization of the patient are practiced whenever possible. Sedation may also be indicated for certain patients.

Maternal Aggression

All female domestic animals that are suckling their young are sensitized to interference with their offspring by strangers. The calmest, old brood mare in the herd may be extremely protective of her new foal. The bitch can be aggressive with strangers and even family members if she perceives a threat to her pups. A sow within earshot of her piglets when they are being restrained can become one of the most dangerous animals encountered. All parties working within a farrowing house must exercise caution, because the vocalization of any young piglet as it is manipulated can make all the sows in the house become sensitized.

> ### Technician Note
> All female domestic animals that are suckling their young are sensitized to interference with their offspring by strangers.

Predatory Aggression

Aggressive activity displayed by chasing and killing prey is observed in predatory domestic animals, such as the dog and cat, and is called *predatory aggression*. This form of aggression does not usually pose a threat to the animal handler, although large dogs may pull the handler down if they feel the urge to chase a cat while on leash.

Territorial Aggression

All domestic mammals have a degree of territorial domain. They will protect the area over which they range from intruders, and they may, in fact, exhibit territorial aggression. Separate groups of horses may share feeding sites and watering holes, but they remain apart from one another and retain control of their own separate home range. The domestic dog regards the yard as its territory or the territory of its pack (the dog's human family). Strangers are treated with suspicion, and this suspicion may lead to barking or attack. Dogs that harass the mail carrier or meter reader are behaving within the norm of canine behavior. The female rabbit is strongly territorial in the captive situation. If a buck is taken to her cage, she will attack him aggressively, often causing serious injury. Thus the doe is always taken to the buck's cage for mating. This female territoriality may be associated with aggression that continues even when the nesting box is empty and can be directed at humans. While the concept of an "attack rabbit" may seem humorous, it becomes less so when reaching into the cage of an old doe and being growled at, struck, and bitten.

Fear-Induced Aggression

When an animal is terrified of an environment and the people in it and is not given an option to avoid the circumstances, it will resort to aggression. Fear is a common cause of aggression in dogs placed under such circumstances. Fear biting is the most commonly encountered type of attack in veterinary hospitals. The attack is not overtly dominant, and the dog is usually giving classic signs of being intimidated: avoiding direct eye contact with the head down, lips pulled back horizontally, ears flattened, and the tail between the legs (Figure 1-1). When the personal space of such a dog is encroached, a sudden attack may ensue. This is fear biting. The attack is usually confined to the proffered hand or forearm, and the purpose is simply to repel the invader.

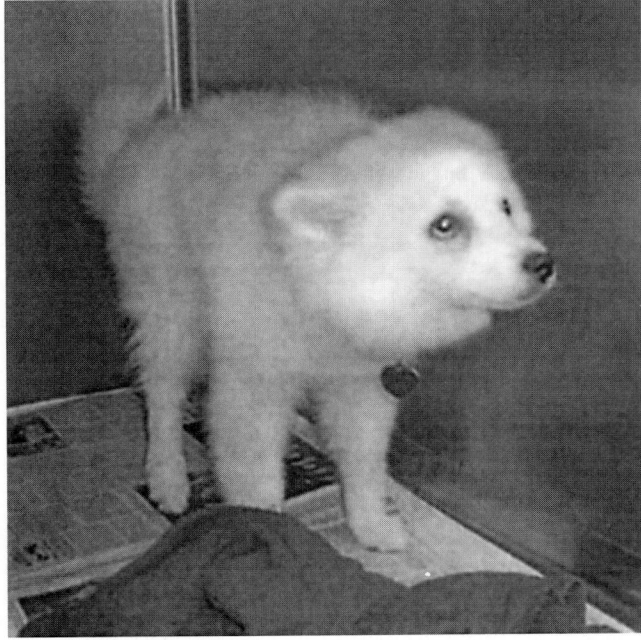

FIGURE 1-1. This dog demonstrates the posture of a classic "fear biter." Note the defensive stare with the ears laid back and the tail between the legs.

Intermale Aggression

Aggression occurring between males can be a problem, particularly when stud animals are being kept. Boars can be extremely vicious when confronting each other, and great care should be taken when handling them. Stallions can become extremely agitated when mixed with another stallion. Bulls spend a great deal of time head butting and pushing one another around to establish the dominance order when they are turned out together.

Dominance Aggression

Certain dogs will establish their authority over a human family, other animals, and strangers because of their heritage as pack animals. Alternatively, a dog may accede to dominance from one family member but attempt to assert itself aggressively with other family members. Such animals are a menace in the clinic, since they will not only fear bite but also attack. Persuasion is of little value in handling these dogs. This type of animal is dangerous, and reliable restraint must be used at all times when handling it.

Typical Behavior of Domestic Animals in Aggression and Avoidance

Cattle

The primary concern when dealing with cattle is bulls, regardless of size. Dairy breed bulls such as the Jersey and Holstein should be considered the most dangerous animal of all the species that veterinary personnel are asked to restrain or handle. They are powerful, unpredictable, and mean spirited. Aggressive behavior is characterized by pawing the ground with the forefeet while holding the head with the frontal area nearly vertical with the ground and snorting. These bulls, after charging and knocking the person down, will make continued attempts to toss the victim, which will lead to goring if the bull still has horns. Bulls may also attempt to kneel on the victim, or continually smash the victim with their foreheads. Little can be done to dissuade or thwart a bull once this activity begins. Front-end loaders and pickup trucks have been used to try to push these animals away from their targets without success. Bulls, particularly the dairy breed types, should always be treated with the utmost respect and with the appropriate means of restraint and containment. The likelihood of a snorting bull, posturing in an aggressive stance, hurting a handler is actually less than one that has been hand raised. The hand-raised bull may appear to be quite gentle and yet when approached may react aggressively. Special handling considerations are made for those who work with semen donors at bull studs. These bulls are selected for the high-quality genetic potentials, and their semen is worth considerable amounts of money. Insensitive handling before and during collection may give rise to reproductive behavior problems leading to decreased collection volumes and significant economic loss.

Aggressiveness in the heifer and cow seems to be directly related to breed and socialization. Dairy cows are generally very docile, probably because they are handled a great deal. Beef cows that have been handled frequently in a quiet, professional manner are very manageable. However, beef cattle that are raised on range with very little human interaction or those that are handled with lots of whipping and shouting tend to be apprehensive and may become quite aggressive. This aggressiveness is compounded when they are nursing calves.

The fight-or-flight distance for a herd of cattle will vary depending on the previous degree and type of contact with humans. The handling of dairy cattle and beef cattle differs greatly. Flight distance for dairy cows is extremely short, with the animal veering off only when directly confronted by the handler. Most dairy cattle are used to a number of different people being around them during milking time and do not resent the introduction of someone new into the herd. This makes handling dairy cows easier for veterinary personnel. Beef cattle have a much longer flight space, which is accentuated when they sense a new presence in a field or pen. It is common for ranchers to be able to walk or drive among their cattle at very close range. When a new pickup or person enters the pasture the cattle's heads come up and they will gradually move further away. If the cattle are approached too quickly, they will break into a disorganized run, which makes them nearly impossible to maneuver. It is important to realize the impact that outsiders have on a herd of beef cattle before trying to handle and examine individuals.

Part of the secret of maneuvering cattle is using a body extension. Canes, stock whips, or wiffle paddles used by a person on foot are viewed by the cattle as an extension of the body. If the cattle can be kept calm, the visual barrier created by these devices allows the handler to maneuver the cattle from pen to pen. If cattle are accustomed to being observed from horseback, maneuvering a herd can be quite easy for one or two riders. Mixing riders and walkers in a pasture is not a good idea and should only be done as a last resort when trying to maneuver a herd of cattle.

Calves

Calves are inquisitive and will become very attentive to the presence of someone new. The calf stretching its head or neck toward the new handler is the usual posture (Figure 1-2). Darting movements will cause the calf to panic, veer, and run away. The approach toward a calf should be slow and deliberate with the hands slightly away from the sides of the body. No loud noises are necessary, and movement of the hands and arms should be kept to a minimum. Using a fence line, or wall, the handler should move to cut off escape routes and negotiate the calf into a corner and then grab it with one arm under the jaw and the other hand should reach and grab the tail.

Cats

Aggressive behavior in cats should never be underestimated. They can be formidable patients in situations of conflict because they will use the claws of all four feet, they have razor-sharp teeth, and when stressed they seem to have a spinal cord that is made much like a Slinky, which allows them to go in many different directions at once. It should be remembered that the cat stalks its prey and runs only short distances to pounce. It is a stealthy aggressor. The true speed of the cat never becomes apparent until it is actively avoiding conflict. When handling cats in any environment, all doors and windows must be closed to prevent escape.

 Technician Note

When handling cats in any environment, close all doors and windows to prevent escape.

Dogs

Overtly aggressive behavior, although not a common problem in dogs, is a significant social problem and one that

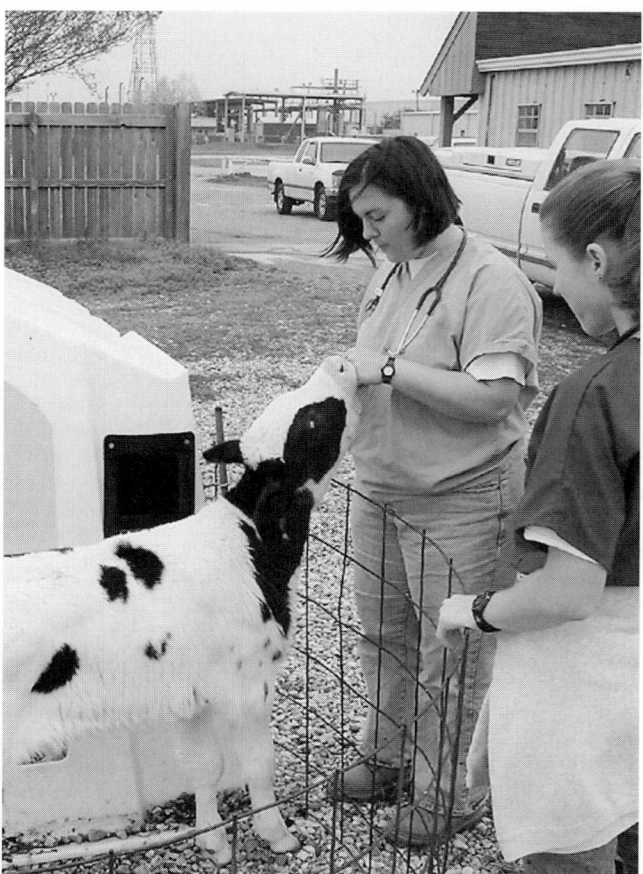

FIGURE 1-2. This Holstein calf demonstrates the curiosity that most bovids have at an early age. It has come up to the new handler without any reservations.

will present difficulties for veterinary personnel. Dominance and submission are important in communication between two dogs in a conflict situation. Fixing the other animal in a direct stare signals dominance. The ears are raised and angled forward. The front end of the body is held high, and the hackles on the back of the neck are raised. The head is held up, and the lips curl to reveal the incisor and canine teeth. The tail will be raised. The clinical stare of veterinary personnel as they examine a dog can be taken as a dominance challenge by a dog.

Lowering the front end of the body and avoiding direct eye contact demonstrate the submissive role. Usually the tail will be held between the legs and the dog may squat and urinate or defecate. The spine may adopt an S shape, and the animal may lie down on its side or back, raising the legs and exposing the undefended belly.

When confronted by a person the dog may demonstrate potential aggression by adopting the dominantly aggressive posture, or it may adopt a submissive stance. The ears will flatten on the back of the head, and the lips may become pulled back at the corners of the mouth into a "grin." The tail is held between the legs. A dog in the active or dominant aggressive posture may attack if the threat is not removed from its fight-or-flight distance. A dog in this posture will bite only if you attempt to encroach on its space. Some dogs may show active aggression only when the owner is present. The protectiveness may actually be possessiveness as the dog defends its own favored object. Removing the owner may resolve the conflict. The opposite may occur when handling dogs that have developed a bond with their usual handlers. These dogs may be quite aggressive without their human partner in the examination room. Retrievers, herding dogs, and guard dogs that tend to associate closely with only one individual may be quite difficult to handle without their owner present.

Certain dogs do not attempt to resolve conflict by dominance or aggression, preferring to avoid it if at all possible. Those that skillfully avoid conflict are described as having a passive defense reflex. Dogs that tend to face conflict are said to have an active defense reflex.

Horses

Blatant aggressiveness in the horse is not common. However, certain horses can be nasty with their aggression. This is most commonly seen in horses that are stalled most of the time. Racehorses and breeding stallions seem to be the worst offenders. Aggressive behavior may be observed on brood mare farms with mares protecting new foals and stallions protecting their band of mares. Lunging forward and biting, kicking with the hind legs, and striking with the front legs characterize the aggressive acts of the horse. Although the field of vision of the horse is nearly 360 degrees, the binocular field of vision is only 60 to 70 degrees in front of the animal. Binocular vision is required for judging distance; therefore vision outside this range requires movement of the head and sometimes the entire body to allow the horse to further investigate what it perceives as the threat.

The approach to a horse should not be made from the blind spot directly behind the horse. The horse, as it detects new objects or people in its environment, will raise its head and observe. If no threat is perceived, the horse resumes its previous activity. If the threat is perceived as real the head turns toward the object, the neck is raised, and the ears will turn toward the object. The nostrils will become dilated to further evaluate the threat. The tail will also become elevated, and the muscles of the torso and lower limbs will become more rigid, ready for fight or flight. Occasionally the horse will snort, further alerting other horses to the presence. Mares with foals will usually nicker, and the foal will move to the other side of the mare. Further encroachment results in rapid movement away from the intruder. If the horse is in a stall it will circle rapidly away, always keeping its hind end toward the intruder.

Technician Note

The approach to a horse should not be made from the blind spot directly behind the horse.

Pigs

Aggressive behavior in the domestic pig has serious economic and physical consequences. Adult boars that are mixed together will circle and threaten each other with grunts and jaw snapping. Fighting commences in the side-to-side position with sideways pushing and slashing at one another with the tusks. Solid panels of plywood should be used to separate the combatants. Commercial pigs are reared in groups, which provide plenty of opportunity for fighting. When new pigs are introduced into a group, fighting will occur especially if living space and trough space are limited. Introducing a sow into an estab-

lished group may induce savage attacks and even deaths. Allowing more space and diversions for the group may reduce aggression in pigs.

Large numbers of unfamiliar pigs adapt better than smaller numbers. There is less fighting, probably because dominance is more difficult to establish in the larger social groups. Avoidance behavior in young pigs in confined areas involves running into corners and huddling, shoving, and climbing over one another. This does not present a problem if small groups are huddled, but larger groups that pile up may produce traumatic lesions and in severe cases death from suffocation.

Remember that the lactating sow can be extremely dangerous because of maternal aggression. When handling suckling pigs, always remove the sow to a secure area out of earshot if possible.

Technician Note

The lactating sow can be extremely dangerous because of maternal aggression.

Sheep

Avoidance behavior in sheep is the basis of maneuvering the flock. When sheep are approached they will flock together and move as a single unit. This herding behavior is well understood by dogs. By carefully controlling their posture, speed of movement, and distance from the flock, the dog uses the sheep's avoidance behavior to maneuver the flock into an enclosure. This is one of the most fascinating and complex interspecies relationships in domestic animal management.

Aggression between rams may lead to injuries between the combatants. Handling these rams may also be difficult because of the willingness of the ram to challenge the handler. Rams are most dangerous when they attempt to head butt and as such should be treated with respect.

Management Ethology

Ethology is the study of animal behavior (see also Chapter 13). Capture, handling, and restraint might be called management ethology, which is the study of animal behavior as a means of determining how best to maneuver and control animals. The approach and handling techniques that are described for each species are in harmony with the typical behavior of the animals that we are asked to restrain, and the physical techniques described are compatible with their anatomy. Humans have great powers of observation, and it is important for students of the animal industries to enhance their powers of observation about animal behavior. Knowledge of body systems and anatomic structure is clearly important, but there is no substitute for alertness, observation, and perception of how the animal is reacting to its environment and to the presence of veterinary personnel. Mental preparation must begin well in advance of any potentially dangerous restraint situation. Confidence and knowledge will be gained over time that ensures the handler of a correct assessment for any situation.

Capture and Restraint of Horses

A cardinal rule when approaching any animal, *especially* a horse, is not to startle it. The handler should always make his or her presence known by talking or calling to the horse. Many horses have learned that being captured leads to work or some sort of unpleasantness, and these types of horses will practice avoidance. Horses also do not like to be closely confined or "squeezed." Close quarters will make many horses anxious, and some will attempt to escape, which may result in injury to the horse and people involved. By calling to the horse the handler begins to have an appreciation of how a particular animal is going to respond.

> ### Technician Note
> A cardinal rule when approaching any animal, especially a horse, is not to startle it.

The normal flight distance of most horses is between 3 and 10 meters (m). Events that occur outside this radius are of little concern to the horse. Once within this area sudden movements or sharp noises may easily startle it. Always be sure that the horse is observing you as you approach. A horse that is looking at you is less likely to be startled than one looking off at some other object. Be aware that if the horse decides to become nervous the first evasive maneuver that it will perform is to wheel away, leaving you facing the hindquarters of the animal.

It should be obvious that approaching a horse from the rear should be avoided if possible. Given the horse's zone of vision and its blind spot, the horse is not likely to see a person directly behind them. A horse's kicking zone extends 1.8 to 2.5 m behind it. The furthest extension of the heels is the most dangerous and is the area of potentially fatal kicks to the head or chest. Horses usually kick to the rear, rather than to the side, but many of them can "cow kick," or kick to the side very well. Therefore it is wise to grant at least 3 m behind and to the side of a horse when dealing with the rear quarters of the horse. The other alternative is to stay in direct contact with the horse as you maneuver about the hind end (Figure 1-3). Staying close to the hindquarters will not allow the full force of a kick and will keep the force of the blow low on the recipient's anatomy. This does not mean that the blow will not be painful or damaging. However, a fractured tibia may be some consolation over a fractured skull. Grasping the tail may discourage some horses from kicking.

The prospective handler should also never stand directly in front of the horse. A horse that becomes agitated may strike out with a front foot and leg at any instant. Agitated horses also may decide to become carnivores at any time and attempt to bite the handler.

The initial approach to the horse is best accomplished from the front and left side (Figure 1-4). The left side in equine terminology is known as the *near side*. This is the side the horse is accustomed to being handled from because of tradition and the fact that most people lead their horses with their right hand. The first point of contact for the handler on the horse should be the withers. The handler should have a slightly outstretched arm that is no higher than the handler's shoulder. The handler should make some low, confidence-building conversation as he or she moves toward the horse. This goes back to the natural behavior of the horse, from mares licking their foals to the social interaction between horses in which they will rub each other on the withers. If the horse moves away, the handler should stop and stay still until the horse has quieted again. Many times if the handler will turn slightly away from the horse and not look directly at it, the horse will turn back to the handler (Figure 1-5). This movement

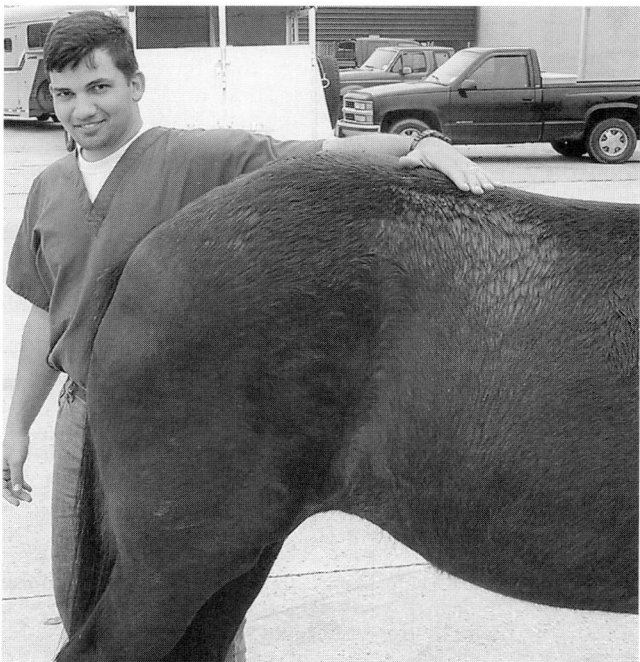

FIGURE 1-3. Note how the handler maintains contact with the horse as he begins to move from one side of the animal to the other. This is especially important since he is in the horse's blind spot.

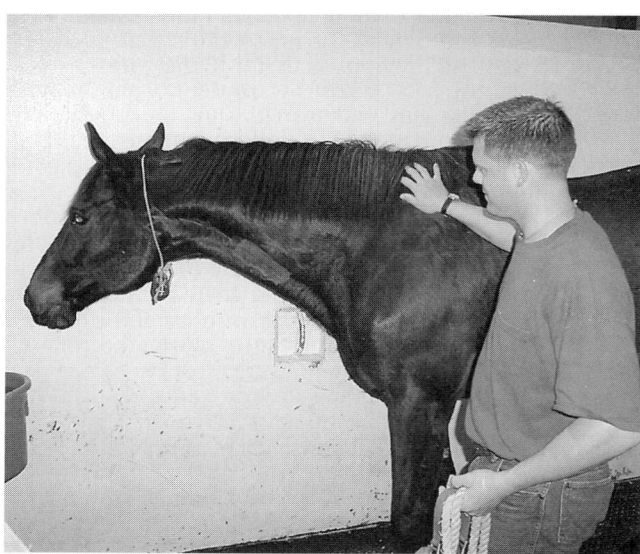

FIGURE 1-4. Initial approach to the horse should be from the left, or near, side. Note the right hand leads to touch the horse at the withers. The left hand holds the halter and lead rope low and to the handler's side.

mimics the communication found in herds of horses when an outsider is finally "welcomed" into the herd. It is always wise to move in slow increments without raising your hands or voice. Presenting the hands in an open and empty manner may help the horse to gain confidence. Sometimes it is beneficial to squat down. This works reasonably well

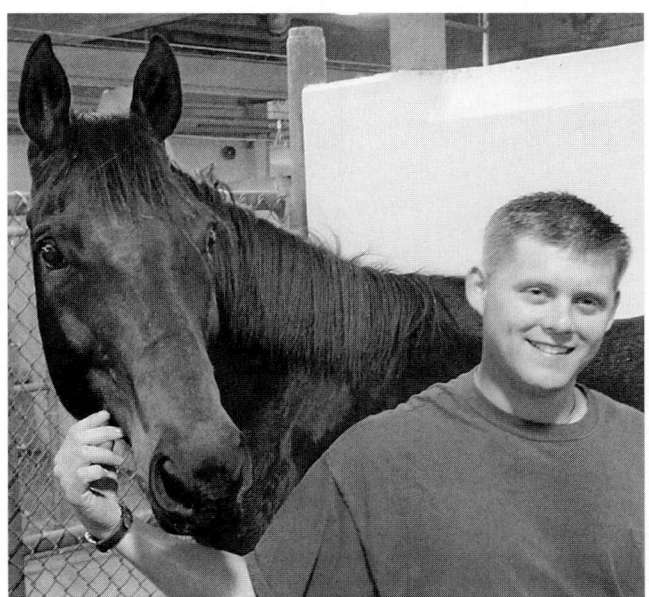

FIGURE 1-5. Note how the horse's ears and head are directed toward the would-be handler, almost as if the horse wants to know what is going to happen next.

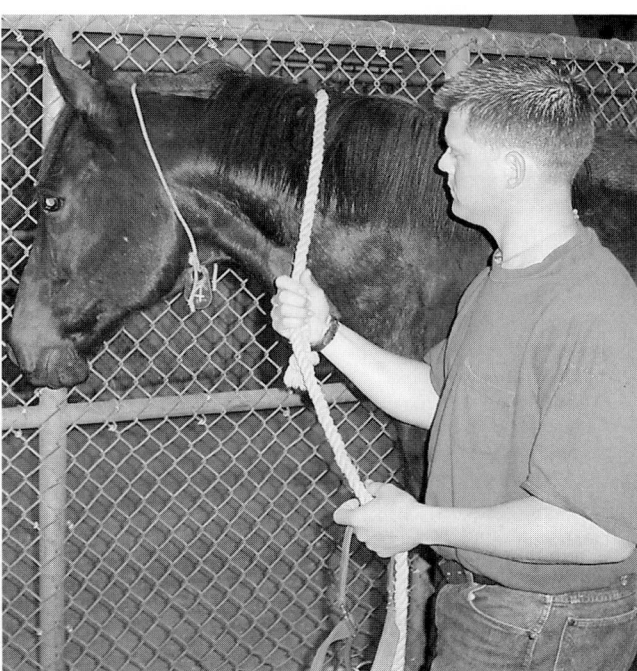

FIGURE 1-6. The use of a small rope looped over the horse's neck will aid in controlling the horse's head and allow the handler to place the halter over the nose.

with young foals and some horses. The shorter stature probably makes the figure less threatening and increases the horse's curiosity. Do not rush toward the horse at any time. Horses will assume you are giving chase and continue to move away, and some can become quite panicked. Once the would-be handler is behind the horse, the horse perceives even more of a threat since it cannot see the presumed intruder.

The approach to halter the horse should also be unhurried and without sudden movements. Keeping the lead rope or halter hidden by your side may assist in the capture of the skittish horse. A small-diameter catch rope may aid in the capture of the horse's neck (Figure 1-6). The rope may be carried up along the neck after gaining the horse's confidence at the withers by a moment of petting. If the horse moves away, attempt to stay with it by moving along side and holding onto the mane. Most horses will have sense enough to know that you mean business if you stay with them at this time.

When the horse is standing quietly, loop a rope around the neck by passing the rope over the horse's neck with the right hand and reaching under the neck to grab the free end with the left hand. When placing the rope over the neck start as low on the back as possible. Remember that slow and steady movements are the key to success. Once the rope is around the neck the horse may be held in the loop and the rope can be maneuvered to the throat-latch area. The halter can then be placed by sliding the nose band over the nose and passing the crown strap to the right hand and then bringing the strap over the horse's head for fastening.

The horse that does not respond to any of the above techniques becomes the biggest problem encountered in a field service practice. The arrival of veterinary personnel may trigger memories of previous contact that the horse does not want to have repeated. The usual reaction is for the horse to move off as far away from the handlers as possible. Of course, the simple solution is to have the horse caught before arrival of the veterinary team. However, this is not always possible. The usual solution to this problem is bribery with a handful or bucket of grain, which will entice the horse to approach or at least be approached. It is best to hold the bribe in the left hand and turn at right angles to the horse so that the neck is within easy reach for petting. As the horse gains confidence with some firm strokes along the shoulder, the right hand can then ease around the neck and allow capture. Many of these horses will attempt to wheel away when the arm is first placed over the neck, and this is where the small rope may be of assistance as a restraint aid. It is desirable to not allow horses to escape the first time because if they do it once they are likely to persist and become even harder to capture the second time. A horse that persists in whirling away becomes a candidate for trapping or, in extreme cases, roping.

Many horses that are impossible to catch in an open field will give up in an enclosed space. However, there are some that become exceptionally nervous in a small area and will kick or try to jump out when approached. The use of another haltered, calm horse within the stall to trap the nervous one will work in a majority of these cases. Similar to catching an unbroken foal, one handler will use the calm horse to trap the other in a corner. Then with slow and steady movements beginning at the withers, the second handler eases up the neck with a rope and makes the loop, which will allow temporary restraint of the nervous horse. A second technique that may be used is to have a solid panel that may be used to "squeeze" the horse into a corner. The panel needs to be sturdy enough to withstand the horse pushing against it and be movable enough to allow the handlers to back away in case the horse "blows up." This should be used as a last resort in attempting to capture the nervous horse. Remember that exciting a horse like this is self-defeating. Excited horses lose whatever sense they have and in fear will go over, under, or through whatever is attempting to contain them.

 Technician Note

Roping horses is the last thing any sane individual wants to do.

It is nearly impossible to rope a horse in a field, and holding on to the horse after it has been successfully roped is also very difficult. Dallying the rope off to the bumper of a truck is not an easy maneuver to accomplish, and then the roper must be able to stay out of the way of the rope as the horse swings back and forth on the other end. If you must rope a horse, it should only be attempted in a small, sturdy enclosure, such as a wooden pen. Do not use a round pen made of pipes. This is an invitation to disaster! It is better to leave the horse uncaught than to have to destroy it because it became hung in pipes and fractured a leg. It is important to keep the horse as quiet as possible and to hide the rope as well as possible. Therefore whirling the rope overhead is not good form, because the sound and sight of the rope will frighten most horses. A low, backhand technique is preferable when roping a horse. The loop is made so that it brushes the ground when the loop and rope are held at waist level (Figure 1-7). A generous amount of excess rope is played out from the coils, which should be held loosely in the off hand. The loop is held with the dominant hand and carried across the body in preparation for the backhand throw. The position of the roper should be about 3 m from a fence such that when the horse is driven past between the roper and the fence the horse will run into the backhand loop. This technique, although admittedly a last resort, can be extremely successful if all parties involved stay calm.

It should be emphasized that gloves should be worn when attempting to rope any animal. After the loop is over the horse's head the coils will come off very quickly. If the horse is charging through at such a rate that the rope cannot be held, release it before being jerked off balance and dragged in the dirt. The loose end of the rope can always be picked up from the ground after the horse has stopped running.

 Technician Note

Gloves should be worn when attempting to rope any animal.

Horses that demonstrate signs of dangerous behavior or viciousness should not be given the opportunity to harm veterinary personnel by their physical proximity. There are alternative means of capture such as tranquilization or anesthesia that do not require being close to the horse. Pole syringes, dart guns, and capture guns, although not common in equine practice, can save handlers from serious injury.

Capture and Restraint of Foals

Newborn foals act from instinct in avoiding strange creatures and will hide behind the dam for safety. Therefore to capture foals is somewhat more difficult and usually re-

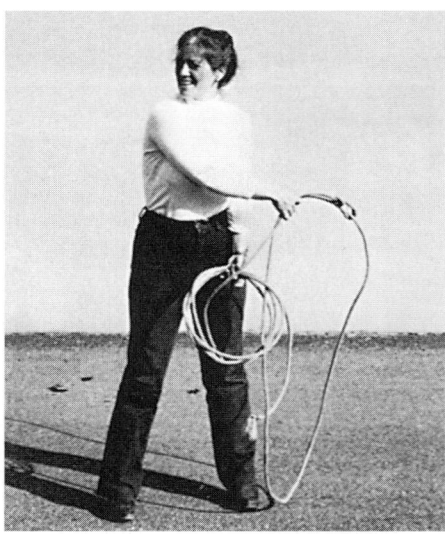

FIGURE 1-7. The method of holding the rope for a backhand throw at a horse.

quires two people. Undoubtedly, these foals will not be halter-broken, and if they are sick or injured they do not need the increased stress that accompanies training to halter. The easiest way to capture a suckling foal is to first catch the mare and back her in a corner of a stout wall or solid fence, allowing her foal to come into the corner between the wall and the mare. The barrier should not have any holes that the foal may try to climb through. Flimsy barriers or barbed wire fences should never be used in an attempt to capture foals. The handler of the mare should realize when the foal starts to struggle against the restraint, it may vocalize in fear and the mare might try to attack those who threaten her foal. The mare handler must be prepared to move the mare to a location away from the foal and handlers immediately following capture of the foal.

The mare should be positioned about the length of the foal away from the corner of the barrier, forming an open box in the corner of the barrier. One person then slowly goes behind the foal and invariably the foal will cower to the hindquarters of the mare (Figure 1-8). The foal should be approached midway between the head and tail with the knowledge that once it senses hands or arms on it, it will try to escape by bolting, rearing, or kicking. Most commonly the foal will bolt forward, into the mare's hindquarters, and the person should grab under the foal's neck and at the tail at this time. The tail should be held from underneath with the palm facing up. Grasping the tail is the most secure way to hold the hindquarters even though the foal may be uncomfortable. It is possible for one person to restrain the foal after this by grabbing the tail and holding it straight up over the back, keeping the other arm under the foal's neck (Figure 1-9). With bigger foals, two people are necessary for restraint, although the technique is similar. The first person advances toward the hindquarters of the foal as previously described and makes the initial contact with the hindquarters of the foal. The mare is then moved forward slightly, and the second person passes behind the mare and grabs under the foal's neck (Figure 1-10). Handlers may have to push the foal against a fence until the foal stops struggling. There is a tendency to lift

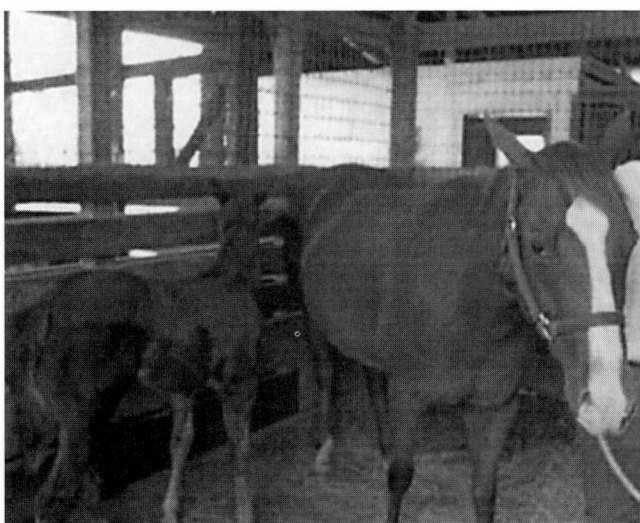

FIGURE 1-8.   The mare is backed into a corner and the foal is driven in beside her to safely capture the foal.

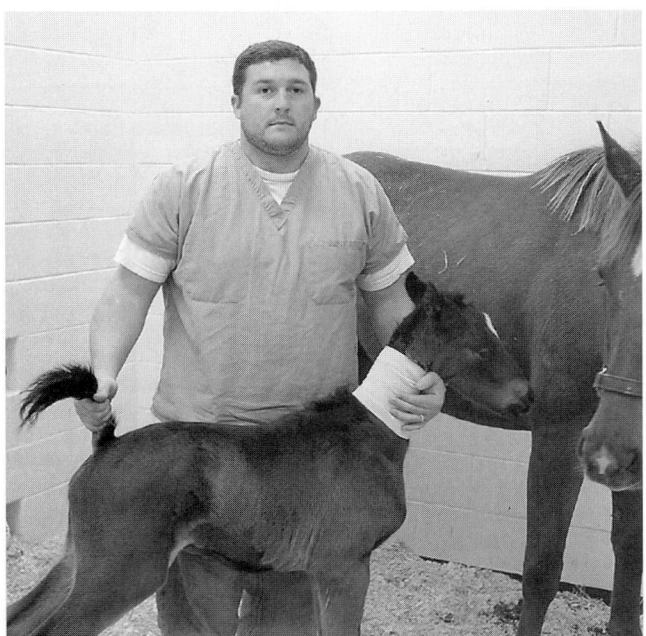

FIGURE 1-9.   The handler must move in swiftly from the side of the foal and capture the tail first and then sweep the arm under the neck of the foal. The mare handler must move her to a safe location at the same time.

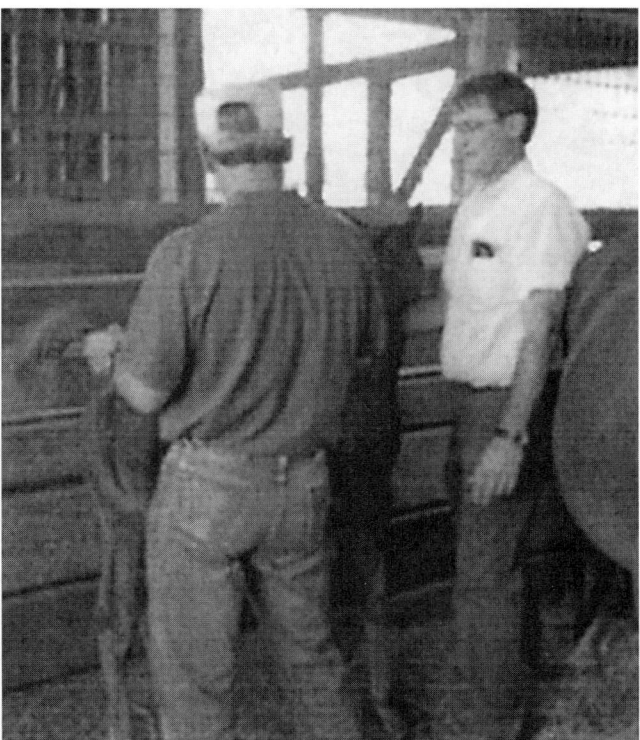

FIGURE 1-10.   Two people may be necessary to capture larger foals. The first enters from the rear, and the second comes around behind the mare and grabs the foal under the neck. The foal is then moved toward a solid wall for support.

small foals off the ground when accomplishing this task, which is poor form. When the foal loses its footing it may become more frightened and struggle more vigorously and batter the shins of the handler.

Attempts to capture foals only by the neck result in a rapid reverse by the foal and subsequent escape. Once a foal escapes, just as with adults, it becomes much harder to capture. Veterinary personnel should not contribute to the negative experiences of a foal. Extra care and gentle techniques should be employed to get the foal to develop trust in people as much as possible.

Following successful capture of the foal it is usually in the best interest of all to position the mare and foal so that they face each other. They should be as close as possible without the mare becoming a nuisance for the procedure being performed. It is generally not recommended to separate the mare and foal because they both will fret until rejoined.

Halter and Leads

The halter is the basic restraint tool for horses, and the lead shank should always be attached to the halter. Horses should never be lead by the halter alone; a lead should always be attached (Figure 1-11). The halter and rope shank may be inadequate for some tasks. Halters that have rings at the side of the nosepiece may be made more effective if a chain lead is passed from one side to the other. The lead is snapped on the side of the halter that is away from the handler after being passed through the loop near the handler, usually on the near side. This arrangement allows finer control of the direction of the horse's nose and, when snapped against the bridge of the nose, reinforces the authority of the restraint because of the discomfort it causes. The chain lead should come in contact with the horse very lightly, if at all, when leading the horse. Only when the horse misbehaves should the chain be used. Constant pressure is worrisome to the animal and does not leave the handler any reserve to use if necessary.

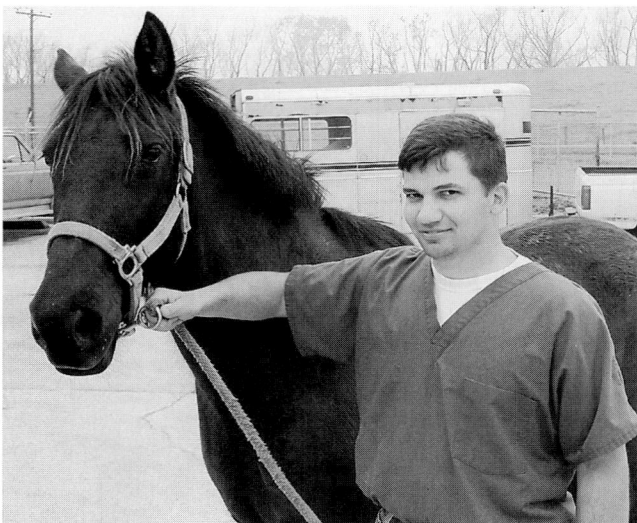

FIGURE 1-11. Halter and lead rope correctly placed on a horse. Note the position of the handler and the position of the arm. This allows the handler ample opportunity to sense impending movements.

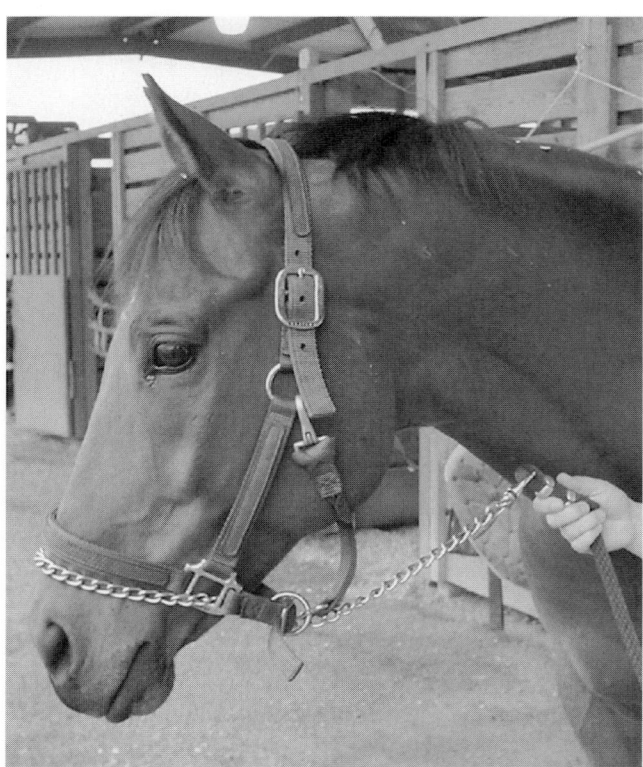

FIGURE 1-12. Lead shank with a chain positioned across the bridge of a stallion's nose to allow for more control.

There are three possible positions for the chain lead on the halter. The least authoritative is under the jaw, which causes a squeeze around the nose. Horses with tender chins or those that are not accustomed to a chain lead may throw their head or lunge backward when the lead is pulled. Horses that sense a squeezing of the nose as a signal to back up must be carefully restrained to respond correctly to this type of lead. It is often necessary to release pressure to allow the horse to stop its reverse. The chain over the nose is very effective in controlling many horses (Figure 1-12). The top of a horse's nose is sensitive, and a pull on the lead with the chain across the nose will make the horse drop the nose and stop forward progress. Very few stallions should be led without this technique. A variation of this technique is to carry the chain across the nose and then to the cheek piece connection of the halter (Figure 1-13). This provides the handler for more control of the horse's head and nose. The most severe method of chain lead restraint is passing the chain over the upper lip and onto the gums of the upper jaw (Figure 1-14). This method works very well with horses that have a bad attitude and need to be reminded about the "chain" of command. When using this technique, it is imperative that the chain is used only when the horse is misbehaving. When used correctly, this method of restraint replaces the use of a twitch and provides the handler with much more stopping power over the horse.

Tying the Horse

A horse should never be tied with a chain over or under the nose. This too is an invitation for disaster. Seldom will it be desirable for a handler to tie a horse in order to perform a procedure. When a horse must be tied the equipment must be strong and sound. The halter, rope, and whatever the rope is tied to must be in premier shape. Snaps on a rope are always suspect because all but the heaviest will break when a horse jerks back on them. If something breaks (the rope, halter, or post) the horse will be free and may have previously learned to pull back as an escape whenever tied.

Another serious problem that can result from the horse pulling back occurs when it goes over backward and sustains head or neck trauma on landing. A horse should be tied to objects that are at the level of its shoulder or higher to prevent it from pawing and getting a foot over the rope. This also prevents the horse from trying to graze and becoming entangled in the tie rope. Horses should also be tied short; only 60 cm of rope should be present from the halter to the post to prevent the horse from having too much play in the rope and getting in trouble (Figure 1-15). Once a horse is tied, care should be taken to avoid hazardous objects arriving into the area that might spook the horse, and the horse should never be left unattended. The shorter the horse is tied, the less likely it is to get into trouble.

One technique that may be used to restrain (or train) a fitful horse is to place a cotton rope around the mid section of the horse just behind the rib cage and then pull it through between the front legs and through the bottom of the halter. This rope is tied slightly shorter than the halter rope. The basis of this technique is that the horse will hit the cotton rope first and feel the pull against its abdomen, causing it to move forward and release pressure on the rope (Figure 1-16).

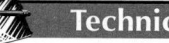
Technician Note

In general, horses should always be held rather than tied for veterinary procedures.

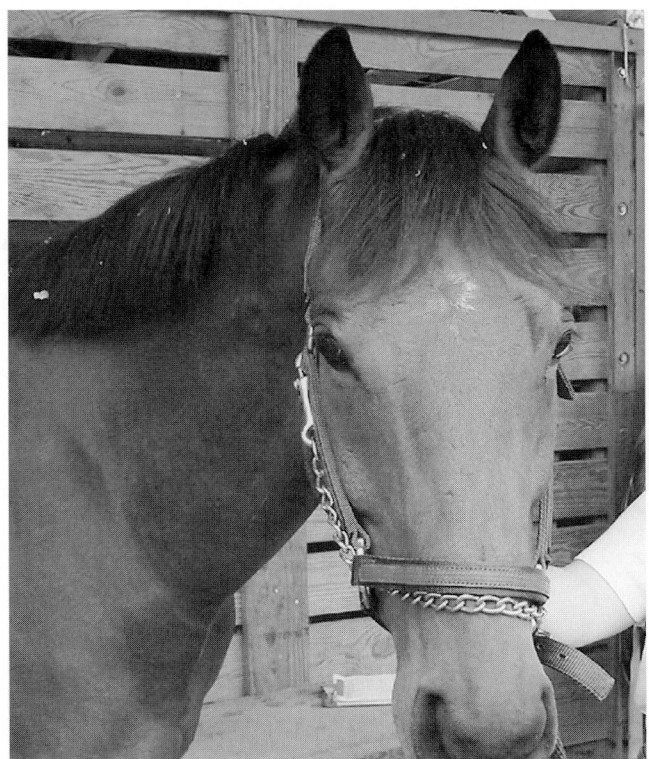

FIGURE 1-13. Lead shank across nose and then to the cheek piece of the halter. This allows the handler much more control of a feisty horse.

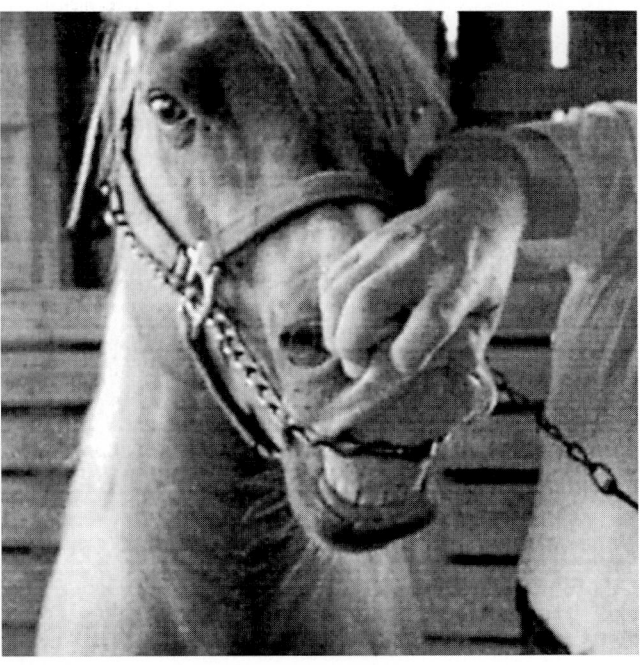

FIGURE 1-14. Lip chain added to the combination for restraint. This technique maximizes the control for the handler and replaces the use of a twitch in many instances.

For veterinary purposes it is generally preferable to hold a horse rather than tie it. Also, it is imperative that the holder stand on the same side of the horse as the veterinarian, so that the head may be directed toward the practitioner rather than the body or hindquarters (Figure 1-17). If the handler is on the opposite side and the handler bails out, the head of the horse follows the handler, leaving the back end of the horse swinging directly into the veterinarian. When the head is controlled and the horse acts up, the worst that will happen is the body of the horse will swing away from both handler and veterinarian. No matter what the circumstances, this technique should be upheld, because in an emergency situation self-preservation of the holder will overcome protection of the practitioner.

The Twitch

The twitch is a nerve-stimulating device that may immobilize horses and can be helpful in equine restraint. Most twitches are applied to the upper lip of the horse. The most innocuous is the humane twitch, which is a hinged pair of long handles that squeeze down over the sides of the lip and may then be secured at the bottom by a thong and snapped back to the halter. The major advantage of this twitch is that once applied it need not be held in place (Figure 1-18). Therefore one person may restrain a horse that is acting up. The disadvantage is that the pressure is fairly mild and most horses ignore it. More traditional twitches rely on a loop and a leverage device. The loop is either of chain or rope and is placed on the lip and tightened by twisting the leverage device. The leverage may

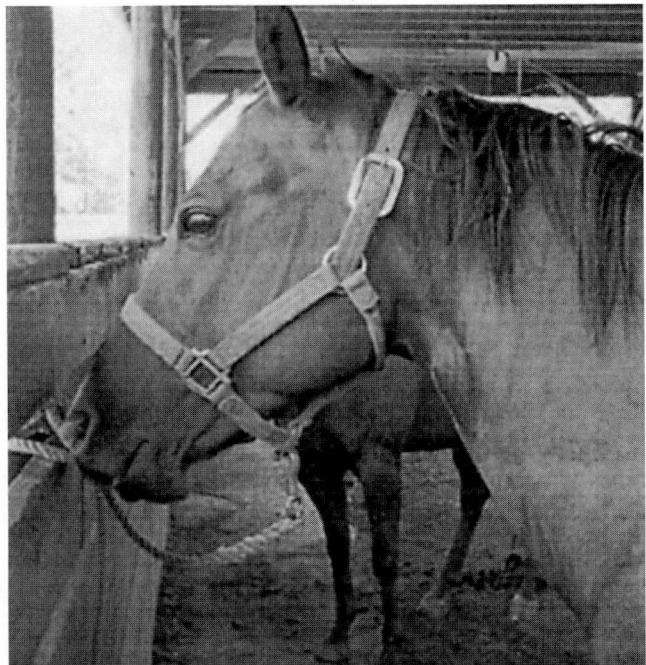

FIGURE 1-15. Properly tied horse at a rail. Note the level of the tie and the short amount of rope between the post and the halter.

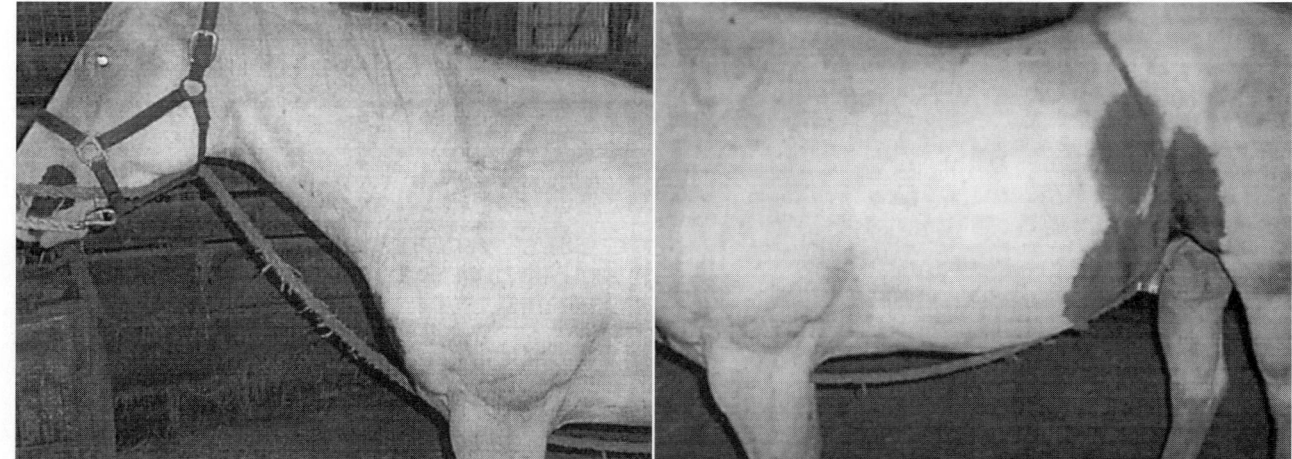

FIGURE 1-16. The technique necessary to place a belly rope on a horse that will not stand tied. **A,** A soft cotton rope is place around the horse's abdomen and then run between the front legs. **B,** The rope is then run down the halter and tied, slightly shorter than the halter rope.

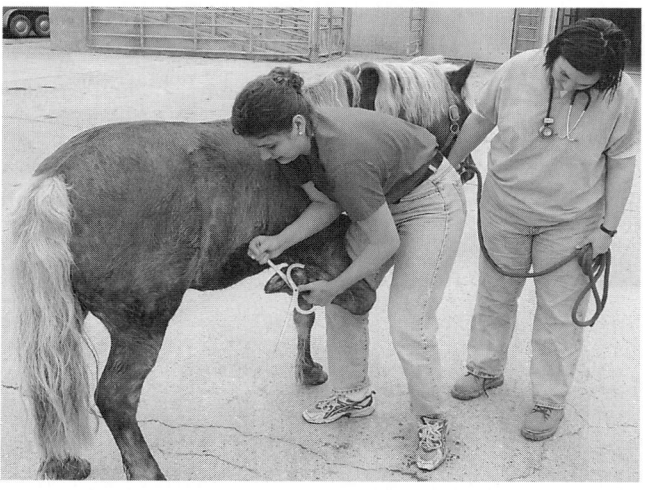

FIGURE 1-17. When handling horses for any procedure it is necessary for the holder and the individual working on the horse to be on the same side of the animal. Note the horse's displeasure demonstrated by the swishing of the tail at the person on the horse's side.

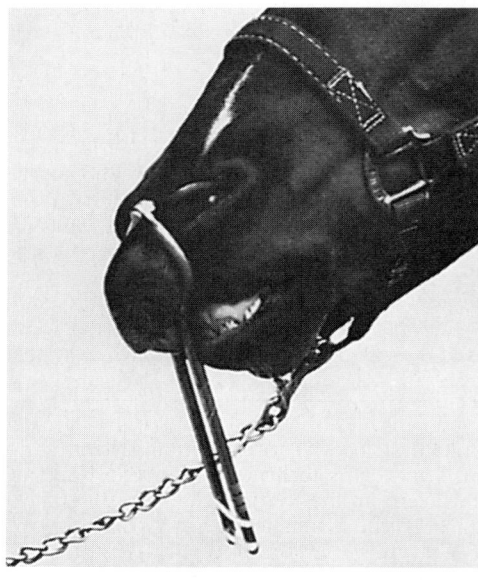

FIGURE 1-18. The humane twitch in place on a horse's lip.

be from a piece of wood or pipe and is about 50 cm long. The loop needs to be seated on the lip behind the heavy gristle pad at the tip and ahead of the nostrils. This area may be hard to find on thick-nosed horses. Horses that have been twitched become quite wise and will throw their heads into the air and tighten their lips when attempts are made to apply the twitch.

Application of the twitch should be done with the calmness and assuredness of the initial capture of the horse. It is best to have an assistant holding the horse by a lead rope when the twitch is applied. The loop should be placed over the thumb and three fingers, leaving the little finger out so that the twitch does not slide down the hand

or arm (Figure 1-19). Grasp the end of the horse's lip, raise the hand with the twitch on it, and slide it onto the horse's nose. The end of the handle should be held in the opposite hand in case the horse throws its head. Twist the end of the handle until the twitch is snug and begins to elongate and distort the shape of the horse's upper lip. The twitch should be tightened until the horse responds by standing still. The average person cannot twist enough to damage the horse's nose. Once the twitch has been applied the person holding it should also be holding the lead rope from the halter. He or she should be positioned on the side of the horse next to the shoulder and should be at the end of the handle of the leverage device (Figure 1-20). In the absence of a twitch it is possible a person with a firm grip can hold the upper lip to accomplish a minor procedure. It should be remembered that horses are able to strike out with their front legs, and twitches may evoke this response. Never stand directly in

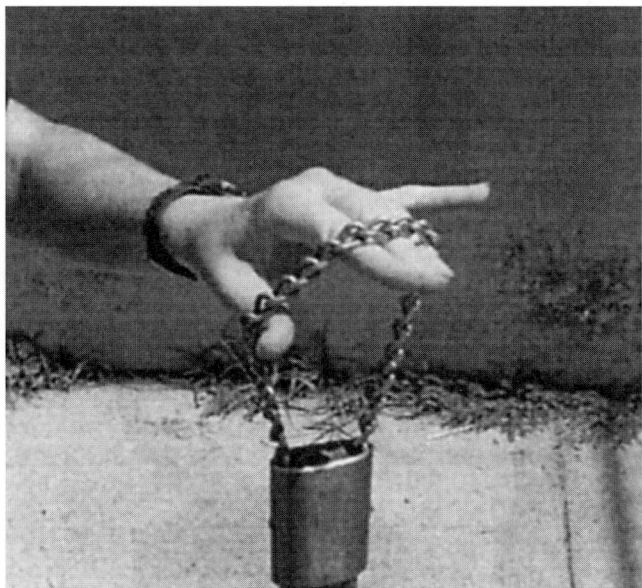

Figure 1-19. The proper placement of the fingers through the loop of chain before placing the twitch on a horse's nose.

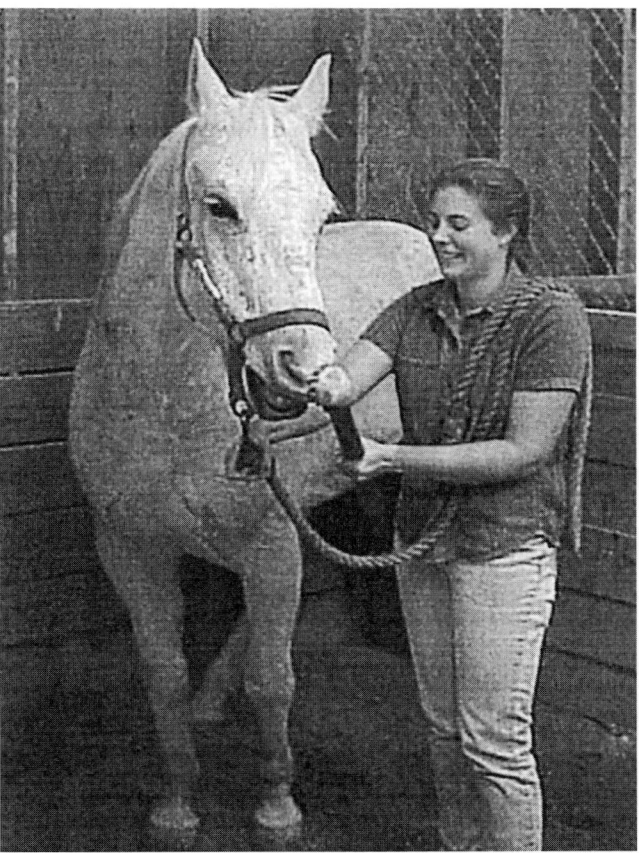

Figure 1-20. This handler demonstrates the proper positioning while holding the twitch and restraining the horse. Note that the horse is backed into a corner and there is still plenty of overhead space.

front of the horse when applying or holding a twitch. As mentioned previously, the lip chain may be an alternative that will produce similar results without having to dodge the flying wooden handle of a twitch or the helicopter feet of a horse that has been stimulated to strike.

Technician Note

Never stand directly in front of the horse when applying or holding a twitch.

A skin twitch may be a more acceptable form of restraint for many owners. This technique may also help for those horses that seem to be very "light" on their front feet, attempting to strike when a regular twitch is applied to their nose. Grabbing the skin of the neck just in front of the shoulder and rolling it around the clenched fist will make many horses stand still (Figure 1-21).

The old cowboy notion of twisting the horse's ear and biting down on it as a means of restraint is poor practice. The supporting structures of the ear may be damaged, and it is extremely common for the horse to become head-shy following ear twisting. Owners are not keen on having this procedure done on their horses, and the handler risks a trip to the dentist after every attempt. Clearly, there are better forms of restraint available.

Lifting the Foreleg
Some horses will stand still if a foreleg is picked up and held. The theory is that with one leg in the air, the horse is less likely to leave the ground with the other three. To lift a horse's foreleg, face the rear and stand next to the horse slightly in front of the leg that is to be lifted (Figure 1-22). Bend from the waist and push your hips slightly into the horse as the hand closest to the horse palpates the suspensory ligament. The suspensory ligament is immediately palmar to the third metacarpal bone. Squeezing the suspensory ligament will cause the horse to flex its fetlock

joint, and cradling the anterior aspect of the fetlock as it flexes will allow the handler to pick up the foot. When holding the foot as a means of restraint, the handler should rotate and face forward with both hands supporting the foreleg (Figure 1-23). To handle the horse's hoof for procedures, the handler should face the rear of the horse. The foreleg should be placed between the handler's legs from the rear and held between the thighs just above the knees, freeing both hands to work on the foot (Figure 1-24).

Lifting the Hind Leg
Lifting the hind leg will only be done as part of an examination procedure, not as a means of restraint. To lift the hind leg, the handler stands near the flank area of the horse and bends from the waist with a hand palpating down the horse's rear limb. A slight lean into the horse will aid in elevating the limb off the ground and the leg should be pulled upward toward the handler. Then the handler should walk under the limb, staying close to the horse's body until the leg is outstretched behind the horse with the foot resting on the inside thigh of the handler. The horse's hock should be at the level of the handler's waist and the tibial region snugly against the side of the back (Figure 1-25). The leg should stay braced in this position without the use of hands. If the horse should resist, the handler's arm should clamp down over the horse's hock joint and attempt to quiet the horse.

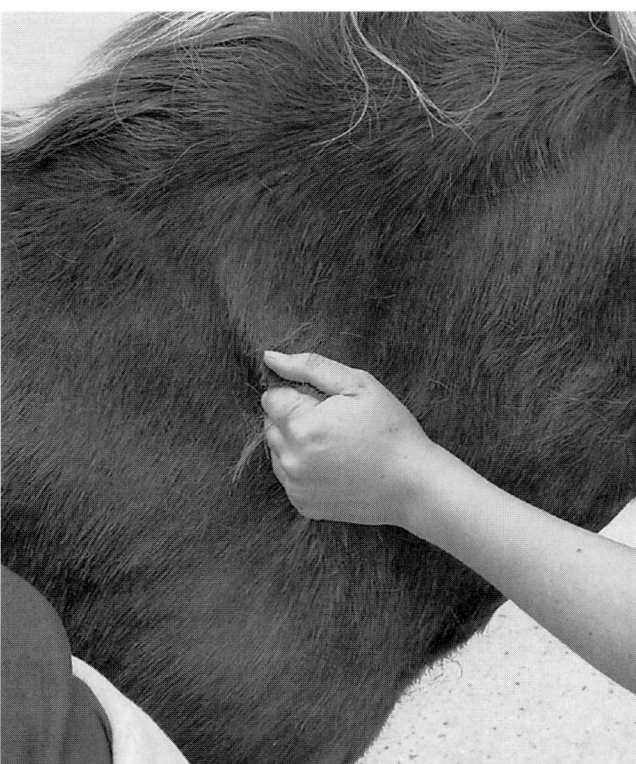

FIGURE 1-21. A skin twitch can be a powerful deterrent to an obnoxious horse. The skin just in front of the scapula is drawn into the clenched fist to accomplish this task.

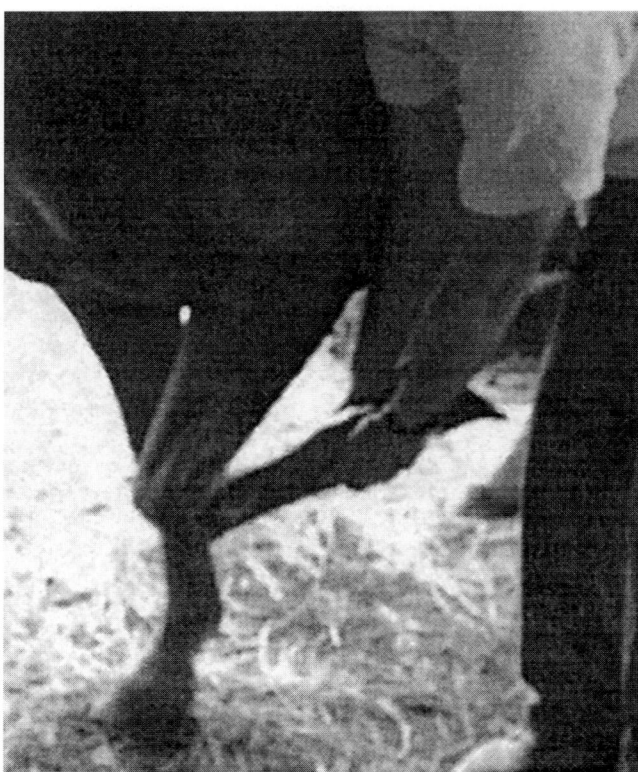

FIGURE 1-23. The handler is positioned properly to restrain the forelimb while a procedure is performed elsewhere.

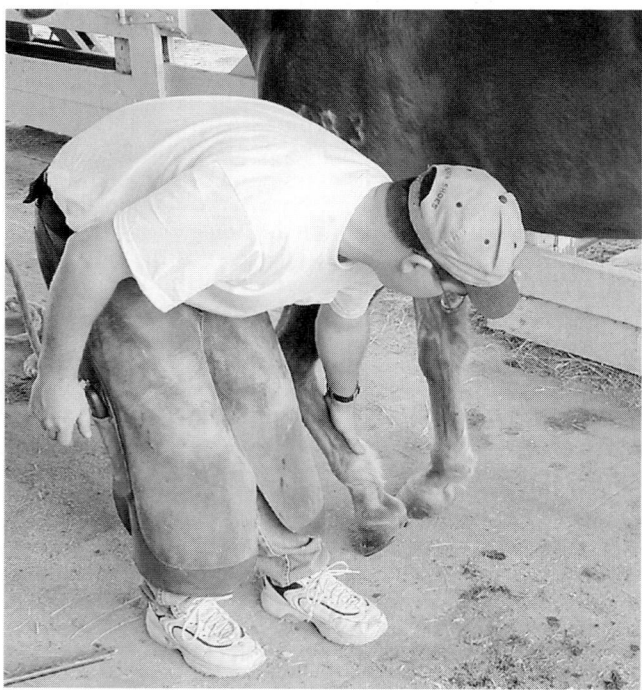

FIGURE 1-22. The proper foot positioning and bending at the waist to pick up a front foot of a horse. The inside hand is placed on the suspensory ligament of the horse's leg.

There are descriptions of how to tie horse's legs up to examine them in the literature, but they have many disadvantages to both horse and handler. A horse with a leg tied up may fall and seriously injure itself. There are too many chemical mediators available in equine practice today to recommend rope restraints for lifting limbs.

Stocks

The use of stocks for fitful horses is clearly the safest way to manage these horses. The best stocks are made of heavy pipes or poles, anchored well to the ground surface, with the horizontal pieces set at the level of the horse's shoulder (Figure 1-26). Stocks are used for many procedures, such as administration of fluids, dental work, nasogastric intubation, rectal palpations, and injections of jittery horses. Many horses will require encouragement to get into the stocks. This can be done safely with voice commands, slight raising of the arms of a second handler standing behind the horse, or a straw broom raised and lowered behind the horse (Figure 1-27). Again, every effort should be made to keep horses calm as they load into the stocks. Some horses have an innate fear of being enclosed. These horses may do anything to get out of a set of stocks. Kicking, jumping, lunging, and striking are all ways in which the horse may try to escape. Therefore it is best to have a quick-release mechanism on the stocks, especially for the rear gate. The rear gate must be closed before tying the horse's head after loading a horse into the stocks. Once a horse is in the stocks, the same principles apply with regard to positioning of the handler. Do not assume that the horse cannot come over the front of the stocks, because

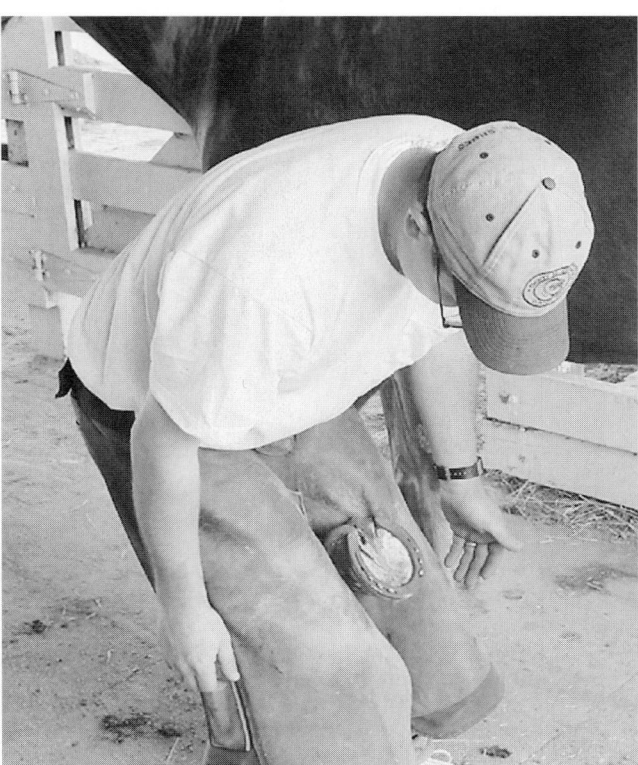

FIGURE 1-24. The hands-free stance while working on front feet. Note that the back is only slightly bent and the knees are directed together to hold the forelimb.

many have done so in the middle of a tantrum. Horses should never be left unattended in the stock.

Technician Note

The use of stocks for fitful horses is clearly the safest way to manage these horses.

The lack of a set of stocks presents a problem with restraint for more noxious veterinary procedures, such as dental work, nasogastric intubation, and rectal palpations. For dental work and nasogastric intubation without stocks, the horse should be backed into the corner of a secure and sturdy area and quieted. Make sure that the ceiling is not so low that if the horse rears it will hit its head. The handler and the veterinarian should be located on the same side of the horse when performing the procedure (Figure 1-28). For palpation without stocks, the horse should be placed along a sturdy solid wall with the handler and veterinarian standing on the same side of the horse. The handler must "read" the horse, and everyone must have a clear idea of where the escape route is located when performing this procedure.

Tail Tie
The horse's tail may be tied during rectal palpations, vaginal examinations, and minor obstetric procedures. This is accomplished by using a small rope or a roll of gauze tied into the hair of the tail. The tail should never be

tied to anything but the horse. Tying the free end around the neck of the horse is best. Should a horse get loose with the tail tied to a stationary object, serious injury could result. The tail tie is a simple quick-release knot using a rope or gauze placed across the tail just below the fleshy portion (Figure 1-29), with the long end tied in a quick-release knot around the neck.

Hobbles
Horses are very seldom hobbled or cast (thrown to the ground with the aid of ropes) since the advent of chemical restraint that is both powerful and short acting. Breeding hobbles are still commonly used on farms that have natural breeding operations. These hobbles prevent a mare from kicking effectively. They are fitted around the hocks with web or leather straps, which are tied to a neck strap or rope after being passed between the forelegs.

The scotch hobble is a means of drawing up the hind leg (Figure 1-30). This technique can be used as a form of restraint for examination of the opposite forelimb. It works by keeping the weight on the hind leg of the side that is being examined. Most often the scotch hobble will be used for holding the hind leg that is "up" out of the way during a castration. A heavy cotton rope should be used to avoid rope burn. A loop is placed around the horse's neck and tied with a bowline before initiation of anesthesia. Once the horse is down in a surgical plane of anesthesia the rope is passed through the loop behind the pastern area and then brought back to the loop. Pulling the end of the rope using the neck loop as a pulley then draws the leg forward. Care must be taken to avoid a rope burn in the pastern area. Some people actually have a leather sheath with two loops on it that is used behind the pastern to allow the rope to slide around the leg without the potential of producing a rope burn.

Restraint of the Down Horse
Control of the head is the key to restraining a horse lying in lateral recumbency, because in order to get up the head must be lifted. Kneeling on the neck near the head will keep most horses down. This should always be done from the back of the horse; in fact, any activities performed on a horse that is down must be done from the back. Approach from the belly side puts the handler in danger of thrashing legs and feet. To keep the horse from damaging the facial nerve and the down eye, the handler should cushion the lateral area of the face and orbital area. This may be done with a towel, inner tube, or foam mat placed under the head. If such a protection is not available and the horse is thrashing its head, pulling up on the nosepiece of the halter will elevate the nose and prevent the horse from moving the head and producing traumatic wounds to the eye and face.

Technician Note

Control of the head is the key to restraining a horse lying in lateral recumbency.

Other Head and Mouth Restraints
Horses will sometimes tear at bandages. Devices are available that may be used to prevent this by restricting the horse's ability to move the head laterally. One such device is the cradle. It is made of wooden slats and leather straps

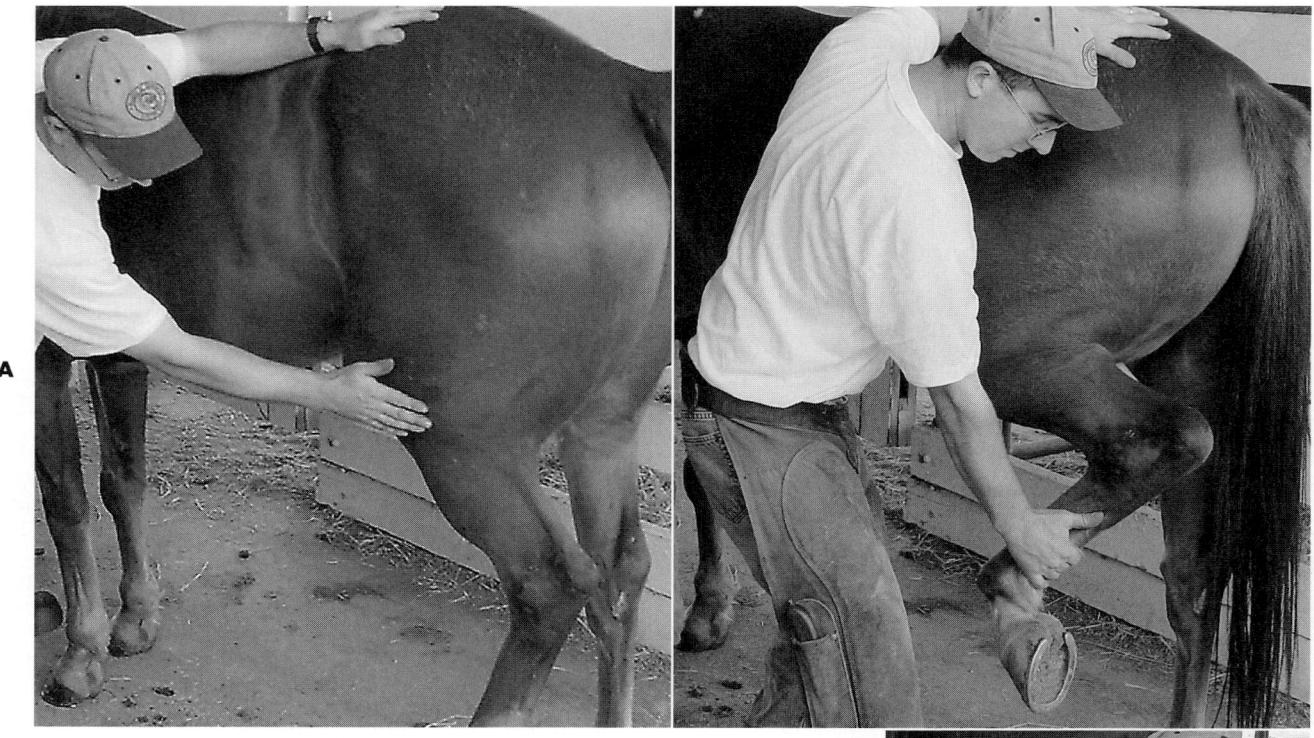

FIGURE 1-25.   Lifting of the hind limb. **A,** The handler stands near the flank and palpates down the limb to give the horse knowledge of his presence. **B,** The leg is then brought forward toward the handler before attempting to go out behind the horse. **C,** The handler then walks in underneath the horse's leg, supporting the tibia on his hip and placing the hoof over the inside thigh to support the lower leg.

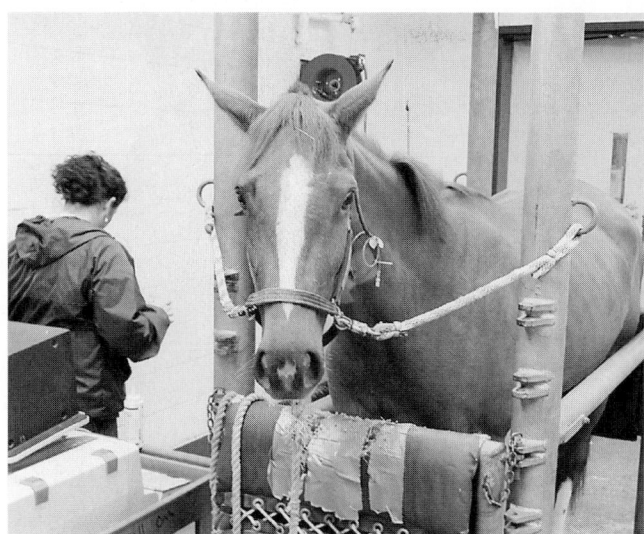

FIGURE 1-26.   This horse is about to enter a set of pipe stocks. Note the height of the side pipes, about the level of the horse's shoulder and stifle joints. This stock is well anchored in cement to avoid unsteadiness once the horse is in the stock.

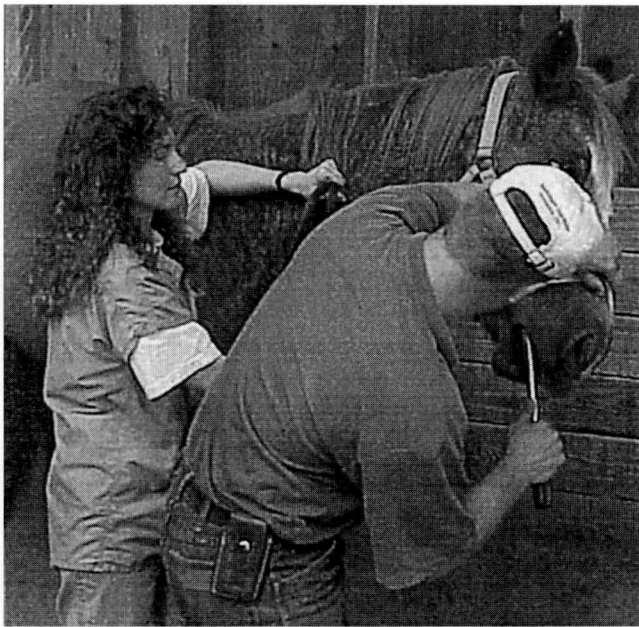

FIGURE 1-28.   This horse is undergoing a dental procedure, and both the handler and the veterinarian are located on the same side of the horse for safety. Note also the solid wall on the opposite side of the horse. This minimizes the opportunities for the horse to become injured.

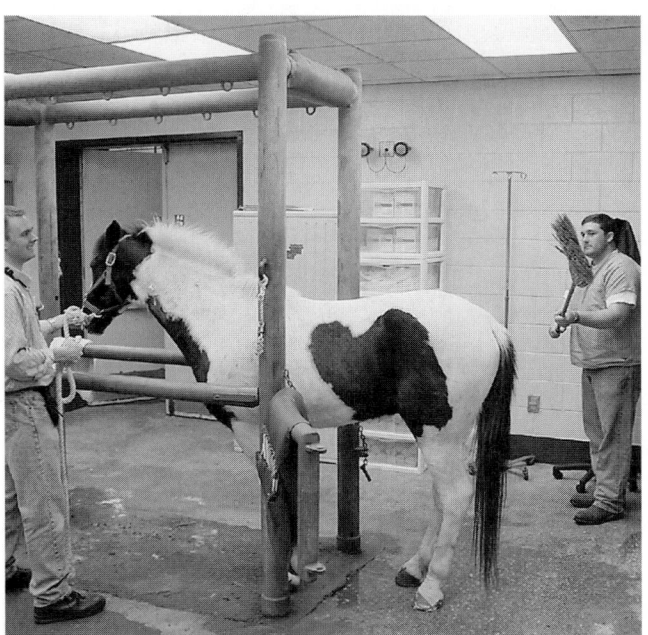

FIGURE 1-27.   The rear end of the horse must always be respected and the back gate must be closed before securing the head of a horse in the stock. The judicious use of the broom helps get many horses to make the final step into the stock.

with a buckle that goes over the horse's neck to secure the cradle and brace the neck in a straight line (Figure 1-31). This device prevents the lateral movement of the neck while allowing the horse to eat and drink. Another method of preventing the horse from chewing at bandages is to

tether the horse to an overhead cable in the stall. Running the cable diagonally across the stall is the usual method. With this technique the horse is able to move about the stall freely but cannot reach far enough laterally to gain access to the bandage.

Horses with severe pain, with neurologic disease, or undergoing anesthesia will frequently throw their heads, crashing into solid objects and mutilating themselves. To prevent this there are foam rubber head protectors made to fit snugly over the head of the horse, much like a helmet (Figure 1-32). The use of these and padded stalls help to prevent self-inflicted trauma.

Wire or plastic muzzles are used frequently on horses that are to be held off feed and to prevent them from eating bedding while still allowing them access to water (Figure 1-33).

Examination of a horse's mouth and dental arcades may be accomplished by standing to the side of the horse's head and placing the hand of the arm more caudal to the mouth over the bridge of the horse's nose. The hand nearest the horse's nose is then inserted into the interdental space (Figure 1-34). The hand must be kept in a vertical position. The fingers are then placed on the lingual surface of the dental arcade, and the thumb palpates the buccal surface. Following dental examination the tongue may be pulled out the side of the mouth through the interdental space. Mouth gags are available to allow for more complete visual examination of horses' mouths. A simple wedge (Figure 1-35), which is pushed up between the upper and lower cheek teeth with the handle hanging out, is commonly used. A variation on this is a round gag, used in a similar fashion to the wedge. There is also a large hinged speculum that fits over the upper and lower incisors and hangs from the halter (Figure 1-36). The mouth can be cranked open using this gag, allowing examinations and procedures to be performed on the caudal cheek teeth. Although this device

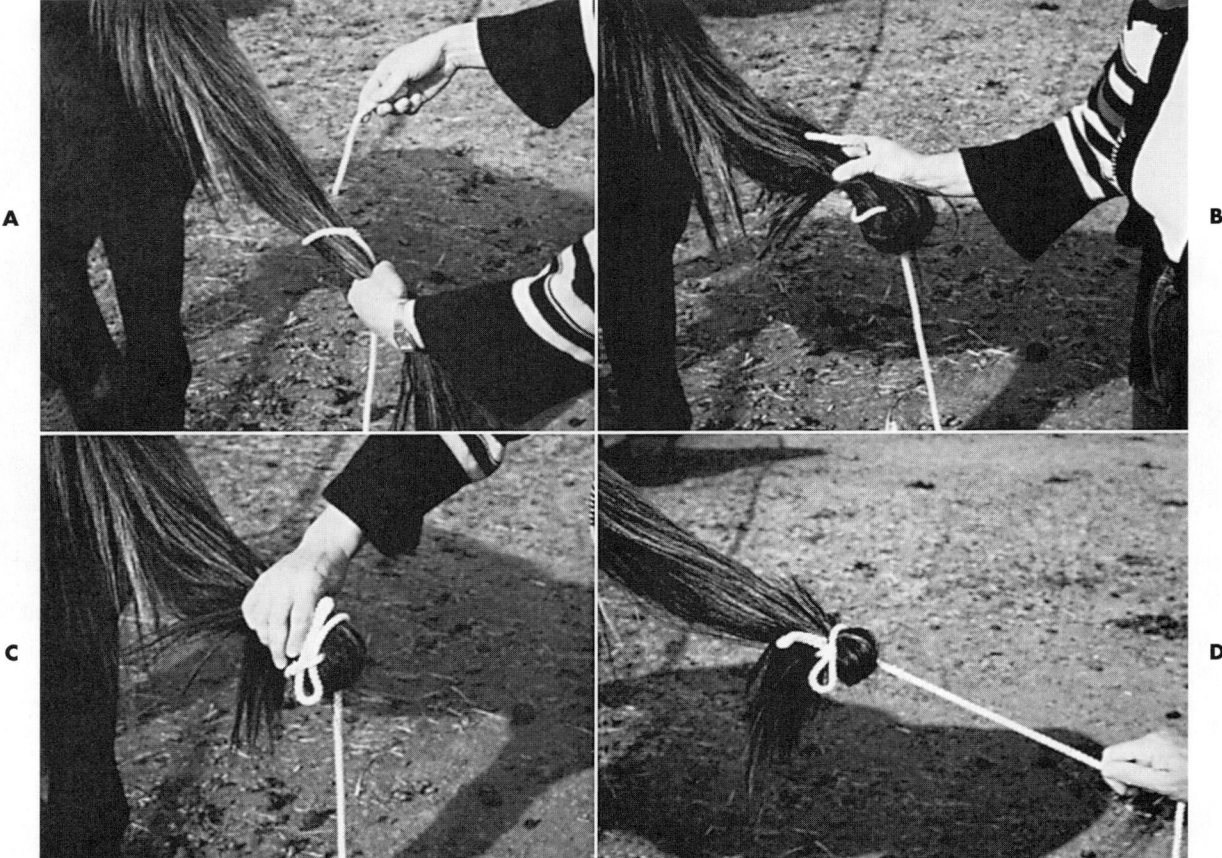

FIGURE 1-29. The steps in making a secure tail tie. **A,** The rope is placed around the tail. **B,** The tail is folded back on itself and on the rope. **C,** The short end of the rope passes over the folded tail, and a loop is pushed through the tail-encircling portion of the rope. **D,** Tension on the long end of the rope makes the knot snug. Pulling the short end of the rope will releae the knot.

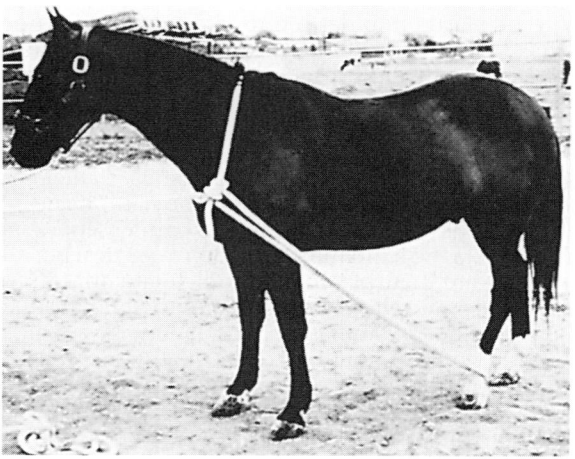

FIGURE 1-30. The scotch hobble on a standing horse.

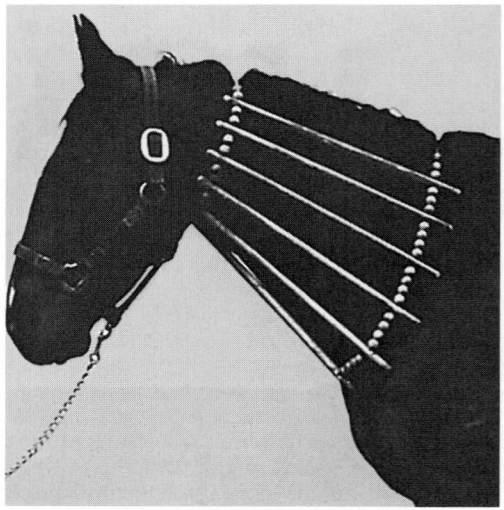

FIGURE 1-31. The horse wearing a neck cradle.

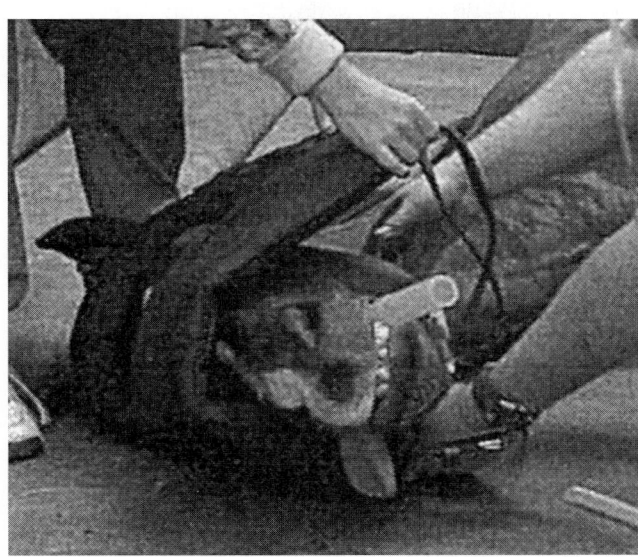

FIGURE 1-32.   The handler is placing a protective foam and rubber helmet over the head of this anesthetized horse to protect the head during recovery from anesthesia.

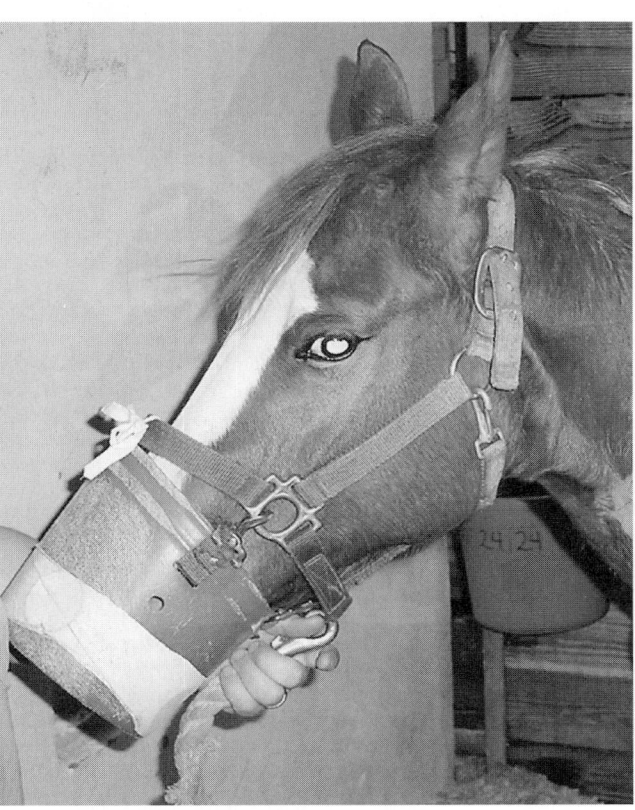

FIGURE 1-33.   This horse is wearing a plastic muzzle to keep it from eating during the perioperative period. The muzzle does have holes to allow the horse access to water.

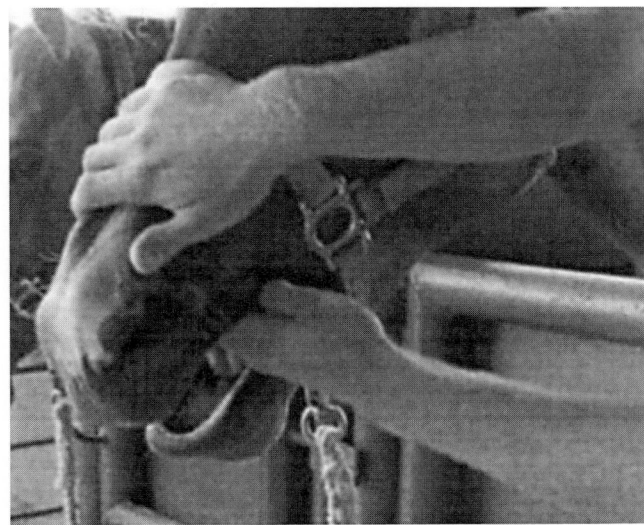

FIGURE 1-34.   The handler is about to perform an oral and dental examination on this horse. It is critical that the examiner keep the hand in a vertical position while checking the teeth because the horse will bite down on a hand placed in a horizontal plane.

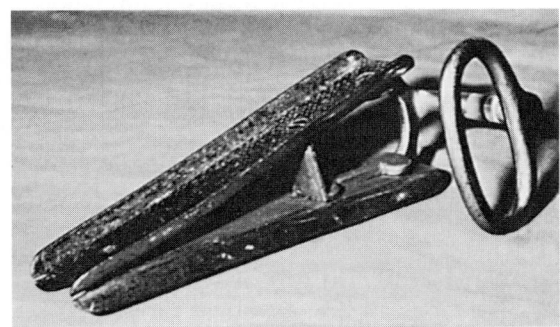

FIGURE 1-35.   The wedge gag. The wedge is slid between upper and lower cheek teeth, and the handle comes out of the corner of the mouth.

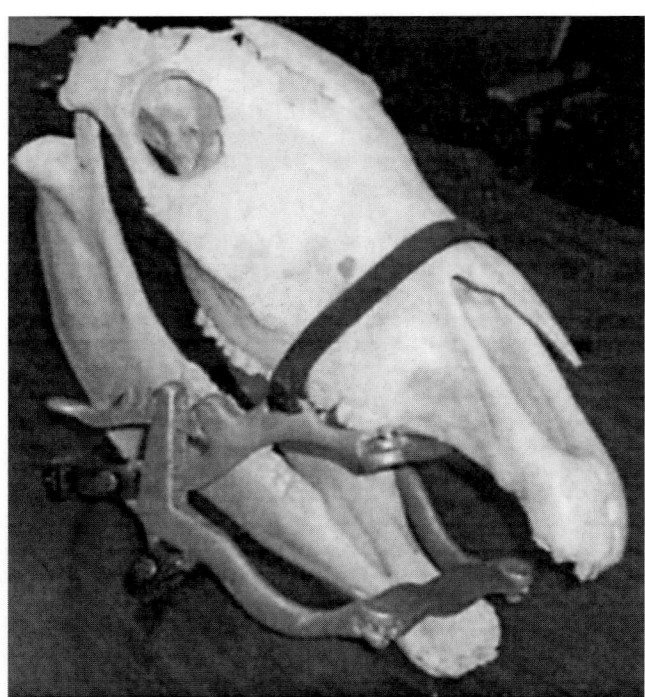

FIGURE 1-36. The position of the hinged speculum inside the horse's mouth to allow for visualization and work on the teeth of a horse.

is effective in getting the mouth open it is heavy and cumbersome for both the handler and the horse. The use of this gag is usually coincidental with sedation of the animal.

Manual and Chemical Restraint

Manual casting of horses has been replaced by chemical restraint and anesthesia. Casting always had inherent danger for both horse and handler. Musculoskeletal damage was always possible when the forefeet of the horse were pulled from under it. Once the horse was cast, the thrashing about caused a variety of injuries.

Chemical restraint is now widely accepted and practiced. Many different agents and combinations of agents are used. These are discussed in Chapter 21. Whenever a horse has been sedated, tranquilized, or anesthetized it is important for veterinary personnel to stay with that horse until it is steady on its feet. Also, when horses are tranquilized, handlers must remember to maintain a safe distance from the horse. When they are under deep sedation, tranquilization, or proceeding through stage 2 of anesthesia, horses may crash into an unwitting handler and cause significant injury to the person. Once the horse is down make sure of the stage of anesthesia before placing restraint ropes or beginning surgical preparations. A slap to the flank of a horse awaiting castration may save damage from the kick of a partially anesthetized colt.

Capture and Restraint of Cattle

Cattle are less difficult to capture than horses. They are also less discriminating than horses about what or whom they step on or run over. Generally, they are not directly approachable for haltering and leading. However, they are easier to drive into pens, alleyways, and chutes. Herds of cattle will vary in the amount of avoidance present. Some herds will allow a person to approach very closely before

moving away. It is preferable to have the herd begin to move when the handlers come within about 12 m of the herd. Cattle are very herd oriented, so they will crowd and bunch together as they are driven, even climbing over other cows if they are driven too hard or fast. This should be avoided because bruising and other injuries are likely to occur.

It must be stressed that herding cattle into weak barriers must be avoided. Most beef cattle will walk through a barbed or smooth wire fence completely unconcerned and unscathed. Sometimes they even leave the wire in place although much looser than it was. Calves become very adept at slipping through the lower strands of pasture fences.

Cattle are usually less spooky than horses about strange surroundings, but they may balk and then bolt suddenly. Generally the balking occurs just as the cattle reach the open gate of a holding corral after being driven off a pasture. The clever cattle rancher avoids placement of strange things at the entrance to a corral, such as dogs, new people, or strange trucks. Veterinary personnel should remain out of sight unless the owner requests assistance in driving cows. Nothing aggravates a rancher more than having all the cows ready to go into the pen and then having them spook at the last instant because something or somebody steps into their sight.

Once cattle are in the corral, they are funneled from larger areas into smaller pens and eventually into an alleyway leading to a chute. Usually there is a system of gates that will allow the handler to block the cattle into these progressively smaller areas. These gates may be used to "cut" calves from cows to facilitate handling. It is best to work larger stock separately from the nursing calves. The handler must be careful in closing gates on a large group of cattle. If they get turned back toward the opening and hit the gate before getting it latched there is a significant chance of injury to the handler.

The alleys leading to the chute should be built just wide enough for one animal in order to prevent attempts to turn around (Figure 1-37). People on foot may follow cattle in an alleyway to drive them toward the chute, but they should always be cautious and ready to climb out of the way. Never enter an alleyway that cannot be easily evacuated. The alleyway is usually arranged so that posts or boards may be slipped behind the cattle to prevent them from moving backward. "Tailing" may be used to push a cow ahead in the alley. Tailing is simply grasping the tail in the middle and twisting it forward onto the cow's back. This provides discomfort to the cow, and the usual and expected response is for the animal to move forward. Never underestimate the ability of a cow to get frightened or balk and begin moving backward. This may cause serious injury to the unwise handler. Cattle prods, wiffle paddles, and electric "hot shots" are available and may be used from outside the alley. Many alleyways will have an elevated walkway that allows handlers to move the length of the alley to assist in moving cattle forward to the chute (Figure 1-38). If an alleyway and chute are not available, the next best solution is to run an individual cow into a gated corner. The handler must then move quickly to get behind the animal and tail it to keep it from backing up. It may be necessary to rope a cow if no other method of restraint is possible, but this is not a technique that is advantageous or desirable in modern veterinary practice.

Once the animal has stopped moving it is then possible to halter it and restrain it by the head. A single, calm cow restrained in a stall may be haltered without resorting to a chute. A bovine halter is all one piece and made from rope,

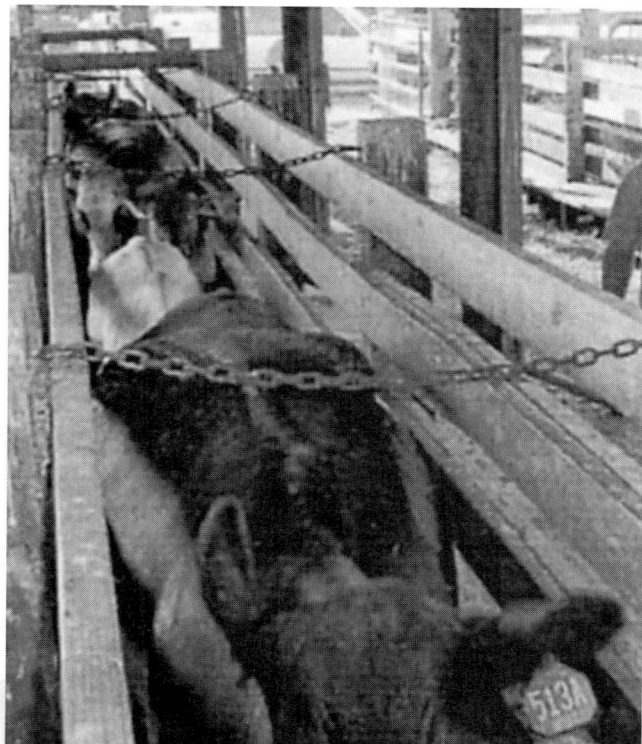

FIGURE 1-37. The alleyway that works best for moving cattle is only wide enough for one cow to pass through. Note that the alley is braced well with support posts and there are chains across the top of the alley to prevent it from spreading.

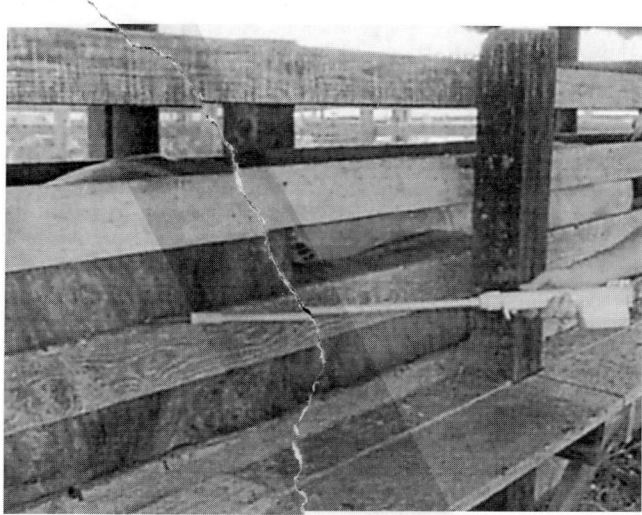

FIGURE 1-38. A "hot shot" with the proper positioning of the handler shown. These devices work well but must be used judiciously to facilitate easy movement of cattle. The walkway that allows for human traffic above the cattle and outside the alleyway is evident just in front of the handler.

as opposed to the equine halter. The halter is placed by loosening the nose loop first and then flipping the crown loop over the animal's ears. Once the crown loop is in place the nose loop may be positioned and the slack in the free end of the rope taken up as the rope comes under the

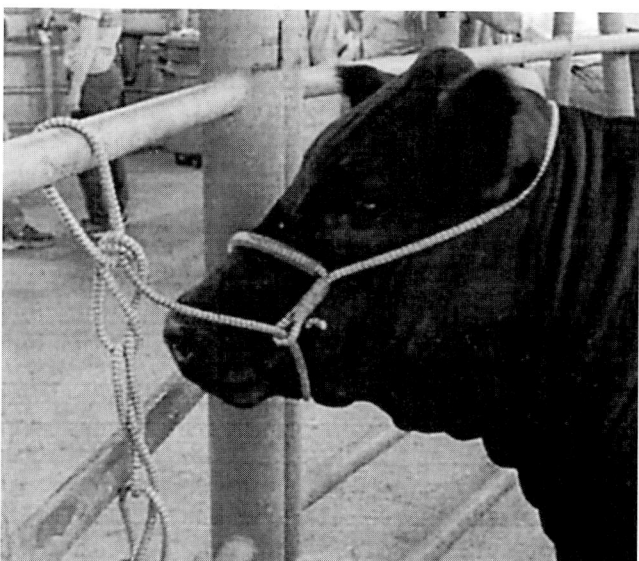

FIGURE 1-39. A rope halter placed correctly and tied to the pipe at an appropriate level to restrain this Angus heifer.

jaw (Figure 1-39). Always keep the cow's head at arm length and bend forward from the waist, because an animal that becomes nervous will throw its head and may catch the handler in a compromised position. Animals with horns may be restrained by placing a loop of rope around the base of both horns and then dallying off to a solid post.

Calves are captured in much the same manner as foals. If the calf is small enough it may be "flanked" and placed in lateral recumbency (Figure 1-40). The dam of the calf deserves respect and must be observed for aggression.

Bulls must always be respected for the aggression that they possess. Extreme caution should be used if driving bulls on foot. The use of feed to entice bulls into a capture area is often necessary. Once the animal is in the enclosed area, gates may be used to squeeze the animal into a position that will allow restraint. Capturing the nose ring using a wire with a hook on the end and then snapping a long lead provide the necessary restraint for most bulls (Figure 1-41).

Technician Note

Extreme caution should be used if driving bulls on foot.

Head Catch

The head catch or chute is the final capture and restraining device for cattle (Figure 1-42). Cattle usually do not willingly put their heads through the head catch. It takes precise timing to close the head catch following the presentation of the head and ears and before the shoulders. Once a bovid gets its shoulders through the head catch, it will escape. Spring-loaded head catches are available, but their use is not as easy as the manufacturers would suggest. Most chutes also can squeeze the animal from side to side after the head is captured. This prevents the animal from moving about during examination. Head catches on manual or hydraulic chutes can be dangerous. Rapidly swinging

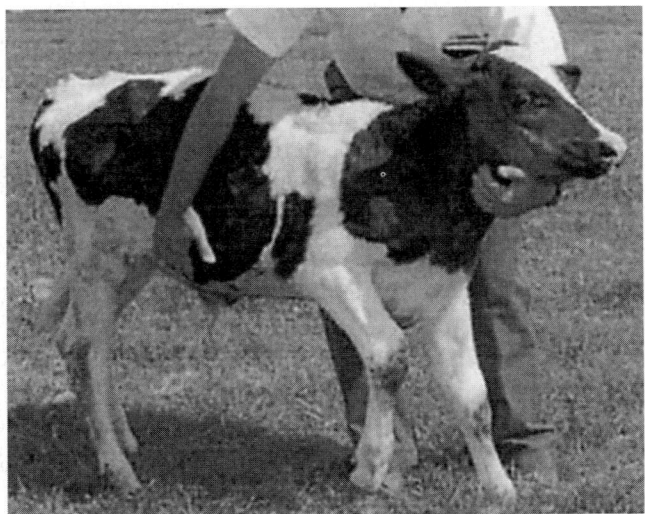

FIGURE 1-40. The proper positioning to "flank" a calf to the ground into lateral recumbency.

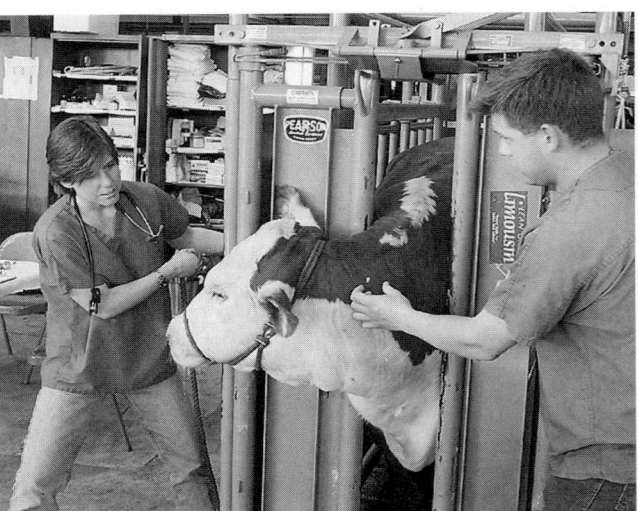

FIGURE 1-42. A chute with a Holstein cow captured inside of it. There are many varieties of chutes, and each has its own handling characteristics. They can be very dangerous if the handler is unfamiliar with the use of the different types of pulls and levers.

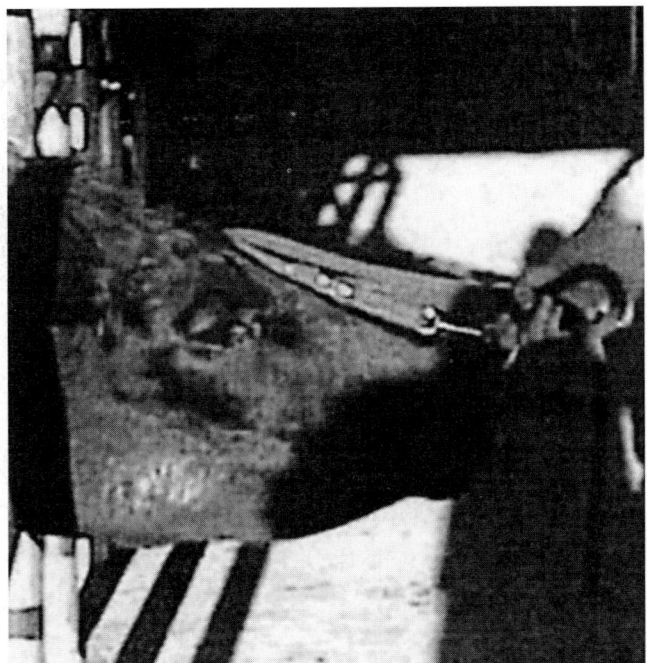

FIGURE 1-41. The handler has a long rope with a heavy snap in the nose ring of this bull and has also elected to hold the ring in his hand. The pipe stock that the bull is in provides additional safety for the handler.

handles or closing panels provide opportunity for the unfamiliar person to get hit. Take time to become familiar with the operation of any chute and head catch before use.

Restraint of the Head

Many different techniques may be used as an adjunct to the head catch to restrain the animal for more invasive proce-

dures than observation. Halters may be applied to pull the head to the side for exposure to the jugular veins. A strong person can grasp over the muzzle and place his or her hands into the mouth to allow for an oral examination. The nasal septum may be pinched between the thumb and forefingers, or nose tongs may be placed in the nose to stabilize the head. The horn or ear should be used to provide leverage for the handler. Care must also be taken to perform these techniques at arm's length to prevent being hit in the head as the animal throws its head up.

Grabbing the animal's tongue and moving it to one side of the mouth allow oral examinations in cattle. The handler makes life easier by grasping the tongue with a towel. Large, metal, hinged speculums may also be used in bovine oral examinations. These are placed and maintained as in the horse. Remember that cattle are not used to being restrained in the first place, and the use of additional hardware on the head may make them dangerous to the handlers should they become panicked or aggravated.

Mouth gags are used in cattle for passage of oral-gastric tubes. The most common type is the Frick speculum (Figure 1-43). This is a stainless steel tube that is placed in the oral cavity, passed over the lingual bulla, and held in place while the tube is pushed through it into the esophagus. Care must be taken to ensure that the tube does not damage the pharyngeal mucosa. Another method that can be used is a block of wood that extends across the animal's mouth and has a hole in the center to allow for passage of the tube. The gag is placed in the interdental space and held by a strap placed behind the head.

Tail Restraint

The tail of a cow can be tied just like that of a horse, with the same precautions necessary about tying the tail to anything other than the cow. The tail of a cow may also be used for driving it as mentioned previously. "Jacking" the tail of a cow will also provide a means of restraint for short procedures. This technique involves pushing straight up and forward on the tail, carrying it vertically in a plane

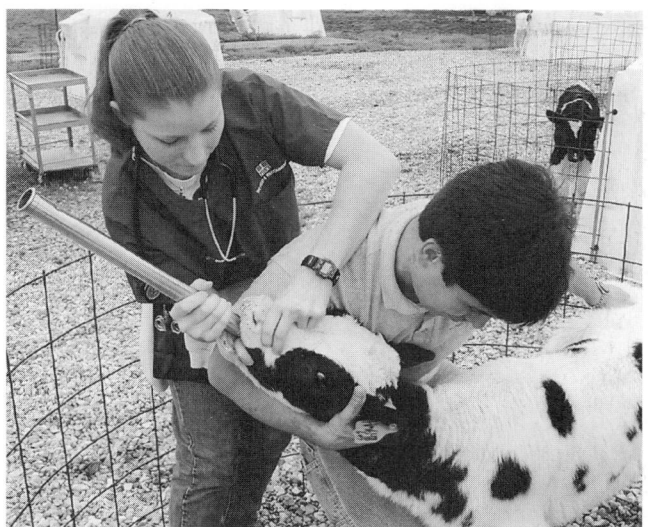

FIGURE 1-43.   The handler is placing a Frick speculum into the oral cavity of this calf. The rear of the calf should be restrained in some manner before attempting this procedure, and great care should be taken to avoid advancing the speculum too far into the pharyngeal region.

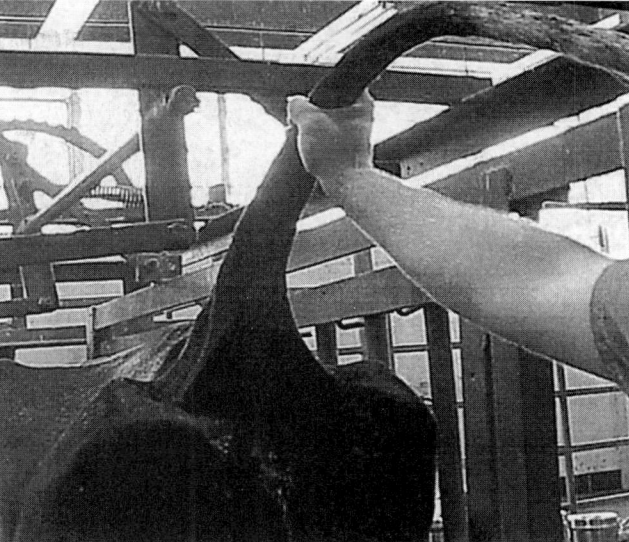

FIGURE 1-44.   The tail "jack" technique. Handlers are reminded to keep the tail on the midline when pushing it forward and to keep their balance when pushing into the cow.

directly over the cow's midline. The handler should remain balanced and have the tail about one third of the way down from the tail head (Figure 1-44). This technique works only when the tail is maintained vertically over the midline of the cow.

Kicking Restraints

Cattle usually kick to the side and forward with a hooking action rather than straight to the rear. Several commercial devices are available to prevent kicking and to restrain the hind legs. Milking hobbles are flat metal hooks with a chain in between that are placed over the tendons of the hind leg just above the hock. The open end of the hooks is to the inside of the leg, and the chain passes around the front of the limbs. Once the hooks are in place, the chain can be drawn up until the hocks are close together.

Pressure on the flank seems to discourage cows from kicking. A device shaped like giant ice tongs may be squeezed over the flank (Figure 1-45), or a rope may be tied snugly around the abdomen just anterior to the udder or prepuce (Figure 1-46).

Lifting Feet

Cattle are very reluctant to lift up their feet, and to accomplish this in a standing animal without assistance requires great effort. The foreleg can be raised with a noose tied around the pastern and the free end of the rope passed over the back of the cow or around an overhead rail or pipe, which will then act as a pulley. The hind leg is more of a problem, because there is no portion of the cow's anatomy that will act as a pulley. The limb may be tied to an overhead beam or rail following placement of a clove hitch around the animal's hock joint (Figure 1-47). Realize that most of the time this will be done in a chute or narrow area and maneuvering space will be limited. However, the use of this procedure will allow for visual and digital examination of the foot and interdigital space of all but the most recalcitrant cattle (Figure 1-48).

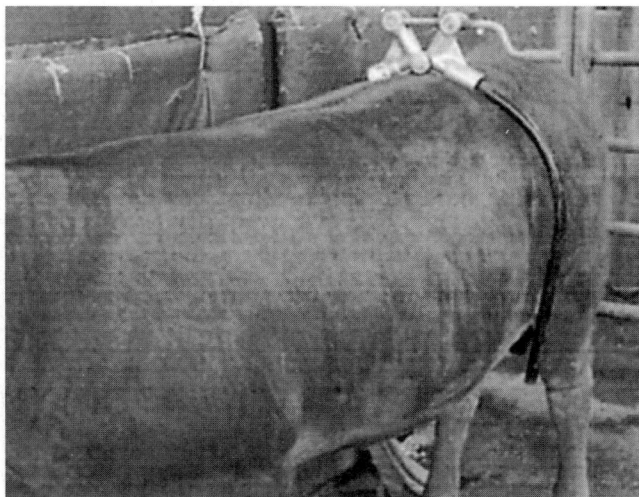

FIGURE 1-45.   This commercially available restraint is known as the Can't Kick Device. The handle on the top turns to move the prongs of the device into the flanks of the cow for restraint and away from the flanks to remove.

Casting

The act of casting a bovid is quite simple. The animal must always be anchored to a sturdy post before placing one of the various rope harnesses on it. Therefore a sturdy halter is the first requirement for casting. The simplest harness technique consists of a noose around the neck, a half-hitch around the girth, and a half-hitch around the flank. Care should be taken to avoid incorporating the udder of a cow, or the testicles of a bull, into the flank rope. The free end of the rope comes off the animal's back with all knots positioned dorsally. Once the harness is secure a strong pull toward the rear of the animal will make it lie down.

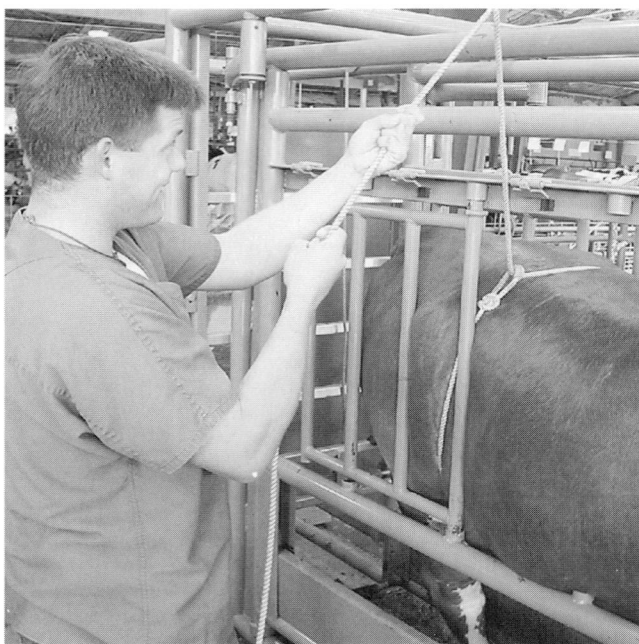

FIGURE 1-46. This technique involves the same concept as the Can't Kick Device but provides more control of the animal by encompassing the entire abdomen. The rope can be cinched down as tightly as needed.

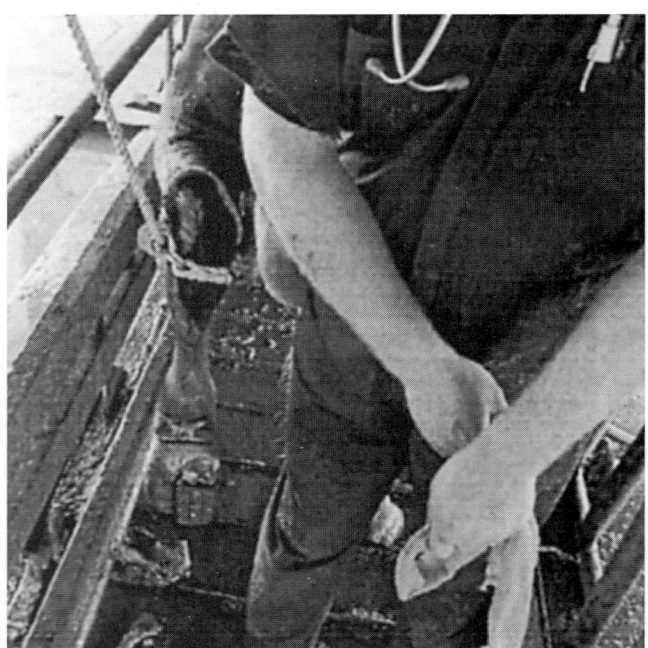

FIGURE 1-48. The person examining the foot and lower leg is not given much room in most chutes. The restraint of the limb by the clove hitch and rope elevation provides a good margin of safety for the examiner.

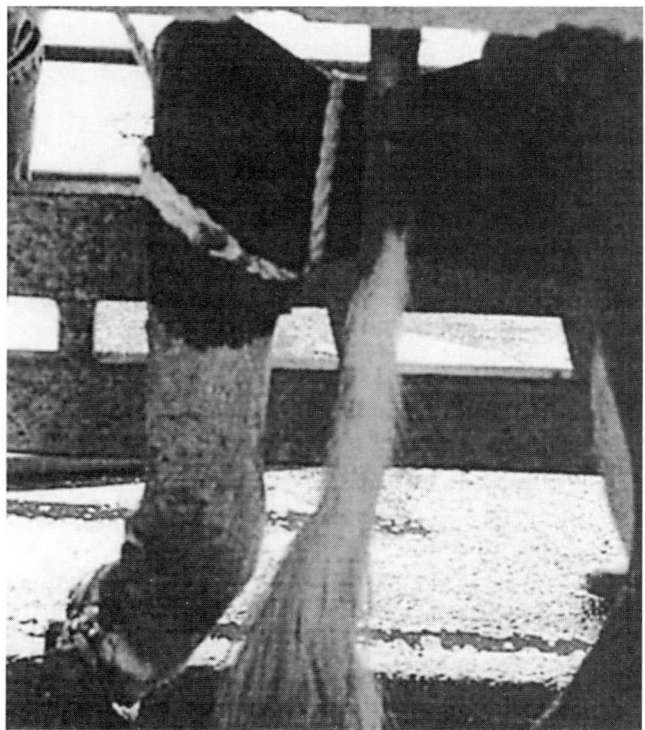

FIGURE 1-47. The hock of this cow is held by a clove hitch that has been placed in a sturdy rope. The rope restraint of the hock allows for the entire hind leg to be elevated by pulling the rope over a beam behind the cow.

One average-sized person can easily cast an adult cow in this manner.

The cow may be rolled onto her back if there are appropriate wedges available to keep her in dorsal recumbency. Square bales of hay may be used to wedge against the animal to keep it in position. The legs should be stretched to the front and rear with stout cotton rope. Cattle in sternal or dorsal recumbency are less likely to bloat than those in lateral recumbency when they are cast. A bovid that must be placed in lateral recumbency should be restrained on its right side. This allows the veterinary personnel to observe the rumen for any signs of bloat that may occur. If the bloat becomes large the procedure should be terminated. Kneeling on the animal's neck may provide additional restraint for cattle in lateral recumbency. Standing cattle that are undergoing any procedure may go down at any time, for unspecified reasons. Therefore restraint of the head should always be with a halter because a rope around the neck may tighten and strangle the cow and the use of nose tongs may lead to ripping out the nasal septum.

Technician Note

A bovid that must be placed in lateral recumbency should be restrained on its right side.

All dairy breed bulls and some beef bulls will have a nose ring. They are easily led with the ring, but care must be taken because the ring may break or pull through the nasal cartilage. Likewise, a bull should not be tied fast by the nose ring. A combination of halter and nose ring may provide the most efficient means of leading a bull.

Chemical restraint is used for cattle; however, it must be remembered that ruminants are exquisitely sensitive to alpha$_2$ agonists, such as xylazine.

Driving Sheep and Goats

Sheep and goats are more herd conscious than cattle and can be driven in bunches. Dogs are an excellent adjunct in working sheep and some goat herds, although goats will occasionally challenge the dogs.

Sheep can be worked in alleyways, and although they tend to climb on and over each other worse than cattle, they do less damage because of their smaller size. Sheep are much more athletic than cattle yet they do not seem to want to climb out of enclosures or go over fences like cattle do when driven hard. Temporary fencing may adequately restrain sheep.

The kids and lambs within a flock may be quite acrobatic, jumping into fences and climbing over structures to avoid being caught. These activities may result in traumatic injuries, and veterinary personnel should be alert to avoid dangerous situations.

Goats and sheep can be caught in small enclosures in the same way as foals or calves are caught, with a hand under the neck and one under the rump. It is important to remember that a sheep or mohair goat must not be restrained by grabbing the wool. The fleece may be damaged, or, in meat animals, a subcutaneous bruise may develop at the site, damaging at least the esthetics of the product.

A useful technique for capturing goats is the use of a shepherd's crook or cane. The goat can be hemmed in toward the fence and then the crook can be placed in the throat-latch area to catch the head. Care must be taken to avoid trauma to the trachea when using this technique.

Technician Note

A useful technique for capturing goats is the use of a shepherd's crook or cane.

Sheep are often set up on their rumps for several different procedures. There are several different ways to end up with the sheep on its rump with its back leaning against the holder who retains a grip on the forelegs (Figure 1-49). The easiest method is for the person to begin on the sheep's left side. Reach under the base of the neck with the left hand and over the back to the right hind leg with the right hand. The sheep is gently lifted off the ground toward the right and upturned, as the right hind leg is lifted to get the animal's weight off it. The right hand moves to the right foreleg as the left hand moves to the left foreleg, and the sheep is held on its rump facing away from the handler. One person can shear a sheep or perform other procedures unassisted with the sheep on its rump by steadying its upper torso between the arms and the lower torso between the legs as the person works.

The method of holding the legs of lambs for docking and castration is the same whether they are held by the handler, laid on a bench, or placed over a fence. The holder grasps the parallel hind and fore leg, bringing the hind leg forward while holding between the hock and fetlock. The fore leg is held just below the elbow.

One person can perform drenching of oral fluids or medicines to a sheep. The sheep is backed into a corner as

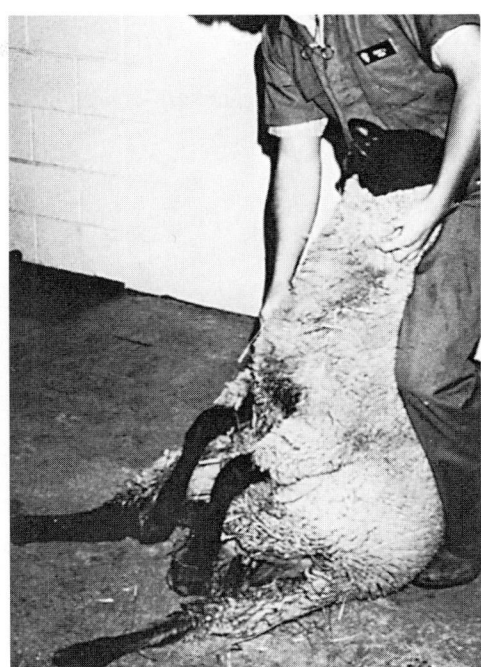

FIGURE 1-49. Holding the sheep set up on its rump.

the handler straddles the sheep above its shoulders, squeezing slightly with the knees. The handler lifts the head by the lower jaw while holding loosely around the muzzle. The dose syringe is inserted into the interdental space on the opposite side of the mouth with the other hand. Do not lift the jaw above a line parallel to the ground surface, and take care to administer the fluid slowly enough so that the sheep can swallow it. The nozzle of the syringe should be inserted well back into the mouth so that the fluid does not dribble out. Caution must be used to keep the animal's head under control so as not to traumatize the pharyngeal mucosa as noted in the bovine section.

Capture and Restraint of Swine

Small piglets can be crowded into corners and then grasped by a hind leg (Figure 1-50). The leg hold should be rapidly changed to holding the pig in both hands around the torso for comfort of the pig. Obviously, this technique is not applicable to adult swine.

Veterinary personnel may be faced with castration of large boars based on owner's perception of when the signs are right. One technique that can be used on market-weight boars is to herd them to a corner and have two handlers grab the nearest hind leg. Following capture, the hind end is then elevated so that the pig is standing on his head in the corner. This technique is not for the feint of heart; it requires coordination and strength of the two handlers to accomplish the task.

Swine can be very aggressive, particularly boars and nursing sows. A fence or panel may be used to "haze" them, and the barrier provides protection to the handler. When the panel is meant to be stationary, take care to push it all the way to the ground and plant it. Pigs will attempt to "root" underneath it. Always be aware of the escape route when entering a pen. Swine are intelligent and individualistic and may be difficult to direct in a large area. They tend to dart through small openings for escape. A

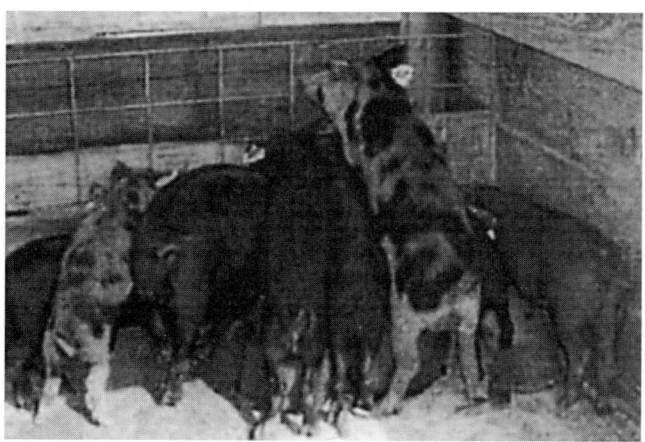

FIGURE 1-50. Piglets pile up in the corner when driven. It is now quite easy to capture one by grabbing onto the hind legs that are presented.

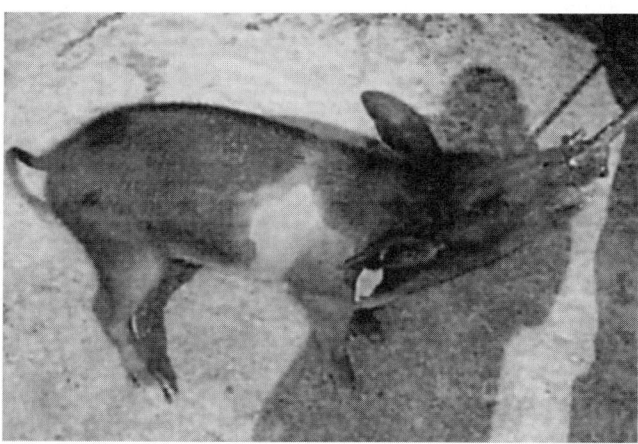

FIGURE 1-51. A handler with a hog snare has captured this pig by the upper jaw, just in front of the cheek teeth. It is obvious that the pig resents this and will resist by pulling back against the snare.

cane is a valuable addition to a handler when attempting to drive and direct swine. Tapping them on the side of the neck and face with the cane while following on foot gives the handler some degree of "steering" capabilities.

Once pigs are inside a small enclosure a snare may be used to catch them. A hog snare is an adjustable metal cable loop at the end of a rigid handle. The usual procedure in capture of the pig is to push it into a corner and then step in, tight to the flank area, and slip the snare loop over the upper jaw from behind. The loop is tightened after it is behind the incisors. The snare has a rigid handle that allows the handler to direct the snout after it is captured. Generally, swine will brace themselves by pulling backward when caught and are immobilized by its use (Figure 1-51). However, the discomfort of the snare usually results in nonstop squealing until it is removed. Handlers are encouraged to wear ear protection when performing any restraint on pigs.

> ### Technician Note
> Handlers should wear ear protection when performing any restraint on pigs.

Pigs can be restrained on their backs in a trough but find it unsettling and complain vocally (Figure 1-52). A sling of canvas with holes for the legs has been used with great success in laboratories and veterinary hospitals to cradle the pigs comfortably for certain procedures. The farrowing crate is the restraint device for sows, which keeps them from lying on their piglets.

Pigs can be restrained for castration or vaccination by holding them off the ground by the hind legs with their backs against the handler's legs. Large pigs will struggle less if their forefeet rest on the ground. Piglets receive oral administration by holding them up by the forelegs and leaning their backs against the handler's legs while they stand on their hind legs.

The pig is an intelligent animal that can be trained to tolerate minor discomforts; unfortunately, the time in-

volved to train swine is often not profitable in agricultural animals. Miniature pigs, kept as pets, are most often seen these days in urban practices. Many of these are spoiled, willful creatures that dominate the household, and their owners are not impressed with rough handling. The support sling is the best method for restraint because it causes the animal no discomfort yet immobilizes well. Many pet pigs are fond of having people scratch their backs and may stand or lie quietly for examination if this is done for them. Holding the pig cradled in the arms of a handler may seem a good idea until the pig struggles. Then the hind foot nearest the body will gouge the holder. Pigs also have powerful jaws and some will bite, especially if in pain. Examination of the mouth can be accomplished by the use of a U-shaped gag, which is placed into the mouth from the front to behind the canines; the gag is then rotated to spread the jaws. Never put fingers into the side of a pig's mouth since the cheek teeth are very sharp.

> ### Technician Note
> Many pet pigs are fond of having people scratch their backs and may stand or lie quietly for examination if their backs are scratched.

Although a miniature pig may live in and control a house, it is still a pig. Pigs vocalize when they are uncomfortable or in pain. Do not be surprised when the cute little pig emits an ear-piercing shriek as it is picked up. This will continue until it is set free. Chemical agents for restraint are highly recommended for use on these animals.

Capture and Restraint of Dogs
Catching Dogs
The only time veterinary personnel should have to catch a dog that is not in a cage or run is if the animal has escaped. In a hospital, dogs are often motivated by fear so personnel should learn to deal with the two types of behavior this produces. Avoidance with submissiveness when cornered

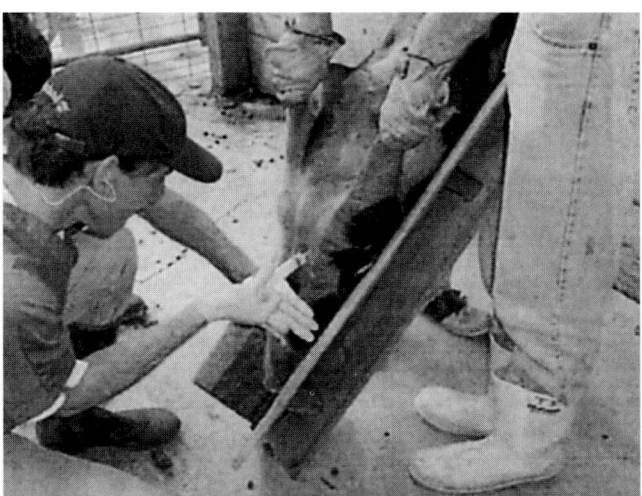

FIGURE 1-52. This pig is being restrained by both hind legs and its back is supported by the V trough. Procedures such as ear notching and bleeding can be done with the pig in this position. Although ear protection is not depicted, the reader should note that the pig will squeal the entire time it is re-strained in this fashion and handlers should wear ear protection.

is one, and the other is avoidance until cornered and then aggression, otherwise known as *fear biting*. Unfortunately, it may be difficult to discriminate between the two until the moment when hands are approaching the dog. It is the rare dog that will not snap at a handler that grabs it as it runs past, yet it is difficult to resist the temptation of doing so as a dog streaks past on its way to freedom.

Dogs that feel they are being chased will run and a person is not going to outrun any but the smallest or most debilitated. It is best to try to keep the dog in sight until there is an opportunity to corner it. Sometimes it helps to have a canine companion to entice the dog to approach. In this situation it will never hurt to have a pocketful of bait to gain the dog's favor. Most dogs respond favorably to voice reassurance, and a higher-pitched voice usually gets better results. With many dogs, squatting in front of them to appear less large and overbearing will help. Moving slowly and deliberately, offer the back of the hand for the dog to sniff, at or below the level of the nose. The response to this action is the first indication of the tendency for the dog to try to bite. Never try to grab the dog's collar or pick it up until some reassurance is given to the animal. Do not confuse a wagging tail with friendliness in a dog with an unknown personality. Watch the ears, eyes, and face. It is not unusual for an aggressive dog to hold the tail erect with a tense, narrow, oscillating motion before biting.

The back of the hand is offered to the dog for two reasons. The first is that it is probably less threatening than the open palm, which may appear to the dog as an attempt to slap. Second, the fingers are out of the way and the dog will be less likely to get the entire hand if it does bite. Caution should be exercised by all handlers in these situations, because dogs bite with lightning speed and the position of the hand may have little to do with the ability to withdraw from danger.

Some dogs are naturally gregarious and trusting and require little in the way of preliminary introduction. The trusting dog will sniff the hand, begin wagging the tail, and

approach for more petting. It is a good idea for the handler to run the hands over the entire dog in a friendly fashion before taking liberties with the body. Evaluating dogs requires knowledge of the relationship of the dog with the owner. Some dogs have trained their owners rather than the opposite, and the handler must forge his or her own relationship with the dog.

Many times dogs act reasonably in an initial examination with the client present and then threaten to bite when approached after the client has gone. When faced with a dog that will bite if given the chance, the sensible approach is to keep your hands and body out of the way. Always remember to keep all outside gates and doors closed when working with difficult animals. The cage door should be held closed as much as possible when trying to catch these animals. They are trouble enough without trying to capture them after they have escaped. Small dogs may be managed by handling with heavy leather gloves. The dog will bite at the fingers of the glove of one hand while the clever handler grabs the animal by the scruff of the neck with the other. Large dogs that want to bite are more troublesome. The first step is to catch them by the neck. A lead rope with a slipknot can be tossed over a dog's head, but sometimes a rope or cable snare similar to a hog snare is required (Figure 1-53). Most dogs will give up when caught by the neck. The truly vicious or confirmed fear biters will continue to attempt to bite and even attack. These animals will require a muzzle or rope with a pole to keep the teeth away from veterinary personnel. Vicious little dogs may be dragged out of cages and held off the ground by a choke rope for a few moments to subdue them. Tracheal damage to the dog is possible, and choking is not a popular event for anyone involved. However, some of these dogs are incorrigible and require force to gain respect.

 Technician Note

Often dogs act reasonably in an initial examination with the client present and then threaten to bite when approached after the client has gone.

A truly vicious large dog is a major challenge. These dogs must always be handled with at least one snare, possibly two if the dog is strong. Once captured, the dog is stretched between the snares for leading. Many of these dogs are used as guard animals, and only one person can handle them. The owner may be able to place the muzzle on the dog before bringing it into the clinic. These dogs must always be treated with respect for their ability to harm the handler.

A dog at large that will not allow approach may require the use of a capture gun or pole syringe. Animal control officers are experienced with the use of these devices and may be able to provide assistance.

Lifting Dogs

Lifting a dog onto the examination table is usually the first step in any examination or procedure. Grasping on either side of the thorax behind the elbows allows the handler to lift small dogs. Putting the arms around the front of the chest and behind the rump will allow a handler to lift a medium-sized dog easily. This technique places the handler in close proximity to the animal's teeth so care must be taken to avoid being bitten by the frightened dog. Large dogs are harder to lift. Their weight may be prohibitive, their bulk makes them awkward, and they are not accus-tomed to being lifted. One person can lift a large dog by

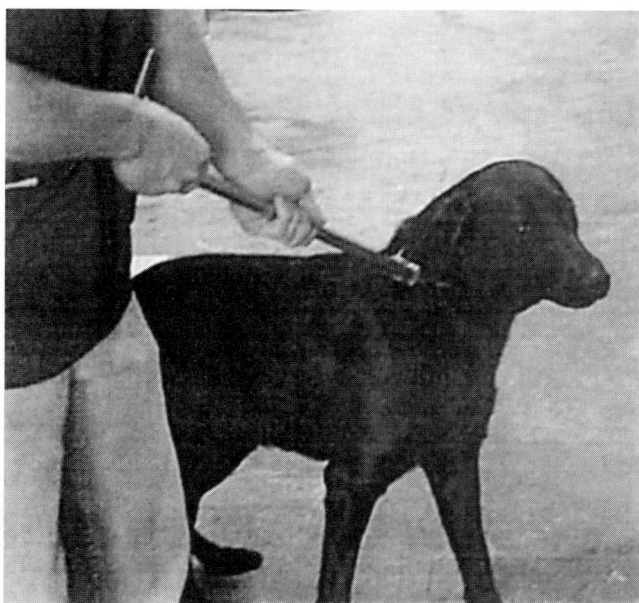

FIGURE 1-53. This dog has been captured with a cable snare. The steel handle allows the handler to keep the dog at a safe distance when maneuvering the animal.

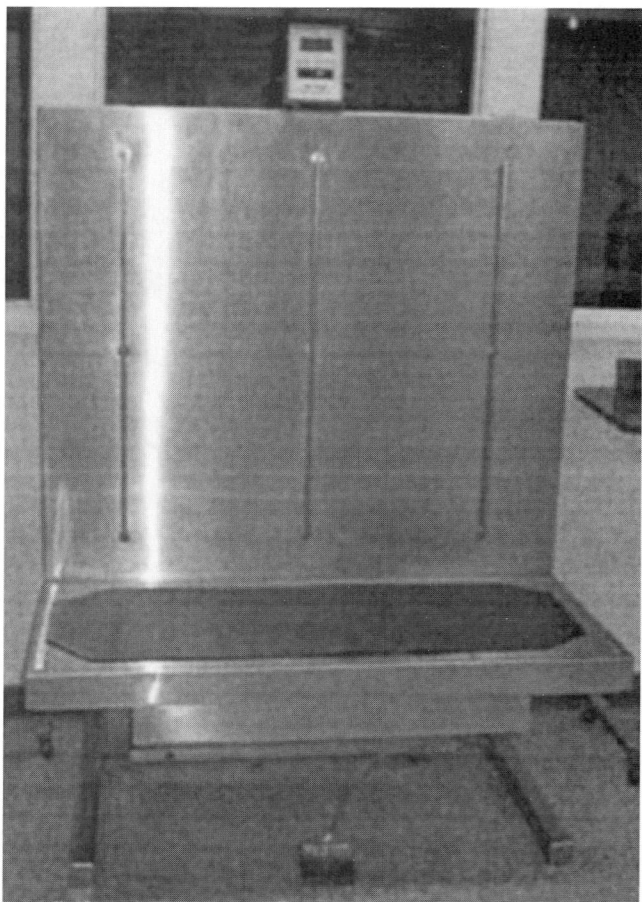

FIGURE 1-54. A stainless steel lift table that also has a self-contained scale. This allows large dogs or those that do not like to be picked up to step onto the table at floor level and then be raised to a comfortable height for examination.

using a forklift technique, placing the arms behind the elbow and in front of the hind legs. If the animal struggles there is danger that it will fall forward or backward. Two people can lift a dog together, if one lifts the forequarters and the other person lifts the hindquarters. Both individuals should be on the same side, away from the table, to accomplish this technique. Some dogs object to being lifted from under the flank area, especially males. If this is the case they definitely need two people to lift them, and the person in back should make sure the placement of the hand or arm is well forward on the abdomen. Many practices now have lift tables that allow dogs to be walked onto the table at floor level and then elevated to a comfortable height for examination (Figure 1-54). Handlers are cautioned that lifting dogs may result in back injury. Lifting with the legs and keeping the back straight will help avoid muscle strains. Large dogs that are nervous about being lifted or react adversely to being on top of a table should be dealt with on the floor.

Never let a dog jump down from a table. Tables and floors have slick surfaces that invite slips and possibly fractures. Lift the dog off the table in the same manner as it was placed.

Technician Note
Never let a dog jump down from a table.

Injured or sick animals pose different problems in lifting. More support is required for patients with fractures or painful abdomens. A stretcher may be required for lifting a badly injured dog. Rational judgment should be used in all instances when lifting is required.

Table Restraint
The degree of restraint required for a dog on the table depends on the procedure. The forequarters and hindquar-

ters must be controlled at all times to prevent the dog from jumping or falling off the table. The form of restraint most commonly used is to have the arms either behind the rump, or under the flank, and in front of the chest pulling the dog inward in much the same manner as lifting. The head may be pulled toward the handler's chest (Figure 1-55). This is adequate restraint on most dogs for examination and intramuscular or subcutaneous injections.

A rectal examination requires only slight adjustments for restraint. The holder's arm should not be behind the dog; rather it can be placed over the dog's back to stabilize lateral movement by drawing the body toward the handler. Sometimes the hand must support the ventral abdomen to prevent the dog from sitting down.

Whenever procedures are done on puppies it is wise to put the bitch into a crate or better, remove her to a kennel outside the room. Care must be taken when removing newborn pups from the bitch for the same reasons discussed previously.

Restraint for Venipuncture
The dog must not be allowed to move during venipuncture because movement results in perivascular placement of the needle. The primary reason for struggling and movement during venipuncture is anxiety. Calm, affectionate

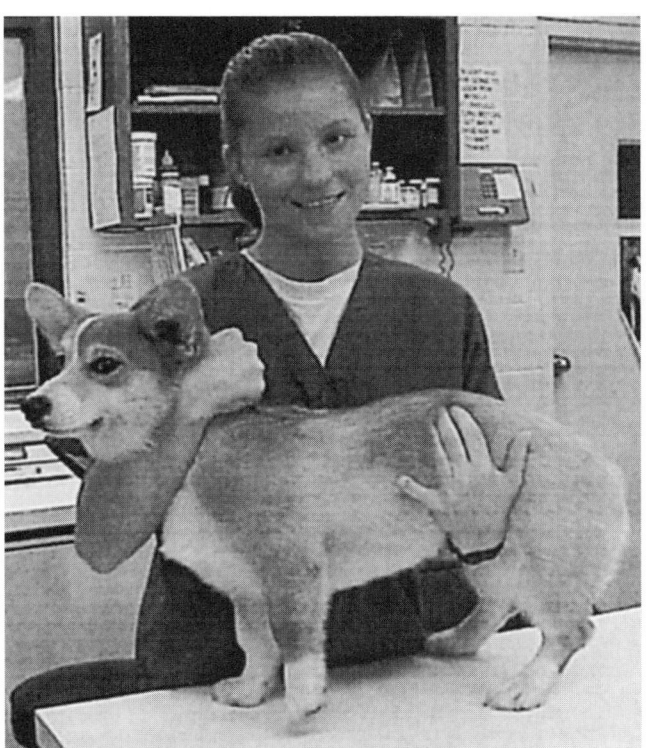

FIGURE 1-55. The handler is providing support for the dog and restraint for examination at the same time. Note the placement of the arms in a forklift position under the neck and in front of the flank. The handler is positioned to draw the animal closer if serious anxiety develops.

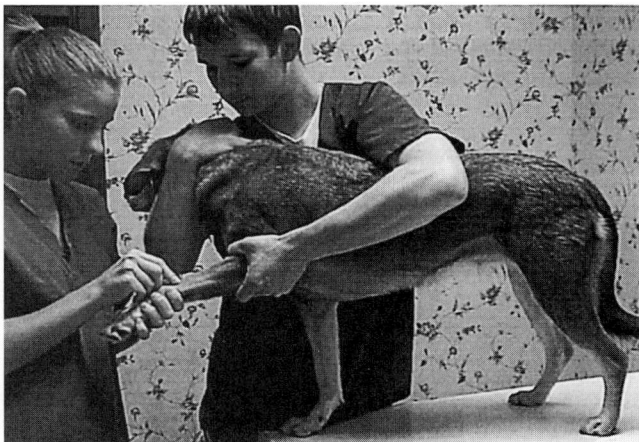

FIGURE 1-56. The correct positioning for obtaining blood samples from the cephalic vein. The handler has the dog well restrained, even though the dog remains standing, and has rolled the vein slightly outward to tighten the skin and provide easy access for the sample. If the dog becomes anxious, the handler will force the dog into sternal recumbency while maintaining the hold.

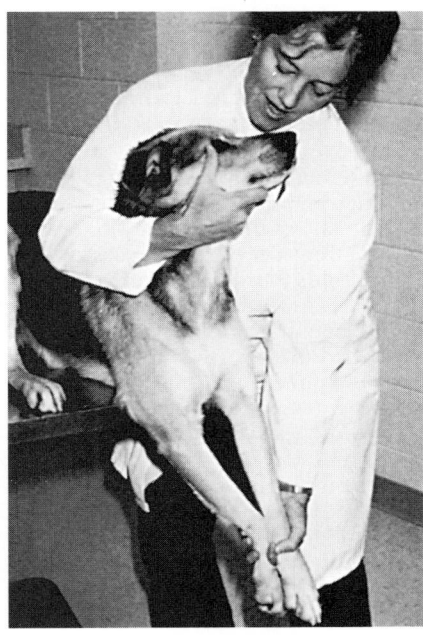

FIGURE 1-57. Method of holding the dog for jugular venipuncture. Note the straight line from the ramus of the mandible to the feet.

handling with petting and soothing words will help alleviate anxiety. The most painful portion of the venipuncture is the piercing of the skin and vessel, which is when the restraint must be most secure. Positioning is the most critical part of a venipuncture to allow for accurate location of the vessel. Diagnostic sampling is discussed in Chapter 3.

The holder must restrain the dog's body, present the forelimb, and occlude the vein to allow it to fill and be recognized under the skin for cephalic venipuncture. To accomplish this, the dog is placed on the table near one end facing the edge. The holder stands beside the table facing the same direction as the dog and nestles the animal on the table under the arm. The handler's forearm, elbow, and upper arm all exert pressure to bring the dog snugly to the handler's side. The hand of the same arm cradles the dog's elbow with the palm and fingers while the thumb clamps down on the cephalic vein (Figure 1-56). To ensure that the vein is under the thumb and on the dorsal surface of the dog's forearm, the holder grasps the limb just below the elbow with the thumb as far inside as possible and rotates the skin outward. The fingers should rest on the table, and the dog's elbow should be pushed slightly forward to stabilize the leg. The elbow should be near the edge of the table to allow good access to the vein.

The free hand is used to restrain the dog's head, and for most dogs this is best accomplished by pressing the head into the chest of the handler by reaching under the neck and placing the hand behind the jaw. The hand may also go around the dog's muzzle to prevent biting when necessary. The holder must release the thumb when the person is ready to perform the injection. Failure to release the

vessel will prevent the substance injected from reaching the general circulation and may result in rupture of the vessel.

Kneeling, or squatting, behind a large dog that is sitting on the floor allows cephalic venipuncture to be performed in the same manner. Most dogs submit to cephalic venipuncture quite readily. Dogs that are gentle may allow cephalic venipuncture while sitting up.

Jugular venipuncture may be necessary in some cases. This is accomplished by placing the dog further forward on the table so the forelegs extend over the edge (Figure 1-57).

The holder stands alongside and puts the arm over the animal as in the cephalic technique, pressing the animal to the table. The hand of the arm over the animal is the one that restrains the head and the hand away from the table restrains the forefeet, with a finger between the feet for a secure grip. The hand on the head grasps the muzzle with the fingers under the jaw, and the thumb is over the nose. Care must be taken when placing the hand to avoid cutting off the animal's ability to breathe. The fingers must not be placed too far caudally on the jaw, which may occlude the jugular vein and make it difficult to locate. The main advantage of this position is to provide a nearly straight plane from the angle of the jaw to the forefeet for easy access to the jugular vein. The dog should be "stretched" to a slight degree to achieve the correct position. Common errors in this position are pulling the forelegs too far forward, which interferes with the angle of entry for the syringe, or pulling the head too far backward, stretching the skin and vessel and collapsing the vein. The correct position of the head should be no more than slightly above 90 degrees from the neck. The head may be directed toward the holder's chest, allowing access to the vessel that is on the side opposite the holder. A large dog can be restrained on the floor with the holder steadying the chest with one hand and the muzzle with the other.

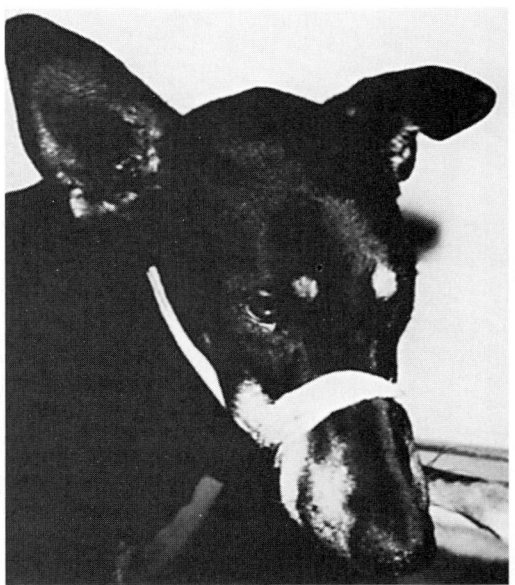

FIGURE 1-58.   The gauze muzzle.

Technician Note

The saphenous vein, located on the lateral aspect of the hind leg, is an alternate venipuncture site for which the dog must be restrained in lateral recumbency.

The saphenous vein, located on the lateral aspect of the hind leg, is an alternate venipuncture site; for this procedure the dog must be restrained in lateral recumbency. To position a dog in lateral recumbency the holder stands behind the dog with one forearm pressed across the animal's neck while that hand holds the forelegs with a finger between the legs. The other forearm presses across the dog's flank, and the hind legs are held in a similar manner. When venipuncture is being performed, only the down leg is held; the person making the puncture stabilizes the other.

Muzzles and Mouth Gags

A dog's mouth can be restrained manually by bringing the hands forward from the rear on both sides of the face. The thumbs are placed on the forehead, and the fingers are looped under the mandibles. The palms of the hands should be below the ears.

Commercial muzzles are made of a variety of materials and come in various sizes. Several sizes should be available. Gauze or rope muzzles can be made if necessary. Nylon rope choke leads are sometimes handy as muzzling devices for snapping dogs. Following capture of the dog a loop of rope made with a single overhand knot is positioned from above the dog's nose until it is in place over the muzzle. This loop should be tightened quickly after it is positioned with the knot on top of the nose. Most dogs will try to push the rope loop off with their forepaw. The first knot must be held snugly while a second knot is made with the ends under the nose. The second knot may be a single overhand, or a square knot may be thrown. The two free ends are then passed behind the dog's head and tied again. This knot is extremely important because it holds the muzzle in place so it must be secure, yet it must be tied in such a manner to allow for quick release should the animal have difficulty breathing.

Gauze roll bandage (7.5 to 15 cm) may be used as a muzzle in the same fashion as the rope (Figure 1-58). Gauze is preferable to rope because it is less slick. However, it also makes a less rigid loop to apply to a recalcitrant dog. The piece of gauze should be cut at least 90 cm long for most dogs. It is important to have sufficient length to begin with, because there may be only one opportunity to muzzle the dog without a significant battle.

Brachiocephalic breeds are difficult to muzzle and can be determined biters. To muzzle them the gauze bandage is first tied around the nose with the first knot tied underneath the jaw. The ends are then passed behind the head and tied with a square knot. Finally, one end is passed over the forehead and under the loop on top of the nose and then tied back to the other side. This keeps the loop from slipping off the top of the short nose.

The mouth of a dog can be examined in a variety of ways. The easiest, if the dog is a willing participant, is to open the mouth with the hands for visual examination. Placing one hand on the upper jaw and the other on the lower and then forcing the lips over the teeth will allow the handler to separate the jaws of the mouth (Figure 1-59). A variety of mouth gags can also be used on dogs. A simple wooden dowel may be pressed toward the back of the mouth to rest between the carnassial teeth. The dowel can be tied in place behind the ears, or it can be held by hand. Stomach tubes may be inserted with the dowel in place. The commercial spring mouth gag has a hole on either end for the canine teeth, and it is inserted on one side of the mouth for a variety of procedures. The disadvantage to this type of gag is that it hangs outside the mouth, is heavy, and can fracture teeth to which it is attached. A syringe case of appropriate size placed over opposing canine teeth makes a lighter and safer gag, especially for use in dental work.

Mobility-Limiting Devices

Self-mutilation and tearing of bandages can be prevented with several devices. The most common is the Elizabethan collar. The concept is to place some type of stiff material extending from the collar area to the dog's nose so that it cannot chew or lick its body. Commercial plastic collars are available, or collars may be fabricated from buckets, large bottles, or heavy plastic sheets. It is most important to

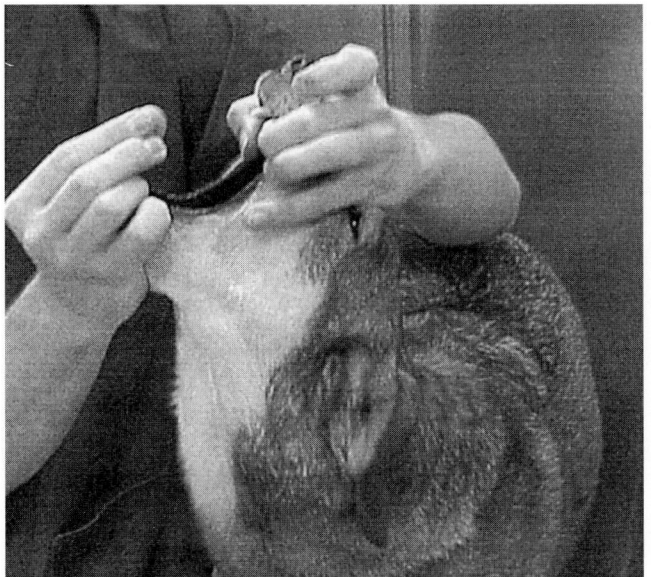

Figure 1-59. Technique for easy examination of the mouth. The lips of the upper jaw are pressed against the teeth by one hand while the lower lips are pressed into the teeth of the lower jaw. Forcing the lips apart then opens the jaw.

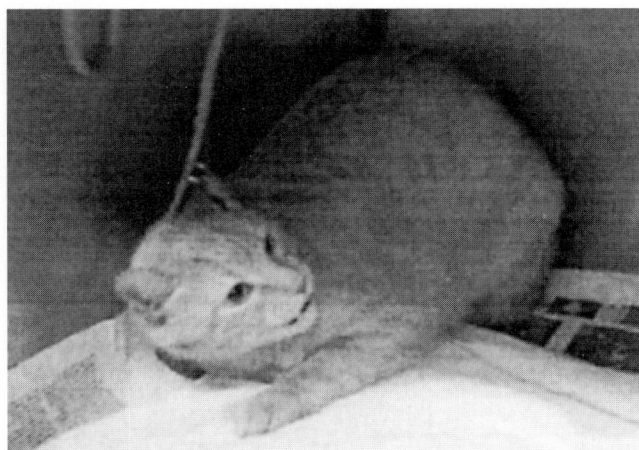

Figure 1-60. Trapped cats will display flattened ears and may hiss and growl before unleashing their claws.

ensure that no sharp edges are present and that the collar is secured to the neck by gauze or the dog's collar. (It is not good for a veterinary practice if the dog traumatizes itself with the collar in a manner greater than the original lesion.) Attention must be given to the ability of the dog to eat and drink following the placement of these devices.

Fastening a pole along the body to a snug collar high on the neck makes another type of device that will limit movement of the head. This would mimic the cradle described for restraint of horses earlier in the chapter. Tape is usually used to keep the device from shifting.

Chemical Restraint
Many drugs are available for chemical restraint and sedation for dogs. The main reason for tranquilization is to remove anxiety, which is one of the major reasons that dogs bite. However, the handler is cautioned that tranquilizing effects vary between dogs and that dogs are still capable of biting even when heavily tranquilized. Chapter 21 gives more information on chemical agents of anesthesia.

Capture and Restraint of Cats
Cats are more apprehensive than dogs with strange people and surroundings. A cat that escapes will search out a hiding place, whereas a dog that escapes will look for room to run away. This may be due to the lower endurance that a cat has for running and the security that cats feel in an enclosed space. A cat that is trapped may well respond with flattened ears, hissing, scratching, and biting at hands and extended fingers (Figure 1-60). Heavy leather gloves may be used to subdue these cats in the same manner as described for small dogs. Grasp the scruff of the neck to lift the cat (Figure 1-61). This may be followed by a rapid "stretch" restraint by also grasping the hind legs. Certain cats are too fast and smart to succumb to the glove technique. These cats may be caught by a neck rope or snare, but they react poorly to a choke compared with the scruff of the neck. One of the easiest ways to catch a cat is to force it into a box pushed into the cage. There are boxes

available that will allow for anesthesia induction after the cat is captured without having to handle the cat at all. All escapes from the box are blocked once the cage is placed in the kennel until the cat is safely inside and the top is closed.

A rope may be used to lasso a cat that is extremely uncooperative. The rope is thrown over the cat and then quickly passed between the cage bars, and the front of the cage is closed. The cat is then brought to the front of the cage with the noose. Next, chemicals may be used to subdue the cat, either by oral spray or injection. If the tail can be hooked and pulled to the cage door while the head is restrained in the noose, the hindquarters will be presented for intramuscular injections. This provides the greatest amount of safety for the handlers.

Carrying Cats
Cats generally feel most secure in close quarters and seldom resist being put into a bag or rolled in a towel. They are best carried from place to place in a cat carrier or small cardboard box with a lid. They can also be carried with one arm if they are not particularly nervous. To carry a cat, its hindquarters are placed under the elbow area and pressed securely to the holder's body with the forearm (Figure 1-62). The cat lies in a sternal position along the forearm while the hand, which has one finger between the legs, holds the forelegs. The cat may still use the hind claws to gouge the abdomen of the holder, who must be ready to grab the scruff of the neck and hold the cat at arm's length if it panics. Quickly grasping the hind legs and pulling away from the scruff of the neck will effectively immobilize almost any cat. This is not a position of comfort for the cat and the cat will object, but it is clearly safer for the holder.

Technician Note
Cats usually feel most secure in close quarters, and they seldom resist being put into a bag or rolled in a towel.

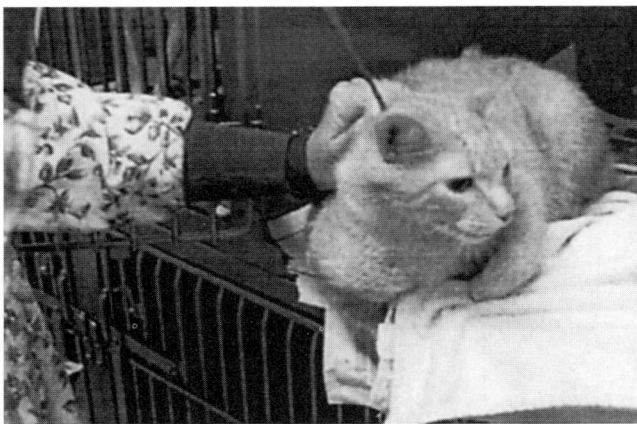

FIGURE 1-61. Capture of the head followed by grasping the scruff of the neck will restrain most cats.

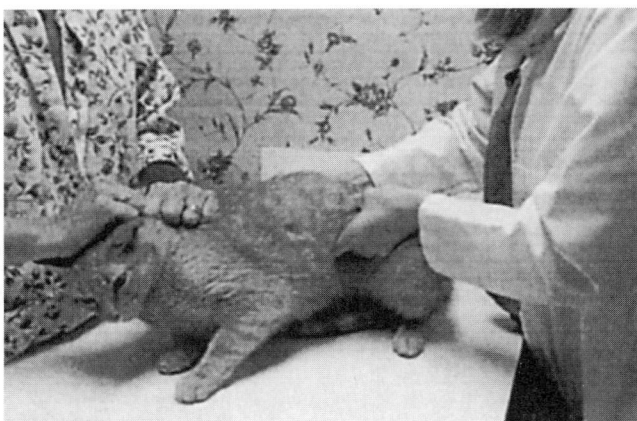

FIGURE 1-63. Restraint for examination of a cat. Note both the handler and examiner have on long-sleeved lab coats.

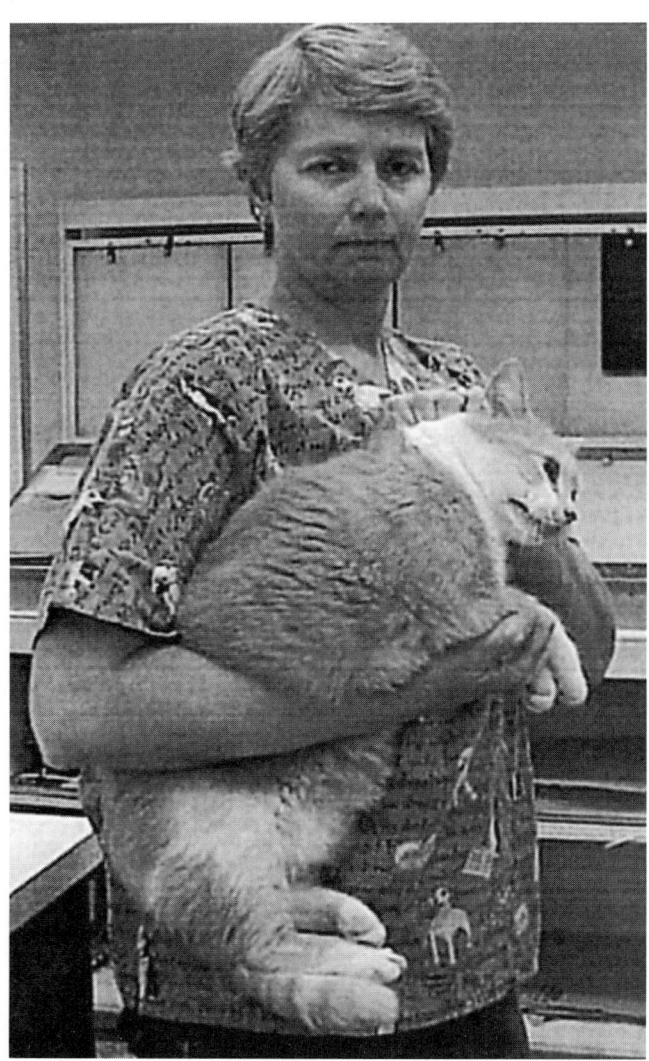

FIGURE 1-62. The proper carrying position for a cat. Note the support given to the abdomen, the grasp of the neck, and the restraint of both front feet.

Restraint for Examination

Table restraint of cats is similar to that of dogs, except that cats tend to use their claws as their first line of defense (if they have them) rather than their teeth. Cats should be allowed supervised movement when it is not necessary for them to be still. Some cats are so terrified that they are best held or cuddled with the head buried under the holder's arm. Cats are not necessarily malicious when they climb onto a person's chest or clamp nails into a forearm, but their actions will hurt if the holder is not prepared. It is a good idea to wear protective gowns or laboratory coats with long sleeves when dealing with cats (Figure 1-63). Cat scratches are potentially dangerous to veterinary personnel, and care should be taken to avoid movements and behavior that will agitate the cat.

Restraint for Venipuncture

Cephalic venipuncture restraint can be applied to cats much as to dogs (Figure 1-64). However, cats will tend to engage their claws and teeth in an effort to get away from the holder. When a cat becomes agitated it seems to lose its spine and develop legs that swirl about like a weed-eater. Once cats develop this attitude they are impossible to hold like dogs, and other restraint techniques must be employed. Jugular venipuncture may be more appropriate for some cats because the hold restrains the head and forefeet more securely than the cephalic technique (Figure 1-65). Wrapping the hind feet with a towel disarms all but the most persistent cat. The head is held with the hand over the top of the head and the jaw or zygomatic arch is grasped with the thumb on one side and two or three fingers on the other side. The other hand then restrains both forelimbs as in the dog.

There are other ways to hold a cat for jugular venipuncture. They involve the cat being placed on its back with the holder occluding the jugular vein and the person using the syringe pushing the chin down toward the table to make the head move backward to get a straight shot at the jugular. The holder can hold two legs in each hand with a finger between the legs while pushing the cat down on the table and using the little finger to press on the thoracic inlet to occlude the jugular vein. A cat can also be rolled in a towel or bag to engage the feet and legs. The holder need only steady the cat on its back and occlude the vessel in this

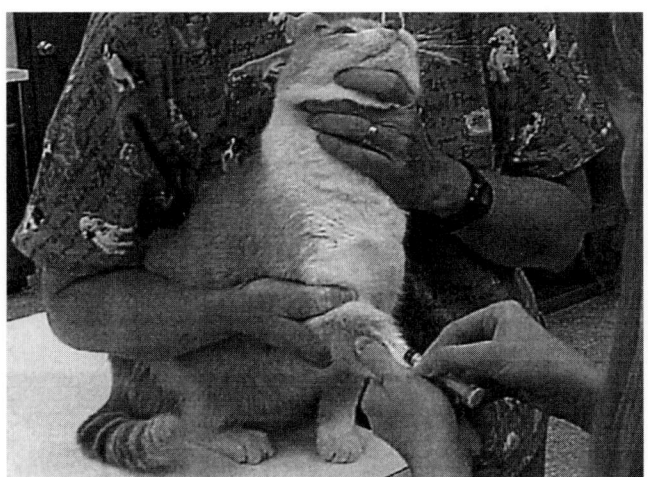

FIGURE 1-64. Proper restraint for cephalic venipuncture in the cat. The head, forearm, and back of the cat are all supported and well restrained by the handler.

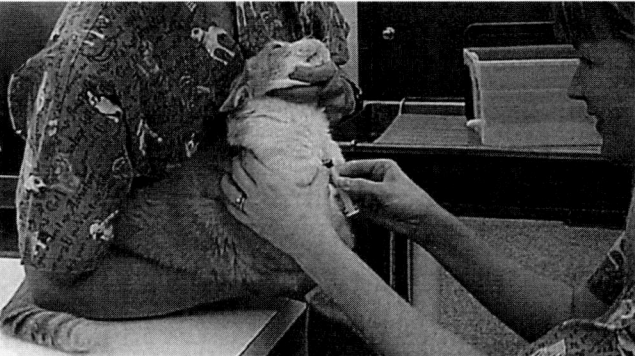

FIGURE 1-65. Restraint for jugular venipuncture in the cat. Note how the hind legs are tucked under the elbow of the handler and the fore feet are extended and held in one hand.

case. Cat bags are made with zippers so a single limb may be withdrawn and used for cephalic venipuncture, and in a similar fashion, there are now restraint boxes made for cats that have different openings to allow for withdrawal of a limb (Figure 1-66).

Stretching a cat in lateral recumbency will provide access to the saphenous vein (Figure 1-67). Most cats do not seem to realize that they can use their fore feet to scratch the hand on the scruff of their neck when they are appropriately stretched. The medial saphenous vein can then be used for venipuncture by holding the hind leg that is up in a flexed position. The little finger can be used to hold off the vein on the down leg for the venipuncture. The person who is performing the venipuncture must restrain the down leg with one hand while handling the syringe with the other.

Bathing
Bathing a cat may be a trying experience for both the cat and the person. Most cats will try to climb up the person's arms to escape standing water or spray. Cats should be bathed on top of a screen suspended over a tub (a metal window screen will suffice) and washed with a light spray of warm water. Almost all cats will clamp their claws into the screen and stand still for the entire bath when using this technique.

Chemical Restraint
The use of chemicals and anesthesia to restrain cats is common. The eyes should be treated with ophthalmic ointments to avoid corneal drying from the lack of blinking when these agents are used. See Chapter 21 for more information on anesthesia.

Restraint of Exotic Animals
Minimal handling of all exotic animals is recommended and must be done efficiently, quietly, and confidently. The best method of learning restraint is by watching an experienced handler. Many clients judge the competency of veterinary professionals on how well they catch and handle the patient. Smooth handling and restraint of their animals reassure clients that the technician is well trained. It is often difficult to quantify the stress factor. The importance

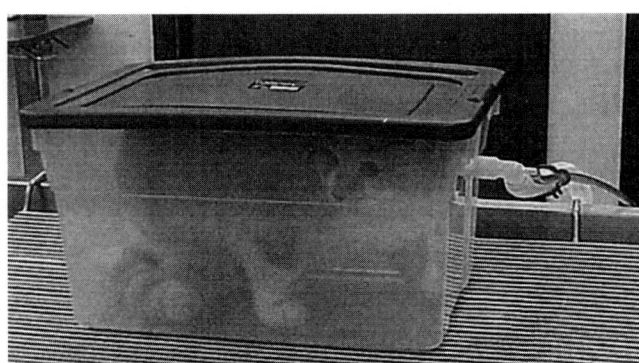

FIGURE 1-66. This cat is being restrained in a capture box that has inlet ports for inhalation anesthesia.

of fast, competent handling cannot be overemphasized. The sights, sounds, smells, and temperatures of the strange environment will stress the exotic animal in a veterinary hospital. As a general rule, the more tame the animal, the better it will tolerate handling. However, do not underestimate the added stress of disease or injury. Do not attempt to learn handling on an exotic animal whose condition is already compromised by disease and trauma. Always discuss the subject of handling and stress with the owner of an ill or traumatized nondomestic pet before handling begins. All treatment and testing material (Culturettes, syringes) must be in place before the animal is restrained to minimize stress. The patient work-up may have to be done incrementally because of the patient's poor physical condition or response to handling.

 Technician Note

Always discuss the subject of handling and stress with the owner of an ill or traumatized nondomestic pet before handling begins.

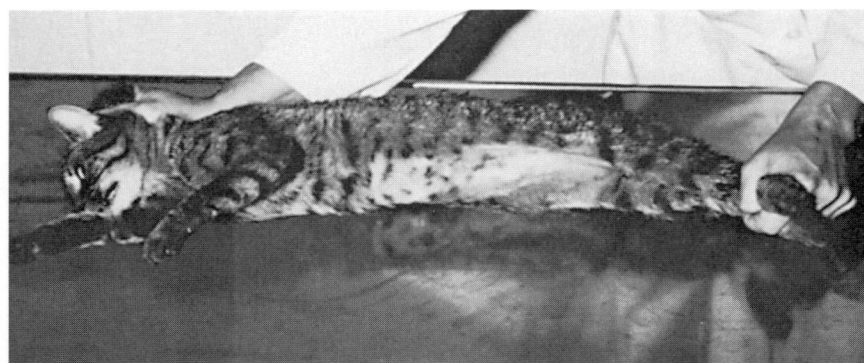

FIGURE 1-67.   Stretching a cat on its side.

Restraint of Birds

Psittacines

When holding and examining a psittacine patient, the medical team should avoid the strong beak, jaws, wings, and feet. The feet usually have sharp, pointed claws. The equipment needed to deal with these patients will include towels or drapes, perches, and nets. Gloves should never be used with psittacine birds. Gloves are not supple enough for handlers to feel the patient within their grasp. Do not use gloves during stressful events with a pet bird because that bird will soon associate the shape of the human hand with negative experiences. The handler should first remove water bowls and perches from the cage. Room lights may be dimmed to take advantage of the bird's inability to rapidly accommodate to changes in lighting. The psittacine bird's primary weapon is the beak; therefore the head should be promptly secured. Placing a towel or drape over the bird's head and securing it are the best way to accomplish this. A wooden perch may be used to give the bird something to bite on other than fingers. The bird cannot bite the catcher if it is chewing on the cage. Once the head is secured, the body is wrapped in the towel, the feet are held, and the bird is held against the holder's body to control the wings. The towel or drape may then be slowly removed from the patient's head for examination, keeping the towel around the wings to secure them from flapping. Commercially available avian restraint boards allow for secure restraint with minimal risk to the patient or veterinary personnel (Figure 1-68).

Passerines

Canaries are the most common passerine species seen in veterinary offices. These birds are easily stressed under normal conditions and are even more sensitive when they are ill. Catching the patient for an examination must be done quickly and efficiently. To catch the passerine patient, all lights should be turned off and the cage door slowly lifted. Grab the patient with one hand, and then turn on the lights. To hold the bird for examination let the bird's head rest between the middle and index fingers while lying on its back. The fingers should not completely encircle the body but should stay on the sides of the bird. Do not put pressure on the breast or the patient may suffocate (Figure 1-69). Care should be taken to hold the head straight so that the thumb does not slip to the anterior part of the neck and occlude the trachea.

Raptorial Species

Birds of prey use their anatomic weapons in a different way. For them, it is of utmost importance to secure the talons. Although many raptors will bite, their jaws are not tremendously strong, and they do little damage with the beak. The mouth is soft except close to the very point of the beak, which the birds use for tearing flesh. The wings should also be considered a weapon and should be properly secured. Equipment needed for restraining raptors includes towels or drapes, gloves of appropriate size and thickness, and hoods. To approach a bird of prey using gloves the handler should be bent down low and approach quietly. Dimming the lights may be a disadvantage for examining a species that hunts at night. The handler should present as little threat as possible to the raptor. As the handler places one hand in front of the raptor's face, the second should be brought in low toward the bird's feet. The upper hand should be held between the handler's face and the bird and may be used to distract the bird. The lower hand should quickly grasp the feet, trying to place the index finger between the bird's feet. The bird is then smoothly and quickly pulled up out of the cage or off the floor so that it does not beat its wings on any surfaces. It is important to hold the bird away form objects such as the examining table or cage. The bird can then be brought into a cradle position, the wings secured between the handler's arm and body, and the hood placed over the head (Figure 1-70).

If hoods are not available, a towel may be draped over the bird's head, which will reduce visual and auditory stimuli and help to calm the bird significantly. An alternative approach to secure a bird of prey may be done with a towel or drape. The handler approaches the bird in the same manner, quietly and low, with the towel or drape spread in front with both hands. The handler moves in slowly until close enough to use the towel as a large glove, completely covering the bird. The handler's hands should contact the bird at the level of the bird's shoulders. It is important to avoid simply throwing the towel because the bird will be able to dodge it or move from under it. The bird is then pressed through the towel with enough pressure to make the bird push up, using its legs on the ground. The handler's hands are then worked downward, alongside the wings, toward the legs, and the legs are grasped at the tarsometatarsus. Once the bird is covered by the towel and its feet secured, the handler then lifts the bird up with the bird's back toward the handler's abdomen. A hood may replace the towel over the head. It is important never to release the feet of a bird of prey until someone else has secured them. A 10- to 15-cm long piece of 2.5-cm (1-inch) wide white cloth tape should be used to secure the talons to prevent accidents (Figure 1-71). If a bird has talons, the legs must be fully extended before the talons can be

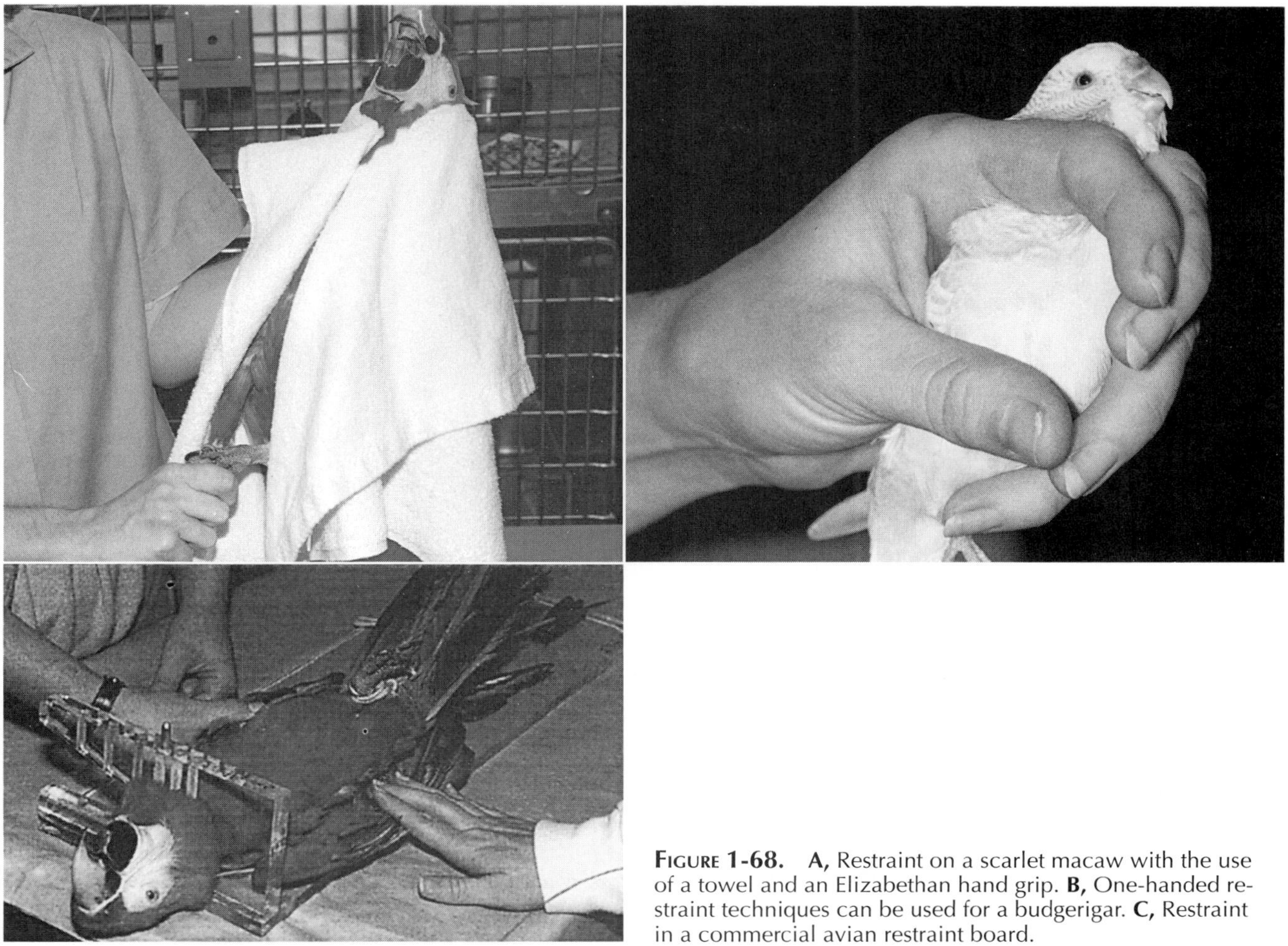

FIGURE 1-68.   A, Restraint on a scarlet macaw with the use of a towel and an Elizabethan hand grip. **B,** One-handed restraint techniques can be used for a budgerigar. **C,** Restraint in a commercial avian restraint board.

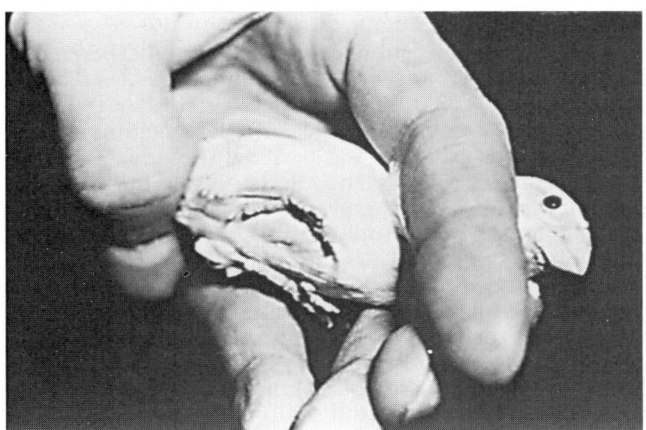

FIGURE 1-69.   The proper technique for restraining a passerine for a physical examination.

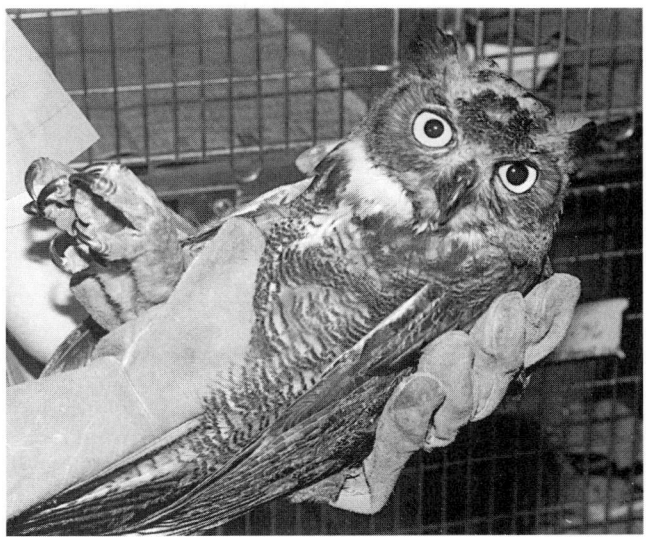

FIGURE 1-70.   The restraint of a great-horned owl with the use of gloves. Note the restraint of the talons.

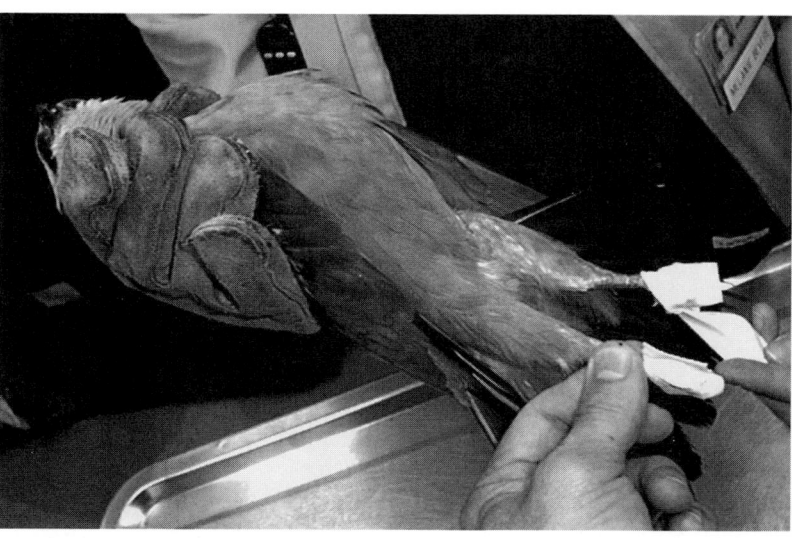

FIGURE 1-71. Taping the talons of raptors using 1-inch white adhesive tape will help protect the technician. Leaving a tab on the end of the taped talon, by folding over the tape, will aid in tape removal at the end of the procedure.

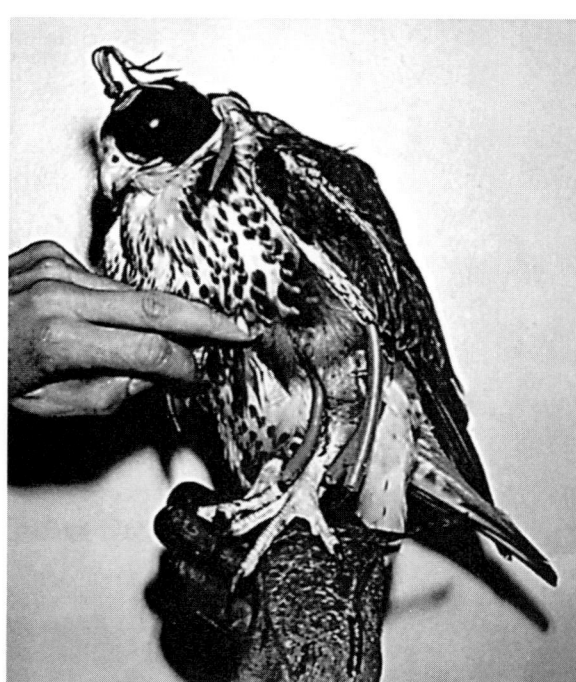

FIGURE 1-72. A falconer restrains a prairie falcon with hood and jesses for examination of an external fixator applied to a tibiotarsal fracture.

removed. Birds of prey under the control of a falconer are a different story because the falconer is often adept at restraining the bird for a physical examination (Figure 1-72).

Two common procedures the veterinary technician is often called on to perform are nail trims and wing clips. Owners request many variations of wing trims. In general, heavier birds (African grey, Amazon parrots) should only have the primary feathers trimmed, while longer, thinner birds (cockatiels) will benefit from most of the primary and secondary feathers being clipped. Both wings should be clipped for a symmetric effect.

Restraint of Reptiles

The veterinary technician should become as familiar as possible with anatomic and physiologic adaptations of reptiles to handle them. Several sources of information are found in the recommended reading list at the end of this chapter. Restraint of turtles or tortoises should be done carefully and with caution. Some species of turtles have a long neck and a sharp powerful beak (rhamphotheca) that can inflict a serious bite to the unwary handler. Some turtles may be able to extend their head and neck nearly to the level of the hindlimbs, two thirds of their body length. Many are quick and therefore should be approached from the rear, with the tail and legs held securely. Simply covering the head, neck, and forelimbs with a cloth towel is usually adequate to prevent injury to the turtle and handler. To prevent an animal from walking during an examination, it may be placed on a broad-based object that will keep the chelonian limbs from touching the examination table surface. The legs may be kept in place by wrapping the shell, with the legs inside, with an elastic bandage. To remove a turtle's head from the shell for examination, straight ovid delivery forceps may be used. Care must be taken using steady, gentle traction without allowing the forceps to touch the eyes. The main force of the forceps' jaws should be applied away from the shell and not onto the head.

Snakes are usually more difficult for the inexperienced handler. Equipment needed may include Plexiglas shields, Plexiglas tubes, tongs, canvas bags or drapes, snake hook, gas anesthetic machine, and plastic bags. Venomous reptiles are not recommended as pets and should be handled only by experienced snake handlers and veterinarians. The general approach to restrain any snake is to immobilize the head and grasp it firmly with the hands at the base of the skull (Figure 1-73). Several methods may be used to immobilize the animal's head initially; a drape, piece of paper, or Plexiglas shield may be used to block the snake's vision while the hands grasp the animal behind the head. The Plexiglas shield can be held in one hand, pressing the head of the snake to the floor, while the other hand grasps the snake at the base of the skull as the shield is slowly moved rostrally off the body. A snake hook may be used to pin the head to the floor.

When a snake hook is used, a suitable soft and resilient

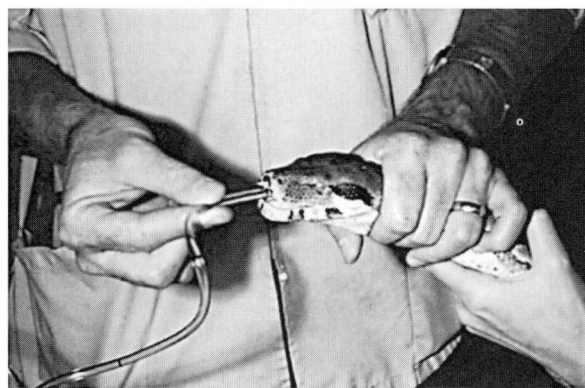

FIGURE 1-73.   These handlers are demonstrating restraint and passage of a stomach tube on a common boa constrictor.

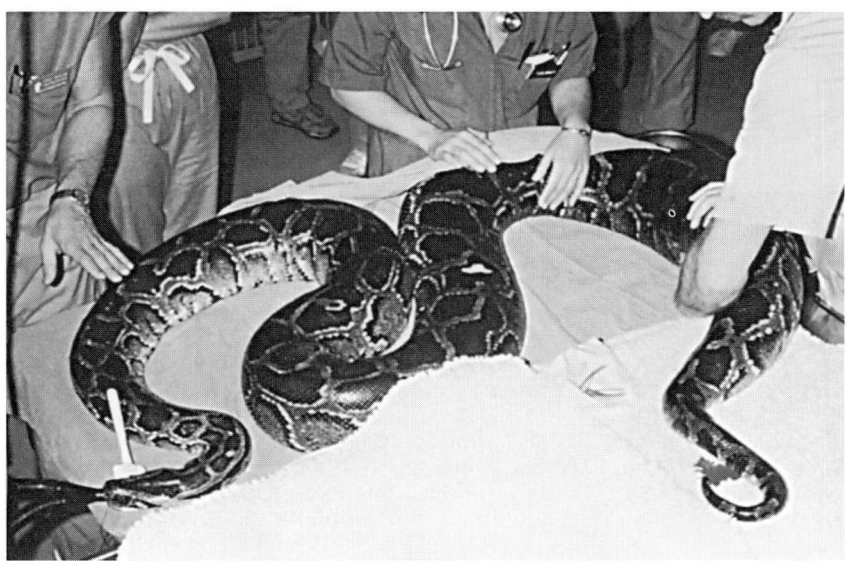

FIGURE 1-74.   Intubation and anesthesia of a Burmese python for deep palpation. The snake is placed inside a large plastic bag filled with isoflurane induced anesthesia.

padded surface is useful to prevent trauma to the snake. A hand then replaces the hook. It is possible to injure a reptile by applying too much pressure with the hook; therefore only experienced technicians should use a snake hook on a client's animals. Most snakes can be easily maintained through hand control at the base of the skull. A few snake species can autotomize their tails as a defense mechanism. Snakes should not be picked up by their tails to prevent skin loss (degloving injury) and automization. Plexiglas tubes may be used in conjunction with a hook or pole. The hook is used to guide the snake into the Plexiglas tube, and the tube should be of sufficiently small diameter to prevent the snake from turning around and coming back out. The aim is to get the snake to crawl up the tube; when it reaches the halfway point the technician grasps the junction of the snake and the tube, trapping the snake's head within the tube. The caudal half of the snake is accessible with this technique. A gas anesthetic unit may be attached to the open end of the tube for further restraint. Plastic tubes are not generally recommended for many elapid snake species (coral snakes, cobras) because of their ability to turn around and injure the handler.

Placing snakes in a plastic bag or box and filling it with anesthetic gases may also induce anesthesia. Following induction, they are intubated and monitored on a gas anesthetic machine with intermittent ventilation (Figure 1-74). Snakes can be easily transported in canvas bags. When handling snakes the body should always be supported, and large species should never be handled alone.

It is always important to remember to wash the hands well before handling reptiles, particularly if the previous patient was a rabbit or rodent, a snake's typical prey, because snakes attack primarily on the basis of smell.

  Technician Note

It is always important to remember to wash the hands well before handling reptiles, particularly if the previous patient was a rabbit or rodent, a snake's typical prey, because snakes attack primarily on the basis of smell.

Lizards and crocodilians may be restrained using a combination of experienced hands, snare poles, towels, drapes, nooses, or Plexiglas shields. All lizards will bite, and some have strong jaws and sharp teeth. Most lizards will also use their claws and tails as weapons. The approach for small to medium lizards is to attempt to block their

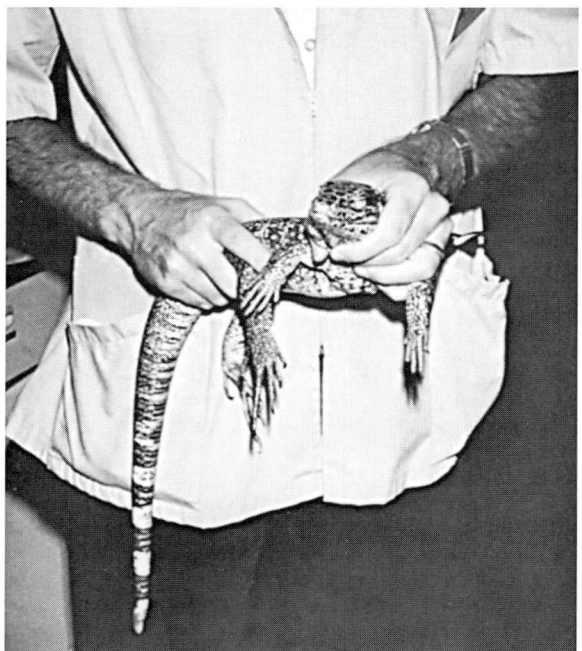

FIGURE 1-75. The proper restraint technique for a large lizard (tegu). One hand is place firmly about the pelvis, and the other is about the shoulders and neck. The tail may be tucked beneath the elbow.

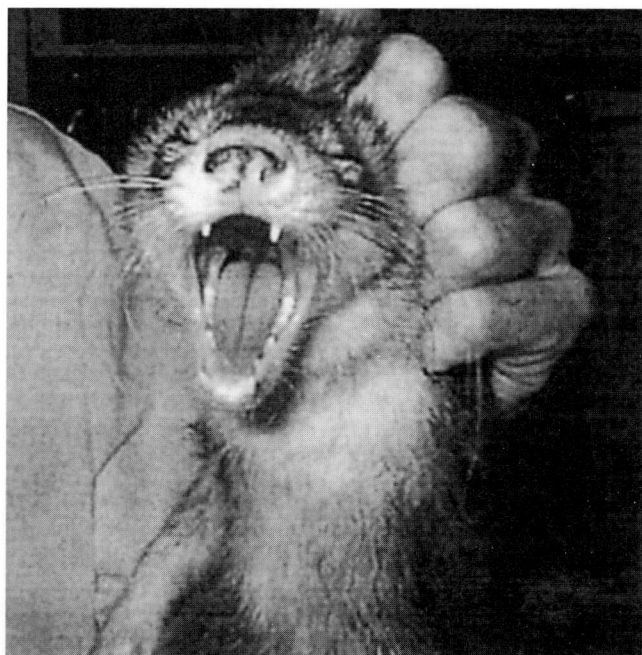

FIGURE 1-76. The proper technique to restrain a ferret. The scruff of the neck is held by one hand, and the other supports the body. Often this technique will elicit a "yawn," at which time the oral cavity may be examined.

vision with a towel or sheet of paper, make a quick grab around the shoulder girdle at the base of the skull with one hand, and restrain the pelvic girdle with the other hand. The tail may then be tucked in against the body, under the arm (Figure 1-75).

A noose made of fine fishing line at the end of a pole may be used for very small lizards. The noose is lowered over the animal's neck, and the pole is quickly lifted with the noose tightened and the animal lifted by the neck. The animal should be restrained and removed from the noose as quickly as possible. For large lizards and crocodilians, it is important to block the animal's vision and then quickly and safely immobilize the head and body simultaneously. This is best accomplished by grasping the animal at the base of the skull or neck with one or both hands and then sitting on the reptile. Two or more people are necessary to accomplish this task, and the mouth should then be taped shut as soon as the reptile is restrained. A noose or rabies pole may be used to help control the mouth before attempting to restrain the head, legs, and tail. Crocodilians, most large lizards, and some chelonians can be immobilized for short periods (up to 30 seconds) by application of gentle, inward pressure on their closed eyes for a few moments. The handler is cautioned that many lizards have tails that detach during stress or trauma. Use extreme caution when grabbing any lizard or reptile by the tail.

Restraint of Ferrets

Ferrets that are not cooperative are a restraint challenge. They belong to the family group that includes weasels, and as such they are quick, agile animals and possess sharp teeth. The ferret's primary weapons are its teeth and when threatened it will not hesitate to bite. Ferrets that are hand

raised can make docile pets in the right circumstances. Proper precautions should be taken when restraining ferrets.

Primary restraint for a ferret is to secure the head and forelegs by gripping the animal by the skin in the dorsal cervical area (the scruff of the neck) (Figure 1-76). The other hand is used to support the bottom of the animal. For the highly aggressive ferret, a towel or drape may be placed over the animal to occlude the vision. The animal's head, neck, and shoulders can then be grasped through the drape or towel. The handler may want to use gloves. Remember, it is not good for any pet animal to associate negative experiences with gloved hands. Once the animal is restrained in this method, the handler may alter the grip on the head to perform a thorough physical examination and other necessary diagnostic procedures. Ferrets may be "stretched" in a manner similar to cats, or they may be grasped with both hands around the forequarters with one hand on the scruff of the neck and the other holding down the forelegs.

Interestingly, ferrets are subject to hypnosis, although it is less likely to be effective when the animal is apprehensive in strange hands. To attempt the hypnosis, the ferret is hung by the scruff with one hand and stroked around the entire length of its torso with the other hand. The susceptible ferret will begin to yawn and its eyelids will droop or close after repeated stroking. The effect is not long lasting and many will be easily startled out of the trance.

Restraint of Llamas

Llamas seem to come in two different styles: those that can be restrained easily and those that never want to be restrained. Driving them into an alley works quite well,

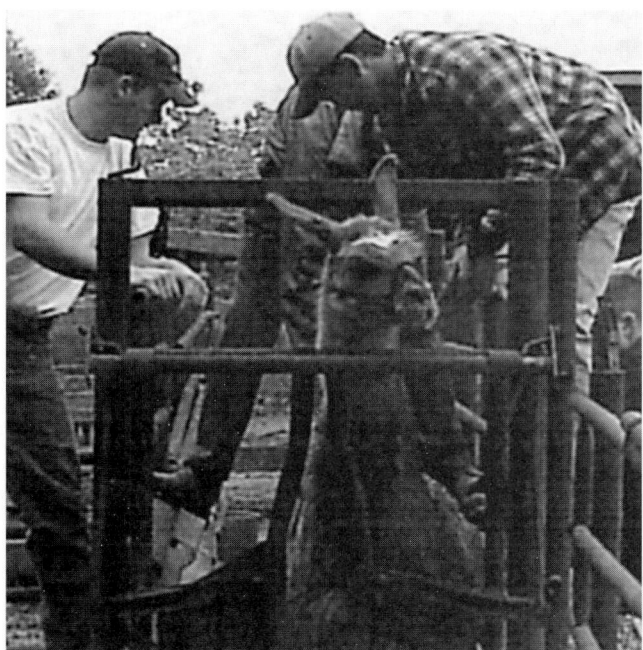

FIGURE 1-77. The capture of a llama in an alleyway. The llama has been haltered and can be led about by the head.

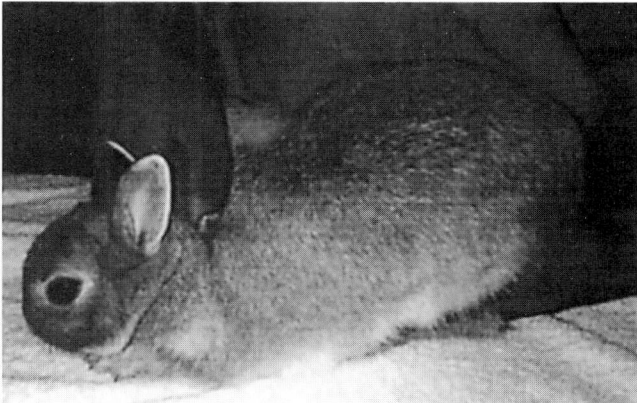

FIGURE 1-78. Proper holding technique for a rabbit undergoing a physical examination.

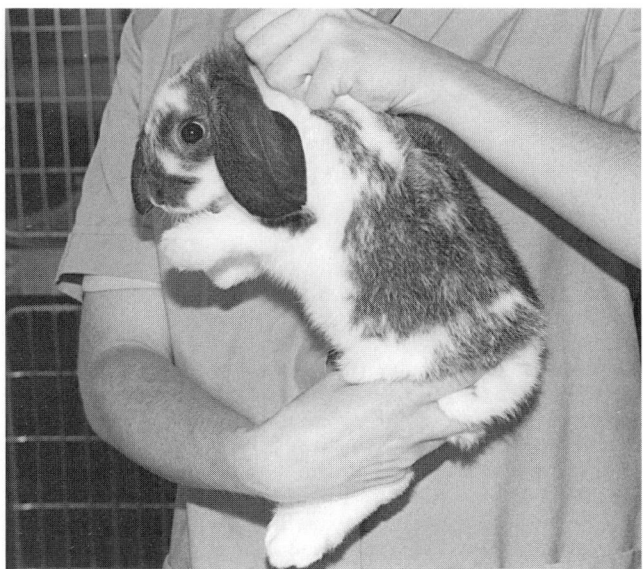

FIGURE 1-79. The proper method of restraint for carrying a rabbit short distances.

and placing a block behind them will allow handlers to approach. Care must be taken to get the block low enough so that the llama does not back under the bar and hurt its back. Llamas will kick, and in most cases they tend to kick more like a horse than a cow, directing the foot straight backward at the perceived threat. The stressed llama will flatten its ears, and many will "spit" in the approximate direction of the threat. The clever handler can slip a loop over the ears and then catch the muzzle in a nose loop to halter a llama (Figure 1-77). Many of them will stand quietly after the halter is placed.

Restraint of Rabbits

Rabbit restraint is important (Figure 1-78). Rabbits have some peculiarities for restraint. Their muscle/skeleton ratio is very high, and their bones are small and light for animals of their size. Rabbits also have extremely powerful hind legs. Restraint of rabbits without controlling their hind legs may precipitate a kicking episode that could result in a "broken back." This terminology is not precise because the bones of the back may not be fractured, but there is definite loss of neural function in the hindquarters that results from trauma to the spinal cord. The hind legs become paralyzed, and bladder and anal tone is lost. The prognosis for recovery is poor in cases of total paralysis. Paralysis may be immediate or delayed depending on the amount of hemorrhage and edema that surrounds the spinal cord.

To avoid this situation the rabbit should never be picked up, carried, or restrained by the ears. To carry a rabbit short distances grasp the nape of the neck skin with one hand while supporting the rear legs with the other (Figure 1-79). The best way to replace a rabbit in a cage is by holding its skin fore and aft, placing it well inside the cage facing outward, and pressing its body down to the floor for a few moments before releasing it. Use of this technique forces the rabbit to turn in its cage before leaping to the safety of

the rear of the cage. The ears should never be used to lift a rabbit of any age. Small plastic pet carriers should be used when carrying rabbits long distances. A towel can be placed around the rabbit to help with restraint when carrying or examining the animal.

 Technician Note

Rabbits should never be picked up, carried, or restrained by the ears.

Rabbits do not like slick surfaces, and losing their footing agitates them. It is best to set them down on something on which they will have good traction, such as a rubber mat, during an examination or treatment. Pressing the rabbit to the table and pulling the hind feet to the rear

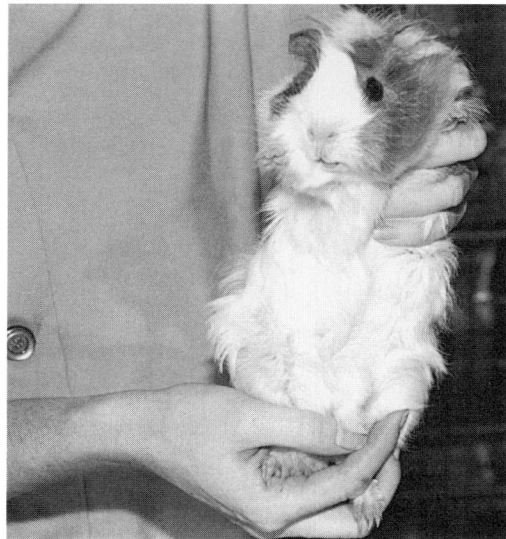

FIGURE 1-80. The proper restraint technique for a guinea pig.

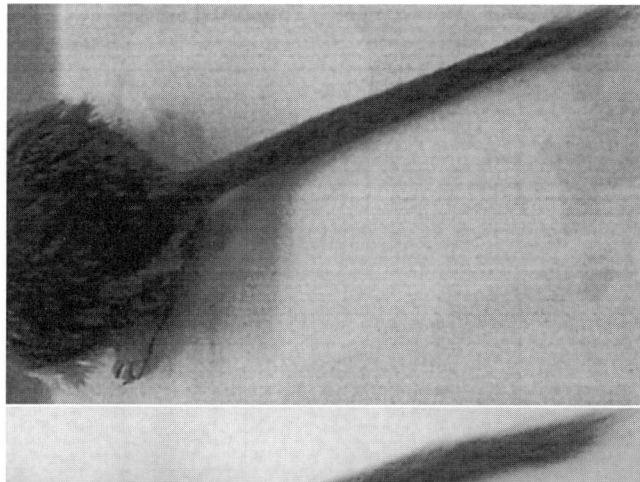

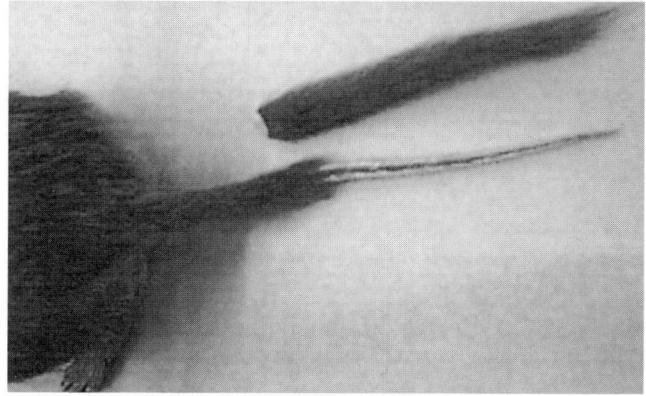

FIGURE 1-81 A, A normal gerbil tail, which should never be used to capture a gerbil. **B,** The skin has sloughed off the tail of this gerbil, which will require a surgical amputation to correct.

allow for trimming of nails, and the forefeet may be trimmed by lifting the foot off the table while the rabbit is held to the surface.

Rabbits have sensitive whiskers and will flinch whenever these hairs are touched or the mouth is approached. To examine the mouth the head must be firmly held. To steady the head for an examination the holder should place the rabbit facing away from his or her body with the forearms pressing down the entire length of the rabbit. The thumbs of the handler are placed behind the ears of the rabbit, and the fingers are used to lift the head from below the mandible. The incisor teeth may be trimmed, aural examinations may be conducted, and ear venipuncture may be performed with the rabbit in this position.

Rabbits may occasionally demonstrate signs of aggression by growling and scratching with the forelegs. Medium-weight gloves will prevent injury to the handler in these cases. Rabbits will seldom bite, so protection against scratches is all that is necessary. Normally, the fight goes out of even the most aggressive rabbit once its forequarters are pressed to the floor and the body is restrained from free movement.

Restraint of Rodents and Small Mammals

Rodents and small mammals can be problematic to examine and treat because restraint without injuring the animal is difficult. These animals are generally very small and may bite when put in a stressful situation. Commercial restraint devices are available for small rodents, but it is difficult to perform a good external examination because of their design. To catch these small animals, a technician can use bare hands or leather gloves. However, the teeth of rodents will penetrate leather gloves, so protection is minimal and may be more psychologic than physical.

Cornering or encircling the animal with both hands will allow the handler to capture a large rodent. Both hands should be used to pick the animal up, with the fingers underneath and the thumbs on top of the body. One hand should be behind the other to support the entire abdomen. Grasping the scruff of the neck and supporting the back legs provide restraint for larger rodents (e.g., guinea pigs,

chinchillas, prairie dogs) (Figure 1-80). A large rodent that is standing on the examination table can also be restrained by wrapping a towel around its torso. Guinea pigs can be quite vocal when restrained. Pregnant guinea pigs develop pendulant bellies and they may be lifted by grasping around the thorax with one hand and around the rump with the other to hold them up. Teeth of the guinea pig may be clipped by holding the head with one or two hands, with the forefinger under the jaw and the thumb behind the head. The guinea pig tolerates being placed upside down in a trough with the legs tied down in the same fashion as swine.

Smaller rodents and mammals are initially restrained by gabbing the tail (mouse, rat) or the scruff (hamsters, sugar gliders, gerbils). Never grab a gerbil by the tail because the skin is easily removed (Figure 1-81). Following skin loss a tail amputation is required. Hedgehogs are covered with sharp spines, and most will require anesthesia to perform examinations or obtain samples for diagnostic procedures. Once restrained, these small patients are held by the scruff, or around the neck with one hand, and the other hand supports the body (Figure 1-82). Hamsters have a great deal of redundant skin from the cheek pouches, and this must be gathered up in the hand to hold them. Most small rodents may be restricted from movement on a surface by placing the hand over them to form a cage, with the head protruding between the first and second fingers (Figure 1-83). If they suddenly become carnivorous and attempt to bite, they may be caught and restrained by driving them

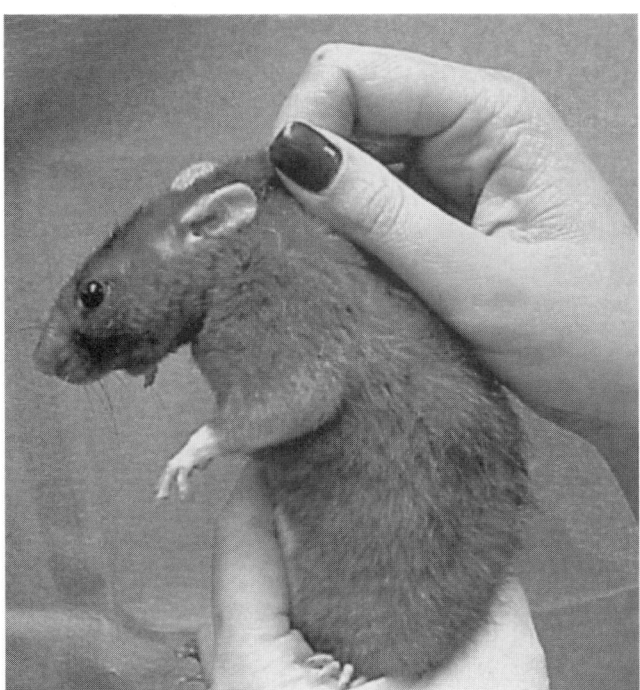

FIGURE 1-82. The proper restraint technique for a rat. Note the gloves on the handler.

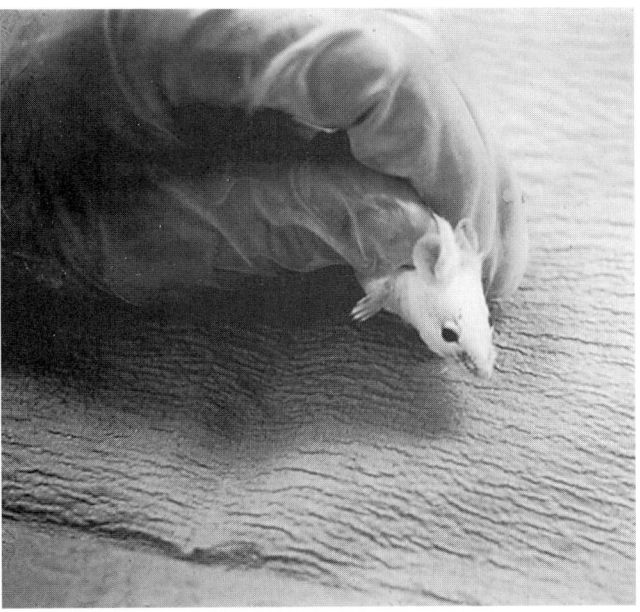

FIGURE 1-83. Proper restraint of a mouse and other small rodents.

into a small can. Rodent restraint tunnels are available in several sizes; usually they are made of Plexiglas and have several ports available for injections.

TRANSPORTATION AND SHIPPING

Cats are often nervous when riding in cars and are usually best transported in carriers. They may be given a tranquilizer if they are excessively nervous, and most tranquilizers will also have an antiemetic effect. Cats and dogs may produce excess saliva when they become nervous, which can be controlled with atropine or a similar drug.

Most dogs and cats do not need tranquilization when shipped on airlines, since they feel secure in their shipping containers if accustomed to them before the trip. Even though the animals may be nervous in their crates, they are probably better off untranquilized in this situation of minimal supervision. Commercial shipping crates of an acceptable size for the dog or cat are useful not only for shipping but also for containment at home. All animals in air freight must be accompanied by a current certificate of veterinary inspection (within 10 days).

Most states require negative results from a Coggins test or brucellosis test for entering horses or cattle. These are recorded on a certificate of veterinary inspection as well as the individual identification of all animals on the trailer.

RECOMMENDED READING

Fowler ME: *Restraint and handling of wild and domestic animals,* Ames, 1978, Iowa State University Press.

Fox MW: *Understanding your cat,* New York, 1974, Bantam Books.

Fox MW: *Understanding your dog,* New York, 1972, Coward, McCann and Geogheagan.

Fraser AF: *Farm animal behavior,* London, 1974, Balliere Tindall.

Hafez ESE: *The behavior of domestic animals,* ed 3, London, 1975, Balliere Tindall.

Hart BL: *Canine behavior,* Santa Barbara, Calif, 1980, Veterinary Practice Publishing.

Kiley-Worthington M: *The behavior of horses in relation to management and training,* London, 1987, JA Allen.

Roberts M: *The man who listens to horses,* New York, 1997, Random House.

2

History and Physical Examination

Ellen Miller

OBTAINING AN ACCURATE HISTORY

Without an accurate history, even the best veterinarian may be unable to solve the problems of a particular patient. The history is the first step in reaching the ultimate diagnosis of the patient's illness. Although obtaining a history can be time consuming, information elicited from the owner may save time and effort later in the diagnostic work-up of a particular problem. For example, a common mistake is the failure to differentiate true vomiting from regurgitation; the diagnostic plans for these two problems are costly and very different. An accurate history will help the veterinarian avoid errors of this kind. In a busy practice, the technician can begin the history-taking process for the veterinarian, freeing up time for the veterinarian to later discuss the primary problem in detail with the client.

The key to history taking is to obtain accurate information by asking the right questions. The specific questions asked will vary slightly depending on the species of animal being evaluated. In this chapter the companion animal is the primary example. However, the principles discussed may be applied to other species. Specific species information concerning exotic animals, equine, and food animals may be found in Chapters 17, 30, and 31, respectively.

Technician Note

The key to obtaining an accurate history is to ask the right questions.

Questions should be unbiased and not intended to lead the client toward a particular answer. For example, instead of asking, "Does Max drink more water than he used to?" it is preferable to ask, "Have you noticed a change in Max's water consumption?" Many people have such a desire to please that they will, without thinking, answer your questions affirmatively. Asking a question in an unbiased fashion forces the client to think. He or she must decide whether there has been a change and, if so, whether the change is positive (more water than normal) or negative (less water than normal). Sometimes, questions need to be asked two or three times but be phrased differently to ensure the owner has understood the question and is consistent with answers. In asking questions, consider the owner's ability to observe the pet. An owner may tell you that the dog does not have diarrhea when he or she does not normally observe the dog defecating and does not know the answer to the question. It may be better to ask, "Do you observe your dog when it defecates?" and if so, "Does your dog have diarrhea?"

Because animal patients cannot talk, the owner must be relied on to provide accurate information. The intelligence of the client and any handicaps that might interfere with the client's ability to observe his or her pet or properly understand or hear the questions must be weighed in the interpretation of answers to those questions.

Signalment of the Animal

The signalment of the animal is the age, breed, and gender, including reproductive status, of that animal. This information is vital in developing a list of the most likely rule-outs for the patient's problem. For example, a young animal is more likely to be vomiting because of an infectious agent, toxin ingestion, foreign body obstruction, or intussusception, whereas an older animal with the same complaint may be more likely to have kidney, liver, or pancreatic disease as the cause of the vomiting. Certain diseases are heritable and occur in particular breeds of dogs and cats. Knowing the breed is the first step in identifying a possible genetic defect. Knowledge of the gender of the patient and whether it is spayed or neutered obviously can help rule out disorders that affect one gender or the other.

Chief Complaint

> ### Technician Note
> The chief complaint is the reason the client presented the patient for evaluation.

The chief complaint is the reason the client brought the animal to be evaluated. Discussing the chief complaint is the most important part of the history-taking process for the client. Although other problems may seem more important, failure to address the chief complaint can annoy the owner and imply that you are not listening. Be sure to spend time on the client's concerns before moving on to other questions. You may say something such as, "That is important information, and I am also interested in your observations regarding...."

History of the Present Illness

This section of the history obtains detailed information regarding the chief complaint and any related problems. Duration, severity, progression, frequency, trigger situations, time of day, and character of the problem must be addressed if applicable. For instance, a miniature poodle that has a dry, honking cough (character) in response to excitement (trigger) two or three times daily (frequency) for longer than 1 year (duration) without progression is likely to have a collapsing trachea at the root of the cough. All these clues will help narrow and prioritize the list of possible causes for the problem. In addition, the severity and progression will help determine the aggressiveness of the diagnostic work-up. The more severe the disease or rapid the progression, the quicker the diagnosis needs to be made.

Past Medical and Surgical History

> ### Technician Note
> Past medical and surgical history can provide valuable information related to the current problem.

The past medical and surgical history can provide very important information related to the presenting problem in certain cases. Does the dog or cat have any medical problems or previous illnesses other than the chief complaint? Not only could the history have a bearing on the current problem, but also it may affect the approach to the new problem both diagnostically and therapeutically. For instance, knowing that a cat received megestrol acetate for a behavioral problem may provide a clue as to the reason for the increased thirst and urination the cat is experiencing. Increased thirst and urination are signs attributable to diabetes mellitus, which can be a sequela to progestogen therapy.

Has the animal ever had surgery, and if so, what type of surgery has it had? For example, a Yorkshire terrier presented with a draining tract from the medial aspect of the right stifle. The past history revealed the dog had surgery to repair a ruptured anterior cruciate ligament in the right stifle 8 months earlier. Based on the knowledge that sutures were most likely used to repair the ligament, it was probable the suture was acting as a foreign body and providing a nidus for infection. The current complaint was solved when the suture was removed. Had the history of the previous surgery not been known, an expensive work-up might have been undertaken.

Environmental History

The type of environment in which the pet lives often helps narrow the list of possible causes for a particular problem. The environment may be primarily indoor, outdoor, or a combination. The animal may live in an outdoor kennel or roam free. All these situations imply potential hazards. An animal that spends the majority of its life indoors is less likely to be traumatized, ingest poisons, or be exposed to infectious diseases (unless in a kennel or cattery situation) compared with an animal that lives outdoors or is free to roam.

Medication History

Information on any medication the animal is receiving is important for reasons that include prioritization of differential diagnoses, potential drug side effects, or drug interactions when additional drugs are prescribed. A dog receiving heartworm preventative is not likely to have heartworm disease as the cause of exercise intolerance if the correct dose is given at the appropriate time intervals. An animal that presents with a history of increased thirst and urination while being treated with corticosteroids may not have a serious problem because these are common side effects of the drug. This knowledge can prevent an unnecessary work-up or help provide an explanation of abnormal laboratory results. An animal receiving corticosteroids for a skin disorder should not be given aspirin or other nonsteroidal antiinflammatory drugs (NSAIDs) at the same time for an acute lameness. If the history of corticosteroid therapy was not known and aspirin or an NSAID was prescribed at antiinflammatory dosages, life-threatening complications, including gastrointestinal ulceration and kidney failure, may result.

Dietary History

It is important to know what type of food and how much food a patient is consuming, especially when dealing with problems of weight loss or obesity, vomiting, diarrhea, and anorexia. For instance, diet must be considered as a potential problem in a dog that has lost weight but has a good appetite. Knowledge of the diet will allow analysis of the digestibility and therefore the availability of nutrients to the animal. If the diet or amount of food the dog is fed is in question, this can be addressed before a costly diagnostic work-up by feeding the dog a high-quality diet in adequate amounts for a period of time and reassessing the body weight to evaluate a response. Another situation in which dietary history is imperative is in regard to the unregulated diabetic animal. A semimoist type of diet with high quantities of simple carbohydrates will cause a postprandial rise in blood glucose, resulting in polyuria and polydipsia.

Dietary history includes questions regarding the potential for toxin, garbage, or foreign body ingestion. Again, answers to these questions may provide crucial information as to the cause of the pet's problem.

> ### Technician Note
> A complete systems review requires that one or two questions be asked about each body system.

Systems Review

The systems review is necessary to ensure a complete history is taken. A systems review requires that one or two

TABLE 2-1	SAMPLE HISTORY QUESTIONS FOR EACH BODY SYSTEM
System	**Question**
General	How is your pet's attitude? Is it interested in the family? Is your pet playful?
Integument	Is your pet scratching, licking, or biting excessively? What do you think of your pet's hair coat?
Respiratory	Is your pet coughing or sneezing? Is there any nasal discharge?
Cardiovascular	Has there been a change in your pet's activity level? Do you exercise your pet regularly, and if so, have there been any changes in the amount of exercise your pet will tolerate? Does your pet cough?
Gastrointestinal	Has there been any vomiting? How is your pet's appetite? Have there been any changes in the stool character?
Genitourinary	Has your pet ever been bred? Has there been a change in the urinating habits of your pet? Do you think your pet drinks the same amount of water as before this problem started?
Musculoskeletal	Have you noticed any lameness?
Neurologic	Does your pet seem alert and aware of its surroundings? Is your pet weak or unable to support weight?
Special senses	Does your pet see sufficiently well? Does your pet hear normally?

questions be asked regarding each body system to identify other problems that the owner may have overlooked or deemed unimportant. These problems, when put together with the chief complaint, may provide evidence to support a specific disease as the cause of the animal's illness. For example, when questioning the owner about water intake in a dog with bilaterally symmetric, nonpruritic alopecia, you find that polyuria and polydipsia are also problems. Because this combination of clinical signs is compatible with hyperadrenocorticism, the diagnostic work-up should include a screening test for this disease. Sample questions for each system can be found in Table 2-1. For ease of remembering, major systems can be listed on a standard history form (Figure 2-1). If a response to any of these questions is positive, then the problem should be pursued with further questions as to the duration, severity, character, and so on.

COMPONENTS OF A COMPLETE PHYSICAL EXAMINATION

A complete physical examination begins with a general impression of the dog or cat, including its attitude, awareness of its surroundings, gait, and general appearance (body weight, condition, appearance of the coat). This portion of the physical examination can begin as soon as you meet the pet and lead it to the examination room. Observe the animal in its new environment. Is it curious and exploring? Is it aware of noises outside the room? Is it totally uninterested in or unable to respond to the new stimuli? Is it favoring any legs when it walks into the room?

It is also appropriate to include measurement of the vital signs, including temperature, pulse, and respirations.

Systems Assessment

The systems assessment is comparable to the systems review section of the history. Each system is examined thoroughly for abnormalities. There is no particular order in which the systems are examined, but a routine pattern should be established by the individual performing the physical examination so no system will be overlooked. Some clinicians prefer to examine the animal from nose to tail, intermingling the systems together, whereas other clinicians will examine each system separately. It does not matter how it is accomplished as long as the examination is complete and thorough. A standardized physical examination form (Figure 2-2) can provide prompting until a routine is developed. The systems can be listed and numbered at the top of the form, with boxes to check if normal or abnormal. Any abnormality can be listed in the space provided by the corresponding system number.

Technician Note

Each of the 10 body systems must be thoroughly examined during the complete physical examination.

Integument

The skin can be examined all at once or during the examination of other systems. Brush the coat with the hand in the opposite direction of the hair growth and observe the skin for redness (erythema) or lesions such as macules, papules, pustules, or crusts. Remember to examine the skin of the extremities and check the nail beds and nails and between the toes. Is there moistness between the toes or brown discoloration indicative of excessive licking in the area? Are the foot pads normal in appearance? Are there areas of hair loss, and if so, where are they located? Is the hair loss symmetric or patchy and random? Is the skin in areas of hair loss normal, or is it hyperpigmented, erythematous, or crusty? What is the general texture of the coat? Is it soft and fluffy like the undercoat hairs, or is it coarse like the guard hairs? Does your hand feel oily or dirty after touching the coat? If lumps are present, are they in the skin or under it? Are they hairless? Is their overall appearance smooth and round or irregular and cauliflower like? Make a note of their size and location on the physical examination form. Are there areas of bruising in the skin? Is the skin excessively thin with tiny wrinkle lines and easily observed blood vessels? Are there blackheads (comedones)? All observations need to be recorded; the significance may be realized later.

Respiratory System

Examination of the respiratory system begins with the nose and throat, including the pharyngeal area. Is there a nasal discharge, and if so, is it unilateral or bilateral? What is the character of the nasal discharge? Does the animal sneeze or cough while being examined? Are the nares of normal size or stenotic as in some brachycephalic breeds? Palpate the bridge of the nose and the frontal sinus above the eyes. Are there any deformities or soft spots? In the oral cavity, examine the pharynx, tonsils, and, if possible, the edge of the soft palate and the epiglottis. Is the palate elongated? Are there any red or ulcerated areas? Are the tonsils normal and in their crypts? Use symmetry to assess for abnormalities.

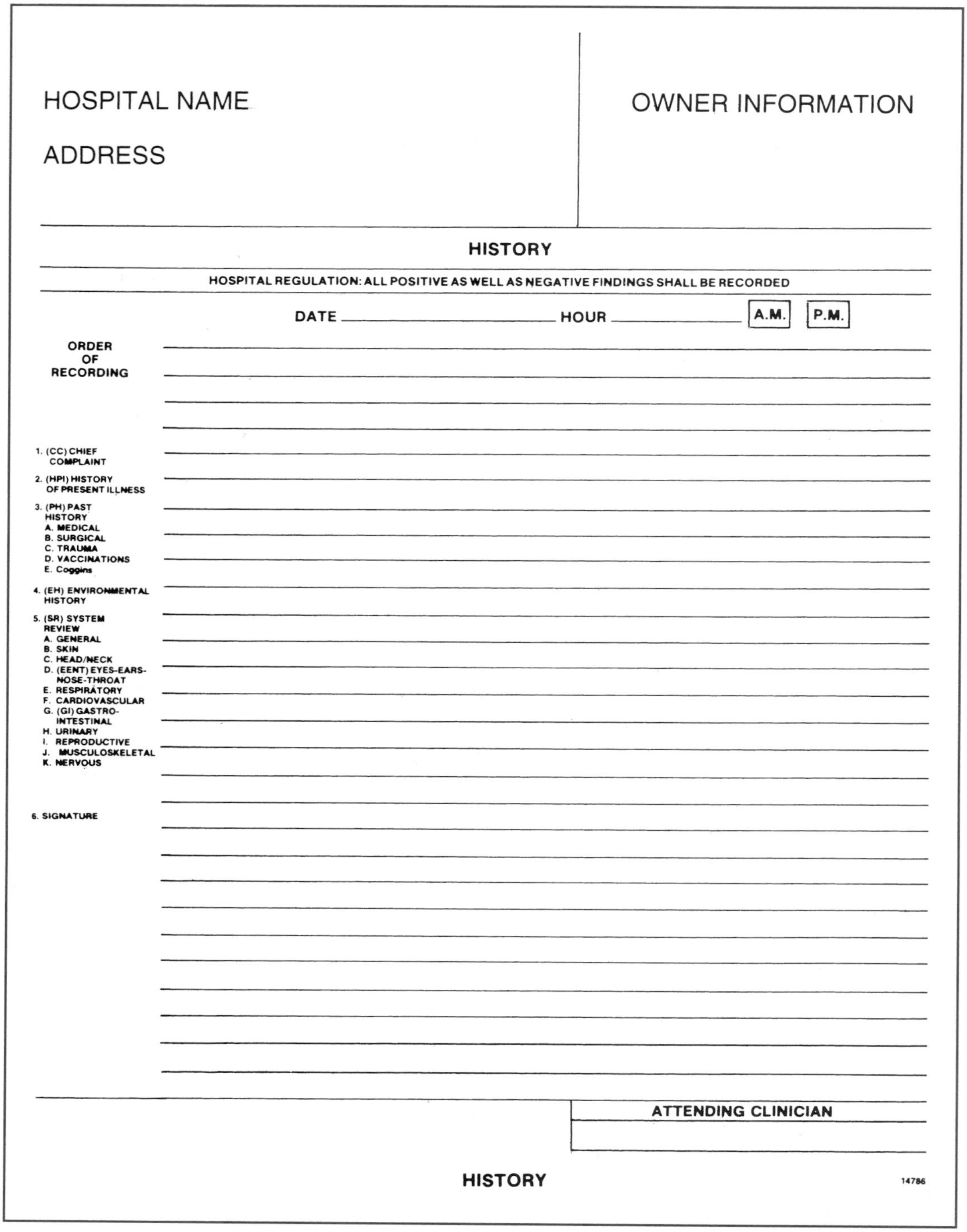

HOSPITAL NAME

ADDRESS

OWNER INFORMATION

HISTORY

HOSPITAL REGULATION: ALL POSITIVE AS WELL AS NEGATIVE FINDINGS SHALL BE RECORDED

DATE _____ HOUR _____ [A.M.] [P.M.]

ORDER
OF
RECORDING

1. (CC) CHIEF
   COMPLAINT
2. (HPI) HISTORY
   OF PRESENT ILLNESS
3. (PH) PAST
   HISTORY
   A. MEDICAL
   B. SURGICAL
   C. TRAUMA
   D. VACCINATIONS
   E. Coggins
4. (EH) ENVIRONMENTAL
   HISTORY
5. (SR) SYSTEM
   REVIEW
   A. GENERAL
   B. SKIN
   C. HEAD/NECK
   D. (EENT) EYES-EARS-
      NOSE-THROAT
   E. RESPIRATORY
   F. CARDIOVASCULAR
   G. (GI) GASTRO-
      INTESTINAL
   H. URINARY
   I. REPRODUCTIVE
   J. MUSCULOSKELETAL
   K. NERVOUS

6. SIGNATURE

ATTENDING CLINICIAN

HISTORY   14786

FIGURE 2-1. A sample standard history form.

Palpate the trachea and larynx. Does the animal cough easily? Are there any swellings or irregularities? Auscultate over the larynx and trachea for any wheezes.

Observe the animal breathe, and note the respiratory rate and pattern. Table 2-2 lists normal ranges for respiratory rates of four species. If the animal is having difficulty breathing, note when the problem is occurring (e.g., inspiration or expiration); this information may be important in the ultimate diagnosis of the problem. Auscultate the lungs in sections or quadrants (Figure 2-3). Normal respiratory sounds can usually be heard in a dog throughout inspiration and through the first third of expiration. The sounds are normally quiet, but with exercise they are louder because of the increased volume of air moving through the airways. The lung sounds of a normal cat often are heard only during inspiration. Feline lung sounds are

PHYSICAL EXAMINATION

(1) GENERAL APPEARANCE ☐ Normal ☐ Abnormal	(2) INTEGU-MENTARY ☐ Normal ☐ Abnormal ☐ Not examined	(3) MUSCULO-SKELETAL ☐ Normal ☐ Abnormal ☐ Not examined	(4) CIRCU-LATORY ☐ Normal ☐ Abnormal ☐ Not examined
(5) RESPIRA-TORY ☐ Normal ☐ Abnormal ☐ Not examined	(6) DIGESTIVE ☐ Normal ☐ Abnormal ☐ Not examined	(7) GENITO-URINARY ☐ Normal ☐ Abnormal ☐ Not examined	(8) EYES ☐ Normal ☐ Abnormal ☐ Not examined
(9) EARS ☐ Normal ☐ Abnormal ☐ Not examined	(10) NEURAL SYSTEM ☐ Normal ☐ Abnormal ☐ Not examined	(11) LYMPH NODES ☐ Normal ☐ Abnormal ☐ Not examined	(12) MUCOUS MEMBRANES ☐ Normal ☐ Abnormal ☐ Not examined

DESCRIBE ABNORMAL: (Use numbers above)   T _____   P _____   R _____   Wt. _____

_____

TEMPORARY PROBLEM LIST	Initial Plan	
	Dx	Rx
(1)		
(2)		
(3)		
(4)		

STUDENT SIGNATURE   CLINICIAN SIGNATURE

PHYSICAL EXAMINATION

FIGURE 2-2. A sample standard physical examination form.

TABLE 2-2	NORMAL RESTING RESPIRATORY AND HEART RATES	
Species	**Respiratory Rate (breaths/min)**	**Heart Rate (beats/min)**
Cat	16-30	160-240
Cow	20-30	50-70
Dog	16-24	70-180 (smaller breeds have higher rates; puppies can have rates up to 220)
Horse	8-12	36-50

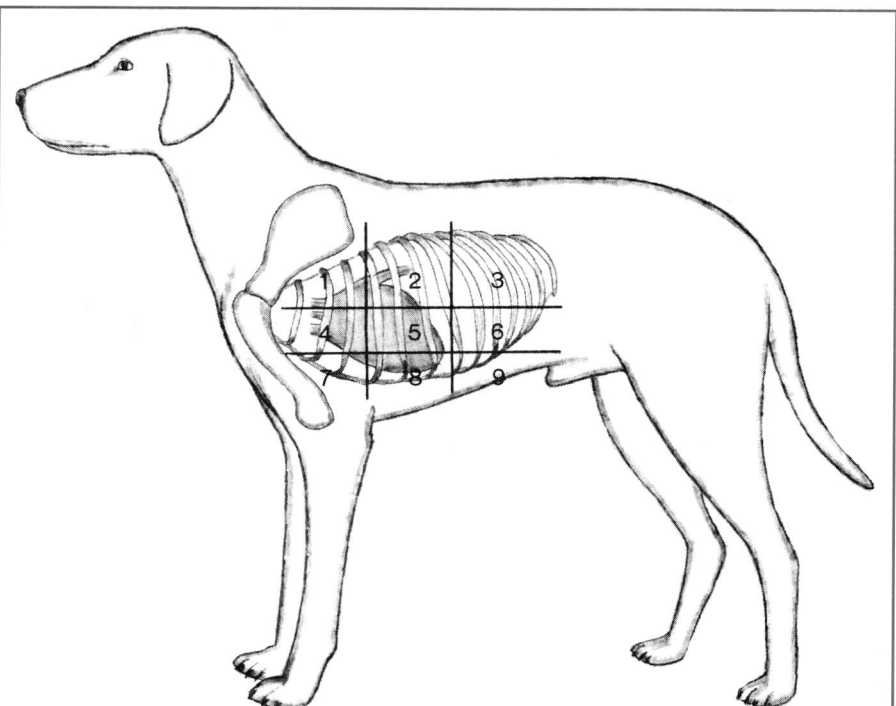

FIGURE 2-3. Division of the lungs into nine quadrants for auscultation and description of location of abnormal lung sounds. (From McCurnin DM, Poffenbarger EM: *Small animal physical diagnosis and clinical procedures,* Philadelphia, 1991, WB Saunders.)

more quiet than canine lung sounds, so loud lung sounds in a cat can be significant. If the animal is panting, all that can be heard is air moving through the large airways and the mouth noises. This is not a true representation of lung sounds, so be sure to close the animal's mouth to listen. Abnormal lung sounds are described as crackles (i.e., short, popping noises) or wheezes (i.e., longer, musical noises). Note the location and timing (expiration or inspiration) of any abnormal noises. The lack of normal respiratory sounds can also be significant and suggests a consolidated lung lobe or a lung lobe that has collapsed because of air or fluid accumulation.

Cardiovascular System

Begin with an examination of mucous membrane color and capillary refill time, blanching the color from the mucous membrane of the oral cavity over the canine tooth on the gingival mucosa or on the inner surface of the labial mucosa. It normally takes 1 or 2 seconds for the pink color to return to the area. The capillary refill time is often prolonged because of poor cardiac output as a result of dehydration or cardiac disease. Examine the jugular furrow in the neck. If the animal is standing, sitting, or lying in a sternal position, it is not normal to see a jugular pulse. Sometimes a jugular pulse can be seen in a normal animal in lateral recumbency. Palpate the femoral pulse, and describe the quality as strong or weak. Does the pulse vary in intensity from pulse to pulse?

Auscultate the heart over the areas described in Figure 2-4. First, note the heart rate and rhythm. Table 2-2 lists the normal rates of four species. If the rhythm is irregular, decide whether the irregularity is related to the respiratory cycle. If the rhythm is irregularly irregular (e.g., no pattern at all), make a note of this. Palpate the femoral pulse while listening to the heart. Is there a pulse for every heartbeat? Next listen for any heart murmurs. Heart murmurs are described on the basis of five parameters: timing, location or point of maximal intensity, quality, grade, and radiation. Box 2-1 describes the various murmurs. These parameters will help the veterinarian generate a list of possible differential diagnoses for the cardiac disease and give the owner some information on prognosis for his or her animal.

Gastrointestinal System

Examination of the gastrointestinal system begins in the oral cavity and includes the teeth, tongue, oral mucosa, and pharyngeal area. Next, palpate the neck for any esophageal masses or foreign objects. Auscultate the abdomen, and note the presence or absence of gut sounds.

Abdominal palpation requires practice and patience to obtain any useful information. In most dogs, a two-handed technique is the best method (Figure 2-5). Stand on either side or to the rear of the dog. Put a hand on either side of the abdomen. The hands should be in a flat but relaxed position. Begin palpating the abdomen in the dorsal, cranial region. With gentle pressure, try to move your hands toward each other. If you move slowly, the animal usually will relax. Do not use the fingertips or the animal will tense the abdominal muscles and palpation will become very difficult. Slowly move your hands toward the ventral, cranial abdomen and feel as structures slip past your fingers. When you have reached the ventrum, move to the dorsal, central region and repeat the same steps. Finally, examine the caudal abdomen in a similar manner. Figure 2-6 illustrates the organs found in the various abdominal quadrants. In a cat or small dog, the one-handed palpation technique is often easier to use (Figure 2-7). The thumb is placed on one side of the animal while the four fingers are placed on the other side of the abdomen. Again, using gentle pressure and a flat hand, begin palpating the dorsal, cranial region of the abdomen and move on to the other

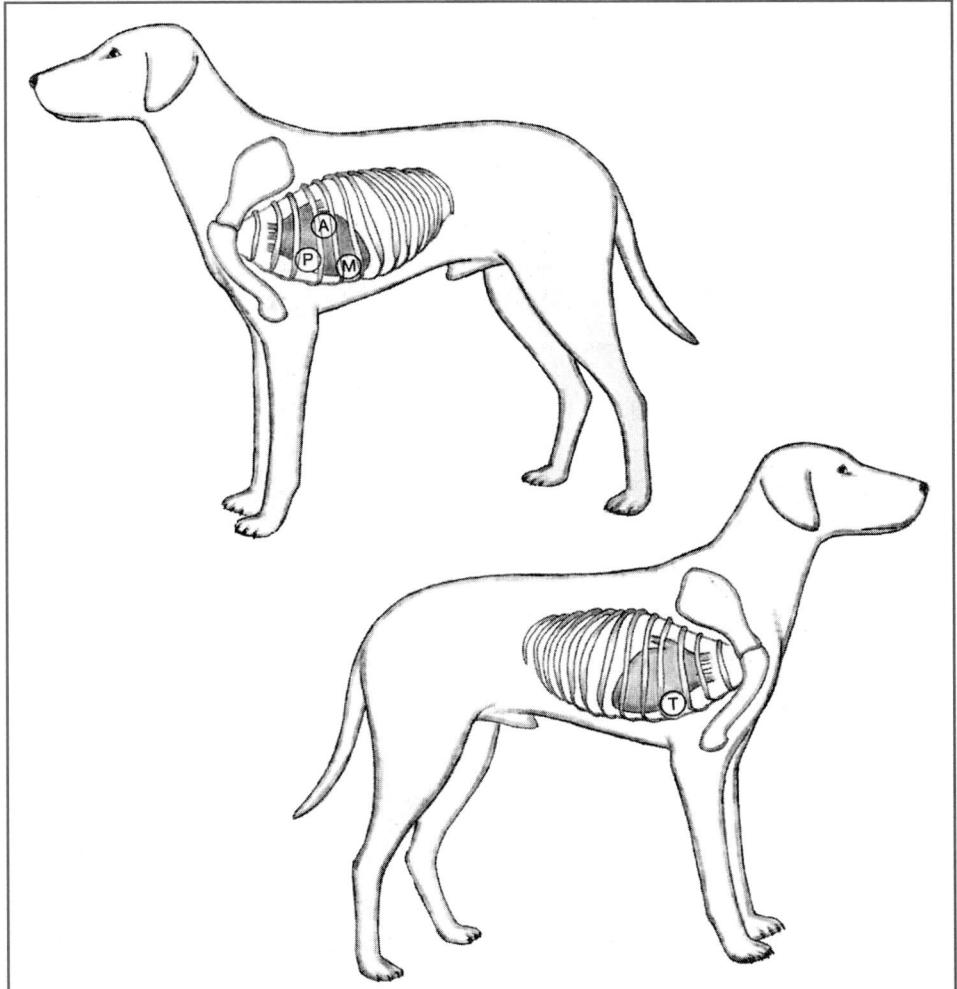

FIGURE 2-4.   Location of heart valves as an aid in the determination of the origin of a heart murmur. *A*, Aortic; *M*, mitral; *P*, Pulmonic; *T*, tricuspid. (From McCurnin DM, Poffenbarger EM: *Small animal physical diagnosis and clinical procedures*, Philadelphia, 1991, WB Saunders.)

Box 2-1   DESCRIPTION OF HEART MURMURS

LOCATION
This is usually the valve area over which the murmur is loudest:
   Aortic
   Mitral
   Tricuspid
   Pulmonic
The location may also be described in relation to chest structures, such as the sternal border.

TIMING
This refers to the part of the cardiac cycle during which the murmur is heard:
   Systole
   Diastole
   Continuous

DURATION
This refers to the duration within systole or diastole in which the murmur is heard:
   Early systole
   Holosystolic (pansystolic)
   Diastole

CHARACTER
This refers to the quality of the murmur:
   Plateau or regurgitant type (same sound for the duration of the murmur)
   Decrescendo, crescendo, crescendo-decrescendo, or ejection type (intensity changes throughout the duration of the murmur)
   Machinery (heard throughout systole and diastole)
   Decrescendo or blowing

GRADE
1/6—Can only be heard in a quiet room after several minutes of listening
2/6—Can be heard immediately but is very soft
3/6—Low to moderate intensity
4/6—Loud but without a palpable thrill
5/6—Loud with a palpable thrill
6/6—Can be heard with the stethoscope bell slightly off the thoracic wall

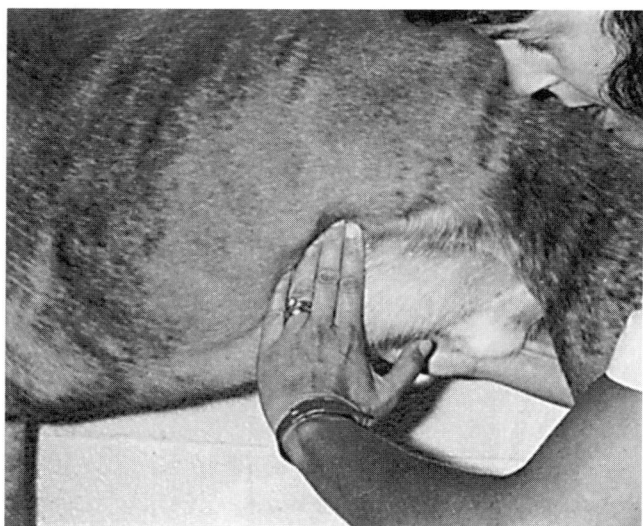

FIGURE 2-5. Two-handed abdominal palpation in the dog. (From McCurnin DM, Poffenbarger EM: *Small animal physical diagnosis and clinical procedures,* Philadelphia, 1991, WB Saunders.)

areas. Often, the four fingers can be used to trap a structure, and the thumb can be moved over its surface to get an idea of the texture, shape, and size of the structure.

With the gastrointestinal tract of a normal animal, you will not identify much except intestines slipping between your fingers. If the animal has recently consumed a meal, the stomach may be palpated behind the ribs as far caudal as the mid abdomen. Note any pain during palpation and where it is elicited. Are there any abnormal structures? If so, what is the shape, size, and consistency? Does the structure seem to have intestines coming from each end as with an intussusception, foreign body, or intestinal tumor? If the abdomen is distended and it is difficult to discern anything, make a note of that.

The perineal area should be examined for evidence of diarrhea caked on the hairs or inflammation of the surrounding skin. A rectal examination can be performed to determine whether any rectal masses, strictures, or enlargements are present. During a rectal examination, the anal glands can be palpated between the thumb and index finger of each side of the anus, ventrolateral to the anal opening.

Urogenital System

The kidneys are readily palpated in the normal cat; however, because of anatomic differences, the right kidney of the normal dog is rarely palpated, and only the caudal pole of the left kidney can be palpated in a small percentage of cases. The kidneys should feel smooth on their surface. Note whether the shape is irregular or if the surface feels generally roughened. The size of the kidneys varies with the size of the animal. In the average 5-kg cat, the kidney is usually 2.5 to 3.5 cm in length and spherical.

The urinary bladder can usually be palpated in the caudal ventral abdomen, depending on its degree of fullness. It will be pear shaped with the small end directed caudally in a dog, whereas it is usually spherical in a cat. It should feel fluctuant or fluid filled. Abnormalities might include a very firm bladder, as occurs with chronic infection, bladder stones, or neoplasia, or a gritty feel when multiple stones are present. The uterus can sometimes be

palpated in the female dog if it is enlarged because of pregnancy, infection (pyometra), or neoplasia. The cervix is dorsal to the urinary bladder and can be palpated during certain stages of the estrus cycle and during pregnancy. It is a firm, tubular structure during these times. The uterine horns can be followed cranioventrally from the cervix.

The urethra can be palpated in the male or female dog rectally on the floor of the pelvis as a turgid tubular structure. In the male dog, the prostate gland can be felt as a widening in the pelvic urethra into a bi-lobed, firm, walnut-sized gland. Note any asymmetry, pain, or irregularities in the prostate and pelvic urethra. The male dog urethra can then be followed distally (caudally) through palpation of the perineal area on the midline. From here it becomes surrounded by penile tissue and is impossible to make out as a separate structure. The penis should be palpated for pain and abnormal shape. Extrude the penis from its sheath and note the color and surface texture.

The testicles of the intact male dog and cat are located in the scrotum in the caudal (cat) or ventral (dog) perineal area. They should be smooth on the surface and symmetric in shape and size. Note any pain on palpation or irregularity in size or shape.

Palpate the mammary chains of the female dog and cat for lumps. Note any pain or swelling. Milk can be expressed from the glands of lactating animals and during the last 1 or 2 weeks of gestation. Examine the milk for color changes; normal milk varies from white to a creamy yellow color.

Musculoskeletal System

Palpate the muscles of the head and limbs, and note any pain or asymmetry. Are the underlying skeletal structures more easy to palpate than normal, indicating atrophy or degeneration of the muscles?

Beginning with the toes, palpate the bones and joints of each limb. Manipulate the joints through their full range of motion, and note any pain response or crepitus (crackling). Firmly palpate the long bones and note any pain response. With your thumb, put firm but gentle pressure on the dorsal spinous process of the thoracic vertebrae one at a time, moving caudally through the lumbar region to the sacrum. Note whether the animal flinches or drops down to move away from the pressure.

Nervous System

The nervous system is technically difficult and time consuming to examine completely. Some knowledge of neuroanatomy, structure, and function is necessary to accurately assess the location and cause of a neurologic problem. Therefore a complete neurologic examination is usually reserved for the patient with known or suspected neurologic disease. The general appearance of the animal, including mental attitude and ability to ambulate, can give information regarding the need for a complete neurologic examination.

The central nervous system can be divided into the brain and the spinal cord for ease of examination and localization of lesions. To assess the brain, the mental status and cranial nerves are examined. Is the animal alert and aware of its surroundings? Does it respond appropriately to stimuli, such as noises or movement? Table 2-3 lists the specific cranial nerves, tests to assess them, and the expected outcomes in the normal and abnormal patient (Figure 2-8).

Localization and characterization of lesions within the spinal cord require assessment of spinal reflexes, postural reactions, and response to painful stimuli. Spinal reflexes

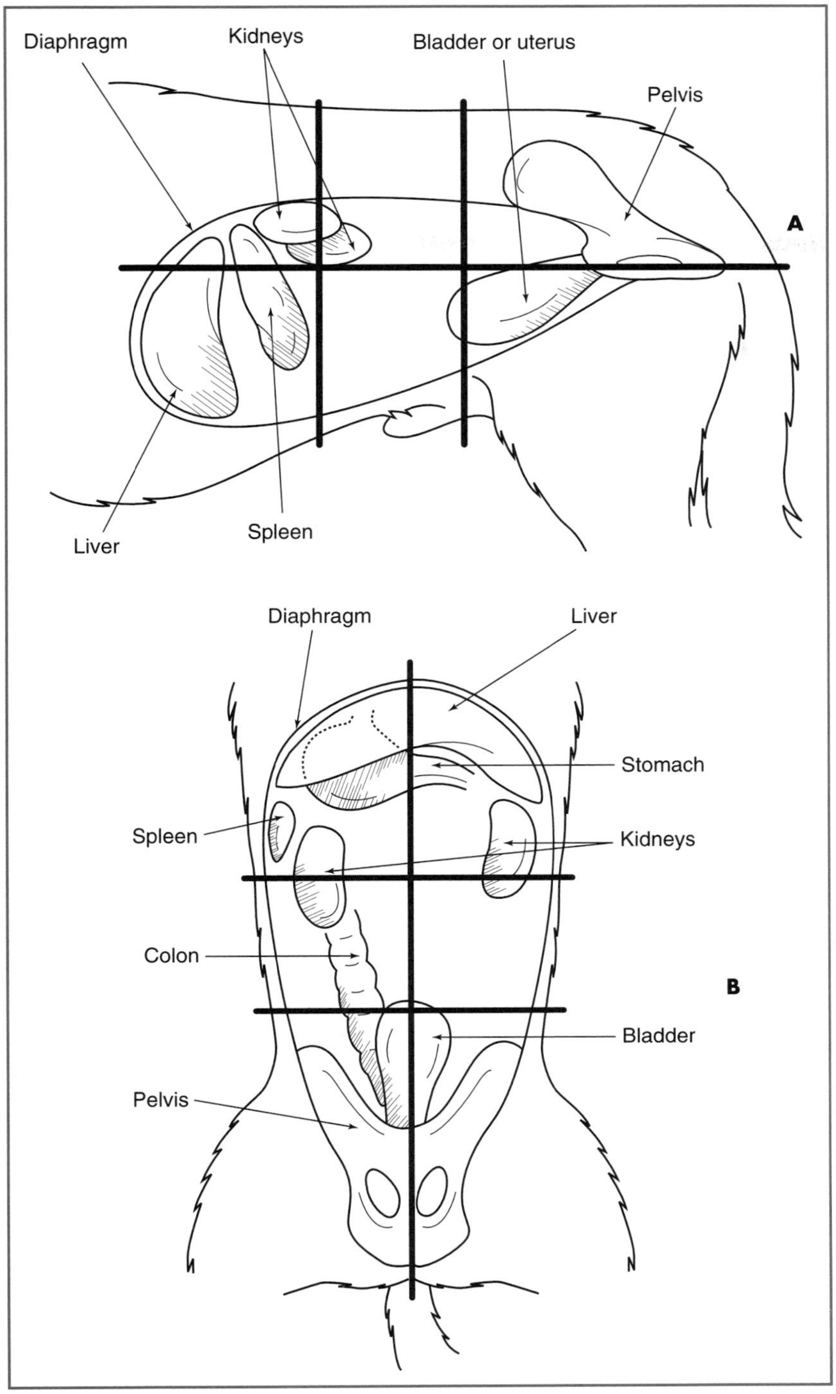

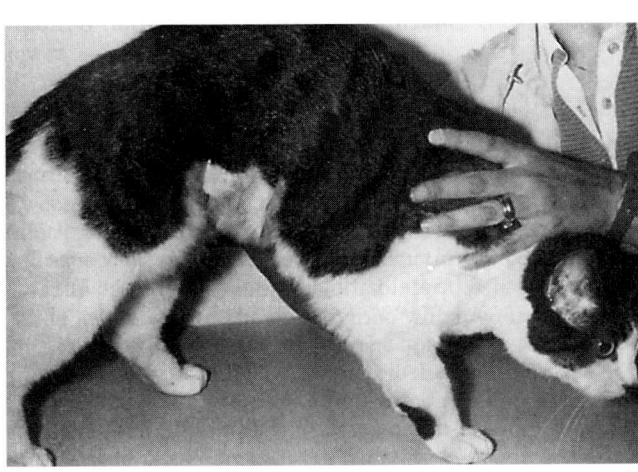

FIGURE 2-6. Location of internal organs within the abdominal quadrants. **A,** Lateral projection. **B,** Ventrodorsal projection. (From McCurnin DM, Poffenbarger EM: *Small animal physical diagnosis and clinical procedures,* Philadelphia, 1991, WB Saunders.)

FIGURE 2-7. One-handed abdominal palpation in the cat. (From McCurnin DM, Poffenbarger EM: *Small animal physical diagnosis and clinical procedures,* Philadelphia, 1991, WB Saunders.)

TABLE 2-3	EXAMINATION OF THE CRANIAL NERVES		
NERVE	**TEST**	**RESPONSE**	
		Normal	**Abnormal**
I. Olfactory	Volatile substance	Sniff, recoil, nose lick	No response
II. Optic	Menace	Blink	No blink
	Pupillary light reflex	Direct, consensual responses present	No direct or consensual responses
III. Oculomotor	Pupillary light reflex	Direct, consensual responses present	No direct response, consensual intact
	Observe eye follow an object	Normal eye movement	Impaired ocular movement in ventral, dorsal, and medial directions
IV. Trochlear	Observe	Normal eye position	Dorsomedial strabismus
V. Trigeminal	Observe	Can close jaw	Jaw drop
	Palpate temporalis	Normal muscle tone	Muscle atrophy
	Corneal reflex	Eye blink	No blink
	Palpebral reflex	Eye blink	No blink
VI. Abducens	Observe	Normal eye position	Medial strabismus
VII. Facial	Observe	Facial symmetry	Lip droop
	Corneal reflex	Eye blink	No blink
	Palpebral reflex	Eye blink	No blink
	Menace	Eye blink	No blink
VIII. Acoustic	Hand clap	Startle response	No response
	Move head horizontally, vertically	Normal nystagmus	No response, resting or positional nystagmus
	Observe	Normal head posture	Head tilt
	Righting response	Normal righting	Unable to right
IX. Glossopharyngeal	Gag reflex	Swallow	No response
X. Vagus	Gag reflex	Swallow	No response
	Oculocardiac reflex	Bradycardia	No response
	Laryngeal reflex	Cough	No response
XI. Accessory	Palpate neck muscles	Normal muscle tone	Muscle atrophy
XII. Hypoglossal	Tongue stretch	Retraction of tongue	No response

From McCurnin DM, Poffenbarger EM: *Small animal physical diagnosis and clinical procedures*, Philadelphia, 1991, WB Saunders, p 115.

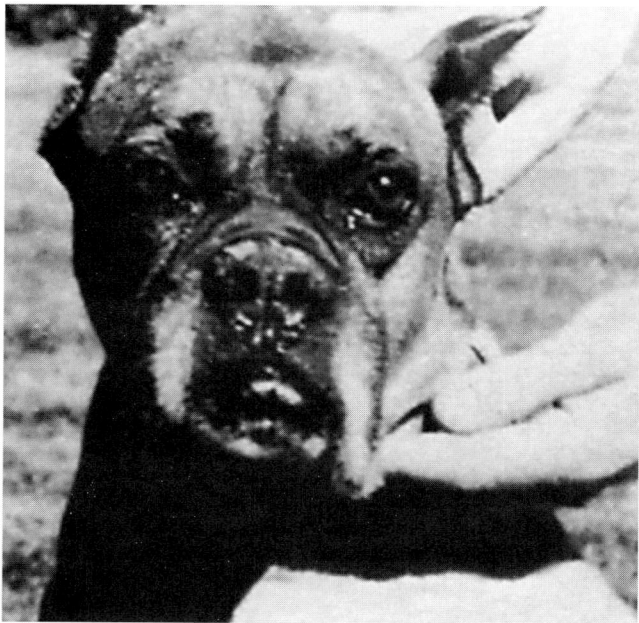

FIGURE 2-8. External ear and head examination showing facial nerve paralysis (note the drooped lip on the left side of the face). (From Oliver JE Jr, Hoerlein BF, Mayhew IG: *Veterinary neurology*, Philadelphia, 1984, WB Saunders.)

are assessed by gentle but firm tapping of a tendon to note the degree of response (contraction) of the muscle. The most common reflexes assessed are the triceps in the front leg (Figure 2-9) and the quadriceps or patellar (Figure 2-10) and gastrocnemius reflexes (Figure 2-11) in the hind limb. The response is graded as in Table 2-4.

Postural reactions include conscious proprioception, wheel-barrowing, hemistanding and hemiwalking, and hopping. The most commonly performed test is the reaction of conscious proprioception, in which the foot is gently turned so that the animal is standing on the top of its foot. Each foot is tested individually. A normal animal will immediately right the foot. A slow or absent response usually indicates spinal cord disease. Wheel-barrowing is performed by holding the animal's rear legs in the air while slowly moving forward; the normal animal will move the front legs forward and maintain an upright position. Hemistanding and hemiwalking require that the front and rear legs on the same side be supported while the animal is required to stand or walk, respectively. A normal animal can stand with ease and walk with minor difficulty. Hopping responses are assessed by holding three of four legs up with the fourth allowed to touch the floor or table. The animal is slowly moved toward the side with the leg down. A normal animal will move the leg laterally to attempt to support weight and maintain balance.

Superficial and deep pain perception is assessed by pinching the skin or bone of the toe area, respectively. The normal response is withdrawal of the leg with some acknowledgment of pain, such as turning to look at the

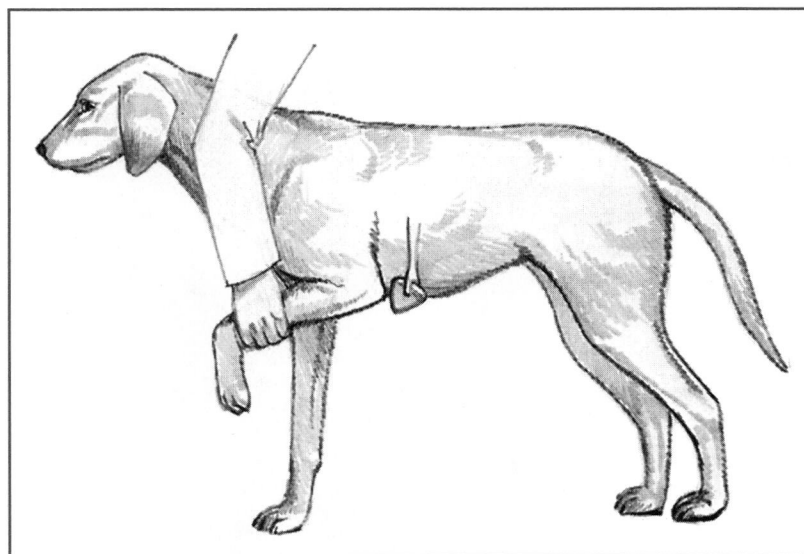

FIGURE 2-9. The triceps reflex can be elicited in lateral recumbency or standing, as shown. (From McCurnin DM, Poffenbarger EM: *Small animal physical diagnosis and clinical procedures,* Philadelphia, 1991, WB Saunders.)

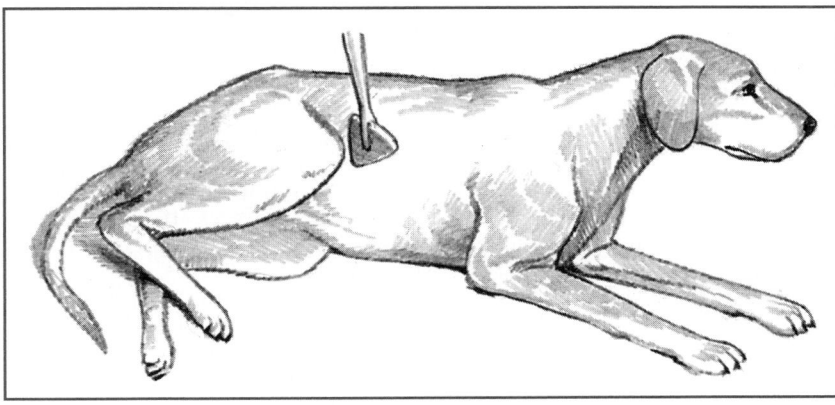

FIGURE 2-10. The femoral, or patellar, reflex. (From McCurnin DM, Poffenbarger EM: *Small animal physical diagnosis and clinical procedures,* Philadelphia, 1991, WB Saunders.)

toe, dilation of the pupils, or a growl or snap. If both responses are absent, the prognosis for recovery is poor.

The *panniculus reflex* is a simple test that aids in the localization of a spinal cord lesion. It is performed by gently pinching the skin of the back just lateral to the midline and watching for a reflex contraction of the skin. Start with the skin near the tail and slowly work forward. The lesion is approximately one vertebra caudal to the location where the first response is elicited.

Last, the anal tone and perineal reflex should be assessed. The anus should be closed and not gaping open. The perineal reflex is tested by gently stimulating the skin around the anus and watching for a "wink," or contraction, of the anal sphincter.

Peripheral Lymph Nodes

The peripheral lymph nodes that can be palpated in the normal animal include the submandibular, prescapular, and popliteal. Usually, the axillary and inguinal lymph nodes will be palpated only if enlarged. Symmetry often is a clue to any abnormalities, so palpate both sides at the same time for comparison.

The submandibular lymph nodes are located at the ventral aspect of the neck near the angle of the jaw. There usually are two on each side just cranial to the mandibular salivary gland. The trick to palpating them is to grab the extra skin of the ventral neck between the thumb and forefingers. Slowly move your hands rostrally, and the nodes should slip through your fingers. In the cat, these nodes are normally pea sized, whereas in the dog, they vary from pea sized (small dogs) to small grape sized (large dogs).

The prescapular lymph nodes lie in the connective tissue just cranial and dorsal to the shoulder joint. Again, it is easiest to grab the skin and muscles and then let the lymph nodes slip through your fingers as you pull your hands cranially. These lymph nodes range from similar in size to slightly larger than the submandibular nodes.

The popliteal lymph nodes can be palpated in the fat pad just caudal to the stifle joint.

Ears

Examination of the ears involves palpation and visual examination of the pinnae, or ear flaps, as well as visual inspection of the external ear canal. Common abnormalities of the ear flaps include hair loss, crusting margins as occur with mange or flea-bite dermatitis, hematomas (blood-filled pockets within the pinna), and skin tumors. The external ear canal should be free of exudate, debris, or hair. If exudate is present, the character of the discharge should be noted (dark brown and flaky as occurs with ear mites, dark brown and malodorous as occurs with yeast infections, or purulent as occurs with bacterial otitis).

If abnormalities are noted on visual inspection or ear

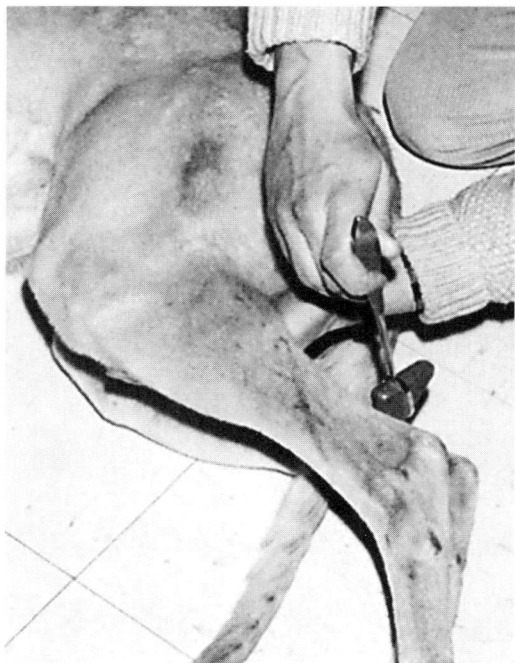

FIGURE 2-11. The gastrocnemius reflex. (From McCurnin DM, Poffenbarger EM: *Small animal physical diagnosis and clinical procedures,* Philadelphia, 1991, WB Saunders.)

TABLE 2-4	GRADING OF REFLEX RESPONSES
Grade	**Description**
0	No response
1	Hyporeflexia (less than normal response)
2	Normal response
3	Hyperreflexia (greater than normal response)
4	Clonus (repetitive response)

disease is the chief complaint, an otoscopic examination should be performed. Holding the pinna up, the otoscope cone is gently inserted into the vertical ear canal (Figure 2-12). While the examiner looks through the otoscope, the otoscope is slowly advanced and rotated 90 degrees to examine the horizontal part of the ear canal. Note any redness, exudate, foreign objects, mites, polyps or tumors, or hemorrhage. The tympanic membrane or eardrum can be visualized at the end of the horizontal canal as a white translucent membrane. Note any color change or lack of translucency, which indicates exudate or hemorrhage in the middle ear.

Eyes

A good ocular examination includes an examination of the external ocular features (eyelids, sclera, cornea, third eyelid

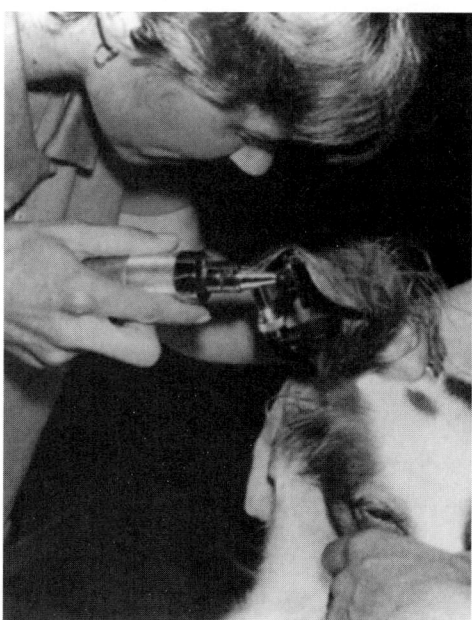

FIGURE 2-12. Examination of vertical canal.

[nictitating membrane]) as well as internal ocular features (anterior chamber, iris, lens), all of which can be visualized without special equipment. First, note the character of any discharge present in or under the eyes. If present, is it watery, mucoid, purulent, or ropy? Examine the eyelid margins for small masses, aberrant eyelashes, and position. Do the eyelids seem to roll inward (entropion) so that the lashes rub on the cornea, or do the eyelids appear to be loose and not in contact with the eye (ectropion)? Is the sclera white or red, as in the inflamed eye? Is the third eyelid in its normal position, or does it appear to be bulging or protruding across the eye? Is the cornea clear or cloudy? If cloudy, note the location of the cloudiness. Does the cornea appear wet? Are there small blood vessels present on the surface of the cornea?

The anterior chamber (portion of the eye in front of the lens and iris) should be clear, allowing easy visualization of the iris. Note any hemorrhage or purulent debris in the anterior chamber. Examine the iris, and compare with the opposite side for symmetry. Are the pupil sizes equal? Are there any brown spots on the iris? Does the iris appear to be tattered? Shine a light in one eye, and note the response in both eyes. Both pupils in a normal animal will constrict when a light is shined in either eye. Carefully record any deviations from normal.

RECOMMENDED READING

McCurnin DM, Poffenbarger EM: *Small animal physical diagnosis and clinical procedures,* Philadelphia, 1991, WB Saunders.

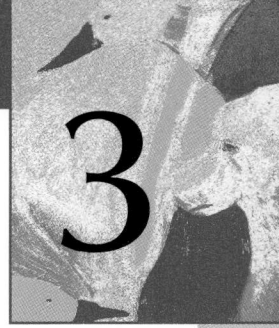

Diagnostic Sampling and Therapeutic Techniques

Tracy J. Jaffe

A veterinary technician proficient in obtaining diagnostic samples and performing a variety of treatment techniques is an invaluable asset to any veterinary practice. Technicians should therefore have expertise in many basic procedures, such as blood and urine collection, intravenous catheter placement, and fluid and medication administration. As the practice of veterinary medicine becomes more specialized, technicians are asked to perform increasingly more advanced diagnostic and therapeutic techniques. Many technicians, for example, are now employed by specialty practices in which performing certain advanced skills has become routine. For this reason, a variety of advanced as well as basic procedures are addressed in this chapter.

BASIC GUIDELINES

Whenever possible, baseline blood or urine samples should be obtained before the initiation of fluid therapy. Administration of fluids and the recent ingestion of a high-fat or high-protein meal may alter blood or urine laboratory values.

All supplies needed for collection of samples and for therapeutic procedures should be gathered ahead of time. Samples should be collected and stored in appropriate containers with the patient's name and hospital identification number printed on the label.

Whenever a needle is inserted through the skin as part of a treatment (e.g., intramuscular injection) or a sampling procedure (e.g., blood collection), the skin should be clean, dry, and free from obvious inflammation and infection. Microbes and other contaminants present on the skin surface may be introduced into the underlying tissue when the needle is inserted. Needles and intravenous catheters from which the protective coverings have been removed should remain sterile and should only be handled at the hub; the shaft, for example, should not be touched or set down on a nonsterile surface.

SMALL ANIMAL SAMPLING AND THERAPEUTIC TECHNIQUES

BLOOD SAMPLE COLLECTION

Venous Blood Sample

Most technicians perform venipuncture on a routine basis either to collect a blood sample for laboratory tests or to inject a drug or medication. Only through experience does one learn to collect a blood sample quickly with minimal trauma to the vessel or stress and discomfort to the patient (Box 3-1). Proper animal restraint is as important as the venipuncture itself.

Venipuncture is performed with either a needle and syringe or a Vacutainer collection system. The method and needle gauge selected depend on the vessel size, blood quantity required, intended use of the sample, and technician preference.

The majority of venipunctures in cats and small dogs are performed with 22-gauge needles. Larger-gauge needles, such as 20- and 18-gauge, may be used in large-breed dogs and in most farm animals. The needle for any venipuncture technique should always be inserted into the vein with the bevel facing upward.

> **Technician Note**
>
> For venipuncture, the needle should be inserted with the bevel facing upward.

Blood collected for coagulation profiles (i.e., activated clotting time, prothrombin time, activated partial thromboplastin time) should be drawn rapidly through a 20-gauge needle. The needle should ideally penetrate the vessel on the first attempt to minimize the amount of

---

BOX 3-1   VENOUS BLOOD COLLECTION

- Attach a 20- to 25-gauge needle to a 1- to 6-ml syringe.
- Occlude the vein with a tourniquet or digital pressure.
- Wipe the skin and hair on top of the vein with an alcohol-soaked cotton ball to help identify the vein.
- Insert the needle with the bevel facing up through the skin and into the vein at a 25-degree angle.
- Slowly retract the syringe plunger, and collect a blood sample.
- Release the pressure on the vein, and release the syringe plunger when a sufficient volume of blood has been collected.
- Remove the needle from the vein.
- Apply digital pressure to the venipuncture site as soon as the needle is remove until hemostasis occurs.

---

tissue fluid that enters the sample; tissue fluid (thromboplastin) may hasten the clotting process.

Smaller, 25- to 28-gauge needles are used with smaller vessels, fragile vessels, or multiple venipunctures. Bihourly sampling to establish a blood glucose curve is a situation in which use of a small-gauge needle is appropriate. The amount of negative pressure applied to aspirate the blood into the syringe must not be excessive. Forceful retraction of the syringe plunger may result in hemolysis of the red blood cells as they pass through the needle, yielding erroneous laboratory values. Application of excessive negative pressure may also cause the vein to collapse.

Just before venipuncture, the hair and skin over the vessel are wiped with a cotton ball saturated with 70% isopropyl alcohol. This helps to remove some superficial skin contaminants, causes vasodilation, and improves visualization of the vein. In animals with dense hair coats, the vessel may be easier to identify if the hair over the vessel is parted with an alcohol-soaked cotton ball or shaved with a clipper. When blood is drawn for bacterial culture, the region on top of the vein is shaved and aseptically prepared. Sterile gloves are worn when collecting blood for culture.

The most frequently used sites for canine blood collection are the cephalic, jugular, and lateral saphenous veins. The cephalic, jugular, femoral, and medial saphenous veins are used for feline venipuncture.

To collect blood from a peripheral vein, introduce the needle into the occluded vessel as far distally as possible. If the initial venipuncture attempt is unsuccessful, reinsert the needle more proximal to the previous entry site. For jugular venipuncture, the initial attempt is made in the caudal third of the jugular vein. Subsequent venipuncture attempts can be made further cranial. If the vessel is damaged in the distal portion of the vein, a more proximal region is still patent and usable for blood collection.

Technician Note

To perform venipuncture on a peripheral vein, introduce the needle into the most distal portion of the vein possible.

After blood is collected the needle is detached from the syringe and the stopper is removed from the collection tube before the blood is transferred into the tube. This

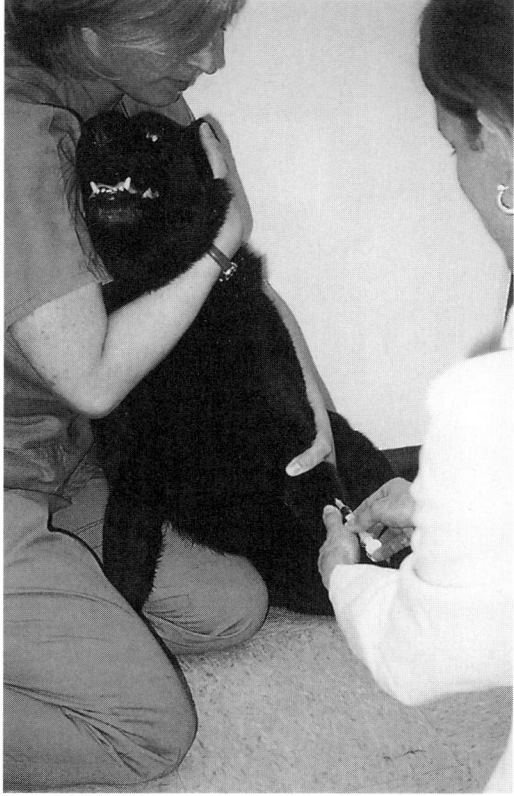

FIGURE 3-1. For venipuncture some large-breed dogs prefer to remain seated on the floor with a foreleg extended.

reduces the amount of hemolysis that may occur if blood is forcefully ejected through the narrow lumen of a needle. If blood is transferred into a tube containing an anticoagulant, such as lavender-topped EDTA tubes, the stopper is quickly replaced and the tube is gently inverted a few times to mix the blood with the anticoagulant. Vigorous shaking can cause hemolysis. The tube containing the anticoagulant should be at least half filled with blood to achieve the appropriate blood/anticoagulant ratio.

Cephalic Venipuncture

To collect blood from the cephalic vein, which is located on the cranial aspect of the foreleg, the animal is restrained in sternal recumbency or in a standing position. Small dogs may be picked up and held in the restrainer's arms with a foreleg extended. Some large-breed dogs prefer to remain standing or seated with a foreleg held in extension. Refer to Figure 3-1.

To perform venipuncture on the right cephalic vein, the restrainer is positioned on the animal's left side. The left hand or arm is placed under the muzzle to pull the head toward the restrainer's body. The restrainer wraps the right arm over the animal's back, extends the right foreleg, and occludes the vein with the thumb at the elbow. Alternatively, a tourniquet may be secured just distal to the elbow joint to occlude the vein if an assistant is unavailable.

Once the patient is restrained, the phlebotomist grasps the leg, places a thumb lateral to the vein, and pulls the skin distally to stabilize the vein. The cephalic vein is wiped with alcohol. A 22-gauge needle attached to a 3-ml syringe

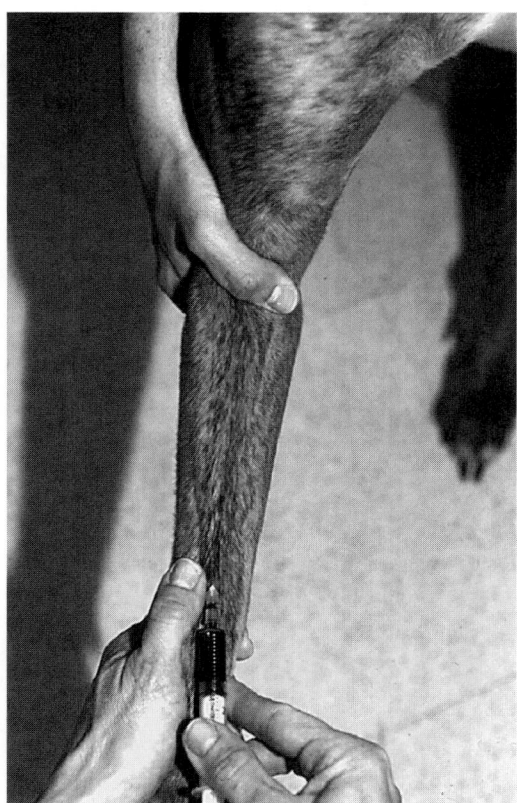

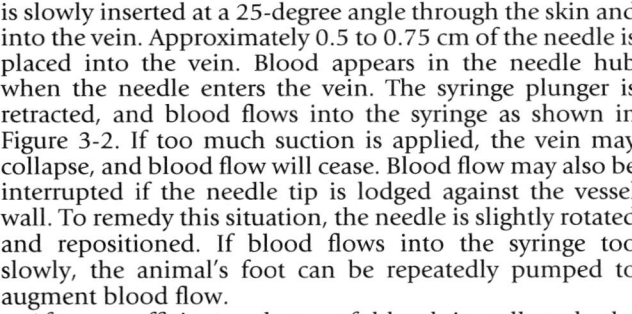

FIGURE 3-2. Restraint of a large-breed dog for venipuncture of the cephalic vein.

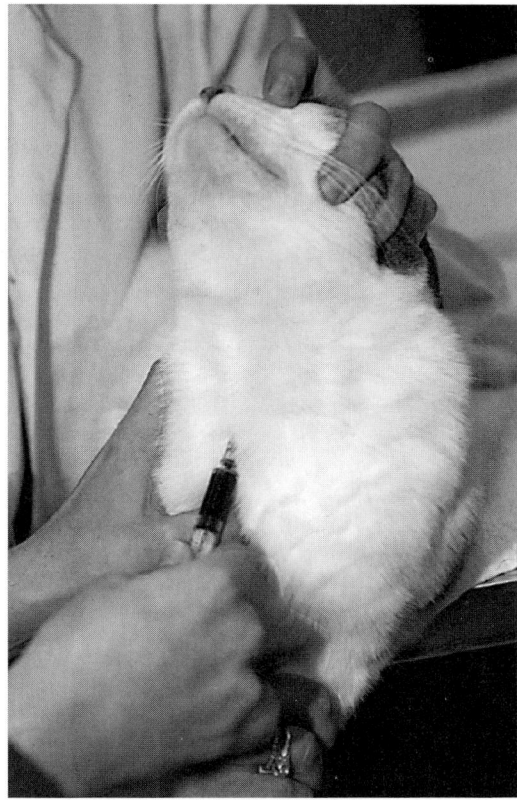

FIGURE 3-3. Venipuncture of the feline jugular vein.

is slowly inserted at a 25-degree angle through the skin and into the vein. Approximately 0.5 to 0.75 cm of the needle is placed into the vein. Blood appears in the needle hub when the needle enters the vein. The syringe plunger is retracted, and blood flows into the syringe as shown in Figure 3-2. If too much suction is applied, the vein may collapse, and blood flow will cease. Blood flow may also be interrupted if the needle tip is lodged against the vessel wall. To remedy this situation, the needle is slightly rotated and repositioned. If blood flows into the syringe too slowly, the animal's foot can be repeatedly pumped to augment blood flow.

After a sufficient volume of blood is collected, the restrainer's thumb or the tourniquet is removed from the vein. The needle is withdrawn, and digital pressure is applied to the venipuncture site for 10 to 20 seconds. Insufficient application of pressure may result in blood leakage from the vessel into the surrounding tissue and the formation of a hematoma. If a hematoma occurs during venipuncture, the needle is promptly removed and a gauze sponge is held firmly over the site until the bleeding subsides. When venipuncture is reattempted, the needle is reinserted proximal to the initial needle entry site or in a different vein.

 Technician Note

The jugular vein is the preferred site for venipuncture if several milliliters of blood are needed.

Jugular Venipuncture

The jugular vein is the preferred venipuncture site if several milliliters of blood are needed. Cats and small to medium-sized dogs are held in sternal recumbency near the edge of a table. Large dogs are restrained in a seated position on the floor.

For left jugular venipuncture, the restrainer stands on the animal's right side. The left arm is draped around the patient's back and holds the patient's body. The holder grasps the front legs just proximal to the elbow. Front legs of the cat or small dog may be stretched downward over the edge of the table. The assistant extends the neck and turns the head slightly away from the jugular vein to be sampled. Overextension of the neck may flatten the vein and should be avoided.

The jugular vein is occluded with the phlebotomist's thumb lateral to the trachea at the thoracic inlet. Once distended, the jugular vein is visualized or palpated as it courses from the thoracic inlet to the angle of the mandible. Wiping the neck with alcohol helps visualize the vein. In cats, water is sometimes used because the smell of alcohol is often repugnant to them. A 20- to 22-gauge needle on a syringe is inserted into the vein at a 25-degree angle with the bevel facing upward as shown in Figures 3-3 and 3-4. Prebending the needle to form a 150-degree angle with the syringe may make feline and small dog jugular venipuncture easier. After a sample is collected, digital pressure in the thoracic inlet is released from the vein and the needle is removed. Pressure is applied to the puncture site for approximately 30 seconds or until the bleeding stops.

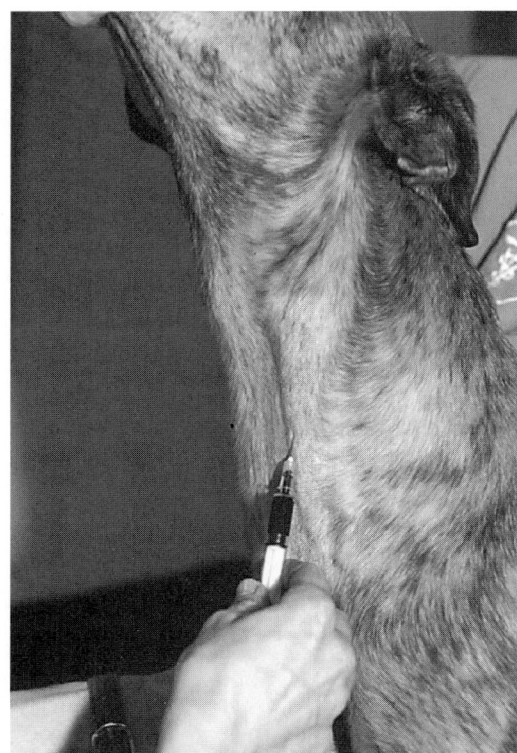

FIGURE 3-4.   Venipuncture of the canine jugular vein.

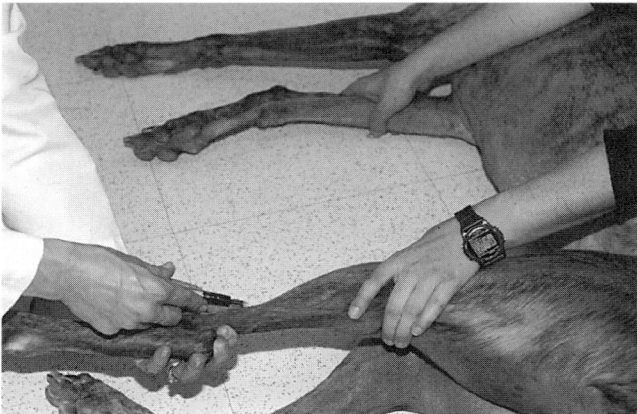

FIGURE 3-5.   Restraint of a dog for venipuncture of the lateral saphenous vein.

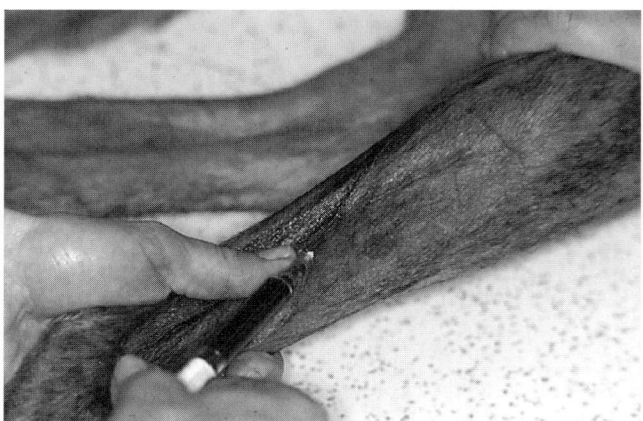

FIGURE 3-6.   The thumb is placed alongside the lateral saphenous vein to stabilize the vessel.

Use of a Vacutainer collection device may make jugular blood collection easier; however, some technicians prefer to use a needle and syringe. The Vacutainer collection system consists of three pieces: a two-way needle, a cylindrical plastic holder, and a glass tube. A needle is twisted into the top of the holder, and a Vacutainer tube sealed with a rubber stopper is held near the base of the holder. After the needle enters the vein the tube is inserted into the base of the holder until the stopper is punctured. Blood is automatically suctioned into the tube until it is three fourths full. The tube is withdrawn from the holder to break the vacuum, and the needle is removed from the vein. If more than one tube of blood is required, the blood-filled tube is replaced with an empty one *without* removing the needle from the vein. The vacuum that draws the blood into the tube will be broken once the needle is withdrawn from the skin.

Lateral Saphenous Venipuncture
The lateral saphenous vein, which is located on the lateral aspect of the hind limb near the hock, is an ideal site for blood collection in the dog. It is often used in aggressive animals when the phlebotomist does not want to be positioned close to the dog's face.

To perform venipuncture of the left lateral saphenous vein, the dog is placed in right lateral recumbency. The restrainer stands at the dog's back, places his or her right forearm across the thorax, and grasps the medial aspect of the right front leg. The left hand grasps and extends the left stifle; this occludes the vein and immobilizes the leg. As seen in Figure 3-5, the phlebotomist holds the left tarsus and pulls the skin taut to stabilize the vessel. Placement of the thumb parallel to the vein helps prevent the vein from rolling when the needle is introduced (Figure 3-6).

Medial Saphenous or Femoral Venipuncture
The medial saphenous or femoral vein, which is located on the medial aspect of the rear leg, is used to obtain small volumes of blood, primarily in feline patients. If the right vein is used, the cat is stretched in right lateral recumbency with the left rear leg abducted. The phlebotomist grasps the tarsus and extends the left leg. The vein is occluded with pressure applied by the restrainer's left hand in the right inguinal region. It is easy to identify the vein after the medial aspect of the leg is wiped with alcohol and the hair is parted over the vessel. Blood is collected with a 22- to 25-gauge needle attached to a 1- or 3-ml syringe. (Figure 3-7). Firm pressure is applied to the puncture site for at least 60 seconds after venipuncture. This is particularly important at these sites because the medial saphenous and femoral veins are prone to hematoma formation.

Marginal Ear Venipuncture
On occasion, the technician will collect blood from a peripheral capillary bed to check for erythroparasitic organisms, such as *Babesia* spp. or *Hemobartonella* spp. This can be accomplished by clipping the quick of a toenail or lacerating the buccal mucosa. A more desirable alternative

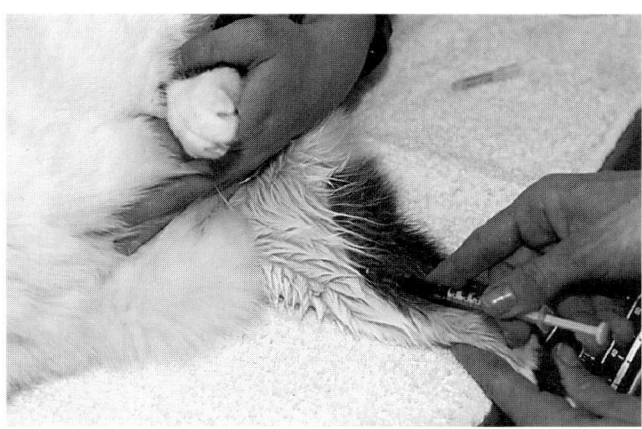

FIGURE 3-7.   Venipuncture of the femoral vein in the cat.

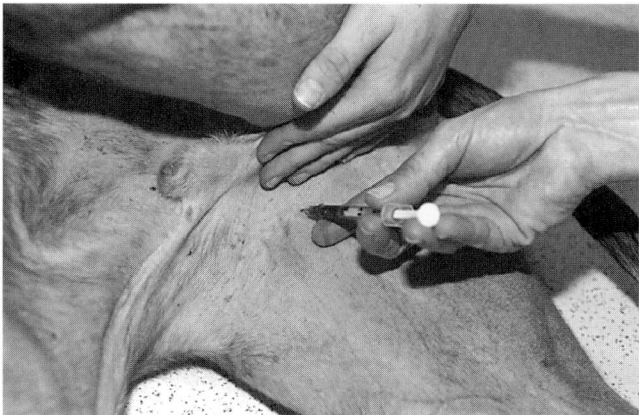

FIGURE 3-9.   Femoral artery blood sample collection.

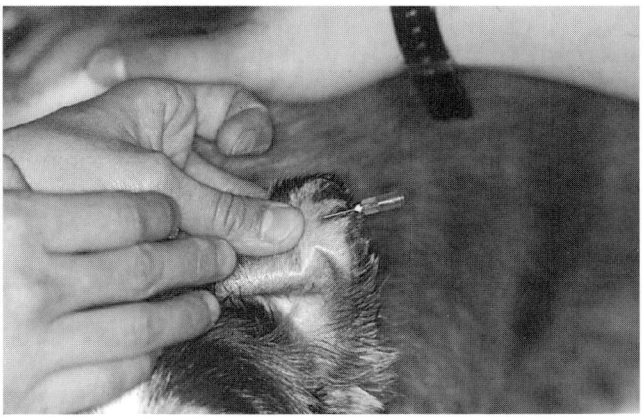

FIGURE 3-8.   Collection of a peripheral capillary sample from the marginal ear vein of the cat.

is to collect a sample from the marginal ear vein (Figure 3-8). The pinna of the ear is swabbed with alcohol to vasodilate the marginal ear vein. A 25-gauge needle is either inserted in the vein or used to nick the vein. Blood is drawn into a heparinized capillary tube and is later smeared into slides for microscopic examination.

Arterial Blood Sample

An arterial blood sample is useful to evaluate the acid-base and blood gas status of an animal. Cost-effective, easy to use arterial blood gas analyzers are becoming increasingly available. It is not necessary to occlude an artery to obtain a blood sample. Femoral and dorsal metatarsal arteries are used to obtain samples in conscious companion animals. When arterial puncture is performed in anesthetized patients, the lingual, brachial, and radial arteries may also be used.

Arterial blood gas samples are collected in a heparinized 1-ml syringe fitted with a 25-gauge, 1.6-cm needle. Arterial blood is generally brighter red than a paired venous sample.

Femoral Artery Sample

To collect a sample from the right leg, the patient is placed in right lateral recumbency with the right rear leg extended and the left rear leg abducted. The mammary glands or prepuce is retracted dorsally to access the femoral artery of the down leg. The inguinal region is wiped with 70% alcohol. Once the arterial pulse is palpated with the fingertips, the needle is introduced into the artery at a 60-degree angle. Gentle suction is applied to the syringe as it is advanced with a slight back and forth action. When the artery is penetrated, blood should rapidly fill the syringe in a pulsatile manner. A sample of 0.25 to 0.5 ml of blood is collected (Figure 3-9). Air bubbles are expelled from the syringe, and the needle is promptly capped with a rubber stopper. Bending the needle in lieu of embedding it in a rubber stopper is not sufficient to maintain an anaerobic environment. Firm pressure is immediately applied to the arterial puncture site for several minutes to prevent hematoma formation.

Dorsal Metatarsal Artery Sample

Blood can be taken from the dorsal metatarsal artery, located on the dorsal aspect of the metatarsus, if the femoral artery is inaccessible or difficult to palpate. The skin is thicker over the metatarsal artery than over the femoral and is more difficult to penetrate. The dog is placed in lateral recumbency, with the hock extended. The dorsum of the metatarsus is shaved and wiped with alcohol. After the arterial pulse is palpated, the needle is introduced into the artery at a 30-degree angle and a blood sample is obtained and handled in the same manner as described for a femoral artery puncture.

URINE SAMPLE COLLECTION

Because urine is often collected for gross and microscopic analysis and/or bacterial culture, the technician should be familiar with the many different methods of collection. For example, urine may be obtained as the patient voids, from manual bladder expression, from catheterization of the bladder, or by cystocentesis.

Routine samples are collected in clean, dry containers, but urine needed for bacterial culture is collected in sterile containers. Samples that cannot be analyzed within 30 minutes of collection should be refrigerated in airtight containers. Once refrigerated, the urine specimens should return to room temperature before urinalysis is performed.

Voided Collection

It is easy to collect a naturally voided urine sample. Voided samples are adequate for routine urinalyses. However, a voided sample is unsuitable for urine culture because the sample may contain bacteria, cells, and debris from hair, skin, or the genitourinary tract. The initial portion of voided urine contains the greatest concentration of contaminants and is usually excluded from collection.

Urine is most easily obtained in the dog by walking it outdoors and catching a voided midstream sample. A collection device is often helpful because many dogs stop urinating when a person gets close to them. These can be improvised by bending a loop in the end of an aluminum rod or straightened metal coat hanger. A paper cup placed in the loop serves as a urine receptacle.

Urine can be collected from a hospitalized animal by placing it on a raised grate in a clean cage. After the animal voids, the urine is collected from the cage floor with a syringe.

Confinement of the animal in a specialized metabolic cage is another means to collect urine. These cages are made of stainless steel and include a grate raised above a slanted cage floor. The floor forms a funnel under which a container is placed for urine collection.

In addition, voided samples can be collected from clean, dry litter pans or pans covered with plastic bags. Cats that prefer to urinate in a litter-type material may require use of specially designed plastic, nonabsorbent pellets, such as NoSorb, CATCO, Tifflin, OH. After the cat urinates in the litter pan, the urine is simply poured out or collected with a syringe.

Manual Bladder Expression

Urine can be collected for routine urinalysis by manual compression of the bladder. Urine expressed from the bladder contains contaminants from the urogenital tract, skin, and hair. Therefore manual expression should not be used to obtain samples for bacterial culture.

Bladder expression may be difficult to perform in some patients, especially males, because transabdominal compression causes the pressure inside the bladder to increase but the urethral sphincter may not relax simultaneously. Manual bladder expression can be done in patients who cannot initiate voluntary urination or completely empty the bladder, such as animals with neurologic impairments.

To express the bladder, support the animal in a standing or lateral position and place a hand on either side of the caudal abdomen. Isolate the bladder between the palmar surfaces of the fingers, and gently apply steady, firm pressure until a stream of urine is produced. It may be possible to express the bladder of cats and small dogs with only one hand.

If urine is not expelled with moderate compression, do not continue to exert pressure. An alternate method of emptying the bladder should be attempted. Care must be taken when attempting to express an overly distended bladder in the presence of urethral obstruction because urethral or vesicular rupture may occur.

Catheterization

Urinary catheterization is performed to collect urine, relieve a urethral obstruction, or empty the bladder (Box 3-2). Although catheterization is performed using aseptic technique, it may induce urethral inflammation and bacterial urinary tract infection. This is particularly problematic in cases where the urinary catheter remains indwelling for prolonged periods. Trauma from catheterization may

---

BOX 3-2   MALE URINARY CATHETERIZATION TECHNIQUE*

- Retract the prepuce to expose the penis.
- Wash the penis and prepuce with warm dilute antimicrobial solution, and rinse well with warm water.
- Lubricate the tip of the sterile urinary catheter with sterile, water-soluble gel.
- Wearing sterile gloves, insert the catheter into the urethra and advance it until the bladder is entered and urine flows through the catheter. If sterile gloves are not worn, keep the catheter in its wrapper and cut a freely moveable paper tab from the tip of the package.
- Use this tab to feed the catheter into the bladder to avoid directly touching the catheter. Do not allow the top edge of the tab to contact any surface.
- Do not force the catheter—if it does not advance easily, remove it and use a catheter with a smaller lumen. If it does not advance easily because of a urethral obstruction, flush a small volume of 0.9% saline into the end of the catheter as it is advanced to attempt to dislodge the obstructing material.
- Once the catheter enters the bladder, attach a syringe to the end and collect a urine sample if needed.
- Attach a closed collection system to the end of the urinary catheter.
- If the catheter is to remain indwelling, secure the catheter in place by inflating the balloon cuff (Foley catheter) or by suturing the tape tab wrapped around the catheter through suture loops placed in the skin of the prepuce. Use 4-0 to 3-0 nylon suture.

*Male cats are sedated.

---

cause an increased number of red blood cells, protein, and transitional epithelial cells in the sample. Urine samples may contain contaminants from the genital region and urethra. Urine obtained by catheterization is acceptable for bacterial culture if a sample cannot be obtained via cystocentesis.

Urinary catheters are temporarily left indwelling in patients at risk of urethral obstruction, such as male cats who have recently had urethral calculi removed. Indwelling urinary catheters are also placed in animals unable to stand to void, those with neurologic impairment that interferes with micturition. Catheterization is also an important part of quantitating urinary output.

The prepuce or vulva should be gently rinsed with warm antimicrobial solution and water and then dried twice daily. Gloves are worn to detach or connect the catheter to extension tubing or a collection system. To create a closed collection system, the catheter is connected, via intravenous tubing, to an empty sterile fluid bag. The bag serves as a urine reservoir. Its contents must be measured and emptied periodically.

Urinary catheters should be inspected for occlusion and adequate urine production every 4 to 6 hours. A normotensive, normovolemic patient with intact renal function should produce 1 to 2 ml of urine per kilogram of body weight per hour. If urine does not accumulate in the collection bag and the bladder is firm and distended, the catheter is probably obstructed. It should be slightly repositioned and inspected for kinks. The bladder can be gently compressed to see if urine will flow through the catheter. As a last resort, a small volume of sterile 0.9% saline can be flushed into the catheter to attempt to relieve the obstruction.

To avoid or limit catheter-induced infection and inflammation of the urinary tract, the catheter should be removed as soon as possible. If catheterization is required beyond 4 days, a new catheter should be placed.

Male Canine

It usually is not difficult to place a urinary catheter in a male dog unless a urethral obstruction exists. A wide range of sizes and types of urinary catheters is available. A 4 to 10 French (Fr) polypropylene urinary catheter is used. If the catheter is to remain indwelling, placement of a softer, flexible feeding tube (Argyle), or a self-retaining Foley catheter (Jorgensen Lab) is a more comfortable alternative.

The dog is placed in lateral recumbency with the upper rear leg abducted. An assistant retracts the prepuce so the tip of the penis is exposed. The prepuce and glans penis are gently washed with warm, dilute antiseptic solution and rinsed with warm sterile saline or water. The package containing the catheter is cut open to expose the distal 3 cm of the catheter. Sterile, water-soluble lubricant or lidocaine ointment is placed on the catheter tip. If sterile gloves are worn, the catheter should be removed from its package. If sterile gloves are not worn, the catheter is kept wrapped so it can be handled aseptically as it is advanced through the urethra.

To place the catheter, the lubricated tip is introduced into the urethra and slowly advanced. The catheter should never be forced. If the catheter cannot be passed, a catheter with a narrower lumen should be used. Resistance may be met when the catheter reaches the os penis or a portion of the urethra that curves around the ischial arch. Steady gentle pressure should overcome this resistance. The catheter can be guided around the flexure of the urethral canal by applying digital pressure on the perineum externally or pressing on the catheter with an index finger placed in the rectum.

Urine should flow into the catheter as it enters the neck of the bladder. The catheter is then advanced 1 cm further. A sterile 20- to 35-ml syringe is attached to the catheter, and urine is slowly aspirated from the bladder. The first several milliliters of urine suctioned from the catheter may contain contaminants and should not be submitted for urinalysis or culture.

If the urinary catheter is not self-retaining (i.e., not a Foley catheter) and it is to remain indwelling, it must be secured. To do this, two 0.75-cm diameter loops are made through the skin on two sides of the distal prepuce using 3-0 or 4-0 nylon suture material. Adhesive tape is folded over on itself to make a "butterfly" around the catheter as it exits from the penis. Suture is passed through one side of the tape and then through the nylon loop in the prepuce. This "chain link" is repeated on the other side of the tape. This secures the catheter to the prepuce so it remains in place. If the catheter needs to be replaced, the suture ring that courses through the tape is cut. Tape is wrapped around the replacement catheter and sutured through the existing loops in the prepuce. When a set of suture loops is left in the prepuce, the urinary catheter can be readjusted or replaced without having to pass another needle through the prepuce.

Female Canine

Catheterization of the female dog is more challenging than in the male. The dog is placed on a table either in standing position, in lateral recumbency, or in sternal recumbency with the hind legs dangling from the end of the table. The vulva is gently washed with a dilute, warm antiseptic solution and rinsed with sterile saline or water. The ventral

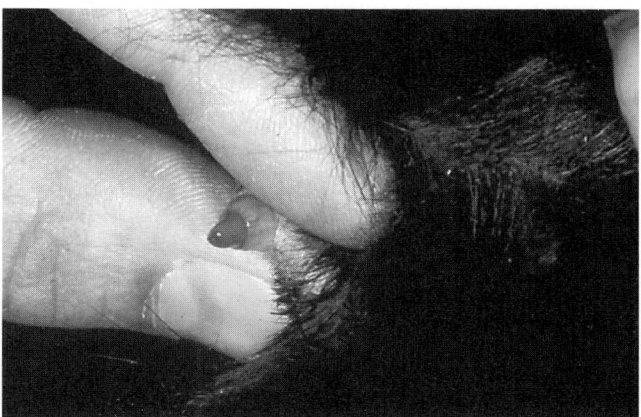

FIGURE 3-10. Retraction of the prepuce to expose the penis for feline urinary catheterization.

vaginal floor is instilled with 1.0 ml of 2% lidocaine. A sterile flexible polypropylene urinary catheter is lubricated with sterile, water-soluble gel at the fenestrated end. Wearing sterile gloves, the technician places a lubricated finger into the vagina and slides it 3 to 5 cm along the ventral floor until the external urethral orifice is identified. The catheter is introduced into the vagina and guided into the urethral orifice by the finger in the vestibule. It is important to avoid inadvertently passing the catheter into the clitoral fossa. The catheter is advanced until it enters the bladder. If "blind catheterization" is not possible, a lighted vaginal speculum or an otoscope fitted with a large speculum is inserted into the vagina and used to visualize the urethral orifice.

If the urinary catheter is to remain indwelling, a soft Foley self-retaining catheter with a removable stylet is used. Once the catheter is placed in the bladder, the cuff is inflated with a few milliliters of water to prevent the tip of the catheter from slipping out of the bladder. The catheter is then taped to the tail to prevent the dog from stepping on it. A urine collection device is placed on the free end of the Foley catheter.

Male Feline

The most common reason to catheterize a male cat is to relieve a urethral obstruction. Catheterization requires the use of a short-acting anesthetic, such as a ketamine-diazepam combination or propofol, either alone or in combination with a gas anesthetic.

The anesthetized or heavily sedated male cat is placed on his side or back with the hind legs drawn forward. As shown in Figure 3-10, the prepuce is retracted to expose the penis. The perineum is prepared aseptically, as described for male canine catheterization, and the penis is extended dorsally so the urethra is parallel to the vertebral column. Sterile gloves are worn and a sterile, lubricated, 3.5 Fr polyethylene or silicone tomcat catheter is passed into the urethra. If resistance is met, the catheter is retracted and then slightly rotated as it is readvanced. If the catheter cannot be easily advanced, a small volume of sterile water or saline is instilled through the catheter. The pressure created often dislodges the obstructing material. Alternatively, saline can be flushed through a 24- or 22-gauge intravenous catheter placed in the urethra. After the obstruction is relieved, a 3.5 Fr catheter is placed to prevent reobstruction.

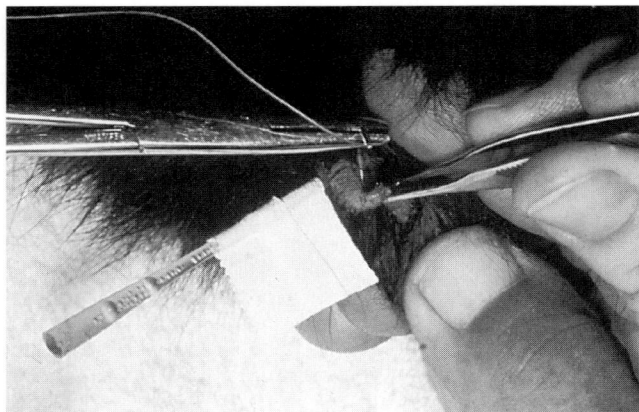

FIGURE 3-11. A urinary catheter is secured in place in a male cat. Tape wrapped around the catheter is sutured to the skin of the prepuce.

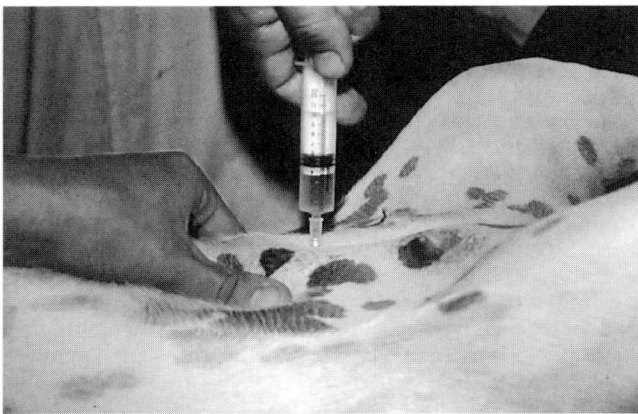

FIGURE 3-12. Collection of a urine sample through cystocentesis in the dog. The bladder is isolated, and urine is aspirated into a syringe.

Once the catheter is in place it is secured with 4-0 nylon in the same fashion as described in the male dog. Refer to Figure 3-11. The cat should be fitted with an Elizabethan collar to prevent removal of the catheter and the urine collection system.

Female Feline

Catheterization of female cats is performed infrequently because of its difficulty, and, as with male cats, it requires sedation. The perineal region is aseptically prepared, and the vulva is pulled caudally. A sterile, lubricated, open-ended 3.5- Fr tomcat catheter is inserted along the midline of the floor of the vagina and into the urethra.

Cystocentesis

Cystocentesis is the percutaneous aspiration of urine from the bladder. It is performed to collect specimens for urinalysis or bacterial culture that will be free of contamination from the distal urethra and genital tract. Cystocentesis is used as a last resort to empty an overly distended bladder when a urethral obstruction prevents urinary catheterization. Recent abdominal surgery or trauma, suspected bleeding disorders, pyometra, or suspected caudal abdominal or bladder tumors are contraindications for cystocentesis.

When cystocentesis is performed, most but not all of the urine should be removed from the bladder. Excessive pressure from a full bladder might lead to extravasation of urine from the puncture site when the needle is withdrawn. On the other hand, removal of the entire volume of urine increases the risk of contact between the needle and the bladder wall, which may result in damage to the bladder.

To perform cystocentesis, the animal is restrained in dorsal or lateral recumbency or in a standing position. The skin of the ventral or lateral abdomen is wiped with 70% alcohol. One hand is used to isolate the bladder. A 22-gauge, 2.5- to 3.75-cm needle attached to a 12- to 20-ml syringe is inserted through the abdominal wall and into the bladder at a 45- to 75-degree angle (Figure 3-12). In male dogs, the prepuce and penis are diverted laterally and the needle is inserted on the ventral midline or slightly paramedian. The syringe plunger is slowly retracted and urine is collected. If blood enters the needle, another cystocentesis attempt should be made with a different needle and syringe. The needle should not be redirected once it is within the abdominal cavity because accidental laceration of viscera may occur. Once a sufficient urine volume is collected, negative pressure is released and the needle is withdrawn.

OTHER COLLECTION PROCEDURES

Fecal Collection

Gross and microscopic examination of feces for intestinal parasites, ova, blood, and mucus is frequently performed in veterinary practice. Samples are most commonly obtained by collecting them from the ground or litter pan after defecation. Alternatively, a lubricated fecal loop or gloved finger can be inserted into the rectum to remove feces. Fresh samples are placed into a sealed container or Ziploc bag. If feces are collected to check for parasites but are not examined for several hours, the sample should be refrigerated or placed in a formalin solution. Samples intended for parasitology examination can be refrigerated for up to 3 days.

Thoracocentesis

The thorax (chest cavity) contains the heart and lungs. Many medical conditions lead to the accumulation of air or fluid in the *pleural space*. This space is located between the lungs and the chest wall. When air or fluid accumulates in the pleural space, the lungs are unable to completely expand. This results in rapid and difficult breathing. *Thoracocentesis* is the process of removing accumulated air or fluid from within the pleural space.

To perform a thoracocentesis, the area between the fifth and twelfth ribs is clipped and surgically prepared with alternating chlorhexidine or povidone-iodine and alcohol scrubs. The thoracocentesis occurs at the seventh or eighth intercostal space, which is located by counting forward from the thirteenth rib. Needles used during the procedure are introduced at the cranial aspect of the rib to avoid penetration of the blood vessels that lie along the caudal aspect. For fluid removal, the needle is inserted in the ventral third of the thorax near the costochondral junction. To remove air, the needle insertion site should be more dorsal.

To perform thoracocentesis, the animal is placed in sternal recumbency or held in a standing position. A 21-gauge butterfly catheter or a 22-gauge needle attached

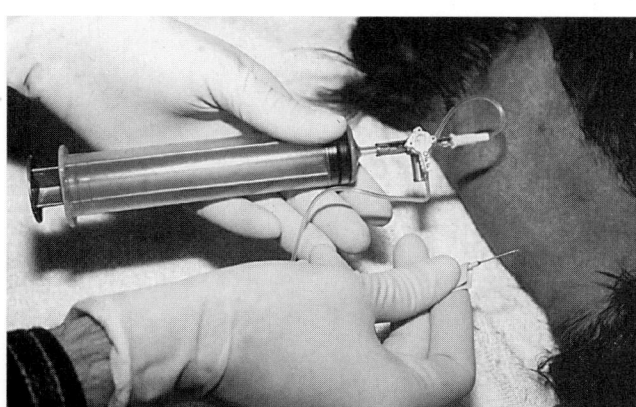

FIGURE 3-13.   Materials used for thoracocentesis of a cat include a 21-gauge butterfly catheter attached to a three-way stopcock and 60-ml syringe.

to extension tubing is connected to a closed three-way stopcock. A 60-ml syringe is also attached to one of the stopcock ports. The needle is directed into the seventh or eighth intercostal space perpendicular to the body wall as shown in Figure 3-13. After the pleural space is penetrated, the needle is directed caudoventrally to avoid puncture of the lung, and the stopcock is opened. Suction is applied with the syringe, and fluid or air is withdrawn from the pleural cavity. If only negative pressure is obtained, the needle is retracted 2 to 3 mm and carefully redirected. Caution should be employed because redirection of the needle may lacerate a lung. If frank blood enters the needle, the needle should be removed. When the syringe is filled, the stopcock valve is closed, and the syringe contents are expelled into a container through the third stopcock port. This process is repeated until no more fluid or air can be removed.

After thoracocentesis, the patient's respiratory pattern is monitored for approximately 2 hours. In addition, the technician must be observant of the stopcock apparatus. If the 3-way stopcock accidentally is opened or any part of the apparatus is disconnected, air could enter the thoracic cavity and cause serious complications.

Abdominocentesis

Similar to thoracocentesis, abdominocentesis is the process of drawing fluid from the abdominal cavity. It is performed for both diagnostic and therapeutic purposes and is an important technique to employ in some emergency and critical care cases, such as those in which abdominal trauma or peritonitis is suspected.

Patients should urinate before abdominocentesis to avoid accidental puncture of the bladder. The patient is restrained in a standing position or lateral recumbency. A 5- to 10-cm area on the ventral abdomen between the umbilicus and bladder is clipped and aseptically prepared. A 20- to 22-gauge, 2.5- to 3.75-cm needle is inserted to the right of the ventral midline 1 to 2 cm caudal to the umbilicus. This right paramedian approach is selected to avoid lacerating the spleen. Fluid is collected as it drips out of the needle hub, or it can be aspirated into a syringe attached to the needle. Sometimes rotation of the needle or insertion of a second needle into the abdomen 2 cm from the first will stimulate fluid flow. If the abdominal effusion is suspected to be compartmentalized, abdominocentesis

can be performed in more than one quadrant, such as in the left and right craniolateral or caudolateral regions.

Abdominocentesis can also be performed with an 18- to 20-gauge, over-the-needle intravenous catheter. After the catheter is inserted into the abdominal cavity, the stylet is removed and a sample is collected.

Gastrocentesis may be performed in an emergency situation. A trochar is inserted into the stomach to *temporarily* relieve pressure in animals with gastric dilation. The skin over the greatest point of abdominal distension is shaved and aseptically prepared. A 14- to 16-gauge needle or trochar is inserted through the abdominal and stomach walls. Gas and fluid will exit the needle once it enters the stomach lumen, but solid ingesta will not fit through the needle. The abdomen is gently compressed with the hands to help evacuate the fluid and gas. The needle is removed after the stomach is decompressed. Gastrocentesis may result in laceration of the stomach or other abdominal organs and the development of peritonitis.

Diagnostic Peritoneal Lavage

Diagnostic peritoneal lavage is performed when abdominocentesis does not provide a sufficient abdominal fluid sample. Warm sterile water or 0.9% sterile saline is injected into the abdomen through an 18- to 20-gauge catheter at a volume of 20 ml/kg of body weight. With the catheter in place, the animal is gently rolled from side to side to disperse the fluid. A sample of abdominal fluid is aspirated through the catheter, and then the catheter is removed. Only a small percentage of the volume of fluid infiltrated into the abdominal cavity will be retrieved.

Transtracheal Wash

A transtracheal wash is performed to obtain fluid samples from the lower respiratory tract for culture or cytology. Light sedation may be required in the dog, but the cough reflex should remain intact.

Percutaneous Technique

The patient is placed in sternal recumbency or a seated position with the head raised slightly. The laryngeal region is clipped and aseptically prepared. A sterile gloved finger is placed on the ventral aspect of the trachea and moved in a cranial direction until the protruding cricoid cartilage is palpated. Just above the cartilage is a flattened, triangular region called the cricothyroid membrane. From 0.5 to 1 ml of 2% lidocaine is injected into the skin, subcutaneous tissue, and cricothyroid membrane.

The needle from an 18-gauge, 20-cm, through-the-needle catheter (ICath, CharterMed, Inc.) is disengaged from the catheter. The catheter is set aside but kept in its protective sleeve. One hand stabilizes the trachea. The needle is inserted at a 90-degree angle through the cricothyroid membrane with the bevel facing downward. Alternatively, the needle can be inserted between any tracheal rings in the cranial third of the trachea.

A burst of air accompanied by a cough occurs when the needle enters the trachea. The needle is repositioned at a caudal 120-degree angle. The catheter is advanced through the needle until it reaches the distal trachea. Placement of the needle with the bevel aimed downward decreases the likelihood of laceration of the catheter as it courses through the needle. The needle is withdrawn through the skin. The catheter, with the stylet removed, is left in place. In large dogs, a sterile 3.5 Fr polyvinyl urinary catheter can be passed through a 14-gauge needle and advanced into the distal third of the trachea in lieu of a through-the-needle catheter (Figure 3-14).

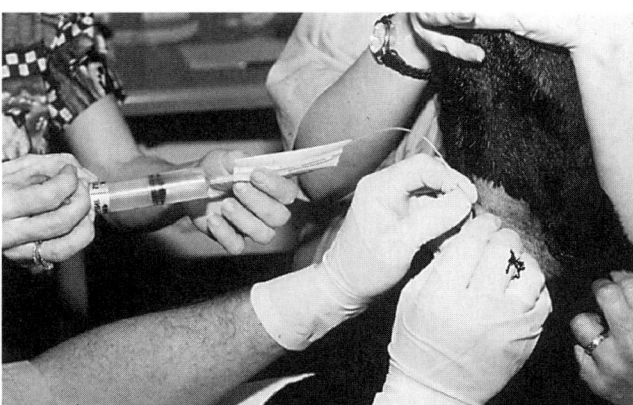

FIGURE 3-14.   Transtracheal wash in a dog with a urinary catheter placed into the trachea.

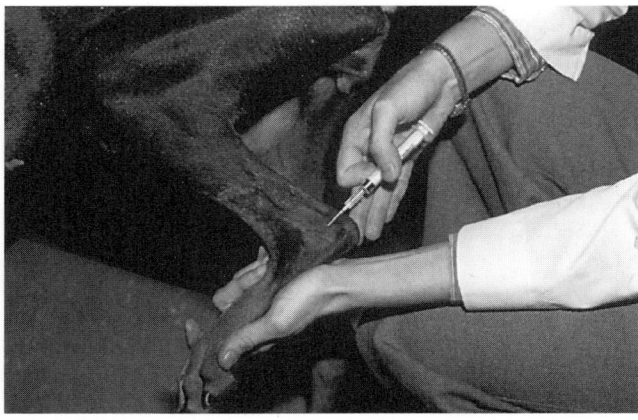

FIGURE 3-15.   Arthrocentesis of the tibiotarsal joint through a caudolateral approach.

A 3-ml syringe is attached to the catheter, and the plunger is retracted. Air is aspirated if the catheter is in the tracheal lumen. If only resistance is felt, the catheter should be repositioned because it may be either kinked, occluded against the tracheal mucosa, or embedded in the tissue surrounding the trachea.

After the catheter is properly positioned in the trachea, the contents of a syringe containing warm, nonbacteriostatic sterile saline, 0.5 to 1.0 ml/kg of body weight, is flushed through the catheter. When the animal coughs, the syringe plunger is immediately retracted several times to collect a sample. Only a small percentage of the volume of fluid infused down the trachea will be reaspirated; the remainder will be absorbed. Additional aliquots of saline are instilled into the catheter and reaspirated until a sufficient sample volume is collected. Catheter position may need to be adjusted during the procedure.

When the transtracheal aspirate is completed, the puncture site is covered with a povidone-iodine ointment-treated gauze sponge and bandaged. Respiration is monitored for 12 to 24 hours after the procedure. The needle insertion site is checked for air accumulation (subcutaneous emphysema) in the tissue surrounding the trachea, which would indicate laceration of the tracheal tissue from the needle.

Technician Note

Only a small percentage of the volume of fluid infused down the trachea will be reaspirated.

Endotracheal Tube Technique

Tracheal aspirates in fractious or very small animals are obtained in a different manner. The animal is lightly anesthetized and intubated with a sterile endotracheal tube. A sterile polypropylene urinary catheter longer than the endotracheal tube is threaded down the tube to just above the tracheal bifurcation. Warm sterile saline is injected through the catheter. When the animal coughs, the sample is aspirated into a sterile 12-ml syringe. The saline injection–aspiration procedure is repeated until a sufficient sample volume is obtained.

Arthrocentesis

Aspiration of fluid from a swollen or painful joint is performed by the veterinarian to help determine the cause of pain or swelling. Synovial fluid is collected for cytologic, bacterial, and biochemical analyses. The technique is reviewed so the technician will be familiar with the site preparation, materials needed, and sample handling.

The anatomy of the joint to be aspirated should be reviewed to determine the appropriate site of needle insertion. For the shoulder, the needle is inserted into the lateral aspect and is directed medially. Aspiration of the elbow is performed from the lateral or caudal aspect. The carpus is tapped from its dorsal surface. The coxofemoral joint is aspirated from its craniodorsal aspect. The stifle is approached from the craniolateral surface, just below the patella. A caudolateral approach is used for tarsal arthrocentesis.

To perform arthrocentesis, the animal is sedated and the skin over the joint is shaved and aseptically prepared. It is often helpful to flex the joint to facilitate needle insertion. The person who performs the aspirate should wear sterile gloves. A 22-gauge needle on a 3- to 6-ml syringe is inserted into the joint space with the needle directed into a bone-free location (Figure 3-15). If the needle contacts bone, it is withdrawn slightly and redirected. After the joint is penetrated, the syringe plunger is retracted to collect the synovial fluid. If blood enters the needle it should be removed.

The color, consistency, volume, and viscosity of the synovial fluid are noted. Normal joint fluid should be clear, pale yellow, and viscous. A fluid drop stretched between the thumb and forefinger should be at least 10 cm long. Fluid is placed on a microscope slide to make a smear for cytologic analysis. A sample is saved for bacterial culture and further laboratory analysis.

Bone Marrow Aspiration

Bone marrow aspiration is performed to evaluate the cells in the bone marrow. It is most commonly performed in patients with nonregenerative anemia, persistent thrombocytopenia, or neoplasia. A complete blood count is done within 24 hours before or after the aspirate so the peripheral and marrow cell populations can be compared. Because aspiration of bone marrow is an uncomfortable procedure, heavy sedation in conjunction with a local anesthetic is recommended.

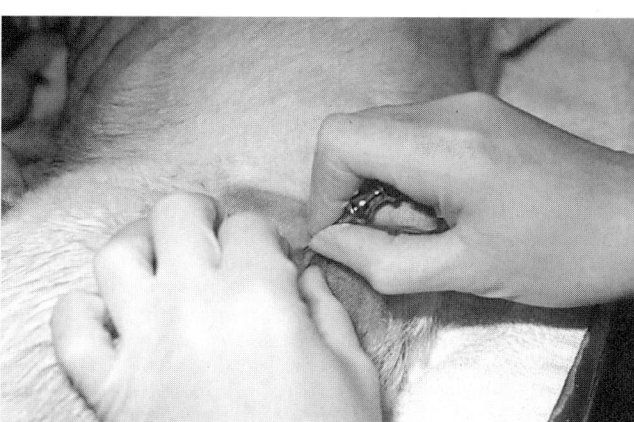

FIGURE 3-16. Technique for placing a bone marrow needle into the ilium of a dog.

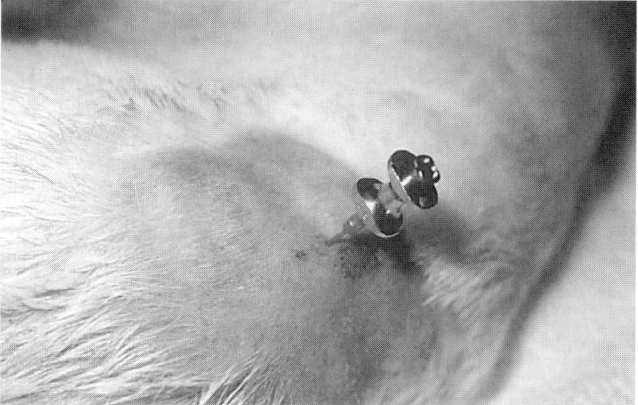

FIGURE 3-17. Bone marrow needle seated in the dorsal aspect of the wing of the ilium. The stylet has been removed after placement.

The most frequently aspirated sites include the ilial wing, humerus, and femur. Patient size and conformation generally determine which site is used.

Aspirates are performed using strict aseptic technique. Hair over the site is shaved, and the skin is surgically prepared. Sterile gloves are worn by the person obtaining the aspirate.

Technician Note

Common sites for bone marrow aspiration include the ilial wing, femur, and humerus.

Ilial Bone Marrow Aspiration
The animal is placed in lateral recumbency or in sternal recumbency with the rear legs drawn forward. The widest portion of the iliac crest region is clipped and aseptically prepared. From 0.5 to 1 ml of 2% lidocaine is infiltrated into the skin, subcutaneous tissue, and periosteum of the bone.

A sterile 15- to 18-gauge bone marrow needle is flushed with an anticoagulant, such as a 2.5% to 3% EDTA solution. A no. 11 scalpel blade is used to make a stab incision through the skin over the iliac crest. One hand is placed on the ilium to stabilize it. The bone marrow needle, with the stylet in place, is introduced through the skin incision and advanced through the application of firm pressure and rotation of the wrist in a clockwise-counterclockwise manner. The needle eventually penetrates the cortex of the bone and enters the marrow cavity (Figure 3-16). If the needle slips off the bone during placement, which may occur if the ilial wings are narrow, the needle is repositioned and another attempt is made.

Once the needle is firmly seated in the bone and the tip is in the marrow cavity, the stylet is removed and placed on a sterile field (Figure 3-17). An anticoagulant-coated, 12-ml syringe is attached to the end of the needle, and negative pressure is rapidly and forcefully applied. One tenth of 1 ml of bone marrow is aspirated into the syringe (Figure 3-18).

The syringe is detached, and a drop of the sample is placed onto a few tilted microscope slides. Marrow particles adhere to the tilted slides, and the excess blood

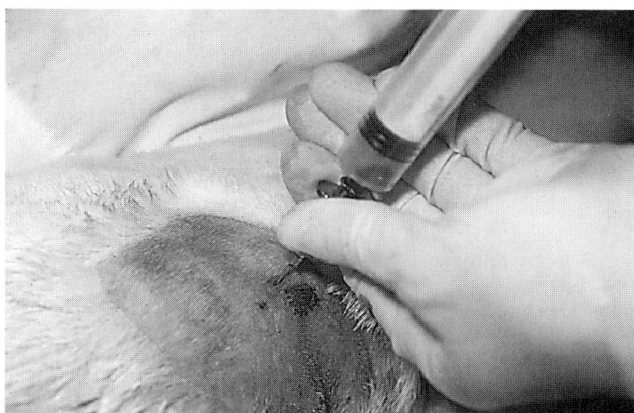

FIGURE 3-18. The bone marrow needle is stabilized as marrow is aspirated from the ilium.

trickles to the end (Figure 3-19). Alternatively, the marrow sample can be emptied from the syringe onto a petri dish. The dish is then tilted to separate the blood from the marrow. The marrow particles are transferred to a slide with the tip of a hypodermic needle. A pull slide is made with each sample. To do this, a glass slide is placed on top of the slide containing the aspirate and the slides are then slid apart to make two slides for cytologic analysis.

If a marrow sample does not enter the syringe when suction is applied, the stylet is replaced and the needle repositioned. Often, the needle simply needs to be advanced an additional few millimeters to position it within the marrow cavity.

After marrow is obtained, the needle is withdrawn, and firm pressure is held on the site until hemostasis occurs. An antibiotic ointment–treated gauze sponge is secured over the aspirate site.

Humeral Bone Marrow Aspiration
The craniolateral aspect of the greater tubercle of the proximal humerus is another bone marrow aspiration site (Figure 3-20). The advantage of this site is that it has less tissue, fat, and muscle overlying the desired bone. Thus

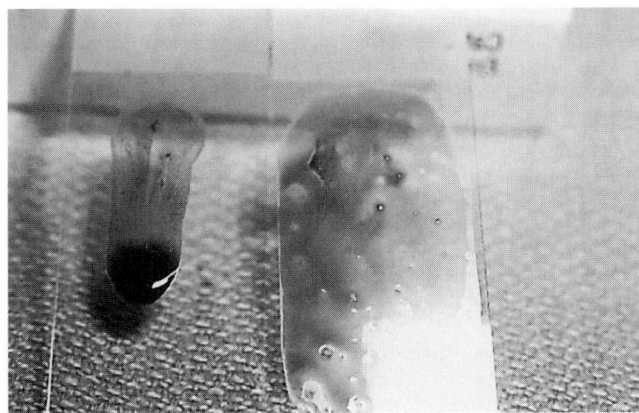

FIGURE 3-19.   Drops of bone marrow are placed on the end of microscope slides, which are tilted to allow blood to run to the other end. A pull smear is made with the bone marrow sample.

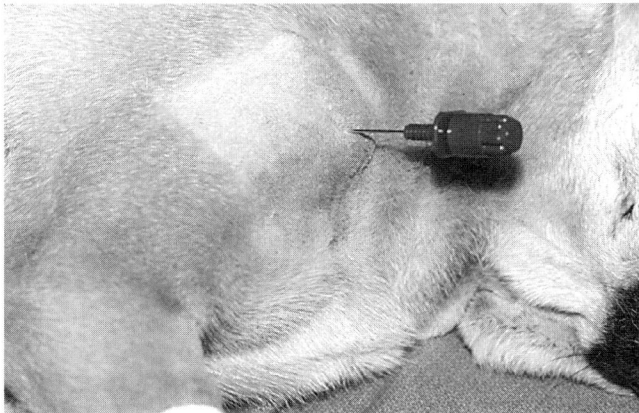

FIGURE 3-20.   Jamshidi bone marrow needle placed into the craniolateral aspect of the proximal humerus to obtain a bone marrow aspirate.

this site is preferred in heavily muscled or overweight dogs when the dorsal iliac crest is difficult to palpate. The humerus is also advantageous to use in animals with narrow ilial wings or in thrombocytopenic patients when hemostasis is a concern.

The animal is placed in lateral recumbency with the humerus to be aspirated positioned on top. The proximal humerus is shaved, surgically prepared, and infiltrated with a local anesthetic. The needle is embedded perpendicular to the humeral shaft as the elbow is held flexed and the shoulder externally rotated. The technique for site preparation, needle placement, bone marrow aspiration, and slide preparation is as previously described for ilial bone marrow aspiration.

Femoral Bone Marrow Aspiration

In small dogs and cats, the femur can be used for bone marrow aspirates. Site preparation, needle placement, marrow aspiration, and slide preparation techniques are the same as described for bone marrow aspiration from the wing of the ilium. Needle placement within the femur is described under the discussion of placement of an intraos-

seous catheter in the section titled Small Animal Sampling and Therapeutic Techniques.

Fine Needle Aspiration

Fine needle aspiration is a quick procedure frequently performed to collect a sample of fluid or tissue cells from a dermal or visceral mass or a lymph node. The skin overlying the tissue to be aspirated is wiped with alcohol to remove superficial contaminants. The mass is stabilized with one hand as a 22-gauge needle is inserted into the center. The needle is redirected once or twice within the tissue and then removed. A syringe containing 1 ml of air is attached to the needle. The syringe plunger is forcefully depressed, and the needle contents are expelled onto a microscope slide. Slides are then prepared with the pull technique described for ilial bone marrow aspiration.

An alternate technique to perform a fine needle aspirate is to use a needle attached to a 3- to 12-ml syringe. The needle is embedded in the mass, and suction is applied to aspirate cells into the needle. During this process, the needle may be redirected once or twice. Negative pressure is released before the needle is withdrawn from the mass. The needle is then detached to allow the syringe to be filled with 1 to 2 ml of air. Subsequently, the needle is reattached and the syringe plunger is depressed so that the contents of the needle are sprayed onto a microscope slide. Slides are made using the previously described pull technique.

Vaginal Cytologic Sampling

Vaginal cytologic sampling is performed to determine the patient's present stage in the estrous cycle for breeding purposes or to collect samples to help diagnose the cause of vaginal disease. To obtain a vaginal smear, the patient is placed in a standing position or lateral recumbency. The vulvar region is wiped with warm water. A gloved hand is used to separate the labia so that a cotton swab can be inserted and rolled against the vaginal wall. The swab is then removed from the vagina and is rolled onto a glass microscope slide for cytologic evaluation.

ADMINISTRATION OF MEDICATION IN THE SMALL ANIMAL

Multiple routes exist for the administration of fluids and medication (Box 3-3). The route used depends on many factors including, but not limited to, patient condition, type of medication or fluid, urgency involved in receiving the fluid or medication, cost, ease of administration, and whether a systemic or local effect is desired.

INTRAVENOUS ADMINISTRATION

Many medications are administered directly into a vein. Intravenous injection is used for drugs or fluids that must rapidly reach high blood levels or would be irritating to tissue or insufficiently absorbed if given by another route (Box 3-4). Certain anesthetics, chemotherapeutic agents, anticonvulsant drugs, and drugs used in cardiopulmonary resuscitation are given intravenously. If an extremely rapid onset of action is required, intravenous or intraosseous administration is the route of choice.

The most frequently used sites for intravenous injection in the dog are the cephalic and lateral saphenous veins. Cats are most often given intravenous injections in the cephalic, medial saphenous, and femoral veins. The jugular vein is used to administer injections in both large and small animals if an intravenous jugular catheter is in place.

Box 3-4	INTRAVENOUS INJECTION

- Occlude the vessel with digital pressure or a tourniquet.
- Grasp the extremity and pull the skin tautly in a distal direction.
- Wipe an alcohol-soaked cotton ball over the hair and skin over a distal section of a peripheral vein.
- Insert a 22- to 25-gauge needle attached to a syringe, with the bevel facing up, through the skin and into the vein.
- Aspirate a small volume of blood into the syringe to ensure the needle is within the vein.
- Release the pressure from the vein.
- Inject the contents of the syringe into the vein.
- Remove the needle, and apply digital pressure to the needle insertion site for 30 to 60 seconds until hemostasis occurs.
- If a hematoma occurs when the needle is inserted, remove the needle and place digital pressure over the hematoma until the bleeding subsides. Make another injection attempt either proximal to the initial site or in a different vein.

To administer an intravenous injection, the vessel is occluded with a tourniquet or digital pressure. Air bubbles are expelled from the syringe before the needle is inserted into the vein. The skin and hair over the vein is swabbed with alcohol, and the needle is then inserted into the vein. Blood will appear in the needle hub when the needle penetrates the vein, but intravenous placement is confirmed by aspirating blood back into the syringe. Pressure is released from the vein, and the syringe contents are injected. The needle is withdrawn, and firm pressure is applied to the venipuncture site until hemostasis occurs.

Intravenous Catheter Placement

When intravenous fluids or drugs must be infused in large volumes, repeatedly, or continuously, a catheter is placed in the cephalic, jugular, or saphenous vein. The technician should be familiar with catheter selection, placement, and maintenance.

The four types of catheters are the butterfly catheter (EZ Set Infusion Set, Becton Dickinson), over-the-needle (OTN) catheter (Angiocath, Becton Dickinson), through-the-needle (TTN) catheters (ICath, CharterMed, Inc.), and single- and multi-lumen guide-wire catheters (MILA International, Inc., or Cook Veterinary Products). If the catheter is to remain indwelling, the over-the-needle, through-the-needle, or guide-wire type is used. Single- or multi-lumen guide-wire catheters are most often placed in the jugular veins in critically ill patients. Detailed instructions for guide-wire catheter placement are available from the manufacturers. Butterfly catheters are used to administer small volumes of fluid and are generally not left indwelling for longer than a few minutes.

Indwelling catheters are placed using aseptic technique to minimize subsequent thrombus formation, phlebitis, and infection. The hair is shaved from the skin on top of the vein, and the skin surface is cleansed a minimum of three times with an antimicrobial solution and alcohol. Ideally, the skin should be in contact with the antimicrobial solution for 2 minutes. If it is necessary to palpate the skin to identify the vein, the area should be rescrubbed or the individual placing the catheter should wear gloves.

Catheters are inspected for irregular surfaces and are usually flushed with heparinized saline (1 unit of heparin per milliliter of 0.9% saline) before insertion. The heparinized saline may prevent development of blood clots within the catheter lumen.

Technician Note

Indwelling catheters are placed using aseptic technique to minimize subsequent thrombus formation, phlebitis, and infection.

Peripheral Vein Catheterization

To place an over-the-needle catheter into a peripheral vein, the skin is aseptically prepared as previously described (Box 3-5). The vessel is occluded with digital pressure or a tourniquet. The extremity is held with the skin pulled tautly to stabilize the vein. A catheter (22-gauge, 2.5 cm long in cats and very young or small dogs; 20-gauge, 2.5 to 3.75 cm long in adult or medium to large dogs) with the stylet in place is aligned parallel with the vein. The tip is inserted through the skin and into the vein at a 20-degree angle in as distal a site as possible. When blood enters the hub of the stylet, the catheter and stylet are advanced an additional few millimeters to ensure the catheter tip is well within the vessel lumen (Figure 3-21). The catheter is then slid off the stylet, which is held stationary, and into the vein. In a patient with sufficient blood pressure, blood will trickle out the end of the catheter if it is within the vein lumen. Digital pressure is removed once the catheter enters the vein. A cap is quickly and tightly placed on the end, and the catheter is flushed with 1 ml of heparinized saline. The saline should pass through the catheter without resistance.

Adhesive tape in 1.3- to 2.5-cm-wide strips is wrapped around the circumference of the catheter and leg to secure the catheter. An antibiotic ointment-treated gauze sponge is taped over the catheter entry site. Tape is placed underneath the catheter cap to isolate it from the skin. It is important that the tape not be applied too tightly or the limb may swell. If this occurs, the catheter should be retaped or removed.

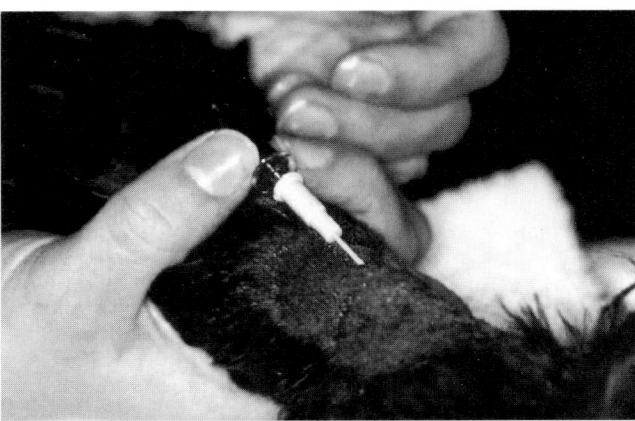

FIGURE 3-21. Technique for placement of an over-the-needle type of catheter into the cephalic vein of a dog.

Box 3-5	INTRAVENOUS CATHETER PLACEMENT IN A PERIPHERAL VEIN

- Flush a 20- to 22-gauge, 2.5- to 3.75-cm over-the-needle catheter with a small volume of heparinized saline.
- Shave and aseptically prepare the skin over the distal portion of the vein.
- Occlude the vein with digital pressure or a tourniquet.
- Align the catheter, with the stylet in place, parallel to the vein.
- Insert the catheter into the skin and vein with the bevel facing upward.
- When blood enters the hub of the catheter, advance the catheter an additional few millimeters.
- Hold the stylet in place and slide the catheter into the vein. Remove the digital pressure or tourniquet as the catheter is advanced.
- Immediately place a catheter cap into the hub of the catheter.
- Inject 1 ml of heparinized saline into the catheter to check patency.
- If the fluid does not inject without resistance the catheter is either kinked, occluded with a blood clot or tissue plug, or extravascular and should be reflushed, repositioned, or replaced.
- If a hematoma occurs during catheter placement, remove the catheter and apply pressure to the hematoma site until hemostasis occurs. Reattempt catheter placement further proximal to the initial entry site or in a different vein.
- Secure the catheter in place with adhesive tape.

Jugular Vein Catheterization

A flexible, 16- to 22-gauge, 20- to 30-cm, through-the-needle catheter is used to catheterize the jugular vein. The size required depends on the size of the animal. Gloves, preferably sterile ones, should be worn to place a through-the-needle catheter in a central (jugular, medial saphenous/femoral) vein.

For jugular catheterization, the ventral surface of the neck is shaved and aseptically prepared. An assistant restrains the patient in lateral recumbency with the front legs pulled caudally and the neck extended. In feline patients, it may be helpful to slightly externally rotate the head. The vein that will be used faces away from the table and is occluded at the thoracic inlet.

The plastic needle guard is removed to expose the catheter needle. The needle is inserted through a fold of tented skin just lateral to the vein in the cranial third of the neck (Figure 3-22, *A*). After the needle penetrates the skin, the needle tip is inserted into the vein. Successful placement is usually denoted by a flashback of blood within the catheter lumen. Once the needle enters the vein, the catheter is fed into the vein through a protective sleeve (Figure 3-22, *B*).

If resistance is met as the catheter is advanced, the catheter is most likely extravascular. The catheter or the patient's head and neck are slightly repositioned and catheter advancement is reattempted. If difficulty in threading the catheter persists, it should be removed and catheterization reattempted at a different site or with a new catheter. The catheter should never be backed out through the introducer needle because the bevel may sever the catheter and create an embolus.

Once the catheter is successfully placed within the vein, the needle is backed out of the skin and covered with the needle guard. Firm pressure is held over the site of skin entry for 30 seconds to control bleeding. The plastic sleeve and stylet are removed, and extension tubing (TPort, Becton Dickinson) prefilled with heparinized saline is firmly placed on the end of the catheter. Approximately 3 ml of heparinized saline is flushed through the catheter to confirm placement within the vein. It should be possible to aspirate blood through a jugular catheter to check patency (Figure 3-22, *C*). In many instances, the animal's head position may need to be adjusted to aspirate blood from the catheter.

A 2.5-cm portion of the catheter is usually left exposed and looped at the skin entry site. If the entire length of a long catheter is inserted into a small patient's jugular vein, the end of the catheter may inadvertently enter the heart. If this occurs, an additional length of catheter can be backed out of the skin.

After placement, the jugular catheter must be secured to the neck. A gauze sponge containing a small amount of antibiotic ointment is taped on top of the catheter entry site and covers any exposed catheter (Figure 3-22, *D*). A long strip of tape is placed longitudinally along the needle guard-hub interface to prevent the catheter from backing out of the needle hub. This strip of tape is also wrapped around the circumference of the neck. Stretch gauze is wrapped several times around the neck to cover the catheter and is taped to the skin at the cranial and caudal borders (Figures 3-22, *E* and *F*). If the patient has a history of vomiting, waterproof tape placed on top of the stretch gauze will help keep the bandage dry. Dogs with jugular catheters should be walked on a harness or leash looped behind one or both front legs to prevent the leash from rubbing against the catheter.

A long, through-the-needle catheter can be placed in a saphenous vein using the same technique as with jugular catheter placement. It is advantageous to use the saphenous vein when the jugular vein is inaccessible or if the patient is vomiting or has a disease affecting the neck (cervical disease). Saphenous catheter placement is not recommended in recumbent animals that cannot stand to void or have diarrhea or fecal incontinence. In such patients, application of an outer layer of waterproof tape will help keep the bandage dry.

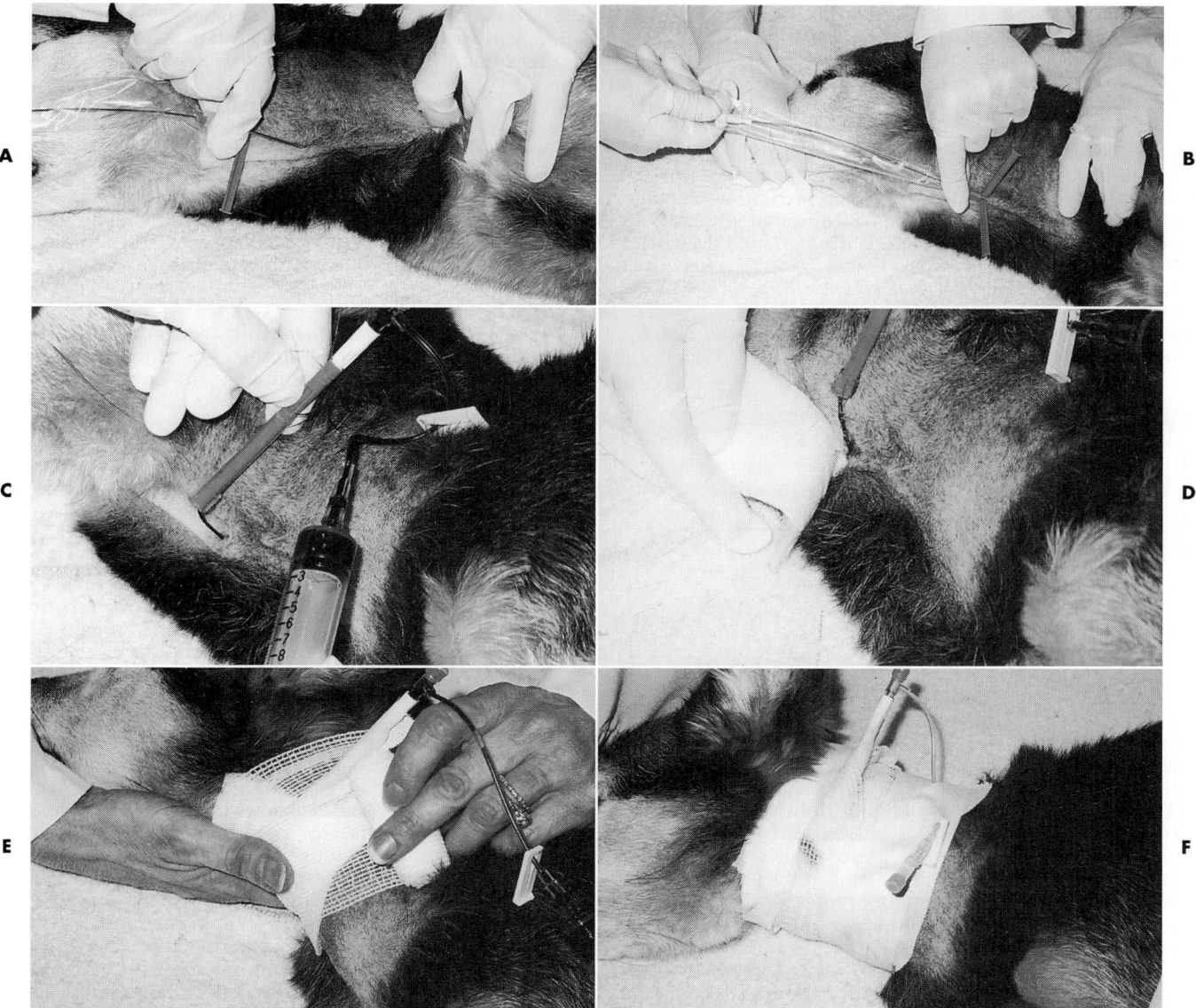

FIGURE 3-22.   A, Needle (with plastic guard folded back) being inserted through skin just lateral to left jugular vein. B, Catheter being fed into the vein through a protective plastic sleeve. C, Needle has been removed from vein and the plastic guard folded back over the needle. The catheter remains in the vein exiting through the needle. The patency of the catheter is checked by aspirating on the syringe. D, An antibiotic ointment is placed on a gauze sponge and applied to the catheter entry site. E, The catheter is secured to the neck with gauze. F, The gauze wrap is covered with waterproof tape.

A long, through-the-needle catheter placed in the jugular or saphenous vein is in direct communication with the vena cava. A major advantage of placement of a long catheter in a central vein is the ability to obtain blood samples directly from the catheter. To collect blood from a long catheter, the "three-syringe technique" is used. The individual, wearing gloves, removes approximately 3 to 5 ml of blood from the catheter with a sterile, heparinized syringe and sets it aside. A second empty syringe is then attached to the catheter, and a blood sample is drawn. The blood from the first syringe is injected back into the catheter, and 2 ml of heparin-ized saline from a third syringe is flushed through the catheter.

Another advantage to the use of a large-gauge, through-the-needle catheter in a central vein is the ability to administer fluids at a more rapid rate than via a short peripheral catheter, which has a narrower lumen. In addition, central venous pressure can be monitored through a catheter placed into the anterior vena cava via the jugular vein or into the caudal vena cava via the saphenous vein. However, through-the-needle catheters are more expensive and require more expertise to place than short, over-the-needle catheters.

Arterial Catheter Placement

Indwelling arterial catheters allow blood pressure monitoring and collection of multiple arterial blood samples. A 22-gauge, 2.5-cm over-the-needle catheter is placed in the dorsal metatarsal artery. The method for arterial venipuncture is previously described in this chapter. Arterial catheter placement technique is similar to that of venous catheter placement except the artery is not occluded. Arterial placement is more uncomfortable than venous catheter placement and is not well tolerated in awake animals. In addition, flushing the arterial catheter may cause the patient some discomfort. *Medications and fluids, with the exception of small boluses of heparinized saline, are never administered via an arterial catheter.* The catheter should be clearly labeled as "arterial" and "not for injection."

Technician Note

Indwelling arterial catheters are placed to allow blood pressure monitoring and collection of multiple arterial blood samples.

Intravenous and Intraarterial Catheter Maintenance

Several important points must be made with regard to maintenance of indwelling intravenous or intraarterial catheters. Catheters should be inspected every few hours and should not be left in place for longer than 72 hours. One exception to the 72-hour rule is catheters placed under strictly aseptic conditions in a central vein, such as those placed to administer total parenteral nutrition (TPN). Such catheters may remain indwelling for longer than 72 hours if catheter or catheter site complications are not noted. The type of material used for catheter construction (i.e., polypropylene, polyvinyl chloride, polyethylene, silicone rubber, polyurethane, nylon, etc.) is also a factor in the determination of the length of time a catheter remains in place. Generally, catheters made of polypropylene and polyethylenes are less likely to stimulate vessel irritation and thrombosis than those constructed of silicone rubber, nylon, polyurethane, and polyvinyl chloride.

The catheter site is checked frequently for pain, redness, swelling, and discharge; if any is noted, the catheter should be removed and a new one placed in a different vein. If catheter-induced bacteremia or septicemia is suspected, the tip of the catheter is submitted for bacterial culture after removal. When swelling is attributed to overly constrictive tape or bandage material and the catheter is still patent, the catheter can be rewrapped more loosely. If the bandage material feels damp, the bandage is removed and the catheter inspected for leakage around the skin entry site and catheter cap. Sometimes blood or fluid leakage is from a loosely applied catheter cap. It is not uncommon to find bandage material wet simply from a spilled water bowl.

From 0.5 to 2 ml of heparinized saline is used to flush venous catheters every 4 to 6 hours and arterial catheters every 2 hours to maintain patency. If a patient is receiving a continuous infusion of fluids, the catheter is generally flushed every 8 to 12 hours. If the catheter does not flush without resistance or if blood cannot be aspirated back into the syringe, the catheter may be bent, be occluded with a blood clot, have a loose catheter cap, or be extravascular.

Catheters should be checked for patency before medication is injected and should be flushed with heparinized saline after drug administration. Nonheparinized saline is used to flush a catheter if the drug is known to precipitate with heparin. When multiple medications are given consecutively, it is important to flush between them to prevent the precipitation that may occur if they mix.

When a catheter is removed, a gauze sponge onto which a small amount of antibiotic ointment is applied is taped over the puncture site. When an arterial catheter is removed, the puncture site is covered with a pressure bandage for 10 minutes followed by a regular gauze bandage.

Intravenous Chemotherapy Administration

Use of chemotherapeutic agents to treat neoplasia is becoming more common in companion animal practices. The veterinary technician should be familiar with chemotherapy administration protocols and safety precautions (see Chapter 10). Because many chemotherapeutic agents are carcinogens, it is advisable to minimize exposure to the drugs during administration. Latex gloves, safety glasses, masks, and nonpermeable, long-sleeved, elastic-cuffed gowns should be worn. Materials used for chemotherapy administration should be disposed of in leak-proof hazardous waste containers. Drug aerosolization is decreased if an alcohol-soaked gauze sponge is placed over the catheter cap when the needle on the chemotherapy drug syringe is inserted into or removed from the catheter.

Intravenous catheters are used to administer cytotoxic solutions, especially those that cause tissue irritation when injected extravascularly. Examples of such drugs, which are termed *vesicants*, include doxorubicin, vincristine, vinblastine, and actinomycin D.

Intravenous chemotherapy catheters must be placed with extreme care. The catheter should be placed in a peripheral vein, and the vessel must be punctured only once during placement. If a "clean stick" is not achieved on the first placement attempt, a different vein should be used. This prevents tissue irritation from drug leakage from the previous puncture site. It is permissible, but not advisable, to place the catheter in the same vein, in a more proximal site, if the initial site has been given time to seal with a clot. Nonheparinized 0.9% sterile saline should be used to flush the catheter when using specific chemotherapy drugs, such as doxorubicin, that precipitate when mixed with heparin.

Catheters used for drug administration should be frequently evaluated for patency. The area proximal to the catheter site should be freely visible to observe for extravasation. Signs that the chemotherapeutic agent has leaked out of the vein include loss of catheter patency, redness or swelling at or proximal to the injection site, or vocalization or signs of discomfort by the patient.

If extravasation occurs, as much of the drug should be removed from the site as possible by aspirating 5 ml of blood back through the catheter. The tissue surrounding the site is infused with saline, corticosteroids, or 2% lidocaine, and either warm or cold compresses are applied depending on the chemotherapy drug used.

When chemotherapy administration is complete, the catheter is flushed with several milliliters of sterile, nonheparinized 0.9% saline. An alcohol-soaked gauze sponge covers the catheter as it is removed from the vein. The skin puncture site is covered with an antibiotic-treated gauze and securely bandaged.

When less than 3 ml of chemotherapeutic drug, such as vincristine, is injected intravenously, a 23- or 25-gauge butterfly catheter is often used. After the drug is administered, the catheter is flushed with several milliliters of saline. The tubing is crimped to prevent fluid from leaking back out of the catheter and the needle is removed from the vein. The needle is covered with an alcohol-soaked gauze pad as it is removed from the skin, and the venipuncture site is bandaged.

SUBCUTANEOUS ADMINISTRATION

The subcutaneous injection is easily and frequently performed and is the most common route for vaccine administration. Although absorption may be slow in obese animals because of the relatively poor vascular supply in fat, subcutaneous injections in general allow for relatively rapid absorption of the injected substance. However, the subcutaneous route is not recommended in severely dehydrated or critically ill patients when immediate absorption is required. In an emergency situation, the intravenous or intraosseous routes provide much faster absorption. The intravenous route is preferred when large volumes of fluid must be administered.

Moderate volumes of isotonic fluids can be injected under the skin to rehydrate animals if intravenous or intraosseous access is unavailable. Approximately 50 to 100 ml of body-temperature fluids can be injected per site, depending on patient size. Owners of patients that may require long-term fluid supplementation at home (i.e., chronic renal disease) can be instructed in how to administer subcutaneous fluids.

The preferred site for most subcutaneous injections is the dorsolateral region from the neck to the hips. The dorsal region of the neck and back should be avoided because of the difficulty in treating any abscesses or masses that may occur after injection. When administering vaccinations, especially to feline patients, the intrascapular region should be avoided because of the incidence of vaccine-induced tumors. Feline vaccinations should be administered in as distal a portion of an extremity as possible (Figure 3-23). The following sites are recommended for feline vaccination: rhinotracheitis-calici-panleukopenia: right front leg; rabies: right rear leg; feline leukemia: left rear leg. Intrascapular injection should also be avoided for insulin injections because of the relatively poor absorption of insulin from that site and fibrosis that may occur with repeated injections. Insulin should be injected in alternating sites along the dorsolateral or ventrolateral aspect of the trunk.

To administer a subcutaneous injection, a fold of skin is tented, and the needle is inserted at the base of and parallel to the long axis of the fold (Figure 3-23). If the needle is inserted perpendicular to the long axis, the needle may penetrate both sides of the skin and the syringe contents may be accidentally deposited on the patient's hair. The syringe plunger is retracted slightly, and the needle hub is checked for blood before injection. If blood appears in the hub, a vessel has been penetrated, and the needle should be removed and reinserted in another location. After injection, the skin is briefly massaged to facilitate drug distribution. If multiple vaccinations or medications are to be administered, the injection sites should be a minimum of several centimeters apart.

Technician Note

Vaccine injection into the intrascapular region should be avoided.

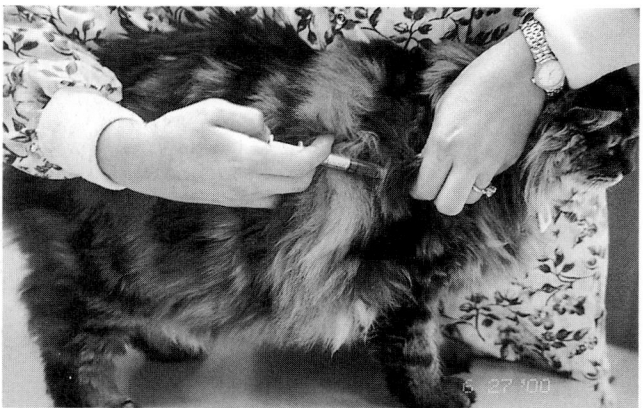

FIGURE 3-23.   Subcutaneous injection made into tented skin on the lateral aspect of the front leg. Note administration of feline vaccination in the intrascapular region is avoided.

INTRAMUSCULAR ADMINISTRATION

The intramuscular route is appropriate for injection of small volumes of medication. Drugs are most often administered in the lumbosacral musculature lateral to the dorsal spinous processes or in the semimembranosus or semitendinosus muscles of the rear leg. Deep lumbar injections in the third to fifth lumbar region are used to administer heartworm treatment (Figure 3-24). Placement of the needle in the lumbosacral muscles is not recommended in very thin animals. When injections are made into the semimembranosus or semitendinosus muscles the needle should enter the lateral aspect of the muscle and be directed caudally to avoid penetration of the sciatic nerve (Figure 3-25). Contact of the needle with the sciatic nerve may cause pain and lameness. Occasionally, the triceps muscles on the caudal aspect of the front legs are used as injection sites. The neck is never used as a site for intramuscular injection.

To make an intramuscular injection, the muscle is isolated between the fingers and thumb and a 22- to 25-gauge needle attached to a syringe is embedded in the muscle. As with subcutaneous injections, the needle hub is checked for blood before administration of medication to make certain a vessel is not inadvertently penetrated. If blood is observed, the needle is removed and inserted in another site. Once placement within the muscle is verified, the drug is slowly injected. The site is massaged for a few seconds after injection to help distribute the substance.

INTRADERMAL ADMINISTRATION

Intradermal injections are performed to densensitize the skin with a local anesthetic or to perform allergy skin testing. Most animals will not tolerate skin testing unless sedated. Hair on the lateral aspect of the trunk is shaved with a no. 40 clipper blade. The skin is carefully wiped with a water-moistened gauze sponge. Vigorous scrubbing or use of an antimicrobial cleaning solution is contraindicated because skin irritation that may occur interferes with testing. To make an injection, a fold of skin is lifted, and a 25- to 27-gauge needle attached to a 1-ml syringe is inserted, with the bevel up, into the dermis. A 0.1-ml volume of allergen is injected. The injection site will appear like a translucent lump if the injection is performed correctly. The skin is then examined for tissue reaction.

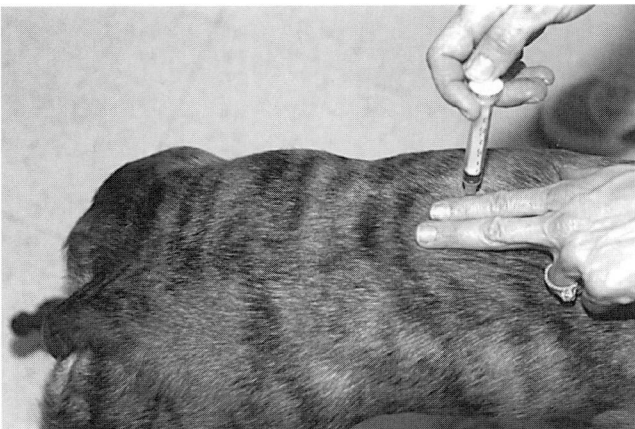

FIGURE 3-24.   Deep intramuscular injection into the lumbar musculature of the dog.

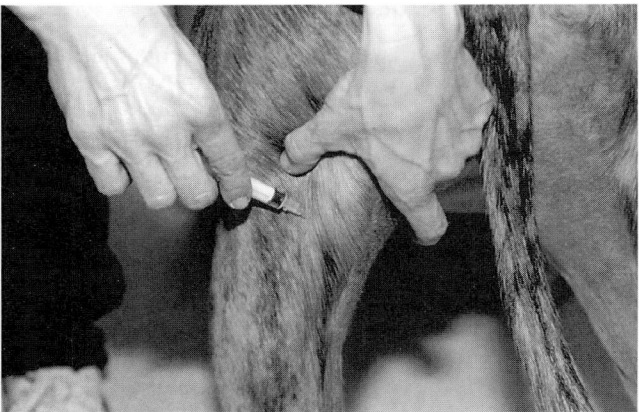

FIGURE 3-25.   Intramuscular injection into the semimembranosus and semitendinosus muscles of the rear leg of the dog.

INTRANASAL ADMINISTRATION

Certain vaccines, such as those for feline infectious peritonitis, feline viral rhinotracheitis-calici-panleukopenia, and *Bordetella bronchiseptica,* are formulated for intranasal (and/or intraocular) administration. The patient's muzzle is held in one hand and elevated slightly. The tip of the vaccine dispenser is placed into the nostril and the dispenser is compressed. Alternatively, the patient's head can be tilted back and the pipette containing the vaccine is squeezed to dispense the liquid onto the plane of the nose. The vaccine runs into each nostril as the animal inhales. This method frequently results in less sneezing after administration than when the dispenser tip is placed directly into the nostril.

Diazepam can be administered intranasally for the immediate treatment of status epilepticus if intravascular access cannot be obtained. Diazepam is absorbed more rapidly into the systemic circulation by the intranasal route than by the intrarectal route.

INTRATRACHEAL ADMINISTRATION

In an emergency situation, such as during cardiopulmonary resuscitation, drugs can be injected directly into the trachea of an unconscious animal. Absorption by this route is extremely rapid.

To perform an intratracheal injection, a polypropylene urinary catheter or rubber feeding tube is inserted into the trachea either directly or through an endotracheal tube. The syringe containing the drug, such as epinephrine, atropine, or lidocaine, is forcefully injected through the urinary catheter or feeding tube. Approximately 10 ml of air or 3 to 10 ml of sterile saline is injected through the catheter or tube immediately afterward to disperse the drug. If a urinary catheter or feeding tube is not available, the drug is sprayed down the endotracheal tube with a syringe and followed by a burst of air. The intratracheal dosage of drugs is usually greater than the intravenous dosage.

 Technician Note

In an emergency situation, such as during cardiopulmonary resuscitation, medications can be injected directly into the trachea because absorption of the drug by this route is extremely rapid.

INTRAOSSEOUS ADMINISTRATION

Needles are placed directly into the bone marrow cavity to deliver fluids, drugs, and blood products when intravenous catheterization is not possible or cannot be performed rapidly. The intraosseous route is often overlooked and may be useful in emergency situations. Medications and fluids quickly enter the central circulation via the intramedullary vessels in the marrow cavity. Intraosseous placement allows rapid fluid delivery to neonates, small animals, and patients with circulatory collapse. Intraosseous needles are removed as soon as intravenous access can be established.

Placement of an intraosseous needle or catheter is contraindicated in septic patients. Catheters should not be placed in bones that are fractured or infected. Skin overlying the insertion site should be free of infection. If the bone cortex is punctured multiple times during insertion attempts, a different bone should be used; fluid that is administered may leak from the bone into the subcutaneous tissue.

Sites for intraosseous administration include the tibia, femur, humerus, and occasionally the ilial wing or ischium. The intraosseous catheter or needle should have a stylet that helps prevent the needle from bending or becoming occluded with a core of bone as it is inserted. Needles used include 15- to 18-gauge bone marrow needles, or specially designed Cook Intraosseous Access Needles. If intraosseous access is needed in a neonate, an 18- to 22-gauge hypodermic needle can be used. If the hypodermic needle plugs with a core of bone, it can sometimes be flushed out with saline. A 22-gauge, 3.75-cm needle can be nested inside an 18-gauge, 2.5-cm needle to serve as a stylet during placement.

Needle placement for the purpose of delivering medications or fluids into the intraosseous space follows the same protocol previously described for needle placement for bone marrow aspiration. To place an intraosseous catheter or needle into the femur, the hip region is shaved and aseptically prepared. The patient is placed in lateral recumbency and the technician stands at the dorsum of the patient. The trochanteric fossa of the femur of the upside leg is identified on the medial aspect of the greater trochanter of the proximal femur.

Approximately 0.5 to 1.0 ml of 2% lidocaine is injected into the skin, subcutaneous tissue, and periosteum over the trochanteric fossa to provide local anesthesia. A stab incision is made through the skin. The femur is grasped, and the hip is held in a flexed position. The intraosseous needle is introduced medial to the greater trochanter and parallel to the femoral shaft. The needle is inserted through the skin incision and into the femur using firm, steady pressure as the wrist is rotated back and forth. Insertion of the needle through a skin incision helps decrease the likelihood that skin contaminants will be carried into the bone. During needle insertion, care is taken to avoid piercing the sciatic nerve, which is posteromedial to the greater trochanter of the femur. When the needle enters the marrow cavity, the needle will feel firmly embedded. Placement can be ascertained through aspiration of bone marrow into a syringe attached to the needle hub.

Once placed, the needle is secured by wrapping a "butterfly" tab of tape around the needle as it exits the skin. The tape is sutured to the skin. A povidone-iodine ointment-treated gauze pad is applied to the skin entry site. A bulky, gauze bandage is placed around the needle for further stabilization. Patency of the intraosseous needle is maintained by flushing every 6 hours with 1 to 2 ml of heparinized 0.9% saline. The needle may remain in place for up to 3 days but is difficult to maintain in an ambulatory patient.

INTRAPERITONEAL ADMINISTRATION

The intraperitoneal route involves placement of substances directly into the abdominal cavity. This route is occasionally used to administer noncaustic fluids, blood products, or medications. It may be used in neonates when intravascular or intraosseous access is difficult to obtain. Specific chemotherapy drugs, such as asparaginase, can be given intraperitoneally. Body temperature fluids may be infused into the abdominal cavity to lavage the abdomen in animals with peritonitis or pancreatitis. Warm or cool fluid intraperitoneal lavage may be used to help treat severely hypothermic or hyperthermic patients.

Substances injected into the peritoneal cavity are absorbed more rapidly than those administered subcutaneously but more slowly than those given by the intravascular or intraosseous route. To administer a drug or fluids into the peritoneal cavity, the ventral abdomen between the umbilicus and the bladder is shaved and aseptically prepared. An 18- to 22-gauge needle or catheter is inserted into the abdominal cavity on the ventral midline a few centimeters caudal to the umbilicus. A syringe is attached and aspirated. If blood or fluid enters the syringe tip, the needle may have punctured a vessel or abdominal organ. The needle is removed, and a new needle is inserted in a different site. If the syringe remains empty when negative pressure is applied, the medication or fluids are injected.

TOPICAL OPHTHALMIC ADMINISTRATION

The topical ophthalmic route of administration is required for medications used to treat ocular diseases or for specific vaccines, such as feline viral rhinotracheitis-calicipanleukopenia (a formulation designed for intranasal/intraocular administration is available). To place medication onto the surface of the eye, good restraint is essential or the medications will be inadvertently placed on the eyelids or face. The tip of the medication dispenser should not contact any surface, including the cornea, because it may become contaminated or scratch the cornea. Eye

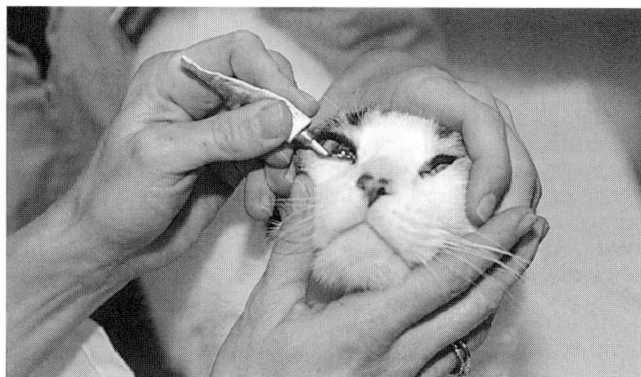

FIGURE 3-26. Ophthalmic ointment is placed on the lower palpebral border in a cat.

medication should be used exclusively by the patient for whom it is dispensed. Sharing ophthalmic medications may transmit ocular infections between patients. If the solution appears to be contaminated (i.e., a clear solution now looks cloudy), contains flecks of material, or has a color change, it should not be used.

To administer substances by the ophthalmic route, the solution or ointment is slightly warmed by holding the container in the palm of the hand for 1 or 2 minutes. This makes administration more comfortable for the patient. The lids are held open with the thumb and index finger of one hand as one drop of medication is deposited onto the sclera. It is helpful to rest the hand holding the medication on the patient's head as the drops are dispensed. To administer ointment, the lids are held open with the thumb and index finger of one hand and a 5-mm strip of ointment is squeezed onto the upper sclera or lower palpebral border (Figure 3-26). The ointment is dispersed across the cornea when the patient blinks. Some technicians find it easier to administer medication if the patient's upper lid is held closed and the medication is placed inside the lower lid.

If multiple topical medications are to be administered into the same eye, they are given a minimum of 3 to 5 minutes apart to allow for sufficient absorption. If both a solution and an ointment are to be applied, the liquid is placed in the eye at least 3 to 5 minutes before the ointment. If the ointment is given first, it may coat the cornea and interfere with absorption of the solution.

AURAL ADMINISTRATION

The ear should be cleared of debris before medication is placed in the ear canal. Precleaning increases the amount of contact between the drug and the epithelium and enhances medication absorption.

To place medication in the ear canal, the pinna is grasped and pulled upward and back toward the head. The tip of the medication dispenser is placed into the vertical ear canal, and the dispenser is squeezed. The base of the ear is then massaged to distribute the medication.

TRANSDERMAL ADMINISTRATION

Certain medications applied topically to the skin have systemic as well as local effects. Many drugs commonly administered by the oral route, such as prednisone or methimazole, can be formulated into an ointment for transdermal application. Other medications, such as nitroglycerin, are manufactured as a cream to be applied directly on the skin.

Medications, such as nitroglycerin, may be absorbed by the individual making the application. Disposable gloves are worn to prevent absorption. A small quantity of ointment is applied to a sparsely haired region, such as the pinna of the ear, the groin, or a shaved area on the ventral thorax. If gloves are unavailable, the ointment can be applied to a small piece of wax paper and wiped onto the skin. The treated area is covered with a light bandage so it will not be accidentally touched. A note is placed on the front of the patient's cage specifying the medication used, the site to which the medication has been applied, and the duration of time that must pass before the application site can be safely touched.

Many topical medications are dispensed in a liquid or aerosol form to control fleas, ticks, mites, heartworms, and intestinal parasites. Depending on the product, the medication is either sprayed on the hair on the entire body or applied to the skin between the shoulder blades. Manufacturer's directions regarding application should be followed closely. Gloves are worn during application, and the site of administration should not be touched for a specified period of time after application.

Transdermal application of analgesics is gaining popularity. One analgesic manufactured in a form specifically for transdermal application is fentanyl citrate. A fentanyl-impregnated self-adhesive patch is placed directly onto a shaved, dry region of skin. The technician should not touch the adhesive side of the patch containing the fentanyl because the medication is absorbed topically. Gentle pressure is applied with the palm of the hand over the patch application site for 1 minute to help the patch adhere to the skin. Each patch can only be applied once—it may not adhere to the skin and deliver the complete dose of fentanyl if it is removed and reapplied. The patch is covered with tape onto which the date and time of placement are recorded.

It is important to place the fentanyl patch in a location in which the animal cannot remove it, such as on the intrascapular region. It should not be applied to skin that will be in contact with a heating pad, heat lamp, or other heat source. The rate of drug delivery is increased when the skin beneath the patch warms and the cutaneous vessels vasodilate.

Topical application of creams (e.g., EMLA Cream, lidocaine and prilocaine) desensitizes the skin so that venipuncture is more comfortable for the patient. This topical anesthetic must be in contact with the skin for at least several minutes (usually 30 to 60) for it to reach its maximum effectiveness.

INTRARECTAL ADMINISTRATION

The mucosa of the large intestine is capable of absorbing medications delivered intrarectally. Medications delivered by this route may have both local and systemic effects. Absorption is most effective when the intestine is free of fecal material. Antiemetic tablets or suppositories can be administered intrarectally to vomiting patients that cannot be medicated orally. A gloved, lubricated finger is used to insert the tablet into the rectum a distance of at least 5 cm. The medication is then gradually absorbed.

Antiseizure drugs, such as diazepam, can be given intrarectally if intravenous or intranasal administration is difficult to perform. A lubricated short rubber feeding tube or urinary catheter is inserted 8 to 10 cm into the rectum. The diazepam is placed into a syringe and injected through the catheter. Several milliliters of warm water are then flushed into the catheter to disperse the drug. Diazepam can also be injected directly into the rectum with a needleless syringe.

Enemas are also administered per rectum. A syringe containing the enema is lubricated and inserted into the rectum. After the enema is injected, the animal should be placed in an area to void, such as outdoors or near a litter box.

Warm water enemas are administered through lubricated plastic tubing inserted through the rectum and into the large intestine. Water is funneled or injected into the end of the tube held in a raised position. The tube is moved back and forth and is slowly advanced up the intestinal tract as fecal material is expelled.

When a medication, such as lactulose, is added to the enema solution, it must be retained within the large intestine for a specified length of time. The solution is injected into a urinary catheter or feeding tube placed into the descending colon. The rectum is held closed with a gloved hand to prevent the enema from exiting. After the allotted time has passed, the catheter is removed and the intestine is evacuated.

ORAL ADMINISTRATION

Administration of medication by direct placement into the oral cavity is frequently and easily performed. Technicians should be adept at giving oral medications to animals and capable of demonstrating techniques to pet owners.

> **Technician Note**
>
> Technicians should be adept at orally medicating animals and able to demonstrate techniques to pet owners.

Oral medications are usually administered in liquid, capsule, or tablet form. Liquids are easy to administer via a dropper or syringe. Pulverized tablets and the contents of capsules can be mixed with a small volume of food, water, or flavored liquid. To administer liquids with a syringe or dropper, the patient's lower lip is pulled out at the commissure. The tip of the syringe or dropper is placed between the cheek and the gums, and small volumes of liquid are injected. The muzzle should be held at a neutral angle and not elevated. Hyperextension of the neck or movement by the patient during administration may result in fluid aspiration into the trachea. If the animal struggles or coughs or if fluid spills out of the mouth, the animal should be allowed to rest before further medication attempts.

A tablet or capsule is most easily administered to a dog if it is hidden in meat, cheese, or a chunk of canned pet food. Cats rarely consume pills hidden in food. Cats will meticulously eat the food that surrounds the pill and leave the medication. If a patient has a diminished appetite it may not consume the entire amount of medication-laced food and will not receive a sufficient dose of medication.

An animal that will not consume baited food is medicated by tilting the head back, prying open the jaws, and placing the pill far back on the base of the tongue (Figures 3-27 and 3-28). The tablet will be expelled if it is not placed far enough back in the pharynx. The technician holds the muzzle closed, rubs under the animal's chin, taps the tip of the nose, or blows air into the nostrils to stimulate the animal to swallow. When the animal licks its nose, it can be assumed that the tablet has been swallowed.

A specially designed device is available to administer tablets to fractious cats and dogs. The tablet is secured in the tip of a plastic rod that is inserted into the back of the mouth. The rod plunger is quickly depressed, and the pill is propelled down the esophagus. Technicians can demonstrate the use of the "pill gun" to owners for administration of medication at home.

Orogastric Intubation

Sometimes it is necessary to administer medication, food, or fluids through a tube passed through the mouth and directly into the stomach. This technique is used to administer activated charcoal solutions or lavage the stomach to treat animals that have ingested toxins. Orphan or weak neonates who cannot nurse can be fed milk replacer via a tube passed through the mouth and into the distal esophagus or stomach. An orogastric tube is also passed to

attempt to decompress a patient with gastric dilation (bloated stomach). Dogs usually permit orogastric tube placement with moderate resistance. Cats, with the exception of neonates, usually require sedation.

The length of 10 to 22 Fr plastic or rubber tube required to extend from the tip of the nose to the thirteenth rib is measured and marked on the tube with tape or ink (Figure 3-29). If the tube is to be placed in the distal esophagus to feed an animal, the distance between the tip of the nose and the eighth rib is marked. Water-soluble gel is used to lubricate the tip of the tube. The animal is restrained in sternal recumbency or in a standing or seated position. A roll of tape, a plastic or wooden speculum with a hole in the middle, or a plastic syringe case with smooth ends is placed behind the canine teeth to hold the mouth open. The muzzle is kept in a normal position and held so the mouth speculum does not become dislodged.

The tube is slowly passed through the speculum (Figure 3-30). Swallowing will be noted as the tube passes over the base of the tongue and into the esophagus. If the animal coughs, the tube may have entered the trachea and should

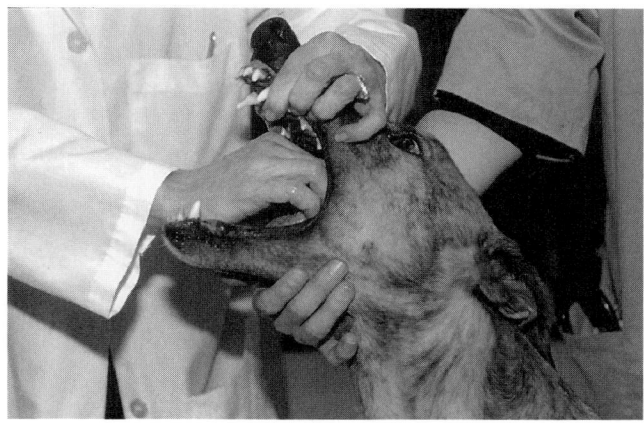

FIGURE 3-27. A dog's muzzle is held open as a tablet is placed into the back of the mouth.

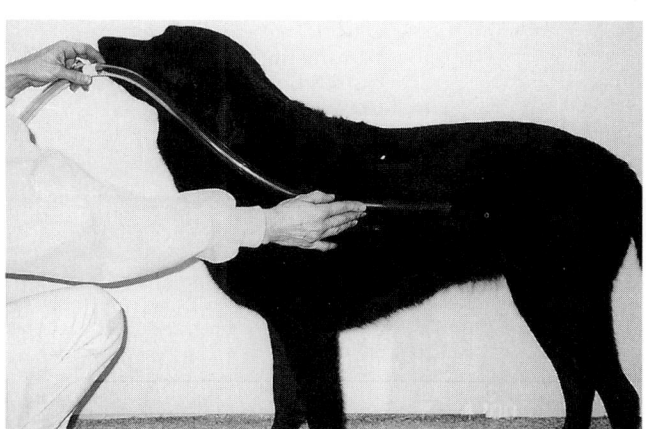

FIGURE 3-29. A length of stomach tube is measured from the nose to the thirteenth rib. It is then marked with tape.

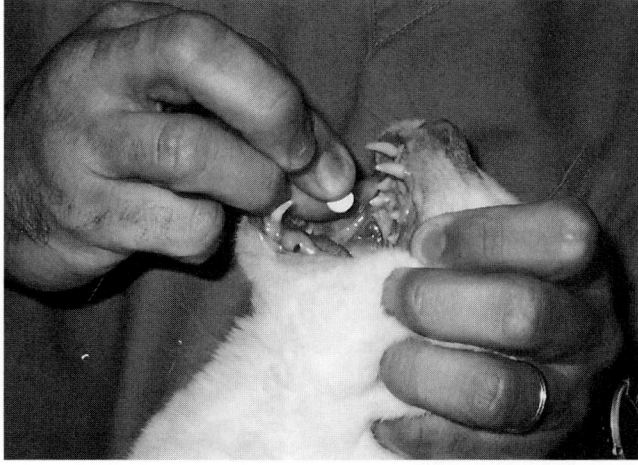

FIGURE 3-28. A cat's neck is hyperextended so the nose points toward the ceiling. The lower jaw is held open as a tablet is placed in the back of the mouth.

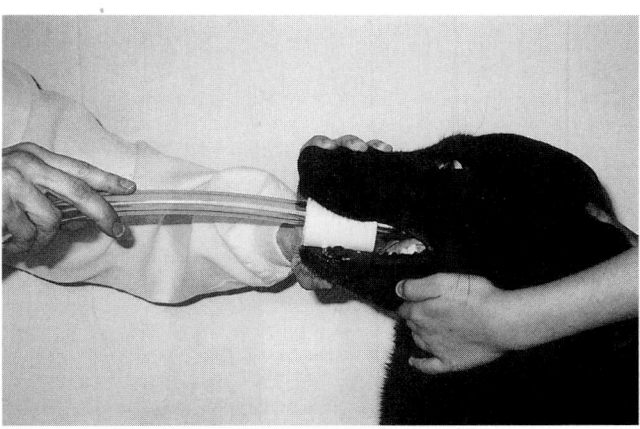

FIGURE 3-30. A roll of tape holds the mouth open as a stomach tube is placed into the oral cavity.

be removed. Once the tube is in the esophagus, it is advanced the premeasured length until it enters the stomach.

Correct placement of the tube in the gastrointestinal tract should always be verified before the introduction of any medications or fluids. Refer to the following section on nasoesophageal tubes for instruction on how to check tube placement.

Fluid is added to the tube with a 60-ml syringe, metal drench pump, or funnel. On completion of fluid administration, the tube is bent to occlude it and withdrawn in a downward direction. This technique prevents a back flow of fluid from entering the trachea.

ENTERAL FEEDING TUBES

Critically ill animals may not be able to normally consume enough calories for proper nutrition and therefore require nutritional support. If the gastrointestinal tract is capable of digestion and absorption, then food slurries, fluid, or medication can be administered via tubes placed directly into the pharynx, esophagus, stomach, duodenum, or jejunum. The technician needs to be familiar with the technique that the veterinarian uses to place enteral feeding tubes and be knowledgeable about tube maintenance.

Nasoesophageal tubes are occasionally used for short-term feeding and the administration of medications. If nutritional support is required beyond 10 days, placement of a gastrostomy tube is preferred (Figure 3-31). If the stomach must be bypassed completely, a duodenostomy or jejunostomy tube is surgically placed.

Enteral feeding tubes should be flushed before and after use with a small volume of warm water to help prevent lumen obstructions. Fluids should always be injected slowly. Before the injection of fluid into a gastrostomy tube, the tube is aspirated with a syringe to make certain the stomach contents have emptied from the previous feeding. If the stomach is still full, the veterinarian should be consulted; the full volume of the next meal should not be instilled into the gastrostomy tube until the previous meal has passed from the stomach. The tube insertion site and tube position are inspected daily to make certain that the tube has not shifted and the skin is free from inflammation, redness, tenderness, or discharge.

Nasoesophageal and Nasogastric Tubes

Nasoesophageal tubes are easy and inexpensive to place in animals that require short-term force-feeding, such as in a severely anorexic cat. These tubes are inappropriate for use in patients that are vomiting or do not have a gag reflex. A 5 to 8 Fr pediatric feeding tube is held up to the animal to determine the appropriate length that is required. For nasoesophageal placement, the distance between the nares and distal esophagus is marked on the tube with ink or tape. Likewise, for nasogastric placement, the distance from the nares to the eighth rib is measured. The patient is held in sternal recumbency, in a seated or standing position. The head is held securely with the neck slightly extended. From 0.5 to 1 ml of 2% lidocaine is infused into one nostril of the dog, or five drops of 0.5% proparacaine is placed into one nostril of the cat. The tip of the tube is coated with xylocaine ointment and placed in the nostril dorsomedial to the alar fold. The tube is advanced into the nostril and directed ventrally. The tube then continues down the ventral meatus and into the nasopharynx. The animal will usually swallow when the tube enters the pharynx.

The tube is placed into the distal esophagus. To check for proper placement, a few milliliters of air are injected into the tube, and the cranial abdomen is simultaneously auscultated. If gurgling sounds are present, the tube has been placed in the gastrointestinal tract. Alternatively, 5 ml of sterile saline may be injected into the tube; if the animal coughs, the tube is in the trachea and should be removed. A radiograph can also be taken to evaluate tube placement.

Suture or tissue adhesive is used to secure the tube to the patient. It should be sutured or glued close to its entrance to the nostril, onto the bridge of the nose, and onto the forehead. The remainder of the tube should be taped to the dorsum of the neck, and the animal should be fitted with an Elizabethan collar to prevent chewing of the tube. A cap is placed on the end of the tube to prevent reflux.

Pharyngostomy Tube Placement

A red rubber feeding tube or silicone pharyngostomy tube ranging in size from 8 to 14 Fr for cats and small dogs and from 14 to 28 Fr for medium-sized to large dogs is used. One end of the tube is flared, and the other is fenestrated. The length of tube needed to span the distance from the angle of the mandible to the distal esophagus is measured and marked on the tube with tape or ink.

Placement of a pharyngostomy tube is performed surgically and requires general anesthesia with endotracheal intubation. The patient is placed in lateral recumbency, and a speculum is placed between the canine teeth to hold open the mouth. The lateral neck area is clipped and aseptically prepped. A gloved index finger is inserted into the mouth and placed between the hyoid apparatus and esophagus. Skin directly over the fingertip is incised with a scalpel blade. A large, curved hemostat is placed through the skin incision and used to bluntly dissect the underlying tissue, muscle, and oral mucosa. The flared end of the

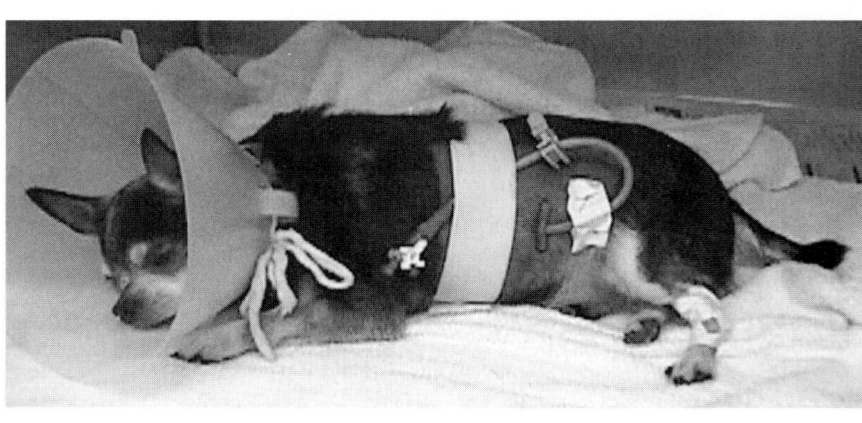

FIGURE 3-31. Gastrostomy tube is placed to feed a postesophageal patient. The Elizabethan collar prevents chewing on the tube or intravenous lateral saphenous catheter.

premeasured tube is brought into the mouth, grasped with the hemostats, and pulled exteriorly through the pharyngostomy site. The fenestrated end of the tube is then directed into the esophagus. Tube placement is checked in the same manner as described for nasoesophageal tubes.

The tube is secured by placing a butterfly tape around the proximal end and suturing the tape to the skin. Alternatively, a Chinese finger-trap suture may be placed around the tube to secure it to the skin. A povidone-iodine-treated gauze sponge should be placed around the skin-tube interface. The tube tip should either be cut so it extends a few centimeters from the skin surface or left long and bandaged over the dorsum of the neck. The exposed tube end is capped with a catheter adapter (ADDTO, Inc.) and a catheter cap (PRN Adapter, Becton Dickinson).

Esophagostomy Tube Placement

Placement of a feeding tube directly into the esophagus to provide nutritional support has proved to be an effective technique. Esophagostomy tubes are better tolerated by patients than are pharyngostomy tubes because they cause less laryngeal irritation and obstruction and are less likely to induce emesis and become dislodged. As such, animals fed via esophagostomy tubes are less likely to aspirate their food than are those fed through pharyngostomy tubes. Placement requires the use of heavy sedation or short-acting anesthesia.

> **Technician Note**
>
> Patients tolerate esophagostomy tubes better than pharyngostomy tubes because they cause less laryngeal irritation and obstruction and are less likely to induce emesis and become dislodged.

A specially designed instrument is available to place esophagostomy tubes, the ELD Gastrostomy Tube Applicator (Jorgensen Laboratories, Inc.). Long hemostats are usually used in lieu of the ELD Applicator by most veterinarians to place esophagostomy tubes; therefore the placement technique using hemostats is given. An instruction sheet detailing the procedure involved in using the ELD Applicator to place an esophagostomy tube is available from the manufacturer.

An esophagostomy tube is placed in the midcervical esophagus on the left side of the neck (Figure 3-32). The animal is placed in right lateral recumbency, and the left

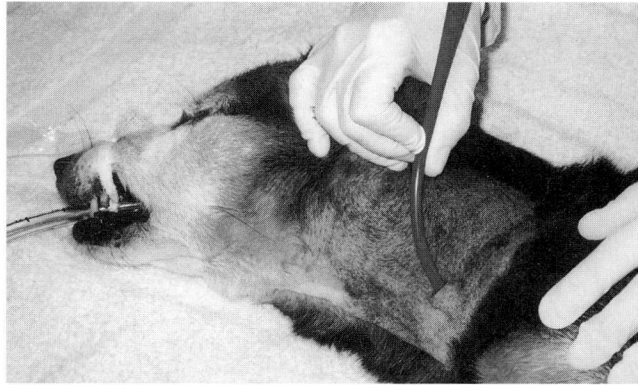

FIGURE 3-32. Esophagostomy tube for enteral feeding is placed into the midcervical esophagus on the left side of the neck.

cervical region is shaved and surgically prepared. The scapulohumeral joint and the angle of the mandible are used as guides to measure the distal and proximal limits of the cervical esophagus. The length of a 20 Fr red rubber feeding tube needed to extend from the skin of the midcervical region to the seventh rib is measured and marked on the tube with ink or tape to place the tube. A pair of extra long curved hemostats is placed into the oral cavity and advanced to the left midcervical region of the esophagus. It is difficult to reach the midcervical region of the esophagus in large-breed dogs when hemostats are used instead of the longer ELD Tube Applicator. The hemostat tips should be palpable on the patient's neck. A stab incision is made with a scalpel blade through the skin and subcutaneous tissue over the tips. The scalpel blade is used to carefully dissect the subcutaneous tissue over the esophagus until the hemostats are able to bluntly penetrate the esophagus. The tips of the hemostats are then brought to the exterior and opened just enough to grasp the fenestrated end of the feeding tube. The hemostats with the attached feeding tube are then withdrawn back through the skin and into the esophagus toward the oral cavity. Once the fenestrated end of the tube reaches the mouth, the tube is bent and redirected back down the esophagus to the level of the seventh rib. Esophagostomy tubes are secured and maintained in the manner described for pharyngostomy tubes. Once esophagostomy tubes are removed, healing occurs by second intention. Stricture of the esophagus at the site of tube placement is minimal after tube removal.

LARGE ANIMAL SAMPLING AND THERAPEUIC TECHNIQUES

VENOUS BLOOD SAMPLE COLLECTION

As with small animals, blood is drawn from large animals to screen for disease and help diagnose the cause of illness. The venipuncture site used depends on the volume of blood needed and the type of restraint available. Venipuncture should not be attempted unless the patient is firmly restrained. The individual that draws the blood or helps with restraint should stand at the side and not in front of the animal. Ideally, cattle and horses should be confined in a chute or stanchion.

Bovine Venipuncture

Blood is collected from cattle from the jugular, coccygeal, or, as a last resort, the subcutaneous abdominal (milk) vein. Either a Vacutainer collection device or a syringe topped with a 16- to 18-gauge, 4-cm needle is used. The skin and hair on top of the vein are wiped with an alcohol soaked gauze before venipuncture to remove superficial contaminants. The vessel is occluded and blood is collected. Digital pressure is applied to the venipuncture site after collection until hemostasis occurs.

> **Technician Note**
>
> Blood is collected from cattle from the jugular or coccygeal vein. The subcutaneous abdominal vein is used on rare occasions.

Jugular Venipuncture

When jugular venipuncture is to be performed, the head is placed in a halter with an attached lead. The head is elevated slightly and drawn to the side opposite the vein to be used. The restraint rope is tied to a stationary object.

The vein is occluded with digital pressure applied to the

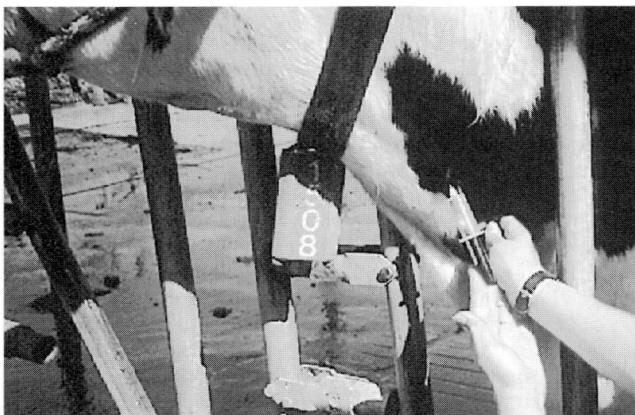

FIGURE 3-33. Bovine jugular venipuncture with a Vacutainer collection device.

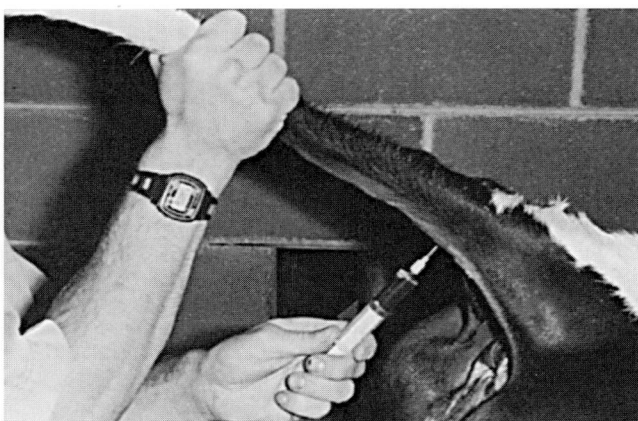

FIGURE 3-34. Venipuncture of the ventral coccygeal vein in the cow.

lower third of the jugular groove. Stroking the groove several times in a downward direction with an alcohol-soaked gauze sponge helps visualize the vein. A needle is placed into the jugular vein at a 45-degree angle. When blood flows out of the needle, the Vacutainer tube is inserted into the needle, and a blood sample is collected (Figure 3-33). When the desired volume has entered the tube, digital pressure is removed. The tube is withdrawn from the needle, and the needle is removed from the vein.

Coccygeal Venipuncture

Blood collection from the coccygeal vein, or "tail vein," is performed when the jugular vein is thrombosed or inaccessible. The coccygeal artery lies close to the vein and should be avoided.

The animal is restrained in a chute, and the tail is grasped and bent toward the back. The ventral surface of the tail is cleaned well with 70% isopropyl alcohol to remove dirt and fecal material. An 18- to 20-gauge, 2.5-cm-long needle with a syringe attached is inserted between the sixth and seventh coccygeal vertebrae, perpendicular to the midline. The needle is inserted until bone is felt and then slowly withdrawn as suction is applied with the syringe. When blood flows into the needle hub, the needle is held in place as a sample is collected (Figure 3-34).

Subcutaneous Abdominal (Milk Vein) Venipuncture

The subcutaneous abdominal vein, located on the mammary gland, can be used as a venipuncture site if the jugular or coccygeal veins are unavailable and only a small volume of blood is needed. Because of the risk of being kicked, the milk vein is only used as a last resort. It is imperative to confine the cow in a stanchion. The technician should stand close to the cow's flank and face toward the cow's head. To collect blood, the skin around the vein is held tautly to stabilize the vein. A 20-gauge, 2.2-cm long needle attached to a 3-ml syringe is inserted into the vein and a blood sample is drawn.

Equine Venipuncture

The jugular vein is used to collect most blood samples from the horse. Many horses can be restrained with a halter and lead rope, but fractious ones may need to be placed in a stock. The restrainer turns the head slightly away from the vein to be sampled. Pressure is placed on the jugular groove in the lower third of the neck to occlude and distend the vein. The vessel is stroked several times in a

downward direction with an alcohol soaked gauze sponge. The method to collect a blood sample from a horse is the same as that previously described in cattle. A 20-gauge, 2.5- to 3.75-cm needle and syringe or Vacutainer collection device is used.

 Technician Note

The jugular vein is used to collect most blood samples from the horse.

In a calm horse, the transverse facial vein of the head is occasionally used to obtain a small volume (less than 1 ml) of blood. The vein courses beneath the facial crest and above the transverse facial artery. A 22- to 25-gauge needle is inserted perpendicular to the skin and into the vein, and blood is collected into a syringe or hematocrit tube.

The external thoracic vein on the cranioventral thorax, the cephalic vein on the medial aspect of the front leg, and the medial saphenous vein on the medial aspect of the rear leg, are alternative sites for blood collection. They are generally only used if the jugular or transverse facial veins are inaccessible.

Porcine Venipuncture

Blood is collected from pigs via the cranial vena cava, external jugular vein, auricular vein, or occasionally the orbital sinus or tail vein. It is more challenging to draw blood from a pig than from most other animals.

Cranial Vena Cava

The right anterior vena cava is used for venipuncture. Because the phrenic nerve courses near the left exterior jugular vein, the left side of the neck should be avoided as a venipuncture site.

To obtain a blood sample from a small pig, the animal is positioned on its back on a 45-degree incline with the head lower than the hips. The head is extended and the front legs are crossed and caudally displaced (Figure 3-35). A 20-gauge, 2.5- to 3.75-cm needle is used in pigs weighing less than 25 kg.

Pigs that weigh more than 25 kg are restrained in a standing position with the front legs parallel and symmetric to each other. An assistant places a hog snare around the maxilla and holds the head slightly elevated in a parallel plane with the body. The individual who takes

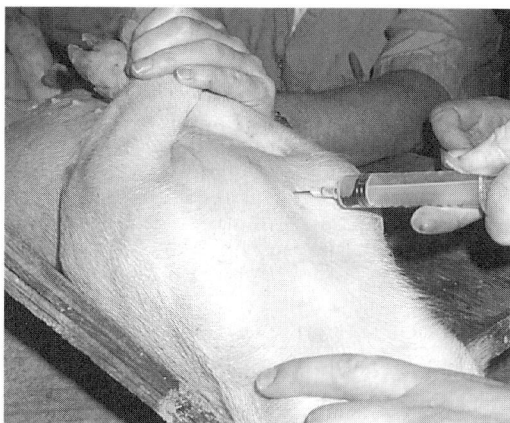

FIGURE 3-35. Venipuncture of the anterior vena cava in a small pig in dorsal recumbency.

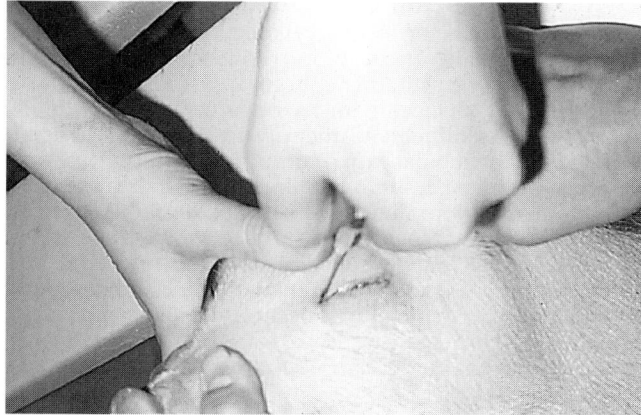

FIGURE 3-37. Small quantities of blood can be collected from the orbital sinus of the pig.

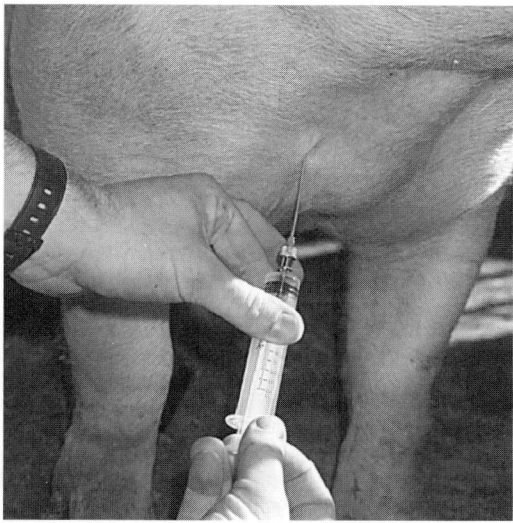

FIGURE 3-36. A blood sample from the anterior vena cava is taken with the needle directed into the jugular fossa just lateral to the manubrium sterni.

the blood sample crouches in front of the right side of the pig. An 18- to 20-gauge, 3.75- to 9.0-cm-long needle with attached syringe is completely inserted into the right jugular fossa just lateral to the manubrium sterni (Figure 3-36). It is placed at a 90-degree angle with the skin of the neck and directed toward the left shoulder. The needle is slowly withdrawn as the syringe plunger is retracted. When blood enters the syringe, the needle is held in place until a sufficient volume is collected.

External Jugular Vein

Blood is frequently collected from the external jugular vein. The needle is inserted near where the internal and external jugular veins merge to become the brachiocephalic vein. A shorter (20-gauge, 3.75-cm-long) needle is used than for cranial vena caval venipuncture, and therefore jugular venipuncture is considered safer for the animal. Because a shorter needle is used and the jugular vein is smaller than the vena cava, the jugular may be more difficult to penetrate in heavier pigs. Venipuncture is per-

formed on the right side of the neck to avoid puncture of the phrenic nerve.

The pig is restrained in a standing position as previously described for vena cava venipuncture. An imaginary horizontal line that passes through the shoulders and manubrium sterni is visualized. A second line is visualized that extends from the manubrium sterni to the scapula at an angle of 45- degrees with the first line. The needle is inserted perpendicular to the skin at the intersection of the second line with the deepest part of the right jugular fossa. The needle is directed caudodorsally and should not be angled toward either scapula. Because the vein is superficial, the syringe plunger should be retracted slightly as soon the needle penetrates the skin. The needle is advanced until blood is aspirated into the syringe. Once a sufficient volume of blood has been collected, the needle is removed.

Auricular Vein

The auricular vein on the dorsal aspect of the pinna is used to collect up to 5 ml of blood. The pig is restrained with a hog snare. A rubber band is placed around the base of the ear to serves as a tourniquet. The ear is held in place and a 20-gauge, 2.5-cm needle attached to a syringe is inserted into the vein. The sample is slowly aspirated into the syringe. When a sufficient volume of blood is collected, the tourniquet is removed and the needle is withdrawn from the vein.

Orbital Sinus

Small quantities of blood can be collected from the venous sinus near the medial canthus of the eye. A 22-gauge needle is inserted into the medial canthus until it contacts bone. The needle is then rotated between the fingers until blood enters the hub (Figure 3-37). A microcapillary tube with the end broken to form a rough point can be used in lieu of a needle. When collection is complete, the needle or capillary tube is removed, and digital pressure is applied over the medial canthus with the head in an elevated position.

Tail Vein

A 20-gauge, 2.5-cm-long needle is occasionally used to collect small volumes (usually less than 5 ml) of blood from the tail vein in adults with intact tails. The vein is located on the ventral midline of the tail.

Ovine and Caprine Venipuncture

The jugular vein is the most accessible site for venipuncture in the sheep and goat. Blood collection is easiest to perform using a Vacutainer collection system, but a 20- to 22-gauge, 2.5-cm needle and syringe can be used. If the jugular vein is difficult to identify in the sheep, wool is pulled over the jugular furrow until the vessel is visualized.

Sheep become passive when tipped up on the rump. For a single-person venipuncture technique, the phlebotomist crouches or stands behind the tipped sheep and slightly moves the head in the direction opposite the vein to be used. One hand occludes the jugular vein, and the other hand holds the Vacutainer collection device or the needle and syringe. The needle is inserted at a 45-degree angle into the jugular vein, and a sample is collected (Figure 3-38).

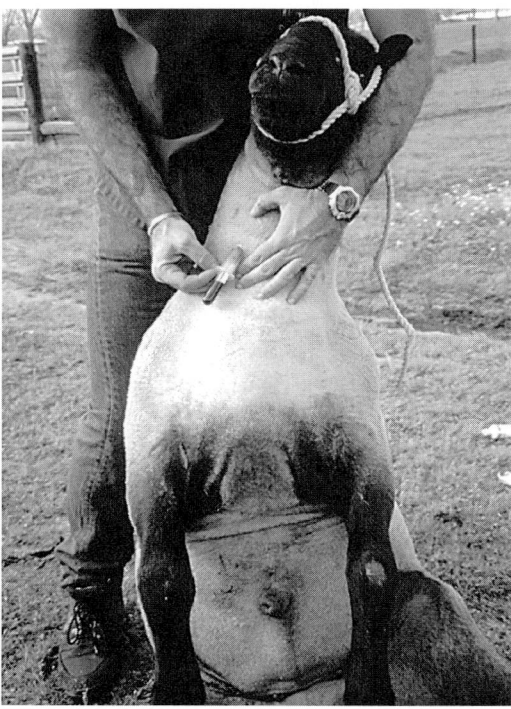

FIGURE 3-38. Sheep placed in a seated position to allow blood to be collected from the jugular vein.

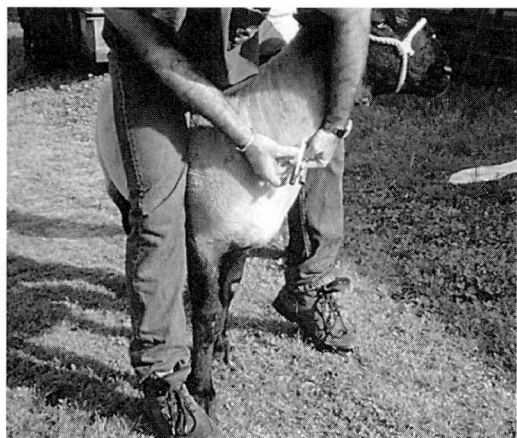

FIGURE 3-39. The venipuncturist straddles the sheep over the shoulders and turns the head to the side to collect blood from the jugular vein.

Blood can be drawn from a standing sheep or goat by straddling it over the shoulders and facing forward. It is helpful to back the animal into a corner to further limit its movement. The venipuncturist holds the sheep's head to the side with the arm that is used to occlude the vein. The other hand is used to collect the blood sample (Figure 3-39).

Although the jugular vein is the easiest site from which to collect a blood sample, the cephalic vein also can be used. The procedure previously described for cephalic venipuncture in the dog can be applied to the sheep and goat.

ARTERIAL BLOOD SAMPLE COLLECTION

Arterial blood samples are obtained to evaluate the respiratory and acid-base status of an animal. Evaluation of blood gas values is most often performed intraoperatively in horses under general anesthesia. Information provided from serial intraoperative blood gases allows the patient's medical status and plane of anesthesia to be monitored more closely.

The carotid and transverse facial arteries are the most frequently sampled arteries in conscious horses. The great metatarsal artery, located on the lateral aspect of the third metatarsal bone, is sometimes used in the foal. When a needle is placed in an artery, bright red blood is expelled from the needle hub in a pulsatile manner. In contrast, if a needle enters a vein, darker red blood will drip out at a slow, constant rate.

The carotid artery lies within in the dorsal aspect of the jugular groove deep to the jugular vein. The artery feels like a cord and a pulse is not palpable. Skin superficial to the artery on the lower third of the right side of the neck is wiped with alcohol. An 18-gauge, 3.75-cm needle is directed into the artery at a 90-degree angle. As the needle in the carotid artery is stabilized with one hand, a heparin-coated syringe is attached and a sample is collected. Bubbles are expelled from the needle and syringe and the needle tip is embedded in a rubber stopper. Firm pressure is held over the needle insertion site for several minutes.

The transverse facial artery is palpated near the lateral canthus of the eye. To collect a blood sample from this site, the skin over the artery is numbed with an injection of 0.25 ml of 2% lidocaine. A 22-gauge, 2.5-cm needle is inserted into the artery. The sample is collected and handled as described above.

A short, over-the-needle catheter can be placed in the artery of an anesthetized patient to monitor intraoperative blood gas values and systemic blood pressure. The catheter can be placed in any of the arteries described above; however, the transverse facial and dorsal metatarsal arteries are most frequently used. The technique for placing and maintaining arterial catheters is previously described in the discussion of intravenous administration of medication in the small animal.

URINE SAMPLE COLLECTION

Urine is collected from large animals to screen for either systemic or urinary tract disease. Urine is routinely collected from race horses for drug analysis. Certain drugs or their by-products can be detected as they are excreted in the urine.

Bovine Urine Collection

Several techniques are used to collect urine from cows. One method to stimulate urination is to stroke the perineum with a piece of straw or your fingers. The tail should not be held aside because it may distract the animal. If stroking the perineum fails to produce a sample, the lips of the vulva can be repeatedly opened and closed to stimulate urination.

Once micturition occurs, a midstream sample is collected in a dry, clean container. If urine is collected for bacterial culture, a sterile specimen cup is used. The initial portion of the stream contains the largest amount of contaminants and should not be included in the sample collected for urinalysis.

Urinary catheterization of the cow is accomplished through use of a sterile flexible or rigid urinary catheter. The perineal region is gently scrubbed with an antiseptic solution and rinsed with warm water. A sterile-gloved, lubricated hand is inserted into the vagina. Fingers are slid approximately 10 cm along the floor of the vagina until the urethral orifice is identified. The catheter is guided into the urethra and advanced until it enters the bladder. Urine will flow through the catheter when it has reached the bladder.

Equine Urine Collection

Catheterization of the mare is performed in a manner similar to that described in the cow. The tail is wrapped to prevent hair from entering the vagina. The vulvar region is aseptically prepared. A sterile-gloved, lubricated hand is placed into the vagina. The urethral opening is located approximately 10 to 12 cm from the ventral commissure of the vulvar lips. The catheter is slid into the urethral orifice and it is advanced 5 to 10 cm until it enters the bladder. Urine should flow into the bladder once it enters the bladder, however, it may be necessary to apply negative pressure with a syringe to stimulate urine flow. The transverse fold of the vagina overlies the opening of the urethral orifice. It is not uncommon to slide the catheter over the transverse fold and miss the urethral orifice beneath it.

Urinary catheterization of the male horse requires tranquilization. Administration of detomidine or a combination of xylazine, butorphanol, and acepromazine sedates the horse and helps extrude the penis from the prepuce. The prepuce and penis are cleansed with warm, dilute antibacterial solution and then rinsed with water. The tip of a sterile, flexible 24- to 28-Fr, 137-cm long urinary catheter is coated with sterile, water-based lubricant. Sterile gloves are worn to grasp the penis and place the catheter, with stylet, approximately 50 to 70 cm into the urethra. It is usually easily advanced through the penile urethra but resistance may be felt as it passes around the ischial arch. At this point, the stylet is gradually withdrawn as the catheter is passed over the pelvis and into the bladder.

When the catheter enters the bladder, urine may flow through the catheter. If is does not, a 60-ml syringe is attached to the catheter and slowly aspirated. If urine still does not flow, a small volume of air can be injected into the catheter or the catheter can be repositioned.

Ovine and Caprine Urine Collection

A 5- to 10-Fr lubricated, sterile canine urinary catheter can be used to blindly catheterize ewes and does. The technique used is the same as described for canine catheterization. Urine can be collected from ewes by holding the nostrils and mouth closed for up to 45 seconds. The ewe will soon struggle to breathe and will urinate. This technique is not highly recommended. A more humane and less stressful way to obtain a urine sample from sheep or goats is to wait until they stand up from a lying down position. They often will urinate when they move from a lying down to a standing position.

Rams and bucks have anatomic obstacles that make urinary catheterization extremely difficult. Urine samples are primarily collected by free catch of voided samples.

FECAL COLLECTION

Feces are collected to examine for intestinal parasites or to culture for organisms such as *Salmonella* spp. Samples can be obtained by simply picking them up from the ground. Alternatively, feces can be manually retrieved from the rectum with a gloved or sleeved hand. The glove or sleeve is turned inside out as it is removed and tied in a knot to store the sample.

RUMEN FLUID COLLECTION

Rumen fluid is collected for analysis in both large and small ruminants. Sometimes rumen fluid is transferred from healthy to sick or weak sheep to inoculate the weak animal's rumen with microorganisms that aid in food digestion.

A medium-size stomach tube lubricated with water-based gel is used to obtain rumen fluid in cattle. Tubes with internal diameters less than 1.5 cm may become obstructed with ingesta and are not recommended for rumen fluid collection.

To perform orogastric intubation, the cow is restrained in a head catch. Nose tongs are placed in the nasal septum to help control head movement. The intubator stands to the animal's side, wraps an arm around the muzzle, and places a speculum into the mouth. One end of the tube is inserted into the speculum, and the other is held in the intubator's mouth. As the animal swallows, the tube is advanced down the esophagus. The intubator blows into the tube to dilate the esophagus, which helps the tube pass through the esophagus and into the rumen.

Placement of the tube within the rumen is confirmed by auscultation of the abdomen as air is simultaneously blown into the tube. Air should be heard bubbling through rumen contents. The distinctive odor of fermented gas will be detected coming from the end of the tube.

Rumen fluid samples are withdrawn from the tube with a dose syringe. The initial fluid portion should be discarded because it often contains an excessive quantity of saliva. This erroneously elevates the pH of the fluid.

When rumen fluid collection is complete, the tube is kinked and removed with a downward motion. This prevents rumen contents from leaking out of the tube and entering the trachea as the tube is withdrawn.

ABDOMINOCENTESIS

Abdominocentesis is performed to obtain samples of abdominal fluid for clinical pathologic evaluation. It is used as a diagnostic technique in horses with suspected peritonitis, colic, chronic diarrhea, weight loss, or fever of unknown origin.

Technician Note

Abdominocentesis is used as a diagnostic technique in horses with colic, chronic diarrhea, weight loss, or fever of unknown origin.

Equine Abdominocentesis

To perform abdominocentesis, the standing horse is restrained in a chute or stanchion. The individual who performs the centesis stands close to the front legs and faces the abdomen to avoid being kicked by the rear legs.

The most dependent site on the ventral midline of the abdomen is clipped and aseptically prepared. Approxi-

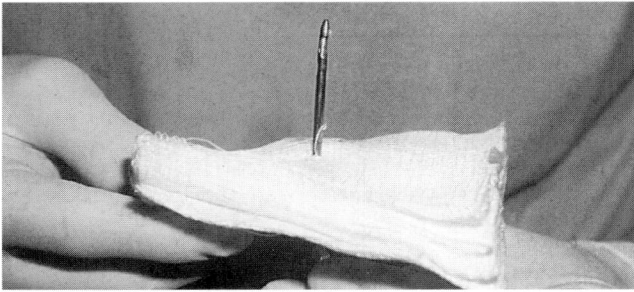

FIGURE 3-40. A teat cannula is pushed through sterile gauze sponges before being inserted into the abdominal cavity to prevent peripheral blood from contaminating the abdominocentesis sample.

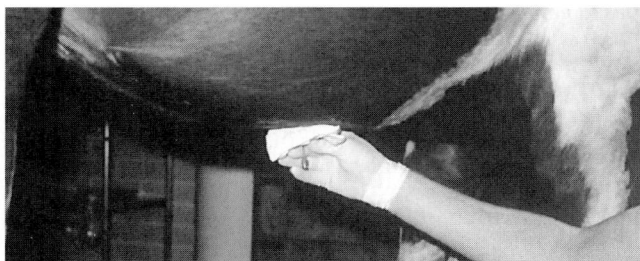

FIGURE 3-41. Abdominocentesis is performed in a horse by passing a teat cannula into the abdominal cavity.

mately 2 ml of 2% lidocaine is infused into the skin and subcutaneous tissue at the abdominocentesis site. Sterile gloves are worn to make a stab incision through the skin with a No. 15 blade. Obvious cutaneous vessels should be avoided. The blade is rotated to form an entrance through which a sterile, 9-cm-long, blunt-ended teat cannula or stainless steel canine urinary catheter may pass. The cannula is pushed through the center of a 4 by 4 sterile gauze sponge and is then inserted through the incision and into the abdominal cavity (Figures 3-40 and 3-41). The gauze prevents blood that drips down the outside of the cannula from contaminating the sample.

The first few drops of fluid that drip from the cannula often contain blood or other contaminants. These first drops should not be included in the collected sample. The sample is collected in sterile tubes with and without anticoagulants. If fluid does not drain, the cannula is rotated or redirected or a syringe is attached to the end and negative pressure is applied.

If a teat cannula is not available, an 18-gauge, 3.75-cm hypodermic needle is used for abdominocentesis in horses and large ruminants, and a 20-gauge, 3.75-cm needle is used in small ruminants. Centesis is performed as previously described except neither a local anesthetic is used nor a blade incision is made prior to needle insertion. If fluid does not flow through the needle, 1 to 2 ml of air is injected to dislodge any particles which might be plugging the needle. Rotation or redirection of the needle or insertion of an additional needle several centimeters away from the initial one may stimulate fluid flow.

Ruminant Abdominocentesis

The site selected for abdominocentesis is determined by which abdominal disorder is suspected. If traumatic reticuloperitonitis is suspected, the centesis site is the ruminoreticular recess. In large ruminants, this recess is in the left

cranial quadrant of the abdomen approximately 5 cm caudal to the xiphoid process and 5 cm to the left of midline. If uterine or small bowel rupture is the concern, centesis is performed 5 cm cranial to the udder and medial to the right flank fold. Care is taken to avoid penetration of the large subcutaneous mammary vessels on the ventral abdomen. Peritonitis in ruminants is often highly compartmentalized; therefore additional sites are tapped if the initial centesis does not yield fluid.

Abdominocentesis in small ruminants is usually performed to diagnose a urinary tract obstruction or a bladder rupture. The needle is inserted approximately 3 cm to the right of the midline in the most dependent part of the ventral abdomen. Insertion at this site avoids accidental rumen puncture. The procedure is as described for large ruminants.

Complications of abdominal paracentesis in horses and ruminants are (1) bowel laceration; (2) introduction of bacteria at the centesis site, resulting in peritonitis or cellulitis; and (3) damage to the xiphoid process if the centesis site is too cranial.

THORACOCENTESIS

Thoracocentesis is performed in large animals, primarily the horse, to drain fluid or air from the pleural cavity. Fluid is submitted for cytologic analysis or bacterial or fungal culture. Light sedation with a combination of xylazine and butorphanol may be required. A 12- or 14-gauge, 6.0- to 7.5-cm teat cannula is used to remove small volumes of air or fluid. If the fluid is thick or large in volume, a wider-bore, 5 to 7.5-cm-long sterile metal bitch urinary catheter or human thoracic drainage cannula is used.

The ventral thoracic region from the fifth to the ninth ribs is clipped and surgically scrubbed. Centesis to remove fluid is performed in the ventral portion of the sixth or seventh intercostal space, 10 to 12 cm dorsal to the olecranon. If air is expected to be withdrawn, the needle is inserted further dorsal in the intercostal space. The needle is inserted along the cranial border of the rib to avoid the intercostal vessels and nerves which run along the caudal border of the ribs. The lateral thoracic vein, which courses subcutaneously over the ventral aspect of the thorax, should also be avoided. From 3 to 5 ml of 2% lidocaine is injected into the skin, subcutaneous tissue, and intercostal muscles down to the parietal pleura. A stab incision is made with a scalpel blade into the anesthetized skin on the cranial aspect of the rib. The cannula, connected to a three-way stopcock with the valve closed, is inserted through the skin incision until it penetrates the pleura. A 60-ml syringe is connected to the stopcock via extension tubing. The stopcock valve is opened, and air or fluid is aspirated into the syringe. After thoracocentesis is completed, the cannula is withdrawn. Skin sutures are usually only needed if the human cannula or canine urinary catheter is used.

TRANSTRACHEAL WASH

A transtracheal wash is performed on occasion to help determine the cause of lower airway disease. It involves the collection of fluid from the lower respiratory tract for cytologic and microbiologic analysis. The following procedure is described for equine and bovine patients. The technique for transtracheal aspiration in small ruminants is similar to that previously described in small animals.

The middle tracheal region is clipped and aseptically prepared. Approximately 2 ml of 2% lidocaine is injected intradermally and subcutaneously over the center of the trachea. A stab incision is made with a scalpel blade through the skin between the tracheal rings. As the trachea is stabilized with one hand, a 12- to 14-gauge needle is inserted, with the bevel facing downward, through the incision and into the tracheal lumen. A burst of air will exit the needle when it penetrates the lumen.

A sterile, 5- or 6-Fr polyvinyl urinary catheter with the tip cut off is threaded through the needle until it reaches the tracheal bifurcation. A syringe is attached to the flared end of the catheter, and the plunger is retracted. Air is aspirated if the catheter is within the tracheal lumen. If air is not aspirated, the catheter is either outside the trachea, bent, or occluded against the tracheal mucosa and the catheter should be repositioned.

Once the catheter is within the tracheal lumen, the needle is withdrawn and the catheter is left in place. Extension tubing connected to a 60-ml syringe filled with sterile 0.9% saline is inserted into the flared end of the catheter. A 30- to 50-ml aliquot of saline is injected into the trachea. Saline is reaspirated and a sample is collected. Approximately 10% of the infused volume will be reaspirated. The catheter may need to be adjusted and redirected during the procedure. Additional aliquots of saline are instilled through the catheter and reaspirated until a sufficient sample volume is obtained.

After the sample is collected, the catheter is removed. The site is covered with an antibiotic coated sterile gauze and wrapped with a bandage for 24 hours. Cellulitis at the tracheal puncture site is the most common complication. If swelling occurs, warm compresses are applied.

ADMINISTRATION OF MEDICATION IN LARGE ANIMALS

INTRAVENOUS ADMINISTRATION

Bovine Administration

The jugular vein is used for intravenous administration of medication or fluids. The haltered animal is restrained in a chute or stanchion with the head elevated and pulled to the side. Digital pressure is placed in the jugular groove to occlude the vein. The skin overlying the vein is wiped with an alcohol-soaked gauze sponge several times in a downward direction to remove superficial skin contaminants and to help identify the vein.

A 16- to 18-gauge, 3.75- to 5.0-cm needle is inserted through the skin and into the vein at a 45- to 90-degree angle with the skin. When blood flows from the end of the needle it is inserted completely to the hub in either an upward or a downward direction. The syringe containing the medication is attached to the needle. Before injection of syringe contents, the plunger is retracted slightly to ensure that blood enters the syringe. The digital pressure is removed from the jugular groove, and the medication is injected. The needle is removed and pressure is placed on the venipuncture site until hemostasis occurs.

 Technician Note

When an animal requires repeated intravenous injections or large volumes of fluids, a catheter is placed in the jugular vein.

When an animal requires repeated intravenous injections or large volumes of fluids, an intravenous catheter is placed in the jugular vein. The procedure for jugular

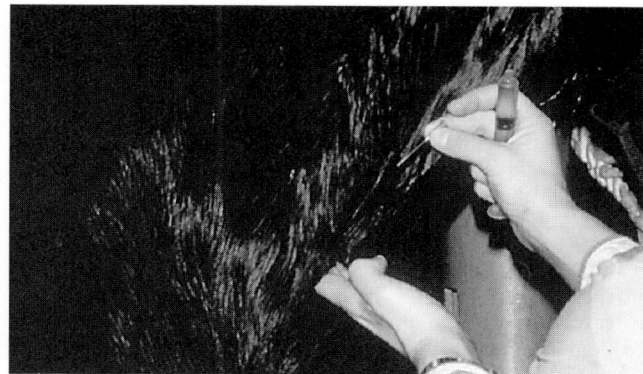

FIGURE 3-42. The needle is placed into the jugular vein to administer intravenous medication to the horse.

catheterization in cattle is similar to that of equine jugular catheterization and will be described in detail in the equine venipuncture section.

The ventral coccygeal vein, on the ventral aspect of the tail, can be used as a site for injection of small volumes of medication. Because of the proximity of the coccygeal vein to the coccygeal artery and the fecal contamination around the tail, the vein is not recommended for injections.

Equine Administration

The jugular vein is used for intravenous injections in the horse. It is large and easily palpated in the jugular groove on the neck. Injection into the right jugular vein is preferred over the left jugular because the esophagus lies in the left jugular groove.

To make an injection into the jugular vein, the vessel is occluded with digital pressure on the jugular groove. The vein is more easily visualized in the proximal third of the neck if the jugular groove is wiped with an alcohol-soaked cotton ball several times in a downward direction.

An 18-gauge, 2.5-cm needle is embedded into the vein, up to the hub, at a 90-degree angle and then directed caudally (Figure 3-42). Blood will trickle constantly from the needle hub if it is in the vein. If the needle inadvertently enters the carotid artery, blood will forcefully spurt out of the hub in a pulsatile manner even when the jugular vein is not occluded. If the needle enters the carotid, it should be removed immediately, and firm pressure applied for several minutes to ensure hemostasis. Use of a large-bore needle and insertion of the needle without the syringe attached decreases the likelihood that an injection of medication will accidentally be given intraarterially.

 Technician Note

If the needle inadvertently enters the carotid artery, blood will eject out of the needle hub in forceful spurts even when the jugular vein is not occluded.

Once it is determined that the needle is placed intravenously and not intraarterially, the needle is stabilized and the syringe attached. The plunger should be retracted slightly to ensure that venous blood flows back into the syringe. Digital pressure on the vein is removed, and the contents of the syringe are slowly injected.

If repeated administration of large volumes of fluid or intravenous medication is required, an intravenous catheter is placed in the jugular vein. Although intravenous catheters can also be placed in the cephalic and lateral thoracic veins, fluids can be administered at a more rapid rate in the larger jugular vein.

To place a jugular catheter, the hair over the cranial third of the vein is clipped and the skin is aseptically prepared. Approximately 1.0 ml of 2% lidocaine is instilled into the skin over the vessel. Latex gloves, ideally sterile ones, are worn to place the catheter. A small incision is made through the desensitized skin with a scalpel blade or 14-gauge needle. The vein is occluded by the application of digital pressure in the jugular furrow.

A 10- to 16-gauge, 13-cm over-the-needle catheter (Angiocath), with a stylet, is inserted through the skin incision and into the vein. (Figure 3-43, *A*). The tip should be at a 45-degree angle pointing downward and parallel with the vein. Blood will appear in the catheter hub when the tip enters the vein. The catheter is advanced an additional 5 mm. It is then laid parallel to the vein as it is slid over the stylet and threaded completely into the vein (Figures 3-43, *B* and *C*). Digital pressure on the vein is released. A cap or extension set is placed on the hub, and the catheter is flushed with heparinized 0.9% sterile saline.

Glue, tape, or suture is used to secure the catheter to the skin. A gauze sponge onto which a small quantity of antibiotic ointment has been applied is placed over the venipuncture site. The catheter is secured with layers of bandage material and adhesive tape wrapped around the neck. (Figure 3-43, *D*).

The catheter site should be checked several times daily for patency and monitored for signs of inflammation or infection. If excessive warmth, redness, firmness, swelling, pain, extravasation of fluid, or discharge is noted around the catheter site, the catheter should be removed and placed in a different vein.

Technician Note

If excessive warmth, redness, firmness, swelling, pain, extravasation of fluid, or discharge is noted around the catheter site, the catheter should be removed and placed in a different vein.

Ovine and Caprine Administration

The injection technique used with goats and sheep is similar to that described in small animals. An 18- to 20-gauge 2.5-cm hypodermic needle is used in adults and a 20- to 22-gauge, 2.5-cm needle is used in lambs and kids.

The jugular vein is the most convenient site for intravenous injection in the sheep and goat. To access the vein, the goat is restrained by a handler who backs the goat into a corner, straddles it over the withers, and turns the head to one side. Restraint in sheep for intravenous injection involves either sitting the sheep up on its rump or straddling the sheep over the withers and stretching the neck laterally. It may be necessary to part the wool or hair to visualize the vein.

Porcine Administration

The auricular vein, located on the dorsal aspect of the pinna, is the most commonly used vein for administration of drugs or fluids. A 19- to 21-gauge butterfly catheter or an 18-gauge over-the-needle catheter can be placed in the ear

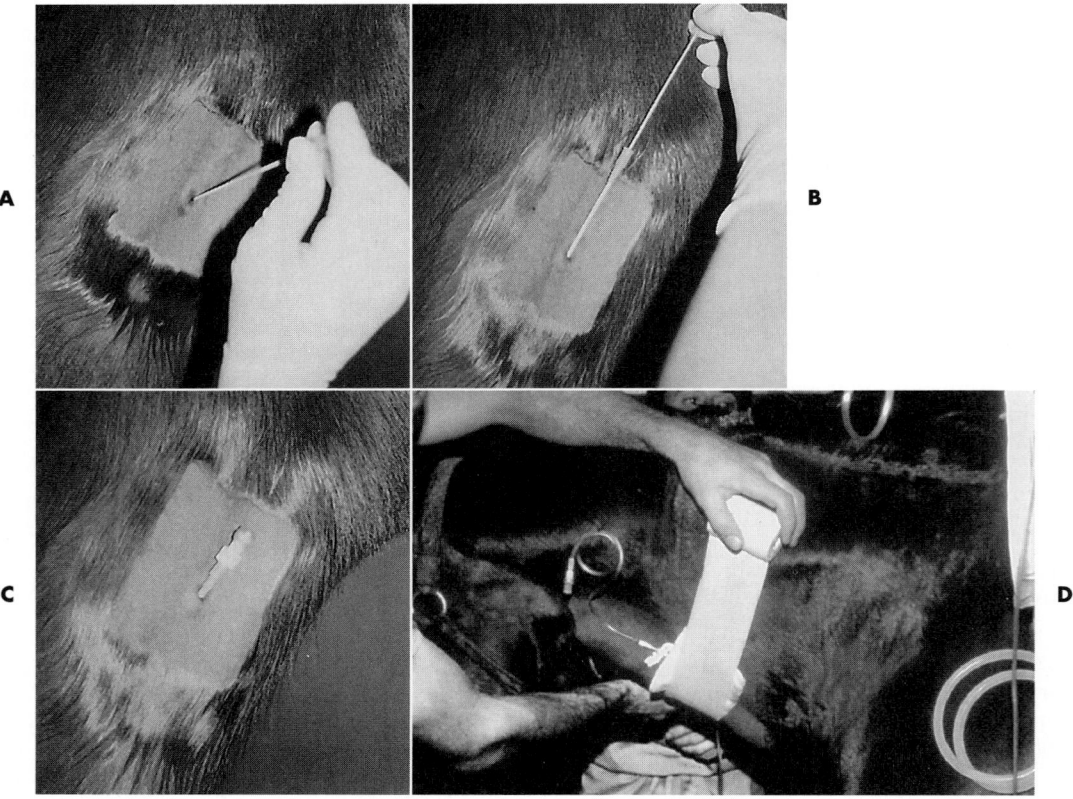

FIGURE 3-43. A jugular catheter is placed in a horse for intravenous fluid therapy. The catheter is secured in place by bandage material that is wrapped around the neck. (*A through C, from Pratt PW: Principles and Practice of Veterinary Technology, St Louis, 1998, Mosby.*)

vein if large volumes of fluid or multiple intravenous injections are needed.

To catheterize the auricular vein, a rubber band tourniquet is wrapped around the ear base to distend the vein. The dorsal aspect of the pinna is aseptically prepared. The catheter is inserted into the vein. After the catheter is threaded into the vein, the tourniquet is released. The catheter is capped, and the hub is affixed to the pinna with quick setting glue. A dry gauze sponge is placed flat against the underside of the pinna to serve as padding. A partially used roll of 5.0-cm-wide tape is placed next to the gauze sponge to support the underside of the pinna. The margins of the ear are bent around the roll of tape. Several strips of adhesive tape are wrapped around the ear to secure the catheter to the pinna.

INTRAMUSCULAR ADMINISTRATION

Bovine Administration

The only muscles recommended for intramuscular injections in cattle are those in the neck. Injection into the gluteal muscle should be avoided because this area is prone to abscessation. Intramuscular injections are performed when the animal is restrained in a stanchion or crowded into a confined area. In cattle and horses, a maximum of 5 to 10 ml, depending on the site and size of the animal, should be administered at each site. It is best to alternate sites if repeated injections are needed over a multiday period.

> **Technician Note**
>
> The only muscles recommended for intramuscular injections in cattle are those in the neck.

The injection site is wiped with 70% isopropyl alcohol to remove gross skin contaminants. A 16- or 18-gauge, 3.75- to 5.0-cm needle is grasped, and a fist is formed with the same hand. The injection site is struck several times with the flat of the fist. The hand is then rotated slightly, and the animal is struck again as the needle is embedded in the skin and muscle. Striking the animal in this manner distracts it and decreases its awareness of the needle insertion. Once the needle is inserted to the hub, the syringe is attached. Before the medication is injected, the plunger is retracted and the hub is checked for blood. If a vessel has been inadvertently penetrated, the needle should be removed and injection made into another location. After injection, the site is briefly massaged to help distribute the injected fluid.

Equine Administration

The neck and rear legs are used for intramuscular injection in the horse. As with cattle, the gluteal region should be avoided because of the difficulty in treating any injection-induced abscesses. The pectoral muscles may be used to make injections, but there is an increased likelihood of inflammation at the injection site. Abscesses that may develop subsequent to injection in the pectoral region are easier to drain than are those in the gluteal muscles.

Intramuscular injections in the neck are given in the indented triangular region bordered by the nuchal ligament, cervical spine, and shoulder blade (Figure 3-44). Medication administered into the nuchal ligament is poorly absorbed. Volumes of up to 10 ml can be injected intramuscularly into the neck. Postinjection muscle tenderness is a relatively common sequela.

The lower half of the semimembranosus and semitendinosus muscles in the caudal aspect of the rear leg are excellent injection sites, but the injector is at risk of being kicked (Figure 3-45). The individual giving the injection stands on one side of the horse and reaches around the rear to inject the opposite leg. If the horse kicks, it usually kicks toward the side of the injection. It is best to stand as close to the horse's body as possible to avoid a kick. It is not always possible to stand on the side opposite the injection. In such a case, the restrainer should stand on the same side as the individual giving the injection and pull the horse's head toward them both. If the horse kicks, it will attempt to straighten itself and spin the rear end away from the injector and restrainer.

Equine intramuscular injections are administered in the same manner as described for cattle except an 18-gauge, 3.75-cm needle is used. The site is tapped with the back of the hand or fist once or twice, and then the needle, without the syringe attached, is inserted through the skin and deep into the muscle.

Ovine and Caprine Administration

Intramuscular injections in the sheep and goat are administered in the semimembranosus and semitendinosus

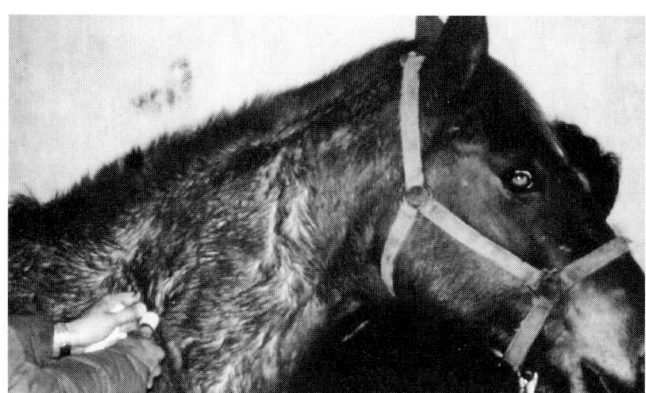

FIGURE 3-44. Intramuscular injection into the cervical muscles in the horse.

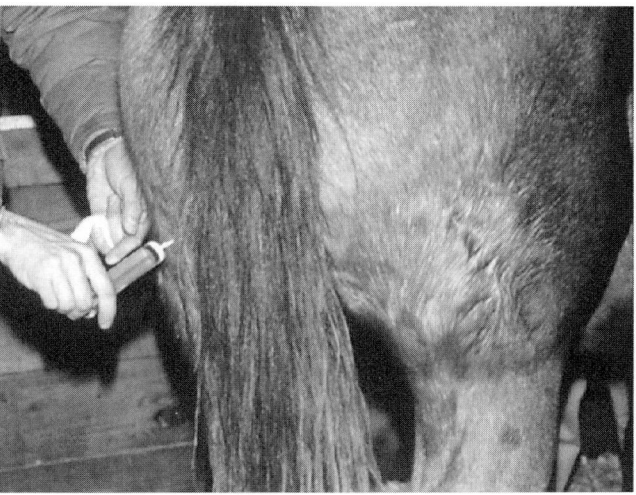

FIGURE 3-45. Intramuscular injection into the semimembranosus and semitendinosus muscles in the horse.

muscles of the rear leg, triceps, neck muscles, or longissimus muscles over the lumbar region. Occasionally the gluteal muscles are used. Goats and sheep do not have sufficient muscle mass for large volume intramuscular injections. A maximum of 5 ml is injected in any single site.

Porcine Administration

Intramuscular injections are made into the cervical muscles or the semimembranosus or semitendinosus muscles of the rear leg. Lameness may occur after injection into the caudal muscles of the rear leg. Use of the muscles of the "ham" for intramuscular injections is avoided in animals intended for use as food because the injection may mark the muscle and downgrade the quality of the meat. Because of the tendency of pigs to store a thick layer of subcutaneous body fat, a needle that is at least 3.75 cm long is needed to penetrate to the muscle. Medications deposited in fat are absorbed much more slowly than are those deposited in the muscle, so the onset of action of the injected substances is delayed.

> ### Technician Note
>
> The use of the muscles of the "ham" for intramuscular injections is avoided in animals intended for use as food because the injection may mark the muscle and downgrade the quality of the meat.

SUBCUTANEOUS ADMINISTRATION

Bovine and Equine Administration

The neck is the site recommended for subcutaneous injections in the horse. Any region on the lateral aspect of the neck or trunk can be used for subcutaneous injections in cattle. The site is wiped with a gauze sponge saturated with 70% isopropyl alcohol to remove superficial skin contaminants. A fold of skin is tented, and an 18- to 20-gauge, 2.5- to 3.75-cm needle with attached syringe is inserted at the base of the tented skin (Figure 3-46). Slight negative pressure is applied by retraction of the plunger to ensure that the needle has not entered a vessel. If placement is satisfactory, the medication is injected under the skin, and

the needle is withdrawn. The area around the site is rubbed to promote distribution of the injected substance.

Ovine and Caprine Administration

The neck and shoulder region is frequently used for subcutaneous injections in the sheep and goat. Axillary or flank subcutaneous injections are made in show animals if the injections contain medications or vaccines, such as clostridial vaccines, that may cause nodular swellings or abscesses. Subcutaneous masses, if located in the prescapular region, may be mistaken by show judges as caseous lymphadenitis. The back or upper flank areas should be avoided as injection sites in goats if the skin will be marketed. Sheep injections should be made when the wool is dry. They have a greater tendency toward injection site reactions if the needle is introduced through wet wool.

Porcine Administration

The skin of pigs is tightly adhered to the body. This limits the volume that can be injected subcutaneously. Subcutaneous injections are made into the lateral side of the neck, immediately posterior to the base of the ear, with a 16- to 18-gauge, 2.5- to 3.75-cm needle.

INTRADERMAL ADMINISTRATION

As in small animals, intradermal injections are made primarily for the purpose of skin testing or to provide local anesthesia. Cattle and sheep are tested for tuberculosis via an intradermal injection into the caudal tail fold (Figure 3-47). Intradermal injections are also used to treat nodular skin lesions and sarcoids. The technique for intradermal injection is as previously described for small animals and can be adapted for use in large animals.

INTRAPERITONEAL ADMINISTRATION

Intraperitoneal injections are usually reserved for treatment of neonatal kids or lambs with umbilical infections or hypoglycemia. The neonate is lifted by the front legs, and a 20-gauge needle with attached syringe is introduced to the left of the umbilicus to a depth of 1.0 cm. The plunger is retracted to ensure that the needle has not penetrated a vessel or an abdominal organ. Once intraperitoneal placement is confirmed, the syringe contents are injected into the peritoneal cavity.

In baby pigs, fluids are usually administered intraperitoneally because of the impracticality of placing an

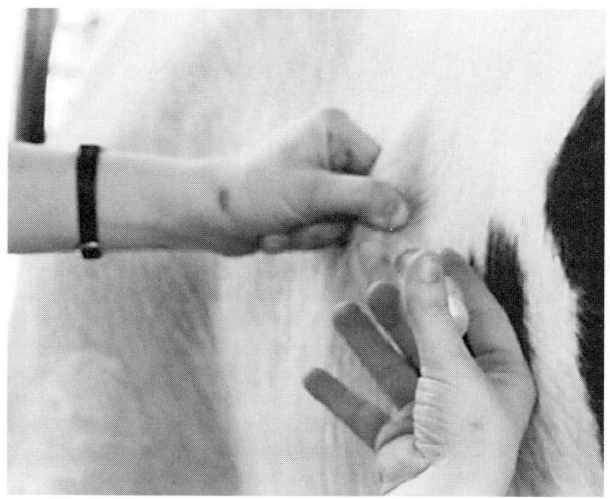

FIGURE 3-46.   To make a subcutaneous injection in a cow, the needle is inserted into the base of a fold of skin.

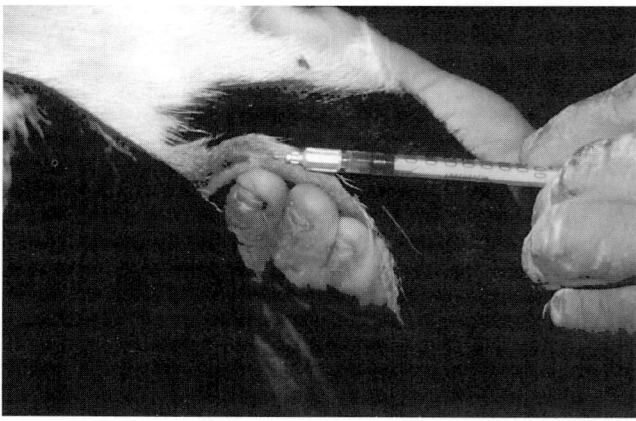

FIGURE 3-47.   Intradermal injection is made into the caudal skinfold to test for tuberculosis in the cow.

intravenous catheter. Fluids should be body temperature, nonirritating, and isotonic. The site of needle introduction is aseptically prepared. To administer intraperitoneal fluids to a baby pig, the pig is grasped by the rear legs, and an 18-gauge, 1.25- to 2.5-cm needle is inserted paramedially between the midline and flank. Intraperitoneal injection in a mature standing pig requires the insertion of a 16- to 18-gauge, 7.5-cm needle.

INTRANASAL ADMINISTRATION

Certain vaccines or local anesthetics are administered intranasally in large as well as small animals. The head is restrained with the nose tilted slightly upward. Excessive nasal exudate is removed from the nostril to be injected. This is best accomplished by cleaning the nares with damp gauze sponges or cotton balls. The needleless syringe containing the vaccine or local anesthetic is injected into the nostril. It is not uncommon for the animal to sneeze out some of the injected substance.

ORAL ADMINISTRATION

The easiest but least reliable method to administer oral medication to a large animal is to mix it with food or drinking water. If the animal detects a different taste or smell it may refrain from ingesting the off-flavored food or water. If the animal is sick, it may have diminished food or water consumption and will not consume the entire medication dose.

Ovine and Caprine Administration
Balling Gun

Administration of tablets to adult sheep and goats can be a challenge. A balling gun is used to help perform the task (Figure 3-48). The end of the gun should be smooth and ideally be made of soft plastic. It should be inspected for sharp edges before each use. Care should be taken not to insert the balling gun too forcefully or too far back into the oral cavity. The tip of the gun should not scrape the roof of the mouth. Improper use can cause trauma to the mouth, pharynx, and esophagus.

To use the balling gun, the animal is backed into a corner and straddled over the shoulders by the handler. The head and neck are held in normal position. A balling gun is placed in the interdental space of the mouth and positioned over the base of the tongue. The bolus is released, and the gun is withdrawn. Observation of the animal after administration is required to ensure that the pill is swallowed.

Dosing Syringe

Small volumes of liquid are administered orally with the use of a 60-ml catheter-tipped syringe, dosing bottle, or dosing syringe. To use a syringe, the tip is introduced into the side of the mouth and over the base of the tongue. The liquid is slowly injected with the head held in a normal position. If coughing occurs, administration should be ceased until the trachea is cleared of fluid. If the animal struggles and becomes upset, it should be allowed to rest before administration is reattempted.

Nasogastric Intubation

A nasogastric or orogastric tube can be used to administer larger fluid volumes, medication, electrolyte solutions, rumen fluid, and colostrum. Nasogastric intubation is generally tolerated better than orogastric intubation (Figure 3-49).

The sheep or goat is restrained in a standing position by a handler who straddles the withers. The nasal passageway is desensitized by the instillation of 0.5 ml of 2% lidocaine into one nostril. A length of flexible plastic or rubber tube needed to extend from the nostrils to the rumen is premeasured and marked. The tube should have a smooth, rounded end and have a sufficiently small diameter to pass through the ventral nasal meatus.

Water-soluble lubricant or water is placed around the tube tip. The tube is inserted into the nostril and slowly advanced into the ventral nasal meatus and nasopharynx. The animal should be observed swallowing the tube as it is advanced. The tube is palpated on the neck as it passes down the esophagus. If the animal coughs, the tube has entered the trachea and should be promptly removed.

Once the nasogastric tube is inserted to the premeasured mark, the placement is checked to ensure that the tube is definitely in the rumen. Air is blown into the end of the tube as an assistant auscults the area over the rumen with a stethoscope. Bubbling is heard as the air passes through the rumen contents. The smell of rumen contents emanates from the end of the tube.

Fluid or medication is flushed through the tube with a dose syringe or drench pump. A bolus of water is generally flushed through the tube after the medication. After the medication and water bolus is administered, the tube is kinked to occlude it. The tube is withdrawn in a downward direction. This technique prevents rumen contents from leaking from the tube and entering the trachea as the tube is removed.

Nasogastric or Orogastric Intubation

Orogastric intubation is performed with the animal restrained in a standing position. The diameter and length of tube needed depends on the size of the animal. A 9.5-mm-diameter foal tube is used with adult sheep and goats. A narrower, 37-cm-long soft rubber feeding tube or metal lamb probe is used to intubate lambs or kids. Because the diameter of the tube used for orogastric intubation is wider than that used for nasogastric intubation, fluids placed into an orogastric tube can be more viscous and can be delivered at a more rapid rate.

A partially used roll of tape is used as a speculum to hold

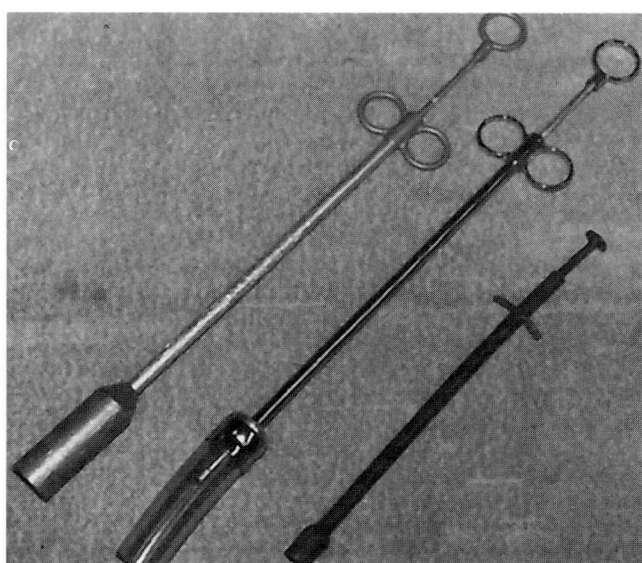

FIGURE 3-48.   Various sizes of balling guns are available. (From Pratt PW: *Principles and Practice of Veterinary Technology*, St Louis, 1998, Mosby.)

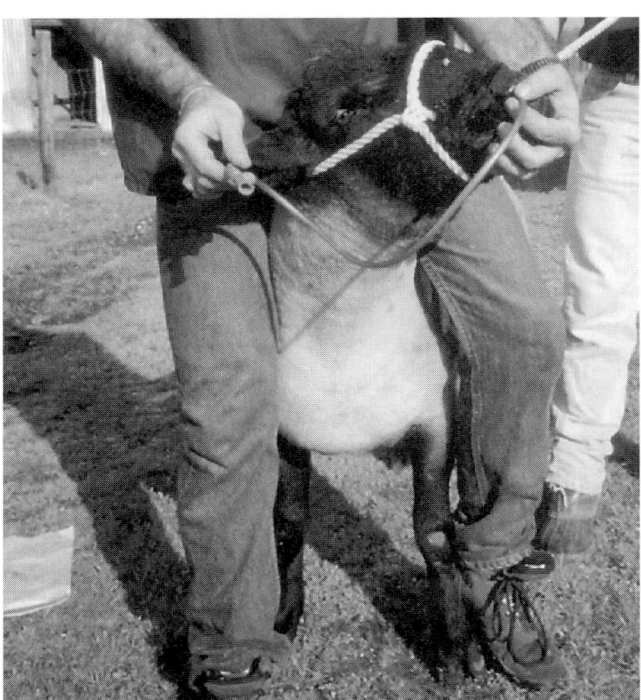

FIGURE 3-49. Nasogastric intubation of a sheep with a stallion urinary catheter.

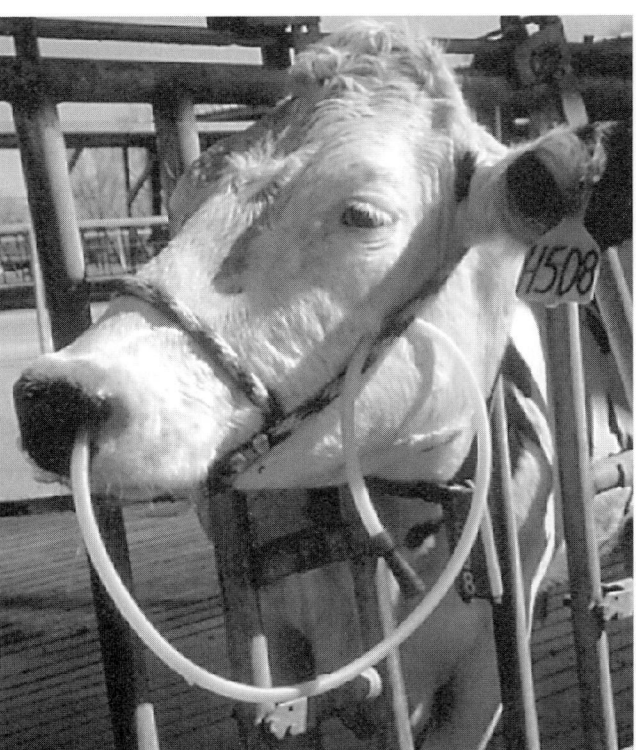

FIGURE 3-50. Nasogastric intubation of a bovine with a foal stomach tube.

the mouth open. The length of orogastric tube needed to span the distance from the tip of the chin to the last rib is marked on the tube. The distal third of the tube is lubricated with water or water-soluble gel. It is placed through the speculum, over the base of the tongue, and into the esophagus. The tube is advanced until it enters the rumen. Placement of the tube in the rumen is verified before any substances are administered.

Bovine Administration

Balling Gun

A balling gun is used to administer medication boluses to cattle. The tip of the gun should be inspected for sharp edges and the mouth emptied of food before the balling gun is inserted. The animal is confined in a head catch. The handler inserts a finger into one nostril and a thumb into the other and pulls the nose dorsally. This causes the animal to open its mouth so the balling gun can be placed over the base of the tongue. Alternatively, a hand can be placed into the interdental space to open the mouth.

Orogastric Intubation

Fluids and medications can be administered to cattle through a stomach tube passed from the nose or mouth directly into the rumen (Figure 3-50). Refer to the discussion of rumen fluid collection for a description of the technique orogastric intubation of large ruminants. The previously described technique for nasogastric intubation of the sheep and goat can be adapted for cattle.

Equine Administration

Syringe Administration

Oral medications are frequently administered to horses. A variety of preparations are available in paste form, includ-

ing anthelmintics, vitamin-mineral supplements, antibiotics, and antiinflammatory agents. Some pastes are available prepackaged in syringes for oral administration. Other pastes must be poured or aspirated into syringes by the technician. Tablets can be pulverized and then combined with water and administered via a syringe or mixed with corn syrup, applesauce, or molasses and added to the feed.

Before oral suspensions are administered, the oral cavity is checked to ensure it is free of food. The head is raised slightly and the syringe is inserted into the interdental space on the side of the mouth. As the plunger is depressed, the syringe contents are slowly emptied onto the base of the tongue. The horse should be sufficiently restrained so that it does not move as the injection is made. If the horse moves, the medication may trickle out of the side of the mouth. The horse should not be permitted to drink water immediately after administration because some medication may be lost into the drinking water.

Nasogastric Intubation

Boluses of medication can also be delivered via nasogastric intubation. This procedure should be performed while under the direct supervision of the veterinarian. A detailed description of the technique used to pass a nasogastric tube is given in Chapter 30.

 Technician Note

Boluses of medication can also be delivered via nasogastric intubation. This procedure should be performed while under the direct supervision of the veterinarian.

INTRAMAMMARY ADMINISTRATION

Intramammary infusion of antibiotics is used to treat or control mastitis. Because potential exists for the introduction of contaminants into the udder during the infusion process, the procedure must be performed aseptically. After the udder is milked out, the teat is cleaned with a dip and thoroughly dried. A separate cloth is used to dry each teat to prevent cross-contamination. The teat is then wiped with 70% isopropyl alcohol and air dried. The teats on the far side of the udder are cleaned before those on the near side.

Teats on the near side are infused before those on the far. The infusion cannula on the antibiotic-syringe is partially inserted into the teat canal. The teat end is grasped and occluded as the udder is massaged to distribute the infused medication. Partial insertion of the cannula into the teat canal delivers fewer contaminants into the udder than does full insertion. Because antibiotic is deposited directly into the streak canal, infection in the canal may be controlled better than when the entire volume of medication is placed in the cistern. Teat dip is reapplied after infusion.

ACKNOWLEDGMENTS

The author wishes to acknowledge the following faculty members of the Veterinary Teaching Hospital and Clinics, School of Veterinary Medicine, Louisiana State University, who assisted in obtaining photographs for the manuscript: Drs. M. ClaxtonGill, J. Taboada, K. Wolfsheimer, D.M. McCurnin, R. McClure, T. Seahorn, and P. Hoyt. The author also wishes to acknowledge the work of Dr. M.J. Lucas and Ms. S.E. Lucas in the second edition of this book.

RECOMMENDED READING

Baldwin K: Placing an intraosseous catheter in the canine trochanteric fossa, *Vet Tech* 12:656-659, 1999.

Crowe DT: Nutritional support for the hospitalized patient: An introduction to tube feeding, *Compend Contin Educ Pract Vet* 12:1711-1720, 1990.

Devitt CM, Seim HB III: Clinical evaluation of tube esophagostomy in small animals, *J Am Anim Hosp Assoc* 33:55-60, 1997.

Ettinger SJ, Feldman, editors: *Textbook of veterinary internal medicine*, ed 5, Philadelphia, 2000, WB Saunders.

Grindem CB: Bone marrow biopsy and evaluation, *Vet Clin North Am Small Anim Pract* 19:669-696, 1989.

House JK, Smith BP, Van Metre DC, et al: Ancillary tests for assessment of the ruminant digestive system, *Vet Clin North Am Large Anim Pract* 8:203-232, 1992.

Bistner SI, Ford RB, Raffe MR: *Kirk and Bistner's handbook of veterinary procedures and emergency treatment*, ed 7, Philadelphia, 2000, Harcourt Health Sciences.

Kopcha M, Schultze AE: Peritoneal fluid. II. Abdominocentesis in cattle and interpretation of nonneoplastic samples, *Compend Contin Educ Pract Vet* 13:703-710, 1991.

Lawhorn B: A new approach for obtaining blood samples from pigs, *J Am Vet Med Assoc* 192:781-782, 1988.

Lucas MJ, Lucas SE: Diagnostic sampling and treatment techniques. In McCurnin DM, editor: *Clinical textbook for veterinary technicians*, ed3, Philadelphia, 1994, WB Saunders.

McCurnin DM, Poffenbarger EM, editors: *Small animal physical diagnosis and clinical procedures*, Philadelphia, WB Saunders, 1991.

Moon PF, Smith LJ: General anesthetic techniques in swine, *Vet Clin North Am Large Anim Pract* 12:663-691.

Orsini JA, Divers TJ: *Manual of equine emergencies*, Philadelphia, 1998, WB Saunders.

Osborne CA, Lees GE, Johnston GR. In Kirk RW, editor: *Current veterinary therapy VII: small animal practice*, Philadelphia, 1980, WB Saunders.

Otto CM, Kaufman GM, Crowe DT: Intraosseous infusion of fluids and therapeutics, *Compend Contin Educ Pract Vet* 11:421-430, 1989.

Pratt PP, editor: *Principles and practice of veterinary technology*, St Louis, 1998, Mosby.

Raskin RE: Bone marrow. In Slatter D, editor: *Textbook of small animal surgery*, ed 2, Philadelphia, 1993, WB Saunders.

Rose RJ, Hodgson DR: *Manual of equine practice*, Philadelphia, 1998, WB Saunders.

Smith MC, Sherman DM editors: *Goat medicine*, Philadelphia, 1994, Lea & Febiger.

Smith BP editor: *Large animal internal medicine*, ed 2, St Louis, 1996, Mosby.

Terry C, Rashmir-Raven A, RL Linford: Placing an intravenous catheter in horses, *Vet Tech* 4:207-212, 2000

Taylor FGR, Hillyer MH, editors: *Diagnostic techniques in equine medicine*, Philadelphia, 1997, WB Saunders.

Tobin E, Hunt E: Supplies and technical considerations for ruminant and swine anesthesia, *Vet Clin North Am Large Anim Pract* 12:531-562, 1996.

Williams CSF: Routine sheep and goat procedures, *Vet Clin North Am Large Anim Pract* 6:737-758, 1990.

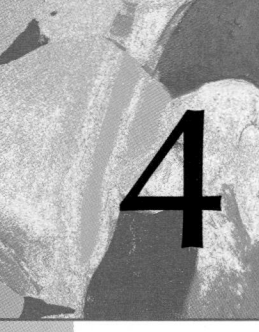

4

Wound Healing, Wound Management, and Bandaging

Giselle Hosgood • *Daniel J. Burba*

The veterinary technician can play an important role in assisting the veterinary surgeon in the management of wounds. The nature of the wound often dictates the method of wound management. To understand the methods of wound management, a knowledge of the physiology of wound healing and the factors that alter wound healing is required. The methods of wound management, the role of bandaging in wound management, and the different types of bandages are then more clearly understood.

WOUND HEALING

A wound is created when an insult, either purposeful, such as surgery, or incidental, such as trauma, disrupts the normal integrity of the tissue. Wound healing is a complex biologic event that is well characterized at the microscopic level, but its regulation at the molecular level is only just beginning to be understood. The process of wound healing begins immediately after the insult and is described in four physical phases: the inflammatory, debridement, repair, and maturation phases (Figure 4-1 and Table 4-1). Wound healing is a dynamic process, and more than one phase of wound healing is usually occurring at any time.

Peptide growth factors appear to play a key role in initiating and sustaining the phases of wound healing (Table 4-2). The platelet appears to initiate the wound healing process through the release of growth factors; the process is then amplified or sustained by wound macrophages, endothelial cells, and fibroblasts. The *inflammatory phase* begins immediately after injury. Hemorrhage fills the wound and cleans the wound surface. The blood vessels constrict immediately to slow hemorrhage, but vasoconstriction lasts only 5 to 10 minutes. The blood vessels then dilate and leak fluid containing clotting elements into the wound. This fluid, combined with blood, causes a blood clot to form. The blood clot stabilizes the wound edges, and fibrin within the clot provides the limited wound strength of this phase. In a sutured wound, the sutures will also provide wound strength at this time. The blood clot will dry and form a scab, which protects the wound, prevents further hemorrhage, and allows healing to progress under its surface. The scab does not provide any wound strength. The blood vessels also leak white blood cells into the wound. This marks the beginning of the debridement phase.

The *debridement phase* begins approximately 6 hours after injury, when white blood cells, namely neutrophils and monocytes, appear in the wound. These cells remove necrotic tissue, bacteria, and foreign material from the wound. The white blood cells, in combination with the fluid that has leaked into the wound, form the exudate commonly associated with wounds.

 Technician Note

There is minimal wound strength during the first 3 to 5 days of wound healing, known as the lag phase.

The *repair phase* begins after the blood clot has formed and necrotic tissue and foreign material have been removed from the wound. The repair phase, which is usually active by 3 to 5 days after injury, is associated with invasion of fibroblasts into the wound. The fibroblasts produce collagen that will mature into fibrous or scar tissue. The repair phase is characterized by a significant increase in wound strength. In contrast, the first 3 to 5 days after injury are associated with a minimal increase in wound strength.

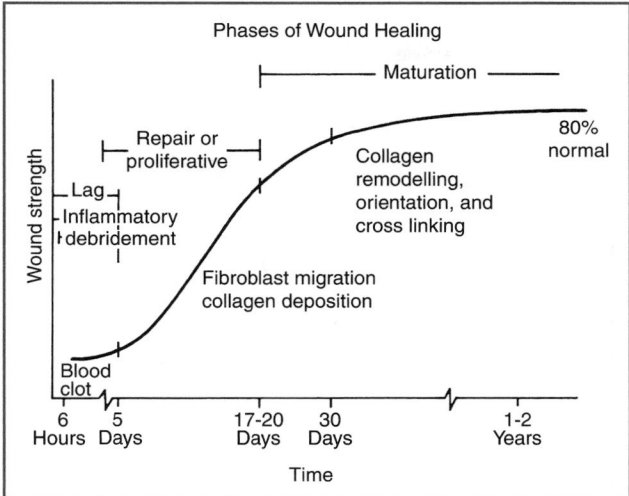

FIGURE 4-1. Schematic representation of the phases of wound healing and associated changes in wound strength.

TABLE 4-1	CHARACTERISTICS OF THE MICROSCOPIC PHASES OF WOUND HEALING
Phase	**Characteristics**
Inflammatory	Begins immediately after injury; characterized by formation of blood clot; platelets stimulate other stages by release of growth factors
Debridement	Part of inflammatory phase; characterized by influx of white blood cells (macrophages, monocytes) into wound; occurs approximately 6 hr after injury; wound healing is sustained by release of growth factors from multiple cell types
Repair (fibroblastic)	Begins 3-5 days after wounding; characterized by invasion of fibroblasts and development of granulation tissue; wound strength increases exponentially
Maturation	Characterized by remodeling of the collagen of the scar and slow gain in wound strength; begins approximately 3 wk after injury and may take weeks to years to complete

TABLE 4-2	CHARACTERISTICS OF SELECTED GROWTH FACTORS AND THEIR ROLE IN WOUND HEALING	
Growth Factor	**Sources**	**Effect on Wound Healing**
Platelet-derived growth factor (PDGF)	Platelets, macrophages, fibroblasts, endothelial cells	Stimulates replication of fibroblasts and vascular smooth muscle
Transforming growth factor β_1 and β_2 (TGF-β_1, TGF-β_2)	Macrophages, lymphocytes, fibroblasts, bone cells, keratinocytes, platelets	Inhibits replication of most cells (keratinocytes, endothelial cells, lymphocytes, macrophages); may inhibit or stimulate fibroblasts; may have a modulating effect on wound healing
Transforming growth factor β_3 (TGF-β_3)	Macrophages	Antiscarring effects
Transforming growth factor α (TGF-α)	Macrophages, eosinophils, keratinocytes	Stimulates replication of epithelial cells, fibroblasts, and endothelial cells; more potent effect on endothelial cells than epidermal growth factor
Epidermal growth factor (EGF)	Almost all body fluids, platelets	Stimulates replication of epithelial cells, fibroblasts, and endothelial cells
Insulin-like growth factor (IGF)	Most tissues, fibroblasts, macrophages	Stimulates replication of fibroblasts, endothelial cells, bone cells, neural tissues, and hemopoietic cells
Fibroblast growth factor (FGF)	Fibroblasts, bone cells, smooth muscle cells, endothelial cells, astrocytes	Stimulates replication of neural tissue, bone cells, muscle cells, and fibroblasts; influences angiogenesis
Keratinocyte growth factor (KGF)	Fibroblasts	Affects epidermal cell motility and proliferation
Vascular endothelial growth factor	Epidermal cells, macrophages	Enhances angiogenesis and increased vascular permeability
Colony-stimulating factor 1	Many cells	Activates macrophages and influences granulation tissue formation

Consequently, the first 3 to 5 days are also known as the "lag phase" of wound healing.

Capillaries appear in the wound at the same time fibroblasts appear. The combination of new capillaries, fibroblasts, and fibrous tissue forms the characteristic red, fleshy granulation tissue that fills the wound, often lying underneath the scab.

Granulation tissue characteristically appears in the wound after 3 to 5 days. Poor granulation tissue is white and has a high fibrous tissue content with fewer capillaries. Granulation tissue is important in wound healing because it fills the tissue defect, protects the wound, provides a barrier to infection, provides a surface for new epithelial cells to form across, and provides a source of special fibroblasts called *myofibroblasts*, which are responsible for wound contraction.

The formation of new epithelium on the wound surface (epithelialization) occurs during the repair phase and begins once an adequate granulation tissue bed has formed. New epithelium is usually visible on a wound in 4 to 5 days. In an incised wound that is sutured, in which the skin edges are close, epithelialization can occur almost immediately (as early as 24 to 48 hours after injury), since there is no defect that needs to be filled with granulation tissue. The normal epithelial cells at the edge of the wound divide and produce new cells that migrate across the granulation tissue. Some hair follicles and sweat glands may also regenerate, depending on the extent of damage. The new epithelium is only one cell layer thick initially and is fragile, but it gradually thickens over time as more cell layers form.

Wound contraction helps to reduce the size of the wound but occurs totally independent of epithelialization. No new skin is formed during contraction. Wound contraction is a result of contraction of the myofibroblasts in the granulation tissue, which pulls the full-thickness skin edges inward. If the skin around the wound is tight and under tension, wound contraction will be limited. Visible wound contraction usually occurs 5 to 9 days after injury.

The *maturation phase* is the final phase of wound healing, during which the wound strength increases to its maximum level because of changes in the scar. Remodeling of the collagen fibers in the fibrous tissue, with alteration of their orientation and increased cross-linking, improves wound strength. The number of capillaries in the fibrous tissue gradually decreases, causing the scar to become paler. The maturation phase begins once collagen has been adequately deposited in the wound and may continue for several years. The wound never regains the strength of normal tissue.

Factors Affecting Wound Healing

Many factors affect wound healing, including host factors affecting the health of the animal, the characteristics of the wound, and external factors directly affecting the wound.

Host Factors

Old animals tend to heal slowly, probably because they are often debilitated and have other ongoing health problems. Animals that are malnourished or have a disease causing low serum protein concentrations below 2 g/dl (e.g., liver disease with poor protein production; kidney disease with excessive loss of protein) will have delayed wound healing and decreased wound strength. In addition, the lag phase of wound healing will be prolonged in these animals.

Wound healing is delayed by certain diseases, such as hyperadrenocorticism or Cushing's disease, in which there is an excess of circulating corticosteroids. Corticosteroids delay all phases of wound healing.

Animals with diabetes mellitus have delayed wound healing and a predisposition to wound infection. Animals with liver disease may have clotting factor deficits in addition to low serum protein concentrations.

Technician Note

Corticosteroids delay all phases of wound healing.

Wound Characteristics

Foreign material in the wound, such as sutures, surgical implants, drains, or extraneous material, can cause an intense inflammatory reaction that interferes with normal wound healing. Soil particles can contain specific infection-enhancing factors.

Compared with a sharp surgical incision, the use of an electroscalpel or electrocoagulation during surgery causes more necrosis at the wound margin, increases the chance of wound infection, and results in a slower gain in early wound strength.

Contaminated tissue becomes infected if the bacteria multiply to a critical number of 10^5 organisms per gram of tissue and then invade the tissue. Whether this occurs depends on the degree of tissue trauma, the amount of foreign material present, the delay between injury and treatment, and the effectiveness of host defenses. Infection stops the repair phase.

Bacterial toxins and associated inflammation directly damage the cells. The wound exudate produced during inflammation can accumulate and separate the tissue, leading to wound infection and delayed wound healing.

Technician Note

Infection stops wound repair.

The blood supply to the wound is obviously important for wound healing and is responsible for delivering oxygen and metabolic substrates to the cells. Damage to the blood supply during surgical treatment should be avoided. Tight bandages that compromise the wound's blood supply should not be used. Movement in a healing wound is also detrimental, because it disturbs the fine cellular structures of the healing tissue. Movement across a wound should be limited. It may be necessary to apply a bandage to the affected limb to reduce movement.

External Factors

Certain drugs and radiation therapy delay wound healing. Corticosteroids depress all phases of wound healing and increase the chance of wound infection. Antiinflammatory drugs (aspirin, phenylbutazone, ibuprofen) have little effect on wound strength but will suppress early inflammation. Prolonged aspirin therapy may delay blood clotting. Chemotherapeutic drugs can have an adverse effect on wound healing, depending on their mechanism of action and the time of administration in relation to the time of injury. Radiation can have a profound adverse effect on wound healing, depending on dose and time of exposure in relation to time of injury.

WOUND CARE

Immediate Wound Care

The wound should be covered with a clean, dry bandage as soon as possible after injury to prevent further contamination and reduce hemorrhage. The bandage should remain in place until definitive treatment is initiated. Antibiotic ointments or powders act only as foreign bodies and delay wound healing and thus should not be applied.

Once the animal is stabilized and other, life-threatening injuries have been treated, the wound can be prepared for treatment. The bandage is removed, and the wound is packed with sterile gauze or filled with a sterile water-soluble lubricant (KY Jelly, Johnson & Johnson, Arlington, TX.) or temporarily closed with sutures, towel clamps, or Michel clips. This allows skin around the wound to be clipped and prepared for aseptic surgery without the introduction of hair into the wound.

Hair from the edges of the wound can be removed by means of scissors dipped in mineral oil to prevent hair from falling into the wound. Once the skin is prepared, the KY Jelly can be flushed out or the sponges removed from the wound.

Wound Lavage

Wound lavage is necessary to remove debris and loose particles and tissue from the wound. It also reduces the number of bacteria in the wound. If infection is suspected, a piece of tissue should be sampled for bacterial culture before lavage. Large volumes of warm, sterile, balanced electrolyte solution are preferred for lavage.

Technician Note

Wound lavage with warm, sterile, balanced electrolyte solution is preferred.

Antibiotics should not be added to the fluid. Soaps, detergents, and antiseptic solutions should not be used, since they damage the tissue. The mechanical action of the lavage is the most important factor for successful lavage. Moderate pressure (7 psi) can be generated with a 35-ml syringe and 19-gauge needle; this method is more effective than pouring fluid over a wound. The syringe can be connected to a bag of fluid with a three-way stopcock to facilitate refilling of the syringe (Figure 4-2). A pulsating, high-pressure (70 psi) stream can be generated by means of a Water Pik (Teledyne, Ft. Collins, CO.) which is even more effective in reducing bacterial population and removing necrotic tissue and foreign material from heavily contaminated wounds.

Wound Debridement

Wound debridement is necessary to remove all contaminated, devitalized, or necrotic tissue, and foreign material from the wound (Table 4-3). This can be performed surgically by excising the affected tissue in layers, beginning at the surface and progressing to the wound depths. Alternatively, the entire wound can be excised *en bloc* if there is sufficient healthy tissue surrounding the wound and vital structures can be preserved. Enzymatic debridement with a commercial solution containing trypsin (Granulex, Smithkline Beecham, Pittsburgh, PA.) can be used for wounds that are not suitable for surgical debridement. Enzymatic debridement is slower and may damage normal tissue.

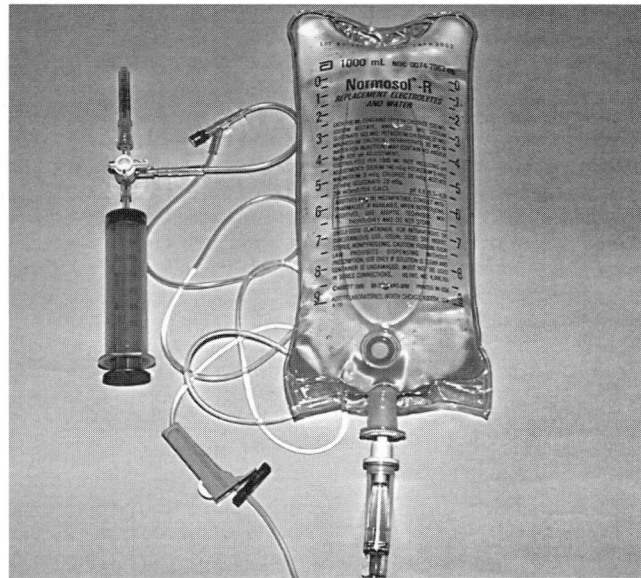

FIGURE 4-2. Connection of a 35-ml syringe and 19-gauge needle to a three-way stopcock and bag of sterile balanced electrolytesolution to facilitate copious lavage of a wound.

TABLE 4-3	METHODS AND INDICATIONS OF WOUND DEBRIDEMENT
Method	**Indications**
Layered debridement	Conservative debridement beginning at superficial layers of wound and progressing to depths; indicated for large wounds with substantial tissue trauma
En bloc	Complete excision of wound; indicated for small wounds in areas with loose skin that can be closed
Enzymatic	Use of trypsin products that dissolve necrotic tissue; very slow method of debridement; indicated in minimally contaminated or traumatized wounds or as an adjunct to surgical debridement

Wound Closure

Selection of one of the four methods of wound closure depends on the nature of the wound (Table 4-4). *Primary wound closure* results in healing by first intention. First intention healing, known as appositional healing, is achieved by the suturing or grafting of a wound soon after injury. Primary wound closure is indicated in fresh, clean, sharply incised wounds with minimal trauma and minimal contamination that are seen within hours of injury. Wounds treated within 6 to 8 hours of injury are treated within the "golden period"; that is, bacteria contaminating the wound have not multiplied to the critical number of 10^5 organisms per gram of tissue and the tissue has not become infected. Wounds treated after the golden period should not be closed, since infection is likely.

Table 4-4	Methods of Wound Closure
Method	**Comments**
Primary closure	First intention healing; closure of a wound with sutures; indicated for fresh clean wounds with minimal contamination or trauma
Delayed primary closure	Closure of a wound before 3-5 days after injury; i.e., before development of granulation tissue; indicated for moderately contaminated or traumatized wounds
Secondary closure	Closure of a wound after 3-4 days; i.e., after granulation tissue has developed in the wound; indicated in severely contaminated or traumatized wounds that require considerable debridement and prolonged wound management; takes advantage of the positive effects of granulation tissue
Second intention healing (contraction and epithelialization)	Wound allowed to heal without surgical closure; relies on contraction and epithelialization; may not be possible or desirable in all wounds

Box 4-1	Factors Important in Wound Management Decision-Making
Time since injury	
Degree of wound contamination	
Degree of tissue trauma	
Thoroughness of initial debridement	
Blood supply of wound	
Animals physical status	
Wound tension and possibility of closure	
Location of wound	

Delayed primary closure is primary closure of a wound 1 to 3 days after injury, before granulation tissue has appeared in the wound. It is indicated for mildly contaminated, minimally traumatized wounds that require some cleansing and debridement or for relatively clean wounds seen 6 to 8 hours after injury. This method allows any local contamination or infection to be controlled before closure.

Healing by contraction and epithelialization is defined as second intention healing and is indicated for dirty, contaminated, traumatized wounds when cleansing and debridement are necessary and when closure may be difficult. Adequate, loose skin surrounding the wound is necessary to allow contraction. Closure by second intention may not always be desirable because the new epithelium is fragile and easily abraded. In addition, contraction may impede normal function, depending on the location of the wound.

Secondary closure results in third intention healing. The wound is sutured at least 3 to 5 days after injury. Granulation tissue will be present in the wound by the time of closure. The granulation tissue helps to control infection in the wound and fills in the tissue defect. Secondary closure is indicated when (1) the wound is severely contaminated or traumatized, (2) epithelialization and contraction will not completely close the wound, or (3) second intention healing is undesirable.

The decision whether to treat a wound primarily or to have it remain open initially and follow up with delayed closure, second intention healing, or secondary closure depends on the (1) time lapse since injury; wounds greater than 6 to 8 hours old should be kept open initially; (2) degree of contamination; wounds obviously contaminated should be kept open initially and thoroughly cleansed; (3) amount of tissue damage; wounds with substantial tissue damage have reduced host defenses, are more likely to become infected, and consequently should remain open initially; (4) thoroughness of debridement; if the initial debridement was conservative, the wound should remain open until definitive debridement is performed; (5) blood supply to the wound; a wound with questionable blood supply should remain open until the extent of nonviable tissue is determined; (6) animal's health; if the animal is unable to endure prolonged surgical debridement, the wound should be kept open and possibly undergo enzymatic debridement until the animal can withstand surgery; (7) closure without tension or dead space; if excessive tension or dead space is present, the wound should be allowed to remain open because dead space allows accumulation of fluid, separation of tissues, and formation of seromas, which may predispose to infection and delay wound healing; and (8) location of the wound; certain locations may not be amenable to closure (e.g., a large wound on a limb) (Box 4-1).

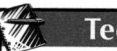 **Technician Note**

Nonadherent bandages are indicated in granulating wounds.

WOUND BANDAGING

Bandaging promotes wound healing by protecting the wound from additional trauma and contamination, by preventing wound desiccation, by preventing hematoma and seroma formation through compression and obliterating dead space, and by immobilizing the wound to prevent cellular and capillary disruption. Bandaging minimizes postoperative edema around incisions and minimizes exuberant granulation tissue formation in open wounds on the lower limb region (below the carpus or tarsus) of horses. In addition, the bandage can absorb wound exudate and debride the wound of foreign material and loose tissue that adheres to the bandage as it is removed. Covering a wound with a bandage promotes an acid environment at the wound surface by preventing carbon dioxide loss and absorbing ammonia produced by bacteria. An acid environment increases oxygen dissociation from hemoglobin and subsequently increases oxygen availability in the wound. The bandage also keeps the wound warm. Higher temperatures improve wound healing and facilitate oxygen dissociation (Box 4-2).

A bandage usually consists of three layers: the primary or contact layer, the secondary or padded conforming layer, and the tertiary or holding and protective layer. The primary bandage layer contacts the wound surface (if present) and may be adherent or nonadherent and occlu-

Box 4-2	BENEFICIAL EFFECTS OF BANDAGING A WOUND

Protects from further contamination
Prevents wound desiccation
Prevents hematoma and seroma formation
Immobilizes the wound and prevents cellular disruption
Minimizes surrounding edema
Absorbs wound exudate and debris
Promotes retention of carbon dioxide and creation of an acid environment, which facilitates oxygen dissociation
Keeps wound warm, which facilitates healing

Box 4-3	STEPS IN BANDAGE PLACEMENT*

Apply anchoring tapes (stirrups)
Apply primary (contact) layer on wound
Apply secondary (padded) layer
Apply tertiary (conforming) gauze layer
Apply splint
Reflect, twist, and adhere tape stirrups to gauze
Apply tertiary (protective) tape

*Some steps may not be indicated.

sive or semiocclusive. Adherent bandages are indicated if some debridement is still necessary. Wounds discharging large amounts of exudate or containing embedded debris are often covered with an adherent, absorbent type of dressing, such as a small stack of gauze pads, disposable baby diaper, or cotton (e.g., combine), in what is called a *dry-dry bandage,* to absorb exudate and allow debris to adhere. The same absorbent material soaked with saline creates a *wet-dry bandage* to "rehydrate" and loosen dried or thick exudate and debris from a wound, facilitating its removal. Nonadherent bandages are required when healthy granulation fills the wound, to avoid disruption of this tissue during removal of the contact layer. Semiocclusive, nonadherent bandages are preferred, because they allow air to penetrate to the wound surface and exudate to escape from the wound surface. Occlusive bandages should not be used if wound exudate is present, since they keep the exudate at the wound surface, and this causes maceration of the wound and adjacent healthy tissue.

The secondary layer is an absorbent, padded, conforming layer of cast padding or roll cotton. The tertiary layer is the holding and protective layer, which uses some form of gauze and elastic or adhesive tape to hold the bandage in place.

Specific bandages and their indications for use in small animal practice are described below. The standard procedure for application of any bandage requires (1) application of anchoring tape strips (stirrups) to the distal portion of the limb; (2) application of a primary bandage layer over the wound, if present; (3) application of the padded secondary layer over the stirrups; (4) application of the gauze tertiary layer; (5) application of the splint; (6) reflection and twisting of the stirrups to adhere to the gauze layer; and (7) application of the protective tertiary layer of tape (Box 4-3). The middle two toes should always be exposed to allow assessment of color, warmth, and swelling. A stockinette can be applied under the secondary layer to help prevent the bandage from slipping. Other modifications are acceptable.

Technician Note

The middle two toes should always be exposed to allow assessment of color, warmth, and swelling.

WOUND BANDAGING IN SMALL ANIMALS

Casts

Fiberglass cast materials are currently used almost routinely because of their light weight, extreme rigidity, rapid setting time, and ventilation and waterproof properties. Casts are indicated for stabilization of certain fractures distal to the elbow or stifle and for immobilization of limbs to protect ligament or tendon repairs. The cast material is applied instead of a tertiary layer; however, minimal padding is suggested to avoid cast loosening and movement and excessive compression (Figure 4-3). It is advisable to monitor animals with casts at least weekly.

Bandages and Splints

The *Robert Jones bandage* is most commonly used for temporary immobilization of fractures distal to the elbow or stifle before surgery. It is a large bulky bandage that provides rigid stabilization because of the extreme compression of the thick cotton secondary layer (Figure 4-4). The Robert Jones bandage is not appropriate for fractures of the femur or humerus.

The *modified Robert Jones bandage,* or simple padded bandage, is a less bulky bandage and is used to reduce postoperative swelling of limbs (Figure 4-5). It provides little or no splinting of the limbs. Less padding is used in the secondary layer, and cast padding is used instead of roll cotton.

Technician Note

The Robert Jones bandage is not appropriate for fractures of the femur or humerus.

A *chest* or *abdominal bandage* is applied in the standard three layers. These bandages should be applied firmly but without constricting the chest or abdomen (Figure 4-6). If an abdominal bandage is used to control abdominal bleeding, the layers are applied more firmly. A rolled towel can be used to reinforce the bandage along the midline and is applied before application of the protective tape. The effectiveness of a compression bandage lasts for only 1 to 2 hours, and it should not remain in place longer than 4 hours.

Distal limb splints can be made with tongue depressors for very small animals, or with aluminum splints, cast material, or thermoplastics (Figure 4-7). They are indicated for temporary immobilization or definitive stabilization of certain fractures of the distal radius and ulna, carpus, tarsus, metacarpals and metatarsals, and phalanges. They can also be used to support a traumatized distal limb. The limb should be well padded to avoid pressure points. The splint should always be placed on the caudal aspect of the limb.

Slings

The *Ehmer sling* is used specifically to immobilize the hindlimb after reduction of craniodorsal coxofemoral luxation and to prevent weight-bearing after surgery on the pelvis. Correct application results in internal rotation and

A **B** **C**

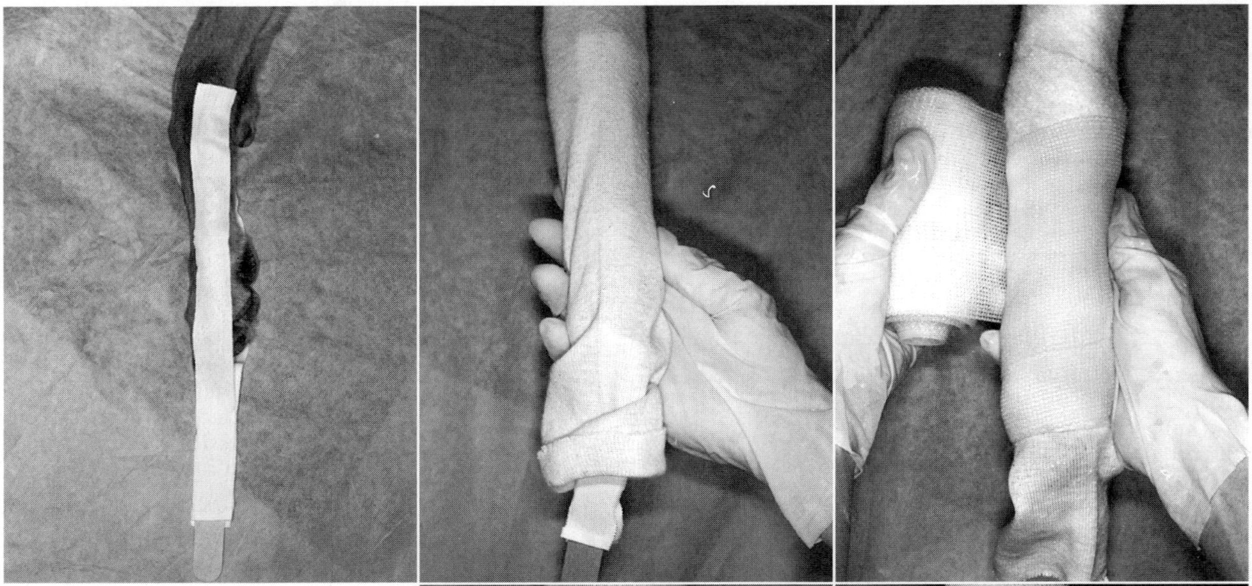

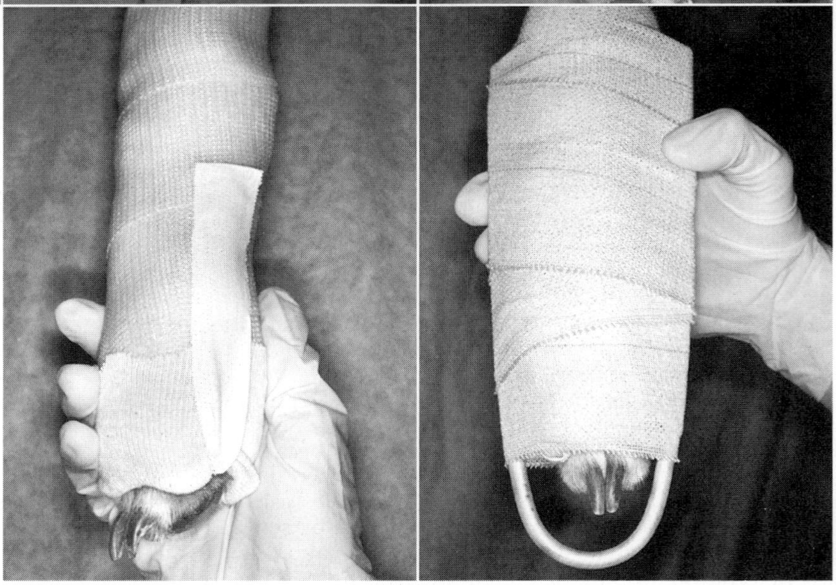

FIGURE 4-3. *Cast.* **A,** Tape stirrups are placed on the lateral aspects of the limb. A tongue depressor is placed between them to prevent adherence of the stirrups to each another. **B,** A stockinette is applied over the limb. A lightly padded, secondary layer is then applied firmly around the leg. **C,** The fiberglass casting material is applied firmly but not tightly to the leg, with care taken to avoid compression of the cast material with the fingers. **D,** The stockinette ends are reflected over the cast, and the tape stirrups are reflected onto the cast. Protective tape is applied over the ends of the cast. **E,** A walking bar can be applied to the cast at this point. The two middle toes are exposed.

D **E**

adduction of the coxofemoral joint (Figure 4-8). Minimal padding is suggested, and the sling is usually applied with adhesive tape alone to prevent slippage.

Technician Note

The 90-90 flexion sling is critical in preventing quadriceps contracture after distal femoral fracture repair in young animals.

The *90-90 flexion sling* is applied with the stifle and hock placed in 90-degree flexion, and no attempt is made to adduct and internally rotate the coxofemoral joint (Figure 4-9). The 90-90 flexion sling is used to prevent stifle joint stiffness and hyperextension caused by quadriceps muscle

contracture after distal femoral fracture repair in young animals. It can also be used as a non–weight-bearing sling to protect other surgical procedures of the hindlimb.

The *Velpeau sling* holds the flexed forelimb against the chest and prevents movement in all joints (Figure 4-10). It is used as a non–weight-bearing sling for the forelimb. The Velpeau sling is indicated after reduction of scapulohumeral joint luxation or to immobilize scapula fractures.

The *carpal flexion sling* is a non–weight-bearing forelimb sling (Figure 4-11). The degree of carpal flexion can be reduced by partially cutting the crisscross of tape formed at the caudal aspect of the carpus.

Hobbles can be applied to the hindlimbs to prevent excessive abduction of the limbs. They are specifically indicated after reduction of ventral coxofemoral luxation and to prevent excessive tension in the inguinal region.

Text continued on p. 114

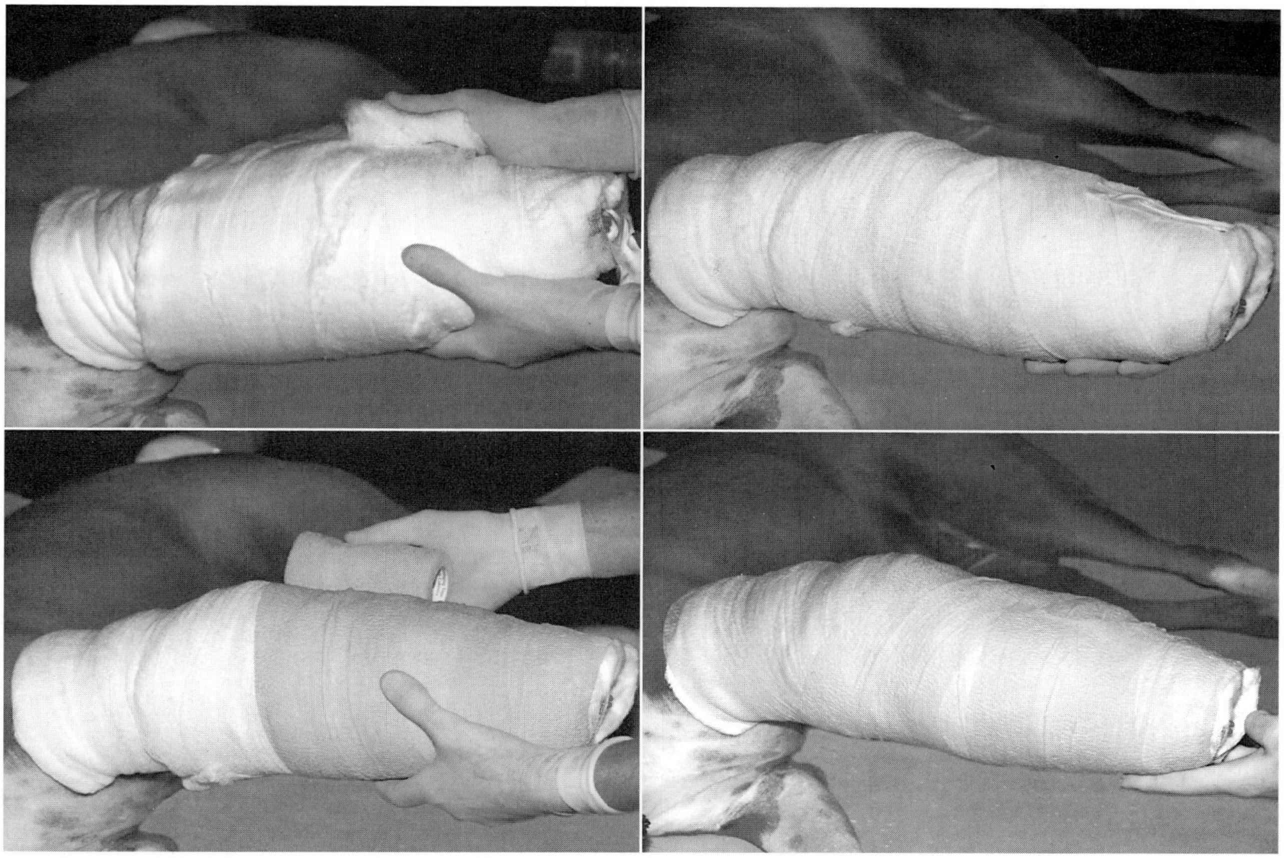

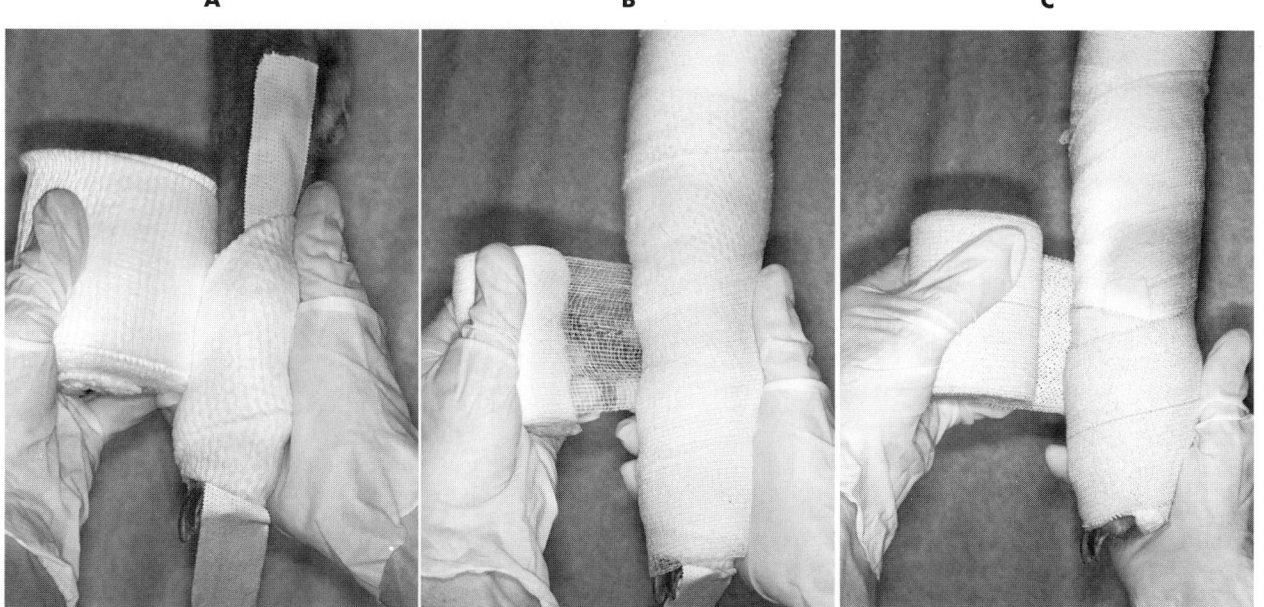

FIGURE 4-4.   Robert Jones bandage. **A,** Tape stirrups are applied, and the limb is wrapped in a secondary layer of roll cotton. **B,** The roll cotton is compressed tightly with a confirming gauze layer. The stirrups are then reflected on top of the gauze. **C,** Protective tape (nonocclusive) is then firmly applied. **D,** The completed bandage should feel solid and "ping" on percussion.

FIGURE 4-5.   Modified Robert Jones or simple padded bandage. **A,** Tape stirrups and a padded secondary layer are applied to the limb. **B,** This is followed by a gauze tertiary layer. **C,** The stirrups are reflected to adhere to the gauze, and the bandage is covered by protective tape.

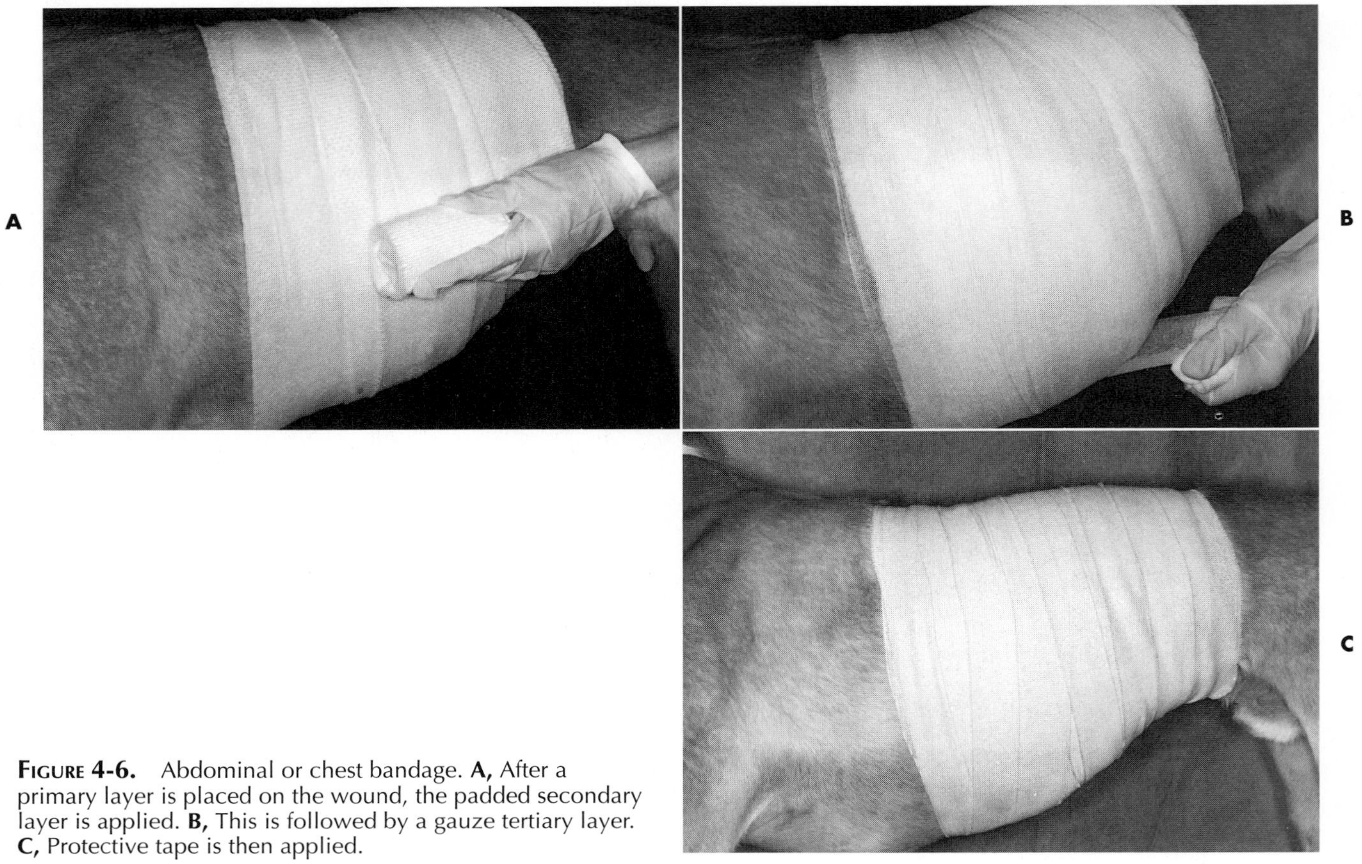

FIGURE 4-6. Abdominal or chest bandage. **A,** After a primary layer is placed on the wound, the padded secondary layer is applied. **B,** This is followed by a gauze tertiary layer. **C,** Protective tape is then applied.

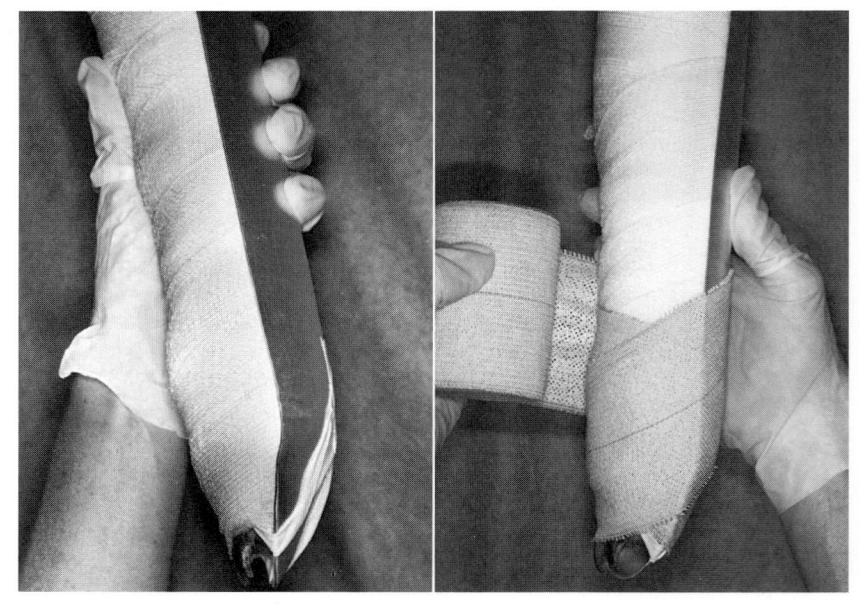

FIGURE 4-7. Splint. **A,** After application of a modified Robert Jones or simple padded bandage (see Fig. 4-5), the splint is applied to the caudal aspect of the ·limb, and the stirrups are reflected onto the splint. **B,** Protective tape is then applied to hold the splint in place.

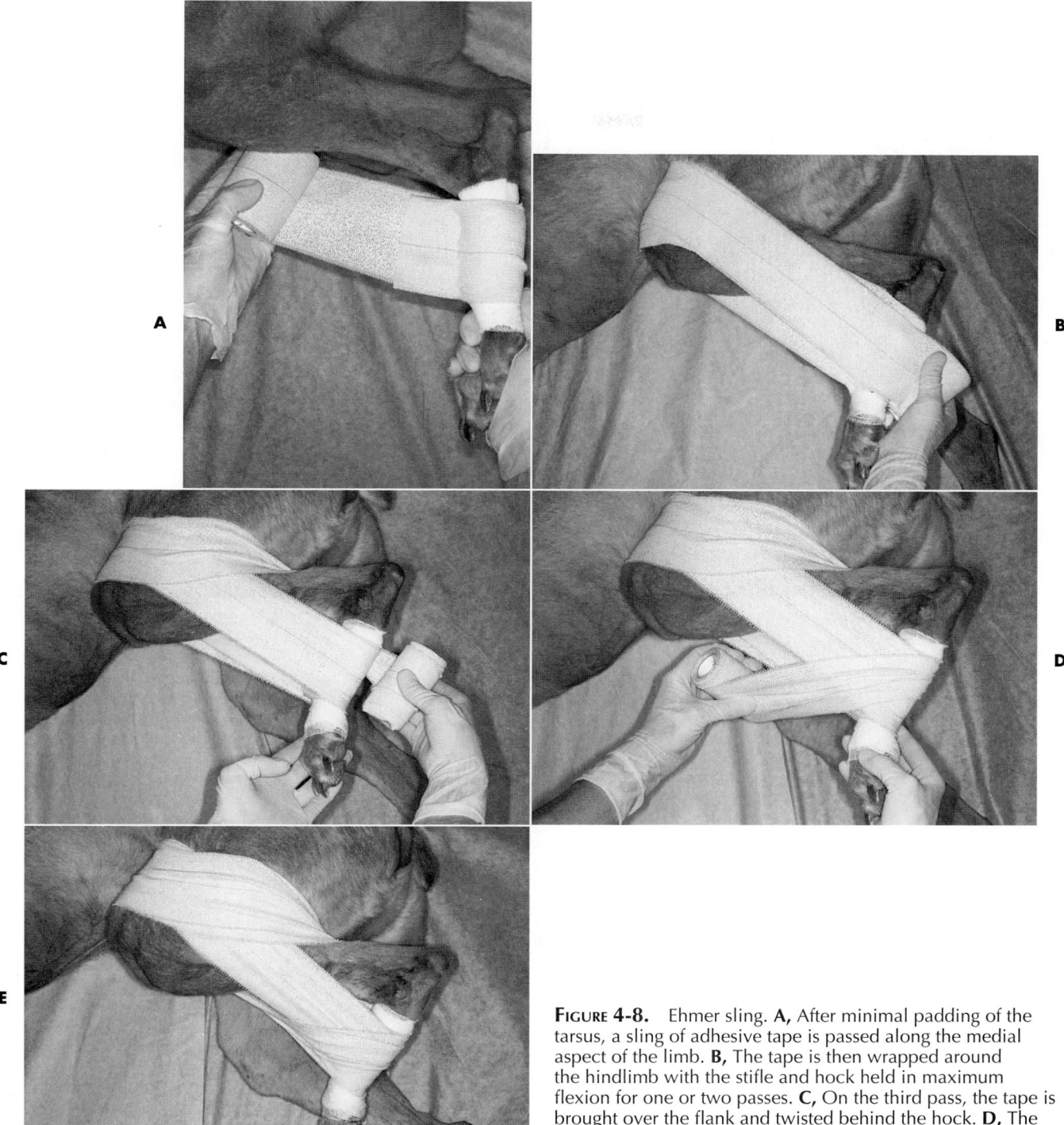

FIGURE 4-8. Ehmer sling. **A,** After minimal padding of the tarsus, a sling of adhesive tape is passed along the medial aspect of the limb. **B,** The tape is then wrapped around the hindlimb with the stifle and hock held in maximum flexion for one or two passes. **C,** On the third pass, the tape is brought over the flank and twisted behind the hock. **D,** The tape is then passed over the front of the metatarsus. **E,** This is repeated for three or four passes.

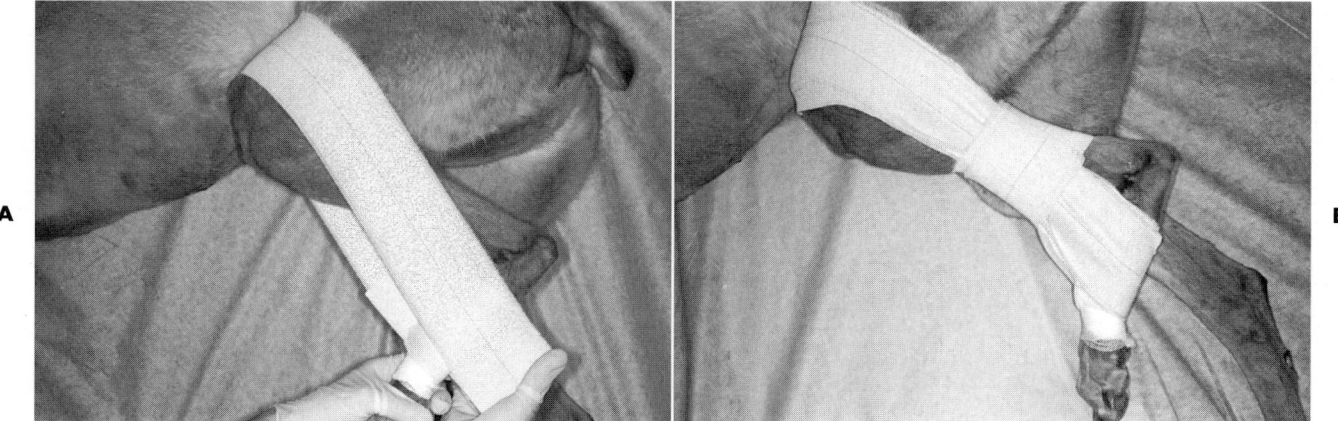

FIGURE 4-9. 90–90-degree flexion sling. After minimal padding of the tarsus, a sling of adhesive tape is passed along the medial aspect of the limb (see Fig. 4-8, *A*). **A,** The tape is then wrapped around the hindlimb with the stifle and hock held in 90-degree flexion. **B,** A second layer of tape is passed horizontally around the tibia to hold the previous layer in place.

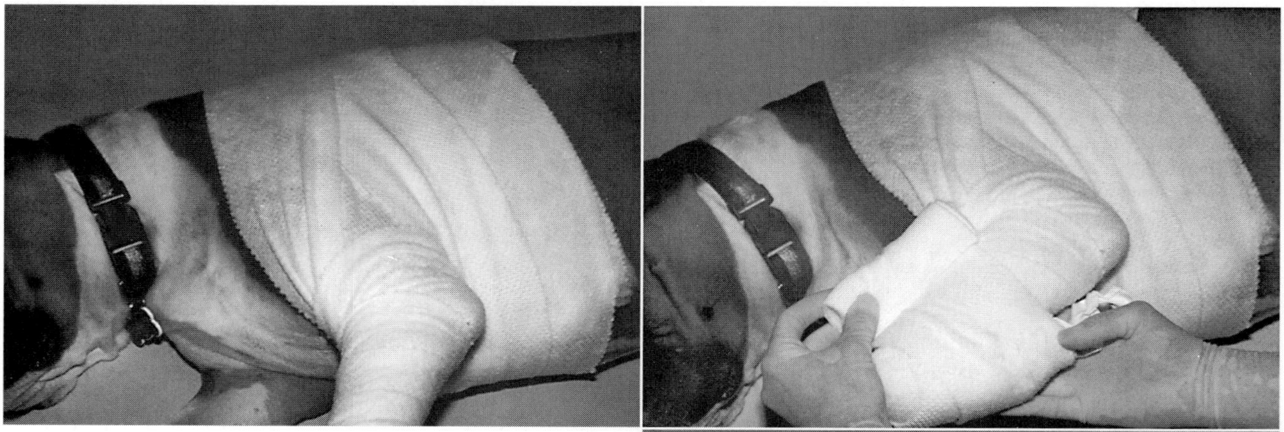

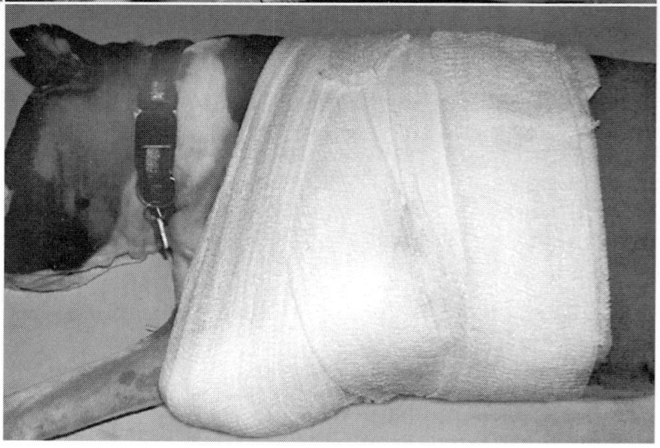

FIGURE 4-10. Velpeau sling. **A,** Stirrups are applied to the forelimb. The entire forelimb and chest are covered with a light padded bandage. **B,** The carpus is then flexed and covered with an additional layer of a light padded bandage. **C,** The flexed carpus and foreleg are then compressed against the chest and held in place with a conforming gauze layer.

Continued

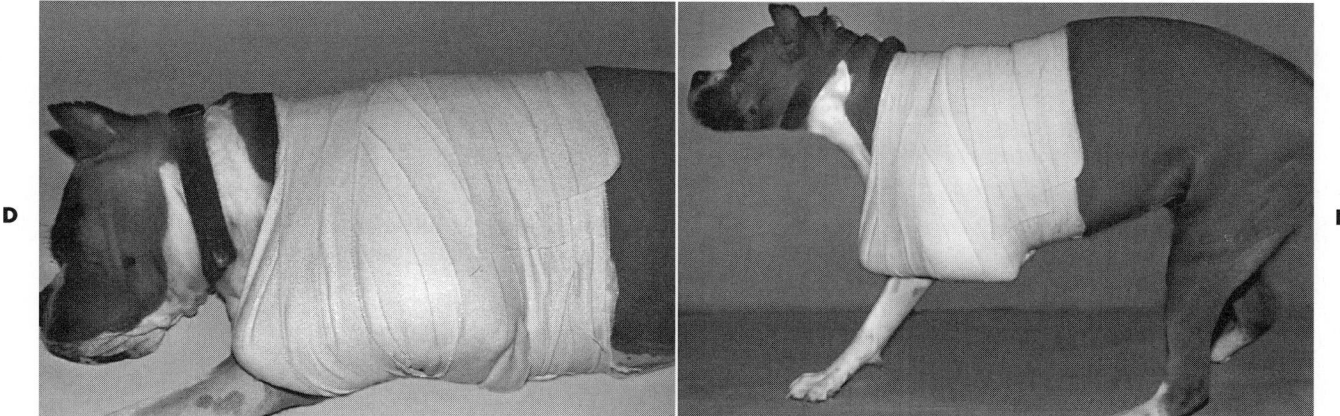

FIGURE 4-10, CONT'D **D** and **E,** The entire leg and chest area are then covered by protective tape (nonocclusive).

FIGURE 4-11. Carpal flexion sling. **A,** Stirrups are applied. With the limb in flexion, a lightly padded bandage is applied. **B,** The stirrups are reflected and protective tape (nonocclusive) is applied. **C** and **D,** One-inch tape is then applied in a figure-of-eight fashion around the carpus to support the carpus. The tape starts at the middle of the carpus and then extends proximally and distally, forming a web of tape behind the carpus.

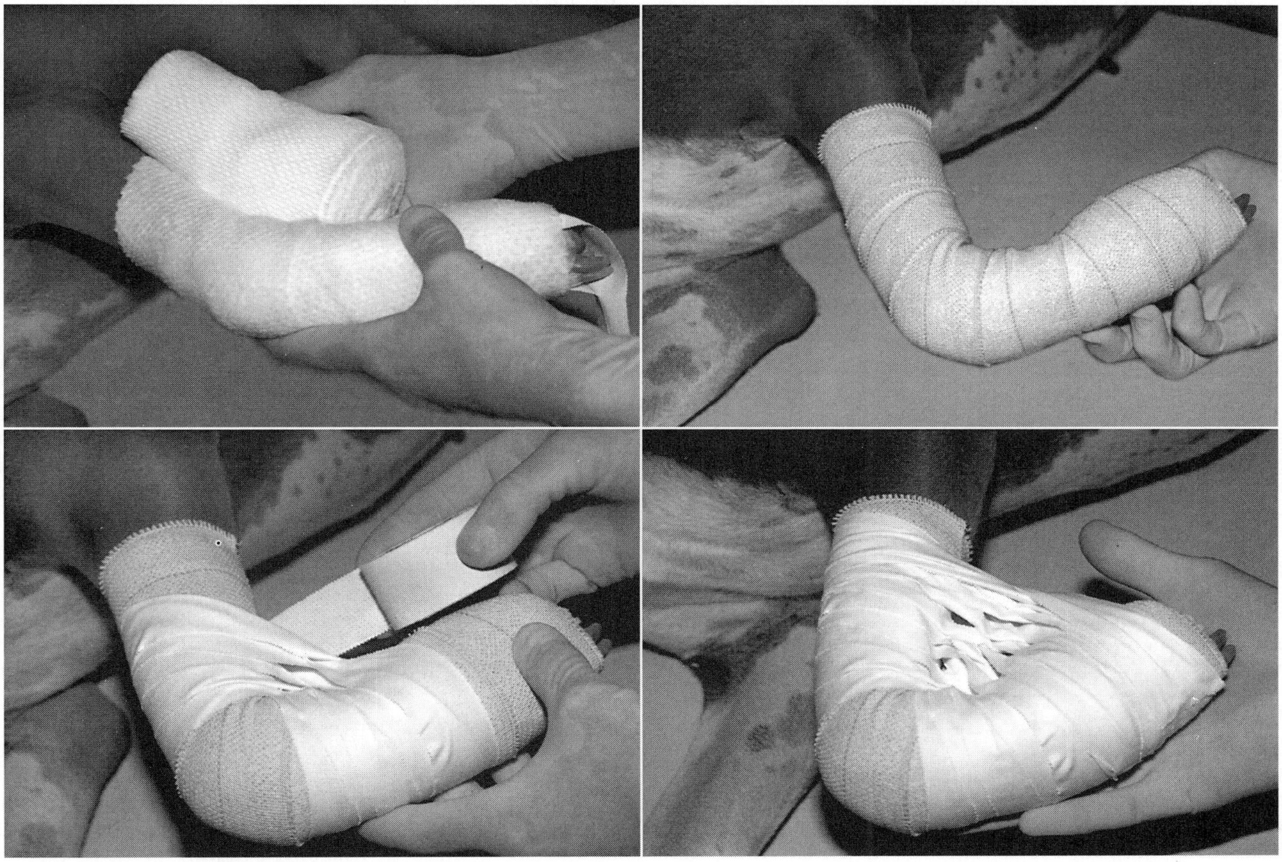

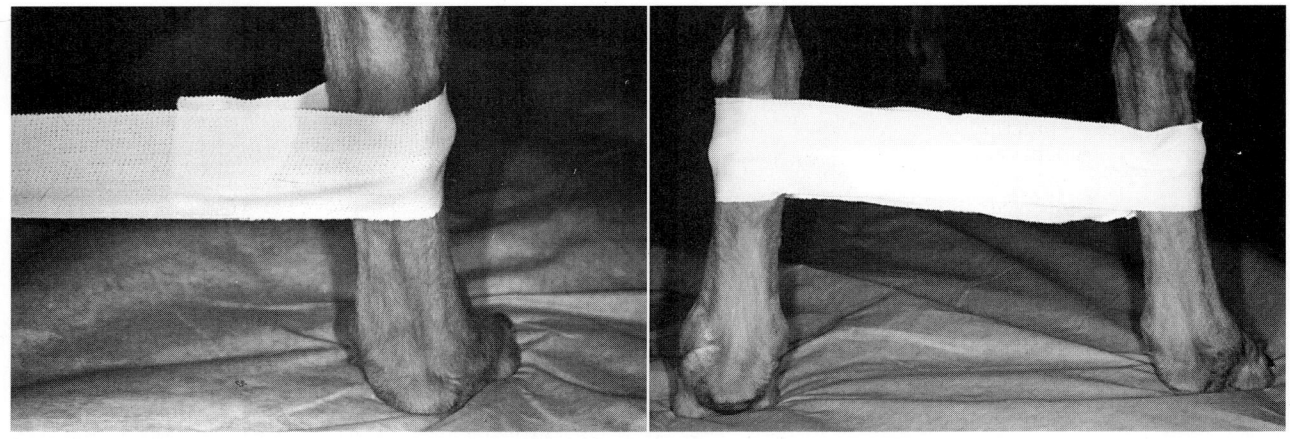

FIGURE 4-12. Hobbles. **A,** Adhesive tape wide enough to cover half of the metatarsal region is placed loosely around the metatarsal region. **B,** The tape is then adhered together between the legs and placed around the opposite metatarsus. The hindlimbs are positioned apart at a distance equal to the width of the pelvis.

They can be used to prevent excessive activity after pelvic fracture repair or for nonsurgical, conservative management of pelvic fractures (Figure 4-12).

Aftercare of Casts, Bandages, Splints, and Slings

Close monitoring of animals with casts, bandages, splints, or slings is extremely important and should be performed daily in the inpatient and at least weekly in the outpatient. Client education for the outpatient is essential. The toes should be monitored daily for warmth, color, and swelling. Abnormal findings indicate a tight cast. Monitoring the bandage for a foul odor that would indicate tissue damage is necessary. Observing for areas of chafing from the cast is important. The animal should be restrained from chewing at the bandage (e.g., by means of an Elizabethan collar), and exercise restriction to short-leash walks is indicated. While the animal is outside, the bandage should be protected from dirt and moisture by application of a plastic bag or other waterproof material. The plastic covering should not remain on for more than 30 minutes, because it prevents the bandage from breathing and the underlying tissue becomes moist and macerated.

SPECIFIC WOUND MANAGEMENT

Characteristics of certain wounds may influence the type of wound management performed. The characteristics of certain wounds and management indications are listed below.

Abrasions

Abrasions are partial-thickness wounds of the epidermis with exposure of the deep dermis. Abrasions can be very painful. Abrasions are associated with minimal bleeding and develop minimal exudate. Healing of abrasions will be enhanced by keeping the wound surface moist and protected rather than allowing a scab to dry on the surface. Application of a nonadhesive, semiocclusive primary layer with a minimal amount of padding and a nonocclusive tertiary layer is indicated. The abrasion will heal by reepithelialization. Bandages should be changed daily and continued until the surface has completely resurfaced with new epithelium.

Lacerations

Lacerations are characterized by sharply incised edges, with minimal tissue trauma. They may be superficial (skin) or deep (tendons, muscle). If tissue is torn away it is called an *avulsion*. Lacerations presented within 12 hours of injury are amenable to minimal debridement of the tissue edges, lavage of the wound, and primary closure. Lacerations presented later than 12 hours after injury may be best treated by *en bloc* debridement of the wound and primary closure. Although uncommon, heavily contaminated lacerations may be best treated by debridement, lavage, and delayed primary or tertiary closure.

Burns

Burns are classified by degree of tissue injury (Table 4-5).

The most common causes of burns in companion animals are fire, cage dryers, prolonged contact with heating pads, heat lamps, spillage of hot liquid, and contact with electrical cords. Unfortunately these causes often result in fourth-degree burns characterized by extensive tissue damage. Animals with more than 50% of the body surface burnt rarely survive.

Animals with fourth-degree burns require intensive management. The large surface area of tissue damage and the extent of the deep tissue damage result in large volumes of fluid, electrolyte, and protein loss through the wound surface. Burn wounds are prone to infection because of the extensive tissue damage, the large surface area exposed to the environment (contamination), and the compromised condition of the animal.

Treatment of an animal with severe burns requires intravenous crystalloid and colloid fluid administration, antibiotic administration, nutritional support, and intensive wound management. Nutritional support is extremely important because the metabolic requirements of the animal may increase up to 200%. The animal is unlikely to take in adequate nutrition voluntarily. Force feeding or enteral feeding through a pharyngostomy, esophagostomy, or gastrostomy tube is indicated.

The wounds must be debrided and managed as open wounds. Any dead skin (eschar) must be removed. Debridement may have to be repeated, particularly for fourth-

TABLE 4-5	CLASSIFICATION OF THERMAL BURNS
First degree	Very superficial burn that involves only the epidermis. Does not blister but becomes erythematous because of dermal vasodilation and is painful. Over 2-3 days the pain subsides and the damaged epidermis desquamates.
Second degree	Superficial burn that involves all layers of dermis. Characteristically forms blisters with fluid collection at the interface of the epidermis and dermis. Blistering may not occur for several hours after injury.
Third degree	Full-thickness burn that involves all layers of the dermis. The surface may appear white or black and appear leathery, firm, and depressed compared with surrounding skin.
Fourth degree	Full-thickness burn that involves not only the dermis, but also subcutaneous fat and deeper structures.

degree wounds, since the extent of the tissue damage may not be evident initially. Burn wounds tend to produce copious, often viscous exudate. Application of a wet-dry primary bandage layer is indicated until healthy granulation tissue is evident. The wet-to-dry bandage facilitates removal of the exudate and some superficial wound debridement. A padded bandage to absorb the exudate with a nonocclusive tertiary layer is required. Ideally, sterile bandage material should be used. Bandages should be changed as often as required to prevent strike through of the bandage by exudate from the wound. Once healthy granulation tissue is apparent in the wound, application of a nonocclusive, nonadherent primary bandage layer is indicated. Coating the wound with salves or lotions is contraindicated because they can be occlusive and keep the exudate at the wound surface. After a healthy granulation tissue wound bed has developed, the wounds are then amenable to tertiary closure or skin grafting.

Puncture Wounds

Puncture wounds are characterized by a small skin opening with often extensive deep tissue damage. Penetrating objects (sticks), gunshots, bite wounds, and insect bites are all types of puncture wounds. Foreign material and bacteria are carried deep into the wound. Puncture wounds should be treated by exploration, debridement, lavage, and primary closure if all the damaged contaminated tissue and all foreign material can be removed from the wound. If the wound remains contaminated, or if there is a large amount of deep tissue damage with resultant dead space in the wound, a drain may be placed. Ideally, a closed suction wound drain that connects to a closed reservoir should be used to reduce contamination of the wound from the environment via the drain. A closed drain also allows the volume and nature of the drainage to be monitored.

Degloving Injuries

Degloving injuries are common injuries seen in small animals, typically the result of being hit by a car and dragged over the road surface. An anatomic degloving injury results in skin and varying amounts of deep tissue (muscle, tendon, ligament, bone) being torn off a limb. A physiologic degloving injury is characterized by an intact skin surface with disruption of the skin attachment and neurovascular supply at the deep fascial level. Necrosis of the detached skin becomes apparent 3 to 5 days after injury.

Degloving injuries require intensive management over a prolonged period of time. Initial debridement, lavage, and management of the open wound are required. It may take several weeks before the wound is covered by a healthy granulation tissue bed. At this time, skin grafting is indicated. Some degloving injuries will completely heal by second intention although the tension on the skin of the distal extremities can be a limiting factor. In addition, the resultant skin contracture and friable new epithelium may not always be a desirable outcome.

Decubitus Ulcers

Decubitus ulcers are the result of compression of soft tissues and skin between a bony prominence and the surface on which an animal is lying. Thin, debilitated animals that are recumbent for long periods are at risk, as are the naturally thin breeds (e.g., Afghans, greyhounds, whippets). The soft tissue and underlying bone of decubitus ulcers may become secondarily infected from environmental microorganisms.

Prevention is the key to management. Adequate soft bedding (water beds) is essential for an at-risk animal. The animal's position should be changed frequently throughout the day. Likely pressure points should be examined daily. Physical therapy and hydrotherapy three or four times per day help to keep the skin clean and promote peripheral circulation. The bedding should be kept clean, dry, and free of excreta. Vulnerable sites can be padded. Maintaining the animal on a high nutritional plane (high protein, high carbohydrate diet) is essential.

For decubital ulcers that have developed, closure of the wound is desirable. Minimal debridement is usually required. Closures often fail since the line of wound closure also overlies the pressure point and tension is often apparent on the wound edges. In some instances, skin flaps may be preferred.

WOUND MANAGEMENT OF HORSES

Wound Care

Basic wound management is no different in large animals than in small companion animals. However, the size and nature of the animal as well as the location of the injury may dictate the way a wound is approached. Thus some additional points will be briefly discussed.

When preparing a wound on a horse, KY Jelly (Johnson & Johnson) or saline-soaked gauze can be used to fill the depths of the wound. Electric clippers are usually used to clip the hair from around the edges of the wound. However, if clippers are not available, the wound edges can be lathered with antiseptic scrub (Betadine Scrub, Purdue Frederick, Norwalk, Conn.), and a straightedge razor or no. 22 scalpel blade (Bard-Parker, Becton-Dickinson AcuteCare, Rutherford, N.J.) can be used to shave the hair (Figure 4-13).

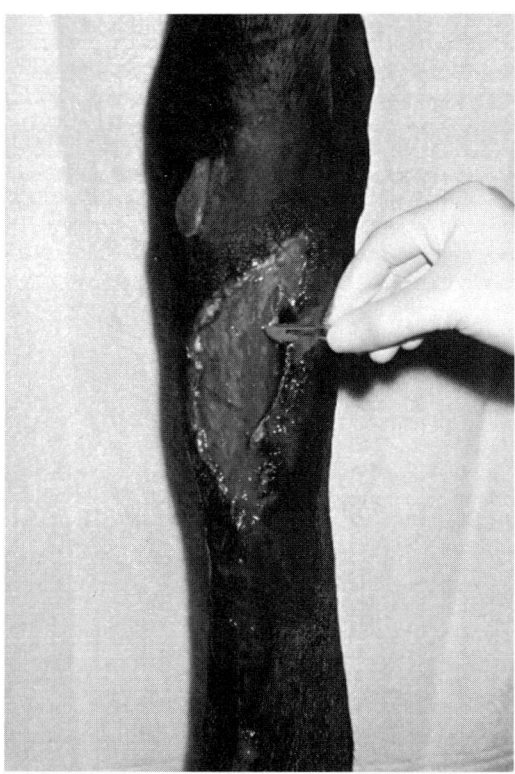

FIGURE 4-13. Once the hair has been lathered with antiseptic (Betadine) scrub, a no. 22 scalpel blade can be used to shave away the hair from the wound edge.

Technician Note

It is important to clip or shave the hair from around a wound.

Various methods can be used to lavage a wound, as described earlier in this chapter. Another available method of wound lavage is the Pulsavac Wound Debridement System (Zimmer, Warsaw, IN.) (Figure 4-14), which is effective in removing debris from wounds. It is equipped with a hand-held spray nozzle that has a trigger to regulate fluid flow. The system can be attached to a vacuum to create suction, which facilitates removal of the lavage solution and debris when the coned head, at the end of the spray nozzle, is placed directly over the wound.

In most cases, local anesthesia with tranquilization or general anesthesia is needed before a wound can be properly treated. If tranquilization is used, local or regional anesthesia is necessary to debride and close the wound. Local infiltration is performed by injecting a local anesthetic, mepivacaine (Carbocaine-V 2%, Pharmacia & Upjohn, Kalamazoo, MI) or lidocaine (Abbott Labs, Abbott Park, IL), approximately 1 cm from the wound edge, subcutaneously around the entire wound. A 22-gauge hypodermic needle is used in most situations and is reinserted repeatedly through the skin, each time at the end of the bleb formed by the preceding injection of local anesthetic (Figure 4-15). In this way, the patient will not react to the succeeding injections. If the wound is located on the distal limb, a ring block or nerve block (e.g., a

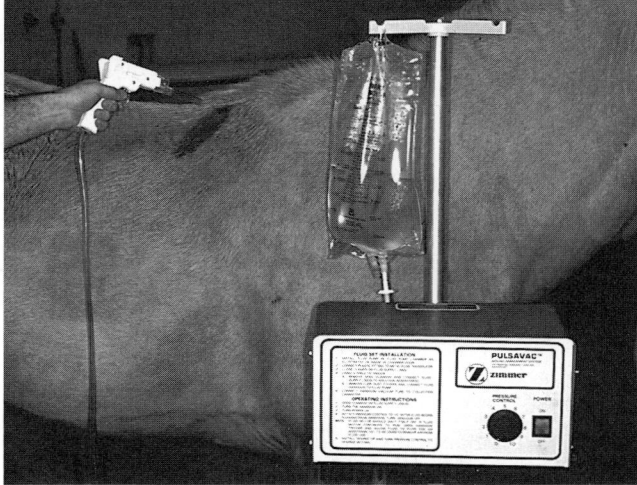

FIGURE 4-14. Pulsavac wound debridement system (Zimmer, Snyder Laboratories) is used to apply a high-pressure (70 psi) stream of lavage solution to a wound, which removes loose debris from the wound.

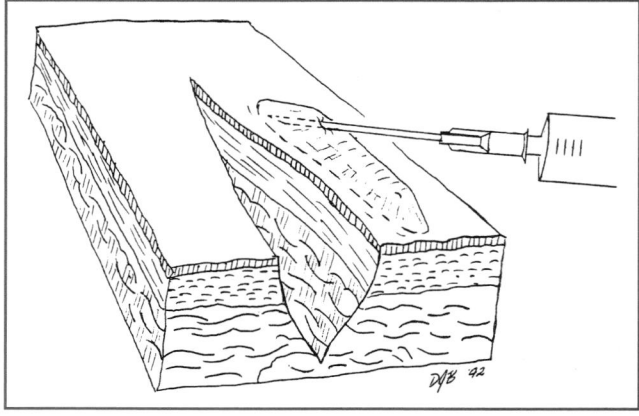

FIGURE 4-15. Proper technique of infiltration of a wound edge with a local anesthetic. The needle should enter through the skin at the point of the last injection.

palmar nerve block) can be used to anesthetize the limb distal to the block.

The same considerations for wound closure in small companion animals apply to large animals as well. It is important to remember that open wounds on the distal aspect of the limb (below the carpus or tarsus) of the horse are notorious for developing exuberant granulation tissue. Exuberant granulation tissue, commonly referred to as "proud flesh," can form rapidly in horses. Various measures must be undertaken to keep exuberant granulation tissue in check, or it can become excessive (Figure 4-16). Methods of controlling granulation tissue include immobilizing the limb (as with a cast), wound bandaging, surgical excision, caustic agents such as equal parts of copper sulfate and boric acid powder, cryotherapy, electrocautery, or topical corticosteroids. Regardless of the decision to allow a wound on the limb of a large animal to heal by first or second intention, a bandage should be placed on the limb.

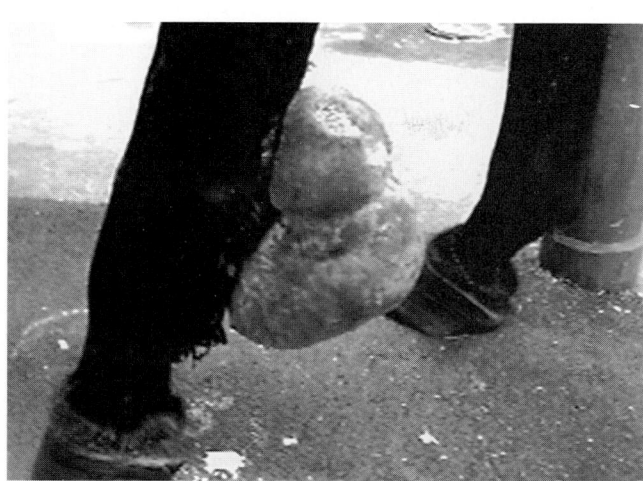

FIGURE 4-16. Excessive exuberant granulation tissue on the plantar aspect of the metatarsus of a horse.

BANDAGING AND CAST APPLICATION TECHNIQUES FOR HORSES

Bandages and casts serve many purposes and can be named for the location and purpose they cover and serve, respectively. Various materials are available for use in a bandage or cast, but the important aspect is their proper application and function. Development of good bandaging and cast application skills is important to ensure proper function of the bandage or cast. The application and purpose of the different types used on horses will be discussed.

Bandages

Lower Limb Wound Bandage

A *lower limb wound bandage* covers a wound on a limb distal to the carpus or tarsus. When the wound is traumatic, after it has been cleaned and debrided, a topical medication is usually applied if it is left unsutured. A nonadhering dressing (Release, Johnson & Johnson; Adaptic, Johnson & Johnson) is then placed directly over the wound. The wound dressing is secured to the limb with rolled conforming gauze (Kling, Johnson & Johnson). The conforming gauze is wrapped around the limb with *light* pressure, overlapping, and without wrinkles to avoid pressure lines, which may cause skin sloughing if applied too tightly. It is wrapped proximal and distal to the wound approximately 2 to 4 cm (Figure 4-17).

The padded layer is applied next. Combine cotton sheets cut from a roll, rolled cotton, layered cotton sheet, quilted leg wraps, or a military field bandage can be used (Figure 4-18). If cotton sheets are available, five are used, folded in half and neatly rolled. The fifth sheet is folded in the opposite direction to the other sheets to conceal the edges. The padded layer is secured to the limb with a roll of conforming gauze (brown gauze, National Health Care Products, Inc., Scottsdale, Ariz.; Kling, Johnson & Johnson). Pressure is applied when wrapping to compress and conform the padding to the limb. The outer shell of the bandage is finished using elastic wrap (Vetrap, Animal Care Products/3M, Minneapolis, Minn.; Ace bandage, Johnson & Johnson), adhesive elastic tape (Elastikon, Johnson & Johnson), or a flannel track wrap. The end of the Ace or track wrap is secured with white tape cut into

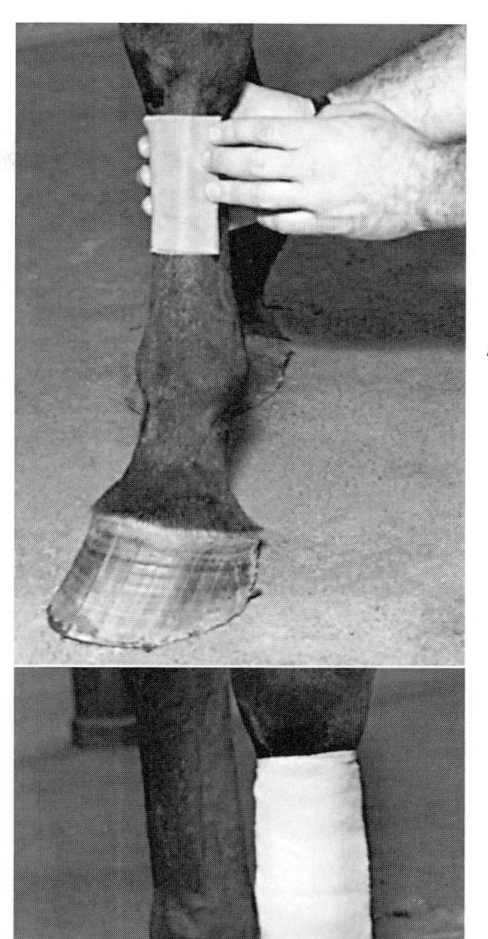

FIGURE 4-17. Application of wound dressing on the distal region of the limb of a horse. **A,** Nonadherent dressing is applied directly over the wound. **B,** Conforming gauze (Kling) is used to maintain a nonadherent dressing over the wound.

strips or placed around the bandage in a "barber pole" fashion (Figure 4-19). Elastikon is placed around the top and bottom of the bandage, with half of the tape sticking to the wrap and half to the skin, to prevent slippage and debris (e.g.,bedding shavings) from getting down inside the bandage.

Lower Limb Support Bandage

This type of bandage is used to provide support of the soft tissues (e.g., ligaments, tendons) of the limb contralateral

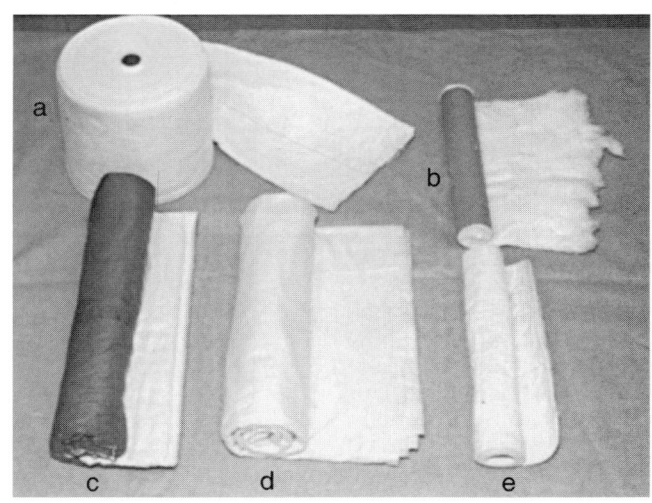

FIGURE 4-18. Various materials can be used for the padded layer in a leg bandage for large animals. *a,* Cotton combine. *b,* Rolled cotton. *c,* Military field bandage. *d,* Cotton sheets. *e,* Quilted leg wraps.

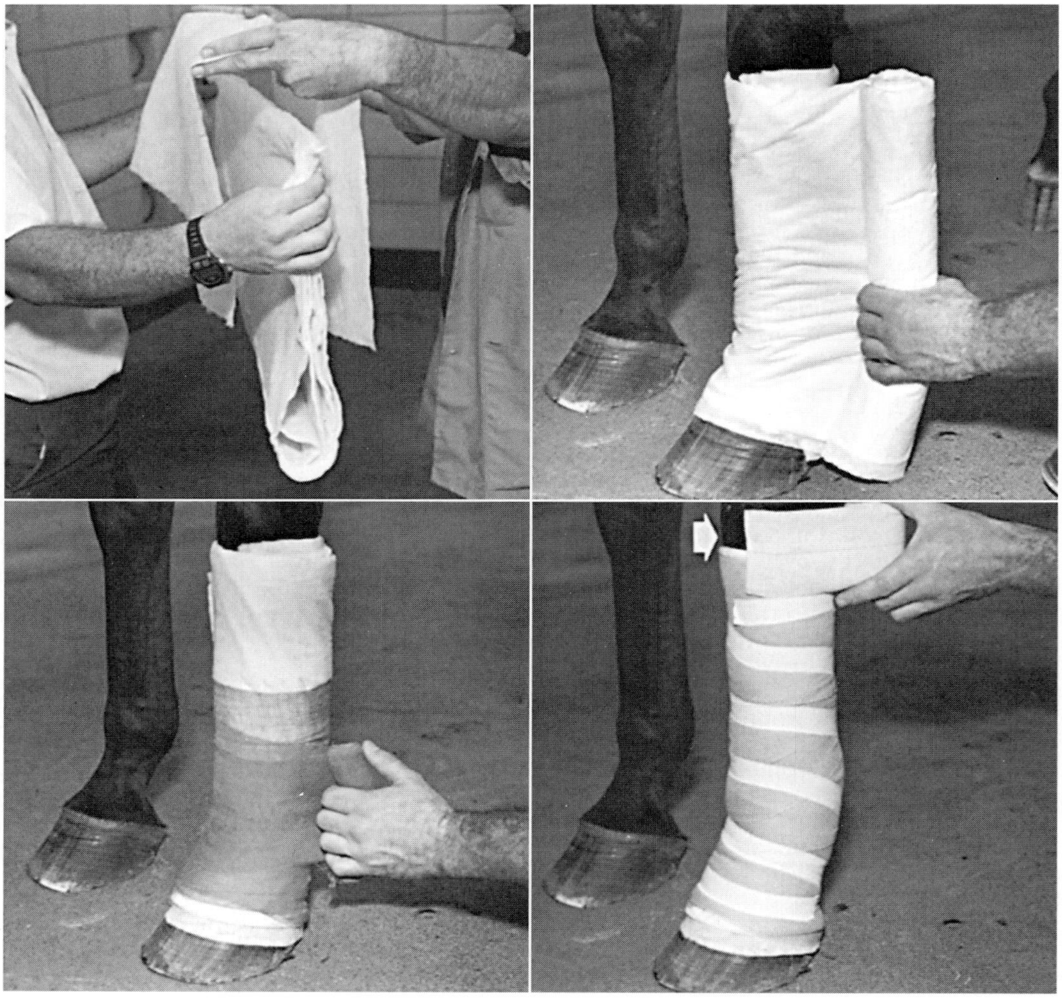

FIGURE 4-19. Application of padded layer of a wound bandage. **A,** The wrap used is constructed by taking five cotton sheets and folding them in half, with the fifth sheet folded opposite the other sheets to conceal the edges. This is then rolled. **B,** Cotton wrap is applied snugly around the limb. **C,** Conforming gauze is used to secure the padded layer to the limb. **D,** An elastic wrap is used to form the outer shell of the bandage. White tape is applied in a "barber pole" fashion to secure the wrap. Wide adhesive tape is used to provide a seal between the skin and bandage *(arrow).*

to the injured leg, which is bearing excessive weight because of decreased weight-bearing on the injured limb. The bandage also minimizes static limb edema in a confined, inactive horse. A support bandage is placed on the lower limb, just like the wound bandage described above except that the underlying wound dressing and inner conforming gauze layer are not used. It is also unnecessary to place wide adhesive elastic tape (Elastikon) around the top and bottom.

Splints

A splint is an addition of a rigid material to a limb bandage to reinforce immobilization of a particular part of a limb. Various materials can be used as the reinforcement, including wooden slats, metal bars, low-temperature thermoplastic, and casting material. However, the most common material used is polyvinyl chloride (PVC) pipe, because of its light weight and strength. The pipe used is 10 cm in diameter and is split in half. It can be bent by heating with a cutting torch to conform to the fetlock angulation. The length and width of the splint vary with the size of the leg and the area being splinted. Depending on the amount of immobilization, splints can be placed the full length of the forelimb or from just below the carpus or tarsus all the way to the ground surface. In most situations, they are placed on the flexor surface of the limb. Splints are used in situations such as extensor or flexor tendon lacerations, flexure deformities in foals, or as needed limb support (as in radial nerve paresis).

A thick bandage is first placed on the limb. It should be long enough to cover the limb above as well as below the ends of the splint. This will prevent pressure sores from developing. Once the bandage is in place, the splint is secured to the limb with adhesive tape (Figure 4-20). Splints should be reset frequently (at least once per day) in foals.

Technician Note

It is important that a bandage cover the limb well above and below the ends of a splint to prevent pressure sores.

Casts

A cast is the most frequently used external coaptation to manage various orthopedic injuries or problems when maximum support and immobilization are required. Casts are commonly used for lower limb problems; however, full-limb application is sometimes indicated in large animals. Indications for use of a cast include lower limb fractures, as an adjunct to internal fixation, tendon lacerations, support of the lower limb during recovery from orthopedic surgery, heel bulb lacerations, and luxations of the tarsus, fetlock, or pastern.

For optimal effectiveness in immobilization, a cast must immobilize the joint proximal and distal to the injury. Full-limb casts must extend up to the elbow or stifle as far as possible. The most frequently used material today is fiberglass. Fiberglass (e.g., DeltaLite, Johnson & Johnson) is appealing because it is lightweight, strong, and relatively easy to apply. However, some veterinarians prefer to use a layer of the traditional plaster of Paris initially under the fiberglass. Plaster conforms well to the contour of the limb, reducing the risk of pressure sores.

Before cast application is begun, several things must be considered. It is important that a limb cast be applied

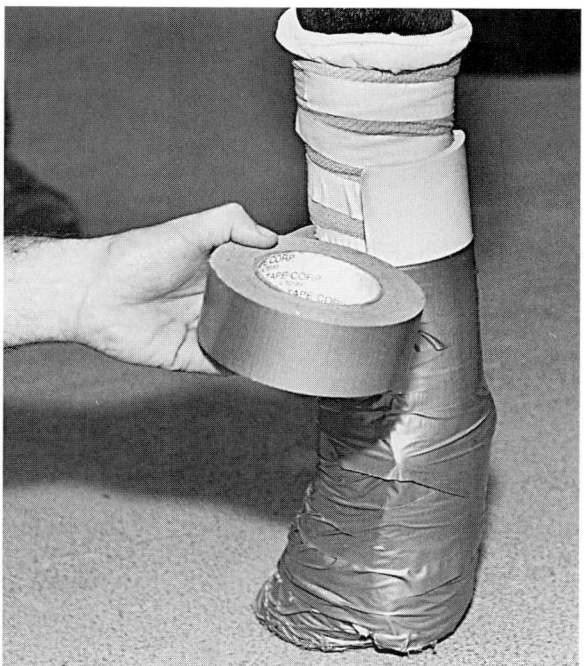

FIGURE 4-20. Application of a lower limb splint. A thick bandage is placed on the limb. The splint (PVC pipe) is positioned along the flexor surface and secured to the bandage with duct tape.

properly or serious problems such as pressure necrosis can occur. Because of its importance, application of a limb cast is described here in detail.

Before the procedure is begun, all the materials needed should be collected: orthopedic stockinette (3-inch), orthopedic felt, towel clamps, white tape (1-inch), wire (approximately 30 cm), $\frac{1}{8}$-inch drill bit and hand drill, broom handle, hoof-trimming equipment, bandage scissors, and cast material (Figure 4-21). It is important that the cast be applied properly, especially if it is to remain on the limb for a prolonged period (4 to 6 weeks).

Generally, it is best to apply the cast with the horse under general anesthesia. The horse is positioned in lateral recumbency so that the limb to which the cast will be applied is uppermost. Debris is cleaned from the sole, the horseshoe removed, and the hoof trimmed. The limb is placed in an extended position perpendicular to the body. Effective support of the leg to maintain the limb in alignment is essential. Traction using wire looped through holes drilled in the hoof can be helpful. Two holes are drilled in the hoof wall 5 cm apart near the toe, in the same direction as that in which a horseshoe nail is driven. The ends of the wire are twisted together to form a loop through which a broom handle is placed to apply traction (Figure 4-22).

The frog can be packed with povidone-iodine (Betadine Solution, Purdue Frederick, Norwalk, Conn.), especially if thrush is present. If a wound is present, a three-layer bandage consisting of a nonadhering dressing, conforming gauze, and adhering elastic tape is used to cover it. The skin must be clean and dry. It can be powdered with talcum or boric acid to help keep the area dry under the cast. The limb is then covered with a double layer of stockinette. The length of the region to receive the cast is measured, and

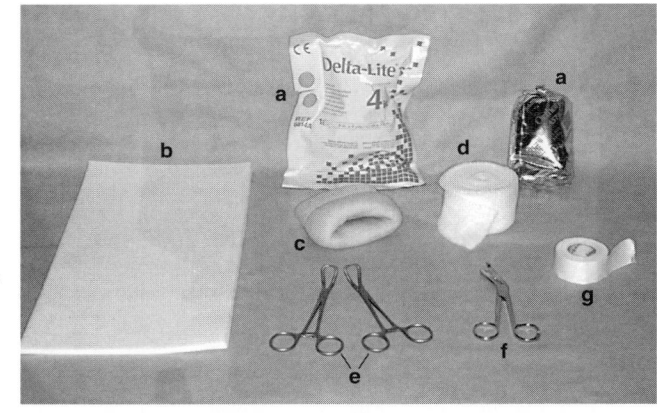
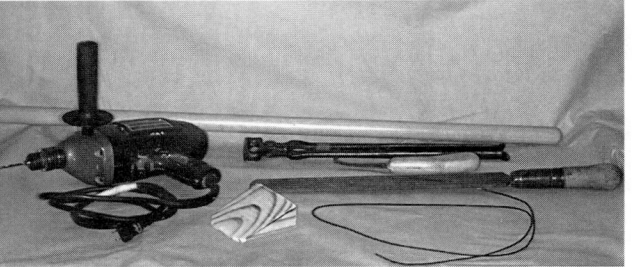

FIGURE 4-21. Materials needed to apply a limb cast on a large animal. **A,** Cast material *(a)*, orthopedic felt *(b)*, orthopedic stockinette (3-inch) *(c)*, cast padding *(d)*, towel clamps *(e)*, bandage scissors *(f)*, and white tape (1-inch) *(g)*. **B,** Wire (approximately 30 cm), 1/8-inch drill bit and hand drill, wooden wedge block, broom handle, and hoof-trimming equipment.

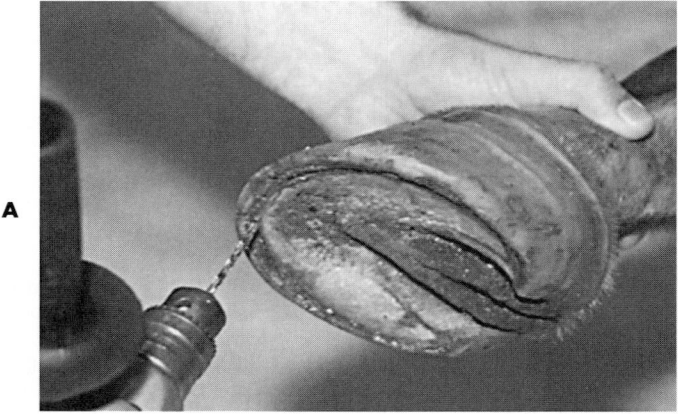
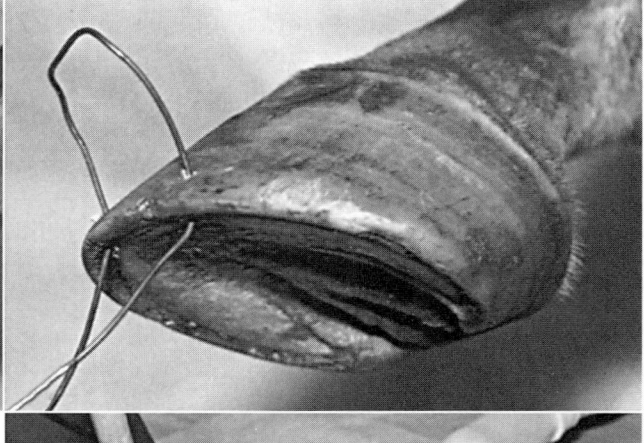
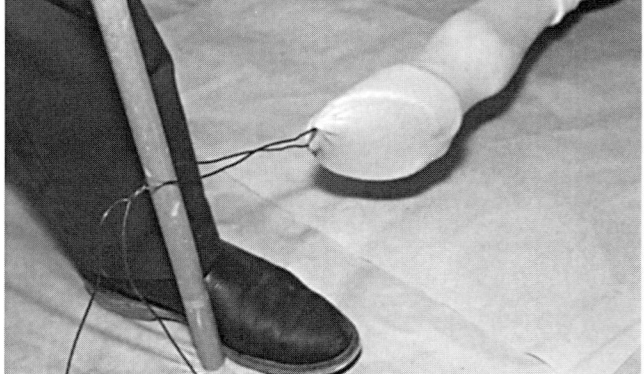

FIGURE 4-22. Traction can be applied to a limb before cast application by drilling two holes in the toe of the hoof, **A,** and threading a loop of wire through the holes, **B,** with a broomstick placed in the loop to apply traction, **C.**

approximately 20 cm is added to this to determine the length of stockinette needed. One end is rolled outward and the other is rolled inward until they meet at the midpoint of the stockinette (Figure 4-23).

The traction wire is threaded through the opening in the stockinette. The broom handle is placed through the wire loop and traction is applied. The outward roll is first unrolled up the leg. A twist is placed in the stockinette just beneath the toe, and the inward roll is unrolled up the leg

(Figure 4-24). Any wrinkles are smoothed out, and towel clamps are used to secure the stockinette to the medial and lateral aspects of the limb, above the area to which the cast will be applied.

A strip of orthopedic felt (5 to 7 cm wide) is placed around the leg at the most proximal limit of the cast. This is held in place with 1-inch white tape (Figure 4-25). Additional padding on the leg should be avoided because this can become compressed, thus allowing the leg to move

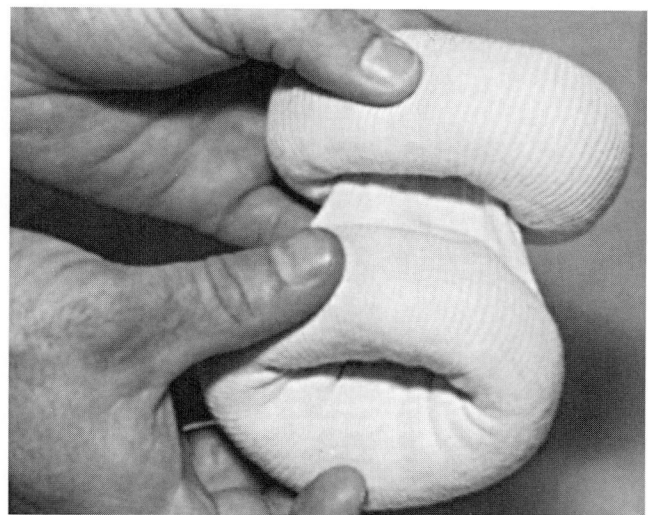

FIGURE 4-23. Orthopedic stockinette used under a cast is pre-rolled. One end is rolled outward and the other is rolled inward until they meet at the midpoint of the stockinette.

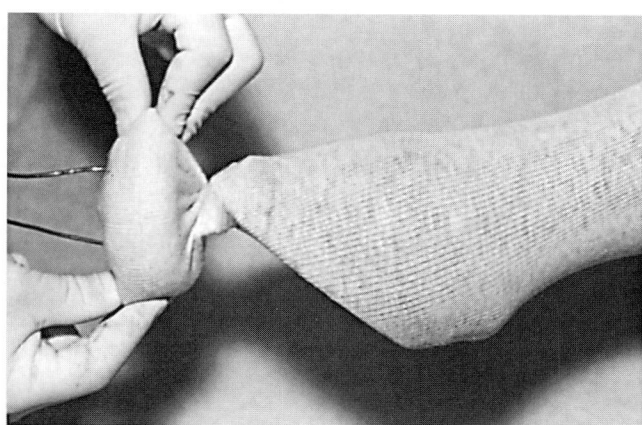

FIGURE 4-24. A twist is placed in the stockinette just beneath the toe, and the inward roll is unrolled up the leg.

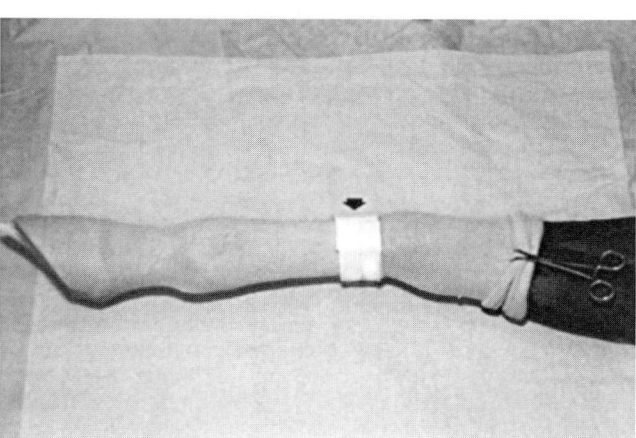

FIGURE 4-25. Before cast material application, the orthopedic stockinette is secured with towel clamps to the medial and lateral aspects of the limb, above the area to receive the cast. A strip of orthopedic felt (5 to 7 cm wide) *(arrow)* is placed around the leg at the most proximal limit of cast. This is held in place with 1-inch white tape.

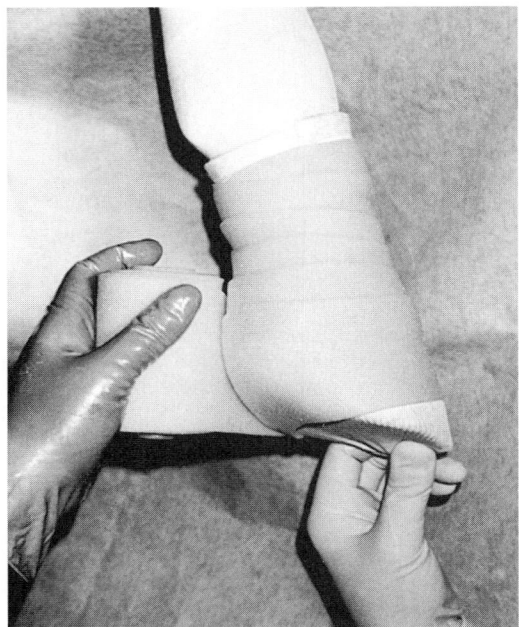

FIGURE 4-26.   A roll of support foam (Custom Support Foam, 3M) can be applied over the stockinette to provide padding under the cast to reduce formation of cast sores.

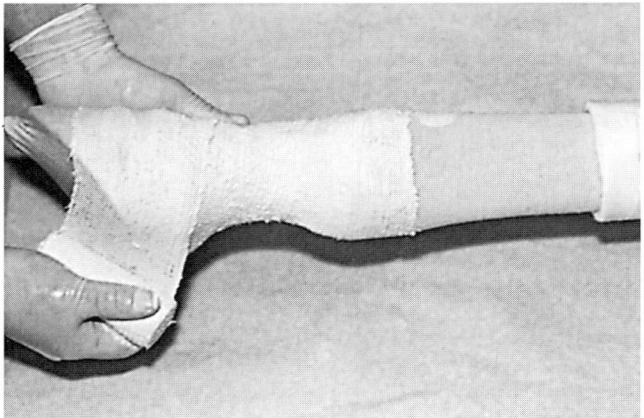

FIGURE 4-27.   Application of the plaster of Paris.

within the cast and cause sores. When a full-limb cast is used, a doughnut pad cut from orthopedic felt is placed over the accessory carpal bone of the forelimb. A thin strip of orthopedic felt is placed over the gastrocnemius tendon and the point of the hock of the hindlimb to prevent the development of pressure sores. A roll of support foam (Custom Support Foam, 3M) can be applied next. Although not necessary, it is applied over the stockinette and was developed to provide padding under a cast to reduce the development of sores (Figure 4-26).

Two layers of 3-inch plaster material are first carefully and snugly applied to the limb. To prevent pressure sores, it is important that these layers be applied without wrinkles. Application of the cast material is usually started at either the proximal or the distal aspect of the limb. We prefer to start distally (Figure 4-27). A roll of plaster is started at the level of the fetlock and worked distally and then proximally. Approximately 1 cm of the orthopedic felt

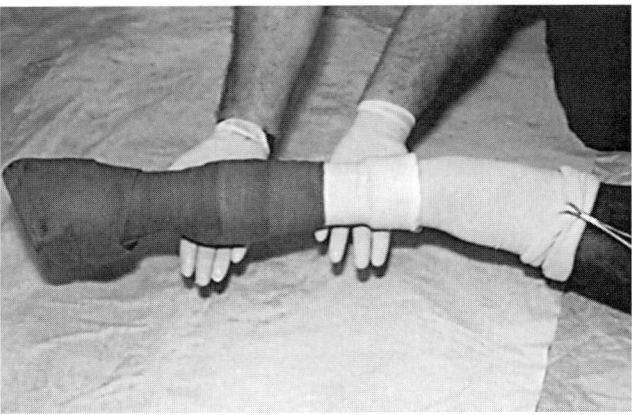

FIGURE 4-28.   As the fiberglass cast material is being applied, an assistant holds the leg out at the upper limb region by resting it on the palms of the hands under the metacarpus/metatarsus region. This method prevents finger impressions from being made in the uncured cast material.

is left exposed above the top of the cast to prevent formation of a sore.

Next the fiberglass cast material is applied. Usually it is easier to begin with 3-inch material because it conforms to the limb better. The cast material is overlapped by one third to one half. As the fiberglass casting material is worked toward the foot, the traction wires are cut, and an assistant holds the leg out at the upper limb region or by resting it on the palms of the hands placed under the metacarpus or metatarsus region. It is imperative to prevent finger imprints in the cast because they could cause a pressure sore to develop (Figure 4-28).

Technician Note

It is very important that the initial layer of casting material be applied to the limb without wrinkles or finger imprints, which may create sores.

More pressure is applied to the succeeding layers of fiberglass. This will allow them to laminate better. Generally, two layers of 3-inch fiberglass cast material are applied, followed by two or three layers of 4- or 5-inch fiberglass. At the time the last roll of cast material is applied, the stockinette is unclamped and the excess is cut off, leaving approximately 4 cm. This 4-cm excess is turned down over the top of the cast and incorporated in the last layer.

A wooden wedge block or a 3-inch roll of wet plaster cast material is placed underneath the heel and also incorporated with the last layer (Figure 4-29). A heel wedge allows the horse to walk more easily while wearing a cast because it decreases the breakover force, reduces pressure on the dorsal proximal limits of the cast at the metacarpus or metatarsus, and allows more even axial weight-bearing down through the cast.

It is best to wear gloves, especially when applying the fiberglass. To save time in identifying the end on a wetted plaster roll, unroll 2 to 3 inches of the plaster material and hold onto it while wetting the roll in a bucket of warm water (Figure 4-30). The excess water is removed by shaking and squeezing the roll. Do not squeeze excessively or excessive plaster will be lost. Fiberglass material is held in a

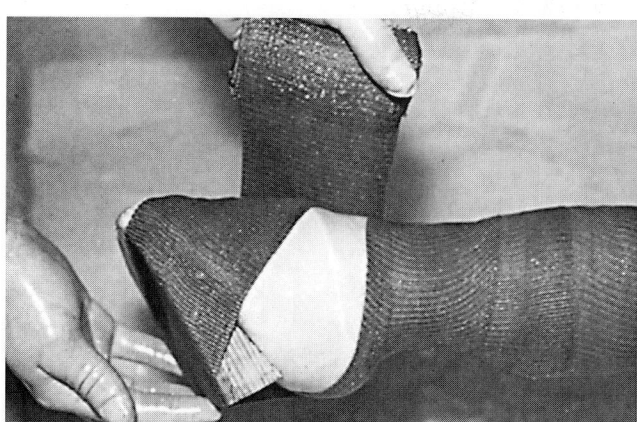

FIGURE 4-29.   A wooden wedge block is placed underneath the heel and incorporated with the last layer of cast material.

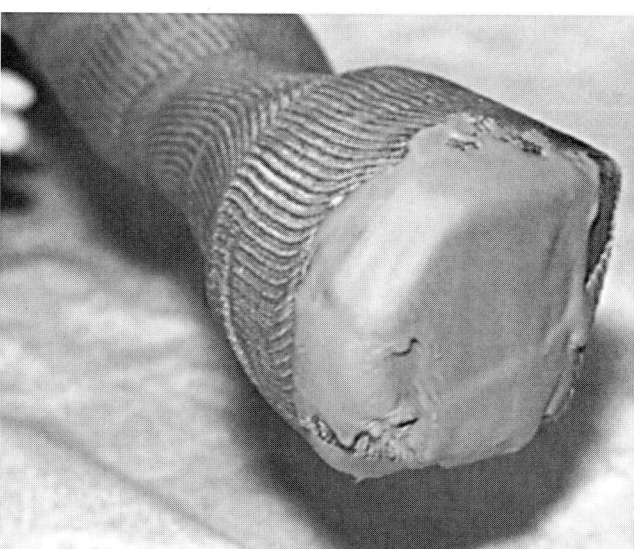

FIGURE 4-31.   The bottom of the cast is protected from wear by capping it with hard acrylic (Technovit).

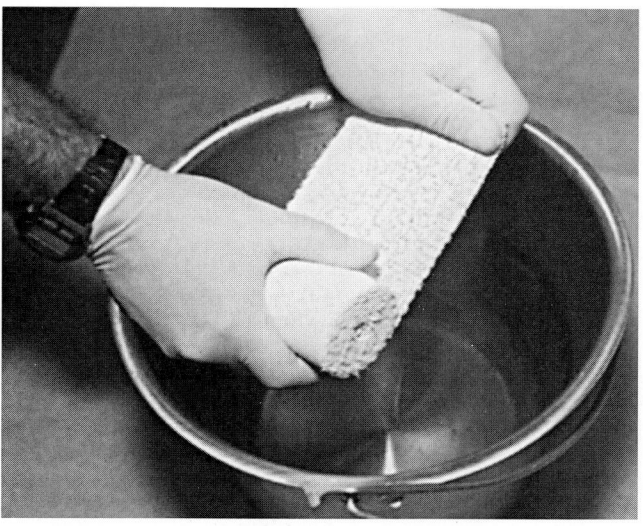

FIGURE 4-30.   The end of the plaster cast material is held away from the roll while it is being moistened.

bucket of clean water until thoroughly wet, and the excess water is shaken out.

When application of the cast is completed, the outer layer is smoothed by running your hand cream–covered gloved hands up and down the cast. Hand cream provides a slick surface, which allows a smooth finish to be placed on the final layer. The hand cream should only be used following the completion of the cast, since it may interfere with curing and bonding of the deeper layers. The bottom of the cast is protected from wear by capping it with hard acrylic (Technovit, Jorgensen Laboratories, Loveland, Colo.) (Figure 4-31). An elastic adhesive tape is placed around the top of the cast and attached to the skin, or a piece of stockinette is pulled over the top and taped to the cast and the limb above the cast to prevent debris (wood shavings) from getting down inside the cast (Figure 4-32).

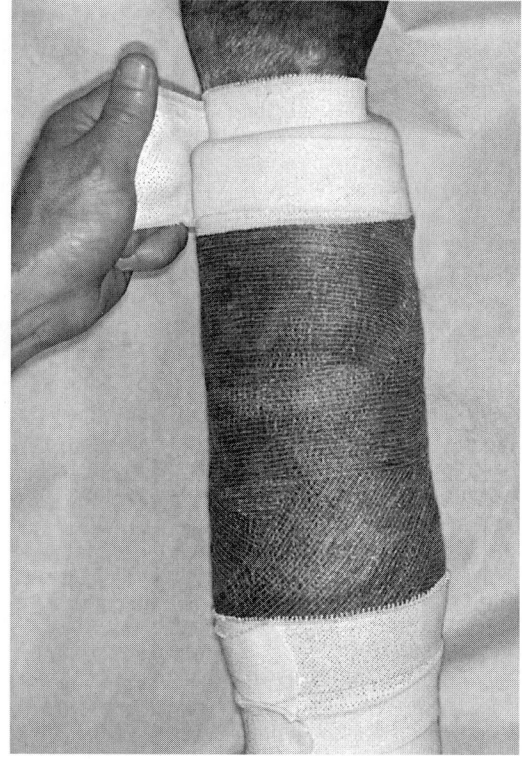

FIGURE 4-32.   Elastic adhesive tape is placed on top of the cast to form a seal between the skin and cast that prevents debris from getting down inside the cast.

Stall confinement is mandatory after cast application. The patient must be monitored daily. Indications for cast change or removal include breakage, increased lameness, swelling, or exudates coming out of the top of the cast. Horses vary in their reaction and tolerance to a cast. If there is any doubt, a cast should be removed and the limb evaluated.

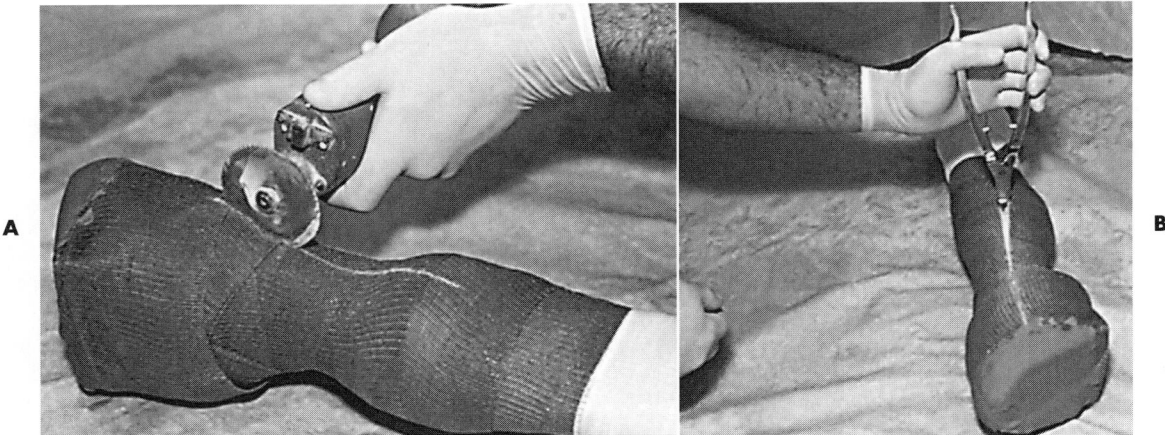

FIGURE 4-33. Removal of a limb cast from a horse. **A,** With a Stryker saw, the cast is split on the medial and lateral surface, and the cut is continued under the foot. **B,** Once the cast is completely cut, the two halves are separated with cast spreaders.

Cast Removal

Removal of a cast is best performed with the animal standing. During cast removal there is a risk of reinjury to the limb in the animal trying to recover from anesthesia. However, general anesthesia is used if the cast is being changed. The cast is split on the medial and lateral surfaces, and the cut is continued under the foot with a Stryker saw (Figure 4-33). With this approach, injury to the flexor and extensor tendons can be avoided. When cutting over bony prominences, one should be careful to avoid lacerating the skin. Once the cast is completely cut, the two halves are separated with cast spreaders. A support wrap is then placed on the limb.

Technician Note

A cast is split on the medial and lateral surfaces to avoid injury to the flexor and extensor tendons.

BANDAGING AND CAST APPLICATION TECHNIQUES FOR CATTLE

The principles applied to limb bandaging and cast application are the same in cattle as in horses, but there are specific techniques related to cattle. Cattle often are not as cooperative as horses, and more restraint is required.

With cattle, a cast can be applied directly over the dewclaws without causing major problems. Sores from motion of the cast can occur in this area because of the inability to closely fit the cast. This can be remedied by placing a pad of orthopedic felt, with holes cut out for the dewclaws, between the dewclaws (Figure 4-34).

Application of a Claw Block

A wooden block is applied to an unaffected claw for various reasons: to alleviate weight-bearing on an adjacent claw if it is fractured or injured or to protect an operated area by raising it higher off the ground after amputation of an adjacent claw. The block is usually made from a piece of wood 5 cm thick and cut to the shape of the sole surface of the claw. Grooves are cut in the ground surface for traction (Figure 4-35).

The claw is first trimmed and debris is removed by means of an electric sander or rasp. This is an important step for effective bonding of the acrylic to the claw. The block is then bonded to the horny surface of the claw with acrylic cement, such as Technovit (Jorgensen Laboratories) (Figure 4-36).

Modified Thomas Splint

Despite advances in external and internal skeletal fixation, modified Thomas splints are still often used in cattle and small ruminants as a means of external skeletal fixation. The modified Thomas splint is often used in combination with internal fixation or a cast. The indications for its use include fractures of the tibia or radius or ligamentous injuries of the stifle. Pressure sores in the inguinal or axillary region are a problem when a Thomas splint is used, despite padding of the metal ring.

Application of a modified Thomas splint in large ruminants does require special equipment, such as a conduit bender, to bend the round rod iron used to construct the splint. The design of the splint varies somewhat among clinicians, but the purpose is the same.

The animal is first placed in lateral recumbency with the affected leg uppermost. A template to fit the individual animal, devised from a nasogastric tube or other similar flexible tubing, is used to construct the ring that will encircle the proximal part of the leg (Figure 4-37). The ring should be large enough not to impinge on any bony prominences. The rod iron is bent in a ring the same size as the template. The variation in design occurs with the extensions that come off the ring to support the animal's limb.

One design has the extensions coming off cranially and caudally to the leg. The extensions of the splint must be shaped to conform to the angles of the hock and stifle. These extensions are also bent away (lateral) from the flat plane of the ring to allow the ventral part of the ring to fit into the axillary or inguinal region. Another design has the extensions coming off the ventral aspect of the ring (Figure 4-38). The ring is then bent so that the extensions are positioned medial to the limb, and to fit the contour of the upper limb (Figure 4-39).

A foot plate is constructed with two threaded rods attached to the extensions of the splint (Figure 4-38). A piece of rod iron can be used instead and bent in a U shape, positioned under the foot, and connected to the

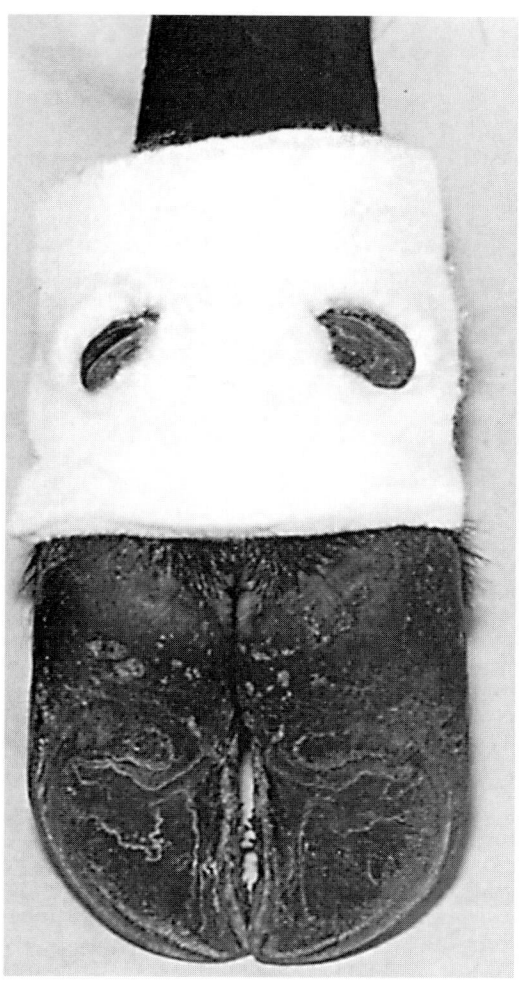

FIGURE 4-34. A piece of orthopedic felt, with holes cut out, can be placed between the dewclaws to reduce pressure sores and motion under a cast.

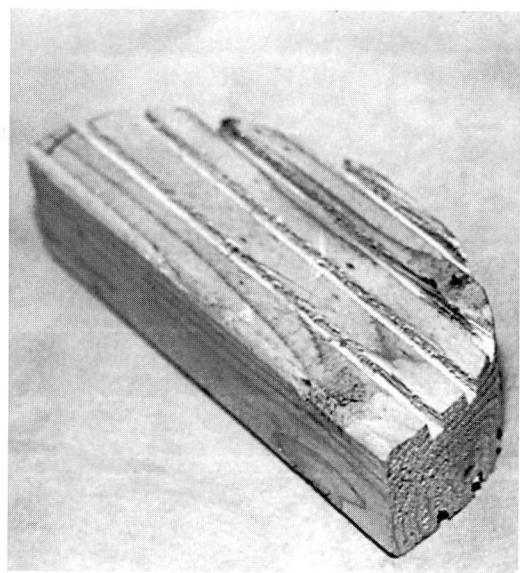

FIGURE 4-35. A claw block made from wood. Grooves are cut in the block to improve traction and bonding.

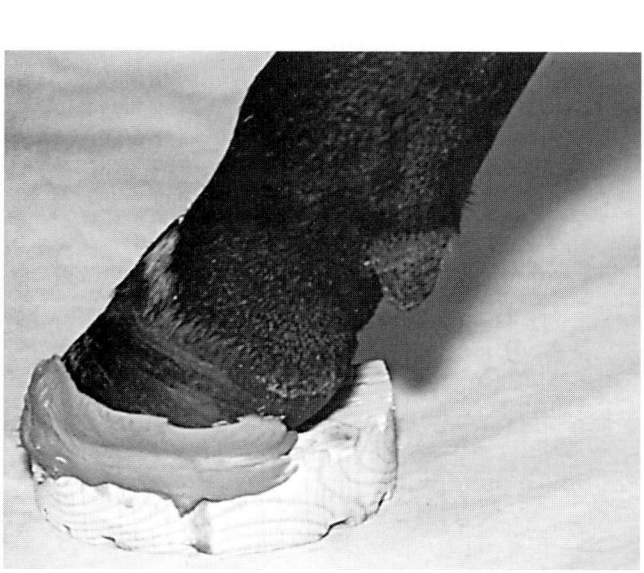

FIGURE 4-36. A wooden block is cemented to the unaffected claw with acrylic.

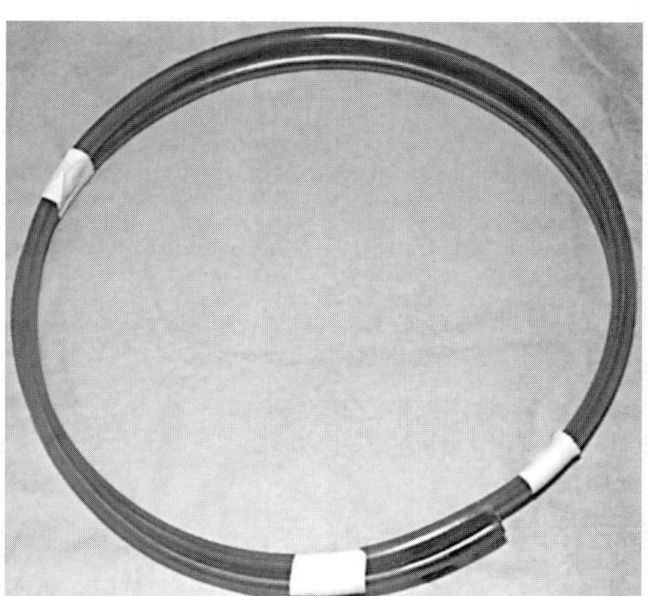

FIGURE 4-37. A nasogastric tube can be used as a template to construct the ring of a modified Thomas splint that will encircle the proximal portion of the leg.

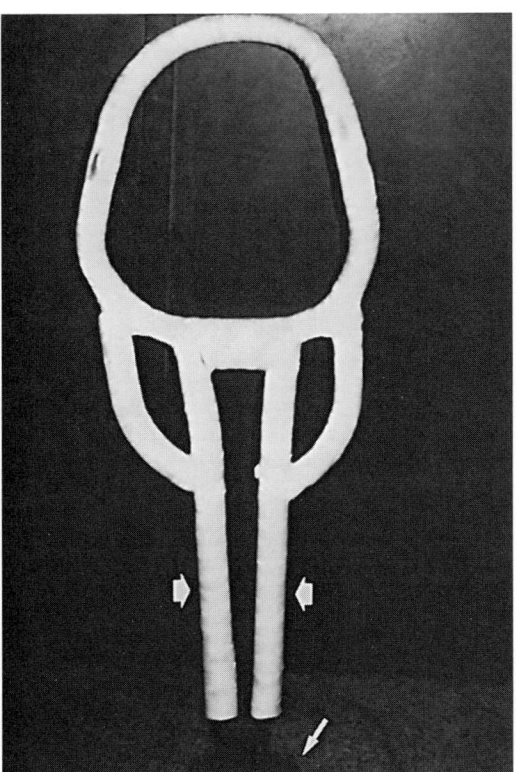

FIGURE 4-38. A modified Thomas splint. Extensions of the splint *(large arrows)* come off the ventral aspect of the ring and are positioned medial to the leg. A plate with threaded rods is constructed to fit under the animal's foot *(small arrow).* (Courtesy Dr. Dwight F. Wolfe.)

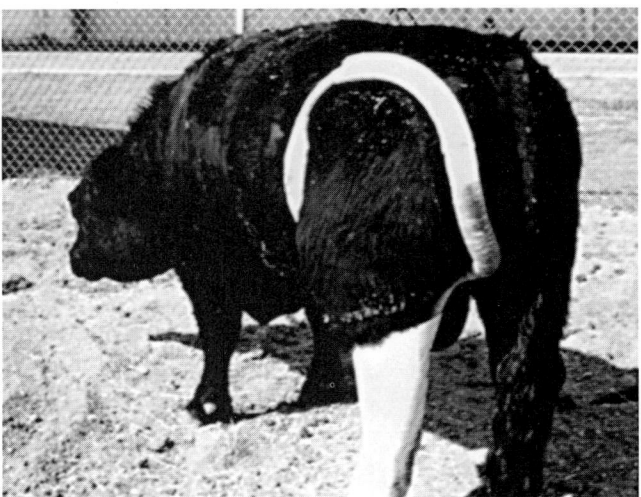

FIGURE 4-39. The limb and modified Thomas splint are covered with layers of cast material and thereby incorporated to stabilize the limb. (Courtesy Dr. Dwight F. Wolfe.)

ends of the extensions of the splint. Some splints are devised with extensions that are threaded so that the length of the splint can be adjusted. The ring is lightly padded with cotton. Holes are drilled into the toes of the hoof wall and wired to the bottom of the splint. A slight amount of traction should be applied to the limb as the splint is applied. Traction should be minimal within the splint, so as not to create excessive pressure in the axillary or inguinal regions, which could interfere with venous drainage or distract the fracture fragments.

Once the splint is in position, the limb and splint are then covered with layers of cast material and thereby incorporated together (Figure 4-39). Cast material should first be placed around the carpus or tarsus to give these areas initial support from bowing medially. The cast material should be applied as proximal as possible.

RECOMMENDED READING

SMALL ANIMAL

Fowler D: Principles of wound healing. In Harari J, editor: *Surgical complications and wound healing in the small animal practice,* Philadelphia, 1993, Saunders, pp 1-32.

Knecht CD et al: *Fundamental techniques in veterinary surgery,* ed 2, Philadelphia, 1981, WB Saunders.

Lozier SM: Topical wound management. In Harari J, editor: *Surgical complications and wound healing in the small animal practice,* Philadelphia, 1993, WB Saunders, pp 63-88.

Mason LK: Treatment of contaminated wounds. In Harari J, editor: *Surgical complications and wound healing in the small animal practice,* Philadelphia, 1993, WB Saunders, pp 33-62.

Swaim SF, Henderson RA: *Small animal wound management,* ed 2, Baltimore, 1997, Williams & Wilkins.

LARGE ANIMAL

Adams SB, Fessler JF: Treatment of radial-ulnar and tibial fractures in cattle, using a modified Thomas splint-cast combination, *J Am Vet Assoc* 183:430, 1983.

Lindsay WA: Wound treatment in horses: healing by third intention, *Vet Med* 83:506, 1988.

Peyton LC: Wound healing in the horse. II. Approach to the treatment of traumatic wounds, *Compend Pract Vet* 9:191, 1987.

Stashak TS: Bandaging and casting techniques. In Stashak TS, editor: *Equine wound management,* Philadelphia, 1991, Lea & Febiger, pp 258-272.

Stone WC: Drainings, dressings, and external coaptation. In Auer JA, Stick JA, editors: *Equine surgery,* Philadelphia, 1999, WB Saunders, pp 104-113.

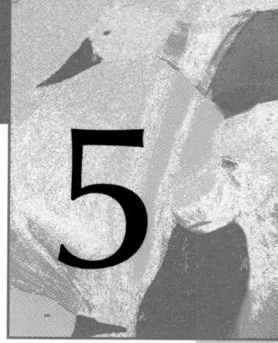

5

Basic Necropsy Procedures

Thomas J. Van Winkle • Perry L. Habecker

A *necropsy* is the examination of an animal, after it has died, to determine the abnormal and disease-related changes that occurred during its life. The term *necropsy* originates from the Greek language and means "viewing the dead." Necropsy is also known as *autopsy*, which is Greek for "seeing with one's own eyes."

Before beginning our discussion of the necropsy, it is important to understand the meaning of terms that are used frequently in this chapter. *Pathology*, for example, is the science and study of disease, especially the causes and development of abnormal conditions. *Gross pathology* refers to pathologic changes in tissue that are visible with the naked eye, whereas *histopathology* refers to pathologic changes in tissue that are microscopic and can be seen with the use of a microscope. *Lesions* are alterations or abnormalities in a tissue (a pathologic change), and the *pathogenesis* is the sequence of events that lead to or underlie a disease.

Necropsies are done for a variety of reasons. For animals they are often done for the following reasons:

- To determine the disease process or processes that led to the animal's death
- To determine the accuracy of the clinical diagnosis
- To evaluate the positive and negative effects of therapeutic measures

In situations in which more than one animal is at risk, such as in multiple animal households, farms, and laboratory animal facilities, the necropsy is also helpful in determining if other animals are at risk for infectious agents, inherited conditions, toxins, or environmental hazards.

To perform a necropsy successfully requires a knowledge of anatomy and gross pathology and a systematic technique for examination of the animal's body. In the necropsy all abnormalities and disease processes should be exposed and described. If needed, appropriate samples are collected for histopathology, cytology, bacteriology, virol-

ogy, parasitology, and toxicology. Descriptions of the gross findings should be recorded and included in a report together with the animal's species, age, gender, and breed (signalment); the history; and the clinical findings. Samples that are submitted to the laboratory for further testing should be packaged with a copy of the report. In addition, the report should be added to the animal's record together with the histopathology and other reports.

 Technician Note

It is important to be sure the owner's permission for the necropsy is obtained and that the animal for necropsy is correctly identified.

Before we begin describing the necropsy procedure there are a number of important things to consider. First, be sure that the owner's permission is obtained before the necropsy is performed. Second, make sure that the animal for necropsy is correctly identified. The species, breed, gender, age, and identifying tags or tattoos should be carefully matched with the information on the owner's permission form and the medical record. This step is critical to avoid performing the necropsy on the wrong animal. In addition, the disposition of the body (cremation, private cremation, burial, etc.) should also be determined before the necropsy if possible. It is also important to perform the necropsy as soon as possible after the animal's death to avoid decomposition (autolysis). If the necropsy must be delayed the body should be refrigerated as soon as possible. Small animals should be placed in thin plastic bags with identification tags secured on both the body and the outside of the bag. Decomposition occurs most rapidly in large obese animals at high temperatures. It is particularly troublesome in large animals that rely on gut fermentation for their nutrients, because the rumen continues to generate heat long after the death of the body. The body should not be frozen, since freezing and subsequent thawing cause many postmortem artifacts.

Technician Note

If the necropsy must be delayed, the body should be refrigerated as soon as possible. The body should not be frozen, because freezing and subsequent thawing cause many postmortem artifacts.

The signalment, history, and clinical findings should be reviewed before the necropsy is started. The record should include the owner's name, address, and phone numbers; other veterinarians involved with the case; the animal's species, breed, age, gender, name or identification; and the hospital record number. The history should include vaccination history, owner's observations of the clinical signs, length of illness, and other animals at risk. The clinical findings should include results of the physical examination, clinical tests (complete blood count [CBC], clinical chemistries, radiographs, etc.), surgical procedures, and the date and time of death or euthanasia.

NECROPSY REPORTS

While the necropsy is being performed, all abnormalities should be described and recorded. A report should be written after the necropsy is completed describing the findings. Tentative conclusions (diagnoses) may be made at the end of the report (refer to Appendix I of this chapter).

All lesions are described and recorded using the following criteria (examples are given in parentheses):

- Location (caudal dorsal left lung lobe, left ventricle, cornea)
- Number (one, two, hundreds)
- Color (red, green, yellow-tan)
- Size (either measurements such as 3 × 5 × 4 cm or weights for liver and heart)
- Shape (round, flat, spherical, stellate)
- Distribution (focal, multifocal, diffuse)
- Consistency (soft, firm, hard, rubbery)
- Odor (sweet, sour, ammonia)

The findings are usually recorded in the order in which they were encountered in the necropsy. Either the present or past tense should be used (not both), and the descriptions should be as specific as possible without drawing conclusions. For example, "there are multiple dark red 1- to 4-mm diameter soft nodules in all lung lobes" rather than "hemangiosarcoma." Based on the descriptions, the veterinarian formulates a morphologic diagnosis, which includes severity, time, distribution, lesion, and anatomic site. An example of a diagnosis might be "severe acute multifocal interstitial pneumonia."

FIXATIVES

Ten percent buffered formalin is the most widely used fixative for the preservation of tissues. This solution may be purchased from a variety of sources and is also easily prepared. It is made by mixing nine parts of water with one part of commercially available formaldehyde solution (37% to 40% HCHO). The addition of 6.5 g of dibasic anhydrous sodium phosphate and 4 g of monobasic sodium phosphate per 1000 ml of solution creates a neutral buffered 10% formalin. This is an excellent general purpose fixative somewhat more desirable than plain (acidic)

10% formalin. The addition of buffers is important because it eliminates the formation of undesirable hematin pigment in tissue sections.

Technician Note

Ten percent (10%) buffered formalin is the most widely used fixative for the preservation of tissues.

For the preservation of whole brains, intact spinal cords, and bones, 50% formalin, made by mixing one part 10% buffered formalin with one part of commercial formaldehyde (37% to 40% HCHO), is superior to the 10% solutions. The stronger 50% solution penetrates and fixes the large tissue mass more rapidly and more thoroughly than 10% formalin. Formalin fixation is usually complete within 24 hours (large brains may take 48 hours). Tissues fixed in 10% formalin are traditionally stored in 10% formalin, but storage in 70% alcohol is superior.

Bouin's fixative is less widely used than 10% formalin, but it is preferred in some instances because it produces less tissue shrinkage and better preservation of cellular detail. Fetal tissues, intestinal epithelium, eyes, testes, endocrine glands, and the inclusion bodies of a number of important diseases are particularly well preserved with this fixative. Bouin's fluid may be purchased from a variety of sources or can be made by mixing 750 ml of a saturated aqueous solution of picric acid, 250 ml of 37% to 40% formaldehyde, and 50 ml of glacial acetic acid. Caution should be taken when handling picric because it is explosive!

Technician Note

All containers of fixed tissue samples should be clearly labeled. Appropriate caution should be used when handling, shipping, and disposing of all fixatives.

FACILITIES AND INSTRUMENTS

Necropsies should be performed in a well-lit, well-ventilated space, ideally outside the usual surgical and treatment areas. The area should be easy to clean and disinfect, have adequate drainage for fluids and water, and be large enough to comfortably move around in. When performing necropsies in the field (outdoors), the appropriate disposal of tissues and the inadvertent spread of disease become particular concerns.

The person performing the necropsy (called the *prosector*) should wear protective clothing, such as a plastic apron, laboratory coat, or scrubs, that can be removed and either discarded or cleaned following the necropsy. Latex or other protective plastic gloves should be worn at all times. In addition, a surgical mask should be worn when dealing with animals that have died from infectious diseases that can be spread through aerosolization. Protective footwear (boots or booties) is appropriate when dealing with larger animals.

Necropsies do not require specialized equipment or instruments. Most can be obtained from surgical suppliers and hardware stores. The following instruments are used in a typical necropsy:

- Necropsy knives (sturdy and that can be sharpened) and honing steel
- Scalpel handle and blades

- Scissors (large and small operating, Mayo, or Metzenbaum work well)*
- Forceps (large and small toothed)*
- Serrated, all-purpose, plastic-handled utility scissors
- Bone-cutting forceps*
- Hacksaw, meat saw, or Stryker saw (for brain removal)*
- Lopping (pruning) shears for cutting ribs and bones*
- String or hemostats for closing off bowel ends
- Labeled plastic buckets or screw-top plastic containers containing formalin*
- Tissue cassettes (for very small tissues) and clip-on laundry tags for identifying tissues
- Labeled, sealable, plastic bags and plastic vials or bottles for refrigerated and frozen samples
- Culturettes for aerobic and anaerobic cultures

Technician Note

All equipment and instruments should be thoroughly cleaned and disinfected following the necropsy. To avoid the spread of pathogens, instruments should be dedicated for necropsy use only.

ANCILLARY PROCEDURES

Before samples are collected for examination in the microbiology, parasitology, and toxicology departments, the diagnostic laboratory should be contacted for specific advice on which samples should be collected, how they should be collected, and how they should be packaged and submitted. This minimizes potential errors and provides the laboratory with the best possible specimens.

Tissues and specimens for bacteriology, mycology, and mycoplasma cultivation are collected aseptically, placed in either Culturettes or sterile containers without preservatives, and submitted to the laboratory *without delay*. Frozen specimens should not be submitted.

Specimens collected for microbiology include the primary site of the disease and its regional lymph nodes. Other samples may include heart, blood, lung, liver, spleen, stomach contents of aborted fetuses, placenta, exudates, synovia, bone marrow, cerebrospinal fluid, brain, and small intestine. When intestine is submitted, a 10-cm segment of intestine is tied off at each end of the intestine to prevent excessive contamination by the internal contents. The instruments used to do this are by necessity heavily contaminated by the microbes exposed at the cut ends. For this reason, intestine should be collected last and should be placed in a separate container from the other tissue samples. Tissue sections of $2 \times 3 \times 1$ cm and fluid specimens of 3 to 5 ml are desirable.

Technician Note

If rabies is suspected the head should be sent to the appropriate laboratory for testing following the guidelines and laws of the state.

Tissues for virus isolation are collected aseptically and either refrigerated in a sterile container or immersed in sterile 50% buffered glycerol in sterile containers, and preserved by freezing. Fresh, refrigerated tissue immersed in virus transport medium (available from the virology laboratory) is the preferred method of tissue submission. Lung, liver, spleen, kidney, and brain are prime specimens. Sections need to be $5 \times 5 \times 10$ mm. Contact the virology laboratory for the appropriate technique. For toxicology, blood, liver, stomach contents, kidney, fat, brain, and urine may be saved. Blocks of tissues $10 \times 5 \times 4$ cm (approximately 200 g), 10 to 20 ml of blood, and 50 to 100 ml of fluids are desirable. They may be frozen.

If rabies is suspected the head should be sent to the appropriate laboratory for testing following the guidelines and laws of the state. A necropsy should only be performed on the rest of the carcass if the brain is found to be negative for rabies.

For cytologic examination, smears are made (after gentle blotting on absorbent paper) by either scraping the cut surface of the specimen with a new scalpel blade and then spreading the scraped material onto a slide or lightly pressing small pieces of tissue against the surface of a clean slide. Several impressions are made across the slide. They are generally submitted unstained to the laboratory, or they can be stained and examined at the time of the necropsy.

NECROPSY PROCEDURE FOR A SMALL MAMMAL

The following procedure is appropriate for dogs, cats, ferrets, rodents, and rabbits. See also Appendix II of this chapter for the steps in the necropsy procedure.

Tissue Collection

It is imperative that tissues being collected for histology are handled carefully before fixation and that they are properly labeled for identification. Tissue sections should not be squeezed, stretched, or rinsed with water, and epithelial surfaces should not be rinsed or rubbed with fingers or instruments before samples are taken for histopathology. Tissues become rigid with fixation, so if there is a need to retain the flatness of the tissue, it can be placed on a piece of cardboard. The tissue will remain adhered to the cardboard after immersion in formalin.

Sections from paired organs may be trimmed differently from one another to distinguish them from one another. For example, the left kidney may be sectioned longitudinally, and the right kidney may be cut transversely. In addition, sections can be labeled with clip-on laundry tags to identify them. If there is any possibility that a section of tissue may lose its identity when mixed with other specimens, the sections should be tagged with clip-on laundry tags. If small in size, the tissues may also be placed in separate labeled containers, such as tissue cassettes. The pituitary of small animals, for example, is well differentiated from other tissues when placed in a small tissue cassette.

Technician Note

It is imperative that tissues collected for histology are handled carefully before fixation and that they are properly marked for identification.

In all cases it is desirable to save sections of critical tissues for histopathologic examination. These include lung, myocardium, liver, spleen, pancreas, stomach, small intestine, kidneys, lymph nodes, whole brain, endocrine organs, urinary bladder, colon, and muscle.

*The size of these items depends on the size of the animal being necroscopied.

Dissection

The method of dissection described here is a standard technique that can be applied to all mammalian species and that is based on two precepts:

- In step-wise fashion, each part of the carcass is examined in situ (as it first appears in the carcass); it is then isolated from the carcass and examined as a whole; finally it is dissected and examined.
- Once a part is taken from the body it is dissected to completion (exceptions include tissues from the gastrointestinal tract, brain, spinal cord, and eyes). Sections for histologic or laboratory examination are collected before further dissection is undertaken.

This method is the opposite of those that call for evisceration now and dissection later, methods that disrupt the entire carcass all at once and that lead to tissues being forgotten or lost. The immediate complete dissection of one part at a time reduces the possibility of lost or forgotten parts and leaves the remainder of the carcass intact. In this way, if the findings in one organ suggest that another part or parts of the carcass should be explored in situ, this is still possible and has not been precluded by previous dissection.

Preliminary Observations

Before the necropsy begins the prosector should review the signalment (species, breed, color, gender, age, weight, animal identification), the clinical history, and the laboratory data available. It is important that the time of death and time of necropsy be recorded. The animal should then be weighed and the weight recorded (in grams or kilograms). All organs that are abnormal in size or shape should be measured and/or weighed.

Technician Note

Before the necropsy begins the prosector should review the signalment (species, breed, color, gender, age, weight, animal identification) of the animal, the clinical history, and any available laboratory data.

External Examination

The exterior of the animal is examined: body conformation, hair coat, skin, nose, mouth (lips, cheeks, gums, teeth, tongue), eyes (eyelids, conjunctiva, cornea, sclera, anterior chamber, iris, lens), ears, mammae, penis, prepuce, scrotum, vulva, anus, and feet. Because the retina undergoes rapid decomposition after death, dissection begins with the eyes. The upper and lower eyelids are examined and excised. The membrana nictitans is grasped with tissue forceps, the globe is lifted, and the soft tissue attachments to the bony orbit are incised with scissors or a scalpel in a 360-degree circle. As the globe is freed from the orbit, care must be taken to avoid excessive tension on the optic nerve. The optic nerve is carefully severed at the optic canal. The excised globe is examined, and then extraocular muscles, fascia, fat, conjunctiva, and membrana nictitans are dissected from the globe. The interior of the eye can be examined by immersing the globe in clear cool water. The sclera is examined, and the unopened globe is immersed in Bouin's fixative or formalin.

Reflection of Skin and Limbs and Examination of Superficial Organs

The animal is placed in left lateral recumbency (on the left side). A midline incision is made beginning at the right axilla and extending cranially to the mandibular symphysis (Figure 5-1). The incision is continued in the opposite direction caudally as a median or paramedian incision, passing between the mammae and around the penis, prepuce, and scrotum, to the perineum (Figure 5-2). The upper forelimbs are reflected by dissection between the scapula and the ribs. Fat, fascia, and superficial muscles are reflected back together with the skin. Skin of the ventral aspect of the neck and throat is reflected. Abdominal skin is reflected, and the hindlimbs are reflected by extending the incision into the coxofemoral (hip) joints. The animal is now placed in dorsal recumbency (on its back) (Figure 5-3).

Skin incisions are extended down the cranial medial aspects of both rear legs, and the skin is reflected. As they are exposed in the dissection, superficial organs are

FIGURE 5-1. The necropsy begins with the animal placed on its left side. A midline incision is made from the mandibular symphysis caudally.

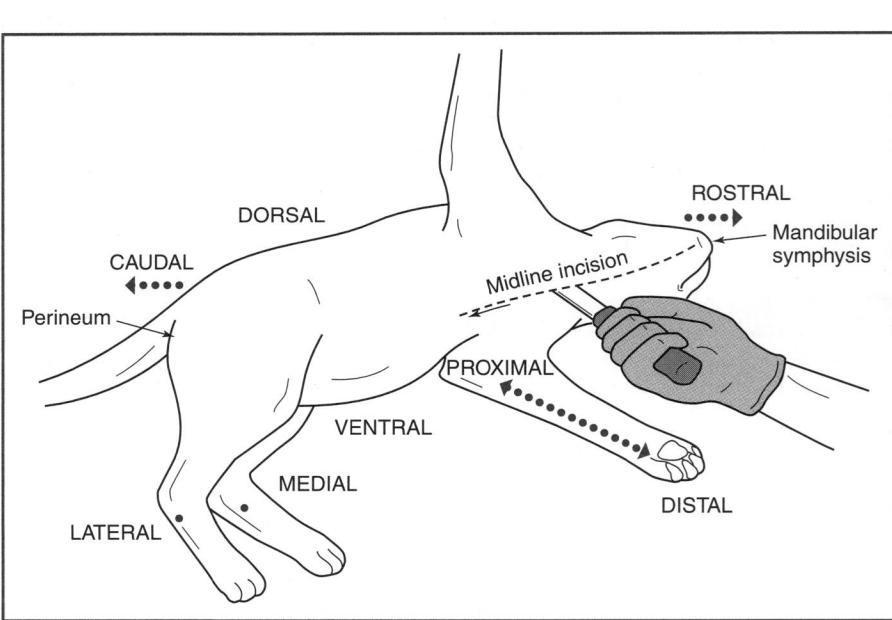

examined and samples from these organs are collected: lymph nodes (mandibular, superficial cervical, prescapular, axillary, inguinal, popliteal), mammary glands, testes, and skin.

In all necropsy examinations, several joints are examined before the body cavities are opened. The coxofemoral joints are opened and examined during the initial incision. The scapulohumeral and stifle joints are also examined on all routine necropsies. The atlantooccipital joint will be examined when the head is removed.

Samples of the sciatic nerve, synovium with patella, and skeletal muscle are collected. Bone marrow samples for impression smears or histopathology should be collected at this time. Generally, marrow is obtained by cracking the upper midshaft femur with pruning shears.

You should at this point have already collected the following: eyes, lymph nodes, testes or mammary glands, skin, synovium, sciatic nerve, skeletal muscle, and bone marrow.

Next, the three major body cavities (peritoneal, pleural, pericardial) are opened. All organs are examined in situ, and any abnormalities are noted. The abdomen is opened by making a midline incision from the sternum to the symphysis pubis and making incisions laterally from the sternum along both caudal costal margins. The abdominal wall is then reflected laterally to expose the abdominal cavity (Figure 5-4).

The diaphragm is now punctured to check for negative pleural pressure, and the diaphragm is cut away from the ventral and lateral rib cage. The ventral rib cage is removed by cutting the ribs bilaterally (on both sides) midway between the costochondral junction and the vertebral column (Figure 5-5). This should be done with utility scissors or pruning shears. Examine the pleural surface of

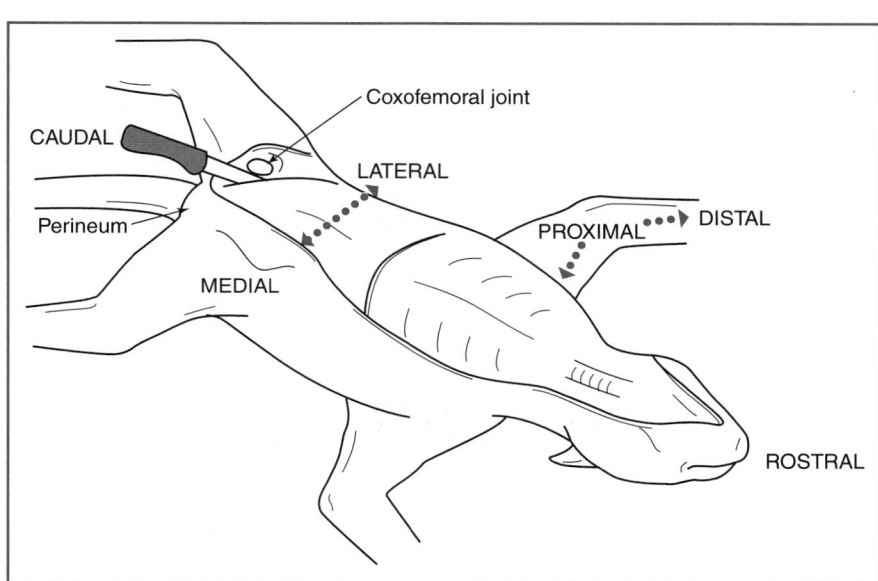

FIGURE 5-2. The front limbs are reflected by making incisions between the ribs and the scapulae. The hind legs are reflected by incising the coxofemoral (hip) joints.

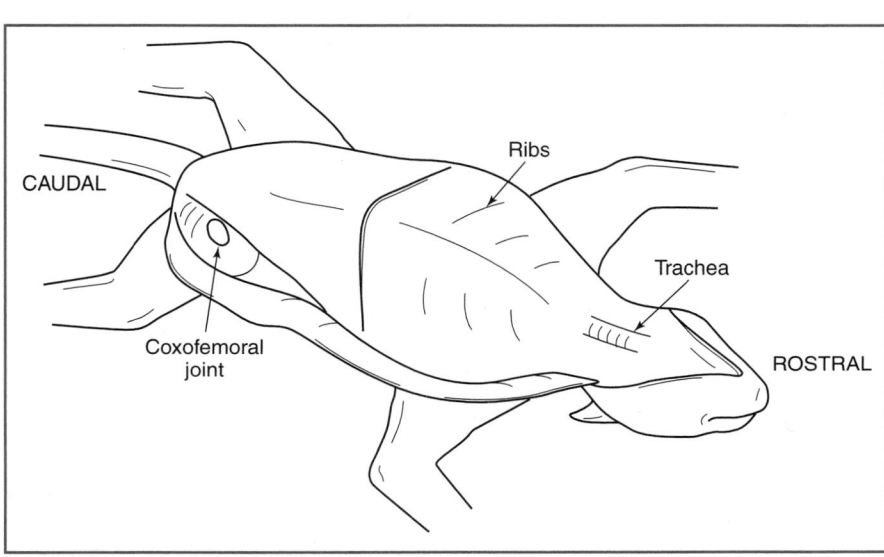

FIGURE 5-3. After all four limbs are reflected, the animal is positioned in dorsal recumbency (on its back).

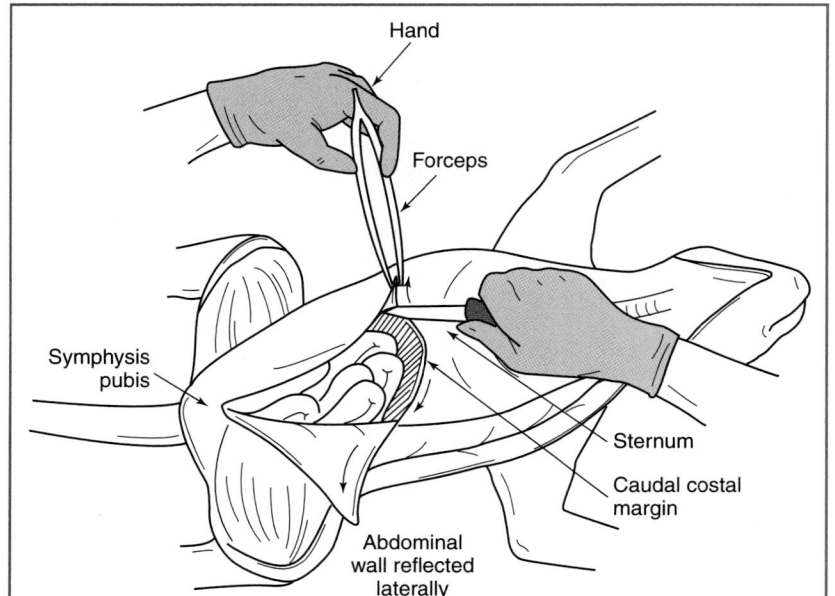

FIGURE 5-4. The abdominal wall is incised with a midline incision. The right and left halves of the abdominal wall are reflected laterally by making incisions from the sternum along both right and left caudal costal margins.

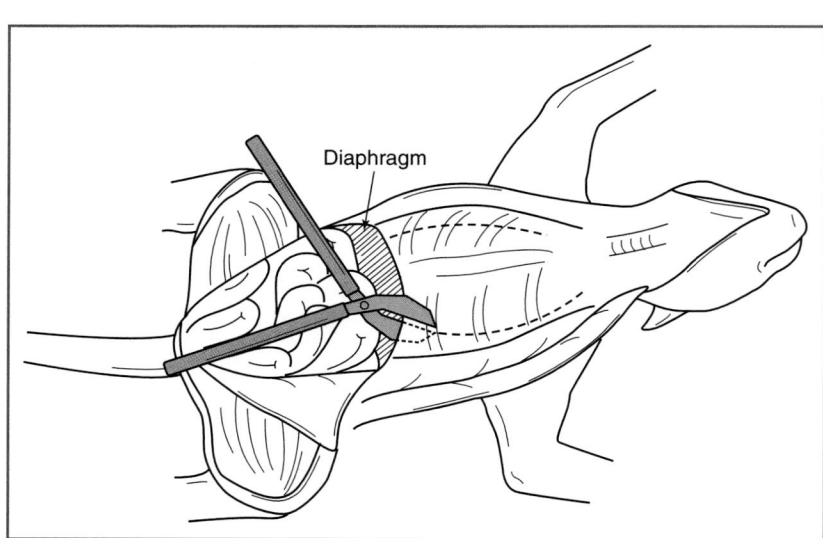

FIGURE 5-5. The ventral portion of the rib cage is removed by cutting the ribs bilaterally (on both sides) with heavy pruning shears.

the rib cage. In young animals the costochondral growth plate may be examined and saved for histopathology. Next, the pericardial sac is opened and the exterior of the heart is examined.

Technician Note

The history and preliminary findings are reviewed with the clinician after all body cavities are opened.

The thyroids, parathyroids, and thymus should be identified at this time and removed. The adrenals should then be identified and removed. The adrenals are sectioned, and the corticomedullary ratio is noted. The mandibular salivary glands, parotid salivary glands, parotid lymph nodes, jugular veins, and parapharyngeal and retropharyngeal lymph nodes are examined.

Examination of Skull and Brain

Remove the tongue from the oral cavity, and reflect the tongue, tonsils, larynx, and esophagus caudally (Figure 5-6). An incision is made through the intermandibular muscles, along the medial surface of the ramus of each mandible, from the angle to the symphysis. The frenulum of the tongue is incised, and the tongue is pulled (or pushed) ventrally between the rami. Using the tongue as a handle, right and left paramedian incisions are extended from the larynx to the thoracic inlet, exposing the length of the trachea and esophagus. It is necessary to cut or disarticulate the hyoid bones dorsal to the pharynx to free the tongue, larynx, pharynx, trachea, and esophagus as a unit.

The spinal cord is transected by an incision into the ventral atlantooccipital joint. Atlantooccipital membranes, ligaments, and joint capsule are transected, disarticulating the head from the vertebral column (Figure 5-7). The skin is removed from the head by leaving it attached to the

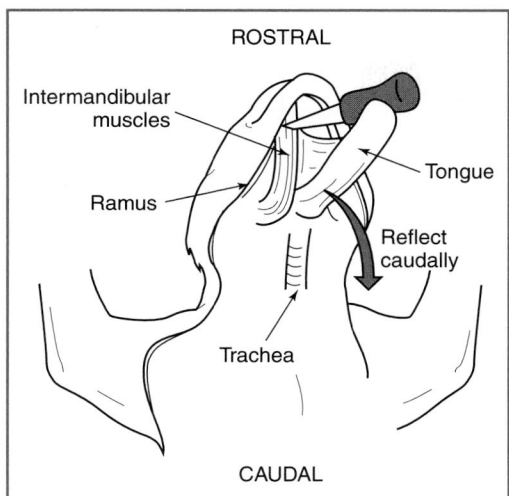

FIGURE 5-6. Examination of the tongue, tonsils, larynx, and esophagus. These are reflected caudally after the intermandibular muscles are incised.

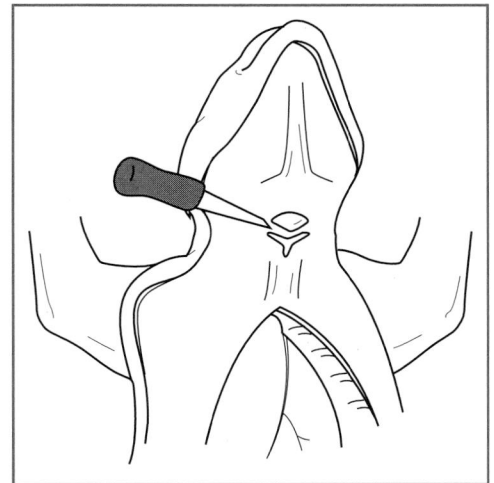

FIGURE 5-7. The spinal cord is transected ventrally by first making an incision into the atlantooccipital joint. The head is disarticulated from the vertebral column.

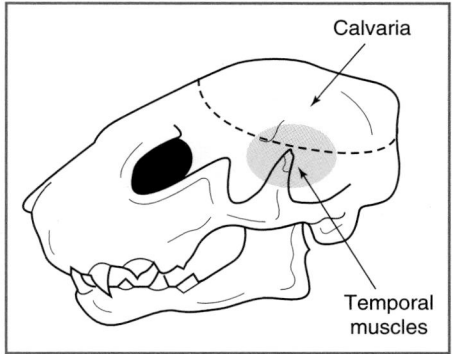

FIGURE 5-8. The temporal muscles are removed to reveal the skull cap, or calvaria.

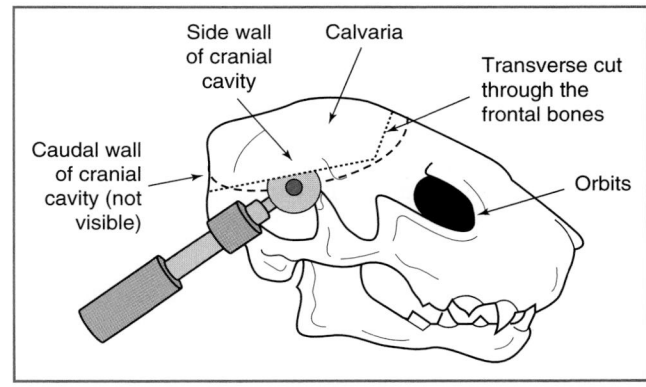

FIGURE 5-9. The cranial cavity is opened by removing the calvaria and caudal wall as a unit.

skin of the body and peeling the head forward out of the skin. The superficial muscles of the head are removed. External ears are opened and examined. Temporal muscles are removed, exposing the calvaria (skull cap) (Figure 5-8).

The calvaria and caudal wall of the cranial cavity are removed from the skull as a unit, exposing the dorsum of the brain. To accomplish this, three cuts are made with a Stryker saw, hacksaw, or meat saw. The first is a transverse cut through the frontal bones. This cut usually is made immediately caudal to the orbits. Care is taken to make the cut just deep enough to transect bone but not deep enough to engage the brain beneath.

The second and third cuts are made through the side walls and caudal wall of the cranial cavity. At 45-degree angles to the longitudinal axis of the skull, they extend from the lateral ends of the transverse cut to the medial

faces of the occipital condyles (Figure 5-9). In very small animals the bone may be broken away piecemeal, progressing cranial from the foramen magnum with scissors, bone-cutting forceps, or postmortem shears. The calvaria and caudal wall, as a unit, are pried loose from surrounding bones and removed. The meninges (the three membranes that cover the brain) and the surface of the brain are examined in situ (Figure 5-10).

To remove the brain the dorsal meninges are removed and the cranial nerves are transected progressing rostrally from the foramen magnum. The brain is examined, tagged, and then immersed in 50% formalin. Brain slicing is postponed until after the brain is fixed thoroughly.

The pituitary gland is removed from its fossa with the brain and examined. The middle ears (tympanic bullae) are opened ventrally using ronguers. In order to examine

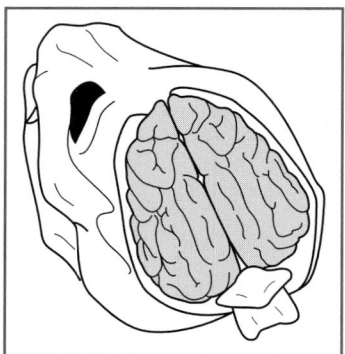

Figure 5-10. The meninges and surface of the brain are examined in situ.

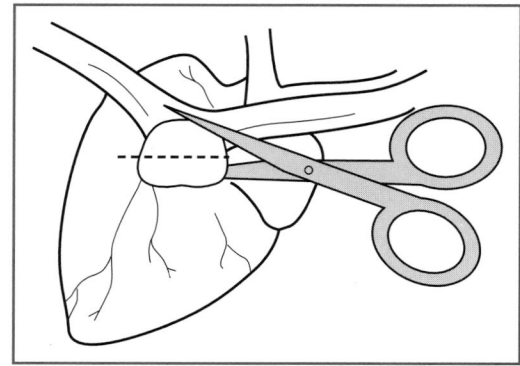

Figure 5-11. Dissection of the heart begins with an incision into the right auricle.

the nasal septum, turbinates, and frontal or maxillary sinuses, the skull is sectioned longitudinally with a saw. The oral cavity is examined.

Dissection and Examination of the Neck and Thoracic Viscera

Now the cervical and thoracic viscera are removed from the body and examined. Using the trachea and esophagus as a handle, the thoracic organs are removed from the body by cutting between the dorsal mediastinum and the vertebral column from the thoracic inlet back to the diaphragm. The dorsal incision is carried above the aorta. At the diaphragm, the aorta, postcava, and esophagus are transected and the throat, neck, and thoracic viscera are removed as a unit. This unit is dissected and examined from tongue to aorta. The tongue is examined and sliced transversely. The pharynx is opened middorsally with scissors, and pharynx and tonsils are examined. The esophagus is opened longitudinally by a middorsal incision. The larynx is opened middorsally with utility scissors or a knife, and the incision is extended through the trachea to the lungs. The lungs are examined and palpated. (For fine fixation, the lung may be "inflated" with 10% formalin gravity-fed into the trachea or bronchi.)

The right side of the heart and pulmonary arteries are examined before the lungs are cut. Hold the heart so that the right side is on the prosector's left and the left side is on the right. The right auricle is incised, and the incision is extended away from the prosector to the far end of the right atrium (Figure 5-11). The incision is then directed downward through the right atrioventricular (AV) valve and along the interventricular septum to the apex of the right ventricle. The incision is then continued up along the interventricular septum through the pulmonic valve into the pulmonary artery (Figure 5-12). The right free wall of the heart is reflected, and the valves and endocardial surfaces are examined. The pulmonary arteries are opened into each lung lobe (Figure 5-13). Air passages and transected lung tissue are examined. Sections of lung are squeezed gently to assess fluid content. Bronchial lymph nodes are examined and sliced longitudinally.

The heart and major vessels are then removed from the lungs. The heart is again held so that the right side is on the prosector's left and the left side is to the right. The left auricle is incised, and the incision is extended away from the prosector to the far end of the left atrium (Figure 5-14). The incision is then directed downward through the left AV

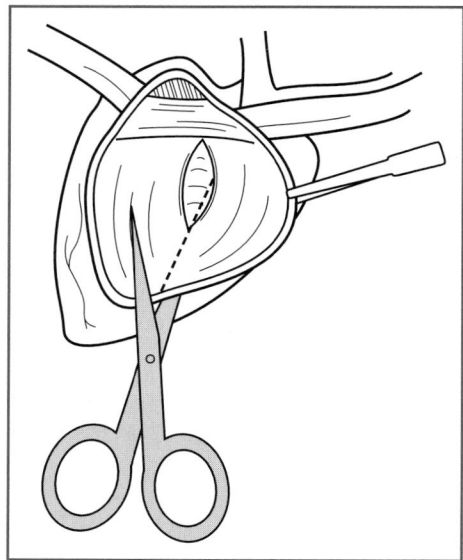

Figure 5-12. The heart is incised through the right atrium and ventricle following the interventricular septum. The incision is then continued into the pulmonary artery.

valve and along the center of the left ventricular free wall to the apex of the left ventricle (Figure 5-15). The aortic valve and aorta are examined by cutting up through the septal leaflet of the left AV valve and into the aorta (Figure 5-16). The valves, endocardium, and endothelial surfaces are then examined. The heart may then be weighed after all major vessels are removed at the base of the heart. Next, the myocardium is sliced longitudinally for examination and samples are collected. Small hearts should be fixed whole after opening.

Abdominal Cavity

Examination of the abdominal cavity begins with examination of the portal vein as it enters the liver and removal of the intestinal tract. The intestine is removed by stripping the mesentery from the small intestine and colon. The duodenum is clamped or tied and transected distal to the tail of the pancreas. The colon is transected at the pelvic inlet, and the intestinal tract is removed and set aside for

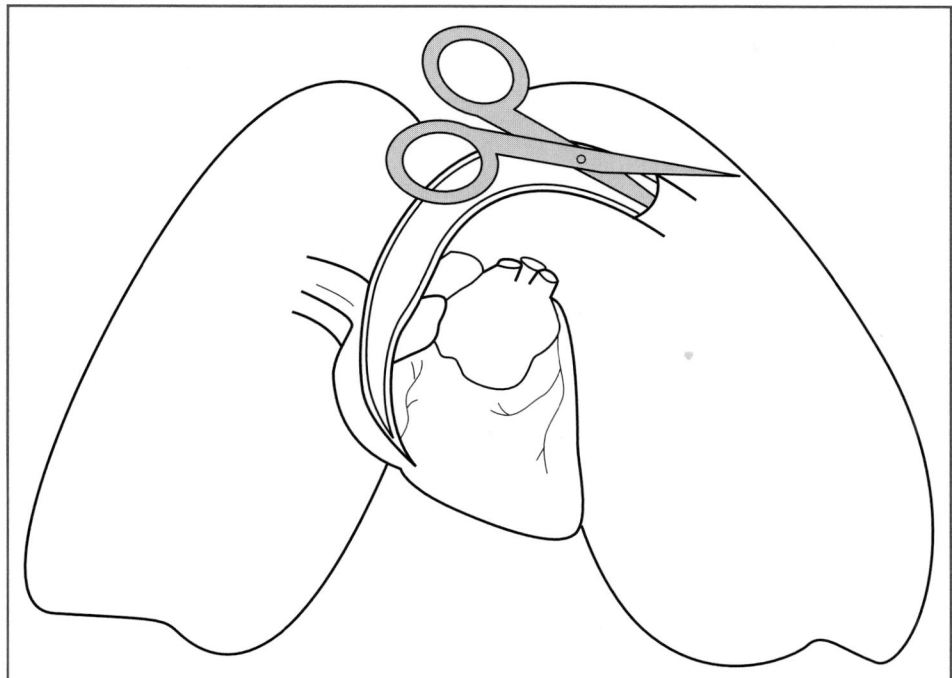

FIGURE 5-13. The pulmonary artery is incised and continued into each lung lobe.

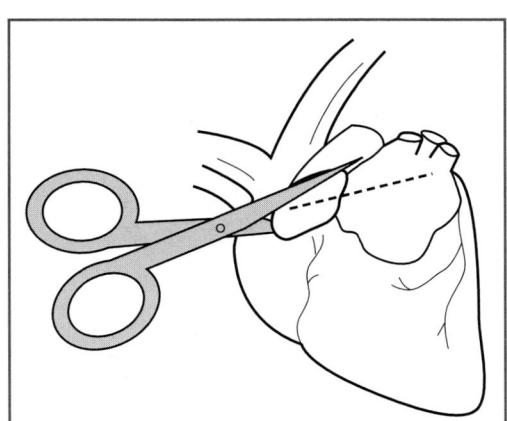

FIGURE 5-14. The second half of the heart is dissected by incising the left auricle and continuing the incision into the left atrium.

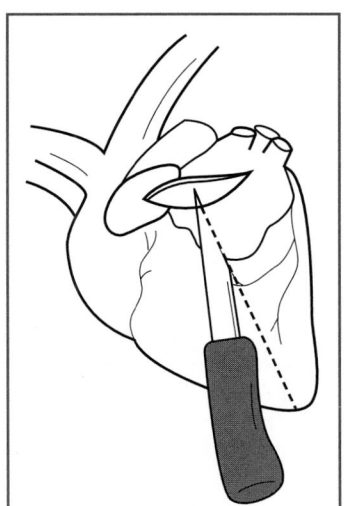

FIGURE 5-15. From the left atrium, the incision is continued through the left atrioventricular (AV) valve into the left ventricle to the apex.

later examination. NOTE: If the animal is thought to have intestinal disease, the intestines are examined now.

The stomach, liver, spleen, pancreas, and duodenum are now removed by cutting the attachments between these organs and the diaphragm and ventral body wall. The spleen is examined and sectioned. The stomach is opened along the greater curvature, and the duodenum is opened. The gallbladder is squeezed to determine patency of the bile duct; the gallbladder is opened; and the stomach, duodenum, and pancreas are dissected from the liver, examined, and sectioned. A section of the right side of the pancreas is collected with the duodenum, and a section of the left side is collected separately. The liver is then examined and sectioned. Multiple slices (approximately 1 cm apart) are made in the liver, and samples are collected from each lobe.

Female Reproductive Tract, Urinary Tract, and Accessory Male Reproductive Organs

To facilitate examination and removal of the urogenital tract, the floor of the pelvis should be removed. This is accomplished by making paramedian cuts through the obturator foramina on the floor of the pelvis. The mesovarium, mesosalpinx, and mesometrium are examined. Ovaries, oviducts, and uterus are freed from mesentery and reflected toward the pelvis.

The left kidney is dissected free from the abdominal wall but remains attached to the ureter. It is sliced longitudinally, and the capsule is peeled from one half of the kidney (Figure 5-17). Examined are the surface, cortex, medulla, and pelvis. The ureters are examined and palpated. If the ureters or renal pelvis is dilated, the ureters are opened from kidney to bladder with scissors. The ureter is cut near the bladder, and the kidney is removed. Sections are taken from the middle of both halves, one with the capsule intact and one with the capsule removed. Any other renal lesions are also collected. The right kidney is now examined in the same manner.

The urinary bladder is incised and opened. Examined are serosa, mucosa, and cut surfaces. Care should be taken not to rub mucosal surfaces. The urethra is opened and examined, and the prostate is examined and sectioned.

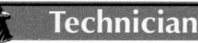

Technician Note

Care should be taken not to rub the mucosal surfaces of the tissues being examined.

Ovaries, oviducts, uterus, cervix, vagina, and vulva are removed from the carcass as a unit. Large ovaries are sliced longitudinally; oviducts are examined and palpated; and uterus, cervix, vagina, and vulva are opened with scissors or knife. Examined are serosa, contents, endometrium, cut surfaces, cervical folds, and luminal surface of vagina and vulva.

Intestinal Tract

The intestinal tract is now examined by laying it out on the table and examining the serosal surface. The tract is then opened from the duodenum through the colon using scissors. The mucosa is examined, and sections are taken from the jejunum, ileum, and colon, including lesions. The mucosa should be handled carefully to avoid artifacts. Once sections are taken the mucosa can be gently rinsed with water to reveal mucosal details.

Abdominal Aorta, Rectum, and Anal Glands

The abdominal aorta is opened longitudinally and examined, and a section is taken for histology. The rectum is opened, and the anal sacs are examined.

Vertebral Column and Spinal Cord

The manner and extent to which the vertebral column is dissected will depend on the history and size of the animal. To examine the vertebral column and spinal cord more extensively, the remaining rib cage, the four limbs, and most of the dorsal spinal musculature are removed from the vertebral column and pelvis. To demonstrate ventral or lateral impingements on the spinal cord of small animals, a dorsal laminectomy is performed. The spinal cord is covered dorsally by the vertebral arches; each arch consists

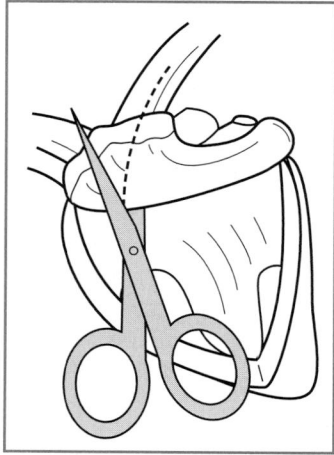

FIGURE 5-16.   The incision is then continued into the aorta.

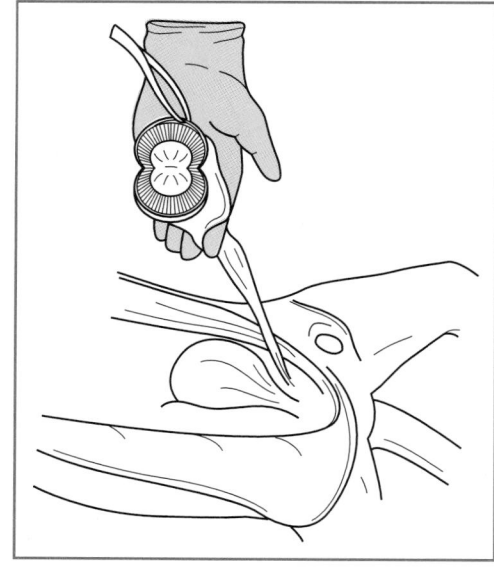

FIGURE 5-17.   The kidney is dissected with a longitudinal incision. The renal capsule is then peeled away to reveal the renal surfaces.

of a right and left lamina, which unite to form the spine. Beginning at the atlas the right and left laminae of each vertebra are cut with bone shears or, in larger specimens, with the Stryker saw. The laminae of atlas and axis are broad and difficult to cut, but the remainder of the vertebrae present little difficulty. Once several dorsal arches have been freed, the connected arches are held as a handle and used to reflect succeeding arches dorsally and caudally. When the entire roof of the vertebral canal has been removed, meninges, spinal cord, and vertebrae are examined in situ. Spinal cord and meninges are removed by cutting spinal nerve roots, and then the floor of the vertebral canal and the intervertebral disks are examined.

NECROPSY VARIATIONS

The following sections describe variations on the basic small mammal necropsy procedure that are useful when dealing with ruminants, horses, pigs, fetal farm animals, birds, and laboratory animals.

Ruminants

Necropsy of ruminants is done with the animal in left lateral recumbency. This positions the rumen on the down side, which facilitates the removal of abdominal organs (Figure 5-18). The right inguinal area is incised, and the coxofemoral joint is penetrated. Muscles near the pelvis are severed, and the right hindlimb is reflected away from the body. The mammary gland is undermined at its body wall attachment and retracted caudally. The mammary glands should remain attached to the body by the perineal skin so that gland position can be maintained when serially sectioned. The right axilla is incised so that the entire forelimb

can be reflected away from the body. The upper half of the trunk is then skinned.

Entry into the abdomen is initiated by cutting the body wall behind the last rib. Cuts along the midline and upper flank permit exposure of the cavity (Figure 5-19). Following an in situ inspection, the omentum is stripped from the forestomachs and double-string ligatures are placed on the duodenum (near the pylorus) and rectum, and a single ligature is placed around the esophagus near the reticulum. This prevents excessive leakage of contents. If the rumen is severely distended with gas, a tiny nick in the wall will relieve gas without excessive contamination. The entire intestinal tract is removed by severing the mesenteric root, and the intestines are opened, examined, and sampled while still attached to the mesentery (Figure 5-20). The dorsal attachments to the rumen are cut, and the forestomachs and abomasum are rolled onto the floor. Ruminoreticular contents should be examined for foreign objects or undesirable plant material.

Because of the size of the chest cavity and difficulty in cutting the ribs in mature animals, the thoracic contents are usually removed via the abdominal cavity. The right side of the rib cage is easily removed with lopping shears in young animals. The diaphragm is incised along its costal attachment, and the ventral mediastinal attachments are severed. The tongue, larynx, and trachea are freed of their attachments and threaded into the thoracic inlet. The entire unit is pulled into the abdomen.

The remainder of the necropsy is similar to that described for the small mammal.

Horse

Left lateral recumbency is the preferred body position. Reflect the right forelimb and right hindlimb as described

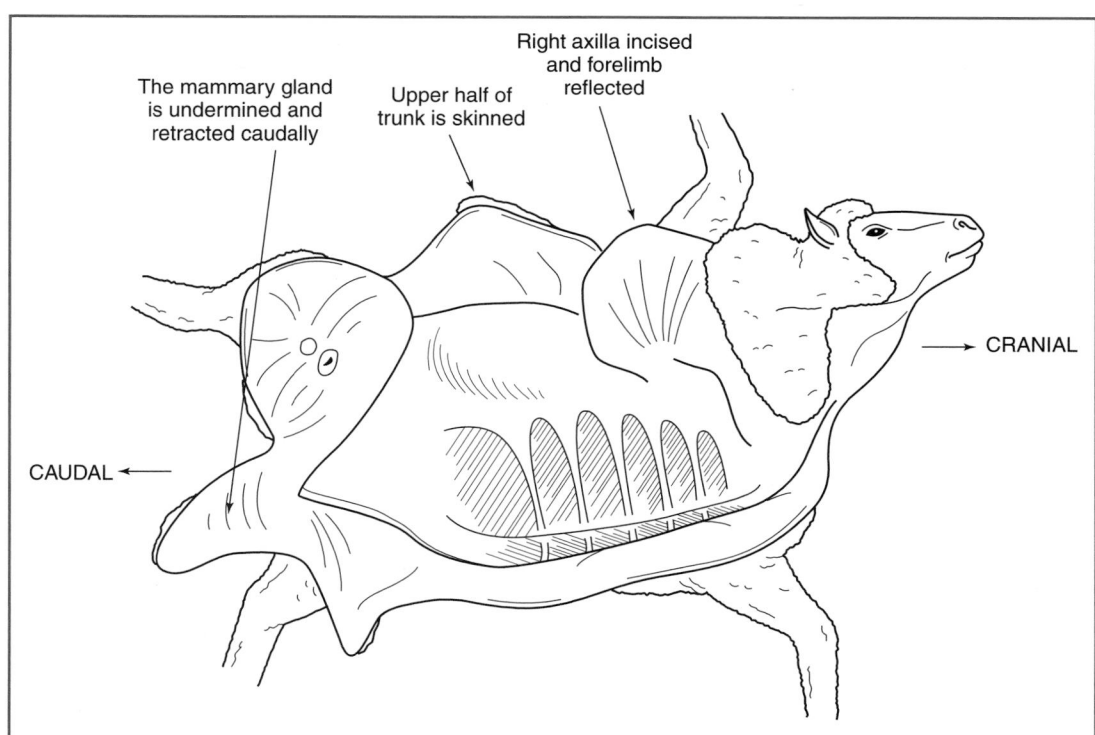

FIGURE 5-18. The ruminant is positioned in left lateral recumbency, which positions the rumen on the "down side." This facilitates access to the abdominal organs.

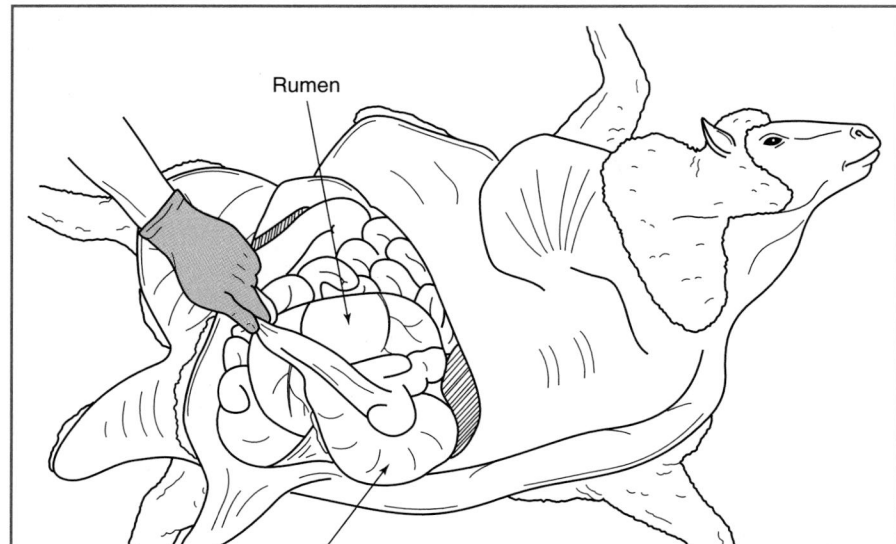

FIGURE 5-19.   Access to the abdominal cavity is achieved by making an incision along the midline followed by cuts along the last ribs.

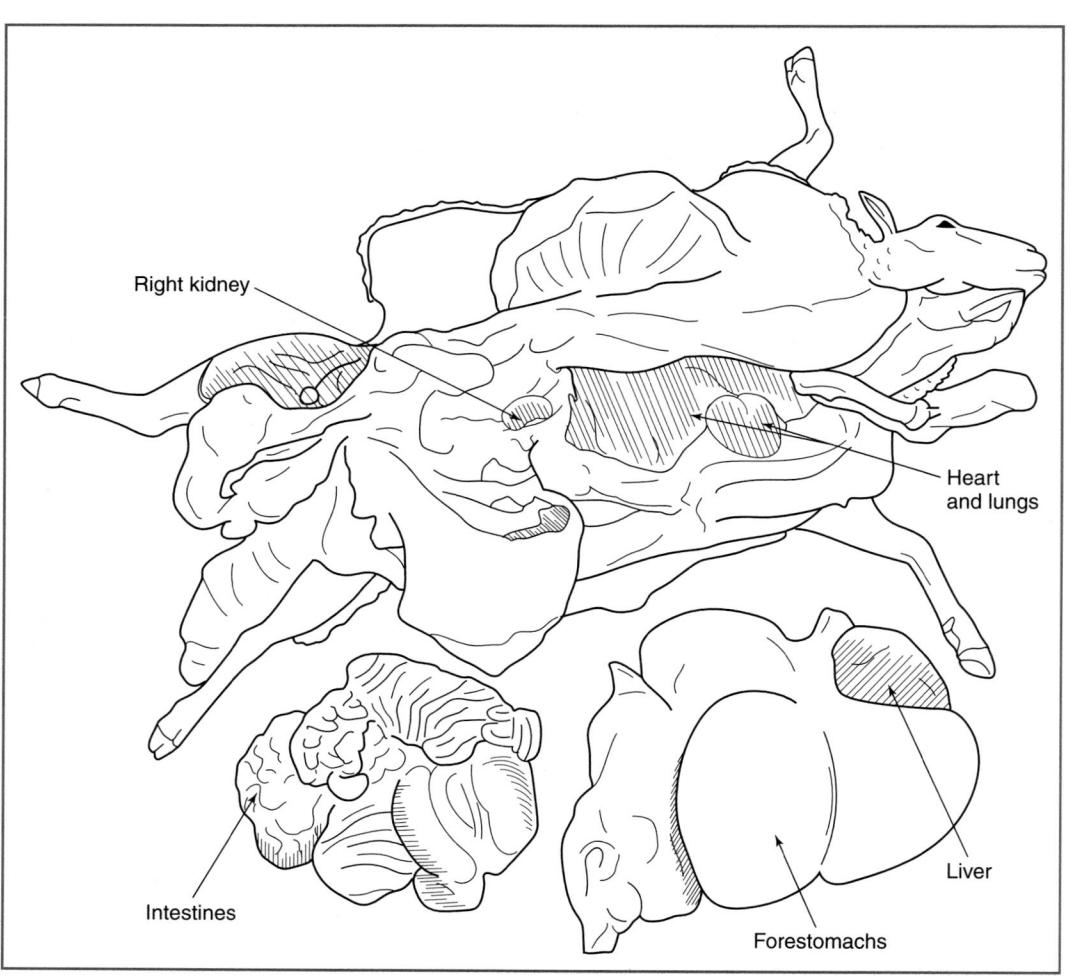

FIGURE 5-20.   After the omentum is examined in situ, it is stripped from the forestomachs. The duodenum, rectum, and esophagus are ligated, and then the entire intestinal tract is removed by severing the mesenteric root.

for the ruminant. Skin the trunk, and enter the abdomen. The intestines are removed in a multistep process:

1. Sever the ileum at the ileocecal junction, and remove the small intestine by cutting along the mesenteric insertion.
2. Cut the duodenum where it wraps around the mesenteric root; a string ligature here will reduce contamination by digesta.
3. Next, remove the small intestine mesentery.
4. Sever the small colon near the pelvic inlet, and detach along the mesocolon.
5. With careful blunt dissection, peel the soft connective tissue and pancreas adhering to the large colon near the mesenteric root. When one's hand can encircle the mesenteric root, the knife is advanced to cut as close to the aorta as possible.
6. The large colon and cecum are sampled and then emptied of their contents. The mucosal surfaces are rinsed and examined.

The remainder of the necropsy is similar to the ruminant and small mammal. Special attention should be given to the guttural pouches and jugular veins.

All joints of the appendicular skeleton should be opened. Joints are best approached from the medial aspect after the skin has been reflected. The coffin joint is the most difficult joint to access, but this is easier if the foot must be split (with a saw) in order to evaluate the hoof wall lamina. Spinal cord removal is extremely tedious without access to a meat-cutter's band saw. Alternatively, the cervical cord can be extracted by disarticulating the cervical vertebrae, one by one. Remove as much muscle as possible before disarticulating at the facets and anulus fibrosus. Sever the nerve roots by advancing a thin, long-handled scissors along the wall of the spinal canal.

Pig

Small mammal procedures apply. Because enteric disease is a frequent reason for necropsy, attention should be focused on collecting the freshest possible gut tissues. It is customary to examine the nasal turbinates of market-weight pigs. This is accomplished with a transverse saw cut of the snout at the level of the second and third premolars. Mature swine have sinus bone covering much of the calvaria. Brain removal is best accomplished by hemisectioning the head.

Fetus

Fetuses are often severely autolyzed, sometimes mummified, because of in utero retention following their death. Nevertheless, sample collection is justified. Fetal membranes (placenta) should be carefully examined and all abnormal-appearing sites sampled. Equine fetal membranes are examined for completeness. Fetuses from cattle and horses are measured (weighed if possible) to estimate gestational age. Standardized charts are in many veterinary textbooks. Crown-to-rump length (the distance from the poll to the tail base along the dorsum) is taken with a flexible tape measure.

The fetus is placed in right lateral recumbency because fetal abdominal organs are most easily sampled from the left side. The left limbs are removed, and the body wall is skinned. The abdominal wall is incised behind the rib and the incision extended along the ribs, sublumbar flank, and midline without touching the underlying viscera or allowing the body wall to drop onto the viscera. The left hemidiaphragm and costosternal cartilage are cut with the tip of the knife, and, similar to the abdominal approach,

the rib cage is retracted without touching the underlying tissues. The ribs usually break along the vertebral column.

Organs are sampled in situ with sterile tools and aseptic technique. The organs of greatest interest for viral cultures are lung, liver, kidney, and lymphoid tissue, such as spleen and thymus. Bacterial cultures are usually taken from stomach fluid, lung, and liver. The body can now be routinely examined for anatomic correctness and sampled for histology. The umbilical stump and brain should always be examined and collected.

Birds

Birds suspected of infectious or zoonotic diseases (psittacosis) should be submitted to a diagnostic laboratory for necropsy. If avian necropsies are done, the prosector should wear protective clothing, gloves, and a mask. The carcass should be wetted by immersing in warm soapy water or disinfectant to decrease spread of infectious agents and reduce irritating aerosolized dander and feathers. After the external examination the bird is placed in dorsal recumbency and the feathers parted along the ventral midline. For small birds the wing may be pinned to a cork board or cardboard for easier dissection. A skin incision is made extending from the beak to the vent, and the skin is reflected. The legs are reflected laterally by cutting into and exposing the coxofemoral joint. The abdomen is opened as in the small mammal necropsy technique, and the sternum and lateral ribs are removed by cutting through the sternum, ribs, coracoid bones, and clavicles using scissors, utility scissors, poultry shears, or pruning shears, depending on the size of the bird. Air sacs and abdominal and thoracic contents are examined, and samples for microbiology are taken if needed.

Technician Note

Birds suspected of infectious or zoonotic diseases (psittacosis) should be submitted to a diagnostic laboratory for necropsy.

For very small birds (small hummingbirds, etc.) the entire carcass can be fixed after the body cavities are opened. For larger birds the joints, nerves, muscles, eyes, brain, and spinal cord can be examined as in the small mammal necropsy technique. The spinal cord in small birds is difficult to remove without damaging it. The entire vertebral column with the spinal cord inside should be collected and fixed after the limbs, head, and muscles surrounding the vertebral column are removed. The vertebral column and spinal cord can be submitted whole and decalcified and trimmed by the pathology laboratory.

In larger birds the thyroid and parathyroid glands, located at the thoracic inlet adjacent to the carotid arteries, are removed. The heart is removed and examined. The entire gastrointestinal tract, liver, pancreas, and spleen are removed beginning with the esophagus. The spleen, liver, and gastrointestinal tract are examined, and specimens are collected as in the small mammal necropsy. The tongue, trachea, and lungs are then removed and examined, and samples are collected. The gonads (only the left ovary is present in birds) and adrenal glands are removed and fixed whole in small birds, and then the kidneys are removed, examined, and sampled.

Laboratory Animals

The necropsy technique for small mammals can be used for most laboratory animals including rodents; however, for evaluation of the health status of laboratory animal colonies more extensive testing is required. Complete health monitoring includes serology, bacteriology, parasitology, and genetic monitoring in addition to gross pathology and histopathology. It is beyond the scope of this chapter to include techniques for blood collection for serology, bacteriologic sampling techniques, techniques for ectoparasite and endoparasite examination, and genetic monitoring. A number of laboratories provide complete diagnostic services and health monitoring for laboratory animals, and these laboratories should be contacted before specimens (either live animals or samples from necropsies) are submitted to them.

Technician Note

The necropsy technique for small mammals can be used for most laboratory animals. However, for evaluation of the health status of laboratory animal colonies, more extensive testing is required.

The technique for small mammals is followed except for the following variations for small rodents. An entire hindlimb can be removed at the coxofemoral joint, the skin removed, and the limb fixed whole for bone, bone marrow, synovium, nerve, and skeletal muscle samples. For very small rodents (mice, hamsters, gerbils) the lungs should be inflated with formalin after the thorax is opened but before the lungs and heart are removed from the thorax. A 5- to 10-ml syringe with a small- to medium-bore needle is filled with formalin. The needle is threaded caudally for a few millimeters from the middle of the trachea, and the trachea is clamped with a hemostat rostral to the needle insertion site. The lungs are gently inflated until they fill the thorax. The trachea is then clamped or tied below the needle insertion site, and the lungs and heart are removed from the chest as before. The heart is often too small to open easily, and before fixation it can be cut longitudinally through the middle of the right and left ventricles.

The intestinal tract can be opened in a few places and then infused with formalin using a 5-ml syringe and a small-bore needle, or the entire tract can be opened up and pinned to cardboard before fixation. The kidney and adrenal gland on each side can be removed as a unit and left together for fixation after the kidney is incised longitudinally to evaluate the pelvis for hydronephrosis. The uterus and ovaries or the testes and seminal vesicles/coagulating gland can be removed along with the urinary bladder and fixed whole without sectioning.

The spinal cord in very small animals is difficult to remove without damaging it. The entire vertebral column with the spinal cord inside should be collected and fixed after the limbs, head, and muscles surrounding the vertebral column are removed. The vertebral column and spinal cord can be submitted whole and decalcified and trimmed by the pathology laboratory.

COSMETIC NECROPSIES

Cosmetic necropsies, although of more limited value than complete necropsies, can be performed when the disease processes are limited to the abdomen and chest. A midline incision is made in the ventral abdomen from the xiphoid to the pubis. The abdominal organs are examined in situ, and the diaphragm is cut away from the ventral rib cage. The colon and ureter are tied off at the pelvic inlet and

transected caudal to the tie. Reaching up through the diaphragm, the trachea and esophagus are grasped at the thoracic inlet and transected. The thoracic and abdominal contents are removed as a unit and dissected and described as in a noncosmetic necropsy. The body cavities are examined. The cavities are filled with paper towels, and the ventral abdominal incision is sutured.

Technician Note

Cosmetic necropsies, although of more limited value than complete necropsies, can be performed when the disease processes are limited to the abdomen and chest.

RECOMMENDED READING

King JM et al: *The necropsy book,* Gurnee, Ill, 2000, Charles Louis Davis, DVM Foundation.
Necropsy examination. In Richie BW, Harrison GJ, Harrison LR, editors: *Avian medicine: principles and application,* Lake Worth, Fla, 1994, Wingers Publishing, pp 355-379.

APPENDIX I
SAMPLE NECROPSY REPORT

Owner:	Brown
Clinic #:	01-34567
Animal name:	Ralph
Clinician:	Smith
Date/time of death:	01/17/01 (9 AM)
Date/time of necropsy:	01/17/01 (11 AM)

This is a 3.0-kg, 7½-year-old, spayed, female seal-point Siamese cross cat in adequate postmortem and emaciated nutritional condition. There is a clipped area on the distal aspect of the right front leg with an electrocardiogram (ECG) lead taped in place. The left antebrachium is clipped, and a catheter is in the left cephalic vein. The ventral cervical area and the ventral and lateral abdomen are clipped. There is very little body fat, and the muscle mass is reduced.

There is approximately 100 ml of yellow stringy fluid in the abdomen. There are multifocal, 2- to 10-mm, yellow-tan clots of fibrin throughout the abdomen and loosely adherent to abdominal organs. There are white-tan, multifocal to confluent, 1- to 5-cm diameter plaques on the surface of the liver, spleen, small intestine, omentum, mesentery, diaphragm, and body wall. The small intestine and colon are dilated (1 to 2 cm in diameter), and the wall of the small intestine is multifocally thickened. In the most severely affected area, at the jejunoileal junction, the serosa is corrugated and the wall is 3 to 5 mm thick. The abdominal and sternal lymph nodes are enlarged (0.5 to 2.0 cm in diameter) and white on the capsular surface. On section, they have a normal lymph node architecture with a thick white cortex.

The lungs are heavy, wet, and red-purple, and they sink in formalin. There is approximately 5 ml of serosanguineous fluid in the pericardium.

GROSS FINDINGS

Lungs: Moderate to severe acute pneumonia, presumptive
Abdomen: Severe fibrinous peritonitis
Small intestine and colon: Severe chronic enteritis and colitis, presumptive

Pericardium: Moderate serosanguineous effusion
Abdominal and sternal lymph nodes: Severe reactive hyperplasia, presumptive

GROSS DIAGNOSIS

- Euthanasia
- Feline infectious peritonitis (FIP)
- Severe enteritis and colitis, presumptive
- Severe pneumonia, presumptive

COMMENT

I am not sure if the changes in the small intestine and colon are due to FIP or some other process. The lung lesion is also not typical for FIP. Impression smears of the peritoneal surface lesions reveal a mixed population of inflammatory cells, including neutrophils, lymphocytes, plasma cells, and macrophages consistent with the diagnosis of FIP.

Samples of lung and small intestine are submitted for bacterial culture. Samples of lymph nodes, small intestine, colon, lungs, liver, and spleen are submitted for histologic examination.

APPENDIX II
NECROPSY PROCEDURE OUTLINE

1. Before you begin dissection be sure you have the owner's permission, correct animal, disposition instructions, body weight, labeled formalin container, instruments, cassette for bone marrow, tag for brain, cardboard for nerve and skin, and an understanding of the clinical history.
2. All routine tissues and all lesions are collected; all lesions are described (measured and weighed if appropriate); and all necessary microbiologic, cytologic, and toxicologic samples are collected for every necropsy.
3. Do the external examination; remove eyes; then place body in left lateral recumbency; and make a midline skin incision extending into axillary and inguinal areas to reflect limbs and extend the incision rostrally to the mandibular symphysis and caudally to the perineum.
4. Dissect/examine, section, and collect (DESC) skin, lymph nodes, salivary glands, and testes or mammary glands. Open the coxofemoral, stifle, and scapulohumeral joints. DESC synovium, skeletal muscle, sciatic nerve, and bone marrow.
5. Open abdomen (midline); puncture diaphragm; open chest (bilateral, cutting ribs) and pericardium; collect microbiologic samples; and examine organs and vessels in situ. (NOTE: Discuss case with clinician at this time.) DESC thyroid, parathyroids, and adrenals.
6. Remove tongue from oral cavity, and reflect the tongue, tonsils, larynx, and esophagus caudally. Cut spinal cord and vertebral column at atlantooccipital joint; remove skin and muscle from calvaria; cut calvaria with Stryker saw in hood; and remove caudal-dorsal calvaria and dorsal meninges. Transect cranial nerves, and remove brain and pituitary. Open tympanic bullae. Section head longitudinally, and examine nasal and oral cavity.
7. Remove tongue, tonsils, esophagus, trachea, lungs, heart, and thoracic aorta together. DESC tongue, tonsils, esophagus, trachea, right atrium, right ventricle, pulmonary arteries, lungs, lymph nodes, left atrium, left ventricle, and thoracic aorta.
8. Remove distal duodenum, jejunum, ileum, colon, and mesenteric lymph nodes together (open later unless critical). Remove liver, duodenum, pancreas, stomach, and spleen en bloc. DESC spleen; open stomach and duodenum; express gallbladder; and DESC liver, stomach, duodenum, and pancreas.
9. Remove floor of pelvis; and DESC right kidney and ureter, left kidney and ureter, urinary bladder, urethra, prostate, ovaries and uterus, cervix/vagina, rectum, anal glands, and abdominal aorta. DESC small intestine, colon, and mesenteric lymph nodes.
10. Remove spinal cord if necessary.

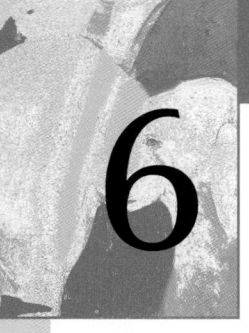

6

PART TWO
Clinical Sciences

Clinical Pathology

Jan L. VanSteenhouse

Accurate clinical pathology data are an invaluable component of the minimum data base used in the diagnosis of diseases in all species. Repetition of selected data also provides a means of monitoring and evaluating the success of chosen treatment regimens. Erroneous data, however, may result in misdiagnoses and be a more serious disadvantage than the lack of data.

Each practice will be faced with the decision of whether laboratory data will be generated within the clinic or be obtained from a reference laboratory. The practice's caseload, availability and turnaround time of a qualified reference laboratory, and experience of the technician are important criteria used to make this determination. Having clinical laboratory data available within 1 hour can be a great advantage to the veterinarian in determining the diagnosis, especially during life-threatening emergencies.

Whether samples are submitted to a reference laboratory or analyzed in the practice, the appropriately trained veterinary technician can be an invaluable asset in ensuring that valid, reliable data are obtained. In either case, knowledge of proper sampling techniques and proper sample handling is essential. The veterinary technician should be familiar with the type and amount of sample to submit for various tests, whether an anticoagulant should be used, and how the sample should be prepared, transported, and stored if it is not immediately analyzed.

It is the veterinary technician's responsibility to have a thorough working knowledge of any in-house analyzer, its sample requirements, its routine maintenance procedures, and basic quality control procedures to ensure accurate laboratory results. The technician should also be familiar with the care and maintenance of all supportive laboratory equipment necessary to keep instruments functioning properly.

Should it be decided that a reference laboratory is more time or cost efficient for an individual practice, it is imperative that the veterinary technician communicate with the personnel of that laboratory. To avoid unnecessary delays and invalid results, the laboratory should be consulted regarding appropriate sample submission for specific tests. Precautions must be taken to ensure that the samples are not damaged or destroyed in transport.

This chapter addresses the more commonly used clinical laboratory techniques and procedures in veterinary hematology, urinalysis, clinical chemistry, and cytology. Techniques and methods are emphasized rather than interpretation. The recommended reading list provides detailed reviews. Laboratory instrumentation and necessary quality control systems for clinical chemistry and hematology are reviewed and summarized. In addition, errors in sampling and sample handling and the consequence of misleading values, which complicate the interpretation of laboratory data, are discussed.

HEMATOLOGY

The basic equipment necessary for hematologic analyses includes a microscope, microhematocrit centrifuge, refractometer, hemacytometer, clean slides, and modified Wright's stain. The benefits of conscientious care and cleaning of these items cannot be overlooked. The complete blood count (CBC) provides the veterinarian with invaluable information regarding the patient's red blood cell (RBC, erythrocyte) mass, white blood cell (WBC, leukocyte) number and distribution, platelet number, and plasma protein. The CBC consists of a PCV (packed cell volume), WBC count, RBC count, hemoglobin determination, RBC indices, platelet count or estimate, total plasma protein determination, and evaluation of the blood smear for RBC morphology and a WBC differential. Hematologic procedures are performed on anticoagulated whole blood. The preferred anticoagulant is ethylenediamine tetraacetic acid (EDTA) because it does not interfere with blood cell morphology and staining. EDTA is commercially available in purple-top Vacutainer tubes in a variety of sizes. Choosing the correct size is essential to obtain accurate results because having a small amount of blood in a large tube will alter some of the values. The various types of sample tubes available and their appropriate uses are listed in Table 6-1.

The morphology of the normal and abnormal blood cells is briefly reviewed, but it is strongly recommended that the technician have on hand and consult the appropriate references listed at the end of this chapter. Table 6-2 contains sample reference ranges for normal hematology values in common domestic species.

Equipment

When choosing a microscope, the laboratory's needs must first be assessed. The fewer "extras" that are included will reduce the requirements for maintenance, service, and repairs. A good-quality binocular microscope with a mechanical stage, an adjustable substage condenser, and good-quality objective lenses will accommodate the needs of any hematology laboratory. The most important aspect, and often the cost determinant, of a good laboratory microscope is the objective lens. Planachromatic lenses are recommended because they provide a flat field of vision with superior optical properties. The entire field will be in focus, resulting in reduced eyestrain and improved microscopic image. The basic laboratory microscope should have 10×, 40× (high dry), and 100× (oil immersion) objective lenses in addition to standard 10× ocular objectives. Many microscopists find an additional 50× oil immersion objective lens useful for evaluation of both blood films and cytology specimens. The manufacturer's manual should provide directions for adjusting the light for optimal intensity (Kohler illumination), which enhances the clarity of the image.

Proper care of the microscope is essential to providing accurate results for an extended period of time. Great care should be taken to follow the manufacturer's directions for proper use, cleaning, and maintenance. The oil immersion lenses require a drop of special immersion oil on the blood film to achieve the appropriate optics. The immersion oil should be wiped from the objective after use to prevent damage to the lens. It is essential that all other objectives be kept free of oil. Lenses should be cleaned with lens paper only. A dust cover should be placed over the microscope when not in use to prevent collection of dust and hairs on the lenses and other surfaces.

Technician Note

No laboratory equipment or instrument, regardless of cost, is any better than the care and maintenance it receives.

A microhematocrit centrifuge is required for determination of the PCV. The centrifugal force generated by the centrifuge separates the cellular components of blood from the plasma. The manufacturer's manual should be consulted for recommended speed settings for the sample being spun. As with all laboratory equipment, the accuracy and functional longevity of the centrifuge are directly related to proper care and use. Safety concerns preclude ever operating the centrifuge without the lid being closed and properly secured. Samples should always be balanced to ensure accurate separation and reduce wear on the motor. Periodic maintenance, such as lubricating the bearings and checking the commutator, should be scheduled according to the manufacturer's recommendations to extend the life of the centrifuge and ensure accurate results.

The refractometer is used to determine the plasma protein concentration by measuring the refractive index of the plasma. Careful cleaning of the sample surface is imperative to prolonging the accuracy and functional life of the refractometer. Several models are available, including one designed specifically for veterinary use (Figure 6-1). The veterinary model is less expensive, has a more shock-resistant casing, and is appropriate for use in veterinary determination of urine specific gravity. Calibration of the zero setting should be checked periodically with distilled water and adjusted according to the manufacturer's manual if necessary.

The Neubauer (recommended) hemacytometer is a small but valuable specialized counting chamber used for determining WBC and platelet counts per microliter of blood (Figure 6-2). It has a special coverglass calibrated for accuracy; regular coverglasses cannot be substituted should it be damaged. Both the hemacytometer and coverslip must be carefully cleaned to avoid scratching the surfaces.

New, clean glass slides are essential for making usable blood films. Slides that are frosted on one end are preferred for labeling purposes.

TABLE 6-1	RECOMMENDED SAMPLE TUBES	
Color of Top	Anticoagulant	Purpose
Purple	EDTA	CBC, platelet counts
Red	None	Chemistries
Tiger (red-black)	Separator gel	Chemistries
Green	Heparin	Electrolytes, stats
Turquoise	Citrate	Coagulation assay

TABLE 6-2	HEMATOLOGY VALUES			
	Canine	Feline	Equine	Bovine
PCV (%)	37-55	3-45	32-48	24-46
Hemoglobin (g/dl)	12-18	8-15	10-18	8-15
Reticulocytes (%)	0-1.5	0-1.0	0	0
WBCs (n/μl)	6000-17,000	5500-19,500	6000-12,000	4000-12,000
Segs (n/μl)	3000-11,400	2500-12,500	3000-6000	600-4000
Bands (n/μl)	0-300	0-300	0-100	0-120
Lymphocytes (n/μl)	1000-4800	1500-7000	1500-5000	2500-7500
Monocytes (n/μl)	150-1350	0-850	0-600	25-850
Eosinophils (n/μl)	100-750	0-750	0-800	0-2400
Basophils (n/μl)	Rare	Rare	0-300	0-200
TP (g/dl)	6.0-7.5	6.0-7.5	6.0-8.5	6.0-8.0
Fibrinogen (mg/dl)	150-300	150-300	100-400	100-600
Platelets (n/μl)	200,000-500,000	300,000-700,000	100,000-600,000	100,000-800,000

n, Number; *PCV,* packed cell volume; *TP,* total protein; *WBCs,* white blood cells.

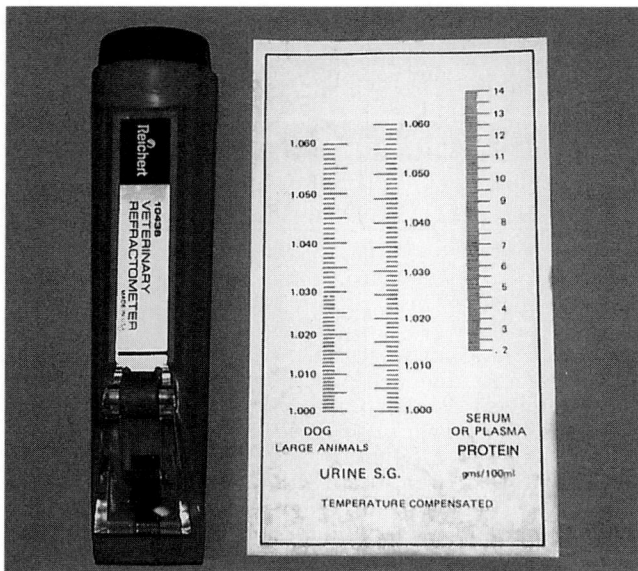

FIGURE 6-1. Veterinary refractometer and reading scale.

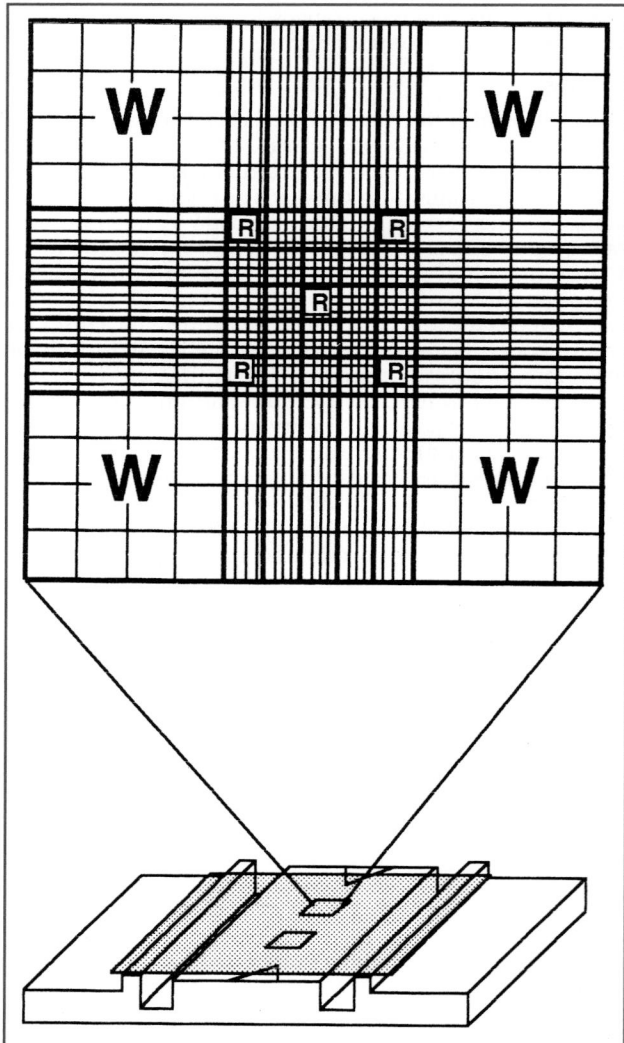

FIGURE 6-2. Neubauer hemacytometer. The large *W*s indicate the squares that are counted for a total white blood cell count with the 1:20 dilution WBC Unopette system. The small *R*s indicate the squares that are counted for a red blood cell count with the RBC Unopette system.

Sample Handling

In general, EDTA is the required anticoagulant for hematology. Be sure to use a tube of the appropriate size for the sample being drawn. It is often difficult to obtain large samples from small dogs and cats; the 2-ml pediatric collection tube is best for a patient of this size. There are collection tubes for smaller volumes (0.5-ml Microtainer tubes, Becton-Dickinson, Rutherford, N.J.). These tubes are excellent for samples from puppies, kittens, and small exotic animal species. Excess anticoagulant resulting from a small amount of blood in a too large tube can erroneously decrease the PCV and increase total protein determined with a refractometer.

Anticoagulated blood samples should be immediately mixed by gentle inversion of the tube. Blood films should be made from well-mixed blood within 15 minutes of obtaining the sample to decrease in vitro morphologic changes in the blood cells. If the practice uses a reference laboratory, unstained blood films should be sent with the EDTA sample. If samples must be held overnight, refrigerate the whole blood but do not refrigerate the blood film. Water will condense on the surface of the blood film if it is placed in the refrigerator and cause lysis of the RBCs. The blood film, as well as cytology slides, should be protected from formalin vapors because formalin will interfere with cell preservation and staining. If samples are being sent out, they should be packaged in separate bags.

Technician Note

Blood films should always be made from fresh blood, before refrigeration, regardless of whether the CBC will be performed in the clinic or sent to a reference laboratory.

Determination of Erythrocyte Numbers

Determination of the PCV, the percentage of total blood volume accounted for by RBCs, is the easiest and most common means of evaluating the RBC mass. This is achieved by filling a plain microhematocrit capillary tube with anticoagulated blood, sealing one end of the tube with a specific clay, and centrifuging the sample in a microhematocrit centrifuge. The spun sample is then applied to a chart to determine the PCV. This method provides a quick and accurate measurement if samples are spun for a standard length of time at a consistent speed. The specific time and speed depend on the particular centrifuge being used. Accuracy also depends on the care and operation of the centrifuge. Blood samples from cattle, sheep, and goats may require centrifugation for a longer time because their smaller RBCs do not pack as well as dog and cat RBCs. The plasma portion at the top of the tube should be evaluated for color and clarity and will also be used for determination of plasma protein. The *hematocrit* provides basically the same information but is obtained by calculation when an automated analyzer is used and thus may be slightly different from the measured PCV. This is most commonly seen in blood samples from collection

TABLE 6-3	UNOPETTE SYSTEMS FOR COUNTING DIFFERENT CELL TYPES			
	Test	Pipette Volume	Dilution	Diluent
	Red cell count	<10 μl	<1:200	<0.85% Saline
	White cell count	20 μl	1:100	3% Acetic acid
	White cell count	25 μl	1:20	3% Acetic acid
	Platelet count	20 μl	1:100	1% Ammonium oxalate
	Eosinophil count	25 μl	1:32	Phloxin

tubes that have an inadequate volume of blood (less than 1 ml in a 5-ml tube or less than 0.5 ml in a 2-ml tube). The excess anticoagulant causes the RBCs to shrink, erroneously decreasing the PCV. When the blood is diluted by the electronic cell counter, the diluent reexpands the RBCs to their true size, providing the true value for the hematocrit.

The actual number of erythrocytes may be determined using an automated cell counter, which is primarily available in reference laboratories. Erythrocyte counts may also be performed manually but are too tedious and inaccurate to be of diagnostic value. RBC counts vary proportionately with PCV and have little to no advantage over PCV. The major advantage of automated cell counters is that they also measure hemoglobin and measure or calculate the RBC indices. Hemoglobin is the protein in RBCs that is responsible for carrying oxygen from the lungs to the tissues.

RBC Indices

RBC indices are commonly provided when automated analyzers are used; these indices include mean corpuscular volume (MCV), mean corpuscular hemoglobin (MCH), and mean corpuscular hemoglobin concentration (MCHC). The MCH is of little value, but the MCV and MCHC are useful in evaluating and determining the cause of anemias (decreased RBC number). MCH and MCHC values calculated with an electronic cell counter will be artifactually affected by hemolysis, Heinz bodies, and lipemia. Samples with these properties therefore cannot be used to determine MCH and MCHC.

Determination of Leukocyte Counts

The total WBC count may be determined manually using the hemacytometer or with an automated cell counter. Either way, it is important that the blood tube be well mixed before the sample is taken. Figure 6-2 diagrams the hemacytometer grid that will be seen microscopically and indicates the areas on the grid to be counted for the WBC count. The glass coverslip is one specifically designed for the hemacytometer and regular coverslips cannot be substituted, so it must be handled and cleaned carefully to avoid damage and should never be used for other purposes. The Unopette dilution system (Becton-Dickinson) is the most accepted method for performing manual WBC counts. A number of Unopette systems are available for counting various cell types (Table 6-3), but the system preferred for counting leukocytes is also used for counting platelets and determining cell counts on samples such as synovial fluid. This system consists of a disposable reservoir containing diluent and an agent to lyse RBCs to accommodate the counting of leukocytes. Each Unopette system comes with detailed instructions for obtaining reliable results and a capillary pipette to draw a specific volume of blood. The interchangeable use of pipettes from another cell-counting system, such as one for RBCs, to

obtain WBC counts will result in significant errors and inappropriately decreased WBC counts.

The accuracy of a manual WBC count depends on adherence to the directions and the proper performance of each step. Care must be taken to accurately fill the capillary tube and wipe off any excess blood on the outside of the tube without touching the tip of the pipette and drawing any of the sample out of the pipette. The blood sample must be carefully transferred to the reservoir with careful mixing to ensure complete delivery of the sample into the diluent. Blood left in the capillary tube or accidentally expelled from the top of the pipette during mixing will result in erroneous WBC counts. It will take practice and may require multiple attempts to completely and accurately fill the hemacytometer chamber. The chambers on both sides of the hemacytometer must be filled for accurate results. Counting both sides and comparing results also serve to check accuracy because the number of cells on one side should closely approximate the number of cells on the other side. Overfilling or underfilling the chamber will cause errors in the final cell count. After charging the hemacytometer chambers, the hemacytometer must be allowed to sit for several minutes to allow the cells to settle. WBCs will be counted using the 10×objective; lowering the condenser on the microscope will increase the contrast, making the cells more prominent and easier to identify and count accurately.

Nucleated RBCs (NRBCs) will be counted along with WBCs by either manual or automated electronic counting methods, thus giving falsely elevated WBC counts. The number of NRBCs encountered on the blood film is counted while performing the differential on 100 leukocytes. The WBC count is then corrected using the following formula if more than 10 NRBCs are counted:

$$\frac{100}{100 + \text{Number of NRBCs}} \times \text{WBC} = \text{Corrected WBC count}$$

For example, if 15 NRBCs are counted while performing the 100-cell differential and the initial WBC count is 30,000/μl, the corrected count is then calculated as follows:

$$\frac{100}{100 + 15} \times 30,000 = 26,087 \text{ WBCs}$$

Increased WBCs are referred to as *leukocytosis*, whereas decreased WBCs are referred to as *leukopenia*. The diagnostic significance of either leukocytosis or leukopenia cannot be appreciated without the WBC differential. The differential is performed by examining the blood film (see Blood Film Evaluation). At least 100 leukocytes are identified and counted according to cell type (as neutrophils, bands, lymphocytes, monocytes, eosinophils, or basophils). The more cells that are counted, the more accurate will be the differential. The percentages of each cell type counted are then multiplied by the total WBC count to give absolute numbers of the cell types present. These numbers are the values used for interpreting changes in the leukogram.

Dramatic increases or decreases in WBC count may also be noted by looking at the *buffy coat*. The buffy coat is the white band of concentrated WBCs between the RBCs and plasma in the microhematocrit tube.

Avian and Reptilian Leukocyte Counts

Unlike mammals, birds and reptiles have NRBCs, which prevents determination of their WBC counts by the methods described. However, the WBC counts of these non-mammalian species may be determined indirectly using another Unopette system for eosinophil determination. This special Unopette is filled with anticoagulated blood, mixed well, and allowed to incubate for approximately 5 minutes to allow uptake of the stain by the cells. If the sample is allowed to stand for a prolonged time, it will result in all the cells taking up the stain and erroneous results. The hemacytometer is filled as for the manual WBC count described, and the red-staining cells are counted in all nine squares of the grid. With proper staining, only the eosinophils and heterophils (nonmammalian equivalent of neutrophils) will be stained. Unlike when performing the mammalian manual count, it is important to keep the microscope condenser up to decrease contrast. If the condenser is down, it will be more difficult to count the heterophils and eosinophils because of RBC interference.

The number obtained does not represent the WBC count but is used in conjunction with the differential to calculate the WBC count. When the differential is completed and the percentages of the various cell types present are known, the WBC count is calculated using the following formula:

$$\text{Cells counted on hemacytometer} \times 32 \times \frac{100}{\%\ \text{Heterophils} + \text{eosinophils}} = \text{WBCs/}\mu 1$$

For example, if 282 cells are counted on one side of the hemacytometer and you have 70% heterophils and 5% eosinophils on the differential, the total WBC count would be as follows:

$$282 \times 32 \times \frac{100}{70 + 5} = 12,032\ \text{WBCs/}\mu 1$$

Platelet Determination

Determination of platelet numbers is important because platelets play an important role in *hemostasis*, or control of blood flow. Several diseases cause decreased numbers of platelets, and these can often be diagnosed and treated before an animal develops a severe bleeding disorder. Similar to WBCs, platelets can be counted manually on a hemacytometer or with an automated cell counter. Feline platelets, in particular, have a tendency to clump, which interferes with obtaining accurate platelet counts; whether the count is done manually or by automation, an erroneously low platelet count can result. For this reason, it is important to always examine the blood film for platelet clumping. In addition, because cats often have relatively large platelets and cat RBCs are small, automated electronic counts are often inaccurate because of the inability to separate the cells by size.

Manual platelet counts can be performed using the same Unopette system and sample used for the manual WBC count. This task can be very tedious, especially if the hemacytometer and coverglass are not properly cared for. Scratches and small dust particles are very difficult to differentiate from platelets. If platelet clumps are present,

the resultant count will be inaccurate. It would be best to obtain another sample with special attention given to ensure a clean venipuncture and adequate mixing of the blood with the anticoagulant. Platelets are identified using the 40× objective and will be easier to see if the condenser is lowered and the light intensity is moderate. The instructions that accompany the Unopette must be followed with regard to the squares of the grid that are counted and the method of calculating the total count.

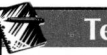

> ### Technician Note
>
> The blood film should always be scanned for platelet clumps, especially in cats, to avoid reporting erroneously low platelet numbers.

When platelet counts are not available or to verify counts obtained manually or electronically, the number of platelets can be estimated from the blood film. While examining the appropriate area of the blood film in which RBCs are spaced in a uniform monolayer, the average number of platelets per 100× oil immersion field in several fields (10 or more) is determined. This average number of platelets multiplied by 15,000 will provide an adequate estimation of the number of platelets per microliter.

Decreased platelet counts can have serious implications for the patient. Therefore, before reporting low platelet counts, all technical problems must be considered. The feathered edge of the blood film must be checked for platelet clumping. The tube of blood from which the sample was taken should be checked for small clots, which could deplete platelets. Either or both of these problems may occur despite the use of an anticoagulant. If neither the blood film nor the tube reveals evidence of platelet aggregation, the low platelet count should be reported as determined. If platelet clumping or clots are found, the sample should be redrawn and the counts repeated.

Blood Film Evaluation

Examination of the stained blood smear is one of the most valuable parts of the complete blood count, and its importance cannot be overstressed. For the sake of time, many technicians are tempted to skip this portion of the CBC, but the numbers alone can be very misleading and result in incorrect diagnoses and inappropriate treatment. Anemias cannot be classified or changes in the WBC accurately interpreted until the differential is completed and the cells are examined for morphologic changes. Examination of the blood film is especially important as an internal quality control when automated electronic cell counters are used. If there appears to be a discrepancy between what the technician sees on the film and the numbers reported by the instrument, the counts should be repeated with special attention given to determining what could be causing the difference. A common cause is that the blood tube was not adequately mixed before sampling for either the count or the blood film. Another common problem is seen, particularly in leukopenic cats, with considerable platelet clumping. The platelet clumps are large enough that they are counted as WBCs in the automated system, resulting in falsely higher WBC counts made by the instrument. With time and experience, the technician will be able to scan the blood film and recognize these discrepancies between the number of leukocytes apparent on the film and the number of WBCs reported by the instrument. As a general rule of thumb, there should be approximately 20 leukocytes per 10× field in a normal canine blood sample.

There are a variety of ways to make quality blood films. New slides should always be used, and they should be handled only by the edges because oils on the slide from fingers will result in poor-quality films. (The reader is referred to Recommended Reading for examples of the different techniques.) What is most important is to try several methods, find the one that is most comfortable, and then practice repeatedly until quality films are consistently produced. A small drop of blood is placed at one end of a slide, and the edge of a second slide is used to spread the drop. It is important to make the film in one even stroke and not use excessive downward pressure. Increased downward pressure on the spreader slide can cause the leukocytes to be carried to the feathered edge and may even cause the cells to rupture or become distorted. In either case the accuracy of the differential will be lessened. The thickness of the blood film can be altered to accommodate samples from severely anemic or dehydrated animals. Increasing the angle between the two slides will concentrate the cells when the PCV is very low. Conversely, decreasing the angle will allow greater spreading of the cells in a concentrated sample (Figure 6-3).

Several modifications of the traditional Wright's stain are available for suitable staining of blood films for veterinary practices. Stat Stain (VWR Scientific, Philadelphia), Diff-Quik (Baxter S/P, McGaw Park, Ill.), and CAMCO Quik Stain (Baxter S/P) are commonly used. They are relatively economical and technically easy to use and maintain. The disadvantages of these stains are few. Polychromatophilic RBCs do not stain as obviously as they do with Wright's stain, and some mast cell and eosinophil granules may be washed out.

It is best to develop a routine when evaluating a blood film and follow the same approach each time to avoid oversights and mistakes. The blood film should first be examined under low power (10×). While scanning on 10×, one can get an impression of the general distribution of nucleated cells (clumped at the edges or spread evenly throughout), estimate the total WBC count (low vs. normal vs. high), and examine the feathered edge of the blood film for aggregates of platelets, the larger leukocytes, neoplastic cells, and microfilaria of *Dirofilaria immitis* or *Dipetalonema reconditum* (Figure 6-4). During the low-power examination, one may identify structures or areas that need a closer look. Last, on low power, one should identify the appropriate area in which RBCs are distributed in a uniform monolayer and the leukocytes are sufficiently spread so that morphologic identification on high power is possible. It is especially important to avoid being too far into the body of the blood film, where the WBCs are rounded and darkly stained. In this area, it is often difficult to differentiate the leukocytes.

The blood film is then studied under high power, generally under oil immersion (100×). The WBC differential is performed at this power. Erythrocytes should be evaluated for morphologic changes and parasites, and platelets should be evaluated for morphology and counted to make the estimated count. These evaluations may be made before or after the differential, but they should be done consistently as part of the routine so they are not overlooked. Platelets are cytoplasmic fragments, so they have no nucleus. They are generally round to oval or spindle shaped with purplish granules and multiple pointed projections (Color Plate I, *B*). They may vary greatly in size, but increased numbers of large platelets may indicate an increased output from the bone marrow (Figure 6-5). After the platelets have been evaluated, the erythrocytes should be studied.

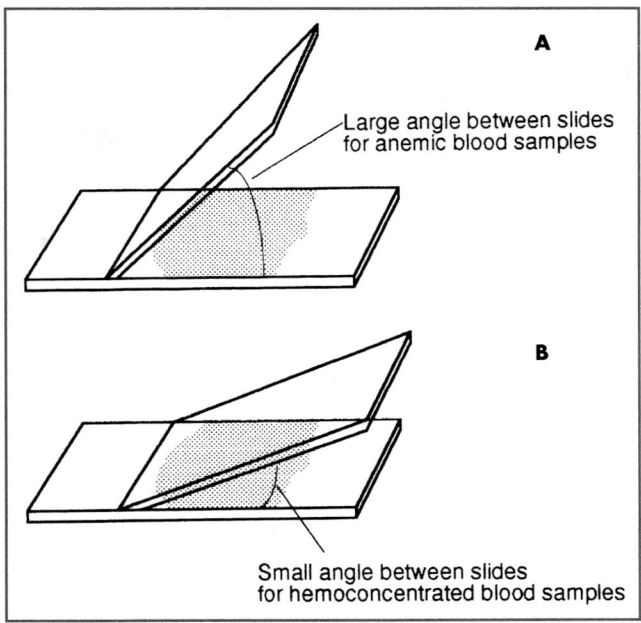

FIGURE 6-3. Difference in slide angle necessary for making blood films from anemic or hemoconcentrated blood. **A,** Large angle for anemic blood. **B,** Small angle for hemoconcentrated blood.

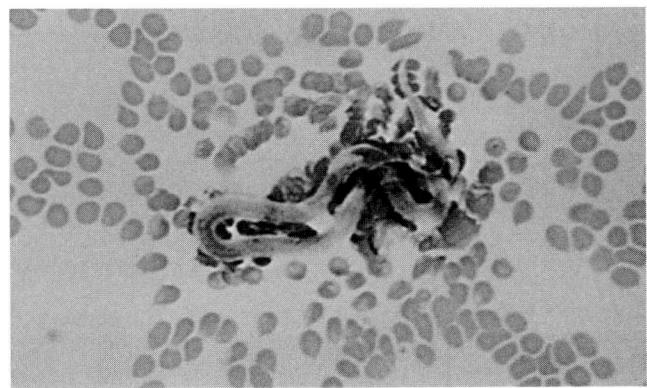

FIGURE 6-4. A microfilaria of *Dirofilaria immitis* at the feathered edge of a canine blood smear. The parasite is about the same width as an erythrocyte. (Courtesy Dr. Mary Anna Thrall.)

Erythrocyte Evaluation

The erythrocytes of most mammals are disk shaped and anuclear. They appear flat with a varying degree of *central pallor* (pale area in center of cell with less hemoglobin) depending on the size. The RBCs of different domestic species differ markedly in size, with those of the dog having the largest diameter (7 μm), followed by the horse, cow, and cat (5.8 μm), the sheep (4.5 μm), and the goat (3.2 μm). Some species have RBCs that vary in size, which is termed *anisocytosis.* Cows normally have more anisocytosis than do other species. In other species, extreme anisocytosis implies either that many of the RBCs are smaller (microcytic), which may indicate iron deficiency, or that many are larger (macrocytic), which may indicate increased production and release of immature cells from the bone marrow in response to anemia. Some poodles normally have larger RBCs than do other dogs. Some Japanese Akita dogs normally have smaller RBCs. These are genetic traits and do not indicate a change in RBC dynamics.

Poikilocytosis is the general term used to indicate changes in RBC shape. *Leptocytes* are RBCs with an increased surface area that makes them highly deformable. Target cells and cells with a transverse fold are two common forms of leptocytes. Because leptocytes can occur for many reasons, they are rarely of any diagnostic significance. Immature polychromatophilic cells often appear as leptocytes.

Acanthocytes are RBCs with a membrane abnormality that causes them to develop multiple, irregularly spaced, club-shaped projections from the cell surface. These must be differentiated from crenated cells, which have numerous rounded, evenly spaced projections. *Crenation* is an artifact resulting from high temperatures or slow drying of the blood film. Acanthocytes may be encountered in normal cattle, but in other species they are often associated with some neoplasms (especially visceral hemangiosar-

coma) or disorders of lipid metabolism. *Schistocytes* are fragmented RBCs formed as a result of the trauma of colliding with intravascular fibrin strands; schistocytes are associated with disseminated intravascular coagulopathy, heartworm disease, and, occasionally, diseases of the spleen or liver that involve fibrin deposition within the vasculature of those organs. *Spherocytes* are RBCs that appear smaller than normal RBCs and exhibit no central pallor (Figure 6-6). Spherocytes are most commonly seen in immune hemolytic anemia and can also be seen after blood transfusions. They are more spherical because bits of their membrane have been removed, making them more rigid and unable to assume the discoid shape more typical of RBCs. They are most easily identified in canine blood, because normal canine RBCs are larger and have a distinct zone of central pallor. In the other species with smaller RBCs, which typically exhibit little or no central pallor, spherocytes are difficult to confirm.

NRBCs, or *metarubricytes*, may be seen in peripheral blood films. An occasional NRBC may be found in a normal animal, but increased numbers are a significant finding and should be reported as the number of NRBCs per 100 WBCs. Care must be taken to avoid confusing NRBCs with lymphocytes. NRBCs of a size similar to small lymphocytes will have more cytoplasm relative to nuclear size and the cytoplasm will be faintly eosinophilic (reddish). Remember to correct the WBC count if more than 10 NRBCs per 100 WBCs are found (see previous discussion of determination of leukocyte counts).

The color of erythrocytes should be noted during examination of the blood film. *Polychromasia* is the term used to describe a variation in the color of RBCs. *Polychromatophilic RBCs* (Color Plate I, *A*) are bluish, although this is not as consistently evident with Diff-Quik stain as it is with Wright's stain. Some polychromasia may be seen in normal, healthy animals, but increased polychromasia in anemias suggests the anemia is regenerative; in other words, the bone marrow is responding to a need for RBCs and releasing immature RBCs. Little or no polychromasia detected on a blood film from an anemic animal suggests the anemia is nonregenerative—the bone marrow is not responding appropriately. Although the presence of polychromasia may be suggestive of a bone marrow response to anemia, confirmation cannot be made without a reticulocyte count.

Polychromatophilic RBCs can be identified as *reticulo-*

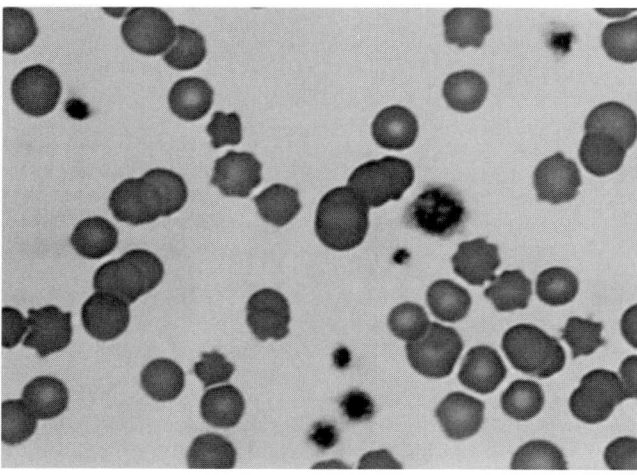

FIGURE 6-5. Feline erythrocytes and platelets. The platelets vary greatly in size.

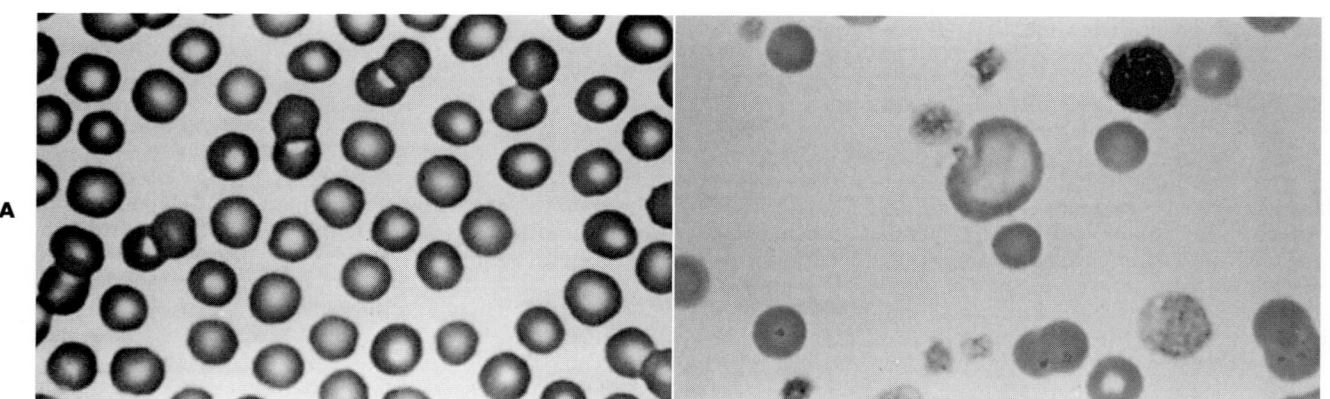

A

B

FIGURE 6-6. **A,** Normal canine red blood cells. Note the distinct central pallor. **B,** Blood from a dog with immune-mediated hemolytic anemia. Note the lack of central pallor in several smaller cells (spherocytes), the large polychromatophilic cell, and a nucleated red blood cell.

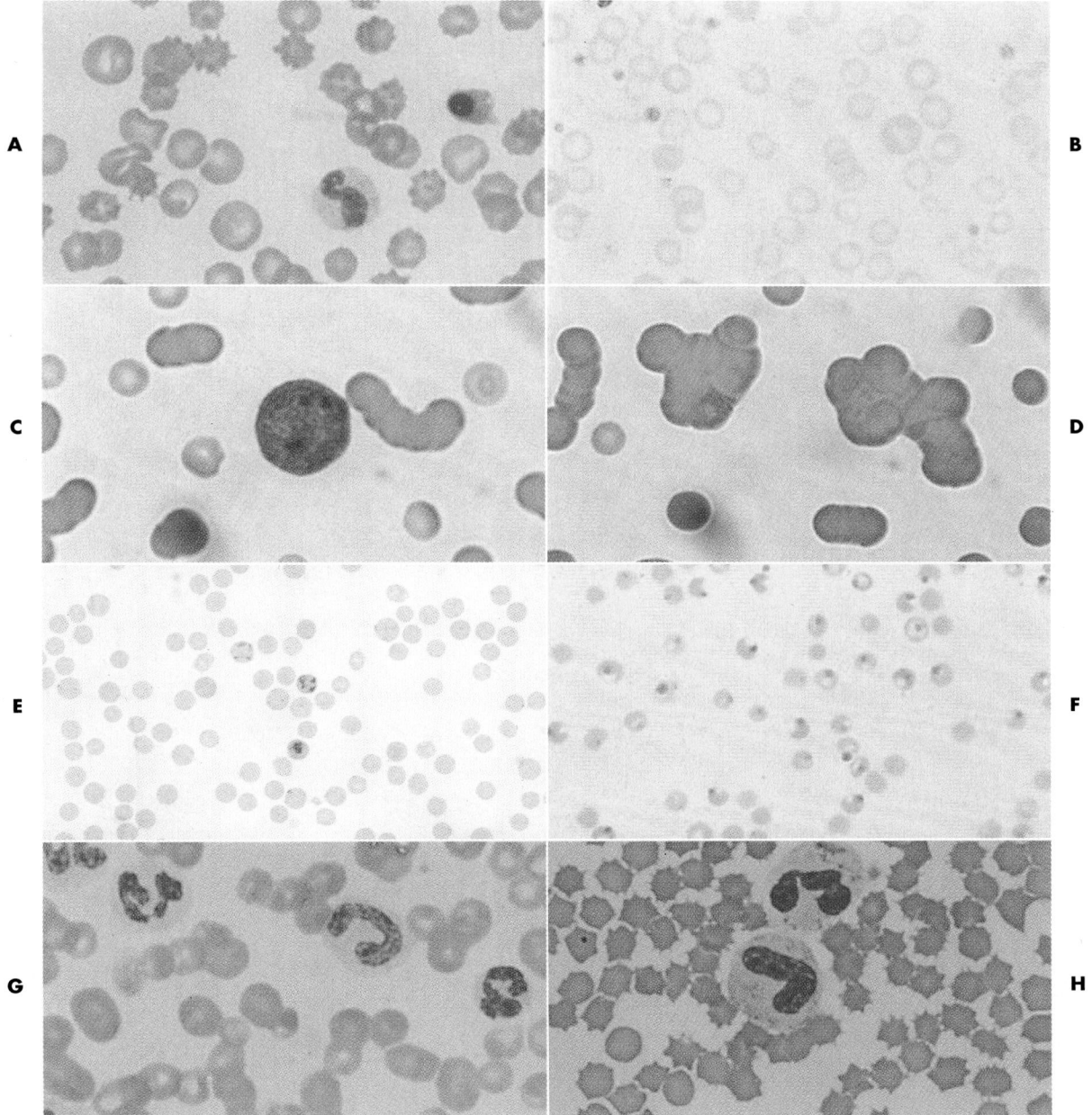

COLOR PLATE I. **A,** Canine blood film displaying several polychromatophilic erythrocytes and one nucleated erythrocyte. A segmented neutrophil is also present. **B,** Canine blood film showing hypochromic erythrocytes with increased central pallor and several distinct platelets. **C,** Feline blood film showing rouleau formation. **D,** Feline blood film showing agglutination. **E,** New methylene blue stain, showing three aggregate reticulocytes. **F,** Feline blood film, new methylene blue stain, showing dark-staining Heinz bodies on the periphery of the erythrocytes. **G,** Canine erythrocytes, segmented neutrophils, and one band neutrophil. **H,** Feline blood film with two toxic neutrophils, one segmented, one band. The toxic changes evident are increased basophilia of the cytoplasm and Döhle bodies.

Continued

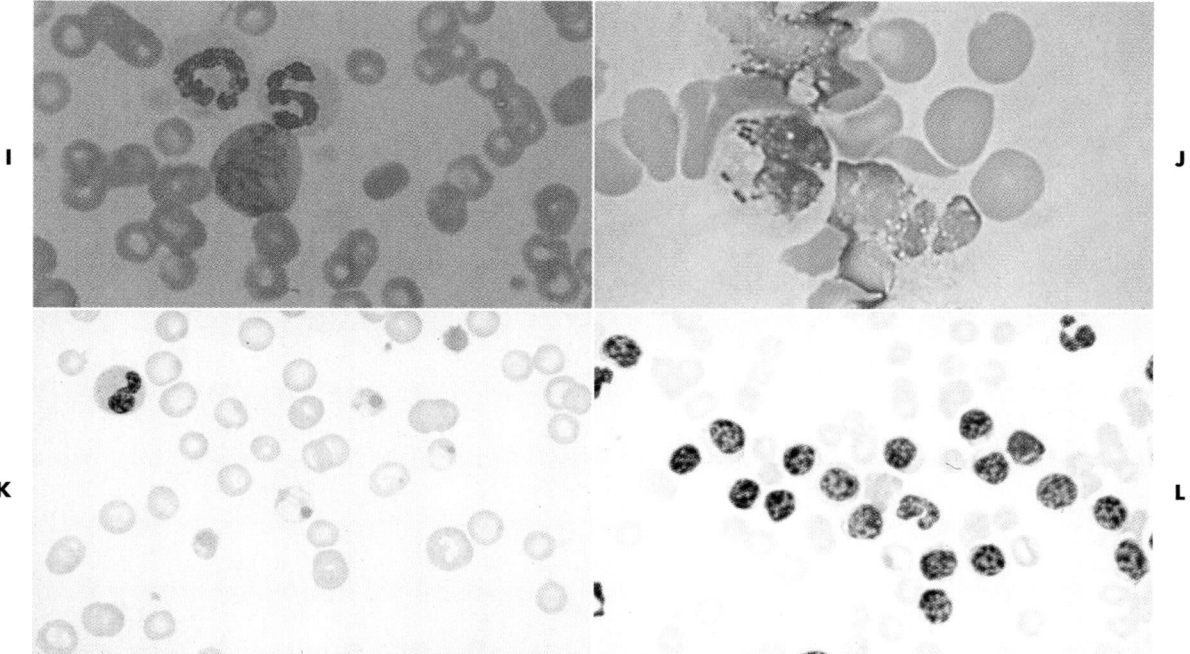

Color Plate I, cont'd. **I,** Canine blood film showing two segmented neutrophils and one monocyte. **J,** Equine abdominal fluid showing a neutrophil with intracellular rod-shaped bacteria. Two smudged cells are also present. **K,** Canine blood film with three distinct viral inclusions in RBCs. **L,** Canine blood smear with small lymphocytes. The excessive number of lymphs is compatible with leukemia.

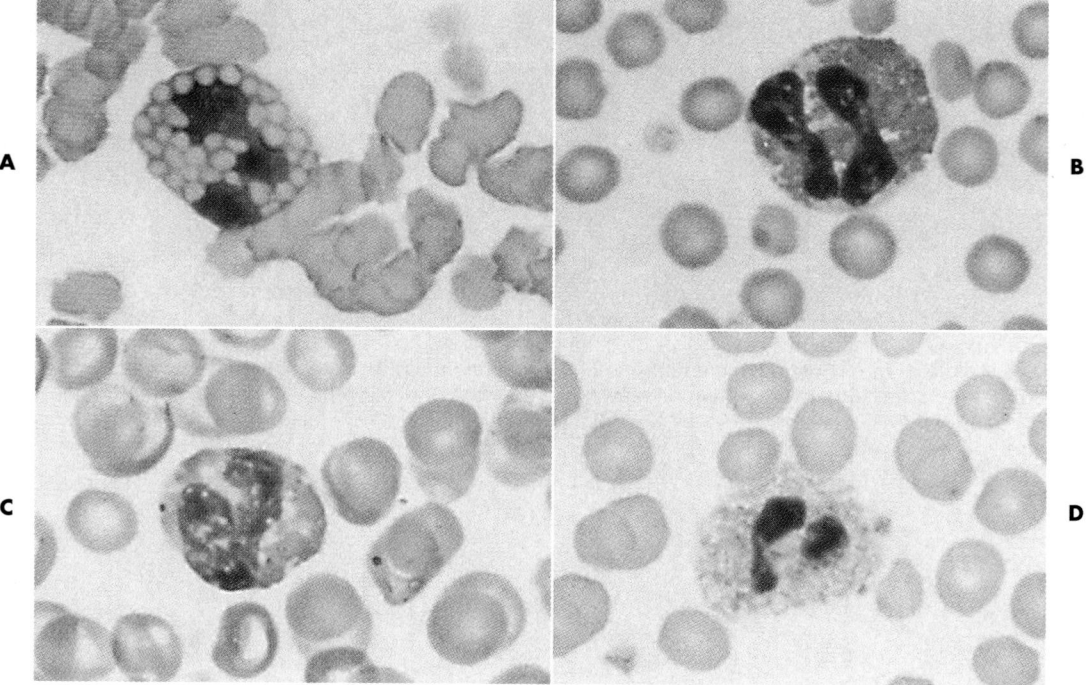

Color Plate II. Species variation in eosinophil granules. **A,** Equine eosinophil. **B,** Bovine eosinophil. **C,** Canine eosinophil. **D,** Feline eosinophil.

cytes (Color Plate I, *E*) when the blood is stained with new methylene blue (NMB). Equal amounts of blood and stain (two to five drops) are mixed in a small tube and left to stand for 5 to 10 minutes. Stain kits (ReticSet, Curtin Matheson Scientific, Houston) are available for reticulocyte counts that do not use liquid stain. Instead, these kits employ stain-coated plastic tubes into which three to five drops of whole blood are placed and then agitated. Whichever method is chosen, a blood film is then made from the mixed sample.

Normal RBCs appear yellowish green with NMB. The reticulocytes will be the same color but will contain deeply basophilic (bluish) dots or strands. Cats have two types of reticulocytes. Only the reticulocytes that have prominent clumps of reticulum (aggregate reticulocytes) are counted. The RBCs with small single dots (punctate reticulocytes) are not included in the count, but their presence should be noted. A reticulocyte count is the number of reticulocytes noted in a count of 1000 RBCs expressed as a percentage (40 reticulocytes of 1000 RBCs = 4% reticulocytes). In dogs and cats, this raw reticulocyte count is then corrected relative to the patient's PCV. This is done by multiplying the raw reticulocyte count by the patient's PCV divided by the normal PCV for that species (45% for dogs and 37% for cats). Increased reticulocytes indicate regenerative anemia. Horses do not release immature RBCs from the bone marrow even when they are severely anemic, so polychromasia and reticulocytosis are not seen in equine peripheral blood.

Hypochromic RBCs have an increased area of central pallor with a narrow, peripheral rim of hemoglobin resulting from an abnormally low amount of hemoglobin within the cell. The most common cause of hypochromasia is iron deficiency. Hypochromasia can be confirmed by a low MCHC provided by automated instruments. True hypochromic RBCs (Color Plate I, *B*) must be differentiated from "punched out" RBCs, which are normochromic but have a more distinct central pallor with a thick dense rim of hemoglobinized cytoplasm. These cells are an artifact of blood film preparation, not a significant pathologic change. Hyperchromasia or increased hemoglobin content in RBCs does not occur.

Rouleaux are groupings of RBCs that resemble stacked coins (Color Plate I, *C*). Marked rouleaux formation is normal in horses and, to a lesser extent, in cats. In dogs, rouleaux formation may occur in inflammatory or neoplastic diseases. It is important to differentiate rouleaux from true *agglutination* (clumping) of RBCs. Agglutinated RBCs tend to appear as clumps rather than as stacked coins (Color Plate I, *D*). Often, agglutination of RBCs can be noted on the side of the blood tube as well as on the blood film. If there is some question in determining whether a blood sample is exhibiting rouleaux or true agglutination, a saline test can be performed. The blood cells are washed by adding one drop of blood to 5 ml of saline and centrifuging for 3 minutes. The supernatant is poured off, the RBCs are resuspended in saline, and a wet mount preparation is made. Rouleaux will disperse, but agglutinated RBCs will remain clumped.

The evaluation of erythrocytes under oil immersion should also include a search for RBC parasites, particularly in cases of anemia. *Haemobartonella felis*, the parasite responsible for feline infectious anemia, appears as small coccoid or rodlike structures on the surface of RBCs. A careful search for *H. felis* organisms should be performed on any anemic cat. These parasites may be very difficult to identify because they can be easily confused with protein and stain precipitates adhered to the cell surface. *Eperythro-*

zoon spp., which are found in cattle, sheep, and swine, may appear similar to *H. felis* or may occur as ring forms on the RBCs. *Anaplasma marginale*, a parasite of bovine RBCs, appears as a small spherical body within the RBC, close to the cell margin. This parasite closely resembles Howell-Jolly bodies but is not as apt to be distributed throughout the cell. Another RBC parasite is *Babesia*, which has various species that can infect any domestic animal. *Babesia* spp. are larger and lighter staining than the previously mentioned parasites, and they tend to occur as piriform structures (often paired) within the RBCs.

Other RBC morphologic abnormalities include *Howell-Jolly bodies, basophilic stippling, Heinz bodies,* and *viral inclusions.* Howell-Jolly bodies are small, often singular, deeply basophilic nuclear remnants that are occasionally seen on normal blood films. Increased numbers of Howell-Jolly bodies can be seen with regenerative anemias. Basophilic stippling is due to staining of small amounts of cytoplasmic ribonucleic acid (RNA) in RBCs. These inclusions are multiple tiny, lightly basophilic dots in the RBC cytoplasm. They can be found in markedly regenerative anemia in dogs and cats but are found more commonly in cattle. Basophilic stippling may also be seen occasionally in lead poisoning. The most consistent finding in lead poisoning is increased numbers of NRBCs with mild to no anemia. Heinz bodies are denatured hemoglobin that has fused to the RBC membrane and appear as refractile projections from the RBC cell membrane (Figure 6-7). These inclusions are most readily seen when the reticulocyte (NMB) stain is applied. They appear as distinct, darkly staining inclusions protruding from the cell surface (Color Plate I, *F*). Distemper virus inclusions may be seen in either RBCs or WBCs. These appear as distinct, spherical eosinophilic inclusions (Color Plate I, *K*).

Leukocyte Evaluation

The WBCs are categorized as granulocytes *(neutrophils, eosinophils, basophils)* and agranulocytes *(lymphocytes, monocytes)*. The granulocytic cells are characterized by *segmented*, or lobed, nuclei and, except for the neutrophil, distinct cytoplasmic granules. The agranulocytes are also referred to as mononuclear cells and do not have segmented nuclei.

NEUTROPHILS. In most species the predominant WBC is the neutrophil (Color Plate I and Figure 6-8). Neutrophils

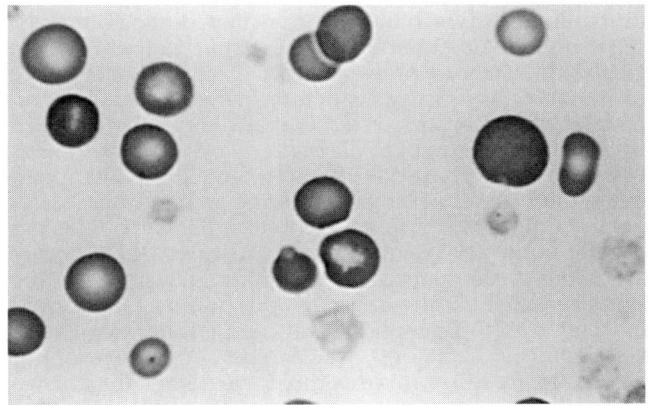

FIGURE 6-7. Feline blood film showing Heinz body formation. Note the small red blood cell with a distinct, pale, rounded projection from its surface (Wright's stain; also see Color Plate I, *F*).

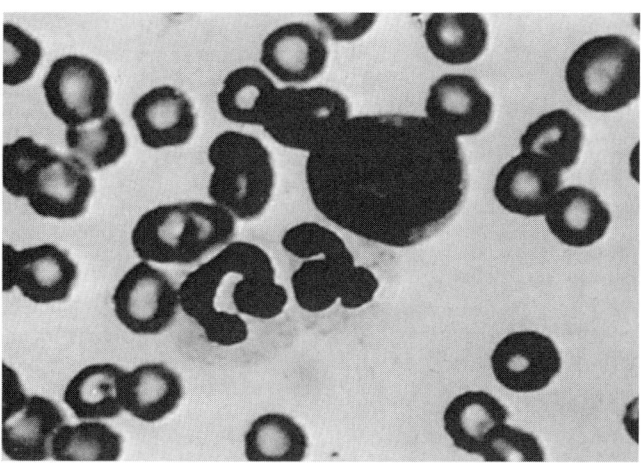

FIGURE 6-8.   Canine blood film. Two segmented neutrophils and a monocyte are present.

have phagocytic and bactericidal capabilities, which means they have an important role in inflammatory conditions. The average time spent by the neutrophil in the blood is only about 10 hours, so it is clear that neutrophil numbers can rise or fall in a matter of hours, depending on the stimuli present. Normal neutrophils have deeply staining, clumped, segmented nuclei (three to five lobes) with relatively clear cytoplasm or, at most, a very faint, almost indiscernible dusting of tiny granules. Equine neutrophils tend to have more distinct nuclear segmentation than canine neutrophils.

Technician Note

Extra care must be taken in differentiating monocytes from toxic band neutrophils, particularly in horses.

An important morphologic change in neutrophils is the appearance of band-shaped nuclei, which indicate the release of immature neutrophils, referred to as *bands*, from the bone marrow. A band nucleus lacks the segmentation seen in the mature segmented nucleus but instead has parallel borders (Color Plate I, *G* and *H*). Even more immature cells, with oval or bean-shaped nuclei, may be seen in cases of extreme tissue demand for neutrophils. Neutrophils, mature or immature, may also show evidence of inflammatory disease as demonstrated by certain cytoplasmic characteristics. *Toxic neutrophils* are characterized by any combination of *Döhle bodies, cytoplasmic vacuolation, basophilia,* and, rarely, cytoplasmic granulation. Cats apparently show toxic neutrophils during many kinds of illnesses (Color Plate I, *H*), but in other species, toxic changes usually imply severe inflammatory disease. Döhle bodies are small, pale bluish-gray irregular inclusions in the cytoplasm that usually indicate mild toxemia. Generalized basophilia of the cytoplasm and cytoplasmic vacuolation are slightly more severe toxic changes. Toxic neutrophils are frequently seen with inflammatory leukograms, characterized by an increased total number of neutrophils *(neutrophilia)* and an increased number of band or other immature neutrophils. In contrast to these cytoplasmic changes, *nuclear hypersegmentation* (nuclei with five or more

lobes) is a normal aging change that implies a nontoxic environment and prolonged circulation of the neutrophil. They are most frequently seen in steroid or stress leukograms, in which neutrophils remain in circulation longer than is normal.

Neutropenia, a decrease in circulating neutrophils, may occur when tissue demand is excessive as a result of severe inflammation exceeding the ability of the bone marrow to supply neutrophils. There may be an increased proportion of immature neutrophils along with the decreased number of neutrophils, which is indicative of the attempt by the bone marrow to meet tissue demands. This can be a very serious, sometimes life-threatening, situation if prolonged because neutrophils are necessary for the body to fight serious inflammation or infection.

EOSINOPHILS.   Eosinophils help to control allergic or anaphylactic hypersensitivity reactions. They are attracted to the sites of these reactions by substances released from sensitized mast cells; therefore eosinophils tend to occur where mast cells congregate. The eosinophil is characterized by a segmented nucleus, colorless to pale blue cytoplasm, and distinct eosinophilic (reddish orange)–staining granules in the cytoplasm.

The morphologic appearance of eosinophil granules varies from species to species, so they can be used to identify the origin of a blood sample. The eosinophils of cats contain numerous tiny rod-shaped granules that may obscure the nucleus. The eosinophil granules of dogs are less numerous and are usually round but may vary considerably in size. Greyhounds often have eosinophils that have degranulated and appear vacuolated. The eosinophil granules of horses are extremely distinctive, being very large and round and a much brighter orange than those of small animals. Bovine eosinophil granules are also bright orange but are much smaller and more numerous than those of the horse and much more uniform in size than those of the dog. Color Plate II illustrates the diversity of eosinophil granules found in various domestic species.

BASOPHILS.   Basophils are relatively rare in blood films but, when present, tend to occur in association with increased eosinophils. Classically, they have dark basophilic (blue) granules, but they also may vary considerably from species to species. Feline basophils tend to have light lavender to almost pink granules rather than the dark purple granules seen in other species. Canine basophils may have few to no granules and must be differentiated from neutrophils on the basis of an elongated nucleus and a more basophilic cytoplasm. Equine and bovine basophils tend to have variable numbers of the more typical dark basophilic granules. Basophils are frequently confused with mast cells because of similar granules, but the basophil nucleus is segmented, and the mast cell nucleus is round or oval.

LYMPHOCYTES.   Lymphocytes are usually small to medium-sized mononuclear cells with a thin rim of light to dark blue cytoplasm and a round, often eccentric, nucleus (Color Plate I, *L*). Their cytoplasm may contain azurophilic (blue) granules. Cattle are notorious for their often large, bizarre-looking lymphocytes. In normal cattle, lymphocytes outnumber neutrophils and may be quite large, with indented (rather than round) nuclei, increased cytoplasm, and perhaps azurophilic cytoplasmic granules. During periods of antigenic stimulation in all species, some of the lymphocytes in the blood film may have extremely basophilic cytoplasm with a pale perinuclear zone (the site of the Golgi apparatus) and possibly azurophilic granules. These cells are referred to as *reactive lymphocytes.*

MONOCYTES. Monocytes (Color Plate I and Figure 6-8) are derived from the bone marrow and circulate in the blood briefly before entering the tissues in which they become *macrophages.* Macrophages phagocytize (ingest) large particles and cellular debris that neutrophils cannot handle. Monocytes have gray-blue, often grainy cytoplasm and a variable-shaped nucleus. The nucleus can be round, oval, ameboid, or lobed. The monocyte is usually larger than the lymphocyte or neutrophil. The most common problem associated with the identification of monocytes is the tendency to confuse monocytes that have a bean-shaped nucleus with a band neutrophil; this is especially a problem when there is toxic change in the neutrophils. The cytoplasm of the monocyte is usually a darker blue than the band neutrophil.

OTHER CELLS. Occasionally, evaluation of the blood film reveals abnormal circulating cell types, such as mast cells, lymphoblasts, myeloblasts, and erythroblasts. The number and type of abnormal cells should be noted because they may indicate leukemia (Color Plate I, *L*) or systemic mastocytosis. Smudge (or basket) cells are degenerated cells appearing as pale eosinophilic nuclear material lacking shape or form (Color Plate I, *J*). These occur when excessive pressure is used in making the film or when old blood is used. A few of these are of little significance, but numerous smudge cells can affect the accuracy of the differential. Blood films with unusual or abnormal cells can be sent to a reference laboratory for evaluation.

ABSOLUTE VERSUS RELATIVE NUMBERS. The numbers obtained when doing the differential are *relative,* or percentages of the whole cell population. These numbers have no diagnostic significance but are used to calculate the absolute numbers of the various WBCs. *Absolute numbers* are the only numbers with diagnostic significance and should always be calculated and reported as such. These are obtained by multiplying the relative percentages by the total WBC count and are expressed as cells per microliter.

Technician Note
Only absolute numbers are significant for interpreting the differential.

Automated Cell Counters

Several instruments available for automated electronic cell counting range in price from $10,000 to $100,000. A basic understanding of the principles of electronic cell counting is useful for the veterinary technician regardless of whether the practice has an in-clinic laboratory. Many practices find it convenient to use human reference or hospital laboratories, but these instruments must be specially calibrated for use with veterinary samples because of the wide variation in blood cell size among the different species. Several instruments have been introduced specifically for veterinary medicine (e.g., Vet ABC-Diff Hematology Analyzer, Heska, Fort Collins, Colo.) that are computer driven with species options and automatically change the instrument settings for multiple species use. The major advantages of electronic cell counters are their speed, accuracy, and reproducibility. In addition to providing RBC and WBC counts, most cell counters will measure hemoglobin and calculate the RBC indices.

The disadvantage of electronic cell counters is their quality control and maintenance requirements. The veterinary technician must be able to recognize when the instruments are not functioning properly and determine the problem. The manufacturer should be willing to train the technician to perform quality control and calibration procedures, keep adequate quality control records, and handle minor adjustments. In addition, the manufacturer should be available for service calls if needed. In some practices, consideration should be given to the purchase of a service contract; this should be discussed before investing in a major instrument.

The operating principle involved in electronic cell counting is based on a type of flow cytometry (the counting of particles as they flow past a detection device). This technology allows the instrument to count blood cells and measure their size. Most instruments use a simple orifice through which an electrical current passes. As particles (e.g., blood cells) move through the orifice, they disrupt the current by increasing the resistance (impedance) proportional to the size of the particle. The instrument is set to detect and count only particles that produce a signal that exceeds a specific resistance or threshold. The threshold settings will determine what particles are counted, based on their size. This principle is important when an instrument is evaluated for use in veterinary medicine. Many instruments developed for human medicine do not accurately count RBCs with a volume of less than 55 femtoliters (fl). The RBCs of the cat, horse, cow, goat, and pig have mean cell volumes below this value.

WBCs from different species also have varying sizes after exposure to RBC lysing solutions. Total WBC counts on some instruments can be falsely decreased in the dog because of their small leukocytes. The reverse is true in the cat. The cat's platelets tend to form large clumps that are counted as leukocytes, thus falsely elevating the WBC count. Close inspection of the blood film will help the technician identify this problem.

Whole blood can be diluted for counting either before introducing the sample into the machine (predilution) or by the instrument as part of the sampling cycle. In the newer instruments, whole blood is aspirated and diluted for the RBC count, and a portion of the sample is lysed to remove the RBCs and allow the WBCs to be counted. The lysed sample is often used for hemoglobin determination.

Quantitative buffy coat (QBC) analysis is another automated cell-counting method that is used in many veterinary practices for measurements of PCV, total WBC count, platelet count, and a limited leukocyte differential. The QBC (IDEXX, Westbrook, Me.) instrumentation consists of large-bore capillary tubes fitted with a free-floating plastic cylinder slightly smaller in diameter than the tube, a centrifuge, and a reading instrument that converts buffy coat band lengths into numeric readings. The tubes are coated with acridine orange, a dye that allows the differentiation of the granulocytes, mononuclear cells (monocytes, lymphocytes), and platelets. Figure 6-9 illustrates the expansion of the buffy coat by the plastic float and where the specific cell layers are found. The QBC instrument is relatively inexpensive compared with the impedance cell counters. It is important to remember, however, that the limited differential obtained should not replace the blood

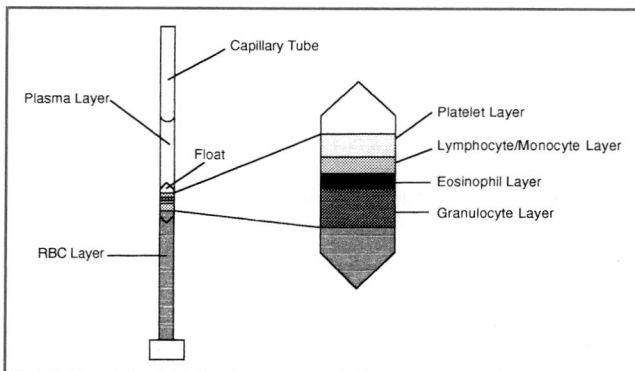

FIGURE 6-9. Illustration of the QBC buffy coat layers that occur through centrifugation. *RBC,* Red blood cell.

film examination; nor should the reticulocyte count be taken at face value.

Technician Note

The differential provided by the QBC instrument is not an adequate substitute for microscopic evaluation of the blood film.

Blood cell morphology is important in evaluating the numbers obtained in the blood cell counts. The QBC instrument cannot tell the technician whether band neutrophils, toxic neutrophils, polychromatophilic RBCs, RBC parasites, or NRBCs are present.

Plasma Protein Determination

Determination of the plasma protein concentration is another standard component of the routine CBC. After noting plasma color and turbidity, break the capillary tube used for measuring the PCV at a point slightly above the *buffy coat* (cream-colored layer of WBCs and platelets just above the RBCs) and allow the plasma to run through the unbroken end onto the prism of a refractometer by capillary action. Lifting the cover and tapping the hematocrit tube on the prism may scratch the surface of the prism. Plasma protein values obtained with a refractometer are accurate as long as the plasma is clear. If the plasma is lipemic, hemolyzed, or otherwise cloudy, the refractive index will be increased and provide an erroneously high protein measurement. Often, the lipemic samples have a very indistinct or unfocused line on the refractometer scale. In contrast to the dilution effect of a small blood sample in a large tube, excess anticoagulant will artifactually increase the plasma protein value obtained.

Determination of plasma *fibrinogen* levels may be useful in the detection of inflammatory processes, particularly in cattle and horses. Two capillary tubes of blood are centrifuged; one is used for the PCV and plasma protein determination, as described. The second tube is placed in a 56° C to 58° C water bath for 3 minutes to cause the precipitation of fibrinogen. The tube is then recentrifuged so the fibrinogen settles just above the buffy coat. The tube is broken above the fibrinogen, and the remaining plasma is placed on the refractometer for protein determination. The difference between protein concentration of the first tube and

protein concentration of the second tube is the fibrinogen concentration.

Fibrinogen is usually expressed in milligrams per deciliter; therefore, if the first tube had a protein concentration of 7.3 g/dl and the second tube has a protein concentration of 6.9 g/dl, the plasma fibrinogen concentration is 0.4 g/dl, or 400 mg/dl. Plasma from cattle with markedly increased fibrinogen may completely coagulate during incubation; when the specimen is respun, the fibrinogen does not settle out, and a fibrinogen value cannot be determined.

Coagulation Testing

Patients will occasionally present with abnormal bleeding tendencies. *Hemostasis,* the maintenance of proper blood flow, depends on vascular integrity, platelet number and function, and several coagulation factors. The coagulation factors are a group of chemicals, enzymes, and cofactors that interact to stabilize a platelet plug and stem the flow of blood. Evaluation of these factors, along with a platelet count, is part of a coagulation profile.

Most of these tests require special instrumentation and are submitted to a reference laboratory; however, sample collection and submission are critical for obtaining valid results. The venipuncture must be accurate to avoid tissue injury, which will invalidate the coagulation assays. In addition to the EDTA tube for the platelet count, blood must be collected in tubes with citrate anticoagulant (turquoise top) for factor assays. Only plastic or siliconized glass should be used in handling these samples because contact with regular glass will invalidate the results. The samples should be centrifuged and the plasma tested immediately or frozen. It is recommended that the reference laboratory always be contacted for additional directions before drawing and submitting samples for coagulation testing.

URINALYSIS

Urinalysis is one clinical laboratory procedure that should be performed as a part of any minimum data base in all veterinary practices but is frequently skipped for a variety of reasons. It is an important diagnostic test that should be done on fresh urine when possible. The techniques involved are simple and require no special instrumentation. Urine samples should be collected into clean glass or plastic containers. In general, no preservatives are necessary. The best time to collect urine for urinalysis is usually in the morning when the animal awakens. Urine that accumulates during the relative inactivity of the night is less likely to be influenced by feeding or exercise. It is generally concentrated, and therefore abnormal constituents, if present, are more easily detected.

Equipment

The equipment necessary for performing the urinalysis is minimal. A supply of clean glass or plastic collection containers, a centrifuge and conical centrifuge tubes, chemical reagent strips, clean glass slides and coverslips, a refractometer, plastic pipettes, and a microscope are all that are required.

Urine Collection

Urine may be collected by several methods. The simplest (if the animal will cooperate) is to catch a free-flow nonsterile sample as the animal voids. If this method is used, the initial stream of urine should not be caught because the first portion may contain cells and debris from the urethra and lower genital tract, resulting in contamination of the sample that may interfere with interpretation. It is better to collect a midstream sample, avoiding the very beginning or the very end of a voided urine sample.

A second method that may be used to collect urine is *cystocentesis*. This procedure involves placing a needle (with a syringe attached) through the ventral abdominal wall into the lumen of the bladder and aspirating urine. Aseptic technique must be used. By performing cystocentesis, secretions and debris of the lower urogenital tract are avoided, and interpretation of urinalysis findings is simplified. Iatrogenic hemorrhage can occur during cystocentesis; therefore it is not unusual to have a widely varying number of RBCs in the sediment of samples obtained by this method.

Another method for collecting urine is by catheterization of the bladder. This procedure must be done as aseptically as possible to prevent introduction of bacteria into the urinary tract. Extreme care should be taken to avoid traumatizing the lining of the urethra with the catheter, or the sample may contain increased numbers of erythrocytes and epithelial cells. Additional information on cystocentesis and catheterization is found in Chapter 3.

Regardless of how the urine sample is collected, it should be analyzed as soon as possible. Many changes begin to occur immediately. Bacteria present in the urine will multiply, cells may degenerate, casts may dissolve (especially if the urine is alkaline), and bacteria that produce urease will convert urea to ammonia, causing the pH to increase. If there is to be any delay in performing the urinalysis, the sample should be refrigerated to slow these processes. However, refrigeration may cause a change in urine specific gravity and interfere with some of the chemistry reactions on the chemistry reagent strip. Before a urinalysis is performed on refrigerated urine, the specimen should be allowed to come to room temperature.

Evaluation of Physical Properties

As with all laboratory procedures, it is wise to follow the same routine protocol with every urine sample analyzed. The physical properties evaluated in most routine urinalyses include color, appearance or turbidity, and specific gravity. After making sure the sample is mixed well, the color (e.g., yellow, gold, red) and appearance (e.g., clear, hazy, flocculent) should be recorded.

Color

Normal urine is yellow to amber, depending on its concentration and constituents. Bright red urine indicates *hematuria* (RBCs in the urine) or *hemoglobinuria* (hemoglobin in the urine). Reddish brown urine usually suggests hemoglobinuria or *myoglobinuria* (myoglobin in the urine); note that these two pigments cannot be distinguished from one another solely on the basis of color. High concentrations of bilirubin or urobilin cause yellowish brown urine that, when shaken, may produce yellowish foam. Whenever an unusual discoloration of the urine occurs, the history of any drug therapy should be evaluated because there are many drugs that can produce abnormally colored urine. It is important to remember urine that is markedly discolored may make it difficult or impossible to interpret color changes when evaluating chemical reagent strips.

Turbidity

Fresh urine is normally transparent, but as it cools, some salts may precipitate, causing the urine to become cloudy. Except for equine urine, fresh urine that is cloudy is often pathologic, and it must be examined microscopically to identify the cause: pus, blood, mucus, bacteria, casts, or

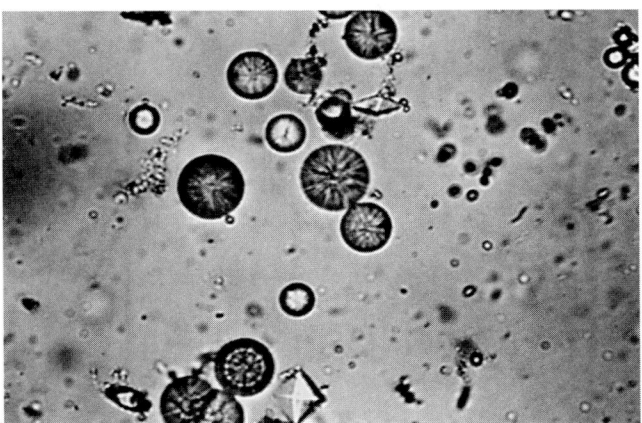

FIGURE 6-10. Photomicrograph of equine urine sediment showing the round calcium carbonate crystals with distinct radiating striations.

crystals. Fresh equine urine is normally cloudy because it contains mucus and calcium carbonate crystals (Figure 6-10). Even clear urine should be examined microscopically because some abnormal constituents may be present in small amounts that may not cause urine to be visually cloudy.

Specific Gravity

Specific gravity (SG) determination is one of the most important parts of a urinalysis. It may be determined before or after centrifugation because the material that settles during centrifugation has little to no effect on SG. The SG value depends on the number and size of particles in solution and is an indicator of the ability of the kidney to concentrate urine. The SG is most accurately determined with a refractometer, which is used for determining plasma protein, and requires only one drop of urine. If the urine sample is turbid, the SG may be determined from the supernatant after centrifugation. Reagent strips for SG are inaccurate.

The normal range for SG is extremely wide: 1.001 to 1.060 in dogs and 1.001 to 1.080 in cats. The major determinant of urine SG is salt concentration because of the large number of particles involved. Protein, in contrast, has little influence on SG, because although the particles are large, they are few in number. Glucose, likewise, has relatively little effect on SG. Both of these components, however, when found in large amounts in the urine, will increase the SG by about 0.001 to 0.002. SG provides a very good indication of how well the kidneys are able to function in maintaining the body's water and osmotic balance. In addition, SG is important in interpreting other tests. Because of the usual inverse relationship between SG and volume, a 2^+ protein in dilute urine (SG <1.012) suggests a greater loss of protein than a 2^+ protein in concentrated urine (SG >1.030).

Isosthenuria is the continued excretion of urine at the SG of glomerular filtrate (1.008 to 1.012). Isosthenuria indicates that the tubules have not attempted to concentrate urine. A single, routine urine sample with an isosthenuric SG is not necessarily abnormal because this is within the normal range and could be a chance occurrence. However, if an animal is dehydrated, azotemic, or uremic, the renal tubules are under pressure to concentrate urine, and under those circumstances, an SG lower than 1.035 in cats, 1.030

in dogs, and 1.025 in large animals indicates that the kidneys are not functioning appropriately.

Chemical Evaluation

Reagent strip chemistries should be performed on unspun urine, unless the urine is very turbid (cloudy). If it is turbid, the chemistry tests may be done after the sample has been centrifuged. Protein, glucose, ketones, blood, and bilirubin in the urine are routinely determined as well as urinary pH. The strips contain pads that are impregnated with reagents and result in a color change when the appropriate urine constituents are present. Although simple to use, proper technique and accurate timing for reading the results are critical. The strips must be properly stored, the urine must be at room temperature and well mixed, and excess urine must be shaken from the strips to obtain valid results. Significantly discolored urine may interfere with the ability to discern colors and color changes on the reagent pads.

Some commercially available strips contain reagent pads for other components, such as leukocytes. These are being evaluated for reliability but are not yet accepted as accurate.

Technician Note

Refrigerated urine samples must be brought to room temperature before chemical analysis is performed.

pH

Urine pH is detected by reagent strips with chemical indicators. The symbol *pH* is used to express the hydrogen ion concentration (acidity) of a fluid. pH 7 is the neutral point. Readings above 7 are said to be alkalotic, and those below 7 are acidotic. In general, dogs and cats tend to have more acidic urine than do cattle and horses. It is imperative that a fresh sample be used because as urine stands it loses carbon dioxide and bacteria that are present may produce ammonia, both of which result in increased alkalinity (raising the pH). The body's acid-base status may affect urine pH, but it is a mistake to use urine pH to evaluate the systemic acid-base balance. Too many other factors influence urine pH; in fact, urine pH may be completely contrary to the body's pH. For example, some cows with metabolic alkalosis have a paradoxical aciduria because the kidney attempts to maintain electrolyte balance at the expense of acid-base balance.

Protein

Most commercial urine reagent strips include a test for *protein*. It is often stated that normal urine contains no protein, but almost all urine contains a small amount of protein, which is due to normal leakage and secretion from the urinary tract lining. However, this normal amount of protein is not detected by routine methods. The strips rely on color changes in tetrabromophenolphthalein blue to detect protein levels that are above a very small amount (>10 mg/dl) present in normal urine. The test reaction is usually graded *trace* or 1+ through 4+, which supposedly corresponds to various protein concentrations. As mentioned, a positive protein reaction in dilute urine implies a greater protein loss than the same level of reaction in a concentrated sample. As with most reagent strip chemistry tests, results are at best only semiquantitative and are subject to several types of error. False-positive values may occur when urine is very alkaline. Second, the strips are more sensitive to albumin than to globulins and therefore can give false-negative readings when proteinuria is caused by globulins. Because the change in color of the reagent strip pad is subjective, different technicians may make different readings on the same urine sample.

Protein loss into urine can be a significant drain on the body's protein stores. One can make a subjective evaluation of the amount being lost by comparing the results with the SG, as previously mentioned; however, a more exact method is to collect all urine produced in a 24-hour period and calculate its total protein content. The collection of 24 hours of urine output generally requires a metabolism cage and is not very practical. The ratio of urine protein to urine creatinine (P/C ratio) in any single sample is a good index of protein loss in the urine. A urine P/C ratio of less than 1.0 is considered normal; more than 2.0 indicates abnormal urinary protein loss; and from 1.0 to 2.0 is suspicious. A urine sample with sediment that indicates inflammation (presence of WBCs) is not suitable for urine P/C ratio. The inflammation must first be successfully treated. If the patient still has proteinuria once all evidence of inflammation is gone, a urine P/C ratio can be requested. Urine P/C ratios are usually done at a reference laboratory because they require a sensitive protein determination.

In interpreting the cause for a positive urine protein test, one must also consider the results of the test for blood and the microscopic examination of sediment. These results may aid in identifying the source of urinary protein. Proteinuria without a positive blood reaction or significant cells indicates glomerular disease, in which defective glomeruli allow passage of albumin into the urine, often resulting in protein readings of 3+ or 4+. There are a few extrarenal factors that may temporarily alter glomerular permeability to protein and result in proteinuria; they include fever, severe exercise, shock, cardiac or central nervous system disease, and the postcolostral period in neonates.

When excessive hemorrhage into the urinary tract occurs, the test for urine protein will be positive and erythrocytes will be seen in the sediment. Possible causes for urinary tract hemorrhage include trauma, neoplasia, and inflammation. Hemoglobin or myoglobin in the urine will cause a positive protein test as well as a positive blood test. In either of these cases, intact RBCs are not a significant part of the sediment.

When proteinuria occurs in conjunction with increased leukocytes in the urine sediment, inflammation of the urinary tract should be suspected. Inflammation rarely causes a urine protein test of more than 2+, unless hemorrhage is associated with the inflammatory process. In some urinary tract infections, bacteria may be seen in the sediment. Determination of the location of the inflammation may depend on the method of collection. With testing of voided samples, the inflammation may be anywhere in the genitourinary tract, whereas if test samples were collected by cystocentesis the inflammation may be localized to the bladder or kidney.

Glucose

In addition to urine protein, a common reagent strip test for urine is the test for glucose. The reagent strips usually use glucose oxidase to detect glucose and for this reason are quite specific for glucose. However, as with all reagent strip tests, they are not quantitative. Tablets that detect glucose are available that are somewhat more quantitative but not specific. The tablets use a copper reduction method that detects many sugars and reducing agents other than glucose.

Normally, urine contains no detectable glucose. Glucose

is filtered by the glomerulus, but the body preserves this energy source by reabsorbing it in the proximal renal tubules. This resorption ability is exceeded once the blood glucose level rises above 180 mg/dl in most species or above 100 mg/dl in the cow. This is the "renal threshold" for glucose, above which it will "spill" into the urine. The primary cause for *glucosuria* therefore is *hyperglycemia.* To confirm this, the blood glucose level should be determined at the same time as the urine glucose. Diabetes mellitus is a common cause of hyperglycemia and glucosuria.

Ketones

A test for urine ketones is included on many reagent strips; tablets are also available. Both use a nitroprusside method that detects acetone and acetoacetic acid but not beta-hydroxybutyric acid, so false-negative results are possible. Ketones will appear in the urine before they build up to a detectable level in the bloodstream, so *ketonuria* may occur before a detectable *ketonemia* occurs. Ketonuria indicates excessive fat metabolism, a deficiency in carbohydrate metabolism, or both but is most commonly seen in conjunction with glucosuria as a complication of diabetes mellitus.

Bilirubin

There are reagent strips and tablets for detecting *bilirubinuria,* both of which use a similar reaction (diazotization), but the tablets are less subject to interference by urine color. The tablets are also highly sensitive, so a 1$^+$ reading, especially in concentrated urine, may not be significant. Both strips and tablets detect conjugated bilirubin and not unconjugated bilirubin. Bilirubin in urine can also be crudely detected by the *foam test.* If a yellowish foam appears when the urine sample is shaken, bilirubin is likely present. Bilirubin may be oxidized on exposure to light, so if there is much delay between obtaining the urine sample and performing the urinalysis, the sample should be protected from light to avoid false-negative results. Many normal dogs, and sometimes cattle, will exhibit bilirubinuria because the kidneys, as well as the liver, have an enzyme that can conjugate bilirubin. This, however, is lacking in cats, and any bilirubinuria is a significant abnormality in cats.

Blood

The designation "blood" is somewhat misleading because this test actually detects intact RBCs, hemoglobin, and myoglobin. Both reagent strips and tablets make use of the peroxidase property of free hemoglobin or myoglobin, which oxidizes orthotoluidine to a blue-colored derivative. If the urine is red and cloudy and erythrocytes are present in the sediment, *hematuria* is the reason for the positive blood reaction.

Hemoglobinuria (hemoglobin pigment in the urine) results in red to brown urine with a positive urine blood reaction and no erythrocytes in the sediment. A positive urine protein test may also be apparent. In contrast to hematuria, hemoglobinuria will be accompanied by *hemoglobinemia,* imparting a pink to reddish discoloration to the serum or plasma.

Myoglobinuria (myoglobin pigment in the urine) will similarly result in red to brown urine with no erythrocytes in the sediment, a positive urine blood reaction, and a positive urine protein test. However, during myoglobinuria, the blood serum or plasma generally remains clear. Myoglobin, which is derived from muscles, is a smaller molecule than hemoglobin and does not bind to serum proteins; thus it is rapidly excreted into the urine before reaching levels sufficiently high to produce discoloration of the serum. Animals with myoglobinuria generally do not show evidence of anemia but have some type of muscle disease, such as exertional myopathy in horses ("tying up" syndrome), trauma, electrical shock, or pressure necrosis from prolonged recumbency. If it is not apparent by clinical signs, hemoglobinuria and myoglobinuria may be differentiated by electrophoresis or a more cumbersome ammonium sulfate precipitation test.

Microscopic Examination

The sediment should be prepared for microscopic examination. Urine sediment examination may reveal extremely useful diagnostic information and be crucial for correct interpretation of the chemical analyses. A few cells and a few casts may be found in normal urine, but increased numbers of various elements indicate certain diseases. A reference is provided for help with sediment evaluation.

Sample Preparation

Pour a standard volume (10 ml is recommended) of urine into a conical-tip centrifuge tube. If the sample available is less than 10 ml, use all that is left after the reagent strip chemistries and SG determinations have been completed. Centrifuge the urine at a slow speed (1500 rpm) for 5 minutes. Higher speeds for centrifugation may disrupt the cells and casts that are present. Decant the supernatant, leaving the sediment in the bottom. Gently tap the tube to resuspend the sediment in the small amount of urine remaining on the sides and in the bottom of the tube. With a small pipette, transfer a drop of suspended sediment to a glass slide and place a coverslip on it. There are commercial stains (SediStain, Clay Adams, Parsippany, N.J.) available for evaluating urine sediments, but with practice and experience they are not necessary.

A phase-contrast microscope is ideal for examining unstained urine sediment. A more practical and highly satisfactory alternative is to lower the condenser of the light microscope and reduce the intensity of the light (as for the manual mammalian WBC count). The slide should first be examined at 10× magnification to obtain an overall impression of how much and what type of sediment is present. The 40× or 45× power (high dry) is then used to make the final identification and count of various components. At least 10 microscopic fields must be evaluated, and the average numbers of various cells and casts per high-power field are reported. The presence and relative amounts of other components are also noted.

Epithelial Cells

Three types of epithelial cells can be found in urine sediment: squamous, transitional, and renal tubular. *Squamous epithelial cells* are very large, with angular borders and small nuclei. They originate from the lining of the distal urethra and vagina or prepuce and are not generally indicative of disease. *Transitional epithelial cells* are medium-sized and oval, spindled, or caudate cells found lining the proximal urethra, bladder, ureters, and renal pelvis. They may occur in groups, especially if the urine was obtained by catheterization. Occasionally, if they are very large and variable, very basophilic, or in large clusters, they should be further evaluated for possible neoplasia. Renal tubular epithelial cells are small, round cells and may indicate tubular degeneration.

Blood Cells

Erythrocytes in unstained sediment appear colorless or yellowish and are round and slightly refractile, with no internal structure. They may be confused with fat droplets, but erythrocytes are fairly uniform in size and do not float in and out of planes of focus as do fat droplets. If there is doubt, a drop of diluted acetic acid will lyse erythrocytes, helping to differentiate them from fat droplets. In concentrated urine, erythrocytes may lose fluid and become *crenated* (shrunken and spiked). In dilute urine, they may imbibe water and swell or even lyse, becoming *ghost cells*. *Leukocytes* in urine sediment are round and granular and larger than erythrocytes but smaller than epithelial cells. The presence of more than five to eight WBCs per high-power field indicates inflammation of the urinary or urogenital tract depending on the method of collection. When this occurs, a careful check for bacteria should be made.

Casts

Casts are another prominent feature of urine sediment. They are elongated structures composed of protein from plasma and mucoprotein from the renal tubules. In general, they form in the distal tubules, in which the urine is more concentrated and acidic. Any structures that happen to be in the tubules at the time the casts form (erythrocytes, leukocytes, or epithelial cells) become embedded in the casts. The presence of increased numbers of casts helps to localize the renal disease to the tubules, but the numbers do not necessarily correlate with the severity of disease. For instance, severe chronic nephritis may be accompanied by just a few casts.

There are five main types of casts, as follows:

1. *Hyaline casts* are colorless, homogeneous, and semi-transparent. They may be difficult to see unless the light is reduced. They indicate mild glomerular leakage.
2. *Cellular casts* contain recognizable cells embedded in the protein matrix. They may be epithelial cell casts that contain sloughed tubular epithelial cells, erythrocyte casts that indicate renal hemorrhage, or leukocyte casts that indicate renal inflammation or pyelonephritis.
3. *Granular casts* are derived from degenerating cells or cellular casts. They are characterized by a nonspecific granular matrix and are designated either coarsely or finely granular, depending on the degree of degeneration. They probably are the most common type of cast found in animals.

4. *Waxy casts* are wide and homogeneous, usually with distinct blunt or squared ends. They indicate a more chronic tubular lesion.
5. *Fatty casts* contain fat globules from degenerating tubular epithelial cells and are most common in cats because of the high lipid content of feline tubular epithelium.

Crystals

Crystals are another major component of urine sediment. Their precipitation and presence depend on urine pH and the solubility and concentration of the substance forming them. Urine crystals that accompany pathologic conditions include *ammonium biurate, monohydrate calcium oxalate, bilirubin, triple phosphate* (struvite, ammonium, magnesium phosphate), and *cystine* crystals. Dihydrate calcium oxalate crystals can be found in normal urine but appear distinctly different from the monohydrate calcium oxalate crystals found with ethylene glycol (antifreeze) toxicity. Figure 6-11 illustrates these two types of calcium oxalate crystals. Bilirubin crystals generally occur in conjunction with bilirubinuria with little to no additional significance. Triple phosphate crystals are often found in alkaline urine when urease-producing bacteria, associated with lower urinary tract disease, are present. Ammonium biurate crystals are dark with very distinct, multiple, irregular protrusions and are often associated with portal caval shunts, a specific liver disorder. Cystine crystals, although sometimes seen in healthy dogs, are also found in a congenital defect of cystine metabolism that leads to cystinuria in dogs. Drugs, such as sulfonamides, may precipitate in the urine of animals, resulting in the formation of crystals.

Microorganisms

Bacteria in unstained urine sediment may be difficult to detect. Rods may appear singly or in chains, but cocci may be lost in brownian movement. For this reason, whenever bacteria are suspected, the sediment should be stained to examine it more thoroughly. Usually, the regular examination of the unstained sediment is completed and recorded first, and then the coverslip is removed and the underlying sediment on the slide is allowed to dry. Once dry, the slide can be stained with Gram's stain or one of the modified Wright's stains, and any bacteria present can be identified. On Gram's stain, the gram-negative, rod-shaped bacteria may be difficult to see among all the pink-staining cellular

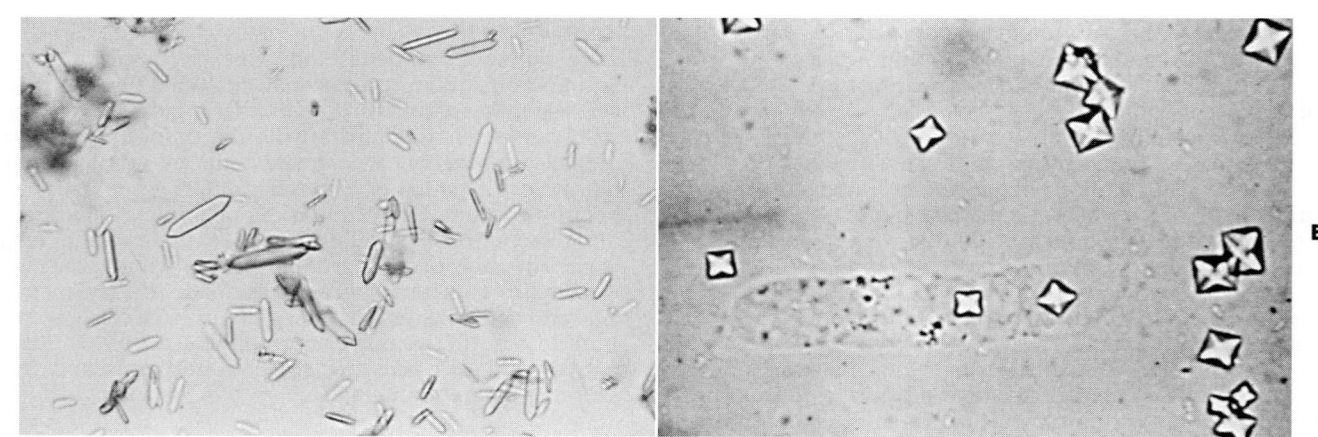

FIGURE 6-11. Photomicrograph of canine urine sediment showing the two forms of calcium oxalate crystals. **A,** Monohydrate form. **B,** Dihydrate form.

debris. With Wright's stain, all bacteria stain dark purple and are relatively easy to find.

Bacteria in a voided sample often are not significant because they may be normal flora from the distal urogenital tract, especially from the prepuce or vagina. Bacteria are significant if they occur in catheterized or cystocentesis samples. Their presence should be correlated with leukocytes in urine because bacteria with no leukocyte response should raise suspicion of contamination of the sample. If bacteria are present in a urine sample, they can multiply as time passes, so this should be taken into consideration when the sample is being analyzed. Rarely, *fungal* organisms are found in urine sediment. The majority of these are insignificant contaminants, although some, such as *Blastomyces*, may be significant.

Miscellaneous Findings

Usually insignificant components of urine sediment include mucus, fat, sperm, and parasites. Mucus appears as narrow, twisted, ribbonlike strands. It is normal in equine urine and can be seen in other species as well because of genital secretions or irritation of the urethra. Fat, as previously noted, takes the form of refractile, variably sized spheres in many planes of focus. Fat is rarely significant. Sperm are commonly seen in male canine urine. Parasites that can occur in urine include the ova of *Stephanurus dentatus*, *Dioctophyma renale*, and *Capillaria plica* and microfilaria of *Dirofilaria immitis*.

CLINICAL CHEMISTRY

Several small relatively inexpensive clinical chemistry instruments have been developed. As with all equipment, veterinary practices must have a demand for them and must be able to justify their expense. Two general types of chemistry analyzers are commonly used: liquid reagent chemistry and dry chemistry. Instruments that use liquid reagents require more technical expertise and time in preparing reagents and monitoring their performance. The dry chemistry instruments are simpler to use and provide consistent performance. The principles of operation differ significantly between the two types of instruments, as does the extent to which specimen quality affects the measurement.

Equipment

Regardless of the decision whether to maintain and operate an in-house chemistry analyzer, veterinary practices will need a sample collection system consisting of either syringes and needles or Vacutainers, plus clean plastic or glass tubes to store or transport samples. A centrifuge and pipettes will be necessary to separate the serum or plasma from the cells.

Clinical Chemistry Instrumentation

The liquid reagent-based instruments use the principle of photometry (the measurement of light transmittance by a solution). Beer's law states that the concentration of a substance in a liquid is indirectly proportional to the amount of light that passes through the liquid. Most instruments have a spectrophotometer to measure the amount of light transmitted. A spectrophotometer consists of a light source directed through a specific path and a photosensitive detector that converts light into electrical energy. Each substance will transmit light at a specific wavelength. To increase the specificity of the measurement, filters are placed between the light source and the sample to allow only a specific wavelength to pass through the

sample. The magnitude of the electrical current produced by the detector corresponds to the concentration of the substance being measured. Solutions that contain a known concentration of specific substances are called *standards* and are used to calibrate the instrument. Each instrument has specific procedures for *calibration*, which should be carefully followed to ensure optimal performance.

The instruments that use dry reagents are becoming more popular for in-clinic use. The major advantage of these instruments is the elimination of liquid reagents, which must be reconstituted or diluted before use. Dry chemistry instruments use reagent slides or cartridges. A specific amount of the patient's sample is added as directed, and the intensity of the color that develops is measured by the principle of reflectance. Light is transmitted to the analyte slide, and the reflected light is conducted to a photodetector. The density of the color formed by the chemical reaction is determined and is proportional to the concentration of the substance being measured. Because this methodology does not depend on reading light transmitted through a liquid as with the spectrophotometer-based instruments, there is less interference from lipemia or hemolysis.

Several dry chemistry instruments are available (e.g., Heska I-STAT, Abaxis VetScan, IDEXX VetTest) that are designed specifically for use with veterinary samples. Examples of chemistry tests available with the Vet Test (Figure 6-12) are listed in Box 6-1. Available tests may vary from analyzer to analyzer, and new tests are often added. The primary advantage of using an instrument intended for veterinary testing is the availability of predetermined reference ranges, which can be used until the laboratory can establish its own values. In most cases with these instruments, little variation occurs from instrument to instrument or operator to operator. Veterinary samples can vary significantly from human samples in the concentration of particular substances. If using an analyzer not specifically for veterinary samples, the limits of the chemistry test (range of values that have a linear relationship within the methodology used) must be adhered to.

Quality Control Programs

It is imperative that any veterinary practice that decides to establish an in-house laboratory make a commitment to quality control. Laboratory instruments will provide valid accurate results only if the samples are handled correctly, a well-maintained instrument is used, and the tests are performed correctly. The importance of routine maintenance and calibration procedures for all instruments cannot be overemphasized. However, even the most sophisticated, accurate, and well-maintained instrument cannot overcome errors in technique or poor sample quality. The technician should be familiar with the principle and limitations of all assays performed in the laboratory. Some of the more common causes for inaccurate results because of technical errors or sample quality are listed in Box 6-2. A quality control program consists of monitoring results of known *control samples* for identification of irregularities in reported values and following generally accepted laboratory procedures. Several textbooks on clinical chemistry and laboratory medicine (see Recommended Reading) provide excellent in-depth reviews of quality assurance programs. The following discussion deals primarily with the basics in monitoring an instrument to ensure the accuracy of reported data.

The three levels of quality control are preanalytic procedures, analytic procedures, and analytic quality monitoring procedures. The *preanalytic procedures* deal with how the

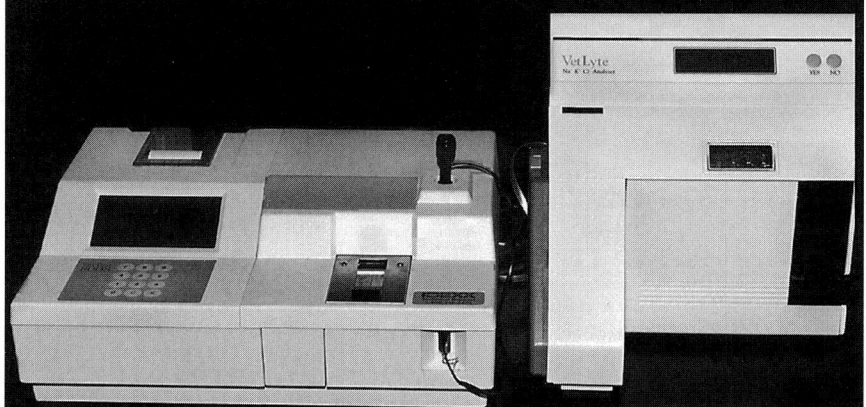

FIGURE 6-12. Vet Test 8008 dry chemistry and Vet Lyte electrolyte analyzer (IDEXX Corp., Westbrook, Me.).

Box 6-1   CHEMISTRY TESTS AVAILABLE ON THE VET TEST 8008
Urea nitrogen
Albumin
Alanine aminotransferase (ALT)
Serum alkaline phosphatase (SAP)
Triglycerides
Calcium
Gamma-glutamyltransferase (GGT)
Amylase
Ammonia
Lactate dehydrogenase (LDH)
Total bilirubin
Uric acid
Creatinine
Total protein
Aspartate aminotransferase (AST)
Cholesterol
Glucose
Creatine kinase (CK)
Magnesium
Lipase
Phosphorus

Box 6-2   COMMON CAUSES FOR INACCURATE RESULTS
Poor-quality or outdated reagents
Failure to calibrate or run controls
Improper pipetting techniques
Improper maintenance of instrument
Lipemic or hemolyzed samples
Allowing serum to sit on clot
Use of inappropriate cuvettes
Power surges or failure

patient is prepared (fasting vs. nonfasting samples), patient and specimen identification, specimen acquisition, and specimen processing. Establishment of standard procedures for each of these steps will decrease the likelihood of samples being misidentified or being of poor quality (hemolysed or lipemic). This aspect of quality control is important even in clinics that send their clinical pathology

samples to a reference laboratory. *Analytic variables* include the analytic methodology, standardization and calibration procedures, documentation of analytic protocols and procedures, and monitoring of equipment while in use. This aspect of quality control is usually well defined by the manufacturer of the instrument and should be followed closely. The final level, *monitoring of analytic quality* using statistical methods and control charts, is the aspect that involves the use of control products and record keeping. This aspect is the responsibility of the technician performing the tests.

 Technician Note

In spite of sales claims, valid results cannot be ensured without inclusion of appropriate control samples and proper calibration.

Controls

Control products are biologic solutions, usually serum based, that have known concentrations of the various constituents or analytes that can be assayed by the instrument. These products should be stable, be available in aliquots to prevent alterations caused by refreezing, and have little vial-to-vial variation. Control products can be purchased from an independent source or from the company that makes the test kit or instrument. Most control products are available as normal, high abnormal, and low abnormal ranges. The control products are analyzed in a manner identical to patients' samples, and the values reported by the instrument are compared with the known values provided with the product.

Many control products are provided in a lyophilized form that requires rehydration with distilled water or a diluent provided by the manufacturer. It is essential that the solution be diluted properly to ensure the concentration of the analytes is correct. Imprecision in diluting the controls will be reflected by values that are not in concert with the known values of the product even though the instrument is working properly. It is highly recommended that volumetric or other precise pipettes be used to dilute the control products (a graduated cylinder is not acceptable).

The control values must fall within a specific acceptable range, which usually encompasses the mean ±2 SD. This

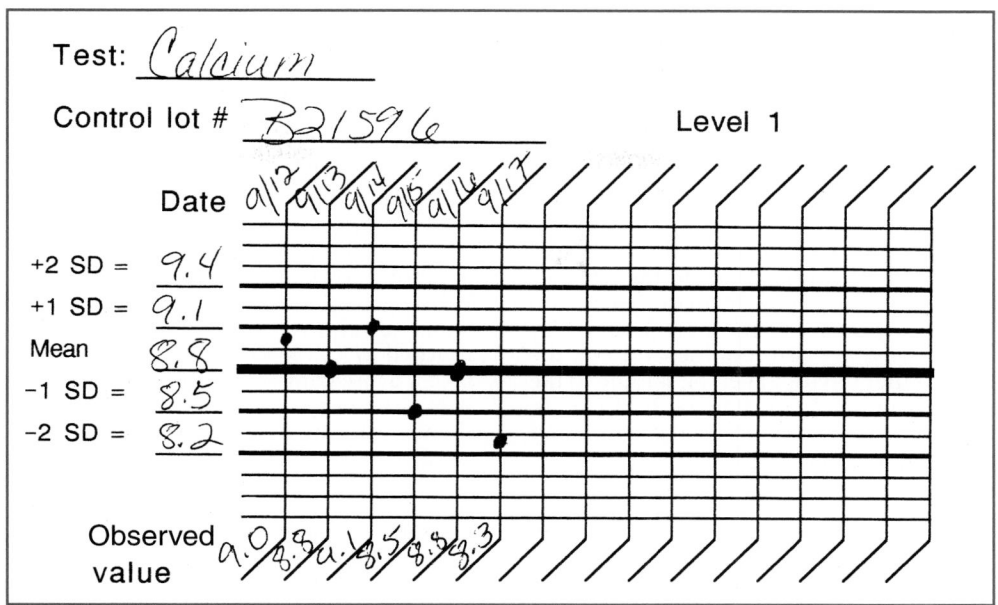

FIGURE 6-13. Levy-Jennings chart illustrating the common procedure used for following the performance of an individual test control serum.

range is established by the manufacturer of the product by repeated assay of the solution. When the instrument reports a control value above or below the established range, there is a problem with the procedure, and test results for that particular sample should not be reported until the problem is identified.

A separate log of the control results should be kept and reviewed periodically. A useful visual display of the instrument's performance for quick inspection and review is the Levy-Jennings chart. Figure 6-13 illustrates the use of the Levy-Jennings chart to keep track of quality control data. By inspection of control data over 1 month, a technician can see the control values gently drift upward or downward, indicating possible deterioration of the control product or a change in the light source intensity. Wide scatter of values outside the range on both the low and high end indicates imprecision on the part of the instrument or technician. It is best to keep the chart close to the instrument, not hidden in a file drawer. Everyone who uses the instrument must be willing to run controls and chart the results. Other useful laboratory records include calibration logs, sample logs, and maintenance logs.

Sample Handling

Sample handling is a critical step in obtaining accurate laboratory data. Several factors can interfere with analysis of a sample. The most common problems in veterinary medicine are hemolysis and lipemia. Difficulty in performing the venipuncture or excess pressure applied to the syringe during collection can cause significant hemolysis. The most common cause of lipemia is collection of a postprandial sample. There are times when both hemolysis and lipemia are unavoidable because they are the result of a disease process.

The effect hemolysis and lipemia will have on laboratory data is method dependent. There are no general rules to assist interpretation of changes caused by sample quality. A good reference laboratory will provide information on how each of its tests is affected by these two changes.

Manufacturers of the instruments and reagents should provide information on how interfering substances such as hemolysis and lipemia affect the methods used in their instrument. Hemolysis will commonly affect inorganic phosphorus and potassium values in horses and some Akita dogs. Lipemia will interfere with any method that depends on optical density read on a spectrophotometer. Some chemistry instruments can compensate for this change. Again, the reference laboratory should be able to indicate which tests are affected. Errors in processing the sample can also cause artifactual changes in laboratory data. It is important to use the appropriate collection tube for the test being performed.

Samples collected for chemistry profiles can be collected in *clot tubes* (red top), which contain no anticoagulant, or in lithium heparin tubes (green top). Blood collected in clot tubes (tubes without anticoagulant) must be allowed to completely clot before the sample can be centrifuged and the serum removed; complete clot formation usually takes about 30 minutes. Clot tubes with activator gels (tiger top) will promote clotting, thus decreasing the time necessary for complete clot formation and facilitating separation of the serum from the RBCs. The sample should not be refrigerated before complete clot formation because this inhibits good serum separation. In addition, a fibrin clot forms above the RBCs if the blood is centrifuged before complete clot formation or at too fast a speed.

Technician Note

Serum must be removed from the clot as soon as possible to avoid inaccurate results.

Blood collected in *lithium heparin tubes* (green top) is excellent for emergency needs because it does not have to clot before it can be separated for analysis. Heparin may interfere with a few chemistry tests, so it is best to check with the reference laboratory before submitting heparinized plasma for chemistry panels. Lithium heparin is also excellent for emergency electrolyte panels. *EDTA (purple top)* is unacceptable for most chemistry tests because it binds calcium to prevent clot formation and thus interferes with many of the assays, particularly those that are enzyme based. In addition, potassium EDTA will markedly increase serum potassium levels.

The necessity of separating serum from the clot as soon as possible cannot be overstressed. Prolonged exposure of serum to the cells will erroneously decrease the glucose, will increase the phosphorus, may increase potassium depending on species (especially in the horse), and may affect some enzyme activities. Do not depend on the reference laboratory courier service to get the sample to the laboratory in time to prevent these changes. It is best to take the time and responsibility to separate the serum and ensure the quality of the sample.

CYTOLOGY

Cytology is the study of cells, specifically involving the microscopic examination of individual cells that have exfoliated from a tissue or structure. Unlike histopathology, cytology is not an evaluation of the architecture of a tissue. In most instances, cytology can be used to differentiate an inflammatory lesion from a neoplastic mass. Sometimes cytologic appearance reveals a very specific diagnosis, and for certain samples, such as bone marrow or mast cell tumors, it may be more helpful than histopathology. It should be emphasized that cytology is an adjunct diagnostic tool and not a replacement for histopathology.

Cytology requires a significant degree of expertise that can be acquired only through experience, especially for cytology of solid masses. Most veterinary practices prefer to send cytology samples to a reference laboratory for evaluation. For this reason, the discussion on cytology is limited to preparation of samples from solid tissues for submission to a reference laboratory and fluid analysis. Veterinary technicians interested in becoming adept at cytology should obtain specific training through continuing education workshops. Excellent reference material is available.

Equipment

One of the advantages of cytology is that it requires no special equipment or supplies other than those used in performing a CBC. A good microscope, clean glass slides, a modified Wright's stain, and a centrifuge for fluid samples will suffice for most cytologic examinations.

Sample Preparation

Most cytology samples of solid masses are obtained through *fine needle aspiration (FNA)*. Cells are aspirated from the mass with a syringe (usually 6 ml) and needle (22 to 25 gauge) inserted into the mass and the application of negative pressure. It is not necessary to aspirate so strenuously that material appears in the barrel of the syringe or even the hub of the needle. Gentle aspiration will usually pull sufficient material into the needle. The sample can then be expelled onto a glass slide. Depending on the consistency of the sample, it can be spread in a manner similar to making a blood smear or by what is referred to as the *squash prep* for more viscous samples. This is done by placing a second slide on top of the slide containing the sample. The weight of the top slide should cause the sample to spread, and then the top slide is pulled off across the bottom slide, resulting in even spreading of the cells.

This method works well for many types of samples, and it may result in fewer broken cells than the traditional technique. It is important not to exert excessive pressure on the top slide or pull the slides apart too rapidly because cells are often fragile, and this will distort or "squash" the cells and make identification difficult if not impossible.

When handling excised pieces of tissue for cytologic study, keep them wrapped in gauze and slightly moistened with saline so they do not dry out. Do not allow any contact with formalin, or even with formalin fumes, until after the cytologic slides have been made and stained. Excised solid masses should be blotted with absorbent paper to remove blood and tissue fluid and then gently touched to a slide to make an impression slide. If the mass is of a dense consistency that does not exfoliate cells easily, it may be necessary to scrape it with a scalpel blade and then spread the material gently and thinly onto the slide. An alternative method is to crosshatch cut the surface of the tissue with the scalpel blade and make an imprint preparation. The crosshatching method is often gentler than the scraping method and preserves the cells better.

If the slides are to be sent to a reference laboratory, it is again recommended that the use of flat slide mailers be avoided because many will arrive shattered. Most reference laboratories prefer unstained slides, which can be stained at the laboratory by means of their standard stain protocol. If a slide has been stained and there are questions pertaining to that slide, it is a good idea to include that slide for comparison purposes.

Fluid Analysis

For fluid analysis, a refractometer and a cell-counting method (e.g., Unopettes and a hemacytometer) are also needed. Once a sample for cytology has been obtained, slides should be made as soon as possible, before the cells degenerate in the fluid. This is especially true of low-protein fluids, such as cerebrospinal fluid and tracheal washings. Many fluid samples can be prepared in the same manner as a blood film, leaving a feathered edge where the largest cells tend to migrate. If the fluid has very few cells, as is the case with cerebrospinal fluid, a direct preparation may not provide sufficient cells for a thorough examination. There are *cytocentrifuges* that are especially designed to make cytologic slides from hypocellular fluids; they are gentler to cells because they spin at a slow speed and have gradual acceleration and deceleration. They also may have a special apparatus that causes cells to be deposited directly onto a slide, with filter paper taking away excess fluid. However, cytocentrifuges are probably impractical for all except the largest practices. As an alternative, these low-cellularity samples can be concentrated similar to the preparation of a urine sediment. The fluid is centrifuged at slow speed, and the slide is prepared from the sediment after the supernatant is decanted or removed with a pipette. It is always advisable to make one or two direct preparations in case the techniques used to concentrate the cells result in too many ruptured cells or other artifacts.

A routine fluid analysis of samples such as abdominal, thoracic, or synovial fluid usually includes a WBC count, which is more appropriately referred to as a total nucleated cell count (TNCC), because some of the cells (mesothelial cells, synovial cells, etc.) may not be derived directly from blood. The TNCC can be performed in the same manner as a WBC count. If there are numerous cells present, these can be counted on an automated instrument, but lower cell counts will require use of the hemacytometer as for a manual WBC count.

Total protein is another helpful parameter in fluid analysis and can be done by refractometer, generally using the supernatant portion of a centrifuged fluid sample. Total erythrocyte (RBC) count is often included in the fluid analysis if done on an automated instrument, but the RBC count alone is rarely helpful in evaluating fluid because of the frequency of peripheral blood contamination of samples. It is more important to check for *erythrophagocytosis* (phagocytosis of RBCs by macrophages) during the cytologic examination because erythrophagocytosis generally implies that the RBCs were present in the fluid before sampling rather than as contaminants.

Fluid samples that have neutrophils as the predominate cell type should be closely evaluated for the presence of bacteria. Bacteria should be present within cells (intracellular) to be considered significant (Color Plate I, *J*). If they are only extracellular, one should consider the possibility of contamination of the sample. If no bacteria are found, it should not be assumed that they are absent. They may be in very low numbers and difficult to find.

Joint Fluid

The analysis of certain fluids includes specific tests that may add more information than routine tests. For instance, the *mucin clot test* is done on synovial fluid by mixing a diluted acetic acid solution (0.1 ml of 7N acetic acid in 4 ml of distilled water) and then adding 1 ml of synovial fluid. Normal synovial fluid contains mucin, which forms a tight white clot in the acetic acid; if the mucin has been digested by bacterial or cellular enzymes, the clot will be less distinct or may not form at all, leaving only hazy or cloudy fluid. Therefore good mucin clot formation usually accompanies normal or noninflamed joints, whereas a poor or absent mucin clot indicates inflammation, infection, or both. The precipitation of mucin in joint fluid by acetic acid precludes the use of the WBC Unopette system because this system contains acetic acid as the diluent in the reservoir. TNCCs on joint fluid should be done using the Unopette system for both WBCs and platelets. The reservoir in this system contains ammonium oxalate, which will not precipitate mucin.

RECOMMENDED READING

GENERAL
Duncan JR, Prasse KW: *Veterinary laboratory medicine/clinical pathology*, Ames, 1994, Iowa State University Press.

LABORATORY EQUIPMENT
Tietz NW: *Fundamentals of clinical chemistry*, ed 4, Philadelphia, 1995, WB Saunders.

HEMATOLOGY
Harvey JW: *Atlas of veterinary hematology: blood and bone marrow of domestic animals*, Philadelphia, 2001, WB Saunders.
Jain NC: *Essentials of veterinary hematology*, Philadelphia, 1993, Lea & Febiger.
Reagan WL et al: *Veterinary hematology: atlas of common domestic species*, Ames, 1998, Iowa State University Press.

URINALYSIS
Graff L: *A handbook of routine urinalysis*, Philadelphia, 1983, JB Lippincott.
Osborne CA, Finco DR: *Canine and feline nephrology and urology*, Philadelphia, 1995, Lea & Febiger.

CHEMISTRY
Coffman JR: *Equine clinical chemistry and pathophysiology*, Bonner Springs, Kan, 1981, Veterinary Medicine Publishing.
Kaneko JJ, editor: *Clinical biochemistry of domestic animals*, New York, 1989, Academic Press.

QUALITY ASSURANCE PROGRAMS
Henry JB: *Clinical diagnosis and management by laboratory methods*, ed 19, Philadelphia, 1996, WB Saunders.

AVIAN AND REPTILIAN HEMATOLOGY
Campbell TW: *Avian hematology and cytology*, Ames, 1988, Iowa State University Press.
Frye FL: *Biomedical and surgical aspects of captive reptile husbandry*, Edwardsville, Kan, 1981, Veterinary Medicine Publishing.

CYTOLOGY
Cowell RL et al: *Diagnostic cytology and hematology of the dog and cat*, ed 2, St Louis, 1999, Mosby.
Menard M, Papageorges M: Fine-needle biopsies: how to increase diagnostic yield, *Compend Cont Ed Pract Vet* 19:738, 1997.

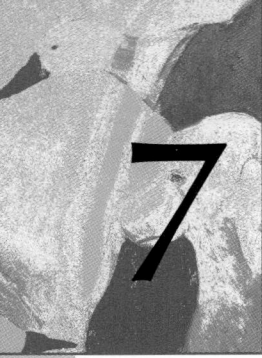

7

Parasitology

Johnny D. Hoskins

Most parasites are capable of causing significant damage to the host. This potential may be a function of the number of parasites present in some cases; in the case of other parasites, location within the host, production of toxins, or interference with normal physiologic processes produces the damage. Clinical signs associated with parasitism may include such disorders as life-threatening anemia, hypoproteinemia, diarrhea, vomiting, and intestinal obstruction, but not uncommonly the damage is more insidious, such as interference with normal weight gain or milk production. Parasitism is most severe in animals younger than 1 year, but it may affect animals of any age.

Ectoparasites (external parasites), including mites, ticks, lice, fleas, chiggers, and myiasis-inducing flies, and endoparasites (internal parasites), including protozoa, trematodes, tapeworms, and nematodes, have representative parasites on or in all animals and in every organ or tissue. Some parasites are host specific, whereas other parasites are capable of infesting or infecting a broad range of animal hosts. Modes of transmission vary considerably from simple, direct transmission to an extremely complex life cycle, involving the use of an intermediate host or transport host or specific environmental conditions. The nematode (wormlike) parasites have five stages in their development. Various nematodes, such as the strongyle nematodes of ruminants and horses, produce an egg that passes through the anus into the environment. A first-stage larva develops within the egg. This free-living larva grows and molts (sheds the skin or cuticle) into a second-stage larva, which then grows and molts into a third-stage larva—the infective larva. The infective larva usually is ingested and develops into a fourth-stage larva and finally into a fifth-stage larva within the host.

Some nematodes have developed modifications from this life cycle. For example, hookworm larvae generally penetrate the skin and circulate in the host's tissue before completing their development in the small intestine. Others, such as roundworms and whipworms, develop into the infective stage within the egg and do not hatch until ingested by the host. Still other important nematodes, for example, *Strongyloides*, have a first-stage larva in the egg when passed. Treatment, including selection of the proper medication and appropriate control in the environment,

always necessitates a thorough knowledge of the biology of each individual parasite.

> ### Technician Note
> The diagnosis of parasitism is not difficult, but timing, choice of technique, and interpretation of the results are often crucial for effective treatment and control.

The following sections provide discussions of specific parasites as they relate to animal host and parasite class within each host. The veterinary technician should become familiar with both the common name and the scientific name (e.g., roundworm = *Toxocara canis*) of the common parasites. Each section contains information on the life cycle, tissue location, treatment, and control for the specific parasite discussed. In addition, a section on diagnostic procedures is presented to outline the most commonly used techniques.

ENDOPARASITES

Parasites of Dogs and Cats
Roundworms (Ascarids)

Toxocara canis, Toxocara cati, and *Toxascaris leonina* are ascarids that are thick, white to cream-colored nematodes. Mature specimens measure about 3.5 to 5 cm for males and 10 to 15 cm for females. Eggs of the *Toxocara* spp. are large, oval, and dark with a thick, rough shell. *Toxascaris leonina* is lighter in color and more egg shaped and has a thick, smooth shell (Figure 7-1). All three species are common in most geographic regions of the United States. The larval stage develops within the egg, and the second stage is the infective larva. Eggs are highly resistant to adverse conditions and, under ideal environmental conditions, become infective in about 2 weeks. Once ingested, *Toxocara* spp. hatch in the small intestine, penetrate the mucosa, migrate through the liver, pass through the heart, and go into the lungs, in which they develop within a short period of time. Larvae are coughed, swallowed, and mature in the small intestine within 4 to 6 weeks.

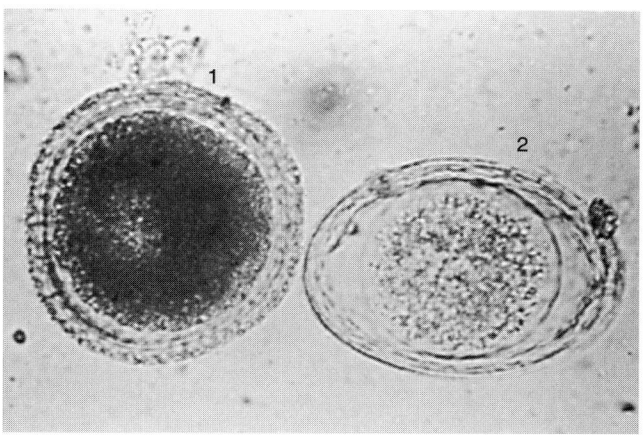

FIGURE 7-1. *1, Toxocara* egg measuring approximately 66 × 42 µm. *2, Toxascaris* egg measuring approximately 85 × 75 µm.

Toxascaris leonina eggs hatch in the small intestine, and the larvae penetrate the intestinal mucosa to develop for about 2 to 3 months and then return to the lumen as adults. In dogs older than 5 weeks, most of the *Toxocara* larvae leave the circulation and are stored in the somatic organs until the dog becomes pregnant. Between the forty-second and fifty-sixth days of gestation, these larvae leave the somatic tissues, cross the placenta, enter the fetal lungs, and remain there until birth. The larvae then complete the cycle already described. Consequently, a high percentage of dogs are infected by the *prenatal* or *transplacental* route. In the pregnant dog and cat, some of the activated *Toxocara* larvae migrate to the mammary glands. These larvae are ingested by puppies and kittens when they first start to nurse. Transmammary infections are more common in cats than in dogs. The eggs of all three ascarids can be ingested by other animals (e.g., mice, chickens) and remain infective in their tissue until eaten by the appropriate host. All three species are readily diagnosed through a number of techniques, and they are amenable to treatment with a number of anthelmintics (Table 7-1). Control is difficult because the eggs are resistant, and control measures necessitate thorough cleansing of kennels, runs, yards, and so forth.

Hookworm

Ancylostoma caninum occurs in dogs, foxes, coyotes, wolves, raccoons, and badgers; *Ancylostoma braziliense* is found in dogs and cats; *Uncinaria stenocephala* occurs in dogs, cats, foxes, coyotes, and wolves; and *Ancylostoma tubaeforme* is found in cats and wild Felidae. Hookworms are all short, thick parasites, with the adult males measuring 6 to 12 mm and the adult females measuring 6 to 20 mm. Hookworms produce a similar strongyle type of egg (Figure 7-2). *Ancylostoma* spp. generally are found in coastal areas of high rainfall, whereas *U. stenocephala* is found in the northeastern United States. All hookworm species have a similar life cycle. Undeveloped eggs pass into the environment, develop, and hatch, releasing a first-stage larva that undergoes a free-living existence until it develops to the third-stage infective larva. Hookworms are capable of establishing themselves in the host after ingestion, but the normal mode of infection is skin penetration. After larvae penetrate, they enter the venous circulation, going ultimately to the lungs, in which they develop for a short

period of time. They are then coughed up and swallowed, and they enter the small intestine and mature. This generally occurs within 4 to 6 weeks.

> **Technician Note**
>
> Hookworms are capable of establishing themselves in the host after ingestion, but the normal mode of infection is skin penetration.

A. caninum has developed the additional modes of *transplacental* or *transmammary infection*. Third-stage larvae penetrate the skin and circulate in the pregnant female host, ultimately crossing the placenta. The larvae also are stored in somatic tissues until the female host becomes pregnant. Most of the somatic larvae activated at the time of pregnancy migrate to the mammary glands of the bitch and are passed on to nursing puppies. Diagnosis is readily performed through identification of the egg by a number of techniques, and these species are amenable to treatment with a number of anthelmintics (see Table 7-1). Control is difficult, especially in warm, humid geographic regions, necessitating regular and thorough cleansing of yards, kennels, and so forth.

Intestinal Threadworm

Strongyloides stercoralis is a nematode that is a parasite of dogs, cats, foxes, humans, primates, and possibly other wild carnivores. Only the female nematode is parasitic, and she reproduces parthenogenetically (without fertilization). Parasitic females live embedded in the mucosa of the small intestine. The eggs develop in utero, and the nematode gives birth to first-stage larvae (Figure 7-3), whose chromosome number determines whether they will develop into a free-living generation before producing larvae destined to be parasitic or become a larval stage possessing a unique chromosome and be destined to develop into third-stage infective larvae. The infective larvae are capable of establishing infection by oral ingestion, after which they penetrate the small intestine and develop there. However, the primary mode of infection is by *skin penetration*. If the larvae use skin penetration, they then penetrate the venous circulation, going ultimately to the lungs to develop for a short period of time. Larvae are then coughed up, swallowed, and penetrate into the mucosa of the small intestine. In immunologically compromised animals, infections may be severe. *S. stercoralis* is widespread in tropical and subtropical regions, as well as in kennels and pet shops, in which environmental conditions are suitable. Diagnosis is not difficult. Frequently, a direct smear of fresh feces is suitable. Treatment is not always satisfactory, and alternate anthelmintics should be considered (see Table 7-1). Control necessitates thorough cleaning of facilities and allowing the facilities to dry.

Whipworm

Trichuris vulpis occurs in the cecum of the dog, fox, and coyote. Like all whipworms, the anterior extremity is slender, and the posterior extremity is thickened, giving *T. vulpis* a whiplike appearance. Males and females are about the same length, measuring 45 to 75 mm. The eggs are characteristic, possessing a thick, brown-yellow shell with a clear polar plug at each end (Figure 7-4). *T. vulpis* is widespread in temperate zones, and the incidence of infection is frequently high. The life cycle is simple and direct. The infective larva develops within the egg. When the egg is ingested, the larvae are released in the intestine,

TABLE 7-1 PARASITICIDES USED FOR TREATMENT AND CONTROL OF INTERNAL PARASITES IN DOGS AND CATS*

Drug	Toxocara, Toxascaris	Ancylostoma, Uncinaria	Strongyloides	Trichuris	Dirofilaria Adults	Dirofilaria Microfilariae	Taenia	Dipylidium	Giardia	Coccidia
Albendazole	+	+	−	+	−	−	+	−	+	−
Amprolium	−	−	−	−	−	−	−	−	−	+
Butamisole hydrochloride	−	+	−	+	−	−	−	−	−	−
Dichlorophen	−	−	−	−	−	−	+	+	−	−
Dichlorophen/toluene	+	+	−	−	−	−	+	+	−	−
Dichlorvos	+	+	−	+	−	−	−	−	−	−
Diethylcarbamazine	+	−	−	−	−	+	−	−	−	−
Epsiprantel	−	−	−	−	−	−	+	+	−	−
Febantel	+	+	−	+	−	−	+	−	−	−
Febantel/praziquantel	+	+	−	+	−	−	+	+	−	−
Fenbendazole	+	+	−	+	−	−	+	−	−	−
Furazolidone	−	−	−	−	−	−	−	−	+	−
Ivermectin	+	+	−	+	−	+	−	−	−	−
Mebendazole	+	+	−	+	−	−	+	−	−	−
Melarsomine dihydrochloride	−	−	−	−	+	−	−	−	−	−
Metronidazole	−	−	−	−	−	−	−	−	+	−
Milbemycin oxime	+	+	−	+	−	+	−	−	−	−
N-Butyl chloride	+	+	−	−	−	−	−	−	−	−
Nitroscanate	+	+	−	+	−	−	+	+	−	−
Oxibendazole/diethylcarbamazine	+	+	−	+	−	+	−	−	−	−
Piperazine salts	+	−	−	−	−	−	−	−	−	−
Praziquantel	−	−	−	−	−	−	+	+	−	−
Praziquantel/pyrantel pamoate	+	+	−	−	−	−	+	+	−	−
Praziquantel/pyrantel pamoate/febantel	+	+	−	+	−	−	+	+	−	−
Pyrantel pamoate	+	+	−	−	−	−	−	−	−	−
Quinacrine hydrochloride	−	−	−	−	−	−	−	−	+	−
Selamectin	+	+	−	−	−	+	−	−	−	−
Sulfadiazine/trimethoprim	−	−	−	−	−	−	−	−	−	+
Sulfadimethoxine	−	−	−	−	−	−	−	−	−	+
Thiabendazole	−	−	+	−	−	−	−	−	−	−

+, Indicated for use; −, not indicated for use.
*Paromomycin, an antibiotic, is being used to manage *Cryptosporidium* infections and resistant *Giardia* infections in dogs and cats.

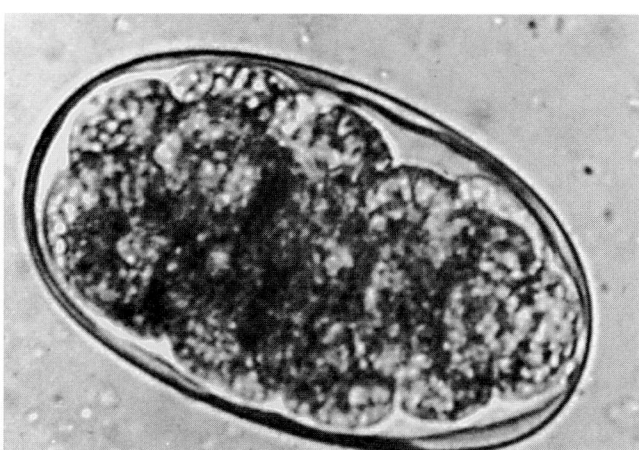

FIGURE 7-2. Strongyle-type egg, as seen in hookworms, measuring approximately 62 × 40 μm.

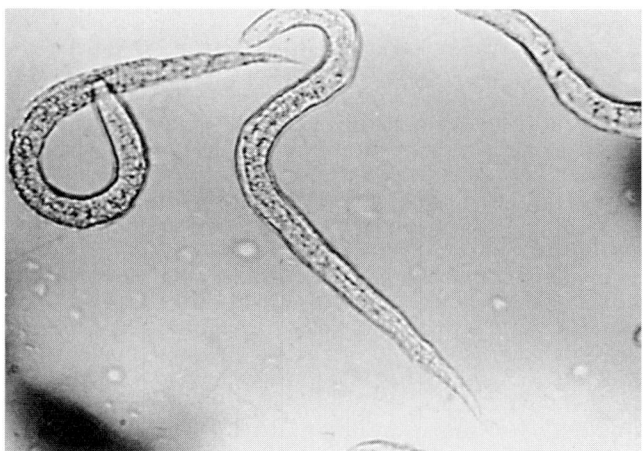

FIGURE 7-3. *Strongyloides* larvae from a dog. Note that the larvae are distorted in appearance because of the flotation solution.

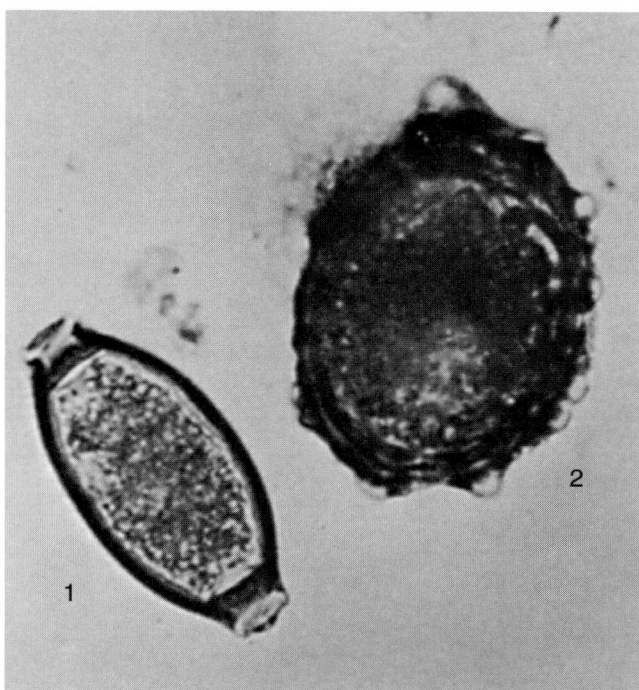

FIGURE 7-4. *1,* Trichurid egg, as seen in whipworms, measuring approximately 80 × 36 μm. *2,* Ascarid egg measuring approximately 60 × 50 μm.

which they penetrate. Larvae develop within 8 to 10 days, return to the surface of the intestine, go to the cecum, and attach and mature in an additional 60 to 80 days. Diagnosis can be effectively accomplished by a number of procedures, but eggs are quite heavy, and interpretation of the severity of infection based on the number of eggs present is not possible. Several treatments are available (see Table 7-1). Control is difficult because eggs are highly resistant to environmental conditions. Sanitation, as applied for ascarids, is the best approach.

Technician Note

The eggs of *Trichuris* spp. are very characteristic, possessing a thick, brown-yellow shell with a clear polar plug at each end.

Whipworm infection is uncommon in cats and wild Felidae in the United States; however, *Trichuris campanula*

has been reported to occur in the United States. Occasionally, *Capillaria* spp. have been found in feces of both dogs and cats. The eggs of *Capillaria* are similar but not as dark in color, and on average the eggs are somewhat smaller than those of whipworms.

Tapeworms

Dogs, cats, the wild Canidae, and some of the wild Felidae are susceptible to infection by a number of tapeworms. The most commonly found tapeworm species are *Dipylidium caninum, Taenia hydatigena, Taenia pisiformis, Taenia ovis, Taenia krabbei, Multiceps serialis,* and *Echinococcus granulosus.* Cats, and some of the wild Felidae, generally are infected with *Taenia taeniaeformis* and *D. caninum.* The species of tapeworms found in dogs and cats depends on their geographic location and the amount of free-ranging activity the animals are given.

Technician Note

Diagnosis of *Taenia* spp. and *Dipylidium caninum* infections is normally done by finding the proglottids in the feces or around the host's anal region or hocks.

All tapeworms have an intermediate host in which the larval stage develops. *D. caninum* uses a flea, in which the larval (cysticercoid) stage develops. *T. hydatigena, T. ovis,* and *T. krabbei* use ruminants—usually sheep, deer, elk, and moose—in which the larval stage (cysticercus) develops in the body cavity (*T. hydatigena*) or muscles (*T. ovis, T. krabbei*). *T. pisiformis* develops in the body cavity of rabbits, and *Taenia serialis* develops in subcutaneous areas or in the muscles of rabbits. The larval stage of *T. taeniaeformis* develops in the liver of mice, rats, and other small

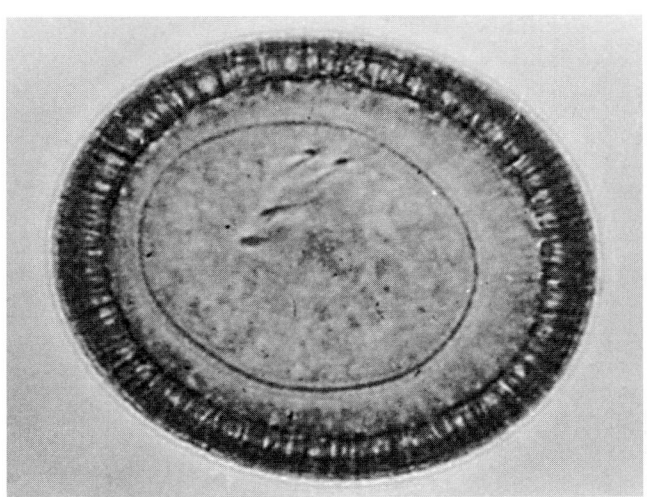

FIGURE 7-5. Typical *Taenia* egg measuring approximately 34 μm. *Dipylidium* eggs appear similar but are contained in packets of 1 to 20 eggs.

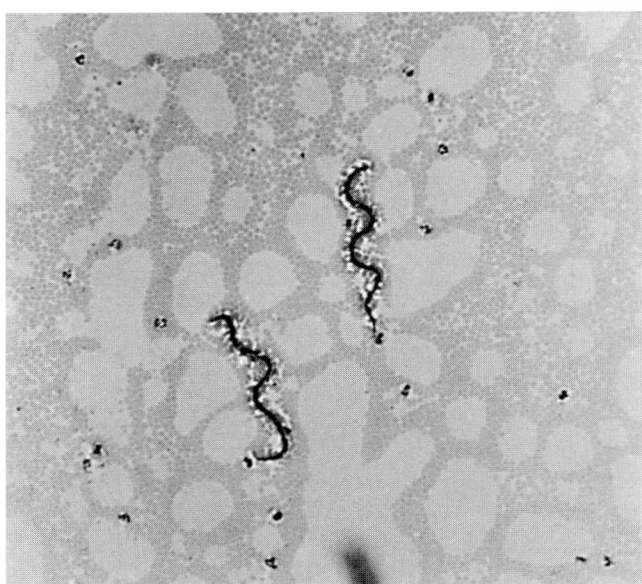

FIGURE 7-6. Stained microfilaria of *Dirofilaria immitis*.

rodents. *E. granulosus* uses ruminants, such as sheep, deer, and elk, and humans as intermediate hosts. The larval stage is a rather large, fluid-filled bladder called a *hydatid cyst* that is easily recognized by its large size (25 to 100 mm in diameter), the presence of numerous small pieces of larval tapeworms (brood capsules) on the inner surface, and the presence of compartments within the body of the cyst in which daughter cysts have grown and fused together.

Diagnosis of *Taenia* spp. and *D. caninum* infections is normally done by finding the proglottids (body segments), or chain of proglottids, around the host's anal region or on their hocks. Although the eggs will float, usually they are not released to mix with the feces (Figure 7-5). *Taenia* spp. have one genital opening per proglottid, whereas *D. caninum* has two, one on either side. Further diagnosis of *Taenia* spp. beyond the genus designation is extremely difficult, requiring morphologic study of the intact parasite.

E. granulosus eggs frequently mix with the feces (unlike *Taenia* spp.), but the eggs are typical *Taenia*-type eggs, possessing a thick, striated shell. *D. caninum* eggs, if seen in feces, occur in packets contained within a thin-walled membrane. A number of treatments are available (see Table 7-1). Control depends on the tapeworm species. *D. caninum* obviously necessitates vigorous control of fleas. For *Taenia* spp., the dog or cat should not have access to the flesh or viscera of the intermediate host.

Heartworm and *Dipetalonema*

Dirofilaria immitis and *Dipetalonema reconditum* are the two filarial nematodes found commonly in dogs and the wild Canidae in the United States. *D. immitis* infections also occur in cats and the wild Felidae, but they are not as common as in dogs. The heartworm, *D. immitis*, occurs primarily in the right ventricle and pulmonary arteries of the host, whereas *D. reconditum* occurs in the subcutaneous tissue. Both nematodes produce a larval form called a *microfilaria*, which circulates in the blood (Figure 7-6). These filarial nematodes are found commonly in areas of the United States where the intermediate hosts occur; however, heartworm is becoming more widespread as infected dogs and cats are brought into areas where the parasite is not normally found.

D. immitis males measure 12 to 20 cm, and the females measure 25 to 31 cm long, whereas *D. reconditum* males are 9 to 17 mm long, and the females are 20 to 32 mm long. Both nematodes need an intermediate host to complete their life cycle. *D. immitis* uses several different species of mosquito, and *D. reconditum* uses the common dog and cat flea. Microfilariae, when ingested by the intermediate host, undergo reorganization and development to the third-stage infective larva. Once infective, they go into the mouthparts of the arthropod and remain there until the arthropod feeds on a susceptible host. *D. immitis* infective larvae enter the tissue for 85 to 120 days and develop into young adults. They then go to the heart and reach sexual maturity in another 60 to 70 days, for a total of 145 to 190 days. *D. reconditum* apparently goes directly into the subcutaneous tissues to develop to sexual maturity.

Technician Note

Diagnosis of heartworm disease in the dog is generally based on identification of microfilaria in the peripheral circulation.

The microfilaria of *D. immitis* is 295 to 325 μm long (average of 313 μm) and 6 to 7 μm in diameter (average of 6.9 μm), whereas the microfilaria of *D. reconditum* is somewhat shorter and more slender, measuring 250 to 288 μm long (average of 276 μm) and 4.5 to 5.5 μm in diameter (average of 4.6 μm).

Various techniques have been used to detect microfilaria, including fresh blood/saline preparation, capillary hematocrit tube, and the Knott, or filtration concentration, test. Fresh blood/saline preparations are helpful in differential diagnosis of *D. immitis* and *D. reconditum* microfilaria. *D. immitis* microfilaria moves in place without directional motion, whereas *D. reconditum* has a directional movement across the microscopic viewing field. Concentration tests are best used for the detection of *D. immitis* microfilaria because they are much more accurate than fresh blood/saline preparations or capillary hematocrit tube tests. Occult heartworm infections (adult heartworms without circulating microfilariae) occur in approximately 25% of dogs and 90% of cats. Several serologic tests are available in commercial kits to test serum of dogs and cats for occult infection. Treatment of *D. reconditum* is unimportant because they are nonpathogenic parasites. The treatment for *D. immitis* necessitates the use of an agent effective for adult heartworms followed by a microfilaricide (see Table 7-1). Control of *D. immitis* necessitates daily or monthly heartworm preventive therapy and mosquito control in enzootic areas.

Giardia

Giardia spp. Are common protozoan parasites of dogs and cats in the United States. A higher incidence of infection occurs among dogs, cats, humans, and beavers than in other animals, such as deer, sheep, moose, and antelope. There are two forms of *Giardia*. The motile trophozoite, which is approximately 12 to 17 μm long and 7 to 10 μm wide, is found in the small intestine. The cyst form (the infective stage) is approximately 9 to 13 μm long (Figure 7-7). When ingested, the cyst wall is digested away in the small intestine, releasing the trophozoite, which immediately divides into two organisms. These organisms attach to the epithelial cells lining the small intestine and continue to multiply by binary fusion over the next 6 to 10 days until a large population exists. At that time, diarrhea develops, and *Giardia* begins to produce cysts. Diagnosis can be accomplished by the direct fecal/saline smear or, more effectively, the zinc sulfate centrifugal flotation technique. Treatment is available (see Table 7-1). *Giardia* is more commonly found among young dogs and cats crowded into kennels and animal shelters. The most effective control procedure is cleanliness and disinfection with quaternary ammonium compounds.

Coccidia

Dogs and cats are hosts for a number of species of *Isospora* (also called *Cystoisospora*), *Cryptosporidium*, and *Sarcocystis*, and the cat is the definitive host for *Toxoplasma gondii*. The incidence and severity of coccidial infection depend on the host's age and immune status, conditions in which the hosts are housed, or their diet and quality of drinking water.

The species of *Isospora* have a direct life cycle; however, some *Isospora* spp. (*Isospora canis, Isospora felis*) can use an intermediate host, such as mice. The life cycle starts with an oocyst in the feces (Figure 7-8). This oocyst must sporulate (develop into the infective form), which occurs in less than 1 week given optimum conditions of warmth and moisture. Once infective, the oocyst encloses two sporocysts, each of which encloses four small, spindle-shaped infective forms called *sporozoites* or a total of eight infective forms in each oocyst. When ingested, the oocyst and sporocyst walls are digested in the intestine, releasing sporozoites to penetrate the intestinal epithelium and enter a cell for subsequent development. Within the intestinal cell, they become spherical and begin to grow to a large size. The nucleus replicates several times, and ultimately thousands of small, spindle-shaped organisms called *merozoites* develop. This asexual process of reproduction is called *schizogony*, and the large structure filled with the merozoites is called a *schizont*.

Once mature, the schizont ruptures, releasing merozo-

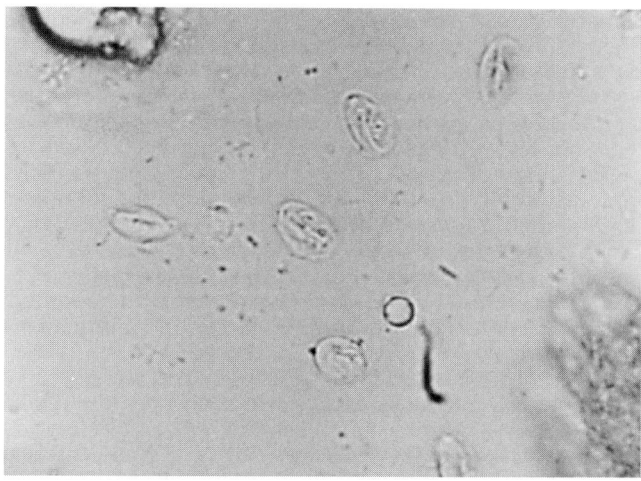

FIGURE 7-7.   Cysts of *Giardia* sp. from a dog fecal flotation using ZnSO₄ at a specific gravity (SG) of 1.18.

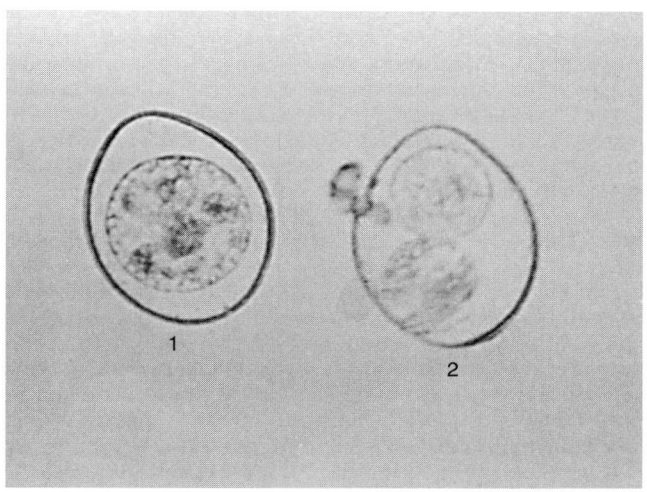

FIGURE 7-8.   Unsporulated oocyst of *Isospora (1)* and sporulated oocyst of *Isospora (2)* measuring approximately 25 × 20 μm.

ites. The next step in the life cycle is species dependent, but usually they move further down the intestine, penetrate a cell, and repeat the asexual process but with smaller schizonts containing fewer merozoites. When released, the merozoites then penetrate a cell, with some of them becoming macrogametes (ova) and some becoming microgametes (sperm). Once fertilization occurs, the oocyst is produced and passes in the feces to begin the life cycle again. Although the life cycle is finite (e.g., only a given number of oocysts can be produced from a single oocyst infection), the reproductive potential is great for some species.

Species of *Cryptosporidium* have essentially the same type of life cycle. *Cryptosporidium* organisms inhabit the respiratory and intestinal epithelium of many hosts, including birds, mammals, reptiles, and fish. Dogs and cats develop intestinal tract infection almost exclusively. Enteroepithelial development is limited to the luminal enterocytes;

extraintestinal tissue cysts do not develop. The enteroepithelial life cycle begins with ingestion of sporulated oocysts by a suitable host. After ingestion of oocysts, four sporozoites are released from each oocyst that penetrate intestinal epithelial cells. Asexual reproduction at the intestinal surface occurs with the production of merozoites that are released and penetrate other cells. Gametogony and sporogony occur, resulting in the production of thin- and thick-walled oocysts. Sporulated, thick-walled oocysts are shed in the feces of an infected host and are immediately infective to a susceptible host. Thin-walled oocysts passed into the intestinal lumen rupture, releasing the sporozoites, which penetrate additional host cells and reinitiate the developmental cycle.

Species of *Sarcocystis* have essentially the same type of life cycle, except the carnivore is the host for the sexual stages (oocyst, sporocyst), and omnivores and herbivores act as hosts for the asexual (schizogony) stage. Infected carnivores pass a thin-walled oocyst, which will rupture, that contains two small, thick-walled sporocysts in which four sporozoites have already developed and are immediately infective to the alternate host. Once ingested, the sporozoites are released and penetrate the epithelial tissue of the intestine. Generally, they enter the circulatory system and begin the first asexual (schizogony) phase in the kidney. The first schizont releases its small, spindle-shaped organisms, which then enter cardiac or smooth muscle, in which they develop into rather large schizonts called *sarcocysts*. When sarcocysts are ingested by a specific carnivore, and most species are specific for each carnivore or herbivore, the small, spindle-shaped organisms penetrate superficial epithelial cells of the intestine and immediately begin the sexual phase, terminating as a thin-walled oocyst about 11 to 14 days after ingestion of the infected flesh.

The life cycle of *T. gondii* is similar to that of *Sarcocystis* with the exception that most animals are suitable hosts for the development of the asexual (schizogony) stages, and only the cat is suitable as a host for the sexual stages. The typical life cycle occurs when a cat ingests the small sporulated oocyst. In the intestine, the parasite goes through two asexual stages and then into the sexual phase, producing oocysts. If, for example, a mouse should eat the oocyst, the first asexual phase occurs in this animal. When a cat eats these schizonts, the parasite goes into one asexual cycle, in the cat's intestine, followed by the sexual cycle. If the first mouse is eaten by another mouse, *Toxoplasma* goes into the second asexual cycle in this mouse. When then eaten by a cat, the parasites go directly into the sexual phase. The asexual cycle can go on indefinitely as animals eat the flesh of infected animals.

Diagnosis of *Isospora*, *Cryptosporidium*, *Sarcocystis*, and *Toxoplasma* is based on recovery of the oocyst or sporocyst (for *Sarcocystis*) by a number of diagnostic procedures. Treatment is seldom administered for *Sarcocystis* infection, but when clinical disease occurs, treatment is recommended for *Isospora*, *Cryptosporidium*, and *Toxoplasma* spp. (see Table 7-1). Control of *Isospora* and *Cryptosporidium* infections requires cleanliness, removal of the animal to clean premises, or both; however, these oocysts are extremely resistant to environmental conditions. Control of *Sarcocystis* is generally not practiced for the carnivore host because *Sarcocystis* is considered nonpathogenic. If control is exercised, the best approach is to prevent consumption of raw flesh from any source, including ground beef. The best control for *Toxoplasma* in cats is to prevent consumption of raw flesh and contact with feces of infected cats.

Parasites of Horses
Roundworm

The ascarid of horses *(Parascaris equorum)* is a creamy white color. The males measure about 28 cm, whereas females are about 50 cm in length. They produce a dark brown, thick-shelled oval to spherical egg that is very resistant to environmental conditions. The larval stage develops within the egg, and the second stage is infective. Development to the infective stage requires about 2 weeks. When the egg is ingested, the larva is released in the intestine, penetrates the intestinal mucosa, enters the circulatory system, and passes through to the liver, heart, and, ultimately, the lungs, in which they develop for a period of time. Subsequently, larvae pass up the bronchial tree, enter the mouth, and are swallowed. They are passed into the small intestine and mature. This entire life cycle requires 10 to 12 weeks. Diagnosis is readily performed using a number of techniques, and these parasites are amenable to treatment by several anthelmintics (Table 7-2). Control is difficult because eggs are extremely resistant to environmental conditions, and the coprophagous habits of foals tend to ensure infection.

Technician Note

The horse ascarid is common throughout the United States, and the incidence of infection, especially among younger horses, is frequently high.

Pinworm

The pinworm of horses, *Oxyuris equi*, is a white to slate gray-colored nematode with a slender, sharply pointed tail. Males are very small, measuring less than 12 mm, and females are 75 to 150 mm long. The eggs are slender and somewhat flattened along one side (Figure 7-9). Frequently, they possess a first-stage larva when deposited. Pinworms are common in horses in the United States. The life cycle is simple and direct. Female parasites living in the cecum pass out through the anal sphincter and deposit masses of eggs on the perineum. Eggs are cemented into masses with a gelatinous material. Eggs drop off, either singly or in masses, landing on ground or feed and become infective within 3 to 5 days. Once ingested, the larvae are released in the small intestine, penetrate the intestinal mucosa, and develop for several days. Larvae then return to the mucosal surface, move to the large intestine, and reach maturity about 50 days after the initial ingestion of the egg. Diagnosis can be performed effectively only by the adhesive tape technique (see the discussion of diagnostic tests). Pinworms are amenable to treatment by a number of anthelmintics (see Table 7-2). Control is difficult because of the coprophagous habits of foals.

Small and Large Strongyles

Strongylus vulgaris, *Strongylus equinus*, and *Strongylus edentatus* are the three species of "large strongyles" of horses. The 40 or more species of "small strongyles" of horses, of which there are several different genera, are blood-sucking nematodes. Strongyles vary in size from less than 12 mm (small strongyles) to 38 to 47 mm (large strongyles). However, some small strongyles, such as *Tridontophorous*, are nearly as large as *S. vulgaris*, the smallest of the large strongyles. All the strongyles produce a similar thin-walled egg containing 4 to 16 brownish cells (Figure 7-9) when deposited and are referred to collectively

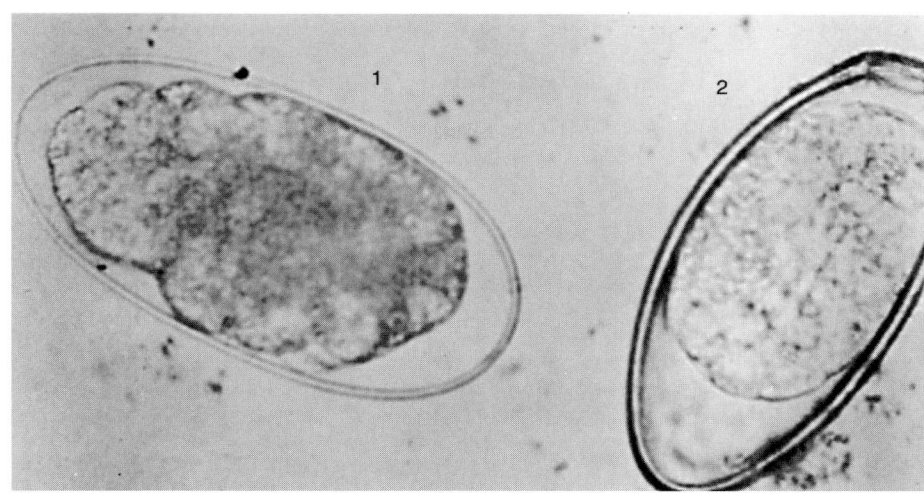

FIGURE 7-9. *1,* Strongyle egg measuring 95 × 50 μm. *2,* Egg of *Oxyuris equi* measuring 90 × 42 μm.

TABLE 7-2	PARASITICIDES USED TO TREAT INTERNAL PARASITES IN HORSES						
				Parasite			
Drug	*Gasterophilus*	*Ascarids*	*Strongylus vulgaris*	*Strongylus edentatus*	*Small Strongyles*	*Pinworms*	*Strongyloides*
Cambendazole	–	+	+	+	+	+	+
Dichlorvos	+	+	+	+	+	+	–
Febantel	–	+	+	+	+	+	+
Fenbendazole	–	+	+	+	+	+	+
Ivermectin	+	+	+	+	+	+	+
Moxidectin	+	+	+	+	+	+	–
Oxibendazole	–	+	+	+	+	+	+
Oxifendazole	–	+	+	+	+	+	+
Phenothiazine	–	–	+	–	+	–	–
Piperazine salts	–	+	–	–	+	+	–
Pyrantel salts	–	+	+	+	+	–	–
Thiabendazole	–	–	+	+	+	+	+
Thiabendazole/ piperazine	–	+	+	+	+	+	+
Thiabendazole/ trichlorfon	+	+	+	+	+	+	+
Trichlorfon	+	+	–	–	–	+	–
Trichlorfon/ phenothiazine/ piperazine	+	+	+	–	+	+	–

+, Indicated for use; –, not indicated for use.

as *strongyle eggs,* a term that refers to the order of nematodes to which this group belongs (order Strongyloidea, the bursate nematodes).

Technician Note

All equine strongyles produce a similar thin-walled egg containing 4 to 16 brownish cells.

All the strongyles are common in horses throughout the United States, and the incidence of infection is generally high. The small strongyles that have been studied have a simple, direct life cycle. The eggs pass in feces, and a first-stage larva develops within the egg. Once developed, the larva hatches and undergoes a free-living existence,

developing and molting to a second-stage free-living larva. It then develops into a third-stage larva that does not feed and awaits ingestion. In ideal environmental conditions, development from the egg stage to the infective larva will occur in less than 1 week. Once the small strongyle is ingested, the larva goes to the cecum, penetrates the cecal mucosa, and develops for 1 to 2 weeks. The larva then returns to the mucosal surface and matures within an additional 1 to 2 weeks. All the species in the genus *Strongylus* have very complex life cycles.

The development of the larval stages for large strongyles in the environment is the same as that for the small strongyles, and once ingested they also penetrate the mucosa of the cecum and develop within a short period of time. *S. vulgaris,* the most important of the large strongyles, leaves the mucosa and by some means goes to the cranial mesenteric artery and its branches and develops in the lumen of the arteries over the next 6 months, becoming a young adult. It then returns to the cecum and matures; the entire prepatent period (the period of time after ingestion and before eggs pass in feces) is about 180 to 200 days. *S. equinus* leaves the cecal mucosa and enters the peritoneal cavity. It then goes to the liver and develops into a young adult. The route taken back to the cecum is incompletely understood, but it may enter the pancreas. The entire prepatent period may be as long as 265 days.

S. edentatus leaves the mucosa and enters the subperitoneal tissue, particularly in the right dorsal flank. Eventually, it enters the venous circulation and goes to the liver. Supposedly, it leaves the liver and about 2 months later migrates in the mesenteries to the perirenal fat for an additional 3 months. It again migrates in the mesenteries to the large intestine, which it penetrates, and develops to maturity in the lumen of the cecum. The entire prepatent period requires 300 to 322 days. Diagnosis of the strongyles can be accomplished by a number of techniques, and they are amenable to treatment by a number of anthelmintics (see Table 7-2). Control is difficult because the parasites are prolific egg producers and development of the larva occurs rapidly. Control is best applied by a treatment and management regimen based on environmental conditions and by limiting the number of horses on the pasture.

Intestinal Threadworm

Strongyloides westeri is a common parasite of horses, principally of foals 2 weeks to 6 months of age, and is widespread across the United States. The life cycle is essentially the same as *Strongyloides stercoralis* of the dog, with the exception that the parthenogenetic female produces a thin-walled egg containing a first-stage larva when deposited (Figure 7-10). Diagnosis can be performed by a number of techniques; however, fresh feces must be used because the eggs will hatch in older feces. Recommended treatments are given in Table 7-2. Control necessitates good hygiene, together with treatment, because the parasite can be transmitted by the transmammary route.

Tapeworms

Anoplocephala perfoliata, *Anoplocephala magna*, and *Paranoplocephala mamillana* are the tapeworms of horses. They are broad, thick, and white and vary in length from about 2.5 cm (*A. perfoliata*) to 75 cm (*A. magna*), although most tapeworms are about 15 cm. The eggs of all species are similar and tend to be amber or have almost no color. The eggs often have a peculiar shape, varying from almost round to somewhat square. The life cycles of all three tapeworms are similar in that the egg is ingested by a free-living mite for further development. In the mite, a small larval form, the cysticercoid, develops to the infective stage within 2 to 4 months. Once ingested by the horse, the larval stage is released from the mite and develops into an adult tapeworm within 6 to 10 weeks. Diagnosis is readily performed by a number of techniques because the eggs mix with the feces. Treatment or control is seldom practiced.

Parasites of Ruminants

Strongyles

Cattle and sheep in the United States are commonly infected by a number of species of strongyle nematodes (order Strongyloidea, the bursate nematodes). Species in the genera *Haemonchus*, *Ostertagia*, *Trichostrongylus*, *Cooperia*, and *Nematodirus* are the most common. These nema-

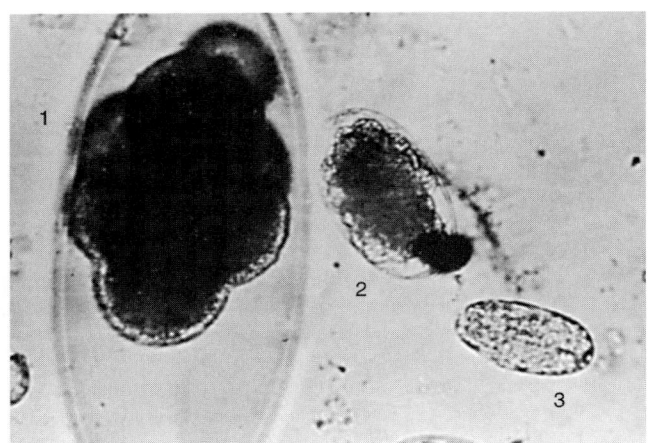

FIGURE 7-10. *1*, Egg of *Nematodirus* measuring approximately 200 × 95 μm. *2*, Strongyle-type eggs measuring approximately 86 × 40 μm. *3*, Egg of *Strongyloides* measuring approximately 52 × 25 μm.

todes vary in size from about 6 mm (*Trichostrongylus*) to about 25 to 30 mm (*Haemonchus*). All except *Nematodirus* produce a similar "strongyle" egg, which is thin walled and contains 4 to 16 brown-colored cells when deposited (Figure 7-10). *Nematodirus* produces an extremely large egg (Figure 7-10). These parasites are widely distributed throughout the United States, but their incidence depends on their ability to develop in the external environment. Some, such as *Haemonchus*, need considerable warmth and moisture, whereas others, such as *Ostertagia*, *Trichostrongylus*, and *Nematodirus*, will withstand colder, drier climates.

The life cycles, although somewhat variable among species, are similar. The first larval stage develops within the egg and hatches to undergo a free-living existence. The larval stage develops within the egg and grows and molts to the third-stage infective form in less than 2 weeks. Once ingested by the host, the larval stage generally penetrates the mucosa in the site it normally inhabits (stomach, small intestine, large intestine) and develops in a short period of time and then returns to the surface of the mucosa and matures. Diagnosis can be effectively performed by most techniques. Several treatments are available (Table 7-3). Control is best practiced by a combination of treatment and pasture management in areas in which there is an abundance of warmth and moisture to promote survival of the larval stages on pastures.

Lungworms

The lungworms of cattle and sheep are *Dictyocaulus viviparus* (cattle) and *Dictyocaulus filaria* (sheep). They are slender, white nematodes; males are 3 to 8 cm long, whereas females are 3 to 10 cm long. Females produce an egg containing a first-stage larva that hatches in the lungs. The first-stage larva passes up the bronchial tree and is swallowed, passing with the feces. Lungworms occur in animals throughout the United States, but their distribution is discontinuous because the larval stages require a certain amount of warmth and moisture to survive. The life cycle is simple and direct. The first-stage larvae live on stored food granules, developing to the third-stage infective form within less than 1 week in optimum environmental conditions. Once ingested, they enter the intestine, penetrate the intestinal mucosa, enter the lymphatic vessels, and develop for a short period in lymph nodes. They

TABLE 7-3   Parasiticides Used to Treat Internal Parasites in Cattle, Sheep, and Goats

Drug	Haemon-chus	Oster-tagia	Tricho-strongylus	Cooperia	Nema-todirus	Strongy-loides	Bunos-tomum	Trich-uris	Oesopha-gostomum	Cha-bertia	Dicty-ocaulus	Monezia	Fas-ciola	Coc-cidia
Albendazole	+	+	+	+	+	–	+	+	+	+	+	+	+	–
Amprolium	–	–	–	–	–	–	–	–	–	–	–	–	–	–
Chlorsulon	–	–	–	–	–	–	–	–	–	–	–	–	+	–
Decoquinate	–	–	–	–	–	–	–	–	–	–	–	–	–	+
Fenbendazole	+	+	+	+	+	+	+	+	+	+	+	–	–	–
Haloxon	+	+	+	+	+	–	+	–	+	+	+	–	–	–
Ivermectin	+	+	+	+	+	+	+	–	+	+	+	–	–	–
Lasolacid	–	–	–	–	–	–	–	–	–	–	–	–	–	+
Levamisole	+	+	+	+	+	+	+	+	+	+	+	–	–	–
Moxidectin	+	+	+	+	+	–	+	–	+	–	+	–	–	–
Monensin	–	–	–	–	–	–	–	–	–	–	–	–	–	+
Morantel tartrate	+	+	+	+	+	+	+	–	+	+	+	–	–	–
Phenothiazine	+	+	+	–	–	–	–	–	+	–	–	–	–	–
Sulfonamides	–	–	–	–	–	–	–	–	–	–	–	–	–	+
Thiabendazole	+	+	+	+	+	+	+	–	+	+	–	–	–	–

+, Indicated for use; –, not indicated for use.

go to the heart, enter the circulatory system, and then go into the lungs to mature in a total of 25 to 30 days. Diagnosis is best performed by use of the Baermann funnel technique. Only a few anthelmintics are considered acceptable (see Table 7-3). Control is best exercised by proper management, ensuring that cattle and sheep do not occupy wet, swampy pastures.

Technician Note
Diagnosis of cattle and sheep lungworms is best performed by use of the Baermann funnel technique.

Tapeworms
Tapeworms in cattle and sheep are *Moniezia expansa* and *Moniezia benedini*. In addition, *Thysanosoma actinioides* occurs in sheep. The *Moniezia* spp. reach lengths of 4 cm, whereas *Thysanosoma* is generally 25 to 30 cm long. *Moniezia* spp. are widespread across the United States, but *T. actinioides* is found only in the western regions. The life cycle of *Moniezia* spp. is the same as for the *Anoplocephala* spp. found in horses, and they use similar free-living mites. The cycle of *T. actinioides* is not known. Diagnosis of the *Moniezia* spp. is readily accomplished by a number of acceptable techniques because the eggs mix with the feces; however, diagnosis of *T. actinioides* can be accomplished only through observation of the pearly white bell-shaped proglottid on the fecal mass. Treatment is seldom applied to *Moniezia* spp. or *T. actinioides*. Control would be difficult, necessitating control of the mites.

Technician Note
The cattle and sheep liver fluke requires the snail as the intermediate host.

Liver Flukes
The common trematodes of cattle and sheep are *Fasciola hepatica* and *Fascioloides magna*. Both trematodes are greenish, flat, and leaflike in shape. *F. hepatica* is about 25 mm long, and *F. magna* is about 50 to 75 mm long. The eggs of both trematodes are very similar and are large and yellow-brown with an operculum, or "lid," at one end (Figure 7-11). *F. hepatica* and *F. magna* are widespread throughout the United States but only in wet, swampy, or subirrigated areas that will support substantial populations of the snail intermediate hosts. The natural hosts for *F. hepatica* are cattle and sheep, but the natural hosts for *F. magna* are members of the deer family. *F. magna* cannot complete its life cycle (by passing eggs into the environment) in cattle and sheep.

The life cycles of both trematodes are similar and quite complex. Eggs passing in the feces must land in water to develop. Inside the egg, a small, ciliated miracidium develops, leaves the egg, and penetrates the tissue of a specific snail, in which it undergoes asexual replication through larval stages called *sporocysts* and *rediae*, ultimately developing into a *cercaria*, which leaves the snail to encyst on vegetation and await ingestion. Once ingested, it goes into the intestine, penetrates through to the body cavity, and penetrates the surface of the liver, in which it wanders for several weeks. *F. hepatica* eventually enters the bile ducts, whereas *F. magna* will form a cyst wall around itself with an opening into a bile duct if it infects members of the deer

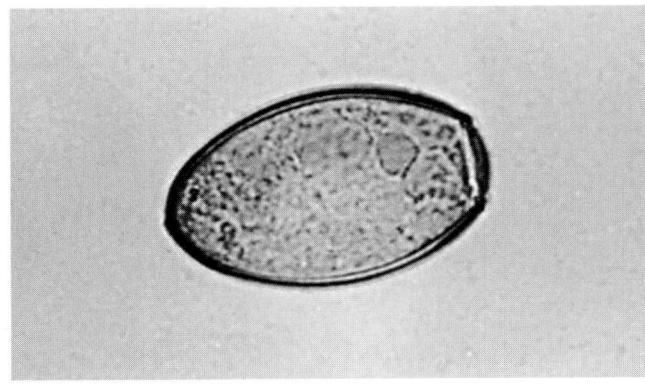

FIGURE 7-11. Egg of *Fasciola hepatica* measuring approximately 130 × 70 μm.

family. In cattle, a calcified cyst is found, whereas in sheep, the parasite continues to wander throughout the liver. The eggs are very heavy and will not float; consequently, a sedimentation procedure is used for diagnosis. Effective treatment is available (see Table 7-3). Control necessitates draining and drying wet, swampy pastures to prevent an overabundance of snails.

Coccidia
Several species of coccidia infect cattle and sheep, and all belong to the genus *Eimeria*. Coccidia are common throughout the United States, and most animals are infected with at least one of the *Eimeria* spp. The severity of the infection depends on the environmental condition (warmth, moisture), stocking intensity, age, and previous exposure. Oocysts of the *Eimeria* spp. sporulate in the environment and reach the infective stage in the same manner as do *Isospora* spp. *Eimeria* spp., however, develop four sporocysts, each of which contains two sporozoites, for a total of eight infective forms per oocyst. The life cycle of *Eimeria* spp. is identical to that of *Isospora* spp., with the exception that an intermediate host is not required. Diagnosis may be accomplished effectively by a number of techniques. A number of treatments are available for the clinical disease (see Table 7-3). Control is difficult because oocysts are highly resistant. Proper management for coccidiosis includes prevention of overcrowding and contamination of feed and water and the use of dry bedding.

Trichomoniasis
Trichomonas foetus is a common protozoan parasite of cattle. This small, flagellated protozoan is equipped with three anterior flagella, an undulating membrane, and a trailing flagellum. Generally, *T. foetus* is a slender, pear-shaped organism. The bull acts as a carrier, with the parasite living on the surface of the penis or in the prepuce. When transmitted by coitus to the cow, the organism develops in the vagina and uterus, causing abortion or fetal resorption. *Trichomonas* multiples by binary fission; consequently, large populations can be generated in a short time. The cows, given a rest through two or three estrous cycles, will usually develop partial immunity. Diagnosis and treatment are performed on the bull. Diagnosis is difficult and complex. Control necessitates resting the cows and allowing immunity to develop, treatment or elimination of infected bulls, and purchase of virgin bulls for breeding.

TABLE 7-4	PARASITICIDES USED TO TREAT INTERNAL PARASITES IN SWINE							
	Parasite							
Drug	Ascaris	Strongyloides	Oesophagostomum	Trichuris	Hyostrongylus	Metastrongylus	Stephanurus	Coccidia
Dichlorvos	+	−	+	+	+	−	−	−
Fenbendazole	+	−	+	+	+	+	−	−
Hygromycin B	+	−	+	+	−	−	−	−
Ivermectin	+	+	+	−	+	+	+	−
Levamisole	+	+	+	−	+	+	+	−
Piperazine salts	+	−	−	−	−	−	−	−
Pyrantel tartrate	+	−	+	−	−	−	−	−
Sulfonamides	−	−	−	−	−	−	−	+
Thiabendazole	−	+	+	−	+	−	−	−

+, Indicated for use; −, not indicated for use.

Parasites of Swine

Stomach Worms

Three stomach worms occur in swine: *Hyostrongylus rubidus*, *Ascarops strongylina*, and *Physocephalus sexalatus*. *H. rubidus* is the most common and the most pathogenic of the three, usually occurring in adult pigs. Its parasitic development is similar to that of *Ostertagia* in ruminants. Diagnosis is based on finding strongyle eggs in the fecal sample, but the eggs can be confused with the eggs of *Oesophagostomum*, which also occurs in pigs. Treatment is given in Table 7-4. *Ascarops* and *Physocephalus* use beetles as their intermediate hosts and are rarely a problem in swine.

Ascaris

Ascaris suum is the large roundworm and is by far the most common parasite encountered in pigs. Its parasitic development is similar to that of *Parascaris* in the horse. *A. suum* is usually more common in pigs under 1 year of age. Diagnosis is based on finding ascarid eggs in fecal samples. Treatment is given in Table 7-4.

Technician Note

Ascaris suum is the large roundworm and is by far the most common parasite encountered in pigs.

Strongyloides

Strongyloides ransomi is found in the small intestine of young swine. Its parasitic development is similar to that of *Strongyloides* in the horse. Diagnosis is based on finding embryonated eggs in fresh fecal samples. Treatment is given in Table 7-4.

Oesophagostomum

Several species of *Oesophagostomum* occur in the large intestine of pigs. Their life cycle is similar to that of *Oesophagostomum* in ruminants. Diagnosis is based on finding typical strongyle eggs in fecal samples. Again, these eggs can be confused with the eggs of *Hyostrongylus* and *Trichostrongylus*. Treatment is given in Table 7-4.

Whipworm

The whipworm of swine is *Trichuris suis*. These worms usually occur in the cecum, and their parasitic development is similar to that of *Trichuris* in dogs. Diagnosis is based on finding typical *Trichuris* eggs in the feces. Treatment is given in Table 7-4.

Lungworm

Three species of *Metastrongylus* occur in the lungs of swine. Earthworms act as the intermediate host for the swine lungworm. Most commonly, the posteroventral part of the diaphragmatic lobe of the lung is involved. Diagnosis is made by finding rough-shelled, embryonated eggs in the feces. Treatment of lungworm infection in swine is given in Table 7-4.

Technician Note

The intermediate hosts for the swine lungworm are earthworms.

Kidney Worms

Stephanurus dentatus is the kidney worm in swine. The adult worms live in the kidneys and perirenal tissue and pass eggs into the urinary bladder. Infection in pigs occurs by ingestion of third-stage larva, ingestion of earthworms containing the third-stage larva, skin penetration, and in utero infection. Although eggs can be identified in urine, diagnosis is usually made at necropsy. Treatment is given in Table 7-4.

ECTOPARASITES

Parasites of Domesticated Animals

The ectoparasites of domesticated animals generally are members of the phylum Arthropoda. There are many different types of ectoparasites, including fleas, mites, lice, ticks, chiggers, bloodsucking flies, and myiasis-inducing flies. Some are host specific, whereas others infect any number of animals. Diagnosis generally is based on the external morphologic appearance, using taxonomic keys. A number of treatments are available (Tables 7-5 to 7-8). Control is often very difficult, sometimes necessitating treatment of the premises and prevention by prohibiting interaction with infected animals (e.g., fleas, ticks, and lice on companion animals).

Fleas

Ctenocephalides canis (Figure 7-12) and *Ctenocephalides felis* are the most common fleas of dogs and cats; *C. felis* is the most common. They are not host specific and will attack other animals and humans. They are widely distributed but are much more common in warm, humid environments. When environmental conditions are favorable, the flea has

TABLE 7-5	PARASITICIDES USED FOR CONTROL OF EXTERNAL PARASITES ON DOGS AND CATS			
	Parasite			
Drug	*Fleas*	*Lice*	*Mites*	*Ticks*
Allethrin	+	–	–	–
Amatraz	–	–	+	–
Carbaril	+	+	+	+
Chlorpyrifos	+	+	+	+
Cythioate	+	–	–	–
D-Limonene	+	+	–	–
Diazinon	+	+	–	+
Fenthion	+	–	–	–
Fipronil	+	+	–	+
Imidacloprid	+	+	–	–
Lime-sulfur	–	–	+	–
Lindane (not legal in United States)	+	+	+	+
Linalool	+	–	–	–
Lufenuron	+	–	–	–
Malathion	+	+	–	+
Methylcarbamate	+	+	–	+
Permethrin	+	+	–	+
Phosmet	+	+	+	+
Pyrethrins	+	+	–	+
Resmethrin	+	+	–	–
Rotenone	+	+	–	+
Selamectin	+	–	+	+

+, Indicated for use; –, not indicated for use.

TABLE 7-6	PARASITICIDES USED FOR CONTROL OF EXTERNAL PARASITES ON HORSES				
	Parasite				
Drug	*Lice*	*Flies*	*Mites*	*Ticks*	*Maggots*
Coumaphos	+	+	–	+	+
Malathion	+	+	+	+	–
Permethrin	+	+	–	+	–
Pyrethrins	+	+	–	–	–

+, Indicated for use; –, not indicated for use.

TABLE 7-7	PARASITICIDES USED FOR CONTROL OF EXTERNAL PARASITES ON CATTLE, SHEEP, AND GOATS											
	Parasite											
Drug	Cattle Grub	Horn Fly	Face Fly	Other Flies	Maggots	Chewing Lice	Sucking Lice	Psoroptic Mite	Other Mites	Ear Ticks	Other Ticks	Sheep Ked
Carbaril	–	+	+	+	–	+	+	–	–	+	+	–
Coumaphos	+	+	+	+	+	+	+	+	–	+	+	+
Chlorpyrifos	–	+	–	–	–	+	+	–	–	–	–	–
Dichlorvos	–	+	+	+	–	–	–	–	–	–	+	–
Famphur	+	–	–	–	–	+	+	–	–	+	+	–
Doramectin	–	–	–	–	–	+	+	–	–	–	–	–
Fenthion	+	–	–	–	–	+	+	–	–	+	+	–
Fenvalerate	–	+	+	–	–	–	–	–	–	+	–	–
Ivermectin	+	–	–	–	–	–	+	+	+	+	+	–
Methoxychlor	–	+	+	+	–	+	+	–	–	+	+	–
Moxidectin	+	+	–	–	–	+	+	+	+	–	–	–
Permethrin	–	+	+	–	–	–	+	–	–	+	–	–
Phosmet	+	+	–	–	–	+	+	+	+	+	+	–
Pyrethrins	–	+	+	+	–	–	–	–	–	–	–	–
Rotenone	–	–	–	–	–	+	+	–	–	–	–	+
Trichlorfon	+	+	–	–	+	+	+	–	–	+	+	–

+, Indicated for use; –, not indicated for use.

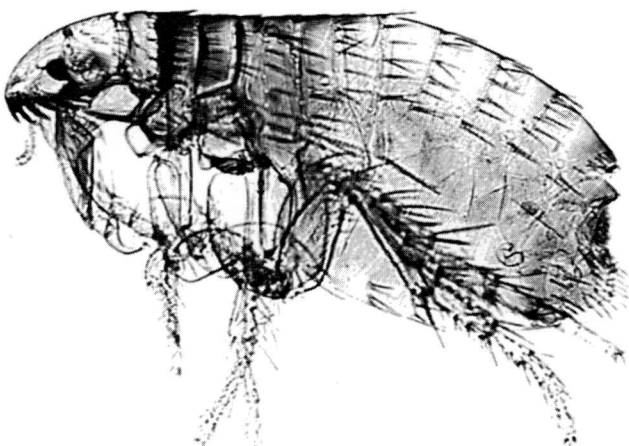

FIGURE 7-12. *Ctenocephalides canis,* the common dog flea.

Drug	Parasite			
	Lice	*Flies*	*Mites*	*Maggots*
Coumaphos	+	+	–	+
Fenthion	+	–	–	–
Ivermectin	+	–	+	–
Malathion	+	–	+	–
Methoxychlor	+	–	–	–
Permethrin	+	+	+	–
Pyrethrins	–	+	–	–

TABLE 7-8 PARASITICIDES USED FOR CONTROL OF EXTERNAL PARASITES ON SWINE

+, Indicated for use; –, not indicated for use.

a great reproductive potential. Fleas thrive at low altitudes in temperature ranges of 65° F to 80° F (18.2° to 26.6° C). Under these conditions, the flea life cycle can be completed, from hatching of an egg to the laying of the next generation of eggs, in as little as 16 days.

Technician Note

The flea life cycle can be completed in as little as 16 days, making control difficult.

The female flea lays her eggs in the fur of dogs and cats. The eggs are not sticky and tend to fall out of the fur and survive in the protected places where a dog or cat sleeps or plays. The eggs will hatch into very small wormlike larvae. The larvae feed on organic debris, especially the dried blood droppings (flea dirt) left by adult fleas. Thus larvae depend on the dog to return time after time to the places at which the eggs dropped off. The larvae molt and form pupae that spin cocoons and then emerge as young and hungry adults in about 3 weeks. An important source of fleas to a dog and cat is these newly "hatched out" young fleas.

Once fleas have had a chance to establish the life cycle in a house and yard environment, no control program will be successful that does not emphasize environmental control. Mechanical cleaning of the house and yard environment should precede any application of insecticides. In general,

the same environmental control methods may be used in households with young dogs and cats as in those with adults. Care should always be taken that animals and people are not directly exposed to insecticides used in household extermination. All effective in-house programs should take advantage of new technologies in flea control. There are insecticides that have truly long residuals (synthetic pyrethroids or microencapsulated products), and there are insect growth regulators (methoprene, fenoxycarb) marketed for preadult flea control.

Advances in outdoor environmental flea control have been less remarkable. At present, the use of insecticides (compounds that contain chlorpyrifos, malathion, or diazinon as their active ingredient) labeled for outdoor flea control is still the best and most economical approach. Such programs will have to incorporate repeated applications at 2-week intervals throughout the flea season, during which temperature and humidity are favorable for flea reproduction.

Technician Note

Flea products containing lufenuron, fipronil, or imidacloprid as the active ingredient should never be administered or used on nursing animals.

All topical insecticides should only be used according to label directions because it is not legally permissible to use or recommend the use of insecticide products beyond label restrictions (see Table 7-5). In general, the use of organophosphate preparations on puppies younger than 16 weeks or on kittens younger than 6 months should be avoided. Any product containing lufenuron, fipronil, or imidacloprid as its active ingredient should never be administered or used on nursing animals. Pyrethrin-based products are generally safe for frequent application; the most effective products are synergized pyrethrin sprays or foams (see Table 7-5). Very small animals and nursing animals sprayed with alcohol-based or other volatile organic solvents may be severely chilled as the solvent evaporates. Water-based sprays are preferable, and small animals and nursing animals should never be thoroughly saturated with a spray. The safest effective products are sprays and foams with microencapsulated pyrethrins. Flea collars that are safe for use on puppies or kittens are not effective in most environments. Topical treatments should be coordinated with in-home environmental flea control (see Table 7-5).

Rabbit Bots and Fox Maggots

Cuterebra spp., the rabbit bot, and *Wohlfahrtia* spp., the fox maggot, occasionally infest dogs, cats, rodents, rabbits, and other wildlife. *Cuterebra* spp. flies usually deposit eggs around burrows or runs. Eggs hatch, and the larvae penetrate the skin of the host, developing to the third stage in subcutaneous tissue without migrating in the host. The larvae then come out of a hole in the skin and pupate in the soil. Females of the *Wohlfahrtia* spp. deposit larvae on the skin of the host, which is usually a young animal. The larvae penetrate and develop in the subcutaneous tissues with limited migration. When they become third-stage larvae, they come out of a hole in the skin and pupate in the soil. Diagnosis of *Cuterebra* is based on the morphologic appearance of the larva, whereas *Wohlfahrtia* spp. diagnosis necessitates using the morphologic appearance of the stigmatal plates and, sometimes, the morphologic appearance of the cephalopharyngeal skeleton. Treatment necessitates surgical removal of the larvae and supportive wound treatment.

Bot Flies

Gasterophilus intestinalis, *Gasterophilus nasalis*, and *Gasterophilus hemorrhoidalis*, the bot flies of horses, are widespread and common, but *G. intestinalis* is the most common. The adult fly cements eggs to the hair of the horse. Either the eggs hatch by themselves and the larvae crawl into the mouth, or the eggs are stimulated to hatch by being licked by the horse. Once in the mouth, the larvae penetrate the mucosa and burrow down the esophagus to the stomach, in which they emerge and develop into the third stage. They usually spend about 10 months as larvae. Ultimately, the larvae pass out with the feces, burrow into the soil, pupate, and later emerge as adult flies, usually in late summer. Diagnosis is based on the type of egg and means of attachment of the spines on each segment (single row, *G. nasalis*; double row, *G. intestinalis*; double row, smaller spines, *G. hemorrhoidalis*). Treatment is generally applied in the fall with a combination of insecticides and anthelmintics or a broad-spectrum compound (see Table 7-2). Control is difficult.

Heel Flies

The heel flies of cattle, *Hypoderma lineatum* and *Hypoderma bovis*, whose larval stages are called *grubs* or *warbles*, are widely distributed wherever cattle are found. Emergence of these flies depends on environmental conditions. For example, they are active in early January in southern Texas and in early August in Montana. When both species are present, *H. bovis* emerges about 1 month later than *H. lineatum*. After emergence, *H. bovis* lays single eggs attached to hair, and *H. lineatum* lays a row of eggs just above the hooves. The larvae hatch from the egg, penetrate the skin, and wander in the subcutaneous tissue for 4 to 5 months. *H. lineatum* then goes to the esophagus for 2 months, and *H. bovis* goes to the epidural fat of the spinal cord for 2 months. Both then go to the subcutaneous tissue along the back for about 2 months. They develop, come out of a hole in the skin, and burrow in the soil, in which they pupate for 1 to 3 months. Diagnosis is generally based on the presence of the lumps (warbles) on the back of cattle; however, species can be diagnosed based on the morphologic appearance of the larvae. A number of treatments are available (see Table 7-7), but they must be applied at a specific time of year.

Technician Note

Diagnosis of *Hypoderma* spp. of cattle is usually based on the presence of lumps on the back of cattle.

Sheep Nasal Fly

The sheep nasal fly (*Oestrus ovis*; often called the sheep nose bot) is common wherever sheep are found. Flies emerge from spring through fall and deposit first-stage larvae around the nasal opening. Larvae then enter the nasal cavity for 2 weeks to 9 months and migrate to the paranasal sinuses for a short time to complete their development. They leave through the nose and pupate in the soil for 15 to 60 days. The life cycle may be completed within 2 to 11 months, depending on environmental conditions. Diagnosis is based on the presence of these larvae in the nose or sinuses. There is no preferred treatment available.

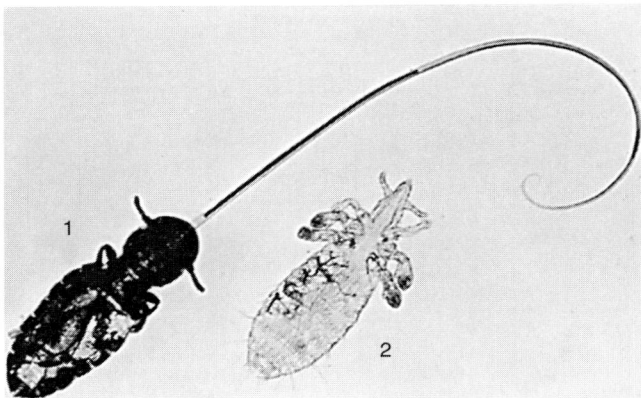

FIGURE 7-13.   *1*, Chewing louse of the order Mallophaga attached to a hair shaft. *2*, Sucking louse of the order Anoplura.

BOX 7-1	LICE ON DOMESTIC ANIMALS

CATTLE
Haematopinus eurysternus, sucking
Linognathus vituli, sucking
Solenopotes capillatus, sucking
Haematopinus quadripertussis, sucking
Damalinia bovis, chewing

SHEEP
Haematopinus tuberculatus, sucking
Linognathus pedalis, sucking
Linognathus ovillus, sucking
Linognathus africanus, sucking
Damalinia ovis, chewing

HORSES
Haematopinus asini, sucking
Damalinia equi, chewing

DOGS
Linognathus piliferus, sucking
Trichodectes canis, chewing

CATS
Felicola subrostratus, chewing

Lice

Domesticated animals commonly are infested with lice of the order Anoplura (sucking lice) (Figure 7-13) and the order Mallophaga (chewing lice). Lice live on the host continuously and infest other animals through direct contact. Lice may be a problem year-round on dogs and cats but are more commonly a problem in the winter months on cattle, goats, sheep, and horses (Box 7-1). Lice deposit an egg, referred to as a *nit*, cemented to the hair or wool of the host. The eggs hatch, and the small larvae are similar to the adult (incomplete metamorphosis). They develop into nymphs and then into adults; the entire life cycle requires 3 to 5 weeks.

Diagnosis is based on the morphologic appearance of the larva, nymph, or adult. Lice of the order Mallophaga have broad heads, and those of Anoplura have pointed heads. Treatment consists of dust, sprays, sponge-on dips, or shampoos, depending on the host and environmental conditions.

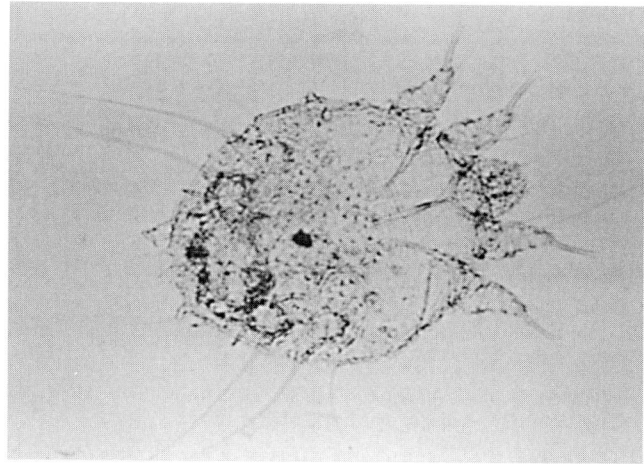

FIGURE 7-14. *Sarcoptes* sp. mite commonly found on dogs and swine.

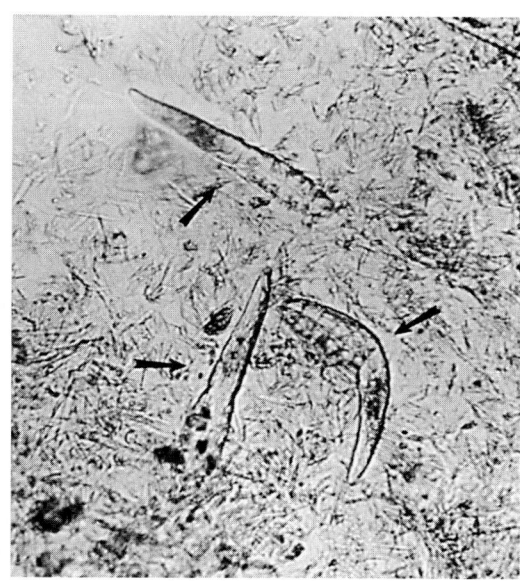

FIGURE 7-15. *Demodex* sp. mite commonly found on dogs.

Mites

The mites commonly found on domesticated animals are given in Box 7-2. Most mites are host specific and even though morphologically similar, subspecies will not cross-infest other hosts. Mites live on the host continuously and infest other animals by contact. The life cycles of these mites are all slightly different because some burrow and others live on the surface of the skin. *Sarcoptes* spp. and *Notoedres cati* females burrow in the skin and deposit eggs. The eggs hatch into six-legged larvae, which develop and molt to eight-legged nymphs, which develop and molt into adults. The entire cycle requires 9 to 17 days.

Species of *Chorioptes, Psoroptes, Psorergates, Otodectes,* and *Cheyletiella* have a similar life cycle except they do not burrow to deposit eggs. *Demodex* spp. generally live in hair follicles. Their life cycle is probably direct, as in the preceding mites, but they can be found in many other tissues of the body.

Technician Note

Mites are usually diagnosed by morphologic appearance of the adult after a skin scraping.

Diagnosis of mites is based on the morphologic appearance of the adult, and it generally requires a thorough skin scraping (Figures 7-14 and 7-15). Sometimes mites, especially *Cheyletiella* and *Demodex*, can be diagnosed by fecal flotation in dog and cat feces because infected animals will bite and lick their skin and ingest mites. Treatment necessitates the use of dust, sprays, sponge-on dips, or shampoos (see Tables 7-5 to 7-8).

Ticks

The ticks found on domesticated animals are not host specific, although they have host preferences, and their distribution is subject to environmental conditions. The species and their host ranges are given in Box 7-3. Ticks are identified as being soft or hard. The most important soft tick is *Otobius megnini,* the spinose ear tick, which lives in the ear of its host. It attaches as a larva, enters the ear, and develops through the larval, nymphal, and adult stages. Adults mate and then drop off. The female deposits eggs and dies.

The hard ticks are generally classified into one-, two-, or three-host ticks. Some, such as *Dermacentor albipictus,* are one-host ticks, attaching as a larva and developing into an adult on that host. Adults drop off, lay eggs, and then die. The three-host ticks attach as larvae, feed, drop off, and molt in the environment to nymphs; reattach to a host, feed, drop off, and molt to adults; and then as adults attach, feed, mate, and drop off to lay eggs and die. *Rhipicephalus sanguineus,* a three-host tick, uses the same host (dog) for all three stages, whereas *Dermacentor venustus* uses small rodents for the larval stage, larger rodents and rabbits for the nymphal stage, and dogs, horses, cattle, and so on for the adult stage. Three-host ticks may

BOX 7-3	TICKS COMMONLY FOUND ON DOMESTIC ANIMALS

OTOBIUS MEGNINI: THE SPINOSE EAR TICK
Most warm-blooded animals

DERMACENTOR ALBIPICTUS: THE WINTER TICK
One-host tick; cattle, sheep, horses, deer, elk, and moose

DERMACENTOR VENUSUTUS (NO COMMON NAME)
Three-host tick; cattle, sheep, horses, wild ruminants, dogs, and humans; immature stages on rodents

DERMACENTOR VARIABILIS: THE AMERICAN DOG TICK
Three-host tick; dogs, primary host; immature stages on rodents

DERMACENTOR NITENS: THE TROPICAL HORSE TICK
One-host tick; horses, donkeys, and mules

AMBLYOMMA AMERICANUM: THE LONE STAR TICK
Three-host tick; cattle, sheep, goats, horses, dogs, cats, and wildlife; nymphs on rodents, larvae often found on birds

AMBLYOMMA MACULATUM: THE GULF COAST TICK
Three-host tick; cattle, sheep, goats, horses, dogs, cats, and wildlife; nymphs on rodents; larvae often found on birds

AMBLYOMMA CAJENNENSE: THE CAYENNE TICK
Three-host tick; mostly horses but also cattle, sheep, goats, and wildlife

IXODES PACIFICUS: THE WESTERN BLACK-LEGGED TICK
Three-host tick; adults feed on deer, dogs, horses, and humans; immature stages found on small mammals, especially white-footed mice

IXODES SCAPULARIS: THE BLACK-LEGGED TICK
Three-host tick; adults feed on deer, dogs, horses, and humans; immature stages found on small mammals, especially white-footed mice

RHIPICEPHALUS SANGUINEUS: THE BROWN DOG OR KENNEL TICK
Three-host tick; usually found on dogs

complete the cycle in a short period of time *(Rhipicephalus)*, whereas other ticks *(Dermacentor)* require 2 years, with 1 year between each stage before reattaching to a host.

Treatment necessitates the use of dusts, sprays, sponge-on dips, collars, or shampoos, depending on the host. Control of *R. sanguineus* requires treatment of the premises and, often, the house or kennel. Control of the other ticks is difficult at best, but the precaution of keeping animals away from infested areas can be practiced.

Myiasis-Producing Flies

Some of the myiasis-inducing flies (those developing in the tissue of animals), such as *Hypoderma*, *Oestrus*, and *Gasterophilus*, are host specific and are discussed according to the appropriate host. Others, such as *Wohlfahrtia* spp. and *Cuterebra* spp., have a more limited host range and are discussed with the hosts usually infested. Blowflies in the genera *Lucilia*, *Calliphora*, and *Phormia*, the flesh flies; species of *Sarcophaga*; and the screw worm fly *Cochliomyia hominivorax* are not host specific and cause problems on several domesticated and wild animals. Blowflies and flesh flies generally deposit eggs (larvae for *Sarcophaga*) on the flesh of dead animals but can use traumatized or soiled areas. The eggs hatch, and the larvae develop through three

larval stages and then drop out of the wound to pupate in the soil. Development of the larvae (maggots) is a function of temperature and varies from 2 to 19 days. Pupation lasts 3 to 7 days. The screw worm fly has essentially the same life cycle but will deposit eggs only in fresh wounds (in living tissue).

Diagnosis is based on the morphologic appearance of the stigmatic plates of the third-stage larvae, except for *Cochliomyia hominivorax*, for which the presence of pigmentation of the tracheal trunks is used for diagnosis. Treatment is usually applied topically (see Tables 7-6 to 7-8). Control measures usually require that procedures such as docking and castration be performed before fly season, dead carcasses be disposed of, and environmental spraying take place.

DIAGNOSTIC PROCEDURES

Fecal Flotation

The nematodes that are parasitic in animals and humans may produce undeveloped eggs, eggs containing larvae, or free larvae. Consequently, special diagnostic procedures often are necessary to determine the parasite with which the animal is infected. For nematodes producing an undifferentiated egg or an egg containing a larva, fresh feces is mixed with a chemical solution of higher specific gravity than water. The chemical solutions most frequently used are sodium chloride, magnesium sulfate, zinc sulfate, sodium nitrate, and sucrose. Eggs in feces mixed with any of the preceding chemical solutions will float to the top and can be removed for examination and identification.

Direct Fecal Smear

The direct smear is best used to aid in the detection of certain protozoan trophozoites found in fecal samples, such as *Trichomonas*, *Giardia*, *Cryptosporidium*, and *Balantidium*. The morphologic appearance and the motility of these organisms can be seen in a direct smear. This method should not be used. The correct procedure is to mix a small quantity of fresh feces with a drop of tap water or physiologic saline solution on a clean microscopic slide. Spread the sample into a thin film, place a coverslip on the slide, and examine it.

Technician Note

Direct smear is not satisfactory to demonstrate eggs of tapeworms, nematodes, and coccidia.

Qualitative Fecal Examination
Willis Technique

A qualitative fecal examination will reveal what parasites are present but not how many. There are a number of procedures for this type of examination, but the most simple technique is the Willis technique. The equipment needed is a sputum vial (or any 48-mm–deep cylinder about 24 mm in diameter), glass microscope slide, coverslip, and tongue depressor. A small amount of feces, about the size of a large pea, is placed in the vial, and sufficient flotation solution is added to cover the feces; then this solution is macerated and mixed. Solution is added until the vial is about half full, and the material is mixed again. The vial is filled with flotation solution until the meniscus bulges slightly, and a clean microscope slide is applied over the vial. This slide is left in place for 10 minutes and then is lifted straight up and turned over, and a coverslip is affixed. Much of the liquid will drain from the slide, but eggs remain firmly attached if the glass is clean. To determine the best level to seek eggs, focus on an air bubble. The chemical solutions most frequently used for this type of examination are sodium nitrate, magnesium sulfate, and sodium chloride.

Disposable Fecal Flotation Kits

Several commercial disposable kits are available that are modifications of the Willis technique. These kits require 1 to 2 g of fecal material, depending on the kit that is used. All the kits have some method for preventing the large particles of fecal material from floating to the top of the vial. As in the Willis technique, a clean microscope slide is placed on top of the vial to collect the eggs that float to the top. It is recommended that the microscope slide be left on top of the flotation vial for 15 to 20 minutes.

Paper Cup Technique

One modification of the Willis technique occasionally used is to mix the chemical solution with a large amount of feces in a paper cup. After thorough maceration, the fluid is strained through two or three layers of cheesecloth (gauze) into a sputum vial. The remainder of the procedure is the same as with the Willis technique. The advantages are that the cup and feces can be discarded, eliminating washing containers, and that cups are handy for field situations. This technique often is used for horses and sheep because of the amount of fiber in the feces. The disadvantages are the same as in the Willis technique.

The advantages of the Willis-type techniques are that they are quick and simple and will provide the observer a qualitative examination for many nematode and tapeworm eggs and some protozoan cysts. These techniques are effective for the recovery of all strongyle-type eggs, as well as eggs of ascarids, *Trichuris, Capillaria,* and *Strongyloides* (egg-producing species only); the protozoan cysts of *Eimeria, Isospora, Cryptosporidium, Sarcocystis,* and *Toxoplasma;* and all the tapeworm eggs that mix with feces. These techniques can be used effectively in horses and ruminants when fragile cysts, larvae, or both are not suspected. However, the disadvantages inherent in these techniques are that they destroy or render unrecognizable fragile cysts and larvae. For dogs, cats, ruminants, and horses in which parasites such as lungworm (any species), *Giardia* spp., *Entamoeba* spp., and *Strongyloides stercoralis* are suspected, another technique—the zinc sulfate centrifugal flotation technique—is recommended.

None of these techniques are suitable for trematode eggs of *Fasciola* and *Fascioloides,* because these eggs are too dense to float, but eggs of *Paragonimus* and *Nanophyetus (Troglotrema)* will float with the use of these techniques.

Zinc Sulfate Centrifugal Flotation Technique

The zinc sulfate centrifugal flotation technique is used almost exclusively for parasites of dogs, cats, and primates. It can also be used for other animals, such as exotic animals or native wild species. The reason it is used for these animals is that the technique is much more versatile, and when examining such animals, a more complete technique is necessary. The technique does not destroy fragile cysts and larvae and is just as effective in recovering the other eggs and cysts as the Willis-type techniques.

Technician Note

The zinc sulfate centrifugal flotation technique is used almost exclusively for parasites of dogs, cats, and primates.

Zinc sulfate, at a specific gravity of 1.18 or 1.20, is usually employed; both specific gravities are effective, but 1.20 is probably best. A small amount of feces (about the size of a large pea) is inserted into a round-bottomed, 10- or 15-ml, plastic centrifuge tube. (Conical 15-ml tubes can be used and are effective, but removal of fecal matter from the tube, especially cat feces, is almost impossible.) The feces should be pushed to the bottom of the tube. Five to ten drops of Lugol's iodine solution are then added, and the mixture is quickly but thoroughly stirred. Sufficient zinc sulfate is then added to fill the tube to approximately half full, and the mixture is thoroughly macerated. Do not let the Lugol's iodine solution remain in contact with feces for more than 1 minute before dilution with zinc sulfate; otherwise, fragile protozoan cysts (e.g., *Giardia*) will distort and rupture.

Fill the tube with zinc sulfate until the meniscus bulges slightly, and then affix an 18-mm × 18-mm or a 22-mm × 22-mm glass coverslip to the top. Be certain to grasp the coverslip at the periphery because human body oils will prevent eggs and cysts from attaching. Gently press the coverslip on the tube, being certain that it makes physical contact without any fecal debris disturbing the seal; otherwise, the centrifuge will "throw" the coverslip.

Place the tube into a swinging head centrifuge and centrifuge for 3 to 5 minutes at 1000 to 1500 revolutions per minute (rpm). When the centrifuge stops, remove the coverslip, place the contents on a clean glass slide, and examine the slide microscopically. The purpose of the Lugol's solution is to stain cysts of *Giardia* and *Entamoeba.* It will also stain tapeworm eggs, larvae, some strongyle eggs, and other findings, but the purpose of the stain is to facilitate recognition of the aforementioned protozoan cysts.

The zinc sulfate technique is excellent for any of the strongyle type eggs—*Strongyloides* (both eggs and larvae), ascarids, hookworms, *Trichuris, Capillaria, Physaloptera,* coccidia, *Entamoeba, Giardia,* all tapeworm eggs that mix with feces, eggs of *Paragonimus* and *Nanophyetus,* and mites such as *Demodex* and *Cheyletiella.* Moreover, the lungworm larvae of dogs and cats, as well as those of ruminants and horses, will float without distortion. The technique cannot be used for *Fasciola* and *Fascioloides* because their eggs are too dense to float in any chemical solution. The technique also is not effective for the trophozoites of rumen or cecal ciliates such as *Balantidium* or the trophozoites of *Trichomonas hominis* (no cyst stage) because they are too fragile for demonstration by any technique other than direct fecal smear.

Formalin–Ethyl Acetate Sedimentation Technique

The formalin–ethyl acetate technique has widespread application in human parasitology and has the advantage that all eggs, cysts, and larvae form sediment and are preserved, regardless of whether they will float. This also is the inherent disadvantage: most other fecal debris likewise is sedimentable.

This technique uses 2% formalin (vol/vol) and ethyl acetate; the remainder of the equipment is the same as in the zinc sulfate technique.

In this technique, a small amount of feces (the size of a large pea) is placed into a small beaker, the beaker is half filled (or filled) with 2% formalin, and the feces are thoroughly macerated. A two- or three-thickness layer of cheesecloth (gauze) is placed over the beaker, and the material is strained into a centrifuge tube. The resulting tube of strained material is filled with 2% formalin and centrifuged at 1000 to 1500 rpm for 1 to 2 minutes. This step is repeated until the supernatant is clear (two or three centrifugations). Approximately half the liquid is poured off, and the fecal matter is dislodged and stirred. Ethyl acetate is added to this half-filled tube. The tube is then stoppered and shaken vigorously. The stopper is removed, and the mixture is centrifuged for 1 to 2 minutes at 1000 to 1500 rpm. When the centrifuge stops, the tube is removed, and an applicator stick is used to gently "ring" the debris at the ethyl acetate–formalin interface (the two liquids are not miscible). The purpose of the ethyl acetate is to trap the lighter debris, removing it from the sediment. Once "ringed," the supernatant is poured off, leaving the bottom 1 to 2 ml of fecal material and formalin. A small amount of this sediment or centrifugate is pipetted onto a microscope slide, a coverslip is affixed, and the material is examined for eggs, cysts, larvae, trophozoites of protozoa, and so forth. A drop of Lugol's solution is added to the periphery of the coverslip and allowed to spread beneath to stain cysts.

The advantages of this technique are that all eggs are present, including trematode eggs, fragile cysts, larvae, and trophozoites of non–cyst-forming (or even cyst-forming) protozoa.

The distinct, and often overwhelming, disadvantage of this technique is that the great majority of debris in the fecal sample (except the very low specific gravity material trapped in the ethyl acetate layer) is in the sediment, making examination extremely difficult. Moreover, the technique is time consuming.

Quantitative Fecal Examination

In many situations, especially in food-producing animals, it is not sufficient just to know whether the animal has parasitizes because most food-producing animals have parasites to some degree. The livestock producer wants to know how severe the infestation is and whether deworming will increase the animals' performance and the net return on their investment. Several procedures are used to perform a quantitative fecal examination for parasitic eggs and larvae. The most common method is described.

Stoll Dilution Technique

A special Stoll flask is available for use with this technique. The flask has two graduations: one at 56 ml and one at 60 ml. However, any 75- to 100-ml flask can be used to substitute for a Stoll flask. The method is as follows:

1. Fill the flask with decinormal caustic soda solution (0.1 N sodium hydroxide) or water to the first graduation.
2. Add feces until fluid goes to the top graduation (4-g displacement).
3. Add several glass beads, place the stop on the flask, and shake until the sample is mixed well. Samples can be stored and soaked overnight or longer in a refrigerator.
4. With a micropipette, transfer 0.15 or 0.075 ml from the thoroughly mixed sample to a clean microscope slide. Cover the fluid with a coverslip, and examine under the microscope, using low power (10×).
5. Examine the entire area under the coverslip, and count the eggs. Next, multiply by the proper dilution factor, either 100 (for 0.15 ml) or 200 (for 0.075 ml) for the eggs per gram of feces.

Stoll Centrifugation Technique

The greatest advantage to the centrifugation modification of the Stoll technique is that it is more sensitive and will detect parasitic eggs when other techniques do not. The method follows.

1. A regular Stoll flask or plastic vial is prepared using 56 ml of water and 4 g of feces. Fill the flask or vial with 56 ml of water to the lower mark. Add feces until the vial is filled to the upper mark (approximately 4 g of fecal material). Mix feces with the water, and when possible, allow feces to soak for 3 to 8 hours. (Mixture should be refrigerated if it stands longer than 2 hours.)
2. Mix thoroughly, and immediately remove 1.5 ml of mixture with a 3-ml syringe.
3. Place the 1.5-ml sample in a 10- to 15-ml test tube, and add flotation solution until a convex meniscus forms at the top of the tube.
4. Place tube in a swing-head centrifuge and place a coverslip on top. Centrifuge at 1500 to 2000 rpm for 2 to 5 minutes.
5. Remove coverslip, and place on a clean microscope slide.
6. Identify and count all the eggs under the coverslip. The count made multiplied by 10 gives the number of eggs per gram. (If more than 50 eggs are seen on the first coverslip and highly accurate results are desirable, the test tube should be topped off with the chemical solution and a second coverslip added before recentrifugation.)

Interpretation of Quantitative Fecal Examination

There is no direct or positive correlation between the number of eggs or larvae found in the feces and the severity of parasitism in the animal. It must also be remembered that during the prepatent period, no eggs or cysts will be seen although the animal may have severe parasitism.

SPECIALIZED DIAGNOSTIC TESTS

Lungworm

The Baermann funnel technique (Figure 7-16) is primarily used to recover larvae of lungworm, although it does have other uses. The funnel consists of a 12.5- to 22.5-cm diameter plastic or glass funnel to which a short piece of rubber tubing is affixed and a centrifuge tube is attached. The funnel is filled with lukewarm tap water, and a screen, gauze, or single layer of facial tissue is lowered into the water. Feces, finely chopped tissues, or culture material is carefully added, and the system is allowed to stand for 24 hours. Larvae filter into the centrifuge tube at the bottom, and the coarse material is held back. The system should not be left for more than 24 hours because the eggs of some nematodes will hatch after this period and so confuse the results. After 24 hours, the rubber hose is clamped, and the centrifuge tube is removed. The bottom 1 or 2 ml of fluid is examined microscopically for larvae.

Microfilaria

Filarial nematodes infect many different tissues of the body and produce an undifferentiated larva called a *microfilaria*. Depending on the species, microfilariae may be found in the blood or the dermis of their host.

Species producing microfilariae that accumulate in the dermis are diagnosed by the *skin maceration technique*. A biopsy of skin measuring at least 12 mm in diameter is finely macerated and allowed to soak for at least 6 hours in physiologic saline solution at approximately 37° C (98.6° F) or about 8 to 10 hours at room temperature (21° C [69.8° F]). At the end of this time, the tissue is strained off,

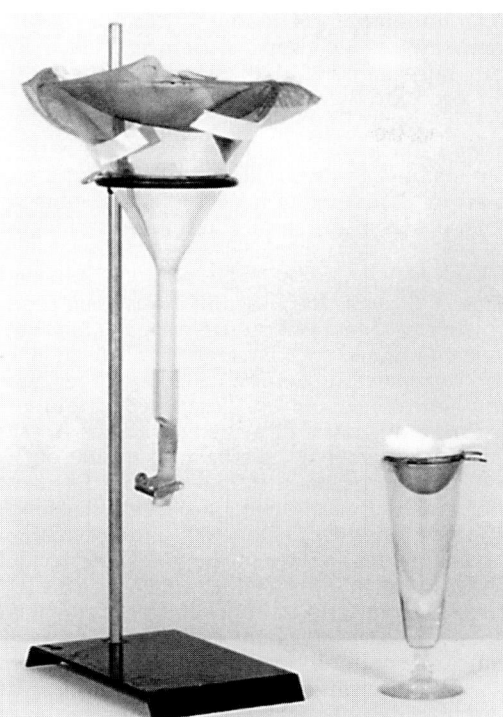

FIGURE 7-16. Baermann apparatus used for recovery of larvae from feces, soil, or minced tissues of an animal.

the liquid is centrifuged, and the bottom 1 or 2 ml is examined for microfilaria. Another method is histologic sectioning of the skin, a procedure that is much more time consuming and not as sensitive as maceration.

For microfilaria of filarial nematodes that occur in the blood, several procedures can be done.

Tests for Blood Microfilaria

DIRECT SMEAR. A thin film of blood is smeared on a slide and dried, and the film is stained with Wright's or Giemsa stain. This is a very poor technique and will work only if microfilariae are numerous.

SALINE PREPARATION. A few drops of freshly drawn blood are mixed with physiologic saline solution, and the resultant preparation is examined microscopically for motile microfilariae. It has the same disadvantages as the direct smear, but when used by technicians experienced in working with microfilaria, it can be very effective.

MICROHEMATOCRIT TECHNIQUE. The microhematocrit tube is examined for microfilariae after centrifugation. Microfilariae will be found at the plasma-blood interface (buffy coat). It has the same disadvantages as the direct smear.

KNOTT TECHNIQUE. Add 1 ml of blood to 9 ml of 2% formalin (or 2 ml of blood in 18 ml of formalin). The mixture is then shaken until hemolysis of the blood occurs; next it is centrifuged at 1500 rpm for 5 minutes. The bottom 0.5 or 1 ml is examined for microfilariae. Microfilariae are preserved, laid straight, and easily measured. Measurements often are necessary to distinguish species and must be done to separate *Dirofilaria* and *Dipetalonema*.

This is the preferred technique for identification of microfilaria.

FILTER TECHNIQUE. Several filter techniques are available commercially for the recovery of microfilaria from the blood. These techniques require 1 ml of blood, which is then mixed with the lysing solution (usually 9 ml) to hemolyze the red blood cells. The mixture is then passed through a plastic chamber containing a filter membrane on which the microfilariae are collected. Next the membrane filter is removed and placed on a clean microscope slide. A drop of stain is placed on top of the membrane, which is covered with a coverslip for examination under the microscope.

> ### ⚡ Technician Note
> The two simplest and most effective techniques to detect blood microfilaria are the filter and the Knott procedures.

The two simplest and most effective techniques described here are the filter and Knott procedures. Both have advantages, depending on the host and parasite.

Pinworms

Pinworms in horses and humans must be diagnosed by the *adhesive tape technique*. With this technique, adhesive tape is folded over a test tube or a smooth, round rod with the adhesive side out. The perianal folds are spread, the tape is applied to the skin in several places, and then the tape is placed on a clean microscope slide with the sticky side down. A few drops of xylene are allowed to seep under the tape to clear the fecal debris, and the slide is examined microscopically for typical pinworm eggs (always flat on one side).

Tapeworms

Most tapeworms occur in the small intestine of their host as adults or, as with *Thysanosoma*, have access to the intestine. All tapeworms use an intermediate host, and because swine, domestic and wild ruminants, or rabbits frequently serve in this capacity, diagnostic procedures for both adult and larval stages must be performed.

ADULT TAPEWORMS. Some adult tapeworms, such as *Moniezia* spp. in ruminants and the anoplocephalids in horses, shed gravid proglottids that are destroyed in the intestine, releasing the eggs to mix with the feces. Any flotation procedures described under nematodes are satisfactory for diagnosis. However, *Thysanosoma* in ruminants and *D. caninum* and *Taenia* spp. in carnivores produce a proglottid that does not break up in the intestine. The proglottid usually passes intact when the animal defecates. Diagnosis necessitates *visual observation* of the proglottid (or chain) on the feces or around the anal region, which is frequently done by observant clients. *Echinococcus* spp. (taeniform tapeworm) in carnivores is an exception in that the eggs usually appear in the feces.

The fish tapeworms found in humans, bears, and wild carnivores shed eggs from the proglottid. Thus the eggs mix with the feces as do *Moniezia* and the anoplocephalids, but this egg is very heavy and will not float; therefore the procedures used for diagnosis of trematodes must be applied (or the formalin–ethyl acetate technique).

LARVAL TAPEWORMS. Most species of tapeworms use arthropods, fish, or mammals as intermediate hosts (an exception is *Hymenolepis diminuta*, which can use an intermediate host but does not need one). Some tapeworms that use mammals as a host have a larva that occurs as a large bladderworm (cysticercus) on the mesenteries or the liver; others produce a small bladderworm that occurs in the muscles. The heavily exercised muscles are the preferred sites for these larvae. Diagnosis may be performed by visual observation of the small bladderworms in the heart, diaphragm, or jaw muscles; by pressing thin slices of tissue between two slides for microscopic examination; by digestion with pepsin–hydrochloric acid; or by histologic section. If the latter technique is used, remember that all tapeworms have small egg-shaped bodies called *calcareous corpuscles* that stain blue or purple with hematoxylin. This will identify the larva as a tapeworm, but it does not identify the species. For species identification, the specific host and the site within the host must be known.

Trematodes

Trematodes (*flukes*) occur in the bile ducts of the liver, parenchyma of the liver, rumen, lungs, small intestine, and other sites, such as skin and oviducts.

Fluke eggs (except *Troglotrema* and *Paragonimus* in the dog) are too heavy to float with the usual chemical solutions available for floating nematode and tapeworm eggs. *Troglotrema* and *Paragonimus* spp. are an exception in that they float with any of the chemical solutions listed earlier.

The diagnostic technique recommended for recovery of fluke eggs, especially liver flukes and fish tapeworm eggs, is to add a small amount of material (one fecal pellet or an equivalent amount) to a centrifuge tube and then add 0.1% detergent. Macerate the feces, shake thoroughly, and then fill with water. Allow to set 5 minutes, decant the supernatant, and repeat the procedure. Continue this until the detergent solution is clear (usually two to five times). The detergent, acting as a wetting agent, separates eggs from fecal debris and allows them to settle. Examine the bottom 1 ml of fluid microscopically for the typical opercular eggs.

Protozoa

Single-celled parasites, such as the helminths, occur in a variety of sites within the animal body. Various species occupy the circulatory system, especially the blood cells; gastrointestinal system (from mouth to anus); and reproductive system. Unfortunately, a variety of techniques must be used for correct diagnosis.

Blood Parasites

Parasites occurring in the blood of an animal, such as *Plasmodium, Haemobartonella, Cytauxzoon, Babesia, Theileria, Leucocytozoon,* or *Trypanosoma,* can be diagnosed by the direct smear technique. The slide is air dried and is then stained with Giemsa or Wright's stain. *Trypanosoma* spp. may not be demonstrable by the direct smear technique; therefore culture in blood agar slants overlaid with liver infusion tryptose medium is the best approach.

Gastrointestinal Protozoa

TRICHOMONAS. *Trichomonas gallinae* from the oral cavity of birds, *Trichomonas equi* from the gastrointestinal tract of horses, and *Trichomonas hominis* from dogs and humans are best demonstrated by direct smear of fresh samples. Lesions suspected of being caused by *T. gallinae* can be scraped (or swabbed), and this material can be mixed with some physiologic saline solution on a clean microscope slide and examined for these typical flagellates. The presence of an undulating membrane is diagnostic. For *T. equi* of horses, one or two drops of fluid expressed from the feces can be examined. If the feces are dry, add saline solution, mix, and then examine a drop.

HEXAMITA MELEAGRIDIS. *Hexamita meleagridis* is the organism responsible for catarrhal enteritis of turkeys and is diagnosed by demonstration of the fast-moving flagellate in the upper part of the small intestine from freshly killed birds.

COCCIDIA. *Eimeria, Isospora,* and *Toxoplasma* produce an oocyst, whereas *Sarcocystis* and *Cryptosporidium* generally produce a sporulated sporocyst, all of which pass with the feces and may be easily demonstrated by either qualitative or quantitative concentration (flotation) techniques.

Sometimes, diagnosis of acute coccidiosis (in sheep or cattle) must be done at necropsy examination. In this situation, a scraping of intestinal mucosa is mixed with physiologic saline solution on a clean microscope slide and examined for schizonts, oocysts, and the small, motile, teardrop-shaped merozoites.

GIARDIA. *Giardia* spp. found in domestic, wild, and laboratory animals ostensibly can be diagnosed by the direct smear technique, but a more effective procedure is the zinc sulfate centrifugal flotation technique. The cysts may be stained with Lugol's solution to make the internal structures easily identifiable.

ENTAMOEBA HISTOLYTICA. The dog is sometimes a transient host for *E. histolytica* and on occasion will show clinical signs of infection. As with *Giardia,* the cyst form is best demonstrated by the zinc sulfate centrifugal flotation technique. Iodine will tint the cyst, facilitating identification. This is an extremely small cyst with four to eight nuclei.

BALANTIDIUM SPP. *Balantidium* is a large ciliate that reportedly causes diarrhea in swine and humans, even though it is usually a commensal organism. Diagnosis is possible by direct smear, observing the large, motile trophozoite, or by the zinc sulfate centrifugal flotation technique, recovering the large cyst. Iodine will stain the sausage-shaped macronucleus as an aid in identification.

HISTOMONAS MELEAGRIDIS. *Histomonas meleagridis* forms a cyst within the egg of the nematode parasite *Heterakis gallinae,* the cecal worm of poultry. In the event of an outbreak of "black head" in turkeys, recovery of the eggs of *H. gallinae* from carrier birds and the presence of pathognomonic lesions in sick turkey poults are sufficient to delineate the cause of the infection as well as the source.

TRICHOMONAS FOETUS. A positive diagnosis of trichomoniasis requires demonstrating the trichomonad from one or more infected animals. There is no serologic or other test based on immunologic reactions that has yet proved practical or specific for trichomoniasis.

Diagnosis in the bull consists of checking the breeding records and determining which bulls are probably infected. After a few days of sexual rest, these bulls should be confined, the preputial hairs clipped, the preputial orifice washed with soap and water and dried, and the bull examined. To collect the smegma sample, a dry plastic insemination pipette is attached to a 10- to 12-ml syringe. The pipette is introduced into the prepuce to its full length. A negative pressure is then created in the syringe, and the pipette is moved vigorously back and forth, scraping the glans penis and preputial membrane. In most bulls, 0.5 to 1 ml of smegma can be collected in the pipette. This material is flushed into a vial containing 2 ml of lactated Ringer's solution or physiologic saline solution. The sample is then layered on Diamond's medium for culturing.

Trichomonas foetus may occur in small numbers; therefore proper handling after collection to avoid extremes of temperature, contact with harmful chemicals, and evaporation must be avoided. It is highly desirable to examine samples within a few hours after collection. Samples should be refrigerated but not frozen if they cannot be cultured immediately. The liquid transport medium (lactated Ringer's solution) is layered on the surface of Diamond's medium and is incubated at 37° C for 48 to 72 hours.

Diamond's medium is very difficult to prepare and is not available commercially but is available from some diagnostic laboratories. Do not use other *Trichomonas* culture media because the great majority will not grow *T. foetus*.

Arthropods

Infestations with ectoparasites means the presence of mites, lice, ticks, chiggers, fleas, or the larval stages of Diptera such as screw worm flies, blowflies, *Hypoderma*, *Gasterophilus*, *Oestrus*, *Cuterebra*, *Cephenomyia* (wild ruminants), or *Wohlfahrtia*. Fortunately, except for mites, the arthropod parasites are sufficiently large that identification is not as difficult as with the other parasites. In general, the host and the site on each host are sufficient.

Mites and Chiggers

Some mites live on the surface of the skin (e.g., *Cheyletiella*, *Otodectes*, *Chorioptes*, *Psoroptes*, and many bird mites), whereas others are burrowing types (e.g., *Demodex*, *Knemidokoptes*, *Sarcoptes*). Consequently, there is no uniform procedure for examination and recovery.

Mites and/or chiggers living under the skin, or even on the surface of the skin, are recovered by deep scraping (sufficiently deep to draw blood) at the periphery of the lesion. Suspected *Demodex* lesions or even any suspected mite or chigger infestation should be clipped of hair and "squeezed" at the time it is scraped to ensure adequate sample collections. This scraped material is then placed on a clean microscope slide that contains mineral oil, covered with a coverslip, and examined with a microscope.

Ticks, Fleas, and Lice

Ticks, fleas, and lice are all of a sufficient size to see with the unaided eye. Ticks and fleas are usually removed and identified. Sometimes lice are difficult to find; therefore a careful examination for nits (louse eggs) attached to the hair may reveal their presence. Accurate louse identification often requires the service of a specialist.

Diptera

The species of Diptera that infest domestic and wild animals are often easily identifiable because they are host or site specific or both (e.g., *Hypoderma*, *Gasterophilus*, *Oestrus ovis*, *Cuterebra*). The larval stages of other dipterous insects are not as easily identified. *Screw worm larvae* can be identified by the presence of two black, pigmented tracheal trunks leading from the spiracular openings of the body. They can be clearly seen in the living third-stage larva with the unaided eye. If a larva does not have pigmented tubules, it is one of myriad blowflies, which can be identified by the pattern of the spiracular openings at the caudal extremity of the body.

The larval stages of *Wohlfahrtia* spp. are parasitic in the very young; skin must be tender for this parasite to penetrate. Identification of the larva is based on the morphologic characteristics of the spiracular plates and cephalopharyngeal skeleton of the third-stage larva.

Preserving Parasitic Samples

Ectoparasites and endoparasites may be adequately preserved in 10% formalin or 70% alcohol. Preservation of tapeworms and flukes for morphologic study is best accomplished by placing the specimen in a dish of water in the refrigerator until it relaxes (overnight) and then replacing this water with cold preservative (10% cold formalin). Preservation of feces can be done with 10% formalin, but this is only satisfactory for some eggs and larvae. Eggs of ascarids, as well as oocysts, will continue to develop. Refrigeration (or even freezing) of feces often is the best approach.

PARASITOLOGY AND PUBLIC HEALTH

Many parasitic diseases can be transmitted between animals and humans (zoonoses). These diseases are always of concern to occupational groups who come into daily contact with a variety of exotic, wild, and domesticated animals. Consequently, the conditions discussed below are those personnel might encounter. Control of most parasitic diseases requires strict attention to personal hygiene and avoidance of contaminated materials. Other zoonosis and public health issues are discussed in Chapter 18.

Cryptosporidosis is caused by *Cryptosporidium* spp. The mode of infection is by direct contact with infected animals and consumption of fecal contaminated water or food. Dogs, cats, calves, lambs, kids, and birds are considered probable sources of infection.

Giardiasis is caused by *Giardia* spp. The mode of infection is by direct contact with infected animals and consumption of fecal contaminated water. Dogs and cats are considered probable sources of infection.

Toxoplasmosis is caused by *Toxoplasma gondii*. Infection can be acquired from sporulated oocysts in cat feces or ingestion of raw or insufficiently cooked meat.

Hydatidosis is caused by infection with the hydatid cyst of the eggs of *Echinococcus granulosus* or *Echinococcus multilocularis*.

Tapeworms are acquired by ingestion of raw or poorly cooked beef (*Taenia saginata*) or pork (*Taenia solium*).

Creeping eruption is caused by penetration of the skin by larval stages of dog and cat hookworm of the genus *Ancylostoma*.

Visceral larva migrans is caused by ingestion of the infective larvae (within the egg) of *Toxocara canis*, especially by very young children.

Strongyloidosis is caused by infection, generally by *Strongyloides stercoralis*, which infects humans, dogs, cats, and foxes.

Trichinosis is caused by infection with *Trichinella spiralis*, generally from consumption of raw or insufficiently cooked pork or bear.

Scabies include the mites that are not strictly host specific and can live for varying amounts of time on alternate hosts. Such mites include *Sarcoptes*, *Notoedres*, or *Cheyletiella*.

APPENDIX

Lugol's Solution

Add 10 g of potassium iodide and 5 g of iodine crystals to 1 L of distilled water and place in a brown (amber) bottle (otherwise it will lose strength). These chemicals do not go into solution readily; heating or preparation several weeks in advance of use is necessary.

Zinc Sulfate

Zinc sulfate at a specific gravity of 1.18 is made by adding 331 g of zinc sulfate to 1 L of distilled water (tap water will suffice). However, because zinc sulfate is hygroscopic, 331 g seldom is adequate, and a hydrometer *must* be used to adjust the specific gravity. To make a solution of specific gravity 1.20, keep adding zinc sulfate until the proper density is obtained.

Ingredients for Willis Technique

GENERAL.   As indicated in the text, the simple flotation technique (Willis technique) of nematode eggs, tapeworm eggs, coccidia, and so forth, which is often used to detect gastrointestinal parasitism in animals and humans, uses concentrated sodium chloride, magnesium sulfate, sodium nitrate, or sugar solutions. All solutions are essentially equally effective, but some (sodium chloride) are more readily available and less expensive than others (sugar). The recipes for each are given below.

SODIUM CHLORIDE.   Saturated sodium chloride has a specific gravity of 1.20. A saturated solution is made by adding 311 g of sodium chloride to 1 L of water. A simple procedure is to keep adding salt to warm or hot water until no more goes into solution. Cool to room temperature. Do not decant the excess salt because this will ensure that a saturated solution is maintained.

SODIUM NITRATE.   Sodium nitrate is used as a saturated solution at a specific gravity of 1.36. It is made by adding 616 g of sodium nitrate to 1 L of water. As with sodium chloride, a simple procedure is to add sodium nitrate to warm or hot water until no more goes into solution.

MAGNESIUM SULFATE.   A saturated solution of magnesium sulfate has a specific gravity of 1.30 and is made by adding 337 g of magnesium sulfate to 1 L of water. As with sodium chloride and sodium nitrate, it can be added to warm or hot water until no more goes into solution.

SUGAR.   Table sugar (cane or beet source) is used at a specific gravity of 1.2 to 1.3 and is made by adding approximately 1500 g of sugar to 1 L of water. As in the preceding recipes, heating the water will facilitate the sugar

going into solution. Between 18 and 20 ml of phenol or formaldehyde must be added as a preservative.

Baermann Funnel

The Baermann apparatus may be used for the recovery of larvae from the feces, soil, or minced tissues of an animal. Although variable results are frequently obtained with this technique, semiquantitative results may be expected from its careful use. Identification depends on the migration of the larvae from the feces, tissues, or soil into water of a warmer temperature, which is brought into contact with the bottom of the material to be examined. Equipment consists of a glass funnel about 25 cm in diameter in which a wire gauze of 1-mm mesh (about 22.5 cm in diameter) is placed. The funnel is joined to a centrifuge tube by means of a rubber tube, the latter being provided with a pinchcock. In use, the assembled funnel is placed in a ring stand. Before use, the funnel is filled with lukewarm water to the level of the wire gauze. The material to be examined is thoroughly broken up and placed on the gauze. Usually within 10 to 15 minutes, larvae may be observed migrating into the water, and a large number may be recovered by drawing the material into the centrifuge tube by means of the pinchcock. The largest yield will be obtained by allowing the material to remain in the funnel for 24 hours before drawing off the larvae.

RECOMMENDED READING

Hoskins JD, Cupp EW: Ticks of veterinary importance. I. The Ixodidae family: identification, behavior, and associated diseases, *Compend Cont Educ Pract Vet* 10(5):564, 1988.

Hoskins JD, Cupp EW: Ticks of veterinary importance. II. The Argasidae family: identification, behavior, and associated diseases, *Compend Cont Educ Pract Vet* 10(6):699, 1988.

Parasitology, *Compend Cont Educ Pract Vet* 14(5):575, 1992.

Sloss MW, Kemp RL, Zajac AM: *Veterinary clinical parasitology*, ed 6, Ames, 1994, Iowa State University Press.

Thienpont D, Rochette F, Vanparijs OFJ: *Diagnosing helminthiasis through coprological examination*, Washington Crossing, NJ, 1979, Pitman Moore.

Williams FW, Zajac AM: *Diagnosis of gastrointestinal parasitism in dogs and cats*, St Louis, 1980, Ralston Purina Co.

8

Clinical Microbiology

Robert L. Jones

The purpose of the clinical microbiology laboratory is to rapidly and accurately provide the veterinarian with information that assists in establishing a diagnosis of infectious disease, formulating specific treatment and preventive programs, and predicting the prognosis and possible complications of the disease. The veterinary technician may have a direct impact on the quality of patient care through a variety of activities ranging from collection of specimens to performing laboratory assays. The sophistication of diagnostic microbiology that is undertaken in a local practice laboratory depends on the size and type of practice, cost of performing tests, and availability of a technician with appropriate diagnostic microbiology knowledge and skills compared with the services available through referral laboratories and their turnaround time for results. Many practices find it cost effective to operate a limited microbiology laboratory that is capable of processing routine bacterial cultures and performing a limited number of diagnostic tests using readily available test kits.

This chapter provides veterinary technicians with a broad overview of clinical microbiology and introduces some of the more common laboratory diagnostic procedures that may be performed. Common procedures that will be discussed include collection and handling of specimens, processing specimens for staining and microscopic examination, bacterial and fungal cultural procedures for isolation and presumptive identification of possible pathogens, antimicrobial susceptibility testing, use of packaged diagnostic kits for detection of microbial antigens and antibody responses, and immunoglobulin quantitation. Emphasis will be placed on those procedures that can be performed in the laboratories of most veterinary practices. For more advanced procedures, the focus will be on applications and interpretations rather than methodology. The problem of nosocomial infections and hospital infectious disease control will be introduced because technicians have a critical role in identifying and solving these problems. This chapter introduces technicians to a variety of diagnostic microbiology activities, but it is not designed to serve as a substitute for detailed technical manuals that should be part of equipping a laboratory.

DIAGNOSTIC METHODS

The choice of methods for examining a specimen in the microbiology laboratory depends on the type of specimen and the pathogen sought. Traditionally, microbiologists have attempted to *isolate agents* in various types of culture systems and then use various identification schemes to characterize them. This is still the most frequently used method in bacteriology. However, there are times when the organism may be difficult to cultivate or may not be viable in the specimen presented to the laboratory. In these cases, demonstration of *specific microbial antigens* in the specimen may be more rapid and cost effective. Immunohistochemical assays that have been introduced into veterinary diagnostics include enzyme immunoassays, latex particle agglutination, and protein A coagglutination procedures. In some diseases, such as botulism and mycotoxicoses, establishing the presence of a *microbial toxin* is necessary, rather than identifying the organism that produces it. Sometimes, a specific *immunologic response* by the patient to an infectious agent can establish the diagnosis. Serum can be tested for the presence of specific antibodies, or skin tests can be performed. Another diagnostic method is *direct examination* of exudates and tissue biopsy specimens. Some microorganisms present such unique morphologic characteristics, host inflammatory responses, and lesions that a preliminary diagnosis can be established without the need for further laboratory testing.

Recent developments in biotechnology are providing new methods for direct detection of infectious agents. *Nucleic acid probes* are considered the next new wave of diagnostic tests. Direct nucleic acid hybridization probe and *gene amplification* protocols are highly specific and can be extremely sensitive. Because these procedures detect the genes (or portions of genes) of organisms and can differentiate closely related organisms based on the presence of a unique genetic sequence, the identified strains are frequently described as genotypes. Deoxyribonucleic acid (DNA) probe assays are particularly well suited for in situ hybridization in tissue in which the location and distribution of the organisms must be determined, identification of slow-growing or difficult-to-isolate organisms, and identification of toxicogenic strains of bacteria that cannot be differentiated from nontoxicogenic strains through the use of conventional methods. Nucleic acid amplification assays use primers and polymerase chain reaction (PCR) to provide specificity and sensitivity to detect as few as one organism or 1 to 10 copies of the specific gene sequence. Because of this exquisite sensitivity, specimen collection and handling procedures are critical. Cross contamination between samples with as little as a single copy of a microbial gene carried on gloves, laboratory bench tops, or aerosolized droplets may result in false-positive test results.

Ultimately, the goal of these molecular techniques is the direct determination of identities and antimicrobial susceptibility patterns of microorganisms in clinical specimens. As the technology for nucleic acid amplification currently stands, application of the procedure is limited to large referral laboratories and research laboratories. Partial or full automation and improved technology will begin to reduce costs and increase access to these assays. Despite their sensitivity, molecular detection procedures will not totally replace conventional culture and serologic procedures because the results of nucleic acid amplification procedures and the results of culture or serology mean different things. Nucleic acid amplification procedures are used to determine whether DNA or ribonucleic acid (RNA) from a particular organism is present in the specimen; they reveal nothing about the viability of the organism (because they can detect DNA from dead organisms) or whether the organism is involved in an infectious process. Culture, on the other hand, clearly demonstrates the viability of the organism, whereas a rise in titer of antibody to a specific organism strongly suggests infection.

COLLECTION OF SPECIMENS

There is tremendous diversity of microbial agents, specimen sources, and samples to be considered in the microbiology laboratory. To compound this fact, specimen selection, collection, and transport requirements may also vary significantly depending on the agent to be detected and the assay to be performed. Therefore it is important that technicians be alert to the potential of receiving and implementing specific instructions about specimen collection and handling for each patient rather than anticipating generic procedures.

Proper Specimen Collection

The goal of specimen collection is to obtain a sample from the patient that is representative of the disease process. Therefore the culture specimen must be from the actual *infection site* (Figure 8-1). It must be collected with a minimum of contamination from adjacent tissues or secretions. Material swabbed from superficial body surfaces (skin or mucous membranes) will usually yield a mixed growth of bacteria, often making it difficult to identify a significant pathogen. Culture specimens recovered from body orifices and draining tracts are frequently contaminated with normal flora. The most useful specimens are those aspirated from normally sterile, closed body compartments after the surface has been aseptically prepared.

Optimal times and *sites* for specimen collection must be observed. Infections by some viruses and mycoplasmas are acute processes that are followed by secondary invasion by opportunistic bacteria; therefore sampling must be performed early in the course of disease. When viruses and bacteria localize in specific tissues, collection should target such sites. Specimens obtained at necropsy for culture

should be collected as soon as possible after the death of the animal (see Chapter 5).

Whenever possible, culture specimens should be obtained before the administration of antimicrobials, especially if the suspected pathogen may be susceptible to the antimicrobial or the antimicrobial may be concentrated at the site of infection. However, the administration of antimicrobials does not necessarily preclude the usefulness of cultures. The antimicrobial drug may be diluted to an ineffective level in culture medium, thereby allowing the pathogen to grow. Antimicrobial-resistant or superinfecting bacteria may still be recovered. In addition, the effectiveness of therapy can be evaluated by determining the relative numbers of bacteria present.

An *adequate quantity* of material should be obtained for complete examination. Aliquots of body fluids (>1 ml), exudates, or pieces of tissue (>3 cm^3) are always more useful than a swab. Smears can be prepared for direct examination, and multiple culture media can be inoculated when adequate material is submitted. Quantitative results can also be obtained if needed.

Appropriate collection devices and specimen handling must be used to ensure optimal survival and recovery of significant microorganisms (Figure 8-2). Sterile swabs are acceptable for transferring most samples from the patient to culture media. If the culture medium is not immediately inoculated, the swab must be placed in a swab transport system (Culturette or CultureSwab, BD Microbiology Systems; Copan Transport Swabs, Copan Diagnostics, Inc.) or into a transport medium. *Transport media* are designed to maintain optimal conditions for survival of the suspected pathogen without allowing overgrowth by contaminating saprophytes. Semisolid transport media, such as Amies transport medium with charcoal for *aerobic bacteria* (growth in the presence of oxygen) or Port-A-Cul tubes (BD Microbiology Systems) for *anaerobic bacteria* (requires absence of oxygen), can preserve specimens on swabs for several days. Swabs should not be placed in nutritive broths before inoculating isolation media because an insignificant nonpathogen may overgrow and prevent recovery of the pathogen. Specimens can be collected in various sterile containers that do not contain preservatives or anticoagulants for transport. If tissues are collected for culture, each piece must be packaged separately in a leak-proof, sterile container.

> ### Technician Note
>
> Transport media can serve as excellent vehicles for submitting a bacterial isolate to a reference laboratory for further characterization. A heavily inoculated swab of the pure culture should be placed in the appropriate medium for shipping rather than submitting an inoculated growth medium.

Each culture specimen container must be *properly labeled*. Identification of the patient by name, species, case number, or owner, as appropriate, should be legibly indicated. If more than one veterinarian works in the practice, the one in charge of the case should be identified so that questions about history and preliminary reports can be communicated efficiently. The source of the specimen should also be included on the label. As discussed later, the source of the specimen will be a significant factor in deciding how to set up the culture, which bacteria to identify, and how to interpret the results. If the culture specimen is to be sent to a referral laboratory, additional clinical history should be

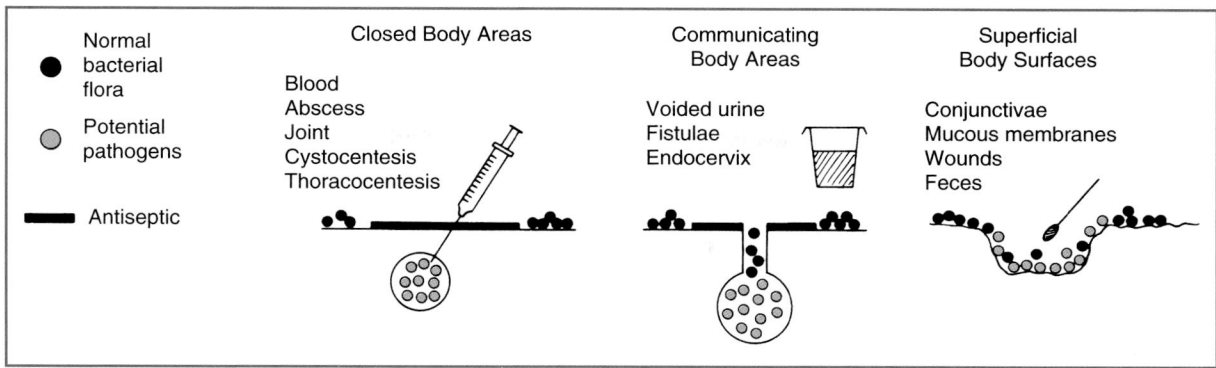

FIGURE 8-1. Methods used to collect bacterial culture specimens and probable sources of contamination.

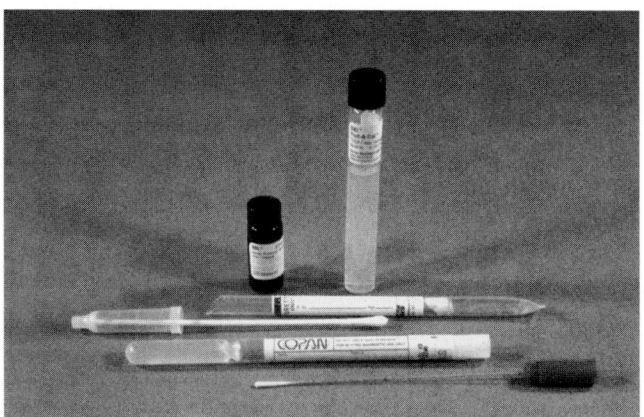

FIGURE 8-2. Copan and Culturette swab transport systems, tube of Amies transport medium with charcoal, and Port-A-Cul anaerobic transport tube. Swabs are used to collect culture inoculum and placed into transport systems or tube of medium for preservation of the viability of bacteria during transportation to the laboratory for culture.

included. Results of previous culture attempts, other laboratory tests, and antimicrobial treatments should be reported, as well as the major clinical manifestations and duration of illness, so laboratory personnel will be able to recognize and identify significant findings.

Special Collection and Handling Procedures

Some groups of microorganisms require special collection and handling for optimal isolation. Anaerobic bacteria must be protected from oxygen. Often, a sterile syringe with a fine-gauge needle (22- to 23-gauge) is the best collection device for aspirating exudates from an infected site. The specimen can be transported to the laboratory in the syringe if air is expressed, the needle is removed to prevent injuries, and the syringe is capped to prevent leakage. Otherwise, the specimen should be transferred to an appropriate anaerobic transport device. Survival and subsequent isolation of anaerobes are enhanced by keeping them in the reduced microenvironment in which they are found. Therefore, as stated previously, exudate and pieces of tissue are better specimens than swabs. If a swab is collected, it must be placed in an appropriate anaerobic transport device. Handling a specimen as if it contains anaerobes will not jeopardize the viability of aerobic

bacteria. Exudates, biopsy material, and tissue should be submitted as quickly as possible to the microbiology laboratory.

In attempts to isolate fungi and mycobacteria, swabs generally are not the best specimens. These agents tend to cause chronic infections, often with small numbers of organisms present. Too few organisms may be present on a swab, or in the case of mycobacteria, they may adhere to the swab, and culture results will be negative.

The more fastidious groups of microorganisms, for example, *Mycoplasma*, *Chlamydia*, *Rickettsia*, and viruses, require special selective transport media. These media are usually formulated to contain antimicrobials that will inhibit the growth of other microorganisms while preserving the viability of the desired agent. Specific transport media and instructions for proper use should be obtained from a referral laboratory that is capable of providing the desired culture service.

PROCESSING SPECIMENS

Each specimen received in the microbiology laboratory should be carefully and individually evaluated, considering anatomic source and condition of the specimen, animal family of the patient, clinical history, and special requests from the veterinarian. Each pathogen has a preferred habitat in which it will grow and specific mechanisms for causing disease. Therefore, for a particular manifestation of disease, there will be a limited number of agents that should be considered as likely pathogens. Table 8-1 lists the most common bacterial species associated with infections of various sites in animals. If the technician can focus the search for pathogens on these most likely agents, results will often be obtained much more rapidly and with less expense.

Condition of the Specimen

If there is evidence that the specimen has become grossly contaminated or dried out, it is of insufficient quantity, there has been excessive delay in receipt, or any other evidence of mishandling is present, an attempt should be made to obtain a second sample. Specimens should be processed the same day they are collected, or they should be held at refrigeration temperatures if a delay is anticipated.

Direct Microscopic Examination

Direct microscopic examination of exudates, impression smears from tissues, or infected body fluids is the most

TABLE 8-1   COMMON BACTERIAL SPECIES ASSOCIATED WITH INFECTIONS

Type of Infection	Canine	Feline	Equine	Porcine	Ruminants
Conjunctivitis	Staphylococcus Streptococcus Pseudomonas	Staphylococcus Pasteurella Chlamydia	Streptococcus Staphylococcus	Streptococcus Staphylococcus	Moraxella bovis Branhamella Streptococcus Staphylococcus Escherichia coli
Central nervous system	Rare	Rare	Streptococcus Actinobacillus Escherichia coli	Streptococcus Escherichia coli	Haemophilus somnus Listeria Escherichia coli Pasteurella haemolytica
Gastroenteritis	Salmonella Clostridium perfringens Campylobacter	Salmonella	Salmonella Escherichia coli Actinobacillus Rhodococcus equi	Salmonella Escherichia coli Brachyspira Clostridium perfringens	Salmonella Escherichia coli Clostridium perfringens Mycobacterium paratuberculosis
Genital tract	Brucella canis Escherichia coli Streptococcus Staphylococcus Mycoplasma	Streptococcus Pasteurella Escherichia coli	Streptococcus Escherichia coli Klebsiella Pseudomonas	Brucella suis Streptococcus Leptospira	Brucella Listeria Arcanobacterium pyogenes Campylobacter Mycoplasma
Mastitis	Staphylococcus	Staphylococcus	Streptococcus	Streptococcus Staphylococcus Escherichia coli Actinobacillus Arcanobacterium pyogenes	Streptococcus Staphylococcus Arcanobacterium pyogenes Nocardia Mycobacterium Escherichia coli Klebsiella
Musculoskeletal	Staphylococcus Escherichia coli Pseudomonas Brucella canis Anaerobes	Rare	Streptococcus Actinobacillus Escherichia coli Rhodococcus equi Staphylococcus	Streptococcus Mycoplasma Escherichia coli Erysipelothrix Arcanobacterium pyogenes	Clostridium Arcanobacterium pyogenes Escherichia coli Streptococcus Erysipelothrix Haemophilus somnus Mycoplasma Chlamydia

Otitis	Staphylococcus Pseudomonas Streptococcus Clostridium perfringens Bordetella bronchiseptica	Rare		Rare Streptococcus	Rare Streptococcus Pasteurella Arcanobacterium pyogenes Haemophilus somnus Arcanobacterium pyogenes Fusobacterium
Upper respiratory	Pasteurella multocida		Streptococcus equi	Bordetella bronchiseptica Pasteurella multocida	Haemophilus somnus Arcanobacterium pyogenes Fusobacterium Pasteurella, Mannheimia Arcanobacterium pyogenes Haemophilus somnus Mycoplasma
Pneumonia	Bordetella bronchiseptica Pasteurella Klebsiella Escherichia coli Mycoplasma Streptococcus Staphylococcus	Rare Pasteurella Chlamydia Bordetella	Streptococcus Actinobacillus Rhodococcus equi Pasteurella Staphylococcus Klebsiella Pseudomonas Bordetella bronchiseptica	Bordetella bronchiseptica Pasteurella multocida Mycoplasma Haemophilus Pasteurella Streptococcus Actinobacillus	Pasteurella, Mannheimia Arcanobacterium pyogenes
Pleuritis	Fusobacterium Prevotella Porphyromonas Actinomyces	Prevotella Porphyromonas Fusobacterium Pasteurella Nocardia	Streptococcus	Actinobacillus	
Skin wounds abscesses	Staphylococcus Streptococcus Pseudomonas Nocardia Actinomyces Fusobacterium	Pasteurella multocida Streptococcus Staphylococcus Anaerobes	Streptococcus Corynebacterium pseudotuberculosis Pseudomonas Dermatophilus Staphylococcus	Streptococcus Staphylococcus Arcanobacterium pyogenes	Arcanobacterium pyogenes Dermatophilus Actinomyces Actinobacillus Staphylococcus
Urinary tract	Escherichia coli Proteus Staphylococcus Streptococcus Klebsiella Pseudomonas	Staphylococcus Escherichia coli	Streptococcus Escherichia coli	Actinobacterium suis Streptococcus	Corynebacterium renale Arcanobacterium pyogenes

important laboratory procedure that can be used for microbiologic diagnosis. It provides immediate information on the types and numbers of microorganisms present as well as the type of host cellular inflammatory response. The likelihood of infection can be determined as can the probable type of agent (i.e., virus, bacterium, or fungus), which in turn determines the nature of the diagnostic assays needed. The most likely pathogen (or predominant organism) may tentatively be identified. This information may be used to provide guidance in selection of optimal culture conditions and as the basis for the interpretation of the significance of subsequent culture results. In some cases it may be all the information the veterinarian needs.

In many situations, Gram's stain is the procedure of choice because it provides differentiation of gram-positive and gram-negative bacteria. However, some bacteria do not stain well with Gram's stain. Gram-negative bacteria may not be well differentiated from the background in exudates and tissue impression smears.

Other tissue stains (i.e., Giemsa and Wright's stains or methylene blue wet mounts) may be more useful for detecting all microorganisms present in the smear. Although these stains are more efficient in demonstrating the presence and morphology of bacteria, they do not provide differentiation of gram-positive and gram-negative bacteria. Careful direct examination may be sufficient for diagnosis without cultures, or it can narrow the diagnostic likelihood to a few bacterial species. This information helps in the selection of optimal culture conditions for identification of suspected pathogens.

Gram's Stain Procedure and Interpretation

The technique for preparing a gram-stained slide is as follows:

1. Prepare a thin smear from tissue exudates or bacterial suspension on a clean slide and allow smear to air dry.
2. Fix material to the slide so that it does not wash off during the staining procedure by passing the slide, right side up, through a flame three or four times.
3. Flood smear with crystal violet solution, and let stand for 1 minute.
4. Wash smear briefly with tap water.
5. Flood smear with Gram's iodine solution, and let stand for 1 minute.
6. Wash with tap water, and decolorize until solvent flows colorlessly from the slide. This usually requires 5 to 10 seconds.
7. Wash briefly with tap water, and flood the slide with safranin counterstain for 30 to 60 seconds.
8. Wash briefly with tap water, blot and air dry, and examine.

The stained smear is best examined using the 100× (oil immersion) objective of the microscope. Gram-positive bacteria retain the crystal violet iodine complex and appear dark-blue or purple. Gram-negative bacteria lose the primary complex, take up the secondary dye safranin, and appear red. Fungi (yeasts) appear gram-positive. Inflammatory cells appear gram-negative, and epithelial cells may appear gram-positive or gram-negative depending on the thickness of the smear. Backgrounds usually appear gram-negative but may appear gram-positive if thick and inadequately washed. Fibrin, mucus, and erythrocytes often stain gram-negative and may mask detection of gram-negative bacteria.

BACTERIAL ISOLATION AND IDENTIFICATION PROCEDURES

Equipment

The equipment and supplies required for the performance of basic diagnostic bacteriology tests depends on the scope of services to be provided. Some of the more common items are as follows: binocular microscope, incubator, anaerobic culture system, staining reagents or kits, specimen collection devices, swabs, transport media, isolation and identification media (Table 8-2), packaged identification systems (Boxes 8-1 and 8-2), and miscellaneous instruments, supplies, and reagents as appropriate for the diagnostic procedures to be performed.

The most expensive item is a good-quality binocular light microscope with a 100× oil immersion objective. Dark-field and phase-contrast options are useful but not essential. Small countertop incubators are available. Important characteristics of a quality incubator include (1) insulated walls to maintain a constant temperature; (2) an adequate seal to maintain a humid atmosphere; (3) a capacity for plates, tubes, and candle jars; (4) a thermometer to check the temperature, which should not fluctuate more than ±2° C; and (5) an adjustable, thermostatically controlled heating element.

Culture Media

Several different media are needed in the bacteriology laboratory for isolation of various microbial agents and for identification of these microorganisms. Both dehydrated and prepared media are readily available today. It is usually much more convenient for small laboratories to purchase prepared media than to prepare their own. In addition, the quality of purchased media will be much more consistent and usually will be quality tested before it is distributed. There are numerous distributors of prepared media throughout the United States. A few national and regional distributors are listed in Box 8-2. Names and addresses of other suppliers can be obtained from local hospitals and by searching the World Wide Web. Some microbiology supply distributors usually have a full line of prepared plates and tubes of media available, as well as the ancillary biochemical reagents, stains, and miscellaneous supplies.

Purpose of Specific Media

Solid media in plates are used for primary isolation of bacteria from clinical specimens. This type of medium allows distribution of the specimen in such a way that *isolated colonies* develop, each representing a single bacterial cell. Some primary isolation media contain inhibitory ingredients that allow them to be *selective* for specific groups of bacteria. MacConkey agar is selective for bacteria that can grow in the presence of bile salts, which is similar to the environment found in the intestines. A *differential* medium contains an indicator system that can distinguish different bacteria, even though both types may grow. The lactose-fermenting ability of bacteria on MacConkey agar is a differential reaction. Table 8-2 lists some of the more commonly used culture media, the indicated use of the media, and selective and differential characteristics.

Inoculation of Media

Before media are inoculated, each tube or plate should be labeled with a distinct identification and the date of inoculation. Plates should be labeled on the bottom with a waterproof marker. Most clinical specimens are collected for culture on swabs. These swabs are used for direct inoculation of primary isolation media. In the labo-

TABLE 8-2	BACTERIOLOGIC PLATE AND TUBE MEDIA FOR THE PRACTITIONER'S LABORATORY	
Media	**Purpose and Inoculation**	**Reactions and Interpretations**
Blood agar plate (trypticase soy agar with 5% sheep blood)	Primary isolation medium for all specimens in which pathogenic bacteria are suspected. Always streak for colony isolation.	Observe growth rates, colony morphologic characteristics, hemolysis. Test selected colonies for Gram's reaction, catalase, and oxidase. Inoculate differential tests and antimicrobial susceptibility tests from well-isolated colonies.
MacConkey agar	A primary isolation and differential plating medium for selection and recovery of Enterobacteriaceae and related gram-negative bacteria. Inoculate by streaking for isolated colonies.	Growth is usually gram negative. Pink to red colonies (with increased redness of the medium) are lactose fermenters (e.g., species of *Escherichia, Klebsiella,* and *Enterobacter).* Colorless colonies (often with a slight change of the medium to yellow) are non-lactose fermenters.
Hektoen enteric agar	A direct plating medium for fecal specimens that is highly selective for *Salmonella.* Inoculate by streaking for isolated colonies.	Disaccharide fermenters are moderately inhibited and produce bright orange to yellow to salmon to pink colonies. *Salmonella* colonies are blue-green, typically with black centers from hydrogen sulfide. *Proteus* colonies may resemble *Salmonella.*
Selenite broth or tetrathionate broth	Enrichment broth for the selective enhancement of growth by *Salmonella* from specimens containing heavy concentrations of mixed bacteria, such as feces. Inoculate relatively heavily, and incubate 18-24 hr.	Subculture to MacConkey agar and Hektoen enteric agar for isolation of *Salmonella.*
Triple sugar iron (TSI) agar slant	A differential medium for detection of carbohydrate (glucose, lactose, sucrose) fermentation and production of hydrogen sulfide. Inoculate by stabbing the butt once with an inoculating needle and by streaking the slant. Incubate with a loose cap.	Yellow color change indicates acidification caused by carbohydrate fermentation. In the butt, glucose fermentation is detected; in the slant, lactose and sucrose fermentation is detected (includes glucose fermentation as an intermediate product). Red color change indicates alkalinization caused by lack of carbohydrate fermentation. Black color indicates hydrogen sulfide production. Results are recorded as slant/butt; A = acid (yellow), K = alkaline (red), or NC = no change.
Christensen's urea agar slant	A differential medium for detection of urease production by an organism. Inoculate by streaking heavily over the slant.	Urease-positive bacteria produce a pink-red color change in the slant and sometimes throughout the butt. Urease-negative bacteria allow the medium to remain the original yellow color.
Motility media*	A test medium for determining if an organism is motile or nonmotile. Inoculate by stabbing the center of the tube with an inoculating needle. Incubate at 35°C for most organisms; incubate at room temperature if *Listeria* is suspected.	Motile organisms migrate from the stab line, flaring out to cause turbidity in the medium. Nonmotile organisms grow only along the stab line; the surrounding medium remains clear.
Indole test media*	A test medium for detecting the ability of bacteria to produce indole as one of the degradation products of tryptophan metabolism. Inoculate, incubate 24-48 hr, then add Kovac's reagent to detect indole.	Development of a red color at the interface of the reagent and the broth within seconds after adding the reagent indicates a positive test.

*Combination media can be purchased that provide for several tests in the same tube, such as SIM (sulfide indole motility), MIO (motility indole ornithine), or MIL (motility indole lysine).

ratory, a sterile swab can be used to transfer inoculum material from liquid and tissue specimens to isolation media. The same swab can be used for inoculation of several media if the least inhibitory medium is inoculated first and the most inhibitory medium is inoculated last; for example, start with blood agar and then MacConkey agar.

Between one fourth and one third of the surface of the agar plates should be inoculated with the specimen. The inoculum is then progressively diluted across the agar by successive steps of streaking with a bacteriologic loop (Figure 8-3). There are several different streaking technique modifications, and any method that yields isolated colonies is satisfactory. With the practice of a light touch to avoid tearing the agar and experience in anticipating the amount of bacterial growth that will occur, slight modifications can be made in technique from one specimen to the next to achieve the best isolation of colonies.

Media dispensed in tubes may be a broth or semisolid agar, or it may be poured as a slant. Broth media can be inoculated with a loop or an inoculating wire by touching the side of the tube just below the surface of the medium. Depending on the purpose of the slant medium, it may require inoculation by stabbing the deep (or butt) portion of the agar (e.g., triple sugar iron [TSI] slants); the slant surface is then streaked from bottom to top (Figure 8-4). When a semisolid medium for motility testing is inoculated, it is important that the inoculating wire is inserted and removed along the same tract within the medium.

Incubation Conditions

Inoculated plates are incubated in an inverted position to prevent condensation of water on the lid. If water drops to the agar surface, it can mix the bacterial growth rather than allowing it to develop as isolated colonies. If tube media have screw tops, they should be left loose during incubation.

Temperature

Cultures should be placed in incubation at an optimal temperature as quickly as possible. The majority of cultures for isolation of pathogenic bacteria are incubated at 35° C. Although optimal growth may occur at other temperatures, in most cases, alternate temperatures are more important for differentiation of bacteria than for primary isolation.

Atmosphere

Most common pathogenic bacteria are aerobes or facultative anaerobes and will grow well in the presence of an atmosphere of air. However, oxygen is toxic to obligate anaerobic bacteria, requiring that a special culture container from which all oxygen has been removed be used for incubation. Two excellent anaerobic systems for the small laboratory are the BioBag Type A environmental chamber and the BBL GasPak anaerobic system (BD Microbiology Systems). Each system consists of a hydrogen generator, a catalyst to facilitate the depletion of oxygen from the atmosphere by combining with the hydrogen, and a sealable container to hold these components and the culture plates. Certain bacteria, such as *Campylobacter*, *Brucella*, *Haemophilus*, and *Mycoplasma* spp., have specialized atmo-

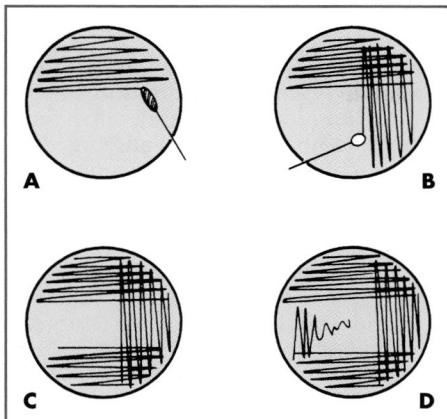

FIGURE 8-3. Plate inoculation and streaking method for isolation of bacterial colonies. **A,** Inoculate with swab, covering one fourth to one third of plate. **B,** Streak lightly, overlapping previous area. **C,** Flame loop, allow it to cool, and streak next area. **D,** Repeat as in **C.**

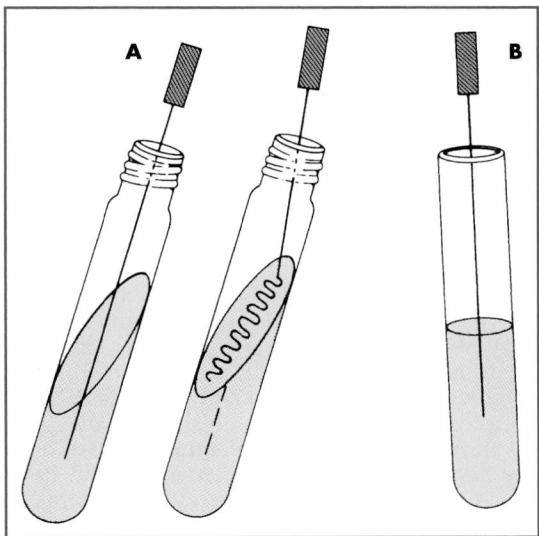

FIGURE 8-4. Inoculation procedure for tube media. **A,** Inoculation of agar slant and butt, such as triple sugar iron (TSI). The inoculation needle is first stabbed into the butt and then removed and streaked over the agar slant surface in a back-and-forth motion. **B,** Inoculation of motility test media. The inoculation needle is stabbed into the medium and withdrawn along the same tract.

spheric requirements and are best forwarded to reference laboratories.

Time

All inoculated plates should be examined after 15 to 24 hours of incubation (overnight). Most cultures will have sufficient growth for evaluation and identification at this time. Culture specimens that contained bacteria on direct microscopic examination but yield negative results after this time or specimens that may be expected to contain slow-growing bacteria should be incubated up to 3 days

before a final negative report is issued. Incubation of primary isolation plates beyond 3 days is rarely indicated unless there is reason to suspect an unusually slow-growing pathogen.

Routine Culture System

The majority of specimens for culture in the veterinary microbiology laboratory can be processed in a routine manner with a minimum of media. The approach presented in this section is not represented as a comprehensive culture system that will successfully isolate and identify all potentially pathogenic bacteria; rather, it is meant as a basic guideline for the veterinary technician who has the opportunity to provide a diagnostic bacteriology service within a private veterinary practice. The system is designed to be cost effective when used for routine aerobic cultures, which will usually account for 80% to 90% of culture requests. Often the veterinarian's immediate objective is for the laboratory to characterize the isolate sufficiently to guide antimicrobial selection or to perform an antimicrobial susceptibility test rather than pursuing definitive identification. The challenge for the technician is to discern when it is better to refer a specimen to another laboratory for more sophisticated diagnostic evaluation.

Primary Isolation Media

Blood agar, containing 5% sheep blood, is the most widely used primary isolation medium because of its ability to support growth of most pathogenic bacteria. It is also a standard medium used extensively for describing colony morphologic characteristics and hemolytic patterns. MacConkey agar is also commonly used as a primary isolation medium. Although it is not always essential, it often provides significant information about bacteria and may provide presumptive identification, or at least group classification, of the isolate. If MacConkey agar is inoculated as a primary isolation medium, rather than used as a differential medium for subcultures, the identification process is often moved forward by 1 day.

In many laboratories, it is customary to include an enrichment broth as part of the primary isolation medium. One of the most common broth media used for this purpose is thioglycolate. This medium can support growth of many anaerobic or facultative anaerobic bacteria that might not be recovered on primary plates incubated aerobically.

Primary growth in a broth medium is frequently difficult to interpret. It must always be compared with a direct microscopic examination because contaminating bacteria from the environment or indigenous flora may overgrow a pathogen in the specimen. Specimens should never be cultured solely in a broth medium for primary isolation. Further discussion of the interpretation of broth subcultures is presented later.

When specific pathogens are sought in specimens, modifications of the basic culture setup can be incorporated into the laboratory routines. Procedures that may enhance the likelihood of recovering specific pathogens are discussed later in this chapter.

Preliminary Evaluation of Cultures

Efficient evaluation of primary cultures requires considerable skill, which is acquired through experience in the microbiology laboratory. Decisions that must be made about isolated bacteria include their possible significance as pathogens, which bacteria require further identification, and what additional tests are needed. As the veterinary technician gains experience in the laboratory and becomes acquainted with common bacterial pathogens, these decisions will become less challenging. Clinically useful results usually only require that identification of bacteria is usually carried to the presumptive level by a few key characteristics rather than to a definitive identification. Only isolates considered to be clinically significant need to be identified. Identification of bacterial growth that results from environmental contamination or indigenous flora is wasted effort.

From the initial examination of primary cultures, considerable information can be obtained to help distinguish which bacteria should be characterized in further detail. The important characteristics of primary cultures to be noted include (1) the number of different types of bacteria isolated, (2) the relative number of each type, (3) the colonial morphologic characteristics of the various isolates, and (4) the changes in the media surrounding the colonies. While making the preliminary evaluation of primary cultures, the technician must keep in mind the source of the specimen. If it was obtained from a normally sterile body site (e.g., joint fluid) and was properly handled, any growth is likely to be significant. If the specimen is from a site normally colonized by microflora (e.g., intestinal tract), interpretation becomes much more difficult. In general, if there is scant aerobic growth of three or more bacteria, the result probably reflects normal flora. Most bacterial infections, other than mixed anaerobic infections, are usually caused by only one or two agents. When a specimen from an infectious process is carefully collected, growth of a single organism in nearly pure culture will often be observed. Therefore the most abundant colony type is usually the most important.

Some general guidelines for selection of significant isolates can be derived from colony morphologic characteristics, although exceptions will always occur. Usually circular, smooth, raised or convex, opaque to gray colonies with an entire edge are more likely to be significant. Large, rough, granular, irregular, spreading, or heavily pigmented colonies are likely to be insignificant unless large numbers are recovered in nearly pure culture.

Technician Note

Some bacterial species characteristically produce hemolysins that can be demonstrated when the bacteria are cultured on blood agar plates, and their hemolysis affects the red blood cells (RBCs) in the zone surrounding the hemolytic colony. The following types of hemolytic activity may be observed:

- *Complete hemolysis:* Complete lysis of RBCs in the medium resulting in a clear, colorless zone surrounding the colony. For *Streptococcus* spp., this is referred to as beta-hemolysis.
- *Incomplete hemolysis:* partial destruction of RBCs with some loss of hemoglobin. Because of streptococcal action on hemoglobin, a zone of greenish discoloration of the agar appears and is known as alpha-hemolysis.
- *Nonhemolytic:* no apparent lysis of RBCs, although there may be some discoloration of media. For *Streptococcus* spp., this is sometimes referred to as gamma-hemolysis.

Changes in the media should be carefully noted. Hemolysis in blood agar is often a good indication of a possible pathogen. Sometimes the hemolytic pattern provides adequate identification, such as the double zone of hemolysis produced by many coagulase-positive isolates of *Staphylococcus*. Pigment production can be an important character-

istic to note on primary cultures. The differential features of MacConkey agar (i.e., ability to grow, lactose fermentation) are important bits of information that can aid in the identification of an isolate. Odors produced by bacteria are difficult to describe adequately but, after experience is gained, become another useful identifying characteristic.

The novice microbiologist may be required to rely on several differential tests for the identification of isolates. As experience is gained and confidence develops, more isolates will be recognized on the primary plates. Knowledge of the more common bacterial species to expect from a specimen (see Table 8-1) will provide a differential list of bacteria to consider so that it is not necessary to face each culture as a complete unknown.

Recording, Interpreting, and Reporting Results

Although it is impossible to devise rigid rules that provide for adequate processing of all specimens, some routines are helpful for observing and recording results of cultures. A laboratory worksheet should be developed for recording all observations. These records should contain sufficient detail so that anyone who works in the laboratory can take over and complete the culture without a special briefing. A worksheet that provides adequate room for a flow chart type of illustration of culture processing and observation is easy to follow (Figure 8-5). These work records may become part of the medical record, so care should be taken to ensure that they are complete and accurate (see Chapter 33).

As an aid to interpreting culture results, the relative abundance of growth of each type of colony should be recorded. A convenient system of recording is a scale of 1+ to 4+, in which each step on the scale represents the number of quadrants of the primary culture plate in which the colony is growing. For example, if the only colonies are in the initial streak lines in which the specimen was inoculated on the plate, growth would be rated 1+. If growth is so abundant that colonies are found in the fourth quadrant (the final streak lines), growth is rated 4+. Any bacterium isolated from broth subculture, but not on primary inoculated plates, is rated 1+, regardless of the abundance of growth on the subculture plate. Bacterial cultures should not be evaluated empirically as positive or negative because this semiquantitative method helps the clinician to interpret the significance of the results. Specimens from most acute bacterial infections that have not been treated with antimicrobials will yield 3+ to 4+ growth. However, because of poor collection technique, mishandling the specimen, presampling antimicrobial therapy, or chronic infections, a smaller number of bacteria may be recovered. The clinician must decide whether these smaller numbers of bacteria are significant. If the culture is from a normally sterile body site, these culture results are often significant.

Indigenous Flora

Specimens cultured from sites populated with an indigenous bacterial flora (often described as normal flora) are more difficult to interpret. Usually these cultures are insignificant if they result in scant growth, especially if it is a mixture of bacteria. To avoid wasting undue time precisely identifying the microflora, the technician should become familiar with the organisms normally found at various body sites (Table 8-3). Many of these bacteria are potential pathogens. If they are identified because of common recognition and are specifically reported while other, less familiar bacteria are overlooked, the report may mislead the clinician by implying undue significance.

DIAGNOSTIC MICROBIOLOGY WORKSHEET

Date _Oct. 14, 2001_ Lab No. _1036_

Patient ID _# 3053 Heidi_

Owner _Smith_

Veterinarian _____

Animal species _Canine_

Specimen _urine – cystocentesis_

_____

Procedures requested:

✓ Aerobic cult

___ Anaerobic cult

___ Fungal cult

✓ Susceptibility

___ Acid-fast stain

___ Other: _____

Direct exam: _>10 gram – neg. rods per field_

Daily log of laboratory activities and observations:

1 – 14 Inoculate   BA   MAC
              10⁻²   10⁻³
1 – 15   TNTC   >100 cfu   Strong
                    hemolytic smooth   lactose –
                        colony   fermenter
              Micro -ID   Susceptibility
                #23431   test
1 – 16 Record susceptibility

SUMMARY OF FINDINGS:

1. _E. Coli   >10⁵   cfu/ml   (hemolytic)_

2. _____

3. _____

Reported by _____JS_____ Date reported _10 – 16 – 01_

KEY REACTIONS

	Isolate:	E. Coli					
	Hrs:	24	48	24	48	24	48
Hemolysis		+					
Gram reaction		−					
MacConkey growth		+					
Oxidase		−					
Catalase							
Coagulase							
TSI							
Urea							
Motility							
Indol							
H₂S							

SUSCEPTIBILITY

ANTIBIOTIC	Code	mm	Int	mm	Int	mm	Int
Amikacin	AN	24	S				
Amox / Clav	AmC	20	S				
Ampicillin	AM	0	R				
Cefotaxime	CTX						
Ceftiofur							
Cephalothin	CF	14	R				
Chloramphenicol	C	0	R				
Clindamycin	CC						
Enrofloxacin	ENO	26	S				
Erythromycin	E						
Gentamicin	GM	24	S				
Kanamycin	K						
Oxacillin	OX						
Penicillin G	P						
Pirlimycin							
Rifampin							
Tetracycline	TE	0	R				
Tilmicosin							
Tobramycin	NN						
Trimeth/Sulfa	SXT	18	S				
Triple Sulfa	SSS	0	R				

FIGURE 8-5. Example of a laboratory worksheet for recording results of various laboratory procedures, including microbial identification and susceptibility tests.

TABLE 8-3	INDIGENOUS FLORA	
Site	**Aerobes**	**Anaerobes**
Skin, ear	*Staphylococcus, Micrococcus,* diphtheroids, and transient environmental and fecal contaminants	
Mouth, nasopharynx	*Micrococcus, Staphylococcus, Streptococcus* (alpha and beta), *Bacillus,* coliforms, *Proteus, Pasteurella, Actinobacillus, Haemophilus,* and *Mycoplasma*	*Bacteroides, Prevotella, Porphyromonas, Fusobacterium, Actinomyces,* spirochetes, and others
Trachea, bronchi, lungs	No residents, only transient contaminants	
Stomach, small intestine	Small numbers of alpha-*Streptococcus*	*Lactobacillus*
Large intestine	*Streptococcus, Escherichia coli, Klebsiella, Enterobacter, Proteus, Enterococcus,* and others	*Clostridium, Fusobacterium, Bacteroides, Porphyromonas, Prevotella,* spirochetes, *Lactobacillus*
Vulva, prepuce	Diphtheroids, *Micrococcus, Staphylococcus,* and fecal organisms	
Conjunctiva, uterus, mammary glands	These areas may occasionally contain small numbers of insignificant bacteria	

Reporting results of cultures from sites with indigenous flora can be a perplexing problem. Often it is better to specify which specific pathogens have been *excluded* by careful cultural examination, such as "no *Salmonella* isolated." Between the extremes of trying to identify everything and reporting "normal flora," the technician and clinician must agree regarding the most useful information expected from a given specimen. Perhaps certain potential pathogens that may be considered significant for the specimen should be carefully sought. In other situations a predominant bacterium can be identified or groups of organisms reported (e.g., coliforms, diphtheroids).

Identification Procedures

Identification of clinically significant bacteria is best accomplished by means of a few rapid tests that can presumptively differentiate organisms. To one who is experienced, such characteristics as colonial morphology, hemolysis, growth on MacConkey agar, and odor may be adequate for presumptive identification. Often, additional differential tests are needed for more precise identification. Figure 8-6 presents a useful approach to identification of unknown isolates when needed.

GRAM'S REACTION.   The first differential characteristic to be considered is the reaction to *Gram's stain*. Gram's stain can be performed on thin smears of bacteria from a single colony (see Gram's Stain Procedure and Interpretation). Potassium hydroxide, 3%, may be used as an alternate and more rapid test for Gram's reaction of isolated colonies. A small drop of 3% potassium hydroxide (no larger than a colony) is dispensed on a slide, and a colony of bacteria is picked from the blood agar plate with a bacteriologic loop and is mixed into the 3% potassium hydroxide. The loop is slowly and gently lifted at 5-second intervals to see whether a viscous gel is sticking to the loop. The formation of any sticky strand that can be lifted with the loop indicates a gram-negative bacterium. The reaction should appear within 20 to 30 seconds. Gram-positive organisms will diffusely mix in the 3% potassium hydroxide. Cellular morphologic characteristics of the gram-positive bacteria are important differential characteristics that require careful examination of a stained smear.

Technician Note

Luxuriant growth on a MacConkey agar plate is presumptive evidence of a gram-negative organism and usually does not need to be confirmed by Gram's stain.

CATALASE TEST.   *Catalase activity* is an important and rapid test for differentiating *Staphylococcus* from *Streptococcus* and *Erysipelothrix* and *Arcanobacterium pyogenes* from other small gram-positive rods. Hydrogen peroxide (3%) is the only reagent needed and can readily be purchased from any drugstore. It should be stored in a dark bottle in the refrigerator. The *slide catalase test* is performed by picking bacteria from the center of a colony with a needle or loop and smearing the bacteria on a clean, dry slide. A drop of hydrogen peroxide is added over the bacteria and immediately observed for bubbling. Lack of bubbling is a negative test. The order of the test procedure must not be reversed or false-positive results can be obtained. If any blood agar is introduced into the test, it can also cause a false-positive result.

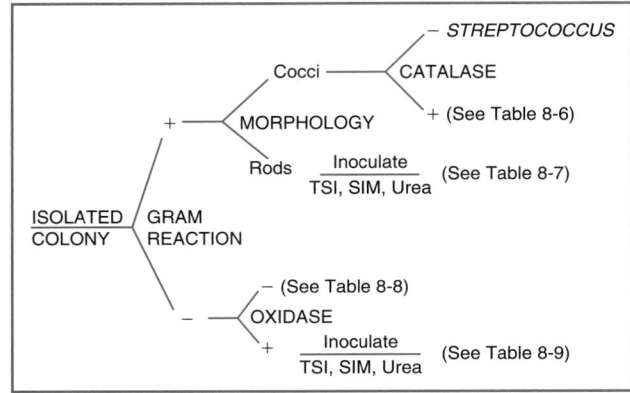

FIGURE 8-6.   General flow chart for identification of common aerobic veterinary bacterial pathogens.

OXIDASE TEST.   *Cytochrome oxidase activity* should be determined for all gram-negative bacteria except strong lactose fermenters, which will be negative. Commercial cytochrome oxidase test reagents are readily available. The reaction is supposed to be clearly visible within a few seconds, but with some reagents the reaction may be delayed for up to 2 minutes for *Pasteurella* and *Actinobacillus*. A heavy inoculum must be used for accurate testing. A wooden stick or platinum loop should be used to pick colonies for testing, because trace amounts of iron from other loops can cause false-positive results.

PRESUMPTIVE IDENTIFICATION.   When Gram's reaction, cellular morphologic characteristics, and catalase and oxidase results have been determined, the bacteria can be tentatively grouped, and differential tests can be selected as indicated in Figure 8-6 for identification.

Isolates of *Streptococcus* are usually characterized by the type of hemolysis they produce. Beta-hemolytic *Streptococcus* is usually considered to be a potential pathogen. Alpha-hemolytic and nonhemolytic *Streptococcus* isolates usually originate from normal flora of skin and mucous membranes and are not considered significant unless they are obtained from normally sterile sites.

Isolates of *Staphylococcus* should be differentiated from *Micrococcus* (Table 8-4), which are considered to be nonpathogenic. Glucose-fermenting ability, determined in TSI agar slants, can be used for differentiation of these genera. If a double zone of hemolysis is observed on the blood agar plate, the bacterium can be identified as a coagulase-positive *Staphylococcus* without need for further testing. All other *Staphylococcus* isolates should be tested for coagulase activity because coagulase activity correlates with pathogenicity. Speciation of coagulase-positive and coagulase-negative *Staphylococcus* spp. may be attempted in special cases if desired.

The small gram-positive rods can be differentiated by inoculating TSI, urea, and sulfide-indole-motility (SIM) medium. The results of these tests, as well as colonial morphology and catalase activity, can identify the isolate (Table 8-5). Individual characteristics of the important pathogens in this group will be discussed later.

Most gram-negative, oxidase-negative bacteria are members of the Enterobacteriaceae family. These bacteria are reactive in biochemical tests and can be identified by one of several different systems. The most rapid and economi-

TABLE 8-4	DIFFERENTIATION OF GRAM-POSITIVE, CATALASE-POSITIVE COCCI			
Organism	Hemolysis	Hyaluronidase	Glucose Fermentation	Coagulase
Staphylococcus aureus	+*	+	+	+
Staphylococcus intermedius	+*	–	+	+
Staphylococcus coagulase–negative sp.	±		+	–
Micrococcus	–		–	–

*Double zones of complete and incomplete hemolysis are frequently observed.

TABLE 8-5	DIFFERENTIATION OF SMALL, NON–SPORE-FORMING GRAM-POSITIVE RODS					
Organism	Motility (22° C)	Catalase	Hydrogen Sulfide in TSI	Urease	Hemolysis	Colony Morphologic Characteristics
Listeria monocytogenes	+	+	–	–	Complete	Very small
Erysipelothrix rhusiopathiae	–	–	+	–	Slow, greenish	Very small
Arcanobacterium pyogenes	–	–	–	–	Complete	Very small
Corynebacterium renale	–	+	–	+	V	Medium size, entire
Corynebacterium pseudotuberculosis	–	+	–	+ (w)	V	Dry, grainy white
Rhodococcus equi	–	+	–	+ (d)	–	Large, mucoid, pink
Other diphtheroids	–	+	–	V	V	V

d, Delayed, may require up to 2 weeks; *TSI*, triple sugar iron (agar); *V*, variable results; *w*, weak.

TABLE 8-6	DIFFERENTIATION OF GRAM-NEGATIVE, OXIDASE-NEGATIVE BACTERIA			
	Growth on MacConkey	TSI	Motility	Identification Method
Enterobacteriaceae	+	A/A, K/A	+*	MicroID or API 20E
Pasteurella, Actinobacillus, Mannheimia	–	A/A, A/NC	–	See Table 8-4†
Pseudomonas	+	K/NC	+	
Acinetobacter	+ (w)	K/NC	–	

A, Acid; *K*, alkaline; *NC*, no change; *TSI*, total sugar iron (agar); *w*, weak.
Klebsiella is nonmotile.
†Negative oxidase results are caused by very weak reactions.

cal methods for differentiating the Enterobacteriaceae family members are the commercially available packaged multitest systems. These systems are discussed later. A few other organisms may be isolated infrequently that are oxidase negative. The most common reason for nonenteric oxidase-negative results is a false-negative oxidase test result. When such results are suspected, further differentiation of oxidase-negative bacteria, as shown in Table 8-6, is necessary.

The most frequently isolated oxidase-positive, gram-negative bacteria of veterinary importance can be differentiated by using three tubes of media (TSI, urea, SIM) as shown in Table 8-7.

DEFINITIVE IDENTIFICATION. The identification procedures discussed in this chapter are presumptive methods. Definitive identification of some isolates may require extensive testing. The cost of such identification in time, media, and specialized techniques is usually not justifiable in a small practice laboratory. Unusual isolates should be forwarded to a referral laboratory for further identification. The isolate should be subcultured to an agar slant medium that does not contain a fermentable carbohydrate, or it should be heavily inoculated onto a swab. The swab can be transported in a transport medium, such as Amies transport medium. Do not attempt to ship agar plates. Invariably, they become contaminated and overgrown, dehydrated, or broken.

COMMERCIAL IDENTIFICATION KITS. Commercial development of kit systems for identification of bacteria has been one of the most important advances in clinical bacteriology. These systems provide a cost-effective method for identification of bacteria in low-volume laboratories. Most kits consist of a number of test compartments arranged in a compact unit. The systems generally involve the use of microtechnique tests in various types of media systems. They may include compartments of solid agar, dehydrated broth, substrate or reagent disks, and supplementary conventional tests. All compartments are inoculated with

TABLE 8-7   DIFFERENTIATION OF GRAM-NEGATIVE, OXIDASE-POSITIVE BACTERIA

Organism	Glucose Fermentation in TSI Agar	Growth on MacConkey Agar	Motility	Hemolysis	Urease	Indole
Aeromonas spp.	+	+	+	+	–	+
Actinobacillus spp.	+	±	–	+ (V)	+	–
Mannheimia haemolytica	+	±	–	+*	–	–
Pasteurella multocida	+	–	–	–	–	+
Pasteurella spp.	+	–	–	–	±	–
Pseudomonas aeruginosa	–	+	+	+	±	–
Pseudomonas spp.	–	+	+	V	V	–
Bordetella bronchise ptica	–	+ (w)	+	–	+	–
Moraxella bovis	–	–	–	±	–	–
Moraxella spp.	–	–	–	–	–	–
Brucella canis	–	–	–	–	+	–

TSI, Total sugar iron; *V*, variable; *w*, weak.
*Hemolysis under the colony.

organisms from an isolated colony or colonies. After the specified period of incubation and the addition of required reagents, the results are recorded as positive or negative for each test. For many of the systems, these reactions have variously weighted values so that the positive results will produce a unique profile number for each combination of positive and negative results. Most systems provide profile directories or registers for identification of the isolate most likely to produce the set of observed reactions.

It is advantageous for the low-volume laboratory to use these systems because they are usually more cost effective than attempting to maintain a large inventory of conventional media. They have a reasonable shelf life (6 to 18 months) and require minimum storage space because of the compact construction. Accuracy is better than conventional media in most small laboratories, because most reactions are easy to interpret and results can be decoded more rapidly than sorting through conventional identification tables. Finally, depending on the specific system, most bacteria can be identified within 4 to 24 hours after isolation.

It is essential that the manufacturer's directions and precautions be carefully observed or misidentification will occur. If the system is limited to oxidase-negative enteric bacteria, only those organisms should be inoculated. Other organisms can still yield a profile number, which will result in an incorrect identification. Problems can also arise from inoculation with an older culture, improper concentration of inoculum, or mixed cultures. As experience is gained, accuracy will be increased.

When selecting one of these systems, factors to consider include the ease of inoculation, manipulations required to add reagents, the availability of interpretive charts or numeric coding devices, and the data base used in development of profile registers. Often it is difficult to discover whether significant numbers of veterinary pathogens are included in the data bases for there to be a reasonable probability of correct identification of unique veterinary pathogens. The most beneficial use of these systems is the identification of members of the Enterobacteriaceae family (see Box 8-1). All enteric identification systems give essentially the same degree of accuracy and reliability of performance. The systems that seem to have gained widest acceptance in veterinary bacteriology include API 20E, MicroID, and Enterotube II. They provide excellent results.

Several packaged kit systems are marketed for identifica-

tion of bacteria other than Enterobacteriaceae (see Box 8-1). Although these systems may provide more definitive identifications of some organisms, they have limited usefulness in small veterinary laboratories. Presumptive identification methods outlined in this chapter are frequently adequate.

The identification kits for yeast and anaerobes are useful for large-volume laboratories, but usually the need for them in the small laboratory is not adequate to be cost effective.

Special Culture Procedures
Blood Cultures

The detection of viable bacteria in an animal's blood has considerable diagnostic and prognostic importance. Blood cultures are indicated for fever of unknown origin, suspected bacteremia associated with endocarditis, arthritis, meningitis, and neonatal septicemias. Blood cultures should be obtained from dogs that have antibodies to *Brucella canis* to aid in confirmation of the diagnosis.

Special care must be taken to avoid contaminating blood cultures with skin microflora. The venipuncture site should be decontaminated using surgical scrubbing procedures (see Chapter 24) and should not be palpated after preparation unless a sterile glove is used. Blood can be obtained by using a syringe and needle or a closed-vacuum bottle system. Often the concentration of bacteria in blood is too low to detect by direct inoculation of plate media. Therefore inoculation of commercially available blood culture media bottles is recommended. Ideally, a sample of 5 to 10 ml of blood should be obtained for culture. Blood samples in anticoagulants, such as heparin and ethylenediaminetetraacetic acid (EDTA), are not acceptable for culture because of the poor survival of some bacteria in the presence of these anticoagulants.

Blood culture bottles should be incubated at 35° C to 37° C for at least 7 days and examined daily for macroscopic evidence of growth. Positive cultures can be recognized by one or more of the following characteristics: turbidity, gas bubbles, fluffy or compact colonies, and hemolysis of the blood. When growth is observed, gram-stained smears and subcultures on plate media should be prepared for examination and identification of the organism. Negative-appearing blood culture broths should be blindly subcultured before being discarded and reported as negative. *Brucella* isolation attempts from blood should be incubated for 2 to 4 weeks before being discarded as negative.

Urine Cultures

Urine is an excellent growth medium for many bacteria because it contains electrolytes, water-soluble vitamins, residual amounts of glucose, and various nitrogenous compounds. Therefore careful attention must be given to proper collection and handling of urine for culture, or a small and insignificant number of bacteria can rapidly multiply to significant numbers. Urine specimens for culturing can be collected in three ways: free catch, catheterization, or cystocentesis (see Chapter 3). The distal urethra and genitalia are colonized with microflora that contaminate free-catch and catheterization specimens. If the skin has been adequately prepared for cystocentesis specimens and the needle does not contact any abdominal organ other than the bladder, any bacteria isolated from the specimen should be significant. To reduce overgrowth with insignificant bacteria that may contaminate urine specimens, cultures should be set up within 2 hours of collection. If cultures cannot be established within 2 hours, the sample must be refrigerated to slow the bacterial growth. Refrigeration begins to fail after 18 to 24 hours. Therefore the best method for identifying urinary tract infections is to establish cultures as soon as possible.

The use of blood agar and MacConkey agar as selective and differential isolation media is recommended for the culture of all urine specimens. There is no need for broth medium for enrichment culturing. The bacteriologic examination of urine specimens collected by methods other than cystocentesis should provide an estimate of the number of microorganisms per milliliter of urine as an aid to interpreting the results. This can be accomplished by inoculating the blood agar plate with a standard dilution loop calibrated to deliver approximately 0.001 ml (Figure 8-7). Each colony that grows represents 10^3 organisms/ml in the specimen; therefore the number of colonies is multiplied by 1000 to obtain the concentration of organisms in the specimen. The number of bacteria can also be estimated through direct microscopic examination of a gram-stained smear of uncentrifuged urine. If one or more bacteria per oil immersion field are observed, usually more than 10^5 organisms/ml should be present in cultures. If more than two types of bacteria are isolated, a second specimen should be collected and cultured to distinguish a mixed infection from contamination or mishandling of the specimen. Bacterial counts can be low because of improper handling of the specimen, dilution from forced fluid therapy, or cystocentesis samples from patients with urethritis that has not become established as a concomitant cystitis.

 Technician Note

The following guidelines can be used for interpretation of urine cultures:

- For a single species, more than 10^5 bacteria/ml indicates significant bacteria.
- Between 10^3 and 10^5 bacteria/ml suggests infection if the urine has been properly collected and neutrophils are present.
- Fewer than 10^3 bacteria/ml suggests contamination or mishandling of the specimen. If there is doubt about interpreting a colony count, the culture should be repeated with a second specimen.

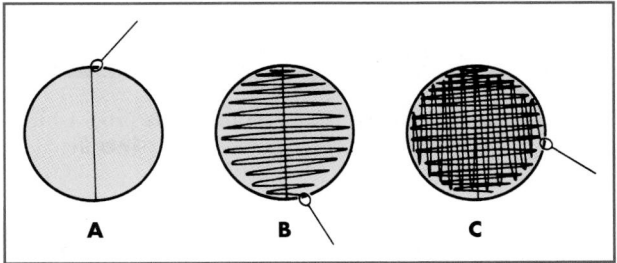

FIGURE 8-7. Procedure for inoculating media for semiquantitative bacterial colony counts when culturing urine. **A,** Primary inoculation with calibrated loop. **B,** Streak at right angles to primary inoculation. **C,** Streak at right angles to previous streak.

COMMON BACTERIAL SPECIES

The bacterial pathogens frequently associated with many infectious processes are listed in Table 8-1. Some of the colony morphologic, growth, and identifying characteristics of these bacteria are listed in Table 8-8. Additional details are given in the following discussion for special isolation and identification techniques. Clinically important characteristics are noted.

Gram-Positive Cocci

Staphylococcus

Staphylococcus spp. are catalase-positive cocci that occur in grapelike clusters. They are frequently isolated from pyogenic lesions, such as wounds, dermatitis, otitis, mastitis, cystitis, and osteomyelitis. They are usually divided into coagulase-positive and coagulase-negative groups. The coagulase-positive species, *S. aureus* and *S. intermedius*, are more important pathogens, and the others are usually considered to be less pathogenic. One of the most important identifying characteristics that should be noted is the development of a double zone of hemolysis (an inner zone of complete hemolysis and a second zone of incomplete hemolysis). This is a common identifying characteristic of most coagulase-positive isolates from animals. Mannitol fermentation is not a reliable correlate of coagulase activity in staphylococcal isolates from animals. Because of a high incidence of acquired antimicrobial resistance, these organisms should be tested for antimicrobial susceptibility.

Streptococcus

Streptococcus spp. are catalase-negative cocci that occur singly, in pairs, or in short chains. Chain formation is more easily demonstrated in broth cultures. *Streptococcus* is the most common bacterial pathogen of the horse and can be found to cause pyogenic infections and mastitis in all species of animals. However, each species tends to be rather host specific. Therefore the streptococcal pathogens of humans rarely cause infections in animals, and animals are usually not reservoirs of human pathogens. Some species cause specific diseases. *Streptococcus equi* ssp. *equi* is the cause of strangles in horses. *Streptococcus agalactiae* is an important cause of bovine mastitis. It can be identified by the CAMP test. Definitive biochemical and serologic (Lancefield typing) testing is usually not clinically important. For clinical interpretation, it is important to evaluate the hemolysis produced on blood agar. Beta-hemolysis (complete clearing) usually correlates well with potential pathogenicity; alpha-hemolysis (incomplete greenish discoloring) and gamma-hemolysis (nonhemolytic) are

TABLE 8-8   IDENTIFYING CHARACTERISTICS OF COMMON VETERINARY BACTERIAL PATHOGENS

	Blood Agar	MacConkey Agar	Other Characteristics
GRAM-POSITIVE			
Staphylococcus	Smooth, glistening, white to yellow pigmented colonies	No growth	Catalase-positive glucose fermenter; Double-zone hemolysis usually indicates coagulase positive; coagulase activity is a useful differential test
Streptococcus	Small, glistening colonies; hemolysis	No growth except some enterococci	Catalase-negative, usually identified by type of hemolysis; beta-hemolytic strains more likely to be pathogens, others are often part of flora; *Streptococcus agalactiae* CAMP-positive
Arcanobacterium pyogenes	Small, hemolytic, streplike colonies	No growth	Catalase negative; slow growth, often requiring 48 hr for distinct colonies; growth enhanced in candle jar
Corynebacterium pseudotuberculosis	Slow-growing, opaque, dry crumbly colonies; usually hemolytic	No growth	Catalase positive; weak urease positive
Corynebacterium renale	Small, smooth, glistening colonies (24 hr); become opaque and dry later	No growth	Catalase positive; urease positive
Rhodococcus equi	Small, moist, white (24 hr); become large, pink colonies; no hemolysis	No growth	Catalase positive, delayed urease positive
Listeria monocytogenes	Small, hemolytic, glistening colonies	No growth	Catalase positive; motile at room temperature
Erysipelothrix rhusiopathiae	Small colonies after 48 hr; greenish (alpha) hemolysis	No growth	Catalase negative, hydrogen sulfide positive
Nocardia	Slow-growing, small, dry, granular, white to orange colonies	No growth	Partially acid fast; colonies tenaciously adhere to media
Actinomyces	Slow growing, small, rough, nodular white colonies	No growth	Require increased carbon dioxide or anaerobic incubation; not acid fast
Clostridium	Variable, round, ill-defined, irregular colonies; usually hemolytic	No growth	Obligate anaerobes
Bacillus	Variable, large, rough, dry or mucoid colonies	No growth	Usually hemolytic; large rods with endospores

usually indications of normal flora of skin and mucous membranes. However, when isolated in nearly pure culture from normally sterile body sites, these organisms can be considered to be clinically significant. Susceptibility to antimicrobials is usually predictable, which means antimicrobial susceptibility testing may be an unnecessary expense.

The enteric group D streptococci have been renamed as *Enterococcus* spp. Urinary tract infections are the most common presentation of these organisms; they occasionally infect wounds and cause bacteremia. They are emerging as significant nosocomial agents and are particularly troublesome because they are likely to be resistant to many antimicrobials.

Anaerobic Cocci

Anaerobic cocci belong to the genera *Peptococcus* and *Peptostreptococcus*. When isolated, these agents are usually associated with mixed anaerobic infections.

Gram-Positive Rods
Spore Formers

Bacillus spp. are common contaminants isolated in the laboratory. They are ubiquitous in soil, water, air, and dust. They are large spore-forming rods that usually grow as large, rough, granular, or spreading colonies. They are usually hemolytic. Occasionally, strains of *Bacillus* will be isolated that react as if they are gram-negative and oxidase-positive. However, they can be identified by the presence

TABLE 8-8	IDENTIFYING CHARACTERISTICS OF COMMON VETERINARY BACTERIAL PATHOGENS—CONT'D		
	Blood Agar	**MacConkey Agar**	**Other Characteristics**
GRAM-NEGATIVE			
Escherichia coli	Large, gray, smooth, mucoid colonies; hemolysis variable	Hot pink to red colonies; red cloudiness in media	Hemolysis frequently associated with virulence
Klebsiella pneumoniae	Large, mucoid, sticky, whitish colonies; not hemolytic	Large, mucoid, pink colonies	Nonmotile; require biochemical tests to differentiate from *Enterobacter*
Proteus	Frequently swarming without distinct colonies	Colorless; limited swarming	
Other enterics	Gray to white, smooth, mucoid colonies	Colorless colonies	Biochemical tests for identification; serotyping indicated for *Salmonella*
Pseudomonas	Irregular, spreading, grayish colonies; variable hemolysis; may show a metallic sheen	Colorless, irregular colonies	Oxidase positive; fruity odor; may produce yellow greenish soluble pigment in clear media
Bordetella bronchiseptica	Very small, circular dewdrop colonies; variable hemolysis	Small, colorless colonies	May require 48 hr for distinct colonies; oxidase positive; rapid urease positive; citrate positive
Brucella canis	Very small, circular, pinpoint colonies after 48-72 hr; not hemolytic	No growth	Oxidase positive; catalase positive; urease positive
Moraxella	Round, translucent, grayish white colonies; variable hemolysis	No growth	Oxidase and catalase positive; often nonreactive in routine biochemical tests; colonies may pit media
Actinobacillus	Round, translucent colonies; variable hemolysis	Variable growth; colorless colonies	Glucose fermenter; nonmotile; urease positive; sticky colonies
Mannheimia haemolytica	Round, gray, smooth colonies; hemolysis under the colony	Variable growth; colorless colonies	Glucose fermenter in TSI; weak oxidase positive
Pasteurella multocida	Gray, mucoid, round to coalescing colonies; no hemolysis	No growth	Glucose fermenter in TSI; weak oxidase and indole positive

TSI, Triple sugar iron (agar).

of spores in stained smears. *Bacillus anthracis* (the agent that causes anthrax) is the important pathogenic species. It is extremely virulent for humans. *Do not attempt to culture it.*

Clostridium spp. are large, spore-forming anaerobic rods. The pathogenic species are noted for their potent toxins and extensive destruction of tissue. Infections may be accompanied by an accumulation of gas (emphysema) in the tissues. Laboratory diagnosis of the toxic diseases (tetanus, botulism, enterotoxemia) and differentiation of the infectious diseases (blackleg, malignant edema, bacillary hemoglobinuria, etc.) require the assistance of reference diagnostic laboratories. Often a gram-stained smear is useful for ruling out clostridial disease or indicating it as a

possibility. *Clostridium perfringens* is occasionally isolated from deep wounds with extensive tissue necrosis, such as compound fractures. The bacterium requires an anaerobic atmosphere for growth and frequently produces a double zone of hemolysis.

C. perfringens is also associated with enteritis and diarrhea in dogs. The presence of enterotoxigenic strains of *C. perfringens* can be presumptively identified in fecal smears by evaluating the smears for the presence of increased bacterial spores because sporulation is associated with the release of enterotoxin. Spores appear as unstained, small, oval structures, and usually are surrounded by a halo of stained bacterial cells unless a specific spore stain is applied.

Small Rods

Corynebacterium spp. are small, club-shaped rods that tend to occur in palisades or in an angular arrangement because of their "snapping" division. Colonies are usually quite small at 24 hours but continue to enlarge and vary markedly by species. Most species are catalase positive. *Arcanobacterium pyogenes* (previously called *Actinomyces pyogenes*) produces a small pinpoint colony, hemolysis, and a negative catalase reaction. Cellular morphologic characteristics must be evaluated carefully to differentiate it from *Streptococcus*. It is the most common pyogenic agent in ruminants. *Rhodococcus equi* is a cause of pneumonia and abscesses in foals. Morphologically, individual cells are coccobacillary and larger than other *Corynebacterium* organisms. *Corynebacterium pseudotuberculosis* causes chronic abscesses in goats and sheep. *Corynebacterium renale* is a cause of pyelonephritis and cystitis in cows. There are many other *Corynebacterium* spp. that are nonpathogenic commensals of the skin; they are frequently referred to collectively as diphtheroids.

Listeria monocytogenes is a small, non-spore-forming rod that is catalase-positive. It is the only small gram-positive rod that is motile at room temperature. It is an infrequent cause of abortion in large animals and septicemia in young animals. In ruminants, it causes an encephalitis known as *circling disease*. The bacteria localize in the pons and medulla (brainstem). Cultures from other parts of the brain may be negative. Isolation may require specific selective and enrichment techniques. The brain is stored in a refrigerator and cultured weekly for up to 12 weeks before the results are considered negative.

Erysipelothrix rhusiopathiae is a pleomorphic rod that is usually slender and small. The colony is small, and an incomplete, greenish hemolysis (alpha like) is produced. The cellular morphologic characteristics must be carefully evaluated to differentiate it from *Streptococcus* because both are catalase negative. A definitive characteristic that differentiates it from other gram-positive rods is the production of hydrogen sulfide. *Erysipelothrix* is most commonly encountered as a cause of septicemic or arthritic disease of pigs, but it is occasionally a cause of endocarditis in dogs.

Filamentous Rods

The Actinomycetaceae family contains several clinically important bacteria that are distinguished by forming branching, filamentous gram-positive rods. Most *Actinomyces* spp. are anaerobic bacteria that may tolerate low levels of oxygen. Therefore some species can be isolated in a candle jar, but the most efficient isolation can be achieved with an anaerobic system. *Actinomyces* spp. colonies are slow to develop, requiring up to 5 days, and are usually raised and irregular in shape. When isolated, they are usually recovered from pyogranulomatous lesions of soft tissue, pyothoraces, or osteomyelitis. *Nocardia* spp. are partially acid fast, which means a modified staining procedure must be used to differentiate them from *Actinomyces* spp. In place of the acid-alcohol decolorizer, only an acid decolorizer is used to demonstrate acid fastness. *Nocardia* spp. are aerobic bacteria with colonies usually appearing after 2 to 5 days of incubation. The colonies are rough and have a dry, granular texture. They adhere tenaciously to the media. *Nocardia* is occasionally isolated from pyothoraces and wounds. It may be a serious mastitis pathogen in some dairy herds. *Dermatophilus congolensis* is another branching, filamentous bacterium. It often has a beaded appearance with transverse and longitudinal divisions. It is an uncommon cause of skin infections of horses and ruminants. The organism can be demonstrated in smears of pus from under the elevated scabs containing tufts of hair. *Streptomyces* spp. are aerobic, filamentous bacteria that are not acid fast. They are abundant in soil and may be isolated as contaminants.

Anaerobes

Anaerobic, gram-positive, non-spore-forming rods belong to the genera *Bifidobacterium*, *Eubacterium*, and *Propionibacterium*. If definitive identification of these organisms is needed, they should be sent to a reference diagnostic laboratory. They are usually isolated in mixed cultures from pyogenic lesions.

Acid-Fast Bacteria

Mycobacteria are mostly small, short rods but are occasionally pleomorphic. They stain poorly with Gram's stain but are acid fast. These bacteria are rarely isolated in veterinary practice laboratories because special procedures and media are usually required. However, preparation of an acid-fast stained impression smear can be a useful diagnostic procedure for making a presumptive diagnosis of mycobacterial infection. Positive findings are significant; however, negative findings have limited predictive value. *Mycobacterium avium* ssp. *paratuberculosis* may be demonstrated in acid-fast stained smears prepared from intestinal mucosa or mesenteric lymph nodes of ruminants. *Mycobacterium avium* infection of birds can frequently be confirmed by examination of acid-fast smears prepared from the liver or intestinal mucosa. Occasionally, abundant acid-fast organisms can be demonstrated in the feces.

Isolation of the zoonotic agents of tuberculosis, *Mycobacterium bovis* and *Mycobacterium tuberculosis*, should not be attempted in a clinic laboratory. Infrequently, a rapid-growing *Mycobacterium* sp. may be isolated from cases of bovine mastitis. The colonies will usually appear at 3 to 5 days of incubation. These organisms should be forwarded to a reference laboratory for definitive identification.

Gram-Negative Bacteria

The Enterobacteriaceae family of bacteria is the largest group of potential pathogens and the most frequently isolated bacteria. The normal habitat of these organisms is the digestive tract and soil; therefore they will usually grow on MacConkey agar and are frequently insignificant contaminants of specimens. They are small gram-negative rods, with some pleomorphism. Some of the common identifying characteristics include oxidase negativity, glucose fermentation, and motility (except *Klebsiella*). Genus and species identification requires numerous biochemical tests, and serotyping is frequently needed to identify pathogenic strains. Acquired antimicrobial resistance from R factors (plasmids) is common in this family of bacteria, making antimicrobial susceptibility testing a necessary clinical evaluation of isolates.

Most non-Enterobacteriaceae, gram-negative bacteria are oxidase positive, and growth on MacConkey agar is variable.

Coliforms

Escherichia coli can frequently be presumptively identified by the strong lactose fermentation reaction it produces on MacConkey agar. Strains causing tissue infections and cystitis are frequently hemolytic. *Escherichia coli* is frequently associated with diarrhea in neonates (especially pigs, calves, and lambs). The pathogenic strains causing diarrhea are best identified by genotyping and other specialized laboratory testing, such as use of the K99 *E. coli* antigen test kit (K99 Pilitest, VMRD, Inc.). However, presumptive evidence of *E. coli* involvement in diarrhea (scours) can be obtained by Gram staining a smear taken from small intestinal mucosa shortly after the death of the animal. If a large number (>25) of gram-negative rods are observed in each oil immersion field, it is a strong indication that *E. coli* is a cause of diarrhea. *Klebsiella* spp. and *Enterobacter* spp. are occasionally involved in infections of the respiratory and urinary tracts and in mastitis. They are becoming more important in veterinary medicine as superinfecting agents after antimicrobial therapy.

Salmonella

Salmonella spp. can cause diarrhea and septicemia in all animals and in humans. When feces are to be cultured, selective and enrichment media should be used to increase the probability of successful isolation of *Salmonella*. Hektoen enteric agar and selenite enrichment broth (see Table 8-2) are recommended. The enrichment broth should be subcultured to both MacConkey and Hektoen enteric agar. Non–lactose-fermenting colonies can rapidly be screened with *Salmonella* polyvalent O antiserum to identify them. To be able to define the epidemiology of salmonellosis outbreaks, the isolates should be forwarded to a reference laboratory for serotyping.

Proteus

Proteus spp. are frequently isolated as specimen contaminants or secondary invaders. They are important pathogens of the urinary tract. Related genera of bacteria that do not swarm on blood agar are *Morganella* and *Providencia*, and they can be readily identified using kits. The swarming *Proteus* spp. sometimes interfere with isolation of other organisms. This problem can be solved by using phenylethyl alcohol (PEA) blood agar plates. *Proteus* and other gram-negative organisms will be inhibited, providing easier isolation of gram-positive organisms.

Other Enteric Organisms

There are many other members of the Enterobacteriaceae family, including *Serratia*, *Citrobacter*, *Edwardsiella*, and *Hafnia*, that are infrequently isolated. Careful clinical evaluation is necessary to determine their significance. Often a repeated culture helps confirm the significance of isolation.

Aeromonas

Aeromonas spp. are oxidase-positive rods that grow on MacConkey agar. They are commonly found in soil, water, and sewage and frequently infect aquatic animals. They are infrequently a cause of septicemia in terrestrial animals.

Actinobacillus

Actinobacillus spp. are oxidase-positive, small rods that usually grow on MacConkey agar. The colony morphologic characteristics are similar to those of *Pasteurella*. *Actinobacillus equuli* is the most frequently isolated species. It produces a very sticky colony. It is frequently the cause of septicemic infections in foals. It can be isolated from most horses as part of the mucosal flora but is generally only an opportunistic pathogen in older horses.

Pasteurella

Pasteurella spp. are usually associated with respiratory infections in most animals. In cats, they are frequently recovered from abscesses. They are small, oxidase-positive coccobacilli. *Pasteurella multocida* produces a characteristic musty odor. Identification can be aided by noting the typically weak glucose fermentation reaction in a TSI tube. *Pasteurella* spp. tend to be nonreactive in most commercial identification kit systems and may be misidentified. Hemolytic strains previously known as *P. haemolytica* have been renamed *Mannheimia haemolytica* for bovine respiratory isolates, and some ovine strains are now called *P. trehalosi*. Antimicrobial resistance is a growing problem in isolates from food animals, thus indicating a need to perform susceptibility tests.

Haemophilus

Haemophilus spp. are often part of the normal flora of mucous membranes. A few species are important pathogens, usually of the respiratory system. They are small coccobacilli that require specially enriched media for growth. They may grow as satellite colonies around *Staphylococcus* on blood agar. In addition to the nutritional growth requirements, an increased concentration of carbon dioxide is necessary. These bacteria are very susceptible to antibiotics and environmental stress factors, such as drying; therefore specimens must be collected and handled carefully or isolation will be unsuccessful.

Pseudomonas

Pseudomonas spp. are common soil and water bacteria. They are usually considered to be opportunistic pathogens of wounds and otitis. Infrequently, they are isolated from the respiratory and urinary tracts. There are many species, but *Pseudomonas aeruginosa* is the most common pathogen. It produces water-soluble yellow-green pigments that diffuse into the medium, and it has a distinctive odor that aids in recognition. Most isolates are quite resistant to antimicrobials and should routinely be tested for susceptibility.

Bordetella

Bordetella bronchiseptica is a small coccobacillus that is frequently recovered from respiratory infections of dogs and is emerging as an important respiratory pathogen of cats. It is associated with atrophic rhinitis in pigs and is infrequently isolated from respiratory infections of other animals. Colonies are slow to develop and may only be pinpointed after 48 hours. Growth occurs on MacConkey agar. It is oxidase positive, urease positive (often within 4 hours), and citrate positive.

Brucella

Brucella spp. are very small coccobacilli that are usually associated with reproductive failure: abortion and infertility. Some species require increased carbon dioxide for growth; however, *Brucella canis* can be isolated in an aerobic atmosphere. Growth is slow, often requiring 3 to 7 days for colonies to be detectable. Suspected *Brucella* isolates should be sent to a reference laboratory for definitive identification because of the regulatory and zoonotic importance of these agents.

Other Gram-negative Rods

A large number of gram-negative bacteria have limited or undetermined clinical importance. Included are bacteria such as *Moraxella*, *Acinetobacter*, *Neisseria*, *Branhamella*, and related pleomorphic coccobacilli. These organisms are commonly found as part of the flora of mucous membranes and are usually secondary, opportunistic pathogens. They are relatively nonreactive in most conventional biochemical tests. Thus identification is usually difficult, even for reference diagnostic laboratories.

Anaerobes

The gram-negative anaerobes *(Bacteroides, Porphyromonas, Prevotella, Fusobacterium)* are frequently involved in mixed infections in abscesses and necrotic tissue. They are normally found in the digestive tract, so infections resulting from contamination of tissues with mucous membrane flora or intestinal contents frequently contain these organisms. Usually Gram's stain of the exudate will indicate that bacteria that do not grow aerobically are present. If obligate anaerobes are isolated, evaluation of the cellular morphologic characteristics provides adequate clinical information. Species identification is rarely important. Taxonomic advances have resulted in the reclassification of some former *Bacteroides* spp. into the genera *Dichelobacter, Porphyromonas,* and *Prevotella.*

Spirochetes and Curved Bacteria

Leptospira spp. cause febrile infections often followed by abortion and infertility. These spirochetes are difficult to isolate and usually die within a few hours while being transported to a laboratory. Darkfield examination of urine may aid in establishing a diagnosis. Most diagnoses are made by serologic testing.

Borrelia burgdorferi is a tick-transmitted spirochete that causes Lyme disease in humans and arthritis and lameness in dogs. Canine borreliosis may be accompanied by high rectal temperature and lymphadenopathy. Detection of serum antibodies to *B. burgdorferi* is the diagnostic test of choice in dogs. Isolation of *Borrelia* by culture is difficult and often nonproductive. Borreliosis is of importance in the United States in dogs and other animals only within areas infested by ticks carrying this agent.

Brachyspira hyodysenteriae (formerly called *Serpulina hyodysenteriae*) is a spirochete that causes dysentery in pigs. Cultural isolation is beyond the capability of most laboratories. Diagnosis of this infection may be made by examining smears of colonic mucosa for numerous large spirochetes.

Campylobacter spp. cause two different types of disease conditions. One group contains important reproductive pathogens, causing abortion and infertility. Because of special needs for enrichment and selective media and a microaerophilic atmosphere, specimens for isolation of *Campylobacter* should be sent to veterinary diagnostic laboratories specially equipped for *Campylobacter* culture. The second group includes important zoonotic enteric pathogens. Most public health and hospital laboratories are equipped to isolate this group. *Campylobacter* spp. are curved gram-negative rods. They can be recognized by darkfield or phase-contrast microscopy by their darting motility.

Helicobacter spp. are helical or curved gram-negative bacteria that colonize the gastric mucosa of humans, dogs, and cats and the intestinal tract of some rodents, birds, and swine. Some species have been associated with gastritis and peptic ulceration, whereas other species are considered to be nonpathogenic flora of the gastric mucosa of animals. They can be detected and identified in histologic sections, by culture in reference laboratories, and by associating strong urease activity in gastric mucus with their presence.

Mycoplasma

Mycoplasma spp. are small bacteria that lack a cell wall and, as a result, are not easily stained and observed in exudates.

Arthritis and pneumonia are the most common mycoplasmal diseases. The role of *Mycoplasma* in urogenital infections is not well characterized. Occasionally strains can be isolated on blood agar plates inoculated with urine from dogs with cystitis. Special media and techniques are required for isolation and identification of most *Mycoplasma.* Therefore arrangements should be made with a reference laboratory for *Mycoplasma* transport media and specimen shipping instructions.

ANTIMICROBIAL SUSCEPTIBILITY TESTING

One of the most important functions of the clinical microbiology laboratory is to provide information that can assist in the selection of appropriate therapy for infectious diseases. All antimicrobial agents have limitations in their spectra of activity. Therefore a universal antimicrobial for all infections is not available. Some organisms are intrinsically resistant to an antimicrobial, whereas others acquire resistance. The most common mechanism for acquired resistance is the acquisition of extrachromosomal pieces of DNA, such as plasmids (R factors) and bacteriophages. As a result, the bacteria are able to produce enzymes that modify or inactivate the antimicrobial, enable the cell to resist accumulation of the drug, or alter target sites and reduce the activity of the drug. Because the acquired resistance traits are not static, the antimicrobial susceptibility pattern *(antibiogram)* is not predictable for many organisms. Therefore susceptibility tests are necessary.

Indications for Susceptibility Testing

Susceptibility testing is indicated for most rapidly growing, aerobic and facultative anaerobic, clinically significant bacteria. Testing should be avoided for isolates representing normal flora and for those bacteria with predictable susceptibility to the antimicrobial of choice. Gram-positive bacteria other than *Staphylococcus* have rather predictable antibiograms; therefore routine testing is not needed. However, susceptibility testing may be indicated if the antimicrobial of choice cannot be safely and economically administered to the patient. Unpredictable resistance patterns are frequently observed with the gram-negative bacteria, thus requiring testing. Most slow-growing and anaerobic bacteria have rather predictable antibiograms, so testing is not necessary. If acquired resistance is found to be a problem in these organisms, special test methods will be necessary for testing them.

In most cases the veterinarian will have started antimicrobial therapy before the laboratory results are available. When the test results become available, therapy can be altered or modified to provide safe, effective, least-cost therapy. In some situations the culture specimen will be from a moribund or dead animal. Susceptibility testing may still be important because it can establish patterns of antimicrobial susceptibility for the organism when encountered in other animals in the herd or region.

Susceptibility Test Methods

The simplest type of susceptibility test is one that tests for the presence of an enzyme that can inactivate an antimicrobial. Penicillin resistance in *Staphylococcus* is acquired by gaining the ability to produce beta-lactamase, an enzyme that inactivates most penicillin derivatives. Sensitive and rapid tests, such as Cefinase (BD Microbiology Systems), are available for detecting this enzyme. If the test is negative, penicillin or a penicillin derivative is usually the drug of choice, and no further testing is needed. If the isolate is producing beta-lactamase, further antimicrobial

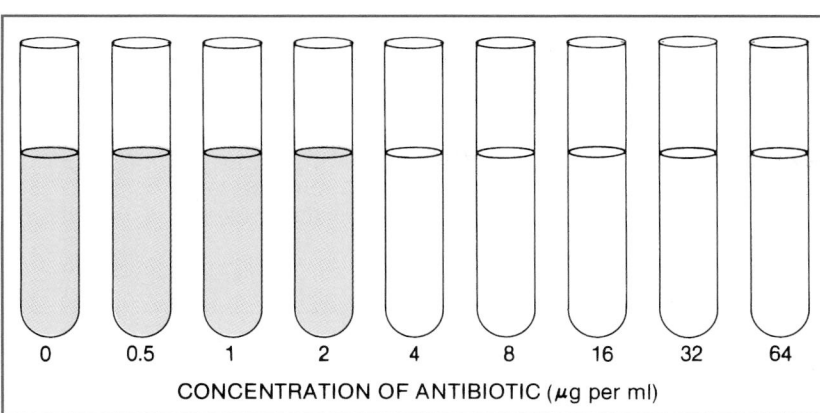

FIGURE 8-8. Broth dilution susceptibility test. The organism grew in broth containing antibiotic in the amounts of 0.5, 1, and 2 μg/ml, but growth was inhibited in the tube containing 4 μg/ml. Therefore the minimal inhibitory concentration is 4 μg/ml.

CONCENTRATION OF ANTIBIOTIC (μg per ml)

susceptibility testing will be needed to select an alternative therapy. A beta-lactamase test can be a very useful part of a mastitis culture procedure to rapidly evaluate the appropriateness of penicillin therapy because it is one of the most frequently administered antimicrobials.

In most cases, tests for antimicrobial inactivating enzymes are not available. Therefore most routine susceptibility tests measure the degree of susceptibility of the isolate to each of several antimicrobials. The broth dilution susceptibility test system is the most precise method and the reference method. This test is performed by introducing a standardized inoculum of an organism into a series of tubes (or wells in a microculture plate) containing serial dilutions of an antimicrobial in medium (Figure 8-8). The lowest concentration of antimicrobial that macroscopically inhibits growth of the organism is the *minimal inhibitory concentration (MIC)*. The MIC of an antimicrobial for a given isolate represents the degree of susceptibility to the drug. If the antimicrobial is going to be used in therapy, the MIC must be achieved at the site of infection to effectively inhibit bacterial growth.

The most commonly used method of antimicrobial susceptibility testing in small laboratories is the *agar diffusion test* using antimicrobial-impregnated paper disks that are applied to the surface of agar that has been streaked with a standardized inoculum. As the antimicrobial is absorbed from the disk into the agar, it begins diffusing in a radial pattern (Figure 8-9). As the antimicrobial diffuses, it becomes more dilute, thereby creating a gradient effect of decreasing concentrations. The bacterial inoculum on the agar begins to grow in all areas except the places in which the antimicrobial concentration exceeds the MIC of the isolate. Zones of inhibition of growth can be observed around the disks. In carefully controlled studies, the diameters of the zones of inhibition have been correlated with MIC values. The results of the diffusion test can then be semiquantitatively interpreted, usually as susceptible, intermediate, or resistant.

The diffusion test is easy to set up, but it requires careful attention to detail to ensure that the results are accurate. Mueller-Hinton agar has been selected as the standard culture medium so that the composition of the agar can be more uniformly controlled. However, this medium will not support growth of some fastidious pathogens, such as *Streptococcus, Listeria, Corynebacterium, Erysipelothrix, Pasteurella*, and some other gram-negative bacteria. For these bacteria, serum or blood enrichment is necessary. Therefore it may be more practical to use blood agar plates for susceptibility tests in low-volume laboratories. Results are

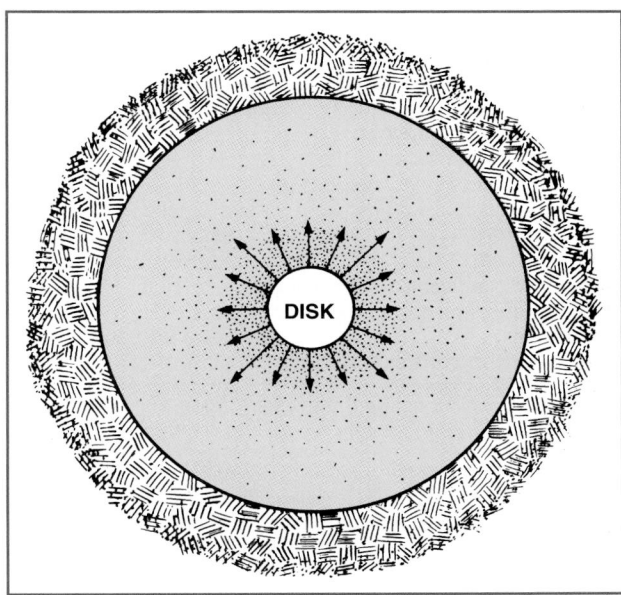

FIGURE 8-9. Principle of antibiotic diffusion in agar from a disk. The concentration of antibiotic is highest near the disk and logarithmically diluted as it diffuses radially into a larger area. At some point, the antibiotic is diluted below the minimal inhibitory concentration for the test organism, which allows the organism to grow. The resulting zone of inhibition is measured and interpreted with the use of Table 8-9.

usually comparable to those obtained with Mueller-Hinton agar; however, false-resistant results will often be obtained on the blood agar when testing sulfonamide activity. Fresh plates with the proper depth of agar must be used to avoid altering the kinetics of antimicrobial diffusion in a shallow or dehydrated plate.

Inoculum density should be standardized to avoid significant variations in zone sizes and misinterpretations. Susceptibility tests should always be performed with a *pure culture* of bacteria. Bacteria in mixed cultures can inhibit growth of slower-growing or fastidious organisms. Therefore, if mixed cultures are tested, antimicrobial resistance of a pathogen may not be detected. Direct susceptibility testing of clinical specimens is discouraged, and, if performed, the results should always be verified by testing isolates in pure culture.

TABLE 8-9   ZONE DIAMETER (MEASURED IN MILLIMETERS) INTERPRETIVE STANDARDS FOR SUSCEPTIBILITY TESTS

Antimicrobial Agent	Disk Content	Susceptible	Intermediate	Resistant
Amikacin	30 µg	≥17	15-16	≤14
Amoxicillin/clavulanic acid (staphylococci)	20/10 µg	≥20		≤19
Amoxicillin/clavulanic acid (other organisms)	20/10 µg	≥18	14-17	≤13
Ampicillin* (gram-negative enteric organisms)	10 µg	≥17	14-16	≤13
Ampicillin* (staphylococci)	10 µg	≥29		≤28
Ampicillin* (enterococci)	10 µg	≥17		≤16
Ampicillin* (streptococci)	10 µg	≥26	19-25	≤18
Cefazolin	30 µg	≥18	15-17	≤14
Cefoxitin	30 µg	≥18	15-17	≤14
Ceftiofur (respiratory pathogens only)	30 µg	≥21	18-20	≤17
Cephalothin†	30 µg	≥18	15-17	≤14
Chloramphenicol	30 µg	≥18	13-17	≤12
Clindamycin‡	2 µg	≥21	15-20	≤14
Enrofloxacin	5 µg	≥23	17-22	≤16
Erythromycin	15 µg	≥23	14-22	≤13
Gentamicin	10 µg	≥15	13-14	≤12
Kanamycin	30 µg	≥18	14-17	≤13
Oxacillin§ (staphylococci)	1 µg	≥13	11-12	≤10
Penicillin G (staphylococci)	10 units	≥29		≤28
Penicillin G (enterococci)	10 units	≥15		≤14
Penicillin G (streptococci)	10 units	≥28	20-27	≤19
Penicillin/novobiocin‖	10 units/30 µg	≥18	15-17	≤14
Pirlimycin‖	2 µg	≥13		≤12
Rifampin	5 µg	≥20	17-19	≤16
Sulfonamides	250 or 300 µg	≥17	13-16	≤12
Tetracycline¶	30 µg	≥19	15-18	≤14
Ticarcillin (Pseudomonas aeruginosa)	75 µg	≥15		≤14
Ticarcillin (gram-negative enteric organisms)	75 µg	≥20	15-19	≤14
Tilmicosin	15 µg	≥14	11-13	≤10
Trimethoprim/sulfamethoxazole**	1.25/23.75 µg	≥16	11-15	≤10

Modified from National Committee for Clinical Laboratory Standards document M31-A, Table 2, pp. 36-39, 1999.
*Ampicillin is used to test for susceptibility to amoxicillin and hetacillin.
†Cephalothin is used to test all first-generation cephalosporins, such as cephapirin and cefadroxil. Cefazolin should be tested separately with the gram-negative enteric organisms.
‡Clindamycin is used to test for susceptibility to clindamycin and lincomycin.
§Oxacillin is used to test for susceptibility to methicillin, nafcillin, and cloxacillin.
‖Available as an infusion product for treatment of bovine mastitis during lactation.
¶Tetracycline is used to test for susceptibility to chlortetracycline, oxytetracycline, minocycline, and doxycycline.
**Trimethoprim/sulfamethoxazole is used to test for susceptibility to trimethoprim/sulfadiazine and ormetoprim/sulfadimethoxine.

Standard antimicrobial disks should be purchased rather than attempting to prepare them from therapeutic drug solutions. It is important to make certain that the disks contain the same amount of antimicrobial as is listed in the interpretation chart (Table 8-9). Otherwise, the results will not correlate with the desired MIC values. All cartridges of disks not in current use should be stored in a –20° C freezer; those currently in use should be kept in the refrigerator to avoid deterioration of the antimicrobials.

Diffusion Test Procedure
Inoculum
Select four or five well-isolated colonies of the same morphologic type from an agar plate culture. Touch the top of each colony with a wire loop, and transfer the growth to a tube containing 0.5 to 1 ml of saline or broth. The turbidity of the bacterial suspension should be equivalent to a MacFarland no. 0.5 standard, which is just turbid enough that a slight change in optical density of the tube is macroscopically visible. Within 15 minutes after preparing the inoculum suspension, dip a sterile nontoxic cotton swab into the suspension and rotate the swab several times

with firm pressure on the inside wall of the tube to remove excess inoculum from the swab. Then inoculate the agar plate by streaking the swab over the entire agar surface. Repeat the streaking procedure two or more times, rotating the plate approximately 60 degrees each time to ensure an even distribution of inoculum.

Test Procedure
Place the appropriate antimicrobial-impregnated disks, selected from the list in Table 8-9, on the surface of the agar. Note that some disks serve as class disks for a group of related antimicrobials, thereby reducing the need for testing each drug individually. The disks should be distributed evenly on the surface of the agar so that they are no closer than 24 mm from center to center. This is best accomplished with a dispensing apparatus. Using a sterile forceps or needle tip, gently press each disk to the agar to ensure complete contact. Because some of the drug begins to diffuse immediately, a disk should not be moved once it has come in contact with the agar. Finally, invert the plates, and place them in the incubator. The inoculated test plate is incubated in an aerobic atmosphere at 35° C for 18 hours.

Measuring Zones of Inhibition

After 16 to 18 hours of incubating a properly inoculated plate, zones of inhibition around the disks should be uniformly circular with a uniformly confluent or almost completely confluent lawn of growth between zones. If only isolated colonies grow, the inoculum was too light, and the test should be repeated. The zone diameters should be carefully measured, including the diameter of the disk, and recorded to the nearest millimeter. The end point should be taken as the area showing no obvious visible growth (not including faint growth of any colonies that can be detected only with difficulty at the edge of the zone of inhibited growth). Large colonies growing within a clear zone of inhibition should be subcultured, reidentified, and retested. Strains of *Proteus mirabilis* and *Proteus vulgaris* may swarm into areas of inhibited growth around certain antimicrobials. The zones of inhibition are usually clearly outlined, and the veil of swarming growth is ignored. With the sulfonamides, organisms may grow through several generations before they are inhibited. Slight growth (80% or more inhibition) with sulfonamides is therefore disregarded, and the margin of *heavy growth* is measured to determine the zone diameter.

Results

Interpret the sizes of the zones of inhibition by referring to Table 8-9, and report results for the organism as susceptible, intermediate, or resistant to each antimicrobial.

Interpretation and Limitations

It is important to understand that antimicrobial susceptibility is not an all-or-none phenomenon. Instead, bacteria have a *degree of susceptibility* as defined by the MIC value. Therefore interpreting diffusion test results as "zone or no zone" is unacceptable. Small zones may represent organisms that can tolerate higher levels of the antimicrobial (high MIC) than can be achieved at the site of infection. The measured diameter of the inhibition zone must be compared with the standards in Table 8-9 to determine if the degree of susceptibility is comparable to the therapeutic level of the antimicrobial. The classification of "susceptible versus resistant" is a practical simplification of the various susceptibilities of organisms in terms of expected clinical response to standard dose therapy.

Although the diffusion test has been accepted as a standard test and is used in most veterinary microbiology laboratories, some limitations should be kept in mind. This test system is not applicable to slow-growing isolates or for use in special atmospheres. In many cases the interpretative criteria (see Table 8-9) are based on assumptions derived from knowledge of pharmacodynamics of antimicrobials in humans and efficacy in treating human pathogens. Dosages, absorption, and distribution of antimicrobials may be significantly different in the various species of animals. Levels of drug in tissues may significantly differ from levels in serum, such as low levels in cerebrospinal fluid. From the chart, a test may be interpreted as susceptible, but the drug may not be able to penetrate to the site of infection. Conversely, ampicillin, for example, is concentrated several-fold in the urine and may exceed the MIC value for an organism that has a small zone of inhibition. Therefore susceptibility test results are not absolute rules for antimicrobial therapy. They should be used as guidelines in selecting therapy in addition to clinical judgment and knowledge of the pharmacokinetics and pharmacodynamics of the antimicrobials.

Some veterinary microbiology laboratories are using microdilution tests to determine the MIC of clinical isolates.

The MIC value can be compared with the levels of drug that can be obtained in the animal for final interpretation.

Technician Note

Susceptible implies that infection caused by the strain may be appropriately treated with the standard dosage of antimicrobial recommended for that type of infection and infecting species, unless otherwise contraindicated.

Intermediate indicates infection caused by a strain with antimicrobial agent MICs that approach usually attainable blood and tissue levels for which response rates may be lower than for susceptible isolates. This category implies clinical applicability in body sites in which the drugs are physiologically concentrated (e.g., quinolones and lactams in urine) or when a high dose of drug can be used (e.g., lactams).

Resistant strains are not inhibited by the usually achievable systemic concentrations of the antimicrobial when normal dosage schedules are used, and/or they may have MICs that fall within the range where specific microbial resistance mechanisms are likely and clinical efficacy has not been reliable in treatment studies.

MYCOLOGY

The fungal agents that technicians will most likely be expected to identify in a clinical laboratory are dermatophytes and some yeasts. Dermatophytes can readily be cultured and identified in local laboratories. The invasive *systemic mycoses* are usually encountered less frequently and require specialized laboratory facilities and procedures for identification.

Dermatophytes

The dermatophytes are keratinophilic (keratin-seeking) fungi that invade hair, nails, and the superficial layers of the skin but not living tissue. They may cause chronic, mild inflammation rather than intense inflammation. Lesions are usually characterized by spreading areas of pruritus and accumulating crusty debris. Lesions can be single or multifocal, and hair loss is variable. Because of the peripherally expanding nature of the lesion, it is also referred to as *ringworm*. Lesions can be markedly different in various species of animals, from a dry, minimally inflamed lesion without hair loss on cats to a large, wartlike crusty lesion on ruminants.

Specimen Collection

Representative bits of hair, scale, or crust should be collected from the area of suspected dermatophyte lesions. Care must be exercised to prevent heavy contamination with saprophytic fungi or bacteria, which can overgrow the culture of the desired pathogen. If the lesion is likely to be contaminated, it should be cleansed gently with 70% alcohol before samples are collected. Various dermatophytes are best recovered from unique parts of the lesion, and so samples of scale, crust, and hair should be selected. Pluck broken, frayed, or distorted stubs of hair within the lesion area. Do not cut off hair to use as the specimen for culture. Brush sampling is the preferred method for obtaining a dermatophyte culture specimen from asymptomatic cats. Use a sterilized (or new) toothbrush to vigorously brush suspected lesions or brush the entire animal for 2 to 3 minutes as if grooming. Then lightly press the brush against the surface of the culture medium several times for inoculation. Avoid pressing too firmly because the agar may tear and subsurface inoculum will not grow well. Crush and separate large pieces of debris when inoculating media. To culture nails suspected of having dermatophytic invasion, make fine shavings with a scalpel. Scatter the specimen over the entire surface of the culture medium. Press the hair and scale onto the agar, but do not bury it into the medium. If samples are not placed directly on culture media, they should be placed in a clean, dry envelope. Do not seal them in a tube or place in transport media. When moisture is allowed to accumulate, bacteria and yeast may overgrow.

Direct Examination

All specimens for fungal culture should be evaluated by direct microscopic examination. Direct mounts can be prepared by mixing a small portion of the material in two or three drops of 10% potassium hydroxide on a microscope slide. Addition of black India ink to the KOH solution will facilitate observation of fungal elements in the specimen. Add a coverslip over the wet mount, and examine for the presence of delicate hyphae in skin scales or for the accumulation of spores on the surface of an infected hair (ectothrix).

Culture Procedure

Sabouraud dextrose agar is the standard medium for isolation of fungi and can be used for the successful isolation of dermatophytes. Selective media, such as Mycobiotic (BD Microbiology Systems), are modified with antibiotics to inhibit bacteria and saprophytic fungi. A selective and differential medium (DTM [dermatophyte test medium]) is probably the most convenient medium available (Synbiotics Corp.; BactiLab, Inc.). The medium contains a phenol red indicator, which turns red as a dermatophyte grows and produces alkaline metabolic products. Occasionally, dermatophytes do not sporulate as well on DTM as on Sabouraud medium, which can hinder identification. This problem can be overcome by using a supplemental medium, such as Rapid Sporulation Medium (BactiLab, Inc.) to enhance sporulation and identification of dermatophytes.

After the agar is inoculated, the cap should be replaced but left loose so that air exchange can occur. The culture is allowed to incubate at room temperature (22° C to 25° C). Placement on an open shelf or counter allows daily observation for up to 2 weeks for growth and color change in the medium. Dermatophytes are identified on the basis of both their gross colony characteristics and microscopic morphologic characteristics. Rate of growth, texture, pattern of growth, color of the colony, and pigmentation of the reverse of the colony should be noted. Most dermatophyte colonies are white or light shades of apricot, yellow, or cream to tan. Darkly colored brown or black fungi are likely to be contaminants. The dermatophytes rapidly change the color of the DTM agar to red, even before a colony is apparent. The red color may appear as early as 3 to 5 days after inoculation and rapidly spreads to most of the agar. Nonpathogenic fungi that grow on the medium do not produce an early color change, although the medium may become red after it is heavily overgrown.

Definitive identification of a dermatophyte and speciation require microscopic examination of wet tape mounts prepared in *lactophenol cotton blue stain*. The slide is examined for microconidia, macroconidia, hyphae structures, and other identifying characteristics. The distinguishing morphologic features of the common dermatophytes are illustrated in most clinical microbiology textbooks.

Systemic Mycoses

The three most important systemic mycoses are coccidioidomycosis, histoplasmosis, and blastomycosis. They are serious zoonotic agents; therefore the small laboratory should not attempt to isolate them in culture systems. All culture work must be carried out in an approved biohazard safety hood. The small laboratory is limited to direct microscopic examination of clinical material. Stained smears and wet mounts are useful diagnostic tools. The size and structural characteristics of these agents in the tissue or yeast phase can serve as specific identifying criteria. If cultures are desired, the clinical material should be inoculated onto isolation media, and the inoculated tubes should be shipped to a reference laboratory. Delays in inoculation of isolation media will result in loss of viability and overgrowth of the sample by contaminating bacteria.

Sporotrichosis is a chronic infection characterized by nodular lesions of the skin or subcutaneous tissues. *Sporothrix schenckii* usually gains entrance by traumatic implantation into the tissue. Therefore there is little danger of contagion except from cats that frequently harbor very large numbers of yeast cells in lesions. The agent can be observed in direct examinations of tissue and exudates or isolated and identified by routine methods.

Yeasts

There are only a few clinical situations in which yeasts are significant veterinary pathogens. In general, animals seem to be much more resistant to yeast infections than are humans. If yeasts are suspected, a direct smear of exudate should be stained for microscopic examination. The best approach to the isolation of yeast is to inoculate blood agar and Sabouraud dextrose agar. The blood agar is incubated at 35° C and the Sabouraud agar at room temperature. Media should be held at least 2 weeks before discarding them as negative. Therefore agar slants in tubes are preferable to plates because they do not dehydrate as rapidly. Culture and identifying methods for the most common pathogenic yeasts are described.

MALASSEZIA PACHYDERMATIS. *Malassezia pachydermatis* is frequently found in cases of external otitis and is emerging as a cause of seborrheic and hypersensitivity reactions associated with dermatitis. It is readily observed in gram-stained smears of exudate as an oval, bottle-shaped, monopolar budding yeast. Isolation in cultures can be difficult but is best attempted by inoculating Sabouraud dextrose agar and incubating it at 35° C in a carbon dioxide incubator.

CRYPTOCOCCUS NEOFORMANS. In direct smears, *Cryptococcus neoformans* may be presumptively identified by its abundant capsular material. Negative staining with India ink provides a black background that outlines the clear capsule for easier observation. It can be isolated on Sabouraud dextrose agar or blood agar. *Cryptococcus neoformans* can be differentiated from other nonpathogenic yeasts because it will grow at 35° C to 37° C and is urease positive. The urease test is performed by inoculating the same urea agar slant that is used for differentiating bacteria.

CANDIDA ALBICANS. *Candida albicans* is a frequently encountered opportunistic fungal pathogen. Infections usually involve mucous membranes. In direct microscopic examinations of wet mounts, unicellular budding yeasts without a capsule are observed. Limited hyphae development may also be observed. *Candida albicans* is readily isolated on Sabouraud dextrose agar or blood agar. Definitive identification can be made by demonstrating germ tube (pseudohyphae) development after 3 to 4 hours' incubation in rabbit serum.

• • •

Other yeasts are isolated much less frequently. It is usually not feasible for small laboratories to attempt to identify these rare isolates. They should be forwarded to a reference laboratory for definitive identification.

VIROLOGY

Laboratory diagnosis of viral diseases depends on the examination of appropriate specimens for evidence of viral infection and then attempting to correlate infection with disease. Because of the nature of viruses and the special laboratory procedures required, most clinical laboratories perform only limited viral diagnostic procedures. Viruses are obligate intracellular parasites. Therefore they are best recovered from living tissue. Detection of viruses in dead tissues is reduced in direct proportion to the length of time since death and the extent of autolysis.

Virus Isolation

Isolation and identification of viruses depend on the inoculation of susceptible living cells for cultivation of the virus. The major methods of providing these living cells include monolayer cell cultures, embryonated hen eggs, and laboratory animal inoculation. These techniques require special laboratory facilities and up to 2 weeks for recovery of a virus. Special care must be taken to ensure that viable virus is delivered to the laboratory for isolation attempts. Therefore specimens should be collected early in the course of infection when viruses are most numerous. At death, virus numbers in the tissues are usually reduced, and there often is extensive secondary bacterial infection. The presence of bacteria in the sample can be damaging to the cells that are being used as recovery hosts for the virus. Therefore specimens should be carefully collected, refrigerated, and promptly delivered to the diagnostic laboratory. Special arrangements should be made with the laboratory personnel so that they can be prepared to process the sample when it arrives. Transport media containing antibiotics and virus-stabilizing agents are often available from viral diagnostic laboratories.

Microscopic Evaluation

In some cases, viral infection can be identified by microscopic examination of infected tissues for the presence of pathognomonic changes or of body fluids for the presence of viral particles. Some viral infections produce distinct changes in host cells, such as the intranuclear inclusions of infectious canine hepatitis, which can provide a definitive diagnosis. Electron microscopic examination of body fluids and washings allows the direct visualization of viral particles. This procedure is often used for diagnosis of respiratory and enteric viral infections because it is rapid and can detect mixed viral infections. The procedure does not require viable viruses, as long as they have retained their structural integrity. Direct electron microscopic examination is limited to cell-free viruses, such as those found in body fluids, rather than examination of infected tissue. Most diagnostic laboratories perform negative-contrast staining; therefore virus identification is limited to morphologic identification. If immunoelectron microscopy procedures are available, the type of virus within a group can be identified.

Antigen Detection

Antigen detection methods are the most frequently used viral diagnostic procedures. Advantages of antigen detection compared with viral isolation include rapid results, less expense, less technically demanding procedures, and less dependence on the presence of viable virus in the sample because most viral antigens remain intact after death of the virus. The most common methods of antigen detection are immunohistochemical staining, hemagglutination, and solid-phase immunoassays. Hemagglutination assays are not easily standardized for use in clinical laboratories.

Immunohistochemical Staining

Examination of selected clinical specimens using a specific antibody labeled with a marker as a probe to identify viral antigen is a rapid and highly reliable diagnostic method. Markers on the antibody can include fluorescent compounds, enzymes, or colloidal gold. The two most important limitations of these procedures are the need for specific antibodies to the viral antigens and a system for detecting the marker. For immunofluorescence, a microscope with an ultraviolet (UV) light source is required.

In the *immunoperoxidase method assay*, the specific antibody is labeled with an enzyme (usually horseradish peroxidase) instead of a fluorescent label. Attachment of the antibody to tissue sections or smears is detected using a chromogenic substrate that is deposited at the site of enzyme-antibody attachment and produces a slide similar to other differential stains. The slide can then be examined by light microscopy. Several of these assays have been developed using monoclonal antibodies to detect viral antigens in tissue, including examination of formalin-fixed specimens.

Colloidal gold immunostaining technology is currently available in the ICT Gold Heartworm Antigen Test (Synbiotics Corp.).

Solid-phase Immunoassays

The use of enzyme immunoassays is based on the excellent ability of this methodology to be adapted to kits that meet practical concerns, such as minimizing reagent cost, reducing technician time required to perform the assay, and simplifying the test protocol. These test systems are frequently referred to by the acronym ELISA (enzyme-linked immunosorbent assay). As a result, several kit systems are available for the detection of antigens from viruses and other infectious agents (Figure 8-10) and for detection of antibodies specific for infectious agents. Three typical configurations of ELISAs are illustrated in Figure 8-11. At present there are several different solid phases commonly used in these assays. The most common solid phase for multiple tests is the microtiter well, but for individual clinical tests, dipstick, immunofiltration, immunomigration, and immunochromatographic formats are more efficient. Immunoassay diagnostic kit manufacturers usually offer technical assistance to kit users. If you have questions about a protocol or test result or are experiencing difficulty in conducting a test after carefully reading and following the manufacturer's instructions, call the company's technical services department and ask for assistance. Most companies provide a toll-free telephone number to facilitate this and will welcome an opportunity to assist you in using their products.

Assays that have been successfully developed for detection of viral antigen include feline leukemia virus (FeLV) in blood (ASSURE/FeLV and WITNESS FeLV, Synbiotics Corp.; SNAP FeLV Antigen Test Kit and Probe Feline

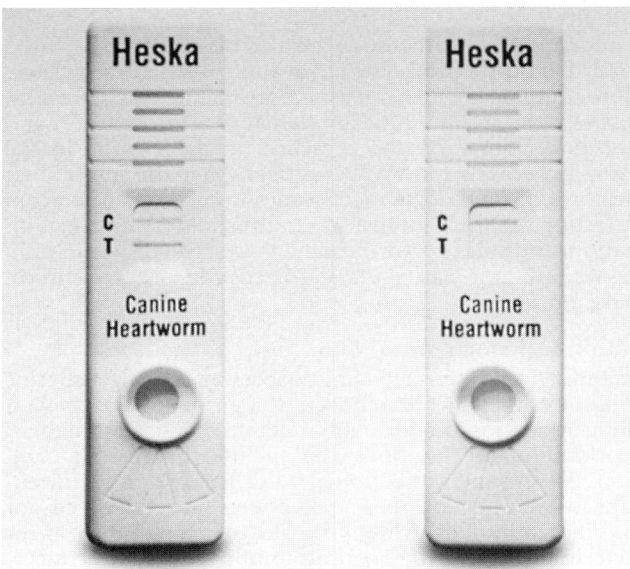

FIGURE 8-10. Solo Step CH lateral flow immunoassay cassette for the detection of antigens produced by canine heartworms in serum. A positive test result has developed in the left cassette, and a negative test result is shown in the cassette on the right.

Leukemia Antigen Test Kit, IDEXX Laboratories, Inc.), FeLV in saliva (ASSURE/FeLV, Synbiotics Corp.), canine parvovirus in feces (ASSURE/Parvo and WITNESS CPV, Synbiotics Corp.; Probe Canine Parvovirus Test Kit and SNAP Parvo Antigen Test Kit, IDEXX Laboratories, Inc.), and influenza virus in respiratory tract specimens (Directigen FluA, BD Microbiology Systems). Kits are also available to detect bacterial antigens (K99 Pilitest, VMRD, Inc.) and heartworm antigens (Solo Step CH, Heska Corp.; SNAP Heartworm Antigen, IDEXX Laboratories, Inc.; ASSURE/CH and WITNESS HW, Synbiotics Corp.).

SEROLOGY

Serologic testing is an important tool in the diagnosis of infectious diseases. Serology is used extensively in the diagnosis of viral infections and in disease surveillance programs. Serologic tests for detecting a specific antibody have been developed for nearly every infectious agent. However, this indirect approach to diagnosing infection on the basis of a host immune response after exposure to an infectious agent has limitations. Serologic tests may vary in their sensitivity and specificity because of the type of test, immunogenicity and cross-reactivity of the antigen, and biologic variation of immune responses by individual animals. Nevertheless, serologic tests often remain the best diagnostic test available. In veterinary medicine, serologic tests are often required by regulatory agencies to prove an animal is not infected or a carrier of a particular infectious agent.

Antibody Response to Infection

The chronology of exposure to an infectious agent and subsequent development of an antibody response are illustrated in Figure 8-12. After exposure, there is a variable period of incubation followed by clinical illness. During the time of clinical illness the animal may be febrile, and this is when the greatest number of microorganisms are present. Therefore it is more likely to transmit the infectious agent, and the best samples can be obtained for recovery of the agent at this time. After a variable period of time from onset of clinical signs (usually after 5 to 10 days), the animal begins to produce antibodies to the agent. Continued production of antibodies after the animal is no longer ill, referred to as the convalescent phase, will cause the titer (serum antibody level) to rise for 1 month or longer.

Interpretation of Serologic Results

The presence of antibodies to a particular organism in an animal serum is not always a simple and absolute diagnosis of current or recent clinical illness caused by the organism. Sources of antibody in the serum of an animal include convalescent antibody after clinical disease or persistent infection, antibody response caused by exposure to an organism without clinical disease occurring, active immune response to vaccination, and passive transfer of maternal antibodies to the neonate. Therefore detection of antibodies in a single serum sample often has limited importance unless the finding can be correlated with other clinical indications of the disease. In most situations, it is necessary to collect two samples—the first one early in the course of the illness (*acute*) and the second one (*convalescent*) at a later time—to demonstrate a change in antibody titer that would indicate recent antigenic stimulation. The change must be at least two dilution increments (usually fourfold), such as an increase from 1:4 to 1:16 or greater, to be considered diagnostically significant. This change in titer is known as a *seroconversion*.

The presence of antibody in serum may be reported quantitatively as a titer or qualitatively as positive or negative. Qualitative tests have less diagnostic value than those tests that report titers, unless the result is negative, in which case the test can exclude some agents from the differential diagnosis unless the serum was collected early in the course of disease. Most qualitative tests, such as immunodiffusion for equine infectious anemia (Coggins' test) and bovine leukosis, are surveillance tests to identify animals who have been exposed and are possible carriers. Occasionally, a single, high-titered serum can aid in establishing a diagnosis, but it always leaves some question of whether the titer increased in association with clinical disease or is a stable, convalescent high titer.

When an animal is exposed to an infectious agent, the first antibodies produced are usually of the IgM class with later antibody production being IgG. Some tests are designed to differentiate these antibody class responses, which can be helpful in confirming a diagnosis. If the antibody response to a virus is of the IgM type, the animal has recently been exposed. If the response is mostly IgG, it was probably exposed several weeks to months previously. Often IgM antibodies are less specific than IgG and may cross-react, resulting in false-positive test results. To prevent this from happening, the test can be modified to exclude IgM reactions.

Serologic tests are frequently relied on as the only diagnostic procedures for abortion cases. Results are often difficult to interpret for two reasons. First, by the time abortion occurs because of infection of the fetus and its subsequent death, the dam is already in the convalescent phase of antibody production, so a seroconversion cannot be demonstrated. Second, the stress of abortion or other clinical illness may trigger reactivation of a latent viral infection. This provides an antigenic stimulus to the animal's immune system and increased antibody production.

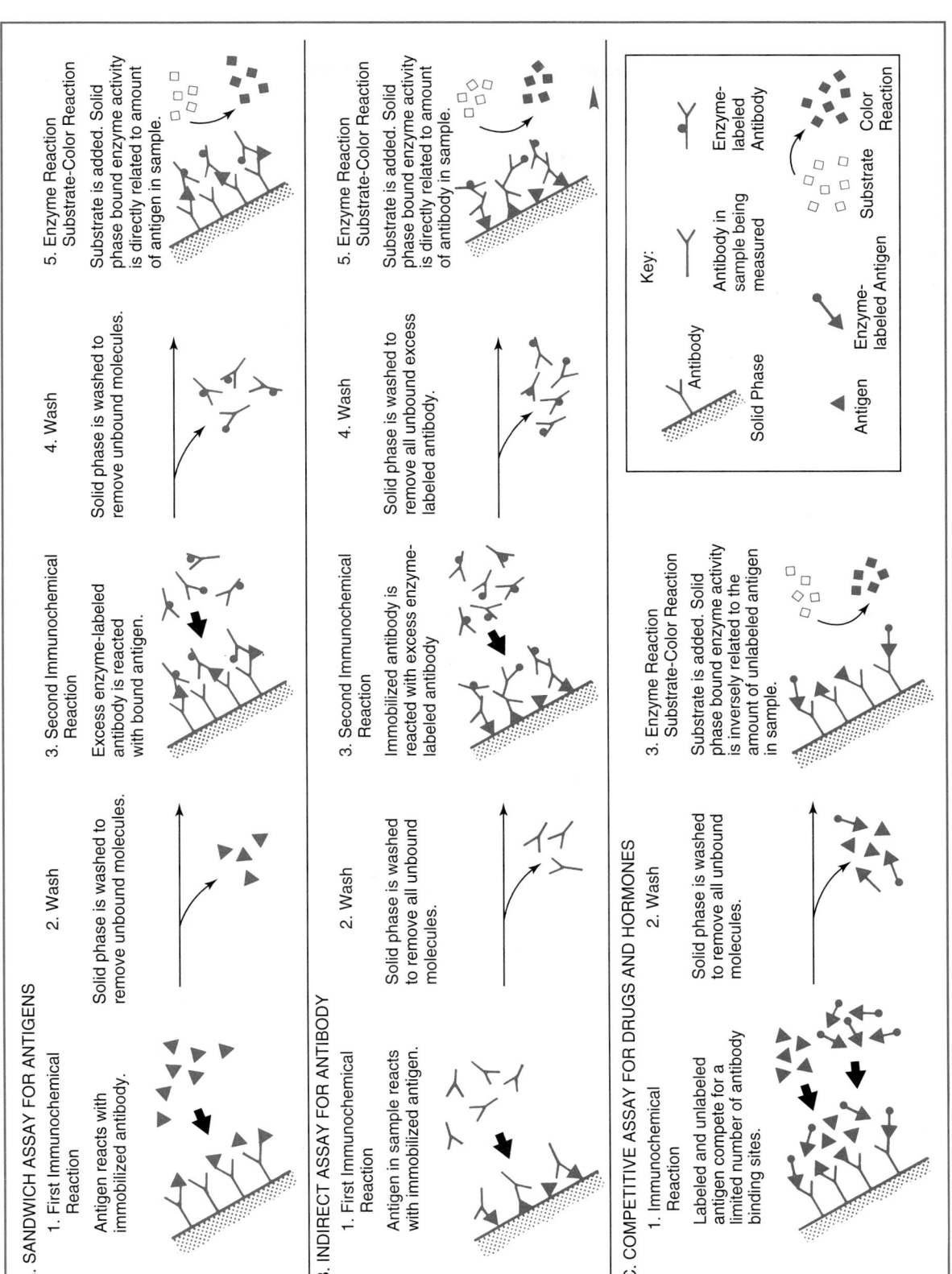

FIGURE 8-11. Enzyme immunoassay configurations and major steps in assay procedures. (Courtesy E.S. Bean and E.T. Maggio, San Diego.)

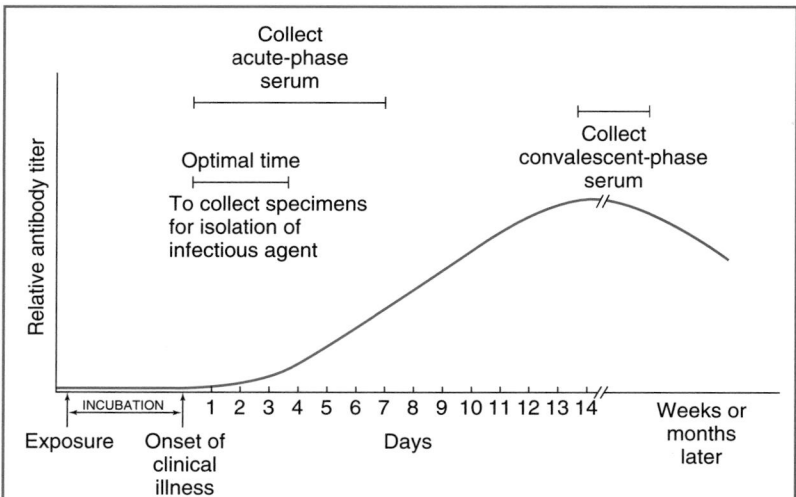

FIGURE 8-12. Antibody response to an infectious disease and optimal times for specimen collection.

However, it is specific for the latent viral infection, not the current clinical illness.

Collection of Serum

Technicians will frequently be responsible for collecting and handling serum samples. Improper methods can reduce the value of test results. The timing of serum collection is important (see Figure 8-12). The first sample should be collected as soon as possible after the animal begins to show signs of clinical illness. If the sample is not collected within the first 5 to 7 days, antibody titers might have already risen. The convalescent sample should be collected at least 10 days after the acute sample. Generally, 14 to 21 days between samples is recommended, but in young animals with a less efficient immune response, up to 4 to 6 weeks may be necessary to demonstrate a seroconversion. The technical procedures of serologic tests are difficult to duplicate exactly; therefore results of tests performed on different days or in different laboratories should not be compared to demonstrate a seroconversion.

Blood should be collected aseptically by venipuncture with a new needle and syringe or evacuated clot tube (Vacutainer tubes and SST Sterile Serum Separation Tubes, BD Vacutainer Systems). Do not use recycled, washed needles, syringes, or tubes. Residual detergent may cause hemolysis or may be toxic to cell cultures used in the test systems. Blood should be allowed to stand at room temperature until a clot has formed; the serum should then be removed from the clot and placed in a new, sterile tube. It may be necessary to separate the serum from the clot by centrifugation to prevent transferring cellular components of the blood. Anticoagulants should not be used to collect plasma because they can be toxic in some test systems. Avoid freezing the whole blood because that will cause hemolysis. The transfer of serum from the original blood tube must be performed aseptically. Contaminating microorganisms can grow rapidly in serum and alter the immunoglobulin molecules. Therefore serum samples (separated from the clot and cells) should be refrigerated until testing is commenced, if within 72 hours. For longer periods of storage, serum may be preserved in a freezer (−20° C). Frozen serum samples should be packaged and shipped with adequate insulation and ice to prevent thawing before arrival at the laboratory. If a second sample will be collected, the first sample should be held until both can be sent to the laboratory together for valid paired testing.

Technician Note

The technical procedures of serologic tests are difficult to duplicate exactly; therefore results of tests performed on different days or in other laboratories should not be compared to demonstrate a seroconversion.

For shipment, the tubes of serum must be carefully labeled and packed so that they will not leak or break. When the environmental temperatures are high, refrigerant and insulating materials should be used to preserve samples during transit.

Serologic Test Procedures

Only a few serologic tests have been standardized and packaged for efficient use in veterinary practice laboratories. When using kits, it is important that the directions be followed carefully because modification of any part of the procedure can cause spurious results. A positive (or known titer) serum and a negative serum should be kept on hand (if not already included in the kit) and included in the test each time it is performed to verify accuracy of the results. Serology (antibody-detecting) kits are available for feline immunodeficiency virus (SNAP FIV Antibody Test Kit, IDEXX Laboratories, Inc.), feline infectious peritonitis (SNAP FIV Antibody Test Kit, IDEXX Laboratories, Inc.), canine borreliosis (Cite Canine *Borrelia burgdorferi* Antibody Test Kit, IDEXX Laboratories, Inc.; LymeCHEK, Synbiotics Corp.), canine brucellosis (D-Tec CB, Synbiotics Corp.), paratuberculosis (Rapid Johne's Test, ImmuCell Corp.), feline heartworm (Solo Step FH, Heska Corp.; ASSURE /FH, Synbiotics Corp.), and canine ehrlichiosis (SNAP *Ehrlichia canis* Antibody Test, IDEXX Laboratories, Inc.). The most frequent mistakes made when performing serologic tests include the use of dirty or contaminated equipment, failure to adhere to instructions (especially incubation times), and unfamiliarity with reading results.

CLINICAL IMMUNOLOGY

Purpose of Evaluating Immune System Function

As the function and complexity of the immune system have been elucidated, an increasing need for laboratory diagnosis of dysfunction of the immune system has been recognized. Clinical immunologic laboratory support has become a well-established part of the diagnostic services and patient care procedures in human medicine. Similar assays are becoming available in veterinary medicine, but very few tests are readily available for use in practice laboratories.

Several types of diagnostic problems present the need for laboratory evaluation of possible immunologic disorders. These disorders can be classified into four types: allergies, autoimmune diseases, immunodeficiencies, and immunoproliferative diseases. In young animals, disorders of the immune system may be observed as developmental defects (sometimes inherited) or may be caused by a failure of passive transfer of maternal antibodies. However, immune function abnormalities can be observed in animals of all ages because of effects of aging, various drugs, or environmental exposure to immunomodulating toxins. A few simple procedures will be discussed in this section. The Recommended Reading list should be consulted for detailed and theoretic discussions of other immune system function assays.

Laboratory Tests for Immunologic Disorders

Allergies are usually diagnosed by physical examination, history, and response to intradermal inoculation of test antigens.

Autoimmune disorders can be diagnosed more efficiently by evaluating lesions obtained by biopsy. Morphologic evaluation, combined with various immunohistochemical staining procedures, provides the most definitive diagnosis. It is best to consult referral laboratories to learn which specimens they are able to analyze and how the sample should be submitted.

Immunoproliferative diseases may result in the production of abnormal amounts or unusual types of immunoglobulin proteins, referred to as *gammopathies*. The techniques of electrophoresis (usually on cellulose acetate) and immunoelectrophoresis are the laboratory tests most frequently used to diagnose these disorders. Abnormalities of routine laboratory tests, such as total protein in serum or urine and A/G ratios, frequently indicate a need for these specialized tests. Because of the infrequent demand for these tests and the cost of electrophoresis equipment, most practices request these services from referral laboratories.

Immunodeficiency or immunosuppressive disorders are the most frequently encountered immune system dysfunctions. Most assays of immune cell function require specialized equipment and procedures that are usually available in only a few reference laboratories. Some cellular function assays require submission of viable cells for evaluation. Recently developed assays are used to detect and quantify receptors on the surface of cells, such as CD18 deficiency in Holstein calves. Assays are being developed in research laboratories for genetic analysis of lymphocytes to detect both immunodeficiency and immunoproliferative dysfunctions. Determination of immunoglobulin levels, as an indication of B-lymphocyte function or passive transfer status, is a readily available laboratory test that will be discussed.

Failure of Passive Transfer

The newborns of most domestic animals depend on absorption of maternal antibodies from colostrum for protection from infectious diseases. Failure of the neonatal animal to obtain and absorb adequate colostral immunoglobulins is frequently associated with increased morbidity and mortality from bacteremia and common neonatal diseases. Determination of the passive transfer status of foals and calves is an important evaluation that can modify patient care. Although total serum protein levels can indicate relative levels of immunoglobulins, this indirect measurement is subject to considerable variability. The reference method for quantitating serum immunoglobulins is the *radial immunodiffusion (RID) test*. The RID test consists of agar containing antisera specific for a particular antigen. In this case, the antigen is a particular immunoglobulin class, such as IgG. Each test requires that quantitated standards be tested at the same time for comparison. Therefore, if single samples are being tested, the cost per sample will be more, and it might be more cost effective to send samples to a referral laboratory. (Commercially produced RID kits for canine, feline, bovine, llama, and equine immunoglobulins are available from Bethyl Laboratories, Inc. and VMRD, Inc.)

Passive transfer status of neonates can be evaluated rapidly and inexpensively in the practice laboratory. Field test kits that incorporate chemical reactions with IgG to produce a turbidity reaction are available for detecting failure of passive transfer in calves, foals, and llamas (VMRD, Inc.).

Several test kits have been developed and marketed for rapid quantification of serum IgG in foals. A semiquantitative latex agglutination test (FOALCHEK, Centaur, Inc.) can be performed with either serum or whole blood. An enzyme-immunoassay test kit (SNAP Foal IgG Test Kit, IDEXX Laboratories, Inc.) measures IgG in serum, plasma, or whole blood. Both of these kits provide accurate results when performed properly and can readily be used in field or clinical laboratories for assessment of passive transfer in foals.

NOSOCOMIAL INFECTIONS

An infection that results from exposure to an infectious agent while the patient is in the hospital is considered to be *nosocomial* (hospital acquired). The nosocomial infection may become clinically apparent during hospitalization or after discharge from the hospital. Infections that are incubating at the time of admission are defined as *community acquired*, even though they become clinically apparent only during hospitalization. In veterinary practices, in addition to nosocomial infections of patients, zoonotic infections transmitted to the staff and clients can be considered part of the biosafety problem.

The incidence of nosocomial infections in veterinary hospitals is not well documented, but it is probably similar to the incidence in human hospitals, which ranges from 3% to 5% of hospitalized patients. The incidence is known to vary with the size and type of hospital and the sophistication of infection control programs. The highest incidence rates are observed in large referral or teaching institutions. The most important institutional risk factors appear to be an increased number of personnel having contact with the patient and an increased mean number of hospitalization days per patient. Therefore these infections are becoming an increasingly significant problem in teaching hospitals and large group practices in which intensive medical and surgical care is available through a large staff. These institutions also tend to care for patients with more critical and chronic diseases. Because these patients have increased susceptibility to opportunistic infection, the occurrence of a nosocomial infection does not necessarily indicate negligence by the hospital staff.

The stressed condition of hospitalized animals often makes them more susceptible to infections than the general population. Factors that predispose an individual animal to nosocomial infection may include extremes of age (old age or neonates), debilitating disease, diagnostic or medical procedures, such as urethral catheterization, immunosuppressive therapy (corticosteroids or cytotoxic drugs), long periods of hospitalization, antimicrobial therapy, presence of other infections, and presence of surgical hardware and drains. For some of the infectious diseases, such as canine distemper, the immunization status of the patient will determine its susceptibility.

Many nosocomial infections are caused by opportunistic microorganisms that infrequently cause infections in healthy animals. However, when the high-risk patient (increased susceptibility) is exposed, the agent can cause disease. Other highly virulent organisms, such as canine parvovirus and *Salmonella*, may cause disease in otherwise healthy patients. The greatest impact on the incidence of nosocomial infections can be made by understanding the sources of exposure and spread of these infectious agents. Microorganisms enter the hospital in or on people, animals, inanimate objects, air currents, and occasionally insects. Within the hospital, they are maintained in or on a variety of reservoirs, including patients with infections, healthy carriers, inanimate surfaces, solutions, food, staff, and insects. From these reservoirs, the potential pathogens may be disseminated by contact or by air to hospital personnel and patients.

The most important vehicles for the spread of nosocomial agents are the hands of hospital personnel. Therefore proper and frequent hand washing is the most important strategy for reducing the rate of nosocomial and zoonotic infections.

Agents of Nosocomial Infections

Bacteria are the most frequent infectious agents involved in nosocomial infections, but viruses, fungi, and protozoa can also be involved. The commonly involved bacteria tend to be somewhat environmentally resistant, and the increasing use of antibiotic therapy precedes an increased level of antibiotic resistance by nosocomial agents. In the presence of limited antibiotic use, penicillin-susceptible, gram-positive cocci of the genera *Streptococcus* and *Staphylococcus* are the most common agents. With increased antibiotic use, penicillin-resistant *Staphylococcus* is frequently detected. Currently, the major problems are with multiple antibiotic-resistant, gram-negative bacilli, such as *Escherichia coli, Salmonella, Klebsiella, Enterobacter, Serratia,* and *Pseudomonas*. Methicillin-resistant staphylococci and vancomycin-resistant enterococci are beginning to emerge as the next wave of serious nosocomial agents. Colonization (growth and establishment) of the body surfaces of the patient by these nosocomial bacterial pathogens is usually a prerequisite to infection. Therefore the patient becomes its own major reservoir of these agents once the organisms are transferred to it during hospitalization. Common reservoir sites are the lower intestinal tract and the nasooropharyngeal area. Antimicrobial chemotherapy is the most important predisposing factor that allows the patient to become colonized because the antimicrobial suppresses normal flora and selects for resistant organisms. The most frequent locations of nosocomial bacterial infections are the urinary and respiratory systems and surgical wounds. Occasionally, infections become bacteremic. Clostridial enterocolitis in dogs has been identified as a nosocomial problem in several large teaching hospitals.

Viral infections are the second most frequent group of nosocomial infections in hospitalized patients but are probably the most important nosocomial infections of outpatients. This is because some of these agents are easily transmitted and are highly infectious to susceptible but otherwise healthy animals. Diseases in this group include canine distemper, canine parvovirus, feline panleukopenia, and respiratory viral diseases of all animals (feline viral rhinotracheitis, equine influenza, infectious bovine rhinotracheitis, canine tracheobronchitis, etc.).

Other viral diseases that are not as contagious can be transmitted to susceptible patients at a veterinary hospital if adequate preventive measures are not followed. The resulting disease would be classified as a nosocomial infection. Examples include transmission of viruses of feline leukemia and equine infectious anemia in blood transfusions.

Fungi have rarely been recognized as nosocomial agents in veterinary medicine. As the awareness level of this problem increases, no doubt more fungal infections will be identified, especially with improved intensive care of immunocompromised patients. Yeasts, such as *Candida albicans*, have occasionally been identified. The dermatophytes do not cause life-threatening infections and are usually overlooked, but they can also be transmitted as nosocomial agents to both patients and hospital staff.

Infection of animals by protozoan pathogens can be acquired in the veterinary hospital. *Cryptosporidium* spp. are relatively resistant to disinfectants and have been the cause of nosocomial enteritis. If litter pans are not properly cleaned, other animals and hospital staff could be exposed to toxoplasmosis. Hemotropic parasites (*Hemobartonella, Anaplasma, Ehrlichia, Babesia*) can be transmitted to other patients in blood transfusions or on surgical instruments that have not been adequately washed and disinfected.

Recognition and Control of Nosocomial Infections

Technicians frequently have the opportunity to be the first persons to recognize a nosocomial infection problem by taking note of an unusual number of isolations of a single pathogen or the appearance of an unusual antibiogram. Excellent diagnostic microbiology laboratory support for accurate identification and antimicrobial susceptibility testing of infectious agents is an essential tool for defining the scope of the nosocomial infection problem.

Measures that can help reduce or control nosocomial infections include sterilization of equipment and supplies, aseptic treatment techniques, isolation practices, judicious use of antimicrobial drugs, diligent hand washing between examining patients, disposal of trash, and establishment of sound housekeeping protocols. These protocols should provide for adequate cleaning, disinfection, and maintenance of patient-care equipment and environmental surfaces, such as cages, tables, floors, and walls.

The control measures that would be necessary to prevent all nosocomial infections are impractical and not economically feasible. Hospitals contain patients with increased susceptibility to infection, and short of total isolation in a controlled environment, few measures are biologically guaranteed. The risk for each patient of acquiring an infection must be individually evaluated. If the risk is sufficiently great, reverse isolation procedures may be indicated to prevent the patient from being exposed to potential pathogens. If active or passive immunizing products are available, their use should be encouraged. Routine immunization programs can effectively prevent many of the viral infections that have been discussed.

Antiseptics, Disinfectants, and Sterilization

The effective use of antiseptics, disinfectants, and sterilization procedures is an important factor in preventing nosocomial infections. Microorganisms vary widely in their susceptibility to germicidal treatments. Bacterial endospores are the most resistant type. In descending order of relative resistance after bacterial spores are mycobacteria, fungal spores, nonenveloped viruses, vegetative fungi, enveloped viruses, and vegetative bacterial cells. The differences in chemical resistance of various vegetative bacteria are relatively minor, except for the mycobacteria, which are relatively resistant to many disinfectants. Other factors that may have a significant effect on the results of disinfection are concentration of the chemical, length of exposure to the chemical, amount of organic matter (soil, blood, feces) present, type and condition (porosity, cracks, etc.) of the material to be disinfected, ambient temperature, and the nature and number of contaminating microorganisms. Good physical cleaning will allow better penetration of crevices and porous material. Generally, the higher the concentration of the chemical agent or the longer a process is continued, the greater its effectiveness. For temperature-based procedures, increasing temperatures will usually increase efficacy.

Veterinary clinics and hospitals should select disinfectants that are registered by the U.S. Environmental Protection Agency (EPA) and labeled as one-step cleaner-disinfectants for use in hospitals. The label should indicate that these products are effective in hard water up to 400 ppm hardness and in the presence of 5% serum. Most nonporous surfaces can be efficiently cleaned and disinfected with the newer combinations of twin chain quaternary ammonium compounds (C_8/C_{10} dimethyl ammonium chloride) and alkyl dimethyl benzyl ammonium chloride. Product labels must always be consulted for proper mixing and diluting instructions and intended applications. Chemical incompatibilities may occur if products are mixed. Therefore do not attempt to combine germicides or alter treatment procedures from the manufacturer's specifications.

Biologic Safety

Potential hazards in the veterinary hospital may be associated with infectious or chemical materials, physical facilities, and animal handling. Management should develop a comprehensive safety program that considers these dangers as well as preparedness for fire, accidents, and other disasters. This discussion will deal primarily with biologic hazards related to infectious agents in the laboratory and hospital.

Each individual has responsibility for protecting himself or herself and others from accidental infection. Laboratory coats should be worn to prevent contamination of street clothes and dissemination of pathogens to homes and families. Disposable examination gloves should be worn when handling heavily contaminated materials. Good hand-washing procedures should become a habit in the laboratory—between procedures if there was a chance of contamination and always before leaving the laboratory. Mouth pipetting should be prohibited in laboratories handling infectious material. Automatic or bulb pipetting devices should be used. Syringes and needles are poor substitutes for pipettes because they tend to favor creation of aerosols that may be inhaled. There is also the inherent danger of self-inoculation when handling syringes and needles. Self-inoculation must be guarded against, both in the laboratory and when inoculating animals. Centrifuge accidents, which may produce infectious aerosols, should be avoided by selecting compatible tubes, performing proper balancing, and not exceeding recommended centrifugal forces.

Good housekeeping procedures that will maintain a neat, uncluttered work area should be adopted. Eating, drinking, and smoking should not be allowed in work areas, even during break periods when there is no laboratory activity.

Immunization of personnel is recommended when they are at increased risk of infection. A minimal prophylactic immunization for all personnel employed in veterinary hospitals and laboratories should include rabies vaccine and tetanus toxoid. Other immunization products may be recommended in areas in which there is an unusually high risk of exposure to a particular infectious agent.

Primary containment equipment and laboratory design features are important factors in biologic safety. Directional airflow should be from clean areas to areas of contamination and should then be exhausted from the building without recirculating. Small veterinary laboratories and hospitals usually cannot justify the cost of biologic safety cabinets for diagnostic procedures. However, some infectious agents are of sufficient hazard that they must be handled only in laboratories with special design features, including biohazard cabinets. Zoonotic pathogens that small laboratories should not attempt to isolate include the agents of anthrax, brucellosis, plague, tuberculosis, tularemia, and systemic mycoses.

The clinical laboratory has a responsibility to decontaminate potentially infectious materials and wastes before they are discarded. Many states have adopted statutes and regulations that stipulate how hazardous waste materials must be handled. Clinical veterinary laboratories are required to comply with these rules as well as EPA and U.S. Occupational Safety and Health Administration (OSHA) requirements. All diagnostic specimens (swabs), inoculated media, viable cultures, glassware, instruments, and equipment should be considered to be contaminated. Decontamination methods should be applied before waste materials are discarded or reusable products are cleansed. The most practical decontamination procedure for most infectious wastes is the steam autoclave. Other methods include physical procedures (incineration, boiling, irradiation), and chemical agents (phenolics, hypochlorites, formaldehyde).

RECOMMENDED READING

Carter CR, Chengappa MM: *Microbial diseases: a veterinarian's guide to the laboratory diagnosis*, Ames, 1993, Iowa State University Press.

Carter GR, Cole JR, Jr: *Diagnostic procedures in veterinary bacteriology and mycology*, ed 5, San Diego, 1990, Academic Press.

Difco manual, ed 11, 1998, Difco Laboratories, Division of Becton Dickinson and Co., Sparks, Md.

Greene CE: *Infectious diseases of the dog and cat*, ed 2, Philadelphia, 1998, WB Saunders.

Hirsch DC, Zee YC: *Veterinary microbiology*, Malden, Mass, 1999, Blackwell Science.

Koneman EW et al: *Color atlas and textbook of diagnostic microbiology*, ed 5, Philadelphia, 1997, JB Lippincott.

Murray PR et al: *Manual of clinical microbiology*, ed 7, Washington, DC, 1999, American Society for Microbiology.

National Committee for Clinical Laboratory Standards: *Performance standards for antimicrobial disk and dilution susceptibility tests for bacteria isolated from animals; approved standard. NCCLS document M31-A*, Wayne, Pa, 1999, National Committee for Clinical Laboratory Standards.

Quinn PJ et al: *Clinical veterinary microbiology*, London, 1994, Mosby.

Research Committee of the National Mastitis Council: *Laboratory handbook on bovine mastitis*, Madison, Wis, 1999, National Mastitis Council.

Rose NR, de Macario EC, Lane HC: *Manual of clinical immunology*, ed 5, Washington, DC, 1997, American Society for Microbiology.

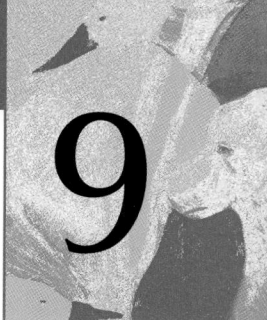

Diagnostic Imaging

Beth Paugh Partington

Radiology and ultrasound are the primary diagnostic imaging techniques available to the veterinarian. However, for the veterinarian to arrive at the correct diagnosis on the basis of a radiographic or ultrasound examination, images of high quality must be available. The responsibility to provide useful diagnostic images usually falls to the veterinary technician.

This chapter deals with the basic but essential information needed to produce x-rays and sonograms of diagnostic quality. It is not the intent of this chapter to offer a course in radiation physics, ultrasound physics, and proper positioning of animals for examination. Excellent textbooks on these subjects have been written and should provide the veterinary technician with the detailed information needed; see Curry et al. (1990), Douglas et al. (1987), Han et al. (2000), Lavin (1999), Morgan (1993), and Ticer (1984). These books should be consulted when the need arises.

This chapter discusses the basic information needed to support and assist the veterinary technician in the area of radiology and diagnostic ultrasound. A short introduction to the use of nuclear imaging, computed tomography, and magnetic resonance imaging is included. Every effort is made to simplify the radiation and ultrasound physics.

RADIOLOGY

Legal Records and Film Identification

Radiographs are part of the medical record and should be clearly labeled as to which animal has been examined. The identification should include the name of the patient and owner or patient identification number, date of the examination, and name of the hospital.

> **Technician Note**
>
> Radiographs are part of the legal medical record and must be correctly identified and carefully labeled.

Several methods of film labeling are available. The most common methods used by veterinarians are leaded num-

bers and letters placed on the cassette at the time of exposure (Figure 9-1, *A*). These show up as white markings on a finished radiograph. Also available is a special graphite-impregnated tape on which the desired information can be written or typed and placed on the cassette, or the information can be taped on a special filter at the time of exposure (Figure 9-1, *B*). One of the better film identification methods is a *light flasher system* (Figure 9-2). It is simple and inexpensive. The required information is typed on a card that is placed in the imprinter. This system requires placing a small, leaded blocker in the upper left-hand corner of the film cassette, which will prevent exposure to that part of the film. The card is placed in the light flasher in the darkroom. The unexposed, left-hand corner of the exposed radiograph is placed underneath the card, and the light is flashed through the card. The information recorded on the card is transferred to the x-ray film and will be developed when the radiograph is processed (Figure 9-3).

One final identification method requires both a film identification camera and special windowed film cassettes. This method allows an individual to type the required information on a 3 × 5 card and place the card into the ID camera. The windowed corner of the cassette is then automatically opened and "flashed" by the camera, and the information is exposed on the x-ray film. The benefits of this system are that the camera will automatically identify the date and time of the examination, it can be done in daylight, and the area on the film in which the identification information is placed is constant (Figure 9-4).

In addition to the legal identification imprinted on the film, it is necessary to identify the part x-rayed at the time of exposure. Leaded right and left markers should be placed on the cassette at the time of exposure to identify the extremity x-rayed or the side on which the animal is positioned for examination (i.e., right or left lateral recumbency). Additional specialty film markers include Mitchell markers, which consist of a plastic bubble containing two to four tiny lead balls that fall toward gravity. These are primarily used in standing radiography of the equine head to assist in identifying fluid levels in paranasal sinuses. Timing markers are used in contrast studies such as upper gastrointestinal studies and excretory urography to identify

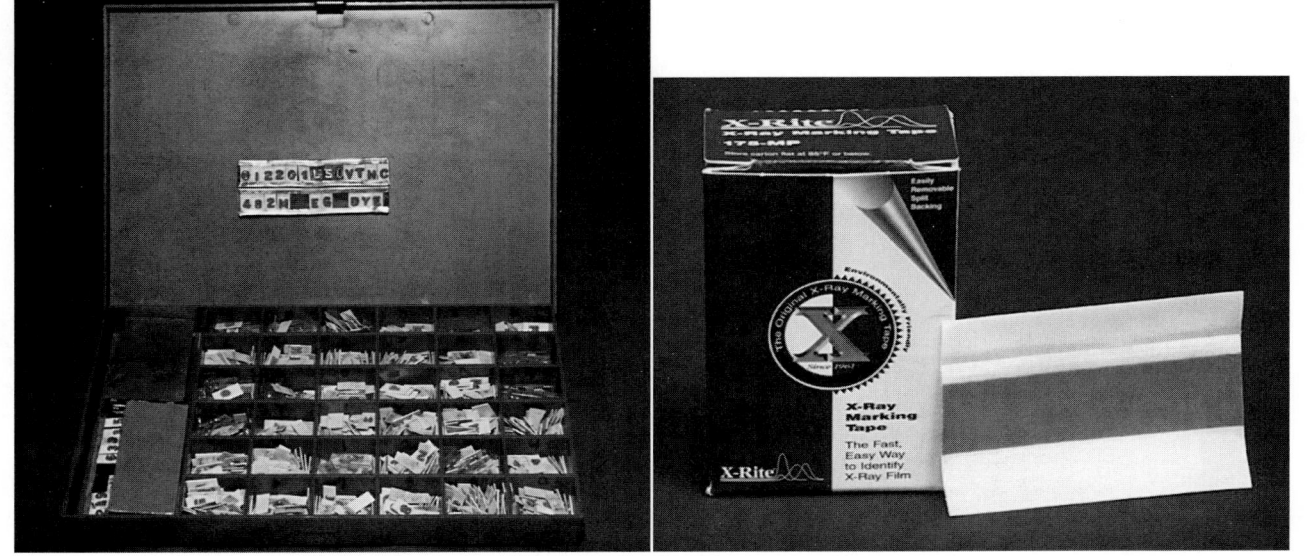

FIGURE 9-1. Film labeling. **A,** Leaded letters and numbers placed on the cassette at the time of exposure. **B,** Radiographic label tape.

FIGURE 9-2. Light flasher. Patient information is printed onto a radiograph with an identification printer. (From Eastman Kodak Co: *The fundamentals of radiography,* ed 12, Rochester, NY, 1980, Eastman Kodak Co, Radiographic Markets Division.)

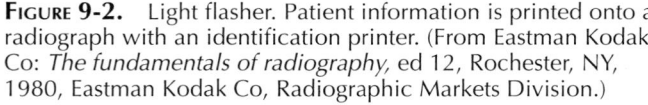

FIGURE 9-3. Film identification as it appears on a radiograph. The identification is flashed onto the film after x-ray exposure with a light flasher system or film identification camera.

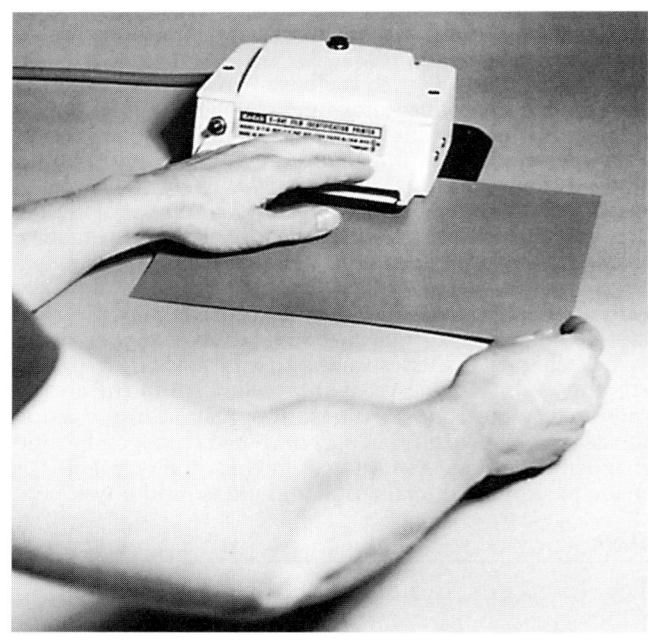

Louisiana State University
Veterinary Teaching Hospital & Clinics
No. 46478   Date 3/20/97
DOB 9/24/84 Owner Partington
Spec. Feline Sex F/S Breed Somali
Animal's Name Emmy
Baton Rouge, Louisiana

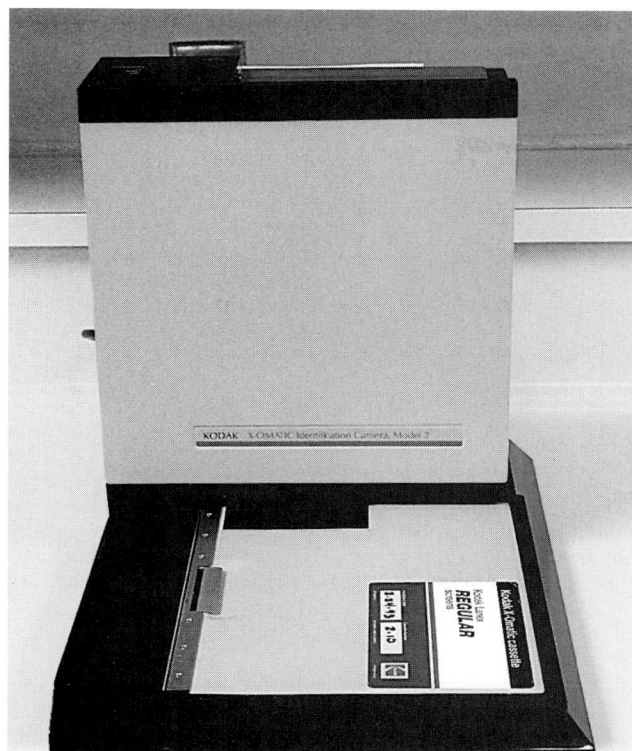

FIGURE 9-4. Film identification camera and special windowed x-ray cassette. Patient information is typed onto a 3- × 5-inch card and inserted into the top of the camera. The special cassette slides into the camera, which opens the window and flashes the identification onto the film.

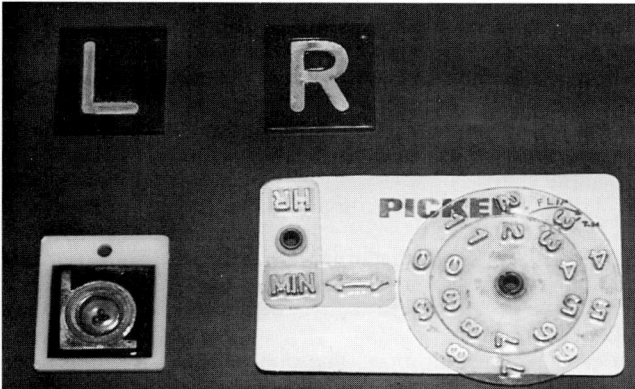

FIGURE 9-5. Leaded letters for film labeling. Left and right markers are used to label extremities and side of recumbency. The Mitchell marker *(lower left)* is used to identify gravitational direction, and the timer marker *(lower right)* is used with contrast studies to identify length of time since contrast medium administration.

when the film was taken in relation to when the contrast medium was administered (Figure 9-5). Front leg versus hindleg and medial versus lateral side identification markers are critical for proper interpretation of equine lower-extremity radiographs.

Filing of the Radiograph

Because a radiograph is part of the medical record, one must be able to retrieve it when needed. The radiographs of each examination should be placed in an x-ray envelope and filed according to the filing system used for other hospital records (i.e., by last name or case number). The following information should be recorded on the envelope: owner's address, animal identification, date, and type of examination. In addition, the radiographic technique used for the examination can be recorded on the envelope to provide an easy reference for follow-up studies.

It would be most advantageous to the veterinarian if the envelope could be coded for use as a self-teaching file. Several color tape systems have been devised to code cases for specific purposes. The system could be refined to include a combination of color to identify species, breeds, system examined, and so on. Morgan (1993) outlined an excellent color-coded system for x-ray retrieval purposes.

PRODUCTION OF X-RAYS

Basic Principles

A basic understanding of x-ray production, radiologic image formation, interactions of radiation with tissue, and radiation protection is essential. For those with little knowledge of physics or mathematics, the idea of having to learn basic radiation physics may be upsetting. However, the aim is not to teach radiation physics but rather to present basic concepts that are useful for those who use x-ray equipment.

X-rays can be defined as nonluminous electromagnetic radiations that are similar to visible light and to radio and television signals but are of much shorter wavelengths. The shorter the wavelengths, the greater is the energy of the x-ray beam. The greater the energy of the x-ray beam, the greater is its penetration.

X-rays are capable of penetrating opaque or solid substances, ionizing gases, and tissues through which they pass and affecting photographic plates and fluorescent screens. Because of these characteristics, x-rays are widely used in medicine for the study, diagnosis, and treatment of certain organic disorders, especially those of internal structures of the body.

Unfortunately, because of their short wavelengths, x-rays are not visible. As a consequence, many veterinarians, physicians, x-ray technologists, and veterinary technicians tend to become careless in the day-to-day use of x-rays by neglecting to use protective equipment or apply basic radiation safety rules.

The X-Ray Tube

Filament and Focusing Cup

The source of x-rays used in diagnostic radiology is the x-ray tube. The generators and transformers used in radiology exist only for the purpose of providing and controlling the amount of electricity reaching the x-ray tube. The x-ray tube is composed of an anode (+) and a cathode (−) enclosed in a vacuum within a glass envelope surrounded by a lead housing. The cathode contains one or two coiled wire filaments within hollowed-out wells or focusing cups. The filaments produce a source of electrons (e−) that are used to produce x-rays (Figure 9-6). The filament is heated to a critical temperature, and the electrons are boiled off and form an e−cloud within the focusing cup. The electrons are then accelerated very rapidly toward the positively charged anode. The collision of the speeding electrons into the anode results in the production of heat and x-rays. The x-rays are directed downward or vertically

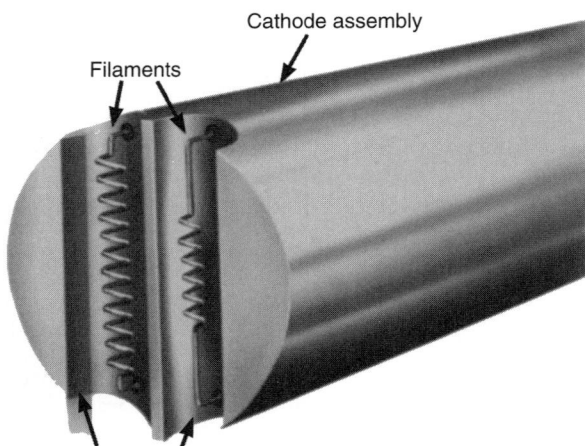

FIGURE 9-6. Cathode assembly showing focusing cups and filaments of two different sizes. Their arrangements produce electron beams that are focused onto narrow rectangles on the target. The smaller filament produces an electron stream of a smaller cross-sectional area and therefore a smaller focal spot. (From Eastman Kodak Co: *The fundamentals of radiography,* ed 12, Rochester, NY, 1980, Eastman Kodak Co, Radiographic Markets Division.)

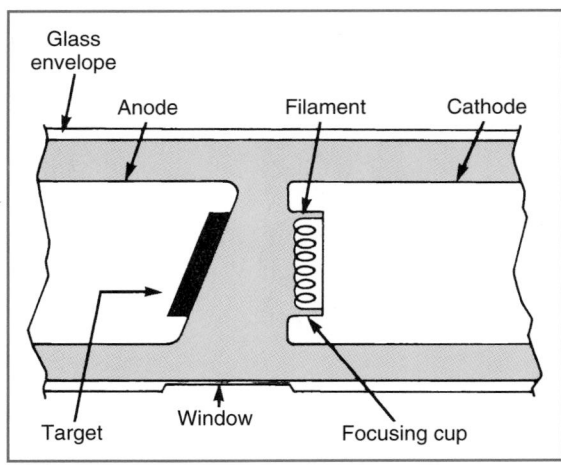

FIGURE 9-7. Stationary-anode x-ray tube. Diagram shows the relation of the anode and cathode. (From Eastman Kodak Co: *The fundamentals of radiography,* ed 12, Rochester, NY, 1980, Eastman Kodak Co, Radiographic Markets Division.)

through the window of the tube by the angle of the anode and the lead shielding of the x-ray tube (Figure 9-7). Two electrical circuits are present in every x-ray tube: a high-voltage, or kilovoltage (kV), circuit and a low-voltage, or milliamperage (mA), circuit. The kilovoltage circuit controls the electrical potential between the anode and cathode. This controls the speed of the electron acceleration and the energy level or penetrability of the resulting x-ray beam. The milliamperage circuit controls the electrical potential across the filament and affects the volume of electrons created and thus the number or volume of x-rays created.

The filament must produce electrons without melting. To this effect, an *alloy of tungsten* is used because it is less brittle and more efficient than pure tungsten for the production of electrons. This alloy has a high melting point and is used for the manufacture of most x-ray tube filaments.

The larger filament contains more tungsten than the small one and therefore can produce more electrons. As a result, the electron beam produced is larger and does not produce as sharp an x-ray picture as the smaller filament. Unfortunately, because of its size, the small filament may melt more rapidly than the larger one if an excess load is placed on it. As a result, the veterinarian and veterinary technician must always be aware of the limits and capabilities of the equipment when selecting which filament (focal spot) to use for a given procedure.

Focal Spot

The smaller filament provides a small target region or focal spot for electrons at the anode. In general, the small filament is used to obtain images of higher quality. However, because of the limited number of electrons provided by a small filament, its use is generally restricted to lower mAs (milliamperage × time in seconds) settings used primarily in tabletop (nongrid) extremity radiography. When higher tube current and shorter exposure time are

desired, the larger filament must be used, although there will be a loss of detail because the focal spot will be larger.

The size of the focal spot is determined by the size of the electron beam that is accelerated within the tube when high-voltage potentials are applied between the electrodes. Thus electrons traveling at an extremely high speed in the vacuum tube are suddenly stopped on the "target" area of the anode. As previously mentioned, the anode target is usually composed of an alloy of tungsten. Tungsten is used because it has the following special properties as a target material:

- High atomic number for the efficient production of x-rays
- High melting point to withstand the large amount of heat generated by the electron beam
- High capacity to transfer heat from the area in which electrons are absorbed
- High density to absorb the electron beam in a small surface area
- Low vapor pressure to maintain the vacuum inside the x-ray tube
- Relatively easy machinability into the appropriate shape at a reasonable cost

Stationary Anode

In early x-ray equipment, stationary anodes were used in most x-ray tubes. This type of x-ray tube is still prevalent in some veterinary hospitals in which older equipment is used, in dental equipment, and in small portable units used extensively in large animal radiology.

In x-ray tubes with stationary anodes, the target area is a small tungsten block about 3.18 mm thick embedded in a large block of copper. The copper is used to absorb and diffuse the tremendous amount of heat generated by the interaction of the electron beam with the target areas. This type of tube is popular and effective in radiography of the extremities of horses and dogs. However, it has limited application for the abdomen and thorax. The stationary anode x-ray tube cannot produce a sufficiently powerful x-ray beam to penetrate thicker body parts. It is also limited in its ability to produce a very rapid x-ray exposure of

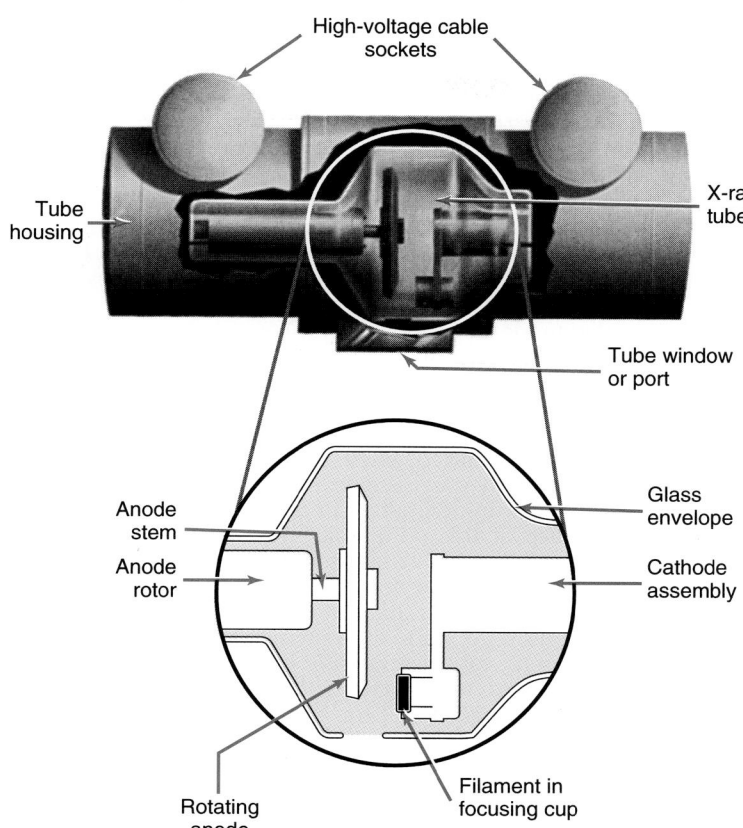

High-voltage cable sockets

Tube housing

X-ray tube

Tube window or port

Anode stem

Anode rotor

Glass envelope

Cathode assembly

Rotating anode

Filament in focusing cup

FIGURE 9-8. Modern rotating-anode radiographic tube. Exploded schematic view demonstrates the relationship of the filament to the rotating target. (From Eastman Kodak Co: *The fundamentals of radiography,* ed 12, Rochester, NY, 1980, Eastman Kodak Co, Radiographic Markets Division.)

sufficient strength for chest radiography to stop respiratory motion (see Figure 9-7).

Rotating Anode

Rotating anodes became popular with the advent of more powerful x-ray machines and the requirement of radiologists to obtain x-ray pictures of higher quality. Rotating anode tubes can use much higher tube currents, shorter exposure times, and focal spots as small as 0.1 mm because the electrons deposit their energy over a larger target region as the anode rotates (Figure 9-8).

The target of a rotating anode is a tungsten alloy bonded to molybdenum or graphite to help diffuse the tremendous heat generated by a high-powered x-ray machine. Rotating anodes are 7.5 to 12.5 cm in diameter. These tubes must dissipate enormous amounts of heat. The apparatus used to rotate the anode and dissipate the heat must be of the highest quality and perfectly balanced to prevent the tube from wobbling. Any imbalance causes the anode to wobble, leading to loss of image quality and eventual tube destruction. Figure 9-9 is a diagram of a rotating anode tube. Some tubes may rotate at speeds varying from 3600 revolutions per minute (rpm) to 10,000 rpm. Rotating anode x-ray machines generally have a two-step exposure switch. The first step of the switch starts the anode rotating, and the second step of the switch activates the high-voltage circuit, resulting in x-ray production. The anode is angled for two reasons. One, the angle directs the x-ray beam vertically to exit the tube window; And, two, it creates a smaller, more compact effective focal spot to create better resolution and produce a higher quality radiograph. The actual focal spot is the target on the anode. The effective focal spot is the tightly packed focused primary x-ray beam

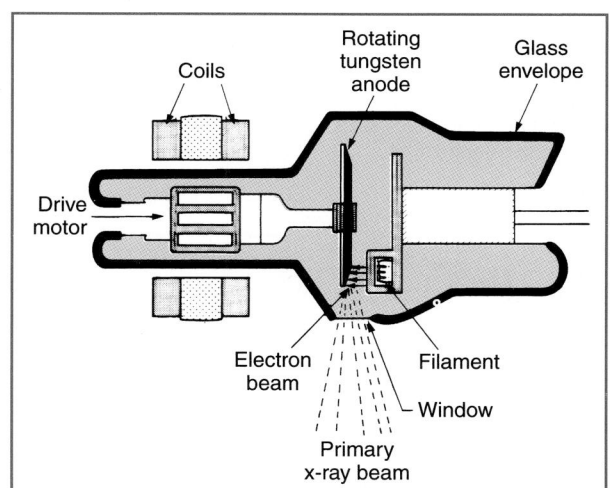

Coils

Rotating tungsten anode

Glass envelope

Drive motor

Electron beam

Filament

Window

Primary x-ray beam

FIGURE 9-9. Rotating-anode tube. Heat is better dissipated by placing the target material at the circumference of a high-speed rotating disk.

that exits the tube window. The actual focal spot is always larger than the effective focal spot (Figure 9-10).

Heel Effect

When an x-ray beam leaves the tube, it has an uneven x-ray photon distribution. This phenomenon is related to the angle of the target areas and the absorption by the anode and target material. As a result of this engineering feature, the x-ray beam is more intense at the side of the cathode than in the center of the beam or on the anode side. This phenomenon is called the *heel effect* (Figure 9-11).

This feature can be used to great advantage in veterinary radiology when x-raying parts of uneven thickness, a common problem in thoracic and abdominal radiography of deep-chested dogs. By placing the thickest part of the patient toward the cathode side of the x-ray tube, a more uniform density can be obtained on the radiograph.

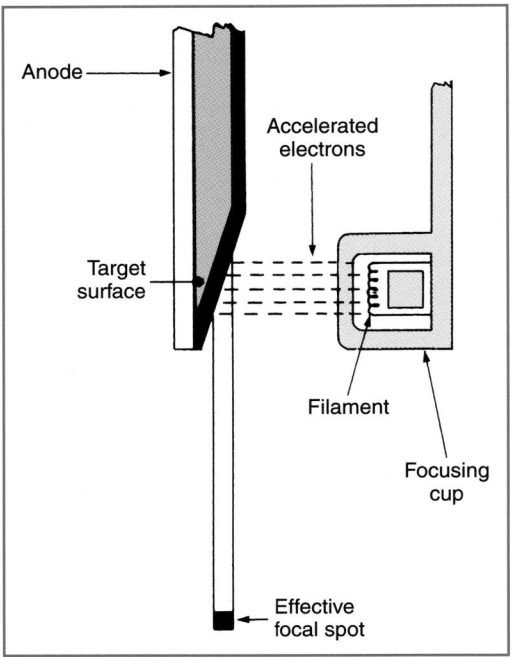

FIGURE 9-10.   Effective focal spot. The surface area is decreased when the target area is constructed at a 20-degree angle to the electron beam.

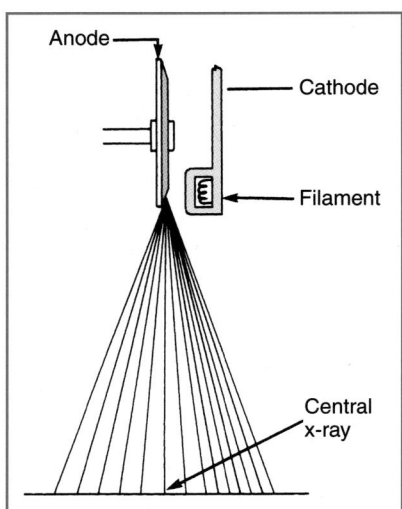

FIGURE 9-11.   Heel effect, which is produced by the uneven intensity of the primary beam. The intensity decreases rapidly toward the anode.

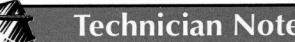
Technician Note

Always place the thickest part of the area being x-rayed toward the cathode side of the x-ray tube.

Tube Rating Chart

A rating chart is provided by all manufacturers of x-ray tubes. The tube rating chart provides important information on the maximum safe exposure time that can be used with specific mA and kV settings. If longer-than-designated exposure times are used, tube damage may occur. The size of the anode focal spot determines the rating of the tube because size controls the amount of energy it can absorb and convert into x-rays and heat.

The Physics of X-Ray Production

X-rays are produced when all the energy packed in extremely rapidly moving electrons comes to an abrupt stop on encountering the target in the x-ray tube. It should be mentioned at this point that most of the energy of the electrons is not converted into x-rays but is dissipated as heat. In fact, 99% of the energy dissipated in the target is lost as heat, and less than 1% is converted to x-ray energy. This explains the elaborate system of heat dissipation built into the x-ray tube described in the previous section.

Two events may occur when electrons approach the atoms of the target: (1) the electrons may miss the atom and its orbital electrons and go through the entire target and eventually be absorbed by the backing material of the target or the lead shielding of the x-ray tube, or (2) the incoming electrons may interact with atoms in the target material and produce x-rays by transferring their energy to these atoms. The faster the electrons travel, the greater is their energy and, therefore, the greater is the energy available for production of x-rays.

Scattered Radiations

In passing through a body of matter, an x-ray becomes attenuated; in other words, its energy decreases gradually. *Scattered radiations* are lower energy x-ray photons that

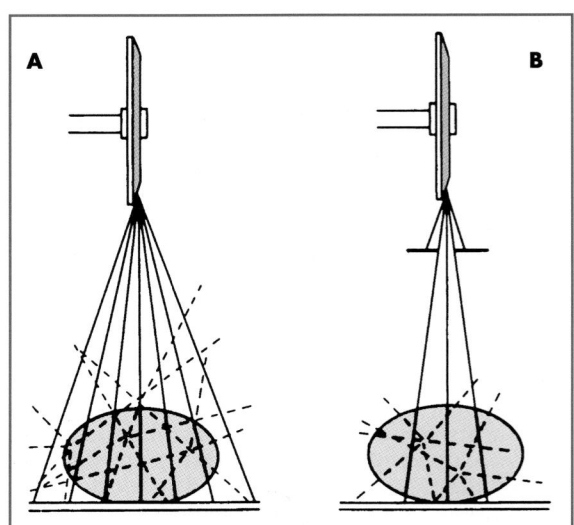

FIGURE 9-12.   Scattered radiations. **A,** Scattered radiations are produced when the primary beam is redirected after interacting with structures in the patient's body. **B,** Reduction in the amount of radiation produced when the primary beam is restricted by a diaphragm or collimator.

have undergone a change in direction after interacting with structures in the patient's body.

Scattered radiations are of concern because they decrease film quality and increase radiation exposure to the person taking the radiograph. Scattered radiations contribute to the overall film blackness or radiographic density but do not contribute to the useful image. This results in reduced subject contrast. Scattered radiations are also the primary source of radiation exposure to technicians manually restraining patients. Scattered radiations are directly increased with increases in the following three factors: kilovoltage, thickness of the part being x-rayed, and size of the field (Figure 9-12).

Careful collimation with beam-limiting devices and close attention to technical factors to avoid retakes are the best ways to decrease radiation exposure from scattered radiations. Several techniques are used to reduce scattered radiations and their effects on the radiograph. Beam-limiting devices, correct kilovolt peak (kVp) settings, compression radiography, and grids are a few devices that can be used to control scattered radiations. They are discussed later in this chapter.

Technician Note

Scattered radiations coming from the area of the patient that is exposed during radiography are the main source of radiation exposure to the veterinary technician.

X-RAY EQUIPMENT

The kind of x-ray unit encountered in a veterinary practice will vary according to the caseload and type of practice. Because one may be working with a large or small animal practitioner, in a large corporate practice, or in a veterinary teaching hospital, it is necessary to be familiar with the several types of x-ray units found in such practices.

Regardless of type and model, most x-ray machines share many features. For small animal radiology, an x-ray machine must have a table on which the animal is positioned (Figure 9-13). For larger animals, hand-held or stationary cassette holders are most often used (Figure 9-14). All x-ray machines must have a control panel to select kilovoltage, milliamperage, and time of exposure. An x-ray machine may have numerous auxiliary meters, buttons, dials, or switches, but kilovoltage, milliamperage, and time of exposure are the three primary factors of x-ray production (Figures 9-15 and 9-16). Many x-ray machines have a common selector control for milliamperage and time of exposure. This mAs dial or setting automatically sets the highest mA station and fastest time to give the requested mAs. Milliamperage × time in seconds (mAs) controls the volume or number of x-ray photons produced. In older machines, mA and time (in fractions of a second) must be set manually to produce a given mAs. The amperage (A) in mAs is always capitalized because it refers to Andre M. Ampere, the physicist credited with discovery of electric currents.

There are basically three types of x-ray machines used in veterinary practice: portable units, mobile units, and stationary units.

Technician Note

Kilovoltage, milliamperage, and time of exposure are the three factors that must be set correctly to produce a properly exposed radiograph.

Portable Unit

As the name implies, portable units can be carried "easily" from one location to another. Weight varies from 6.75 to

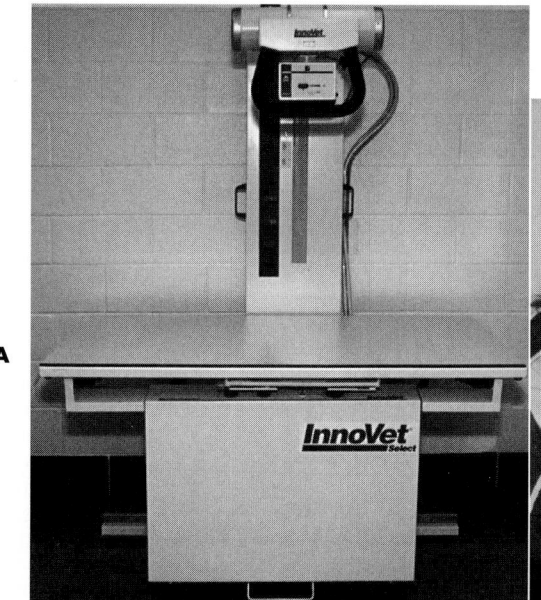
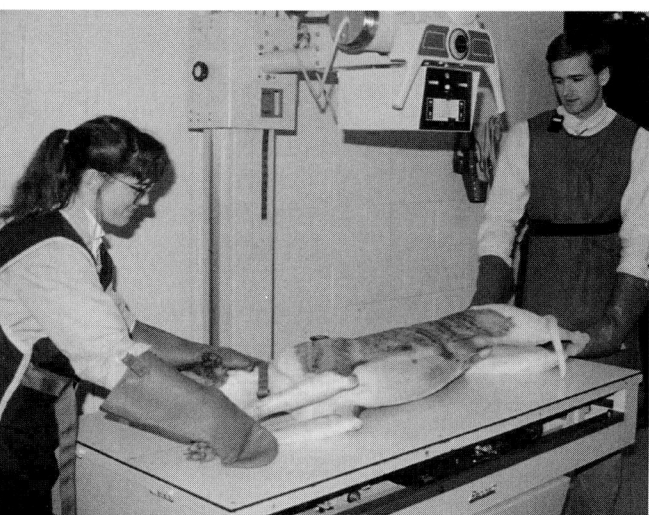

FIGURE 9-13.   A, 300-mA x-ray machine commonly used in small animal practice. **B,** Canine patient correctly positioned on an x-ray table for a lateral thoracic radiograph.

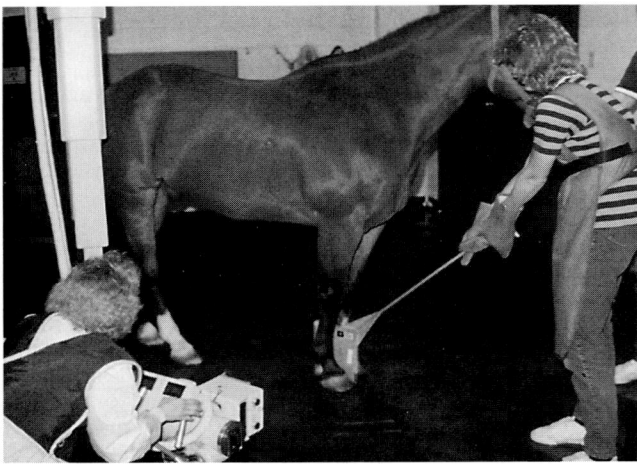

FIGURE 9-14. Large animal radiography unit using special film cassette holders for equine extremities.

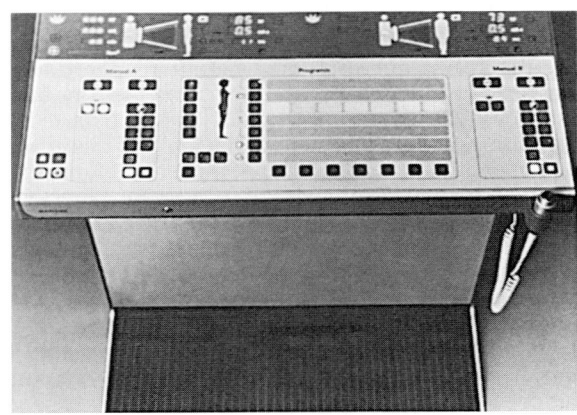

FIGURE 9-16. Operator control console used in some of the larger veterinary clinics and several veterinary teaching hospitals.

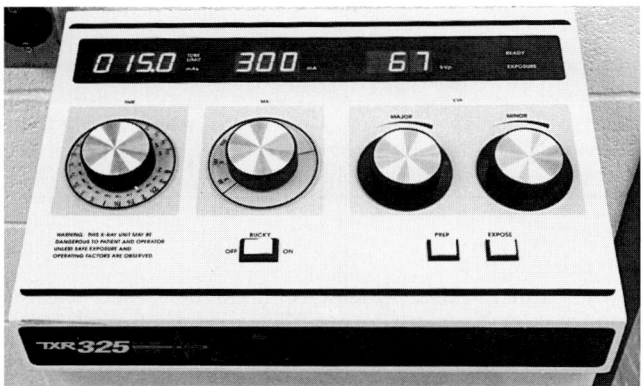

FIGURE 9-15. Typical instrument panel of an x-ray machine used by veterinarians showing multiple dials for selection of milliamperage, time, and kilovolt peak (kVp).

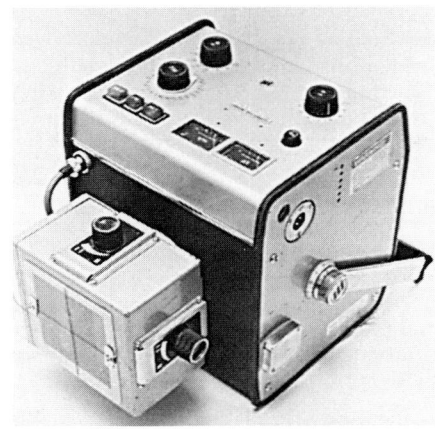

FIGURE 9-17. Portable x-ray unit. Such units are commonly used in large animal practices, mostly for the examination of extremities. This particular unit has a lighted collimator, which is an added safety device.

20.25 kg or more. They are generally used on blocks or custom-made stands. From the safety aspect, these units should never be hand held. This recommendation applies especially to lighter models that have less shielding. Hand holding an x-ray machine not only places the operator in close proximity to the x-ray tube but also decreases film quality because of tube motion during exposure.

Common characteristics of portable units include the following:

- A single focal spot of about 1.2 mm, stationary anode tube, and single filament, although a few models have two filaments and focal spot sizes
- Collimation varying from lead adapter plate to adapt to film size to lighted collimator with adjustable field size
- Tube output varying up to 90 kVp at 10 mA, usually with settings at 10, 20, and 30 mA and at 70, 80, or 90 kVp
- Electronic timer ranging from 0.01 to 10 seconds
- Electrical input of 110 V with an adapter to 220 V

Some models may use 12 DC (direct current) or operate on an automobile battery with converter (Figure 9-17).

Mobile Unit

Mobile units are medium-powered, wheel-mounted units that can be moved around the hospital. In many small animal practices, these units are used as a fixed unit and remain in one room. They are also popular in a mixed practice, in which the same unit can be used for both large and small animals.

These units are powered by 220-V or 110-V outlets. The 220-V units require more extensive electrical wiring, especially if the same units must be used at several locations. These units are equipped with a long, heavy power cord that can be a problem when working with large animals. The 110-V units are usually lighter and therefore easier to move around, and the power cord is smaller, which can be an advantage when taking x-rays of equine extremities. However, these units are usually less powerful than the 220-V units (Figure 9-18).

Stationary Unit

Stationary units are more powerful and are found in most small and large animal hospitals. A typical stationary small animal unit is pictured in Figure 9-13. Custom large

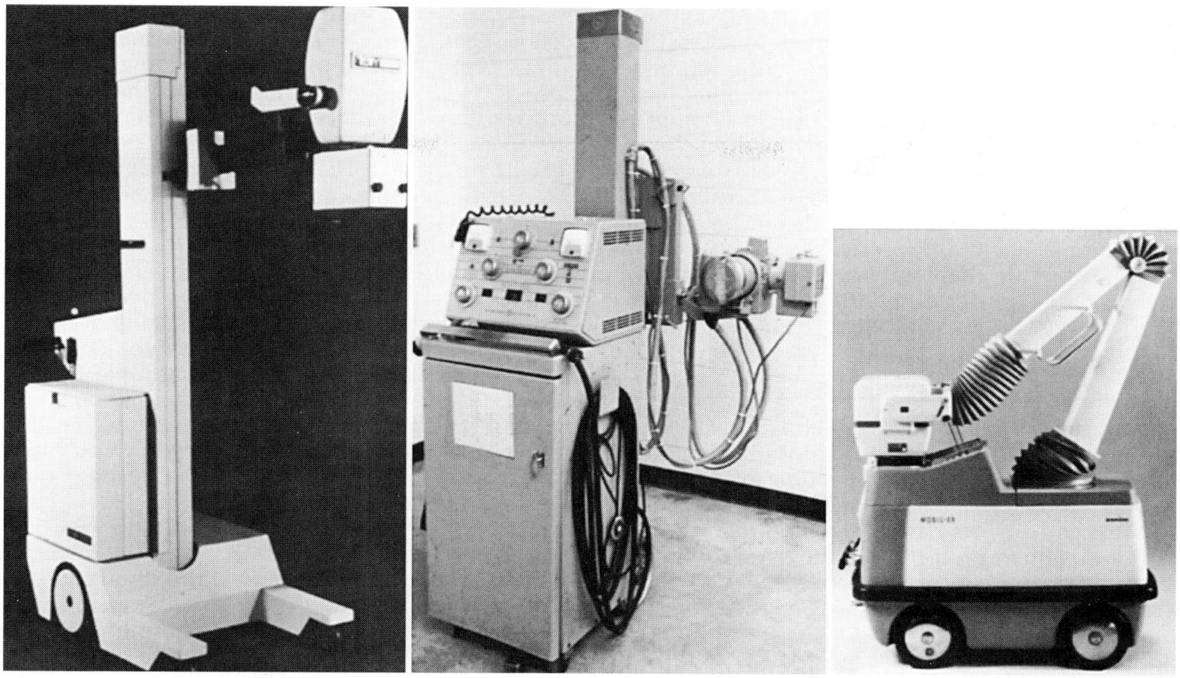

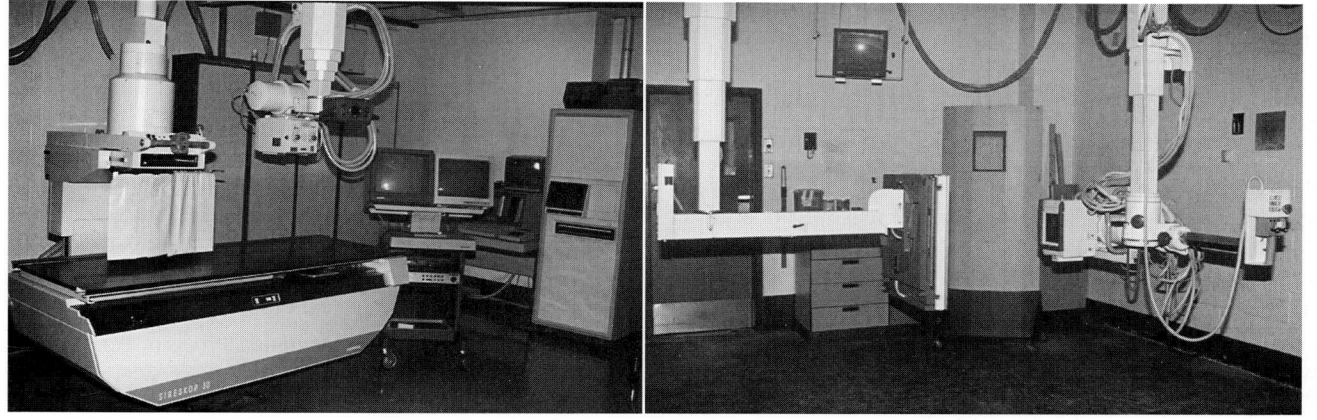

FIGURE 9-18. Three types of mobile units that are used in veterinary practice. These units can be used for both large and small animal radiology in mixed practices.

FIGURE 9-19. Stationary units. **A,** Radiography/fluorography (RF) used for special procedures, such as angiography, in a few large and small animal hospitals and several veterinary teaching hospitals. **B,** High-powered stationary large animal unit that includes a ceiling-suspended x-ray unit and a Potter-Bucky suspension system. The two units can be interlocked when needed for a fixed focal spot–film distance.

animal units and radiography/fluorography (RF) rooms are common in all veterinary teaching hospitals. Some of these units are among the most powerful diagnostic x-ray units installed in the United States.

They vary in size from 300 mA, 100 kVp up to 2000 mA, 150 kVp. They can be powered by single-phase or three-phase generators. The x-ray tube may be suspended from the ceiling or attached to a floor-stand support. The tube can rotate 90 degrees in all directions and usually has a heavy-duty collimator (Figure 9-19).

Stationary units commonly seen in small animal veterinary practices are of the 300 to 500 mA type with an exposure time of 1/60 second to 1/120 second. All these units can hold a cassette tray under the table with or without a Potter-Bucky grid. Some units have an image intensifier unit for fluoroscopic study or a fixed fluoroscopic screen.

Fluoroscopy

Fluoroscopic units are more suited to the study of moving structures and dynamic processes than are x-ray films. Although films exposed close together in time provide some information about these structures and processes, an image that is continuous in time is required for maximum information. The presentation of a continuous image is called *fluoroscopy,* and it involves directing the x-ray beam through the patient and onto an image intensifier. The image intensifier amplifies the x-ray coming through the patient, thus reducing the amount of radiation needed for the continuous exposure. The resulting images can be videotaped for analysis, and the tapes can be stored as part of the permanent medical record. The use of fluoroscopy is usually confined to gastrointestinal studies and myelography and is essential to heart and vascular studies. A fluoroscopic unit can be a very useful piece of equipment, but it is rarely used in veterinary medicine because of economic reasons. For a more extensive discussion of fluoroscopy, review the chapter discussing this subject in Curry et al. (1990), Douglas et al. (1987), Eastman Kodak Co. (1980), Lavin (1999), and Morgan (1993).

EXPOSURE FACTORS

The veterinary technician is responsible for selecting an x-ray technique that will provide a diagnostic radiograph. The factors that must be selected are time of exposure, milliamperage, and kilovoltage. As previously mentioned, most recent x-ray machines have a common dial for time of exposure and milliamperage, called the mAs setting. The selection of each factor is based on an accurate technique chart. How to prepare a technique chart is discussed later in this chapter.

Other factors that enter into the production of a diagnostic radiograph are focal-film distance, type of intensifying screen, type of x-ray film, and tabletop versus grid technique. All these variables are discussed in greater detail.

Milliamperage

The milliamperage setting controls the quantity of electrons boiled off at the filament in the x-ray tube. It is a *quantity factor*, because it controls the amount of x-rays that will be produced at the target area. Most diagnostic units used in small animal radiology are operated at settings from 50 to 300 mA. The smallest portable x-ray unit commonly used in large animal practices may use current flow as low as 10 or 20 mA, whereas the larger units used in small animal hospitals and veterinary teaching hospitals may have a current flow of 2000 mA.

Adjustments of the milliamperage setting control on an x-ray machine will control the amount of x-ray produced. When one increases the milliamperage setting, radiographic density, or film blackness, increases; conversely, when one decreases the milliamperage setting, a reduction in radiographic density, or a lighter film, results.

Exposure Time

The exposure time regulates the number of electrons that flow from the cathode to the anode per exposure. Ultimately, it regulates the quantity of x-ray reaching the film and therefore the film density. By increasing the milliamperage setting, one can reduce the time of exposure for a given film density. Conversely, if a lower milliamperage setting is selected, a longer time of exposure will be needed to obtain the same film density.

As an example to illustrate this concept, an exposure made at 100 mA and $1/10$ second should produce a film of equivalent density to an exposure made at 200 mA and $1/20$ second. In both cases the mAs factor (mA × time) is the same and is equal to 10 mAs. It should be remembered that shorter exposure times reduce the problem of motion, which may result in loss of detail. For this reason, a thoracic radiograph on a dog or cat should be taken at $1/20$ to $1/60$ second to prevent blurring of the radiograph as a result of respiratory motion.

Kilovoltage

Kilovoltage is a *quality factor* that regulates the energy of the x-ray beam. This setting regulates the voltage applied between the anode and cathode in the x-ray tube. The higher the voltage, the greater is the energy of the x-ray beam and therefore the greater is the amount of tissue that can be penetrated. The kilovoltage setting most often used in diagnostic radiology varies from 40,000 to 150,000 V (40 to 150 kV).

The kilovoltage setting increases the scale of contrast on a radiograph. The scale of contrast refers to the number of shades of gray that can be seen. In general, the greater the scale of contrast, the higher is the quality of the x-ray film because small differences in soft tissue density are better seen. Higher kilovoltage settings are used for soft tissue examination, such as thoracic examinations, and lower kilovoltage settings are used for bony structures. Increasing the kilovoltage will also increase radiographic density, or film blackness, because of increased patient penetration with the higher energy x-ray beam.

Focal-Film Distance

The focal-film distance refers to the distance between the target in the x-ray tube and the surface of the x-ray cassette. This factor is usually kept constant from one exposure to another. It is usually kept at a distance of 70 to 85 cm for large animal radiology and 90 to 105 cm for small animal radiology.

It is important to keep the focal-film distance constant from one exposure to the next because it has a significant influence on exposure factors. An increase in distance decreases the number of x-rays reaching the film very rapidly. If one doubles the focal-film distance, the number of x-rays reaching the film will be reduced by a factor of four. This is often referred to as the *inverse square law*, which states that the intensity of the x-ray beam at a given point is inversely proportional to the square of the distance from the x-ray source.

It is sometimes necessary to change the focal-film distance to obtain proper positioning. This simple calculation will help choose the proper mAs setting when the distance is changed:

$$\text{Old mAs} \times \frac{\text{New distance}^2}{\text{Old distance}^2} = \text{New mAs setting}$$

For example, if an x-ray taken at 10 mAs at 100 cm must be taken at 50 cm, by using the formula given, the new mAs setting can be calculated as follows:

$$10 \text{ mAs} \times \frac{50^2}{100^2} = 2.5 \text{ mAs}$$

This new mAs setting should produce an x-ray of similar radiographic density to the original setting of 10 mAs.

Technique Chart

A technique chart is an essential component for obtaining diagnostic x-ray examinations in a consistent way. A technique chart must be formulated for each x-ray machine because there are differences in output with each machine (even those made by the same manufacturer). Therefore one should never use an x-ray chart formulated for another x-ray machine without making appropriate changes. If one selects exposure factors from a good technique chart, consistent radiographic examinations of diagnostic quality will be obtained. In addition, there will be a saving of x-ray films because waste from repeated exposures will be avoided.

Several types of technique charts can be formulated.

Each type must be formulated with the goal of using the maximum potential of a particular x-ray machine. Perhaps the most popular type of technique chart used by veterinarians is a variable kilovoltage chart. A variable mAs chart is probably more appropriate for the most powerful x-ray machines. However, a combination of variable kilovoltage and mAs technique charts is best. Such charts take into consideration the need to adapt a technique chart for different body systems, such as a thoracic and abdominal study, as well as examination involving the musculoskeletal system.

This chapter cannot discuss appropriately every type of technique chart. The principle of how to prepare a variable kilovoltage technique chart, along with an example of such a chart (Table 9-1), is given. For a more extensive discussion of how to prepare different technique charts with examples of each, please refer to the discussion this topic by Han et al. (2000), Lavin (1999), Morgan (1993), and Ticer (1984).

Formulation of a Technique Chart

A technique chart is formulated by a series of trial-and-error exposures. It is necessary, however, to standardize as many variable factors as possible before starting trial exposures. Factors such as the type of cassette and intensifying screen, type of x-ray film, and the focal-film distance must be constant, and a grid should be used if available. The darkroom procedures must be standardized to include fresh solution and developing time recommended by the manufacturer based on the temperature of the solution. It is most important to understand that all these factors should be constant because the technique chart will be valid only under the conditions of formulation. If, for example, cassettes and intensifying screens in a veterinary practice are of different age or speed, the film density for a given technique will be different from one study to the next, although the same factors are used.

For trial exposure, a normal dog with a lateral abdominal measurement of 8 to 10 cm should be selected. A trial exposure at a setting of 65 kV at 2.5 mAs is suggested. Two exposures are made at this setting. In selecting the mAs setting, the shortest possible time of exposure for a given mAs setting is selected. The two films are then developed according to standard technique and are examined for proper "diagnostic" density. If the films are either overexposed or underexposed, a second series of exposures is made by halving or doubling the mAs setting. The films are again processed and examined for diagnostic quality. All films should be examined and compared with each other for consistent density between exposures. The best film is selected. If one of the techniques selected is completely satisfactory, a technique can be formulated starting with the factors that produced the "diagnostic" film. If, however, none of the films are totally satisfactory, a fourth series of exposures is started in which the kilovoltage setting is decreased or increased until an excellent film is obtained.

Because there is an increase in scattered radiation with an increase in thickness of a part to be x-rayed, it is recommended that a grid be used for thicknesses greater than 10 cm. If a grid of 8:1 ratio is used, it will necessitate a doubling of the mAs setting technique over the formulated technique. At this point, however, it is recommended that

TABLE 9-1	VARIABLE kV TECHNIQUE CHART FOR AN X-RAY MACHINE OF 300 mA, 125 kV, 1/120-SECOND TIMER WITH FFD OF 40 INCHES					
Thickness (cm)	kV	mA	Seconds	mAs	Grid 8:1
4	48	300	$1/120$	2.5	No
5	50	300	$1/120$	2.5	No
6	52	300	$1/120$	2.5	No
7	54	300	$1/120$	2.5	No
8	56	300	$1/120$	2.5	No
9	58	300	$1/120$	2.5	No
10	63	300	$1/60$	5	Yes
11	65	300	$1/60$	5	Yes
12	67	300	$1/60$	5	Yes
13	69	300	$1/60$	5	Yes
14	71	300	$1/60$	5	Yes
15	73	300	$1/60$	5	Yes
16	75	300	$1/60$	5	Yes
17	77	300	$1/60$	5	Yes
18	79	300	$1/60$	5	Yes
19	81	300	$1/60$	5	Yes
20	84	300	$1/60$	5	Yes
21	87	300	$1/60$	5	Yes
22	90	300	$1/60$	5	Yes
23	93	300	$1/60$	5	Yes
24	96	300	$1/60$	5	Yes
25	99	300	$1/60$	5	Yes
26	102	300	$1/60$	5	Yes
27	105	300	$1/60$	5	Yes
28	99	300	$1/30$	10	Yes
29	102	300	$1/30$	10	Yes
30	105	300	$1/30$	10	Yes

FFD, Focal-film distance; kV, kilovolts; mA, milliamperes; mAs, milliamperes per second.
Radiographs were taken with Kodak Lanex Regular screens and Kodak TML x-ray film.

the accuracy of the technique chart be checked by making a few trial exposures of larger dogs using a grid.

The technique chart is formulated by subtracting 2 kV for each decrease in centimeter of thickness and adding 2 kV for each increase in centimeter of thickness. One should keep in mind that a doubling of the mAs setting is necessary at thicknesses greater than 10 cm if a grid is used. At 80 kV and higher the increase in kilovoltage should be in steps of 3 kV for each increase in centimeter thickness until the limit of the machine is reached.

Table 9-1 illustrates a variable kilovoltage technique chart formulated for an x-ray machine of 300 mA, 125 kV, and $1/120$ second minimum time of exposure. Remember, however, that this is only an illustration of how to formulate a technique chart and should not be used with any one x-ray machine without adaptation to that particular machine.

IMAGE FORMATION

When an x-ray beam penetrates a body system and reaches an x-ray film, a latent image is produced that will be revealed when the film is processed chemically. Several factors are involved in the formation of a high-quality latent image. This section discusses the factors that enter into the formation of an x-ray image.

X-Ray Cassette

Cassettes (film holders) used in veterinary medicine are of two types. The *nonscreen* type is a direct-exposure *cassette* in which the film is placed in a cardboard cassette or a plastic film holder (Figure 9-20). The nonrigid system must be light-proof and is used when great detail is needed for an examination. The disadvantage of this type of cassette is that it will require an exposure time in excess of 26 times the normal exposure time of a regular par screen cassette system. Nonscreen exposures should be used only when the animal is under general anesthesia or heavy sedation to stop motion and no personnel are required for restraint in the radiology room. Nonscreen exposures are used primarily for intraoral occlusal studies of the nasal cavity and dental arches.

The second type is the more conventional *image intensifying screen,* which is placed in a *rigid cassette* (Figure 9-21). It is important that the hinges of the cassette be of the highest quality to ensure excellent and uniform contact between the x-ray film and the intensifying screen and to prevent light leakage that could fog or darken the film. Various materials are used in the manufacture of x-ray cassettes. Most cassettes have a solid front made of either plastic or light metal. Recently, carbon fiber (mostly graphite) also has been introduced. Such cassettes are excellent and may reduce the amount of x-rays needed to make an exposure by as much as 20%. The cassette back may be made of steel and can sustain moderate patient weight without being damaged. Sometimes a small area of about 7 × 3 cm is shielded from the primary beam for the purpose of film identification (see Figure 9-4).

Cassettes are expensive and should be handled with care. When dropped, they may warp, or if the cover is forced, the hinges may be damaged, resulting in a cassette that does not close properly. If the film contact is not perfect along the surface of the cassette, distortion of the x-ray image will occur. The surface of the cassette should be kept clean at all times to avoid creating film artifacts.

Intensifying Screens

Intensifying screens are the smooth shiny white inner surfaces of the film cassette. They are made of layers of tiny crystals bonded together on a plastic support and covered with a protective coating. These crystals fluoresce, or emit light, after exposure to x-rays. The screens are placed in the inner surfaces of the cassette, and the x-ray film is sandwiched between. Because film is more sensitive to light exposure than to radiation exposure, the use of fluorescent intensifying screens dramatically decreases the amount of radiation needed to produce a film of diagnostic radiographic density. Screens allow much lower mAs settings, which decrease loss of detail as a result of motion, decrease patient radiation exposure, and help to prolong x-ray tube life. In addition, intensifying screens increase radiographic contrast and therefore improve radiographic detail.

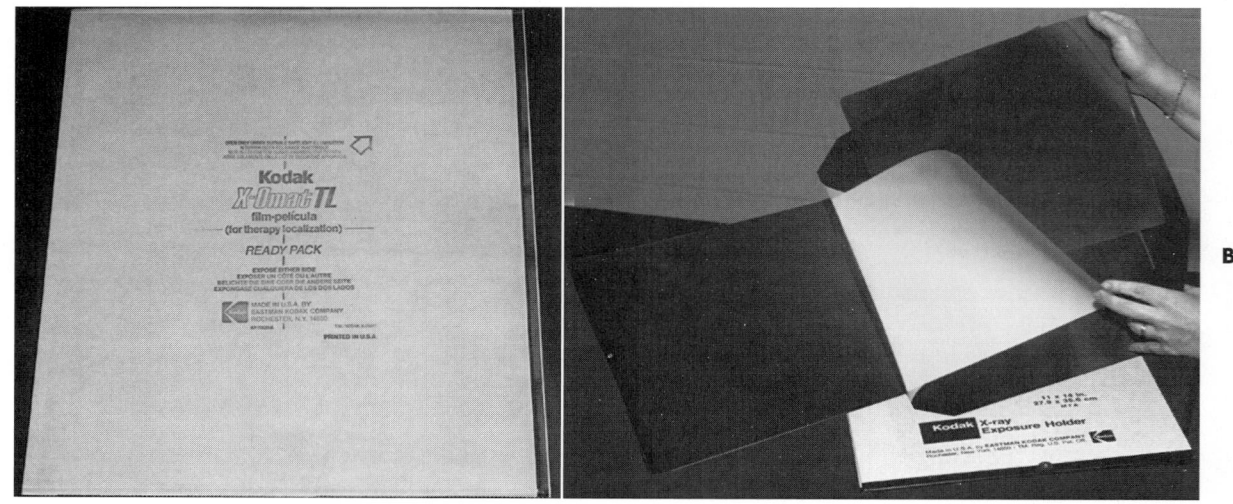

FIGURE 9-20.   Nonscreen film. **A,** Ready pack film with a special emulsion for direct exposure. **B,** X-ray exposure holder for regular screen film. Such a cassette necessitates exposure time in excess of 26 times the normal exposure time of a regular par screen cassette system. (From Eastman Kodak Co: *The fundamentals of radiography,* ed 12, Rochester, NY, 1980, Eastman Kodak Co, Radiographic Markets Division.)

Intensifying screens are mounted in pairs in an x-ray cassette (Figure 9-22). They are made of four components:

- A backing of cardboard or plastic, most commonly a Mylar material
- Reflecting layers, such as titanium dioxide, that reflect light from the active layer back toward the x-ray film
- An active layer of light-emitting phosphor, such as calcium tungstate or rare earth material, that produces the fluorescence that exposes the film following absorption of x-rays
- A plastic coating that reduces static electricity and provides a protective covering that can be cleaned

The screens must be cleaned on a regular basis—at least monthly or whenever screen artifacts are noted on a radiograph. It is best to use a cleaning product recommended by the manufacturer for this purpose. If this is not available, a 70% alcohol solution will work (Figure 9-23). It is essential that the surface of the screen be thoroughly dry before inserting an x-ray film or closing the cassette; otherwise, the film will stick to the screens and permanently ruin them. Any stain on the surface of the screen will interfere with transmission of light from the screen to

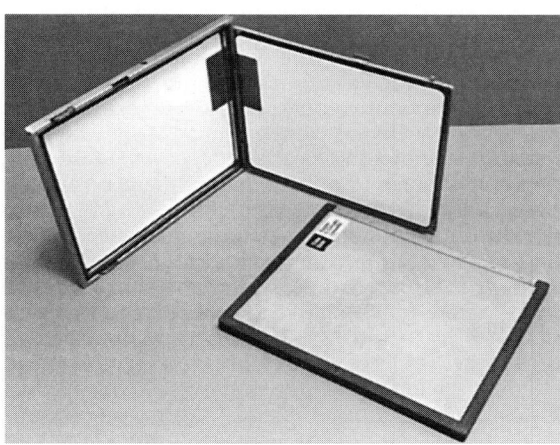

FIGURE 9-21. Open and closed rigid film cassette with image intensifying screens.

the film and cause an artifact. The technician must be very careful not to spill or splash darkroom chemicals onto the surface of the screens, or they may be ruined. It is for this reason that emphasis is placed on the maintenance and cleanliness of screens.

Screen Speed

The speed of a screen pertains to its ability to convert absorbed x-ray energy into visible light. Screen speed is a relative term that refers to the amount of radiation required by that screen to produce a film of diagnostic radiographic density. A fast screen requires less radiation than a regular, medium, or par screen to produce the same degree of blackness on the radiograph. The faster the screen, the poorer is the radiographic detail or resolution. Fast screens have a thicker phosphor layer and larger crystals to increase x-ray absorption and light production. Slower or detail screens have smaller crystals and are less efficient at light conversion but produce a radiograph of greater detail and resolution. Detail screens are also called *fine screens* and generally require four times the amount of radiation as a medium or par screen. Regular screens are intermediate in speed between par or medium and fast screens.

The original phosphor used in intensifying screens was calcium tungstate. This phosphor produces light in the blue spectrum and is commonly found in veterinary hospitals that have acquired used cassettes and screens from local human hospitals. Improved rare earth phosphors introduced in 1975 emit light in the green spectrum and are able to produce the same degree of radiographic detail as calcium tungstate screens with less radiation exposure. Table 9-2 shows the relative speed of various calcium tungstate and rare earth screens. Rare earth screens are more efficient because they absorb more x-ray photons per crystal and produce more light per absorbed photon. These properties of rare earth screens have definite advantages in veterinary medicine and include the following:

- Reduced exposure time
- Reduced motion artifacts
- Decreased tube voltage, resulting in improved contrast
- Decreased tube current, which prolongs the life of the tube
- Reduced production of heat in the x-ray tube
- Reduced patient radiation dose

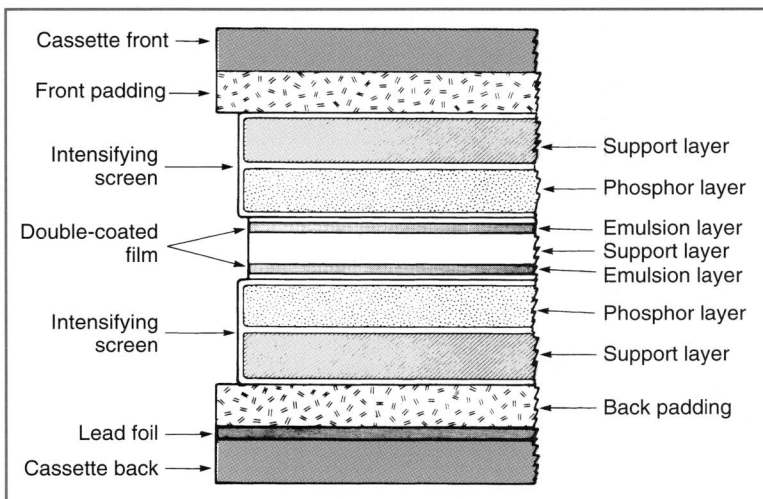

FIGURE 9-22. Cross section of a cassette intensifying screen system.

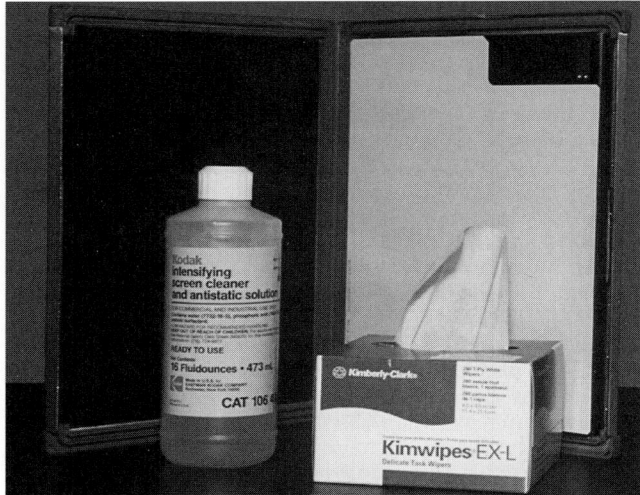

FIGURE 9-23. Open film cassette with a single intensifying screen (shiny white surface), used for detail extremity radiography. Screens should be handled carefully and cleaned regularly with approved solutions.

TABLE 9-2	RELATIVE SPEED OF CALCIUM TUNGSTATE* AND RARE EARTH† SCREENS	
Screen Type		**ASA Film Speed**
Fine-detail calcium tungstate		30
Par calcium tungstate		100
Fine-detail rare earth		150
Regular calcium tungstate		200
Fast calcium tungstate		250
Medium rare earth		300
Regular rare earth		400
Fast rare earth		600

*Kodak X-O$_{MAT}$ with X-O$_{MAT}$ RP film.
†Kodak Lanex with T MAT L film.

Technician Note

Rare earth screens are advantageous for veterinary radiography because they require fewer x-rays to produce a diagnostic radiograph. Lower exposures mean less patient and technician dose, fewer retakes because of patient motion, and longer x-ray tube life.

The main disadvantage of rare earth screens at this time is their cost, which is much greater than regular calcium tungstate screens. They have a definite place in large animal radiology because of their speed. This is an important factor when they are used with the smaller, low-capacity portable x-ray units. Table 9-3 presents an example of a technique chart that can be used with a small, portable x-ray unit in combination with the rare earth screen.

There is a misconception in veterinary medicine that intensifying screens last forever. This is not true. Screens have a predictable lifetime and gradually wear out with repeated use. Most rare earth screens are worn out after 10 to 12 years of regular use. The radiograph produced with a very old screen will have a white speckled pattern most notable in the black areas on the film. This artifact is called *screen craze.* Most screens have a company name and screen number printed on the edge. By calling the manufacturer, the technician can find out the age of the screen and the best type of film to use with that particular screen.

X-Ray Film

Because the recording medium for most x-ray examinations is photographic film, some basic principles of photography must be understood.

An x-ray film is prepared from a suspension of light and x-ray-sensitive granules embedded in a gelatin emulsion coated over a polyester base. The sensitive granules are usually silver bromide crystals of different sizes. The gelatin matrix is protected by a thin covering called the *T coat.* Just like the image-intensifying screens, the sensitive crystals come in various sizes. Images of exceptional detail can be recorded on films containing very fine crystals. In faster films the crystals are larger, which results in a loss of detail, which is compensated for, however, by possible shorter time of exposure. Because of the shorter time of exposure, faster films may sometimes provide better image detail because the images contain fewer motion artifacts.

X-ray film can be separated into two categories: *screen film* (Figure 9-24) and *nonscreen film.* Screen film is sensitive primarily to the wavelengths of light emitted from intensifying screens. Nonscreen films are designed for direct exposures to x-rays and are relatively insensitive to visible light from screens. Nonscreen films provide superb detail and are especially good for intraoral examination of the nasal cavity, dental studies, and bony extremities. Because this type of x-ray film is exposed by x-rays only, it has the disadvantage of needing very long exposure times to obtain necessary film density (Figure 9-25). Patients should be under general anesthesia and no personnel should be in the room during nonscreen film exposures.

Screen-type films are less sensitive to direct ionizing radiation but are very sensitive to visible light. This type of film requires less exposure to produce a radiograph because of its sensitivity to the fluorescence emitted by the intensifying screens. Remember that screens produce a specific color or spectrum of light. The film used should be matched in sensitivity to the light spectrum of the screen.

Rare earth screens do need special x-ray films to produce an optimal radiograph. Every x-ray film manufacturer produces a rare earth type of x-ray film. There is great confusion because of the endless names and types of combinations of x-ray film and image-intensifying screens available on the market. Again, please refer to Douglas et al. (1987) and Morgan (1993) for a more elaborate discussion of this important topic.

Technician Note

Be sure the x-ray film you are using is maximally sensitive to the spectrum of light your screens are emitting.

Grids

When x-rays enter a patient, some pass straight through to the film cassette, but a great many are scattered or redirected along a different path before exiting the patient. The purpose of a grid is to control the scatter radiation before it reaches the x-ray cassette. A grid is constructed of a sheet of lead strips interfaced with radiolucent spacers made of plastic or aluminum. These strips are encased in an aluminum protective cover for durability. Grids come in various

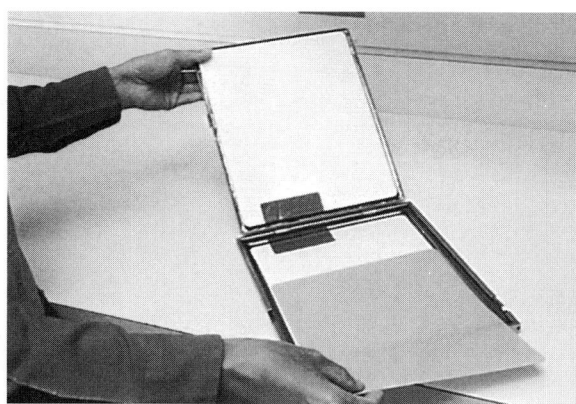

FIGURE 9-24. Screen film manufactured for the special purpose of being used with image-intensifying screens. Such film, when used with the proper combination of screen, will drastically reduce x-ray exposure time.

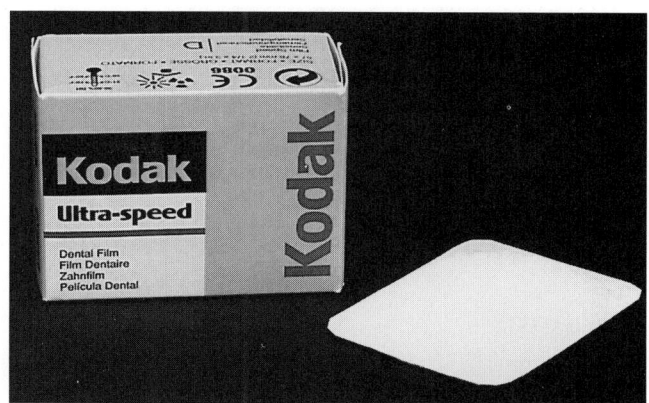

FIGURE 9-25. Prepackaged nonscreen film that can be used for dental and occlusal intraoral radiographic examinations. This type of film requires long exposure times because of the lack of intensifying screens. Patients should be under general anesthesia, and the technician should make the exposure from outside the room or behind a radiation safety barrier.

TABLE 9-3	TECHNIQUE CHART FOR PORTABLE X-RAY UNIT OF 10 mA AT 90-kV, 15 mA AT 80-kV, AND 20 mA AT 70-kV CAPACITY USING KODAK CASSETTE WITH RARE EARTH SCREEN OF REGULAR SPEED*					
Examination	**Size**	**View**	**kVp**	**Time (sec)**	**Distance (cm)**	
Fetlock	Foal	DP or obliques	80	0.02	60	
	Large adult		80	0.04	70	
Carpus	Foal	DP or obliques	80	0.02	70	
	Large adult		80	0.04	70	
Tarsus	Foal	Lat	80	0.02	70	
		DP	80	0.04	70	
	Adult	Lat	80	0.04	70	
		DP	80	0.08	70	
Stifle	Adult	Lat	80	0.1	70	
		CdCa	90	0.25	70	

DP, Dorsoplantar or dorsopalmar; *kV*, kilovolts; *mA*, milliamperes; *kVp*, kilovolt peak; *Lat*, lateral; *CdCa*, caudocranial.
*For a more complete treatment of cassette and image-intensifying screens, refer to Douglas et al. (1987) and Morgan (1993). Both have excellent discussions of all types of screens available on the market today.

sizes similar to x-ray cassettes and are usually placed directly over the cassette between the animal and the cassette (Figure 9-26).

The purpose of a grid is to allow only the primary x-ray beam to pass through and prevent scattered radiations from reaching the film. The grid is constructed in such a way as to absorb all radiations that do not pass between the lead strips. This arrangement may absorb most scattered radiations if grids of high ratios are used. However, it has the disadvantage of absorbing part of the primary x-ray beam and therefore requires greater exposure time to obtain a given film density. Figure 9-27 illustrates how a grid absorbs scattered and secondary radiation and prevents it from reaching the film.

Grids are made of different ratios and number of strips per 2.5 cm. The ratio varies from 5:1 to 16:1 and from 60 lines (strips) per 2.5 cm to 120 lines per 2.5 cm. The higher the ratio and the number of lines per 2.5 cm, the more radiation is absorbed by the grid. The ratio of a grid refers to the relation between the height of the lead strips and the width of the radiolucent spaces. For example, if the height of the lead strip is 12 times greater than the thickness of the space, the grid ratio will be 12:1, and if it is 10 times greater, the ratio will be 10:1. The greater the ratio, the more efficiently the grid absorbs scattered radiations. Figure 9-27, *A*, illustrates the ratio of a 5:1 grid.

The grid is most useful when x-raying parts of the body in which scattering is considerable, which in practice includes all thick parts of the body (e.g., thorax, abdomen, skull) and those joints and bones in excess of 10-cm thickness. The grid lines are visible on the resulting film, but this is made up for by the increased resolution of the image on the radiograph.

Grids may be *parallel* or *focused*. A parallel grid is one constructed with strips parallel to each other. A focused grid is one in which the lead strips and spacers are gradually angulated from the center to the periphery of the grid. The distance from the point of convergence, or focal point, is referred to as its focal distance, or radius. The advantage of a focused grid is that it allows unobstructed amounts of radiation to pass through it at the center and at the edge of the grid as long as the radiations are parallel to

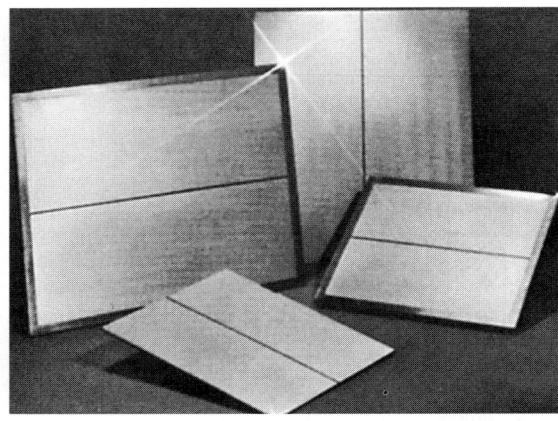

FIGURE 9-26. Various sizes and types of grids commonly used in veterinary radiology of large and small animals.

the axis of the lead strips. Such grids can be used only at a specific focal-film distance specified by the manufacturer. If distances above or below the focal distance are used, grid cutoff will occur, which means that part of the primary beam will be absorbed by the grid. For veterinary work, a grid with a ratio of 8:1 at 103 lines per 2.5 cm is recommended.

Potter-Bucky Diaphragm

One other type of grid encountered in veterinary hospitals is the *Potter-Bucky diaphragm.* This is simply a movable grid. The movement of the diaphragm is timed to suit a particular exposure, and the grid moves across the film during the exposure so that the grid lines are not shown on the resulting film. When using a movable grid, the exposure time must be increased by a factor of four or the kilovoltage increased by about 20%. Usually, Potter-Bucky diaphragms are positioned under the table and electronically linked to the timer of the x-ray machine (Figure 9-27, *B*).

Another method to reduce scattered radiation is the *air gap technique.* It is a simple technique that consists of increasing the distance between the patient and the surface of the cassette. With this technique, the amount of scattered radiations produced is not reduced, but fewer scattered radiations reach the film because of the increased distance between patient and film. With the air gap technique, it is not necessary to increase the exposure factors, as must be done with a grid. However, this technique will decrease the sharpness of the image because of increased subject-to-film distance. It is also less effective at high kilovoltage settings, because the higher energy scatter occurs in a forward direction. This technique is used most commonly in veterinary radiology for magnification purposes and for equine thoracic radiography.

Technician Note

Always use a grid between the patient and the film cassette when the body part being x-rayed is greater than 10 cm thick.

THE DARKROOM

The importance of the darkroom in radiography cannot be overemphasized. Radiography unquestionably begins and ends in the darkroom, in which films are loaded into

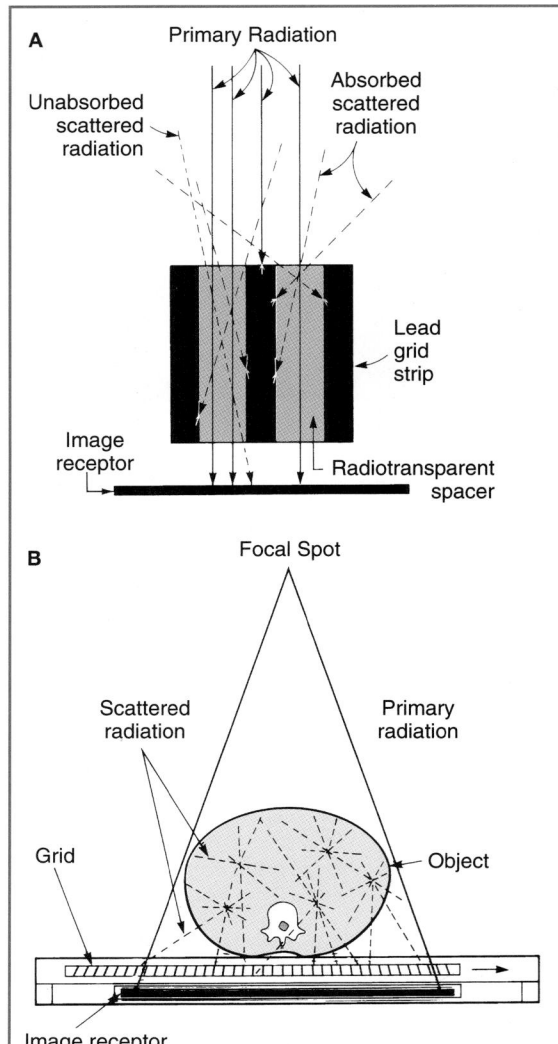

FIGURE 9-27. Cross section of a grid. **A,** Diagram of a small section of a grid showing how a large proportion of the scattered radiation is absorbed and image-forming primary radiation passes through to the image detector. **B,** Diagram of focused Potter-Bucky diaphragm being moved toward the right. (Modified from Eastman Kodak Co: *The fundamentals of radiography,* ed 12, Rochester, NY, 1980, Eastman Kodak Co, Radiographic Markets Division.)

cassettes ready for exposure and returned for processing into a finished radiograph. Most mistakes made in veterinary radiography are related to the processing of radiographs. It is necessary to keep the darkroom very clean and light proof. It is also essential for the technician to have a thorough knowledge of x-ray darkroom technique and of conventional or automatic processing. The chemicals should be changed, replenished, maintained, and mixed according to the strict directions of the manufacturer.

Equipment

A darkroom need not be spacious. For most veterinary practices, a small room of about 240 × 240 cm is adequate. However, it is essential that this room be made totally

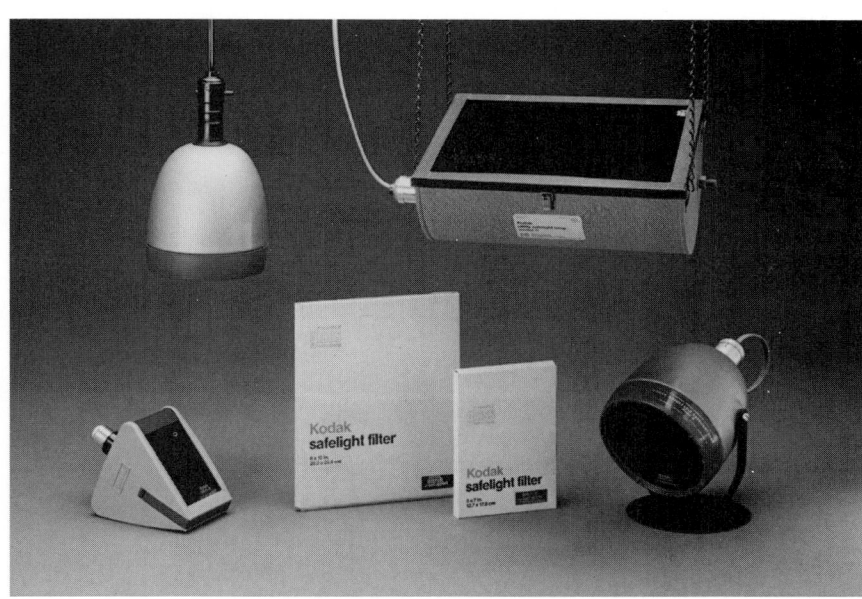

FIGURE 9-28. Several examples of darkroom safelights and packaged safelight filters. The filters must be matched to the light sensitivity of the film being used in the darkroom and must not be cracked or incompletely sealed by the filter holder.

dark. If there is a window in the room, there is no reason not to open it for ventilation when the room is not in use; however, the window should be light proof when closed. One can easily check if a darkroom is light proof by turning off all lights, including the safelight, closing the door tightly, and slowly turning around in the center of the darkroom, looking for any light leaking into the room. It is important also that a lock be placed on the door to avoid its being opened while films are being processed. A darkroom need not be completely dark, because a safelight can be used during film processing. A safelight is a light bulb shielded by a plastic filter that stops any light the film is sensitive to from penetrating the filter and entering the room. It is important, however, that the safelight does not exceed the wattage recommended for the type of filter used; otherwise, the exposed films will be "fogged," or partially exposed, and the quality of the radiographs compromised. The proper type of light filter must be used in the darkroom. Orange, red, or yellow filters may be used with most x-ray films, but with the rare earth type of x-ray film, a special red filter must be used (Figure 9-28). As a principle, it is important to keep in mind that no films should be exposed to the safelight any longer than necessary. It is important to work rapidly but carefully when processing x-ray films and loading and unloading films in the cassettes.

There should be a worktable in the darkroom for loading and unloading cassettes, located as far away from the processing tanks as possible so that liquid or dry chemicals will not be spilled on it. Above or below the bench there should be shelves to store film hangers and unexposed films and cassettes. It is necessary to keep x-ray film in a cool, dry place protected from extraneous x-rays.

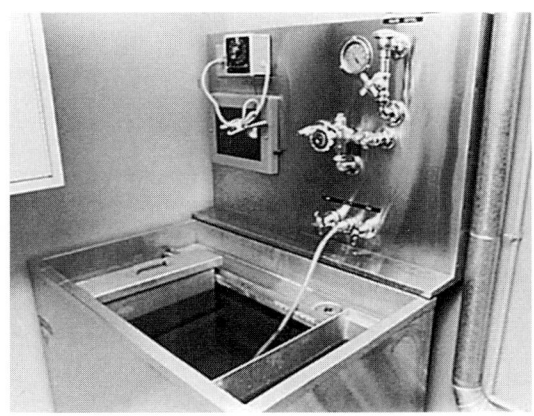

FIGURE 9-29. Processing tanks holding the developer *(left)*, screening water to wash the films *(middle)*, and fixer *(right)*. There is a mixing valve that maintains the solutions at a constant temperature.

Hand Processing Equipment

The processing equipment should include a developing tank, rinsing tank, and fixer tank. The tanks should be big enough to accommodate several 35- × 42.5-cm films at the same time. Running water in the rinsing tank is ideal. If it is not available, the water should be changed frequently. Development and fixer solutions should be changed every 90 days regardless of use and more frequently if radiograph volume is high. The tanks should ideally be made of stainless steel for ease of cleaning (Figure 9-29).

In certain areas of the United States, it will be necessary to heat up or cool down the solutions during certain times of the year. This may be accomplished with an electric heater or a cooling device. During the heat of the summer, it may be necessary to add ice to the washing water to keep the solutions at the proper temperature. An inexpensive way to keep the solution temperature constant in processing tanks is by installing a good quality shower-bath mixer valve. This type of valve is sufficient and economic enough

---

Technician Note

Remember that all film and safelights are not created equal. Make sure the wavelength or color of light to which your film is sensitive is completely blocked by your safelight filter.

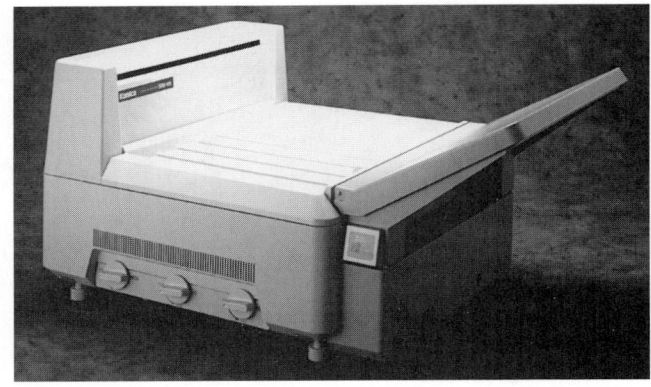

FIGURE 9-30. Smaller tabletop automatic film processor used in many newer veterinary hospitals. (Courtesy Konica Medical Imaging, Wayne, NJ.)

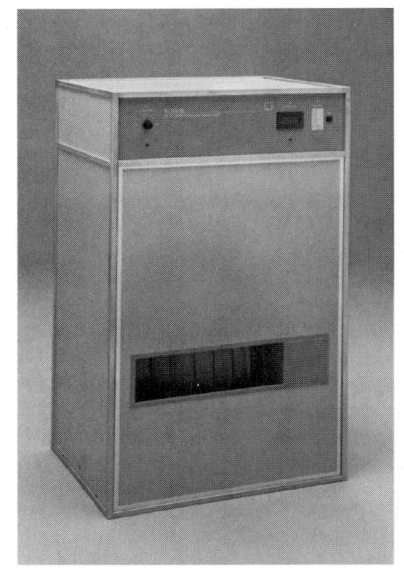

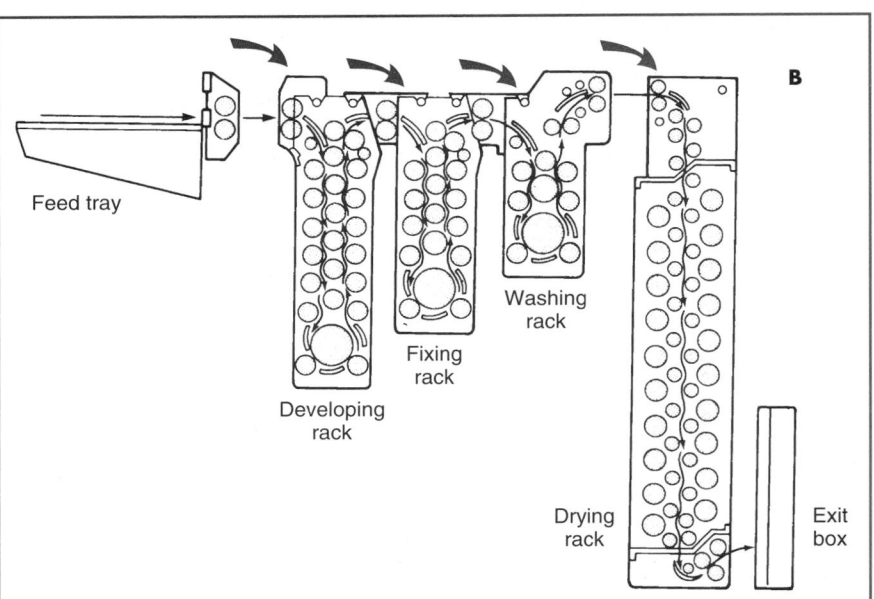

Feed tray

Washing rack

Fixing rack

Developing rack

Drying rack

Exit box

FIGURE 9-31. Automatic processor. **A,** Kodak X-OMAT processor (a 90-second processor). **B,** Diagram of a typical automatic x-ray processor.

to maintain the solution at a constant temperature in a low-volume practice. It is also important to have separate stirring rods made of stainless steel, plastic, or rubber and to mix the solutions thoroughly every day before starting the processing of films. Good ventilation is necessary to keep the room dry and avoid accumulation of volatile chemicals.

Automatic Film Processors

There are several makes and sizes of automatic processors on the market. In recent years, many veterinary hospitals have invested in automatic processing systems. There are small-capacity, 90-second processor units that can be installed in most darkrooms without remodeling (Figure 9-30). The larger processor units necessitate some remodeling because the input tray must be in the darkroom and the output side must be out of the darkroom. This usually necessitates some structural and plumbing modifications (Figure 9-31).

As with manual processing tanks, it is necessary to maintain fresh solution and ensure that the solutions are flowing properly within the processor. Automatic processors may speed up and standardize film processing but

require similar, if not more, maintenance compared with manual processing tanks. It is important to provide ventilation in the darkroom when automatic processors are used. Usually, a good-quality, light-tight exhaust fan installed in the ceiling is adequate.

Film Storage

X-ray films must be handled and stored properly for maximum usefulness. The film must be protected from light, x-radiations, gamma radiations, heat, moisture, and pressure. All these hazards may result in film fogging and decrease radiograph quality. As previously mentioned, the darkroom can fulfill this function if the room is kept clean and free of moisture. It may be helpful if the x-ray films are kept in their original boxes and placed in a cabinet. Special bins to store x-ray films can be purchased, but they are an unnecessary expense if proper care is used in storage (Figure 9-32).

Cassette Loading and Unloading

Care must be taken when transferring x-ray film from its box to the x-ray cassette to avoid static electricity, bending, creasing, or scratching. The film should be handled carefully,

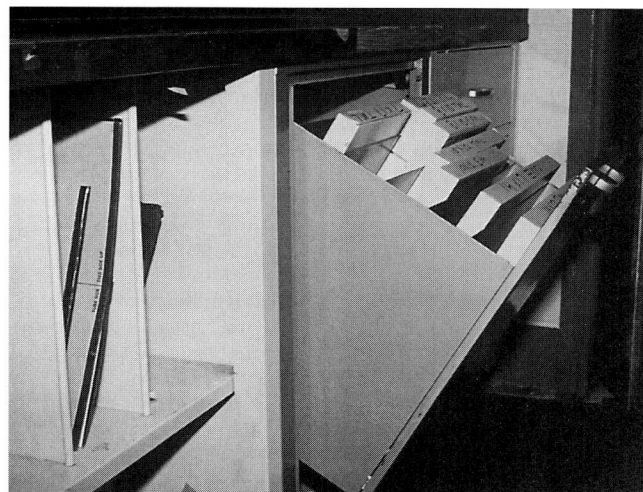

FIGURE 9-32. Film storage bin commonly used in darkrooms; it is designed to store open x-ray box films to load x-ray cassettes.

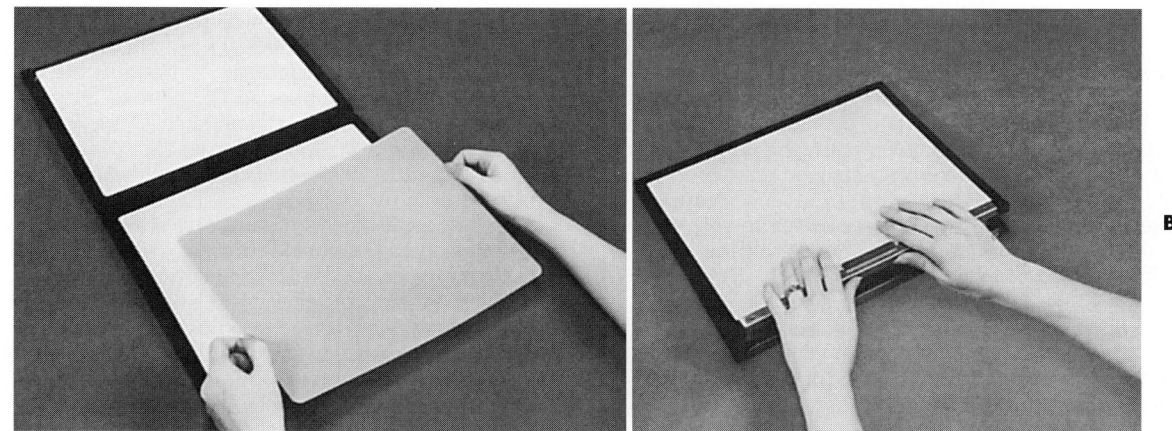

FIGURE 9-33. **A,** When loading a cassette, use both hands to avoid kink marks and carefully place the film into the cassette. **B,** The cassette must be closed and latched gently. (From Eastman Kodak Co: *The fundamentals of radiography,* ed 12, Rochester, NY, 1980, Eastman Kodak Co, Radiographic Markets Division.)

held only by the corners, and pulled from the box in a continuous and slow motion (Figure 9-33). The film should be carefully placed in the cassette, making sure the edges do not extend over the edge of the film cassette. Great care should also be taken in removing x-ray film from the cassette to prevent damage or soiling of the intensifying screen.

Hanging X-Ray Film
When exposed films are placed on a film hanger after exposure, they must be handled carefully. The films should be handled *only* by the corners and clipped to the stationary bottom clip first and then to the flexible top clip. It is most important to have dry hands when handling exposed, nonprocessed films. Any developer or fixer solution touching the film will create an artifact on the processed film (Figure 9-34).

Developing X-Ray Film
As previously mentioned, processing solutions (developer and fixer) should be stirred before inserting the film. When the film is placed in the developer, it should be agitated up and down a few times to remove air bubbles from the

surface of the film. The film should be developed for 5 minutes at 20° C (68° F). If the temperature is above or below 20° C, the developing time should be adjusted according to the directions of the manufacturer. Rapid (3-minute), high-temperature film development or sight processing is not recommended because of decreased radiograph quality.

In the developing solution, the chemicals reduce the exposed silver halides in the x-ray film to metallic silver, which is black. Gradually through the developing process, the latent image is revealed. The film is then removed from the developer tank and quickly rinsed in the central water bath. It is then placed in the fixer solution, which stops the development process and preserves the film. The film should remain in the fixer for approximately twice the development time. The film is then placed in the central rinse tank for about 15 to 20 minutes. Films can be dried in a special air-circulated film dryer box or allowed to hang until dry in a well-ventilated, dust-free area. For a more complete discussion of the chemistry of x-ray processing, please refer to the Eastman Kodak publication *The Fundamentals of Radiography* (1980).

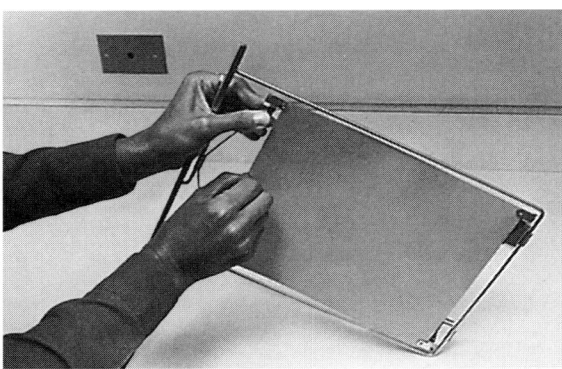

FIGURE 9-34. When hanging x-ray films, they should be handled by the corners only and should be clipped first to the stationary bottom clip and then to the flexible top clip.

Silver Recovery

In larger veterinary practices, the silver contained within the x-ray film emulsion may be removed and recovered. Most of the silver that is not exposed to x-rays is not converted to metallic silver and accumulates within the fixer solution. Silver recovery units can be attached to the fixer solution to remove the silver by an electrolytic process. This, however, is only economic for the larger-volume veterinary hospital. The silver can also be recovered from exposed and nonexposed x-ray film. A few companies specialize in recycling x-ray film for silver recovery. This could be the source of a small bonus at the time an x-ray file is purged of the old cases on file.

RADIOGRAPHIC FILM QUALITY

It is of utmost importance to produce radiographs of excellent quality to arrive at a radiographic diagnosis. A film of good diagnostic quality should have excellent detail, correct scale of contrast, and optimal density. Each of these film characteristics is briefly discussed.

Detail

Radiographic detail refers to the degree of sharpness that defines the edge of an anatomic structure. It is the best possible reproduction of an organ. Detail is influenced by every possible factor, but some are more influential than others.

The focal-film distance is one important factor in the loss of detail. If the focal spot is too close to the part x-rayed, there will be magnification and lack of distinction at the margins of the structures. Therefore it is important to keep the focal-film distance as long as possible without significantly reducing x-ray beam intensity. Most veterinary hospitals have radiographic technique charts that use a focal-film distance of 36 to 48 inches (80 to 110 cm).

Movement in veterinary radiology is a constant problem, especially with older units that have a minimum exposure time of $1/10$ second. It is difficult to produce diagnostic films of the thorax with a unit that does not have a minimum time of exposure of at least $1/30$ second and ideally $1/120$ second. With large animals, movement is a constant problem with a small, portable unit. This is why rare earth screens are becoming so popular in veterinary medicine; they have the advantage of requiring a much shorter exposure time.

The size of the focal spot is another important factor that regulates detail. The larger the focal spot, the poorer the detail. Because most equipment in veterinary medicine has a rather large focal spot of 0.8 mm or more, loss of detail may be significant, especially with older units that have focal spots of 1.2 to 2 mm. Therefore it is important to place the part to be x-rayed as close as possible to the x-ray film. If the part is too far from the film, there will be magnification and distortion, resulting in a loss of detail. This is especially important in large animal radiology.

Other exposure factors that affect detail are poor film-screen contact and overexposed or underexposed radiographs that often result from an improper technique chart or carelessness. Poor radiographic processing causes more ruined radiographs than all other factors combined. All processing errors affect detail. It is therefore important to standardize the developing process by following exactly the instructions of the manufacturer.

Radiographic Contrast

Radiographic contrast refers to the density or opacity difference between two areas on a radiograph. High contrast means the opacity differences are large and there are fewer shades of gray. High-contrast radiographs are very black and white. Latitude refers to the range of different opacities on the radiograph. Long-latitude radiographs have a much larger number of shades of gray, but the difference or contrast between each shade is small. High-contrast radiographs are preferred for spine and extremity films. Long-latitude, low-contrast radiographs are preferred for thoracic films.

Kilovoltage is the exposure factor that has the greatest influence on radiographic contrast. The higher the kilovoltage, the greater the latitude and therefore the greater the number of shades of black, gray, and white. The absorption of the x-ray beam at high kilovoltage is more uniform among the various tissues in the body, resulting in less contrast. Therefore, for thoracic examinations, a high-kilovoltage technique is recommended. For skeletal studies, a lower-kilovoltage technique is recommended.

Other factors reducing contrast are scattered radiations (which can be markedly improved by the use of a grid), light leakage, and rapid, high-temperature processing techniques.

Radiographic Density

Radiographic density refers to the degree of blackness of the film. It is the result of the amount of light that was transmitted to the x-ray film after interaction of the crystals in the intensifying screens with the x-ray beam. When a film is properly exposed, the anatomic part x-rayed will have good contrast with good differential absorption of the x-ray beam by the various tissue densities. Therefore the part should be clearly seen but should not be so dark as to overexpose the anatomic structures to the degree that they are difficult to differentiate from the background film density. The thickness and density of the anatomic part x-rayed do affect density. The thickest part will absorb more radiation, sometimes as much as denser tissues of lesser thickness.

The primary factor affecting density is the milliamperage times seconds (mAs) setting. As discussed above, the mAs factor is a quantity factor that regulates the amount of x-rays produced. If more x-rays reach the film, more light will be emitted by the screens, and the film will be darker. Therefore it can be stated that high mAs settings will increase film density and low mAs settings will reduce film density.

Box 9-1	TECHNICAL ERRORS

INCREASED FILM DENSITY
Too high mAs or kV settings
Too short focal-film distance
Wrong measurement of anatomic part
Equipment malfunction
Speed of intensifying screen too fast

DECREASED FILM DENSITY
Too low mAs or kV settings
Too long focal-film distance
Wrong measurement of anatomic part
Speed of intensifying screen too slow

BLACK MARKS OR ARTIFACTS
Film scratches
Crescent mark from rough handling
Static electricity (linear dots or tree pattern)
Top of film black, resulting from exposure to light while still in box
Defective cassette that does not close properly, exposing margins of film to light

WHITE MARKS (ARTIFACTS)
Dirt or debris between the film and screen
Defect or crack in screen
Contrast medium on tabletop, skin, or cassette

GRAY FILM
Film accidentally exposed to radiation (scattered, secondary, or direct)
Lack of grid for examination of a thick part
Outdated film
Film stored in too hot or too humid place

DISTORTED OR BLURRED RADIOGRAPH
Motion: patient, cassette, or machine
Too great focal-film distance, causing magnification and distortion
Poor film-screen contact
Poor centering of primary x-ray beam

LINEAR ARTIFACTS
Gridlines
Grid out of focal range
Primary beam not centered
Grid upside down
Grid damage, causing distorted gridlines

MISCELLANEOUS ARTIFACTS
Cone cut, causing underexposed margins
Target damage, resulting in inconsistent film density: requires tube replacement
Double exposure
Blank film: faulty equipment, nonexposed film processed

kV, Kilovolts *mAs;* milliamperes times seconds.

Another factor that affects film density is the kilovoltage setting. At a higher kilovoltage, the x-ray tube is more efficient in producing x-rays and therefore increases the energy level of x-rays produced. If all other exposure and development factors are kept constant, increasing the kilovoltage will increase the radiographic density. This effect is more apparent at lower-kilovoltage settings for a given part than at higher-kilovoltage settings.

The distance from the focal spot to the surface of the film is another important factor in film density. If everything remains constant but the distance, a given examination could be markedly overexposed if the distance is reduced, or it could be underexposed if the distance is increased. This effect can be dramatic because the intensity of the radiation is reduced or increased as the square of the distance is changed. This effect was discussed in the section regarding inverse square law. It does emphasize the need for consistency and accurate measurement of the focal-film distance.

Magnification

Magnification is a technique rarely used in veterinary practices, but it is popular in veterinary teaching hospitals. Magnification is based on the principle that a larger image of an anatomic structure can be obtained if the distance between the object and the film is increased. Generally, the object to be magnified is placed halfway between the film cassette and the focal spot of the x-ray tube. This results in an x-ray image twice as large as the actual anatomic structure. However, to obtain diagnostic films, it is necessary to have a very small focal spot. A focal spot of 0.3 mm or smaller is needed for radiographic magnification. If larger focal spots are used, the advantage of direct magnification is lost because of the blurring at the margin of an organ produced by the larger focal spot. This technique would be useful to veterinarians, especially for studies of extremities in small dogs and cats and for studies of the skull.

Technical Errors and Artifacts

Several errors can be made in handling x-ray films or in setting up a technique for an examination. In general, these errors will reduce the quality of the radiograph and in certain cases may nullify its diagnostic value. Boxes 9-1, 9-2, and 9-3 are intended to help the technician identify the cause of errors and take corrective measures. Box 9-1 deals with technical errors other than those occurring as a result of film processing. Boxes 9-2 and 9-3 deal with errors caused by poor film processing.

The advent of automatic processing equipment has helped tremendously in eliminating many errors made in hand tank processing techniques. It has standardized film processing and made it easier to trace the cause of processing mistakes, which are usually mechanically related. Even with automatic processors, many mistakes can be made and must be recognized and corrected to obtain the best possible radiographs.

Several other mechanical failures may occur with automatic processors. It is important to keep the processor clean at all times. It is especially important to wash the roller assembly thoroughly at least once each week. Processors are sophisticated machines that must be serviced regularly by professionals. It is unreasonable and cost ineffective for a veterinarian to expect the technician to service the processor. However, it is the responsibility of the technician to be able to recognize processor problems and correct them when possible. It is also the technician's responsibility to keep the processor clean at all times and to ensure that fresh developer and fixer solutions are provided as needed.

Box 9-2   FILM PROCESSING MISTAKES IN WET TANKS

INCREASED FILM DENSITY
Film overdeveloped
Temperature of solution too high
Wrong concentration of developer
Defective thermometer

DECREASED FILM DENSITY
Film underdeveloped
Temperature of solution too low
Exhausted developer
Contamination of developer
Developer too diluted or improperly mixed
Failure to add replenisher solution as needed
Defective thermometer

FOGGED FILMS
Light leakage in darkroom from defective safelight, door, windows; around processor pipes; or turning lights on in darkroom before film is cleared
Film exposed to radiation from any source: through wall if storage room adjacent to x-ray room, cassette left in x-ray room while exposure made
Overdeveloped film
Contaminated developer

YELLOW RADIOGRAPH
Fixation time too short
Exhausted fixer solution

WHITE SPOTS
Defective screens: pitted, scratched
Dust or grit on surface of film
Fixer on film before processing

BLACK SPOTS
Drops of developer solution on film before processing
Films stacked together in fixer

AIR BUBBLES
Film not agitated when placed in developer; air bubbles form on surface of film

RETICULATION
Solutions have uneven temperature from bottom to top of tanks
Need to stir up solution to even up temperature in tanks
Weak fixer or lack of hardening solution

BRITTLE RADIOGRAPHS
Drying temperature too high
Drying time too long

MISCELLANEOUS MISTAKES
Film wet: too short drying time
Grit on films: dirty tanks and solutions
Corner marks: wet or dirty fingers on hangers
Sticky film: film washed or dried improperly
Static electricity: low humidity and rough or too fast handling of films
Scratches: careless handling

Box 9-3   COMMON TECHNICAL ERRORS WITH AUTOMATIC PROCESSORS

INCREASED DENSITY
Temperature of developer too high
Overreplenishment
Light leak from cover or in darkroom
Speed too slow
Faulty thermostat

Decreased Density
Temperature of developer too low
Underreplenishment
Exhausted developer, necessitating thorough cleaning of tanks every 6 months
Faulty thermostat

PROCESSING STREAKS
Crossover rollers dirty
Dirty wash water
Air tubes need cleaning

SCRATCHES ON FILM
Guide shoes misaligned or dirty
Dryer air tubes mispositioned

WET OR DAMP FILM
Thermostat malfunction
Dryer temperatures too low
Insufficient air venting
Film not hardened sufficiently

FILM OVERLAP
Film fed too rapidly into processor
Tension on rollers too high

RADIATION SAFETY

Since 1970 there has been a tremendous growth in the use of x-ray equipment by veterinarians. There are few diagnoses in medicine or surgery that cannot be aided by the use of diagnostic radiology. It therefore behooves technicians to be aware of the hazard of using x-rays or any other type of ionizing radiation.

It is the responsibility of the veterinarian to ensure that proper radiation safety measures are observed in the hospital. It is also the veterinarian's responsibility to instruct the technician in the proper use of the equipment and to ensure that the design of the x-ray room meets state regulations.

All animal tissues are sensitive to radiation; that is, absorption of radiation doses above a certain minimum roentgen value will change or alter the tissue. The following tissues (not in order of sensitivity) are most readily affected by ionizing radiation: skin, lymphatics, hemopoietic and leukopoietic (blood-forming tissues), breast, thyroid, bone (especially the epiphysis or growing centers), and the germinal epithelium or gonads. These tissues are sensitive to all forms of ionizing radiation. All animal species are affected, including humans, even though there are different degrees of sensitivity among species. The more rapidly dividing tissues are affected most by radiation.

Technicians should remember that one of the best protective devices at their disposal is the ability to avoid retakes. Careful attention to patient positioning, thickness measurements, setting techniques, and film processing will decrease radiograph retakes and reduce technician and patient radiation exposure. See Chapter 35 for additional radiation safety information.

Radiation Filtration

The x-ray beam is a composite or spectrum of x-ray photons of various energy levels. The kVp setting is the highest energy level within the beam, but there are photons of all levels from the kVp on down. The useful portion of the x-ray beam (the portion that passes through the patient to interact with the film and screens) is the upper two thirds of the energy levels. The lower third of the x-ray beam energies is too weak to pass through the patient. This radiation is called *soft radiation*. It is of no use for image formation and only causes increased radiation exposure of the patient. Aluminum has a marked effect on filtration of softer (lower energy level) x-rays. Insertion of 1 or 2 mm of an aluminum filter into the path of the primary beam at the portal of the x-ray tube is essential to filter out or absorb the soft x-rays that are a component of all x-ray beams in the diagnostic range. By absorbing these soft radiations, the filter reduces the amount of radiation absorbed by the patient. Increased aluminum filtration also generally improves latitude and detail by improving the quality of the x-ray beam.

Radiation Measurement

To understand radiation safety and radiation dose units of measurement, it is necessary to define a few terms commonly used in the measurement of radiation exposure.

Roentgen

The roentgen (R) is defined as a unit of radiation exposure that will liberate a charge of 2.58×10^{-4} coulombs per kilogram of air. Roentgens are a measure of radiation exposure or x-ray machine output and are generally evaluated with an ionization chamber placed below the primary x-ray beam. As an example, 1 roentgen is the approximate exposure to the body surface for an anteroposterior radiograph of the abdomen for an average adult human.

Rad

The unit of absorbed dose of ionizing radiations is called a *rad*. It is the energy imparted by ionizing radiations to a unit mass of irradiated material and is equal to 100 ergs/g of tissue. The number of rads deposited in tissue per roentgen of radiation exposure varies with the energy of the x-ray beam and with the composition of the absorber.

Rem

Rem is an abbreviation for rad equivalent man; it is the product of the dose in rads and the relative biologic effectiveness of the radiation used. This unit of measurement makes allowance for the fact that the effect of radiation on different tissue varies with the type of radiation or relative biologic effectiveness. A rem is equal to the absorbed radiation dose in rads multiplied by a quality factor:

$$Rem = Rads \times Quality\ factor$$

Because the quality factor for diagnostic radiation is 1, for all practical purposes in veterinary practice 1 rem = 1 rad. For larger particles of radiation, such as neutrons, protons, and alpha particles, the quality factor increases from 3 to 20. These larger, more dangerous particles of radiation are not emitted from diagnostic x-ray machines.

Maximum Permissible Dose

The maximum permissible dose (MPD) should be of great interest to the veterinary technician because it is the maximum dose of radiation a person is allowed to receive during occupational exposure over a certain time. This dose is 0.1 rem for an average weekly dose or 3 rem over 13 weeks, 5 rem per year, and a maximum accumulated dose of $1(N - 18)$ rem, where N is age in years. The $N - 18$ says that an individual should not have occupational exposure to radiation before the age of 18 years. The technician should remember that the MPD is the dose that the U.S. Nuclear Regulatory Commission has determined should not harm the person receiving it during her or his lifetime. The MPD is maximum occupational exposure allowed by law; technicians should try to keep radiation exposure as low as possible by carefully following radiation safety practices.

Personal Monitoring

To protect the staff from overexposure, the radiation that each person receives can be measured on a *film badge*. A film badge is a container that holds a special film designed to record a wide range of exposures. The film holder incorporates several different types of metal filters that permit differentiation of the type of ionizing radiation exposures. This badge should be worn outside the apron on the collar at the level of the thyroid gland (Figure 9-35). Film badges can be exposed by heat, pressure, and chemical fumes. The film badge should be taken care of and stored outside the radiology area so that the amount of radiation it detects is actually the amount to which the person was occupationally exposed.

Radiation monitoring badges come in several forms: rings, clips, and wrist badges. Several companies offer a badge service. These badges are mailed back to the company and analyzed on a monthly or quarterly basis.

Film badge readings are reported in millirem (mrem), or 1/1000 rem. The annual MPD equals 5000 mrem. Techni-

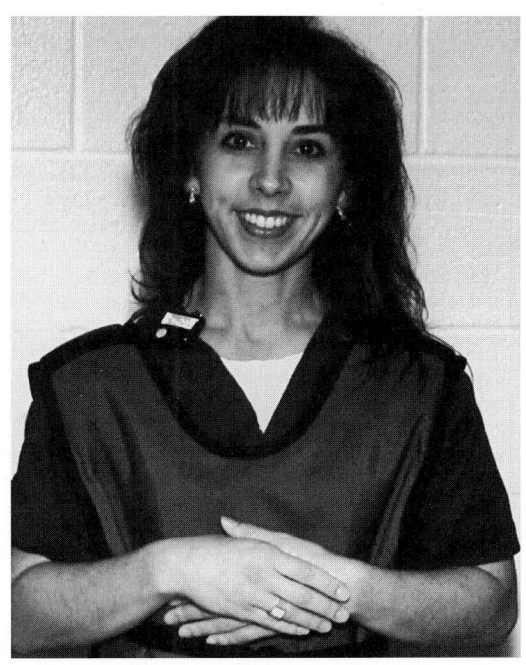

FIGURE 9-35. Each technician working in radiology should have a film badge to measure occupational radiation exposure. The film badge should be worn outside the lead apron at the level of the upper neck. This technician, who works in a very busy radiology section, also wears a ring badge inside her lead gloves to measure dose to the hands.

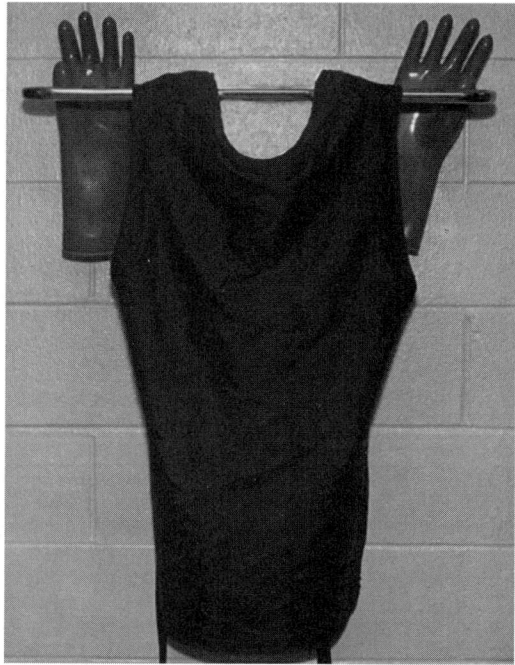

FIGURE 9-36. A collimator is used to limit the size of the x-ray beam to the part to be examined. By coning down on an area, the amount of scattered and secondary radiation can be drastically reduced.

cians using x-ray machines should insist that the veterinarian for whom they work provide them with a radiation monitoring device.

Protection Practices

- Always use a collimator and always use the smallest possible aperture that will cover the anatomic area of interest (Figure 9-36).
- Make sure there is an aluminum filter at the portal of the x-ray tube. This is to protect the patient, not the technician.
- Make sure the proper exposure factors are used to avoid retakes.
- Make sure the animal is positioned properly the first time—again to avoid retakes.
- Never permit any part of your body to be in the path of the primary x-ray beam.
- Always wear an apron and gloves when holding an animal or an apron alone if one has to be in the room when an exposure is made. The apron should have 0.5-mm lead equivalent minimum to ensure good protection from secondary and scattered radiations (Figures 9-37 and 9-38).
- Use accessory equipment designed to reduce radiation exposure, such as cassette holders, restraining devices, and positioning devices (Figure 9-39).
- Anesthesia or tranquilization of the patient should be used every time an animal cannot be controlled easily and adequately for a given examination.
- Only required personnel should be in the examining room at the time of exposure. A pregnant woman should not be in the room, nor should anyone less than 18 years of age.
- Use good, fast screens to reduce the mA settings as much as possible.

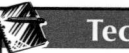

Technician Note

When working in radiology, always remember the "big three" of radiation safety: time, distance, and shielding.

Radiation safety is a frame of mind. It is a habit, and it requires awareness of the danger of radiation. It is easy to

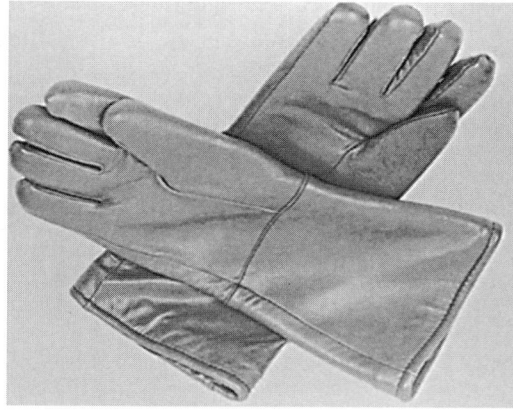

FIGURE 9-37. Apron and gloves on a stand. It is important to keep the apron on a stand and the gloves well aerated when not in use to increase the useful life of the apron and gloves. The apron should have a minimum of 0.5 mm of lead equivalent.

FIGURE 9-38. Lead gloves should have a minimum of 0.5 mm of lead equivalent; 1 mm of lead equivalent is ideal. They should always be worn when restraint is needed for examination.

become careless with radiation because it is invisible, tasteless, and odorless and produces no external stimulation at diagnostic levels. Technicians should always remember that although invisible, radiations are dangerous to one's health. X-ray effects are cumulative. The ionization that results from continued exposure to x-rays and other high-energy rays constitutes the cumulative effect. They can destroy all living tissue if the absorbed doses are high enough. Secondary radiations are less harmful than primary radiations but are still extremely harmful. Therefore

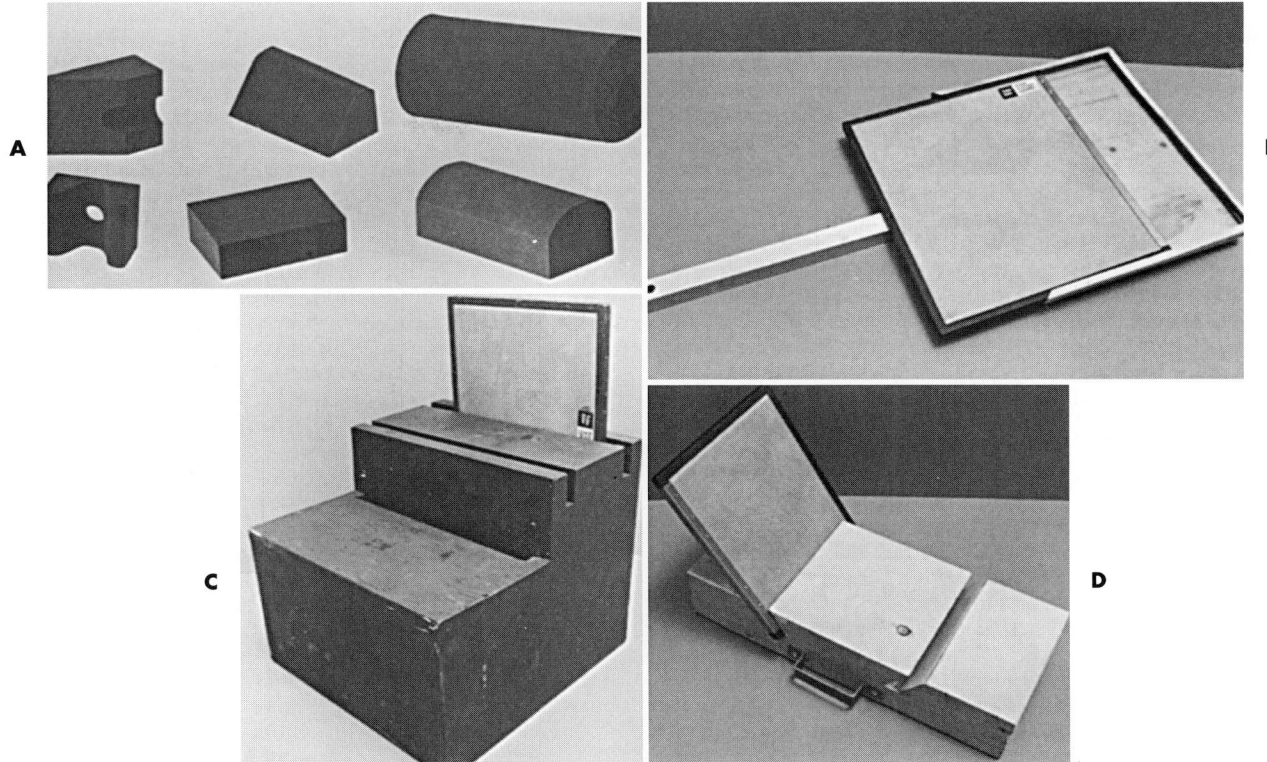

FIGURE 9-39. A number of commercially available positioning devices can be used to help position animals and reduce the time needed to perform the examination. **A,** Various foam devices used to position small animals. **B,** Cassette holder for large animal examinations. **C,** Block for examination of large animal foot. **D,** Block for examination of large animal fetlock and pastern joints.

carelessness has no place in radiology. Remember the big three methods of radiation protection: *time, distance, and shielding.* Time means avoiding retakes; do it right the first time. Lower the time of exposures; keep the mAs as low as possible to still produce diagnostic radiographs. Distance means staying as far away as possible from the patient and x-ray beam. Shielding means always wearing an apron and gloves. It is important to take care of one's apron and gloves. Hang them carefully after use, and do not allow the apron to be folded. Careless use causes creases and cracks to develop in the gloves and aprons and reduces their effectiveness.

RADIOGRAPHIC CONTRAST AGENTS

In radiology, *contrast* means density difference. In many radiographic examinations, there is insufficient natural or inherent contrast of the anatomy to make a diagnosis; this is especially true in gastrointestinal, urogenital, and spinal cord disease. The addition of positive or negative contrast medium can increase the radiographic density difference between anatomic structures and increase the likelihood of correct image interpretation. In veterinary medicine, four types of contrast media are used:

- Radiolucent gases: air, nitrous oxide, carbon dioxide
- Insoluble inert radiopaque medium: barium sulfate
- Soluble ionic radiopaque medium: iothalamate, diatrizoate
- Soluble nonionic radiopaque medium: iohexol, iopamidol

Radiolucent gases absorb very small amounts of radiation, resulting in images of greatly reduced radiographic opacity. These agents are used primarily in double-contrast gastrograms, double-contrast cystograms, and rarely, pneumoperitoneography. Contraindications for their use are primarily in patients with severe hemorrhagic cystitis, in which there is an increased likelihood for gas absorption into the circulation. Nitrous oxide and carbon dioxide are considered safer than room air because their increased solubility is less likely to cause serious air embolization.

Barium sulfate has a high atomic number and absorbs a large amount of radiation, resulting in greatly increased radiographic opacity. It is used almost exclusively for upper and lower gastrointestinal examinations. Barium sulfate is inert, nonabsorbed, and fairly soothing to the gastrointestinal tract. It coats the gastrointestinal mucosa better than organic iodides, improving visualization of the luminal surface. Barium sulfate is available in powder, paste, or liquid solutions. Micropulverized, solubilized barium sulfate solutions are vastly superior to powdered barium sulfate products because of the increased uniformity in mucosal coating. Contraindications for use include patients with severe constipation or upper or lower bowel perforations. As with all oral contrast media, care should be used in patients with known aspiration pneumonia or a high likelihood of aspiration.

Soluble radiopaque ionic contrast media include iothalamate and diatrizoate. The negatively charged iothalamate and diatrizoate are benzoic acid derivatives with three iodine molecules. They are coupled with positively charged sodium or meglumine to form a soluble salt. The high atomic number of iodine increases radiation absorption and increases radiographic opacity. These products can be used orally for gastrointestinal examinations; intravascularly for venous or arterial studies and excretory urography and in the peritoneal tract, bladder, and urethra; and intraarticularly and in draining wounds for fistulography and in salivary ducts for sialography. Ionic organic iodides should not be used in the respiratory tract or intrathecally for myelography. Because ionic iodides are essentially a hyperosmolar salt solution, they can result in an increase in intravascular fluid volume when used intravascularly followed by an osmotic diuresis. The hyperosmolarity can cause diarrhea when used orally. Because of these properties, these agents are contraindicated in dehydrated patients or patients with a known iodine sensitivity.

The newest class of positive contrast agents contains the nonionic organic iodines, represented by iohexol, iopamidol, iotolan, and, historically, metrizamide. These agents can be used like ionic organic iodines but have the advantage of not dissociating into positively and negatively charged ions in solution. This allows the agents to be used intrathecally (in the cerebrospinal fluid space around the spinal cord) for myelography as well as everywhere ionic iodides can be used. These contrast agents are still hyperosmolar but much less so than the ionic organic iodides. They appear to have a lower incidence of side effects or contrast reactions but have the disadvantage of increased cost.

Organic iodides (both ionic and nonionic) may cause serious contrast reactions, or side effects, when given intravenously, intraarterially, or intrathecally. These reactions are much less likely when the agents are used orally. Contrast reactions include nausea and vomiting, hypotension, cardiac arrest, and anaphylaxis. These reactions occur very infrequently, but it is advised to have a catheter in place when using these agents and rapid access to fluids, oxygen, endotracheal tubes, and cardiovascular arrest resuscitation drugs during organic iodide contrast procedures. Do not leave these patients unattended after contrast administration. For a thorough discussion of contrast media and contrast procedures, see Douglas et al. (1987), Han et al. (2000), Lavin (1999), Morgan (1993), and Thrall (1998).

Common Contrast Media and Applications
Esophagus
CONTRAST AGENTS. Barium sulfate, weight/volume (w/v) suspension 100%, is used alone and diluted to evaluate an enlarged esophagus or as a thick paste if the esophagus is not enlarged. Barium mixed with food may be more appropriate for diagnosis of esophageal strictures. Oral organic iodides (ionic or nonionic) are used when perforation of the esophagus is suspected.

PROCEDURE. No special preparation is needed. Ideally, the study is done using fluoroscopy. If this is not available, the exposure must be made when the animal swallows. The barium is administered with a syringe into the buccal pouch.

Stomach and Small Bowel
(Upper Gastrointestinal Studies)
CONTRAST AGENTS. Three kinds of contrast agents are used for upper gastrointestinal studies: barium sulfate 25% to 30% w/v, oral iodines, and negative contrast, including air, carbon dioxide, and nitrous oxide. Barium sulfate is the most commonly used agent for upper

gastrointestinal studies when perforation is not suspected. Negative contrast media are used in combination with barium sulfate for double-contrast studies. Oral iodinated products are given when perforation is suspected because barium sulfate will not be resorbed once it leaks into a body cavity.

PROCEDURE. Food should be withheld for 24 hours, and warm water enemas should be administered about 2 to 3 hours before the gastrointestinal study. Acepromazine (Ayerst Laboratories) can be used without adverse effects on gastrointestinal motility.

DOSAGE. The dosage for barium sulfate is 10 ml/kg and for oral Hypaque or Gastrografin, 3 ml/kg.

FILM SEQUENCE. The survey film consists of a ventrodorsal (VD) and a lateral (Lat) view. Immediately after administration of contrast medium, four films should be taken to completely evaluate the stomach: a VD, a dorsoventral (DV), and both a right and left lateral. At 15, 30, and 60 minutes, the film sequence consists of VD and right lateral. These same views are taken at various intervals until contrast reaches the large bowel. The timing sequence will vary with the patient and the suspected disease process.

Large Bowel (Lower Gastrointestinal Study, Barium Enema)
CONTRAST AGENTS. Barium sulfate 10% to 15% (w/v) or iodinated preparations, such as Gastrografin or oral Hypaque, are used for the lower gastrointestinal studies.

PRECAUTIONS. Barium sulfate should not be used when a perforation is suspected. A barium enema should not be performed for 48 hours after taking a biopsy of the colon or rectum.

PREPARATION. The patient is fasted for 24 to 48 hours and may be given a gastrointestinal cleansing agent such as GoLytely (Braintree Labs). Warm water enemas must be given before the examination because it is essential that the entire large bowel be cleansed before a barium enema is performed. A Bardex (French; Bard Hospital Division, C.R. Bard) catheter and barium container are needed for the study.

PROCEDURE. The animal should be anesthetized. The balloon-tipped catheter is inserted into the rectum, and the cuff is inflated to form a firm seal against the colonic wall. The barium or iodine is placed in the colon by gravitational flow. A 15% w/v barium sulfate solution is used for barium enemas. The dose is 5 to 10 ml/0.45 kg of body weight. Ideally, the study is done using fluoroscopy. Radiographic views needed are Lat, VD, and right and left VD oblique views. After completion, the barium is evacuated, and air is injected to obtain a double-contrast study of the large bowel.

Urinary Tract
CONTRAST AGENTS. Several kinds of contrast studies are available for study of the kidneys. However, because the *intravenous pyelogram* (IVP) is the one most used in practice, this discussion is limited to it.

An IVP, or excretory urogram, is performed by injecting contrast medium intravenously. Ionic organic iodide products are most commonly used. A meglumine diatrizoate and sodium diatrizoate preparation is probably the most popular contrast product used for IVP examinations. The standard dose of contrast is 800 mg of iodine per kilogram, which may be increased by 50% in patients with poor renal function.

COMPLICATIONS. The most common complications encountered with an IVP are vomiting, anaphylactoid reactions, and hypotension. Vomiting is a transient reaction of short duration and is not serious in nature. Care should be taken that the animal does not aspirate during the procedure. Anaphylactoid reactions are rare but must be attended to immediately. It is necessary to have epinephrine available for immediate administration whenever an IVP is done. Hypotension is rare, but when it occurs, it can be life threatening and may lead to renal failure.

CONTRAINDICATIONS. The only serious contraindication is dehydration or iodine sensitivity.

PROCEDURE. The animal should fast for 24 hours, but water should be available to avoid dehydration. Enemas should be given when needed, at least 2 to 3 hours before the IVP. VD and Lat films should be taken before the examinations. Films should be taken in the VD and Lat positions immediately after injection of the contrast medium and at 5 and 15 minutes after injection. When needed, follow-up studies at 20 or 25 minutes after injection may be indicated.

Urinary Bladder

CONTRAST AGENTS. Ionic organic iodide contrast materials are most desirable for retrograde cystography. Nonopaque contrast materials, such as air, carbon dioxide, and nitrous oxide, are used in addition to organic iodides for double-contrast cystography. Do not use barium sulfate.

PROCEDURE. The colon should be cleansed. Depending on the breed and size of the animal, different catheters may be used. A Foley catheter, tomcat catheter, or soft flexible male catheter may be needed. In addition, a syringe and three-way valve are needed. Two types of cystography are commonly performed in veterinary practice: positive-contrast cystography and double-contrast cystography. Positive-contrast cystography is used to detect leaks or rupture of the lower urinary tract after trauma. Ionic organic iodide contrast at concentrations of 10% to 15% is injected retrograde into the urinary bladder at 5 to 15 ml/kg of body weight. Double-contrast cystography is used to detect all other forms of urinary bladder disease. A catheter is placed into the urinary bladder, and all urine is removed. Next, 3 to 10 ml of organic iodide contrast is injected, followed by carbon dioxide or room air at 5 to 15 ml/kg of body weight. Because of the variability of urinary bladder volume, it is best to fill the bladder to palpable turgidity. Lateral and oblique VD radiographic views are most helpful.

Urethrography

CONTRAST AGENTS. Ionic organic iodide compounds at 20% concentration are best for urethrography.

PROCEDURE. A balloon-tipped catheter (Foley type) is placed into the distal urethra. The cuff is inflated for a snug fit to prevent contrast from leaking around the catheter. Contrast, 10 to 20 ml, is hand-injected rapidly. The x-ray is taken during injections of the last few milliliters. A Lat view and two oblique (O) views should be taken during the separate injections of the contrast material.

Spinal Cord

Myelography is the contrast examination most frequently performed to localize and characterize spinal cord lesions. Myelograms are always performed with the animal under general anesthesia. Nonionic iodinated contrast medium is injected into the subarachnoid space (cerebrospinal fluid space) at the cisterna magna (skull-C1 space) or in the caudal lumbar spine area (L4-L6). Myelography is most commonly performed before surgical intervention.

CONTRAST AGENTS. Two nonionic contrast agents are currently in wide use in veterinary medicine: iopamidol (Isovue, Bracco Diagnostics) and iohexol (Omnipaque, Sanofi Winthrop). The dose of contrast medium ranges from 0.25 ml/kg for cervical evaluation with a cisternal injection to 0.45 ml/kg for cervical evaluation from a lumbar injection. The concentration of iodine should be between 240 and 300 mg/ml, and injection volume should not exceed 15 ml.

CONTRAINDICATIONS. Infection of the spinal cord and meninges and when the disease is to be treated medically only are contraindications.

PROCEDURE. Survey films should be taken first. The site of injection should be aseptically prepared. Spinal needles of 20 to 22 gauge and 3.75 to 8.75 cm should be available because the size of the animal may vary considerably and some dogs may be so obese that even an 8.75-cm needle is short! Carefully collimated films are taken in the VD and Lat positions immediately after administration of the contrast medium.

POSITIONING

Proper positioning is essential to obtain diagnostic radiographic examinations. It is again the responsibility of the veterinary technician to properly position the animal. It is not the intent of this chapter to discuss positioning at length. Please refer to the excellent treatment of this topic by Butler et al. (2000), Douglas et al. (1987), Han et al. (2000), Lavin (1999), Morgan (1993), and Ticer (1984).

Principles of Positioning

To achieve proper positioning, it is useful for the technician to remember that two views at right angles are necessary to obtain a diagnostic study. This principle applies to all examinations in small animals and to extremities in large animals. The exceptions to this rule are thoracic examinations and spinal examinations in the horse and in cases of trauma or in debilitated animals when only lateral views can be taken without causing undue stress to the animals.

Another principle to remember is the importance of centering the primary beam on the lesion itself, when known. This is especially important in orthopedic cases in both small and large animals. For example, fracture healing may look very different when the x-ray beam is centered over the fracture line as opposed to a short distance away from it. Costly errors have been made by veterinarians who removed supporting devices before the correct time. These errors occurred because fractures may have appeared healed when the primary beam was centered away from the fracture line itself.

It is also important, when performing a radiographic examination, to use an x-ray film that is sufficiently large to completely cover the system to be examined. When x-raying very large dogs it may be necessary to use two films for the abdomen: one for the cranial abdomen and one for the caudal abdomen, which is generally taken at a lower kilovoltage peak. For extremities, the primary beam should be directed at the lesion. It is good to have a radiograph large enough to include the proximal and distal joint to obtain a good spatial anatomic relationship of the lesion.

These principles are basic but essential. Proper positioning is obtained through practice. These topics are well illustrated and discussed in the references mentioned. A positioning reference textbook should be available in the radiology room of every veterinary practice.

RESTRAINT

The importance of restraint to achieve proper positioning cannot be overemphasized. It is part of radiation safety. Without proper restraint, many examinations should not be undertaken. In some cases, attempting to make examinations without restraint would be life threatening with large animals and dangerous with certain small animals.

There are many types of restraints; some are mechanical or manual, and some are chemical. For the purpose of radiation safety, manual restraint should be avoided as a routine procedure. When it is essential to be in the room with the animal, one should wear a protective lead apron and gloves, and the x-ray beam should be limited to the system to be examined by coning devices or by adjusting the collimator.

Mechanical restraint comes in various forms. A number of commercial devices designed for animal positioning are available, varying in price from a few dollars to several hundred dollars. One of the most useful and inexpensive devices to use in the dog is a simple muzzle, which often has a calming effect on an animal (see Chapter 1). Sandbags and sponges can also be used to obtain excellent positioning. When the animal is positioned properly, it is most important to take the radiograph rapidly, since one can hope for only a few seconds of restraint before the animal moves.

Chemical restraint can be achieved with tranquilizers, analgesics, or anesthesia (see Chapter 21). Chemical restraint has contributed greatly to the progress made in radiology by allowing positioning that would otherwise be impossible to achieve. For example, complete examination of the skull should not be attempted without anesthesia. Every time total immobility or relaxation is required for proper positioning, general anesthesia should be used. Most spinal examinations will prove nondiagnostic unless the examination is done with the animal under anesthesia. In several circumstances, tranquilization is adequate to control most animals. Tranquilizers are excellent to control frightened or aggressive dogs and cats. They are also most useful for controlling large animals.

Again, good positioning is essential in producing diagnostic x-ray films. It takes time to learn and become proficient at achieving every position needed for a variety of examinations in large and small animals. However, most organs can be x-rayed with proper techniques, equipment, and accessory devices and the use of mechanical or chemical restraint or both.

DIAGNOSTIC ULTRASOUND

Ultrasound imaging is becoming an essential diagnostic tool in veterinary practice. It is portable, does not require the use of ionizing radiation, and is noninvasive, well tolerated by patients, and accepted by clients. As ultrasound equipment becomes affordable, the only problem

with its introduction into practice is the long learning curve associated with its use. Recent veterinary graduates are more familiar with the uses and indications for ultrasound, because veterinary schools have integrated ultrasound into the curriculum. All new veterinary technicians are encouraged to familiarize themselves with the basics of diagnostic ultrasound, but remember that ultrasound is user dependent. The image and interpretation are only as good as the person doing the examination.

Ultrasound Basics

Sound is a mechanical pressure wave made up of a series of compressions and rarefactions transmitted through a medium. Sound waves are characterized by their wavelength or distance between compressions, their frequency in cycles per second, and their velocity or speed of transmission (Figure 9-40). These characteristics are integrated by the following formula:

$$\text{Velocity} = \text{Wavelength} \times \text{Frequency}$$

For simplicity, assume that the speed of sound in the body is 1540 m/sec. Therefore, as the frequency of sound increases, the wavelength decreases. Shorter sound waves produce increased image resolution but decreased patient penetration. The frequencies used in veterinary diagnostic ultrasound generally range from 2.5 to 12 megahertz (MHz). A hertz (Hz) is 1 cycle per second. Therefore typical ultrasound frequencies will range from 2 to 12 million cycles/sec, or 2.5 to 12 MHz. Audible sound will range from 20 to 20,000 Hz.

Real-time, gray-scale ultrasound is based on the *pulse-echo principle*. A short pulse of sound, usually 2 or 3 cycles long, is produced from the transducer and transmitted into the patient. The sound wave strikes an echogenic surface in the patient and returns some of the sound to the transducer. The strength of the returning sound wave determines the brightness of the image, and the time it takes for the sound to travel into the patient and back to the transducer determines where the echo will be seen on the screen. Remember that the time it takes for a sound wave to traverse a distance and be reflected back is a function of the distance between the sender and reflector and the speed of the sound wave in that medium. For all practical purposes, the speed of sound in small animal tissues is constant at 1540 m/sec.

Ultrasound production and reception are based on the *piezoelectric effect*. A piezoelectric crystal will change shape or thickness when subjected to a voltage pulse. Rapid pulses of electrical energy are transformed into mechanical energy or sound waves by the vibrating crystal. Returning

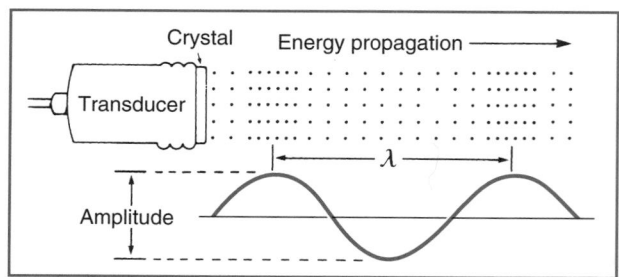

FIGURE 9-40. Sound wave with a wavelength = λ. *Closely spaced dots,* compressions; *widely spaced dots,* rarefactions. The amplitude is proportional to the loudness.

sound waves cause the crystal to vibrate, and that mechanical energy is transmitted into electrical energy by the transducer. This electrical signal is transformed into the gray-scale image on the screen. The transducer acts as both the sound transmitter and the receiver. The operating frequency of the transducer is partially determined by the thickness of the piezoelectric crystal. The thinner the crystal, the higher the transducer frequency. The transducer transmits sound 0.01% of the time. It receives returning sound waves 99.9% of the time.

Ultrasound-Tissue Interaction

To better understand the ultrasound image, it is important to understand the interaction of ultrasound within tissue. As the sound wave proceeds through the body, it is progressively attenuated or weakened. This *attenuation* limits the depth of penetration of the sound wave and therefore limits the depth of structures that can be effectively imaged. The ultrasound beam is attenuated or weakened by absorption, reflection, scattering, refraction, and diffraction. Reflection is a redirection of the sound beam back to the transducer and is the basis of the diagnostic image. Absorption is sound energy converted to heat within the tissues. Scattering is the intertissue microreflection of sound, which is responsible for much of the echo texture of various organs. Refraction and diffraction are the bending of the sound beam as it crosses areas of differing tissue densities. Refraction attenuation is important in the generation of several ultrasound artifacts.

Sound reflection or echo production forms the basis of the ultrasound image. An echo is produced whenever the ultrasound beam crosses an acoustic interface. An acoustic interface is the boundary between two tissues of differing acoustic impedances, or Z. See the following equation:

Acoustic impedance (Z) = Density (P) × Speed of sound transmission (C)

or

$$Z = P \times C$$

If we assume the speed of sound in soft tissue to be constant at 1540 m/sec, then the main factor that influences acoustic impedance is the density or composition of tissue. Thus the more different two adjacent tissues are, the greater will be the echo reflection between them. This is why very homogeneous populations of cells (lymphoma, lymph nodes, regenerative liver nodules) produce few echoes and are generally hypoechoic (darker). If the acoustic interface difference is small, only a small percentage of sound will be reflected. If the difference is large, a large portion of sound will be reflected. Most soft tissues have a Z, or acoustic impedance, within 1% to 2% of liver.

INTERFACE	% REFLECTION
Fat-muscle	0.94
Fat-bone	49.00
Tissue-air	100.00

From looking at this list one can see the acoustic impedance (Z) between fat and muscle is very low, whereas the acoustic impedance between fat and bone and between soft tissue and air is very high. This property is why ultrasound cannot be used to image through bone or gas. Too much of the sound beam is reflected back from bone and gas interfaces because of the large change in tissue density.

Patient Preparation

Patient preparation is important because 100% of the sound is reflected when the ultrasound beam intersects air.

Hair traps air, which is how it insulates the animal, but if one tries to pass ultrasound through hair, the majority of the ultrasound beam is reflected before it ever enters the animal. A careful close clip of the area to be examined, as well as removal of dirt and scales, will improve the ultrasound image. A generous volume of ultrasound gel is also beneficial to displace air and couple the transducer to the skin (Figure 9-41). Small animals are placed in a padded V-trough table on their backs for abdominal examination and in lateral or sternal recumbency for cardiac examination. Most small animals tolerate abdominal and cardiac examinations well and rarely require tranquilization. A special cardiac table with large and small holes in it is very helpful for echocardiography. The animal is placed in lateral recumbency with the chest area over the appropriate-size hole, which allows for better ultrasound transducer access (Figure 9-42). Large animal examinations are done in the standing tranquilized animal. Again, close clipping, especially for tendon examinations, is critical for an optimal examination.

Ultrasound Display Modes

The returning echo can be displayed in several ways. *A-mode,* or *amplitude mode,* displays the returning echoes as spikes from a baseline. The echo depth is determined by its location along the baseline. The echo intensity is displayed by the height of the spike. A-mode ultrasound machines are used predominantly in ophthalmology and have little value in veterinary practice.

B-mode, or *brightness mode,* forms the basis for two-dimensional imaging. The returning echoes are displayed as dots on the image screen. The brightness of the dot is a function of the strength of the returning echo. The placement of the dot is a function of the time it took for the echo to return to the transducer. The cross-sectional image is formed through data storage. The sound beam is automatically swept across the patient while the transducer is held steady and moved slowly over the area of interest. The rapid collection of images is called *real time.* This permits direct observation of moving structures, such as a beating heart or puppy motion. With B-mode real-time equipment, images are displayed in gray scale. Gray scale is a technique in which the various echo strengths are displayed in numerous shades of gray from black to white, similar to a black and white television picture.

M-mode, or *time-motion (TM) mode,* is produced by passing a narrow sound beam across a body part. Each echo interface is presented as a dot. The motion of the body part is displayed by sweeping the image across the screen or image recorder. M-mode can be thought of as a very thin sector of B-mode displayed as a function of time. M-mode is primarily used for echocardiography. Ideal ultrasound equipment for veterinary practice would be a real-time B-mode scanner with M-mode capabilities (Figure 9-43).

The selection of appropriate transducers is critical when purchasing ultrasound equipment. Transducers vary in type, size, style, shape, and frequency (Figure 9-44). Linear array transducers are made with several piezoelectric crystals stacked side by side. The crystals are fired in rapid sequence to produce a rectangular cross-sectional image. The major drawback for older linear array transducers is their large footprint or contact area. It is difficult to use these transducers for intercostal cardiac studies and for subcostal studies in the cranioabdominal area in small animals. Linear array transducers are primarily used for transrectal reproductive examinations in cattle and horses. Newer microcase, small-footprint linear array transducers are used very effectively for small animal imaging.

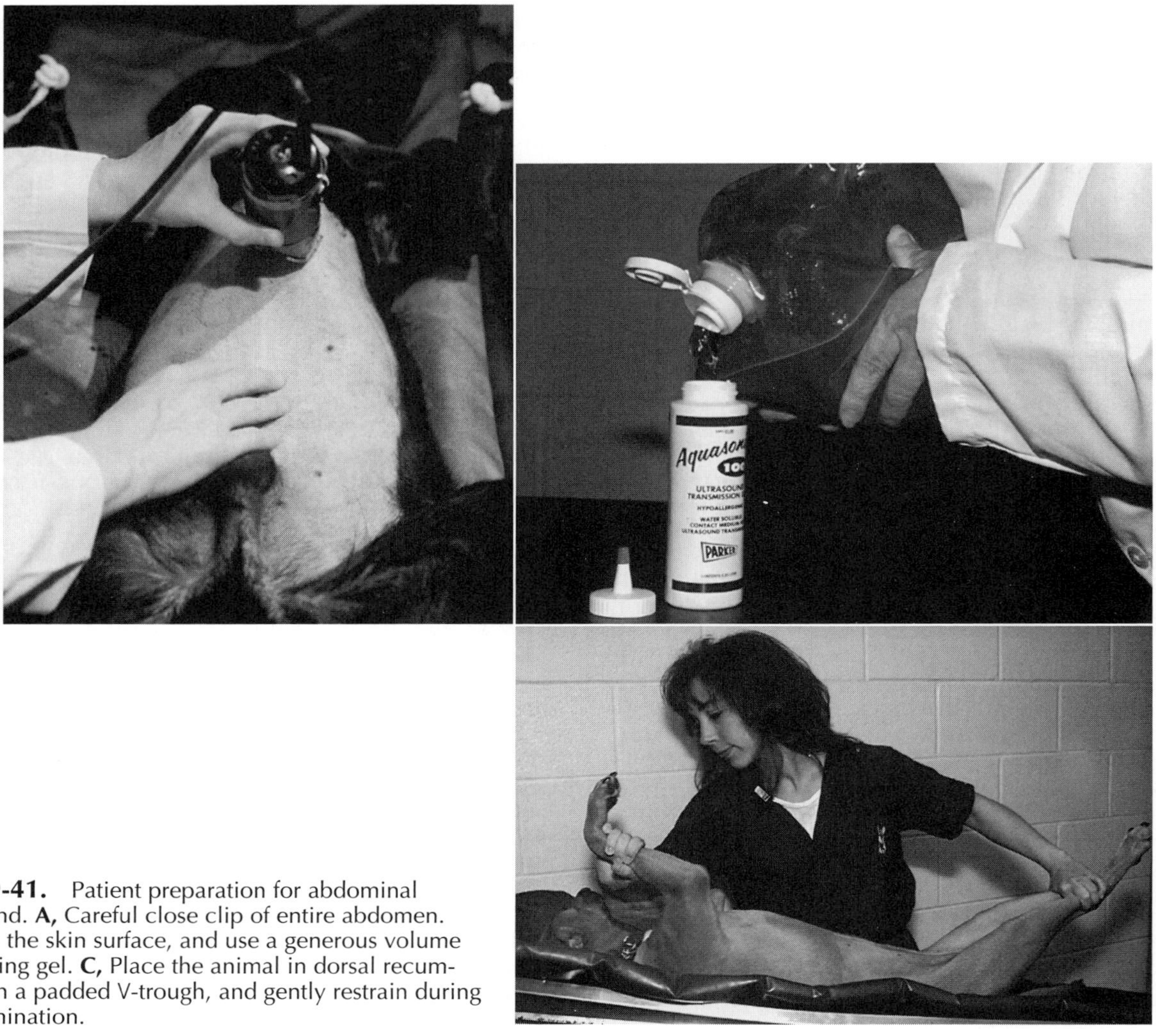

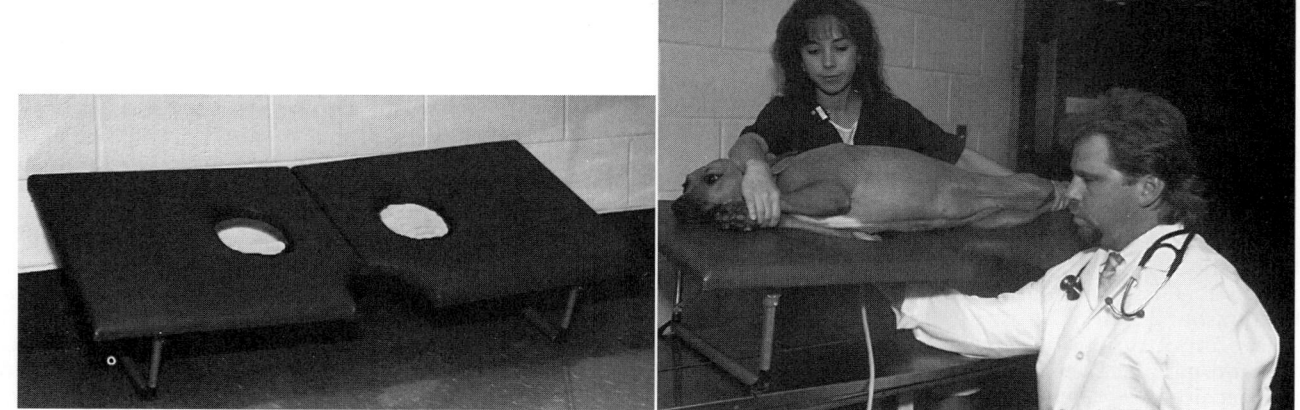

FIGURE 9-41.   Patient preparation for abdominal ultrasound. **A,** Careful close clip of entire abdomen. **B,** Clean the skin surface, and use a generous volume of coupling gel. **C,** Place the animal in dorsal recumbency on a padded V-trough, and gently restrain during the examination.

FIGURE 9-42.   **A,** Small animal cardiac ultrasound table. **B,** Patient properly positioned and restrained for echocardiography. The dog's cardiac notch is placed over the table hold so the sonographer can access the chest from beneath the table.

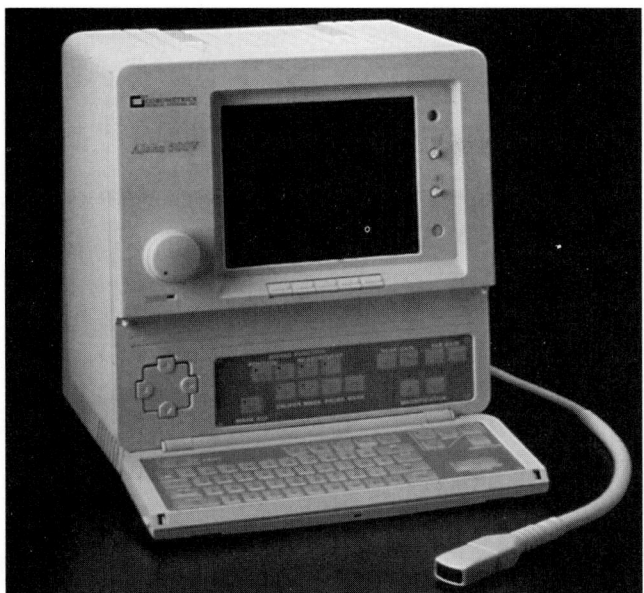

FIGURE 9-43. Portable, real-time, gray-scale, dedicated veterinary ultrasound unit that can be used on both large and small animals.

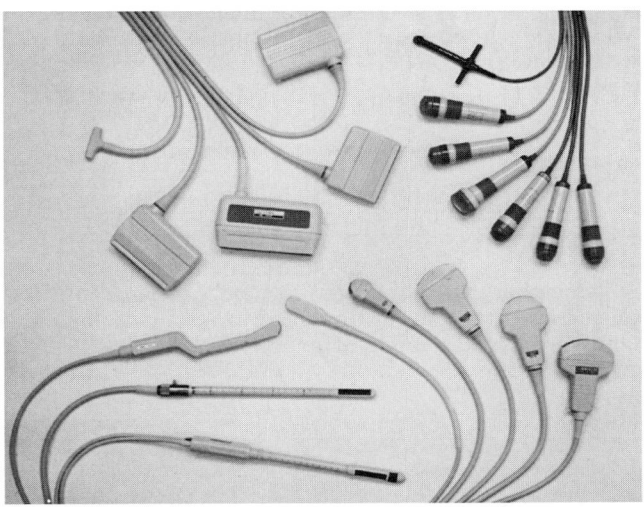

FIGURE 9-44. Several types of ultrasound transducers available for veterinary use. The transducers in the upper left are linear array, upper right are sector scanners, lower right are phased array, and lower left are transrectal and transvaginal transducers.

Sector scanners produce a triangular field. The crystal is swept across the area by mechanical or electronic means, and the transducer generally has a small contact area. Newer, more expensive transducers may incorporate annular array and dynamic focusing technology. These transducers form the ultrasound beam by adding together many small beams from an array of small crystals. Dynamic focusing allows the operator to place any portion within the beam into maximum resolution without having to change transducers.

Deciding what frequency of transducer to use is easy. Use as high a frequency transducer as possible to maximize

resolution while still allowing penetration to the needed depth. Remember that the higher the frequency of the transducer, the shorter will be the sound wavelength and the better will be the resolution. However, as the frequency increases, the depth of sound beam penetration decreases. For abdominal ultrasound in small dogs (15 kg or less) and cats, a 7.5-MHz transducer is ideal. For middle-size to large-breed dogs, a 5-MHz transducer works well. A guide for selecting a transducer is as follows:

High frequency:	Increases resolution
	Increases attenuation
	Decreases penetration
Low frequency:	Decreases resolution
	Decreases attenuation
	Increases penetration

> ### Technician Note
> Use as high a frequency transducer as possible to maximize resolution while allowing penetration to the necessary depth.

The ultrasound equipment controls vary from machine to machine, but the concept of *time-gain compensation* (TGC) is fairly universal. The echoes coming from acoustic interfaces close to the transducer are stronger than the echoes returning from farther away from the transducer. Time-gain amplification compensates for the progressive attenuation with depth in the ultrasound beam. TGC is operator dependent and is set for the best-looking uniform image. TGC controls most often are a series of slide pods on the front of the machine. The top pod is the near field of the image, and the lowest pod is the far field or bottom of the image.

The Ultrasound Image

As one begins using ultrasound, the need increases to restudy anatomy. The ultrasound image is a thin cross-sectional slice through the body in a new or different orientation. It will help to use a standard image orientation, which places the head or front of the animal on the left in the sagittal or longitudinal view and the animal's right on the left of the screen on the transverse or axial view.

Ultrasound terminology is easy to remember. *Echogenicity* refers to the strength or amplitude of the returning echoes. A structure that is *sonodense* or *echogenic* (bright) produces echoes. A structure that is *anechoic* or *sonolucent* (dark) produces few or no echoes. A structure is *hyperechoic* (brighter than) if it produces more echoes than adjacent structures. A structure is *hypoechoic* (darker than) if it produces fewer echoes than surrounding structures. An *isoechoic* (same as) structure has a level of echogenicity similar to that of adjacent structures. Remember that echogenicity is a relative term. Any structure can be made bright by adjusting machine control settings. Compare organs at the same depth and control settings to avoid misinterpretation of relative echogenicities.

Ultrasound Artifacts

Most people fail to take the time to fully understand ultrasound artifacts. They ignore artifacts because by definition an artifact does not contribute useful image information. This is not true of ultrasound artifacts. Ultrasound artifacts provide accurate clues to what makes up the ultrasound image.

Reverberation Artifact

Reverberation artifact occurs when the ultrasound beam hits gas or air. Because of the large drop in acoustic impedance (soft tissue/air interface), all of the ultrasound beam is reflected back to the transducer. A portion of the reflected beam bounces off the transducer surface and reenters the patient. It hits the air interface a second time, and the same thing happens again. This occurs repeatedly and appears on the screen as a set of bright parallel lines that are the same distance from each other. Each parallel line represents the distance between the transducer and the gas interface. Reverberation artifact can also be referred to as *dirty shadowing* or *comet tails* (Figure 9-45).

Shadowing

Shadowing artifact occurs because of inadequate sound beam penetration through a highly reflective or sound-absorptive substance. Acoustic shadowing is an area of darkness or hypoechogenicity that occurs deep to very dense material, such as bone, calcium, or calculi. Very small objects cast an acoustic shadow only if they are within the focal zone or narrow portion of the ultrasound beam.

Acoustic Enhancement

If the ultrasound beam passes through an area with few tissue interfaces (low attenuation region), the emerging ultrasound beam will have more intensity than would be expected and will be brighter or more echogenic distal to the nonattenuating structure. The best example of this is the normal gallbladder surrounded by the hepatic parenchyma. The liver tissue distal or deep to the gallbladder appears brighter than adjacent hepatic tissue (Figure 9-46). This artifact is seen deep to fluid-filled structures and is also referred to as *through transmission.*

Refraction, or Edge Artifact

Refraction is a hypoechoic band or stripe at the margin of a curved structure caused by the refraction or bending of the sound beam. The sound beam is deflected from its true path and never returns, with an effect similar to shadowing. Edge artifact is helpful to identify very smooth round structures, such as early pregnancy vesicles.

Mirror-image Artifact

The ultrasound machine places the returning echo on the viewing screen as a function of the time it took the echo to return. If the sound wave reverberates within a highly echogenic structure before returning to the transducer, the image will be duplicated on the screen distal to the original image. This is most commonly seen as a duplication of the gallbladder in mirror image on the other side of the diaphragm.

Slice-Thickness Artifact

If the width of the ultrasound beam cuts through both the edge of a cystic structure and solid tissue, the solid tissue may look as if it is layered within the cyst. This artifact is responsible for the erroneous appearance of debris within the urinary bladder and gallbladder, although no debris is present. The erroneous appearance is the result of volume averaging of tissue by the ultrasound machine.

The Ultrasound Examination

A complete ultrasound examination requires at least 20 to 30 minutes to perform. When ultrasound is used for a quick answer to a question such as pregnancy versus pyometra, the examination will be shorter. When using ultrasound for abdominal disease diagnosis, a complete examination should be performed every time.

It is important to have a thorough understanding of the normal appearance of the various abdominal organs before trying to identify the abnormalities associated with disease. The ranking of small animal abdominal organs from least echogenic (darkest) to most echogenic (brightest) is as follows:

Least echogenic	Renal medulla
	Liver
	Renal cortex
	Spleen
	Prostate
Most echogenic	Renal sinus fat

Remember that echogenicity is a relative term, and one must compare organs at similar control settings and similar depths to avoid misinterpretation.

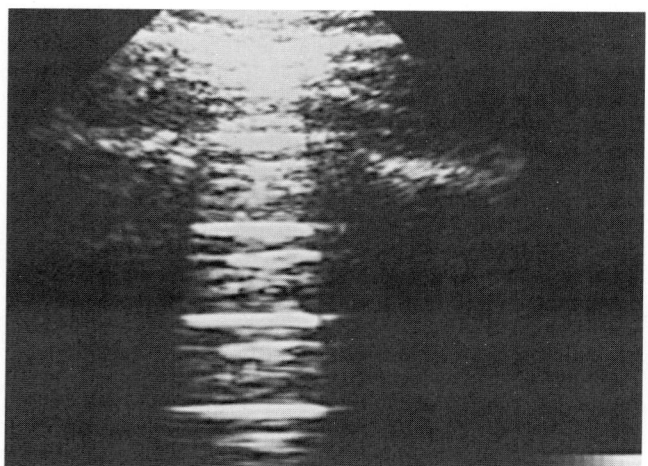

FIGURE 9-45. Reverberation artifact from the air-filled lung of a normal horse. The parallel, evenly spaced echogenic bands represent reverberation between the transducer and pleural surface.

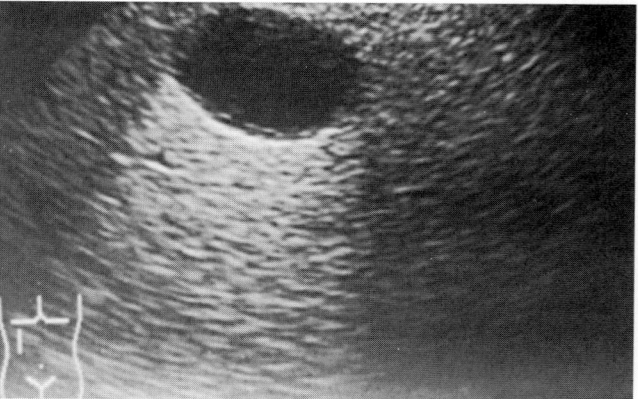

FIGURE 9-46. Bright echogenic band beneath the gallbladder represents acoustic enhancement. The ultrasound beam is not attenuated as much as it traverses the fluid-filled gallbladder as it is in the surrounding liver.

Clinical Use

The clinical application of ultrasound in veterinary medicine has exploded during the past 10 years. Equipment designed for use in people is readily adaptable for use in veterinary medicine, and several companies are producing dedicated veterinary ultrasound machines. Both 5- and 7.5-MHz sector scanners are most popular for small animal and nonreproductive large animal imaging. The 3- and 5-MHz linear array transducers are extensively used for transrectal large animal reproductive ultrasonography. Traditional cardiac and solid abdominal organ examinations remain the mainstay, but ultrasound is used to answer hundreds of clinical questions in a wide variety of species. The following section lists common ultrasound applications in both large and small animals.

Uses of Ultrasound in Large and Small Animals
- Tendon injury evaluation and response to surgery or therapy
- Diagnosis of tendon sheath infections, adhesions, and foreign bodies
- Evaluation of joint effusions, intraarticular injury, osteomyelitis, and neoplasms
- Congenital and acquired cardiac disease and response to therapy
- Pleural effusion, pleuritis, and pleuropneumonia
- Soft tissue neck, thyroid, parathyroid, tongue, and mediastinal disease
- Hepatic, renal, splenic, adrenal, urinary bladder, gallbladder, and biliary disease
- Abdominal and peripheral vascular malformations
- Peritoneal and pleural fluid assessment and sampling
- Abdominal masses of unknown origin
- Intestinal foreign bodies, intussusceptions, infiltrative disease, and neoplasia
- Testicular and prostate evaluation and location of retained testicles
- Pregnancy diagnosis, fetal evaluation, twin removal, and complete fertility evaluations
- Soft tissue neoplasia, granulomas, abscesses, and foreign bodies
- Umbilical infections and persistent and patent urachus
- Ocular and orbital evaluation
- Vascular thrombosis and catheter foreign body evaluation
- Guidance for fine needle aspiration, drain placement, biopsy, and culture

NUCLEAR MEDICINE

Many veterinary schools and several progressive specialized veterinary practices have nuclear medicine capabilities. Nuclear medicine can be divided into therapeutic and diagnostic procedures. Currently, veterinary therapeutic nuclear medicine involves the administration of radioactive iodine (^{131}I) for the treatment of hyperthyroidism and thyroid tumors. Diagnostic nuclear medicine involves the administration of radionuclides to the animal and detection of the electromagnetic radiation emitted from the animal with a gamma scintillation camera. Radionuclides are atoms with an unstable nucleus that undergoes radioactive decay. Radioactive decay is the transformation or disintegration of an unstable nuclide by spontaneous emission of electromagnetic radiation. Electromagnetic radiations that are of nuclear origin are termed *gamma rays*, in contrast to diagnostic radiations (x-rays), which originate from the electron cloud that surrounds the nucleus.

Diagnostic nuclear medicine does not generate visual images equivalent to those of diagnostic radiology but detects functional or physiologic, pharmacologic, and kinetic data from the patient in image or numeric data form. Figure 9-47 shows a standard gamma scintillation camera, control panel, and nuclear medicine computer. Common clinical uses of veterinary nuclear medicine include bone scanning to detect tumor metastasis to bone and radiographically undetectable bone injury or infection, lung scanning to detect pulmonary embolism and as a pulmonary function test, renal scans to assess kidney perfusion

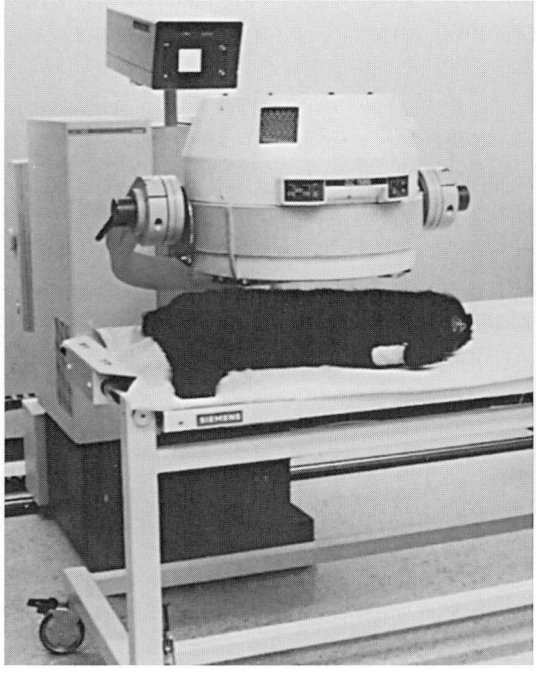
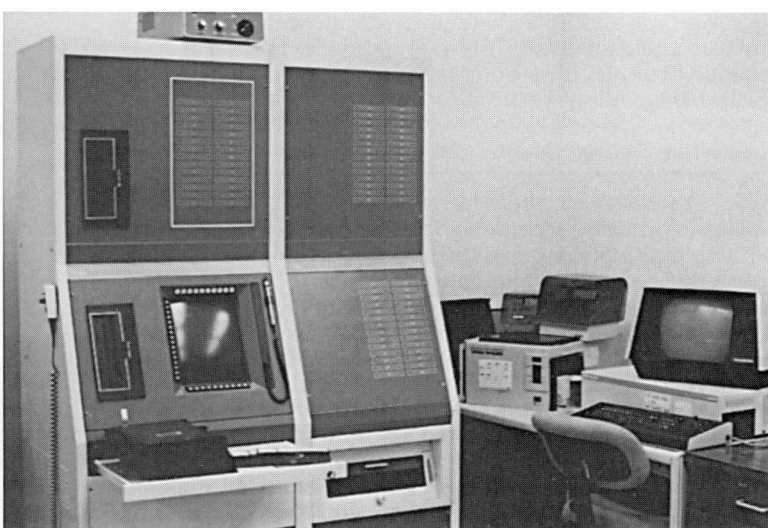

FIGURE 9-47. A, Gamma scintillation camera in position over a dog during a whole-body bone scan to check for metastatic neoplasia. **B,** Control panel monitor, nuclear medicine computer, and matrix camera.

and function, and thyroid scans for the characterization of hyperthyroid patients and to detect metastasis. Other, less common nuclear medicine studies include hepatobiliary scanning, brain scans, labeled white blood cell scans for the detection of occult infection, lymphoscintigraphy, nuclear angiography, and scans to detect an unknown focus of blood loss.

The most commonly used radionuclide is technetium 99m (^{99m}Tc). This agent is commercially available from a disposable technetium generator. Technetium is administered in an ionic form as ^{99m}TcO$_4$ (pertechnetate) or bound to a specific organ-localizing pharmaceutical agent before administration. Technetium is the radiopharmaceutical of choice because it has a 6-hour physical half-life ($T_{1/2}$) and emits a 140-keV gamma ray, which is appropriate for most imaging studies. The radioactive or physical half-life of a radionuclide is the time required for the number of radioactive atoms to decrease by 50%.

Radiation safety practices are important with nuclear medicine. When working in a practice that uses nuclear medicine, one should insist on receiving comprehensive instruction in radiation principles and safety. This chapter is meant only as an introduction.

The primary route of radionuclide administration to veterinary patients is intravenous. Latex examination gloves should be worn, and careful injection techniques should be performed to ensure the entire dose is delivered intravenously and not perivascularly. This is especially important in equine bone scans for which a large dose of radionuclide is administered. The routes of excretion of the radioactive imaging agents vary with the agent used. Technetium is primarily excreted in urine, with a lesser amount in the feces. Animals should be housed in a separate restricted area of the hospital, and their stool and urine should be carefully collected and held for decay until the levels are below exempt quantities. Always wear latex examination gloves, and limit contact with patients to only that necessary for their care. Never eat or bring eating utensils (coffee cups, spoons, etc.) into a nuclear medicine area. The dose of radiation to the patient is small, but repeated physical contact or accidental ingestion of radionuclides may be harmful to the nuclear medicine technologist. Animals should be held until they pose no radiation threat to their owners or the population at large. This is generally 3 to 10 physical half-lives of the radiopharmaceutical, depending on specific state regulations.

COMPUTED TOMOGRAPHY

In the past 10 years, there has been an expansion of the diagnostic imaging techniques available to veterinary patients. Most veterinary schools and several specialty practices have access to computed tomography (CT) scanning. A CT scan is obtained by passing a very thin x-ray beam transaxially through the patient and measuring the x-ray attenuation at multiple sites in a thin slice of the patient's anatomy. The computer then reconstructs the transmitted x-ray data into a cross-sectional image on a video monitor. The image can then be captured on film or videotape or stored for later use on magnetic tape. The advantage of CT over standard radiography is the greatly improved radiographic contrast, spatial resolution, and cross-sectional anatomic presentation. The most common use of CT in veterinary medicine is head and spinal examinations for neurologic disease. CT allows the veterinarian a noninvasive look inside the patient's skull (Figure 9-48).

When a CT scan is performed, the patient is placed in VD or DV position on the long narrow movable CT table. The

table then moves the patient through the circular gantry that houses the x-ray tube and detectors (Figure 9-49). The table moves in a measured stepwise fashion. During each table step, the CT scanner obtains a single cross-sectional slice of data. The patients need to be heavily sedated or under general anesthesia to prevent any motion and must be positioned perfectly straight. Most studies are performed twice on the same animal. The first study is performed without contrast, and the second is performed after intravenous iodinated contrast administration. Urographic contrast agents are commonly administered at a dose of 800 mg of iodine per kilogram of body weight. Contrast will highlight vascular structures, and some neoplasms will have a characteristic contrast enhancement pattern. Besides brain studies, CT can be used to identify and characterize musculoskeletal, thoracic, and abdominal disorders.

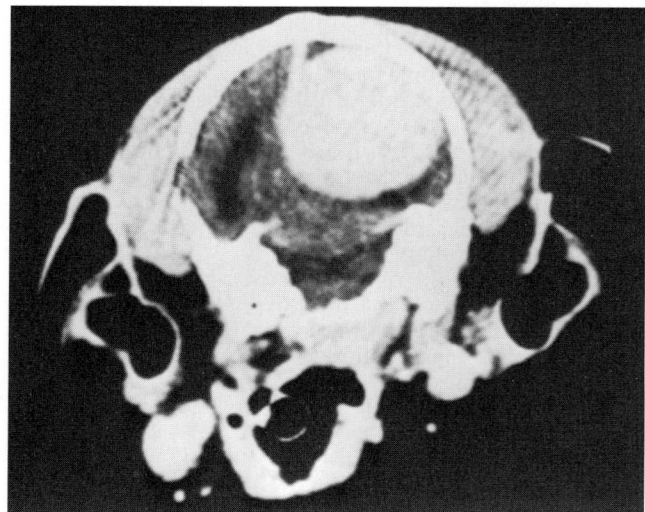

FIGURE 9-48. Computed tomogram of a dog brain showing a large contrast-enhancing brain tumor (meningioma) in the central cerebrum.

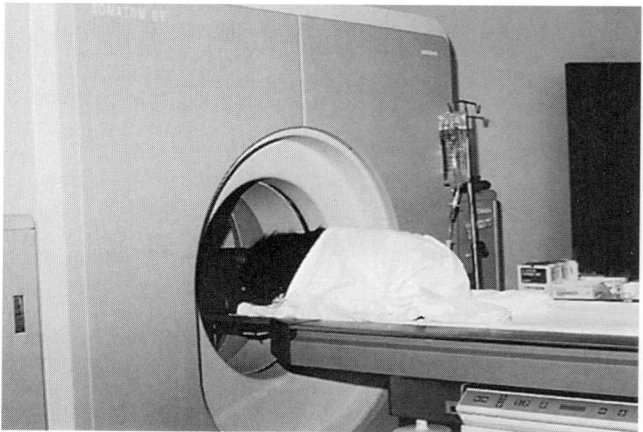

FIGURE 9-49. Dog in position for a brain computed tomogram (CT). The large circular gantry houses the x-ray tube and detectors. The table moves the patient through the gantry in precise, measured, incremental steps.

MAGNETIC RESONANCE IMAGING

The newest imaging modality to be used in veterinary medicine is magnetic resonance imaging (MRI). MRI is similar to CT in that the image is a thin slice of cross-sectional anatomy made up of a matrix of volume elements. MRI differs from CT in that it uses no ionizing radiation to create the image. Instead, the MRI represents the intensity of a radio wave signal from tissue in which

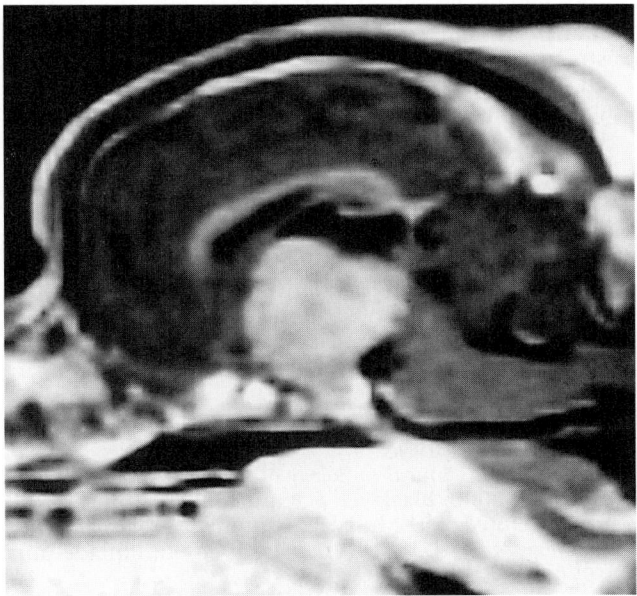

FIGURE 9-50. Sagittal T1 postgadolinium contrast magnetic resonance image of a dog with a large enhancing pituitary macroadenoma.

hydrogen nuclei have been disturbed by a characteristic radiofrequency pulse. MRI is superior to CT in image resolution, anatomic definition, and sensitivity to tissue composition differences. Because of this, MRI is vastly superior to CT for imaging of the brain and spinal cord and is currently used primarily for head and spine evaluation. Figure 9-50 is a sagittal canine brain MRI of a patient with a large contrast-enhancing pituitary tumor.

Two general types of MRI units (also called *magnets*) are used in veterinary imaging: low field strength, or resistive, magnets and high field strength, or superconductive, magnets (Figure 9-51). Magnetic field strength is measured in tesla (T). Low field strength magnets are 0.4 T or less, and high field strength magnets are 0.6 T and above. The most typical superconducting magnet has a field strength of 1 or 1.5 T. Regardless of the type of magnet used, the technician needs to be aware of several safety measures and patient management concerns peculiar to MRI.

As with CT, almost all MRI is done off the clinic premises in an imaging center, a mobile truck–based MRI unit, or a human hospital. Only a few veterinary teaching hospitals have in-house MRI units. Therefore everything needed to anesthetize, resuscitate, and recover a patient needs to be taken to the imaging site. Most practices that perform off-site imaging have a large tackle box or physician's bag filled with all necessary drugs, fluids, catheters, intravenous access lines, syringes, needles, tape, gauze, and endotracheal tubes. It often helps to do a mock run or pretend case before a clinical case to ensure everything is correctly packed. Imaging centers and hospitals appreciate clean, odor-free, and flea and tick-free veterinary patients. It is a good idea to bathe the patient within 24 hours of the examination if possible and to ensure the patient's bowel and bladder are evacuated before entering the hospital or imaging center.

A serious problem with MRI is the strong magnetic field (Figure 9-52). One cannot use anything made of ferromagnetic metal in or around the magnet. The magnetic field will rapidly and forcefully pull these objects into the

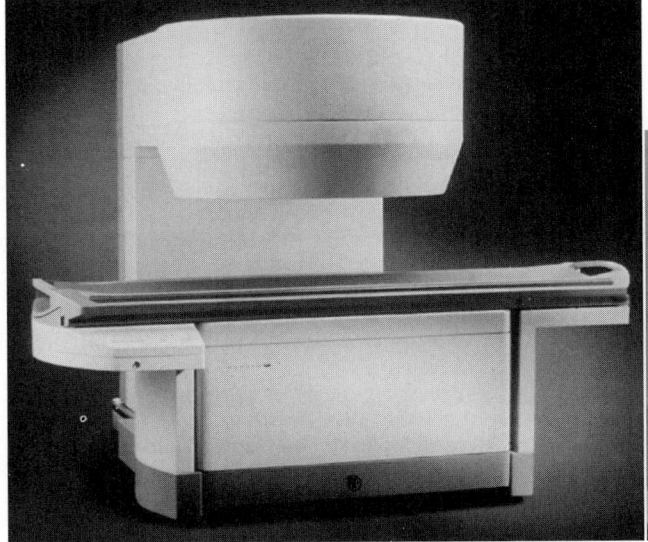 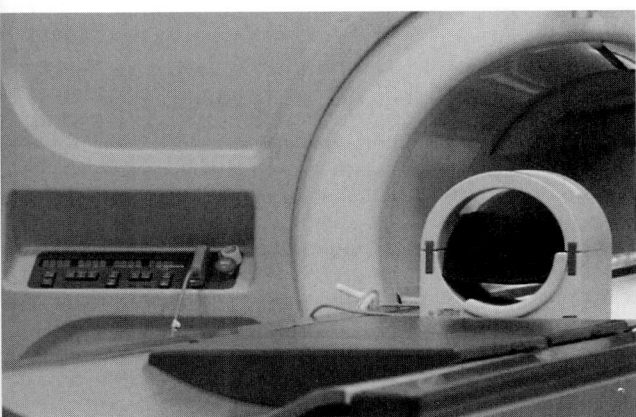

FIGURE 9-51. **A,** An open or low field strength MRI scanner. These machines are easier to position and monitor the patient but may require longer scan times. **B,** Superconductive or high field strength MRI scanner. The smaller circular structure on the table is a human knee coil often used to image small animal brains. The closed MRI gantry is the larger circular structure adjacent to the control panel.

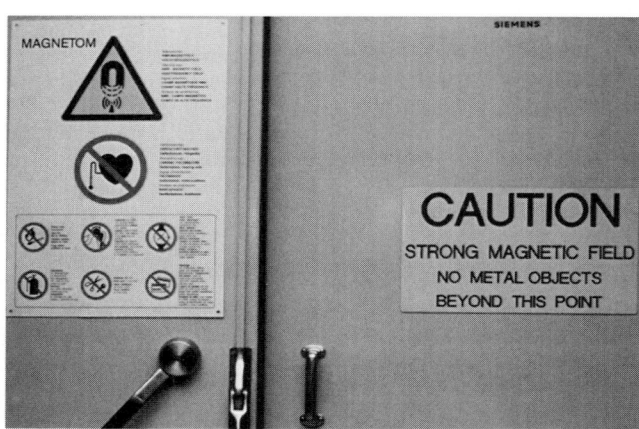

FIGURE 9-52. Warning signs positioned at the entrance to an MRI scanner. The technician must realize that the MRI magnet is always turned on and the high magnetic field may extend beyond the scanner room door. Never bring anything metallic into the MRI suite.

magnet, potentially injuring anything in its path. This generally includes the gas anesthesia machine, oxygen tank, intravenous poles, clipboards, ink pens, leashes, collars, and beepers. There are nonmagnetic products available for use during MRI, but they are generally prohibitively expensive for most veterinary hospitals. The exception is an aluminum oxygen tank. Because of this limitation, anesthesia is generally performed with injectable drugs and heavy tranquilization. Patients must be absolutely still for MRI; any motion will severely degrade the image, so they must be under fairly deep injectable anesthesia. This is sometimes complicated since it is often difficult to carefully monitor the animals during the examination because of the narrow tubular shape of some magnets and the inability to use mechanized monitoring devices. Patients that cannot tolerate deep injectable general anesthesia with minimal monitoring are not good candidates for an MRI. MRI examinations generally take 45 to 60 minutes to perform and are done with and without intravenous contrast, similar to CT examinations, but with a paramagnetic contrast agent (usually gadolinium pentetic acid [DTPA]). Organic iodide contrast will not work for MRI examinations.

Besides anesthesia and monitoring difficulties created by the high magnetic field, personal precautions must be taken. It is important to remember that even though no images are being produced and the MRI technician is not at the controls, the magnet is still on at full power at all times. Credit cards and watches may be permanently damaged if carried too close to the high magnetic field. Any device that delivers a radio frequency signal cannot be close to an MRI; these include but are not limited to televisions, radios, and pager transmitters. In addition, technicians with cardiac pacemakers, aneurysm or intracranial hemaclips, neural stimulators, metallic fragments within the orbits, hearing aids, or intrauterine devices should not be in charge of patient care during an MRI.

REFERENCES

Butler JA et al: *Clinical radiology of the horse,* ed 2, Oxford, England, 2000, Blackwell Scientific Publications.

Curry TS, Dowdey JE, Murry RC: *Christensen's introduction to the physics of diagnostic radiology,* ed 4, Philadelphia, 1990, Lea & Febiger.

Douglas SW, Herrtage ME, Williamson HD: *Principles of veterinary radiology,* ed 4, East Sussex, England, 1987, Balliere Tindall.

Eastman Kodak Company: *The fundamentals of radiography,* ed 12, Rochester, NY, 1980, The Company.

Han CM, Hurd CD, Kurklis L: *Practical guide to diagnostic imaging: radiology and ultrasonography,* ed 2, St Louis, 2000, Mosby.

Lavin LM: *Radiography in veterinary technology,* ed 2, Philadelphia, 1999, WB Saunders.

Morgan JR: *Techniques of veterinary radiography,* ed 5, Ames, 1993, Iowa State University Press.

Thrall DE: *Textbook of veterinary diagnostic radiology,* ed 3, Philadelphia, 1998, WB Saunders.

Ticer JA: *Radiographic technique in veterinary practice,* ed 2, Philadelphia, 1984, WB Saunders.

RECOMMENDED READING

Butler JA et al: *Clinical radiology of the horse,* ed 2, Oxford, England, 2000, Blackwell Scientific Publications.

Curry TS, Dowdey JE, Murry RC: *Christensen's introduction to the physics of diagnostic radiology,* ed 4, Philadelphia, 1990, Lea & Febiger.

Douglas SW, Herrtage ME, Williamson HD: *Principles of veterinary radiology,* ed 4, East Sussex, England, 1987, Bailliere Tindall.

Eastman Kodak Company: *The fundamentals of radiography,* ed 12, Rochester, NY, 1980, The Company.

Green RW: *Small animal ultrasound,* Philadelphia, 1996, Lippincott-Raven, ch 1-3.

Hall EJ: *Radiobiology for the radiologist,* ed 4, Philadelphia, 1993, Lippincott-Raven.

Han CM, Hurd CD, Kurklis L: *Practical guide to diagnostic imaging: radiology and ultrasonography,* ed 2, St Louis, 2000, Mosby.

Lavin LM: *Radiography in veterinary technology,* ed 2, Philadelphia, 1999, WB Saunders.

Morgan JR: *Techniques of veterinary radiography,* ed 5, Ames, 1993, Iowa State University Press.

Nyland TG, Mattoon JS: *Veterinary diagnostic ultrasound,* Philadelphia, 1995, WB Saunders.

Rantanen NW, McKinnon AD: *Equine diagnostic ultrasonography,* Baltimore, 1998, Williams & Wilkins.

Stashak TS: *Adam's lameness in horses,* ed 4, Philadelphia, 1987, Lea & Febiger.

Thrall DE: *Textbook of veterinary diagnostic radiology,* ed 3, Philadelphia, 1998, WB Saunders.

Ticer JA: *Radiographic technique in veterinary practice,* ed 2, Philadelphia, 1984, WB Saunders.

10

Veterinary Oncology

G. Neal Mauldin • Glenna E. Mauldin

Geriatric medicine has become a major part of routine veterinary practice. As the population of pet animals ages, veterinarians should expect to see an increase in the number of dogs and cats with neoplastic diseases. Some studies estimate that 40% to 50% of dogs and cats older than 10 years will develop a potentially life-threatening cancer. Many owners will wish to pursue the diagnosis and treatment of these tumors and thus will create an increased need for veterinarians who specialize in oncology. Some forms of cancer therapy, such as chemotherapy, can be performed easily in private practice with a minimum of specialized equipment. Other types of cancer treatment, such as radiation therapy, require referral to an institution that has the appropriate radiation facilities. Regardless of the treatment being offered, oncology nurses and technicians can play a critical role in the treatment of companion animals diagnosed with cancer.

Significant advances have been achieved by studying tumor behavior and the response of tumors to various treatment protocols in animals. The contributions to both human and animal health that can be made through cancer research in animals are countless and can be rewarding to the veterinarians and technicians participating in these clinical research programs. The importance of the human-animal bond has also gained wide recognition in veterinary medicine, and the emotional aspect of treating cancer in animals cannot be ignored. Many clients have had previous experience with cancer in their own lives, which leads to increased anxiety and fear when their pet is diagnosed with cancer. The veterinarian and technicians treating the veterinary cancer patient must be compassionate and recognize the emotional needs of the client, as well as provide quality medical care to the animal. Box 10-1 gives the names and addresses of organizations for cancer information and treatment.

As part of the veterinary health care team, the veterinary technician's role in providing appropriate case management, quality patient care, and client support is vital. Knowledge of the basic principles of oncology will help the technician to understand the diagnostic and therapeutic approach to cancer therapy and to become an active participant in the treatment of the veterinary cancer patient.

BOX 10-1 ORGANIZATIONS FOR CANCER INFORMATION AND TREATMENT

VETERINARY

Veterinary Cancer Society
Barbara J. McGehee
Executive Director
1303 Ramona Ave.
Spring Valley, CA 91977
http://www.vetcancersociety.org

HUMAN

American Cancer Society
National Home Office
1599 Clifton Road, NE
Atlanta, GA 30329
1-800-ACS-2345
http://www.cancer.org

National Cancer Institute
Public Inquiries Office
Building 31, Room 10A31
31 Center Drive
MSC 2580
Bethesda, MD 20892-2580
301-453-3848
http://www.nci.nin.gov

ONCOLOGY

Oncology is the study of cancer. In general, cancer is defined as an uncontrolled growth of cells on or within the body. Virtually any type of normal cell may undergo the changes that eventually result in the development of cancer. Other terms that are commonly used to describe cancer include *tumor, mass, neoplasm,* and *growth.* Tumor growth may cause clinical signs as a result of the following: destruction of tissue and impairment of normal organ function either directly or indirectly; pain, inflammation, and infection; and systemic symptoms that are indirectly associated with the cancer (called *paraneoplastic syndromes*).

> ## Box 10-2 EXAMPLES OF PARANEOPLASTIC SYNDROMES AND ASSOCIATED TUMORS
>
> ### HYPOGLYCEMIA
> Hepatocellular carcinoma
> Insulinoma
> Leiomyosarcoma
>
> ### HYPERCALCEMIA
> Lymphoma
> Apocrine gland adenocarcinoma of the anal sac
> Parathyroid tumors
> Multiple myeloma
>
> ### POLYCYTHEMIA
> Renal carcinoma
>
> ### DISSEMINATED INTRAVASCULAR COAGULATION
> Hemangiosarcoma
> Thyroid carcinoma
>
> ### ANEMIA
> Multiple tumors
>
> ### HYPERPROTEINEMIA
> Multiple myeloma
> Lymphoma
>
> ### FEVER
> Multiple tumors

Modified from Ogilvie GK. In Withrow SJ, MacEwen EG, editors: *Clinical veterinary oncology*, Philadelphia, 1989, JB Lippincott, p 30.

Paraneoplastic syndromes are abnormal systemic conditions that occur in locations other than the site of the tumor itself. Often these abnormalities are caused by the production of hormones and other substances synthesized by the tumor (Box 10-2). Thus the clinical signs caused by cancer are not necessarily restricted to one organ system. Rather, they affect the entire animal systemically and can affect all organ systems and tissues at once.

Tumors can be either *benign* or *malignant*. The cells that make up benign tumors exhibit unchecked growth but do not destroy local tissue. However, benign tumors can impair tissue function by their presence. For example, a dog with a large lipoma in the axilla (underarm) may have decreased ability to use the front leg. Some benign tumors can cause significant problems. Most meningiomas (tumors of the meninges surrounding the brain and spinal cord) are histologically benign. However, they can cause severe neurologic dysfunction and death if not identified and treated in a timely manner.

The cells in malignant tumors exhibit uncontrolled growth and are capable of local tissue destruction. They also have the potential for metastasis. *Metastasis* is the process by which cancer cells spread from a primary tumor to secondary locations, such as lung, lymph node, and visceral sites (e.g., liver). The mechanisms of metastasis are not fully understood and vary among different types of tumors. However, the basic metastatic process can be summarized as follows: cancer cells leave the primary tumor, enter lymphatic or blood vessels, travel to distant tissues, become established, and subsequently grow to form secondary tumors.

In addition to being classified as benign or malignant, tumors can be categorized according to their tissue of origin and their histologic features (Table 10-1). Carcinomas, for example, arise from epithelial tissues, including skin, mucous membranes, glandular structures, and organs such as liver or kidney. Carcinomas generally spread through both the lymphatic system and bloodstream, so regional lymph node and lung metastases are commonly seen. Sarcomas, on the other hand, arise from mesenchymal tissues, such as cartilage, connective tissue, or bone. These tumors generally spread via the bloodstream and rarely metastasize through lymphatics. Thus pulmonary metastases are relatively more common with sarcomas, but local lymph node involvement is rare.

The prefix of a tumor's name indicates the specific tissue of origin. For example, an osteosarcoma is a sarcoma originating from bone. The suffix of the name generally indicates whether the tumor is benign or malignant, for example, fibroma (benign) versus fibrosarcoma (malignant). However, exceptions to this rule include *melanoma*, *insulinoma*, and *thymoma*, all of which are malignant tumors. More than 100 histologic types of cancer exist, and each may require special treatment and carry a different prognosis. It is also important to realize that the incidence and behavior of cancer in dogs is often quite different from cats.

Additional methods to further classify tumors and to help in predicting behavior and prognosis include the tumor's *grade* and *stage*. Established grading systems categorize tumors of the same histologic type according to shared microscopic features. For example, the cells in a low-grade soft tissue sarcoma have well-defined cellular architecture (well differentiated), with few mitotic figures in the nuclei (slow cell division), and exhibit minimal invasion of surrounding normal tissue. The cells in a high-grade soft tissue sarcoma have poorly defined cellular architecture (undifferentiated), exhibit numerous mitotic figures (rapid cell division), and exhibit aggressive invasion of surrounding normal structures. Well-established and reliable grading systems exist for some tumor types, such as canine mast cell tumors and soft tissue sarcomas, but other canine and feline tumors do not yet have well-developed criteria for grading.

A tumor is staged according to the physical characteristics of the tumor and the extent of disease. The World Health Organization's staging system is known as the TNM system, and it categorizes tumors according to the attributes of the tumor at the primary site (T), whether there is involvement of regional lymph nodes (N), and whether the tumor is present as metastases at distant sites (M). Defined subclassifications, represented as numbers following the T, N, and M (e.g., $T_3N_1M_0$), describe the size and extent of the tumor in these locations. Evidence of clinical signs of illness is usually designated "a" (denoting healthy) or "b" (denoting sick).

The exact cause of most cancers is not fully understood. Carcinogenesis is the process by which normal cells become transformed into cancer cells. In general, two events must take place before malignant transformation can occur: *initiation* and *promotion*. During the first event (initiation), the cell is exposed to a factor or factors that rapidly and irreversibly alter its deoxyribonucleic acid (DNA). Promotion, which follows initiation, is a prolonged process during which initiated cells are stimulated by an agent or agents to evolve into tumor cells. Under favorable conditions, a single transformed cell can proliferate and eventually develop into an invasive cancer. Factors with carcinogenic potential include inherited genetic defects, hormones, viruses, diet, immune system dysfunction, trauma, chronic inflammation, radiation, and a wide variety of chemical factors. It is unfortunate that identification of a simple cause and effect relationship between a specific carcinogenic factor and subsequent tumor development in an exposed or affected individual is extremely difficult. The

TABLE 10-1	CLASSIFICATION OF TUMORS IN ANIMALS		
	Tissue Type	**Benign**	**Malignant**
	CONNECTIVE TISSUE		
	Bone	Osteoma	Osteosarcoma
	Cartilage	Chondroma	Chondrosarcoma
	Fibrous tissue	Fibroma	Fibrosarcoma
	Fat	Lipoma	Liposarcoma
	Smooth muscle	Leiomyoma	Leiomyosarcoma
	Skeletal muscle	Rhabdomyoma	Rhabdomyosarcoma
	Blood vessels	Hemangioma	Hemangiosarcoma
	HEMOLYMPHATIC TISSUE		
			Lymphomas
			Multiple myeloma
	EPITHELIAL TISSUE		
	Skin	Papillomas	Squamous cell carcinoma
	Sebaceous glands	Adenomas	Adenocarcinomas/carcinomas
	Sweat glands	Adenomas	Adenocarcinomas/carcinomas
	Ceruminous glands	Adenomas	Adenocarcinomas/carcinomas
	Mammary glands	Adenomas	Adenocarcinomas/carcinomas
	Nasal mucosa	Adenomas	Adenocarcinomas/carcinomas
	Gastrointestinal mucosa	Adenomas	Adenocarcinomas/carcinomas
	Biliary tract	Adenomas	Adenocarcinomas/carcinomas
	Urinary tract	Adenomas	Adenocarcinomas/carcinomas

Modified from Dubielzig RR. In Withrow SJ, MacEwen EG, editors: *Clinical veterinary oncology*, Philadelphia, 1989, JB Lippincott, p 19.

cause of cancer is multifactorial and complicated. Although cancer prevention is the ultimate goal of research, much work remains to be done before it becomes a reality.

DIAGNOSTIC APPROACH IN THE CANCER PATIENT

Through early diagnosis and appropriate treatment of cancer, the prospects for cure or tumor control are greatly improved. The most dangerous approach in a canine or feline patient with a suspected tumor is to advise the owner to "just watch it." The American Veterinary Medical Association (AVMA) has published a list of the early warning signs of cancer:

Abnormal swellings that persist or continue to grow
Sores that do not heal
Weight loss
Loss of appetite
Bleeding or discharge from any body opening
Offensive odor
Difficulty eating or swallowing
Hesitation to exercise or loss of stamina
Persistent lameness or stiffness
Difficulty breathing, urinating, or defecating

Although not every animal with one or more of these clinical signs has cancer, a geriatric patient showing these signs should be carefully evaluated for neoplastic disease. A consistent diagnostic approach and biopsy are essential for establishing the correct diagnosis.

History, Physical Examination, and Minimum Data Base

The first steps in evaluating a canine or feline patient with suspected cancer are to obtain an accurate history from the client and to perform a thorough physical examination. No diagnostic test can equal the valuable information gained from a complete history and physical examination. The history should include the owner's conception of the primary problem, the observed or perceived clinical signs, the duration of those signs, any treatments administered, and the response to those treatments. Concurrent or past medical problems should be characterized in detail. Owners should also be questioned regarding routine health maintenance, including vaccinations, parasite control, and diet. Knowledge of the signalment (age, breed, gender) of an animal may assist in the diagnosis of some cancers. Certain tumors, for example, occur more frequently in a particular species, breed, gender, or age-group. Most companion animals that develop cancer are middle aged to geriatric. The average age at the time of diagnosis is 6 to 15 years. However, it is essential to remember that the age of the animal should never be a deterrent to aggressive treatment. The patient's physiologic age, as determined by careful evaluation of cardiovascular, renal, and hepatic function, is more important for predicting treatment-associated risk than the chronologic age.

After a complete history is taken, a detailed physical examination should be performed to evaluate each organ system (see Chapter 2). This approach allows assessment of the primary problem, as well as concurrent diseases. Lymph nodes, especially those close to the cancer, should be palpated for enlargement. Evidence of local tumor invasion, spread to draining lymph nodes, or distant metastases is important in defining the extent of the patient's cancer. Any skin or subcutaneous masses detected on the patient's body should be measured and their location recorded in the medical record.

A minimum data base should be gathered next. This generally consists of a complete blood count (CBC), serum chemistry diagnostic profile, urinalysis (UA), and thoracic radiographs. The CBC is used to assess abnormalities in the red blood cells, white blood cells, and platelets. The biochemical profile should be evaluated for the presence of problems involving electrolytes, liver enzymes, creatinine, blood urea nitrogen (BUN), and serum protein concentrations. The UA permits further assessment of renal function. Urine for urinalysis should be obtained by cystocentesis whenever possible. Voided samples are often contaminated by debris washed out of the urethra, which makes microscopic evaluation of the urine sediment unreliable. However, cystocentesis should be avoided in animals with bleeding disorders, as well as those suspected of having bladder cancer. Transitional cell carcinoma is by far the most common form of bladder cancer in the dog, and cells exfoliating from this tumor during cystocentesis will readily transplant into normal abdominal tissues. The specific gravity of urine should always be determined before the patient receives fluid therapy, because intravenous administration of fluids may lower the specific gravity.

Technician Note

All blood samples should be obtained through venipuncture of the jugular veins if possible. Peripheral veins should be spared in the event that repeated catheterization for anesthesia or chemotherapy administration is indicated. Lack of venous access can be a frustrating problem in a small animal patient requiring multiple intravenous chemotherapy treatments. Some chemotherapy agents, such as the drug doxorubicin, can cause severe tissue damage if even a small amount is administered outside the vein. For this reason, an intravenous catheter must be placed whenever chemotherapy is administered.

Radiography

Radiology plays an important role in the diagnosis and staging of cancer (see Chapter 9). The lungs are a common site for the development of metastases from certain malignant tumors. Chest radiographs should be obtained when the animal is in right lateral *and* left lateral recumbency, as well as in a ventrodorsal or dorsoventral position, to accurately evaluate all lung fields for metastatic nodules. Views in two planes are necessary for all radiographic examinations, in order to localize any lesions that may be present. The use of the additional lateral view improves the ability to visualize both lung fields by allowing the "up" lung to be expanded and filled with air, thereby enhancing the radiographic appearance of any nodule that may be present. Radiographs of the abdomen or other anatomic structures may also be indicated based on physical examination findings or to investigate the most likely sites of involvement for the patient's specific cancer.

In addition to radiography, other imaging techniques are now commonly used to assist in the clinical evaluation of the small animal cancer patient. Ultrasonography, for example, is a noninvasive method that may be employed to examine the architecture of specific organs or masses found in the thoracic cavity or abdomen. Computed tomography (CT) scans, magnetic resonance images (MRIs), and nuclear medicine scans are additional noninvasive imaging techniques that are available at many universities and some private referral hospitals. Each provides different methods by which to assess virtually any area of the body. CT scans and MRIs play an increasingly important role in staging the extent of cancer in cats and dogs and also in the formulation of treatment plans, particularly when radiotherapy is indicated.

Cytology

Cytology is the study of individual cell morphology for the purpose of obtaining a clinical diagnosis (see Chapter 6). It is an effective screening tool and can be particularly valuable in differentiating neoplasia from inflammation or infection. Results of the cytologic examination may also indicate the need for a tissue biopsy to obtain a definitive diagnosis. Every skin or subcutaneous mass that is identified during the physical examination should be evaluated by either cytologic or histopathologic examination and not assessed simply by gross appearance.

Adherence to the proper techniques for collecting and preparing cytology samples is essential for obtaining accurate results. Failure to collect sufficient cells or distortion of cellular architecture through poor handling techniques will make a reliable cytologic diagnosis impossible. Tumors that are easily diagnosed by cytologic examination are generally composed of cells that exfoliate or shed easily. These loose cells can then be processed onto glass slides with minimal distortion to their architecture (e.g., mast cell tumors, many carcinomas). A positive cytologic report is highly suggestive of neoplasia and warrants further investigation (biopsy or surgical removal). A negative cytologic report must be interpreted with caution, because a false-negative finding is possible when sample acquisition or preparation was improperly performed. Samples for cytologic examination are easily gathered in many different ways: by fine needle aspiration of the mass itself or accessible lymph nodes, by thoracocentesis or abdominocentesis, by impression smears of small biopsy samples or ulcerated lesions, or by needle biopsy of bone marrow. These procedures can be performed quickly, with minimal discomfort to the animal. Except in the case of bone marrow aspiration, anesthesia or sedation is generally not necessary.

Fine Needle Aspiration

Samples for cytologic evaluation of cutaneous tissue masses and lymph nodes are obtained by fine needle aspiration (FNA). Improvements in ultrasound and fluoroscopic instrumentation have also allowed FNA to be used safely for the collection of samples from within body cavities. For external masses, a 6- or 12-ml syringe, a 22-gauge needle, and clean glass slides, preferably with a frosted edge to allow labeling of the slide, are needed to perform the procedure.

To perform an FNA, the lesion is swabbed with alcohol and stabilized between the clinician's fingers. The needle is then inserted into a representative area. The needle may be inserted with or without the syringe attached, and several core samples are obtained by redirecting the needle several times without exiting the skin (Figure 10-1). Small portions of the needle contents are then squirted onto a series of clean glass slides, and a second clean slide is used to smear the preparation.

Slides should be labeled with a lead pencil on the frosted edge of the slide before staining. The solvents used during the staining process will wash off most types of ink, including indelible ink. Identification of the slides should include the animal's name and patient identification number, as well as the specific location of the mass that was aspirated. The slides are then air dried and sent to a qualified veterinary cytologist for evaluation, along with a complete and detailed description of pertinent clinical and historical information.

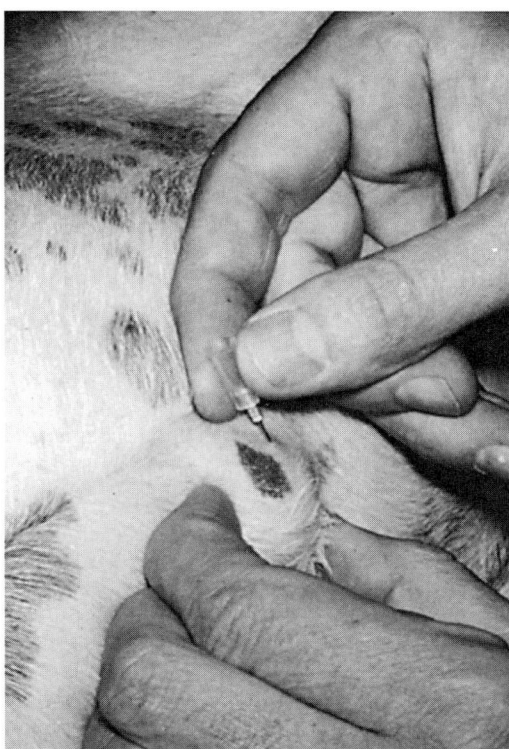

FIGURE 10-1. Fine needle aspiration of a cutaneous mass. A 22-gauge needle is inserted into the mass. The needle is redirected several times to obtain a good sample of cells. A syringe is then attached to the hub of the needle, and the contents are expelled onto clean glass slides.

Technician Note

Stain some of the prepared cytology slides for preliminary in-house review, saving the best and most representative slides for outside laboratory examination. Slides that are evaluated in-house must be fixed with an appropriate stain. The most common stains available include Wright's stain, new methylene blue, and Romanovsky's stains, such as Diff-Quik (American Scientific Products). Not all stains perform equally well under all circumstances. For instance, the characteristic granules diagnostic of mast cells may stain poorly or not at all when using Diff-Quik stains.

Bone Marrow Aspiration

Evaluation of the cellular elements in bone marrow is sometimes indicated when abnormalities exist in the erythrocyte, leukocyte, or thrombocyte cell lines in the peripheral blood. Examination of bone marrow is also necessary to accurately determine the stage of certain tumors, such as lymphoma, multiple myeloma, and mast cell tumor. The most common technique used to collect a sample from the bone marrow is aspiration biopsy using a 16- or 18-gauge bone marrow needle (see Chapter 6). If this method fails to retrieve sufficient cells, a core sample can be obtained by means of a Jamshidi bone marrow biopsy needle (American Pharmaseal Co.).

The preferred sites for biopsy of the bone marrow are the iliac crest, proximal humerus, and trochanteric fossa of the proximal femur. It is important to remember that marrow in the long bones is replaced by fatty tissue as an animal ages and that the most representative sample in a geriatric dog or cat will usually be obtained from a flat bone. Some dogs will tolerate bone marrow aspiration after infiltration of the overlying skin with a small amount of local anesthetic alone; most cats require sedation.

Histopathology

Obtaining a definitive histopathologic diagnosis is perhaps the most important step in the overall diagnostic plan for the cancer patient. The results of histopathology determine the treatment plan and prognosis and thus influence the owner's decision whether or not to treat. It is crucial that every mass that is removed be submitted for histopathologic examination, regardless of its gross appearance.

An advantage of histopathology over cytology is that the pathologist receives a larger sample that is less likely to be distorted by procurement and processing techniques. Individual tumors can exhibit significant cellular heterogeneity and may contain areas of necrosis, fibrosis, and inflammation, as well as neoplastic cells. Because of this variation in cellularity, entire masses or multiple sections of large tumors should be submitted for evaluation. All the tissue samples submitted are then examined to determine cell type, histologic grade, and surgical margins.

Biopsy Techniques

Common methods used to obtain biopsy tissue include needle core biopsy, incisional biopsy, and excisional biopsy.

Needle Core Biopsy

Specialized needle biopsy instruments can be used to quickly and easily collect core samples of tissue through small (1- to 2-mm) skin incisions. The TruCut needle (Travenol Laboratories) is most commonly used for biopsy of cutaneous or subcutaneous masses; adaptations of this type of needle can be used for ultrasound- or fluoroscope-guided needle core biopsy of masses and organs within body cavities. These needles obtain a 1- to 1.5-cm sliver of tissue approximately the same diameter as that of a pencil lead.

The biopsy site is clipped and prepared for minor surgery. The mass is stabilized between the clinician's fingers, and a small incision (1 to 2 mm) is made in the skin using a scalpel. The infiltration of a local anesthetic into the incision site precludes the need for sedation or anesthesia in most cases. The needle is introduced, and a sample is obtained (Figure 10-2). The tissue sample is gently removed from the needle blade and placed in 10% buffered neutral formalin. Impression smears of this tissue can also be made by rolling the sample across a clean glass slide before placing it in formalin.

Samples of bone lesions can be obtained in a similar manner with use of a closed needle core biopsy technique. General anesthesia is necessary for this procedure, which is performed with a trephine bone biopsy instrument or a Jamshidi bone marrow biopsy needle (American Pharmaseal Co.). These instruments are used to retrieve multiple core samples of bone. A potential complication of bone biopsy is pathologic fracture of bone already weakened by tumor infiltration. A smaller-gauge Jamshidi needle is preferred to minimize this risk, and in addition only one cortex of the bone is penetrated, leaving the opposite cortex intact. Sterile technique is used to prepare the biopsy site. Knowledge of normal anatomic landmarks is necessary to locate the lesion within the bone and also to avoid

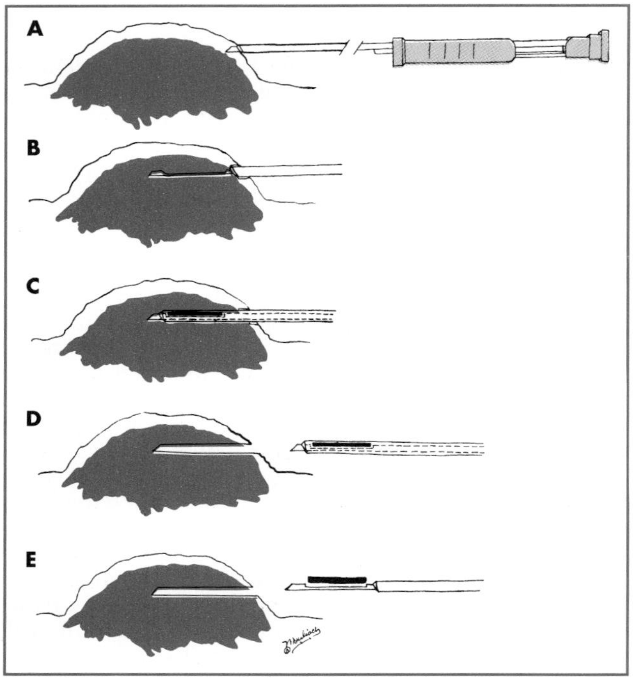

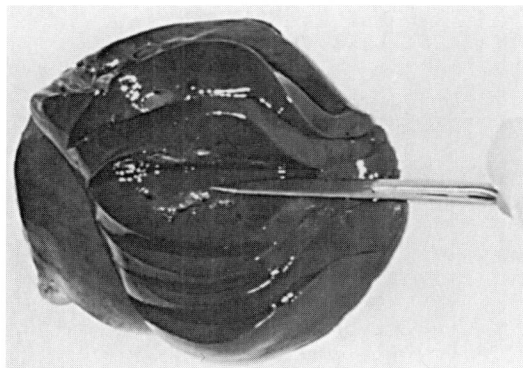

FIGURE 10-2. Mechanism of action of TruCut biopsy needle used for typical nodular biopsy. **A,** With the instrument closed, the outer capsule is penetrated. A small skin incision is made with a no. 11 blade to allow insertion of the instrument. **B,** The outer cannula is fixed in place, and the inner cannula with specimen notch is thrust into the tumor. The tissue to be excised then protrudes into the notch. **C,** The inner cannula is now fixed, and the outer cannula is moved forward to cut off the biopsy specimen. **D,** The entire instrument is removed, with the tissue sample contained within. **E,** The inner cannula is pushed forward to expose the tissue in the specimen notch.

FIGURE 10-3. A large mass is sliced (loafed) into 1-cm sections. A 1-cm thick base connecting all the slices is left to help orient the pathologist.

accidental penetration of nearby joints, nerves, or vessels. Two radiographic views of the bone containing the lesion should be available to facilitate its localization.

Incisional Biopsy

An incisional biopsy involves making a small skin incision and removing a wedge of tissue from an underlying tumor. It is useful for obtaining more tissue than can reasonably be collected by needle core biopsy. This is especially important when cancer cells are intermixed with many necrotic or inflammatory elements that can complicate subsequent histopathologic evaluation.

Contamination of the biopsy tract with tumor cells is a potential complication when using both the needle core biopsy and incisional biopsy techniques. For this reason, it is important that biopsy specimens be obtained through small incisions and with minimal disruption of the surrounding tissue. In addition, the biopsy incision should be made with consideration of the eventual definitive surgery so that the biopsy tract is removed with the tumor. Thus it is best for one surgeon to perform both the definitive surgery and the biopsy.

Excisional Biopsy

Excisional biopsy involves the complete removal of a mass for biopsy. Margins of normal tissue surrounding the

tumor are included in the excision. Depending on the results of the histopathologic examination, this method of biopsy may be all that is required for both diagnosis and treatment. However, a second surgery or adjuvant therapy may be indicated if the tissue margins are not free of cancer cells.

Biopsy Preparation

Once a biopsy specimen has been obtained, it should be handled gently so as not to distort the cellular architecture. Evaluation of the surgical margins is extremely important for determining the success of surgical resection and assessing whether further treatment is indicated. The edges or surfaces of the resected tissue that need to be most carefully evaluated for presence of tumor should be marked to enable the pathologist to easily identify them. The use of commercially available tissue "paints" has been shown to be extremely helpful in marking surgical margins. Paint will not distort the tissue and can be used to mark the entire margin. The paint will be present as a peripheral colored line when the tissue is examined under the microscope. If tumor cells are in contact with the paint-labeled margin, then tumor cells probably remain within the patient, indicating the need for further surgery or other additional treatment.

After the margins have been marked, biopsy specimens should be placed in 10% buffered neutral formalin solution for fixation. The volume ratio of formalin to tissue for initial fixation is approximately 10:1. The tissue should be no thicker than 1 cm to allow effective penetration of the formalin. If it is thicker, it can be cut in the same manner as a loaf of bread to allow the formalin to penetrate. However, one edge should be left intact so that the pathologist understands the original orientation of the mass (Figure 10-3). Once the sample has been sufficiently fixed, it can be transferred to doubled or tripled plastic bags, or commercial mailers, with less formalin (1:1 ratio) for transportation to the laboratory.

A detailed information sheet should accompany the sample to the laboratory. Information that should be recorded includes the clinic and veterinarian's name, the owner's name, the animal's name and signalment, the site of the biopsy, and a brief but detailed clinical history, including pertinent treatments and the suspected diagnosis. Any margins requiring evaluation should be recorded as well. For some tumors, such as mast cell tumors, a histologic grade may also be requested to help predict tumor behavior.

The pathologist is responsible for identifying the tumor type and providing information regarding completeness of surgical margins and histologic grade. However, the pathologist is limited by the quality of the sample submitted and the amount of information provided. It is ultimately the responsibility of the attending clinician to assess whether the pathologist's diagnosis accurately reflects the clinical presentation of the patient.

THERAPEUTIC OPTIONS

Once a diagnosis has been made, the available therapeutic options can be assessed. The clinician, technician, and client should discuss together the various choices for diagnosis and treatment with respect to the prognosis, benefits, potential complications, and cost. When speaking to the client, it is important that the clinician speak in simple terms that are easily understood. Information handouts are helpful to explain commonly performed procedures such as amputation, mastectomy, and the care and monitoring of incisions and bandages. Handouts can also be used to explain the nature, method of action, and expected side effects of common chemotherapy drugs.

There are three primary treatment options for canine and feline cancer patients: surgery, chemotherapy, and radiotherapy. A single modality is recommended for some patients, whereas multimodality protocols combining more than one type of treatment are preferred for others.

Surgery

Traditionally, surgery has been the treatment of choice for most types of localized cancer in dogs and cats. Surgery is certainly the best method for removing solitary masses, but its benefits may be limited by damage to important nearby structures. In addition, patients whose tumors have a systemic component, such as a metastatic carcinoma or lymphoma, should undergo surgery as a diagnostic or palliative procedure only. Aggressive resection and reconstruction should not be considered if long-term disease control is not possible. In such instances, combining surgery with other modalities (adjuvant therapy) or using other modalities in place of surgery is necessary. Thus, to provide the best possible care, the oncologic surgeon must understand and be familiar with all the potential therapy options.

Successful surgical resection of malignant cancer requires an aggressive approach. The tumor must be removed completely with a minimum of cosmetic and functional loss to the patient. A concerted attempt is made during resection to avoid incising the tumor and contaminating the surgical field with neoplastic cells. Cells released in this manner may implant in the wound and result in local recurrence. Instead, surgical resection should be performed in the normal tissues surrounding the mass so that a generous margin of normal tissue is removed together with the tumor.

Extensive surgical resections and prolonged surgery times may be necessary in patients that are severely debilitated from cancer or other concurrent disease. These cases require careful perioperative planning and monitoring so that complications are avoided. It is the mutual responsibility of the clinician and technician to make sure that the patient has had a complete presurgical evaluation and that the surgical team is aware of any complicating conditions. The anesthetic protocol must be tailored to the needs of the individual patient. It is best to perform major surgeries early in the day, so that the animal receives optimal monitoring from a full staff during the recovery period. Preparation for surgery should include clipping wide areas around surgical sites to accommodate extensive resections should they be necessary. A thorough surgical scrub follows clipping. Perioperative antibiotics may be indicated if a prolonged operative period or potential contamination during surgery is anticipated. Intravenous fluids, regional analgesics (epidural anesthesia or local anesthesia in regional nerves), and the parenteral use of analgesic agents also provide for an improved recovery in most patients (see Chapter 22).

Another type of surgery used to treat cancer is cryosurgery. This involves the use of a cold source (usually liquid nitrogen) to freeze superficial cancers that are usually less than 2 cm in diameter. After freezing, the treated tissue dies and sloughs away, leaving a wound that later heals. There may be permanent discoloration or loss of hair associated with this process. Cryosurgery is useful for small, superficial lesions, such as eyelid, skin, and anal masses. A disadvantage of cryosurgery is that the completeness of tumor removal cannot be determined because there is no tissue to submit for margin evaluation. Cryosurgery should not be used to treat large, invasive masses or in cases where a definitive histologic diagnosis has not yet been obtained.

The goal of surgery may be curative or palliative. Palliative surgery involves tumor resection in order to improve the patient's quality of life despite known metastasis or an otherwise poor long-term prognosis. An example would be a dog with an ulcerated or painful mass (e.g., mammary gland tumor or osteosarcoma) that has metastasized but the metastatic lesions do not yet cause clinical signs. In this case, surgical resection of the mass may improve the patient's quality of life but will not prolong survival. Ultimately, the patient will succumb to progressive metastatic disease.

Chemotherapy

Chemotherapy is generally defined as the treatment of cancer with chemical agents. Chemotherapy provides a means of delivering antitumor therapy to the whole body. It is therefore most appropriate for patients who have systemic, as opposed to local, neoplastic disease. There are four primary indications for chemotherapy in canine and feline patients. It is the most effective single treatment for some types of cancer, such as lymphoma, and offers the best opportunity for attaining remission. Chemotherapy is often recommended after surgical removal of malignant tumors to prevent the development of metastases and to inhibit local regrowth of tumor at the primary site. Canine osteosarcoma is routinely treated in this way. Certain chemotherapeutic agents, known as radiation sensitizers, are sometimes administered in conjunction with radiotherapy. These drugs increase the efficacy of radiotherapy. Cisplatin and doxorubicin are examples of radiation sensitizers. Finally, chemotherapy is occasionally used as a single modality for the treatment of cancers that are not amenable to surgical resection or radiotherapy or for tumors that have already metastasized. In most cases of this type, the goal of treatment is not to induce remission but rather to temporarily improve the patient's quality of life by reducing pressure, bleeding, or pain.

Chemotherapeutic agents are categorized into groups based on their mechanism of action. However, regardless of category, the majority of chemotherapeutic agents are cytotoxic and result in tumor cell death by injuring either the cell's DNA or its protective cellular membrane. Drugs that disrupt DNA typically target cells that exhibit rapid cell turnover, a characteristic of many neoplastic cells. It is unfortunate that chemotherapeutic agents may have similar effects on normal cells within the body that have high turnover, such as the cells of the gastrointestinal tract, the bone marrow, and hair follicles. This is the basic mechanism responsible for many of the toxicities classically associated with chemotherapy: nausea, vomiting, diarrhea, bone marrow suppression, and hair loss.

The dose and timing of drug administration are predetermined to achieve maximum cancer cell destruction while minimizing the damage to normal cells that causes patient toxicity. Protocols that include a number of different drugs are preferred over single drug protocols, because drugs that have complementary mechanisms of action and balanced toxicities can be combined. Chemotherapy drug dosages are generally based on the surface area of the body (meters squared) in the dog and on body weight in the cat. A meter-squared dosing chart that can be used in both dogs and cats is included in Chapter 23.

In most cases, suppression of the bone marrow causing a decrease in the circulating neutrophil count is the toxicity that determines the highest dose of chemotherapeutic agent that will be tolerated by the patient. The interval between doses is determined in part by the time necessary for the bone marrow to recover from the previous treatment. The time at which the neutrophil count is at its lowest following the administration of a chemotherapy drug is known as the *nadir of leukopenia*. It is important to be familiar with the nadir of leukopenia for the different chemotherapeutic agents used in veterinary oncology and to understand that the greatest effect on an animal's bone marrow is likely to occur several days after the chemotherapy is administered. The nadir of leukopenia occurs approximately 7 to 14 days after drug administration for most chemotherapeutic agents, but for some drugs it is longer. Two critical questions to ask the owner of a systemically ill pet that is receiving chemotherapy are what drug was last administered and when that treatment was given.

Chemotherapeutic agents have the potential to be teratogens (they may cause defects in a developing fetus), mutagens (they may cause injury to chromosomes), and carcinogens (they may cause DNA damage that ultimately leads to the development of a second cancer). The risks from chronic low-dose exposure are unknown, but no safe level of exposure has been identified. Since 1994, the U.S. Occupational Safety and Health Administration (OSHA) has required employers to protect their employees from occupational health hazards, such as handling chemotherapeutic agents. The veterinary community must recognize, promote, and institute policies and procedures that facilitate the safe mixing, handling, and administration of these drugs. Use of a biologic safety cabinet is optimal when reconstituting chemotherapy agents.

Technician Note

Protective gloves, mask, clothing, and eye shield, as well as appropriate and standardized drug-handling procedures, must be routine whenever using chemotherapeutic agents.

There are many important nursing considerations with respect to the administration of chemotherapeutic drugs

---

BOX 10-3   NURSING CONSIDERATIONS FOR THE ADMINISTRATION OF CHEMOTHERAPEUTIC AGENTS

CONCERNS BEFORE DRUG ADMINISTRATION

Admitting
1. Patient status
   a. History since last chemotherapy
   b. Physical examination
2. Appropriate diagnostics submitted
   a. Blood work
   b. Radiographs

Treatment Plan
1. Verification
   a. Drug and dosage
   b. Blood work
2. Appropriate catheterization
   a. Necessary equipment assembled
   b. Vein selection
   c. Aseptic technique
   d. Completely clean stick
   e. Intravenous challenge with saline bolus before and after drug administration
3. Appropriate protective equipment for person mixing and administering drugs
4. Appropriate protective equipment for person restraining patient
5. Knowledge of drug toxicities
6. Emergency protocols established
   a. Treatment of extravasation
   b. Treatment of anaphylaxis
   c. Treatment of chemical spill
7. Client informed of potential toxicities

CONCERNS DURING DRUG ADMINISTRATION
1. Extravasation of drug
2. Anaphylactic reaction
3. Patient comfort

CONCERNS AFTER DRUG ADMINISTRATION
1. Hematologic toxicity
2. Nonhematologic toxicity
3. Appropriate medications prescribed
   a. Chemotherapy drugs
   b. Antibiotics
   c. Other medications
4. Treatment documentation
   a. Patient medical record
   b. Future treatment plan
   c. Client information handouts

From Dickinson K: Unpublished data. Comparative Oncology Unit, Colorado State University Veterinary Teaching Hospital, May 1996.

(Box 10-3). Toxicities such as myelosuppression (Box 10-4), extravasation (Table 10-2), and anaphylaxis (Box 10-5), as well as issues associated with nursing staff and owner exposure, are well documented. Additional potential patient toxicities include alopecia, gastrointestinal upset, sterile hemorrhagic cystitis, renal failure, cardiac toxicity, and neurotoxicity. Taking all necessary precautions to minimize risks to both the patient and the veterinary health care team is essential. Several references exist in the veterinary literature that will assist in the development of appropriate hospital policies for the safe dosing, mixing, handling, and administration of chemotherapeutic agents (see Recommended Reading).

After each treatment, the patient should be monitored for signs of toxicity. Clients should be given detailed

---

BOX 10-4 MYELOSUPPRESSIVE CHEMOTHERAPEUTIC DRUGS COMMONLY USED IN VETERINARY MEDICINE

HIGHLY MYELOSUPPRESSIVE
Doxorubicin
Cyclophosphamide
Carboplatin

MODERATELY MYELOSUPPRESSIVE
Melphalan
Chlorambucil
Cisplatin

MILDLY MYELOSUPPRESSIVE
L-Asparaginase
Vincristine
Corticosteroids

Modified from Ogilvie GK. In Withrow SJ, MacEwen EG, editors: *Small animal clinical oncology*, ed 2, Philadelphia, 1996, WB Saunders.

BOX 10-5 HYPERSENSITIVITY POTENTIAL OF CHEMOTHERAPEUTIC DRUGS

HIGHEST REPORTED INCIDENCE*
L-Asparaginase
Paclitaxel (Taxol)
Cisplatin
Melphalan (intravenous)
Anthracycline antibiotics (doxorubicin, daunorubicin)

CASE REPORTS
Etoposide (VP16)
Methotrexate
Cytarabine
Cyclophosphamide
Chlorambucil
5-Fluorouracil
Mitoxantrone
Bleomycin
Dacarbazine (DTIC)
Vinca alkaloids (vincristine, vinblastine)

Modified from Oncology Nursing Society: *Cancer chemotherapy guidelines: module—recommendations for the management of vesicant extravasation, hypersensitivity and anaphylaxis*, Pittsburgh, 1992, The Society.
*Reports of greater than 5% incidence in the literature.

TABLE 10-2 CHEMOTHERAPEUTIC DRUGS CLASSIFIED AS VESICANT OR IRRITANT AGENTS

Generic Name	Brand or Other Name
VESICANT*	
Dactinomycin	Actinomycin D
Doxorubicin	Adriamycin
Vinblastine	Velban
Vincristine	Oncovin
IRRITANT†	
Carmustine	BCNU
Cisplatin	Platinol
Dacarbazine	DTIC
Mitoxantrone	Novantrone

Modified from Oncology Nursing Society: *Cancer chemotherapy guidelines: module—recommendations for the management of vesicant extravasation, hypersensitivity and anaphylaxis*, Pittsburgh, 1992, The Society.
*An agent causing tissue destruction or necrosis on extravasation.
†An agent causing pain, inflammation, and blotches at injection site.

---

handouts describing known toxicities for each agent and the associated clinical signs. If the hospital staff or the client detects any abnormalities, the animal should be reevaluated. If chemotherapeutic agents are administered properly and the client is carefully educated regarding the potential risks, toxicity can be minimized and the patient will maintain an excellent quality of life during therapy.

Radiotherapy

Ionizing radiation can also be used for cancer therapy. Radiation causes cell death by disrupting the DNA of the cell or by destroying important molecules required by the cell. Cell death occurs when the cell is so injured that it can no longer repair itself or divide. Radiotherapy can be used alone or in combination with surgery, chemotherapy, or hyperthermia. It is most appropriately prescribed for the treatment of localized cancers and will not be effective in controlling systemic disease. Most radiotherapy protocols involve the administration of multiple small doses (fractions) on a Monday, Wednesday, and Friday schedule or a Monday through Friday schedule, usually for 15 to 21 fractions. Because radiation targets DNA, like chemotherapy, it is most effective against tumor cells with rapid rates of turnover. Similarly, radiotherapy side effects are seen in normal tissues within the irradiated field that also have a high rate of cell turnover.

The potential side effects of radiation are divided into delayed and acute effects. Delayed side effects of radiotherapy develop months to years after treatment and usually involve permanent changes, such as necrosis or fibrosis of normal tissues. Acute effects are seen during the latter stages of a course of radiotherapy and, although they may require additional nursing care, are temporary. The most common acute effects of radiation occur because the rapidly dividing cells of the skin and mucosal linings are extremely radiation sensitive. The growth characteristics of these cells are similar to those of cancer cells. Thus the damage to acutely responding normal tissues mimics damage to neoplastic tissue. For this reason, the acute toxicities of radiotherapy should never be permitted to limit the dose delivered. If radiotherapy is temporarily discontinued to provide time for the repair of acutely injured normal tissue, then tumor tissue will also be allowed to repair.

A frequent acute side effect of irradiation of oral or nasal tumors is mucositis of the oral cavity. Tea or warm water flushes can decrease the discomfort associated with this condition. Irradiation of skin may also induce a desquamative dermatitis or loss of the superficial layers of the epidermis. With regular flushing and use of analgesics as needed, these conditions will resolve within 2 to 3 weeks. The use of oil-based or occlusive topical creams should be avoided, and self-trauma such as licking must be prevented. Hair loss or change in color may be permanent, and the owner should be made aware of this possibility before the initiation of radiation treatments.

Technician Note

The use of oil-based topical creams for the treatment of radiation-induced desquamative dermatitis should be avoided. Self-trauma must also be prevented when dealing with acute radiation dermatitis.

EUTHANASIA

Unfortunately, veterinary cancer therapy does not always result in a cure. In many cases, the most reasonable goal for both client and clinician is a long disease-free interval and improvement or preservation of quality of life. Euthanasia is an important component of pet cancer management. Euthanasia is the best option for some clients at the time of diagnosis; for others, this choice is made after therapy has been instituted and has failed. In either situation, electing to euthanize a pet is an extremely difficult decision and one with which the client must be completely comfortable. Euthanasia should only be performed after careful consideration of all available options.

The veterinarian and technician must be prepared to provide medical information and expertise, as well as nonjudgmental emotional support and compassion to both the client and patient. Much of the emotional support comes from the technical staff. Clients may feel inhibited when talking to the veterinarian but can sometimes talk more freely with a nurse or receptionist. Technicians need to be aware of the important role they play in veterinary medicine, not only in providing treatment for the patient, but also in supporting the needs of the client. Good communication skills and compassion will be as important as the specific medical treatment provided to many canine and feline cancer patients (see Chapter 20).

RECOMMENDED READING

Couto CG: Management of complications of cancer chemotherapy, *Vet Clin North Am Small Anim Pract* 20(4): 1037, 1990.

Morrison WB: Chemotherapy safety. In Hahn KA, Richardson RC, editors: *Cancer chemotherapy: a veterinary handbook*, Baltimore, 1995, Williams and Wilkins.

Morrison WB: *Cancer in dogs and cats: medical and surgical management*, Baltimore, 1998, Williams and Wilkins.

Oncology Nursing Society: *Cancer chemotherapy guidelines: modules 1-5, recommendations for cancer chemotherapy*, Pittsburgh, 1992, The Society.

Ringlein JW: Principles of oncology nursing and management of nausea and vomiting. In Skeel RT, editor: *Handbook of cancer chemotherapy*, Boston, 1987, Little, Brown.

U.S. Department of Labor, Occupational Safety and Health Administration: *Hazard communication standard. 29 CFR 1910.1200, amended February 9, 1994*, Washington, DC, 1994, US Government Printing Office.

U.S. Department of Labor, Occupational Safety and Health Administration: *Instruction CPL 2-2.20B CH4, directorate of technical support*, Chapter 21. Controlling occupational exposure to hazardous drugs, Washington, DC, 1995, US Government Printing Office.

Withrow SJ, MacEwen EG: *Small animal clinical oncology*, ed 2, Philadelphia, 1996, WB Saunders.

Ziegfeld CR, editor: *Core curriculum for oncology nursing*, Philadelphia, 1987, WB Saunders.

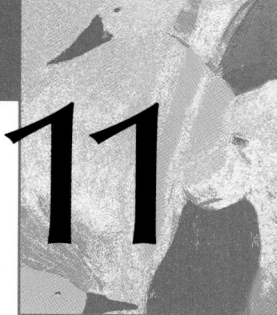

Preventive Health Programs

Johnny D. Hoskins • Susan C. Eades • Marjorie S. Gill

In veterinary practice, preventive health programs are an integral part of providing for the general health needs of dogs, cats, horses, cattle, small ruminants, and swine. Regularly scheduled vaccinations alone do not represent a comprehensive preventive health program. Vaccinations are only one component of a preventive health program that attempts to meet the general health needs of an animal.

The time and effort invested in a preventive health program are rewarding not only to the animal but also to its owner or owners and those persons attending to the health needs of the animal. The veterinary technician can provide direct assistance to the consulting veterinarian by ensuring that the general goals of the preventive health program are met.

PREVENTIVE HEALTH PROGRAM FOR DOGS

For most dogs, a preventive health program usually begins when they are first presented to the veterinary hospital or clinic at 6 weeks of age. A general outline of one preventive health program and its implementation for dogs is presented in Box 11-1.

Physical Examination

Clinical evaluation of a dog initially focuses on taking a complete case history and performing the physical examination (see Chapter 2). Basic information about the animal, such as breed, age, and gender, as well as owner concerns or complaints, is essential to the case history. After obtaining the case history, the physical examination should be conducted in a systematic manner. Body weight as part of the physical examination is recorded for several reasons. First, the weight provides information needed for dispensing medication; and second, it is an immediate indicator of the nutritional status of the animal. The body weight of a growing puppy steadily increasing at each office revisit is an indication that the puppy is receiving adequate nutrition (see Chapter 14).

Vaccinations

In general, vaccinations for the prevention of canine distemper, canine parvovirus type 2 disease, and rabies are the most important (see Box 11-1). In addition to regularly scheduled canine distemper, canine parvovirus type 2, and rabies vaccinations, other vaccinations can be incorporated into the preventive health program, as detailed below.

Canine Distemper Vaccine

Canine distemper (CD) is a viral disease of dogs and other carnivores; it has worldwide distribution. Since effective vaccines have become available, CD has been well controlled in domestic and zoo carnivores. Unvaccinated dogs and many feral species are susceptible to CD virus and can carry and spread the disease. The natural hosts include all animals in the Canidae family (e.g., dingo, fox, coyote, wolf, jackal), the Mustelidae family (e.g., ferret, mink, skunk, badger, marten, weasel, otter), and the Procyonidae family (e.g., raccoon, panda, kinkajou, coati).

After exposure to CD virus, it spreads rapidly to epithelial cells and the central nervous system. These animals develop fever, depression, anorexia, ocular and nasal discharges, and signs related to disease of the respiratory and gastrointestinal tracts. The ocular and nasal discharges initially are serous and later become mucopurulent. Coughing is a frequent manifestation of the respiratory disease, and, on physical examination, a mild breathing problem and increased lung sounds may be detected. Diarrhea and occasional vomiting reflect gastrointestinal tract involvement. The condition almost invariably deteriorates from this point, and weight loss and dehydration develop. Eventually, animals become moribund and die with or without convulsions or other evidence of neurologic disease.

| Box 11-1 | GENERAL OUTLINE OF A PREVENTIVE HEALTH PROGRAM FOR DOGS |

I. First office visit for health program—usually at 6 wk of age
   A. Conduct a general physical examination, and record body weight
   B. Check for external parasites and dermatophytes, and initiate appropriate therapy
      1. Fleas, ticks, ear mites (Otodectes cyanotis)
      2. Mange mites, especially Demodex canis and Sarcoptes scabiei
      3. Dermatophytes, particularly Microsporum spp. and Trichophyton mentagrophytes
   C. Conduct fecal examination including both direct smear and flotation
   D. Initiate administration of heartworm preventive management
   E. Administer an anthelmintic for hookworms and roundworms and, if tapeworms are present, administer praziquantel or epsiprantel
   F. Vaccinate with DA₂PL-PC* and, possibly, with kennel cough vaccine,† canine Lyme borreliosis vaccine, and Giardia vaccine
   G. Advise on nutrition and routine grooming
   H. Provide owner with client education pamphlets on topics such as the following:
      1. Identification, treatment, and control of fleas, ticks, and ear mites
      2. Benefits of preventive management for canine heartworm disease
      3. Management of normal and abnormal puppy behaviors
      4. Skin, nail, and ear care
      5. "How to" on grooming and nutrition
   I. Fill in the puppy's health record for the owner

II. Second office visit for health program—usually at 9 wk of age
   A. Conduct a general physical examination, and record body weight
   B. Check for external parasites and dermatophytes, and initiate appropriate therapy
      1. Fleas, ticks, ear mites (O. cyanotis)
      2. Mange mites, especially D. canis and S. scabiei
      3. Dermatophytes, particularly Microsporum spp. and T. mentagrophytes
   C. Conduct fecal examination including both direct smear and flotation
   D. Adjust dosage of heartworm preventive according to body weight
   E. Administer an anthelmintic for hookworms and roundworms and, if tapeworms are present, administer praziquantel or epsiprantel
   F. Vaccinate with DA₂PL-PC* and, possibly, with kennel cough vaccine, canine Lyme borreliosis vaccine, and Giardia vaccine
   G. Adjust nutrition according to health needs, and, if needed, change the grooming procedures
   H. Provide owner with client education pamphlets on topics such as the following:
      1. Identification, treatment, and control of fleas, ticks, and ear mites
      2. Benefits of preventive management for canine heartworm disease
      3. Dental, skin, nail, and ear care
      4. "How to" on grooming and nutrition
      5. Management of normal and abnormal puppy behaviors
      6. Exercise and its importance
   I. Fill in the puppy's health record for the owner

*This refers to the use of a vaccine to protect against the following: D—canine distemper; A₂ (canine adenovirus type 2)—infectious canine hepatitis; P—canine parainfluenza; L—leptospirosis; P—canine parvovirus type 2 disease; and C—canine coronavirus disease.
†This refers to the use of vaccine to protect against canine Bordetella bronchiseptica–induced disease. Puppies may be vaccinated with either an intranasal vaccine or a parenteral vaccine.

Vaccination is the preferred method of preventing CD. Active immunity can be induced in dogs with live-virus vaccines and heterotypic-virus vaccines. Tissue culture–adapted live–CD virus vaccines are highly effective if the recommended full doses are administered. The splitting of vaccine doses is never recommended. A heterotypic vaccine has been introduced to overcome the problem related to maternal CD antibody. Measles virus stimulates production of measles virus antibodies but not CD virus antibodies in dogs with low levels or without maternal CD antibodies. When dogs are vaccinated with measles virus and later challenged with virulent CD virus, the CD virus replicates. Because of an anamnestic response, however, the CD virus does not spread to epithelial or neural tissues, and dogs recover rapidly. Because of the uncertain immune status of puppies between 6 and 12 weeks of age, a combined CD and measles virus vaccination can be used. If puppies have lost their maternal CD antibody, CD virus vaccine is preferred. If maternal CD antibody is still present, however, the measles virus vaccine will have some effect when CD virus vaccine would not.

Canine Parvovirus Vaccine

Canine parvovirus diseases are relatively new diseases in the general dog population. Canine parvovirus type 2 (CPV-2) was initially described in the United States in 1978 and is the contagious enteric disease that most dog owners fear. Retrospective analyses of sera showed that CPV-2 did not exist in the general dog population before 1978. In 1967, a related parvovirus called canine parvovirus type 1 (CPV-1; also referred to as minute virus of canines) was first isolated from the feces of military dogs. The CPV-1 is not the same canine parvovirus as the CPV-2. CPV-1 infection results in clinical disease only in puppies from birth to 21 days old. Affected puppies usually present with diarrhea, vomiting, dyspnea, and constant crying. Sudden death has also been observed. Lesions are restricted to the villi of the small intestine, lungs, and myocardium. The canine parvovirus vaccine used to protect dogs against CPV-2 does not protect puppies from CPV-1 infections.

Susceptible animals to CPV-2 enteritis are of any breed, age, and gender, although young dogs are significantly more severely affected. Vomiting is often severe and is followed by diarrhea, anorexia, and rapid onset of dehydration. The feces appear yellow-gray and are streaked or darkened by blood. Elevated body temperature and leukopenia may be present, especially in severe cases. The CPV-2 enteritis may progress rapidly, with shocklike death occurring as early as 2 days after the onset of illness. In severe cases, shock and disseminated intravascular coagulation

Box 11-1	GENERAL OUTLINE OF A PREVENTIVE HEALTH PROGRAM FOR DOGS—CONT'D

III. Third office visit for health program—usually at 12 wk of age
   A. Conduct a general physical examination, and record body weight
   B. Check for external parasites and dermatophytes, and initiate appropriate therapy
      1. Fleas, ticks, ear mites (O. cyanotis)
      2. Mange mites, especially D. canis and S. scabiei
      3. Dermatophytes, particularly Microsporum spp. and T. mentagrophytes
   C. Conduct fecal examination, including both direct smear and flotation
   D. Adjust dosage of heartworm preventive according to body weight
   E. Administer an anthelmintic for hookworms and roundworms and, if tapeworms are present, administer praziquantel or epsiprantel
   F. Vaccinate with DA$_2$PL-PC* and rabies vaccines and, possibly, with kennel cough vaccine,† canine Lyme borreliosis vaccine, and Giardia vaccine
   G. Adjust nutrition according to health needs and, if needed, change grooming procedures
   H. Provide owner with client education pamphlets on topics such as the following:
      1. Identification, treatment, and control of fleas, ticks, and ear mites
      2. Dental, skin, nail, and ear care
      3. "How to" on grooming and nutrition
      4. Management of normal and abnormal puppy behaviors
      5. Recommendations for spaying and castration
      6. Exercise and its importance
   I. Fill in the puppy's health record for the owner

IV. Subsequent visits for health program—usually annual visits‡
   A. Conduct a general physical examination, and record body weight
   B. Check for external parasites and dermatophytes, and initiate appropriate therapy
      1. Fleas, ticks, ear mites (O. cyanotis)
      2. Mange mites, especially D. canis and S. scabiei
      3. Dermatophytes, particularly Microsporum spp. and T. mentagrophytes
   C. Conduct fecal flotation and occult heartworm examination, or all tests, for intestinal and heartworm infection screen
   D. Adjust dosage of heartworm preventive according to body weight
   E. Administer an anthelmintic according to fecal examination findings
   F. Vaccinate with DA$_2$PL-PC* and rabies and, possibly, with kennel cough vaccine,† canine Lyme borreliosis vaccine, and Giardia vaccine
   G. Adjust nutrition according to health needs and, if needed, change grooming procedures
   H. Provide owner with client education pamphlets on topics such as the following:
      1. Identification, treatment, and control of fleas, ticks, and ear mites
      2. Dental, skin, nail, and ear care
      3. "How to" on grooming and nutrition
      4. Management of normal and abnormal behaviors
      5. Exercise and its importance
   I. Fill in the dog's health record for the owner

‡A fourth office visit may be desirable at 15 wk of age for an additional parvovirus-2 vaccine booster in some puppies, especially high-risk breeds such as Doberman pinscher, rottweiler, Labrador retriever, and other presumed high-risk breeds.

are often responsible for the death of the animal. The recovery may be prolonged by secondary complicating factors, such as bacteria, parasites, or other viruses.

Attenuated and killed CPV-2 vaccines are available that produce high, long-lasting levels of immunity while being safe when used either alone or in combination with other canine vaccine components. All attenuated CPV-2 vaccines produce vaccine-virus shedding in the feces but at lower levels compared with dogs infected with and shedding virulent virus. Despite the shedding potential, the attenuated CPV-2 vaccines are safe for puppies and do not cause fetal infection; however, use in pregnant animals has not been recommended. Bitches should be vaccinated at least 1 month before conception to avoid any adverse effects that might occur. By vaccination of the bitch before conception, a high level of maternal immunity may be induced to help protect puppies in utero or during the first weeks of life against CPV-2 disease.

Rabies Vaccine

Rabies is acute infectious encephalitis characterized by altered behavior, aggressiveness, progressive paralysis, and in most species, by death. The rabies virus is usually present in the saliva of infected mammals, and in nature it is usually transmitted by a bite. Rabies most commonly affects the dog, cat, fox, skunk, raccoon, bobcat, coyote, bat, mongoose, and other small carnivorous mammals that are mainly responsible for the transmission of the disease.

Three phases of clinical signs are recognized in dog rabies: the prodromal, excitative, and paralytic. The term *furious rabies* refers to the syndrome in which the excitative phase is predominant; *dumb rabies* refers to those cases in which the excitative phase is extremely short or absent, and the disease progresses quickly to the paralytic phase. The prodromal phase is often difficult to recognize. Changes in behavior and temperament may be seen. The animal may become restless, snap at imaginary objects, and vocalize at the slightest provocation. During this phase, there may be a slight rise in body temperature. Mydriasis, a sluggish corneal reflex, and some loss of appetite may be noticed. The prodromal stage usually lasts 2 or 3 days and sometimes only a few hours.

The excitative phase is usually not difficult to recognize when affected dogs become aggressive. It may last 1 to 7 days, but it can be so short that it passes unrecognized and the typical aggression is never noticed. In the excitative phase, animals become increasingly restless and nervous. At the onset they may hide in dark places. Photophobia and hyperesthesia may become apparent. Chewing, biting, and swallowing unusual things such as sticks, straw, and stones are typical. Subsequently, the animal becomes more irritable and aggressive. During the excitative period, a dog may run as much as 20 miles per day. It may attack any animal encountered. Self-mutilation is very common. In most cases there is a characteristic change in the voice, caused by paralysis of the laryngeal musculature. Swallowing may become difficult, resulting in drooling. Convulsions and incoordination occur toward the end of this phase. If the animal does not die during a convulsion, it goes into the paralytic stage, becomes comatose, and dies. The total course may last as long as 10 days.

Paralytic rabies may be difficult to recognize. Paralysis of the pharynx and masseter muscles makes it impossible for the animal to eat or drink. Following paralysis of the head and neck, the animal's entire body becomes paralyzed. Coma and death follow within 2 to 4 days of generalized paralysis. The animal with dumb rabies appears thin and dehydrated. The initial signs include drooling and slight protrusion of the tongue. The body temperature is usually normal or subnormal. If the animal has been unable to close its mouth for a while, the tongue and buccal mucosa may become red-brown and leathery. The animal's pupils may be dilated, or one or both pupils may be constricted. Strabismus may be unilateral or bilateral and either divergent or convergent. The congested third eyelid may protrude over much of the cornea. Poisoning is often suspected in rabid dogs, especially when they are found several days after their disappearance.

Inactivated rabies virus vaccines are currently licensed and available for preexposure vaccination of dogs against rabies. All rabies vaccines are administered in 1-ml doses intramuscularly at one site in the thigh or subcutaneously. The vaccines are licensed for immunization of dogs 3 months of age and older. Dogs vaccinated between 3 and 12 months of age should receive a second dose 1 year later. The vaccines are licensed for 1- to 3-year effective immune periods. Accidental human exposure to licensed rabies vaccines for animals is not considered a hazard for humans.

Canine Adenoviruses Vaccine

Infectious canine hepatitis (ICH) is caused by one of two recognized canine adenoviruses. The virus that causes systemic ICH is known as canine adenovirus type 1 (CAV-1). ICH is an uncommon disease in today's dog population. Certain strains of canine adenovirus have a strict affinity for the epithelial cells lining the respiratory tract and fail to produce infectious hepatitis in dogs. This strain of canine adenovirus infection is now known as canine adenovirus type 2 (CAV-2). Signs of CAV-2 infection includes a fever that usually develops first and persists for 1 to 3 days after an incubation period of 5 or 6 days for susceptible dogs and a harsh, dry hacking cough of 6 or 7 days' duration that may progress to a fatal pneumonia. Other signs include depression, anorexia, some difficulty in breathing, muscular trembling, and serous nasal discharge. In some dogs the nasal discharge become mucopurulent.

Products currently available for vaccination are attenuated virus strains of CAV-1 or CAV-2. Such vaccines have proven to be excellent immunizing agents, either alone or combined with attenuated canine distemper virus. The amount of virus required to immunize a puppy is the same as that required for an adult, regardless of breed, and all current vaccines are standardized to ensure efficacy. Attenuated live virus (CAV-1) vaccines will occasionally cause immune-mediated corneal and iridal reactions 1 to 3

weeks after vaccination. The corneal edema disappears spontaneously and without sequelae if managed conservatively. Attenuated CAV-2 is now approved to replace CAV-1 in vaccines so postvaccination corneal opacity should no longer constitute a major problem. CAV-1 protects dogs against CAV-1 and against CAV-2, and CAV-2 protects dogs against CAV-2 and against CAV-1. Consequently, the currently available vaccines for ICH protect dogs against both types of canine adenoviruses.

Infectious Tracheobronchitis Vaccine

Infectious tracheobronchitis (kennel cough) is a bacterial (Bordetella bronchiseptica) or viral (parainfluenza virus) respiratory disease in dogs that is characterized by spontaneously induced coughing, which usually suddenly appears after being recently boarded or exposed to another coughing dog. Kennel cough is extremely contagious. Vaccination can be an effective means for preventing or at least reducing the incidence of infectious tracheobronchitis in dogs of all ages. Intranasal vaccination, in particular, provides rapid, long-term immunity against B. bronchiseptica and parainfluenza virus infection and disease. Puppies can be vaccinated intranasally as early as 2 to 4 weeks of age without interference from maternal antibody, and the vaccine is safe to use in pregnant bitches during all trimesters. One dose is effective for 1 full year. Adult dogs can receive a one-dose intranasal vaccination at the same time as their puppies or at the time they receive their annual vaccinations. Puppies being prepared for shipment or entering a boarding kennel or veterinary hospital should be vaccinated at least 1 to 2 weeks before admission or shipping. Other infectious tracheobronchitis vaccines available include inactivated B. bronchiseptica parenteral vaccine. Parenteral vaccines are administered as two doses 2 to 4 weeks apart. When dogs younger than 4 months of age are being vaccinated, they should be revaccinated after reaching the age of 4 months. Initial vaccination of puppies with parenteral vaccines is recommended at or about 6 to 8 weeks of age.

Canine Leptospirosis Vaccine

Canine leptospirosis had previously been characterized in natural infections into hepatonephric syndromes caused by two organisms: Leptospira interrogans serovars canicola and icterohaemorrhagiae. These serovars typically produced acute hemorrhagic diathesis, subacute icterus, or subacute uremia. Widespread use of a bivalent vaccine against L. canicola and L. icterohaemorrhagiae has led to a significant decreased incidence of leptospirosis in the general dog population. However, environmental and reservoir changes in canine leptospirosis have introduced other Leptospira organisms into the general dog population, such as L. grippotyphosa, L. pomona, L. hardjo, and L. bratislava, emerging as the most commonly identified serovars recognized in infected dogs. Currently, only one manufacturer has canine leptospirosis vaccine that contains the serovars icterohaemorrhagiae, canicola, grippotyphosa, and pomona in its product.

Canine Coronavirus Vaccine

Canine coronavirus (CCV) causes highly contagious viral enteritis and spreads rapidly through kennels of susceptible dogs. The primary source of infection is infectious fecal material. The incubation period is short, about 1 to 4 days. Dogs can have CCV and CPV-2 infections simultaneously. Other enteric microflora, such as Clostridium perfringens, Campylobacter spp., and Salmonella spp., may increase the severity of the enteric illness. Animals usually present with a sudden onset of diarrhea and sometimes vomiting. The fecal material is characteristically orange in color, is very malodorous, and infrequently contains blood. Loss of appetite and lethargy are also common signs. Fever is not constant, and leukopenia is not a recognized feature. CCV vaccines are available for protection against CCV infection. The manufacturers recommend that the CCV vaccine be included as part of the routine vaccination program.

Canine *Giardia* Vaccine

Enteric infections with *Giardia* spp. are extremely common in dogs younger than 6 months and in immunocompromised dogs. Recurrent diarrhea problems are usually the primary presenting complaint. The *Giardia* vaccine acts at the intestinal level against both the trophozoite and cyst forms of the *Giardia* spp. The *Giardia* vaccine is most effective when dogs are continuously exposed to contaminated *Giardia*-laden water.

Canine Lyme Borreliosis Vaccine

Canine Lyme borreliosis is caused by the pathogenic strains of *Borrelia burgdorferi*. The organism has been recovered from many different tissues of infected ticks, and simply crushing an infected tick between unprotected fingers has been reported to lead to human infection. *B. burgdorferi* infections in dogs cause fever, depression, anorexia, stiffness, and most important, joint pain and swelling. Joints frequently involved include the carpus, digits, shoulder, elbow, tarsus, and stifle joints. Many affected dogs will have multiple episodes of lameness with intervals between episodes of 1 to 23 months. Lymphadenopathy and renal disease have also been seen in dogs with Lyme borreliosis. Canine *B. burgdorferi* vaccine, available as killed bacteria and recombinant products, provides protection against canine Lyme borreliosis. According to the manufacturers currently marketing canine *B. burgdorferi* vaccines, puppies 9 to 12 weeks of age or older should receive two doses administered at 2- to 3-week intervals; with annual revaccination a single dose is recommended.

Heartworm Preventive Therapy

Puppies can be started on a heartworm preventive program, using ivermectin, milbemycin oxime, or selamectin at 6 to 8 weeks of age. Heartworm preventive products that contain ivermectin (Heartgard 30 and Heartgard 30 Plus, MSD AGVET) should be administered orally at the recommended minimum dose level of 6 μg/kg of body weight at monthly dosing intervals. A heartworm preventive product that contains milbemycin oxime (Interceptor, Ciba Animal Health) should be administered orally at the recommended minimal dose level of 0.5 mg/kg of body weight at monthly dosing intervals. A heartworm preventive product that contains selamectin (Revolution, Pfizer Animal Health) should be topically applied on the skin at the recommended minimum dose level of 6 mg/kg of body weight at monthly dosing intervals. Heartworm preventive products of any type should be started in heartworm areas 1 month before the beginning of mosquito season and continue until 2 months after the season's end.

Routine Dog Care

The external ear canal of dogs may accumulate cerumen (wax), exudate, or debris as a result of inflammation or a foreign body, such as a grass awn, which requires foreign body removal and cleaning. Certain dog breeds, particularly poodles, Bedlington terriers, and Kerry blue terriers, also may accumulate excessive hair in the external ear canal. The initial step in the treatment of any external ear problem is complete and thorough cleaning of the entire external ear canal. Frequently, thorough cleaning requires the administration of a short-acting general anesthetic or heavy tranquilization. The first step in ear canal cleaning is to remove any hair that is present, and if excessive wax is present, instill a cerumenolytic agent, such as dioctyl sodium succinate, to soften the wax. Remove excessive wax and debris by using a soft rubber bulb syringe and a dilute disinfectant solution to lavage the external ear canal. Use balls of cotton and cotton applicator sticks to carefully wipe the wax from the external ear canal. Suspend some of the debris in mineral oil, and smear on a microscope slide to be examined under low power for the presence of ear mites.

Gently clean the horizontal ear canal with extreme caution to prevent damage to the eardrum (also known as the tympanic membrane) or the packing of debris deep into the horizontal portion of the ear canal. If the ear canal contains exudate, obtain a sample for cytologic smear and bacterial culture before instrumentation and cleaning. The least affected external ear canal should be cleaned thoroughly before the worst ear canal. If bacterial growth is observed, the technician should obtain antibiotic sensitivity. If the cytologic smear reveals the presence of yeast, initiate appropriate treatment for yeast infection. Some veterinarians prefer to use pulsating streams of water from a dental hygiene apparatus to clean the external ear canal. Add approximately 5 ml of povidone-iodine or chlorhexidine solution to approximately 236 to 384 ml of warm water. Apply the stream of water in a rotating motion and directed parallel to the external ear canal. Catch the excess water and debris in an ear irrigation basin or similar vessel. An inexpensive alternative is the use of a rubber bulb syringe to manually loosen debris and aid in flushing the ear canal. This technique is not recommended if the tympanic membrane is not intact. Regardless of the technique employed to clean the external ear canal, another ear canal examination should be performed to evaluate the completeness of the ear cleaning. Once the ear canal is sufficiently clean, carefully dry the canal with clean cotton swabs, and instill the initial dose of prescribed ear preparation.

Nail trimming is an important general care technique. Excessive nail length results in altered walking and the potential accentuation of lameness problems. Excessively long nails are more likely to be traumatically torn away from their attachment site. Untrimmed nails can also become ingrown, usually into the animal's foot pads, resulting in cellulitis or abscess formation. A sturdy, durable nail trimmer is required for nail trimming. Common types of nail trimmers are made by Resco and White. In order to avoid cutting nails too short in dogs, hold the cutting surface of the nail trimmer parallel to the plantar surface of the digital foot pads, and cut the nail in that plane. Because many animals resent handling of their feet for nail trimming, it is a good practice to routinely give a nail trim to any animal anesthetized or tranquilized for any procedure. If the owner is receptive, it is desirable to provide instructions in the proper technique of nail trimming so that this routine task can be done at home.

Owner Education

Owner education pamphlets on a variety of dog-related topics can be sent home with the owner each time the dog is seen for the preventive health program. Generally, only one or two well-written owner education pamphlets are given to the owner at the end of each office visit.

Veterinarians and veterinary technicians are in an excellent position to provide meaningful owner educational services and thus make owners more aware of their dogs and the associated responsibilities of dog ownership. By offering consultative advice and providing owners with educational pamphlets, the veterinary technician not only assists owners who are seeking medical treatment for their dogs but serves a vital role in educating people in the community.

PREVENTIVE HEALTH PROGRAM FOR CATS

For most cats, a preventive health program begins when they are first presented to the veterinary hospital or clinic at 8 to 10 weeks of age. A general outline of one preventive health program and its implementation for cats is presented in Box 11-2.

BOX 11-2   GENERAL OUTLINE OF A PREVENTIVE HEALTH PROGRAM FOR CATS

I. First office visit for health program (usually at 8-10 wk of age)
   A. Perform a general physical examination, and record body weight
   B. Check for external parasites and dermatophytes, and initiate appropriate therapy for the following:
      1. Fleas and ear mites (*Otodectes cyanotis*)
      2. Mange mites, especially *Notoedres cati, Demodex* spp., and *Cheyletiella* spp.
      3. Dermatophytes, particularly *Microsporum* spp. and *Trichophyton mentagrophytes*
   C. Perform fecal examination, including both direct smear and flotation
   D. Administer anthelmintics, such as pyrantel pamoate for roundworms and hookworms and praziquantel or epsiprantel for tapeworms (if present)
   E. Vaccinate with FVRC-P,*† *Chlamydia,‡* FeLV§ (possibly test for FeLV/FIV before initial FeLV vaccination), FIP,|| *Bordetella,* and *Giardia* vaccines
   F. Advise on nutrition and routine grooming
   G. Provide owner with client education pamphlets on topics such as the following:
      1. Identification, treatment, and control of fleas, ticks, and ear mites
      2. Benefits of vaccination for FeLV infection
      3. Management of normal and abnormal cat behaviors
      4. Grooming "how to" and nutrition
   H. Fill in kitten's health record for the owner
II. Second office visit for health program (usually at 12-14 wk of age)
   A. Perform a general physical examination, and record body weight
   B. Check for external parasites and dermatophytes, and initiate appropriate therapy for the following:
      1. Fleas and ear mites (*O. cyanotis*)
      2. Mange mites, especially *N. cati, Demodex* spp., and *Cheyletiella* spp.
      3. Dermatophytes, particularly *Microsporum* spp. and *T. mentagrophytes*
   C. Perform fecal examination, including both direct smear and flotation
   D. Administer anthelmintics, such as pyrantel pamoate for roundworms and hookworms and praziquantel or epsiprantel for tapeworms (if present)
   E. Vaccinate with FVRC-P,* *Chlamydia,‡* FeLV,§ rabies, FIP,|| *Bordetella,* and *Giardia* vaccines
   F. Adjust nutrition and grooming procedures
   G. Provide owner with client education pamphlets on topics such as the following:
      1. Identification, treatment, and control of fleas, ticks, and ear mites
      2. Benefits of vaccination for FeLV infection
      3. Dental, skin, nail, and ear care
      4. Management of normal and abnormal cat behaviors
      5. Exercise and its importance
      6. Recommendations for spaying, castration, and declawing
   H. Fill in kitten's health record for owner
III. Subsequent visits for health program (usually annual visits)
   A. Perform a general physical examination, and record body weight
   B. Check for external parasites and dermatophytes, and initiate appropriate therapy for the following:
      1. Fleas and ear mites (*O. cyanotis*)
      2. Mange mites, especially *N. cati, Demodex* spp., and *Cheyletiella* spp.
      3. Dermatophytes, particularly *Microsporum* spp. and *T. mentagrophytes*
   C. Perform fecal examination (fecal flotation)
   D. Administer an anthelmintic according to fecal examination findings
   E. Vaccinate with FVRC-P,* *Chlamydia,‡* FeLV,§ rabies, FIP,|| *Bordetella,* and *Giardia* vaccines
   F. Adjust nutrition and grooming procedures
   G. Provide owner with client education pamphlets on topics such as the following:
      1. Identification, treatment, and control of fleas, ticks, and ear mites
      2. Benefits of vaccination for FeLV infection
      3. Dental, skin, nail, and ear care
      4. Management of normal and abnormal cat behaviors
      5. Exercise and its importance
      6. Recommendations for spaying, castration, and declawing
   H. Fill in cat's health record for owner

FeLV, Feline leukemia virus; *FIV,* feline immunodeficiency virus; *FIP,* feline infectious peritonitis.
*FVRC-P refers to the use of a vaccine to protect against feline viral rhinotracheitis (FVR); feline calicivirus infection (C); and feline panleukopenia (P).
†Cats being prepared for shipment or entering a boarding kennel or veterinary hospital or clinic should be vaccinated at least 1-2 wk before admission or shipment.
‡The vaccine currently available apparently produces effective protection only against *Chlamydia psittaci* infections. As with other vaccines for respiratory ailments, complete protection is not afforded; however, clinical signs of conjunctivitis or upper respiratory tract disease, if they do occur, can be restricted to short courses and are mild.
§Refers to the use of a vaccine to protect against FeLV infection. FeLV and FIV are administered subcutaneously in healthy kittens or older cats as two doses, with the second dose given 3 or 4 wk after the first. Annual revaccination with a single dose is recommended.
||The Primucell-FIP Vaccine (Pfizer Animal Health) is administered intranasally to healthy cats. Primary vaccination with two doses should be given with the second dose administered 3-4 wk after the first, and single-dose annual revaccination is recommended.

Physical Examination

Clinical evaluation of a cat initially focuses on taking a complete case history and performing the physical examination (see Chapter 2). Basic information about the animal, such as breed, age, and gender, as well as owner concerns or complaints, is essential to the case history. After obtaining the case history, the physical examination should be conducted in a systematic manner. Body weights as part of the physical examination are recorded for several reasons. First, the weight provides information needed for dispensing medication; and second, it is an immediate indicator of the nutritional status of the animal. The body weight of a growing kitten steadily increasing at each office revisit is an indication that the kitten is receiving adequate nutrition.

Vaccinations

In general, vaccination for the prevention of feline panleukopenia, feline viral rhinotracheitis, feline calicivirus infection, and rabies are the most important (see Box 11-2). In addition to regularly scheduled feline panleukopenia, feline viral rhinotracheitis, feline calicivirus infection, and rabies vaccinations, other vaccinations can be incorporated into the preventive health program, as detailed below.

Feline Panleukopenia Vaccine

Feline panleukopenia (FPL) is a highly contagious parvoviral disease that is characterized by an explosive, short course and a moderate to high mortality. The FPL virus causes fever, anorexia, diarrhea, weight loss, and leukopenia. This is the canine parvovirus infection of cats. There are many excellent vaccines for immunization of cats against FPL. If these are used correctly and at the proper age, cats should be completely protected against FPL. Several slightly different programs for the immunization of cats against FPL have been presented during the past few years. The safest recommendation is to start the vaccination program at an early age and to vaccinate kittens at frequent intervals until they are at least 16 weeks of age. This might prove beneficial in certain circumstances, such as in catteries or colonies, in which kittens could be vaccinated at 6 weeks of age, followed by repeated vaccinations at 3-week intervals until the cats are 16 weeks old. However, most kittens presented to the veterinarian are vaccinated with a minimum of two or possibly three vaccinations, with yearly or every 3 years revaccination using a single dose of vaccine.

Feline Viral Rhinotracheitis Vaccine

Feline viral rhinotracheitis (FVR) is a highly contagious viral disease of cats characterized by sudden onset of conjunctivitis, lacrimation, and nasal discharge accompanied by sneezing. The FVR vaccines may be obtained as a single vaccine or in combination with feline calicivirus vaccine. The FVR vaccines produce significant protection against FVR disease following vaccination and, as such, should be part of the routine vaccination program. The FVR vaccines are administered subcutaneously or intramuscularly to kittens at 9 weeks and again at 12 weeks of age, with yearly or every 3 years revaccination using a single dose of vaccine.

Feline Calicivirus Vaccine

Feline calicivirus-induced respiratory infections occur among cats in about the same frequency as FVR. Fever, lacrimation, and serous nasal discharges that soon become purulent first manifest the disease. The fever tends to fluctuate after its initial appearance. Sneezing, anorexia, and depression are common. Ulceration of the glossal epithelium or the palatine mucosa occurs with FCV infection and may be the only sign of infection. The FCV vaccines may be obtained as a single vaccine or in combination with feline viral rhinotracheitis vaccine. The FCV vaccines produce significant protection against FCV disease following vaccination and, as such, should be part of the routine vaccination program. The FCV vaccines are administered subcutaneously or intramuscularly to kittens at 9 weeks and again at 12 weeks of age, with yearly or every 3 years revaccination using a single dose.

Rabies Vaccine

Rabies is an acute infectious encephalitis characterized by altered behavior, aggressiveness, progressive paralysis, and in most species by death. The rabies virus is usually present in the saliva of infected mammals, and in nature it is usually transmitted by a bite. Rabies most commonly affects the dog, cat, fox, skunk, raccoon, bobcat, coyote, bat, mongoose, and other small carnivorous mammals that are mainly responsible for transmission of the disease. Three phases of clinical signs are recognized in cat rabies as in dog rabies: the prodromal, excitative, and paralytic. For more details concerning rabies refer to the section entitled Rabies Vaccine earlier in the chapter.

Inactivated rabies virus vaccines are currently licensed and available for preexposure vaccination of cats against rabies. All rabies vaccines are administered in 1-ml doses intramuscularly at one site in the thigh or subcutaneously. The vaccines are licensed for immunization of cats 3 months of age and older. Cats vaccinated between 3 and 12 months of age should receive a second dose 1 year later. The vaccines are licensed for 1- to 3-year effective immune periods.

Feline *Chlamydia* Vaccine

Although feline chlamydiosis is not as prevalent as feline viral rhinotracheitis or feline calicivirus infections, it is evident that in some cat populations chlamydial infection is contributing to persistent conjunctivitis and upper respiratory tract disease. The vaccines currently available produce effective protection only against *Chlamydia psittaci* infections. As with other vaccines for respiratory ailments, complete protection is not afforded; however, clinical signs of conjunctivitis or upper respiratory tract disease, if they do occur, can be restricted to short courses and are mild. Vaccines for feline chlamydiosis can be obtained from several manufacturers in various combinations with the more traditional feline vaccine components.

Feline Leukemia Virus Vaccine

Domestic cats may become infected with several retroviruses, including feline leukemia virus (FeLV) and feline immunodeficiency virus (FIV). The FeLV and FIV cause a large number of diverse disease syndromes, including lymphoreticular and myeloid neoplasms, anemias, immune-mediated disorders, and an immunodeficiency syndrome somewhat similar to human acquired immunodeficiency syndrome (AIDS). Excretion of FeLV occurs primarily by way of salivary secretions, although the virus is also present in respiratory secretions, blood, milk, feces, and urine.

Several FeLV vaccines are currently available to protect cats of all ages against FeLV infection. The vaccines are administered subcutaneously in healthy kittens or older cats as two doses, with the second dose given 3 or 4 weeks after the first. Annual revaccination with a single dose is recommended. According to the manufacturers, the vaccines cause no interference with simultaneous vaccinations against rabies, panleukopenia, and respiratory viruses. The vaccines also do not affect red blood cell or white blood cell counts, weight gain, reproductive capability, or FeLV testing in kittens vaccinated as young as 6 weeks of age. In viremic cats, vaccines may produce minimal antibody responses and cats remain viremic, but they are not harmed by the vaccination. No FIV vaccine is available yet.

Feline Infectious Peritonitis Vaccine

Coronavirus infection is of significant importance in the world's cat population. As many as 80% to 90% of cats are affected within individual catteries and multiple-cat households. Cats are susceptible to infection with several different strains of feline coronavirus. Depending on which strain of feline coronavirus is involved, clinical signs may range from asymptomatic infection to gastrointestinal disease of varying severity to widespread fibrinous serositis and disseminated vasculitis commonly referred to as feline infectious peritonitis (FIP). In FIP disease, young cats may be seen with nonspecific signs, such as nonresponsive fever, anorexia, lethargy, chronic weight loss, and pale mucous membranes. Icterus may be seen in cases with severe liver involvement. Recurring episodes of diarrhea and constipation may be observed. Progressive abdominal distention occurs from an accumulation of ascitic fluid in the peritoneal cavity.

A first-generation, temperature-sensitive FIP virus (TS-FIPV) vaccine that affords protection against FIP virus challenge has become available (Primucell-FIP Vaccine, Pfizer Animal Health). This TS-FIPV vaccine contains attenuated whole coronavirus and is recommended by the manufacturer to be administered intranasally to healthy cats. Primary vaccination with two doses should be given, with the second dose administered 3 to 4 weeks after the first, and annual revaccination with a single dose is recommended. Cats vaccinated twice intranasally with the TS-FIPV vaccine have not developed a febrile response, nor have they had any blood dyscrasia indicative of FIP disease. Likewise, vaccinated pregnant cats, dexamethasone-suppressed cats, feline leukemia virus-infected cats, and feline enteric coronavirus-infected cats have not shown a febrile response or any blood dyscrasia.

Feline *Bordetella* Vaccine

Feline *Bordetella bronchiseptica* (FeBb) is a primary respiratory pathogen in cats of all ages and breeds. FeBb should be considered in instances of feline upper respiratory infection and pneumonia. Even cats not showing signs of respiratory disease can be significant carriers of FeBb organisms. FeBb is readily transmitted from cat to cat, especially those living in multiple-cat environments. Proper husbandry, good nutrition, parasite control, and control of other respiratory infections can help reduce the risks of a cat contracting FeBb. A FeBb-specific vaccination can also help prevent acute infections. This vaccine is the only licensed product available for protection of cats against FeBb infection. The FeBb vaccine is safe in kittens as young as 4 weeks old and will not cause any serious disease or pneumonia through its use. The vaccine is also safe in pregnant queens.

Feline Fungal Vaccine

Common flaky skin lesions referred to as ringworm are usually caused by *Microsporum canis*. A *M. canis* killed fungal vaccine that affords protection against ringworm-induced skin lesions is available. The vaccine is used in cats 4 months of age and older as an aid in the prevention and treatment of clinical signs of disease caused by *M. canis*. Vaccination has not been demonstrated to eliminate *M. canis* organisms from infected cats. Primary vaccination

with two doses should be given, with the second dose administered 3 to 4 weeks after the first; revaccination with a single dose every 6 months is recommended.

Feline *Giardia* Vaccine

Enteric infections with *Giardia* spp. are common in cats younger than 6 months and in immunocompromised cats. Recurrent diarrhea problems are usually the primary presenting complaint. The *Giardia* vaccine acts at the intestinal level against both the trophozoite and cyst forms of the *Giardia* spp. The *Giardia* vaccine is most effective when cats are continuously exposed to contaminated *Giardia*-laden water.

Vaccine-Associated Sarcomas

Epidemiologic evidence has shown a strong association between administration of inactivated feline vaccines, specifically FeLV and rabies, and subsequent soft tissue sarcoma development at vaccine sites. The prevalence of sarcoma development after vaccination has been reported as 1 case per 10,000 vaccines administered. Sarcomas are believed to develop in areas of prolonged inflammation produced by the vaccine products. Although epidemiologic studies have failed to identify specific brands of FeLV or rabies vaccines involved, this may be due to the relatively low incidence of sarcomas found, large numbers of brands of FeLV and rabies vaccines administered to cats, or other factors. The vaccine component most commonly thought to be associated with local postvaccinal inflammation is the vaccine's adjuvant. Adjuvants of different types are used in many but not all inactivated feline vaccines.

Recommendations include a change in vaccination site location, decreased use of polyvalent vaccines, use of nonadjuvanted vaccines, and not overvaccinating. The most important recommendation for prevention of vaccine-associated tumors would appear to be not to overvaccinate. The National Vaccine-Associated Sarcoma Task Force studying vaccine site tumors recommends that no vaccine be given in the interscapular space, that rabies vaccine be administered in the distal right rear leg, that FeLV vaccine be administered in the distal left rear leg, and that all other vaccines be administered in the right shoulder. It appears that intramuscular administration and subcutaneous administration both result in local inflammation and sarcoma production. Subcutaneous sites are recommended for all vaccines because they will result in earlier detection of these sarcomas. The reasoning behind this is not based on prevention but rather earlier diagnosis and potentially a higher cure rate when treated surgically.

It is also recommended that any vaccine site lumps present after 3 months from the time of vaccination be removed but only after a biopsy. A biopsy will determine the magnitude of the surgery, such as lumpectomy versus extensive tissue removal. Do not excise the mass before biopsy. Attempts at simple excision of these tumors are seldom curative and ultimately lead to local recurrence with a more difficult second attempt. Rear leg amputation has a higher rate of cure than surgery in the interscapular space for vaccine-associated sarcomas. Most chemotherapeutic attempts result in partial responses, but some complete responses have been observed with these drugs. Although the vast majority of vaccine-associated tumors are only locally invasive, approximately 1 out of 20 will metastasize to the lungs or other sites.

Heartworm Preventive Therapy

Kittens can be started on a heartworm preventive program using ivermectin at 6 to 8 weeks of age. A heartworm preventive product that contains ivermectin (Heartgard for

Cats, MSD AGVET) should be administered orally at the recommended minimum dose level of 24 µg/kg of body weight at monthly dosing intervals. Heartworm preventive products of any type should be started in heartworm areas 1 month before the beginning of mosquito-season and continue until 2 months after the season's end.

Routine Cat Care

The external ear canal of cats may accumulate cerumen (wax), exudate, or debris as a result of inflammation or ear mites, which requires cleaning. The initial step in the treatment of any external ear problem is complete and thorough cleaning of the entire external ear canal. Remove excessive wax and debris by using a soft rubber bulb syringe and a dilute disinfectant solution to lavage the external ear canal. Use balls of cotton and cotton applicator sticks to carefully wipe the wax and debris from the external ear canal. Suspend some of the debris in mineral oil and smear on a microscope slide to be examined under low power for the presence of ear mites.

Gently clean the horizontal ear canal with extreme caution to prevent damage to the eardrum (tympanic membrane) or the packing of debris deep into the horizontal portion of the ear canal. If the ear canal contains exudate, obtain a sample for cytologic smear and bacterial culture before instrumentation and cleaning. Remember that the least affected external ear canal should be cleaned thoroughly before the worst ear canal. If bacterial growth is observed, obtain antibiotic sensitivity. If the cytologic smear reveals the presence of yeast, initiate appropriate treatment for yeast infection. Once the ear canal is sufficiently clean, carefully dry the canal with clean cotton swabs, and instill the initial dose of prescribed ear preparation.

Nail trimming is an important general care technique. A sturdy, sharp nail trimmer is required for nail trimming. Common types of nail trimmers are made by Resco and White. In cats, expose the nails by grasping the paw between the thumb and index finger and slide the skin on the dorsum of the paw away from the nails. Once the nails are exposed, trim them. Because many animals resent handling of their feet for nail trimming, it is a good practice to routinely give a nail trim to any animal anesthetized or tranquilized for any procedure. If the owner is receptive, it is desirable to provide instructions in the proper technique of nail trimming so that this routine task can be done at home.

Owner Education

Owner education pamphlets on a variety of cat-related topics can be sent home with the owner each time the cat is seen for the preventive health program. Generally, only one or two well-written owner education pamphlets are given to the owner at the end of each office visit.

Veterinarians and veterinary technicians are in an excellent position to provide meaningful owner educational services and thus make owners more aware of their cats and the associated responsibilities of cat ownership. By offering consultative advice and providing owners with educational pamphlets, the veterinary technician not only assists owners who are seeking medical treatment for their cats but also serves a vital role in educating people in the community.

PREVENTIVE HEALTH PROGRAM FOR HORSES

A preventive health program for horses should be designed to meet the specific needs of the individual animal or herd. Such programs generally vary from one stable to another and from one veterinary practice to another depending on expected exposures, management styles, and personal preferences of attending veterinarians and horse owners. An example of one preventive health program for horses is outlined in Box 11-3.

Physical Examination

New additions to a stable or an established herd should be Coggins' test–negative for equine infectious anemia (EIA) and quarantined for 1 month before entering the general population. During this time, the first physical examination for the preventive health program can be performed. The physical examination should be completed in a manner that will gain the confidence of the new horse and allow the veterinarian to establish the current health status and soundness of the animal. These observations are then recorded in a permanent medical record at the stable.

In addition to recording the rectal temperature, respiratory rate, and heart rate before and after light exercise, the thorax should be thoroughly auscultated. The horse should be weighed or the body weight estimated with a thoracic tape, both to establish a weight baseline and for future reference in calculating doses. Both eyes should be completely examined for soundness. A dental examination should reveal incisor malocclusion and abnormal wear of the cheek teeth. Similarly, the musculoskeletal system and skin should be examined. Physical examination should be repeated at 2- to 3-month intervals as part of the preventive health program for horses of all ages. Obtaining a history and performing a physical examination are discussed in Chapter 2.

Vaccinations

A variety of vaccines approved for use in healthy horses can be obtained from manufacturers as individual components or in various combinations. Table 11-1 lists some vaccines currently available.

Horses that are immunologically naive or that have an unknown immunization history should receive an initial immunization, which is then followed in 4 weeks by a second immunization.

Technician Note

Horses that are immunologically naive or have an unknown immunization history should receive an initial immunization followed in 4 weeks by a second immunization.

Further booster vaccinations can be administered as indicated by the risk of exposure and the veterinarian's experience with the vaccine. In rare instances, anaphylactoid reactions associated with the use of any vaccine can occur. These life-threatening crises must be handled quickly. Accordingly, it is essential that epinephrine be available for the treatment of anaphylactoid reactions. Other complications, such as fever, lameness, and swelling, or abscess formation at the injection site, may also occur with the routine use of these vaccines. The horse owner should always be apprised of these possibilities before any vaccine is administered. Common diseases and vaccines used as an aid in disease prevention are discussed below.

Tetanus Vaccines

Tetanus, or lockjaw, is a disease characterized by muscular rigidity that may culminate in death from respiratory arrest or convulsions. Tetanus is caused by the toxins produced by the anaerobic bacterium *Clostridium tetani*. Active im-

Box 11-3   GENERAL OUTLINE OF A PREVENTIVE HEALTH PROGRAM FOR HORSES

FIRST QUARTER: JANUARY-MARCH

All Horses

Deworm at least every 8 wk. Exercise care in choice of anthelmintics for mares in the third trimester. Begin deworming foals at 2 mo of age.

Trim feet every 6 wk. More frequently in foals requiring limb correction.

Dentistry: check twice yearly and float teeth as needed. Remove wolf teeth in 2-yr-olds and retained caps in 2-, 3-, and 4-yr-olds.

Immunize for respiratory disease: influenza, strangles, and rhinopneumonitis.

In southeastern United States immunize for equine encephalitis.

Stallions

Perform complete breeding examination. Maintain stallions under lights if being used for early breeding.

Pregnant Mares

Immunize with tetanus toxoid, and open sutured mares 30 days prepartum. Develop a colostrum bank. Ninth-day breeding only for mares with normal foaling history and normal reproductive tract. Wash udders of foaling mares.

Open Mares

Maintain under lights if being used for early breeding. Perform daily teasing. Perform reproductive tract examination during estrus. Mares should not be too fat but in gaining condition during breeding season.

Newborn Foals

Dip navel in disinfectant.

Carefully, give a cleansing enema at birth.

Administer tetanus prophylaxis if indicated by history.

Perform immunoglobulin test at 12-24 hr.

SECOND QUARTER: APRIL-JUNE

All Horses

Deworm at least every 8 wk.

Trim feet every 6 wk. Do not forget the foals and yearlings.

Dentistry: check teeth and remove or float teeth as needed.

Immunize for equine encephalomyelitis. Administer appropriate vaccine boosters.

Stallions

Maintain an exercise program.

Monitor the semen quality.

Broodmares

Palpate at 21, 42, and 60 days after successful breeding.

Foals

Creep-feed the foals, and provide free-choice minerals. Immunize at 3 mo of age.

Group foals by gender and size when weaned.

THIRD QUARTER: JULY-SEPTEMBER

All Horses

Deworm at least every 8 wk. Clip and sweep the pastures.

Trim feet every 6 wk. Continue corrective trimming on foals.

Dentistry: check teeth and remove or float teeth as needed.

Stallions

Maintain an exercise program.

Broodmares

Administer rhinopneumonitis boosters to pregnant mares according to manufacturer's labeled directions. Administer appropriate vaccine boosters to foals and yearlings.

Check condition of mare's udder at weaning, and reduce amount of feed given until milk flow is reduced.

Foals

Administer all appropriate immunizations. Provide free-choice minerals. Maintain a protein supplement in creep feeders.

FOURTH QUARTER: OCTOBER-DECEMBER

All Horses

Deworm at least every 8 wk. Select anthelmintics appropriate for season.

Trim feet every 6 wk. Continue corrective trimming on foals.

Dentistry: check teeth and remove or float teeth as needed.

Stallions

Continue exercise program.

Check immunizations.

Perform breeding examination.

Broodmares

Confirm pregnancy.

Begin treating open mares.

Check immunizations.

---

munity to tetanus is produced by administration of a tetanus toxoid, which is a purified, inactivated toxin of *C. tetani.*

Tetanus antitoxin is produced by hyperimmunization of donor horses with tetanus toxoid. Administration of antitoxin to unvaccinated horses induces immediate protection, which lasts approximately 2 weeks.

Equine Encephalomyelitis Vaccine

Equine encephalomyelitis is a viral neurologic disease of horses caused by eastern, western, and Venezuelan viruses.

These viruses are maintained in nature by bird and animal reservoirs and are transmitted to horses by biting insects. Venezuelan equine encephalomyelitis occurs in South and Central America but has not been diagnosed in the United States for several years. The trivalent vaccine is commonly used for horses in states bordering Mexico to create a buffer zone, which may prevent spread of Venezuelan equine encephalomyelitis into the United States. The clinical signs of equine encephalomyelitis may be as subtle as fever and partial anorexia or as severe as marked depression, convulsions, and death. Death rate varies

TABLE 11-1   EQUINE VACCINES

Vaccine	Manufacturer	Type	EEE	WEE	VEE	EVA	A/1	A/2	EHV-1	EHV-4	TT	TAT	Rb	St	Anx	PHF	Bot	Rota
Anthrax vaccine	Colorado Serum	–													X			
Arvac	Fort Dodge Animal Health	MLV				X												
		I	X	X							X							
Bot Tox-B	Neogen	I			X												X	
Caphalovac VENT	Bayer	I	X	X	X						X							
Double EFT	Fort Dodge Animal Health	I	X	X			X	X			X							
Double EFT + EHV	Fort Dodge Animal Health	I	X	X			X		X	X	X							
Double ET	Fort Dodge Animal Health	I	X	X							X							
Encephaloid IM	Franklin	I	X	X														
Encephaloid I.M.	Fort Dodge Animal Health	I	X	X														
Encephalomyelitis vaccine	Colorado Serum	I	X	X														
Encevac with Havlogen	Bayer	I	X	X														
Encevac-T with Havlogen	Bayer	I	X	X							X							
Encevac-T + Havlogen	Bayer	I	X	X							X							
Encevac TC-4 with Havlogen	Bayer	I	X	X			X	X			X							
Encevac-TC-4 + Havlogen	Bayer	I	X	X			X	X			X							
Equicine II with Havlogen	Bayer	I					X	X			X							
Equigard	Boehringer Ingelheim	I							X	X								
Equigard-Flu	Boehringer Ingelheim	I					X		X	X								
Equiloid	Fort Dodge Animal Health	I	X	X							X							
Equiloid	Franklin	I	X	X							X							
Equine Rotavirus Vaccine	Fort Dodge Animal Health	I																X
Equivac EHV 1/4	Fort Dodge Animal Health	I							X	X								
EWT	Schering-Plough	I	X	X			X				X							
EWTF	Schering-Plough	I	X	X			X				X							
Flu Avert I.N.	Heska	I						X										
Flumune	Pfizer Animal Health	I					X	X										
Flumune EWT	Pfizer Animal Health	I	X	X			X	X			X							
Fluvac	Fort Dodge Animal Health	I					X	X										
Fluvac	Franklin	I					X	X										
Fluvac EHV-1/4	Fort Dodge Animal Health	I					X	X	X									
Fluvac EHV 4/1	Franklin	I					X	X	X	X								
Fluvac EWT Plus	Fort Dodge Animal Health	I	X	X			X	X			X							
Fluvac EWT	Franklin	I	X	X			X	X			X							
Fluvac Plus	Fort Dodge Animal Health	I					X	X										
Fluvac-T	Fort Dodge Animal Health	I					X	X			X							
Inflogen 3	Fort Dodge Animal Health	I					X	X			X							
Inflogen-3 + EHV	Fort Dodge Animal Health	I					X	X	X	X								
Mystique	Bayer	I														X		
Mystique II	Bayer	I												X		X		
PHF-Vax	Schering-Plough	I														X		

Continued

TABLE 11-1   EQUINE VACCINES—CONT'D

Vaccine	Manufacturer	Type	Vaccine Components															
			EEE	WEE	VEE	EVA	A/1	A/2	EHV-1	EHV-4	TT	TAT	Rb	St	Anx	PHF	Bot	Rota
PHF-Vax + 4	Schering-Plough	I	X	X			X	X			X					X		
Pinnacle I.N.	Fort Dodge Animal Health	M												X				
Pneumabort-K + 1b	Fort Dodge Animal Health	I							X									
Pneumabort-K + 1b	Franklin	I							X									
Potomacguard	Fort Dodge Animal Health	I														X		
Potomacguard	Franklin	I														X		
Potomacguard EWT	Fort Dodge Animal Health	I	X	X							X					X		
Potomacguard EWT	Franklin	I	X	X							X					X		
Prestige + Havlogen	Bayer	I							X	X								
Prestige II + Havlogen	Bayer	I					X	X	X	X								
Prodigy + Havlogen	Bayer	I							X									
Rabguard-TC	Pfizer Animal Health	I											X					
Rabvac 3	Fort Dodge Animal Health	I											X					
Rhino-Flu	Pfizer Animal Health	MLV, I					X	X	X									
Rhino-Flu	Pfizer Animal Health	MLV					X	X	X									
Rhinomune	Pfizer Animal Health	MLV							X									
RM Equine Ehrlichia + Imrab	Merial	I											X			X		
RM Equine EWTF	Merial	I	X	X			X	X			X							
RM Imrab 3	Merial	I											X					
RM Imrab Bovine Plus	Merial	I											X					
Strepguard with Havlogen	Bayer	I												X				
Super-Tet with Havlogen	Bayer	I									X							
Tetanus Antitoxin Equine Origin	Bayer	Antitoxin										X						
Tetanus toxoid	Fort Dodge Animal Health	I									X							
Tetanus toxoid	Colorado Serum	I									X							
Tetanus toxoid	Franklin	I									X							
Tetanus toxoid—concentrated	Colorado Serum	I									X							
Tetanus toxoid—concentrated	Professional Biological	I									X							
Tetmune EW	Pfizer Animal Health	I	X	X							X							
Tetnogen	Fort Dodge Animal Health	I									X							
Tetnogen-AT	Fort Dodge Animal Health	Antitoxin										X						
Tetanus antitoxin	Sanofi	Antitoxin										X						
Tetanus antitoxin	Fort Dodge Animal Health	Antitoxin										X						
Tetanus antitoxin	Professional Biological	Antitoxin										X						
Tetanus antitoxin	Coopers Animal Health	Antitoxin										X						
Tetanus antitoxin	Colorado Serum	Antitoxin										X						
Triple E	Fort Dodge Animal Health	I	X	X	X													
Triple EFT	Fort Dodge Animal Health	I	X	X	X		X	X			X							
Triple EFT + EEV	Fort Dodge Animal Health	I	X	X	X		X	X	X	X	X							
Triple ET	Fort Dodge Animal Health	I	X	X	X						X							
Unitox	Bayer	I									X							

Anx, anthrax; *A/1*, Equine influenza myxovirus A–equi 1; *A/2*, equine influenza myxovirus A–equi 2; *Bot*, botulism; *EEE*, eastern equine encephalomyelitis; *EHV-1*, equine herpesvirus 1; *EHV-4*, equine herpesvirus 4; *EVA*, equine viral arteritis; *I*, inactivated; *MLV*, modified live virus; *PHF*, Potomac horse fever; *Rb*, rabies; *Rota*, rotavirus; *St*, strangles; *TAT*, tetanus antitoxin; *TT*, tetanus toxoid; *VEE*, Venezuelan equine encephalomyelitis; *WEE*, western equine encephalomyelitis.

with the type of virus infection, but it may range from 19% to 90%.

The equine encephalomyelitis vaccines currently used for active immunization are inactivated virus vaccines. They should be administered annually before the season of the biting insects. In areas where winter freezes are not common, semiannual vaccinations may be advisable. In endemic areas, frequent boosters (every 2 to 4 months) are recommended.

Equine Rhinopneumonitis Vaccine

Equine herpesvirus (EHV) has caused sporadic infections and death in horses throughout the world. Four distinct equine herpesviruses have been identified: EHV-1, EHV-2, EHV-3, and EHV-4. EHV-1 and EHV-4 cause rhinopneumonitis. EHV-1 has been exclusively associated with the neurologic form of rhinopneumonitis, and it is also responsible for late-gestation abortions, stillbirths, and weak neonatal foals that fail to survive. EHV-4 is most frequently associated with upper respiratory tract disease in young horses and rarely is a cause of abortion.

Until recently all herpesvirus vaccines were prepared from EHV-1 virus. Vaccination of foals and young horses to prevent EHV-4 infections relied on the induction of cross-reactive antibody to EHV-1. The resulting immunity was short-lived and requires revaccination at 2- to 3-month intervals. New vaccines have been introduced that contain both EHV-4 and EHV-1 and are approved for use in the prevention of respiratory infection.

Pregnant mares should be vaccinated during the fifth, seventh, and ninth months of gestation using an inactivated EHV-1 vaccine. Total protection from abortion cannot be achieved.

Equine Influenza Vaccine

Equine influenza has a worldwide distribution and is frequently seen in mobile populations of horses. Disease outbreaks usually occur in horses 1 to 3 years of age after mixing with infected horses at the racetrack or show ground. Equine influenza may also occur in older horses, but the clinical signs are mild. Infection is characterized by fever, depression, anorexia, muscle soreness, and coughing.

The equine influenza viruses of importance in the United States are A/1 and A/2. Currently available vaccines contain inactivated virus that includes both A/1 and A/2 strains. Intranasal vaccines may increase protection via local immunity to A/2 strains. The duration of protective immunity from vaccination is short-lived, requiring revaccination every 2 to 3 months during periods of exposure (showing and racing).

Strangles Vaccine

Strangles is a respiratory disease caused by infection with the bacterium *Streptococcus equi*. Strangles is easily transmitted through direct contact with mucopurulent discharges from infected horses or from contaminated fomites, such as feeding utensils, buckets, or other equipment. Strangles is characterized by sudden onset of fever and upper respiratory catarrh, followed by acute swelling and abscess formation in submaxillary, submandibular, and retropharyngeal lymph nodes.

Technician Note

Strangles is easily transmitted through direct contact with mucopurulent discharges from infected horses or from contaminated fomites.

Several inactivated subunit M protein vaccines and one inactivated whole-cell bacterium are available for intramuscular injection as an adjunct to the prevention of strangles. All these vaccines may cause postinjection reactions or abscesses at the site of administration. Because of these side effects, vaccination for strangles is performed only in immunologically naive horses with a high likelihood of exposure. Vaccination is not 100% effective for preventing disease but does often reduce the severity and incidence of disease. Most recently, live strangles vaccine for intranasal administration has become available.

Equine Viral Arteritis Vaccine

Equine viral arteritis infection may cause subclinical to severe disease and death. The disease is characterized by fever, depression, nasal discharge, lacrimation, coughing, and limb swelling. Several attenuated live-virus vaccines have been developed. Only one serotype of virus appears to be relevant to the protection of horses. The vaccine induces partial to complete protection against the clinical signs of disease, but virus replication will still occur after virus challenge.

Potomac Horse Fever Vaccine

Potomac horse fever (equine monocytic ehrlichiosis) is caused by *Ehrlichia risticii*. It is most prevalent in eastern states, particularly near large waterways, but has been identified in many regions of the United States and in other countries. Although not proven, aquatic insect vectors and snails are as the tick is believed to be involved in disease transmission. An approved vaccine is now available for use in the prevention of Potomac horse fever, and its use should be considered in areas where the disease is known to occur.

Botulism Vaccine

The currently available equine vaccine is a *Clostridium botulinum* type B toxoid. The most common application for this vaccine is vaccination of mares 30 days before foaling for prevention of shaker foal syndrome in areas of high incidence. However, *C. botulinum* type C is an important pathogen in some regions of North America.

Anthrax Vaccine

Anthrax vaccines for use in horses are currently available but are not widely used except where a genuine risk is identified.

Rabies Vaccine

An approved rabies vaccine is available for use in horses. Routine preexposure immunization should be considered in areas where wildlife rabies is epizootic.

Dental and Hoof Care

Many directional instructions from rider or driver reach the horse through the mouth. If the bit causes pain, the instructions given to the horse may be compromised. Wolf teeth cause extreme pain in some horses, especially with broken snaffle, overdraw checks, and gag bits. The mouth of the young horse should be examined, and if wolf teeth are present, they should be removed before training begins. Deciduous premolars that are retained and enamel points on cheek teeth may also cause pain in the mouth that interferes with normal feeding and willing response to the bit. In addition, the cheek teeth should be checked visually or by palpation for evidence of abnormal wear, such as wave mouth, step mouth, or shear mouth. Of course, all dental examinations should include inspection for malocclusion.

The role of the veterinarian and veterinary technician in hoof care is largely advisory and can be given via owner education pamphlets.

> **Technician Note**
>
> The role of the veterinarian and veterinary technician in hoof care is largely advisory and can be given via owner education pamphlets.

Frequent hoof cleaning helps in the prevention of thrush. Keeping the hooves trimmed short and maintaining the correct hoof-pastern axis also helps to prevent excess stress on tendons and ligaments of the limb. In foals that are born splay-footed or pigeon-toed, frequent hoof trimming can often correct these conformation problems.

Parasites

It is well accepted that the athletic horse cannot perform at its genetic peak potential if handicapped with a heavy parasite load. Likewise, the pet horse may not maintain its well-kept appearance if burdened with external or internal parasites. Therefore close attention to parasite control is extremely important in a preventive health program. Complete records are essential to ensure that each horse is being adequately treated. If all horses pastured together are not dewormed at the same time, the parasite control program will be ineffective. Pastured horses should be dewormed every 60 days or more often. Fecal flotations should be evaluated on 10% of the herd immediately before and 7 days after dewormer administration. Egg counts greater than 200 eggs/g before deworming indicate that the interval between treatments is too long. The presence of ova after treatment indicates resistance. Horses that never eat grass may not require deworming as often. Feed additives are available that are lethal to developing housefly and stable fly larvae in treated horse feces (but not effective against existing adult flies). These types of feed additives are to be used with caution, because they are organophosphate larvicides with possible side effects if used concomitantly with other pharmaceutical products. Chapter 7 contains additional information on parasitology.

Nutrition

Horses have evolved as forage eaters, and their digestive system is able to handle most forages, such as grass and hay, efficiently. Further, metabolic diseases (e.g., laminitis, azoturia) are less likely to occur in horses fed diets composed primarily of roughage rather than grain. Therefore the horse's diet should contain mostly high-quality roughage with just enough grain supplement to maintain body weight. The amount of grain in the diet should increase as the amount of work performed increases. A complete vitamin and mineral supplement is usually added to the diet to ensure that the proper balance of vitamins and minerals is received. All guesswork can be removed from ration planning if there is a feed analysis laboratory in proximity. Equine nutrition is discussed in Chapter 15.

Sanitation

Advice on sanitation may be communicated orally to the horse owner or given via owner education pamphlets. The fact that diseases are effectively spread from sick horses to susceptible horses via shared feed and water buckets, bits, twitches, chain shanks, trailers, and clothing is sometimes overlooked. Water and feed buckets should be cleaned and sanitized on a regular basis. Proper manure disposal is also important in preventing the spread of infectious diseases and in controlling flies and internal parasites.

PREVENTIVE HEALTH PROGRAM FOR CATTLE

Preventive health programs for beef and dairy cattle are generally based on recommendations of the consulting veterinarian and the specific needs of the herd and the herdsman. Accordingly, the development of a vaccination program should be based on several factors. First, it is important to have a knowledge of disease conditions present within a given herd and of the disease conditions present in the surrounding area. This should be based on accurate diagnosis or previous diagnoses of diseases in the specific herd and surrounding herds. Second, it is necessary to be familiar with the management procedures present on a farm that allow for a vaccination program designed around the working patterns of the herd; this is especially true for a cow-calf operation. Third, the population variances within a herd should be known. Vaccine choices and the frequency of their use can vary depending on such factors as open versus closed herds, source of new replacement cattle, and feeding practices. General approaches to preventive health programs for beef and dairy cattle are presented in Tables 11-2 and 11-3, respectively.

Vaccinations

Vaccines that may be included in preventive health programs for beef and dairy cattle can be obtained from manufacturers as individual components or in various combinations. Table 11-4 lists some vaccines currently available. Diseases for which vaccines are more frequently used in these preventive health programs are detailed below.

Campylobacteriosis (Vibriosis) Vaccine

Campylobacteriosis is a venereal disease of cattle caused by the bacterium *Campylobacter fetus* subsp. *veneralis*. Infection of a cow's genital tract often causes early embryonic death resulting in temporary infertility, repeat breeding, delayed conception, and a prolonged calving interval. The *Campylobacter* organism may be transmitted during coitus or by artificial insemination with contaminated semen. Systemic vaccination can cure as well as prevent *Campylobacter* infection. Vaccination of breeding stock is highly recommended.

Trichomoniasis Vaccine

Trichomoniasis, caused by *Tritrichomonas foetus,* is a venereal protozoal disease of cattle that manifests as infertility, relatively early abortion, or pyometra. It causes virtually no systemic illness, so its presence within a herd may go undetected for long periods, resulting in substantial economic losses. The bull serves as an asymptomatic carrier, and the organism may be spread by natural breeding or artificial insemination with contaminated semen. Inactivated protozoal vaccines are now commercially available to aid in prevention of the disease in known problem herds.

Leptospirosis Vaccine

Leptospirosis is a common bacterial disease of cattle that may cause hemolytic anemia, nephritis, decreased milk production, and late-term abortion. Abortion is probably the most economically significant effect of the disease. Regular vaccination of breeding animals for leptospirosis is strongly encouraged. Heifers should be vaccinated two or three times at monthly intervals before breeding and again

TABLE 11-2	GENERAL OUTLINE OF A PREVENTIVE HEALTH PROGRAM FOR BEEF CATTLE

COW-CALF HERD RECOMMENDATION*

At Birth
Ingestion of colostrum within the first few hours after birth is an important factor in baby calf survival. Immunize with oral bovine rotavirus and coronavirus enteric disease vaccine if a calf diarrhea problem exists in the herd.

1- to 3-Mo-Old Calves
Immunize with a seven-way clostridial diseases product. Deworm with commercial product that is safe for calves.

Preweaning Calves
Deworm with broad-spectrum commercial dewormer, and immunize as follows:

Immunizing Vaccine	Age for Vaccine Administration
Brucella abortus, strain RB-51 (calfhood vaccination—replacement heifers only)	4-12 mo
Clostridial diseases:	5-6 mo
Clostridium perfringens types C and D, C. chauvoei, C. novyi, C. septicum, C. sordellii	
IBR and PI-3 respiratory diseases (inactivated vaccines only)	5-6 mo, booster at 12-13 mo
BVD (inactivated vaccines only)	5-6 mo, booster at 12-13 mo
BRSV	5-6 mo, booster at 12-13 mo

Weaning Calves
Deworm with broad-spectrum commercial dewormer, and treat for lice and grubs. Castrate the bull calves. Immunize with Pasteurella (optional) and Haemophilus (optional) vaccines.

Prebreeding Replacement Heifers
Deworm with broad-spectrum commercial dewormer, and treat for lice. Immunize as follows:

Immunizing Vaccine	Time of Vaccine Administration
IBR and PI-3 respiratory diseases	10-12 mo
Clostridial diseases:	10-12 mo
C. perfringens types C and D, C. novyi, C. septicum, C. sordellii, C. chauvoei	
BVD	10-12 mo
BRSV	10-12 mo
Leptospirosis	10-12 mo
Campylobacteriosis	10-12 mo

Prebreeding Cows
Deworm with broad-spectrum dewormer, and treat for lice. Immunize for leptospirosis and campylobacteriosis.

Precalving Cows
Immunize as follows:

Immunizing Vaccine	Time of Vaccine Administration
IBR and PI-3 respiratory diseases (inactivated vaccines only)	Before calving
BVD (inactivated vaccines only)	Before calving
BRSV	Before calving
Bovine rotavirus and coronavirus enteric diseases	Before calving
Escherichia coli enteric disease	Before calving
Clostridial diseases:	Before calving
C. perfringens types C and D, C. chauvoei, C. novyi, C. septicum, C. sordellii	

Bulls
Deworm annually with broad-spectrum dewormer, and treat for lice and grubs. Immunize as recommended for prebreeding replacement heifers annually (see the above section).

FEEDLOT RECOMMENDATIONS†

On Arrival into the Feedlot
Deworm with a broad-spectrum dewormer, and immunize for IBR, PI-3, BVD, BRSV, and clostridial diseases (use seven-way vaccine). Inactivated IBR, PI-3, and BVD vaccines are the safest.

Three-Four Wk After Arrival into the Feedlot
Implant a commercial implant product. Treat for lice and grubs. Administer booster immunizations if necessary. Abort the heifers if necessary. Castrate and dehorn if necessary.

BRSV, Bovine respiratory syncytial virus; BVD, bovine virus diarrhea; IBR, infectious bovine rhinotracheitis; PI-3, parainfluenza-3.
*Other optional vaccines that may be incorporated into the immunization program, depending on individual herd needs and diseases endemic to the area, include anthrax and anaplasmosis.
†Other optional vaccines that may be incorporated into the immunization program, depending on individual herd needs and diseases endemic to the area, include Haemophilus somnus, Pasteurella spp., leptospirosis, and anthrax.

TABLE 11-3	GENERAL OUTLINE OF A PREVENTIVE HEALTH PROGRAM FOR DAIRY CATTLE*

CALVES

At Birth

Immunize with bovine rotavirus and coronavirus enteric disease vaccine,† and administer *Escherichia coli* enteric disease vaccine orally.

Weaning Age (about 2 mo) to Breeding Age (about 15 mo)

Immunizing Vaccine	*Age for Vaccine Administration*
Brucella abortus, strain RB-51 (calfhood vaccination—replacement heifers only)	4-12 mo
Clostridial diseases:	2-4 mo, booster in 2 wk
Clostridium perfringens types C and D, *C. chauvoei, C. novyi, C. septicum, C. sordellii*	
IBR and PI-3 respiratory diseases	4-6 mo, booster at 12-13 mo
BVD	6-8 mo, booster at 12-13 mo
BRSV	6-8 mo, booster at 12-13 mo
Leptospirosis	4-6 mo, booster in 2 wk
Campylobacteriosis	4-6 mo, booster at 12-13 mo

FRESH COWS AND HEIFERS

Immunizing Vaccine	*Time of Vaccine Administration*
IBR and PI-3 respiratory diseases (inactivated vaccines only)	30 days postpartum
Bovine virus diarrhea (BVD) (inactivated vaccines only)	30 days post partum
BRSV	30 days postpartum
Leptospirosis	30 days postpartum
Campylobacteriosis	30 days postpartum

DRY COWS AND BRED HEIFERS

The goal of dry cow immunization is to provide optimal protection for the newborn calf.

Immunizing Vaccine	*Time of Vaccine Administration*
Leptospirosis	At time of dry-off
Bovine rotavirus and coronavirus enteric diseases†	At time of dry-off, booster in 2-3 wk
Escherichia coli enteric disease†	At time of dry-off, booster in 2-3 wk
Clostridial diseases:	At time of dry-off, booster in 2-3 wk
C. perfringens types C and D, *C. chauvoei, C. novyi, C. septicum, C. sordellii*	

BRSV, Bovine respiratory syncytial virus; *BVD*, bovine virus diarrhea; *IBR*, Infectious bovine rhinotracheitis; *PI-3*, parainfluenza-3.

*Other vaccines that may be incorporated into the vaccination program, depending on individual herd needs and diseases endemic to the area, include *Haemophilus somnus, Pasteurella* spp., *Salmonella* spp., *Clostridium haemolyticum,* anthrax, and anaplasmosis.

†Use if problem of neonatal calf diarrhea exists on the farm.

at midgestation of the first pregnancy. Because leptospirosis bacterins produce immunity of fairly short duration, annual (prebreeding) or twice-annual (prebreeding and midgestation) boosters should be given.

Brucellosis Vaccine

Brucellosis is caused by the organism *Brucella abortus.* Infection in the cow can result in late-term abortion, usually around 5 months or more into gestation, and shedding of the *Brucella* organisms in the milk. In bulls, infection results in orchitis, impaired fertility, and shedding of *Brucella* organisms in the semen. Brucellosis is a serious human health hazard, and known *Brucella*-positive reactors must be culled from the herd and vaccination of replacement heifers performed. *B. abortus* strain RB-51 vaccine is a live bacterial product that confers long-term, cell-mediated protection. Vaccination of females only is accomplished using a strain RB-51 live culture vaccine. Age of vaccination of heifers is critical and usually determined by federal and state regulations. Vaccination is only undertaken by accredited veterinarians or state or federal animal health representatives. Care must always be exercised when using *B. abortus* vaccine, because accidental injection,

ingestion, or exposure through broken skin or mucous membranes can result in human brucellosis (undulant fever).

Anthrax Vaccine

Anthrax is caused by the bacterium *Bacillus anthracis* and is characterized by septicemia and sudden death. Often, affected animals are simply found dead without any prior signs of illness. Typically, the dead animal exhibits blood oozing from body orifices, failure of blood to clot, and absence of rigor mortis. Differential diagnosis of sudden death in cattle may include anthrax, lightning strike, clostridial diseases, and anaplasmosis. Vaccination for anthrax is recommended 4 weeks before anticipated exposure in those areas where the disease has historically been a problem.

Clostridial Vaccines

Clostridial infections are caused by bacteria that live as spores in the soil. These spores may be ingested by cattle as they graze or may enter the body via wound contamination. The more common clostridial infections encountered in cattle are described briefly in the following paragraphs.

Text continued on p. 289

TABLE 11-4 CATTLE VACCINES

Vaccine	Manufacturer	Type	Anthrax	BRSV	Brucella spp.	BVD Type I	BVD Type II	Campylobacter	Clostridium chauvoei	Clostridium haemolyticum	Clostridium novyi	Clostridium perfringens C and D	Clostridium septicum	Clostridium sordellii	Coronavirus	Escherichia coli	Fusobacterium	Haemophilus somnus	IBR	Leptospira spp.	Moraxella bovis	Papillomavirus	Pasteurella haemolytica	Pasteurella multocida	PI-3	Rabies	Rotavirus	Salmonella	Staphylococcus spp.	Tetanus Toxoid	Tritrichomonas
4 Once	Bayer Corporation	MLV/K		X		X													X				X	X	X						
7-Way	Aspen	K							X		X	X	X	X																	
7-Way/Somnus	Aspen	K							X		X	X	X	X				X													
Absolute M	AgriLabs	K																					X	X							
Alpha 7/MB	Bio-Ceutic	K							X		X	X	X	X							X										
Alpha 7	Boehringer Ingelheim	K							X		X	X	X	X																	
Alpha-7/MB	Anchor	K							X		X	X	X	X							X										
Alpha-CD	Anchor	K										X																			
Alpha-CD	Bio-Ceutic	K										X																			
Anthrax Spore Vaccine	Colorado Serum	Live	X																												
Bar Somnus-2P	Anchor	K																X					X	X							
Bar Somnus	Anchor	K																X													
Bar-4 Somnus	Anchor	K																X					X	X	X						
Bar-4	Anchor	K																	X				X	X	X						
Bar-Vac 7/Somnus	Anchor	K							X		X	X	X	X				X													
Bar-Vac 7+Redwater (8-Way)	Anchor	K							X	X	X	X	X	X																	
Bar-Vac CD/T	Anchor	K										X																		X	
Bar-Vac-7/MB	Boehringer Ingelheim	K							X		X	X	X	X							X										
BovEye	Pfizer Animal Health	K																			X										
Bovi-K 4	Pfizer Animal Health	MLV/K		X		X													X						X						
Bovine 3	Durvet	MLV				X													X						X						
Bovine 4	Durvet	MLV/K		X		X													X						X						
Bovine 4KL	Durvet	MLV/K		X		X													X						X						
Bovine 8	Durvet	MLV/K				X													X	X					X						
Bovine 9	Durvet	MLV/K				X		X											X	X					X						
Bovine Past H-1	Durvet	K																					X								
Bovine Pili Shield	Grand	K														X															
Bovine Rhinotracheitis-Parainfluenza3 Vaccine	Colorado Serum	MLV																	X						X						
Bovine rhinotracheitis-virus diarrhea-parainfluenza-3 vaccine	Colorado Serum	MLV				X													X						X						
BoviShield 3	Pfizer Animal Health	MLV				X													X						X						
BoviShield 4	Pfizer Animal Health	MLV		X		X													X						X						

BRSV, Bovine respiratory syncytial virus; *BVD*, bovine virus diarrhea; *IBR*, infectious bovine rhinotracheitis; *K*, killed (inactivated); *MLV*, modified live virus; *PI-3*, parainfluenza-3.

Continued

TABLE 11-4 Cattle Vaccines—cont'd

Vaccine	Manufacturer	Type	Anthrax	BRSV	Brucella spp.	BVD Type I	BVD Type II	Campylobacter	Clostridium chauvoei	Clostridium haemolyticum	Clostridium novyi	Clostridium perfringens C and D	Clostridium septicum	Clostridium sordellii	Coronavirus	Escherichia coli	Fusobacterium	Haemophilus somnus	IBR	Leptospira spp.	Moraxella bovis	Papillomavirus	Pasteurella haemolytica	Pasteurella multocida	Pl-3	Rabies	Rotavirus	Salmonella	Staphylococcus spp.	Tetanus Toxoid	Tritrichomonas
BoviShield 4+L5	Pfizer Animal Health	MLV/K		X		X	X												X	X					X						
BoviShield BRSV	Pfizer Animal Health	MLV		X																X											
BoviShield IBR	Pfizer Animal Health	MLV																	X												
BoviShield IBR-BRSV-LP	Pfizer Animal Health	MLV/K		X															X	X											
BoviShield IBR-BVD	Pfizer Animal Health	MLV				X													X												
BoviShield IBR-BVD-BRSV-LP	Pfizer Animal Health	MLV/K		X		X													X	X											
BoviShield IBR-P13-BRSV	Pfizer Animal Health	MLV		X															X	X					X						
BRD-1	Franklin	K				X																									
Breed-Back-10	Bio-Ceutic	MLV/K				X		X										X	X	X					X						
Breed-Back-10	Anchor	MLV/K				X		X										X	X	X					X						
BRSV Vac	Bayer Corporation	MLV		X																											
BRSV Vac 3	Bayer Corporation	MLV		X															X						X						
BRSV Vac 4	Bayer Corporation	MLV		X		X													X						X						
BRSV Vac 9	Bayer Corporation	MLV/K		X		X													X	X					X						
BRSV Vac F3Lp	Bayer Corporation	MLV/K		X		X													X	X											
Brucella abortus vaccine (strain RB-51)	Professional Biological	Live			X																										
Calf-Guard	Pfizer Animal Health	MLV													X												X				
Campylobacter fetus bacterin—bovine	Colorado Serum	K						X																							
CattleMaster 4	Pfizer Animal Health	MLV/K		X		X													X						X						
CattleMaster 4+L5	Pfizer Animal Health	MLV/K		X		X													X	X					X						
CattleMaster 4+VL5	Pfizer Animal Health	MLV/K		X		X		X											X	X					X						
CattleMaster BVD-K	Pfizer Animal Health	K				X																									
Cattle-Vac 4	Durvet	K		X		X													X						X						
Cattle-Vac 4-Somnus	Durvet	K		X		X												X	X						X						
Cattle-Vac 8	Durvet	K				X													X	X					X						
Cattle-Vac 9	Durvet	K		X		X													X	X					X						
Cattle-Vac 9-Somnus	Durvet	K		X		X												X	X	X					X						
C-D Toxoid	Anchor	K										X																			
C&D Toxoid	Aspen	K										X																			
Clostri Shield BCD	Grand	K										X																			
Clostri Shield C	Grand	K										X																			
Clostridial 7-Way	AgriLabs	K							X	X	X	X	X	X																	

Continued

Product	Manufacturer	Type	Clostridial 7-Way plus Somnumune	Clostridial 8-Way	Clostridium chauvoei-septicum bacterin	Clostridium chauvoei-septicum—Pasteurella haemolytica-multocida	Clostridium chauvoei-septicum-novyi-sordellii bacterin	Clostridium perfringens types C&D—tetanus toxoid	Clostridium perfringens types C&D toxoid
Conquest 5K (oil base)	Aspen	K							
Conquest-1+3	Aspen	MLV/K							
Conquest-4K+H.S.	Aspen	K							
Conquest-4KW	Aspen	K							
Conquest-4KW+H.S.	Aspen	K							
Conquest 5K+VL5 (oil base)	Aspen	K							
Conquest-8K	Aspen	K							
Conquest-9K	Aspen	K							
Conquest-9K+H.S.	Aspen	K							
Conquest-4K	Aspen	K							
Cow-Vac 9	Aspen	MLV/K							
Defensor	Pfizer Animal Health	K							
Discovery-4+PH/somnus	Franklin	K							
Discovery-3	Franklin	K							
Discovery-3 VL5	Franklin	K							
Discovery-3L5	Franklin	K							
Discovery-4	Franklin	K							
Discovery-4L5	Franklin	K							
Discovery-4+PH	Franklin	K							
Discovery-4+somnus	Franklin	K							
Discovery-4L5+PH	Franklin	K							
Discovery-4L5+somnus	Franklin	K							
E. coli Bac	AgriLabs	K							
Electroid 7 vaccine	Schering-Plough	K	X	X					
Electroid D	Schering-Plough	K		X					
Elite 4-HS	Anchor	K							
Elite 4-HS	Bio-Ceutic	K							
Elite 4	Anchor	K							
Elite 4	Bio-Ceutic	K							
Elite 9-HS	Anchor	K							
Elite 9-HS	Bio-Ceutic	K							
Elite 9	Boehringer Ingelheim	K							

TABLE 11-4 Cattle Vaccines—cont'd

Vaccine	Manufacturer	Type	Anthrax	BRSV	Brucella spp.	BVD Type I	BVD Type II	Campylobacter	Clostridium chauvoei	Clostridium haemolyticum	Clostridium novyi	Clostridium perfringens C and D	Clostridium septicum	Clostridium sordellii	Coronavirus	Escherichia coli	Fusobacterium	Haemophilus somnus	IBR	Leptospira spp.	Moraxella bovis	Papillomavirus	Pasteurella haemolytica	Pasteurella multocida	Pl-3	Rabies	Rotavirus	Salmonella	Staphylococcus spp.	Tetanus Toxoid	Tritrichomonas
ENDOVAC-Bovi	Immvac	K																										X			
Express 4-HS	Anchor	MLV/K		X		X												X	X						X						
Express 4-HS	Bio-Ceutic	MLV/K		X		X												X	X						X						
Express 4	Anchor	MVL/K		X		X													X						X						
Express 4	Bio-Ceutic	MLV/K		X		X													X						X						
Fermicon 7/Somnugen	Bio-Ceutic	K							X		X		X	X				X													
Fermicon CD/T	Bio-Ceutic	K										X																		X	
Fermicon CD	Bio-Ceutic	K										X																			
Fermicon-7+Haemolyticum (8-Way)	Bio-Ceutic	K							X	X	X	X	X	X																	
Fortress 7	Pfizer Animal Health	K							X	X	X	X	X	X																	
Fortress 8	Pfizer Animal Health	K							X	X	X	X	X	X																	
Fortress CD	Pfizer Animal Health	K										X																			
Fusion 3	Merial	MLV/K				X													X						X						
Fusion 4	Merial	MLV/K		X		X													X						X						
Herd-Vac 3	Bayer Corporation	MLV				X													X						X						
Herd-Vac 3 S	Bayer Corporation	MLV/K				X												X	X						X						
Herd-Vac 4	Bayer Corporation	MLV/K		X		X												X	X						X						
Herd-Vac 4KL	Bayer Corporation	MLV/K		X		X													X						X						
Herd-Vac 8	Bayer Corporation	MLV/K				X													X	X					X						
Herd-Vac 9	Bayer Corporation	MLV/K				X		X											X	X					X						
Heritage 2	Bayer Corporation	MLV				X													X												
Heritage 1	Bayer Corporation	MLV																	X												
Horizon 1+Vac 3	Bayer Corporation	MLV/K		X		X													X						X						
Horizon 10	Bayer Corporation	MLV/K		X		X		X											X	X					X						
Horizon 4	Bayer Corporation	MLV/K		X		X													X						X						
Horizon 9	Bayer Corporation	MLV/K		X		X													X	X					X						
IBL vaccine	Aspen	MLV/K				X													X	X					X						
IBP vaccine	Aspen	MLV				X													X						X						
IBP-L5 vaccine	Aspen	MLV/K				X													X	X					X						
IBP-RS vaccine	Aspen	MLV		X		X													X						X						
IBP-RS-L5 vaccine	Aspen	MLV/K		X		X													X	X					X						
IBP-SomnuMune vaccine	Aspen	MLV/K				X												X	X						X						

Product	Manufacturer	Type
IBR Plus 4-Way	Merial	MLV/K
IBR vaccine	Aspen	MLV
IBR-BVD-PI3/Somnugen 2-P	Bio-Ceutic	MLV/K
IBR-BVD-PI3/Bar Somnus 2-P	Anchor	MLV/K
IBR-PI3/Bar Somnus 2-P	Anchor	MLV/K
IL vaccine	Aspen	MLV/K
IP-RS vaccine	Aspen	MLV
I-Site	AgriLabs	K
J Vac 4L5	Merial	K
J Vac	Merial	K
J Vac L5	Merial	K
J-5 bacterin	Pharmacia & UpJohn	K
Journey 3	Merial	MLV/K
Journey 4	Merial	MLV/K
Lepto 5	AgriLabs	K
Lepto 5	Bayer Corporation	K
Lepto 5	Durvet	K
Lepto 5	Merial	K
Lepto 5	Premier Farmtech	K
Lepto 5 vaccine	Aspen	K
Lepto Shield 5	Grand	K
Lepto-5	Colorado Serum	K
Leptoferm-5	Pfizer Animal Health	K
LeukoTox	A.A.H.	K
LeukoTox 1	A.A.H	K
Leuko-Tox M	A.A.H.	K
Leuko-Tox MTD	A.A.H.	K
Lysigin	Bio-Ceutic	K
MastiGuard	Bayer Corporation	K
Maxi-Guard Pinkeye bacterin	Addison	K
Nasalgen IP vaccine	Schering-Plough	MLV
Ocu-guard MB	Anchor	K
Ocu-guard MB	Bio-Ceutic	K
Odyssey-3 L.V.	AgriLabs	MLV
Odyssey-3 L.V.+V.L.5	AgriLabs	MLV/K
Odyssey-3 L.V.+SomnuMune	AgriLabs	MLV/K
Odyssey-3 L.V.+K. BRSV	AgriLabs	MLV/K
Odyssey-3 L.V.+Lepto 5	AgriLabs	MLV/K
Odyssey-4 L.V.K.	AgriLabs	MLV/K
Once PMH	Bayer Corporation	MLV
OneShot	Pfizer Animal Health	K
P.H. Bac 1	AgriLabs	K
Papillomune	Biomune	K
Pasteurella haemolytica multocida bacterin	Colorado Serum	K

283

Continued

TABLE 11-4 CATTLE VACCINES—CONT'D

Vaccine Components

Vaccine	Manufacturer	Type	Anthrax	BRSV	Brucella spp.	BVD Type I	BVD Type II	Campylobacter	Clostridium chauvoei	Clostridium haemolyticum	Clostridium novyi	Clostridium perfringens C and D	Clostridium septicum	Clostridium sordellii	Coronavirus	Escherichia coli	Fusobacterium	Haemophilus somnus	IBR	Leptospira spp.	Moraxella bovis	Papillomavirus	Pasteurella haemolytica	Pasteurella multocida	PI-3	Rabies	Rotavirus	Salmonella	Staphylococcus spp.	Tetanus Toxoid	Tritrichomonas
Piliguard E. coli-1	Schering-Plough	K														X															
Piliguard Pinkeye + 7	Schering-Plough	K							X		X	X	X	X							X										
Piliguard Pinkeye-1	Schering-Plough	K																			X										
Pinkeye Shield XT4	Grand	K																			X										
Pinkeye-3	Aspen	K																			X										
Pneumosyn-H	Franklin	K																					X								
Pneumosyn-H + somnus	Franklin	K																X					X								
PolySal B	A.A.H.	K																										X			
PregGuard 9	Pfizer Animal Health	MLV/K				X		X											X	X					X						
Premier 8	Bayer Corporation	K				X													X	X					X						
Premier 4	Bayer Corporation	K		X		X													X						X						
Premier 4-SomnuTech	Bayer Corporation	K		X		X												X	X						X						
Premier 9	Bayer Corporation	K		X		X													X	X					X						
Premier 9-SomnuTech	Bayer Corporation	K		X		X												X	X	X					X						
Presponse HM	Fort Dodge Animal Health	K																					X	X							
Presponse SQ	Fort Dodge Animal Health	K																					X								
Pre-Vent 6	AgriLabs	K						X												X											
Pro-Bac 1	A.V.L.	K																					X								
Pro-Bac 3	A.V.L.	K																					X	X				X			
Pro-Bac 3R	A.V.L.	K																X					X	X							
Pro-Bac 4	A.V.L.	K																X					X	X				X			
ProSystem 3	Intervet	K														X															
Pulmo-guard PH-1	Anchor	K																					X								
Pulmo-guard PH-1	Bio-Ceutic	K																					X								
Pulmo-guard PH-M	Anchor	K																					X	X							
Pulmo-guard PH-M	Bio-Ceutic	K																					X	X							
Pyramid 4+Presponse SQ	Fort Dodge Animal Health	MLV/K		X		X													X				X		X						
Pyramid MLV 3	Fort Dodge Animal Health	MLV				X													X						X						
Pyramid MLV 4	Fort Dodge Animal Health	MLV		X		X													X						X						
Pyramid IBR	Fort Dodge Animal Health	MLV																	X												
Quadraplex/Somnugen	Bio-Ceutic	K																X					X	X	X						
Rabdomun vaccine	Schering-Plough	K																								X					
Rabguard-TC	Pfizer Animal Health	K																								X					

Product	Manufacturer	Type
Redwol with Spur	Bayer Corporation	K
Reliant 3	Merial	MLV
Reliant 4	Merial	MLV/K
Reliant 8	Merial	MLV/K
Reliant IBR	Fort Dodge Animal Health	MLV
Reliant IBR/BVD	Merial	MLV
Reliant IBR/BVD/Lepto	Merial	MLV/K
Reliant IBR/Lepto	Merial	MLV/K
Reliant IBR/PI3	Merial	MLV
Reprotec-T	Franklin	K
Reprotec-TVL5	Franklin	K
Respishield 4	Merial	K
Respishield 4 L5	Merial	K
ResProMune 4+VL5	AgriLabs	K
ResProMune 10	AgriLabs	K
ResProMune 4 IBP-BRSV	AgriLabs	K
ResProMune 4+SomnuMune	AgriLabs	K
ResProMune 8 IBP-Lepto 5	AgriLabs	K
ResProMune 9	AgriLabs	K
Resvac 4/Somubac	Pfizer Animal Health	MLV/K
Resvac BRSV/Somubac	Pfizer Animal Health	MLV/K
RM Imrab 3	Merial	K
RM Imrab Bovine Plus	Merial	K
RXV Alliance 4	RXV	MLV/K
RXV Alliance IBP	RXV	MLV
RXV Alliance IBP+Somnus	RXV	MLV/K
RXV Alliance IBP+Lepto 5	RXV	MLV/K
RXV Antidote One PHM	RXV	MLV
RXV HerdVac 4KL	RXV	MLV/K
RXV Rescue 3K-L 5 Vac	RXV	K
RXV Rescue 4K Vac	RXV	K
RXV Rescue 4K-L 5 Vac	RXV	K
RXV Rescue 4K-Somnus Vac	RXV	K
RXV Rescue 4K-L5 Somnus	RXV	K
RXV Vac Alliance Cow-Vac 9	RXV	MLV/K
RXV Vac Alliance SommuMune	RXV	K
RXV Vac IBR-BVD-PI3	RXV	MLV
RXV Vac Lepto 5	RXV	K
RXV Vac Vibrio-Lepto 5	RXV	K
Salmo Shield T	Grand	K
Salmo Shield TD	Grand	K
Salmonella dublin-typhimurium bacterin	Colorado Serum	K
ScourGuard 3 (K)/C	Pfizer Animal Health	K
ScourGuard 3 (K)	Pfizer Animal Health	K

Continued

TABLE 11-4 CATTLE VACCINES—CONT'D

Vaccine Components

Vaccine	Manufacturer	Type	Anthrax	BRSV	Brucella spp.	BVD Type I	BVD Type II	Campylobacter	Clostridium chauvoei	Clostridium haemolyticum	Clostridium novyi	Clostridium perfringens C and D	Clostridium septicum	Clostridium sordellii	Coronavirus	Escherichia coli	Fusobacterium	Haemophilus somnus	IBR	Leptospira spp.	Moraxella bovis	Papillomavirus	Pasteurella haemolytica	Pasteurella multocida	PI-3	Rabies	Rotavirus	Salmonella	Staphylococcus spp.	Tetanus Toxoid	Tritrichomonas
Siteguard G	Schering-Plough	K							X	X	X	X																			
Siteguard MLG vaccine	Schering-Plough	K							X	X	X	X	X	X																	
Somato-Staph	Anchor	K																											X		
Somato-Staph/Lepto-5	Anchor	K																		X									X		
Somnu Shield	Grand	K																X													
Somnu Shield XT	Grand	K																X													
SomnuMune	AgriLabs	K																X													
SomnuMune	Aspen	K																X													
SomnuTech	Bayer Corporation	K																X													
Somubac	Pfizer Animal Health	K																X													
StayBred VL5	Pfizer Animal Health	K					X													X											
Super-Tet with Havlogen	Bayer Corporation	K																												X	
Syn Shield	Grand	K		X																											
Tetanus toxoid—concentrated	Colorado Serum	K																												X	
Tetanus toxoid—concentrated	Prof. Biological	K																												X	
Tetanus toxoid—unconcentrated	Colorado Serum	K																												X	
Tetguard	Boehringer Ingelheim	K																												X	
Tetnogen	Fort Dodge Animal Health	K																												X	
Titanium 3	AgriLabs	MLV				X	X												X												
Titanium 3+BRSV LP	AgriLabs	MLV/K		X		X	X												X	X											
Titanium 4	AgriLabs	MLV				X	X												X						X						
Titanium 4 L5	AgriLabs	MLV/K		X		X	X												X	X					X						
Titanium 5	AgriLabs	MLV		X		X	X												X						X						
Titanium 5 L5	AgriLabs	MLV/K		X		X	X												X	X					X						
Titanium BRSV 3	AgriLabs	MLV		X															X						X						
Titanium IBR	AgriLabs	MLV																	X												
Titanium IBR-LP	AgriLabs	MLV/K																	X	X											
Triangle 1	Fort Dodge Animal Health	K				X																									
Triangle 3	Fort Dodge Animal Health	K				X													X						X						
Triangle 3V5L	Fort Dodge Animal Health	K				X		X											X	X					X						
Triangle 4 2 ml dose	Fort Dodge Animal Health	K		X		X													X						X						
Triangle 4+HS	Fort Dodge Animal Health	K		X		X												X	X						X						

286

Product	Manufacturer	Type																		
Triangle 4+PH/HS	Fort Dodge Animal Health	K	X	X										X	X				X	X
Triangle 4+PH-K	Fort Dodge Animal Health	K	X	X										X	X			X	X	X
Triangle 8	Fort Dodge Animal Health	K		X										X	X				X	X
Triangle 9	Fort Dodge Animal Health	K	X	X										X	X				X	X
Triangle 9+HS	Fort Dodge Animal Health	K	X	X									X	X	X				X	X
Triangle 9+PH-K	Fort Dodge Animal Health	K	X	X									X	X	X		X	X	X	X
TrichGuard	Fort Dodge Animal Health	K			X															
TrichGuard V5L	Fort Dodge Animal Health	K													X					
Trichontrol	Pfizer Animal Health	K																		
Trichontrol VL5	Pfizer Animal Health	K			X									X	X					
TriVib 5L	Fort Dodge Animal Health	K			X									X	X					
TSV-2	Pfizer Animal Health	MLV											X	X					X	
Ultrabac 7	Pfizer Animal Health	K				X	X	X	X											
Ultrabac 7/Somnubac	Pfizer Animal Health	K				X	X	X	X		X									
Ultrabac 8	Pfizer Animal Health	K	X	X		X	X	X	X											
Ultrabac CD	Pfizer Animal Health	K					X													
Vib Shield	Grand	K			X															
Vib Shield L5	Grand	K			X									X	X					
Vib Shield Plus	Grand	K			X															
Vib Shield Plus L5	Grand	K			X									X	X					
Vibo-5/Somnugen	Bio-Ceutic	K			X					X				X	X					
Vibo-5	Bio-Ceutic	K			X									X	X					
Vibralone-H-L5	Bayer Corporation	K			X			X						X	X					
Vibri-Lep-5	Franklin	K			X									X	X					
Vibrin	Pfizer Animal Health	K			X															
Vibrio/Leptoferm-5	Pfizer Animal Health	K			X									X	X					
Vibrio-Lepto 5	AgriLabs	K			X									X	X					
Vibrio-Lepto 5	Bayer Corporation	K			X									X	X					
Vibrio-Lepto 5	Durvet	K			X									X	X					
Vibrio-Lepto 5	Premier Farmtech	K			X									X	X					
Vibrio Lepto 5 (oil base)	Aspen	K			X									X	X					
Vibrio-Lepto 5 vaccine	Aspen	K			X									X	X					
Vibrio-Lepto-5	Anchor	K			X									X	X					
Vibrio-Lepto-5/Somnus	Anchor	K			X								X	X	X					
Vira Shield 3	Grand	K	X	X										X	X					
Vira Shield 2	Grand	K	X	X																
Vira Shield 2+BRSV	Grand	K	X	X			X													
Vira Shield 3+VL5	Grand	K	X	X	X									X	X				X	
Vira Shield 4	Grand	K	X	X										X						X
Vira Shield 4+L5	Grand	K	X	X									X	X	X				X	X

Continued

287

TABLE 11-4 CATTLE VACCINES—CONT'D

Vaccine	Manufacturer	Type	Anthrax	BRSV	Brucella spp.	BVD Type I	BVD Type II	Campylobacter	Clostridium chauvoei	Clostridium haemolyticum	Clostridium novyi	Clostridium perfringens C and D	Clostridium septicum	Clostridium sordellii	Coronavirus	Escherichia coli	Fusobacterium	Haemophilus somnus	IBR	Leptospira spp.	Moraxella bovis	Papillomavirus	Pasteurella haemolytica	Pasteurella multocida	Pl-3	Rabies	Rotavirus	Salmonella	Staphylococcus spp.	Tetanus Toxoid	Tritrichomonas
Vira Shield 5	Grand	K		X		X	X												X						X						
Vira Shield 5+L5	Grand	K		X		X	X												X	X					X						
Vira Shield 5+Somnus	Grand	K		X		X	X											X	X						X						
Vira Shield 5+VL5	Grand	K		X		X	X	X											X	X					X						
Vision 7 Somnus with Spur	Bayer Corporation	K							X		X	X	X	X				X													
Vision 7 with Spur	Bayer Corporation	K							X		X	X	X	X																	
Vision 8 with Spur	Bayer Corporation	K							X	X	X	X	X	X																	
Vision CD•T with Spur	Bayer Corporation	K										X																		X	
Vision CD with Spur	Bayer Corporation	K										X																			
Volar	Bayer Corporation	K															X														
Wart Shield	Grand	K																				X									
Wart vaccine	AgriLabs	K																				X									
Wart vaccine	Colorado Serum	K																				X									

Infections with *Clostridium chauvoei* (the causative agent of blackleg), *Clostridium septicum* (the causative agent of malignant edema), and *Clostridium sordellii* primarily affect striated muscles. The spores of these organisms are deposited in muscles by the circulation after ingestion or via wound contamination. When conditions of reduced oxygen tension within these muscles exist (e.g., trauma during handling, transporting, butting, or riding), the spores vegetate and the resulting organisms multiply. Toxins released by the multiplying organisms rapidly destroy the muscles and cause death through destructive effects on vital organs. Death may occur suddenly, as early as 12 hours after onset of infection.

Infections with *Clostridium novyi* type B and *Clostridium haemolyticum* (also known as *Clostridium novyi* type D) primarily affect the liver. These spores are usually ingested and travel by the circulation to the liver, where they remain latent until some form of liver damage occurs that allows the spores to vegetate and the resulting organisms to multiply. Predisposing conditions that may activate the spores in the liver include liver flukes, migrating parasites, abscesses, bacterial hepatitis, fatty infiltration, and various hepatotoxins. Potent toxins produced by the multiplying bacteria are absorbed systematically and cause death through destructive effects on vital organs and blood vessels. Death may occur suddenly, as early as 24 hours after onset of infection.

Infections with *Clostridium perfringens* types B, C, and D affect primarily the gastrointestinal tract. These organisms are normal inhabitants of the gastrointestinal tract of cattle and tend to proliferate under conditions of reduced oxygen tension created by consumption of large quantities of concentrate feed or when sudden changes in feed occur. With favorable conditions, the organisms multiply rapidly and produce toxins that can cause several intestinal lesions leading to a hemorrhagic, necrotic enteritis and sudden death, particularly in young animals.

> ### Technician Note
> Clostridial infections causing sudden death commonly occur in cattle; therefore routine vaccination is highly recommended.

Because these clostridial infections commonly occur in cattle, routine vaccination for clostridial infections is highly recommended.

Anaplasmosis Vaccine

Anaplasmosis in the United States is a common rickettsial disease of cattle and is caused by the intraerythrocytic parasite *Anaplasma marginale*. Affected red blood cells are destroyed by the liver and spleen, resulting in a severe anemia. Clinical signs caused by an acute anemia may include pale mucous membranes, weakness, depression or aggressive behavior, and increased heart and respiratory rates. Anaplasmosis often causes sudden death and must be differentiated from anthrax and the clostridial diseases.

Currently there is no vaccine commercially available for prevention of anaplasmosis. It is anticipated that a vaccine will be available again within the next several years.

Bovine Respiratory Disease Complex Vaccines

There are several viruses and bacteria that are widespread in the cattle population and are considered to be the major contributors to the bovine respiratory disease complex.

Multiple infections may occur with these viruses, and secondary infections with these bacteria often exacerbate the primary diseases produced.

Parainfluenza-3 (PI-3) virus causes a mild respiratory disease that is often associated with shipment of cattle to the feedlot (and thus commonly referred to as *shipping fever*). Clinical signs may include fever, serous to mucopurulent nasal discharge, coughing, increased respiratory rate, weakness, depression, and weight loss.

> ### Technician Note
> Respiratory virus infection in cattle marks the beginning of "shipping fever" and often leads to severe secondary bacterial pneumonia.

Infectious bovine rhinotracheitis (IBR) virus causes high fever, nasal discharge, conjunctivitis, increased respiratory rate, coughing, dyspnea, and severe hyperemia of the muzzle (commonly referred to as *red nose*).

Bovine virus diarrhea (BVD) virus can cause respiratory disease and is often confused with or obscured by the other viruses of this complex. In addition to the respiratory disease, the virus may also cause a mild transient diarrhea and may be associated with abortions and birth of malformed or weak calves if the primary infection occurs during pregnancy. The chronic form of BVD, known as *mucosal disease*, often results in ulcerative lesions throughout the alimentary tract, causing persistent diarrhea and usually death. In general, attenuated (modified live virus) vaccines containing IBR or BVD should *not* be administered intramuscularly to pregnant cows or to calves nursing pregnant cows because abortion may result. Intranasal attenuated IBR vaccines *are* safe, however, for pregnant cows or calves nursing by pregnant cows.

Bovine respiratory syncytial virus (BRSV) has been recognized in recent years as a major viral component of the bovine respiratory disease complex. Infection typically causes anorexia, coughing, increased respiratory rate, serous ocular and nasal discharge, fever, pulmonary edema and emphysema, and subcutaneous edema of the neck and throat. Death may occur rapidly, as early as 48 hours after onset of infection.

The bacteria *Pasteurella multocida* and *Pasteurella haemolytica* are normal inhabitants of the bovine respiratory tract and therefore are common secondary bacterial invaders in cases of primary viral pneumonia in cattle. In addition, these bacteria contribute to a primary fibrinous pneumonia and pleuritis that are readily apparent at necropsy. Clinical signs associated with these *Pasteurella* organisms may include fever, coughing, dyspnea, mucopurulent nasal discharge, depression, anorexia, and, in severe cases, death.

The bacterium *Haemophilus somnus* is another bacterial pathogen that can be a part of the bovine respiratory disease complex. It ranks second to *P. haemolytica* as the most frequent isolate from acute cases of fibrinopurulent pneumonia. *H. somnus* infection often develops as a septicemia, which can progress to fibrinous pleuritis, pericarditis, polyarthritis, or thromboembolic meningoencephalitis (also known as TEME or sleeper's syndrome).

Many vaccines are currently available for these virus- and bacterium-induced bovine respiratory diseases. The vaccines contain these agents in various combinations and in the attenuated (modified live virus) or inactivated forms. Their routine use will depend on the needs of the herds and herdsman.

Enteric Disease Vaccine

Bovine rotavirus and coronavirus as well as enterotoxigenic bacterial strains of *Escherichia coli* are often isolated from calves with diarrhea. These organisms may occur in combination or with other bacterial, viral, or protozoal pathogens. The combination of enterotoxins produced by *E. coli* and the cytopathogenic effects of rotavirus and coronavirus induces secretion of large amounts of fluid and electrolytes into the lumen of the gut, resulting in diarrhea, dehydration, and, in severe cases, death. Vaccines are currently available for immunization of pregnant heifers or cows before calving. Some of these vaccines are also designed for oral administration to the newborn calf.

Moraxella Vaccine

Moraxella bovis is the principal cause of infectious bovine keratoconjunctivitis (IBK). Infection may result in characteristic clinical signs, including epiphora, blepharospasm, photophobia, corneal ulcers, corneal edema, and chemosis. Healing may occur at any stage, but occasionally, with or without appropriate treatment, an affected cornea may perforate, resulting in loss of vision. Several inactivated vaccines are now available for protection against infection by *M. bovis.*

External and Internal Parasites

Control of external parasites, especially lice and grubs, may be achieved with repeated applications of approved insecticidal sprays or pour-on products or with the use of ivermectin. Many commercial products are currently available for effective treatment of lice and grubs. Always follow the manufacturer's labeled instructions completely, and closely observe the slaughter and milk withdrawal times when using these products. Some products are not recommended for use in Brahmans, Brahman crosses, or exotic cattle breeds.

The most common internal parasites of beef and dairy cattle are the barber's pole worm (*Haemonchus* spp.), the brown stomach worm (*Ostertagia* spp.), the bankrupt worm (*Trichostrongylus* spp.), the hookworm (*Bunostomum* spp.), Cooper's worm (*Cooperia* spp.), the intestinal worm (*Nematodirus* spp.), the nodular worm (*Oesophagostomum* spp.), the lungworm (*Dictyocaulus* spp.), and the liver fluke (*Fasciola* spp.). In general, it is a good idea to deworm calves at least once before weaning and again at weaning. Cows, heifers, and bulls should be dewormed as needed. Many commercial dewormers are currently available. Product choice depends on the parasite or parasites diagnosed by fecal examination within a herd and the resistance patterns of those parasites. Cattle raised in locales where liver flukes exist should be treated in the spring and/or fall. Chapter 7 contains additional information on parasitology and specific drug therapy.

Several commercial implants are currently available for beef cattle that are designed to improve feed efficiency and increase feed savings. Most implants contain anabolic agents, such as estradiol, progesterone, testosterone, zeranol, or combinations of these agents. The type of implant and its scheduled use depend on the gender and age of calves implanted as well as the needs of the herdsman. Ruminant nutrition is discussed in Chapter 15.

Management Recommendations for Dairy Calves

The ultimate goal in raising replacement heifers is to produce a healthy heifer that will calve and enter the milking herd by 24 months of age (see Table 11-3). Probably the single most important factor in successful rearing of baby calves is to see that the calves ingest colostrum soon after birth. If the calf does not nurse on its own shortly after birth, the herdsman should administer at least 2 L of warm colostrum to the calf within the first hour. During the first 3 days of life, continue to feed colostrum at 10% of the calf's body weight daily, split into two feedings (e.g., a 40-kg calf should receive 2 L of colostrum twice daily).

After this time, the calf can be switched to whole milk or a good-quality commercial milk replacer administered at 10% of its body weight daily divided into two feedings. For the neonatal calf, it is important to use a milk replacer that contains 20% to 22% crude protein, all of which is milk derived, and 18% to 20% crude fat. Fresh water should be provided at all times, and grain (18% to 20% protein) and hay should be offered as a free choice beginning at 7 to 14 days of age.

Calves should be housed in individual huts until weaned. Separating calves helps to control direct transmission of disease, prevents postfeeding sucking among calves, reduces stress of competition, and allows for assessment of individual feed intake and fecal consistency. Most dairy calves should be weaned by 50 to 60 days of age.

PREVENTIVE HEALTH PROGRAM FOR SWINE

An effective and economical preventive health program is an essential part of successful swine production.

 Technician Note

An effective and economical preventive health program is an essential part of successful swine production.

Preventive health programs should be individually designed by the consulting veterinarian and based on the specific needs of the swine herd and the producer. The preventive health programs should include immunization programs for disease prevention, well-proven methods of external and internal parasite control, recommendations for appropriate nutrition, and improvements in general management and sanitation procedures. Box 11-4 presents a general approach to preventive health programs for swine herds and its implementation.

Vaccinations

Vaccines that may be incorporated in preventive health programs for swine herds can be obtained from manufacturers as individual components or in various combinations. Table 11-5 lists some vaccines currently available. Diseases for which vaccines are commonly used in preventive health programs are described below.

Leptospirosis Vaccine

Leptospirosis is an important bacterial disease that affects domestic animals as well as humans and wildlife. Leptospirosis in swine is characterized by poor production, anemia, kidney disease, and abortions. Abortions are especially common after infection during late pregnancy. Routine vaccination of the breeding swine (e.g., gilts, sows, boars) 2 to 4 weeks before breeding has proved to be effective in its prevention. Because immunity is short-lived, semiannual revaccination is generally recommended.

Porcine Parvovirus Vaccine

Porcine parvovirus (PPV) is believed to be the most common cause of infectious reproductive failure in swine. Infection of pregnant sows and gilts can result in stillbirths,

---

Box 11-4 GENERAL OUTLINE OF A PREVENTIVE HEALTH PROGRAM FOR SWINE

PREBREEDING RECOMMENDATIONS FOR BOARS

Purchase boars 60 days before intended use. Quarantine new boars for 30 days, then allow fence line contact with gilts and sows for 30 days before breeding. Immunize boars for leptospirosis and erysipelas. Treat for external and internal parasites before breeding.

PREBREEDING RECOMMENDATIONS FOR SOWS AND GILTS

Immunize for leptospirosis, porcine parvovirus infection,* and pseudorabies* 2-4 wk before breeding. Flush gilts by increasing feed (energy) intake before breeding to increase ovulations. Treat for external and internal parasites before breeding.

PREFARROWING RECOMMENDATIONS FOR SOWS AND GILTS

Limit feed intake to about 4 lb per head per day or feed according to condition to avoid overweight sows or gilts at farrowing. Immunize for colibacillosis,* atrophic rhinitis, erysipelas, TGE, porcine rotavirus infection,* and *Clostridium perfringens* type C* according to manufacturer's labeled instructions. Treat for external and internal parasites before farrowing with approved products.

FARROWING RECOMMENDATIONS

Gradually increase feed intake so lactating swine are receiving full feed at peak milk production. (Rule of thumb: Feed daily 1 lb of feed for every pig being nursed [e.g., a lactating sow with a litter of 12 pigs should receive at least 12 lb of feed daily].)

GENERAL RECOMMENDATIONS FOR PIGS

At Birth
Perform newborn pig procedures (e.g., clip needle teeth, dock tails, castrate, ear-notch, and inject iron dextran).

One Wk of Age
Immunize for TGE,* rotavirus,* and atrophic rhinitis.

Four-Five Wk of Age
Weaning occurs at this time. Immunize for atrophic rhinitis, erysipelas, and *Actinobacillus* infection.*

Six-Eight Wk of Age
Treat for external and internal parasites with approved products.

Older Than Eight Wk of Age
Repeated treatments for external and internal parasites with approved products may need to be done during the growing-finishing period.

*Dependent on problems in the individual swine herd.

---

mummified fetuses, embryonic death, and infertility (formerly referred to as SMEDI). Prebreeding vaccination is recommended in swine herds experiencing PPV infections.

Transmissible Gastroenteritis Vaccine

Transmissible gastroenteritis (TGE) is a common viral disease of swine. TGE affects swine of all ages but is most devastating to pigs younger than 10 days of age. Clinical signs in very young pigs may include anorexia, vomiting, profuse watery diarrhea, and dehydration, which often progress to death. Older swine can exhibit similar but milder symptoms, and death is rare.

Vaccination of prefarrowing sows and gilts may be necessary for herds in which TGE has been diagnosed as a cause of neonatal diarrhea. In addition, vaccination of pigs within the first week of life may assist in the prevention of postweaning scours.

Porcine Rotavirus Vaccine

Porcine rotavirus infection causes a gastroenteritis that may be characterized by vomiting, watery diarrhea, dehydration, and death in young pigs. It is generally difficult to differentiate porcine rotavirus infection from TGE. Porcine rotavirus infection commonly occurs in both nursing and weaned pigs, and many swine herds have serologic evidence of its presence. Vaccination of prefarrowing sows and gilts, nursing pigs, and pigs 7 to 10 days before weaning is recommended for the prevention of postweaning scours in herds where porcine rotavirus infection has been diagnosed as a cause of enteric disease in young pigs.

Clostridium perfringens Type C Vaccine

The bacterium *Cl. perfringens* type C can cause enteric disease in young pigs. In peracute infection, there is a rapid onset of bloody diarrhea and death within the first 2 days of life. Acutely infected young pigs usually develop a red-brown liquid feces and die within 2 days after onset of enteric disease. The subacute infection may result in persistent diarrhea, emaciation, and death after 5 to 7 days of age. In chronic infections, a gray mucoid diarrhea occurs that lasts for about 7 days. Some of these patients will die, whereas others survive and typically become chronic poor doers.

Vaccination of prefarrowing sows and gilts effectively assists in the control of *C. perfringens* type C infections in nursing pigs.

Neonatal Porcine Colibacillosis Vaccine

Neonatal porcine colibacillosis is caused by bacterial enterotoxigenic strains of *E. coli*. The results are diarrhea, dehydration, and, in severe cases, death. Vaccination of healthy, pregnant sows and gilts provides good protection against neonatal colibacillosis in their nursing pigs.

Bordetella, Pasteurella, Actinobacillus, and Mycoplasma Vaccines

Bordetella bronchiseptica is considered to be the major cause of atrophic rhinitis in swine. In young pigs, atrophic rhinitis is characterized by acute rhinitis that results in destruction of the nasal turbinates. Destruction of the turbinates leads to impaired filtering of air in the nasal passages, decreased rate of weight gain, and increased incidence of respiratory infections, including pneumonia. Vaccination of pregnant swine and nursing pigs can often reduce the incidence of clinical atrophic rhinitis. *Pasteurella multocida* is a common bacterial pathogen of the respiratory tract of swine. In combined infections, *P. multocida* and *B. bronchiseptica* can cause a more severe form of atrophic rhinitis than in cases where either agent occurs alone. Several inactivated vaccines containing *P. multocida* are currently available.

Actinobacillus pleuropneumoniae, the most common causative agent of respiratory disease in swine, causes a severe and often fatal disease affecting swine of all ages. Manifestations of the disease are fibrinopurulent bronchopneumonia and fibrinous pleuritis. Acute *Actinobacillus* infections can cause death within 12 hours after the onset of clinical signs (e.g., coughing, cyanosis, blood-tinged nasal discharge). However, some animals may die suddenly without development of clinical signs. Chronic infections are usually subclinical and are characterized by decreased performance and an extended finishing period.

Text continued on p. 297

TABLE 11-5 SWINE VACCINES

Vaccine	Manufacturer	Type	A pleuropneumoniae	Bordetella	Clostridium perfringens	Escherichia coli	Encephalomyocarditis	Erysipelothrix	Haemophilus parasuis	Influenza	Leptospira spp.	Mycoplasma	Parvovirus	Pasteurella multocida	PRRS	Pseudorabies	Rotavirus	Salmonella	Serpulina (Treponema)	Streptococcus spp.	T.G.E.	Tetanus Toxoid
Argus SC	Bayer Corporation	MLV																X				
AR-P+D	Schering-Plough	K		X										X								
AR-Pac-P+ER	Schering-Plough	K		X				X						X								
AR-Pac-PD+ER	Schering-Plough	K		X				X	X					X								
AR-Parapac+ER	Schering-Plough	K		X				X	X					X								
AR-Parapac	Schering-Plough	K		X				X						X								
Atrobac 3	Pfizer Animal Health	K		X										X								
A.V.M. Intra/Vac	Cuprem	MLV		X																		
Borde Shield 4	Grand	K		X				X						X								
Borde-Cell	AgriLabs	MLV		X																		
Bordetella bronchiseptica intranasal vaccine	MVP	MLV		X																		
BratiVac	Pfizer Animal Health	K									X											
BratiVac-6	Pfizer Animal Health	K									X											
Breed Sow 7	AgriLabs	K						X			X		X									
Breed Sow 6	AgriLabs	K									X		X									
C&D Toxoid	Aspen	K			X																	
Clostri Shield C	Grand	K			X																	
Clostridium Bac with Imugen II	Bayer Corporation	K			X																	
Clostridium perfringens types C and D toxoid	Colorado Serum	K			X																	
Clostridium perfringens types C and D—tetanus toxoid	Colorado Serum	K			X																	X
Durvac Parvo-Lepto 5	Durvet	K									X		X									
Durvac P-Strep	Durvet	K	X																	X		
Durvac S. suis	Durvet	K																		X		
Durvac-Salmonella	Durvet	K																X				
E. coli Bac	AgriLabs	K				X																
E-Bac	Bayer Corporation	K						X														
EMC Vac	Bayer Corporation	K					X															
Emulsibac SS	MVP	K																		X		
Emulsibac HP	MVP	K	X																			
ENDOVAC-Porci	Immvac	K																X				
Enterisol Coli	Boehringer Ingelheim/NOBL	K				X																
Enterisol Coli C	Boehringer Ingelheim/NOBL	K			X	X																
Enterisol SC-54	Boehringer Ingelheim/NOBL	MLV																X				
Enterisol Coli E	Boehringer Ingelheim/NOBL	K				X		X														
Equisimillis Shield	Grand	K																		X		
ER Bac/Leptoferm-5	Pfizer Animal Health	K						X			X											

Product	Manufacturer	Type														
ER Bac	Pfizer Animal Health	K						X								
Ery Shield	Grand	K						X								
Ery Shield+L5	Grand	K		X				X								
Ery Vac 100	Arko	MLV						X								
Ery Vac 500	Arko	MLV						X								
Erycell	Grand	MLV						X								
Erysipelas	Durvet	K						X								
Erysipelas bacterin	AgriLabs	K						X								
Erysipelothrix rhusiopathiae bacterin	Colorado Serum	K						X								
EVA	Pfizer Animal Health	MLV						X								
FarrowSure B	Pfizer Animal Health	K		X				X	X							
FarrowSure B-PVR	Pfizer Animal Health	MLV/K		X				X	X						X	
FarrowSure PRV	Pfizer Animal Health	MLV/K		X				X	X						X	
FarrowSure	Pfizer Animal Health	K		X				X	X							
Haemo Shield P	Grand	K									X					
Ingelvac DART	Boehringer Ingelheim/NOBL	K								X						
Ingelvac HP	Boehringer Ingelheim/NOBL	K									X					
Ingelvac HPE	Boehringer Ingelheim/NOBL	K						X			X					
Ingelvac HPME	Boehringer Ingelheim/NOBL	K						X		X	X					
Ingelvac PRRS MLV	Boehringer Ingelheim/NOBL	MLV										X				
Ingelvac PRRS-HP	Boehringer Ingelheim/NOBL	MLV/K									X	X				
Ingelvac PRRS-HPE	Boehringer Ingelheim/NOBL	MLV/K						X			X	X				
Ingelvac PRRS-HPME	Boehringer Ingelheim/NOBL	MLV/K						X		X	X	X				
Ingelvac PRV-G1	Boehringer Ingelheim/NOBL	MLV											X			
Lepto 5	Bayer Corporation	K	X	X	X	X	X									
Lepto 5	Durvet	K	X	X	X	X	X									
Lepto 5	AgriLabs	K	X	X	X	X	X									
Lepto 5 Vaccine	Aspen	K	X	X	X	X	X									
Lepto Shield 5	Grand	K	X	X	X	X	X									
Lepto-5	Colorado Serum	K	X	X	X	X	X									
Leptoferm-5	Pfizer Animal Health	K	X	X	X	X	X									
Lepto-Parvo	Boehringer Ingelheim/NOBL	K	X	X	X	X	X		X							
Litter Guard LT	Pfizer Animal Health	K													X	
Litter Guard	Pfizer Animal Health	K													X	
LitterGuard LT-C	Pfizer Animal Health	K													X	X
M+Pac	Schering-Plough	K								X						
Maxi/Guard Nasal Vac	Addison	MLV												X		
MaxiVac FLU	SyntroVet	K												X		
M-Pac	Schering-Plough	K								X						
Myco Shield	Grand	K								X						
Myco Silencer	Bayer Corporation	K								X						
Mycogard	Bayer Corporation	K								X						
Nitro-Sal	Arko	MLV														X
Para Shield	Grand	K							X							
Parapac	Schering-Plough	K							X							
Parapleuro Shield P	Grand	K						X			X					
Parapleuro Shield P+BE	Grand	K						X			X					

K, Killed; *MLV*, modified live virus; *PRRS*, porcine reproductive and respiratory syndrome; *TGE*, transmissible gastroenteritis.

Continued

TABLE 11-5   SWINE VACCINES—cont'd

Vaccine Components

Vaccine	Manufacturer	Type	A pleuropneumoniae	Bordetella	Clostridium perfringens	Escherichia coli	Encephalomyocarditis	Erysipelothrix	Haemophilus parasuis	Influenza	Leptospira spp.	Mycoplasma	Parvovirus	Pasteurella multocida	PRRS	Pseudorabies	Rotavirus	Salmonella	Serpulina (Treponema)	Streptococcus spp.	T.G.E.	Tetanus Toxoid
Parasuis Bac	Bayer Corporation	K							X													
Parvo Lepto 5	Bayer Corporation	K									X		X									
Parvo Shield	Grand	K											X									
Parvo Shield L5	Grand	K									X		X									
Parvo Shield L5E	Grand	K						X			X		X									
Parvo-Vac/Leptoferm-5	Pfizer Animal Health	K									X		X									
Pilimune	Bayer Corporation	K				X																
Pleuro Ban E	A.A.H.	K	X					X														
PleuroGuard 4	Pfizer Animal Health	K	X	X				X						X								
Pleuromune with Imugen II	Bayer Corporation	K	X																			
Pleuromune-S with Imugen II	Bayer Corporation	K	X																	X		
Pneu Pac	Schering-Plough	K	X																			
Pneu Pac-ER	Schering-Plough	K	X					X														
Pneu Parapac	Schering-Plough	K	X						X													
Pneu Parapac+ER	Schering-Plough	K	X					X	X													
Pneumosuis III	Pfizer Animal Health	K	X																			
Poly-Sal P	A.A.H.	K																X				
Porcimune vaccine	Schering-Plough	K				X																
Porcimune B vaccine	Schering-Plough	K		X		X																
Porcine Pili Shield	Grand	K				X																
Porcine Pili Shield+C	Grand	K			X	X																
Prefarrow Strep Shield	Grand	K																		X		
Prevail MycoPlex	Aspen	K										X										
Prevail Para Pleuro Bac+3DT	Aspen	K	X	X				X	X		X			X								
Prevail Parvoplex 6-Way+E	Aspen	K						X			X		X									
Prime Pac PRRS	Schering-Plough	MLV													X							
ProSystem 1	Intervet	MLV																			X	
ProSystem 2	Intervet	MLV															X					
ProSystem 2*1	Intervet	MLV															X				X	
ProSystem 2*1*4*3	Intervet	MLV/K			X	X											X				X	
ProSystem 2*1*4*3/B*P*E	Intervet	MLV/K		X	X	X		X						X			X				X	
ProSystem 2*4*3	Intervet	MLV/K			X	X											X					
ProSystem 3	Intervet	K				X																
ProSystem 4*3	Intervet	K			X	X																
ProSystem 5	Intervet	K																	X			
ProSystem B*P*E	Intervet	K		X				X						X								
ProSystem B*P*E/4*3	Intervet	K		X	X	X		X						X								
ProSystem B*P*M	Intervet	K		X								X		X								

Product	Manufacturer	Type
ProSystem Ery	Intervet	K
Prosystem M	Intervet	K
PRRomiSE	Bayer Corporation	K
PRV/Marker Gold	SyntroVet	MLV
PRV/Marker Gold-Maxi FLU	SyntroVet	MLV/K
PR-Vac Plus	Pfizer Animal Health	MLV
PR-Vac	Pfizer Animal Health	MLV
PR-Vac-Killed	Pfizer Animal Health	K
ReproCyc PLE	Boehringer Ingelheim/NOBL	K
ReproCyc PRRS-PLE	Boehringer Ingelheim/NOBL	K
RespiSure	Pfizer Animal Health	K
Rhini Shield TX4	Grand	K
Rhinicell	Grand	MLV
Rhinicell+E	Grand	MLV
Rhinobac 3	Pfizer Animal Health	K
Rhinogen CT 5000	Bayer Corporation	K
Rhinogen CTE 5000	Bayer Corporation	K
Rhinogen CTSE	Bayer Corporation	K
Rhinogen PE	Bayer Corporation	K
Rhusigen Vaccine	Schering-Plough	K
Rotamune with Immungen II	Bayer Corporation	K
Rota-Vac TGE	Pfizer Animal Health	MLV
RXV Vac Lepto 5	RXV	K
Salmo Shield C	Grand	K
Salmo-Bac	AgriLabs	K
Salmonella bacterin	Pfizer Animal Health	K
Salmo-Shield 2	Grand	K
Score	Bayer Corporation	K
Scourmune	Schering-Plough	K
Scourmune-C	Schering-Plough	K
Scourmune-CR	Schering-Plough	K
Scourmune-CRT	Schering-Plough	MLV/K
ScourShield	Pfizer Animal Health	MLV/K
Sow Bac CE	Bayer Corporation	K
Sow Bac-E	Bayer Corporation	K
Sow Bac E Toxoid	Bayer Corporation	K
SS Pac	Schering-Plough	K
Strep Bac with Imugen II	Bayer Corporation	K
Super-Tet with Havlogen	Bayer Corporation	K
Suvaxyn AR/E/EC-4	Fort Dodge Animal Health	K
Suvaxyn AR/T	Fort Dodge Animal Health	K
Suvaxyn AR/T/E	Fort Dodge Animal Health	K
Suvaxyn E	Fort Dodge Animal Health	K
Suvaxyn E 250 dose	Fort Dodge Animal Health	K
Suvaxyn EC-4	Fort Dodge Animal Health	K
Suvaxyn GestaFend 8	Fort Dodge Animal Health	MLV/K

Continued

TABLE 11-5   SWINE VACCINES—cont'd

Vaccine Components

Vaccine	Manufacturer	Type	A. pleuropneumoniae	Bordetella	Clostridium perfringens	Escherichia coli	Encephalomyo-carditis	Erysipelothrix	Haemophilus parasuis	Influenza	Leptospira spp.	Mycoplasma	Parvovirus	Pasteurella multocida	PRRS	Pseudorabies	Rotavirus	Salmonella	Serpulina (Treponema)	Streptococcus spp.	T.G.E.	Tetanus Toxoid
Suvaxyn HerdFend PrVgpl-	Fort Dodge Animal Health	MLV														X						
Suvaxyn L	Fort Dodge Animal Health	K									X											
Suvaxyn L+B	Fort Dodge Animal Health	K									X											
Suvaxyn LE+B	Fort Dodge Animal Health	K						X			X											
Suvaxyn P	Fort Dodge Animal Health	K											X									
Suvaxyn PL	Fort Dodge Animal Health	K									X		X									
Suvaxyn PLE	Fort Dodge Animal Health	K						X			X		X									
Suvaxyn PLE+B	Fort Dodge Animal Health	K						X			X		X									
Suvaxyn PLE+B/PrVgpl-	Fort Dodge Animal Health	MLV/K						X			X		X			X						
Suvaxyn RespiFend APP	Fort Dodge Animal Health	K	X																			
Suvaxyn RespiFend HPS	Fort Dodge Animal Health	K							X													
Suvaxyn RespiFend MH	Fort Dodge Animal Health	K										X										
Suvaxyn RespiFend MH/HPS	Fort Dodge Animal Health	K							X			X										
Swine Master F.P.	AgriLabs	K	X	X					X					X								
Swine Master M Plus	AgriLabs	K							X			X		X								
Swine Master 8	AgriLabs	MLV/K		X	X	X		X				X		X			X				X	
Swine Master B-P+D/M	AgriLabs	K		X								X		X								
Swine Master B-P-E+D/C-E	AgriLabs	K		X	X	X		X						X								
Swine Master B-P-E+D	AgriLabs	K		X				X						X								
Swine Master H/P	AgriLabs	K	X																			
Swine Master M	AgriLabs	K										X										
Swine Master-R.T.	AgriLabs	MLV															X				X	
Swine Master-R.T.C.E.	AgriLabs	MLV/K			X	X											X				X	
Tetanus toxoid	Fort Dodge Animal Health	K																				X
Tetanus toxoid	Franklin	K																				X
Tetanus toxoid—concentrated	Colorado Serum	K																				X
Tetanus toxoid—concentrated	Professional Biological	K																				X
Tetanus toxoid—unconcentrated	Colorado Serum	K																				X
Tetguard	Boehringer Ingelheim	K																				X
Tetnogen	Fort Dodge Animal Health	K																				X
TGE Cell	Grand	MLV																			X	
TGE Shield	Grand	K																			X	
TGE Vaccine	Pfizer Animal Health	MLV																			X	
TG-Emune Rota with Imugen II	Bayer Corporation	K															X				X	
TG-Emune with Imugen II	Bayer Corporation	K																			X	
Toxivac AD	Boehringer Ingelheim/NOBL	K		X										X								
Toxivac AD+E	Boehringer Ingelheim/NOBL	K		X				X						X								
Toxivac EC	Boehringer Ingelheim/NOBL	K		X		X		X						X								
Toxivac Plus Parasuis	Boehringer Ingelheim/NOBL	K		X		X		X	X					X								
WeanVac 3	Pfizer Animal Health	K	X	X				X														

Mycoplasma hyopneumoniae is the most common cause of chronic pneumonia in swine. The disease is not usually evident until pigs are 3 to 6 months old. It is characterized by a chronic, nonproductive cough, often induced by exercise. The greatest economic loss from the disease is decreased growth rate; for every 10% of lung affected by pneumonia, average daily gain is reduced by 5.3%. Morbidity is variable and mortality is low in uncomplicated cases. Secondary bacterial infections may exacerbate clinical signs.

Porcine Reproductive and Respiratory Syndrome Vaccine

Porcine reproductive and respiratory syndrome (PRRS) is also known as swine infertility and respiratory syndrome (SIRS), mystery swine disease, and blue ear disease. It is recognized as a viral disease of swine that causes respiratory problems in all ages of pigs as well as reproductive problems in breeding swine. Clinical signs include transient, mild anorexia; lethargy; and fever in grower-finisher pigs and breeding animals. Cyanosis of the ears (blue ear disease), vulva, tail, abdomen, or snout is occasionally reported. Viral infection of breeding gilts or sows may result in premature farrowings with small, weak, or stillborn piglets and an increased incidence of fetal mummies. Respiratory distress ("thumping") and open-mouth breathing in suckling and weanling pigs may occur. The virus tends to increase the incidence of secondary respiratory infections in young pigs. Chronic infection in nursery and grower-finisher pigs may result in decreased growth rate and feed efficiency and increased morbidity and mortality as a result of secondary infections. A vaccine for PRRS has recently been approved.

Erysipelas Vaccine

Erysipelas is caused by the bacterium *Erysipelothrix rhusiopathiae* and can occur as acute septicemia, skin discoloration (commonly known as *diamond skin disease*), chronic arthritis, and vegetative endocarditis. Erysipelas is extremely common among swine herds, and therefore routine vaccination of gilts and sows before farrowing and of pigs at weaning is highly recommended.

Pseudorabies Vaccine

Pseudorabies is a viral disease of swine that is characterized by fever, vomiting, encephalitis, and sudden death in nursing pigs, and abortion, stillbirths, or mummies in pregnant swine. Vaccines are currently available, but their use is limited by state regulations.

Streptococcus Vaccine

Streptococcus suis is a primary cause of meningitis and septicemia in postweaning pigs. It has also been associated with pneumonia and arthritis in pigs and abortion and infertility in sows and gilts. Animals with peracute cases may die suddenly, whereas those with less severe cases exhibit central nervous system (CNS) signs often followed by death. *S. suis* can pose a significant human health hazard. Available vaccines may help to reduce the losses caused by *S. suis.*

Encephalomyocarditis Vaccine

Encephalomyocarditis (EMC) virus primarily infects the heart and brain of swine. Mortality can be up to 100% among pigs less than 1 week old. Although mortality from EMC declines as pigs mature, older pigs do become clinically ill. Not all weaned pigs with EMC infections show clinical illness, and a normal-appearing pig may die suddenly, especially if excited or forced to exercise. A very small lesion in the cardiac conduction system can result in death. There is a vaccine available that markedly reduces gross and microscopic lesions caused by EMC virus in weaned pigs. Vaccination is recommended in herds experiencing problems with EMC virus.

External and Internal Parasites

Control of external parasites, especially lice *(Haematopinus suis)* and mange mites (*Sarcoptes scabiei* var. *suis*), may be done with repeated applications of approved insecticidal sprays or pour-on products or with the use of ivermectin. Treatment of external parasites should be done at the same time as treatment for internal parasites; however, always read the manufacturer's labeled instructions, because some types of sprays and pour-on products cannot be used concomitantly with dewormers or may not be used safely in pregnant or young nursing swine.

The most common internal parasites of swine are the roundworm *(Ascaris suum)*, the whipworm *(Trichuris suis)*, the threadworm *(Strongyloides* spp.), the nodular worm *(Oesophagostomum* spp.), the lungworm *(Metastrongylus* spp.), the red stomach worm *(Hyostrongylus rubidus)*, and the kidney worm *(Stephanurus dentatus)*. Many commercial dewormers are currently available. Product choice should depend on the parasites diagnosed by fecal examinations within a herd, convenience of administration, and cost effectiveness. In general, it is a good idea to deworm adults before breeding, sows and gilts before farrowing, and pigs once or twice after weaning and once during the growing-finishing period. Chapter 7 contains additional information on parasitology and specific drug therapy.

PREVENTIVE HEALTH PROGRAM FOR SMALL RUMINANTS

In North America, sheep and goats are managed under a wide variety of conditions, including extensive range operations, semiconfinement, total confinement, and hobby farm systems, and as backyard pets. Meat-producing goats have gained popularity in recent years. One primary task of the small ruminant veterinarian and veterinary technician is to educate the producer about the value of careful observation, animal identification, and record keeping for improvement of herd and flock health and productivity. With adequate information, the veterinarian and veterinary technician can then make sound recommendations concerning nutrition, vaccination, parasite control, and management geared to the needs of a particular herd or flock.

Vaccinations

The number of vaccines licensed for use in small ruminants is limited. The veterinarian's first choice should be a licensed vaccine used in accordance with label instructions; however, products licensed for use in other species (particularly in cattle) frequently are considered to be effective in sheep and goats. Use of vaccines depends on the disease incidence within a given herd or flock, but vaccination for enterotoxemia and tetanus should be included in every herd and flock health program (Table 11-6).

Enterotoxemia Vaccine

Toxins produced by *Clostridium perfringens* types C and D may cause enterotoxemia in young sheep and goats. The organism is present in the gastrointestinal tract of healthy animals but may overgrow and produce potent toxins in the presence of rich ingesta and bowel stasis. Enterotoxemia is most likely to occur in young animals nursing from

TABLE 11-6   OVINE VACCINES

Vaccine	Manufacturer	Type	Bacteroides nodosus	Bluetongue	Brucella ovis	Campylobacter	Chlamydia	Clostridium chauvoei	Clostridium haemolyticum	Clostridium novyi	Clostridium perfringens C and D	Clostridium septicum	Clostridium sordellii	Corynebacterium	Fusobacterium	Parapoxvirus (orf)	Pasteurella haemolytica	Pasteurella multocida	Rabies	Tetanus toxoid
7-Way	Aspen	K						X		X	X	X	X							
Bar-Vac 7+Redwater (8-Way)	Anchor	K						X	X	X	X	X	X							
Bar-Vac-CD/T	Anchor	K									X									X
Bluetongue vaccine	Colorado Serum	MLV		X																
Campylobacter fetus bacterin—ovine	Colorado Serum	K				X														
Case-Bac	Colorado Serum	K												X						
Caseous D-T	Colorado Serum	K												X						X
C-D toxoid	Anchor	K									X									
C & D toxoid	Aspen	K									X									
Chlamydia psittaci bacterin	Colorado Serum	K					X													
Clostri Shield BCD	Grand	K									X									
Clostri Shield C	Grand	K									X									
Clostridial 7-Way	AgriLabs	K						X	X	X	X	X	X							
Clostridial 8-Way	AgriLabs	K						X	X	X	X	X	X							
Clostridium chauvoei-septicum bacterin	Colorado Serum	K						X				X								
Clostridium chauvoei-septicum novyi-sordellii bacterin-toxoid	Colorado Serum	K						X		X		X	X							
Clostridium chauvoei-septicum—Pasteurella haemolytica-multocida bacterin	Colorado Serum	K						X				X					X	X		
Clostridium perfringens types C & D—tetanus toxoid	Colorado Serum	K									X									X
Clostridium perfringens types C & D toxoid	Colorado Serum	K									X									
Covexin 8 vaccine	Schering-Plough	K						X	X	X	X	X								X
Defensor	Pfizer Animal Health	K																	X	
Electroid 7 vaccine	Schering-Plough	K						X	X	X	X	X								
Electroid D	Schering-Plough	K									X									
Enzabort Eae-Vibrio	Colorado Serum	K				X	X													
Fermicon CD	Bio-Ceutic	K									X									

Product	Manufacturer	Type	1	2	3	4	5	6	7	8	9
Fermicon CD/T	Bio-Ceutic	K				X					X
Fermicon-7+Haemolyticum (8-Way)	Bio-Ceutic	K		X	X	X	X	X			
Footvax 10 Strain	Schering-Plough	K	X								
Ovine ecthyma vaccine	Colorado Serum	Live							X		
Ovine Tetanus Shield	Grand	K									X
Pasteurella haemolytica multocida bacterin	Colorado Serum	K								X	
Prorab-1	Intervet	K								X	
Rabdomun vaccine	Schering-Plough	K								X	
Rabguard-TC	Pfizer Animal Health	K								X	
Ram epididymitis bacterin	Colorado Serum	K						X			
Redwol with Spur	Bayer Corporation	K			X						
RM Imrab 3	Merial	K								X	
RM Imrab Bovine Plus	Merial	K								X	
Siteguard G	Schering-Plough	K				X					
Siteguard MLG vaccine	Schering-Plough	K		X	X	X	X				
Super-Tet with Havlogen	Bayer Corporation	K									X
Tetanus toxoid	Fort Dodge Animal Health	K									X
Tetanus toxoid	Franklin	K									X
Tetanus toxoid—concentrated	Colorado Serum	K									X
Tetanus toxoid—concentrated	Professional Biological	K									X
Tetanus toxoid—unconcentrated	Colorado Serum	K									X
Tetguard	Boehringer Ingelheim	K									X
Tetnogen	Fort Dodge Animal Health	K									X
Ultrabac 7	Pfizer Animal Health	K		X	X	X	X				
Ultrabac 8	Pfizer Animal Health	K		X	X	X	X				
Ultrabac CD	Pfizer Animal Health	K				X					
Vision 7 with Spur	Bayer Corporation	K		X	X	X	X				
Vision 8 with Spur	Bayer Corporation	K		X	X	X	X				
Vision CD T with Spur	Bayer Corporation	K				X					X
Vision CD with Spur	Bayer Corporation	K				X					
Volar	Bayer Corporation	K					X				

K, Killed; *MLV,* modified live virus.

dams that are heavy milk producers or in animals receiving heavy grain rations as in feedlot situations. It is for this reason that the disease is called *overeating disease*. Enterotoxemia is easily prevented by vaccination of the dams before lambing and kidding and vaccination of lambs and kids several times at 2- to 4-week intervals beginning at 6 to 8 weeks of age. Vaccination for enterotoxemia is effective and should be a part of all herd health programs.

Tetanus Vaccine

Tetanus is caused by a toxin produced by the anaerobic organism *Clostridium tetani*, a bacterium that may be carried into wounds or surgery sites. Clinical signs may include muscular stiffness (sawhorse stance), difficulty in swallowing (lockjaw), prolapse of the third eyelids, labored breathing, and exaggerated response to external stimuli. Because small ruminants are particularly susceptible to infection, vaccination for tetanus at the time of vaccination for enterotoxemia is vital (combination products are available). In addition, booster vaccination is recommended any time an animal is wounded or has undergone any surgical procedure (e.g., dehorning, castration, tail docking).

Contagious Ecthyma Vaccine

Contagious ecthyma (sore mouth, orf) is a viral infection of goats. Kids are primarily affected but may spread the disease to the udder of the doe. Clinical signs include papules, vesicles, pustules, and scabs on the lips, muzzle, eyelids, oral cavity, udder, teats, and feet. Affected kids usually exhibit a decrease in feed consumption, and some kids become depressed, anorectic, and febrile. Contagious ecthyma is transmissible to humans, and so it is advisable to wear gloves when handling infected animals. Effective live-virus vaccines are available but are not recommended for closed herds that are not experiencing contagious ecthyma. Proper precautions, such as wearing gloves during vaccine administration and disposal of contagious ecthyma vaccine containers, are necessary to prevent risks to human health.

Foot Rot Vaccine

Bacteroides nodosus is the primary causative agent of foot rot in sheep. It is a highly contagious disease and is probably the most common disease of sheep in the United States, causing more economic loss than any other disease. Lameness in one or more feet is the most obvious clinical sign. The development of foot rot is facilitated by wet environmental conditions. A vaccine is available that, when combined with regular foot trimming and foot baths, significantly reduces the incidence of disease within a flock.

Bluetongue Vaccine

Bluetongue is a viral disease of ruminants; however, clinical disease is largely restricted to sheep. Clinical signs may include oral ulcers; edema of the face, lips, muzzle, and ears; excessive salivation; cyanosis of the tongue (thus the name); and lameness caused by coronitis. Teratogenic effects include abortions, stillbirths, and weak, live "dummy lambs." An attenuated live-virus vaccine is available for prebreeding vaccination of healthy sheep and goats; vaccination of pregnant females may produce teratogenic effects.

Campylobacteriosis (Vibriosis) Vaccine

Campylobacteriosis is caused by *Campylobacter fetus* subsp. *fetus* and *Campylobacter jejuni*. The principal clinical sign with this disease is abortion, which usually occurs in the last 6 weeks of pregnancy. Losses from abortion may be substantial in individual flocks. Vaccines for *Campylobacter* alone or in combination with *Chlamydia* are now available for prevention of abortion in sheep.

Chlamydia Vaccine

Chlamydia psittaci, the cause of enzootic abortion of ewes (EAE), is a major cause of abortion in sheep and goats. Abortions or stillbirths with placentitis usually occur in the fourth or fifth month of gestation; other animals in the flock or herd may concurrently show signs of arthritis or pneumonia. Vaccines for *Chlamydia* alone or in combination with *Campylobacter* are now available for prevention of abortion in sheep.

Foot Care

Foot rot is one of the most common diseases of sheep and goats.

Technician Note

Foot rot is one of the most common diseases of sheep and goats.

It is highly contagious, and infection can result in lameness in a significant number of animals within a herd or flock. Frequent foot trimming combined with foot baths, foot soaks, or vaccination, or a combination of these, is important in the control of the disease. Repeated foot soaking alone is an economic, practical, and effective treatment for foot rot in large commercial operations where hoof trimming is impractical. Products typically used for foot baths or foot soaks include zinc sulfate, copper sulfate, and formalin (care must be taken to prevent sheep from drinking solutions high in copper). There is some evidence of genetic susceptibility to development of foot rot in sheep; therefore culling animals with recurring infections may be helpful.

Nutrition

Sheep and goats should be fed a good-quality commercial feed labeled for that particular species. Feeding horse or cattle feeds to small ruminants may result in copper toxicity because the copper levels in those feeds are much higher than normally tolerated by sheep and goats. Feed commercial feeds according to the manufacturer's recommendations and based on the needs and use of the animal. Good-quality roughage may be fed free choice. Because castrated lambs and kids (wethers) are predisposed to the development of urinary calculi, it is advisable to feed a diet of good-quality roughage or pasture and no grain. If grain must be fed, it is advisable to supplement their feed with salt and a urinary acidifier, such as ammonium chloride (see Chapter 15).

External and Internal Parasites

There are few effective anthelmintics labeled for use in small ruminants. Most small ruminant veterinarians use cattle dewormers for the treatment of external and internal parasites in sheep and goats. Products commonly used include avermectins, fenbendazole, albendazole, and levamisole. Caution should be exercised when using these products in lactating does and animals intended for slaughter. Recommendations for extra label use of these products and suggested milk and slaughter withdrawal times may be obtained from the Food Animal Residue Avoidance Data Bank.

Frequency of deworming varies according to several factors, including concentration of animals in a given area and environmental conditions. Severe gastrointestinal parasitism can be life threatening, especially in subtropical climates, where it may be necessary to deworm small ruminants as often as every 3 to 4 weeks during the hot, humid summer months. Pasture management and careful rotation coupled with strategic deworming are critical to effective parasite control. Routine fecal examinations, either individual or composite samples, may be useful to determine the frequency of deworming and the effectiveness of various anthelmintics. See Chapter 7 for more information.

RECOMMENDED READING

DOGS AND CATS

Hoskins JD: Canine viral diseases. In Ettinger SJ, Feldman EC, editors: *Textbook of veterinary internal medicine*, vol 1, ed 5, Philadelphia, 2000, WB Saunders.

Hoskins JD: Pediatrics: puppies and kittens, *VetClin North Am Small Anim Pract* 29:837, 1999.

Hoskins JD: Update on feline coronavirus disease. In August JR, editor: *Consultations in feline internal medicine*, ed 3, Philadelphia, 1997, WB Saunders.

Hoskins JD: Viral infections. In Morgan RV, editor: *Handbook of small animal practice*, ed 3, Philadelphia, 1997, WB Saunders.

Hoskins JD, editor: *Veterinary pediatrics: dogs and cats from birth to six months*, ed 3, Philadelphia, 2001, WB Saunders.

Hribernik TN, Hoskins JD: Rickettsial infections. In Morgan RV, editor: *Handbook of small animal practice*, ed 3, Philadelphia, 1997, WB Saunders.

HORSES

George LW: Diseases of the nervous system. In Smith BP, editor: *Large animal internal medicine*, St Louis, 1990, Mosby.

Martens JG, Martens RJ: Equine herpesvirus type 1: its classifications, pathogenesis, and prevention, *Vet Med* 86:936, 1991.

Messer NT, IV: The use of biologics in the prevention of infectious diseases. In Smith BP, editor: *Large animal internal medicine*, St Louis, 1990, Mosby.

Wilson JH, Erickson DM: *Neurological syndrome of rhinopneumonitis. Proceedings of the American College of Veterinarians Internal Medicine Forum*, New Orleans, May 30-June 2, 1991, p 419.

CATTLE

Aldridge B, Garry F, Adams R: Role of colostral transfer in neonatal calf management: failure of acquisition of passive immunity, *Compend Contin Educ Pract Vet* 14:265, 1992.

Baker JC, Velicer LF: Bovine respiratory syncytial virus vaccination: current status and future vaccine development, *Compend Contin Educ Pract Vet* 13:1323, 1991.

Heinrichs AJ: Milk replacers for dairy calves. I, *Compend Contin Educ Pract Vet* 16:1605, 1994.

Larson BL: Immunization to decrease pregnancy wastage in beef cattle. II, Available vaccines, *Compend Contin Educ Pract Vet* 18:571, 1996.

Smith BP: *Large animal internal medicine*, ed 2, St Louis, 1996, Mosby.

Spire MF: Immunization of the beef breeding herd, *Compend Contin Educ Pract Vet* 10:1111, 1988.

SWINE

Christianson WT, Joo HS: Porcine reproductive and respiratory syndrome: a review, *Swine Health Prod* 2:10, 1994.

Cowart RP: *An outline of swine diseases*, Ames, 1995, Iowa State University Press.

Fedorka-Cray PJ et al: *Actinobacillus (Haemophilus) pleuropneumoniae*. I, History, epidemiology, serotyping, and treatment, *Compend Contin Educ Pract Vet* 15:1447, 1993.

Primm ND, Friendship RM, Hall WF: Deworming strategies for swine. II, Anthelmintics and their use in the control of endoparasites, *Compend Contin Educ Pract Vet* 12:889, 1990.

SMALL RUMINANTS

Council report: vaccination guidelines for small ruminants (sheep, goats, llamas, domestic deer, and wapiti), *J Am Vet Med Assoc* 205:1539, 1994.

Robinson A, Wolf C: American Association of Small Ruminant Practitioners survey of biologic usage, *Symposium on Health and Disease of Small Ruminants*, pp 197-214, 1991.

Zajac AM, Moore GA: Treatment and control of gastrointestinal nematodes in sheep, *Compend Contin Educ Pract Vet* 15:999, 1993.

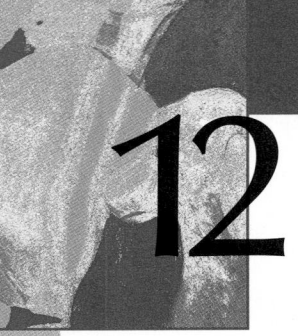

12

Neonatal Care of Puppy, Kitten, and Foal

Johnny D. Hoskins • Jorge De la Calle

Caring for the ill puppy, kitten, or foal from birth to young adulthood is often complicated by age-related changes in the body systems. These age-related changes occur because the normal development of specific body systems continues well after birth. Thorough clinical evaluation of the ill puppy, kitten, or foal may include the case history, physical examination, routine laboratory tests, electrocardiogram (ECG) (lead II rhythm strip), and possibly radiography.

PUPPY AND KITTEN

Physical and Laboratory Examination

The physical examination of a sick puppy or kitten should be conducted in a systematic manner. Additional information on the physical examination is found in Chapter 2. The first skill used in the examination is careful observation of the animal's responses, specifically noting the puppy's or kitten's general condition, mentation, posture, locomotion, and breathing pattern. Next, the body temperature, respiratory and heart rates, capillary refill time, and body weight should be recorded. After completing the observation and vital sign collection phase, the clinician should assess the function of specific body systems (Box 12-1).

Veterinarians often use a commercial laboratory facility for routine tests, such as hemograms, serum chemistry profiles, and urine analyses. However, collections from puppies and kittens younger than 6 weeks of age often do not yield adequate samples for testing by these laboratories. As an alternative, the veterinarian can use in-house laboratory tests, including microhematocrit for the packed cell volume (PCV), blood film examination of erythrocyte and leukocyte morphology, blood glucose and urea nitrogen (BUN) by reagent strip for whole blood, urine evaluation by reagent strip for urinalysis and a urine sediment examination, and total plasma solids and urine specific gravity by refractometer. The results of these few tests may

be sufficient to confirm illness or assist in case management of an illness.

An ECG can be used to diagnose life-threatening arrhythmias and conduction disturbances in puppies and kittens; however, ECG identification of right- or left-sided chamber enlargement or hypertrophy and alterations in mean electrical axis (MEA) usually is not attempted. The ECGs of young kittens normally have smaller amplitude P waves and QRS complexes than puppies in all leads. Any ECG lead with easily recognizable P waves and QRS complexes can be used to identify arrhythmias.

Real-time, gray-scale ultrasonography is the newest diagnostic tool to be used in puppies and kittens to identify selected abdominal and cardiac diseases. Ultrasonography usually is tolerated better by puppies and kittens and is safer for personnel than routine radiography. For ultrasonography in most puppies and kittens, a 5-MHz ultrasound transducer or, preferably, a 7.5-MHz transducer is required. The higher the transducer frequency, the better is the image resolution but the greater is the ultrasound beam attenuation in soft tissue. Linear array transducers used transrectally for reproductive examination are inadequate for imaging in most puppies and kittens.

Most echocardiography is performed in puppies and kittens that are 6 weeks of age or older. Echocardiography, whether obtained by the M-mode, two-dimensional, contrast, or Doppler echocardiographic technology, has facilitated evaluation of puppies and kittens with congenital heart disease by improving the diagnostic accuracy and lessening the stress and risk to animals. For echocardiography in puppies and kittens, a 7.5-MHz transducer is preferred. Heart lesions readily identified with M-mode or two-dimensional echocardiography include pericardial effusion, valvular vegetations, chamber size, myocardial hypertrophy, and abnormal cardiac motion.

Contrast echocardiography may be helpful in confirming a right-to-left shunting lesion. Doppler ultrasonography is becoming increasingly available. Doppler imaging

Box 12-1	PHYSICAL EXAMINATION OF PUPPY AND KITTEN

HEAD AND ORAL CAVITY

Check for malformations of the skull, cleft lip, stenotic nares, or cleft palate. The mucous membranes should be light pink and moist. The teeth, if present, should be examined for early occlusion.

EARS

External ear canals open between 6 and 14 days after birth and should be completely open by 17 days. When ear canals first open, cytologic examination shows an abundance of desquamative cells and some oil droplets. A thorough otoscopic examination can be made in kittens older than 4 wk of age.

EYES AND EYELIDS

The eyelids separate into upper and lower eyelids at 5 to 14 days after birth. Menace reflex may not appear until 3 to 4 wk of life. Reflex lacrimation begins when the eyelids separate; therefore evaluation of tear production by Schirmer's tear test can be done thereafter. Pupillary light responses are present after the eyelids open but may not be evident until 21 days of age.

NOSE

Check appearance and patency of the nostrils and the presence of fluids (mucus, pus, blood, milk, clear discharges).

THORAX

Check the thoracic wall, whether symmetric or deformed, and auscultate the thorax using a stethoscope with a pediatric chest piece (2-cm bell; 3-cm diaphragm). The heart rate approximates 220 beats/min and the respiratory rate is from 15 to 35 breaths/min during the first 4 weeks of life; they become similar to adults thereafter. The normal heart rhythm of puppies and kittens is a regular sinus rhythm. Heart sounds are localized to the left cardiac apex (left fifth to sixth intercostal space, ventral third of thorax), the left cardiac base (left third to fourth intercostal space above the costochondral junction), or the right cardiac apex (right fourth to fifth intercostal space opposite the mitral valve area). Heart murmurs are the most common type of abnormal sound heard, and frequently they are functional murmurs and not murmurs associated with congenital heart disease. Absence of lung sounds or audible asymmetry may indicate abnormalities within the thorax or lungs.

ABDOMEN

Unless the liver margins extend beyond the ribs, the liver is not enlarged. The spleen normally is not palpable unless it is enlarged. Both kidneys are palpable in all kittens. The stomach may feel like a large, fluid-filled sac if it is full. The intestines are palpable as soft, slightly fluid or gas-filled structures that are freely movable and nonpainful. The urinary bladder can be gently squeezed to determine resistance to urine outflow.

SKIN AND UMBILICUS

The skin should be inspected for wounds, state of hydration, and condition of foot pads. The skin and hair coat should also be examined for evidence of bacterial infection, external parasites, or dermatophytosis. The umbilicus should be carefully inspected for evidence of inflammation, infection, or abnormalities of the abdominal wall. The umbilical cord normally drops off by 2 to 3 days of age.

LIMBS, TAIL, ANUS, AND GENITALIA

Check the limbs for deformities or absence of long bones, number and position of toes and pads, position of limbs at rest and during movement, presence of soft tissue (bruises, swelling, wounds), and condition of joints (deformities, range of mobility). The tail is inspected for length, mobility, and deformities. The anus should be evaluated for patency, redness, and signs of diarrhea, and the genitalia should be checked for position and appearance.

NERVOUS SYSTEM

Suck reflex is present at birth and disappears by 3 wk of life. Eliminative behaviors are controlled for first 3 to 4 wk of life by anogenital reflex.

---

of high-velocity, retrograde, or turbulent flow through valves or intracardiac communications provides useful diagnostic and prognostic information in puppies and kittens with congenital heart defects. Interpretation of echocardiography from puppies and kittens requires an awareness of the growth pattern and developmental anatomy of the heart during the first year of life. After birth, there is a decrease in right ventricular mass relative to the left ventricle and to body weight, a decrease that occurs by the third week of life in puppies.

Additional information on ultrasound and radiology can be found in Chapter 9.

A finely tuned technique chart is necessary if good-quality radiographs are to be produced for all body parts of young puppies and kittens. Kilovoltage must be greatly reduced for radiography of a young puppy or kitten because of minimal absorption of x-rays by partially mineralized bones and because of the thinness of soft tissue body parts. A general guideline for reducing kilovoltage is to reduce the radiographic exposure to about one half of that used for adult dogs and cats of the same thickness. Extrapolations to thinner dogs and cats can be made based on the fact that each 1 cm of soft tissue is the equivalent of 2 kVp at values equal to or less than 80 kVp. Most radiography of young puppies and kittens will be performed in the 40- to 60-kVp range; therefore a change of 4 to 6 kVp doubles or halves the film exposure.

Technician Note

Kilovoltage must be greatly reduced for radiography of a puppy or kitten.

An additional step that can be helpful in producing maximum-quality radiographs in young puppies and kittens is to use a single high-detail intensifying screen within the cassette. The single screen should be adhered to the back inner surface of the cassette. The screen should be a rare-earth, high-detail type. The emulsion side of the x-ray film must be positioned toward the screen.

The development of computer equipment that can average electrical signals by extracting low-amplitude, time-locked potentials from random background electrical activity has provided procedures for noninvasive evaluation of the auditory and visual system. Recording of the brain stem auditory-evoked response (BAER) is the best objective procedure for assessment of hearing in puppies and kittens. The electrical potential from the cochlea, cochlear nerve, and brain stem in response to an auditory stimulus is recorded. The BAER approximates functional maturity by 4 to 6 weeks of age. If there is no response at all in puppies or kittens older than 6 weeks of age, the cochlea is not functioning, as may occur with congenital deafness.

The electroretinogram (ERG) is the electrical recording of retinal response to light. The ERG approximates functional maturity by 5 to 10 weeks of age. If there is no response at all after 10 weeks of age, the retina is not functioning, as may occur in retinal blindness from congenital or acquired causes. The visual-evoked response (VER) provides an objective evaluation of the central visual pathways. The VER is the cortical electrical activity that occurs in response to a light stimulus administered to the eye. The VER approximates functional maturity by 6 weeks of age. If there is an altered VER after 10 weeks of age, central visual pathways may not be functioning, as may occur in central blindness from congenital or acquired causes.

Newborn Puppies and Kittens

Newborn puppies and kittens are for all practical purposes completely helpless. They rely on their mother for warmth, food, elimination, cleanliness, and protection. They are incapable of thermal regulation for the first 6 days of life and require an external heat source to stay warm for 1 to 3 weeks of life. They nurse from the mother every 1 to 2 hours for the first week, and the mother licks their external genitalia both to stimulate urination and defecation and to clean them after every feeding. Five to fourteen days after delivery, the puppies' and kittens' eyes open but have limited vision; 1 or 2 days later their external ear canals open. By 18 days of age they begin to move around and explore their environment.

Keep puppies and kittens in a small box with sides high enough both to keep them inside and to prevent drafts. Raise the bottom of the box off the floor and cover it with a padded, disposable, or washable flooring such as indoor-outdoor carpeting and disposable diapers or cotton towels to keep the box as warm and dry as possible. Materials that become slippery when wet, such as newspapers, should not be used as bedding. Covered hot water bottles or heating pads set on the lowest setting may help keep the environmental temperature stable. Never set heating pads on higher settings, because severe burns can result. A puppy's or kitten's rectal temperature should be maintained at 96° F to 97° F for the first week of life and at 97° F to 100° F for the second, third, and fourth weeks. Do not cover the entire floor of the box with a heating pad; the puppy or kitten must be able to get away from the heat source if it gets too warm. A ticking clock placed in the box may help to keep puppies and kittens quiet.

Principles of Orphan Animal Care

Hand-raising orphan puppies and kittens requires a great deal of time and effort. The ideal solution to the problem of caring for a motherless puppy or kitten is to locate a lactating mother that will accept the puppy or kitten and raise it with its own. When a foster mother is not available, it is necessary to hand feed the puppy or kitten until about 4 to 6 weeks of age but leave the puppy or kitten if possible with litter mates between feedings during this time so it can interact with other puppies and kittens and thereby learn appropriate social behavior. If neither of the previous options is possible, total care of the puppy or kitten must

be undertaken. Puppies and kittens are usually mature enough to be sold between 6 and 8 weeks of age.

Successful rearing of orphaned puppies and kittens requires providing them with a suitable environment; the correct quantities and quality of nutrients for different stages of growth; a regular schedule of feeding, sleeping, grooming, and exercise; and the stimulus that provokes urination and defecation.

Newborn puppies and kittens are unable to effectively control their body temperature. They gradually change, during their first 4 weeks of life, from being largely poikilothermic to being homeothermic. That is, for the first week of life their body temperature is directly related to the environmental temperature, and a steady ambient temperature of 86° F to 90° F is needed. Over the next 3 weeks, the ambient temperature can be gradually lowered to 75° F. Humidity should be maintained at 55% to 60%. It is equally important that sudden changes of environmental conditions be avoided and that disturbances be minimized outside of socialization, exercise, and hygiene activities.

Feeding orphaned puppies and kittens that still require mother's milk can be rewarding. The most obvious alternative to a mother rearing her own young is for another nursing mother to act as a foster mother. If a foster mother is not available, it is necessary to hand feed the puppies or kittens a replacement food that is a prototype of nutritive substance formulated to meet the optimum requirements of the puppy or kitten. Mother's milk is the ideal food. Various modifications of homemade and commercially prepared formulas simulating mother's milk have been used with good success. Several homemade or commercially prepared formulas for rearing puppies and kittens may be used (Box 12-2).

Commercially prepared milk formulas are preferred, because they more closely compare to mother's milk. These formulas generally provide 1 to 1.24 Kcal of metabolizable energy per milliliter of formula. The caloric needs for most nursing-age puppies and kittens is 22 to 26 Kcal per 100 g of body weight. Therefore the average puppy or kitten should daily receive approximately 13 ml of formula per 100 g of body weight during the first week of life, 17 ml of formula per 100 g of body weight during the second week, 20 ml of formula per 100 g of body weight during the third week, and 22 ml of formula per 100 g of body weight during the fourth week. These amounts of formula should be given in equal portions three or four times daily. For the first 3 weeks of life, the formula should be warmed before each feeding to about 100° F or to a temperature near the animal's body temperature.

After each feeding, the abdomen should be enlarged but not overdistended. When a milk formula is used, less than the prescribed amount should be given per feeding for the first feedings. The amount is then gradually increased to the recommended feeding amount by the second or third day. The amount of milk formula is increased accordingly as the puppy or kitten gains weight and a favorable response to feeding occurs. Puppies should gain 1 to 2 g/day/lb (2 to 4 g/day/kg) of anticipated adult weight for the first 5 months of their lives. The kitten should weigh at birth 80 to 140 g (most weigh around 100 to 120 g) and gain 50 to 100 g weekly.

When preparing the formula, always follow the manufacturer's directions for its proper preparation, and keep all feeding equipment scrupulously clean. A good way of handling prepared formula is to prepare only a 48-hour supply at a time and divide this into portions required for each feeding. Once formula is prepared, it is best stored in the refrigerator at 4° C (39.2° F).

Box 12-2   TYPES OF FORMULAS FOR PUPPIES AND KITTENS

COMMERCIAL PREPARED MILK FORMULA FOR PUPPIES OR KITTENS
- Begin Milk Replacer for Puppies (Performer Brand)
- Begin Milk Replacer for Kittens (Performer Brand)
- Esbilac Powder for Puppies (Pet-Ag Inc.)
- Esbilac Liquid for Puppies (Pet-Ag Inc.)
- GME Powder for Puppies (a goat milk formula; Pet-Ag Inc.)
- Kittylac Powder for Kittens (Lander Corp.)
- KMR Liquid for Kittens (Pet-Ag Inc.)
- KMR Powder for Kittens (Pet-Ag Inc.)
- Multi-Milk for Multi-Animals (milk replacer for animals with lactose intolerance; Pet-Ag Inc.)
- Nurturall Liquid for Puppies (Veterinary Products Laboratories)
- Nurturall Powder for Puppies (Veterinary Products Laboratories)
- Nurturall Liquid for Kittens (Veterinary Products Laboratories)
- Nurturall Powder for Kittens (Veterinary Products Laboratories)
- Veta-Lac Powder for Puppies (Vet-A-Mix)
- Veta-Lac Powder for Kittens (Vet-A-Mix)

HOMEMADE PREPARED MILK FORMULA FOR PUPPIES
- 120 ml of cow's or goat's milk
- 120 ml of water
- 2-4 egg yolks
- 1-2 tsp vegetable oil
- 1000 mg of calcium carbonate

HOMEMADE PREPARED MILK FORMULA FOR KITTENS
- 90 ml of condensed milk
- 90 ml of water
- 120 ml of plain yogurt (not low fat)
- 3 large or 4 small egg yolks

The easiest and safest way to feed prepared formula to nursing-age puppies and kittens is by nipple bottle, dosing syringe, or tube. Nipple bottles made especially for feeding orphan puppies or kittens or bottles equipped with preemie infant nipples are preferred. When feeding with a nipple bottle, hold the bottle so that the puppy or kitten does not ingest air. The hole in the nipple should be such that when the bottle is inverted, milk slowly oozes from the nipple. It may be necessary to enlarge the nipple hole with a hot needle to get milk to ooze from the bottle when inverted. When feeding, squeeze a drop of milk onto the tip of the nipple and then insert the nipple into the puppy's or kitten's mouth. Never squeeze milk out of the bottle while the nipple is in the animal's mouth; doing so may result in laryngotracheal aspiration of the milk into the lungs. In addition, prepared formula should never be fed to a puppy or kitten that is chilled or that does not have a strong sucking reflex. Only when the sucking reflex is present should nipple-bottle feeding be attempted.

Tube feeding is the fastest way to feed orphaned puppies or kittens. Most owners can do it easily with a little training. The following may be used: a no. 5 Fr. infant feeding tube for puppies or kittens weighing less than 300 g, a no. 8 to 10 Fr. infant feeding tube for puppies or kittens weighing over 300 g, or an appropriately sized, soft, male urethral catheter. Once weekly, mark the feeding tube clearly to indicate the depth of insertion to ensure gastric delivery; that is, the distance from the last rib to the tip of the nose can be measured and marked off on the feeding tube as a guide. Never feed into the distal esophagus. When feeding, fill a syringe with warm prepared formula and fit it to the feeding tube, being sure to expel any air in the tube or syringe. Open the animal's mouth slightly, and with the animal's head held in the normal nursing position, gently pass the feeding tube to the marked area. If an obstruction is felt or coughing occurs before reaching the mark, the tube is in the trachea. If this does not happen, slowly administer the prepared formula over a 2-minute period to allow sufficient time for slow filling of the stomach. Regurgitation of formula rarely occurs; but if it does, withdraw the feeding tube and interrupt feeding until the next scheduled meal.

A vital aspect of tending orphaned puppies and kittens is to simulate, after feeding, the mother's tongue action on the anogenital area that provokes reflex micturition and defecation. Application of this stimulus has to be taken over by the person tending the puppies or kittens. The necessary result can be achieved by swabbing the anogenital area with moistened cotton or dry, soft tissue paper to manually stimulate reflex elimination. It is sometimes possible to effect the same response simply by running a forefinger along the abdominal wall. This stimulation should be regularly provided after each nipple-bottle feeding or tube feeding. After they reach about 3 weeks of age, puppies and kittens are usually able to relieve themselves without simulated stimulation.

Most puppies and kittens benefit from gentle handling before feeding to allow for some exercise and to promote muscular and circulatory development. In addition, at least once per week the orphaned puppy or kitten should be gently washed with a soft moistened cloth for general cleansing of the skin, simulating the cleansing licks of the mother's tongue.

As mentioned before, the orphaned puppy or kitten should be encouraged to begin eating solid food at 3 or 4 weeks of age, respectively. Once the animals are eating satisfactorily from a bowl, gradually reduce the amount of prepared formula being given until only the puppy or kitten food designed for growth is being fed, at least three times daily.

Puppies and kittens should be checked for gastrointestinal parasites at 3 weeks of age, and they require fecal rechecks when they return for their vaccinations. Heartworm preventive medication should be started at 6 to 8 weeks of age in areas where heartworms are endemic. The initial vaccination series consists of one injection of a multivalent vaccine given at 6 weeks of age and two boosters given at 9 weeks of age and 12 weeks of age. Puppies and kittens whose immune status is uncertain may receive an additional injection of multivalent vaccine as early as 2 weeks of age. The rabies injection is given at 3 months of age in most states.

Causes for Neonatal Care

Puppies and kittens commonly present for severe illnesses or rearing as an orphan during the period between birth and 12 weeks of age. Illnesses may have been acquired in utero, during the birth process (0 to 2 weeks of age), or in the postweaning period (6 to 12 weeks of age). Illness during the postweaning period is primarily caused by infectious (bacterial, viral, protozoal, parasitic) diseases or malnutrition potentiated by weaning stress, exposure to pathogenic organisms in the immediate environment, or diminished local or systemic immunity. In general, most puppy and kitten illnesses will occur because of congenital anomalies, nutritional diseases resulting from improper diets fed to the mother or her young, abnormally low birth weights, traumatic insults during or after the birth process (dystocia, cannibalism, maternal neglect), neonatal isoerythrolysis, infectious diseases, and other miscellaneous factors.

Malnutrition

Malnutrition occurs when basic nutritional requirements for the puppy or kitten are not being met. Malnutrition is especially common during the time when the young depend entirely on the mother. Several factors can contribute to malnutrition in the nursing puppy or kitten. The puppy or kitten may ingest insufficient or inadequate milk because the mother dies; the mother may disown her young; a larger litter may be born than can be cared for properly; and partial or complete lactation failure by the mother as a result of mastitis, metritis, or underdeveloped mammae may occur. In addition, puppies and kittens may be born underdeveloped, be so weak and sick that they cannot suckle, or have a congenital anomaly that precludes adequate milk intake. Failure to provide an adequate growth diet at 3 to 4 weeks of age can also result in malnutrition.

Immediate recognition of a malnourished puppy or kitten is usually based on their smaller, lighter appearance; feeble attempts to feed; or inability to attain adequate weight gain for its age. High-pitched, constant crying and inactivity with an accompanying weak sucking reflex are advanced indications that the nursing puppy or kitten is receiving insufficient or inadequate milk. Reduced body tone and muscle strength may be evident on handling. A coexisting congenital anomaly that is not immediately life threatening may be detected on physical examination as well.

Technician Note

Hypoglycemia and dehydration occur quickly when the puppy or kitten is not adequately fed.

The management of malnutrition in the nursing puppy or kitten generally requires that the proper nourishment be provided. Complications that are frequently encountered during the management of malnutrition are diarrhea, dehydration, hypoglycemia, and hypothermia. If diarrhea occurs during feeding of adequate amounts of commercial milk replacement formula, immediately reduce the amount of solids intake to one half of that offered. This can be done by diluting 1:1 the milk replacement formula with water or preferably with a mixture of equal parts of Ringer's solution and 5% dextrose in water solution. As the condition of feces improves, gradually increase the amount of solids to the recommended level. Hypoglycemia and dehydration occur quickly when the malnourished puppy or kitten is not adequately fed. Milk replacement formula should not be fed to a weak and severely chilled puppy or kitten that possesses a diminished sucking reflex or in which body temperature is below 35° C (95° F). Giving an equal mixture of warm Ringer's solution and 5% dextrose/water solution parenterally or administering orally a warm nutrient-electrolyte solution every 15 to 30 minutes until the puppy or kitten responds can help to alleviate or prevent dehydration and mild hypoglycemia.

Bacterial Infections

When bacterial infections overcome the ability of the puppy's or kitten's immune system to provide adequate protection, life-threatening illnesses such as neonatal sepsis occur. The bacterial invasion of the bloodstream that regularly occurs in puppies and kittens after birth would rarely be of any consequence in healthy adults. However, when overwhelming bacteremia develops in puppies and kittens 4 to 16 weeks of age, the severity of the illness usually influences survival. Factors predisposing puppies and kittens to septicemic conditions include coexistence of inadequate nutrition and thermoregulation, viral infections, parasitism, and developmental and heritable defects of the immune system.

Bloodstream invasion usually occurs by the more common bacteria, such as *Staphylococcus, Escherichia, Klebsiella, Enterobacter, Streptococcus, Enterococcus, Pseudomonas, Clostridium, Bacteroides, Fusobacterium,* and *Salmonella* spp.; of these, gram-negative bacilli most often occur. Sources from which gram-negative bacilli enter the bloodstream include gastrointestinal tract and peritoneal infection, respiratory tract infection, skin and wound infection, and urinary tract infection.

Signs of Neonatal Illness

The clinical manifestations of neonatal illness do not always allow specific identification of the cause. Further, many puppies and kittens have unusual or a wide variety of clinical presentations, which may not be immediately recognized as being associated with a specific illness. Death can occur so suddenly that noticeable signs are virtually absent. More typically, however, puppies and kittens will cry a lot and show signs of restlessness, weakness, hypothermia, diarrhea, altered respiration, hematuria, failure to thrive, and cyanosis, and in advanced stages, they may slough parts of their extremities.

The diagnosis of a neonatal illness is usually based on the case history and physical findings. Ideally, a complete blood count, plasma chemistry profile, urinalysis, urine and/or blood culture, and culture of suspected sources of infection are obtained. When dealing with neonatal sepsis, it is imperative to conduct a thorough search for the primary source of infection and collect appropriate bacterial culture samples before initiating antimicrobial therapy.

The hemograms of septicemic puppies and kittens are usually characterized by a normochromic normocytic anemia. Thrombocytopenia and mild to moderate neutrophilia with a left shift may be present. Another laboratory finding that is consistent with, but by no means specific for, neonatal sepsis is hypoglycemia. The remaining laboratory values from the plasma chemistry profile and urinalysis may reflect a specific organ failure.

Management of Neonatal Illness

Early, prompt care for the ill puppy or kitten is required for satisfactory results. Because many neonatal diseases may cause sudden death, puppies and kittens suspected of having a severe illness should be treated immediately. In most instances, rewarming, fluid replacement, and antimicrobial therapy are started empirically. Severely ill puppies and kittens may also require glucose therapy if hypoglycemia is present (Box 12-3).

Technician Note

Rewarming, fluid/glucose replacement, and antimicrobial therapy are the hallmarks of management for the ill puppy or kitten.

BOX 12-3	MANAGEMENT OF SEVERELY ILL PUPPY AND KITTEN

1. External warming procedure
   a. Use circulating hot water blanket and hot water bottle
   b. Take at least 20 to 30 min for gradual warming of the patient
   c. Turn the patient every hour
   d. Record rectal temperature every hour (preferred temperature, 37.7° C [100° F])
2. Parenteral fluid therapy
   a. Use multiple-electrolyte solution supplemented with 5% dextrose solution
   b. Supplement fluids with potassium chloride solution if plasma potassium concentration is less than 2.5 mmol/L
   c. Administer warm fluids slowly by intravenous or intraosseous route
3. Glucose replacement therapy
   a. Administer 5% dextrose solution intravenously or intraosseously, to effect
   b. Administer 10% dextrose solution, 1 to 2 ml/kg, to the patient that is profoundly depressed or having seizures
   c. Maintain plasma glucose concentration at 80 to 200 mg/dl for euglycemia
4. Antimicrobial therapy
   a. Collect bacterial culture samples (whole blood, urine, exudate, feces) before initiation of antimicrobial therapy
      (1) For blood culture, collect 1 ml of whole blood aseptically and inoculate blood directly into enriched tryptic or trypticase soy broth, dilute the whole blood 1:5 to 1:10 in enriched broth, and examine broth for bacterial growth 6 to 18 hr later

      (2) For urine culture, collect urine by cystocentesis and culture it by standard methods
      (3) For exudate and fecal cultures, collect and culture by standard methods
   b. Begin empiric treatment with antimicrobial agent(s) immediately after collection of appropriate bacterial culture samples
   c. Adjust dosage and dosing interval of antimicrobial agent(s) selected
   d. Administer antimicrobial agent by intravenous or intraosseous route
5. Provide oxygen and nutritional therapy
   a. Administer oxygen by mask or intranasal catheter to counteract tissue hypoxemia
   b. Encourage food intake once patient is normothermic and adequately hydrated
6. Monitor effectiveness of medical management
   a. Observe for improvement in patient's general demeanor
   b. Regularly assess cardiopulmonary status (it is extremely easy to overhydrate the severely ill puppy or kitten, and so attentive monitoring of breathing pattern is helpful for early recognition of overhydration)
   c. Weigh patient three or four times per day to record weight gain
   d. Observe for moistness of mucous membranes and clearness of urine in assessing for adequate hydration (healthy puppies and kittens have clear, colorless urine when normally hydrated; any color to the urine usually indicates dehydration)

The beta-lactam antimicrobial agents are considered to be the first choice in the treatment of septicemic puppies and kittens. The beta-lactam antimicrobial agents include the penicillins, the cephalosporins, and the combination of beta-lactam antimicrobials and beta-lactamase inhibitors. Unfortunately, clinical information necessary for appropriate dosing of antimicrobial agents in septicemic puppies and kittens is not always available. Drug distribution, especially in puppies and kittens younger than 5 weeks of age, differs from that of adults because of differences in body composition, such as lower total body fat, higher percentage of total body water, lower concentrations of albumin, and a poorly developed blood-brain barrier. Because of these differences, modifications of dosing amounts for adults, as much as 30% to 50% reduction of the adult dose, or changes in dosing frequency may be necessary when antimicrobial agents are administered to septicemic puppies and kittens.

Further, fluid replacement therapy and antimicrobial agents should be administered intravenously or intraosseously in severely ill puppies and kittens because systemic absorption after oral, subcutaneous, or intramuscular administration may not be reliable. Most drugs ingested by the lactating bitch or queen appear in her milk; the amount generally is 1% to 2% of the mother's dose. Therefore severely ill puppies or kittens should never be treated by treating only the lactating mother.

FOAL

The critically ill foal is perhaps the most intensively managed of all veterinary patients. The most important factor influencing a foal's survival is undoubtedly diligent nursing care. Successful foal management requires a team approach, and competent veterinary technical support has become the foundation of the team. The skills required of equine neonatal technicians are extensive. Assessment of the foal should attempt to identify factors relative to the dam that increase the foal's risk of being diseased. This chapter provides only an overview of these skills, and individuals with aspirations in this area should consult other textbooks that focus on equine and human neonatal care. See Recommended Reading at the end of this chapter. Additional clinical training can be obtained in most university teaching hospitals that have a foal neonatal care unit.

The High-Risk Mare

Early recognition of high-risk mares is an important management consideration, allowing early identification of high-risk foals. The most common conditions that place mares in this category include cachexia, advanced age, poor general state of health, vaginal discharge, poor perineal conformation, previous foaling difficulties, and prolonged transport during late gestation. Any concurrent diseases in the mare, but especially those affecting the cardiovascular system, compromise the fetus.

Mares should be evaluated for these risk factors. Some of them may be avoided just by proper management of the pregnant mare. Others may be closely monitored to prevent further potential problems. Once a mare is classified as high risk, evaluation of the viability of the fetus should be performed. Such evaluation includes rectal and ultrasonographic examination. Pregnant mares with no identifiable risk factors do not require prepartal evaluation of the fetus. On the other hand, mares classified as high-risk dams should be evaluated for viability.

The evaluation begins with a rectal examination. The fetus should be gently stimulated by ballottement and in response will often move. Even when high-risk mares require evaluation of the fetus, multiple rectal examinations may have a deleterious effect. The next step consists of transabdominal ultrasonographic examination, in which the heart rate, aortic diameter, and activity of the fetus may be evaluated, as well as uteroplacental contact and thickness.

The heart rate should become detectable at approximately 160 days of gestation. The heart rate average is 120 beats/min. However, it is highly variable during late gestation, from 80 to 160 beats/min. Fetal heart rate decreases over the course of gestation and becomes less variable. A low-frequency probe (e.g., 2.5 MHz) is required to image the fetal heart.

The uroplacental thickness should be 8 to 16 mm, and fluid should not be detectable between the placenta and uterine wall. If fluid is present between these two structures, it may be the result of placentitis or hemorrhage with consequent premature placental separation. Based on these findings, the uteroplacental unit should be monitored closely for further separation, and induction of labor may be an option at this point.

There are several methods to determine and predict parturition. However, just a few reliable methods can be found. Historically, gross appearance of the mammae, such as enlargement of the glands and presence of "wax" on the surface of the teats, has been used as a reliable method, and it is still valid today. Nevertheless, as many as 15% of mares may fail to exhibit this sign. One of the most consistent and significant changes before parturition is the rapid rise in colostral calcium. The levels of calcium in precolostrum can be determined by practically any laboratory or even just by the use of hard water test kits. Levels of calcium above 10 to 12 mmol/dl are considered to be significant enough to predict parturition within 1 day. Even when calcium levels seem to be the most reliable method to date to predict parturition, it is subject to false-negative and false-positive results.

The High-Risk Foal

The term *high-risk foal* refers to the foal that is not necessarily ill but at high risk of becoming ill. Sick foals generally appear normal for the first 24 hours of life and then quickly decompensate. Because survival depends on early recognition of disease, during the period of vague clinical signs, foals at high risk of becoming ill are assumed to be abnormal and are treated accordingly. During the initial examination, physical, historical, and laboratory factors that may classify the foal as high risk are identified.

The classic early signs of disease in the foal are lethargy, depressed suck reflex, depressed appetite, increased recumbency and sleeping, and decreased affinity for the mare. Historical factors relative to the foal that increase its chance of being high risk include the presence of twins, abnormal birth behavior (see Physical Examination), abnormal phys-

ical findings, failure of passive transfer, and shortened gestational length.

Technician Note

Incomplete skeletal ossification is common in immature foals and can result in crushing injury to the carpal and tarsal bones during normal weight-bearing. Foals exhibiting signs of immaturity should undergo carpal and tarsal radiography to identify this condition so proper supportive therapy can be instituted.

The equine gestational length may range from 315 to 365 days, with an average of 341 days. Prematurity refers to foals that are born before 320 days of gestational age. Physical signs of prematurity include low birth weight, weakness, delayed postpartal standing, soft pliant lips and ears, flexor tendon laxity, prominent forehead, soft silky hair coat, and incomplete ossification of the carpal and tarsal bones. Any of these physical abnormalities will categorize the foal as high risk. The terms *prematurity*, *dysmaturity*, and *immaturity* are often used incorrectly. Dysmature foals are of a gestational age more than 320 days with physical signs of prematurity. Immaturity is a blanket term encompassing all foals with physical signs of prematurity regardless of gestational age. It is noteworthy that miniature horse foals normally have a prominent forehead. Technicians working with foals should remember that external signs of immaturity correlate with immaturity of other body systems and greater susceptibility to disease and injury. For example, foals with a soft silky hair coat are likely to have incomplete skeletal ossification, which can result in crushing injury to the carpal and tarsal bones by simple weight-bearing. Individuals involved with foal care should be aware of the fragile nature of the equine neonate and take appropriate precautions.

Physical Examination

Recognizing high-risk foals requires familiarity with normal peripartal history and behavior. After birth, the normal equine neonate will exhibit a suck reflex in 20 minutes, stand within 1 to 2 hours, and nurse within 2 to 3 hours. Foals should urinate within 10 hours of birth and pass meconium, the dark first feces, by 24 hours of age. The mare should pass her placenta within 4 to 6 hours of delivering the foal.

The physical examination of the foal begins at a distance. The awake foal should be alert and easily aroused by stimuli in its environment. The respiratory rate is 20 to 40 breaths/min at birth, increasing to 60 to 80 breaths/min within 1 hour. The respiratory rhythm is regular in the awake state but may be irregular while the foal is sleeping. The degree of inspiratory and expiratory effort should be noted. Foals should develop a strong bond with their mare by 1.5 hours of age. Foals nurse an average of seven times per day. Head bobbing while searching for the udder is normal. Within 24 hours of birth the normal foal should be strong, alert, and capable of running.

As the examination continues, the foal's body systems should be thoroughly evaluated. Because the foal has its own list of common diseases (Table 12-1), special attention should be directed toward their early identification. The heart rate is 40 to 80 beats/min within 5 minutes after birth, increasing to 130 at 6 to 60 minutes and stabilizing at 90 to 100. The heart rate will increase to 130 or higher on exertion (e.g., when standing). Normal rectal temperature ranges from 37.2° C to 38.9° C (99° F to 102° F). The

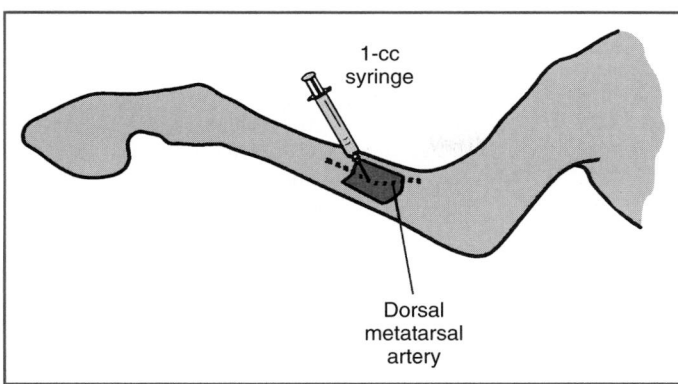

FIGURE 12-1. Location of dorsal metatarsal artery for collection of arterial blood samples in the foal.

TABLE 12-1	DISEASES OF FOALS
Body System	**Diseases**
Infectious	Septicemia/bacteremia, pneumonia, meningitis, omphalophlebitis, nephritis, septic arthritis, osteomyelitis, septic peritonitis
Gastrointestinal	Meconium impaction, gastric and duodenal ulceration, enteritis, peritonitis, intussusception, intraluminal obstruction, volvulus, cleft palate, prognathism, brachygnathism, atresia coli, atresia recti, atresia ani
Respiratory	Respiratory distress complex, pneumonia, meconium aspiration, persistent pulmonary hypertension
Cardiovascular	Ventricular septal defect
Musculoskeletal	Flexural deformities, angular limb deformities, incomplete skeletal ossification, osteochondrosis, physitis, rib fracture
Urogenital	Patent urachus, rupture of the ureter, bladder, urethra or urachus, umbilical hernia, scrotal hernia
Immunologic	Failure of passive transfer, combined immunodeficiency
Hematologic	Neonatal isoerythrolysis, anemia
Neurologic	Neonatal maladjustment syndrome, brain and spinal hemorrhage, epilepsy
Ocular	Corneal ulcer, entropion, ectropion
Miscellaneous	Hypoxemia, hypoglycemia, hypothermia

integument should be inspected for decubital ulcers, urine, and fecal scalding.

Evaluating cardiovascular stability begins by palpating. The arterial pulse is easily identified at the facial artery, which courses beneath the ramus of the mandible; the brachial artery, located at the medial aspect of the elbow; and the great metatarsal artery, which is palpable on the lateral aspect of the third metatarsal bone (Figure 12-1). This latter vessel is ideal for the collection of arterial samples for blood gas analysis. The foal should not have pulse deficits, jugular distention, or a jugular pulse. Cardiac auscultation generally reveals a grade II to VI machinery or holosystolic murmur at the left heart base, which abates by 72 hours after birth. Rarely, the murmur may continue for 30 to 60 days. This murmur is suspected to be associated with closing of the ductus arteriosus. Rate and rhythm of the heart should also be assessed. The capillary refill time should be less than 2 seconds. Mucous membranes of the mouth, eyes, nares, vulva, and urethra should be pink and moist. Cyanotic, jaundiced, or injected membranes are abnormal. All membranes should be closely inspected for ulceration or petechiae. It should be noted that membrane color is not an adequate assessment of oxygenation in the foal. Adequate oxygenation can only be assessed by means of arterial blood gas analysis.

A complete auscultation of the lung fields should be performed. The respiratory tract is a major route for expo-sure to organisms causing septicemia. The boundaries of the equine lung begin at the seventeenth intercostal space at the level of the tuber coxae and slope in an arc to an area just above the olecranon.

Technician Note

All high-risk foals should undergo thoracic radiography at admission even if thoracic auscultation is normal.

A foal's lung sounds are normally harsh, making evaluation subjective. An elevated respiratory rate, which exacerbates harsh lung sounds, can occur with many systemic diseases in the absence of lung disease. The slightest wheeze or crackle should be taken seriously. Note that auscultation is extremely insensitive for the detection of lung disease in the foal. The chest should be carefully examined for possible rib fractures. Because pneumonia and other lung diseases can be ruled out only by radiographic examination of the thorax, all high-risk foals should have thoracic radiographs performed on admission.

In examining the gastrointestinal system, the passage of meconium should be ensured because meconium impaction is the primary cause of neonatal colic. Foals should have fecal matter on the thermometer. If none is present, the possibility of a nonpatent gastrointestinal system (atresia ani, atresia coli) in a foal that exhibits abdominal pain or straining to defecate should be considered. Diarrhea is a significant finding because the gastrointestinal system is a second major route for exposure to bacterial organisms causing septicemia. Borborygmi should be detectable by auscultation. Abdominal distention or "pings" noted on auscultation are abnormal findings. The mouth is examined for cleft palate and abnormal dentition. Foals with clefts in the soft palate often require endoscopic examination to identify the abnormality.

The musculoskeletal evaluation needs to focus on two major types of diseases: infectious and noninfectious. Infectious diseases involving joints or growth plates need to be considered as emergency situations, since they will have a direct detrimental effect on the animal's future performance. All palpable joints should be carefully evaluated for signs of swelling, heat, or pain. Musculoskeletal infectious diseases should be suspected in foals with abnormal gait or reluctance to move.

Noninfectious diseases include multiple abnormalities. However, just incomplete skeletal ossification and some congenital or traumatic defects should be considered as emergency situations for which immediate therapy needs to be established.

The urogenital system is another area for intense examination. For many years, the significance of the umbilicus as a major route of infection has been recognized. The umbilical stump, palpable outside the abdomen, consists of remnants of the urachus (which connected to the bladder in utero), one umbilical vein, and two umbilical arteries. Within the abdomen, the umbilical vein courses forward to the liver, and the umbilical arteries travel caudally entering the wall of the bladder. The umbilicus is closely inspected for infection, increased size, and moistness, which suggests patency. Because the predominance of the umbilical structures is within the abdomen, thorough examination requires ultrasonic imaging. The umbilical, inguinal, and scrotal areas are palpated for hernias and distention. Abdominal distention or pitting edema of the perineal or inguinal areas may indicate impatency of the urinary tract. Because of its liquid diet, the normal foal passes dilute urine frequently.

The neurologic system of the foal is relatively unique compared with that of the adult horse. When the foal stands for the first time, it assumes a base-wide stance and, as it tries to ambulate, takes exaggerated steps. Exaggerated response to visual, auditory, and tactile stimuli and exaggerated jerky movements are normal. The recumbent foal will normally have hyperreflexive spinal reflexes even as severe as myoclonus (rhythmic muscle contraction) when one is eliciting the patellar reflex. The normal foal also exhibits a crossed extensor reflex (extension of a limb in response to squeezing the opposite limb) for as long as 4 weeks. When restrained, the standing foal initially struggles and then falls limp into the arms of the person restraining it, as if sleeping. Loosening the restraint causes the foal to support its weight again.

During the neurologic examination, the eyes must not be neglected. Foals do not have a menace reflex for 2 weeks after birth. When excited, the pupillary light reflex of the foal may be slow. The presence of entropion or ectropion should be noted because such conditions and associated corneal ulceration are common. The eyes are carefully examined for corneal abrasion and ulcers, uveitis, hyphema (blood in the anterior chamber), hypopyon (purulent exudate in the anterior chamber), and congenital cataracts.

Laboratory Examination

The hematologic values and serum chemistry values of the foal differ somewhat from those of the adult horse (Table 12-2). The ranges provided are from the laboratory of the University of Florida, College of Veterinary Medicine. Because of interlaboratory variations in technique and equipment, reference ranges should be established at each laboratory. The packed cell volume (PCV) of the normal foal is greater than that of the adult during the first 24 hours of

TABLE 12-2	SELECTED LABORATORY VALUES OF THE EQUINE NEONATE		
Age	**PCV (%)**	**RBC (× 10⁶/μl)**	**Plasma Protein (g/dl)**
Presuckle	40-52	9.3-12.9	4.5-5.9
≤12 hr	37-49	9.0-12.0	5.1-7.6
1 day	32-46	8.2-11.0	5.2-8.0
1 day-1 mo	28-46	7.2-11.6	5.1-7.9
Adult	31-47	5.9-9.9	6.2-8.0
	Serum Protein (g/dl)	**ALP (IU/L)**	**GGT (IU/L)**	**SDH (IU/L)**
Presuckle				
<12 hr	4.0-7.9	152-2835	13-39	0.2-4.8
1 day	4.3-8.1	861-2671	18-43	0.6-4.6
1 day-1 mo	4.4-7.76	137-1462	8-169	0.6-8.4
Adult	5.5-7.9	64-214	5-28	0.5-3.0
	Glucose (mg/dl)	**Creatinine (mg/dl)**	**BUN (mg/dl)**
Presuckle			
<12 hr	108-190	1.7-4.2	12-27
1 day	121-233	0.4-4.3	9-40
1 day-1 mo	101-221	0.4-2.1	2-29
Adult	57-96	0.9-2.0	12-24

Data from Koterba AM, Drummond WH, Kosch PC: *Equine clinical neonatology*, Philadelphia, 1990, Lea & Febiger; University of Florida, College of Veterinary Medicine.
ALP, Alkaline phosphatase; *BUN*, blood urea nitrogen; *GGT*, gamma glutamyl transferase; *PCV*, packed cell volume; *RBC*, red blood cell (count); *SDH*, sorbitol dehydrogenase.

life and falls into the low normal range of the adult from 2 weeks to 1 year of age. Total red blood cell count (RBC) for the foal remains above that of the adult from birth through 1 year of age. Band neutrophils are uncommon in the normal foal and more than 100 to 150 cells/μl should be considered abnormal. Plasma protein concentrations of the foal are expected to be much lower than those of the adult before absorption of colostral immunoglobulins, but as noted, the normal range of plasma protein concentration in the foal after suckle remains below that of the adult horse. Serum protein concentrations follow a similar trend.

Serum concentrations of alkaline phosphatase (ALP), gamma glutamyl transferase (GGT), sorbitol dehydrogenase (SDH), alanine transaminase (ALT), and glucose in foals are consistently higher than those in adult horses. ALP elevation is attributable to increased bone, intestine, and liver activity. The GGT and SDH activities are attributed to a greater liver activity, perhaps associated with greater liver mass relative to body mass in the foal. ALT changes are of questionable clinical significance because this enzyme is not organ specific in the horse. Foals' higher serum glucose concentrations are attributed to their frequent feeding behavior. Serum creatinine and urea nitrogen may be elevated above levels of normal equine adults during the first 36 to 72 hours of life. Creatinine and urea nitrogen values fall below the normal adult values by 1 to 3 days after birth. Urine specific gravity is also low throughout the neonatal period, with values ranging from 1.001 to 1.012.

Admitting the Sick Foal

The labor involved in admitting, monitoring, and treating a sick foal is intensive. A team approach to the diagnostic work-up and management of the foal is integral to success. For this reason, management of the severely compromised neonate has been most successful in a specialized neonatal intensive care unit.

Technician Note

Initial management of the foal should identify and treat the three most immediate life-threatening conditions of compromised foals: asphyxia, hypoglycemia, and hypothermia.

Three conditions are immediately life threatening in the compromised foal: asphyxia, hypoglycemia, and hypothermia. Initial management of the foal should address these problems before proceeding to less-threatening problems. Ambulatory foals should be gently restrained during work-up to minimize stress. Recumbent foals should be examined on a well-padded, warm (25° C [77° F]) surface. As the foal is examined, nasal insufflation of oxygen is warranted if the foal is showing respiratory distress. Although it is ideal to collect blood gas samples before oxygen insufflation and begin intravenous fluid administration after collecting samples for blood culture, the stability of the patient should alter the order of admission protocol as needed.

Once initial parameters are recorded, heat lamps and circulating water blankets are applied if the foal's rectal temperature is less than 37.8° C (100° F). Foals should be warmed slowly to prevent cardiovascular collapse and thermal burns. Heating blankets and heat lamps should not exceed 39.4° C (103° F). Foals are extremely susceptible to burns, and electric dry heat pads are not recommended. Next, a peripheral vein is prepared for venipunc-

ture under sterile conditions. The cephalic vein is ideal, because the jugular vein should be used only for venous catheterization. Blood is collected for aerobic and anaerobic blood culture, complete blood count (CBC), fibrinogen, serum chemistry, electrolyte analysis, and assessment of passive transfer. Once initial blood cultures are collected, a venous catheter is placed if warranted. An arterial blood gas sample is collected. A second set (and possibly a third) of blood cultures is collected in 15 minutes to 1 hour. Appropriate fluid therapy is administered.

Technician Note

Venous catheters and lines must be placed and maintained under conditions of rigid asepsis.

Venous catheters are a primary iatrogenic portal of infection and *must* be placed and maintained under conditions of *rigid asepsis*. Always clip hair, and use sterile solutions to scrub liberally for catheter placement. Wear sterile gloves. Use an extension set on the catheter, and wrap the secured catheter with a sterile dressing. The fluid of choice and rate of administration for initial therapy depend on the foal's glucose, electrolyte, and hydration status. As a rule of thumb, 0.45% sodium chloride with 2.5% dextrose solution is a safe initial fluid in the dehydrated foal. The normal maintenance fluid requirement in the equine neonate is 80 to 120 ml/kg/24 hr or 150 to 225 ml/hr for the average 45-kg foal. Shock fluids can be administered at 20 ml/kg/hr for short periods. Concentrations of dextrose solution from 5% to 10% are warranted in the severely hypoglycemic foal but should be administered with the understanding that hyperglycemia can be detrimental. Bolus dosing of 25% to 50% dextrose solution is not advised.

Once the foal is stabilized, it is weighed, thoracic radiographs are performed, and therapy is determined. Additional diagnostic measures that may be warranted include abdominal ultrasound and radiographs, transtracheal aspiration, arthrocentesis, cerebrospinal fluid collection, urinary catheterization, fecal collection, abdominocentesis, nasogastric intubation, and gastroduodenal endoscopy.

Routine Perinatal Therapy

Certain aspects of neonatal care are common to all foals regardless of their risk category. At birth, the umbilicus should be allowed to tear on its own. A dilute (2% to 3.5%) iodine solution should be applied to the umbilical stump. This treatment should be continued four times per day for 1 week or until umbilical disease abates. Foals from mares that were not vaccinated with tetanus antitoxin in the last 4 to 6 weeks of gestation should receive 1500 IU of tetanus antitoxin intramuscularly. On some farms, an enema is routinely administered after birth. If the foal has not defecated within 24 hours or is straining to defecate, a pediatric Fleet enema or warm, soapy water enema can be administered. This should be done with great care and generous lubrication, because the rectal mucosa of the foal is fragile.

Failure of Passive Transfer

Foals are born without appreciable quantities of circulating protective immunoglobulin. The mare's first milk contains colostrum rich in immunoglobulins that the foal must ingest and absorb for adequate immunologic protection. Because the gastrointestinal cells that allow absorption of these immunoglobulins are lost soon after birth, the foal must ingest the colostrum by 6 hours of age. Inadequate absorption of colostrum is termed *failure of passive transfer* and is thought to be associated with increased susceptibility to infection.

Assessing adequate passive transfer is an integral portion of the initial work-up. Although there is some debate over what constitutes adequate passive transfer, most neonatal clinicians agree that high-risk foals should have serum immunoglobulin G (IgG) concentrations greater than 800 mg/dl. IgG levels are generally measured 18 to 24 hours after birth to allow time for absorption of ingested colostrum. Several tests that quantify IgG are available, each with advantages and disadvantages. At this time, the time-honored gold standard is the radial immunodiffusion (RID) test. Although this appears to be the most accurate test, the expense, limited availability, and 24-hour testing time preclude its use in routine screening. The concentration immunoassay technology (CITE) test is perhaps the most commonly used screening test because it is quick, accurate, easily performed, and readily available. Of the rapid test methods (zinc sulfate turbidity, latex agglutination, CITE), CITE is the only test that has sensitivity in the 800 mg/dl range.

Ensuring adequate passive transfer is an integral part of treatment for all equine neonates regardless of their disease process. When an immunoglobulin deficit is detected, it can be replaced by one of two methods. The first, oral administration of colostrum from a donor, is ideal but is not generally useful because most foals are too old to absorb colostrum by the time a deficit is detected. Foals should receive 1 to 2 L of colostrum by 12 to 16 hours of age and have IgG levels measured 16 to 20 hours later. Failure of passive transfer after 24 hours is treated with intravenous administration of plasma from an appropriate donor. Commercial plasma is available and is expensive. Plasma is administered via a sterile intravenous catheter. A general rule of thumb is that 1 L of plasma raises the IgG level of the 45-kg foal by 200 mg/dl.

Antimicrobial therapy should always be based on isolating infected organisms and antimicrobial sensitivities. Special considerations need to be made regarding physiologic features of the neonate, such as reduced hepatic activity and renal immaturity. Nevertheless, antibiotic therapy should be instituted as soon as sepsis is suspected, without waiting for culture results. In general, a combination of a penicillin and an aminoglycoside provides adequate coverage.

Nutrition

The currently accepted minimum energy requirement of the compromised equine neonate is 180 Kcal/kg/day. Achieving this level via the enteral route (using the gastrointestinal tract) is practically impossible, and accordingly many compromised foals require parenteral (intravenous) nutrition to achieve sufficient energy intake. At this time, adequate nutrition is assessed based on weight gain. The healthy 45-kg foal should gain 1.4 to 1.6 kg/day.

Some foals require assistance or encouragement to nurse from their mare. Every effort should be made to feed foals from their mare. Foals that are unable or unwilling to nurse from their mare can be allowed to nurse a bottle or bucket if they maintain a suck reflex. Without a strong suck reflex, the foal will require an indwelling nasogastric tube for feeding. Enteral feeding is ideal because it is physiologic, inexpensive, and simple, and it stimulates gastrointestinal maturity. The primary complication associated with enteral feeding is aspiration pneumonia. Before each use of a nasogastric tube, its position within the stomach or

Box 12-4	CALORIC DENSITIES OF SELECTED MILK REPLACERS FOR FOALS
Foal Lac (Pet-Ag Inc.): 260 Kcal/pint
Mare's Match (Land O Lakes): 221 Kcal/pint
Nutri-Foal (Ross Laboratories): 345 Kcal/pint	

distal esophagus must be ensured. Recumbent foals must be placed in sternal recumbency during and for 30 minutes after feeding to prevent regurgitation and aspiration of milk.

Mare's milk is the best source of enteral nutrition for the foal. When available, mare's milk should always be used. To prevent mastitis, the mare's udder and caretaker's hands should always be cleaned before milking and teat dip should be applied after milking. Several alternatives to mare's milk are available, but all have their drawbacks. Preparations formulated for enteral nutrition of other species are generally not suitable for the foal. Goat's milk is palatable but causes some metabolic abnormalities and should not be utilized alone for extended periods. Goat's milk has a caloric density of 276 Kcal/pint. Milk replacers are readily available and inexpensive but unpalatable and notorious for causing gastrointestinal upsets. Goat's milk can be added to milk replacers to improve palatability. Milk replacers, when fed according to labeled directions, underestimate the caloric requirements of foals by 50% to 70%. Quantities to be fed should be calculated daily based on caloric requirement and the foal's body weight. Box 12-4 lists the caloric density of several milk replacers.

When feeding foals, all utensils should be thoroughly cleaned and disinfected before and after use. Once reconstituted, milk should be kept refrigerated. The preparations should be discarded after 2 hours at room temperature. Foals will not nurse from commercial cow nipples but do quite well with a lamb's nipple. Orphan foals should be bucket fed as soon as possible to limit human imprinting, which can become dangerous as the foal matures. Enteral feeding should be started gradually. Begin at 50 to 100 ml every 30 to 60 minutes. If the foal tolerates these feedings, the volume of milk may be gradually increased, and timing of feedings may be spaced to every 2 hours. Many high-risk foals will not tolerate enteral nutrition, and feeding should be discontinued if regurgitation, abdominal distention, colic, or severe diarrhea occurs. Foals receiving less than 100 Kcal/kg/day should be considered candidates for parenteral nutrition.

Monitoring and Nursing Care

Once the foal has been admitted and initially examined, diligent monitoring is critical. The objective of frequent monitoring is to detect subtle changes in body parameters that signify a worsening or improvement in the foal's status. The primary complications that occur in foals are the development of alternative resistant nosocomial infections, alternate sites of infection (arthritis, osteomyelitis), corneal ulcers, decubital ulcers, and malnutrition. Frequency of monitoring varies with the severity of the patient's illness. Parameters should always be recorded on a flow sheet. Table 12-3 lists parameters that should be monitored and is basically a thorough, foal-oriented physical examination with the addition of blood pressure, blood gas, and ventilator monitoring as warranted. Pay close attention to the catheter site for evidence of jugular distention, heat, pain, or swelling. Box 12-5 suggests exam-

TABLE 12-3	MONITORING IN THE CRITICALLY ILL FOAL
Body System	**Parameters Monitored During Physical Examination**
Cardiovascular	Pulse: rate, rhythm, strength
	Heart rate, rhythm, and murmurs
	Mucous membranes: color, CRT, petechiae, injection, hyperemia
Respiratory	Breathing: rate, effort, pattern
	Chest excursion
	Lungs: auscultation, percussion
Thermoregulatory	Body temperature: warmth of extremities
Gastrointestinal	Feces: volume, consistency
	Borborygmi: frequency, character
	Abdominal distention, signs of colic and gastric reflux
Urinary	Urination: frequency, volume
	Umbilicus: monitor for patency and signs of infection
Musculoskeletal	Joints: lameness, warmth, distention
	Tendon and ligament laxity
	Angular limb deformity
Integument	Decubital ulcers; urine and fecal scalding
Ocular	Cornea: abrasions, ulcers, edema
	Anterior chamber: hypopyon
	Lids: entropion
	Sclera: injection, petechiae
Nervous	Mental status, attitude, behavior
	Posture and muscle tone
	Gait: limb proprioception
	Cranial nerve and spinal reflexes

From Koterba AM, Drummond WH, Kosch PC: *Equine clinical neonatology*, Philadelphia, 1990, Lea & Febiger.
CRT, Capillary refill time.

BOX 12-5	TRENDS OR CHANGES IN CONDITION THAT OFTEN WARRANT INTERVENTION

1. Trends
   a. Increasing or decreasing body temperature
   b. Increasing or increasingly irregular respiratory rate
   c. Increasingly rapid (>120 beats/min), slow (<60 beats/min), or irregular heartbeat
   d. Weakening peripheral pulses
   e. Blood gases
      (1) *Decreasing* Pa_{O_2}: if foal is receiving oxygen therapy, check flow rate and pressure gauge for any disconnections or plugs in tubing; consider the amount of struggling and length of time in lateral recumbency; if there are no equipment problems, consider worsening pulmonary function
      (2) *Increasing* Pa_{CO_2}, particularly with increased effort of breathing: suggests foal's respiratory system may be failing
      (3) *More negative base excess:* implies worsening metabolic acidosis; cause should be determined
2. Seizure activity
3. Colic
4. Decreased nursing activity
5. Gastric reflux
6. Diarrhea or constipation, excessive straining to defecate
7. Abdominal distention
8. Lack of, or reduced, urination
9. Eye abnormalities, most commonly corneal ulcers
10. Pitting edema, most commonly observed in subcutaneous tissues of ventral abdomen and legs, may indicate fluid overload, impaired renal function, infection, or capillary injury

Modified from Koterba AM, Drummond WH, Kosch PC: *Equine clinical neonatology*, Philadelphia, 1990, Lea & Febiger.

---

ination parameters that warrant closer attention by the attending clinician.

The hallmarks of nursing care for the foal are cleanliness and tender loving care. Working with foals is as much an art as a science. Standing foals are generally restrained against a wall with one hand under the neck and the other under the rump. The recumbent foal can be a challenge to restrain. Techniques are described, but the reality is usually different. Restraint should be safe for the foal, handlers, and associated intravenous lines and equipment.

If more than one foal is being treated, care must be exercised to avoid cross contamination. All injections are made through skin that is clean after alcohol swabbing of the area has dried. Intramuscular injections are limited to the semimembranosus region and should not be given in the neck or gluteal region. Fluid lines should be changed daily. Once disconnected, fluid lines are contaminated and should be replaced. Multidose vials and catheter caps should be disinfected before needle insertion. Needles and syringes are *not* reused. All intravenous ports should be capped with injection caps. Catheters should be flushed with heparinized saline every 4 hours. The interval for catheter change depends on the type of catheter material and the status of the vein. The commonly used Teflon catheters should be removed and placed in an alternate vein *at least every 72 hours.* Silastic and polyurethane catheters are available and, because of their lower thrombogenicity relative to Teflon, can remain in place for several weeks if they receive the proper care. These catheters are expensive but quickly become cost-effective over a time course that would require several Teflon catheter changes.

The foal should be kept clean, dry, and warm, and milk should be warmed before being fed. All joints should be placed through passive range of motion several times per day. Because of the adverse effects of lateral recumbency on lung pathologic conditions and ventilation, foals should be maintained in a semisternal position with their thorax and forelimbs in sternal recumbency and their hips and rear limbs in lateral recumbency. This position can be achieved through the use of wedge-shaped pads or sandbags positioned at the level of the elbows and thorax.

If this position cannot be maintained, the recumbent foal should be turned from side to side every 2 to 4 hours. Foals should be encouraged to stand and ambulate. This effort may range from the handler's suspending the foal and encouraging it to bear weight to the handler taking the foal for casual short walks in the fresh air.

Summary

Working with compromised foals is an exhausting endeavor. Despite intensive labor, many high-risk foals will still die, usually taking with them a piece of each team member who has worked so hard to save them. Attention to detail must be unrelenting, and with the help of diligent, highly skilled technicians, more will survive.

RECOMMENDED READING

PUPPY AND KITTEN

Boothe DM, Tannert K: Special considerations for drug and fluid therapy in the pediatric patient, *Comp Contin Educ Pract Vet* 14:313, 1992.

Dow SW, Papich MG: Keeping current on developments in antimicrobial therapy, *Vet Med* 86:600, 1991.

Hoskins JD: *Veterinary pediatrics: dogs and cats from birth to six months,* ed 3, Philadelphia, 2001, WB Saunders.

FOAL

Clabough DL: Disease of the equine neonate, *J Equine Vet Sci* 8:5, 1988.

Drummond WH: Bridging the gap between the human and equine neonate. In Rossdale PD, editor: *The application of intensive care therapies and parenteral nutrition in large-animal medicine,* Deerfield, Ill, 1986, Travenol Labs.

Koterba AM: IV fluid therapy and nutritional support in the sick neonate, *Equine Vet Educ* 3:33, 1991.

Koterba AM, Drummond WH, Kosch PC, editors: *Equine clinical neonatology,* Philadelphia, 1990, Lea & Febiger.

Madigan JE, editor: *Manual of equine neonatal medicine,* ed 2, Woodland, Calif, 1991, Live Oak.

McKinnon AO, Voss JL: *Equine reproduction,* Philadelphia, 1993, Lea & Febiger.

Reed MS, Bayly MW: *Equine internal medicine,* Philadelphia, 1998, WB Saunders.

13

Animal Behavior

Suzanne Hetts

Most veterinary technicians do not need to be convinced how important applied animal behavior is to veterinary medicine. However, as further proof, recent studies have shown that behavior problems are one of the most common reasons that dogs and cats are surrendered to shelters and that dogs who have been to basic training classes are less likely to be surrendered, whereas most dogs in shelters have not had basic training (Patronek et al., 1996a, 1996b; Salman et al., 1998). In addition, when owners received advice about behavior problems that was either not helpful or not tried, that in turn put their pets at greater risk for surrender.

WHY BEHAVIOR WELLNESS?

Most of the emphasis on continuing veterinary education in animal behavior has been on problem resolution techniques. Lectures on resolving separation anxiety, aggression problems in both dogs and cats, and fears and phobias are common in veterinary technician continuing education programs. However, problem resolution skills are arguably the most advanced and complex and require the most education and experience. Problem resolution services are also usually the most problematic for veterinary professionals to profitably implement. Although technicians may either want to or feel an obligation to help owners resolve problems, veterinary practice owners may feel the time they spend trying to help owners is a financial drain. Practitioners may not know what to tell owners or how to resolve problems, and they may not know who in the community can be trusted to refer clients for behavioral assistance.

Comparatively less effort has been invested in intensely focusing on preventing normal behaviors from becoming problems and on early identification of problems when they first develop. Yet at least one study suggests that many owners who relinquish their pets have tolerated problems for months or years, often unable to find effective help in resolving the problem (DiGiacomo et al., 1998). Most dogs who are surrendered to shelters are under 3 years of age (New et al., 1999), and some types of problems, most notably aggression, often seem to develop when the pet is around 2 years of age. Thus there seems to be, in many cases, a window of opportunity for prevention and detection of problems that is not being taken advantage of to the fullest extent possible.

Owners often ignore or tolerate problems such as inappropriate elimination, phobias, or family pets not getting along until either the problem worsens or there is a lifestyle change that makes resolution of the problem a priority. Problems are usually much more difficult to resolve at these stages than had intervention been obtained earlier. For both general practice veterinary professionals, including technicians, and pet owners, then, focusing on preventing problems, detecting them early, and providing appropriate intervention and referral when they do occur is more beneficial than a narrow focus on problem resolution, which is often sought at a crisis moment.

WHAT IS BEHAVIOR WELLNESS?

Problem prevention, early detection or assessment of developing problems, and resolution services and appropriate referrals to behavioral consultants are the three basic components of a behavior wellness program. If given sufficient education in behavior wellness and proper direction and support from the veterinarian, veterinary technicians can be the most strategically positioned individuals on the veterinary health care team to deliver many services within a behavior wellness program.

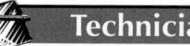

Technician Note

The technician is often the first person owners ask about why their pets behave the way they do.

The technician is often the first person owners ask about why their pets behave the way they do, how to prevent problems, and what to do once their pets' behavior has become a problem. This can be used to everyone's benefit in the implementation of a behavior wellness program. In addition, practice management consultants are emphasizing the importance of veterinarians delegating health care tasks to their support staff when such tasks do not require the veterinarian (Wood, 1997). Increased use of techni-

---

Box 13-1   BENEFITS OF A BEHAVIOR WELLNESS PROGRAM

- The technician's job can be more rewarding and interesting.
- The technician and the clinic will better understand and meet both the clients' and the patients' needs. It is clear from the studies of animal shelters that the need for behavioral services is not being met.
- A behavior wellness program can help to make a visit to the clinic less stressful and more enjoyable for patients. This in turn can result in better health care for the pet. Many owners put off visiting the veterinarian if they know from past experience that this will be stressful and unpleasant for the animal.
- Pets become safer and easier to handle, and fewer staff members are bitten.
- A behavior wellness program increases the number of client visits per year.
- A program adds a significant dollar amount to the bottom line each year.
- A program attracts and retains top of the line staff: the most motivated and best educated.
- A program decreases frustration in dealing with problem owners and problem pets because the technician can now provide them with services that can *prevent* pets from becoming difficult patients.

---

cians in history taking, nutrition, prophylactic dental services, and general client education has set precedents that provide the veterinary technician with a unique opportunity to play a leading role in behavior wellness programs as well. Doing so can have a number of positive benefits to the technician, to the clinic, and to pets and their owners (Box 13-1).

IMPLEMENTING A BEHAVIOR WELLNESS PROGRAM

First Step: A Change in Perspective

The veterinary technician might have a number of different reactions when owners ask questions about behavior.

If behavior is a particular interest of the veterinary technician, he or she may spend quite a bit of time with owners, attempting to give them the information they seek. Depending on the question and the technician's background, he or she may feel comfortable and qualified to discuss owners' questions or not quite sure what to tell the owners. Some technicians even use their personal time, for which they are not compensated, to talk to owners about behavior.

The veterinary technician may feel pressured and resentful of the time spent answering behavioral questions and perhaps not feel that it is within one's job description. The technician might also have other assigned tasks to complete, and spending time talking to an owner about behavior will put him or her behind schedule.

The veterinary technician might have experienced both reactions, in different situations, depending on other responsibilities, directions received from the practice owner, how and when the owner approaches with a question, and the type of question being asked.

A behavior wellness program requires that the technician not only *react* to questions when they are asked, but also take a *proactive* approach and make behavior a part of every nonemergency appointment. This means initiating discussions about the pet's behavior, whether the owner does or not. Veterinary technicians who do not take the

lead in asking questions about behavior are missing the point of behavior wellness. Owners are unlikely to initiate discussions about behavior unless a problem exists, which means missed opportunities for prevention and early detection that are at the core of behavior wellness.

Interviewing Skills: Asking Good Questions

Initiating discussions requires excellent interviewing skills. Such skills are important not only in behavioral wellness but also in any medical history taking the technician does. The first important interviewing skill is to be able to ask nonleading, open-ended questions so that the question does not lead the client into a particular answer and so that a response requires more than a yes or no; for example, "Is your pet showing any problem behavior?" or "Do you have any questions about setting up a litterbox?" A client could answer both questions "no" and yet have a 6-month-old dog who growls when people come too close to the food dish (the owner thinks this is normal and therefore not a problem) or have located a new kitten's litterbox in the basement on a cement floor next to the furnace (the owner sees nothing wrong with this placement and thus has no questions). More productive questions might be, "Does your dog ever growl at you or not want you to do certain things to him?" and "Would you describe in detail for me the characteristics of your cat's litterbox?" The technician should try to not only obtain concrete descriptions about the animal's behavior but also discover what procedures the owners are using to raise and train the pet. One goal is to evaluate these procedures and provide more appropriate alternatives when necessary.

Interviewing Skills: Interpersonal Communication

For owners to give good information about their pets, they need to feel comfortable talking to the veterinary technician. They need to know that he or she is not just "going through the motions" in interviewing them but is genuinely interested in them, their pets, and what they have to say. Even on a busy day a harried technician can make a good impression and encourage clients to open up, while at the same time keeping the conversation on track, by using a few simple communication skills.

PUTTING CLIENTS AT EASE BY SITTING DOWN. Conducting the behavioral interview sitting down puts the technician and client at the same level and also helps relieve any tension or nervousness. The technician who remains standing gives the impression of being in a hurry or less approachable. Having clients sit down helps to relax them and put them more at ease.

 Technician Note

When talking to clients, the technician should face them in order to communicate that they are the focus of one's attention.

USING ACTIVE LISTENING SKILLS. When talking to clients, the technician should face them in order to communicate that they are the focus of one's attention. If the technician's body is directed elsewhere, the message is that his or her attention is as well. The technician can keep an open body posture by trying not to cross legs or arms, hold a clipboard or folder at chest or face level, or stand behind a barrier such as an examination table. Doing so sends the message that the technician is not completely open to hearing the client. Maintaining casual eye contact by looking at the client from time to time, rather than burying one's face in papers, enhances communication. Looking up while still being able to take notes takes practice, but it is a skill worth developing. The technician can acknowledge what the client is saying by giving frequent feedback without interrupting, by Nodding the head, and by saying "OK," "Hmmm," "I see," or other neutral, quick statements to let the client know the technician is engaged in the conversation. A warm or neutral tone of voice rather than an abrupt or abrasive one is also helpful.

Obtaining Behavioral Descriptions, Not Interpretations

Owners often describe their pets' behavior in relatively vague terms, such as "He goes crazy at the door!" Consider the following three examples of what this statement might actually mean. When the doorbell rings the dog does the following:

- Barks, growls, runs to the door, and lunges up at it
- Wildly jumps up, grabs his ball, races to the door, tail wagging, with a "happy face," and thrusts his wet, slimy ball into the visitor's hand
- Barks, shies away from the door, continues barking, hides behind the owner when answering the door, and will not allow visitors to get near him

These are just three of many possible things that "He goes crazy at the door!" might mean. This illustrates the importance of obtaining behavioral *descriptions* not interpretations. The technician should not be reluctant to continue to probe for additional information until certain what a client is attempting to describe. It may require repeated questioning to obtain a description that provides a mental picture of the behavior in question. The technician should use good communication skills so that clients understand he or she is genuinely attempting to clarify information rather than harassing them with repeated questions. He or she can paraphrase the client's description of the pet's behavior and then ask if this is correct. This gives the client an opportunity to agree or provide additional information.

Technician Note

The first component of a behavior wellness program is problem prevention.

Problem Prevention Component

The first component of a behavior wellness program is problem prevention. The approach to preventing behavior problems requires a bit of explanation. On the one hand, there is not sufficient scientific information available about all behavior problems to document that specific procedures prevent specific problems. On the other hand, problem prevention can be approached from the standpoint that if pet owners were provided with accurate behavioral information and management procedures they could realistically implement, then the following could potentially be prevented:

- Normal behaviors that can become problems during normal behavioral development (house soiling as a result of inadequate house training or litterbox set-up; destructive behavior as a result of normal chewing, play, and investigative behavior)

- Nuisance behaviors, such as dogs jumping up on people or cats getting on counters
- Social behavior problems stemming from a lack of socialization

To maximize the effectiveness of problem prevention information, sufficient time should be allotted for the prevention session and the information given must be well organized, easy to understand, and relevant as well as behaviorally accurate. A thorough discussion of prevention methods for the above three categories could take at least 30 minutes. The best time to conduct problem prevention appointments is the first veterinary visit after a new animal has been added to the family. This means problem prevention appointments should be done for adult dogs and cats new to the household as well as for puppies and kittens.

Practice management experts continue to advocate that veterinarians focus their time on those services and activities that require their unique expertise. Technicians can conduct many procedures that are commonly required in the practice, such as blood drawing and routine dental procedures. Imparting information on preventing problem behaviors is another service technicians who are trained in behavior can perform. Technicians are usually best positioned to have the first contact with the client during a scheduled appointment. This initial contact can, with the support of the veterinarian, be structured as time devoted to problem prevention or behavior assessment, another component to behavior wellness to be covered later in this chapter.

Realistic Expectations

Part of problem prevention is helping owners set realistic expectations of their pets' behavior and of pet ownership. For example, any pet owner should be told to expect to lose something of value to a pet's house soiling or destructive behavior or to illness-related damage (diarrhea stains on the couch cushions). Most people expect some problem behaviors from puppies and kittens, but surprisingly many owners do not expect their 8- or 9-month-old cat or dog to still be prone to chewing and destructive play behaviors. Clients who have recently acquired adult animals often make the erroneous assumption that their new pets are already "trained" and they will not have to worry about house training, chewing problems, and so on. Adult animals new to the home, however, should be treated just like a puppy or kitten for the first few weeks in order to prevent problems as a result of owner expectations that were too high and pets who needed training and supervision while making the adjustment to their new homes. In addition to expecting to lose something of value, other general client education areas when a new pet joins the household are as follows:

- The necessity of "pet proofing" the house
- The necessity of initial constant supervision, regardless of age (required for a longer time with puppies and kittens than with older animals)
- Importance of socialization for both dogs and cats
- Necessity of providing sufficient outlets for social play, object play, and physical exercise
- Discouraging anthropomorphic interpretations related to spite, jealousy, and revenge

Principles of Problem Prevention

Problem prevention principles (Hetts, 1999) organize information about prevention into logical sections or components. Having a means to organize information makes it easier to develop problem prevention handouts on a variety of problems and may also ensure better coverage of the pertinent content. The information given to clients during problem prevention appointments should focus on the following principles:

- Eliciting and reinforcing appropriate behavior
- Preventing or minimizing inappropriate behavior
- Meeting the pet's behavioral and developmental needs
- Minimizing the use of punishment and using it correctly when necessary

Each of these principles will be discussed in some detail.

> ### Technician Note
> Animals need to be taught and encouraged to perform desirable behaviors.

Eliciting and Reinforcing Desirable Behavior. Eliciting desirable behavior is perhaps the most important component of all. Animals need to be taught and encouraged to perform desirable behaviors. A simple idea the technician can share with owners is to *catch the pet doing something right.* He or she can remind owners of the simple principle that behaviors that result in pleasant consequences are likely to be repeated. This is a very powerful tool and one that owners seldom devote enough effort to. Most owners are entirely too focused on ways to punish or discipline undesirable behavior. Whenever the dog eliminates outside, the cat plays with its own toys, the puppy is lying down quietly, or the kitten is resting on a chair, owners should reinforce these behaviors. Reinforcement may consist of a tidbit, presentation of a new or favorite toy, petting, or any other event the pet finds rewarding. Verbal praise alone, especially when an owner is first establishing a relationship with a new pet, is often not adequate reinforcement. Praise usually first needs to be paired with petting, play, or food for a time in order to take on sufficient reinforcement value.

In addition to catching a pet doing something right,

owners may also need to encourage or elicit the right behavior. In some situations, such as encouraging cats to use the litterbox, this is integrally connected to meeting the pet's behavioral needs, which will be discussed later. With other behaviors, such as teaching a dog to sit rather than jump on people at the door, the dog can usually be successfully lured into position using a tidbit (Figure 13-1).

Technicians may also find it necessary to educate owners about the value and acceptability of using food in training. Both food and toys are very powerful ways to elicit and reinforce behavior when used correctly. The owner controls access to both, so the old adage that "a dog should work for me, not for food" is a useless argument. To not make the pet dependent on the food in order to perform the desired behavior, the following steps need to be completed:

- The food must be changed from being a lure to elicit the behavior to only being available as a reinforcer after the behavior has been performed.
- The food should be used as a reinforcer first on a continuous schedule to establish the behavior and subsequently on an intermittent, unpredictable schedule to maintain the behavior (petting or praise should always be used).
- All cues that the pet can use to predict whether or not food is available must be phased out.

> ### Technician Note
> The fewer opportunities animals are given to engage in undesirable behaviors, the less likely such behaviors are to become habits.

Preventing or Minimizing Inappropriate Behavior. The fewer opportunities animals are given to engage in undesirable behaviors, the less likely such behaviors are to become habits. A cat that begins to eliminate on the carpet because the litterbox does not meet its behavioral needs may quickly develop a surface preference for carpet. If a puppy

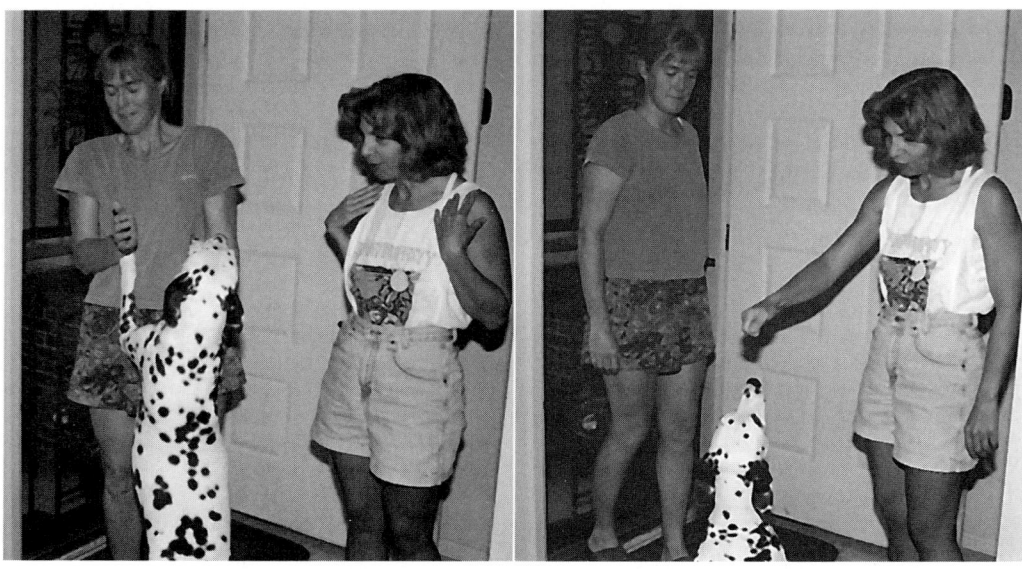

FIGURE 13-1.   The lure-reward method of encouraging a dog to sit rather than jumping on people.

gets used to pulling on the leash while walking, this can quickly become a habit, making loose leash walking more difficult to teach. Playing with a kitten with hands and feet rather than its toys can result in a cat who bites hands that move quickly. With these and other normal behaviors, not allowing the pet to make a "mistake" or perform undesirable behavior by appropriately managing the pet's environment is a big step in preventing problems.

The technician should instruct owners that, in addition to catching the pet doing something right, it is up to them to manage the pet's environment to prevent bad habits from developing. Constant supervision of puppies and adult dogs new to the household is an absolutely critical component of house training and also prevention of normal puppy destructive behavior. Supervision can be accomplished in a number of ways, including crate training, baby gates to keep the pup in either a puppy-proof area or in the same room with the owner, or tethering the dog to the owner or an object near the owner using a leash and collar. Supervision of cats and kittens may mean closing doors to certain parts of the house.

MEETING THE PET'S BEHAVIORAL AND DEVELOPMENTAL NEEDS. The types of behaviors mentioned previously that easily lend themselves to problem prevention tend to be normal behaviors. A prevention approach acknowledges the pet's need for normal behaviors such as elimination, chewing, playing, and greeting people and finds ways to allow the pet to express them in acceptable ways. This is a much more effective approach than focusing on suppression of normal behaviors, which is not realistic and does not meet the pet's behavioral needs.

A good example of the importance of meeting the pet's behavioral needs is in the creation of a cat-friendly litterbox. Many litterbox problems develop because the areas the cat is soiling have characteristics that meet the cat's behavioral preferences for elimination better than the litterbox area. Figure 13-2, for example, shows a litterbox that is deficient in several areas, as follows:

- Dirty
- In an area where the cat is unlikely to spend much time

- Next to noisy appliances
- On a cold cement floor
- Not easily accessible

Compare with a clean litterbox (Figure 13-3) located in a quiet, private area but easily accessible and in a more central part of the house. Which box is the cat most likely to use? Cat owners, especially novice ones, often need a significant amount of education about what cats need in the way of a litterbox. Helping cat owners set up a litterbox that is likely to meet the behavioral preferences of most cats can go a long way toward preventing many litterbox problems. Litterbox characteristics that should be discussed in a problem prevention appointment are listed in Box 13-2.

Meeting a dog's behavioral needs by providing an appropriate location for elimination is another important part of the house-training process (the importance of reinforcement and supervision was discussed previously). Providing a desirable elimination location for dogs may be a less complicated process than for cats. Many dogs also seem to prefer soft surfaces, such as grass, so a gravel-covered pen may not be acceptable to all dogs, and a small section of grass may need to be added. Some dogs do not like braving weather extremes (wet and cold for small, short-coated dogs or hot and humid for heavy-coated dogs), so an outside area that is somewhat protected from the weather is an important consideration. In addition, like cats, dogs tend to develop preferences for where and on what they like to eliminate early in life. These early preferences have a large influence on later behavior. Consequently, urban dogs who will be expected to eliminate on city streets and curbs should be introduced to these surfaces early on.

Both puppies and kittens normally spend an enormous amount of time in various kinds of play, so providing sufficient outlets for appropriate playful behavior is another important aspect to meeting the pet's behavioral needs. Young, and to a lesser degree adult, animals need time for social play with their owners or other animals and for object play with toys. A variety of toys that allow for chewing, chasing, stalking (cats), and retrieving (dogs) should be provided. Owners who do not realize they must be prepared to devote time to playing with their pets may become frustrated with their pet's "hyperactivity"

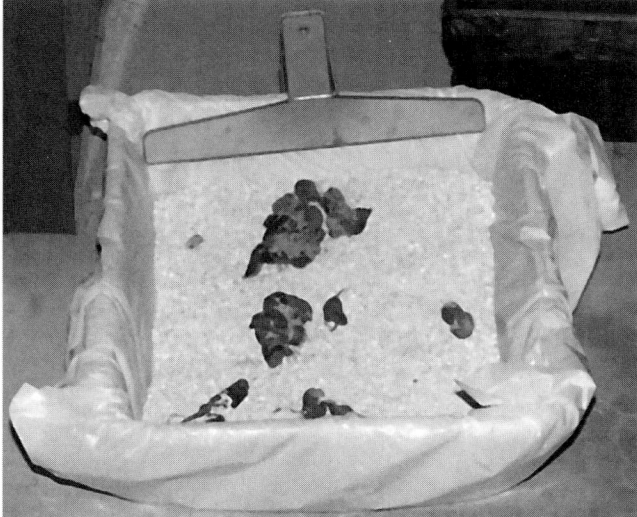

FIGURE 13-2. A litterbox that will not meet the behavioral needs of most cats.

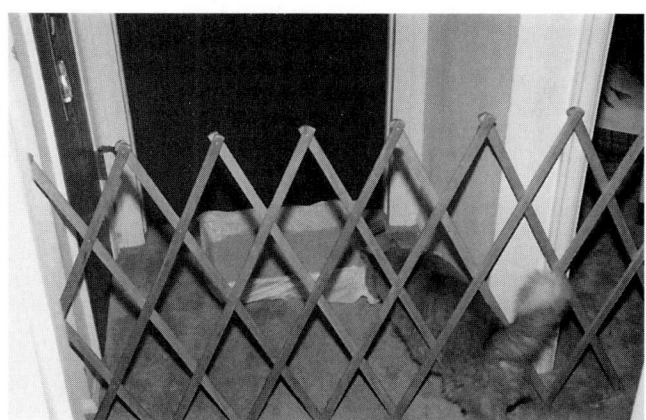

FIGURE 13-3. A cat-friendly litterbox.

Box 13-2	IMPORTANT LITTERBOX CHARACTERISTICS TO DISCUSS WITH OWNERS

1. Type and number of boxes
   a. Size—average, smaller, larger
   b. Cover or not—start without unless a good reason to cover
2. As many boxes as cats
3. Litter
   a. Type—the finer the better
   b. Depth—1½ to 2 inches generally
   c. Unscented preferred
4. Liners or not
   a. Some cats may dislike
   b. Ease of cleaning may result in cleaner litterbox
5. Location
   a. Where in house
      (1) Balance privacy with accessibility
      (2) Avoid startling noises or other stimuli
   b. Where in room
      (1) Ability to see and be protected
      (2) Escape routes—more than one
      (3) Access routes—easy to access, no obstacle courses
      (4) Comfortable surface—soft and warm generally
   c. Multiple boxes not adjacent to one another
   d. Away from food, water, and resting places
6. Cleaning
   a. Scoop at least daily
   b. Litter always appears dry and clean
   c. Wash with mild, odor-free cleaners—no dried urine or feces on box
   d. Self-cleaning litterboxes can be an option for some owners

or pestering behavior that results from not having this need for play and physical activity met.

Technician Note

Punishment becomes only a small part of problem prevention.

MINIMIZING PUNISHMENT AND USING IT CORRECTLY WHEN NECESSARY. When the other principles are followed, punishment becomes only a small part of problem prevention. First, it is important to know there are two kinds of punishment—positive and negative. In learning theory terminology, positive and negative do not refer to good or bad, but instead to adding something or taking something away. Thus positive punishment is the addition, or presentation, of something unpleasant immediately following an undesirable behavior. In contrast, negative punishment is taking away, or removing, something pleasant immediately following an undesirable behavior. For example, a positive punishment (and not recommended!) is kneeing a dog in the chest when it jumps on someone. A negative punishment is turning one's back, walking away, and ignoring the dog. This is negative punishment because the dog wants attention (something pleasant) and by jumping up it loses any opportunity to obtain that attention. There are many situations in which negative punishment can be

applied instead of positive punishment, including the following examples:

- Dog barks at the owner to get attention—owner leaves the room.
- Dog paws at person who is petting her—person stops petting and walks away.
- Dog attempts to dash through door before being given permission—owner shuts door and walks away.
- Dog will not release toy for owner to throw—owner walks away and refuses to play with dog.
- When told to sit, dog lies down instead—owner withholds tidbit.
- Dog barks at people near its crate—owner throws blanket over the crate until dog is quiet (the enjoyable opportunity to see and bark at people is taken away).

Because negative punishment does not involve the application of aversive stimuli, it is very often preferred over positive punishment when a particular behavior needs to be decreased. For punishment to be used effectively and humanely, several criteria must be met. These criteria are particularly important when considering the use of positive punishment, because it involves the use of aversive, or unpleasant, stimuli. Criteria for effective punishment are as follows.

Immediate Punishment. Any punishment must be delivered within a very few seconds after the undesirable behavior. Any longer delay prevents the punishment from being relevant to the target behavior and increases the likelihood that the pet has performed another behavior before the punishment is delivered. "Guilty looks" that dogs display when owners attempt to deliver punishment after the fact are nothing more than submissive behaviors. Dogs display these behaviors either in reaction to owners' threatening behavior when they are scolding their dogs or when dogs can predict that punishment is likely. Some dogs learn to discriminate that when the owner comes home and there is a mess somewhere in the house (trash overturned, feces on the floor, a torn-up couch cushion), bad things will happen to them. If the owner comes home and there is no mess, nothing bad happens and the dog displays normal greeting behaviors.

Consistent Punishment. All occurrences of the undesirable behavior must be punished in order for punishment to be most effective. If an owner catches the dog misbehaving some of the time but not all of the time, it is likely the behavior will continue because the dog continues to play the odds that it will not be punished.

Punishment Delivered at an Intensity Likely To Be Effective. Animals will learn to tolerate higher levels of aversive stimuli if they are presented with gradually increasing intensity than if a moderately intense stimulus is used initially. For example, an owner might gently tell his or her dog "no," which is not sufficient to stop the misbehavior. The owner may then gradually say "no" in increasingly threatening tones until it is necessary to scream at the dog to get him to stop the behavior. In contrast, an owner who says "no" in a more firm, authoritative tone of voice initially would be more likely to successfully stop the misbehavior and not have to scream. Unfortunately, many aversive stimuli that are intense enough to inhibit behaviors also can elicit fearful and aggressive responses.

Remote Punishment Rather Than Interactive. Punishment that comes from the owner has several potentially undesirable outcomes. First, the pet often learns that a behavior will be punished *only* in the owner's presence. This leads owners to anthropomorphically conclude the pet "knows better" because he only does the behavior

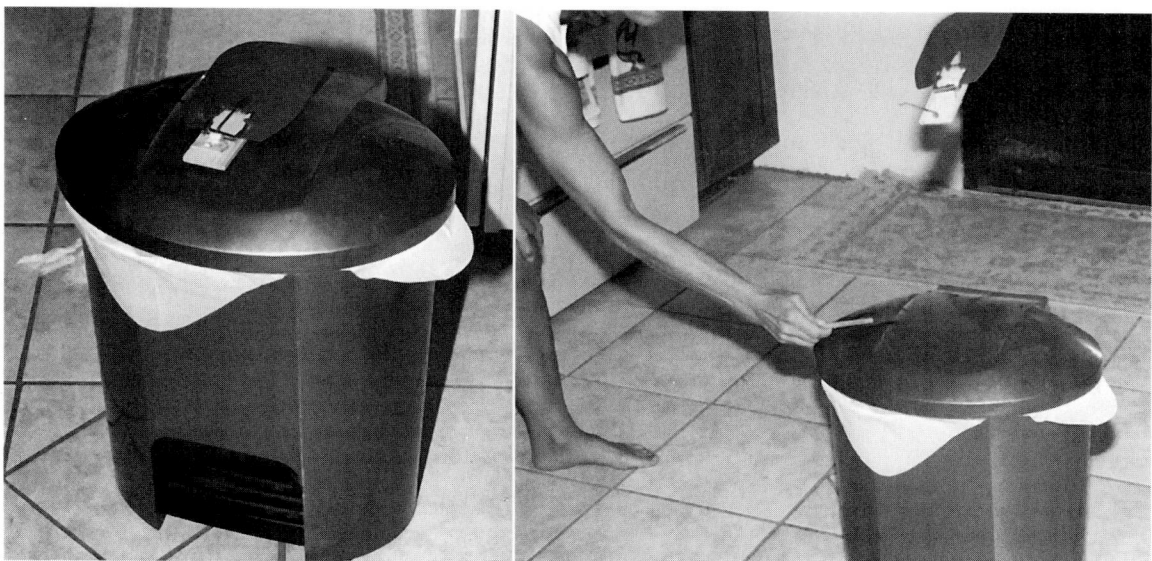

FIGURE 13-4. A Snappy Trainer is a modified mousetrap that safely startles the pet. When triggered by the pet's touch, it snaps into the air but is unable to snap closed on the pet's body.

when the owner is not present. The cat thus does not scratch the stereo speaker or the dog does not lift his leg on the couch when the owner is home but does so when the owner is at work. Second, owner-delivered punishment, especially if it is severe (scruff shakes, rollovers, hitting) or does not meet the other criteria, can result in the pet being afraid of or aggressive toward the owner, and has a negative impact on the human-animal bond. Remote punishments or booby traps are more likely to be immediate and consistent. Examples of remote punishers are as follows:

- Citronella antibark collar (ABS, Inc.)
- Snappy Trainer (Interplanetary Pet Products, Inc.) (Figure 13-4)
- Motion detector
- Citronella boundary system in which a collar the dog wears delivers a citronella spray if the dog crosses the boundary
- Hand-held noisemaker, such as an air horn or ultrasonic device (these require activation by the owner, who must be able to covertly, immediately, and consistently do so)

Keep in mind that, by definition, punishment decreases the frequency of the behavior it follows. If an owner has repeatedly attempted to punish a behavior but the pet is still showing the behavior at the same frequency, then the behavior has not really been punished. A general guideline for owners is that if positive punishment has not been successful after three to five applications, it probably will not be. If undesirable behaviors are occurring on a frequent basis, then problem resolution skills rather than a problem prevention approach are necessary. Problem prevention takes a *proactive* approach by not allowing undesirable behaviors to occur and become a habit.

Technician Note

An animal that is stressed or fearful is more likely to bite or scratch.

Preventing Problem Behaviors at the Clinic

Visiting the veterinary clinic is very stressful for some pets and consequently for their owners. An animal that is stressed or fearful is more likely to bite or scratch. This not only makes the animal more difficult to handle, but also puts technicians and other veterinary professionals at risk of being injured and sometimes can prevent the pet from receiving the best medical care. It is therefore to everyone's benefit to take a problem prevention approach and help patients become more relaxed while at the veterinary clinic. Once pets have a bad experience, it can make it more difficult to handle for all future visits to the clinic. Creating positive associations with the clinic when a puppy or kitten comes in for the first appointment is the ideal place to start, but this is not possible when dealing with adult animals new to the veterinary practice. In either case, however, a proactive approach and using a knowledge of behavior and learning can make patients easier to handle. Boxes 13-3 and 13-4 provide information on interpreting the body postures of dogs and cats. This allows the technician to better interpret the pet's emotional state and make better predictions about what she is likely to do next. Using the behavior assessment tools that will be discussed in the next section will also provide the technician with information that can be used to determine what sorts of procedures the pet may not tolerate well *before* one attempts them. The following protocols provide a place to start in preventing problem behaviors in both dogs and cats at the veterinary clinic.

Dogs and Puppies

ESTABLISHING A POSITIVE EXPECTATION IN THE WAITING AREA. Technicians and other staff members should approach the dog and offer a tidbit (assuming this will not interfere with the reason for the visit) from an open palm, not feeding from the fingers. A nonthreatening approach should be used, as described in Table 13-1.

If the dog attempts to avoid the technician (backs away, attempts to hide), displays fearful body postures (Box 13-3), or displays threatening behaviors (growls, barks,

BOX 13-3	READING AND INTERPRETING CANINE BODY POSTURES*

Offensively threatening dogs will usually show one or more of the following:
- Standing up tall with a stiff body posture, oriented toward the subject of the threat
- Piloerection (erection of the hair) on the back
- Tail straight up in a vertical line (may be wagging slowly)
- Ears up and forward or pricked forward
- Direct eye contact or staring
- Teeth bared with vertical retraction of the lips
- Barking or growling

Fearful or submissive dogs will usually show the following (dogs in pain may show these characteristics as well):
- Crouched body posture or lying down, especially rolled over on the back exposing the belly; will usually try to move away from the source of the fear
- Tail tucked between the legs
- Ears pinned back against the skull
- Eyes wide open to expose the sclera; avoidance of direct eye contact
- Lips may be retracted, exposing the teeth in a submissive grin
- Whining, whimpering, or yelping
- Shaking, panting, urinating, or defecating

Defensive dogs will usually show a mixture of threatening and fearful characteristics:
- Crouched body posture
- Piloerection possible
- May or may not be directly oriented toward the subject of the threat
- Tail usually down
- Ears possibly pinned back
- Eyes not directly staring; may look away from subject of threat, or alternate between staring and avoidance of contact
- Teeth bared in horizontal retraction of lips
- May be growling, barking, or whining and whimpering

Dogs experiencing conflicting emotional or motivational states will show the following:
- Displacement (irrelevant) behaviors, such as frequent yawning, licking of the lips, grooming, or sleeping
- Ambivalent behaviors—alternating between different motivational states, such as fear and friendliness or submission and defensive threat
- Redirected behaviors—behaviors directed at other animals or people not directly involved with the animal; redirected aggression is particularly dangerous for others in the area if a dog is aggressively motivated but cannot get to the original target

*For additional information on observing and interpreting canine and feline body postures, the videotape *Canine behavior: body postures,* available from ACT Programs, 918 N. Elm, Denton, TX 76201, 800-357-3182, is an excellent resource.

BOX 13-4	READING AND INTERPRETING FELINE BODY POSTURES

Offensively threatening cats will show the following:
- Standing, hips higher than the shoulders, tail down
- Direct eye contact or staring
- Ears out to side of head
- Growls or hisses

Fearful cats will show the following:
- Crouched body posture or lying down
- Ears flat against the head
- Looks away or avoids eye contact
- Tries to get away or hide
  NOTE: Cats do not show submissive behavior.

Defensive aggressive cats will show the following:
- Standing up, back arched, tail up or down (Halloween cat)
- Ears pinned flat against the head
- Eyes dilated; may or may not look directly at person
- Growls or hisses

TABLE 13-1	POSTURES TO AVOID WHEN APPROACHING FEARFUL OR UNFAMILIAR DOGS

Postures to Avoid	Appropriate Postures
Direct eye contact	Look at the floor, off to the side, or above the dog's head
Frontal approach	Turn the side of the body toward the dog or approach at a slight angle rather than head on
Reaching toward or over the dog's head or neck	Allow the dog to approach, let the dog sniff a hand held at the side of the body, pet the dog from under the chin
Leaning forward, over the dog's body	Bend at the knees, or stand straight up

face of undesirable behavior is not operant reinforcement of the behavior but instead is classical conditioning of a desirable emotional state.

For unruly dogs, a more assertive approach can be used (facing the dog, making eye contact) and the dog required to sit, go down, or perform any trick it knows (e.g., shake hands) before receiving the tidbit. Any undesirable behavior (jumping up, barking) should be ignored (no verbal correction, turning away from the dog, moving out of its reach, breaking eye contact) *without* repeating the command more than twice. The tidbit can be used to lure the dog into a sit or down position if necessary. Attempting to push the dog away or touching her to "help" her into the desired position (sit, down) will usually be counterproductive. If the dog jumps up, it is *never* appropriate to step on the dog's feet, squeeze the paws, or knee her in the chest.

Using these techniques also models good dog handling and teaching skills to the owner. Dogs who refuse to eat the treats are probably highly stressed or anxious. The technician can try a more tempting tidbit and make a note of this response for the veterinarian. A behavioral check sheet that reports the results of these reception area interactions should be filled out by the technician and made available to the veterinarian before examination room contact.

prolonged eye contact), the treat should be dropped on the floor, near the dog, with no other attempts at interaction (no talking to the dog, looking in the dog's direction, or any of the "don'ts" listed above) as the technician continues walking past the dog and owner. Multiple repetitions from the same person and from more than one staff member will help the dog to generalize before being taken into the examination room. Giving the dog a tidbit in the

CREATING A GOOD FIRST IMPRESSION IN THE EXAMINATION ROOM. The technician should ignore the dog when he or she first walks in and not attempt to approach the owner if the dog is close by. The technician should continue with duties while continuing to ignore the dog for a few minutes. During this time, the technician observes the dog's body postures and how he reacts to movements (shifting positions on the chair, reaching for something, standing up, etc.). The technician will be much better prepared to interact with the dog if he or she has some sense of the dog's social behavior and emotional state before doing so. One can look for offensive and defensive postures, displacement behaviors (yawning, grooming, lip licking) that can indicate stress and anxiety, and also a lack of friendly behavior. The latter may be the most difficult to read. The technician should beware of dogs that stare or watch him or her closely without any other behavioral responses (no tail wags, no avoidance responses, no fearful or threatening behavior, etc.).

Next, the technician can attempt a friendly interaction by talking to the dog using the nonthreatening approach described above and carefully observing its reaction. The next move depends on the dog's reaction. The handling variations described above can be used. If a fearful dog refuses to approach, the technician can try a "Hansel and Gretel" trail of treats, starting from the dog's location and moving toward him or her. If the technician or another staff member has identified a fearful or threatening animal from the reception room interactions, the technician may want to toss two or three small tidbits toward the dog while walking into the room (or as the dog and owner walk in as discussed below).

Initial friendliness in response to nonthreatening social interactions is not always predictive of how a dog is going to react to restraint and more threatening interactions (touching feet, opening the mouth, looking in the eyes and ears, etc.), so it is important not to jump to conclusions or go too fast when initiating more direct handling procedures. An examination room check sheet on the dog's behavior should be completed by either the technician or the veterinarian and made part of the patient's record.

TAKING A PREVENTIVE (PROACTIVE) APPROACH RATHER THAN A REACTIVE ONE. In the examination room, if the dog is fearful, it may be helpful for the technician to sit on the floor or a low chair, at a distance the dog considers safe, and begin the Hansel and Gretel technique while the veterinarian begins talking to the owner and taking the history. If the technician can entice the dog to approach and can conduct some gentle, nonthreatening touching that is paired with tidbits, this may help the dog to better tolerate the upcoming examination. During this brief counterconditioning and desensitization session, the technician can offer a tidbit with one hand (not from the fingers but from an open palm) while doing one of the following:

- Touching the dog's collar
- Touching or reaching toward the dog's feet
- Lifting an ear
- Touching a hip
- Running a hand down the dog's back

Touching potentially sensitive areas has thus been paired with something positive for the dog, helping to decrease fear or anxiety. Although it could be argued that this requires additional staff time, it may require less time for one technician to conduct handling exercises that may allow the dog to tolerate procedures than the three or more

staff members it will take to restrain the dog that becomes unmanageable.

An even broader view of the preventive approach is for these types of handling exercises to be conducted the first and every time a puppy comes to the clinic and for owners to be encouraged to do the same thing at home, mimicking the technician's behavior that they have observed in the clinic. Another type of proactive approach involves dogs who, from past experience, are known to be threatening, aggressive, or generally difficult to handle. The veterinarian can instruct the technician to educate owners on how to accustom their dog to tolerate a muzzle for short periods. Basket muzzles are usually better tolerated by the dog than the sleeve type. A well-fitting basket muzzle should not come off. Because these may be difficult for owners to obtain, the clinic may consider offering them for sale. The dog can then be muzzled at home or in the car before arriving at the clinic.

MANAGING THE ENVIRONMENT. Dogs who are very fearful, highly reactive, agitated (barking, lunging [even if friendly, not threatening] to the end of the leash), or threatening or aggressive may be helped by getting them into an examination room as soon as possible and away from other people and animals. Structural barriers (or even using plants or rearranging the seating layout) can also be used in the reception area to create individual areas. If the clinic's location and weather permit, even suggesting the owner take the dog around the building for a walk or wait in the car is better than allowing the dog to sit in the reception area and become more and more agitated. Allowing the dog to become agitated before the examination sets the stage for the potential of redirected aggression.

Technician Note

Many dogs who are fearful or aggressive respond better if they are allowed to approach a person, rather than the other way around.

Many dogs who are fearful or aggressive respond better if they are allowed to approach a person, rather than the other way around. This means that it may be better if the technician and the veterinarian are in the examination room first, so the dog is approaching them (coming into their space) rather than vice versa. If the technician has already placed a problem dog in the examination room, one strategy might be for the technician to take the dog out of the room to the scale to be weighed. While the dog is gone, the veterinarian can enter the room, sit down, and be prepared to toss several tidbits to the dog when she reenters the room. Fearful dogs may tolerate handling better if examined on the floor rather than the table. It may also help to use a rug or nonslip mat to provide better traction. The dog who is slipping and sliding will feel out of control and probably become more fearful.

Threatening and Aggressive Dogs in the Clinic

There are two issues in threatening situations: the technician's safety and well-being and the dog's safety and well-being. Good behavior skills should minimize the occurrence of those situations in which emergency restraint has to be used for safety reasons. The minimal amount of physical restraint necessary for the technician's safety is the maximum that should be used. For example, if a dog snaps, it is usually appropriate to stop and muzzle it rather than "stringing it up." Additional information on animal restraint is found in Chapter 1.

It should be remembered that the goal of restraint and force is to keep personnel safe while performing necessary procedures. The goal of restraint and force is *not* to "teach the dog a lesson" or to teach him not to be fearful or aggressive. The former will only make things worse, and it is not possible to accomplish the latter in the context of a medical interaction in the veterinary clinic.

The technician should keep in mind that using physical force may allow one to do what needs to be done at the time, but the price may be creating a dog who becomes increasingly difficult or even impossible to handle during future visits. This may happen after only *one* bad experience. If the owner is present, it may also cost the practice a client. Consider this analogy: if a child or elderly relative became difficult to handle in a medical setting, would a client appreciate that person being dealt with roughly? For the family, the pet, like children and elderly persons, represents the most vulnerable and helpless members of the family.

It is best to assume an attitude of cautious calm (Hetts, 1999), as follows:

- Respect the dog and its ability to injure, without being overly fearful.
- Although a knowledge of breed *tendencies* is helpful, be careful that breed *biases* do not result in approaching or handling the dog in a manner that could be counterproductive.
- Have confidence in your ability to accurately observe, interpret, and react accordingly to the dog's body postures and other communication signals without being overconfident or feeling invincible.
- Know what can be done to avoid being bitten or getting in a confrontation with the dog.
- Know when to back off (or use proper restraint) if you do not think you can accurately interpret the dog's intentions or when you realize that the dog will bite if you persist.

THINGS THAT ARE NOT HELPFUL.　The following behaviors are not helpful:

- Forcing the issue
- Punishment
- Increased restraint
- "Dominating" the dog, showing it "who's boss"
- Not knowing when to back off
- Taking the dog's behavior personally and becoming angry and impatient
- Not allowing "reassurance" to be used appropriately (can be used successfully in some circumstances to calm the dog down)

Instead, consider the following options.

- **Use of a Gentle Leader.** Some dogs are intimidated when wearing a Gentle Leader (Premier Pet Products). This has been referred to as a calming effect, but a better term is probably behavioral suppression. Other dogs, however, become somewhat panicked when the Gentle Leader is first put on and try frantically to take it off. This is one reason to encourage the use of the Gentle Leader early on; if the dog is accustomed to it, the technician will have greater control of the dog in the clinic.
- **Backing off and trying again later.** Some people believe that if they back off when a dog attempts to bite, that the dog has "won." Although it may be true that the

aggressive behavior has "worked" for the dog in that situation, because it has resulted in people leaving her alone, having the behavior reinforced is probably less of a problem than forcing the issue and escalating the situation until the dog and possibly the technician are out of control. If the situation permits (e.g., if the procedure does not have to be performed immediately), it may be most helpful to put the dog in a cage, cover the front with a towel, and allow the dog to calm down. Perhaps allowing another technician or staff member to handle the dog later may be better. Certain dogs and certain people have personality conflicts just as people do.

Technician Note

If the dog is intimidated and frightened by being on the examination table, the technician can try conducting the procedure on the floor.

- **Changing the environment.** If the dog is intimidated and frightened by being on the examination table, the technician can try conducting the procedure on the floor. If the dog is slipping on the floor, a nonskid rug can be brought in for it to stand on.
- **Changing the interaction.** The technician can start with an easier version of what needs to be done that the dog will tolerate. For example, if the dog resists having her feet touched, the technician can begin by stroking the legs while offering a tidbit and gradually work up to touching the feet.

MUZZLING THE DOG.　Rather than struggling to control the dog with a leash and collar, because of concern that she might turn her head and snap, the dog can be muzzled. With a muzzle on, the technician will be less concerned with the need for tight restraint and the dog may calm down the less tightly it is restrained.

Cats in the Clinic

Once cats become emotionally aroused, they may stay aroused for hours. The technician's goal is to keep them as calm as possible for as long as possible. If the veterinary practice has a joint reception room for dogs and cats, the technician may suggest that owners leave their cats in the car (weather permitting) when they are checking in at the desk. Another alternative is to immediately provide the owner (as soon as she or he walks in the door) with a towel or blanket to drape over the cat's crate to minimize the cat's opportunity to become frightened by unfamiliar sights. If the waiting room is noisy or crowded, try to get the cat placed in a quieter examination room as quickly as possible. With cats who have a history of being difficult to handle, allowing the cat and owner to wait in an empty office or other place rather than a disruptive waiting area would be preferable.

Before the cat and owner are brought to the examination room, Feliway can be applied to the examination table. Feliway (Abbott Laboratories) is a synthetic analog of the cat's facial pheromones and is said to have a calming effect on cats when they are in unfamiliar surroundings. (This product has received mixed reviews and may work best to *prevent* the cat from becoming aroused, rather than to calm it once aroused.) Before attempting to take the cat out of the carrier, assess the cat's arousal level. What does the cat do if the carrier is moved, if she is touched with a pen or other harmless object (not a finger!) through the wires or air holes of the carrier? Is the cat vocalizing? The cat's body postures are described in Box 3-4.

Once the cat and owner are settled in the examination room, several techniques can be applied, depending on the cat's arousal level and what type of medical or examination procedures will be required during the appointment. If the cat resists coming out of the carrier, rather than reaching in and pulling her out, the technician can either take the top off the plastic airline carrier by removing the screws or tilt the carrier so that the cat slides out. If the cat does not need to be handled immediately but merely put in a cage or given an injection, the carrier can be put directly in the cage with the carrier door left open, so the cat can come out on its own. Once the cat is in the larger cage, a Plexiglas shield can be used to push and hold the cat to the rear of the cage and the injection administered through holes in the shield. This avoids having to handle the fractious cat at all until it is medicated. Another option is to put the opening of the carrier directly into a large canvas cat bag. Some cats will crawl into the bag because it appears to be a darker, safer hiding place than the carrier. The cat can then be handled through the zippered opening of the bag. Some cat bags with frames allow the cat to be put into the bag directly from a standard cage. (Bag and shield available from ACES, 800-338-ACES; Crestline, CA.)

Cats are probably less likely to respond to food treats than are dogs. Play toys can be tried, as long as the play does not overly excite the cat, making it more likely to redirect aggression toward a person who then tries to handle her. As with dogs, the technician should not attempt to start interacting with the cat initially; instead, let the cat become accustomed to his or her presence in the examination room before attempting to interact. Inexperienced staff members should not stick their fingers through the carrier to try to make friends with the cat unless the cat is making the first move by putting its paw out through the carrier. The technician can allow the cat to approach and sniff a finger, either when in the crate (keeping the finger outside the crate!) or out of it, as an initial greeting.

Technician Note

Most cats do not like to be stroked and patted in the same way dogs do.

Most cats do not like to be stroked and patted in the same way dogs do. When initially touching the cat, restrict petting to the head between the cat's ears and the cat's cheeks. Scent glands are located in these areas, and many cats seem to enjoy having them rubbed or being given the opportunity to rub up against a stationary hand. Do not pat the cat along the side or stroke it from head to toe until she seems calm and tolerant and the owner has told you the cat enjoys this kind of touching.

If the cat becomes impossible to handle during an examination or other procedure, if time permits, one can try backing off, put the cat in a cage, cover the door with a blanket, and try again later. With the next attempt the technician should be prepared with a cat bag or net, rather than engaging in another wrestling match.

Behavior Assessment Component

Early detection of behavior problems is another component of behavior wellness. When problems cannot be prevented, detecting them soon after they appear and making sure that owners obtain effective, qualified assis-

tance in a timely manner may prevent problems from reaching the crisis stage in which the pet's continued presence in the home is at risk.

Performing behavior assessments will likely also require another shift in perspective. A recent study found that as few as 25% of veterinarians routinely discuss behavior issues with clients, 17% never do, and only 11% of veterinarians thought it was their responsibility to initiate discussions about behavior problems with clients (Patronek, Dodman, 1999). A behavior wellness approach *requires* that veterinary professionals take the initiative to inquire about the pet's behavior patterns. If they do not, the situation may progress to full-fledged problem status, in part because owners often do not interpret certain behaviors as early warning signs of potential problems such as the following:

- The dog leaves the room and avoids an infant whenever the infant is placed on a blanket on the floor. The owner may not understand this is an indication the dog is fearful, a behavior that could escalate to growling and snapping when the infant reaches the crawling or toddler stage.
- The cat often urinates right next to the litterbox. The owner tolerates and never mentions this behavior because it occurs on cement in the unfinished basement. The owner may not have the foresight to see that when he or she decides to finish the basement, this can turn into the cat urinating on the new carpet.
- A dog owner who is a teacher has been home all summer with a new puppy. She or he thinks it is cute that the puppy cries, paws, and becomes very distressed at the door when the owner steps outside for a short time to get the mail or mow the yard. The owner does not view this behavior as an indication of a potential separation anxiety problem when she or he goes back to work in the fall.

The important point in these examples is that the owners would never think to discuss these behaviors with the technician because they do not see them as problems or potential problems. Several studies (DiGiacomo et al., 1998; Scarlett et al., 1999), as well as my personal experience, indicate that pet owners surrendering their pets to a shelter had often experienced some lifestyle change that either prevented them from continuing to tolerate the problem or, as in the examples above, resulted in the same behavior changing from being acceptable to viewed as a problem. The goal of a behavior assessment is to detect these situations and identify problems or potential problems early so they can be resolved in a timely manner.

Behavior Assessment Tools

Behavior assessments should include several components. Box 13-5 provides a sample of an assessment tool that inquires about the frequency of common undesirable behaviors. If the questionnaire reveals these behaviors have occurred recently, even infrequently, it provides a starting point for a conversation to obtain more detail about the nature of the problems.

A second component to a behavior assessment includes questions about the daily management of the pet, questions about the pet's typical behavior patterns, and potential changes in the family's lifestyle. Box 13-6 provides an example of Part 2 of an assessment tool. A recent study found that dogs who were confined in a crate, left outside, or confined to a small part of the house on a routine basis were at greater risk of surrender to a shelter than those who had free run of the house (Patronek et al., 1996a).

Box 13-5	BEHAVIOR ASSESSMENT TOOL, PART 1: OWNER QUESTIONNAIRE ABOUT UNDESIRABLE BEHAVIORS

Since the last clinic visit (or in the past month, or since you've owned the pet if this is the first visit):

1. How often has your pet soiled (eliminated, gone to the bathroom) in the house?
   - ☐ always/almost always
   - ☐ most of the time
   - ☐ some of the time
   - ☐ rarely or never

2. How often has your pet damaged things, either inside or outside the house?
   - ☐ always/almost always
   - ☐ most of the time
   - ☐ some of the time
   - ☐ rarely or never

3. How often has your pet been overly active (hyperactive)?
   - ☐ always/almost always
   - ☐ most of the time
   - ☐ some of the time
   - ☐ rarely or never

4. How often has your pet been too noisy (barked, whined, meowed, cried)?
   - ☐ always/almost always
   - ☐ most of the time
   - ☐ some of the time
   - ☐ rarely or never

5. How often has your pet shown fear of people, other animals, noises, or objects?
   - ☐ always/almost always
   - ☐ most of the time
   - ☐ some of the time
   - ☐ rarely or never

6. How often has your pet growled, hissed, snapped, threatened, or attempted to bite people, including family members?
   - ☐ always/almost always
   - ☐ most of the time
   - ☐ some of the time
   - ☐ rarely or never

7. How often has your pet growled, hissed, snapped, or threatened other animals?
   - ☐ always/almost always
   - ☐ most of the time
   - ☐ some of the time
   - ☐ rarely or never

8. How often has your pet attacked or started a fight with other animals?
   - ☐ always/almost always
   - ☐ most of the time
   - ☐ some of the time
   - ☐ rarely or never

9. How often has your pet escaped from the house or yard?
   - ☐ always/almost always
   - ☐ most of the time
   - ☐ some of the time
   - ☐ rarely or never

Box 13-6	BEHAVIOR ASSESSMENT TOOL, PART 2: PET'S MANAGEMENT AND BEHAVIOR PATTERNS AND FAMILY'S LIFESTYLE

1. Does your pet have free run of the house when you are gone, or is she kept crated; left outside, in the basement, or in the garage; or confined to a small part of the house on a regular basis? If the pet is confined, why?
2. Is your cat allowed outside? When and for how long? Supervised/leashed/confined or not?
3. Is your pet recently spending more time outside because its behavior inside the house has become more of a problem?
4. Are you planning a move to a different house?
5. Will the composition of your family change in the near future (new baby, marriage, divorce, children moving home, etc.)?
6. Will any young children reach the crawling or walking stage in the near future?
7. Will any family member's schedule undergo a significant change in the near future (e.g., resuming/leaving work, school, hours/shift change at work)?
8. Is there anything you (or any other family member) are afraid or reluctant to do with or to your pet, such as clipping nails, taking food or toys away, rolling it over, touching its body in certain places, disciplining it, or walking by or disturbing it when resting?
9. How does your pet get along with the children in the family?
10. If you have multiple pets, how does each pet get along with the others?
11. How does your pet react when visitors (adults and children) come to your house?
12. How does your pet react to unfamiliar animals (dogs, cats, small mammals, birds)?
13. How does your pet behave when left alone? How does the pet react to your departure?
14. What things is your pet afraid of? How does she behave when afraid?
15. How does your pet respond to handling, mild restraint, and petting?

Similarly, cats who were allowed outside were also at greater risk (Patronek et al., 1996b). Thus it may be very important to find out where the pet spends most of its time. Because lifestyle changes affect the pet's behavior and can be potential triggers for all kinds of problems, a behavior assessment should include this information. Last, this component inquires about the pet's reaction to common situations not covered in the first part of the assessment.

Technician Note

Veterinary professionals should make behavior assessments a routine part of every pet's ongoing health care.

Schedule for Administering Behavior Assessments
Veterinary professionals should make behavior assessments a routine part of every pet's ongoing health care. An assessment could be administered at 3- to 4-month inter-

vals if the pet is being seen more frequently for medical reasons or during every appointment if the pet is seen at intervals longer than 4 months. With the support of the veterinarian, trained technicians are best positioned to conduct behavior assessments before the start of the medical appointment. The behavior assessment should be made part of the pet's permanent record, and the technician should discuss the results with the veterinarian. If answers to the questions in Part 1 are "some of the time" or greater, if lifestyle changes have or will occur, or if "red flags" surface in the client's descriptions of the pet's normal behavior patterns, the practice should have procedures in place to develop an action plan to see that these important behavioral issues are addressed. An action plan could include an in-house behavior consultation, referral to a behavior consultant or dog trainer for obedience classes, dissemination of educational materials, or behavior management products sold or recommended.

Follow-up for Behavior Assessments
Technicians can also be responsible for conducting behavioral follow-up telephone calls, just as many currently do for medical cases. After routine surgeries, suturing, or

dental procedures, technicians are often given the responsibility of calling clients to inquire about the pet's status and progress. Behavior issues deserve the same type of follow-up. Technicians can call the client to determine if the pet owner followed through with the suggested referral, implemented any training or behavior modification techniques that were suggested, or purchased behavior management products that were recommended. Very few veterinary practices have routine procedures in place to follow up on behavioral problems in the same way they follow up on medical problems.

> ### Technician Note
> Behavioral problems should be approached from the same model as medical problems: diagnosis, treatment, and follow up.

Problem Resolution Component

Problem resolution is not something to be taken lightly or attempted with an off-handed, try this, try that approach. Behavioral problems should be approached from the same model as medical problems: evaluation, diagnosis, treatment, and follow-up; or put another way: analysis, behavior modification, and follow-up. Attempting to treat a behavioral problem without knowing the cause or motivation for the behavior can be just as disastrous as attempting to treat a medical condition without a diagnosis. For example, surgery would not be considered for a limping dog until it was determined why the dog was limping; similarly an antibark collar should not be recommended for a barking dog until the reason for the barking is determined.

Technicians should always look to the veterinarian for guidelines as to their role in providing problem resolution information to clients. Owners often ask technicians questions about their pets' behavior even before they ask the veterinarian. If the veterinary technicians and the veterinarians in the practice are working together to determine the technicians' role in providing information, it may be helpful to consider the disadvantages to jumping into problem solving without adequate preparation.

Dangers of Problem Solving Without Adequate Preparation

Attempting to problem solve without being prepared is not helpful to the technician, the client, or the pet. Behavioral consulting requires being knowledgeable about animal behavior and animal learning, having sufficient time to obtain a behavioral history and explain detailed recommendations to clients, and being available to follow up after the initial consultation. Attempting to problem solve without sufficient preparation can have the following unwanted consequences.

OWNER'S FRUSTRATION.   Behavioral problems are frustrating, and many pet owners can quickly lose patience. If owners are investing their time to implement recommendations yet see no results, their frustration level may quickly increase. In one case an owner was advised to confine her cat in a large crate with litterbox, food, and water for 1 month to "retrain" the cat to use the litterbox. The cat, of course, used the box reliably while confined. On being released from confinement, the cat walked over to the other side of the room and urinated on the carpet. Both the owner and the cat were frustrated, and the cat was surrendered to an animal shelter. What makes cases like this sad is that most litterbox problems can be resolved with proper intervention.

TECHNICIAN'S AND PRACTICE'S CREDIBILITY.   If clients discover from other sources that the information the veterinary technician provided was not accurate, appropriate, or helpful, they may lose faith in the technician and the veterinary practice. Consider this example. An owner's dog was barking excessively when left home alone. The owner was told to sneak back and throw a can of coins at the dog to reprimand the barking. When the problem was later diagnosed as a separation anxiety problem and the owner told that this approach would probably exacerbate the problem and increase the dog's anxiety, she no longer trusted the veterinarian who gave her inappropriate information and took her dog to another practice instead.

LIABILITY FOR INJURIES.   A technician who advises a pet owner to handle his or her pet in a certain way that elicits an aggressive response from the animal may be legally liable for injuries that result. In one case, an owner was advised to give her dog a scruff shake when it did not obey her commands. When her dog failed to get off the bed when told to, she grabbed the dog by the neck as instructed, and the dog promptly bit off her finger. The owner sued the trainer who had given this instruction, and the case was settled out of court in her favor.

WORSENING PROBLEM.   A playful kitten was pouncing on its owner's ankles as he sat in a chair. He was told to grab the kitten by the scruff of the neck, throw her into a room by herself, and leave her there for several hours. The kitten did not learn to stop pouncing on the owner's ankles. Instead, she learned that whenever her owner reached for her, she needed to defend herself. She began to hiss, scratch, and bite whenever the owner tried to touch her. The problem had escalated from simple play-motivated aggression, which might well have resolved on its own, to a much more difficult, defensive aggressive behavior problem.

Self-assessment

As technicians work with the veterinarian to determine what their role in problem resolution will be, the self-assessment questions in Table 13-2 may help guide decisions. Can the technician arrive at a behavioral diagnosis, or cause, for the behavior by knowing what questions to ask in a thorough behavioral history? If the technician cannot answer yes to most of the questions in Table 13-2, then problem solving may not be an appropriate role at this time.

> ### Technician Note
> Typically, veterinarians want to evaluate the potential that medical causes might be contributing to the pet's behavioral problem before making a referral.

Referring Behavior Cases

WHEN TO REFER.   Technicians are often put in the role of referring clients to behavioral consultants or dog trainers without sufficient direction from the veterinarian. Veterinarians and technicians should work together to develop guidelines for when it is appropriate for a technician to make the referral. Technicians should not take it on themselves to make the referral without these guidelines. For

TABLE 13-2	SELF-ASSESSMENT BEFORE PROBLEM SOLVING
Question	**Case Example**
Can I take a behavioral history about this problem? Do I know what questions to ask to determine the type of problem that is causing the behavioral symptom?	Excessive barking can be caused by separation anxiety and territorial behavior (among other things). Can I obtain a behavioral history that will distinguish between these two problems?
Will my recommendations for resolving the problem address the specific type of problem rather than merely treating the symptom? If not, is there a rationale that makes the symptomatic approach appropriate?	Constructing a higher fence to resolve an escaping problem is a symptomatic treatment. The reason for escaping is ignored. If the higher fence keeps the dog in the yard without additional problems, this may be sufficient. However, if the escaping is motivated by separation anxiety, other symptoms of the problem are likely to be seen. Can I determine when a symptomatic approach is appropriate and when it is not?
Am I familiar with a variety of possible problem resolution methods, only a few of which are based on aversive techniques?	One approach to destructive chewing is to give off-limits items an unpleasant taste. Am I familiar not only with other ways of discouraging unacceptable chewing but also with even more ways to *promote* acceptable chewing behavior?
Do I have the time to complete all the components of a behavior case that includes analysis (diagnosis), treatment (devising and explaining a plan), and following up?	Obtaining a history and explaining a treatment plan to an owner may require several hours, certainly more than 10 or 15 minutes. Follow-up contacts can occur over several months. Can I realistically expect to have sufficient time to handle the case properly?

From Hetts, S: *Pet behavior protocols: what to say, what to do, when to refer*, Lakewood, Colo, 1999, AAHA Press.

example, owners often call the veterinary practice when the cat is urinating outside the litterbox, the dog bit a neighborhood child, or the dog is lifting his leg on the furniture, and ask for advice. It should be the veterinarian's decision as to whether the pet should be seen at the clinic before the owner is referred for a behavioral consultation, either in-house or to an outside consultant. Typically, veterinarians want to evaluate the potential that medical causes might be contributing to the pet's behavioral problem before making a referral. Many behavioral consultants will not accept a referral until this has been done.

TYPE OF REFERRAL. The first decision that needs to be made is whether the dog should be referred for behavioral consulting or to an obedience class. Obedience classes are helpful when dogs are unruly and not responsive to verbal directions from the owners. Jumping up, door dashing, pulling on the leash, and not coming when called are all examples of undesirable behaviors that can be improved through a good obedience class. Obedience classes, however, do not resolve problems such as separation anxiety, excessive barking, house soiling, destructive behavior, or aggression. These types of problems require behavioral consultations that include analysis and subsequent modification of the problem behavior. When the decision is made to refer a cat for a behavioral problem, obviously the owner should be referred to a behavioral consultant knowledgeable and experienced in cat behavior.

EVALUATING BEHAVIORAL CONSULTANTS AND DOG TRAINERS. Technicians can be very helpful to the veterinary practice by assisting with the evaluation of behavioral consultants and dog trainers the practice may be considering using for referral resources. Veterinarians know that clients' experiences with referrals, both good and bad, will reflect directly back on the veterinary practice. Because there is such great variation in the qualifications and methods of behavioral consultants and dog trainers, it is incumbent on the veterinary practice to evaluate the credentials and competency of the people to whom it refers clients. This can be a time-consuming process, but one that can benefit greatly from using the skills of trained technicians.

The technician who has been given the assignment of gathering information about individuals in the community who offer behavioral consulting services should keep in mind that anyone can use the professional titles of animal behaviorist, behavioral consultant, dog behaviorist, cat behaviorist, and so on, regardless of background and training. Although there is a veterinary board specialty in behavior and the Animal Behavior Society professionally certifies academically trained behaviorists who meet its criteria, relatively few individuals are certified in this manner, and it is likely that one is not located near a particular veterinary practice. Because some of these individuals provide behavioral consultations by telephone, this is an option that is always available, regardless of the location of the veterinary practice. In addition, many people with a wide variety of backgrounds who are not certified offer behavioral consulting services. Obtaining information about the consultant's educational and experiential background and observing a consulting appointment are critical tasks the veterinary practice can assign to the technician before agreeing to refer its clients to a noncertified consultant. The veterinarian can then make an informed decision as to who he or she feels is best qualified to provide consulting services to the practice's clients.

Although there is no widely accepted professional certification or training programs for dog trainers, the National Association of Dog Obedience Instructors (NADOI) does endorse its member trainers. Members must meet criteria for different levels of endorsement. The Association of Pet Dog Trainers promotes the use of dog-friendly training methods and is in the process of developing a certification program for humane training. In addition, guidelines for humane dog training are being developed and will be available through the American Humane Association.

| Box 13-7 | GUIDELINES FOR EVALUATING A DOG TRAINER OR BEHAVIORAL CONSULTANT |

FINDING AND WORKING WITH DOG TRAINERS

- Look for trainers who rely on teaching methods that use positive reinforcement for the right response rather than punishing the wrong one.
- Observe an obedience class without your dog. Are the dogs and people having a good time? Talk with a few participants, and see if they are comfortable with the trainer's methods. If someone will not let you sit in, do not enroll.
- Do not allow trainers to work with your dog unless they tell you first exactly what they plan to do.
- Do not be afraid to tell a trainer to stop if she or he is doing something to your dog you do not like.
- If a trainer tells you to do something that you do not feel good about, do not do it! Do not be intimidated, bullied, or shamed into doing something that you believe is not in your dog's best interest.
- Avoid trainers who offer guarantees about results. They are either ignoring or do not understand the complexity of animal behavior.
- Avoid trainers who object to using food as a training reward. Food is an acceptable positive reinforcement training tool.
- Avoid trainers who use *only* choke chains. Head collars are humane alternatives to choke chains and pinch collars.
- Look for trainers who treat both people and dogs with respect, rather than an "I'm the boss" attitude.

FINDING AND WORKING WITH BEHAVIORAL CONSULTANTS

- Look for academic training in the science of animal behavior, as well as hands-on experience.
- Certification by a professional organization tells you the individual has met the requirements for education, experience, and professional ethics.
- Look for people who recognize the importance of *you* working through the problem with your pet rather than sending it somewhere to be "fixed."
- Membership in a professional organization suggests communication with colleagues and a means to keep current on new information.
- Ask for professional references, such as former clients, colleagues, or veterinarians who refer cases.
- A knowledge of positive reinforcement methods, behavior modification techniques such as counterconditioning and desensitization, how to use food appropriately, and humane products such as head collars is a must.
- Look for people who treat you with respect and are not abrupt and abrasive.
- Avoid people who guarantee problem resolution. Animals are complex, and no one knows everything there is to know about them.
- Avoid quick fixes. This approach does not do justice to you, your pet, or the problem.

Technicians can be designated to observe several obedience classes and, ideally, participate in the class with a dog, before the veterinary practice agrees to refer clients to any given trainer. Box 13-7 provides basic recommendations for assessing behavioral consultants and trainers.

HOW TO MAKE THE REFERRAL. If it is decided that the technician will at times be making the referral to a dog trainer or behavioral consultant, most veterinarians would want the technician to conduct those referrals in a professional manner. This means that the client should be told what to expect from the referral. From previous evaluation of the consultant or trainer, the technician will know what kinds of services are offered and what fees are charged. Provide the client with this information rather than referring the client for "tips" or "advice." It frustrates the client and the behavioral consultant if the client expects a "25 words or less" solution free of charge, which is what using words such as tips and advice implies. How the technician makes the referral will have a significant impact on clients' perceptions of behavioral consulting and how likely they are to follow through with an appointment. If clients get the impression that this is a trivial referral, they are also unlikely to take it seriously or believe that a behavioral consult can successfully help them change their pets' behavior. Similarly, clients will not take the importance of training classes seriously if the suggestion is made in an offhanded manner, rather than as an important component of a behavior wellness or problem prevention program.

SUMMARY

This chapter has discussed the important role that technicians can play in making behavior wellness an integral part of the practice of veterinary medicine. A focus on behavior wellness rather than on resolving complex behavioral problems makes sense for technicians and the veterinary practice. It also fills a need for pets and their owners that is too often going unmet. More effective problem prevention and early detection of problems when they do occur have a great potential to keep pets out of animal shelters and prevent euthanasias for behavioral problems. Behavior wellness programs can be applied to any species of companion animal by inserting species-typical behavioral information. It is hoped this chapter can motivate technicians to seek additional continuing education in animal behavior so they can make greater contributions to behavior wellness.

REFERENCES

DiGiacomo N, Arluke A, Patronek G: Surrendering pets to shelters: the relinquisher's perspective, *Anthrozoos* 11:41, 1998.

Hetts S: *Pet behavior protocols: what to say, what to do, when to refer*, Lakewood, Colo, 1999, AAHA Press.

New JC et al.: Moving: characteristics of dogs and cats and those relinquishing them to 12 US animal shelters, *JAAWS* 2:83, 1999.

Patronek GJ, Dodman NH: Attitudes, procedures, and delivery of behavior services by veterinarians in small animal practice, *JAVMA* 215:1606, 1999.

Patronek GJ et al.: Risk factors for relinquishment of dogs to an animal shelter, *JAVMA* 209:572, 1996a.

Patronek GJ et al.: Risk factors for relinquishment of cats to an animal shelter, *JAVMA* 209:582, 1996b.

Salman MD et al.: Human and animal factors related to the relinquishment of dogs and cats in 12 selected animal shelters in the United States, *JAAWS* 1:207, 1998.

Scarlett JM et al.: Reasons for relinquishment of companion animals in US animal shelters: selected health and personal issues, *JAAWS* 2:41, 1999.

Wood F: Boost your passive income, *Vet Econ*, 1997.

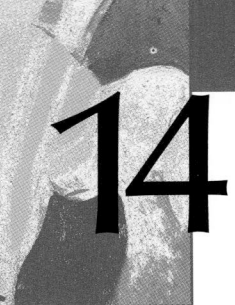

14

Companion Animal Clinical Nutrition

Philip Roudebush • Susan A. Berryhill

The veterinary technician plays an important role in educating clients about proper nutrition for their pet. For this reason, technicians should be knowledgeable about the diverse nutritional demands of healthy companion animals and understand the medical indications for specially prescribed diets in clinically ill animals. The information most commonly sought by clients is what to feed and how to feed it. However, nutritional deficiencies or excesses (particularly excesses) can also be problematic for clients when managing their pets. The nutritional assessment and specialized feeding of anorectic and hospitalized patients represent another area in which the technician plays a major role. In addition, the technician assists with the education of pet owners during important transitional feeding periods, such as when a discharged patient is being changed from a hospital diet to a home diet. Veterinary technicians who are able to provide nutritional counseling to clients and who share their knowledge about nutrition with co-workers increase the quality of care provided to patients, strengthen bonds with clients, and increase profitability for the practice.

This chapter defines nutrients and their use, distinguishes nutrients from ingredients, and suggests nutrient intake levels for pets and horses. Determination of food dosage for pet animals, true feeding costs (cost per calorie or cost per day), and quality assessment guidelines for horse forages and prepared animal foods are also discussed. A summary of companion animal clinical nutrition familiarizes the reader with dietary therapy. Basic assisted feeding techniques for hospitalized animals are also described.

OVERVIEW OF NUTRITIONAL OBJECTIVES AND PRINCIPLES

Nutritional goals differ sharply between agricultural and companion animals. As in human nutrition, the goal of feeding companion animals is to maximize the length and quality of life by reducing nutritional risk factors that work against wellness. The other aspect of well-pet nutrition is to match the nutritional intake with the life stage of the animal. For example, an adult dog should be fed an adult maintenance food rather than an all-purpose food formulated to meet the needs of puppies.

ENERGY-PRODUCING NUTRIENTS

A nutrient is any substance ingested to support life (Figure 14-1) and may be classified as an energy-producing nutrient or a non–energy-producing nutrient. Energy-producing nutrients are sugars, fatty acids, and amino acids. Although nutritionally different, each possesses a common availability and structure of hydrocarbon, making them suitable as metabolic "fuels." Digestion, assimilation, and metabolism of nutrients produce the chemical energy for the "fire of life." The energy released for the metabolism of food fuels the formation of storage molecules, such as adenosine triphosphate (ATP). The energy is stored in the chemical bonds that make up the ready-to-use molecules. When ATP is broken down the energy is released and used for cell maintenance, reproduction, repair, heat production, muscle contraction, and the synthesis of new tissue.

> **Technician Note**
>
> A nutrient is any substance ingested to support life and may be classified as an energy-producing nutrient or a non–energy-producing nutrient.

Carbohydrates: Sugars, Starches, and Fibers

Carbohydrate is a general biochemical classification that includes sugars, starches, and fibers. Sugars are numerous and include monosaccharides and disaccharides and more complicated sugar molecules. Multiple sugars can bond and link to form complex sugar polymers. Polymerized

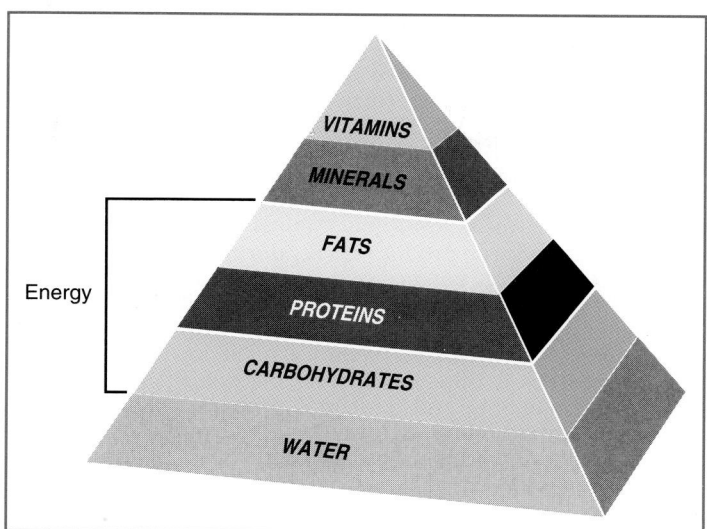

FIGURE 14-1. Six basic classes of nutrients are important for life sustenance. Carbohydrates, fats, and proteins may be used for energy but also serve as structural components.

sugars include starches and fibers. The starch or fiber type depends on sugar species and type of polymer linkages. Glucose (a monosaccharide blood sugar) and lactose (a disaccharide milk sugar) are two important animal sugars. Glycogen is an animal-specific starch and can quickly depolymerize to release its glucose content. Glycogen storage in the body is limited.

In the plant kingdom, starches and fibers (Box 14-1) are numerous and diverse. Feed grain starches are an energy source of fundamental importance to animals. Cellulose and other fibers are structural elements of grass, plants, and wood. Mammals lack fiber-degrading enzyme systems, so fiber is not digestible by the monogastric mammal; however, fiber is digestible by bacteria and protozoan microbes in the rumen, cecum, and large intestine of animals. Short-chain fatty acids result from fiber digestion, and these are transformable to glucose. Fiber thus serves as a major energy source for grazing animals. Debates over the environmental impacts and costs of cattle grazing and feedlot finishing sometimes ignore the creation of high-quality animal-source protein from inedible plant tissues. In simple-stomached animals, fiber reduces digestibility and effective caloric density yet maintains dry matter bulk. This effect finds applications in reducing caloric density for weight control foods. Fermentation of fiber occurs to some degree in the large intestine of simple-stomached animals. Some metabolic and gastrointestinal (GI) tract transit disorders also respond to increased levels of fiber in the food.

Technician Note

Mammals lack fiber-degrading enzyme systems, so fiber is not digestible by the monogastric mammal.

Lipids, Fatty Acids, Fats, and Oils

Fatty acids are building block components of vegetable and animal fats. The type and distribution of constituent fatty acids determine the physical, nutritional, and biologic characteristics of the fat or oil. Lipids have one to three molecules of fatty acids, are highly digestible, and have twice the caloric density of a similar quantity of carbohydrate or protein. Fat imparts significant food flavor that

Box 14-1	CARBOHYDRATES
SOLUBLE	**FIBER**
Starches	Pectin
Sugars	Lignin
	Cellulose
	Mucilage
	Gum

Box 14-2	ESSENTIAL FATTY ACIDS
CATS	**DOGS**
Linoleic	Linoleic
Alpha-linolenic	Alpha-linolenic
Arachidonic	

often improves its acceptability and palatability. Fat also facilitates digestion and assimilation of fat-soluble vitamins (A, D, E, K). The technician will see literature referring to types of fatty acids. The length of the carbon chain *backbone* identifies a fatty acid as *long-chain, medium-chain,* or *short-chain.* Short-chain fatty acids (1 to 8 carbon atoms in length) from rumen fluids and gases are important sources of energy. Long-chain fatty acids (12 to 20+ carbon units) are the most common components of dietary fats and oils.

Technician Note

The length of the carbon chain *backbone* identifies a fatty acid as *long-chain, medium-chain,* or *short-chain.*

The degree of hydrogen saturation (numbers of hydrogen atoms per carbon atoms) is variable, and the terms *saturated, unsaturated,* and *polyunsaturated* therefore denote hydrogen content. Positioning of double-bond carbon to carbon linkages within the fatty acid (Box 14-2) leads to further subclassifications. *Omega-6* and *omega-3* fatty acids designate some of these positioning features. Examples of

Box 14-3	ESSENTIAL AMINO ACIDS
Arginine	Methionine
Histidine	Phenylalanine
Isoleucine	Threonine
Leucine	Tryptophan
Lysine	Valine
	Taurine (essential in cats only)

omega-6 (n-6) fatty acids include linolenic acid and arachidonic acid. Examples of omega-3 (n-3) fatty acids include alpha-linolenic and eicosapentaenoic acid (EPA). The ratio of omega-6 to omega-3 distribution and/or amount of these fatty acids has different biologic effects in several body systems and has increasingly important therapeutic applications in clinical nutrition.

Amino Acids and Protein

Amino acids (Box 14-3) are the building blocks for plant and animal protein. Gastric and intestinal digestion subdivides protein into progressively smaller peptide units. The peptides undergo further digestion to yield the amino acids that are assimilated. The amino acid pool is then available for protein synthesis. The turnover and depletion of the pool determine the current amino acid requirement. Growth and lactation increase requirements more than maintenance and exertional work or exercise.

Technician Note

Amino acids are the building blocks for plant and animal protein.

Amino Acids as Energy Sources

Amino acids can serve as energy nutrients as well as the synthesis substrate for new protein. Any amino acid intake beyond withdrawal from the circulating pool is metabolized into energy. This is because there is no way to store extra amino acids from excess dietary protein as new viscera or muscle. Conversion of extra amino acids into energy is a several-step process. Removal of the amino (nitrogen-containing) group from the hydrocarbon skeleton of the amino acid is the first step. The conversion of the hydrocarbon skeleton into ATP, CO_2, and water is the second step. The nitrogen content must be eliminated as the third step. In addition to being "expensive energy," the metabolism of excess amino acids increases liver and kidney processing and excretory requirements for the urea and organic acid waste byproducts.

Essential Amino Acids

All 22 amino acids are necessary for synthesis of new protein. Since the body synthesizes 12 amino acids, an *essential* amino acid is one requiring supply from oral intake. The quantity and distribution of essential amino acids in a protein are important features determining a protein's biologic quality. All proteins are not of equal worth, and an ideal protein contains the exact essential amino acid distribution profile to meet a specific requirement. When profiles are not ideal (the case in practical diets), a higher protein digestibility and a higher biologic quality of protein better fulfill amino acid requirements with more efficiency and lower total nitrogen content than a low-quality protein. A limiting amino acid is one cause of decreased protein quality. When an otherwise high biologic value protein has a missing essential amino acid and therefore a more limited quality, the full potential of the biologic value of the protein is restored when the limiting acid is added. This is one reason why mixed animal and plant protein sources are often complementary to each other in food formulation.

Amino Acids as Emergency Fuels

Amino acids can produce energy during starvation or other negative energy balance situations. As starch and fatty acid stores are depleted, amino acids are mobilized from skeletal muscle and visceral proteins to provide glucose for energy. *Gluconeogenesis* (chemical breakdown of protein for glucose) is a valuable survival mechanism but "wastes" vital circulating and structural proteins. Loss of muscle mass and strength is a common clinical observation during anorexia and illness or injury, and muscle atrophy is a fundamental signal to the technician that protein is supplying energy.

Protein Requirements

Clients often inquire about the best protein intake for animals. Crude protein quantity (on the label) is the usual concern, and clients assume that more is better. However, a high protein number is not always the defining criterion for food quality. Chemical analysis for crude protein measures only total nitrogen content. The essential-to-nonessential amino acid profile, protein digestibility, and amino acid bioavailability are neither measured nor stated. Lower quantities of a higher biologic quality protein usually represent a higher-quality food and a more appropriate nutritional objective.

In cats, gluconeogenic amino acids are a major source of energy, and cats are specifically adapted to high protein intake. Herbivores evolved eating seasonal grasses and plants and have rumen or cecal microbes capable of synthesizing a portion of the amino acid requirement.

NON–ENERGY-PRODUCING NUTRIENTS

Water

Water is the most important nutrient. Water quality issues matter greatly to animals. In horse husbandry, the provision of an accessible and potable water supply is a fundamental issue. Dehydration from heavy sweat and prolonged work can be compensated for in animals by periodically watering them while they are working if that is possible. Frozen water can result in dehydration of animals, and a functioning stock tank heater or ice breaking is needed for horses in prolonged freezing weather. Dehydration is a common and frequently major clinical problem in sick patients unwilling or unable to eat and drink.

Technician Note

Water is the most important nutrient.

Minerals

More than 18 mineral elements are believed to be essential for mammals. *Macro* and *micro* describe two mineral intake levels. Calcium, phosphorus, magnesium, sodium, potassium, chlorine, and sulfur are dietary macrominerals (Tables 14-1 and 14-2).

Macrominerals are constituents of bone and structural proteins, and they participate as cofactors and catalysts in

TABLE 14-1	MINERAL CATEGORIES		
Macrominerals*		**Microminerals†**	
Sodium and chloride NaCl		Zinc Zn	Copper Cu
Potassium K⁺		Selenium Se	Iron Fe
Phosphorus P		Manganese Mn	Boron B
Magnesium Mg²⁺		Iodine I	Molybdenum Mo
Calcium Ca²⁺		Fluorine F	Cobalt Co
Sulfur S		Chromium Cr	

*Measured in %.
†Measured in ppm or mg/kg.

TABLE 14-2	MINERAL FUNCTIONS AND EFFECTS OF DEFICIENCY AND EXCESS		
Mineral	**Function**	**Deficiency**	**Excess**
Calcium	Constituent of bone and teeth, blood clotting, muscle function, nerve transmission, membrane permeability	Decreased growth, decreased appetite, decreased bone mineralization, lameness, spontaneous fractures, loose teeth, tetany, convulsions, rickets (osteomalacia: adults)	Decreased feed efficiency and intake, nephrosis, lameness, enlarged costochondral junctions, effect on bone and cartilage maturation
Phosphorus	Constituent of bone and teeth, muscle formation, fat, carbohydrates and protein metabolism, phospholipids and energy production, reproduction	Decreased appetite, decreased feed efficiency, decreased growth, dull hair coat, decreased fertility, spontaneous fractures, rickets	Bone loss, urinary calculi, decreased weight gain, decreased feed intake, calcification of soft tissues, secondary hyperparathyroidism
Potassium	Muscle contraction, transmission of nerve impulses, acid-base imbalance, osmotic balance, enzyme cofactor (energy transfer)	Anorexia, decreased growth, lethargy, locomotive problems, hypokalemia, heart and kidney lesions, emaciation	Rare Paresis, bradycardia
Sodium chloride	Osmotic pressure, acid-base balance, transmission of nerve impulses, nutrient uptake, waste excretion, water metabolism	Inability to maintain water balance, decreased growth, anorexia, fatigue, exhaustion, hair loss	Occurs only if there is inadequate good-quality water available; causes thirst, pruritus, constipation, seizures, and death; chronic amounts may complicate hypertension
Magnesium	Component of bone, intercellular fluids, neuromuscular transmission, active component of several enzymes, carbohydrate and lipid metabolism	Muscular weakness, hyperirritability, convulsions, anorexia, vomiting, decreased mineralization of bone, decreased body weight, calcification of aorta	Urinary calculi
Iron	Enzyme constituent: activation of O_2 (oxidases, oxygenases), O_2 transport (hemoglobin, myoglobin)	Anemia, rough hair coat, listless, decreased growth	Anorexia, weight loss, decreased serum albumin concentrations, hepatic dysfunction, hemosiderosis

From Hand MS et al, editors: *Small animal clinical nutrition*, ed 4, Topeka, 2000, Mark Morris Institute, p 67.   *Continued*

many biochemical reactions. When minerals circulate as ionized cation or anion electrolytes, they participate in osmotic fluid balance, nerve conduction, muscle contraction, blood clotting, blood pH buffering, and numerous other physiologic processes (Table 14-2).

Food provision of the macrominerals is expressed as parts per hundred (percent). Deficiency of macromineral intake produces serious clinical effects, but these are uncommon with proper feeding of appropriate foods. Deficiency most frequently follows anorexia, starvation, or poor-quality food. For example, calcium deficiency frequently develops when inappropriate homemade foods

are prepared for dogs, cats, and reptiles. Excess macromineral intake results from supplementation or poorer quality foods high in mineral-containing ingredients, such as meat and bone meal. Owner supplementation leads to excess total intake when a food is already adequate in macrominerals. The technician most commonly encounters this situation among well-intentioned, but uninformed, purebred animal hobbyists. For example, when adequate calcium and vitamin D in foal or puppy foods are supplemented for "support" of rapid skeletal growth, a resulting hypercalcemia may actually inhibit normal bone growth and cartilage maturation.

TABLE 14-2	MINERAL FUNCTIONS AND EFFECTS OF DEFICIENCY AND EXCESS—CONT'D		
Mineral	**Function**	**Deficiency**	**Excess**
Zinc	Constituent or activator of 200 known enzymes (nucleic acid metabolism, protein synthesis, carbohydrate metabolism), skin and wound healing, immune response, fetal development, growth rate	Anorexia, decreased growth, alopecia, parakeratosis, impaired reproduction, vomiting, hair depigmentation, conjunctivitis	Relatively nontoxic. Reported cases of Zn toxicity from consumption of diecast Zn nuts or pennies
Copper	Component of several enzymes (oxidases), catalyst in hemoglobin formation, cardiac function, cellular respiration, connective tissue development, pigmentation, bone formation, myelin formation, immune function	Anemia, decreased growth, hair depigmentation, bone lesions, neuromuscular, enzootic ataxia, aortic rupture, reproductive failure	Hepatitis, increased liver enzyme activity
Manganese	Component and activator of enzymes (glycosyl transferases), lipid and carbohydrate metabolism, bone development (organic matrix), reproduction, cell membrane integrity (mitochondria)	Decreased growth (rare in dogs and cats), impaired reproduction	Relatively nontoxic
Selenium	Constituent of glutathione peroxidase and iodothyronine-5-deiodinase, immune function, reproduction	Muscular dystrophy, reproductive failure, decreased feed intake, subcutaneous edema, renal mineralization	Vomiting spasms, staggered gait, salivation, decreased appetite, dyspnea, "garlicky" breath, nail loss
Iodine	Constituent of thyroxine and triiodothyronine	Goiter, fetal resorption, rough hair coat, enlarged thyroid glands, alopecia, apathy, myxedema, lethargy	Similar to deficiency, decreased appetite, listlessness, rough hair coat, decreased immunity, decreased weight gain, goiter
Boron	Regulates parathyroid hormone, influences metabolism of Ca^{2+}, P, Mg^{2+}, and cholecalciferol	Decreased growth, decreased hematocrit, hemoglobin, and alkaline phosphate	Similar to deficiency

From Hand MS et al, editors: *Small animal clinical nutrition,* ed 4, Topeka, 2000, Mark Morris Institute.
Ca, Calcium; *P,* phosphorus; *Mg,* magnesium.

Microminerals

Important microminerals (trace minerals) include iron, manganese, copper, iodine, and selenium. Dietary requirements for these minerals are in parts per million (mg/kg) instead of the percent levels for macrominerals. Hemoglobin, thyroxin, and many enzymes and cofactors contain micromineral constituents. Trace mineral deficiency and intoxication syndromes are potentially important in all species. Iron-deficient intake and chronic blood loss lead to depleted iron stores. Trace mineral deficiency can also result from bioavailability reductions from a competitive inhibition of assimilation. High calcium and/or phytate content may reduce bioavailability of zinc, copper, and other minerals, and zinc-responsive dermatoses are seen in dogs fed inferior, high-mineral foods.

Technician Note

Important microminerals, or trace minerals, are iron, zinc, manganese, copper, iodine, and selenium.

Vitamins

Vitamin (from *vital amine*) describes essential dietary cofactors that participate in many biochemical reactions. Vitamins have both common and chemical names. Vitamins are classified as fat soluble (A, D, E, K) or water soluble (all B and C) based on water solubility and route of excretion. Vitamins are not energy nutrients, and intake in excess of requirements does not improve performance. However, vitamins are often ascribed mystical performance enhancement values, and the "more is better" philosophy is frequently encountered. In the world of performance athletes, in which vitamin megatherapy is routinely encountered, abusive oversupplementation levels of fat-soluble vitamins may lead to toxic syndromes (Table 14-3). Vitamins C and E act as biologic antioxidants. Supplementation in food at levels above those known to meet minimum requirements may help avoid oxidative stress or injury to tissues.

Nutrients Versus Ingredients

The terms *nutrient, ingredient, formula,* and *nutrient profile* are easily confused and sometimes used interchangeably.

TABLE 14-3	VITAMINS		
Vitamin	**Function**	**Deficiency**	**Toxicity**
Vitamin A	Component of visual proteins, differentiation of epithelial cells, spermatogenesis, immune function, bone resorption	Anorexia, retarded growth, poor hair coat, weakness, increased cerebrospinal fluid pressure, eye disorders, aspermatogenesis, fetal resorption	Cervical spondylosis (cat), retarded growth, anorexia, erythema, long-bone fractures
Vitamin D	Ca^{2+} and P homeostasis, bone mineralization and resorption, insulin synthesis, immune function	Rickets, osteoporosis, osteomalacia	Hypercalcemia, calcinosis, lameness, anorexia
Vitamin E	Biologic antioxidant, maintains membrane integrity	Sterility (males), steatitis, anorexia, dermatosis, immunodeficiency, myopathy	Minimally toxic, increased clotting time reversed with vitamin K
Vitamin K	Allows blood clotting protein formation	Prolonged clotting time, hemorrhage, hypoprothrombinemia	Minimally toxic, anemia (dogs), none described in cats
Vitamin B complex	Multiple metabolic reactions, component of energy-producing biochemical reactions that produce energy and allow proper function of tissues and organs	Retarded growth, diarrhea, emaciation, ataxia, anemia, dermatitis	Low toxicity, except niacin in the cat, which can cause convulsions and death
Vitamin C	Synthesized from D-glucose in dogs and cats; synthesis of collagen proteins and carnitine, biologic antioxidant	Deficiency symptoms have not been described in normal dogs and cats	None described in dogs and cats
Choline	Component of membranes, neurotransmitter	Fatty liver (puppies), thymus atrophy, decreased growth rate, anorexia	None described in cats or dogs
Carnitine (vitamin-like nutrient)	Transports long-chain fatty acids into the cell	Hyperlipidemia, cardiomyopathy, muscle asthenia	None described in cats and dogs

From Hand MS et al, editors: *Small animal clinical nutrition,* ed 4, Topeka, 2000, Mark Morris Institute.
Ca, Calcium; *P,* phosphorus.

Nutrients are fundamental energy and metabolic substrates and cofactors such as lysine, glucose, or zinc. *Ingredients* are the raw materials used to manufacture a finished product. The *formula* selects and apportions ingredients. The *nutrient profile* describes the resulting quantitative distribution of the individual nutrients within the finished formula. These definitions are important in client education efforts when nutrient profile becomes confused with ingredients. In particular, some pet food advertising focuses on the presence of a particular ingredient as a brand point of difference. However, at the absorptive surface of the small intestinal mucosa, the ingredient of origin for a digested nutrient is immaterial. Importance should be placed on the nutrient value of the ingredient.

Technician Note

Nutrients are fundamental energy and metabolic substrates and cofactors such as lysine, glucose, or zinc. *Ingredients* are the raw materials used to manufacture a finished product.

Additives and Preservatives

Additives are nonenergy, nonnutrient components added to protect nutrient stability or enhance acceptability. Clients sometimes question additives and preservatives from the standpoint of necessity and food safety. The technician will need an opinion on the subject of natural versus synthetic additives in particular.

Colors, flavors, palatability enhancement digests, emulsifying agents, stabilizers, thickeners, and dough conditioners are examples of additives. Preservation of the nutrient profile is an important need achieved by both physical and chemical means. Dehydration is an important form of food preservation as seen in dried meats, dry pet food, and dry hay. Drying can protect nutrients for months. Canned pet foods involve the use of heat sterilization, an anaerobic environment, and a physical vacuum as a preservative and antioxidant system. Chemical preservatives are additives that retard oxidation, discoloration, or spoilage.

Organic acids or inorganic salts, such as common table salt, have a preservative effect through their antimicrobic activity (salted meats). Humectants are a preservative additive that binds water to inhibit mold and fungal growth. Chemicals that inhibit oxygen's destruction of vulnerable bonds are antioxidants. These agents primarily protect fatty acids and fat-soluble vitamins from rancid oxidation and loss of potency. Over the food's shelf life, a significant percentage of an antioxidant is "consumed" doing its job. Additives protect product quality and have good safety records based on years of application in animal agriculture and in pets (Mumma et al., 1986). One may question the need for coloring additives.

ESTIMATING ANIMALS' ENERGY REQUIREMENTS

Energy requirement estimates are used to calculate feeding quantity. There are several predictive equations for energy requirements based on the animal's species and physiologic requirements. The daily energy requirement is simply the calories needed to maintain neutral weight for the animal's current activity and environment. This number is a range affected by several activity and environmental factors (Figure 14-2). Work, lactation, and growth further modify energy requirements, and such multiples over maintenance are sometimes called *production energy requirements.*

Predictive equations are useful, but judging the body composition and condition is the key issue for energy balance assessment. The guideline for maintenance energy requirements is simply "to feel but not see the ribs" in a scheme of body condition scoring (BCS) (Figure 14-3).

COMPANION ANIMAL NUTRITION

Feeding Dogs

Dogs are highly social pack animals and cooperative team hunters. Wild-type feeding is both hierarchic and competitive, with intrapack feeding order maintained by the alpha-dominant animal. Food intake in wild canids is distinctly omnivorous, although pet food advertising emphasizes the carnivorous aspects of intake ("meatier is better"). Wild dogs eat intestines and intestinal contents of herbivorous prey, as well as organs and flesh. Many domesticated dogs will eat vegetables, grains and pastas, meat, processed foods, various dairy products, and even fruit. Dental and digestive anatomy and nutritional biochemistry further document the dog as omnivorous, and it is fair to say domesticated dogs can adapt well to a varied dietary intake. However, when domesticated dogs eat grass or feces, owners complain that the pet is not behaving as a carnivore. Although such ingestive behavior is natural, behavior modification (e.g., the use of cayenne pepper sauce on the feces) may reduce the objectionable activity.

Canine Pediatric Nutrition

Puppies usually nurse soon after birth. Postsurgical nursing of the bitch who has undergone cesarean delivery should specifically note colostrum production by the dam and intake by puppies before discharge from the hospital. Colostrum provides fluid for vital postpartum circulatory expansion and maternal immunity factors (globulin antibodies) for absorption by the intestine. Most puppies are healthy and are capable and active in nursing. Most mothers are lactating well and attentive to the litter; therefore no assistance is needed from the technician or owner. The possible exception is extremely small, toy-breed puppies for whom frequent, assisted hand feeding for several weeks after birth may be needed to preclude hypothermia and hypoglycemia. When there is concern about lactation, a quick indicator for quality and quantity, in addition to examining the milk itself, is to weigh the puppies. A normal growth rate for puppies is 2 to 4 g/day/kg of anticipated adult weight. Weight gain below this rate accompanied by restless, hungry-seeming puppies is a sign of feeding distress.

Raising Orphan Puppies

Neonatal puppies unable to nurse require a canine milk replacement formula. Canine milk is higher in protein and

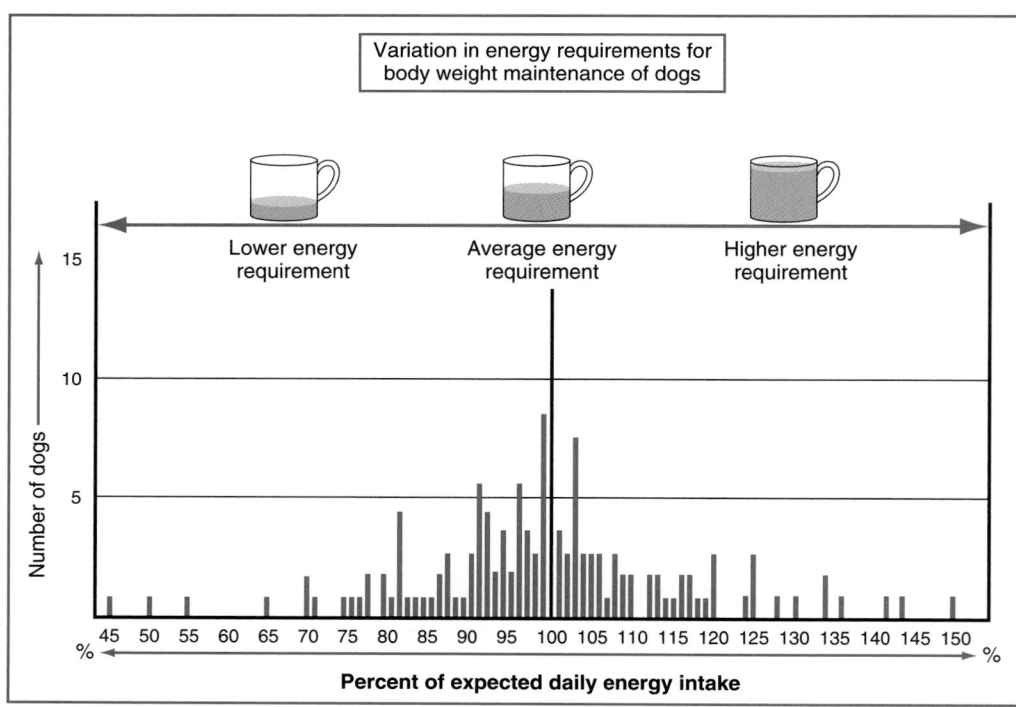

FIGURE 14-2. Variation in canine energy requirements. Note that some dogs require more energy and some less energy than the expected amount. Similar differences are also noted in cats.

lower in lactose than bovine milk, so water, not cow's milk, should be used to mix formula. The orphan formula dose is initially 15% of the puppy's weight per day divided into several doses. Food dose adequacy is usually evidenced by the puppy's becoming content and going to sleep after feeding. Assisted feeding of neonates is by feeding syringe and a flexible, rubber feeding tube (Figure 14-4). If there is adequate nursing vigor, one may substitute a pet nurser system (Figure 14-4). At litter discharge from the hospital, the technician should pretest flow rate from all nipples dispensed and give explicit instructions for sanitation and formula mixing. When the puppy reaches 2 to 3 weeks of age, the food dose approximates 25% of the body weight divided into four to six daily feedings.

BODY CONDITION SCORING SYSTEM

Body condition assessment will assist the veterinary technician in determining if the puppy or kitten is growing appropriately and if the correct amount of food is being offered. Proper growth can reduce risk for obesity and growth related skeletal disease.

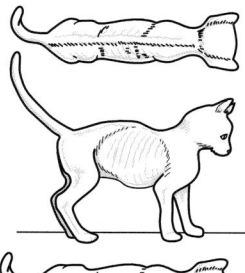

1. VERY THIN

The ribs are easily palpable with no fat cover. The tailbase* has a prominent raised bony structure with no tissue between the skin and bone. The bone prominences are easily felt with no overlying fat. In animals over six months, there is a severe abdominal tuck when viewed from the side and an accentuated hourglass shape when viewed from above.

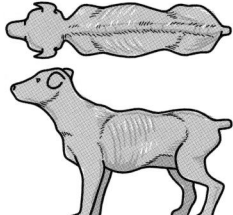

2. UNDERWEIGHT

The ribs are easily palpable with minimal fat cover. The tailbase* has a raised bony structure with little tissue between the skin and bone. The bony prominences are easily felt with minimal overlying fat. In animals over six months, there is an abdominal tuck when viewed from the side and a marked hourglass shape when viewed from above.

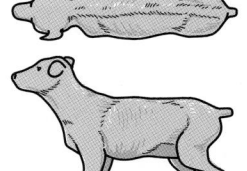

3. IDEAL

The ribs are palpable with a slight fat cover. The tailbase* has a smooth contour or some thickening and the bony structures are palpable under a thin layer of fat between the skin and the bone. The bony prominences are easily felt with a slight amount of overlying fat. In animals over six months, there is an abdominal tuck when viewed from the side and a well proportioned lumbar waist when viewed from above.

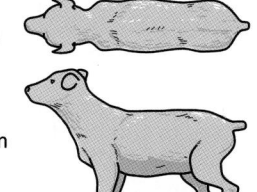

4. OVERWEIGHT

The ribs are difficult to feel with moderate fat cover. The tailbase* has some thickening with moderate amounts of tissue between the skin and bone. The bony structures can still be felt. The bony prominences are covered by a moderate layer of fat. In animals over six months, there is little or no abdominal tuck or waist when viewed from above. Abdominal fat apron present in cats.

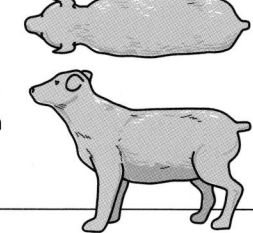

5. OBESE

The ribs are very difficult to feel under a thick fat cover. The tailbase* appears thickened and is difficult to feel under a prominent layer of fat. The bony prominences are covered by a moderate to thick layer of fat. In animals over six months, there is a pendulous ventral bulge and no waist when viewed from the side. The back is markedly broadened when viewed from above. Marked abdominal fat apron present in cats.

*Tailbase evaluation is done only in dogs.

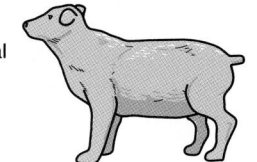

FIGURE 14-3. Body conditioning scoring system.

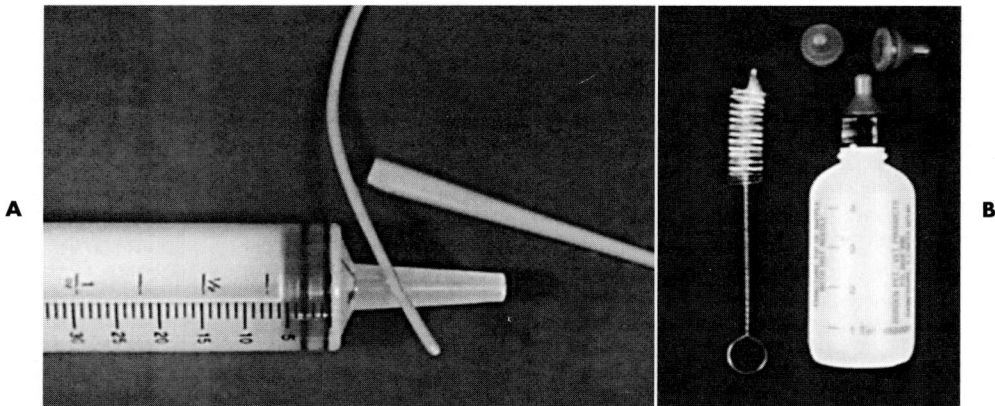

FIGURE 14-4.   A, Orphan puppies and kittens are raised on species-specific milk replacement. Tube gavage with flexible feeding tube and a catheter-tip syringe is an easy and safe technique in neonatal puppies and kittens. **B,** Pet nursers are used in neonates with adequate sucking vigor. Always test the flow and temperature of formula in advance and sanitize equipment between uses.

 Technician Note

The orphan formula dose is initially 15% of the puppy's body weight per day divided into several doses.

Box 14-4	OBESITY-PRONE DOG BREEDS

Beagle
Labrador
Sheltie
Cocker spaniel
Golden retriever
Cairn terrier
Scottish terrier
Dachshund
Basset hound
Cavalier King Charles spaniel

Weaning Puppies

Peak lactation occurs at 4 weeks, and weaning concludes at 6 to 8 weeks. Begin introducing puppies to semisolid gruel made from 2 parts of water to 1 part of a high-quality, dry, canine growth/lactation pet food. Three weeks of age is a suitable time to introduce a semisolid gruel, except for toy breeds and weak animals. Mash the mixture with a fork, and place the gruel in a shallow pan. Gruel ingestion inevitably follows a play period and begins acclimating the puppies to intake of particulate solids. At 5 weeks of age, puppies are reducing their intake of mother's milk and consuming significant amounts of gruel. The ratio of water can be reduced as the puppies approach total weaning onto dry or moist foods.

Feeding Growing Dogs

Absolute and relative nutritional requirements change rapidly during a puppy's growth. Rate of growth, as well as final adult size, is obviously and dramatically different between various dog breeds. Nutrient guidelines for small- and medium-breed versus large- and giant-breed dogs are listed in Table 14-4. Most growing puppies eat four or five times daily during the postweaning period, but meal frequency declines as gastrointestinal capacity increases. The quantity of food can be determined in several ways, and Figure 14-5 demonstrates some model calculations for establishing a food dose. The methods of feeding puppies require specific consideration. The *ad libitum* (ad-lib) feeding method allows excess nutrient intake in many puppies. When the puppy overconsumes energy and calcium, developmental bone disease may surface. This is especially evident in rapidly growing members of the large and giant breeds. Unfortunately, some growth-type pet foods contain excessive calcium even at appropriate levels of dry matter intake. Energy overconsumption, by itself, was studied in two groups of Labrador retriever puppies. One group ate ad lib, and the second group was limited to 75% of the ad-lib quantity. Serial pelvic radiography for 2 years showed significant reductions in hip laxity in the meal-limited group. To help control the risk to normal orthopedic development of large-breed and giant puppies, a specific nutrient profile has been developed to control the potential overconsumption of energy and macrominerals while supplying growth levels of protein and vitamins.

Roly-poly puppies also risk current and future obesity. The technician should emphasize the risk of juvenile overfeeding as a part of the client education program. This is especially true when the animal is a member (or cross breed) of obesity-prone breeds (see Box 14-4).

Feeding Adult Dogs

A primary objective in feeding the adult dog is finding the energy requirement and food dose that maintains a neutral energy balance (see Figure 14-5). Nutrient guidelines for adult dogs are found in Table 14-4. In adult dogs, ad-lib feeding is commonly associated with overconsumption and problems with obesity. However, ad-lib feeding is less labor intensive for animal colonies and kennels. Late detection of anorexia and timid animals not having adequate intake are potential problems with this method. When dogs are individually penned or can eat from self-feeders, these problems are eliminated.

Individual meal feeding is best whenever possible (Figures 14-6 to 14-8). In the time-restricted method, feed from one to three times daily with ad-lib consumption for 5 to 15 minutes. If the dog consistently leaves a little food in its dish and also maintains an ideal body condition, the

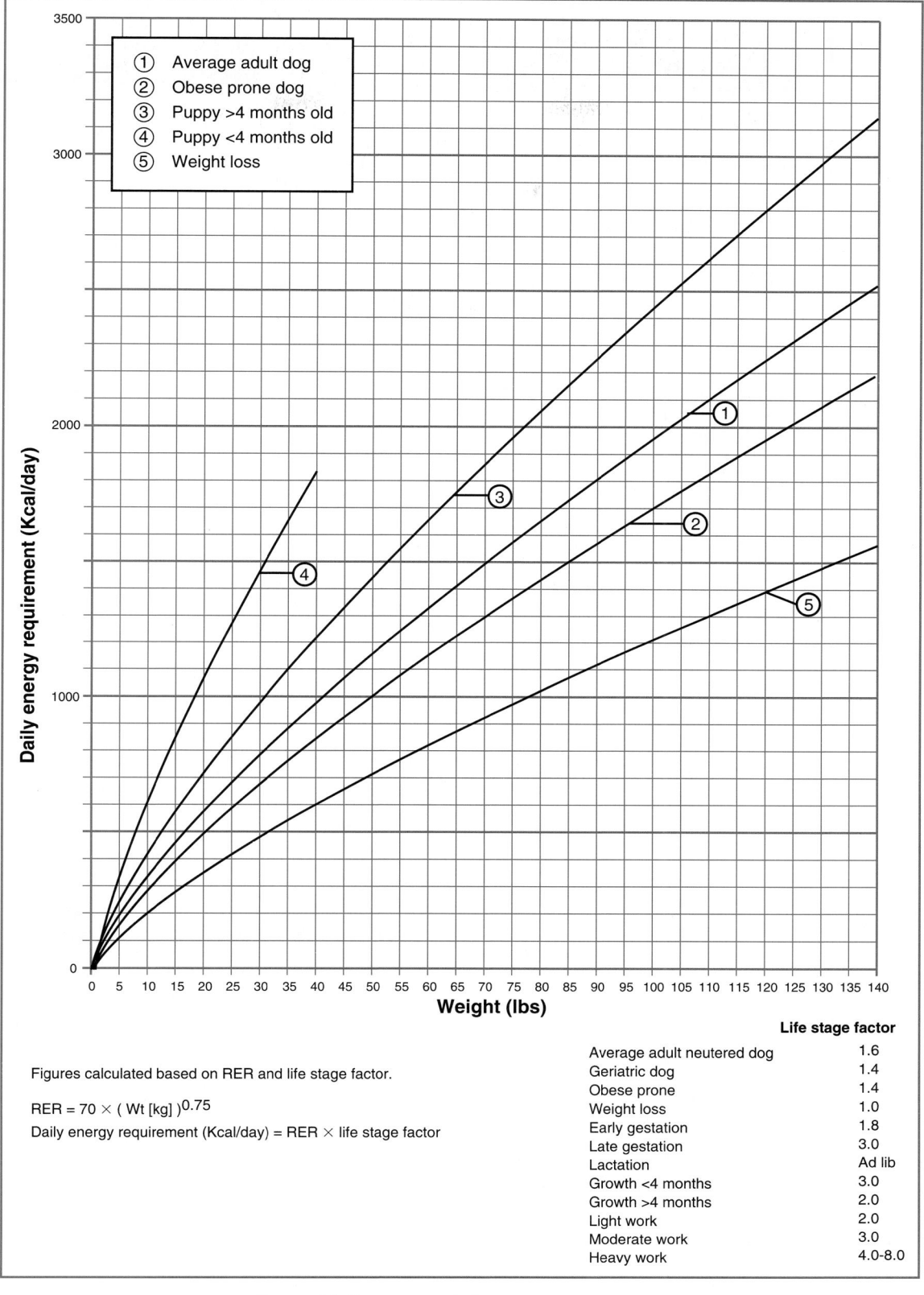

FIGURE 14-5.   Canine daily energy requirements.

TABLE 14-4   NUTRIENT GUIDELINES FOR WELLNESS*

Life Stage	Energy Kcal ME/g	Protein	Fat	Fiber	Calcium	Phosphorus	Sodium
				% Dry Matter			
DOG							
Growth/reproduction	3.5-5.0	22-35	10-25	5 max	0.7-1.7	0.6-1.3	0.35-0.6
Large-breed growth	3.0-4.0	22-35	8-12	10 max	0.7-1.2	0.6-1.1	0.3-0.6
Adult maintenance	3.5-4.5	15-30	10-20	5 max	0.5-1.0	0.4-0.9	0.2-0.4
Obesity prone	3.0-3.5	15-30	7-12	5-17	0.5-1.0	0.4-0.9	0.2-0.4
High energy	>4.5	22-34	26 min	5 max	0.5-1.0	0.4-0.9	0.2-0.5
Geriatric†	3.5-4.5	15-23	7-15	10 max	0.5-1.0	0.2-0.7	0.15-0.35
CAT							
Growth/reproduction	4.0-5.0	35-50	18-35	5 max	0.8-1.6	0.6-1.4	0.3-0.6
Adult maintenance	4.0-5.0	30-45	10-30	5 max	0.5-1.0	0.5-0.8	0.2-0.6
Obesity prone	3.3-3.8	30-45	8-17	5-15	0.5-1.0	0.5-0.9	0.2-0.6
Geriatric†	3.5-4.5	30-45	10-25	10 max	0.6-1.0	0.5-0.7	0.2-0.5

Max, maximum; *min*, minimum; *C*, cup.

*Nutrients are expressed as % dry matter. Energy is expressed as Kcal metabolizable energy (ME) per gram dry matter.

†Older animals require frequent body condition scoring. Feed intake adjustment may be required to maintain an ideal body condition because some older individuals tend to be heavy and others tend to lose weight.

Average Caloric Content of Pet Foods

Dog food (generic, private label, grocery)

Dry	350 Kcal/C
Soft-moist	275 Kcal/C
Canned	500 Kcal/14- to 15-oz can

Cat food (generic, private label, grocery)

Dry	300 Kcal/C
Soft-moist	250 Kcal/C
Canned	180 Kcal/5.5- to 6.5-oz can

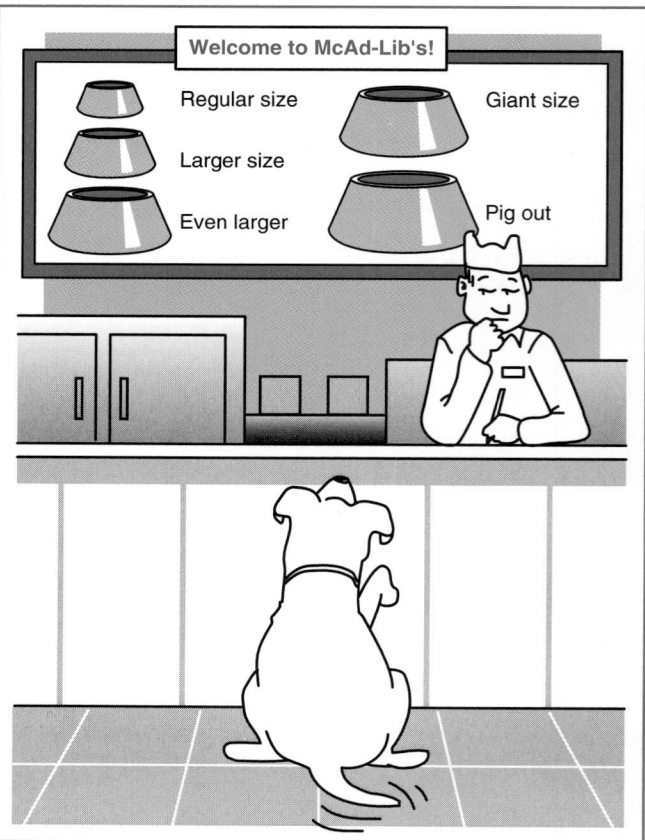

FIGURE 14-6.   Ad-lib feeding means an excess of food, at all times, for self-feeding.

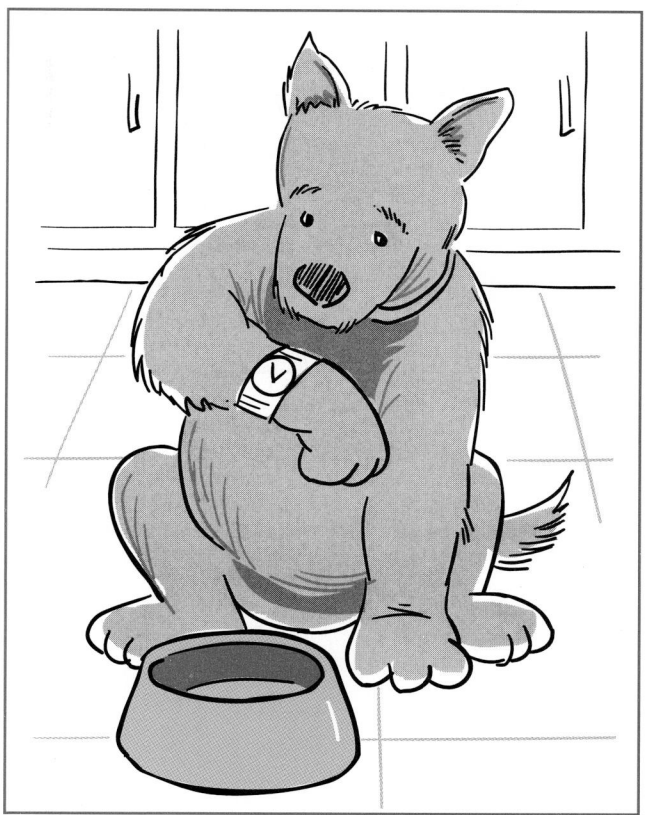

FIGURE 14-7. Time-controlled feeding provides an unrestricted food quantity in a set period of time.

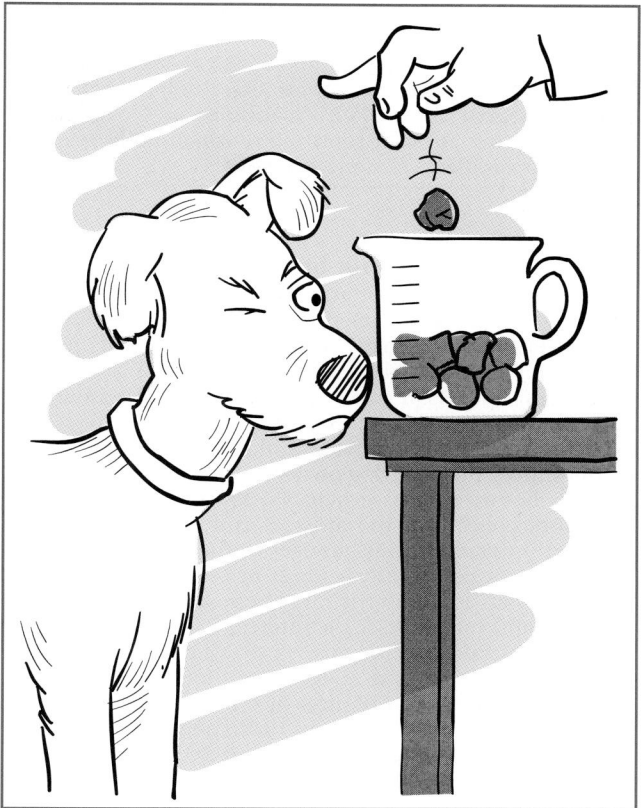

FIGURE 14-8. Portion-controlled feeding involves the measurement of pet food and providing it in a quantity that maintains optimum body condition.

Box 14-5	FEEDING DO'S AND DON'TS	
DO'S		**DON'TS**

DO'S
- Provide fresh water.
- Feed for control of calorie intake.
- Feed for ideal weight and body condition.
- Feel but do not see ribs.
- Provide a consistent food, and ritualize the time and place of feeding.
- Use life-stage feeding concepts by correlating diet to pet's life stage.
- Feed treats with nutrient profile and caloric density considerations.

DON'TS
- Provide stagnant or frozen water.
- Allow excess calorie consumption.
- Feed obesity-prone dogs on an ad-lib or free-choice basis.
- Rotate flavors or brands on a frequent basis.
- Make rapid transitions.
- Use growth/lactation foods for adult maintenance.
- Supplement a balanced/high-quality food.
- Allow competitive eating.

conclusion must be that the animal is self-regulating its food intake at its energy requirement. Time-restricted feeding works well for many dogs and their owners; however, some dogs ravenously overeat during the allotted time. In dogs that overeat, try volume-restricted meal feeding by serving a calculated food dose. To determine the daily volume, divide the energy requirement by the food's caloric density. Then feed one half to one third of the daily volume two or three times per day. An average caloric density guideline for pet foods is listed in Table 14-4. Other aids for food dose calculations are suggested feeding amounts on labels, food dose calculators, and technical information from manufacturers (Box 14-5). Maintenance pet food is recommended for the average house pet.

It should also be recommended that table foods be eliminated or used in moderation (10% or less). Fat trimmings quickly unbalance a base diet and lead to finicky behavior and predisposition to obesity. Avoid feeding animal bones because sharp fragments may wedge between teeth, lacerate the esophagus, or cause gastrointestinal obstruction or constipation. Nylon bones and chew toys are safer substitutes for natural bones but still cause problems in some individuals. Table 14-4 lists guidelines for assessing pet foods used in life-stage feeding.

Technician Note

Avoid feeding animal bones because sharp fragments may wedge between teeth or lacerate the esophagus or cause gastrointestinal obstruction or constipation. Nylon bones and chew toys are safer substitutes for natural bones, but still cause problems in some individuals.

Feeding Adult Dogs With Increased Energy Needs

Increased energy is important in working dogs and stressed animals. Supply extra energy by using pet foods of increased fat, caloric density, and digestibility. This permits dry matter intake and gastric fill to remain at familiar, nonexcessive levels. Increasing the quantity or frequency of a regular food is a secondary option.

The technician can provide a high-quality client service by reminding hunting dog owners to aerobically condition animals before extensive field work. Aerobic training before work conditions the muscles and cardiovascular system and induces enzyme changes in the muscle that allow more efficient use of fatty acids as muscle fuel. The aerobic use of fatty acids spares the rate of consumption of muscle glycogen and can increase the interval to exhaustion. When aerobic conditioning begins, convert the dog to more calorie-dense food and suggest feeding the majority of daily calories after completion of training to help prevent hunting dog hypoglycemia. Unfortunately, the more obvious feeding recommendation would seem to be the reverse, namely, feeding before work. However, insulin release follows glucose assimilation after the meal's digestion, allowing a high rate of glucose transfer into the cells. If the animal simultaneously begins hard work, the combination of the two glucose-consuming activities may precipitate hypoglycemia. If animals show consistent signs of hunting dog hypoglycemia, even after conditioning, they may be fed 10% to 15% of the daily calorie dose as a light feeding at 2-hour intervals during work. Clients should also be reminded of the importance of adequate water intake throughout the work period.

Feeding During Pregnancy and Lactation

Early and midterm pregnancy is a nutritional nonevent, but requirements increase modestly during the last third of gestation. Recommend a growth/lactation formula to meet the increased requirements. Lactation markedly increases energy, protein, and mineral requirements. After whelping, the bitch returns to her regular body weight and eats to service increased needs (Figure 14-9). Expect food intake to rise rapidly by 50% the first week and by 200% to 400% by the fourth week of lactation. This level of demand is equivalent to those of heavily pulling sled dogs, and the loss of fat and even muscle is common during lactation. This potential underfeeding situation can be helped by allowing ad-lib intake of a high-quality growth/lactation pet food. Supplements are *not* needed for normal animals when high-quality pet foods are used.

Technician Note

Expect food intake to rise rapidly by 50% the first week and by 200% to 400% by the fourth week of lactation.

Weaning the Litter

Food intake should be terminated for 24 hours to help the bitch slow and stop her milk production. The food intake

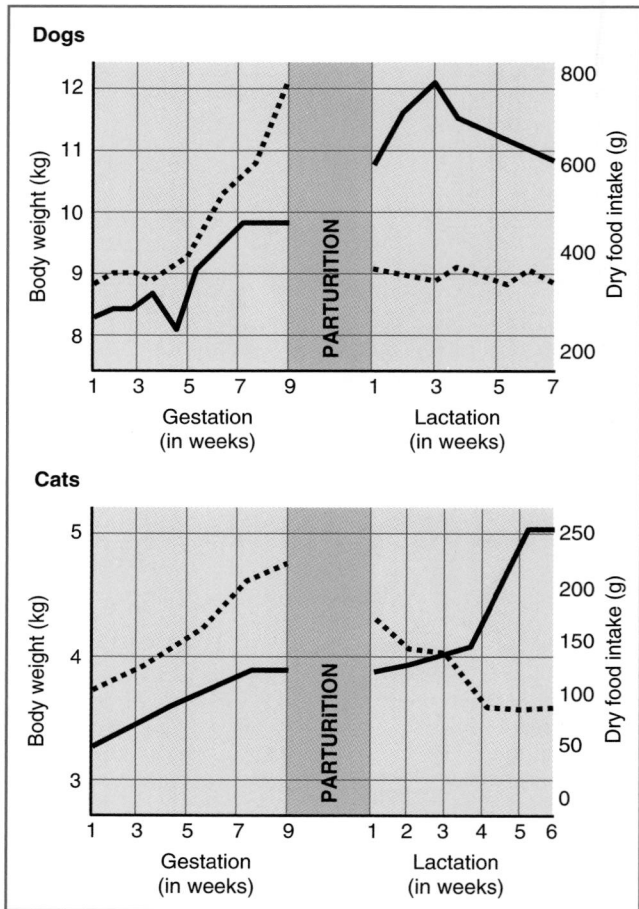

FIGURE 14-9. The pattern of normal weight gain during gestation and loss in the postpartum and lactation periods differs between cats and dogs. *Solid line* indicates food intake. *Dashed line* indicates body weight.

can be resumed using maintenance foods at one third of the customary maintenance level. On the second day use two-thirds feeding and full intake on day three. When lactation quickly dries from acute calorie deprivation, the bitch will more readily reject the puppies' attempts to continue to nurse.

Obesity-Prone Animals

Definition, Causes, and Health Risks of Obesity

Malnutrition of obesity is at epidemic proportions. Canine and feline obesity estimates are 25% to 30%. Obesity means body composition with a ratio of too much fat to lean tissue. (*Overweight* is not always an accurate measurement for *overfat*.) There are several known causes for obesity, and as a confidant of the owner the technician is vital in the crusade to prevent and treat this epidemic.

Technician Note

Canine obesity estimates are 30%, with feline obesity as high as 40%.

One cause for obesity-prone animals is overfeeding a young animal. A positive calorie balance during juvenile growth may induce increased numbers of fat cells (hyper-

TABLE 14-5	NUTRIENT CHARACTERISTICS OF HUMAN SNACK FOODS*					
Food	Serving Size	Kcal/Serving	Kcal/g	Protein (g)	Fat (g)	Sodium†
Cow's milk (3.5%)	1 C = 244 g	150	0.6	8	8	122/81
Whole egg (boiled)	1 egg = 50 g	79	1.6	6.1	5.6	69/87
Ice cream (vanilla, 10% fat)	1 C = 133 g	266	2.0	4.8	14.3	116/43
American cheese	1 oz	93	3.3	5.6	7	337/362
Cottage cheese (low fat, 2%)	1 C = 226 g	203	0.9	31	4.4	918/452
Gelatin	1 C = 280 g	162	0.6	3.2	0	108/67
Hot dog	8/lb = 57 g	180	3.2	6.9	16.3	585/325
Bologna (beef)	1 slice = 23 g	72	3.1	2.8	6.6	226/313
Big Mac	1 sandwich = 200 g	570	2.9	24.6	35	979/172
Peanut butter (smooth)	2 T = 32 g	188	5.9	9	5.4	234/124
Popcorn (w/ butter)	3 C = 37 g	192	5.2	2.8	11.5	273/142
Corn chips	1 oz	153	5.5	1.7	8.8	218/142
Potato chips	1 oz	148	5.3	1.8	10.1	133/90
Pretzels	1 oz	110	3.9	3.0	1.2	543/493

All values from Pennington JAT: *Food values of portions commonly used*, ed 15, New York, 1989, Harper & Row.
C, Cup; T, tablespoon.
*Metabolizable energy for humans.
†Sodium content per serving/sodium content per 100 Kcal.

plasia). Once formed, these fat cells are present for life and have minimal volumes of triglyceride content below which they cannot shrink (Crane, 1991). Therefore a lifelong predisposition for excess weight develops. Needless adipocyte hyperplasia is prevented by using meal feeding for puppies, kittens, and foals.

A second cause of obesity is genetic predisposition. Several lines of evidence establish genetic inheritance as influential on the resting metabolic rate (Crane, 1991). This means "easy keepers" with less food intake required.

Third, a declining lean body mass and declining activity level are part of the normal aging process. Decreases in energy requirements may be considered in a geriatric feeding program (Markham, Hodgkins, 1989). However, some older pets may also become thin.

Fourth, animals may overeat just because the food is palatable. Volume-restricted meal feeding and control of the intake of treats will be needed when this situation is identified.

Fifth, multianimal households or other group-feeding situations may provoke competitive eating. The control measures are volume-restricted feeding and separation of the competitive animals by time or place of feeding. Most owners can engineer these circumstances with a little thought and coaching.

Sixth, surgical neutering of males and females alters metabolism, deregulates satiety, and increases the desire to feed. One may suggest less calorically dense foods concurrent with postneuter suture removal. This seems especially prudent in obesity-prone breeds of dogs.

Health Risks of Obesity
An animal whose body fat exceeds 20% to 30% of its body weight is obese. Obesity may increase the risk for a number of diseases, exacerbate existing disease, and decrease the animal's life span. Obese dogs have a higher risk for cardiovascular disease, may experience elevated blood pressure, and are less tolerant of environmental extremes. Overweight animals also have a higher risk for degenerative joint disease. Obese dogs have a higher risk of certain types of cancer. Other health problems associated with obesity are dyspnea, dystocia, and dermatologic problems. An obese patient should always be evaluated for underlying endocrine diseases, such as hyperadrenocorticism, hy-

pothyroidism, and diabetes mellitus. Obesity has been shown to be a predisposing factor for hepatic lipidosis in cats. Because obesity is such a common disease, clients should understand the negative impact to their companion of additional unwanted pounds.

Diagnosis and Treatment of Obesity
One can assess the quantity of the patient's fat by examining the subcutaneous deposits visually and by palpation over the ribs, groin, and tail head. Radiographs of the abdomen and thorax will also reveal fat accumulations. Weighing only indirectly measures body composition, but using ideal weight tables for purebred animals is useful. Body condition scoring (see Figure 14-3) is a visual and useful method for combining various assessment criteria into an opinion regarding the pet's body composition and relative fatness. Obesity is best prevented but can be treated by caloric restriction and exercise. Specific treatment requires teamwork among the owner, the veterinarian, and the technician.

Weight control is rarely as easy as it sounds, but long-term success in weight reduction can be achieved in practice. However, success is precious, and some practices focus most strongly on identifying those clients most able or most likely to be educated and motivated. In monitoring any treatment program, the veterinary technician is of fundamental importance as educator and cheerleader. Part of the dietary management program is building awareness of extraneous contributions of calories, such as treats, including both human snack foods and commercial pet treats (Tables 14-5 and 14-6).

Feeding the Geriatric Animal
The definition of *geriatric*, as it pertains to the dog, is not precise because of breed variability in the natural life span and because "miles as well as years" influence the wear and tear of physiologic aging. As a generality, toy and small-sized breeds are geriatric at 7 years, medium-sized dogs at 6 years, and large and giant breeds as early as 5 years of age.

Loss of reserve capacity of organ function is universal with normal aging. Chronic progressive renal disease is common in older dogs and cats. There is no proven cause for or prophylactic strategy against the scourge of renal aging. However, the progressive loss of renal reserve ulti-

TABLE 14-6 **DOG AND CAT TREATS**

Treat	Manufacturer	Weight (g/treat)	Calories (Kcal ME)	Protein (g)	Fat (g)	Fiber (g)	Calcium (mg)	Phosphorus (mg)	Potassium (mg)	Sodium (mg)	Magnesium (mg)
DOG TREATS											
Milkbone (small)	Nabisco	5	16	1.1	0.3	0.1	71	54	30	21	7
Beggin Strips Orginal Bacon Flavor	Purina	10.3	29	1.7	0.6	0.1	44	49	33	65	11
Bonz	Purina	20.4	66	3.1	1.3	0.3	241	155	86	53	24
Purina Biscuits (medium)	Purina	10.2	37	2.5	1.3	0.2	114	106	91	29	21
Meaty Bone (medium)	Heinz	18.2	64	2.3	1.8	0.4	8	55	71	116	20
100% Natural Treats	Heinz	7.6	26	1.3	0.5	0.1	17	49	48	41	15
Snausages (beef flavor)	Heinz	6.6	17	1.5	0.6	0.1	61	46	98	44	7
Pup-Peroni Jerky Snack Sticks	Heinz	6.6	21	1.8	1	0.1	55	44	59	73	7
Original Jerky Treats	Heinz	6.8	22	2	1.3	0.1	35	35	71	140	7
Fiber Formula Biscuits (medium)	Stewart	10.1	26	1.5	0.3	1.7	63	37	NA	7	NA
Science Diet (adult maintenance)	Hill's	5	17	1.1	0.5	0.2	29	29	29	11	4
Science Diet (light)	Hill's	5	15	0.8	0.3	0.6	29	29	38	11	7
Science Diet (senior)	Hill's	5	16	0.8	0.4	0.4	30	27	28	7	5
Prescription Diet	Hill's	5	15	0.8	0.3	0.8	28	21	36	5	6
CAT TREATS											
Pounce (with tuna)	Heinz	1.5	3.7	0.32	0.13	0.01	13.5	11.3	1:1.2	9.2	1.2
Pounce Hairball Treatment	Heinz	1.0	2.9	1.7	0.4	0.2	2	6	7	5	0.6
Whisker Lickin's (Kluckers)	Purina	1.1	3	0.32	0.12	0.01	9	10.7	1:0.84	6.2	0.7

From Hand MS et al, editors: *Small animal clinical nutrition*, ed 4, Topeka, 2000, Mark Morris Institute.
ME, Metabolizable energy; *NA*, not applicable.

mately reduces the animal's capability to excrete phosphorus, urea, and other metabolic waste byproducts of protein metabolism. Controlling excesses of intake during the geriatric period does no harm even in the absence of clinical signs of renal failure. Therefore the recommendation to avoid excessive protein, phosphorus, and sodium chloride seems medically prudent.

In renal failure, the veterinarian will prescribe specific intake restrictions of protein, phosphorus, and sodium and, perhaps, other measures to control hyperphosphatemia. Cats have elevated potassium requirements during renal insufficiency and renal failure. Many animals with renal insufficiency and failure will be in their geriatric period of life.

Calorie control may begin or be continued in some older animals. On the other hand, other older animals may have inadequate calories because of systemic illness, dental or oral pain, failing sight and smell, or progression of finicky tastes or fixed food addictions. Blanket feeding recommendations based solely on age are unwise without consideration of the individual. Pet foods specifically intended for seniors emphasize moderate energy density with good palatability and reductions of some excess nutrients, as found in all-purpose pet foods.

Feeding Cats

Cats are not "small dogs" and are physically, physiologically, and behaviorally adapted as solo-hunting, carnivorous predators. Use of amino acids as important energy sources translates into cats having twice the protein requirement of the more omnivorous dog. The percentage of total dietary calories originating from an ideal protein source (biologic value of 100%) is 8% in adult cats but 4% in adult dogs. Other feline specific requirements include taurine as an eleventh essential amino acid (McDonald et al., 1984). Animal origin types and/or sources of vitamin A, niacin, pyridoxine, and arachidonic acid (a fatty acid) are other feline-specific requirements. Feeding dog food to cats for convenience or economy is ill advised. If the technician encounters this dietary history, the veterinarian should be alerted for educational intervention. Figure 14-10 summarizes energy requirements for cats in differing life stages and lifestyles.

Feeding Kittens and Adult Cats

One must confirm adequate colostrum intake for all kittens. Like puppies, the orphan kitten can be raised by tube gavage or nurser administration of queen's milk replacement. Kittens are weaned later than puppies—generally at 7 to 9 weeks. Growth-sustaining kitten foods are then meal fed two or three times daily until the kitten is 10 months of age.

As adults, feral cats have nibbling eating patterns because they hunt mice and other small animals most of the night and part of the day. Nibbling minimizes the effect of the postprandial alkaline tide—a physiologic event that alkalinizes the urine after meal feeding. This may help to protect against urinary crystalluria, but twice-daily meal feeding is practical and works well for indoor cats.

A consistent feeding product and schedule should be recommended during adult maintenance. Decreased finickiness results from this approach, but flavor rotation is a perspective of some owners in response to the large number of cat food flavors present on supermarket shelves. Flavor rotation is unnecessary for variety, and a transient "newness" factor increases food intake when the new flavor is introduced. The result is the owner's perception of doing the cat a favor (expressed as increased intake). However,

weight homeostasis may be upset by frequent flavor rotation.

Commercial feline treats are usually clones of dry cat food (see Table 14-6). As such, they are appropriate for treating when given in moderation and dietary restriction is not needed. Some cat owners prefer "natural" treats, such as raw or cooked poultry necks, oxtails, or liver. Although little harm results from the use of such treats in moderation, finicky behavior and nutritional imbalance are potential hazards. Liver contains an inverted Ca/P ratio (1:17), and potentially toxic levels of vitamin A (hypervitaminosis A) can occur with long-term use.

Hairballs occur commonly in cats because of their normal grooming behavior and sharp barbs on the tongue, which enhance hair ingestion. Hairballs are periodically regurgitated from the oropharynx or esophagus or vomited from the stomach, or they pass into the intestinal tract, where they are voided in the feces. Owners observe periodic gagging, retching, and regurgitation or vomiting of hair and mucus. Hairballs are often tubular and usually do not contain food or bile. Although hairballs do not usually cause significant clinical disease, they are a nuisance for many cat owners. Many laxatives, lubricants, treats, and foods are available for routine management of these problems. Laxatives and lubricants should be used intermittently because large daily doses may interfere with normal digestion and nutrient absorption. Several complete and balanced moderate-fiber foods are now available for control of hairball problems in cats.

Feeding Cats in Gestation and Lactation

There are significant differences in food intake between the bitch and the queen during the initial stages of lactation (Figure 14-9). The queen apparently will forgo postpartum hunting to attend her kittens. As a solitary hunter, she hunts less and uses the body fat stored during gestation to support her lactation. The practical significance is that clients may question low food consumption in their new mother cat. Such clients are advised that the queen will eat heavily, as expected, by the third week of lactation.

Feline Lower Urinary Tract Disease

Domestic cats are thought to have evolved from desert-adapted ancestors. Urine specific gravity greater than 1.070 indicates excellent ability to concentrate dissolved urinary solutes as a water conservation mechanism. High solute concentration may favor formation of urinary crystals (crystalluria). Specific minerals dissolve into solution or precipitate as solids at specific urine pH levels. Controlling urine pH and other nutritional risk factors to reduce crystalluria requires a knowledge of the crystal to be inhibited. This is because struvite and oxalate, the two most common stones, form most readily in alkaline and acidic urine, respectively. Maintaining a physiologic urine acidity (pH 6.2 to 6.4) and keeping magnesium intake at nonexcessive levels are prudent risk control measures for struvite crystalluria. Maintaining a more alkaline urine pH (6.4 to 6.8) while avoiding excess calcium, sodium, and magnesium is a prudent risk control measure for calcium oxalate crystalluria.

It is an oversimplification to state that controlling urine mineral concentrations or pH always controls feline lower urinary tract disease (FLUTD). This is because the FLUTD syndrome is multifactorial and not all causative agents or combinations of contributory factors are presently known. The term *idiopathic FLUTD* is used for cats with naturally occurring lower urinary tract disease for which a specific cause (e.g., bladder stones) is not identified after

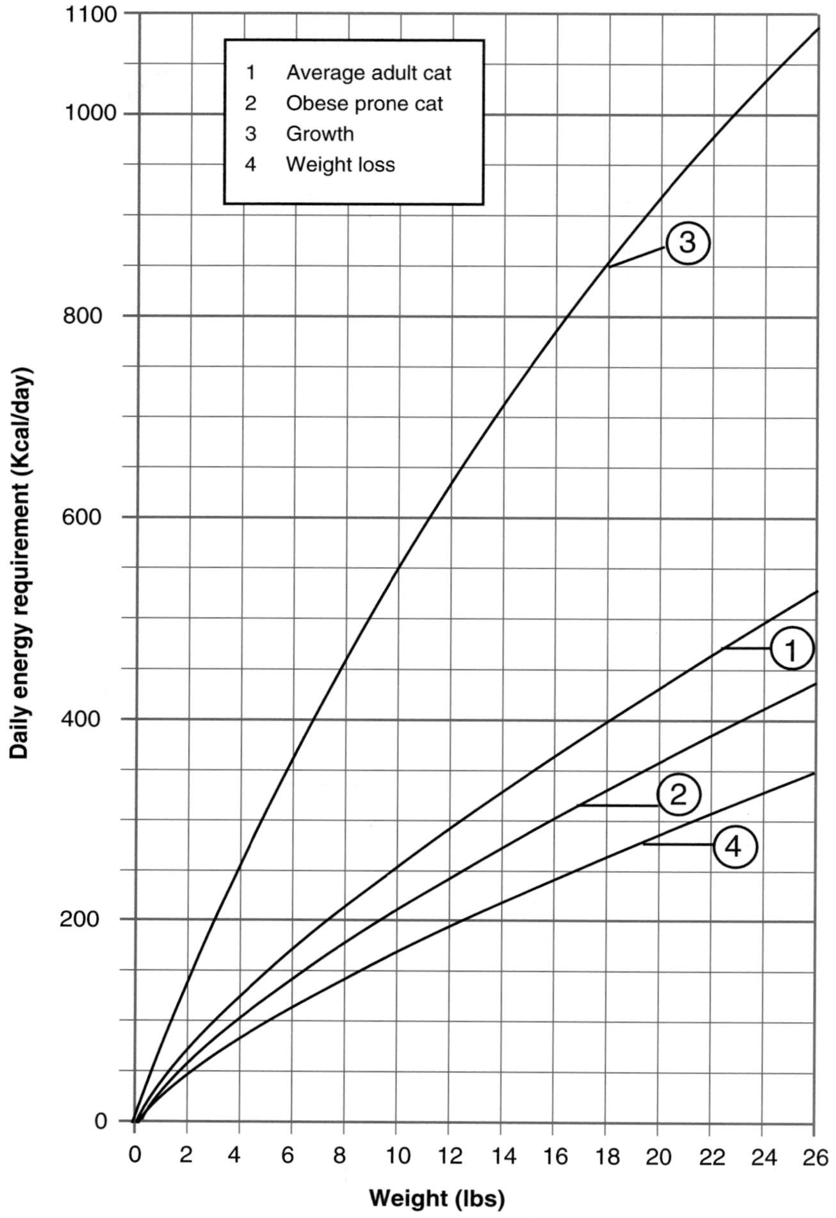

FIGURE 14-10. Feline daily energy requirements.

Legend within figure:

1   Average adult cat
2   Obese prone cat
3   Growth
4   Weight loss

Y-axis: Daily energy requirement (Kcal/day)
X-axis: Weight (lbs)

Figures calculated based on RER and life stage factor.

$RER = 70 \times (\text{Wt [kg]})^{0.75}$

Daily energy requirement (Kcal/day) = RER × life stage factor

	Life stage factor
Average adult neutered cat	1.2
Geriatric cat	1.1
Obese prone	1.0
Weight loss	0.8
Early gestation	1.6
Late gestation	2.0
Lactation	Ad lib
Growth	2.5

appropriate evaluation. Potential causes of idiopathic FLUTD include viral infection, stress, and neurogenic inflammation. Idiopathic FLUTD is not well understood; however, water seems to be a key factor in controlling the recurrence of the disease. Canned and other high-moisture foods increase total urine volume and are the preferred products for cats with idiopathic FLUTD.

Technician Note
The FLUTD syndrome is multifactorial, and not all causative agents or combinations of contributory factors are presently known.

PET FOOD ASSESSMENT

Many clients ask for recommendations about food form, specific brand information, and differences among brands. Some owners will inquire about the suitability of home cooking, feeding from the table, and using high percentages of table foods. Although various homemade foods can be suitable for maintenance, most practices recommend commercial pet foods. The nutrient content, safety, and overall quality of commercial foods are good.

Complete and balanced pet food is fundamental to suitability and quality, whether homemade or commercially prepared. A *complete* food contains all nutrients in a bioavailable form. *Balanced* means that nutrient concentrations are proportioned to total energy density. In combining these two definitions, the animal fulfills all nutrient requirements when consuming its energy requirement if it consumes a complete and balanced food. If nonenergy nutrient requirements can be met in this fashion, feeding becomes as easy as calculating energy requirements. However, balance is a relative term, and two foods can be stated to be balanced with very different nutrient profiles. This situation occurs because official guidelines for energy requirements are published as ranges or a minimum number. Therefore any nutrient value within the range or above the minimum can be said to be balanced.

A second general assessment is whether a pet food is specific purpose or all purpose. Formulations noting different nutritional requirements for growth, maintenance, reproduction, hard physical exertion, and the senior life stage are specific-purpose foods, and the nutrient profile can be more sharply focused to the specific need. All-purpose products, by definition, accommodate all physiologic situations. Because all-purpose foods support growth and lactation, they can be fed to all animals with no one needing to explain their proper use. Thus all-purpose foods are commonly sold in mass market settings and include generic, private label, and grocery brands. This includes many pet foods perceived as specific for adult maintenance because there is no reference to puppy or kitten on the label.

Dry Matter Nutrient Content and Forms of Pet Food

Nutrient concentration is expressed *as is (as fed)* or on a *dry matter* basis. Using dry matter removes the confusing effects of differing moisture levels (Figures 14-11 to 14-14). The veterinary technician most frequently needs to convert an as-fed (with moisture) basis to a dry-matter basis (moisture removed). The illustrations calculate protein on a dry-matter basis for a canned and dry pet food. Manufacturers or their technical information (e.g., published product literature) can be consulted for dry matter nutrient levels.

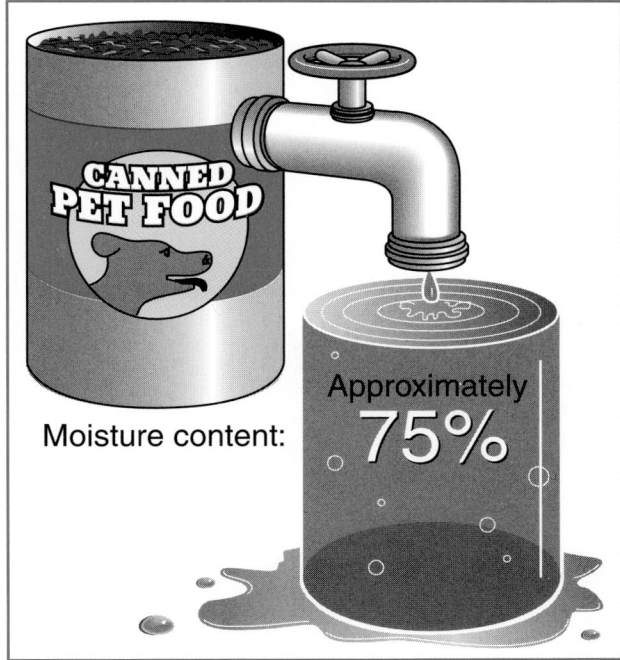

FIGURE 14-11.   Moisture content in canned pet food.

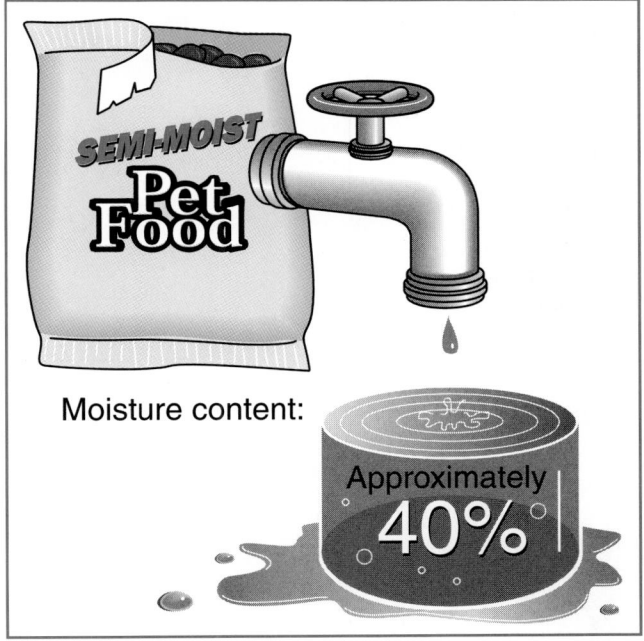

FIGURE 14-12.   Moisture content in semimoist pet food.

Differing moisture content characterizes four different pet food forms. New owners are often interested in pet food form when making food selection for a new pet.

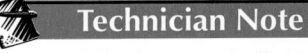
Technician Note
Canned foods are typically 70% to 83% water.

DRY
Pet Food
Moisture content:
Approximately
10%

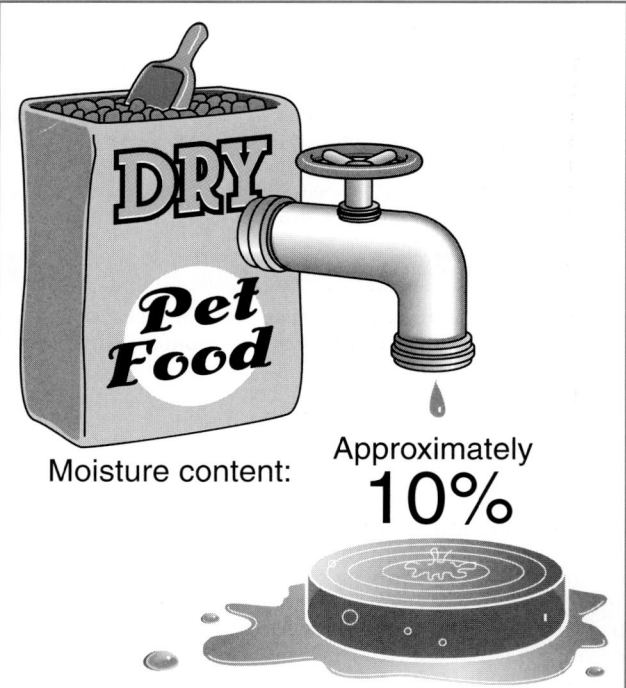

Figure 14-13. Moisture content in dry pet food.

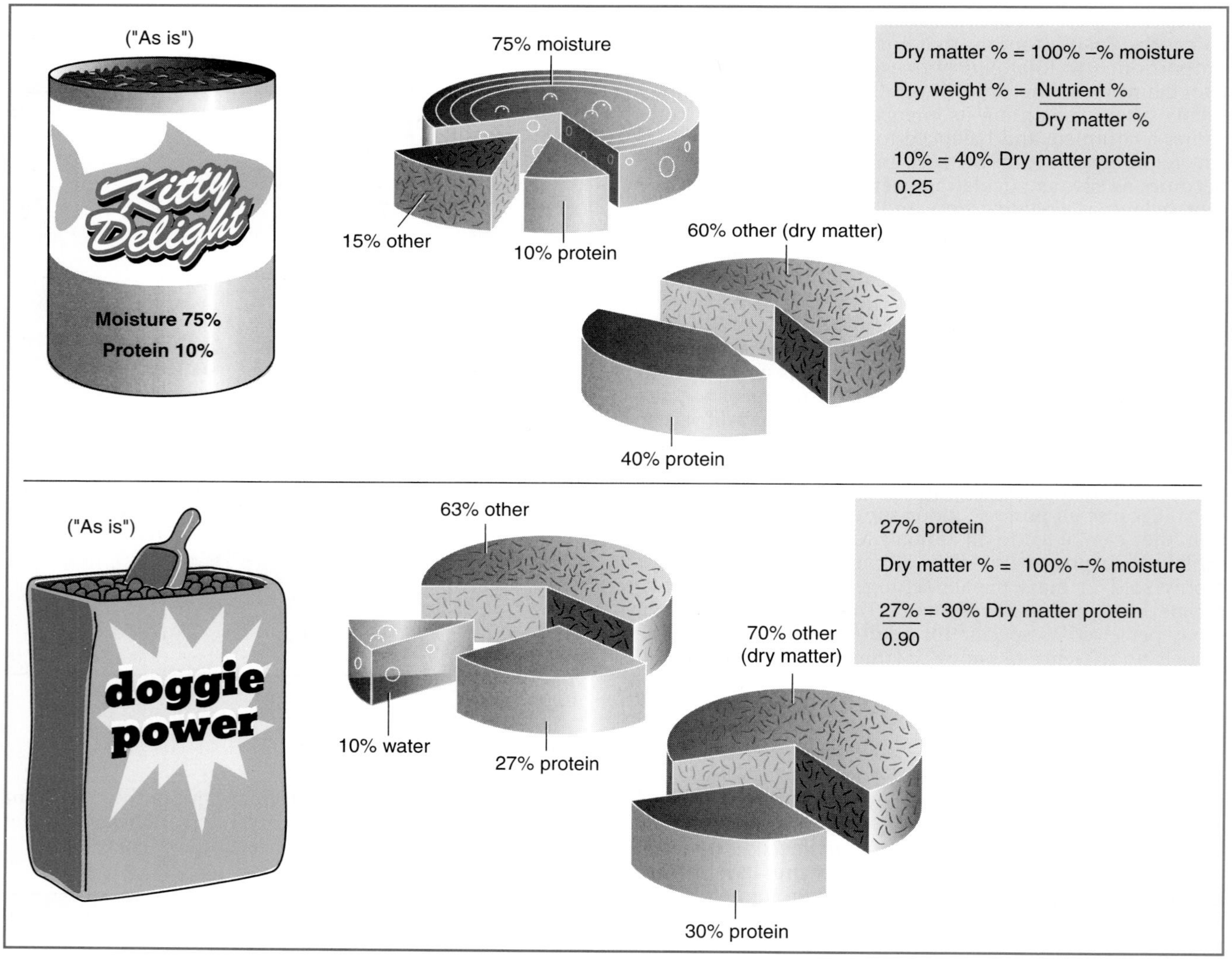

("As is")
Kitty Delight
Moisture 75%
Protein 10%
75% moisture
15% other
10% protein
60% other (dry matter)
40% protein
Dry matter % = 100% –% moisture
Dry weight % = Nutrient % / Dry matter %
10% / 0.25 = 40% Dry matter protein
("As is")
doggie power
63% other
10% water
27% protein
70% other (dry matter)
30% protein
27% protein
Dry matter % = 100% –% moisture
27% / 0.90 = 30% Dry matter protein

Figure 14-14. Dry matter analysis.

Canned foods are typically 70% to 83% water and have three forms: a ration loaf, an all-meat appearance, and processed meats and flours bound into a jellied matrix by gums or alginates. The high palatability of canned foods results from a high content of water, protein, fat, and the inherent flavor of animal source tissues. Moist foods are expensive on a per-calorie basis, because fresh and frozen meat and byproduct ingredients are more costly than equivalent meals and flours. In addition, the can's total dry matter (where the nutrients are) is diluted with water and the package is costly. These features have major implications for the overall cost of feeding over time.

Questions arise regarding the use of moist foods as a combination mixer with dry foods. This is an acceptable practice and the compromise some owners seek in the tradeoff between higher palatability at lower cost. As the ratio of moist food increases in a mix, the palatability and percentage of fat and protein calories usually increase as well. Finally, some owners use "gourmet" pet food as desserts or treats.

Technician Note

Dry pet foods typically have a moisture content of 6% to 12%.

Dry pet foods typically have a moisture content of 6% to 12%. In making dry pet food, dry ingredients are mixed and moistened into a dough. The dough is kneaded, cooked, and extruded into an air-expanded particle. These steps are equivalent to the baking of bread. Although dry pet foods have less average palatability than the moist

---

Box 14-6	COST OF FEEDING

The cost of feeding on a per-day basis is a better measure of value than the unit cost of the can or package.

Pet owners usually compare the cost of pet foods on the price per unit (e.g., price per bag or price per can) rather than the true cost of feeding (cost per day or cost per year). It is easy to compare the price per unit when evaluating two different pet foods, but more difficult to compare the true cost of feeding. The following example demonstrates that veterinarians and their health care team members need to discuss the true cost of feeding with pet owners when clients are concerned about the price of a particular food.

MOIST CAT FOOD

A 4.5-kg, three-year-old neutered male cat is diagnosed with lower urinary tract disease due to struvite urolithiasis. A moist veterinary therapeutic food (Food A) is recommended to help prevent further episodes of struvite urolithiasis. The cat's owner is concerned about the "high cost" of the veterinary therapeutic food, but would be willing to use Food A if it costs the same as what she now feeds her cat (Food B, a gourmet grocery brand). This calculation shows that the veterinary therapeutic food costs markedly less to feed than the cat's current food.

	FOOD A	FOOD B
Cost/can	$1.46	$0.50
Size of container	425 g	100 g
Cost/gram	$0.003	$0.005
Feeding amount (300 kcal/1,255 kJ)	214 g	350 g
Cost/day	$0.74	$1.75
Cost/year	$270	$639

---

forms, they have the advantage of lowest *true cost* compared with moist foods (Box 14-6). There are also significant differences between the true costs of feeding dry foods and the impression that foods that are "expensive" on a cost-per-pound basis may actually be more economical. Dry pet foods are the predominant source of calories in North America because of convenience and cost and are the only form suitable for ad-lib feeding.

Neither dry foods nor hard baked treats replace regular dental prophylaxis. Further, clean teeth are found in dogs eating moist food and calculus-encrusted teeth occur in dogs eating dry food.

Water may be added to improve the acceptability/palatability of a dry pet food. The addition of water is the objective in dry pet foods that feature a self-originating "gravy." If more palatability is required for a dry food, use a moist food or canned palatability enhancement mixer.

Certain bacteria (e.g., *Bacillus cereus*) are found in soil, grains, cereal products, and other foods. These bacteria may be found in small numbers in dry pet foods and are normally of no health significance. However, they can rapidly increase in numbers when moisture levels are raised (e.g., adding water or moist foods to dry pet food) at room temperature. These bacteria can produce a potent toxin that causes vomiting and diarrhea. Therefore pet owners should be warned not to add water to dry pet foods and leave them exposed to high ambient temperatures for prolonged periods. Dry pet foods with added water or mixed with moist foods are usually safe if consumed within a few hours.

Technician Note

Pet owners should be warned not to add water to dry pet foods and leave them exposed to high ambient temperatures for prolonged periods. Dry pet foods with added water or mixed with moist foods are usually safe if consumed within a few hours.

Technician Note

Semimoist foods typically have a 25% to 35% water content.

Semimoist foods typically have a 25% to 35% water content. This pet food form had considerable popularity in the 1970s but has declined in recent years. An intermediate moisture level and sweetness produce palatability between that found in canned and dry forms. Humectant preservatives and cellophane wrapping allow reasonable shelf life. Antimicrobial additives help prevent spoilage or bacterial proliferation. Semimoist foods have readily available soluble sugars and simple carbohydrate sources and are not recommended in diabetic animals or other animals in which blood sugar control needs to be regulated.

When the dry and semimoist forms are mixed, a hybrid form of "soft dry" results. The advantages of the dry food are enhanced by the extended palatability from the semimoist fraction.

Homemade Foods

Feeding commercially prepared pet foods offers several advantages over feeding homemade foods, including convenience, cost, and consistency. Most commercial foods are easier to use, are less expensive, and provide better nutritional balance. Nevertheless, many owners prefer to prepare homemade foods. In doing so, they feel less guilty and have the impression of preparing a "real meal" that is more natural and traditional.

It is possible to achieve the same nutrient balance with a homemade food as with a commercially prepared food. However, this largely depends on the accuracy and competence of the veterinarian or animal nutritionist formulating the food and on the compliance and discipline of the owner. Most homemade recipes have been crudely balanced using the average nutrient content of specific foods and computer formulation. Unlike commercial foods, few of the numerous published homemade recipes for dogs and cats have been tested to document performance over sustained periods, including tests for palatability, digestibility, and safety. Therefore veterinarians and veterinary technicians should encourage regular dietary histories and patient monitoring for pets fed homemade foods.

Veterinary technicians should be willing to assess an existing homemade food recipe, offer nutritionally adequate recipes, or make appropriate formula substitutions for clients. Homemade formulations can be checked for nutritional adequacy and adjusted using the following "quick check" guidelines:

1. *Do five food groups appear in the recipe?*
   a. A carbohydrate/fiber source from a cooked cereal grain or potato
   b. A protein source, preferable of animal origin, or, if more than one protein source is used, one source should be of animal origin
   c. A fat source
   d. A source of minerals, particularly calcium
   e. A multivitamin and trace mineral source
2. *Is the carbohydrate source a cooked cereal or potato and present in a higher or equal quantity than the meat source?* The carbohydrate/protein ratio should be approximately 1:1 for cat foods and 2:1 to 3:1 for dog foods.
3. *What is the type and quantity of the primary protein source?* The overall protein quality in a homemade food can generally be improved by using an animal-source protein. Skeletal muscle protein from different animal species has very similar amino acid profiles. Thus there is no great advantage to feeding one meat source over another.
4. *Is the primary protein source lean or fatty?* The fat content of different cuts of meat varies. When the specified protein source is lean, an additional animal or vegetable fat source should compose 2% to 5% of the formula.
5. *Is a source of calcium and other minerals provided?* A homemade food is almost never spontaneously balanced in minerals; most homemade foods require a specific calcium supplement.
6. *Is a source of vitamins and other nutrients provided?* Supplements providing vitamins, microminerals, fatty acids, taurine, and other specific nutrients of concern for cats and dogs should be used in homemade recipes.

Patients that eat homemade foods should be brought in for regular veterinary examinations and nutritional reviews (at least two visits per year). The technician should ask the client to record and submit a 3- to 5-day food history as part of the evaluation.

Digestibility and Stool Quality

Digestibility is an important but often misunderstood concept. Feeding a food with higher digestibility may allow animals to consume less of this food to meet their energy

---

Box 14-7	FOOD DIGESTIBILITY

$$\frac{\text{Nutrient food} - \text{Nutrient feces}}{\text{Nutrient food}} \times 100\% = \text{\% Nutrient digestibility}$$

needs. Highly digestible foods may be more economic to feed than a less expensive food with lower digestibility. Digestibility of a food is determined by a mathematical equation comparing the amount of a nutrient in the food and the amount of the same nutrient in the feces (Box 14-7). Above-average digestibility can be defined as protein, fat, carbohydrate, and energy digestibility more than or equal to 85%, 90%, 90%, and 85%, respectively. Foods higher in fiber will be lower in digestibility.

Many owners are interested in the volume and firmness of feces their pet excretes. Cat owners will be concerned with odor, and dog owners will be concerned with ease of clean up. The quantity and texture characteristics of feces relate to the amount of dry matter eaten and its digestibility (Figure 14-15).

Palatability (Box 14-8) is also an important factor in pet foods.

Market Categories

Understanding market objectives for a product may assist with some aspects of pet food quality assessment. Generic (white label) and private label (a grocery chain's own brand) foods are made at contract feed mills using least-cost formulation methods. Market emphasis is low cost. Nationally advertised and distributed (popular) brands predominate in grocery stores and mass merchandise outlets. These foods are also least-cost formulated and are marketed for their high palatability and anthropomorphic appeal. Flavor, shape, color, ingredient, and brand name proliferation characterize these products, allowing them to engage the largest amount of shelf space.

Specialty brand pet foods are often sold in veterinary hospitals and pet superstores and regular stores. Fixed, specific formulations and high-quality ingredients characterize this category. Although differences in nutritional philosophy may be noted among different manufacturers, these brands are consistent in the overall objective of emphasizing a philosophy of optimum nutrition.

Dog and Cat Treats and Supplements

Giving treats is an enjoyable aspect of the human-companion animal bond. Treats include almost anything in the owner's kitchen from the healthy items to items high in salt and calories (see Tables 14-5 and 14-6). Because treats may be a substantial source of calories and protein, it is important to inquire about treat intake if a patient's disease requires regulation of dietary intake. Diabetes mellitus, urolithiasis, obesity, cardiac failure, and renal failure are a few clinical examples.

Supplements and treats are not interchangeable terms, concepts, or products. A supplement adds something to improve a nutrient profile or to treat deficiency. When used to correct a diagnosed deficiency, supplements have a therapeutic role. More commonly, however, they affect the balance of an otherwise adequate food intake or create an unnecessary excess. When foods are of poor quality, the use of supplements probably will not correct the fundamental reasons for quality deficits. Nutritionally and economically, the prudent choice is to use a higher-quality food and skip attempts to supplement a poor product into adequacy.

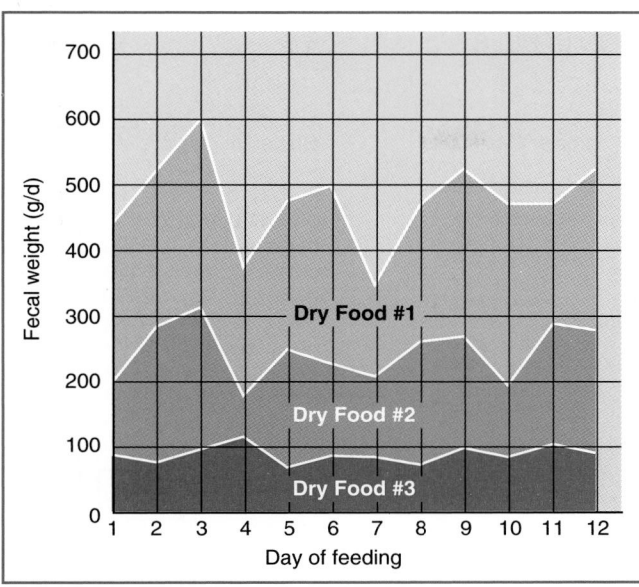

FIGURE 14-15. Increased digestibility and caloric density have an inverse relationship to fecal volume. Food 1 was a lower-energy food and produced voluminous stool volume with difficult cleanup characteristics. Food 3 featured high digestibility and was energy dense, and stool cleanup was quick and nonmessy.

Box 14-8	PALATABILITY FACTORS

Moisture
Odor
Fat/protein levels
Temperature
Texture
Cats: Shape (dry food)
   Acidity

Reading Pet Food Labels in the United States

Label information and ingredient description are controlled in the United States by the Association of American Feed Control Officials (AAFCO). Pet food labels must contain the net weight; product designator (e.g., cat food); maker or distributor; a list of guaranteed analyses for crude protein, fat, fiber, and moisture; a list of ingredients; a nutritional adequacy statement; and feeding instructions if the food is complete and balanced (Figure 14-16). Many labels contain much more information, such as calorie content and product attributes.

There is considerable information regarding food quality and a few potential pitfalls requiring awareness when reading labels. The first is that guaranteed analysis states only maximal and minimal levels. Because feed labels are a legal contract between manufacturer and consumer, the guaranteed nutrient levels are conservative and may be far different from the actual analysis. Instead of using the numbers from guaranteed analysis, one can find a better source of data on nutrient content in the typical or average analysis supplied by a manufacturer. Further, the ingredient list descends by weight since the ingredients were added on an as-is basis. This often means water-containing ingredients are listed high in the ingredient ordering when a dry ingredient actually predominates on a dry-matter basis.

Nutritional Adequacy Statement

The nutritional adequacy statement may be as simple as *totally nutritious* or *complete and balanced,* or the statement may be more elaborate. The technician should interpret the method used to determine the nutritional adequacy statement. The statement "formulated to meet the AAFCO dog food nutrient profile" (or similar wording) indicates only a laboratory analysis for a minimal chemical content. Such testing is not an animal feeding performance trial and says nothing about adequacy, bioavailability, or excesses.

The AAFCO Animal Feeding Test statement (see Figure 14-16), however, indicates that a representative product was used in animal feeding tests and performed at a defined level. Thus the consumer knows that living animals have been test fed, and the technician should recommend products with the "feeding test" claim rather than the "formulated" statement when there is a choice. A nutritional adequacy statement is not needed on treats or snacks intended for intermittent feeding.

The Percentage Rules

The designator and modifying wording on pet food labels contain considerable information regarding content of the named ingredient in a product. According to AAFCO rules, when a label statement identifies only one ingredient, at least 70% of the total product will consist of that named ingredient (e.g., beef). When modifying words accompany the named ingredient, the amount of the named ingredient that must be present declines to 10% for moist foods and 25% for dry foods (chicken *dinner,* fish *entree,* liver *stew,* etc.). When a named ingredient is modified by the word *with* (e.g., with beef), the total portion of the named ingredient declines to 3%. When the term *flavor* is used (e.g., cheese flavor), the named flavor must be detectable only by the animal. The designator *food* (e.g., dog food) means that there are no rules regarding minimal content of ingredients. Indirectly, the technician may gather further quality information about a product through understanding these nuances of pet food labeling.

Technician's Role

The technician is in a position to assess pet food and livestock food quality by far better means than reading even the most informative of labels. That method is the direct assessment of an animal's performance. Feeding performance in daily use defines the real gold standard of quality assessment.

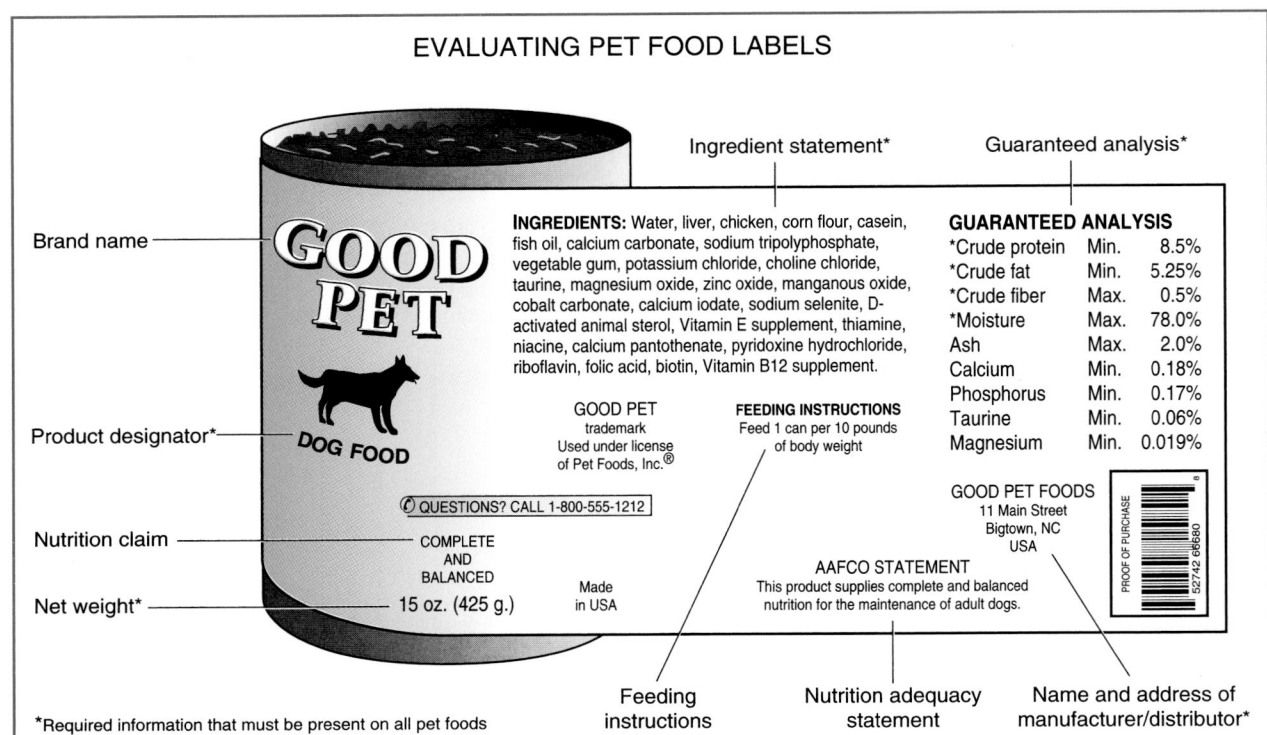

FIGURE 14-16.　A pet food label is the contract between the manufacturer and the consumer. Labels provide information required by law and may have optional information, such as feeding directions.

Feeding Costs for Dog and Cat Foods

There are substantial variations in actual daily feeding costs (see Box 14-6). When cost comparisons are calculated, a pet food perceived as expensive may actually be cheaper on the per-calorie and actual feeding cost basis. Unfortunately, unit price comparison rather than feeding cost information influences the purchasing decision.

CLINICAL NUTRITION

Thy food is thy remedy.

Hippocrates

Clinical nutrition is a veterinary medical subspecialty with the objective of modifying the cause, progression, or end-stage effects of illness by applying specific nutrient profiles. The application of prophylactic or therapeutic dietary management is the expression of this objective. Purpose-specific dietary management has a long history of efficacy, but the use of altered nutrient profiles should be justified by professional diagnosis, judgment, and monitoring.

Technician Note

When cost comparisons are calculated, a pet food perceived as expensive may actually be cheaper on a per-calorie and actual feeding cost basis.

Numerous nutrient profiles support various prophylactic and therapeutic applications in small animal patients. Examples are as follows: high protein/low carbohydrate;

high protein/fat/micronutrient; low protein/high nonprotein calorie; low fiber/high digestibility; fiber enhanced; low sodium; very low sodium; low mineral; low fat/high fiber/low calorie; low copper; and restricted/novel protein sources. Specific effects on urine pH and restriction of urinary solutes such as magnesium are attained from specific formulations. Nutrient control objectives are fulfilled with either hospital-formulated/owner-cooked feedings or commercially prepared formulas. Table 14-7 summarizes objectives and nutrient profiles for selected applications. Table 14-8 is a diary for use in taking food intake histories at home for animals with suspected food allergy or intolerance.

Feeding Hospitalized Small Animal Patients

Malnutrition is a major clinical problem for patients unable or unwilling to eat. To complicate the food deficit, hypermetabolic energy requirements often follow significant illness or injury. A state of accelerated starvation and lean tissue catabolism follows protein-calorie malnutrition. Decreased immune function, delayed wound healing (rate and strength), loss of muscle and visceral mass, delayed general recovery, and increased mortality all result from protein calorie malnutrition (Box 14-9). The veterinary technician is critical in daily cage-side nutritional management. A "wait until ready to eat" passivity is not beneficial, and no patient has yet been starved into wellness. Even when the patient is overweight, an acute hospitalization is not the setting for weight reduction.

Technician Note

The veterinary technician is a critical individual in daily cage-side nutritional management.

Text continued on p. 357

TABLE 14-7   SUMMARY OF SMALL ANIMAL CLINICAL NUTRITION*

Disease	Objectives	Considerations	Product†	Comments
Allergy, food				
Dog	Reduce antigen ingestion	Novel highly digestible protein source or protein hydrolysate Reduce total protein content Simplify food Distilled H_2O	Prescription Diet Canine d/d or Canine z/d	8 to 10-wk trial period Avoid treats, snacks, access to other food sources, chewable medications, supplements
Cat		Same as dog except Control Mg^{2+} intake Provide taurine Control urine pH	Prescription Diet Feline d/d or Feline z/d	
Anemia	Support RBC production	↑ Iron, cobalt, and copper ↑ B complex vitamins ↑ Protein	Prescription Diet Canine p/d Feline p/d	Cat foods are suitable for dogs in acute care settings
Anorexia	Prevent protein/caloric malnutrition Stimulate appetite	Establish fluid/electrolyte balance Acid-base balance ↑ Protein and fat ↑ Micronutrients	Prescription Diet Feline/Canine a/d Canine p/d Feline p/d	
Ascites	Reduce fluid retention	Restrict sodium chloride	Prescription Diet Canine h/d, k/d Feline h/d, k/d	h/d = marked salt restriction k/d = moderate salt restriction
Bone loss and fracture healing	Correct deficiency of energy and protein	↑ Protein ↑ Energy Avoid supplementation	Prescription Diet Canine p/d Feline p/d	Extra dietary calcium does not increase rate of fracture healing
Cancer	Increase longevity and quality of life	↓ Soluble carbohydrate ↑ Fat and n-3 fatty acids ↑ Arginine	Prescription Diet Canine n/d Canine/Feline a/d	Use in conjunction with chemotherapy or other forms of cancer therapy
Colitis	Normalize gastrointestinal motility Rebalance microflora Provide local healing factors	Feed small meals 3-6 times/day Control dietary antigens Vary levels of dietary fiber	Prescription Diet Canine w/d, i/d, d/d Feline w/d, d/d	
Constipation	Normalize gastrointestinal motility Maintain stool water Maintain stool bulk	>10% fiber	Prescription Diet Canine w/d Feline w/d	No table scraps or bones Increase exercise Encourage water intake Cats: keep litter box clean
Copper storage disease	Restrict copper intake	<1.2 mg copper/100 g dry diet	Prescription Diet Canine l/d	No table scraps or treats
Debilitation	Restore tissue, plasma, and nutrients	↑ Protein ↑ Fat ↑ Macronutrients and micronutrients	Prescription Diet Canine/Feline a/d	Assist feed if needed
Developmental orthopedic disease	Reduce rapid growth	↓ Fat and energy density ↓ Calcium	Prescription Diet Canine p/d Large Breed	Avoid calcium-phosphorus supplements
Diabetes mellitus	Even rate of glucose absorption Consistent caloric intake	>10% fiber ↓ Soluble carbohydrates	Prescription Diet Canine w/d Feline w/d	Weigh animal frequently and note in medical record

Mg, Magnesium; *RBC,* red blood cell.

*Nutrients in table are expressed on a dry weight basis.

†Other North American therapeutic brands with wide distribution include CNM (Purina), VMD, Medi-Cal, and IVD Select Care (Heinz), Eukanuba Veterinary Diets (Iams), and Waltham Veterinary Diets (Mars).

Continued

TABLE 14-7 SUMMARY OF SMALL ANIMAL CLINICAL NUTRITION—CONT'D

Disease	Objectives	Considerations	Product	Comments
Diarrhea, acute	Normalize gastrointestinal tract motility and secretion	Withhold food for 1-2 days Feed small amounts 3-6 times/day ↓ Fiber ↓ Sugar ↑ Digestibility	Prescription Diet Canine i/d Feline i/d	Electrolyte disturbances and dehydration are common
Eclampsia	Provide Ca/P in correct quantity and ratio prepartum	High digestibility of diet Balanced minerals/vitamins	Prescription Diet Canine p/d Feline p/d	Avoid supplementation
Flatulence	Decrease aerophagia Avoid food fermentation	Avoid milk or milk products Feed small meals 3-6 times/day ↑ Caloric density	Prescription Diet Canine i/d Feline i/d	Feed in a flat, open dish Avoid vitamin or fatty acid supplementation Separate competitive eaters
Gastric dilatation/bloat (postoperative)	Prevent gastric distension	Avoid exercise before and after feeding ↑ Digestibility of diet Small frequent feedings	Prescription Diet Canine i/d	Diet form or type is *NOT* related to risk of occurrence or recurrence
Heart failure Dogs	Control Na$^+$ retention	↓ Na$^+$ intake Maintain energy and protein intake ↑ B complex vitamins	Prescription Diet Canine h/d Canine k/d	Prescription Diet k/d has moderate Na$^+$ restriction
Cats		↓ Na$^+$ intake ↑ Taurine Control Mg^{2+} levels	Prescription Diet Feline h/d Feline k/d	Avoid high Na$^+$ treats and water (see Table 14-5)
Hyperlipidemia	Control fat intake	↑ Fiber intake ↓ Fat intake	Prescription Diet Canine w/d Feline w/d	Common in schnauzers Consider fat in treats, table foods, and supplements
Hyperthyroidism (cats)	Support increased energy need	↑ Energy intake ↑ Vitamins and minerals ↑ Protein	Prescription Diet Feline a/d	Monitor for evidence of concurrent renal disease
Liver disease (fat tolerant)	Reduce protein metabolism Maintain liver glycogen Prevent ammonia toxicity	↑ Digestible energy Protein restriction High biologic value proteins Control Na$^+$ intake	Prescription Diet Canine l/d Feline l/d	May feed small meals (4-6 times/day)
Lymphangiectasia	Decrease dietary fat	↓ Intake of long-chain triglycerides Control protein levels Consider medium-chain triglycerides	Prescription Diet Canine w/d or r/d	Medium-chain triglyceride oils and powder can increase caloric density
Obesity	Maintain intake of all nutrients except energy	↓ Energy digestibility Replace digestible calories with indigestible bulk Increase bulk to control hunger Added carnitine	Prescription Diet Canine r/d Feline r/d	Requires professional advice and teamwork with veterinary technician and client

Condition	Goal	Nutritional factors	Product	Comments
Oral disease: gingivitis (gum inflammation), periodontitis (loss of tooth attachment)	Control accumulation of plaque, stains, and calculus; Maintain gingival health	Food that promotes chewing and mechanical cleansing of teeth	Prescription Diet Canine t/d, Feline t/d	Many treats make dental claims but are not effective
Pancreatitis, acute (recovery phase)	Control pancreas secretions	↓Fat; ↑Digestibility; Feed small meals 3-6 times/day	Prescription Diet Canine i/d, Feline i/d	Frequent, small meals
Pancreatic exocrine insufficiency	Reduce requirements for digestive enzymes	↓Fiber; ↓Fat; Highly digestible carbohydrates; ↑Caloric density	Prescription Diet Canine i/d, Feline i/d	Pancreatic enzymes complement highly digestible food
Renal failure	Reduce signs of uremia; Slow progression of disease	↓Protein (↑biologic value of protein); ↑Nonprotein calories; ↓Phosphorus and sodium; Increase B complex vitamins	Prescription Diet Canine k/d, Canine g/d, Canine u/d, Feline k/d, Feline g/d	Small meals 4-6 times/day; Conversion to a protein-restricted diet may take 7-10 days; Water available at all times
Canine urolithiasis (struvite): Treatment	↑Urine volume; ↓Urine pH; Restrict Mg^{2+}, NH_4^+, PO_4	↓Protein; ↓PO_4, Mg^{2+}; ↓Na^+; ↓Urine pH (5.9-6.1)	Prescription Diet Canine s/d	Evaluate and treat urinary tract infection; Average duration of stone dissolution is 36 days; follow-up via radiography
Prevention	Maintain physiologic level of urinary solutes and urine pH	Control protein excess; ↓Ca^{2+}, P, Ma^{2+}; ↓Sodium mildly; ↓Urine pH (6.2-6.4)	Prescription Diet Canine c/d	Monitor urine sediment for crystalluria and infection
Canine urolithiasis (ammonium urate): Prevention		↓Protein; ↑Nonprotein calories; ↓Nucleic acids; ↓Ca^{2+}, P, Mg^{2+}, Na^+; ↑Urine pH (6.7-7.0)	Prescription Diet Canine u/d	Drugs plus diet may be successful treatment; Monitor urinary crystalluria; Prevention may require long-term drug treatment
Canine urolithiasis (calcium oxalate and cystine): Prevention	↓Urinary concentration of calcium oxalate or cystine	↓Protein; ↑Nonprotein calories; ↓Ca^{2+}, P, Na^+, Mg^{2+}; ↑Urine pH (6.1-7.0)	Prescription Diet Canine u/d	Treatment by surgical removal; Prevention by dietary management ± drugs

Na, sodium; *P,* phosphorus; *Ca,* calcium.

Continued

TABLE 14-7 SUMMARY OF SMALL ANIMAL CLINICAL NUTRITION—CONT'D

Disease	Objectives	Considerations	Product	Comments
Feline urolithiasis (struvite): Treatment	↑ Urine volume ↓ Urine pH (5.9-6.1) Restrict Mg^{2+}, Ca^{2+}, PO_4	↑ Caloric density ↓ P and Ca^{2+} Mg^{2+} >20 mg/100 Kcal ↑ Na^+ Urine pH (6.2-6.4)	Prescription Diet Feline s/d	Dissolution is complete 1 mo after negative radiographs Recurrence is high if prevention is not implemented
Prevention	Maintain physiologic levels of urinary solutes and urine pH	Mg^{2+} >20 mg/100 Kcal (0.1% DMB) ↓ P ↑ Caloric density Urine pH (6.2-6.4)	Prescription Diet Feline c/d-s	In obesity, use calorie-restricted diets that maintain urine pH 6.2-6.4 (Prescription Diet w/d is suggested)
Feline urolithiasis (calcium oxalate): Prevention	↑ Urine volume ↓ Urinary Ca^{2+}, oxalate ↑ Urine pH	↓ Protein ↑ Nonprotein calories ↓ P, Ca^{2+}, Na^+ Mg^{2+} <20 mg/100 Kcal	Prescription Diet Feline c/d-oxl	Monitor urinary crystalluria
Vomiting	Minimize gastric secretion Gastrointestinal rest	↑ Digestibility ↑ Caloric density	Prescription Diet Canine i/d Feline i/d	Frequent, small meals

Ca, Calcium; *DMB*, dry matter basis; *Mg*, magnesium; *Na*, sodium; NH_4, ammonium; *P*, phosphorus; *PO*, phosphate; *RBC*, red blood cells.

TABLE 14-8	DIARY FOR DIETARY ELIMINATION TRIAL						
Day	Date	Food Offered	Food Consumed	Other Items Ingested*	Clinical Signs (scale 0-5 and comments)†	Feces (scale 1-5 and comments)‡	Other Observations
1							
2							
3							
4							
5							
6							
7							
8							
9							
↑ (Continue 10 through 58) ↓							
59							
60							

*Other Items Ingested
List other ingested items, such as the following:
- Rawhide chews
- Chewable vitamin supplements
- Chewable medications
- Commercial treats or snacks
- Fatty acid supplements
- Table foods
- Fresh food
- Access to other food sources (e.g., dog eating cat food or cat eating an animal it has captured outdoors)

† Clinical Signs
- 0 = No clinical signs
- 5 = Severe clinical signs
  - Itching (scratching, rubbing face, chewing, licking, head shaking)
  - Hair loss
  - Skin lesions (scabs, scales, bleeding, red skin, pimples)

‡ Feces Assessment
1 = Liquid feces that have lost all form
2 = Soft feces with no form
3 = Soft feces that form a pile
4 = Mixture of soft and firm feces with a cylindrical shape
5 = Firm feces with a cylindric shape

Presence of mucus or fresh blood
Number of bowel movements per day

From Hand MS et al, editors: *Small animal clinical nutrition,* ed 4, Topeka, 2000, Mark Morris Institute.

Patient Selection for Assisted Feeding

The technician frequently uses *subjective global assessment* (SGA) to determine nutritional status. SGA considers the dietary history, the body's condition scoring system (see Figure 14-3), and the current morbidity index of the illness or injury. Body scoring is done by physical examination, with 0 = cachexia and 5 = obesity. Albumin, total protein, and other markers for malnutrition decline with energy deprivation and protein-calorie malnutrition. However, these objective indicators change too slowly to be functional prognosticators, and the use of SGA permits functional, early clinical recognition of nutrient depletion and negative nitrogen balance. The most important outlook for the hospital is an awareness of the critical "need to feed" and the need to do so early. These steps reduce catabolism and improve responses to virtually all other therapy.

Indications for nutritional support include recent weight loss of more than 10%, absent or poor food intake for more than 2 days, acute illness or injury, acute muscle wasting, and heavy gastrointestinal or urinary system losses of protein or electrolytes. The technician assesses daily needs and progress in conversation with the veterinarian and by the daily patient progress notes. The clinical signs, the patient's desire and ability to eat, and response to therapy can all rapidly change.

Enteral Versus Parenteral Feeding

Parenteral nutrition (PN) is an intravenous nutrition technique whose objective is complete bypass of the seriously impaired gastrointestinal tract. PN technique is the controlled infusion of special feeding fluids of concentrated dextrose, amino acids, special fat emulsions, and micronu-

Box 14-9	BENEFITS OF NUTRITIONAL SUPPORT IN THE DEBILITATED ANIMAL

PROTEIN
- Helps maintain lean body mass
- Provides amino acids to support metabolism
- Promotes wound healing
- Enhances immune function
- Provides a source of fuel for muscle

FATS
- Primary source of energy
- Provides essential fatty acids
- Modulates immune function
- Promotes wound healing

VITAMINS AND MINERALS
- Enhances cellular and humoral immunity
- Enhances the ability to taste and smell
- Provides antioxidants

trients. Maintaining enterocyte function is important to reduce PN complications of bowel atrophy and bacterial translocation across the intestine into the circulation (bacteremia). Even during PN, partial enteral intake supports the enterocyte cells of the small intestinal mucosa.

Enteral feeding is more physiologic, safer, and cheaper than parenteral nutrition. Therefore feeding by mouth or tube is used if the gastrointestinal tract can absorb nutrients. Contraindications to enteral nutritional feeding are the need for complete gastrointestinal secretory rest and a high risk of aspirating vomitus.

Methods of Assisted Enteral Feeding

Coax feeding, appetite stimulation with drugs, forced oral feeding, and various tube administration techniques are four separate enteral feeding methods. These techniques are reviewed in Table 14-9. The benefits of nutrient provision in the debilitated animal are presented in Box 14-9.

TABLE 14-9	OPTIONS IN ENTERAL FEEDING

Feeding Method	Objective	Technique	Advantage	Disadvantage
Owner hand feeding	Overcome partial anorexia	Hospital visit; bring favorite foods	Familiarity with food preferences should be explored	No effect in full anorexia
Temptation	Overcome partial anorexia	Use an unfamiliar food of high odor	New odor may stimulate food exploration	No effect in full anorexia
Force feeding pet foods	Overcome partial anorexia	Bolus of moist food; mouth held to force swallowing	Food is complete and balanced	High handling stress Probably limited calorie intake
Forced feeding (calorie pastes)	Overcome partial anorexia	Administer flavored pastes from tube	Moderate handling stress	Pastes not complete food Limited calorie intake Severe protein restriction
Assisted feeding	Achieve full caloric intake	Oral syringing of specific formula	User and patient friendly Moderate handling stress High calorie intake	Learned aversion if nauseous
	Overcome partial anorexia		Food given at rate for comfortable swallowing	
Orogastric	Achieve full calorie intake	Intubate esophagus/ stomach	Rapid administration No tube clogging Best for short-term use	High handling stress Intolerance to repeated feedings
Nasoesophageal	Bypass oral cavity and swallowing Achieve full caloric intake	Indwell 6-10 Fr. tube in nostril	Ease of intermediate use	Sedation/topical anesthesia Liquid food only
Pharyngostomy	Bypass oral cavity and swallowing Achieve full caloric intake	Indwell 16-28 Fr. tube in pharynx	None	General anesthesia required Mechanical interference with laryngeal function Possible gagging and vomiting Possible esophagitis

Continued

> ## Technician Note
>
> *Parenteral nutrition* (PN) is an intravenous nutrition technique whose objective is complete bypass of the seriously impaired gastrointestinal tract.

The technician must carefully monitor all assisted feeding methods for the stress associated with restraint and monitor all feeding tubes for mechanical blockage or kinking. This is a critical monitoring obligation for small-bore tubes. Water is flushed through the tube to clear debris after each feeding. Capping the tube prevents air from entering the catheterized viscus between uses. It is preferable for the same person to feed, since this may allow quicker notation of flow and resistance changes in the tube.

It is also important to monitor gastrointestinal tolerance during the refeeding of the animal. The objectives of repletion feeding may be at odds with the patient's best interests when serious vomiting and diarrhea follow feeding.

Steps in Enteral Alimentation Calculations and Food Selection (Figures 14-17 to 14-19)

1. Calculate resting energy requirement (RER) as follows:
   RER = 70 × Body weight (kg)$^{0.75}$
2. Most hospitalized veterinary patients have metabolic rates very near their RER. Therefore initially feeding patients at RER is a rational and safe recommendation. Regular nutritional assessment of the patient is strongly recommended to adjust initial feeding rates.
3. The proportion of fat, carbohydrate, and protein in foods fed to hospitalized patients should be similar to that which the liver is estimated to be using from body stores. By the fifth day of food deprivation or longer, patients should receive the majority (greater than 50%) of their calculated RER as fat. For dogs, use a food that provides protein of at least 4 to 6 g/100 Kcal; for cats, use a food that provides at least 6 to 8 g/100 Kcal.
4. Consider physical form and other nutritional characteristics before the final selection of feeding products. Note that oral calorie paste supplements are extremely deficient in protein and that meat baby foods are neither complete nor balanced. Five percent dextrose does not provide adequate calorie concentrations and is devoid of protein. Table 14-10 summarizes the nutrient profile of selected enteral products used in small animal patients.
5. Establish the food dose, administration rate, and feeding schedule. A conservative rate of patient refeeding is needed after prolonged anorexia or gastrointestinal disease. Controlling the size and frequency of the per-feeding dose by giving small frequent feedings can be a critical factor in improving patient tolerance. Calorie and volume intake at RER levels may require a 3-day transition period.

TABLE 14-9	OPTIONS IN ENTERAL FEEDING—CONT'D			
Feeding Method	**Objective**	**Technique**	**Advantage**	**Disadvantage**
Esophagostomy	Bypass oral cavity, pharynx, and swallowing. Achieve full caloric intake	12-18 Fr. tube in left lateral cervical esophagus	Easy to maintain and install. Easy to "eat around the tube". Minimal risk of esophageal stricture	General anesthesia required
Gastrostomy	Bypass proximal gastrointestinal tract for full or partial caloric intake	16-28 Fr. tube placement at laparotomy. Percutaneous endoscopic placement. Nonendoscopic placement	Well-tolerated long term. Effective and efficient	General anesthesia required. Gastrocutaneous fistula forms in 5 days. Wait 24 hr to use
Gastroduodenostomy	Bypass stomach	Duodenum cannulated via tube gastrostomy	Achieve full caloric intake	Loss of mechanical and chemical phases of gastric digestion. May require endoscopic equipment
Jejunostomy	Bypass stomach and duodenum	10 Fr. tube through submucosal tunnel. Anchor bowel and tube to body wall	Achieve full or partial caloric intake. Predigested foods required to maximize nutrient delivery and minimize digestive work	Water transfer to gut lumen may cause cramping and diarrhea

ENTERAL FEEDING WORKSHEET

1. Calculate resting energy requirement (RER)

   RER = (70) x (kg) $^{0.75}$

   70 X [Body weight (kg)] $^{0.75}$ = [RER (Kcal/day)]

2. Choose a veterinary-specific critical care formula

3. Calculate volume of diet required

   [Name of diet choosen]

   [RER (Kcal/day)] ÷ [Kcal/ml] = [ml formula/day]

4. Number and volume of feedings

   [ml formula/day] ÷ [Number feedings/day] = [ml formula/feeding]

FIGURE 14-17. Calculations for the daily food dose are done by dividing the patient's Kcal requirement by the Kcal/ml energy content of the food (see Table 14-10). The daily amount (milliliters) of food is usually divided into small portions that are given frequently.

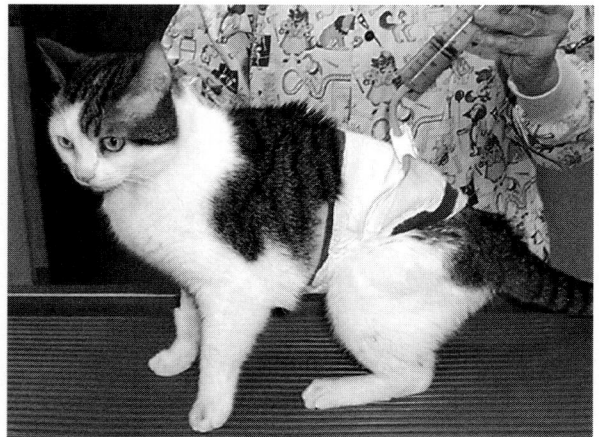

FIGURE 14-18. Feeding for convalescence, repletion, and recovery should extend past hospital discharge. This cat is anorectic and has received blended pet food by tube gastrostomy for several months. Most owners can be coached in food preparation for tube feeding techniques.

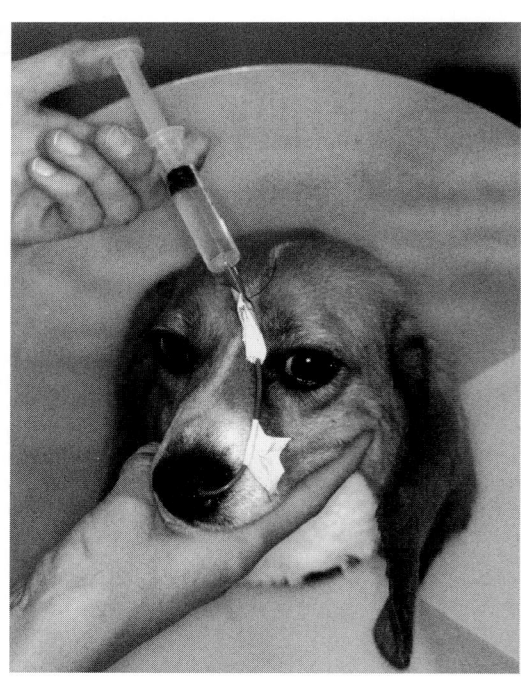

FIGURE 14-19. This dog is receiving a liquid pet food by small-bore nasoesophageal tube feeding. This technique is convenient for short-term feeding (several days).

TABLE 14-10	COMPOSITION OF ENTERAL VETERINARY FORMULAE				
			Energy Distribution		
Product	Caloric Content (Kcal/g)	Protein Content (g/100 Kcal)	% Protein Calories	% Fat Calories	% CHO Calories
VETERINARY PRODUCTS (CANNED)					
Prescription Diet					
Feline p/d*	0.8	10.1	36	56	8
Feline k/d*	0.8	6.0	23	49	28
Feline c/d-s*	0.6	9.9	36	43	21
Feline l/d	1.05	7.2	25	45	30
Canine k/d†	0.6	3.1	11	48	41
Canine p/d†	0.8	1.9	23	51	26
Canine n/d†	0.8	7.8	27	57	16
Canine i/d†	0.7	5.8	23	30	47
Canine/Feline a/d	1.3	8.8	35	53	12
Purina CV-Formula Feline	1.4	8.7	32	50	18
Eukanuba Maximum Calorie Canine/Feline	2.0	7.4	29	66	5
Select Care Canine Development	0.9	8.0	28	30	42
Select Care Feline Development	1.0	10.4	36	54	10
VETERINARY PRODUCTS (LIQUID/PASTE)					
CliniCare Canine	1.0	5.5	20	55	25
CliniCare Feline	1.0	8.6	30	45	25
CliniCare RF Feline	1.0	5.6	22	57	21
NutriCal paste	4.6	0.3	1	62	37
HUMAN POLYMERIC FOODS					
Jevity	1.1	4.2	17	29	54
Pulmocare	1.5	4.2	17	55	28
Osmolite HN	1.1	4.2	17	29	54
Sustacal	1.0	6.1	24	21	55
HUMAN MONOMERIC					
Peptamen	1.0	4.4	16	33	51
Vital HN	1.0	4.1	15	9	74
SUPPLEMENT					
Promod (protein)	1.5 Kcal/ml	23.6	0	0	0
Casec (protein)	4.0	30.7	0	100	0
MCT oil (medium triglycerides)	8.3 Kcal/ml	0	0	100	0
Vegetable oil	8.5 Kcal/ml	0	0	100	0
Baby food (turkey)	1.0	14.6	58	42	0

CHO, Carbohydrate.
*½ Can (202 g) + ¾ C (170 ml) water.
†½ Can (209 g) + ¾ C (170 ml) water.

FEEDING PET BIRDS

Dietary-induced diseases frequently occur in companion and aviary psittacine and passerine birds for several reasons. First, until recently, specific nutritional requirements for these birds were unknown. Thus investigators and veterinary practitioners tended to extrapolate the well-known nutrient needs of poultry to other avian species. Although these nutrient needs generally apply, specific nutritional differences of domestic chickens and other avian species have been reported. For example, riboflavin deficiency in broiler chicks manifests itself clinically as curled-toe paralysis, which is not observed in cockatiel chicks. Cockatiels lack pigmentation (achromatosis) in their primary feathers as a result of riboflavin deficiency. Although differences of this type exist experimentally, many prepared foods overcome these differences by supplying levels of nutrients well in excess of the minimum requirement for chickens.

Second, and more important, many people think that all-seed diets (particularly diets composed of only one seed type, such as millet or sunflower) and diets composed of or heavily supplemented with fruits, vegetables, and other human foods are complete foods for birds. In reality, most commercially available seeds are deficient in certain limiting nutrients (e.g., specific amino acids, vitamins, trace minerals, and macrominerals, such as calcium and sodium). Also, seeds are not the primary or natural diet of most species of companion birds. For example, one study revealed that when given the opportunity, the endangered Puerto Rican parrot (*Amazona vittata*) consumed 7 species of fruits, seeds, and leaves (new foliage), the fruiting structures of 44 species of trees (in addition to bark), and 7 species of canopy vines. Thus seeds compose only a small part of their total diet in the wild.

In addition, evidence suggests that increased protein may be needed during certain points in the reproductive cycle. In the wild, insects supply these increased needs. It is difficult for bird owners to meet these special needs by feeding only seed mixtures.

However, perhaps the most common cause of dietary-induced diseases in companion birds is the practice of adding fruits and vegetables sold for human consumption to commercially prepared foods or supplemented seed mixtures. The most readily available fruits and vegetables contain primarily water, carbohydrates, and fiber. They are severely deficient in protein, vitamins, and minerals when compared to the nutrient recommendations for psittacine and passerine birds. Thus fruits and vegetables primarily dilute key nutrients present in nutritionally balanced commercially prepared foods. Birds often preferentially eat fruits and vegetables because of their high water content instead of dry extruded or pelleted foods and seed mixtures. In fact, birds often select food items based on water content, texture, color, or taste, rather than nutrient content, resulting in very imbalanced nutrient intakes.

This common feeding practice leads directly to the third reason captive birds develop nutritional deficiencies, which is the tendency of individual birds to select specific food items from a variety of offerings. Because malnourished birds often tend to overeat the food items presented to them, it is unclear whether this is a cause or an effect of malnutrition. It does lead to the popular misconception that birds are able to preferentially balance their diets. As a result, individual birds may become habituated or fixated on a specific food item (e.g., sunflower, safflower, or millet seeds or grapes or oranges); yet these specific items are usually deficient in several essential nutrients.

The patient history should minimally include a list of foods offered daily. In addition, clients should be encouraged to provide a sample of any commercially prepared foods they feed.

If the food offered is commercially prepared, examine the label for nutrient information or guarantees. The primary nutrients of concern are protein and calcium. Many foods commonly fed to companion birds are composed primarily of carbohydrates and fat. The label of an acceptable commercially prepared food should list a protein guarantee of at least 12%. From the list of ingredients on the label, determine if a source of calcium is included in the food. Seeds commonly contain more phosphorus than calcium. Thus an added calcium source, such as calcium carbonate, dicalcium phosphate, bone meal, ground limestone, or ground oyster shells, helps balance the calcium/phosphorus ratio of bird foods.

The food should not be used for long-term feeding if its label contains no nutrient information or is just a list of ingredients such as seeds or dried fruit. The following discussion describes common strategies used to feed birds.

Foods appropriately balanced with carbohydrates, proteins, fats, vitamins, minerals, and water are essential for all birds. Stewardship of confined birds must address good nutrition at several levels: the daily satisfaction and health of the bird as well as the long-term contributions to growth, maturation, defense against disease, and reproductive health (the hallmark of good nutrition).

Three methods of providing nutrients and achieving these objectives are commonly used: commercially prepared foods, seeds and seed mixtures, and homemade mixed foods.

Commercially Prepared Foods

The benefits of using commercially prepared, nutritionally complete foods become obvious when the feeding of birds kept as companions is compared with the feeding of other companion animals. Prepared foods supply more than 90% of the nutrients for companion dogs and cats in North America and can contribute markedly to the health of these animals. The gradual transition from diets composed primarily of human food, including table scraps, to commercially prepared complete and balanced foods for dogs and cats has taken about 50 years. The same transition will undoubtedly occur in a much shorter time for pet birds as the number and quality of products available increase.

The major benefits of commercially prepared foods are nutrient balance and convenience (Figure 14-20). Manufacturers commonly formulate commercial foods using sound scientific principles following established nutrient recommendations. Although adherence to these recommendations and ingredient quality may vary among manufacturers, an extruded or pelleted diet supplies all the nutrients in one particle. Such formulations help prevent alteration of nutrient balance by uninformed owners who feed imbalanced seeds or human foods or by birds that consume different quantities of imbalanced foods that are fed separately.

A potential disadvantage of feeding commercial foods is that testing protocols for nutritional adequacy have not yet been established for avian foods, as they have been for commercial canine and feline foods. Nevertheless, the probability of producing a nutritional imbalance by feeding a commercial avian food is much less than when seeds or human foods prepared by uninformed owners are fed to birds.

Seeds and Seed Mixtures

Seeds are a popular, convenient, inexpensive method of providing nutrients to companion birds (see Figure 14-20), but they are not necessarily the best or even the most natural food for pet birds. A recent renaissance in the pet bird food industry has taken into account the long forgotten holistic views of habitats and natural history of many avian species. Interesting facts have come to light. Food selection in birds is predominantly a learned behavior. Nestling birds accept the appropriate foods brought to them by their parents and once fledged observe where and how to obtain these foods for themselves. In a pet industry where captive breeding and isolation of companion birds are the norm, individual birds have little or no experience with their natural environment or natural food sources and may not have the opportunity to observe feeding behaviors of other birds. Although hundreds of years of domestication in some species have altered feeding behaviors, the associated physiology of nutrient assimilation and use have not changed markedly. The types of seeds present in most commercial mixes are not native to areas where most pet bird species originate. Although seeds may have been used opportunistically in the wild, they would not have been available in large quantities. Considering all these facts, seeds are no more of a natural food than any other method of providing nutrients for companion birds.

Other disadvantages of all seed diets are that the diet can be altered easily by uninformed owners or birds can consume certain seed types, avoiding others, resulting in an imbalanced nutrient intake. With these disadvantages in mind, seeds are much less desirable than commercially prepared foods for feeding companion birds.

As mentioned, seeds are a common element in many pet bird diets. A well-balanced seed mixture can supply essential nutrients such as fats, carbohydrates, and some minerals. However, seeds are rarely if ever an appropriate sole nutritional source because they provide inadequate levels of protein, vitamins, and minerals. There are numerous commercially available seed mixtures that vary greatly in

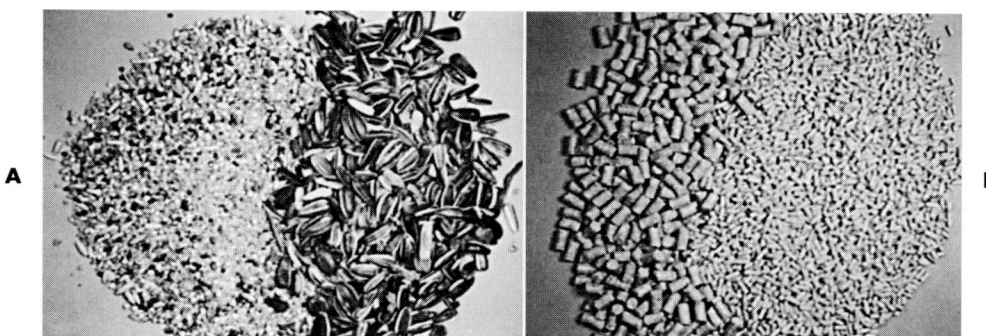

FIGURE 14-20.   A, Seeds are an important part of many avian diets. However, high-oil seeds and nuts, such as sunflower seeds and peanuts, may cause addictions and nutritional imbalance. Oil seeds are deficient in protein relative to calorie content and in calcium and micronutrients. **B,** Complete and balanced avian foods are available as fortified seed mixtures and extruded and pelleted foods.

type and quality. Individual seed types are also sold in most stores; thus formulating seed mixtures is a common practice. The availability of individual seed types promotes nutrient imbalance when uninformed owners create a mixture based primarily on the price and physical appearance of the seeds. Thus creation or use of homemade seed mixtures should be discouraged.

Commercial mixtures for a particular group of birds may vary greatly in seed types and proportions from one company to another, indicating the lack of scientific sophistication involved in preparing seed mixture diets. Seed mixtures may contain protein, vitamin, and mineral supplements in pellet or crumble form. This is the manufacturer's attempt to overcome the nutrient imbalances inherent in a seeds-only diet. The assumption is that birds will consume all the seeds and supplement pellets and thus have a nutritionally balanced diet. Unfortunately, this assumption is not always reality. If seed mixtures containing supplements are used to feed confined birds, the owner should be advised to leave the food in front of the bird until the entire mixture has been eaten before giving the bird more of the mixture. This practice will ensure that the bird consumes the entire diet, not a nutritionally imbalanced, isolated segment. Because individual birds may not accept some components of a supplemented seed mixture, consuming them irregularly or not at all, an imbalanced nutrient intake is much more likely to occur when a supplemented seed mixture is the sole dietary form fed.

Bird owners feed a variety of live foods as supplements to seeds and seed mixtures. When research showed that even strict seed eaters opportunistically eat insects as a protein source at certain periods in their reproductive cycle and to improve their condition for migration, insect foods became commercially available.

White worms (*Enchytraes* larvae) are available commercially and can be kept for long periods, much like earthworms, in a cool, damp moss and leaf litter substrate. These worms are especially useful to provide when parent birds are brooding and feeding their young. Ant pupae, which bird fanciers have relied on heavily for their avian diets, are now available commercially in large outlets and by mail order. Water shrimp (*Daphnia* spp.) are relished by some species and greatly enhance red pigments in their plumage. Aphids that feed on members of the rose family concentrate the same pigments and may be more appropriate for small passerine birds. Moth larvae, commonly known as waxworms, and beetle larvae, called mealworms,

supply extra protein and fat, especially at the onset of the breeding season. Care should be taken to restrict the intake of these insects, or birds will rapidly gain weight and become obese.

Homemade Mixed-Food Diets
A wide variety of homemade mixed-food diets have been suggested as alternatives for birds that will not accept commercially prepared foods or seed mixtures even with added fruits and vegetables. These diets can result in excellent feathering and appropriate body mass for the species, with no discernible signs of nutritional deficiency, if prepared carefully from scientifically developed recipes. These diets often contain varying amounts of ingredients such as seeds, nuts, cooked eggs, low-fat yogurt or cheese, vegetables, fruits, grains, bread, pasta, multigrain cereals, legumes, seed mixes, pelleted or extruded psittacine diets, vitamin supplements, and calcium supplements (Table 14-11). When converting birds to a new homemade diet, have the client offer a mixture containing all the ingredients at one time. This practice usually prevents preferential selection of certain ingredients. Although larger parrots have difficulty eating small seeds such as milo or oat groats, a seed mixture containing 30% hulled safflower, 30% milo, 30% oat groats, and 10% peanuts works well for smaller birds.

Although homemade mixed-food diets may provide adequate nourishment, most companion bird owners are unwilling to devote the time necessary to adequately prepare these diets. In addition, owners must be willing to regularly observe which food components are being consumed to prevent birds from developing or reverting to preferential selection of specific ingredients.

Water
Although feeding a well-balanced food is essential, it is easy to overlook the single most important dietary component: water. As with all animals, water is absolutely essential for birds. Water acts as a food carrier and aids in digestion. Some foods are high in water content, but others require free water for efficient digestion and absorption. Some avian species are more physiologically adept at extracting water from their foods. Budgerigars in the wild, for example, are capable of absorbing sufficient water from seeds and green foods to allow them to go without water for many days. This observation, however, is not an experiment to be undertaken by the pet owner. Birds should

TABLE 14-11   SUGGESTED DIET FOR MAINTENANCE OF ADULT CAGED BIRDS

	Canary	Budgerigar	Cockatiel	Conure	Amazon/African Gray Parrot	Macaw/Cockatoo
OFFER DAILY						
Whole-grain bread cubes or primate biscuit	1/4 T	1/2 T	1 T	1 1/2 T	2 T	4 T
Fresh dark green or yellow vegetables	1/2 T	1 T	2 T	4 T	3 T	1/2 C
Protein source (cheese, hard-cooked eggs, egg, meat, mature legumes)	1/4 Size of pea	1/2 Size of pea	Size of pea	1/4 t	1/2 t	1 T
Dry seeds (two 15-min periods) (sunflower)	0	0	1 T	2 T	2 T	4 T
Small seeds (canary, niger, poppy, rape, millet, safflower, hemp)	Ad-lib	Ad-lib	Ad-lib	Ad-lib	Ad-lib	Ad-lib
2 TO 3 TIMES WEEKLY						
Fruit (cantaloupe, apricot, apple)	1/8 t	1/8 t	1 t	1/12 Apple	1/12 Apple	1/6 Apple
Citrus fruit	0	0	0	1/12 Orange	1/12 Orange	1/6 Orange
Fresh corn on the cob	3 or 4 Kernels	1/8 Piece	1/4 Piece	1/2 Piece	1/2 Piece	1 Piece
Peanuts	0	0	0	1	2	4
ADD TEMPORARILY FOR NEW BIRDS						
Vitamin A (from 10,000 IU capsule)	1 Drop/wk	2 Drops/wk	3 Drops/wk	1 Drop/day	1-2 Drops/day	4 Drops/day
Yogurt	Drop	Few drops	1/4 t	1/4 t	1/2 t	1
ALWAYS AVAILABLE						
Calcium/mineral supplements (cuttlebone, mineral treat block, oyster shell, calcium lactate)						

Modified from Harrison GJ, Harrison LR: *Clinical avian medicine and surgery*, Philadelphia, 1986, WB Saunders.
C, Cup; T, tablespoon; t, teaspoon.

never go for more than a few hours without access to fresh clean water. Studies have shown that canaries will die within 48 hours if water is withheld.

Water makes up more than 50% of a bird's body weight. Because birds have no sweat glands, water intake plays an important role in thermoregulation. Breeding females may require increased amounts of water for egg production and for heat regulation while incubating eggs.

Water should be provided in containers that are easily accessible but not located in a place that can collect feces, feathers, or food particles. For this reason, water bowls should be attached to the wall of enclosures, near or above food bowls. They should not be so large as to invite bathing.

Changing Foods

Unless commercially prepared, nutritionally complete foods are fed, birds fed free choice may develop a habituation to a single type of food (monophagism). This fixation may result in single or multiple nutrient deficiencies. After a deficiency occurs, the owner is faced with changing the food. This can be a formidable challenge depending on the age and species of the bird. Changing foods is generally easier with younger birds and with smaller parrots such as cockatiels and conures. Cockatoos, macaws, and African gray parrots are more resistant to change. Most passerine birds switch to new foods easily.

Totally changing the diet should not be attempted if the bird is sick or under stress (e.g., recent acquisition, change in environment, exposure to temperature extremes, molting). Conversion to a new balanced food may take from weeks to months depending on the degree and length of habituation. Ninety percent of healthy cockatiels can be converted to a new food within 7 days.

A variety of strategies can be used to convert birds to a new food. If one of the following approaches is unsuccessful, an alternative one should be tried:

- Gradually add the new food to the current diet, increasing the amount of the new food over days to weeks. Remember that texture and color are important; therefore adding a food that the bird really likes (e.g., brown sugar, carrots) may make the conversion much easier.
- Unless the new food is extruded or pelleted, warming or cooling the food may make a difference in acceptance. The food should be warmed to no hotter than 40.6° C (105° F). Microwave ovens should be used cautiously because the interior of the food may be much hotter

than the exterior. Alternatively, food can be cooled to refrigerator temperatures (2° C to 4° C [35° C to 40° F]).
- Try offering the bird a soft food, such as baby cereal, fruits or vegetables, cooked oatmeal, or cream of wheat. Birds like the texture of these foods. Then gradually add a prepared diet to these mixtures.
- If a bird is hand-trained or hand-reared, feeding outside the cage is often helpful (Box 14-10). Alternatively, place the new food item in the cage at a strategic locations (e.g., by a mirror or favorite toy or attached to the cage bars).
- Have the owner eat what he or she wants the bird to eat. Some birds mimic their owners by eating foods they see their owners eat.
- Begin feeding a new food every other day. For larger birds, remove the seeds on that day. If a smaller bird (e.g., a budgerigar, canary, or finch) has not eaten the new food by late afternoon, offer seeds to prevent hypoglycemia overnight. Alternate-day feedings will also prevent excessive weight loss. Increase feedings to 4, then 5, then 7 days per week.
- Remove all seeds before retiring for the night. In the morning, offer a commercially prepared complete food with new food items instead of the seed. Do not add seed until noon. This strategy presents no danger to the birds because the previous seed or seeds are available later in the day.

The bird's physical condition and body weight should be monitored during the conversion period to prevent starvation. Keep in mind that most birds eating all seeds or junk food (e.g., potato chips, peanuts, candy) may be overweight or even obese. If a bird loses excessive body condition during the conversion period, as determined through weighing, it may refuse to eat the previously fed food. Gavage or tube feeding for 1 to 3 days will be required to stimulate the bird to eat.

All these strategies have been successful in enticing companion psittacine birds to eat a more balanced diet. Occasionally, however, individual birds cannot be converted. These birds may require specialized water and food supplements to overcome serious vitamin and mineral deficiencies. In some cases when conversion is unsuccessful, the bird may need to be hospitalized away from the owner. At the hospital, a rigorous dietary protocol can be implemented that may be successful once the behavioral influences of the owner are eliminated. In multiple-bird households, owners will have an easier time converting birds to a new food if at least one bird has been converted and the other birds can observe it eating the new food.

Client education is crucial to the success of food conversion, especially with companion birds. Owners should be advised to be persistent and patient during this process.

Nutritional Disease of Pet Birds

Nutritional disease is common in pet birds. Box 14-11 lists human foods that can add diversity to the diet of compan-

---

Box 14-10	HAND-FEEDING HATCHLINGS

SCHEDULE
- Birth: every 2 to 3 hr
- 3 wk: four times per day
- 4 wk: three times per day

FOOD DOSE
- Distend crop
- Fill again when empty

DIET
- Liquid slurry of 25% dry matter (250 g of dry food powder and 750 g of water)

COMMERCIAL FORMULAS

GROUND PRIMATE BISCUITS

HOMEMADE DIETS

Box 14-11	FEED DIVERSITY

Cheerios
Pellets, crumbles, crimps
Cooked vegetables
Bananas
Peanut butter

BOX 14-12	NUTRITIONAL DEFICIENCIES

Vitamin A (squamous metaplasia, hyperkeratosis)
Iodine (hypothyroidism)
Vitamin E (encephalomalacia)
Zinc (failure to thrive)
Selenium (muscular dystrophy)

TABLE 14-12		ESTIMATING HORSE WEIGHT	
Girth Circumference		Body Weight	
(in)	(cm)	(lb)	(kg)
64.5	163.8	800	363.6
67.5	171.5	900	409.1
70.5	179.1	1000	454.5
73.0	185.4	1100	500.0
75.5	191.8	1200	545.5
77.5	196.9	1300	590.9

ion birds. Box 14-12 gives nutritional deficiencies of birds and the resulting conditions.

Technician Note

Dietary-induced diseases frequently occur in companion and aviary birds.

EQUINE NUTRITION

Nutrients for Horses

Nutrients of concern for horses are water, energy, protein, calcium, phosphorus, and vitamin A. Although all animals require access to good-quality water on an ad-lib basis, this is especially true for an animal capable of copious sweating (Carson, 1993). Hot, exhausted horses should rest and perhaps consume some hay while cooling. A waiting period of 30 minutes should occur before allowing water after heavy exercise.

Horses evolved eating grass and other range forages. Not surprisingly, grass and hays serve well as a foundation for feeding all horses. *Good-quality* grass or legume hay, free-choice water, calcium, phosphorus as needed, and trace mineralized salt are the only foods needed by the adult horse at maintenance.

Technician Note

The role of grain and protein meal concentrates is to complement forages during periods of higher than maintenance nutrient demand.

Grain and protein meal concentrates complement forages during periods of higher than maintenance nutrient demand. Unfortunately, some horse feeding programs overlook quality forages and focus on elaborate programs of concentrate supplementation. The technician attending performance horses will also encounter a wide variety of owner- and trainer-selected supplements. These are diverse and may well match the current nutritional fad. Time-proven horse feeding programs emphasize simplicity and quality forage feeds.

Equine food dose calculations are based on the horse's weight; a simple and frequently used method is to calculate an amount of feed per 100 lb of horse. Therefore a horse weight tape is a simple and inexpensive tool worth having and using (Table 14-12). For example, a 6-year-old, 1000-lb light-breed gelding is at rest in a backyard paddock. The animal receives only 1 hour per week of light work. This horse is considered to be at maintenance activity requiring 1.5% of the horse's body weight (BW) per day as dry matter (Figure 14-21). This means that 15 lb of a good-quality hay will suffice in addition to salt and water. If a 6-inch hay "flake" weighs 5 lb, then feeding three per day (one in the morning and two in the evening) can be suggested as a food dose. Table 14-13 summarizes different dry matter intake levels for various activity and physiologic states (Figure 14-22). As in small animals, equine overfeeding is a problem, and a routine portion of all horse evaluations is body condition assessment.

Some hays or hay/grain combinations need calcium and phosphorus supplementation. Most commonly, a source of phosphorus is added when a good legume hay is the sole source of nutrition. Powdered mineral supplements are often mixed with hay or loose rock salt and provided as part of the diet. Nutrient intake objectives and feeds to meet these are found in Table 14-14.

The microminerals zinc, manganese, iron, copper, cobalt, and sometimes iodine, found in trace-mineralized salt blocks, can also be provided ad lib in a location protected from rain (Figure 14-23).

Technician Note

Routine horse feeding problems include overgrazed pastures, ingestion of sand and weeds, underfeeding as a result of poor-quality forage, too much grain, too fine a grind in pelleted feeds, various nutrient imbalances, and toxic supplementation.

Routine horse feeding problems include overgrazed pastures, ingestion of sand and weeds, underfeeding because of poor-quality forage, too much grain, too fine a grind in pelleted feeds, various nutrient imbalances, and toxic supplementation. Unfortunately, horses are not routinely or easily weighed in the typical setting, and changes in condition may be insidious. Accidental engorgement of grain may precipitate colic or founder with morbid or even tragic results.

Feeding Sick Horses

Hospitalized horses develop the same protein-calorie deficits, hypermetabolic stress, and catabolic wasting states as small animals. These have identical negative clinical effects, and early interventional feeding is vital in equine critical care. Major gastrointestinal tract (colic) surgery is especially challenging in the perioperative period. The animal needs a feed rich in protein, calories, and micronutrients but has reduced gastrointestinal motility. The veterinarian will focus closely on when gastrointestinal motility returns. Homogenized, moistened alfalfa pellet mashes are high-protein, high-energy, and nonirritating repletion formulas. These may be given as slurries through nasogastric

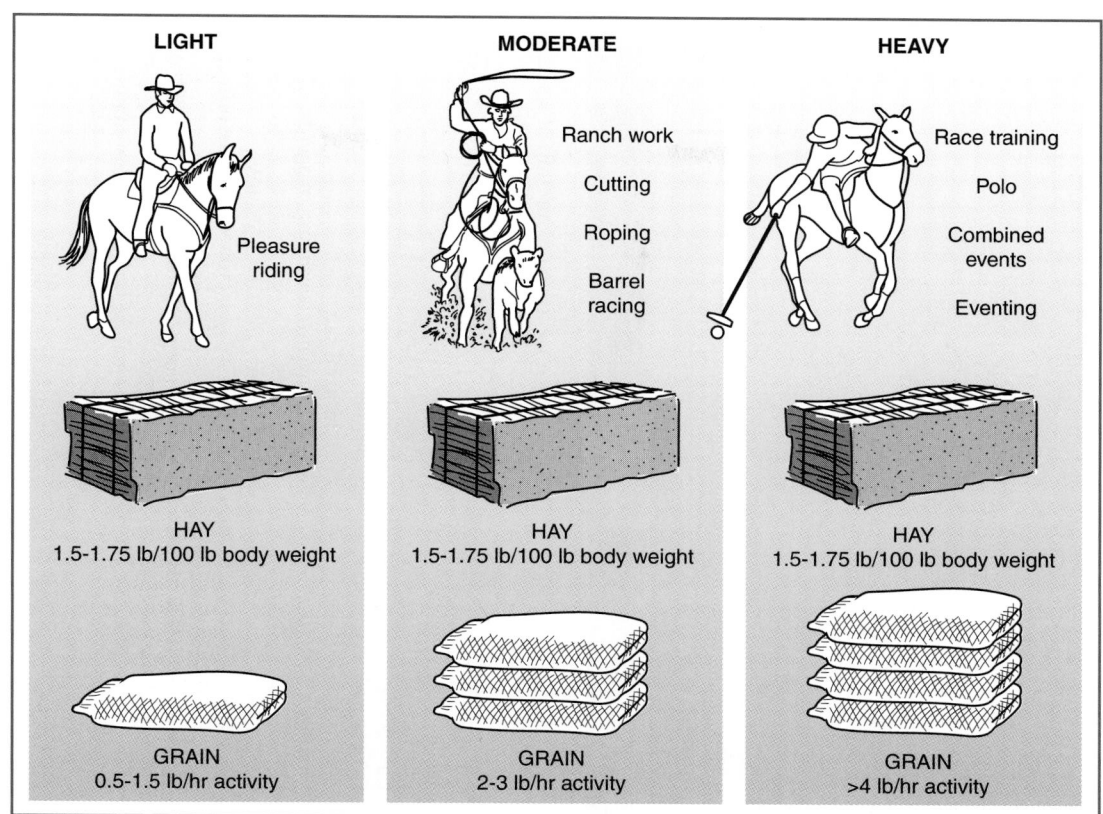

FIGURE 14-21. Adjusted feeding based on an activity level. Maintenance feed levels can be based per 100 lb of weight. Supplemental feeding over maintenance should be based on the level and duration of work.

TABLE 14-13	BARNYARD METRICS
Volume	**Weight (lb)**
HAYS	
Brome, 6-in flake	4-5
Alfalfa, 6-in flake	5-6
1 QUART	
Oats (whole)	1
Corn (whole)	1.7
Beet pulp	0.6
Bran	0.5

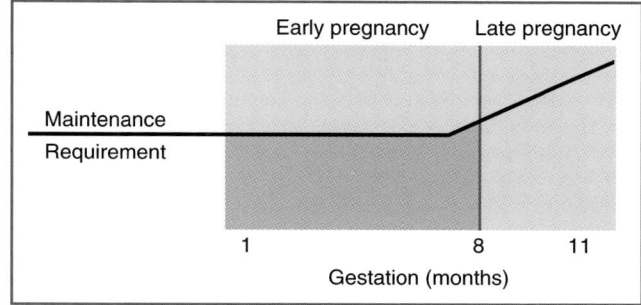

FIGURE 14-22. Early gestation is not "eating for two," and the mare should be fed for maintenance. In the last trimester of pregnancy, requirements increase for energy, protein, and minerals.

tubes and are often enriched with nutriment modules. Liquid enteral formulas based on mare's milk replacement and commercial equine critical care formulas are available and well tolerated. These formulas should be given in small frequent feedings via indwelling nasogastric tubes.

Assessing Forages and Grains for Horses

The veterinary technician can assess the quality of water, pastures, and hays (Figure 14-24).

A feed-bunk rule for horses is not to exceed a 50:50 ratio of concentrate to roughage. Oats and corn are the two most common feeds, and noting their relative energy content is important. Various horse grains, mixed concentrate supplements, and several totally complete extruded or pelleted horse feeds will be encountered on horse calls

(Figure 14-25). If horses consume only complete extruded or pelleted feeds, an issue may be an adequate roughage intake. The sudden onset of fence chewing when only a complete pelleted food is used suggests the need for at least some long-stem or coarse chopped hay.

Forage quality varies greatly by soil quality, species of grass, season of year, rainfall, overgrazing, pasture rotation, weed control, and the presence of toxic weeds. Laboratory analysis of forages for moisture, energy, protein, fiber, and macrominerals is fundamental in assessing roughage nutri-

TABLE 14-14   NUTRIENT SUPPLY FOR HORSES*

Age	Energy	Protein	Vitamins and Minerals	Comments
Nursing foals	Supplement mare's milk if foal is very thin	>16%	Ca²⁺ >0.85% P >0.5% Cu >25 mg/kg	At 2-3 mo of age, begin 1 lb concentrate mixture/mo of age/day Adequate Ca²⁺, P, trace minerals in grain mix If creep feeding, mix 50:50 chopped hay to grain Wean at 4 mo
Weaning	Adequate to feel but not see the ribs	15%	Vitamin A 50 IU/kg BW Ca²⁺ 0.7% P 0.4%	Dry matter intake = 3% of BW Free-choice good roughage and trace mineral salt 1 lb concentrate mix/mo of age/day: 7-9 lb mix
Yearling	Adequate to feel but not see the ribs	13%	Vitamin A 50 IU/kg BW Ca²⁺ 0.5% P 0.3% Vitamin A 50 IU/kg BW	Dry matter intake = 2.5% BW Free-choice good roughage, trace mineral salt 1 lb concentrate mix/mo of age/day: 7-9 lb max Feed as mature horse at 90% of mature weight
Adult *Maintenance*	Adequate to feel but not see the ribs	8.5%	Ca²⁺ 0.3% P 0.2% Vitamin A 50 IU/kg BW	Dry matter = 1.5% BW 1½-1¾ lb roughage/100 lb BW Free-choice trace mineral salt
Adult *Working* *Light* (pleasure ride)	Add 0.5-1.5 lb of grain/hr of activity/day	8.5%	Ca²⁺ 0.3% P 0.2% Vitamin A 50 IU/kg BW	Amortize grain supplement over the week

Moderate (ranch work, roping, cutting, jumping, barrel racing)	Add 2-3 lb of grain/hr of activity/day	8.5%-10%	Ca²⁺ 0.3% P 0.2% Vitamin A 50 IU/kg BW	
Heavy (race training, polo)	Add 4 or more lb of grain/hr of activity/day	8.5%-10%	Ca²⁺ 0.3% P 0.2% Vitamin A 50 IU/kg BW	Dry matter = 1.75% BW
Adult reproduction *Mares*	Feed at maintenance until late pregnancy	8.5%-10%		
Late pregnancy	Needs 20% more energy	11%	Ca²⁺ 0.5% P 0.35% Vitamin A 50 IU/kg BW	Feed 1½-1¾ lb grass hays/100 lb BW with addition of ½-¾ lb grain or concentrate mix/100 lb BW Free-choice trace mineral salt–mineral Ca²⁺/P mix
Last 3 wk of pregnancy	Needs 30% more energy		Needs 100%, more Ca²⁺ and P Vitamin A 60 IU/kg BW	1¾-2 lb legume hay/100 lb BW Free-choice trace mineral salt–mineral Ca²⁺/P mix
Lactation	Allow 75% energy increase at peak lactation	14%	Ca²⁺ 0.5% P 0.35% Vitamin A 60 IU/kg BW	Dry matter = 1.75%-2.0% BW free-choice grass hay Add 1½-2 lb/100 lb BW of concentrate Add Ca²⁺/P mix and trace mineralized salt At weaning, stop concentrate; return to maintenance forage
Stallions	Feed for maintenance			

BW, Body weight; *Ca,* calcium; *Cu,* copper; *P,* phosphorus.
*Free-choice, potable water should be available at all times.

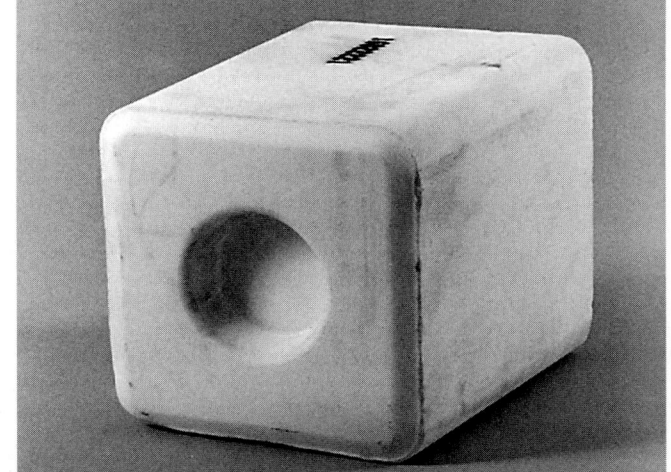

FIGURE 14-23. Additional sodium chloride and adequate intake of trace minerals can be provided with plain or trace mineralized salt blocks.

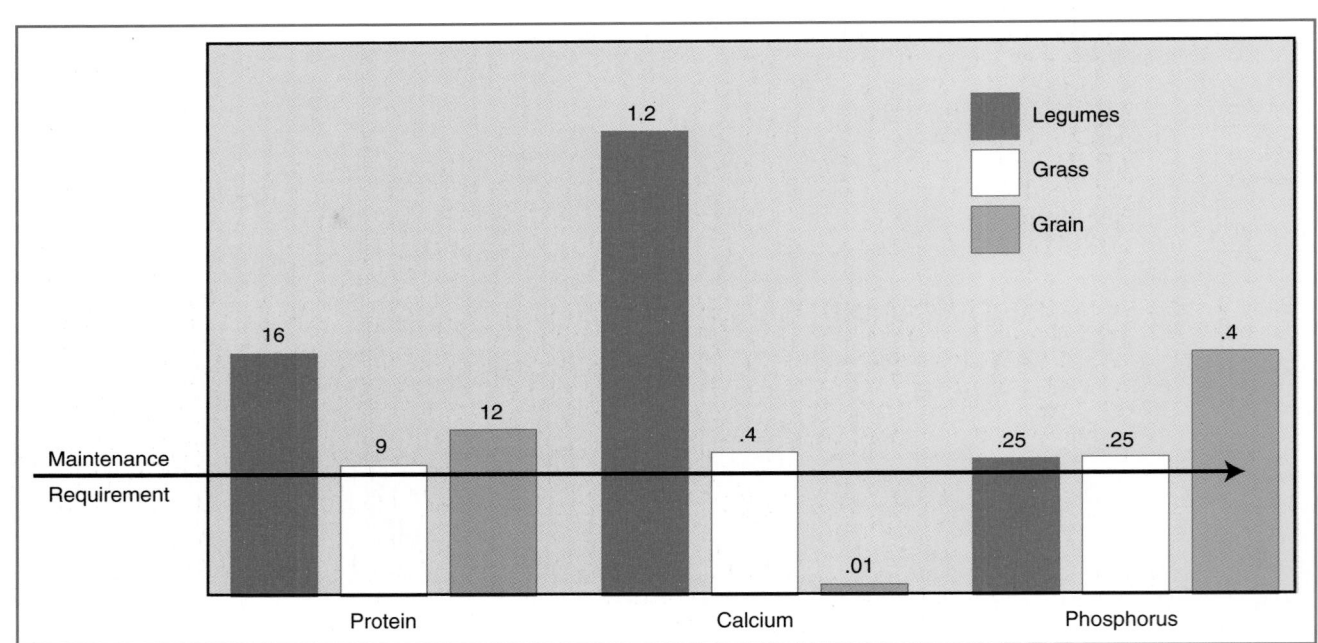

FIGURE 14-24. High-quality grass and legume hays, water, and salt suffice for equine maintenance. However, a source of supplemental phosphorus benefits some hay and can be provided as mineral mix.

ent content. Hay analysis is free (or inexpensive) from regional agriculture extension services. When hay analysis is unavailable, one can make some conclusions about hay quality from a physical inspection. Observe the leafiness and the leaf/stem ratio. This is important because two thirds of the energy and three fourths of the protein reside in leaves (Figure 14-26). Smaller and more flexible stems suggest the correct maturity for grass and legume hays. Fully developed seed heads in grass hay and flowers in alfalfa mean overmaturity. Greenness (chlorophyll and beta-carotene), presence of weeds, mold, foreign material, rain damage, poor curing, and mechanical mishandling are

other visual qualities to be checked in forage assessment. An additional discussion of feed analysis can be found in Chapter 15.

ACKNOWLEDGMENT

The authors and editors wish to acknowledge the exceptional contributions of Dr. Stephen W. Crane and Sheila R. Grosdidier, who authored large portions of this chapter for the previous two editions of the book. Their original contributions served as the foundation for the material appearing in this edition.

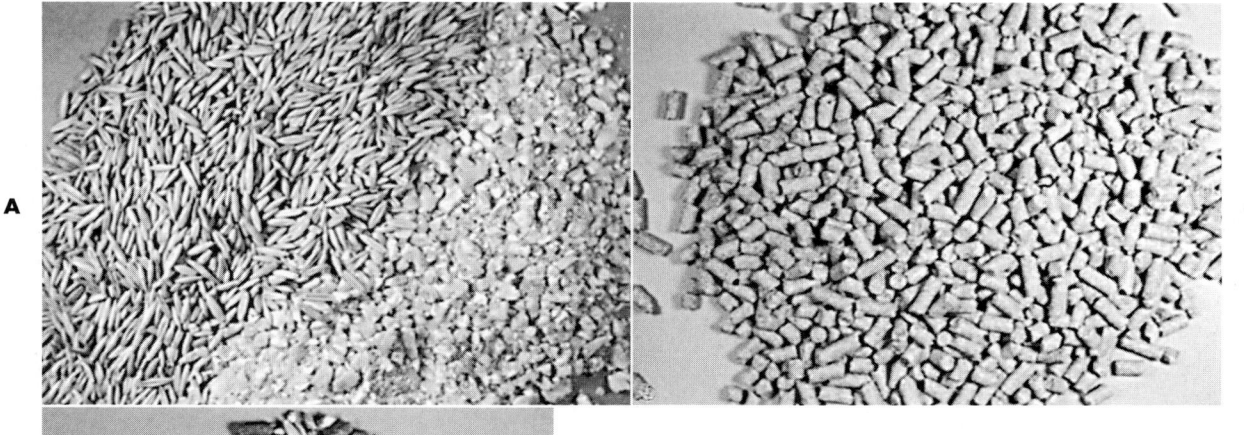

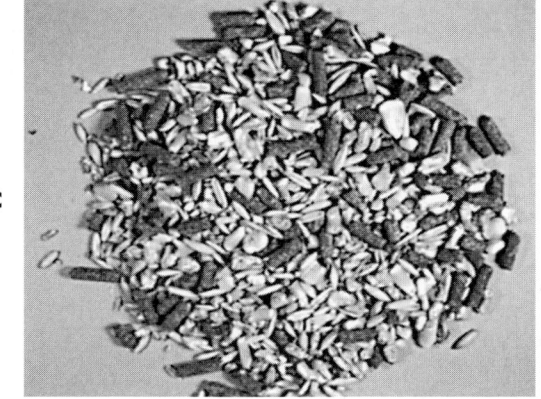

FIGURE 14-25. A, Grain and protein-meal concentrates complement the forage foundation of equine feeds. Concentrates are needed when significantly more energy or protein is required. Oats *(left)* and corn are two popular concentrate grains. On an equal volume basis, corn provides twice the energy of oats. This difference should be made clear to owners who usually feed by volume (coffee can) and may switch between the two grains. B, Pelleted horse foods are an expensive convenience but may lack the chewing or gastrointestinal fullness effects associated with long-stem roughage. Some horses chew or gnaw wood when consuming only complete foods. C, Complete horse feeds may be mixed from grain, forages, and mineral mixes and then pelleted or extruded. Complete feed can be used as a hay supplement or as the total diet when hay is unavailable.

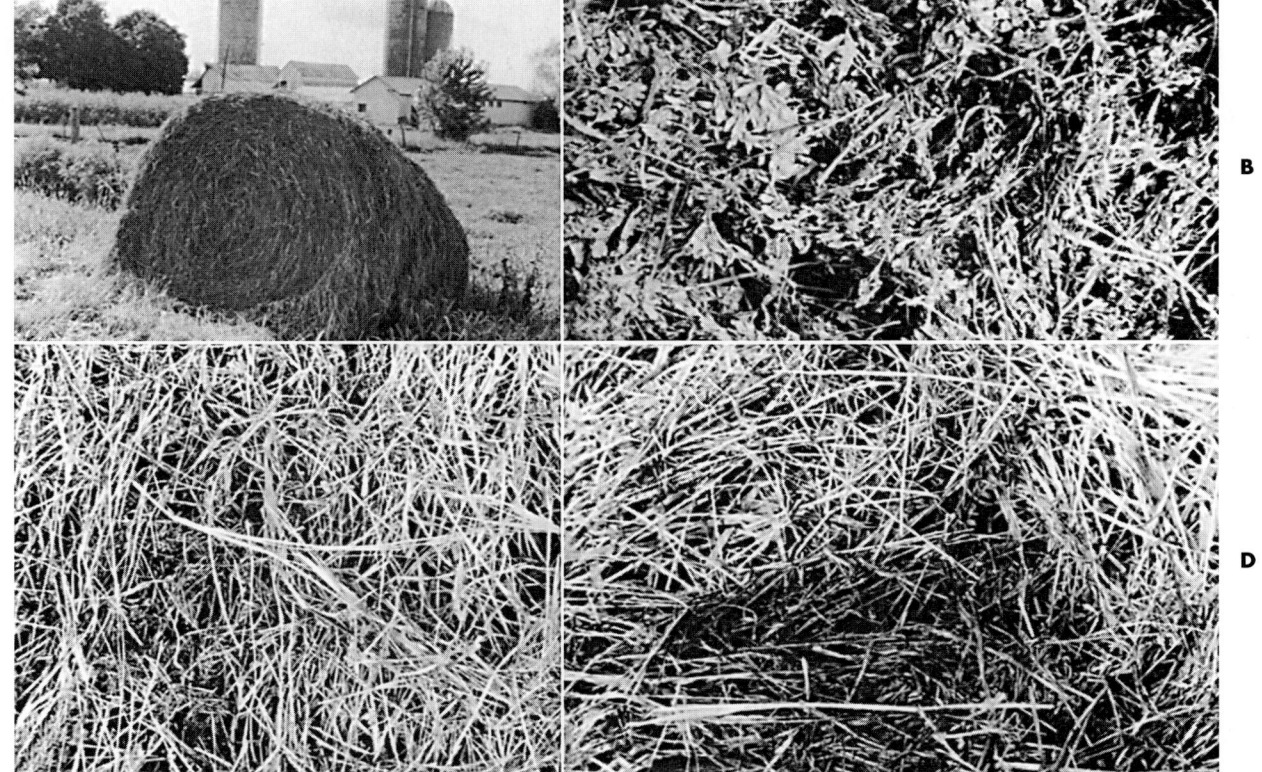

FIGURE 14-26. A laboratory analysis for protein, energy, and macrominerals gives objective guidelines to forage quality and is available from agricultural extension services. Hay quality depends on the species of forage (legume vs. grass), maturity, cutting number, curing, handling, storage **(A),** and age when fed. B, High-quality alfalfa hay is not overmature and has a high proportion of leaves to stems. Leaves contain two thirds of the energy and three fourths of the protein. Flexible, tender stems, light green color, and absence of molds and dust are seen in good legume hay. C, Poor-quality alfalfa hay has reduced leaf numbers and tough stems. Seed heads in a grass hay and flowers in alfalfa hay indicate overmaturing at the time of cutting. D, A hay contaminated by mold *(dark areas)* is usually unpalatable and possibly dangerous.

REFERENCES

Carson TL: Water quality for livestock. In Howard JL, editor: *Current veterinary therapy: food animal practice*, ed 3, Philadelphia, 1993, WB Saunders.

Crane SW: Occurrence and management of obesity in companion animals, *J Small Anim Pract* 32:275, 1991.

Markham RW, Hodgkins EM: Geriatric nutrition, *Vet Clin North Am* 19:165, 1989.

McDonald ML et al: Essential fatty acid requirements of cats: pathology of essential fatty acid deficiency, *Am J Vet Res* 45:1310, 1984.

Mumma RO et al: Toxic and protective constituents in pet food, *Am J Vet Res* 47:1633, 1986.

RECOMMENDED READING

Bonagura JD: *Current veterinary therapy*, XIII, Philadelphia, 2000, WB Saunders.

- Management of anorexia, pp 69-74
- Nutritional assessment of pet food labels, pp 74-80
- Parenteral nutrition products, pp 80-84
- Mechanical devices for percutaneous placement of gastrostomy tubes: use of Eld applicator, pp 94-87
- Refeeding syndrome, pp 87-89
- Microenteral nutrition, pp 136-140
- Hypoallergenic diets for dogs and cats, pp 530-536
- Essential fatty acids, pp 538-542
- Esophageal feeding tubes, pp 597-599
- Dietary sensitivity, pp 632-637
- Nutritional management of diarrheal diseases, pp 653-658
- Nutritional management of liver disease, pp 693-697
- Nutritional management of heart disease, pp 711-716
- Summary of dietary recommendations in urinary diseases, pp 841-846

Hand MS et al, editors: *Small animal clinical nutrition*, ed 4, Topeka, 2000, Mark Morris Institute.

- Small animal clinical nutrition: an iterative process, pp 1-19
- Nutrients, pp 21-107
- Introduction to commercial pet foods, pp 112-126
- Making commercial pet foods, pp 127-146
- Pet food labels, pp 147-161
- Making pet foods at home, pp 163-181
- Food safety, pp 183-198
- Health maintenance programs for dogs and cats, pp 201-211
- Normal dogs, pp 213-260
- Normal cats, pp 291-347
- Assisted feeding in hospitalized patients: enteral and parenteral nutrition, pp 351-399
- Obesity, pp 401-430
- Dental disease, pp 475-504
- Developmental orthopedic disease of dogs, pp 505-521
- Renal disease, pp 563-594
- Feline lower urinary tract disease, pp 689-718
- Feeding small exotic mammals, pp 943-960
- Feeding reptiles, pp 961-977
- Feeding passerine and psittacine birds, pp 979-991
- Neonatal, pediatric and orphaned puppy and kitten care, pp 1012-1019
- Comparative analysis of milks and milk replacers, pp 1064-1072
- Feeding orphaned and injured birds, mammals, amphibians and reptiles, pp 1101-1121

Lewis LD: *Equine clinical nutrition: feeding and care*, Philadelphia, 1995, Williams & Wilkins.

Robinson NE: *Current therapy in equine medicine*, ed 4, Philadelphia, 1997, WB Saunders.

15

Concepts in Livestock Nutrition

William D. Schoenherr

Optimal nutrition has often been identified as the most expensive element in achieving full productivity and profitability in livestock (Ensminger, 1990). The veterinary technician must have a strong fundamental knowledge of nutrient needs and be able to identify potential for problems and increase the client's understanding of essential feeding philosophies. The client who has the greatest need for this type of information is not the large intensive livestock farmer who normally has feeds professionally formulated for optimum production. Most often, the questions will be from clients who run small operations, have family members raising livestock for 4H or FFA projects, or possess a "hobby farm." With these needs in mind, this chapter focuses on common nutritional problems and sound principles to help the veterinary technician provide meaningful, relevant information.

Various nutritional disorders can be very similar to a vast array of diseases and may not be easily identified by the livestock producer as a nutritional disorder until the problem becomes chronic and additional assistance is sought. Therefore it is essential to get a complete history, including a detailed feeding regimen, on any livestock patient who is exhibiting signs of illness.

Dramatic enhancements have occurred in large animal nutrition, including studies that have increased understanding of the specific nutrient needs of livestock to maximize the genetic potential for efficient production, successful breeding, and generation of high-quality, lean meat. Future research will continue to improve our understanding of animal physiology and lead to improvements in livestock production (Table 15-1).

NUTRIENTS

Nutrients are ingested to support life. Livestock producers want to obtain the most desirable results from the nutrients their animals consume at an economical rate and with an advantageous financial return. Ingested nutrients are either retained by the animal or excreted in the urine and feces. Retained nutrients are used for a wide array of body functions, such as homeostasis; replenishment and development of tissues; reproduction; and milk, wool, and meat production.

Maintenance nutrient requirements (MNRs) are the levels of nutrients needed to sustain body weight without gain or loss (Box 15-1). The MNR is the minimum level of dietary need; usually the vast percentage of published requirements are higher than this standard. As a general rule, one half of consumed and absorbed nutrients are used to fulfill MNRs. Individual variation results in fluctuation from this standard; be sure to evaluate need against all information to achieve most accurate results.

Feeding standards are available listing the amounts of nutrients required by different species for specific productive purposes, such as maintenance, growth, finishing, lactation, work, wool, or eggs. The most widely used feeding standards in the United States are those published by the National Research Council (NRC), and they are established for beef cattle, dairy cattle, sheep, goats, swine, and poultry (see Recommended Reading). Periodically, the

Box 15-1	ELEMENTS THAT INFLUENCE NUTRIENT REQUIREMENTS OF LIVESTOCK

Body size
Health status
Stress
Environment
Exercise
Behavior
Genetics
Reproductive status
Gender
Breed

TABLE 15-1 **Feeding Problems in Ruminants**

Disease	Symptoms	Cause	Prevention	Comments
Bloat	Distension of the left flank and then the right flank Hypersalivation Profuse burning ↑ Froth or gas accumulation in the rumen Respiratory distress Cyanosis Death	↑ Change in pasture with heavy fertilizer Genetics Bacterial overgrowth Overeating	Feed coarse grasses or dry forage before turnout to quick-growing pastures Avoid straight pastures Keep stock on pasture continuously rather than sporadically Allow full access to water and salt	Watch legume exposure for all ruminants
Enterotoxemia (overeating disease)	Death is often the first symptom Circling Progressive weakness Head butting Convulsions	Often occurs in faster-growing juveniles *Clostridium perfringens* Excess consumption of high-energy feeds or lush pasture or heavy milk supply	Vaccination with *Clostridium perfringens* type D for lambs and types C and D for breeding ewes	Primarily sheep and goats; sometimes cattle If outbreak occurs, consider enterotoxemia antiserum for 21-day protection in lambs
Fescue toxicosis (fescue foot)	↓ +/− Lameness Necrosis of tail end Milk production Abortion	↑ Change in parasitized animal ↑ In malnourished animal Endophyte fungus *Acrenonium coerophalum*	Avoid heavy parasitism and malnutrition Use fungus-free fescue seed for planting	Cattle and sheep mostly Highest occurrence in fall and winter in all fescue pasture
Grass tetany (hypomagnesemia)	Disorientation Paddling Convulsions Muscle twitching	Most common in cows 4 yr and older ↑ Occurrence during early lactation in heavy milking cows Pastures with ↓ Mg^{2+} and ↑ K^+ and ↓ Ca^+ availability	Start providing Mg^{2+} 30 days before high-risk times ↑ Mg^{2+} in lactating and older cows and ewes Highest risk spring, winter, and fall Molasses supplement with Mg^{2+} may be required	Stress front weather, movement, or environment increases risk
Milk fever (parturition, paresis, or hypocalcemia)	↓ Appetite Nervous behavior Collapse Wrenching of head toward back	Postcalving in high-producing cows ↓ Blood Ca^{2+}	Feed ↑ P, ↓ Ca^{2+} 14 days before parturition Feed balanced Ca^{2+}/P rations Vitamin D intake 1 wk before parturition Avoid obesity	Watch Ca^{2+} and P levels in dry periods

Condition	Clinical signs	Causes	Prevention/Treatment	Comments
Displaced abomasum	↓ Appetite ↓ Milk production Diarrhea, discolored feces	Pregnancy Lack of bulk in diet Sudden jarring of fresh cows Poor muscle tone	Avoid acidosis or alkalosis Eliminate or reduce moldy or mycotoxin-laden feeds	Occurs most frequently in high-producing, heavily fed dairy cattle near parturition
Ketosis	Occurs: 14-50 days after parturition in cattle 2 wk before parturition in sheep ↓ Milk production ↓ Appetite Sugary-acid breath ↓ Body weight Frequent urination Trembling Collapse	Mycotoxin exposure ↑ Chances in multiple births with ewes and does Rapid loss of body fat and low availability of carbohydrates in diet	Maintain lean body condition and avoid excess fat ↑ Energy intake before parturition and ↓ after parturition Avoid sudden changes in the physical nature of the feeds	Ewes at risk before lambing Cows typically at risk after calving
Thiamine-deficiency polio	Decreased vision Incoordination Acute death Excitable	Thiamine deficiency Overgrazing Feeding lambs in rich pasture	Cause not fully discovered ↓ Grain intake while ↑ roughage quality, 1 wk before ↑ Animals' intake of high-energy diets	Primarily feedlot and young cattle under 2 yr old Goats may be affected while nursing young
Rickets	In young animals, enlarged joints Painful gait Leg bowing	Incorrect Ca^{2+}, P, vitamin intake	Provide balanced Ca^{2+}, P, and vitamin D diets	
Urinary calculi Urolithiasis	Difficult urination Bloody urine	↑ Increase in feedlots High K^+ consumption, ↑ P, ↓ Ca^{2+}	Readily available water Balance P/Ca^{2+} ratio	Males have ↑ risk
Water belly	Kicking at abdomen Rupture of bladder	Vitamin A deficiency Excess silicate intake	Avoid vitamin A deficiency ↑ Salt availability Balanced ratios	
White muscle disease	Irregular gait Hunched-back appearance Heart irregularities Death	Selenium deficiency Geographic distribution: ↓ Se in many areas of United States and Canada	↑ Se to dietary intake in known deficient areas	Most common in most rapidly growing individuals in flock or herd

From Naylor JM et al: *Large animal clinical nutrition*, St Louis, 1991, Mosby; McDonald P et al: *Animal nutrition*, New York, 1995, Longman Scientific and Technical; Maynard LA et al: *Animal nutrition*, ed 7, New York, 1979, McGraw-Hill; Ensminger ME et al: *Feeds and nutrition*, Clovis, Calif, 1990, Ensminger Publishing.

feeding standards are updated and published by a committee appointed by the NRC.

> ### Technician Note
> MNRs are the level of nutrients needed to sustain body weight without gain or loss.

Digestion (the process of protein, carbohydrate, and fat breakdown into absorbable nutrients) is accomplished by both chemical and physical methods. It is essential to remember that it is not the alfalfa hay, corn, or oats that is actually used by the cells of livestock but rather the digested and absorbed nutrients, such as amino acids, sugars, fatty acids, minerals, and vitamins, that present at the cellular level. The quality, quantity, and cost of nutrients that can be provided by the feedstuff are of primary importance when choosing ingredients for farm animal feeding.

PROTEIN

Protein is the principal constituent of organs and soft tissues. It is constructed of building blocks called *amino acids* that are linked together in a chain. The arrangement of amino acids in the chain and the length of the chain are two factors that help to determine the composition of the protein. There are 10 essential and 12 nonessential amino acids. Essential amino acids must be supplied in the diet because the animal body cannot synthesize them fast enough to meet its requirement. Amino acids consist of nitrogen, carbon, oxygen, and sulfur. The deconstruction or deamination process releases these elements into the body system and results in either their elimination from the body or their use as energy.

> ### Technician Note
> Protein is a common component of plants, with highest constituency in the seed and leafy portions.

Animal feeds (Box 15-2) are identified often by crude protein content, but the measurement rarely illustrates the quality or utilization potential of the protein. A feed can possess a high protein content, yet the *biologic value* of that protein is low. Protein biologic value is the percentage of true absorbed protein that is available for productive body functions. Conceptually, it is the "amino acid grade card," since it defines the available amino acids. In general, proteins of animal origin have greater biologic value than do proteins of plant origin. The higher the biologic value, the better is the protein used for productive purposes. Protein quality is also measured as *protein efficiency ratio*, which is the number of grams of body weight gain per unit of protein consumed (McDonald, 1995).

Animal and plant proteins vary greatly in their distribution of amino acids and biologic value. When combined in correct proportions with other protein (e.g., animal protein), proteins that individually have very poor biologic value (e.g., corn) may yield a biologic value similar to that of a single high-quality protein. The quality of proteins depends on disallowing overprocessing of feeds, overheating in storage, and form of the feed (Nash, 1985) (Figure 15-1).

Protein Use by Ruminants

Rumen digestion facilitated by microbes has the ability to convert most feed protein into peptides and amino acids,

Box 15-2	RELATIVE IMPORTANCE OF LIVESTOCK FEEDS (% OF TOTAL TONNAGE FED)	
Pasture/grasslands	40.0%*	
Corn	23.3%	
Hay	12.2%	
Grains/high-protein feeds	16.9%	
Silage/miscellaneous	7.6%	

From the U.S. Department of Agriculture (USDA) Economic Research Service, 1983-1984.
*Varies significantly by season and pasture quality.

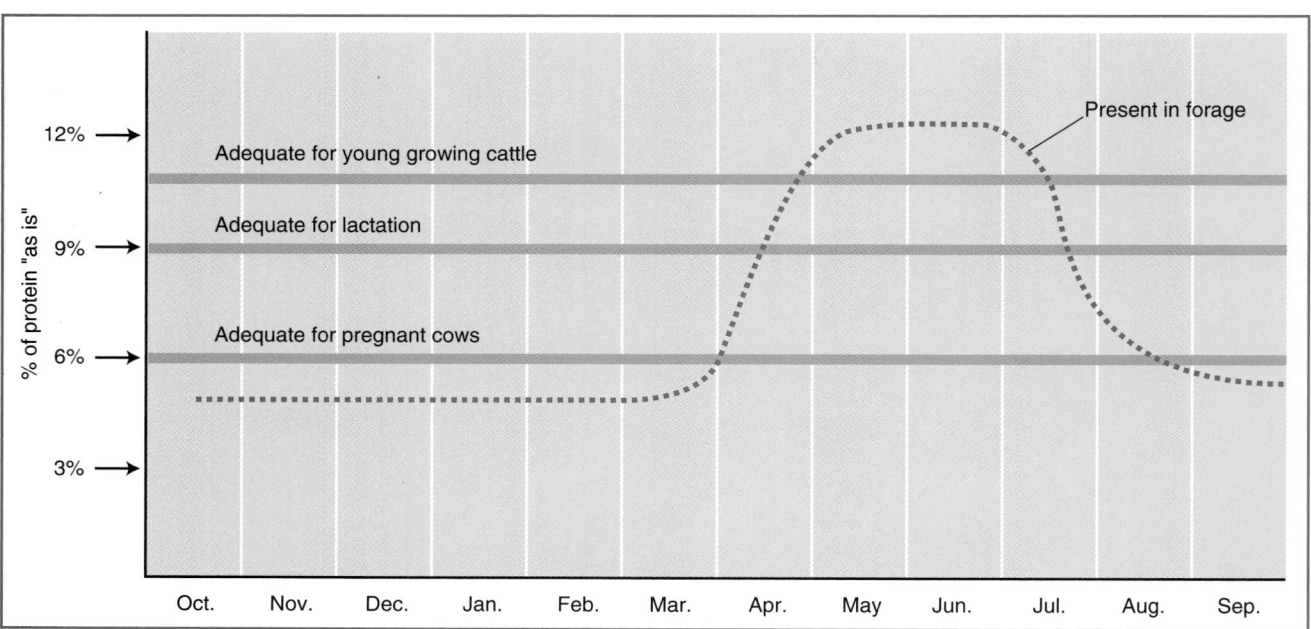

FIGURE 15-1.   Nutrient content of forage varies with pasture quality and season.

many of which are further degraded into ammonia, organic acids, and carbon dioxide. The ammonia released on microbial degradation of feed protein will be removed from the rumen by absorption through the rumen wall or used by the microorganisms for synthesis of microbial protein. Microbial protein synthesized by the microorganisms results in a fairly constant protein quality supply to the lower digestive tract. The protein quality from moderate to poor feeds will usually be improved by rumen metabolism, whereas the opposite may occur with high-quality protein feeds. The rumen microbes also have the ability to convert nonprotein nitrogen sources into microbial protein. Typical nonprotein nitrogen sources include urea, ammonium salts, ammoniated byproducts, or free amino acids and are best used judiciously because an excess or an imbalanced intake can be toxic (Church, 1984).

FATS

Fats provide dietary energy; serve as a source of heat, insulation, and protection for the animal body; and provide essential fatty acids. Fat has 2.25 times more energy per gram than protein or carbohydrates. Fats also aid the absorption of fat-soluble vitamins. Linoleic, linolenic, and arachidonic fatty acids are considered essential, even though linoleic acid is capable of being converted to arachidonic acid. However, the process to make these conversions is arduous and inefficient, and as such, arachidonic acid should be considered conditionally essential (McDonald, 1995).

Technician Note

Fat has more energy per gram than all other nutrients.

CARBOHYDRATES

Carbohydrates (Box 15-3) are the primary energy source in livestock rations. They are less expensive and more readily available than proteins or fats. Most feedstuffs of plant origin are high in carbohydrate content, especially cereal grains. Carbohydrates must be broken down into simple sugars for absorption from the digestive system. This requires digestive enzymes generated by the host or by microflora inhabiting the digestive system of the host. The carbohydrate-splitting enzymes are effective in splitting most complex carbohydrates into simple sugars except those with the beta linkage, as found in cellulose (fiber). Microflora in the rumen of ruminants and the cecum of some nonruminants, such as the horse or rabbit, produce an enzyme so that these species can use fiber for energy. Carbohydrates are commonly categorized into animal feeds as concentrates (grains, high-starch compounds) and forages (grass, hays, legumes). There are no minimum or maximum requirements for carbohydrates; rather, intake is defined in conjunction with energy need.

Technician Note

Carbohydrates are the primary energy source in livestock rations.

Feedstuff Energy

The largest function of feed is to provide energy for body processes. Total digestible nutrients (TDNs), gross energy, digestible energy, metabolizable energy, and net energy are all different measures of feed energy value.

TDN is a general measure of the nutritive value of a feed. Digestibility coefficients are used to compute the content of total digestible nutrients. The usefulness of TDN as a measure of feed energy is limited in that it does not take into account energy losses in urine, combustible gases, and heat. The discrepancies can be large for forage-based feeds, because they tend to overestimate the energy available for productive purposes. TDN is expressed as a percentage of the ration or in units of weight and not as an actual caloric number.

Gross energy (GE) is the total energy (Box 15-4) potentially available in a feed consumed by an animal. All energy values used in the following scheme are expressed in kilocalories (kcal) or megacalories (Mcal) per unit of weight. During digestion and absorption, a portion of the GE escapes the body in the form of undigested food residue in the feces. Subtraction of the energy lost in the feces from the consumed GE accounts for energy that was digested and absorbed, or *digestible energy (DE)*. The measurement of DE uses the same elements as TDN and gives similar energy values to feed. Energy that is digested and absorbed by the body is not used with 100% efficiency; a portion of the absorbed energy is lost in the urine and as combustible gases. Accounting for these energy losses leads to a step beyond DE or TDN, *metabolizable energy (ME)*. The energy values for ME are used widely in the formulation of equine and poultry feeds. One further refinement in this energy scheme is accounting for heat lost from the body during metabolism of the nutrients. *Net energy (NE)* represents the actual portion of energy available to the animal for use in maintaining body tissues or during pregnancy or lactation. NE values are used extensively in the beef, dairy, and sheep industry.

MINERALS AND VITAMINS

Minerals and vitamins are needed in small amounts compared with other nutrients but play integral roles in many metabolic processes. Minerals are divided into two categories: microminerals and macrominerals (Box 15-5). The list of minerals and vitamins and their functions are given in Tables 15-2 to 15-4.

WATER

Water is the cheapest and most abundant nutrient. It makes up 65% to 85% of an animal's body weight at birth

Box 15-3	CATEGORIES OF CARBOHYDRATES

Fiber-forages: Structural carbohydrates, cellulose, hemicellulose
Sugars (molasses, growing plants): Glucose, sucrose, fructose
Starches: Stored carbohydrates, grains

Box 15-4	VARIABLES AFFECTING ENERGY REQUIREMENTS

Activity
Environment
Body size
Life stage
Reproductive status

and 45% to 60% of body weight at maturity. Water is derived metabolically from the breakdown of organic nutrients in the animal tissues or drinking water or obtained from foodstuffs (Figure 15-2). Because water is the largest constituent of the animal, deprivation of water of only a few percentages of body weight is life threatening. Clean, fresh water should be readily available to maintain a zero water balance (Table 15-5).

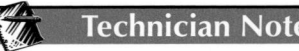

Technician Note

Water is the cheapest and most abundant nutrient.

DAIRY CATTLE

The dairy industry is successfully using many different production systems. Systems are based on geographic area and feedstuff availability. The traditional pasture system continues to be used in areas with readily available land, whereas dry lot systems are more popular in urban and suburban areas (Figure 15-3).

Regardless of the dairy production system, two feeding

Box 15-5   MINERAL CATEGORIES

MACROMINERALS*	MICROMINERALS†	
Salt (sodium chloride; NaCl)	Zinc (Zn)	Copper (Cu)
Potassium (K)	Selenium (Se)	Iron (Fe)
Phosphorus (P)	Manganese (Mn)	Silicon (Si)
Magnesium (Mg)	Iodine (I)	Molybdenum (Mo)
Calcium (Ca)	Fluorine (F)	
Sulfur (S)	Chromium (Cr)	Cobalt (Co)

*Measured in kg.
†Measured in ppm or μg.

TABLE 15-2   MACROMINERALS FOR FOOD ANIMALS

Minerals	Use	Toxicity	Deficiency	Sources
Calcium	Nerve transmission Clotting cascade Cardiac function Muscle contraction Milk production	Calcium kidney stones ↑ Calcium deposition into soft tissue ↑ Blood calcium level ↓ Absorption of Zn, Mg, Fe, Cu	↓ Quality of bone/teeth ↓ Milk production Osteomalacia Osteoporosis Hypocalcemia (tetany) Rickets	Alfalfa Milk Fish by-products Soybean meal Bone meal Dicalcium phosphate supplement
Phosphorus	Milk secretion Building muscle Teeth/bone development Acid-base balance Protein metabolism	↓ Absorption of Ca Urinary stones if Ca is low	Similar to Ca Osteomalacia Rickets Hematuria Pica ↓ Breeding ↓ capability	Meat meals Soybean oil meal Wheat bran Bone meal Monosodium phosphate supplement
Sodium	Muscle contraction Absorption of carbohydrates Part of sweat and bile Osmotic pressure Acid-base balance Water balance	↑ Toxicity with ↓ H_2O intake Staggering Blindness Hypertension Neurologic disorders	↓ Breeding capability Cravings: urine drinking ↓ Growth rate ↓ Milk production Weight loss ↓ Appetite	Molasses Meat by-products Salt/mineral blocks Monosodium glutamate supplement
Potassium	Heart function Insulin secretion Acid-base balance Muscle development	↓ Heart rate ↓ Mg use Exaggerated when ↓ Mg and H_2O restricted	↓ Growth Excess NaCl depletes K Irregular gait Pica ↓ Weight	Molasses Forages Soy byproducts Carrots Potassium gluconate supplement
Chlorine	Water balance Osmotic pressure Acid-base balance HCl production in stomach	↑ When water is restricted Rare	↓ Appetite ↓ Growth Alkalosis ↓ Respiratory rate Muscle cramps Convulsions Alfalfa	Meat meals Molasses Salt blocks (NaCl) Potassium chloride supplement
Magnesium	Cellular energy metabolism Alkalinizer Nerve impulse relaxant Bone and teeth	Rare	↑ Grass tetany ↑ Body temperature Respiratory rate Hypersalivation Death	Meat/bone meal Molasses Wheat bran Alfalfa supplements
Sulfur	Carbohydrate metabolism Insulin production Hair and wool production	Hydrogen sulfide gas production	↓ Growth ↓ Hair/wool production	Meat meal Yeast Whey Supplements

TABLE 15-3	MICROMINERALS FOR FOOD ANIMALS			
Minerals	**Use**	**Toxicity**	**Deficiency**	**Sources**

Zinc	Skin
	Hair
	Bone maintenance
	Synthesis of protein
	Development of
	  reproductive organs
		↓ Growth
		Anemia
		Bone changes
		↑ Appetite
		Stiff gait
			↓ Growth
			↓ Appetite
			Bone irregularities
			↓ Wound healing
			Wool and hair loss
			Parakeratosis
				Meat meal
				Corn gluten or germ
				  meal
				Wheat by-products
				  supplements

Selenium	Vitamin and sparing-
	  tissue damage
	Fatty acid oxidation
		Weight loss
		Blind staggers
		Lameness
		Anemia
		Paralysis
			White muscle disease
			  (sheep)
			Liver necrosis (pigs)
				Poultry/fish meals
				Wheat by-products
				Cereals
				Oil seed meals

Manganese	Bone/cartilage growth Clotting cascade Metabolism of nutrients	Nontoxic	↓ Growth Lameness Reproductive disorders	Wheat Grass/alfalfa/hay Corn Sorghum supplements
Iodine	Hormone production Influence growth Muscle tissue development Milk production Nutrient metabolism	Horse: Hyperparathyroidism Goiter ↓ Utilization of iodine	↓ Hair quality ↓ Growth Reproductive problems Abortion	Molasses Meat/bone meal Oats Wheat Iodized salt Soybean meal
Fluorine	Bone Teeth	↓ Feed use ↓ Hair/wool quality Deformed teeth/bone	Rare	Fish meals Present in most foods

Chromium	Synthesis of some fatty
	  acids
	↑ Insulin use
	Stabilizes DNA
	  and RNA
		Rare	Hyperglycemia
			  glucosuria
			↓ Fat metabolism
				Wheat
				Potatoes
				Corn
				Vegetable oil
				Supplements

Copper	Pigment of hair/wool
	Reproduction
	Skeletal structure
	Hemoglobin
	  construction
	Absorption of iron
		Although rare,
		  sometimes seen in
		  sheep ingestion of
		  copper foot bath
		Gastroenteritis
		Hypersalivation
		? Appetite
		Thirst
			Swayback (lambs)
			↓ Wool quality
			Lameness
			Anemia
			Diarrhea
				Safflower oil
				Molasses
				Grass hays
				Cotton seeds
				Mineral mix

Iron	Hemoglobin
	  production
	Muscle oxygenation
	Enzyme activation
		Irregularity in red
		  blood cell
		  production
		Reproductive disorders
			Anemia
			Pica
			Diarrhea
			↓ Hair coat quality
			↓ Iron in milk
				Fish/meat meals
				Safflower
				Alfalfa
				Corn gluten meal
				Supplements

Silicon	Skeletal development	Calculi formation	Skeletal abnormalities	Meat by-products Grains

Molybdenum	Metabolism of fats,
	  carbohydrates,
	  proteins
	Growth promotion
	Enamel production
		Diarrhea
		↓ Weight
		↓ Hair quality
		↓ Reproduction
			Rare	Grass/alfalfa/hay
				Meat meal
				Corn
				Oats
				Wheat

Cobalt	Formation of vita- min B$_{12}$	Rare	↓ Skin/hair coat quality Abortion ↓ Milk ↓ Appetite	Soybean meal Meat/poultry meal Corn Wheat Molasses

TABLE 15-4	VITAMINS FOR LIVESTOCK			
Water Soluble	**Function**	**Toxicity**	**Deficiency**	**Sources**
B COMPLEX				
Biotin	Metabolism of carbohydrates, fats, proteins Enzyme activities	No known toxicity	↓ Growth ↓ Hair quality Lameness ↓ Reproduction	Young grasses Safflower meal Soybean meal supplements
Thiamine (vitamin B_1)	Coenzyme of energy metabolism Peripheral nerve function Maintenance/assistance of appetite	No known toxicity	Heart irregularities ↓ Body temperature	Wheat Millet Oil seed meals Oats Supplements
Pyridoxine (vitamin B_6)	Nitrogen metabolism Fat and carbohydrate metabolism	Nontoxic	Anorexia ↓ Growth Eye discharge Anemia	Green pastures Meat/fish meals Corn gluten meal Safflower meal Alfalfa
Cobalamin (vitamin B_{12})	Red blood cell formation Maintenance of nerve tissue DNA synthesis	Nontoxic	↓ Coordination (blackleg: pigs) ↓ Reproduction	Fish/meat meals Whey Brewer's yeast supplements
Niacin	Growth ↓ Cholesterol levels Release of energy from fats, proteins, carbohydrates	Nontoxic	↓ Growth ↓ Appetite Diarrhea Unthriftiness	Wheat barley Yeast supplements
Folic acid	Construction of hemoglobin Manipulation of protein Choline synthesis	Nontoxic	Anemia Diarrhea ↓ Growth	Soybean meal Alfalfa Wheat Meat/fish meal Supplement
Pantothenic acid	Metabolism of fats, protein, carbohydrates Hemoglobin production Maintenance of normal blood levels	Nontoxic	Neurologic disorder Goose stepping (swine) ↓ Hair quality Enteritis	Wheat bran Alfalfa Safflower meal Supplements
Riboflavin (vitamin B_2)	Metabolism of amino acids and fatty acids Retinal pigment Adrenal function	Nontoxic	↓ Growth Moon blindness (horses) Anemia Unthriftiness ↓ Reproduction (swine)	Alfalfa Green pastures Sweet/white clover Supplements
Vitamin C	Absorption of iron Metabolism of folic acid Antioxidant Teeth/bone integrity	Rare in food animals	↓ Wound healing Hemorrhage Enlarged joints Ulcerated gums	Green pastures Hay Potatoes

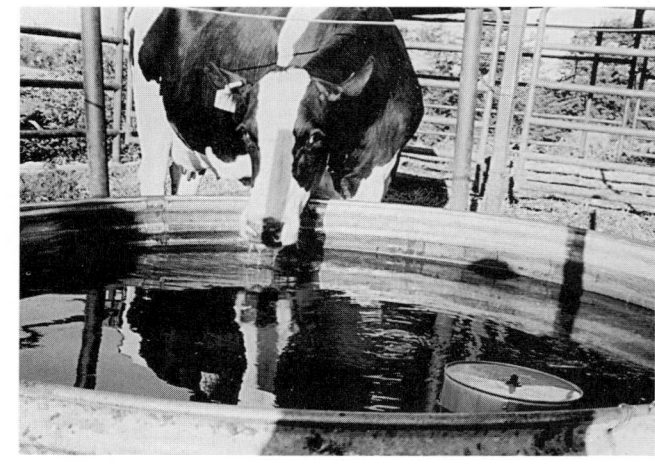

FIGURE 15-2. It is essential that fresh water is readily available to dairy cows to obtain maximum milk production. This watering system maintains an agitator to keep water from becoming stagnant.

TABLE 15-5	WATER CONSUMPTION GUIDELINES	
Species	**Weight (lb)**	**Consumption (gal/day)**
SWINE		
Pigs	30-125	0.3-2.0
Feeder pigs	126-200	2.0-3.2
Finisher pigs	201-250	3.2-4.0
Sow/boar maintenance	150-400	1.3-3.5
	401-600	3.5-5.2
Sow: late gestation	250-400	4.5-5.0
	401-600	5.0-7.5
Sow: lactation	250-400	5.5-6.5
	401-600	6.5-9.8
SHEEP		
Lambs	20-50	0.4-0.6
Feeder lambs	50-110	0.5-1.4
Finisher lambs	111-125	1.4-1.8
Ewes: grain and hay intake*		
Maintenance	150-300	0.3-1.2
Lactation	150-300	0.5-2.4
Rams: grain and hay intake	150-300	0.3-2.0
CATTLE		
Calves	100-200	1.2-2.5
	201-400	2.5-4.9
Developing steers/heifers	401-600	4.5-6.2
	601-800	6.0-8.2
	801-1000	8.0-9.8
Finishing steers		
Pasture	1001-1200	8.5-10.2
Maintenance	800-1000	3.6-4.6
	1001-1200	4.4-7.2
	1201-1400	5.0-7.2
	1401-1600	6.0-9.0
Cows: late gestation	800-1000	4.4-5.5
	1001-1200	5.3-6.6
	1201-1400	6.4-7.9
	1401-1600	7.7-9.5
Beef cows/heifer lactation	800-1000	6.7-15.6
	1001-1200	8.3-18.8
	1201-1400	10.0-21.8
	1401-1600	11.7-25.0
Dairy cows/heifer peak lactation†	800-1000	14.8-20.6
	1001-1201	18.5-24.3
	1201-1400	22.5-28.8
	1401-1600	28.0-32.2
	1601-1800	30.5-36.0

*Intake is influenced dramatically by factors found in table. Table is intended as a guideline.
†Dairy cattle intake varies on milk production more than beef cattle.

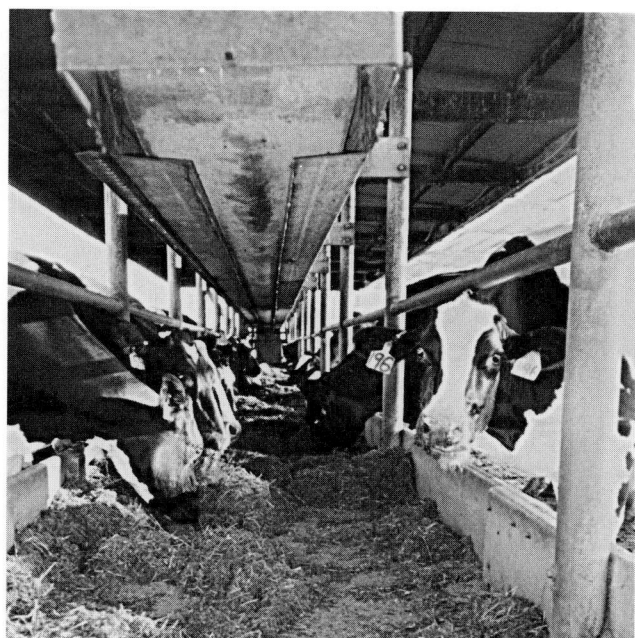

FIGURE 15-3. Large quantities of forage are ingested by dairy cows on a daily basis and are paramount to fulfillment of energy requirements.

good feeding program is necessary for profitable milk production. Nutrient requirements for lactation are large and often several times the MNR (Figure 15-4 and Tables 15-6 to 15-8). Water is also important for dairy cows (Boxes 15-6 and 15-7).

Technician Note

Feed represents 50% of the total costs of milk production.

Energy

Carbohydrates (forage, concentrate) are the major energy source for lactation, followed by fats and proteins. Carbohydrates constitute 50% to 80% of energy on a dry matter basis of many forages and grains. Forages possess a significant fiber content that is broken down by the microbial population in the rumen and used as energy (Figure 15-5).

Although the rumen capacity of the dairy cow is considerable, she cannot eat sufficient forage to meet her extensive nutrient needs during lactation. Estimated daily intake for forages is based on body weight and forage quality. A guide for estimating consumption of forage (dry matter basis) fed on a free-choice basis is in Box 15-8 and Table 15-9.

If cows are allowed to consume all the forage they want, they will not have sufficient rumen capacity to consume enough concentrate to meet the energy requirements needed for lactation. In general, most dairy farmers try to feed forage at a rate of 1.75% of body weight. The concentrate fed with the forage will vary with the kind of forage offered (a high-protein concentrate will be needed with a low-protein forage) and the availability and cost of the feedstuffs. The concentrate provides more energy and usually is higher in protein than the forage. Fat utilization varies with age, environment, and reproductive status.

programs predominate. Total mixed ration (TMR) is the practice of weighing and blending all feedstuffs into a complete ration. Each bite consumed by the cow contains all the required levels of nutrients needed. The other program is a forage and grain diet fed separately. The animals are provided hay free choice at all times, silage is offered once or twice per day, and feed concentrates are fed twice daily.

Feeding, more than any other single factor, determines the productivity of lactating dairy cows. Feed represents about 50% of the total cost of milk production. Therefore a

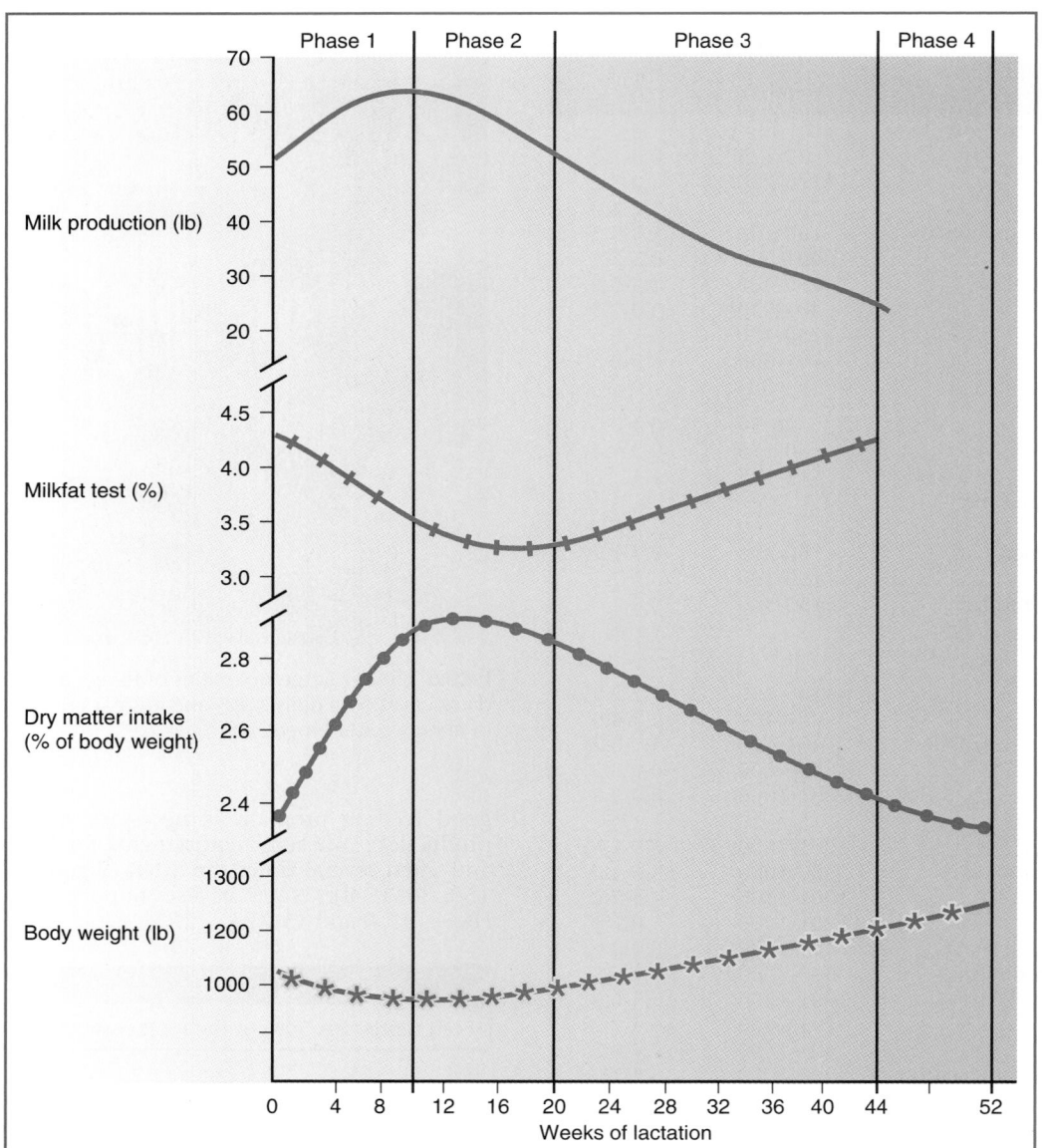

FIGURE 15-4.   Milk production varies during a typical 52-week production phase. Disparity is also observed in milk fat content, dry matter intake requirements, and body weight.

TABLE 15-6	DAILY FEEDING CONSIDERATIONS IN DEVELOPING FEMALE DAIRY CATTLE*				
Weight (lb)	NE (Mcal)†	Total Crude Protein (%)	Minerals‡		
			Ca²⁺	P	
200-399	6.4-11.5	16-18	15-18	9-15	
400-599	11.5-15.4	12-16	18-23	13-15	
600-799	15.4-19.5	12-14	23-24	15-17	
800-999	19.5-23.9	12-14	24-26	17-18	
1000-1199	23.9-28.4	12-14	26-28	18-19	
1200-1399	28.4-33.8	12-14	28-30	19-21	

*Ranges shown in table are to be used as guidelines, recognizing that variations can occur as a result of breed, milk production levels, butter fat content, rate of gain, and lactation cycle.
†Net energy (NE) expressed in megacalories (Mcal).
‡Ca^{2+}/ phosphorus ratio needs to be maintained from 0.43% to 0.66%; levels above 0.95% to 100% can result in decreased performance and metabolic abnormalities.

TABLE 15-7	DAILY GUIDELINES FOR LACTATING DAIRY COWS*					
					Minerals‡	
Weight (lb)	Milk Yield (lb)	NE (Mcal)†	Total Crude Protein (%)		Ca^{2+}	P
800	15-45	13.1-21.6	12-16		40-77	25-49
	45-60	21.6-25.8	16-17		77-96	49-61
	61-75	25.8-34.0	16-18		96-115	61-78
1000	20-40	14.9-20.3	12-16		44-70	29-44
	41-70	20.3-25.6	16-18		70-114	44-73
	71-90	25.6-36.3	16-18		114-146	73-86
1200	20-40	17.0-23.7	12-16		50-81	33-52
	41-60	23.7-30.3	16-18		81-110	52-70
	61-80	30.3-37.0	16-18		110-139	70-87
1400	50-75	27.7-35.7	15-17		95-131	62-83
	76-100	35.7-43.7	16-18		131-165	83-104
	101-125	43.7-51.7	16-18		165-200	104-126
1600	60-90	31.0-40.0	15-17		108-146	69-92
	91-120	40.0-48.3	16-18		146-184	92-116
	121-150	48.3-57.0	16-18		184-221	116-137
1800	60-90	40.9-44.6	16-18		121-164	78-104
	91-120	44.6-54.4	16-18		164-207	104-131
	121-150	54.4-64.1	16-18		207-249	131-157

*Mineral values assume that balance has been established. Variations occur with breed, lactation phase, milk yield, and age. This table is designed to be used only as a guideline. Feed to maintain body condition. Table assumes a 4% milk fat content of lactation.
†Net energy (NE) measured in megacalories (Mcal).

TABLE 15-8	DAILY NUTRIENT CONSIDERATIONS FOR DAIRY CATTLE*					
		Total Crude	Minerals (g)		Vitamins (1000 IU)	
Weight (lb)	ME† (Mcal)	Protein (g)	Ca^{2+}	P	A	D
FEMALES: 60 DAYS BEFORE GESTATION						
800-1000	13.8-16.4	850-925	24-30	16-18	30-35	12-14
1000-1200	16.4-19.2	925-1000	30-35	18-22	35-42	14-17
1200-1400	19.2-21.5	1000-1100	35-42	22-26	42-48	17-19
1400-1600	21.5-23.6	1100-1200	42-45	26-30	48-56	19-22
DAIRY BULLS						
1000-1300	14.3-17.8	775-900	16-20	10-12	17.00-21.00	2.7-3.3
1301-1500	17.8-19.7	900-1000	20-24	12-15	21.00-25.25	3.3-3.9
1501-1700	19.7-21.6	1000-1125	24-28	15-18	25.25-29.50	3.9-4.6
1701-1900	21.6-23.5	1125-1225	28-32	18-20	29.50-33.75	4.6-5.3
1901-2100	23.5-25.3	1225-1325	32-36	20-22	33.75-38.00	5.3-5.9
2101-2300	25.3-27.0	1325-1425	36-40	22-25	38.00-42.50	5.9-6.6
2301-2500	27.0-28.8	1425-1520	40-44	25-28	42.50-46.60	6.6-7.3
2501-2700	28.0-30.4	1520-1610	44-48	28-30	46.60-50.90	7.3-7.9
2701-2900	30.4-32.1	1610-1700	48-52	30-32	50.90-55.10	7.9-8.6

*Ranges shown in table are to be used as guidelines recognizing that variations can occur because of milk production levels, butter fat content, rate of gain, and lactation cycle.
†Metabolizable energy (ME) measured in megacalories (Mcal).
‡Ca^{2+}/phosphorus ratio needs to be maintained from 0.43% to 0.66%; levels above 0.95% to 100% can result in decreased performance and metabolic abnormalities.

BOX 15-6	FACTORS AFFECTING WATER INTAKE

Dry matter intake
Reproductive status
Activity
Type of feeding regimen
Environment
Weight
Age
Rate of gain

BOX 15-7	IMPORTANCE OF WATER

- For digestion, absorption, and utilization of nutrients
- For production requirements
- Watering methods
  - Free water always available
  - Twice daily watering
- Cleanliness
  - Water heaters in winter to prevent freezing
  - Troughs kept clean

Fat intake during lactation can be 5% to 6% of total energy intake. Excessive dietary fat intake can negatively affect rumen microbial activity, depressing fiber utilization (Shirley, 1986).

Protein

Restriction of protein or energy during lactation can lead to reduced milk production and increased reproductive problems. Protein is supplied by the forage or concentrate and should be added at levels to ensure that minimum protein requirements are met (see Tables 15-6 to 15-8). Protein intake that exceeds the requirement is used as energy at a premium value. Protein is an expensive nutrient and is not an economic source of energy. Most cows are fed a high-protein legume hay, such as alfalfa, and grain, which should supply most or all the protein needs during lactation. Nonprotein nitrogen supplied as urea also can be an

effective feedstuff to supply protein equivalents in dairy rations.

Minerals and Vitamins

Milk is composed of 0.7% minerals on a dry weight basis. The average cow will lactate 140 lb of mineral as a portion of the milk produced per year. Balanced mineral intake is essential; mineral requirements for lactation are given in Tables 15-6 to 15-8.

Rumen microorganisms can synthesize the water-soluble vitamins, whereas vitamin K is the only fat-soluble vitamin readily synthesized by microorganisms. The supplementation of water-soluble vitamins or vitamin K normally is not necessary in rations for ruminants.

Forages of good quality and properly harvested normally contain adequate levels of vitamin E and the precursor of vitamin A, carotene. Vitamin A is stored for extended periods in the body. Vitamin D is synthesized through ultraviolet radiation by the skin or added to a dairy ration as sun-cured forage or a vitamin supplement.

Although water-soluble vitamins are synthesized by the rumen microflora, some evidence indicates that supplemental thiamin, choline, and niacin may be beneficial in cows undergoing heavy stress or various disease states. Daily requirements for vitamins for lactating dairy cows are found in Table 15-8.

DAIRY CALVES

Newborn calves require the mother's colostrum within the first 72 hours of life to acquire energy and maternal immunity from disease. Peak benefits of colostrum intake are realized within the first 24 hours postpartum. Optimally, the first milking colostrum should be given to the calf at 10% to 12% of the calf's weight with at least one half administered within 4 to 6 hours after birth. Colostrum can be successfully frozen and used at a later date as well as diluted equally with water should diarrhea occur because of the richness of the colostrum. The initial sucking of the calf will create a bypass of the rumen, allowing the milk to go directly into the abomasum. This ability will decrease as the calf ages and the rumen becomes functional. Calves normally start on milk replacers and then are offered calf starters within the first week of life. Calf starter rations are commonly fed until about 3 months of age at a rate of 5 to 7 lb of calf starter per day. During the first week of life, a forage source should be added to diet selection as well as free-choice water. Calves are typically weaned at 4 to 8 weeks of age and accustomed to solid food.

BEEF CATTLE

Feeding represents almost three fourths of the cost of production of beef cattle (Neumann, 1977). Beef producers control their profitability by obtaining optimal nutrient intake with least cost feed formulation. Profitability hinges on the ability to balance utilization of resources, such as pasture and feedlot, with the production of high-quality finishing animals generated by the breeding herd. Beef production usually is divided into two primary areas: cow-calf production and finishing cattle.

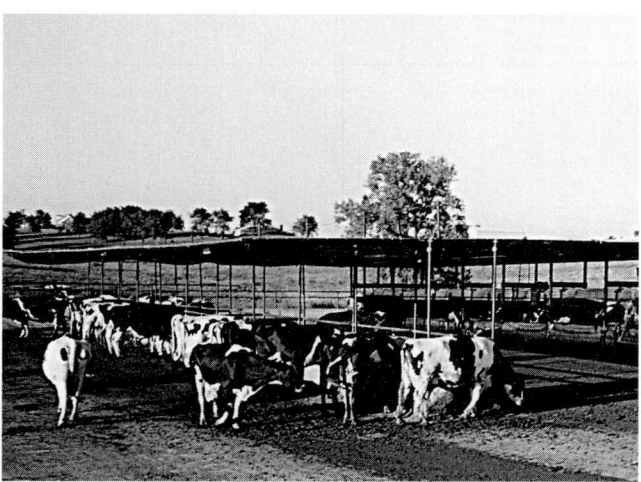

FIGURE 15-5. Shaded feeding area that has a misting system to allow the cows a cool, comfortable environment that facilitates maximum feed intake and utilization.

Box 15-8	FACTORS AFFECTING DRY MATTER INTAKE
Stage of lactation	
Body condition	
Quality of feed	
Environment	
Size of cow	
Milk production	
Feeding regimen	
Age	

TABLE 15-9 FORAGE QUALITY

Forage Quality	Daily Intake (% Body Weight)
Excellent	3.0
Good	2.5
Average	2.0
Fair	1.5
Poor	1.0

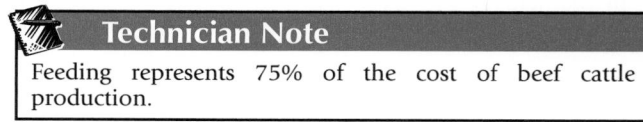

Technician Note

Feeding represents 75% of the cost of beef cattle production.

COW-CALF PRODUCTION

Breeding Herd

A live calf from each cow each year should be the goal of the profitable cow-calf producer. Nutrition has a large impact on the beef breeding herd. Cows gaining weight just before and during the breeding season have a shorter period between calving and the first estrus period and typically have higher conception rates.

Energy

Carbohydrates are the major energy source for beef cows, followed by proteins and fat. Forages commonly fed to beef cows possess a significant fiber content that is broken down by the microbial population in the rumen and used as energy.

Technician Note

Carbohydrates are the major energy source for beef cows.

Feeding beef cows can be very economic because high-quality forage or pasture can supply all energy needs with no need for energy supplementation from grains or fats. In the summer, pasture normally will supply adequate energy for the cow. If pasture is inadequate, supplemental energy should be provided in the form of silage or hay. In the winter, pregnant cows are fed wintering rations (a combination of forages, grain, and a protein source supplemented with vitamins and minerals) to meet energy needs with minimal weight gain. Cows in good condition are more tolerant to the stresses of winter and require less maintenance energy per unit of weight than do cows in poor condition.

Protein

Most pasture, silages, and forages contain adequate levels of protein (Box 15-9) to meet the needs of the breeding cow. If low-grade roughages (e.g., cobs, straw, stalks) are fed over extended periods of time, the ration must be supplemented daily with 1 to 1.5 lb of a 35% to 45% crude protein supplement. A review of deficiency and toxicity signs can be found in Box 15-10 and 15-11.

Box 15-9	TYPICAL GRAIN: NUTRITIONAL OVERVIEW
20% (or less) protein
18% (or less) crude fiber
Variable moisture
85% (or less) carbohydrate
6% (or less) fat
75%-80% TDNs (total digestible nutrients)

Box 15-10	SIGNS OF UNDERNUTRITION
↓ Growth
↓ Hair/skin quality
Skeletal irregularities
↓ Reproductive capabilities
↓ Immune function
Death

Box 15-11	PROTEIN DEFICIENCY AND TOXICITY IN CATTLE
Deficiency
↓ Appetite
Weight loss
↓ Growth
↓ Reproductive capability
↓ Milk production
Toxicity
Ammonia: Avoid >40% excess protein or nonprotein nitrogen (NPN) intake

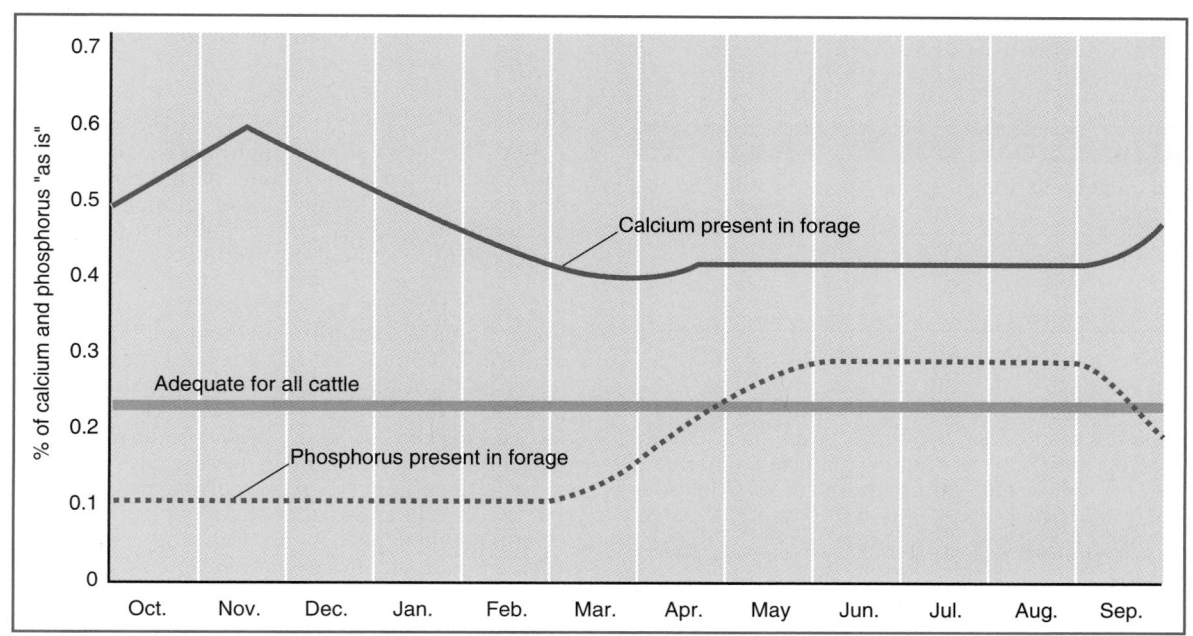

FIGURE 15-6. Calcium and phosphorous availability varies greatly during the seasons of the year and should be supplemented if inadequate amounts are present in livestock forage sources.

Box 15-12   FEEDING CONSIDERATIONS FOR CALVES

DAIRY CALVES
Days 1-3: Colostrum from dam
Days 4-7: Transition to milk replacer or other liquid feed;
   begin offering starter and free-choice water
Days 5-84: Starter and free-choice water through weaning;
   begin offering forage

BEEF CALVES
Ensure calf nurses within 2 hr of birth to obtain vital
   colostrum
Ensure that calf continues to thrive and that cow does not
   show signs of mastitis or decreased milk production

ORPHANS
Can sometimes be grafted to another cow
Ensure that colostrum has been administered
Feed like dairy calves

Minerals and Vitamins

Mineral supplementation will be necessary and is usually offered on a free-choice basis when animals are on pasture (Figure 15-6). Trace-mineral salt blocks and granular salt are popular methods of offering minerals and salt to animals on pasture. Good-quality pasture and roughages are adequate in vitamins A and E with ample levels to meet the needs of breeding cows. Supplemental vitamin A should be provided when low-grade roughages or long-stored hays are used as a major source of energy in wintering rations. There are mineral mixes that contain a stabilized form of vitamin A.

Calves

The basic food for calves consists of the mother's milk (Box 15-12) plus access to pasture or forage fed to the cows. Many cow-calf producers offer calves a highly palatable creep feed to supply additional nutrients, leading to improved weaning weights and decreased weight loss by nursing cows. Creep-fed calves will weigh 30 to 50 extra pounds by weaning time. The greatest response to creep feeding is found when pasture is short or quality is poor. Beef calves generally are weaned at 7 to 8 months of age.

Technician Note

Creep-fed calves can weigh 30 to 50 more pounds by weaning time.

FINISHING CATTLE

The *finishing* of cattle refers to the time in the growth phase of growing cattle when they are fed to produce beef that is desirable to the food consumer. Most finished cattle are between 1 and 2 years of age and weigh more than 1000 lb. The goal of the finishing feeding program is to maintain maximum feed intake and gain without causing digestive upsets (Table 15-10).

Energy

High-energy diets are used to increase weight gain, improve the carcass characteristics, and decrease the cost of energy compared with diets high in fiber. Total dry feed intake commonly will be 2% to 3% of the animal's body

TABLE 15-10   DAILY NUTRIENT CONSIDERATIONS FOR BEEF CATTLE*

Weight (lb)	Net Energy (NE; Mcal)	Total Protein (lb)	Minerals (g) Ca²⁺	Minerals (g) P
GROWING/FINISHING†				
300-400	3.0-3.6	0.75-1.5	10-42	6-8
401-500	3.7-4.4	0.90-1.9	11-40	8-18
501-600	4.4-5.0	1.0-2.0	12-38	9-19
601-700	5.0-5.6	1.1-2.1	13-36	11-19
701-800	5.6-6.2	1.3-2.1	14-34	12-20
801-900	6.2-6.8	1.4-2.2	15-33	14-20
901-1000	6.8-7.3	1.5-2.3	16-37	16-22
1001-1100	7.3-7.5	1.6-2.3	19-35	18-23
1101-1200	7.5-7.8	1.7-2.4	20-34	20-24
1201-1300	7.8-8.4	1.8-2.4	20-32	20-24
YEARLING HEIFERS, EARLY TO LATE GESTATION				
700-800	8.0-8.6	1.3-1.6	19-28	19-22
801-900	8.6-9.1	1.4-1.7	21-28	15-19
901-1000	9.1-9.8	1.5-1.7	20-23	14-20
1001-1100	9.8-10.3	1.5-1.7	23-25	18-20
1101-1200	10.3-10.8	1.6-1.8	25-27	20-21
1201-1300	10.8-11.4	1.6-1.8	26-28	21-23
1301-1400	11.4-12.0	1.8-2.0	26-28	23-24
LACTATING COW/HEIFER				
800-900	10.0-14.0	2.0-2.4	23-35	19-20
901-1000	10.4-14.5	1.9-2.5	24-36	19-20
1001-1100	11.0-15.0	2.0-2.6	25-38	20-22
1101-1200	11.5-15.5	2.0-2.7	27-39	22-23
1201-1300	12.0-16.2	2.1-2.3	23-41	23-25
1301-1400	12.5-17.0	2.2-2.9	30-42	25-26
BREEDING BULLS				
1300-1500	9.3-10.3	2.0-2.2	23-31	22-25
1501-1700	10.3-11.3	1.7-2.2	23-31	22-25
1701-1900	11.3-12.3	2.0-2.2	26-29	26-29
1901-2100	12.3-13.3	2.0-2.3	27-33	27-33

From National Research Council: *Nutrient requirements of beef cattle*, ed 8, Washington, DC, 1990, National Academic Press.
*Values represent guidelines, and individual variations dictate the constant appraisal of body condition to ensure desirable results.
†Assumes medium- to large-frame steers.

weight. The feed contains high levels of grains to supply readily available energy. Cattle fed these rations are more prone to develop digestive upset (rumen acidosis), founder, or liver abscesses and require more attention and management to avoid these problems.

Protein

Protein requirements (9% to 14%) are greatly affected by age, size of animal, and growth rate. Young cattle require higher levels of protein (as a percentage of the diet) than do older cattle. Protein sources cost more than feed grains, but experienced finishing cattle producers know that a protein deficiency is more expensive than a slight protein excess in the ration. When protein is deficient, energy is not well used, and performance suffers.

Supplemental protein for finishing cattle can be provided by natural protein sources or nonprotein nitrogen (e.g., urea). Nonprotein nitrogen sources are used most efficiently by cattle consuming relatively high levels of grain. A normal range of urea intake for many finishing rations is 0.10 to 0.15 lb per animal per day.

Box 15-13	SALT USE IN CATTLE

RULE 1: SUPPLY
3-5 lb in each spring and summer month
1-1.5 lb in each fall and winter month

RULE 2: AVAILABILITY
Make salt available at all times

RULE 3: ROTATION
Continue to rotate salt
Manger throughout pasture

Box 15-14	COMMON SHEEP BREEDS

WOOL BREEDS	MEAT BREEDS	COMBINATION BREEDS
Rambouillet	Suffolk	Polypay
Merino	Dorset	Texel
Debouillet	Hampshire	Tunis
Columbia	Shropshire	Leicester
Targee	Southdown	Cheviot
	Oxford	

Box 15-15	ENERGY INTAKE VARIABLES IN SHEEP

Breed size
Gender
Reproductive status
Weaning age
Multiple birth
Age
Environment
Stress
Shearing
Forage quality

Minerals and Vitamins

Calcium is often added to the high-grain diets fed to finishing cattle. Generally, when forage (especially legumes) constitutes more than 25% of a finishing ration, additional calcium is not required. Grain contains adequate levels of phosphorus to meet the needs of finishing cattle. Finishing rations are balanced to contain a calcium/phosphorus ratio of 2:1 or higher. Salt is added to diets or fed on a free-choice basis to finishing cattle to meet the sodium requirement (Box 15-13). The less forage that is formulated into the diet, the more need there is for trace-mineral supplementation.

High-quality forages contain adequate amounts of vitamin A precursors and vitamin E. Generally, finishing rations are supplemented with 20,000 to 30,000 IU of vitamin A daily because they contain high levels of grain. Vitamins E and D are added to finishing rations when the feed ingredients are devoid of these vitamins or the production practices merit their inclusion (see Table 15-10).

SHEEP

Feeding represents the single largest cost of production for all types of sheep operations. Sheep producers control their revenue by offering feeds that support optimum production, are cost effective, and minimize nutrition-related problems. Sheep production is divided into two principal areas: the breeding flock and lamb production.

Breeding Flock

Ewes are the foundation of the sheep operation; they produce lambs and generate wool (Box 15-14). These two cash crops can be influenced greatly by feeding management. The mature ewe (3 to 8 years of age) needs only sufficient feed to maintain her normal weight from the time her lambs were weaned until 15 weeks (21-week gestation) into her next pregnancy, assuming not much weight was lost during lactation. Pasture is adequate to meet her nutrient needs during this period of production (see Figures 15-1 and 15-6 for reviews of nutrient composition of pasture).

Energy

The energy requirements of the ewe largely depend on the stage of the reproductive cycle (Box 15-15). During the first two thirds of the pregnancy, energy requirements are close to those required for MNR, and good pasture or hays can supply all the energy needs (Box 15-16). In the last trimester, energy requirements increase, and forages must be supplemented with grains. Poor care during the last trimester of pregnancy leads to lambing problems, lower wool output, and depressed milk production. A common problem attributed to poor nutrition in ewes is lambing paralysis or ketosis. Feeding inadequate forages with little

or no grain can create a deficiency of usable carbohydrates during the last trimester of pregnancy in ewes carrying twins or triplets and can lead to paralysis and coma in the mother. Prevention is the least expensive route to avoid pregnancy disease in the breeding flock. Energy requirements are highest during lactation and proportional to the number of lambs the ewe is nursing (Figure 15-7).

Technician Note

A common problem attributed to poor nutrition in ewes is lambing paralysis or ketosis.

Protein

Adequate protein intake ensures good wool production and reproductive function (Box 15-17). The most limiting amino acid for the maturation of wool is methionine; protein ingested by the breeding flock must contain adequate levels of this amino acid. Most pasture, silages, and forages contain adequate levels of protein and amino acids to meet the needs of the breeding flock. If low-grade roughages (e.g., cobs, straw, stalks) are fed over extended periods of time, the ration must be supplemented daily with a protein supplement.

Minerals and Vitamins

Trace-mineral salt blocks and granular salt represent popular methods of offering minerals (Box 15-18) and salt to ewes on pasture. Sheep store copper quite well in various organs and tissues and develop toxicity symptoms to copper more rapidly than other livestock. Care should be taken to avoid exposing sheep to high levels of copper in their trace-mineral source.

Good-quality pasture and roughages are adequate in vitamins A and E with ample levels to meet the needs of the breeding flock. Supplemental vitamin A should be provided when low-grade roughages or long-stored hays are used as a major source of energy in wintering rations.

Box 15-16	ADVANTAGES AND DISADVANTAGES OF PASTURE FEEDING LIVESTOCK

ADVANTAGES
- Provides exercise
- Uses land unsuitable for other purposes
- Decreases diseases transmitted through close contact with other animals
- Decreases feed costs
- Good-quality pastures can provide quality feedstuffs

DISADVANTAGES
- Dependent on soil quality (deficiencies result in poorer quality pasture)
- Large acreage often needed to support animal's energy requirements
- Land may be made valuable for other uses

Box 15-17	VARIABLES IN PROTEIN REQUIREMENTS OF SHEEP

Breed size
Reproductive status
Age
Body condition
Ratio of protein to energy
Nonprotein nitrogen availability

Box 15-18	FEEDING GUIDELINES FOR NONPROTEIN NITROGEN (NPN) USE IN SHEEP

- Balance NPN within total nutritional profile. Feed continuously after 3- to 6-wk transition.
- Avoid sporadic availability.
- Maintain nitrogen/sulfur ratio at not more than 10:1.
- Restrict use to not more than 1.0% dry matter, with one third of total nitrogen ration as NPN.
- Avoid excess intake and possible toxicity.
- Watch NPN levels when they coincide with high roughage intake.

From Ensminger ME et al: *Feeds and nutrition,* Clovis, Calif, 1990, Ensminger Publishing; Maynard LA et al: *Animal nutrition,* ed 7, New York, 1979, McGraw-Hill; McDonald P et al: *Animal nutrition,* New York, 1995, Longman Scientific and Technical; Naylor JM et al: *Large animal clinical nutrition,* St Louis, 1991, Mosby.

Box 15-19	MILK REPLACEMENT FOR LAMBS

OPTIMAL REQUIREMENT
25% to 30% fat
20% to 25% protein derived from milk product
<30% lactose derived from milk product

FEEDING
Provide ration immediately
Ration should be 20% to 24% protein, high in vitamins and minerals, well balanced, and ground fine
NOTE: Avoid cow's milk (too high in lactose)

From Ensminger ME et al: *Feeds and nutrition,* Clovis, Calif, 1990, Ensminger Publishing; Maynard LA et al: *Animal nutrition,* ed 7, New York, 1979, McGraw-Hill; McDonald P et al: *Animal nutrition,* New York, 1995, Longman Scientific and Technical; Naylor JM et al: *Large animal clinical nutrition,* St Louis, 1991, Mosby.

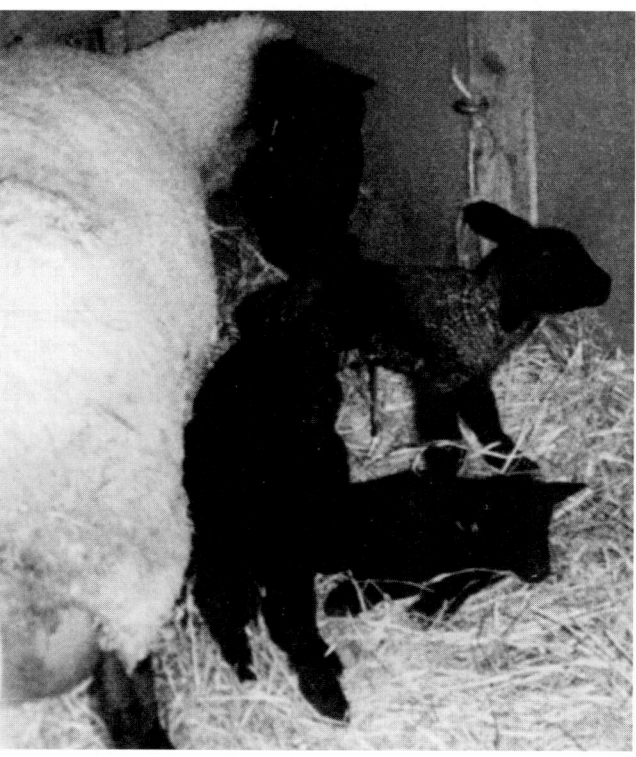

FIGURE 15-7.   Energy requirements of the ewe will vary depending on the number of lambs she must nurse.

Lambs

Lambs must be nursed with colostrum milk within the first hour after birth to improve survivability. Colostrum milk provides immunologic protection and energy for the newborn lamb. The lamb must consume at least 6 to 8 oz of colostrum to receive immunologic protection. Lambs are weaned successfully at 8 weeks of age or earlier.

Technician Note

Lambs must receive colostrum within the first hour after birth to have immunologic protection.

Lambs also can be successfully weaned from their mother at 1 day of age and offered a milk replacer (Box 15-19). They should be weaned from the milk replacer at 3 to 4 weeks of age and transitioned to a high-quality, palatable solid feed. Postweaning rations (until lambs reach 50 lb) should be high-quality protein (16% to 20% crude protein), high energy, and well fortified with vitamins and minerals (Figure 15-8).

Grower (50 to 85 lb) and finisher (more than 85 lb) rations for lambs are normally formulated to contain 15% to 16% and 13% to 14% protein, respectively. A simple ration of shelled corn, long alfalfa hay, and supplement (protein, calcium, vitamins, trace minerals) can be fed to growing-finishing lambs (Figure 15-9). Research does not clearly indicate the need for vitamin additions to rations for early lambs, but it has become a common practice to fortify the rations with vitamins A, D, and E (Table 15-11).

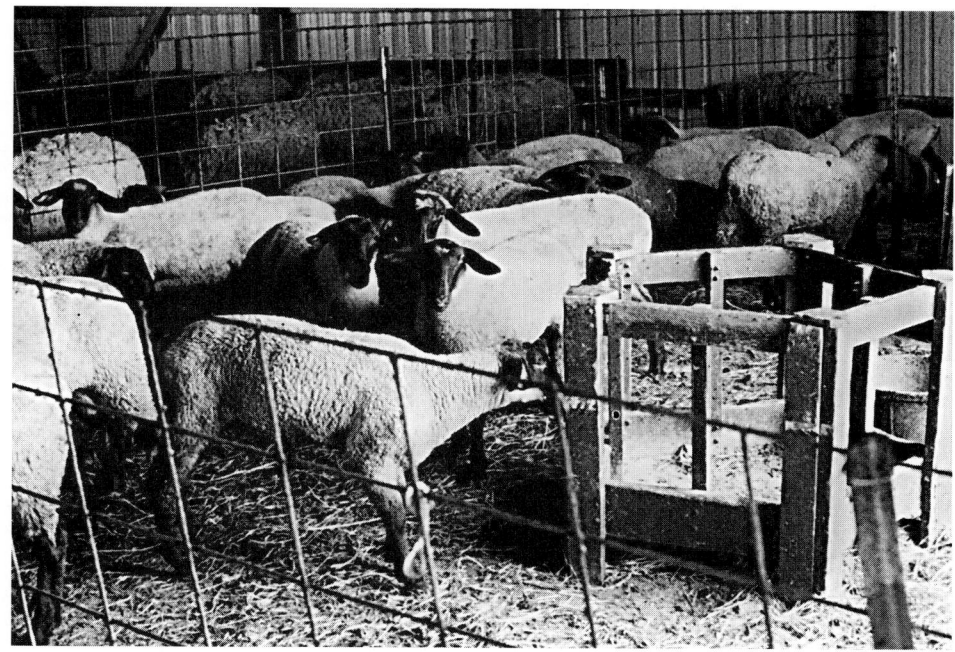

FIGURE 15-8. Optimal feed regimens in the grower-finisher lamb crop will provide excellent results.

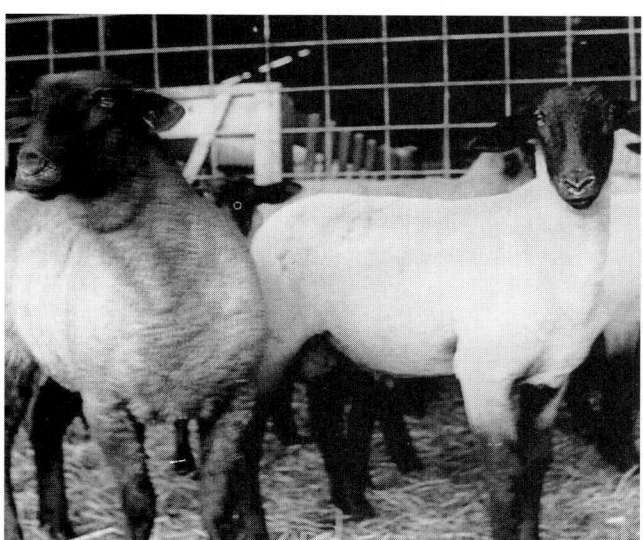

FIGURE 15-9. Growing-finishing lambs.

Large, fast-growing lambs are susceptible to overeating disease (enterotoxemia), which can cause death. This disease is caused by toxins produced by *Clostridium perfringens* and appears to be related to overeating by lambs of a ration high in grain (see Chapter 31). A vaccination with bacterin or toxoid can be used for lambs older than 2 months of age and will virtually eliminate symptoms of overeating disease.

SWINE

The swine industry has changed dramatically over the past 25 years. Most pigs are raised in confinement to reduce labor requirements for the owner and to improve the

environment for the animal (Figure 15-10). The genetic base of the swine industry has changed to a more prolific breeding herd and better-muscled, faster-growing offspring. Feed still constitutes 60% to 70% of the cost of raising swine. Few swine are grazed on pasture; most are fed complete high-grain rations in self-feeders or are limit fed if in the breeding herd. The production of pigs normally is divided into three distinct areas: the breeding herd, starter pigs, and growing-finishing pigs.

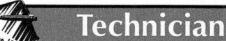

Technician Note

Feed constitutes 60% to 70% of the cost of raising swine.

Breeding Herd

For profitable production of swine, the sows must be bred, gestate 114 days, nurse a litter for 21 to 35 days, rebreed within 10 days after weaning, and continue the cycle for five to seven litters. Nutrition plays a key role in allowing this to occur, especially during lactation (Table 15-12).

Energy

After breeding and for the first two thirds of gestation, energy intake is limited to 6000 to 7000 Kcal ME (metabolizable energy) per day. The total amount of feed is increased during the last third of gestation, providing 9000 to 10,000 Kcal ME per day, which contributes additional energy to the developing fetuses during this last stage of gestation. Overfeeding energy during gestation has a direct negative impact on lactation feed intake, which can impair lactation performance.

In lactation, the goal of the swine producer is to encourage as much energy intake by the lactating female as possible (15,000 to 20,000 Kcal ME per day). Sows are often fed twice per day to ensure fresh feed and improved energy intakes. Frequently, fat is added to the lactation ration to improve palatability and energy density. Sows peak in milk production between the second and third

TABLE 15-11	DAILY NUTRITIONAL CONSIDERATIONS IN SHEEP						
		Daily Consumption	Total Crude	Minerals (g)		Vitamins	
Weight (lb)	ME (Kcal)*	(as Fed) (lb/day)	Protein (lb/day)	Ca²⁺	P	A (1000 IU)	E (IU)
WEANED LAMBS TO FINISHING							
20-40	1.3-2.6	1.2-2.9	0.35-0.45	4.9-6.5	2.2-2.9	.47	12
41-60	2.6-3.2	2.9-3.4	0.45-0.48	6.5-7.2	2.9-3.4	.95	24
61-80	3.2-3.8	3.4-3.7	0.48-0.51	7.2-8.6	3.4-4.3	1.40	21
81-100	3.8-4.0	3.7-4.1	0.51-0.53	8.6-9.4	4.3-4.8	2.30	25
101-Finish	4.0-4.2	3.8-4.1	0.53	8.2-9.4	4.5-4.8	2.80	25
EWE LAMBS							
Early							
80-100	2.9-3.0	3.4-3.7	0.35-0.36	5.2-5.5	2.7-2.8	3.0-3.1	21
101-120	3.0-3.1	3.7-3.9	0.35-0.36	5.2-5.5	2.8-3.0	3.1-3.4	22
121-140	3.1-3.2	3.7-3.9	0.35-0.36	5.5	3.0-3.3	3.4-3.7	24
141-160	3.1-3.3	3.9-4.1	0.35-0.36	5.5	3.3-3.4	3.4-3.7	26
Late							
80-101	5.0-5.4	3.7-3.9	0.41-0.44	6.4-7.8	5.0-5.4	3.1-3.9	22
101-120	5.4-5.8	3.0-4.1	0.44-0.45	7.8-8.1	5.4-5.8	3.9-4.3	24
121-140	5.8-6.2	4.1-4.4	0.45-0.48	8.1-8.2	5.8-6.2	4.3-4.7	26
141-160	6.2-6.3	4.4-4.7	0.46-0.48	8.1-8.2	6.2-6.3	4.3-4.7	27
Lactation							
80-100	2.9-3.0	5.1-5.7	0.67-0.71	8.4-8.7	5.6-6.0	4.0-5.0	32-34
101-120	3.0-3.1	5.7-6.1	0.71-0.74	8.7-9.0	6.0-6.4	5.0-6.0	34-36
121-140	3.1-3.2	6.1-6.7	0.74-0.77	9.0-9.3	6.4-6.9	6.0-7.0	36-38
Ewes: Maintenance to Early/Mid							
110-130	2.4-2.6	2.4-2.9	0.21-0.27	2.0-3.2	1.8-2.5	2.35-2.80	18-20
131-150	2.6-2.7	2.5-3.1	0.27-0.29	2.5-3.5	2.4-2.9	2.80-3.30	20-21
151-170	2.7-2.9	2.9-3.7	0.29-0.31	2.8-3.8	2.4-3.3	3.30-3.75	21-22
171-190	2.9-3.1	3.0-3.9	0.31-0.33	2.9-3.9	2.8-3.4	3.75-4.25	22-24
Ewes: Late Gestation (Last 30 Days)/Lactation							
100-130	4.0-6.0	4.1-5.9	0.43-0.45	5.6-6.9	4.8-5.2	4.25-5.10	24-27
131-150	4.2-6.6	4.4-6.1	0.45-0.47	6.9-9.1	5.2-6.6	5.10-5.95	26-28
151-170	4.4-7.0	4.7-6.3	0.47-0.49	7.6-9.5	6.6-7.4	5.95-6.80	28-30
171-190	4.7-7.5	4.9-6.6	0.49-0.51	8.5-9.6	6.8-7.8	6.80-7.65	30-33

*ME (metabolizable energy) is measured in megacalories (Mcal), 1 Mcal = 1000 kilocalories.

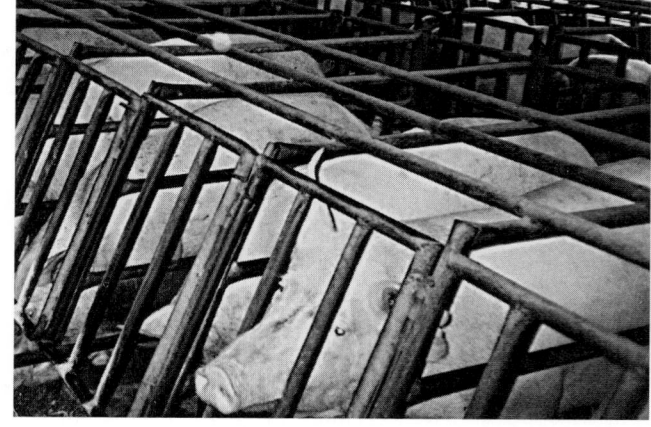

FIGURE 15-10. Sows are commonly kept in a farrowing containment pen to prevent injury to the piglets and ensure ready access to milk by the piglets.

TABLE 15-12	COMPLETE FEED RATION CONSIDERATIONS IN SWINE			
Stage Weight	Protein (%)	Complete Ration Fed (lb)	Comments	
Weaning pigs (12-20 lb)	20-24	Free feed	Use if weaned early and transitioning to solid feed	
Starter pigs (up to 40 lb)	18-20	Free feed		
Feeder/finisher pigs (40 lb to 220-250 lb finishing weight)	13-18	Free feed*	May be limited in feed after 125 lb	
Gilts and sows				
Breeding/maintenance	11-14	4-6	Increase amount to maintain body	
Gestation	11-14	4-6	condition and last month of gestation	
Lactation	14-20	10-15	through weaning	
Boars	14-16	4-7	Increase in breeding season	

*See text on feeding methods.

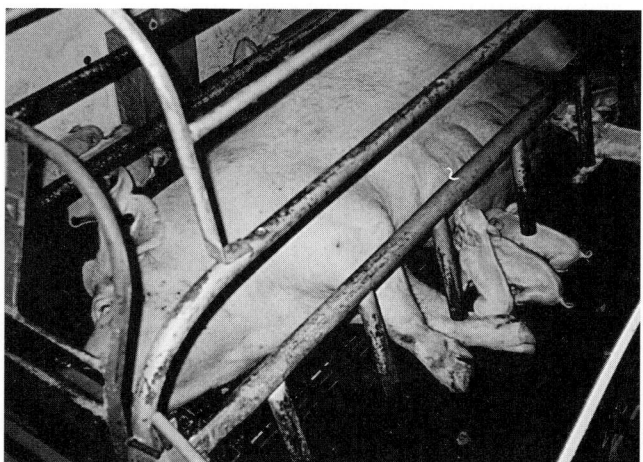

FIGURE 15-11.   Sow nursing piglets in containment of pen.

weeks of lactation, and they should be full fed to support the production of milk. A rule of thumb for feeding lactating sows is to offer 4 to 5 lb of the base ration plus 1 additional pound for every pig nursing (Figure 15-11).

Technician Note
Sows are often fed twice daily to ensure adequate energy intake.

Protein
The protein requirements during gestation are relatively low (11% to 12% crude protein; 0.5 lb of protein per day). The development of the fetuses and reproductive tissue requires small amounts of protein each day.

During lactation, sows require higher levels of protein intake to support milk production (2 to 3 lb of protein per day), which is accomplished by feeding a ration with a higher protein content at a greater intake level. Sows not fed adequate levels of protein or energy during lactation will support milk production with loss of body tissue stores. Sows can lose more than 100 lb in weight during lactation if not fed proper amounts of energy or protein.

BOX 15-20	PREVENTION OF IRON-DEFICIENCY ANEMIA IN BABY PIGS

- Allow access to soil that has not been in contact with other pigs.
- Inject 100-200 mg iron before 72 hr of age.
- Paint sows' teats lightly with iron solution periodically.
- Encourage prestarter ration creep feeding early.
- Provide iron supplementation in creep feeder.

Minerals and Vitamins
Minerals and vitamins need to be supplemented throughout the life of pigs. The breeding herd is normally fed diets fortified with the minerals calcium, phosphorus, salt, zinc, iron, copper, iodine, selenium, and manganese. Calcium and phosphorus are kept in a balance of 1:1 to 2:1 for all stages of production. Low levels of calcium and phosphorus in the breeding herd rations can lead to fractures and lameness in the female.

Sow's milk is virtually devoid of iron, and anemia of nursing pigs will occur unless they are supplemented with another source of iron (Box 15-20). The two most common ways to supply additional iron are (1) an injection of iron (150 to 200 mg) as iron dextran or other iron-carbohydrate complexes at 3 days of age and (2) an oral iron solution given at 3 days of age or swabbed onto the dam's udder several times during lactation.

The vitamins supplemented in breeding herd diets are the fat-soluble vitamins A, D, E, and K and the water-soluble vitamins thiamin, riboflavin, niacin, pantothenic acid, B_6, B_{12}, choline, biotin, and folic acid. Adequate additions of these vitamins ensure proper development of the fetus in gestation and milk production in lactation (Box 15-21).

Technician Note
Sow's milk is devoid of iron, and nursing pigs will develop anemia unless they are supplemented with iron.

Starter Pigs
Pigs are commonly weaned at 3 to 5 weeks of age and remain in the starter phase until they weigh 40 to 50 lb (Figure 15-12). The earlier the age at weaning, the more complex is the ration required to help in the transition

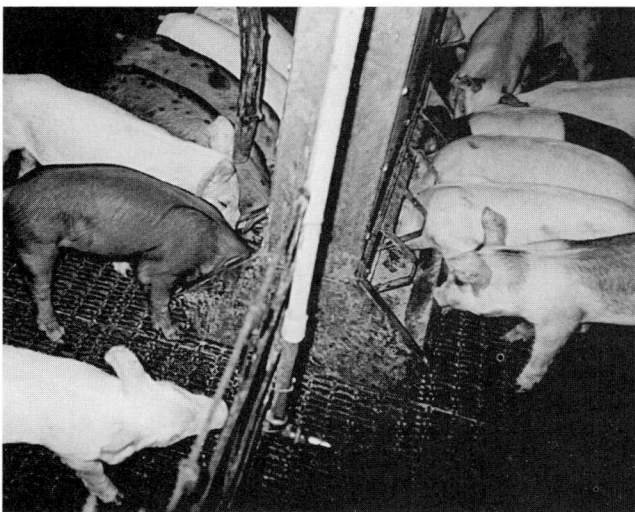

FIGURE 15-12. Grower-finisher pigs are fed large quantities of complete rations to obtain the most desirable carcass quality. *Bottom left,* pig is using an automatic watering system to fulfill water requirements at will.

| Box 15-21 | ORPHAN PIGLET FEEDING |

HOMEMADE REPLACER
32 oz whole cow's milk
Water-soluble antibiotics
1 raw egg
16 oz half-and-half

DIRECTIONS FOR FEEDING PIGLETS
Give 2 oz per feeding per piglet every 3 hr
Feed in a shallow, clean feeding pan
Be sure that all piglets are eating
Give iron supplementation as needed
Start creep feeding at 7 days of age

---

from mother's milk to solid food. Starter diets (20% to 24% protein) are very complex and nutrient-dense complete feeds and therefore often purchased from a commercial feed manufacturer. The highest-quality ingredients are used to make starter diets and include milk products, fishmeal, spray-dried blood products, oats, corn, and fat. Vitamin and mineral supplementation levels are high in starter diets. These feeds typically are pelleted and quite costly (see Table 15-12).

As the pig ages, the complexity and nutrient density of the starter ration decrease, leading to a lower-cost formula. In the last 2 or 3 weeks of the starter period, crude protein decreases to 18% to 20%, and the diet is often offered as a ground feed.

Growing-Finishing Pigs

Growing-finishing diets have been modified to complement the changes in the genetic base of modern swine. The leaner pigs require higher levels of protein and consume less energy than previous generations (see Table 15-12).

Energy

Complete grower-finisher rations are based on cereal grains and frequently have fat added to increase caloric

intake. Fibrous feed ingredients often are not used or are used sparingly to prevent depressions in caloric intake. Corn, wheat, sorghum, and barley are the more popular cereal grains used to supply energy and comprise 60% to 85% of the ration.

Protein

Contemporary swine nutrition does not concentrate on the protein content of feeds but on the amino acid levels. Lysine typically is the first limiting amino acid in swine formulas. Amino acid levels decrease as a percentage of the diet throughout the growing-finishing phase.

Amino acid levels are matched to muscle growth throughout the growth period to maximize lean tissue growth. Underfeeding of amino acids depresses muscle deposition, and overfeeding amino acids leads to excess, which is costly.

Typical protein sources in growing-finishing diets are soybean meal, meat and bone meal, and synthetic amino acids. When protein sources are expensive, synthetic amino acids can replace a portion of the protein source with no loss in performance. The most commonly available synthetic amino acids are lysine, methionine, threonine, and tryptophan.

Minerals and Vitamins

Growing-finishing swine are fed diets fortified with the minerals calcium, phosphorus, salt, zinc, iron, copper, iodine, selenium, and manganese. Calcium and phosphorus are kept in a balance of 1:1 to 2:1 throughout this period. Deficiencies of phosphorus will depress growth performance as the animal grows.

Riboflavin, niacin, pantothenic acid, and vitamin B_{12} are the water-soluble vitamins most likely to be deficient in swine diets formulated with grains and plant protein. The fat-soluble vitamins A, D, E, and K also should be added to growing-finishing rations.

REFERENCES

Church DC: *Livestock feeds and feeding,* Corvallis, Ore, 1984, O and B Books, pp 19-31, 89-93, 189-234.

Ensminger ME: *Swine science,* Danville, Ill, 1990, Interstate Printers and Publishing, pp 416-441, 506–534.

McDonald P et al: *Animal nutrition,* ed 7, New York, 1995, Longman Scientific and Technical Publishing, pp 91-134.

Nash MJ: *Crop conservation and storage,* Oxford, England, 1985, Pergamon Press, pp 85-101.

Neumann AL: *Beef cattle,* New York, 1977, John Wiley & Sons, pp 187-221.

Shirley RL: *Nitrogen and energy nutrition of ruminants,* Orlando, 1986, Academic Press, pp 54-79.

RECOMMENDED READING

Cunha TJ: *Swine feeding and nutrition,* New York, 1977, pp 201-208.

Garmsworthy PC: *Nutrition and lactation in the dairy cow,* London, 1988, University Press, pp 246-254.

Haresign DJ: *Recent developments of pig nutrition,* London, 1985, Butterworth, pp 368-386.

Jones DH, Wilson AD: Nutritive quality of forage. In Hacker ED, editor: *The nutrition of herbivores,* Sydney, 1982, Academic Press, pp 106-119

Kruesi WK: *Sheep raiser's manual,* Charlotte, Vt, 1985, Williamson Publishing, pp 23-26, 67-72, 90-111.

Linciciome DR: *Sheep: applied and basic research information,* Scottsdale, Ariz, 1983, International Goat and Sheep Research, pp 85-99.

Lloyd LE et al: *Fundamentals of nutrition,* ed 3, San Francisco, 1978, WH Freeman & Sons, pp 456-501.

Machlin LJ: *Handbook of vitamins,* New York, 1984, Marcel Dekker, pp 29-54.

Maynard LA et al: *Animal nutrition,* ed 7, New York, 1979, McGraw-Hill.

Menzies CS: *United States sheep and goat industry,* Ames, Iowa, 1982 CAST Report, pp 12-31.

National Research Council: *Nutrient requirements for beef cattle,* ed 7, Washington, DC, 2000, National Academic Press.

National Research Council: *Nutrient requirements for dairy cattle,* ed 6, Washington, DC, 1989, National Academy Press.

National Research Council: *Nutrient requirements for sheep,* ed 6, Washington, DC, 1985, National Academy Press.

National Research Council: *Nutrient requirements for swine,* ed 10, Washington, DC, 1998, National Academic Press.

Naylor JM, Ralston SL: *Large Animal Clinical Nutrition,* St Louis, 1991, Mosby, pp 21-42, 460-468, 267-274.

Pond WG: *Swine production and nutrition,* Westport, Conn, 1984, AVI Publishing pp 91-96.

Taylor RE: *Beef production and the beef industry,* Minneapolis, 1984, Burgess Publishing, pp 389-404.

Tribble LG, Stansbury WF: *Swine report,* Dallas, 1985, Texas Technical University.

Webster J: *Calf husbandry: health and welfare,* London, 1984, Collins, pp 71-78.

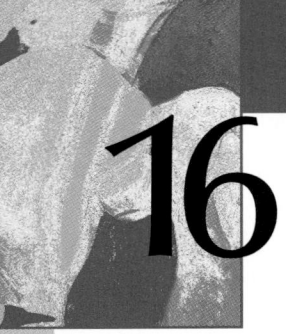

16

Animal Reproduction

Carlos R.F. Pinto • Bruce E. Eilts • Dale L. Paccamonti

The events that occur in the process of reproduction in domestic animals are elegant processes of checks and balances that ultimately result in the birth of a newborn that will carry the genes for the next generation. This chapter will provide a generic overview of female and male reproductive events, followed by more in-depth reviews of the most important aspects of reproduction in the canine, feline, bovine, porcine, ovine, caprine, equine, and camelids.

GENERAL FEMALE REPRODUCTION

There are two embryologic tubular systems present in the early embryo that will become either the male genitalia or the female genitalia. If an animal has XY chromosomes it will become a male and one tubular system will persist, and if it has XX it will become a female and the other tubular system will persist. Because there are two systems, many potential abnormalities can occur when sections of the systems fail to regress or fail to develop fully. An example of embryonic malformation would be the hermaphrodite, which has developed both male and female gender organs.

The normal stages of reproduction are proestrus (the time leading to estrus), estrus (the time of mating), and diestrus (the time when pregnancy is being established). In most species, pregnancy is the normal event, because that ensures species survival. However, if pregnancy does not occur, the female will return to a sexually active state to entice mating with a male. If pregnancy is not established the events will recur, thus forming a cycle of proestrus, estrus, diestrus, proestrus, estrus, diestrus, and so forth. The other normal events in the reproductive life of an animal are puberty, the time of first ovulation, pregnancy, and anestrus, a time when the animal is not undergoing any reproductive events. The name given to these recurring events is the estrous cycle. **(Note that estrus is spelled estrous when it is an adjective, as in estrous cycle).**

The brain is the initiator of the reproductive cycle. Neural input from higher brain centers results in the release of gonadotropin-releasing hormone (GnRH) from the hypothalamus. The GnRH is released from neurons in the hypothalamus into the hypophyseal-portal vessels. It then enters the anterior pituitary, causing release of the gonadotropins, follicle-stimulating hormone (FSH), and luteinizing hormone (LH).

Technician Note

The brain is the initiator of the reproductive cycle.

FSH and LH are large, complex hormones that are stored within granules inside cells in the anterior pituitary. These two hormones are glycoproteins, a complex of carbohydrates and proteins. Because the gonadotropins are extremely large, complex hormones, they cannot be synthesized. The complexity and protein nature of the gonadotropins make them antigenic, and exogenous administration of these drugs derived from other species can induce antibody formation.

The beginning of an estrous cycle in most females starts with GnRH from the hypothalamus causing the release of FSH from the anterior pituitary (Figure 16-1). The FSH is released into the bloodstream and is carried to the ovaries where it initiates its follicle-stimulating action. The FSH causes the growth of ovarian follicles. Ovarian follicles are structures on the ovary that contain the egg, or oocyte (Figure 16-2). All the oocytes that will be present for the life of the female are present on the ovary at birth, and most of the follicles contain no fluid. Some follicles are selected to grow and start to develop fluid around them (an antrum) in a process that is independent from FSH stimulation. Once a follicle has reached the antral stage, action of the FSH causes rapid growth of the follicle. The follicle wall is composed of two layers, the thecal cell layer and the granulosa cell layer. As the follicle grows, it produces the steroid hormone estrogen. Estrogen is the hormone that causes the outward signs of estrus (sexual receptivity) when the female is in estrus. The oocyte within the follicle also begins to mature, so it will be ready for fertilization after ovulation. As the follicle grows and reaches maturity, the granulosa cells also produce a protein hormone called *inhibin*. Inhibin inhibits further FSH release, so that only a

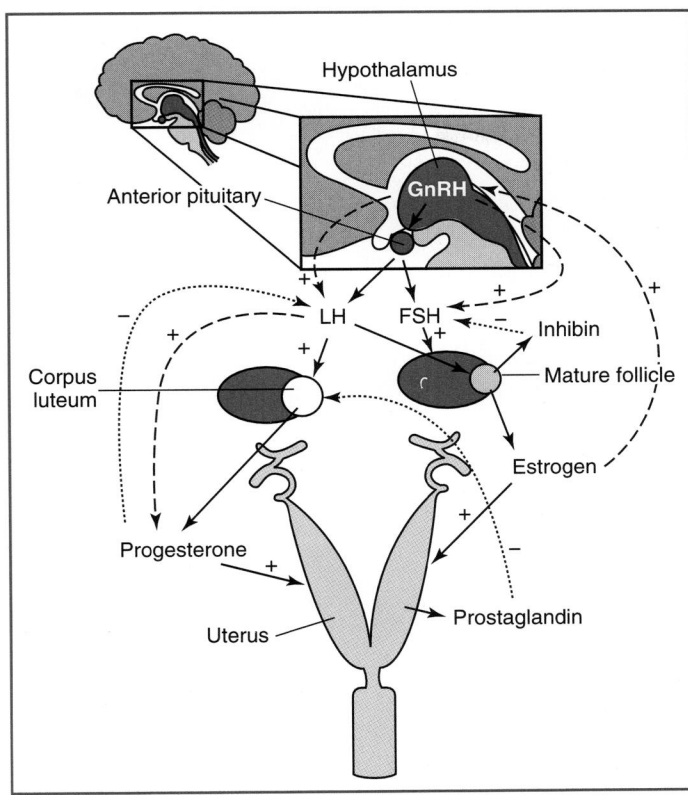

FIGURE 16-1. The general hormonal control of female reproduction. Pulsatile GnRH causes FSH to be released from the anterior pituitary. FSH causes follicular growth and maturation where estrogen is produced. Inhibin from the follicle feeds back on the anterior pituitary and causes less FSH to be released. A surge of estrogen from the follicle causes GnRH release from the hypothalamus, which causes an LH surge. LH causes ovulation of the follicle and the formation of a corpus luteum, which produces progesterone. If a pregnancy signal is not secreted by the early embryo (bovine, equine, ovine, caprine) prostaglandin is released from the uterus, goes to the corpus luteum, and causes luteolyis (luteal death). The cycle then starts over with follicular growth.

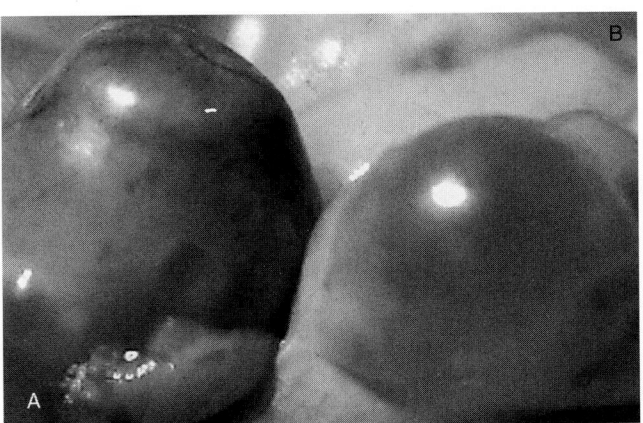

FIGURE 16-2. A bovine corpus luteum, *A,* and follicle, *B,* on the ovaries.

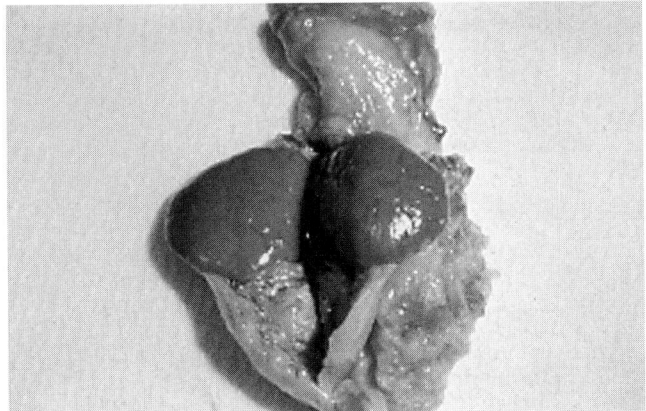

FIGURE 16-3. A cut section of a bovine corpus luteum.

species-specific number of follicles are chosen for final growth and maturation (depending on the species, this may be one or more).

The estrogen surge produced by the developing follicle stimulates the release of GnRH from the hypothalamus, which causes release of LH from the anterior pituitary. At the ovary, LH causes the mature follicle to ovulate. Ovulation is the release of the oocyte into the oviduct. After ovulation the follicle transforms into a corpus luteum, or yellow body. The corpus luteum (Figure 16-3) has been transformed by the LH surge to produce only progesterone. Progesterone is the hormone that maintains pregnancy.

The pregnancy actually begins in the oviduct. The oviduct is often called the *uterine tube* and consists of three segments: the infundibulum, the ampulla, and the isthmus (Figure 16-4). When ovulation of the oocyte occurs, it is picked up by the dilated end of the oviduct called the infundibulum. The oocyte is then transported through the ampulla to the junction of isthmus and ampulla. In most species, this is where fertilization occurs. Fertilization is the joining of the oocyte, which has half the chromosome complement, with the sperm cell, which has the other half of the chromosome complement, thus forming the embryo that has both the maternal and paternal chromosome complement. The embryo normally

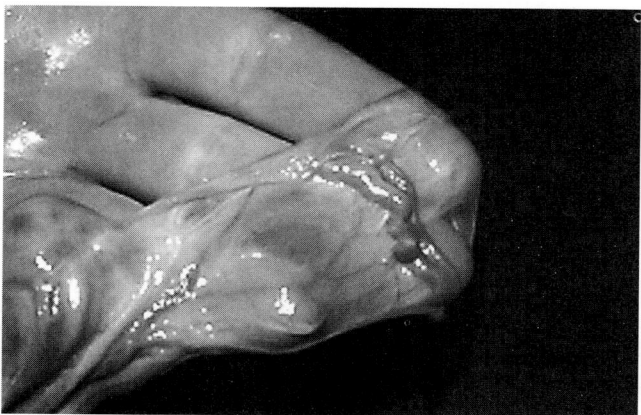

Figure 16-4. A bovine oviduct showing the fingers inserted in the infundibulum.

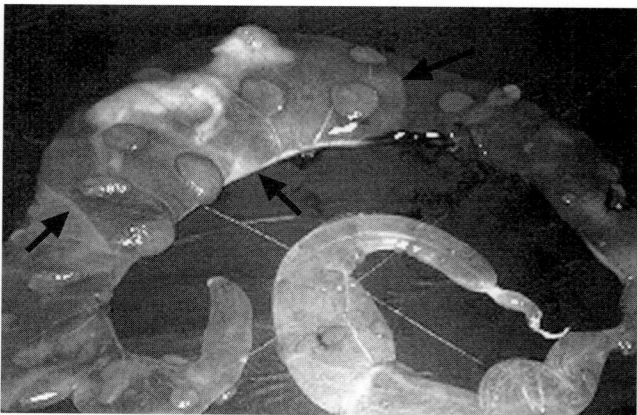

Figure 16-5. A bovine fetus within the amnion *(arrows)*, which is within the chorioallantois.

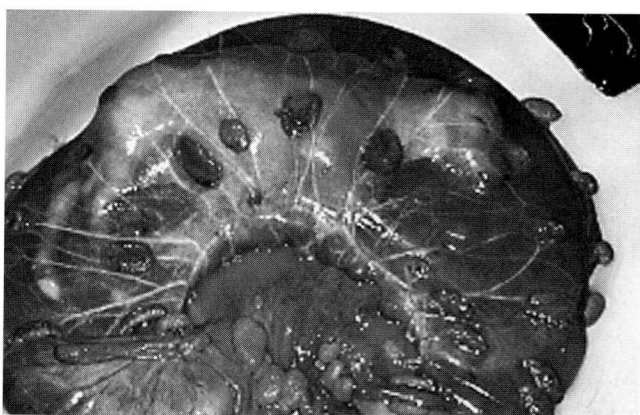

Figure 16-6. Bovine placentomes *(P)* on the chorioallantois.

stays within the oviduct for several days before it moves into the uterus.

If the oocyte is not successfully fertilized, the corpus luteum still develops and maintains progesterone production for a time that is consistent within each species. This time of progesterone domination is called *diestrus*. It is the early embryo in most species that signals to the uterus/ovary that pregnancy has been established. If the signal for pregnancy is not received by the uterus, most species (not the dog and cat) will initiate an ending of diestrus, so the animal can return to estrus and have another chance to become pregnant. In most species this occurs when the hormone prostaglandin is released from the uterus. The prostaglandin is a small molecule derived from arachidonic acid. When prostaglandin is released, it binds to receptors on the corpus luteum and lyses it. Since the corpus luteum is the source of progesterone, once the corpus luteum is destroyed by the prostaglandin, progesterone concentrations in the blood fall. When progesterone is not present, there is a rise in FSH that allows new follicles to grow. This time of growing follicles after the death of the corpus luteum is called *proestrus*. As the animal enters proestrus the follicles grow, estrus follows and the LH surge causes ovulation, and a corpus luteum forms. Therefore the animal has estrous cycles until pregnancy is established.

Once the embryo is in the uterus, it must establish itself as a viable pregnancy before prostaglandin destroys the corpus luteum. Different species have different mechanisms to do this. Each species appears to have a relatively unique substance produced by the early embryo that prevents the corpus luteum from being destroyed by prostaglandin released from the uterus. Dogs and cats appear rather unique in that their corpora lutea (plural for corpus luteum) appear to have preprogrammed life spans without any endogenous destruction by prostaglandins if they are not pregnant.

As pregnancy progresses the early embryo changes from an embryonic disk and a yolk sac of nutrients to a complex structure that includes the fetus and placenta. The placenta forms from specialized cells on the embryo. These cells develop into the chorion and allantois. The amnion is a fluid-filled sac that immediately surrounds the fetus, whereas the chorion and allantois fuse to form a chorioallantois. Therefore the fetus has two fluid-filled sacs surrounding it (Figure 16-5). The chorion attaches to the uterus and has the function of transferring nutrients from

the uterus to the fetus. The structure of the placenta varies from species to species (Figures 16-6 and 16-7). The ruminants have many individual attachment areas called *placentomes*. Dogs and cats have a zone of the placenta that attaches to the uterus. Horses and pigs have a more generalized attachment (diffuse) of the placenta to the uterus. In some species, such as the ewe and horse, the placenta produces the progesterone that maintains the pregnancy instead of the corpus luteum.

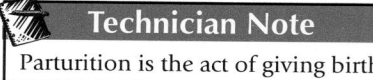

Technician Note

Parturition is the act of giving birth.

Parturition is the act of giving birth. The only domestic species in which the entire parturition mechanism is completely understood is sheep; other species are hypothesized to be similar. As gestation progresses, the fetal hypothalamus and pituitary mature enough to cause the fetal release of corticotropin-releasing hormone from the hypothalamus, which causes the fetal adrenal to produce high concentrations of cortisol. The high cortisol concentrations cause a change in placental production of progesterone to estrogen and a release of prostaglandin from the uterus. These hormones cause the cervix to dilate and the uterus to contract, thereby forcing the fetus out. Parturition is nor-

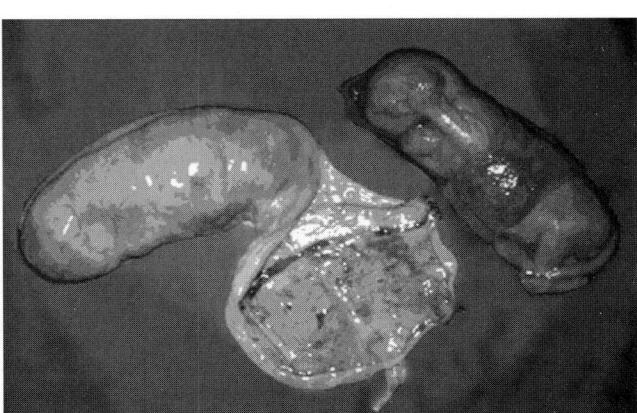

FIGURE 16-7. A canine puppy with the zonary placenta surrounding it.

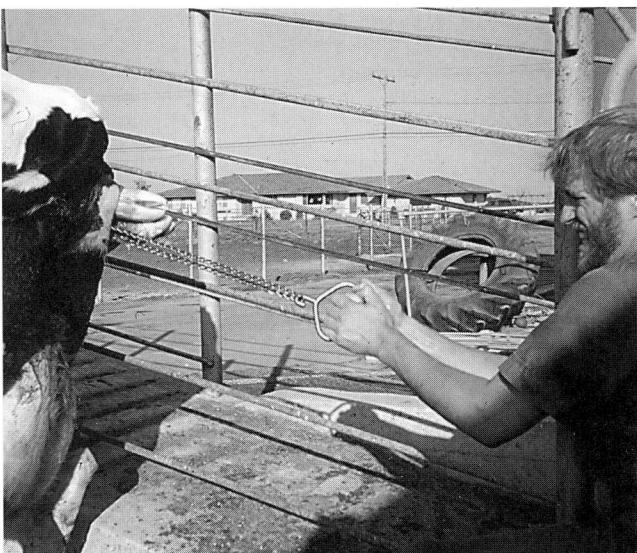

FIGURE 16-8. Chains placed around the legs of a bovine calf in a normal delivery position.

mally divided into three stages: I, II, and III. Stage I is the preparatory stage. Maternal pelvic ligaments relax and the cervix softens, preparing for delivery. Behaviorally, the female becomes restless and prepares to give birth. The expulsion of the fetus is stage II (Figure 16-8). Stage III is the expulsion of the placenta. The timing of the events of parturition varies by species. A summary of the length of the estrous cycle and the length of gestation is found in Table 16-1.

CANINE REPRODUCTION

The estrous cycle of the bitch has four phases: proestrus (9 to 10 days average), estrus (9 to 10 days average), diestrus (57 to 58 days average), and anestrus (2 to 5 months average) (Figure 16-9). Interestrus consists of diestrus and anestrus combined and therefore usually lasts 4 to 7 months. Interestrus periods of less than 4 months are associated with infertility.

During proestrus, the bitch is attractive to male dogs but will not allow mating. The vulva appears swollen, and a serosanguineous discharge is present. Estrogen, which is rising during proestrus, causes the epithelial cells in the vagina to cornify. Vaginal cytology is a common tool used to follow a bitch's cycle. To prepare a vaginal cytology slide, moisten a long cotton swab and pass it through the vulva and vestibule (Figure 16-10). The canine vagina is nearly vertical at the entrance. To get a swab into the cranial vagina once past the vulvar lips, direct the swab nearly vertical (toward the anus) until it will go no further. Redirect the swab horizontally, and twirl it to obtain a sample. Roll the swab on a slide and stain the slide using a modified Wright's or Giemsa stain. Noncornified cells have a rounded cytoplasm and a large stippled nucleus. Cornified cells have a more angular-shaped cytoplasm, and the nucleus is either pyknotic or not apparent. The percentage of cornified cells increases approximately 10% per day, reaching 90% to 100% (full cornification) by the onset of estrus (Figure 16-11).

Estrus is the period of receptivity when the bitch will allow mating. During estrus, the vulvar swelling typically decreases slightly and the bloody discharge changes to straw colored, although a bloody discharge may continue throughout estrus. Vaginal cytology is fully cornified, and the background of the slide is clear. No white blood cells should be present. Occasionally, bacteria may be seen on the slide.

The end of estrus, or the first day of diestrus, is typified by an abrupt decline in the percentage of cornified cells. This day is important to detect because whelping can be accurately predicted from day 1 (D1) of diestrus. Day 1 of diestrus also correlates well with the LH peak (8 days before D1) and ovulation (approximately 6 days before D1).

To maximize fertility, viable sperm must be present when the oocyte is ready to be fertilized. If the male is readily available, mating every other day is usually practiced. If performing artificial insemination and male availability is not limited, breeding three times per week (e.g., Monday, Wednesday, Friday) for as long as the vaginal cytology is fully cornified provides equally good results. However, when the number of breedings is reduced to one or two during a single estrus, such as with frozen or fresh cooled semen, timing insemination to coincide with ovulation becomes critical. Ovulation occurs approximately 2 days after the LH surge. The bitch ovulates immature oocytes that require 2 to 3 more days for maturation. Mature oocytes are then viable for another 2 to 3 days. Therefore the fertile period is 4 to 8 days after the LH surge, with peak fertility occurring 5 to 6 days after the LH surge.

Technician Note

The bitch ovulates immature oocytes that require 2 to 3 more days for maturation.

To best estimate the day of ovulation, hormone assays should be used. Vaginal cytology does not give a very precise prediction of ovulation. The LH peak may occur anywhere from the same day of, or up to 2 days after, full cornification. Unlike most species, serum progesterone rises before ovulation in the bitch. Therefore progesterone is useful to predict the LH surge because the increase in serum progesterone is closely associated with the LH peak. Before the LH surge, serum progesterone is less than 1 ng/ml. On the day of the LH surge, serum progesterone

TABLE 16-1   SUMMARY OF THE LENGTHS OF THE ESTROUS CYCLE AND GESTATION PERIODS IN DOMESTIC ANIMALS

Species	Puberty	Estrous Cycle Length	Estrus Duration	Ovulation	Optimal Breeding (Fresh/Frozen)	Gestation
Canine (Dog or bitch)	6 months	No true cycle. Estrus is 2 times/year	9 days	2-4 days after onset of cytologic estrus	Days 3 and 5 or 4 and 6 after LH peak/ Day 5 or 6 after LH peak	57 days from first day of cytologic diestrus or 63 days from ovulation or 65 days form LH peak
Feline (Cat or Queen)	6-12 months	Seasonally polyestrous and depends if ovulation occurs seasonally polyestrous	8 days	Induced ovulators After coitus	After third day of estrus and every > 2 hours apart for at least 3 breedings/–	65 days
Equine (Horse or mare)	18 months	21 days (diestrus is consistently 15 days)	4-7 days	1-2 days before end of estrus	(within 48 hours of ovulation) At ovulation	330 days
Bovine (Cow)	12 months	21 days	18-20 hours	12-18 hours after end of estrus	12 hours after end of estrus	283 days
Caprine (Goat or doe)	6-9 months	21 days	24-36 hours	24 -30 hours after onset of estrus	18-24 hours after onset of estrus	150 days
Ovine (Sheep or ewe)	6-9 months	17 days	24-48 hours	24 -30 hours after onset of estrus	12-30 hours after onset of estrus	150 days
Porcine (Pig or sow)	5-6 months	21 days	2 to 3 days	Day 2 of estrus	24 and 36 hours after onset of estrus (12 and 24 in gilts)/–	114 days
Llama	10-12 months	Induced ovulators	1-36 days (induced ovulators)	Induced ovulators	Induced ovulators	344 days
Alpaca	10-12 months	Induced ovulators	1-36 days (induced ovulators)	Induced ovulators	Induced ovulators	344 days

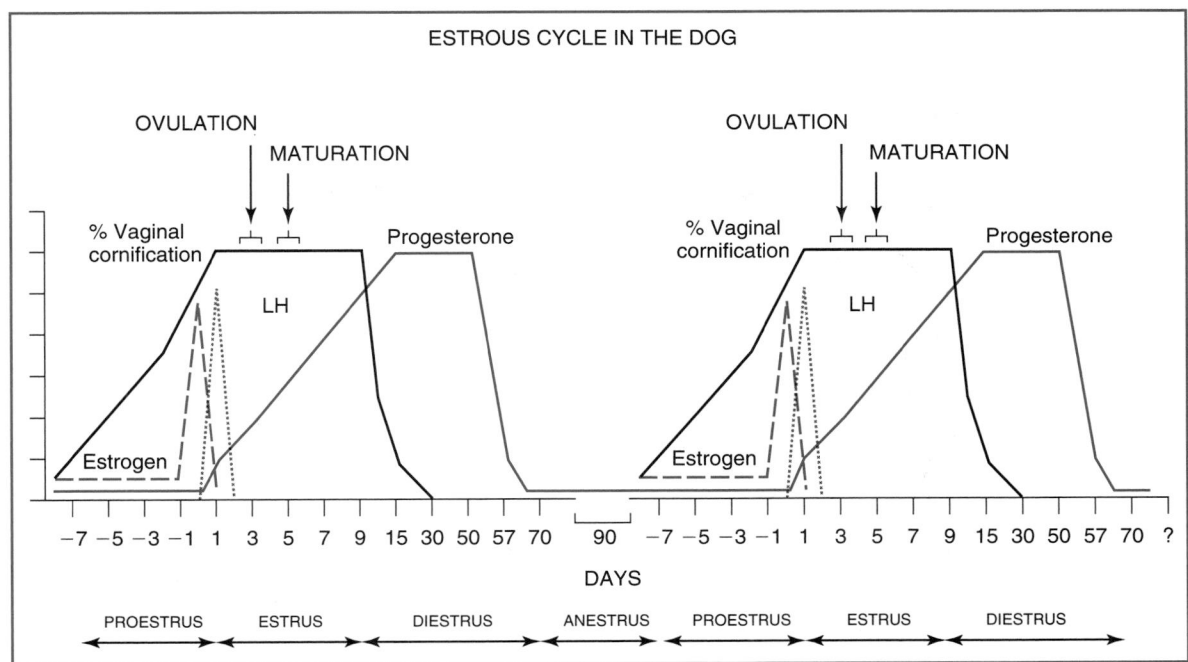

FIGURE 16-9. The canine estrous cycle. Proestrus lasts around 9 days. During proestrus the vaginal cornification increases around 10%/day, and estrogen peaks at the end of proestrus. There is 100% vaginal cornification throughout a 9-day estrus. On day 2 or 3 of estrus the LH peaks. At the same time the LH peaks, progesterone starts to rise. About 2 days after the LH peak, ovulation occurs, followed by a 24-day maturation of the oocytes. At the start of diestrus, the vaginal cornification abruptly declines to less than 50% cornified. Diestrus lasts about 57 days and is characterized by high progesterone. At the end of diestrus, progesterone declines and the bitch enters a 90-day anestrus. The cycle then starts over again.

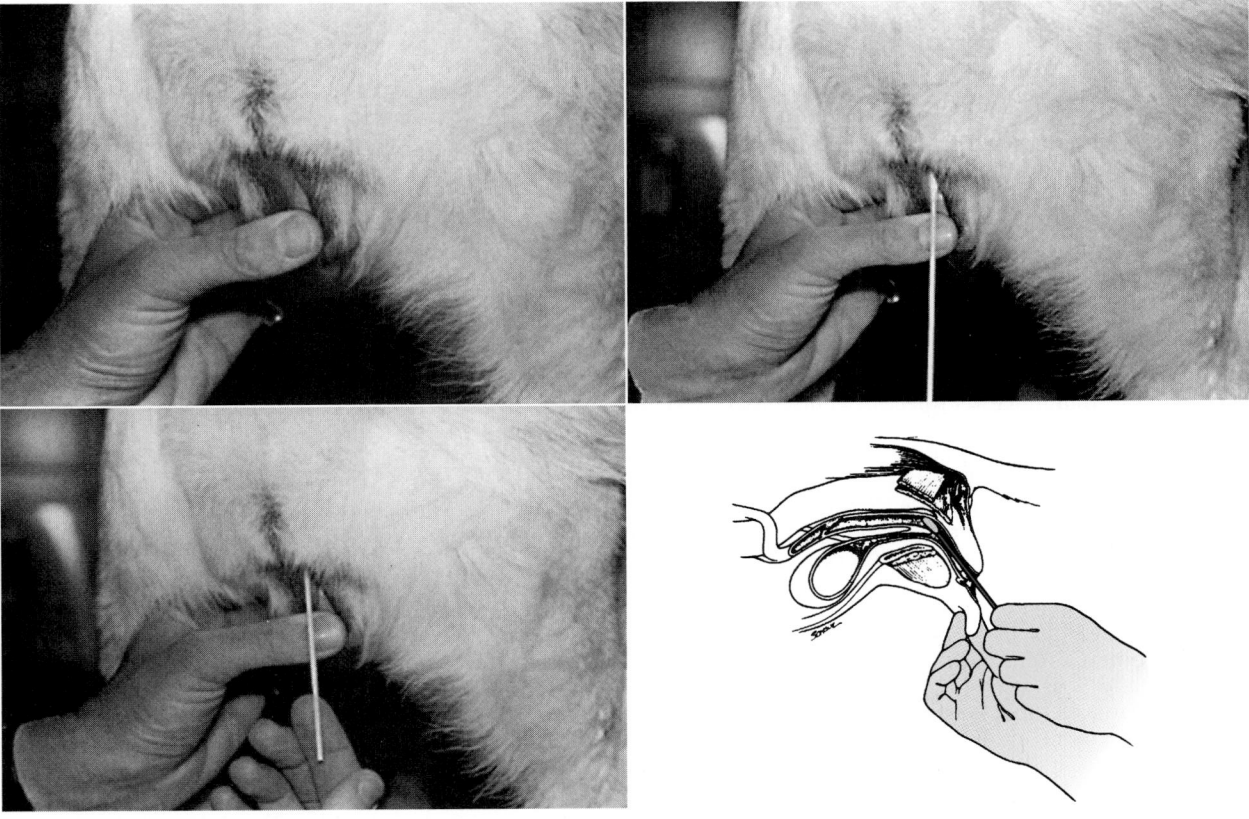

FIGURE 16-10. Vaginal cytology preparation. (From Feldman EC, Nelson RW, editors: *Canine and feline endocrinology and reproduction*, ed 2, Philadelphia, 1987, WB Saunders.)

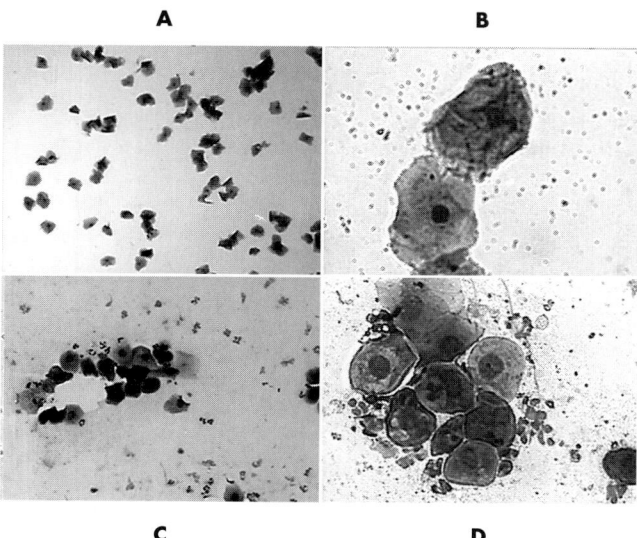

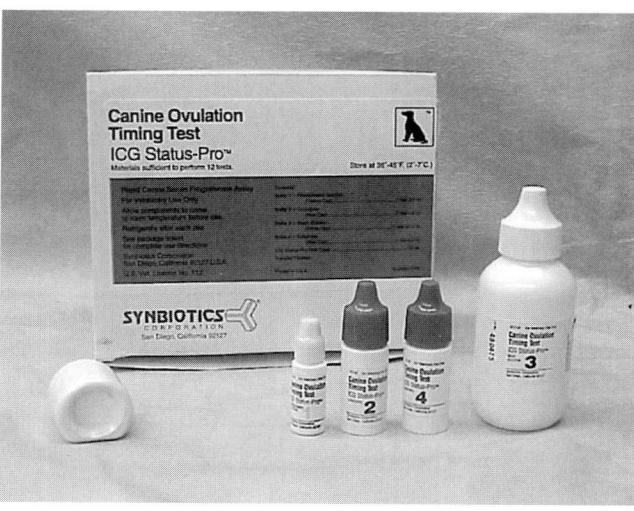

FIGURE 16-11.   **A,** A low power and, **B,** a high power view of a vaginal cytology sample of a dog in estrus. **C,** A low power and, **D,** a high power view of a vaginal cytology sample of a dog in diestrus.

FIGURE 16-12.   A commercially available kit to perform qualitative progesterone analyses.

rises to 1.5 to 2.0 ng/ml and after that continues to rise during diestrus or pregnancy. By identifying this initial rise in progesterone, the day of the LH surge can be estimated and insemination performed during the period of peak fertility. Although LH can be measured semiquantitatively with in-house test kits, the peak only lasts 1 day so serum must be tested daily. Progesterone assays provide some advantages because after the initial rise (on the same day as the LH surge) progesterone continues to rise so the day of initial rise can be estimated even if a day is missed.

In-house, semiquantitative kits for progesterone analysis are available (Figure 16-12). The in-house tests are easy to perform, and results are available in about 20 minutes. Some aspects of the tests require attention to detail to achieve meaningful results. The kits need to be at room temperature before use, and the manufacturers recommend the kits be placed at room temperature for approximately 2 hours before use. If the test is run using a cold kit, results will be incorrect, often giving a false-high progesterone. Blood should be allowed to clot at a cool temperature (in the refrigerator), and cells should be separated from serum or plasma as soon as possible (within 20 minutes of collection is the manufacturer's recommendation). If serum is allowed to remain in contact with the red blood cells, progesterone will be bound by them and test results will be artificially low. Hemolyzed or lipemic samples may also cause erroneously low results. Serum samples may also be frozen for analysis later. If a laboratory is available that can give rapid turnaround time and provide quantitative results, this is preferable when breeding with frozen semen or any time breedings are limited.

If only two breedings are to be performed, such as with fresh cooled semen, insemination should be performed on either days 3 and 5 or days 4 and 6 after the LH peak or initial rise in progesterone, keeping in mind that viability of fresh chilled semen is reduced and timing of insemination is more critical. The viability of frozen semen is reduced even further and timing is even more critical. When frozen semen is used, usually a single surgical insemination is conducted. Surgical insemination with

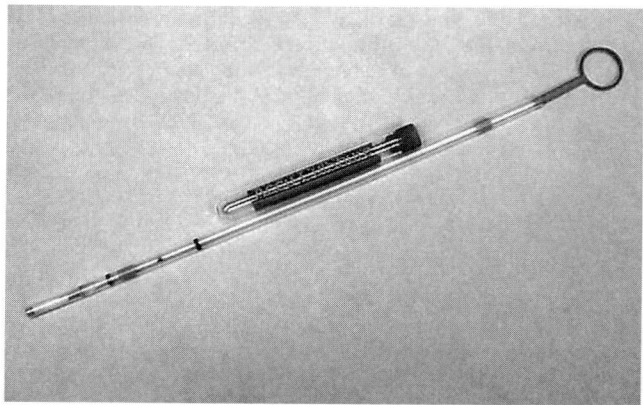

FIGURE 16-13.   A guarded canine vaginal culture swab.

frozen semen should be performed on day 5 or 6 after the LH peak or initial rise in progesterone.

Vaginal Cultures

Vaginal cultures can be taken from the bitch for various reasons including prepubertal or postpubertal vaginitis, postparturient discharge, discharges during pregnancy, postabortion discharge, and prebreeding in normal or infertile bitches. Vaginal cultures are best performed with a guarded swab (Figure 16-13) to avoid contamination as the culture swab is passed through the vestibule. If a culture is to be performed as part of a prebreeding examination, and the client needs a negative culture before breeding, then the performance and interpretation of the culture become critical. Bacteria, including mycoplasma, can be cultured from the vagina of the majority of fertile and infertile bitches. Once a culture has been obtained, it must be interpreted. If the culture was obtained as part of a work-up for a clinical problem, a pure culture is probably significant. However, a vaginal culture as part of a prebreeding examination, and in the absence of clinical signs, often produces results of little significance.

Pregnancy Diagnosis

Pregnancy diagnosis can be performed by palpation, hormone assay, ultrasonography, or radiography. Palpation can be performed during a 7- to 10-day window beginning around day 21 after D1. After approximately day 30 post-D1, the embryonic vesicles become confluent and the ability to diagnose pregnancy by palpation is lost until late in gestation. Ultrasound can be used after approximately day 20 post-D1, possibly earlier, depending on the machine and probe used, until parturition. Radiography can be used after day 45 post-D1. An in-house assay for relaxin is available and is reliable after about day 24 of gestation (Figure 16-14). When pregnancy testing, it is very helpful to know the day of progesterone rise or day 1 of diestrus to be able to estimate gestation length. Whereas gestation length seemingly can be as short as 55 days or as long as 70 days when timed from breeding, it is a reliable 57 to 58 days when timed from day 1 of diestrus. Because a bitch is receptive to the male for 9 or 10 days, timing from breeding is quite variable, resulting in errors (false-negative results) when examining for pregnancy or predicting whelping.

Technician Note

Pregnancy diagnosis can be performed by palpation, hormone assay, ultrasonography, or radiography.

Parturition and Dystocia

Stage I of whelping averages 6 to 12 hours but can be as long as 36 hours. The bitch is usually restless and may show nesting behavior. She often appears nervous, pants, and may tremble or shiver. Body temperature drops to 99° F about 24 hours before stage II in approximately 85% of bitches. This temperature drop is related to the abrupt decline in progesterone and can be useful for the dog owner to signal that whelping is imminent. To be reliable, the temperature should be taken at the same time each day, preferably in the morning before any activity. Stage II, when the bitch pushes the puppies out, lasts approximately 20 to 60 minutes per puppy (Figure 6-15). However, no more than 2 hours should elapse between each delivery. Stage II usually lasts a total of 3 to 6 hours but may be as long as 24 hours total. The presentation of the puppies is 60% anterior in the bitch. A blackish-green discharge is normal during parturition and comes from the site of placental attachment to the uterus.

Guidelines for recognizing dystocia (difficult birth) are strong continual contractions for 30 minutes without progress; weak, infrequent contractions for 2 hours without progress; or a prolonged interval between puppies. If any of these criteria is met, veterinary examination is warranted. Ultrasound can be used to assess fetal viability, but radiography is the only reliable method to accurately determine the number of pups in utero, their relative size, and their position.

Postpartum Problems

The bitch has the longest postpartum uterine involution period of the domestic species. A nonodorous hemorrhagic vulvar discharge is normal for 8 to 10 weeks after whelping and does not indicate metritis. Clients are often concerned when a bloody discharge persists for that length of time but

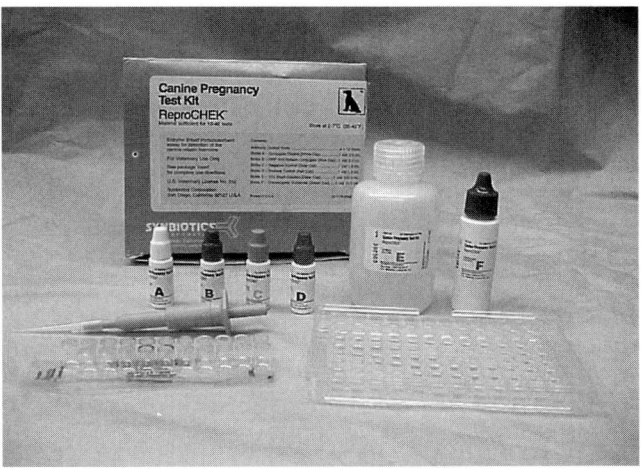

FIGURE 16-14. A commercially available kit to measure canine relaxin to determine pregnancy in a bitch.

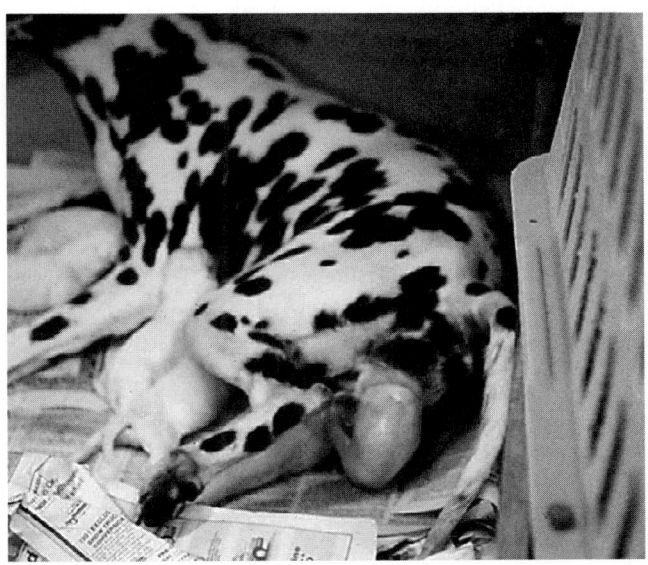

FIGURE 16-15. A puppy being delivered during a normal canine parturition.

should be reassured that it is normal. When the discharge persists for a prolonged period, such as 12 weeks or more, the bitch is considered to have subinvolution of the placental sites (SIPS). Treatment in these cases can be medical (ergonovine), surgical (ovariohysterectomy), or conservative (monitoring).

Indications that a bitch is suffering from postpartum problems include signs of discomfort, such as crying and whining by the pups caused by the lack of attention from the dam. Metritis is characterized by a foul-smelling vaginal discharge. Retained placenta results in a green discharge. Clinical signs of mastitis in the dam include fever, lethargy, and swollen mammary glands. The glands may be discolored as well. In many cases of metritis or mastitis, the pups will need to be hand fed or at least supplemented.

Eclampsia, or hypocalcemia, is characterized by tremors and excitation and is more common in smaller breeds. It most commonly occurs in the postpartum period. It is a true emergency. Hyperthermia and convulsions may require sedation or short-term anesthesia in addition to calcium treatment.

Pseudopregnancy

All bitches experience a 57- to 58-day period of elevated serum progesterone after estrus, whether pregnant or not. As progesterone declines at the end of a nonpregnant diestrus, many bitches, even if not pregnant, will experience mammary development, lactation, and maternal behavior. Clients may be concerned that the bitch is uncomfortable, or the behavioral changes may be unacceptable. With time, clinical signs will fade and the bitch will return to normal. Alternatively, hormonal treatment with mibolerone or cabergoline can be used. Treatment with a progestogen, such as megestrol acetate, is contraindicated because signs of pseudopregnancy will return when therapy is halted.

Pyometra (uterine infection) can be a life-threatening situation in the bitch. It is progesterone related, usually occurring during diestrus, and may follow inappropriate estrogen therapy. The bitch may or may not have a vaginal discharge depending on whether the cervix is open or closed. A bitch with pyometra is often lethargic, depressed, and febrile and exhibits polyuria and polydipsia. A leukocytosis is found on complete blood count (CBC). Palpation or ultrasonography reveals an enlarged, fluid-filled uterus. If the breeding potential of the bitch is to be preserved, medical treatment with prostaglandin, cabergoline, and antibiotics is indicated; otherwise, surgical treatment (ovariohysterectomy) is usually recommended.

Technician Note

A bitch with pyometra is often lethargic, depressed, and febrile and exhibits polyuria and polydipsia.

Mismating

It is not unusual to have a client bring in a dog that has been bred accidentally or escaped while in estrus and request that she be "mismated" (aborted). In the past, few options were available other than estradiol cypionate (ECP), ovariohysterectomy, or allowing her to whelp. The use of ECP is not without risks. If given late in estrus or at the beginning of diestrus there is a significant risk of pyometra. Another very serious potential complication with the use of ECP is aplastic anemia. Further, many bitches presented for mismating may actually not have been bred or will not become pregnant. In one report, more than half of the bitches presented for pregnancy termination were not pregnant and therefore would have been treated needlessly. For these reasons, and the availability of suitable alternatives, the use of ECP for mismating is no longer recommended. In many cases, the preferred method is to wait until such time as pregnancy diagnosis can be performed. If the bitch is pregnant, therapeutic options include prostaglandin, cabergoline, bromocriptine, or dexamethasone.

Prostaglandin effectively terminates pregnancy and is safe in dogs if used properly. Prostaglandin should be given subcutaneously, rather than intramuscularly. Further, a single dose will be ineffective in lysing the corpora lutea so multiple small doses are used, usually two or three times per day for 5 to 7 days. Side effects include vomiting, diarrhea, and urination. An uncommon complication is

cardiovascular collapse. Therefore an intravenous catheter is often recommended during the initial phases of treatment in case fluid therapy is necessary.

An alternative to prostaglandin is cabergoline (or a related compound, bromocriptine). Both are dopamine agonists, and administration will result in progesterone decline and pregnancy loss. Bromocriptine may be associated with vomiting, whereas cabergoline causes few side effects.

Dexamethasone is an attractive alternative to the previously mentioned drugs. It is administered orally, so it can be given at home. With any of these drugs, it is important to monitor pregnancy loss and continue therapy until abortion is complete. In addition, if the pregnancy is advanced when therapy is begun, it is important to inform the client that fetal discharge may be observed.

Brucellosis

Canine brucellosis, although typically thought of as a disease characterized by abortion and infertility, may manifest itself in a variety of ways. Although usually considered a venereal disease, *Brucella. canis* is also spread through oronasal routes. Aborted fetuses and vaginal discharges are rich sources of *B. canis* organisms. Infected males shed the organism in their urine in addition to their semen. Transmission can occur between adult dogs in the absence of aborted material or sexual contact.

Because *B. canis* is an intracellular organism, the disease is extremely difficult to treat effectively and cures are nearly impossible to achieve. No treatment has been found that is 100% effective in achieving a cure, although serum titers may decrease. Because of the nature of the disease and the potential for spread, euthanasia is commonly recommended for breeding animals in a kennel situation. A less drastic choice for pets is neutering and antibiotic therapy, although persistent infection is still likely.

Because of the finality of neutering or euthanasia, a correct diagnosis is imperative. Unfortunately, many testing methods result in a high incidence of false-positive results and can be regarded as screening tests only. For example, antibodies against antigens of *Pseudomonas aeruginosa*, *Bordetella bronchiseptica*, and some *Staphylococcus* spp. can cause a false-positive result in a brucellosis test. Therefore a positive reaction on a screening test does not mean a dog is infected but does suggest the need for further, more definitive diagnosis.

The in-house screening test (D-Tec CB, Synbiotics) is very rapid and very sensitive. False-positive results are very common (20% to 50% of positive dogs do not have brucellosis, and some breeds, such as English sheepdogs, have exceptionally high false-positive rates) (Figure 16-16). A negative result is highly accurate, provided infection did not occur within 3 to 4 weeks before testing. Screening tests can give a false-negative result when a dog is infected for less than 4 weeks or is chronically infected and has recently received antibiotic treatment. If a dog is positive on the in-house test, samples should then be submitted to a diagnostic laboratory for further testing with a more specific test.

FELINE REPRODUCTION

Although most species have an LH surge that causes ovulation during every estrous cycle, the queen must have vaginal stimulation to induce an LH surge. The queen is therefore an induced ovulator. Because the queen does not necessarily ovulate during each estrous cycle, there are unique aspects in the queen's estrous cycle that are not seen in other species. When a queen comes into estrus, there are three potential outcomes after estrus: the queen can ovulate and become pregnant, the queen can ovulate and not become pregnant, or the queen may not ovulate (Figure 16-17). Each of these outcomes results in a different series of subsequent events and time sequences for return to estrus. The outcomes also depend on the season of the year, because queens are seasonal breeders.

Technician Note

The queen is an induced ovulator.

Seasonality

Most queens have estrous cycles during the spring and are considered long-day breeders. This may be masked by the fact that most domestic cats are kept indoors under artificial lighting. The artificial lighting may be sufficient to stimulate estrous cycles all year long. The season and effect of artificial lighting must always be taken into account when discussing the queen's estrous cycle.

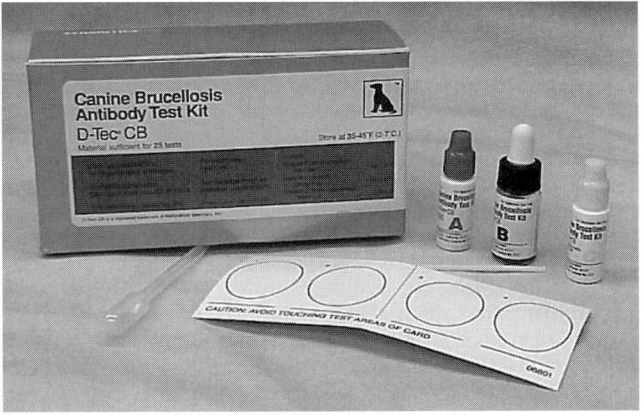

FIGURE 16-16. A commercially available kit to check for *Brucella canis.*

Estrous Cycle

Proestrus in the queen is only 1 to 3 days long and may not be apparent. Estrus in the queen lasts 8 to 10 days, and the queen shows very distinctive outward signs of estrus. These signs include rolling and assuming an exaggerated lordosis when petted. The lordosis results in an elevation of the queen's hindquarters. These signs are so intense that many queens in estrus are presented for neurologic problems. Unlike other species that automatically enter a diestrus period of progesterone domination after estrus, the queen must have adequate vaginal stimulation to ovulate. The vaginal stimulation must come after the third day of estrus, and there must be multiple stimulations at least 2 to 3 hours apart to induce an LH rise sufficient to cause ovulation. Even if breeding does occur, vaginal stimulation will not necessarily be adequate to elicit a sufficient LH rise to cause ovulation.

If the queen ovulates and becomes pregnant, the gestation period is 63 to 66 days after mating. After parturition the queen undergoes an anestrous period of variable duration. Anestrus is a time when nothing is happening on the ovaries and the queen does not come into estrus. Postpartum anestrus may be as short as 2 weeks or as long as 6 weeks. Depending on the season and/or lighting conditions, the queen may then return to proestrus or go into seasonal anestrus.

If a queen is bred, ovulates, but does not become pregnant, a diestrus (or pseudopregnancy) of approximately 40 days follows the estrus. During diestrus the queen has high concentrations of progesterone produced by the corpora lutea on the ovaries that prevents the return to estrus. These corpora lutea apparently have a finite life span and cannot be lysed with exogenous prostaglandin. After a nonpregnant diestrus, a short anestrus occurs. This anestrus is approximately 2 weeks long. Again, depending on the season and/or lighting conditions, the queen may return to proestrus or enter a seasonal anestrus.

If the queen is not bred or is bred and has insufficient stimulation to cause an LH surge, ovulation will not take place. If there is no ovulation, the follicles on the ovary regress. At this time there are no structures on the ovaries (follicles or CLs), so this is called *anestrus*. This is a transitory anestrus so a better term is *interestrus*. Depending on the season and/or lighting conditions, the interestrus may be 3 to 14 days or may extend into a long seasonal anestrus.

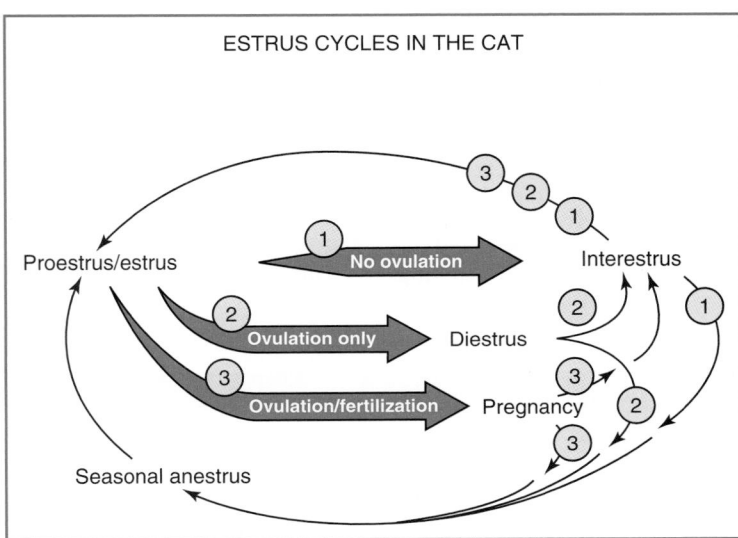

FIGURE 16-17. The feline estrous cycle. Depending on the season and if ovulation occurs, the queen can do one of six things on entering an 8-day estrus. If ovulation is not induced *(1)*, the queen can go into a 2- to 14-day interestrus or seasonal anestrus. If the queen ovulates but is not pregnant *(2)*, a 36-day diestrus followed by either a 2- to 14-day interestrus or seasonal anestrus can occur. If the queen ovulates and is pregnant *(3)*, a 65-day pregnancy followed by either a 2- to 6-week interestrus or seasonal anestrus may occur.

Technician Note

Pregnancy can be diagnosed in the queen from 16 to 30 days postcoitus by abdominal palpation, after 14 days postcoitus to term by ultrasound, and after 43 days by radiography.

Pregnancy can be diagnosed in the queen 16 to 30 days postcoitus by abdominal palpation, after 14 days postcoitus to term by ultrasound, and after 43 days by radiography. Palpation must be done within a time frame, because the gestational sacs are too small before day 16 and they become too confluent after day 30 to distinguish. Ultrasound can detect if the fetus is alive by seeing the fetal heartbeat, but it is difficult to count the number of fetuses and to estimate their size. Radiography is the best method to count the number of conceptuses and to estimate their size, but fetal mineralization of the skeleton must be adequate to detect them radiographically.

Common Reproductive Problems

Queens are generally very fertile and have few infertility problems. Because most pet queens have ovariohysterectomies performed at an early age, few of these queens are seen for reproductive problems.

The most common questions arise from the irritating clinical signs that accompany estrus in the queen. Queens that have not undergone ovariohysterectomy are often presented for prolonged estrus. Although cystic ovaries do occur in queens, they are not often the cause of the prolonged estrus. More commonly, a queen with persistent estrus is undergoing normal estrus, with a very short 1- to 2-day interestrus, followed by another estrus. This makes it seem like the queen is in constant estrus, when in fact there are normal periods of estrus and interestrus occurring. Treatment for this condition is either ovariohysterectomy or induction of ovulation.

Ovulation can be induced by vaginal stimulation with a cotton swab, glass rod, or thermometer. The stimulations must meet the same criteria as breeding to be effective: the vaginal stimulation must come after the third day of estrus, and there must be multiple stimulations at least 2 to 3 hours apart to induce an LH rise sufficient to cause ovulation. An alternative to vaginal stimulation is the administration of GnRH or human chorionic gonadotropin (hCG). The GnRH will cause an endogenous release of LH from the anterior pituitary, thereby resulting in ovulation. The drug hCG has LH action and will directly cause ovulation. After ovulation induction, estrus will not be shortened; however, the queen will then enter diestrus and interestrus phases, so estrus will not recur for approximately 2 months. There are no drugs approved to control the estrous cycle in the queen.

Another common complaint is the queen that comes into estrus after ovariohysterectomy. It is important to document the presence of extra ovarian tissue by hormone analysis. This is most easily done using the same techniques to induce ovulation. If the queen goes out of estrus and has high progesterone, then extra ovarian tissue must be sought surgically. If not, then the adrenals may be the source of the estrogen causing the signs of estrus.

Parturition in the queen can last as long as 36 hours. The following criteria can be used to diagnose dystocia (abnormal birth): 20 minutes of intense labor with no kitten, 10 minutes of intense labor when a kitten is present, acute depression, or the presence of fresh blood for more than 10 minutes. If any of these criteria is noted, it is advised that the queen be examined. Although most queens do not

have problems queening, an examination and radiographs will help rule out if a cesarean delivery is required.

The normal pospartum discharge is red-black, nonodorous fluid that can be seen as long as 3 weeks after queening. If the queen appears depressed or the kittens are dying, the queen should be examined for mastitis or metritis.

Technician Note

The normal pospartum discharge is red-black, nonodorous fluid that can be seen as long as 3 weeks after queening.

Pyometra in the queen presents with similar signs as seen in the bitch, including depression and vaginal discharge. Bitches with pyometras tend to be older, whereas queens can be any age.

EQUINE REPRODUCTION

Mares are seasonally polyestrous, meaning that during the breeding season they cycle repeatedly. The natural breeding season centers around the period of long day length. Under natural conditions, mares begin cycling in late March or early April and continue until September or October. Some mares may continue to cycle year round. In the northern hemisphere, many breed associations have designated January 1 as the birth date for all horses born in a given year. This means that a horse born in January and a horse born in June will both be considered 1 year old the following January when they are actually 12 months and 7 months old, respectively. This is a large difference for horses competing as 2 year olds. Therefore there is a great deal of pressure to have foals born early in the season (January or February). Unfortunately, many mares are not cycling at this time. The most cost-effective method to stimulate earlier cyclicity is to "trick" the mare into perceiving that the days are lengthening by providing artificial lighting and mimicking a 16-hour daylight period. This should be started by December 1 to get the most benefit. A 200-watt bulb in a 12- × 12-foot stall is sufficient. For an outdoor situation, eight 1000-watt metal halide flood lights at a height of 20 feet will provide sufficient light for an 84- × 66-foot paddock. Artificial lighting should be added in the evening, rather than in the morning. Turning the lights on earlier in the morning is less effective than leaving them on later in the evening.

During the breeding season, the mare's estrous cycle averages 21 to 22 days in length. Diestrus, the period when a corpus luteum is present and producing progesterone, is a consistent 15 days in length, based on hormone levels (Figure 16-18). During this time, the mare will tease "out," resisting the stallion's advances by kicking, squealing, pinning her ears back, and clamping her tail between her legs. Based on behavioral signs, diestrus is shorter (approximately 14 days) because she does not tease "out" until 1 day or so after ovulation. Estrus, or the period of receptivity, is shown by teasing "in." The mare squats, urinates, lifts her tail, and "winks" (everts her clitoris) on approach of the stallion.

Technician Note

Estrus, or the period of receptivity, is shown by teasing "in."

Between the noncycling period (anestrus) and the cycling period, a period called *transition* occurs. Transition

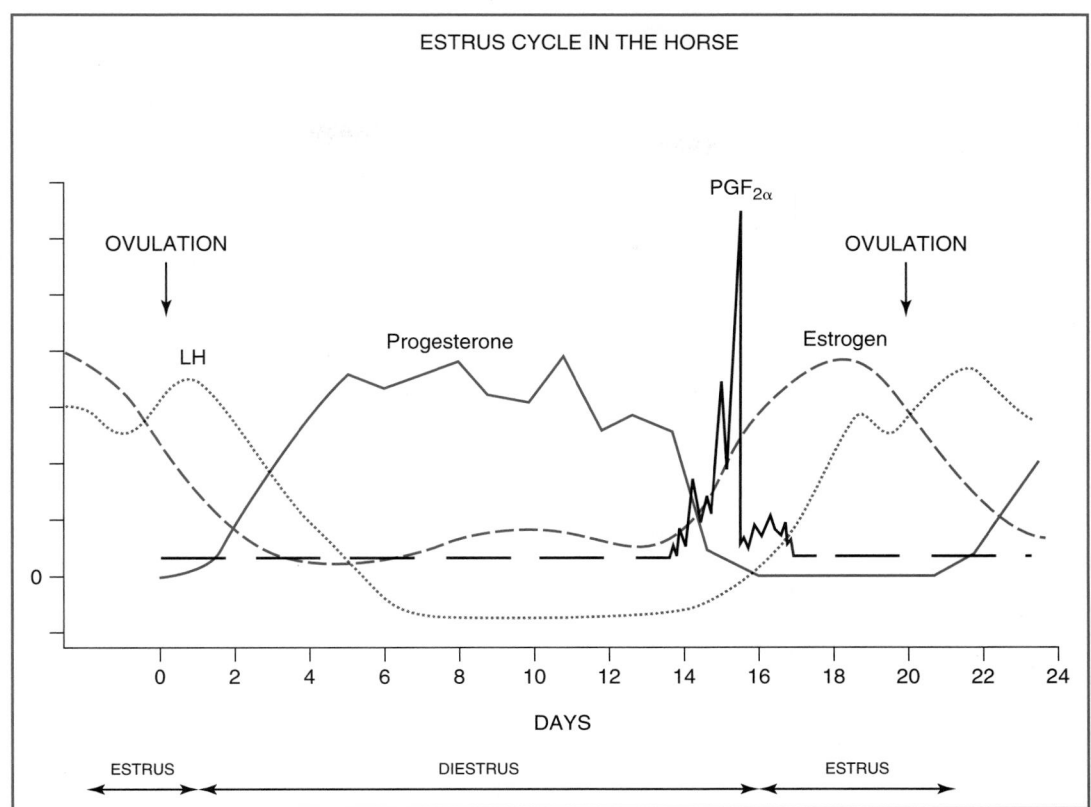

FIGURE 16-18. The equine estrous cycle. Estrus is 5 to 7 days long, and LH peaks after ovulation. Diestrus begins around 2 days after ovulation. Progesterone is high throughout a 14- to 15-day diestrus. If a pregnancy signal is not secreted by the early embryo by day 15 or 16, prostaglandin is released from the uterus, goes to the corpus luteum, and causes luteolysis (luteal death). The cycle then starts over.

varies in length and is characterized by irregular periods of estrous behavior but without ovulation. A mare may exhibit estrous behavior for 2 or 3 days, then stop for a few days, and then begin again. Alternatively the mare may exhibit estrous behavior continuously without ovulation for 3 weeks or more. Although follicles may be present during these periods, they do not ovulate. The transitional period is a physiologically normal occurrence. Although cyclicity can be induced earlier in the year, a transitional period will still precede the onset of cyclicity. Awareness of this can help to reduce needless breedings and help mare owners understand this sometimes aggravating period. Administration of altrenogest, a synthetic progestogen, will stop the estrous behavior and is often used during transition.

During the breeding season, the duration of estrus is variable (4 to 7 days). Estrus tends to be shorter near the peak of the breeding season (June) and longer farther away from June, such as March or September. Follicular development can be monitored by palpation per rectum and ultrasonography during estrus to decide optimal breeding time.

Breeding Soundness Examination

Breeding soundness examinations are commonly performed at the sale or purchase of a mare or when a mare fails to become pregnant after breeding. A typical breeding soundness examination consists of rectal palpation, ultrasonography, vaginal speculum examination, uterine cul-

ture/cytology, and a uterine biopsy. During the ultrasonographic examination, structures on the ovaries, and more importantly, features of the uterus can be observed. Fluid-filled structures such as follicles (Figure 16-19) and endometrial cysts will be black. Corpora lutea have a variable appearance, ranging from a rather homogeneous gray to a "spider web" trabecular pattern with a brighter thick-walled circumference. An important indication of the stage of the estrous cycle is the ultrasonographic appearance of the uterus. During diestrus it has a homogeneous hyperechoic appearance, but in estrus it has a very characteristic appearance caused by edema in the endometrial folds. It has been described as looking like the spokes of a cartwheel, an orange slice, or pizza (Figure 16-20).

Vaginal speculum examination, uterine culture/cytology, and uterine biopsy are performed aseptically. First wrap the tail with a clean tail wrap or gauze. Prepare a clean bucket with clean water and add small (approximately 10 cm × 10 cm) pieces of cotton. Rather than placing disinfectant in the bucket, it is preferable to place the soap on the cotton itself before scrubbing the vulva, thereby leaving clean water to rinse the vulva. Otherwise, disinfectant residues may remain on the vulva and be carried into the vagina, with a potential spermicidal or tissue-irritating effect. The vulvar labia should be scrubbed in a manner similar to that for surgical preparation, that is, from the center of the area being cleaned to the perimeter and repeated until clean. Check the inside of the labia during the procedure to be sure no feces have

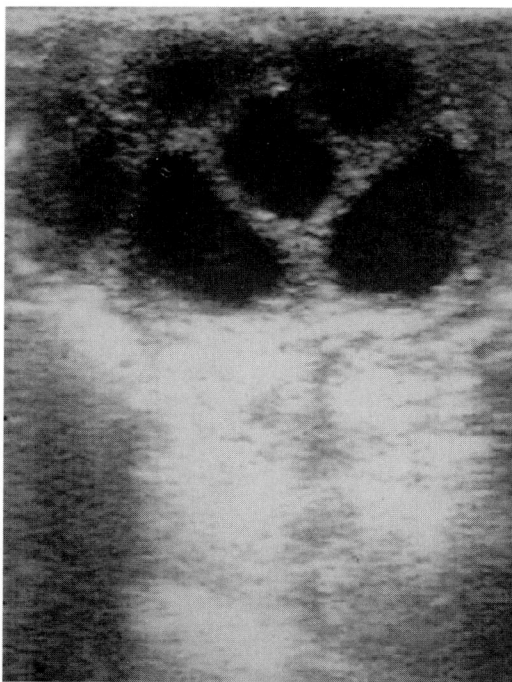

FIGURE 16-19. An ultrasound image of the black appearance of multiple follicles on an equine ovary.

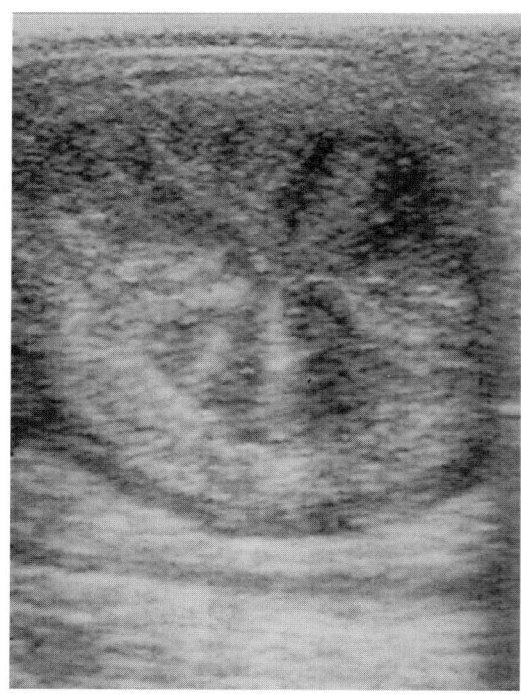

FIGURE 16-20. The sliced-orange ultrasonographic appearance of the uterus of a mare in estrus.

entered as a result of the palpation and ultrasonography procedures.

A vaginal speculum examination can discern trauma to the cervix; discharge emanating from the uterus, cervix, or vagina; urine pooling in the cranial vagina; and other conditions associated with subfertility. After aseptically preparing the vulva, a small amount of sterile lubricant is placed on the end of a speculum, the labia are parted, and the speculum is placed into the vagina. A light source is then used to look through the speculum and examine the vagina and cervix (Figure 16-21).

The next procedure usually performed is a uterine culture/cytology. The importance of performing a cytologic examination in conjunction with the culture cannot be overstated. Without a cytologic specimen, it is impossible to differentiate between an infectious process and a contaminant resulting from improper sampling or mare preparation. When obtaining a culture/cytology specimen only guarded swabs should be used. After aseptically preparing the vulva, a sterile sleeve is used to introduce the culture/cytology instrument into the vagina, through the cervix, and into the uterus. After the swab is withdrawn, the sample can be used to prepare a cytology specimen. Stain the cytology slide using a modified Wright's or Giemsa stain. The slide should contain numerous epithelial cells and be examined for inflammatory cells, primarily neutrophils. A positive cytology slide will contain numerous inflammatory cells, whereas a negative slide will not. Bacteria isolated from a culture with a negative cytology finding can be considered contaminants. In fact, an argument can be made to not submit the culture if the slide is negative. However, if the slide is positive, not only do culture results reveal the causative agent but also sensitivity results aid in making a therapeutic choice. Excess lubricant

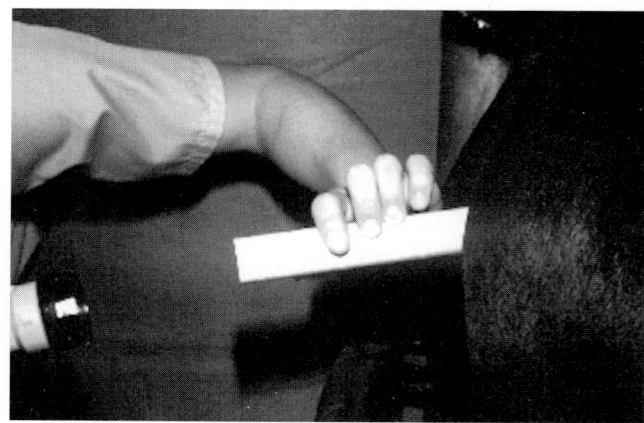

FIGURE 16-21. A vaginal speculum examination being performed on a mare using a disposable speculum.

used during the procedure can interfere with interpretation by staining darkly and obscuring the field.

The next, and often final, step in the breeding soundness examination is to obtain an endometrial biopsy. Again, as with the previous procedures, it is done in an aseptic manner. The closed instrument is carried into the uterus, wearing a sterile sleeve (Figure 16-22). The instrument is held in the uterus while the hand is withdrawn and placed in the rectum. The instrument is then opened to permit endometrial tissue to enter the jaws and then closed to snip off a piece of endometrium. The tissue is next placed in fixative and processed through a laboratory.

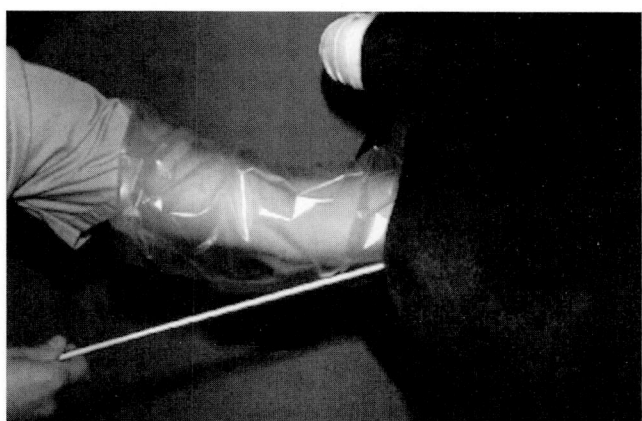

FIGURE 16-22. A uterine biopsy instrument being inserted through the vagina and cervix into the uterus.

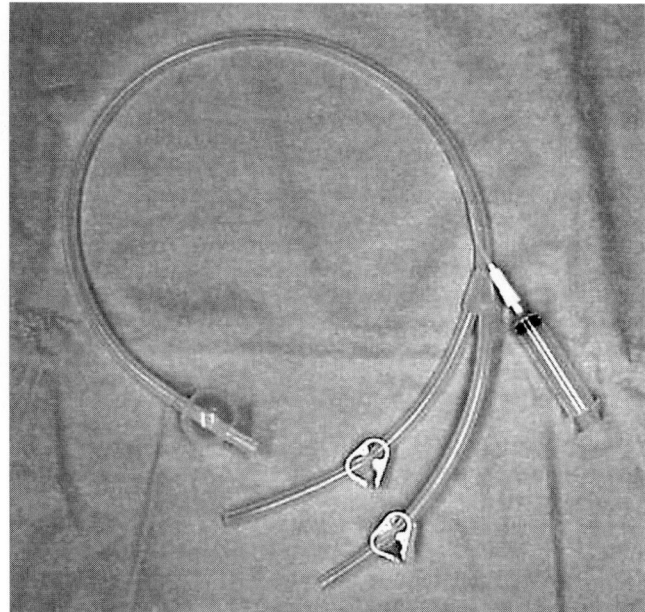

FIGURE 16-23. A large-bore catheter used to lavage a mare's uterus.

Artificial Insemination (Uterine Infusion)

Breeding a mare by artificial insemination (AI) is a relatively simple procedure. It is an aseptic procedure, and the same procedure is used for AI as for uterine infusion. A sterile sleeve is donned and a sterile pipette carried through the vagina and cervix into the uterus. The semen or intrauterine medication is then deposited directly into the uterus.

Postbreeding Treatments

In addition to oxytocin or cloprostenol injections, common postbreeding treatments include intrauterine infusion of antibiotics and uterine lavage. Intrauterine infusion is performed in the same aseptic manner using sterile equipment as artificial insemination.

Uterine lavage is performed using a large-bore catheter with an inflatable cuff (Figure 16-23). The catheter is placed in the uterus, and the cuff is inflated and seated against the internal cervical os to provide a good seal. Sterile saline, usually 1 L at a time, is infused into the uterus and then retrieved. This is repeated until the saline retrieved is clear. This procedure helps to clear the uterus of debris.

Pregnancy

Diagnosis

Pregnancy diagnosis is usually done with the aid of ultrasonography 2 weeks after ovulation. With experience, the characteristic ultrasonographic appearance of the conceptus at various stages can be easily recognized and used to evaluate its growth and health (Figure 16-24). The term *conceptus* refers to everything derived from the fertilized ovum, including the fetal membranes and fluids as well as the embryo or fetus. Fetal sexing is most commonly performed between 60 and 70 days by identifying the position of the genital tubercle.

Hormonal methods for pregnancy diagnosis exist. They can be useful in cases where rectal palpation is not feasible, such as with very small miniature horses or wild, fractious mares. Pregnant mares will test positive for equine chorionic gonadotropin (eCG), formerly called pregnant mare serum gonadotropin (PMSG), from 35 days until approximately 120 days of gestation. False-positive results happen if fetal death occurs during that period. Another hormone used for pregnancy testing is estrone sulfate. The benefit of

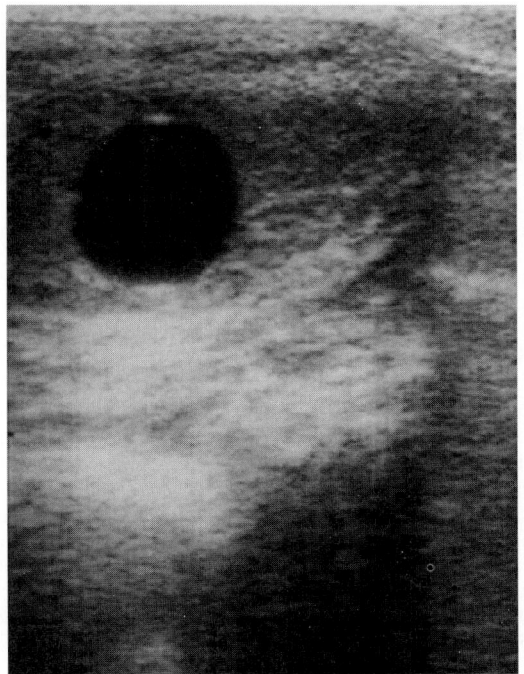

FIGURE 16-24. An ultrasound of the black appearance of a 14-day pregnancy in an equine uterus.

estrone sulfate, compared with eCG, is that it is produced in high quantities by a viable fetoplacental unit beginning around 60 days of gestation. If the pregnancy is lost, estrone sulfate drops off rapidly so false-positive results are uncommon.

Vaccinations

Equine herpesvirus can be a significant cause of abortion in horses. Vaccines are available, and a good program consists of vaccination at 5, 7, and 9 months of gestation. Either a killed or modified live vaccine may be used. Repeated vaccinations at these intervals are necessary each time a mare is pregnant in order to provide good protection. In addition, it is advisable to minimize stress and is important to keep pregnant mares separated from new additions to the herd or horses that have a lot of outside contact.

It is also recommended to give an annual booster for flu, encephalitis, and tetanus at 10 months' gestation. This practice will help to ensure good-quality colostrum and increase the level of protection provided to the foal by passive transfer of antibodies through the colostrum. Additional information on preventive health programs is found in Chapter 11.

Parturition

Gestation length in mares is generally quoted as 330 to 340 days. However, there is a wide variation in normal gestation length, ranging from 320 to 400 days. It is important to remember that the fetus determines gestation length. For this reason, chemical induction of parturition based on gestation length alone is risky and can result in the birth of premature foals. The decision to induce parturition is based on the following criteria: (1) gestation length greater than 330 days, (2) relaxation of pelvic ligaments, (3) presence of colostrum in the udder, (4) relaxation or softening of the cervix, and most importantly (5) milk calcium more than 400 ppm with milk potassium higher than sodium. The electrolyte changes are very well correlated with fetal maturity and are the best way to assess readiness for birth. Calcium can be measured with a water hardness test kit, but be sure to use one that measures only calcium, not just divalent cations. Magnesium, another divalent cation present in colostrum, rises slowly as parturition approaches and can interfere with interpretation of the results. Milk calcium greater than 400 ppm and potassium less than sodium can occur in cases of placentitis or twins, so induction of parturition should not be considered unless potassium is greater than sodium, along with the increase in calcium.

Parturition

Parturition is a very rapid process in horses. In the normal course of events, as the mare begins labor (stage I) she will lie down, get up, roll, and so forth. During these maneuvers, the foal is getting into the correct position. Finally at the end of stage I, the chorioallantois ruptures ("water breaks"), signaling the onset of stage II. Usually within 10 minutes a bluish white membrane (amnion) appears at the vulvar opening. Within another 10 minutes the feet will protrude through the vulva, still within the amnion. After another 10 minutes the head protrudes and delivery will be completed soon thereafter (Figure 16-25).

Technician Note

Parturition is a very rapid process in horses.

A red membrane protruding from the vulva, the chorioallantois, is an indication of premature placental separation, or "red bag." This is an emergency, and the chorioallantois must be ruptured manually and delivery assisted or the foal will quickly die.

If the guidelines for the time frame of delivery are not

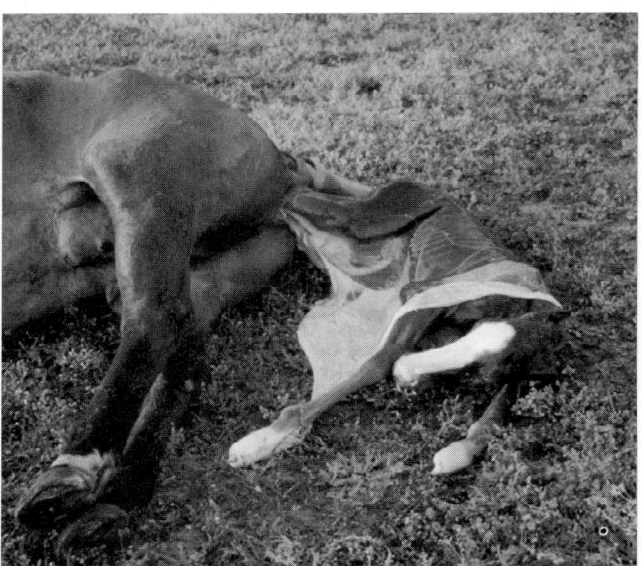

FIGURE 16-25. A foal being delivered by a mare.

being met, examination for possible dystocia is indicated. It is critical to perform any obstetric manipulations in as clean a manner as possible and with sufficient good-quality obstetric lubricant. Failure to adhere to guidelines of strict cleanliness and ample lubrication invites complications in the postpartum period and can compromise future fertility.

Postpartum Problems

Mares do not experience postpartum problems as commonly as cows, but when they do, they can be life threatening. A retained placenta for more than 6 hours' duration deserves veterinary attention. Various methods, such as large-volume saline distension or oxytocin therapy, can be used to stimulate placental release. Manually detaching the placenta should not be done because of the potential for causing damage to the uterus and hemorrhage. Systemic antibiotics, antiinflammatories, and tetanus toxoid are usually administered in cases of retained placenta more than 6 hours in duration.

Technician Note

A retained placenta for more than 6 hours' duration deserves veterinary attention.

Postpartum metritis, often a sequela to retained placenta or contamination during obstetric procedures, can lead to septicemia and laminitis. As a result, treatment should not be delayed in a postpartum mare that has a foul-smelling vaginal discharge or is febrile or depressed.

Hormone Use in Mares

Prostaglandin

Prostaglandin $F_{2\alpha}$, and its analog cloprostenol, can be used to lyse a corpus luteum and return a mare to estrus. It is effective beginning about 5 or 6 days after ovulation, when the corpus luteum has matured sufficiently to respond. Mares will return to estrus in 2 to 7 days after prostaglandin administration. Prostaglandin should not be used to induce parturition because of the high incidence of premature placental separation, dystocia, and fetal death.

Human Chorionic Gonadotropin

Human chorionic gonadotropin (hCG) is used to induce ovulation in mares that have a follicle 35 mm or larger. Dosages commonly used range from 2000 to 3500 IU given intravenously, and ovulation can be expected to occur in 36 to 48 hours in approximately 80% of mares. Although concerns about antibody production have been expressed, no correlation between antibodies and failure to induce ovulation has been shown. Nevertheless, some mares fail to ovulate after receiving hCG repeatedly.

Deslorelin

An alternative to hCG for ovulation induction is an analog of GnRH, deslorelin (Ovuplant, Fort Dodge Animal Health). Ovulation occurs within approximately the same time frame as with hCG. However, deslorelin appears to be more effective on slightly smaller (30-mm) follicles than hCG and failure of the mare to ovulate is reportedly less common.

Progestins

Altrenogest (Regu-Mate, Intervet) is a progesterone-like compound that is administered orally. It is used primarily for pregnancy maintenance and estrous cycle control. Its use for pregnancy maintenance is empiric in that true progesterone deficiency as a cause of pregnancy loss has not been documented. However, anecdotal reports of mares failing to maintain pregnancy unless supplemented with altrenogest are not uncommon. Because the fetoplacental unit eventually takes over progestogen production, altrenogest therapy can usually be discontinued at about 4 months' gestation.

The other reason to use altrenogest is estrous cycle control. Altrenogest mimics progesterone in the mare. Therefore mares given altrenogest act as if they were in diestrus. Altrenogest can be used for estrus synchronization in embryo transfer programs and to manipulate the estrous cycle to prevent or control the onset of estrus in performance mares. Altrenogest is also used in mares in late gestation when there is concern about possible impending abortion. Through its action, uterine motility is inhibited, thereby supporting maintenance of pregnancy.

Oxytocin

A common cause of infertility is persistent mating-induced endometritis. An inflammatory response to sperm cells normally occurs after breeding, whether by natural service or artificial insemination. This inflammatory response is necessary to remove excess semen and debris and to prepare the uterus for pregnancy. Uterine clearance mechanisms, such as uterine motility and lymphatic drainage, are critical in this process. Infertility results when uterine clearance mechanisms fail and fluid remains in the uterus after breeding. Ultrasound examination 12 hours or more after breeding should reveal no fluid in the uterus. If fluid is still present, oxytocin therapy (20 IU intravenously or intramuscularly) should be instituted. Oxytocin is very effective in aiding uterine clearance and can be given as often as every 2 or 3 hours.

Oxytocin is also the only drug available to safely and reliably induce parturition. If the mare has met the criteria and is ready to give birth, a small dose (10 IU intravenously) of oxytocin is sufficient to initiate parturition. Lower doses result in a more natural process, whereas higher doses result in a faster and more forceful delivery.

Domperidone

Domperidone is a dopamine antagonist used to alleviate the effects of fescue toxicosis and stimulate lactation. It has also shown some promise to stimulate cyclicity in mares with lactational anestrus and may be beneficial in hastening the onset of cyclicity in the spring, but this has not yet been well documented.

BOVINE REPRODUCTION

The cow is a nonseasonal polyestrous species, meaning that cows have estrous cycles all year around. The entire estrous cycle averages 21 days long, but it can be as short as 18 days and as long as 24 days (Figure 16-26). Estrus lasts 18 to 20 hours but may be shorter in hot, humid weather because of heat stress. Estrus is the time the cow is in "standing heat" and will stand with all four legs firmly braced to be mounted by a bull or another cow. Ovulation occurs 12 to 18 hours after the end of estrus. Estrus is followed by metestrus, which is 3 to 5 days long and is the time of luteal development. A bloody discharge from the vulva may be noticed in nearly half of all cows and heifers 1 or 2 days after they are in estrus. This is no indication of fertility or infertility but merely a sign that the individual was in estrus 1 or 2 days earlier. During metestrus, a corpus hemorrhagicum (CH) is formed at the site of ovulation. This structure will develop into a corpus luteum over the next few days. However, during metestrus the CL is not yet mature and not yet susceptible to the luteolytic action of prostaglandin. The next phase is called *diestrus* and lasts from day 5 or 6 until day 17 of the estrous cycle and is the time that the mature corpus luteum ("yellow body") is present and producing progesterone. During diestrus there are waves of follicular growth that are important in understanding a cow's response to estrous cycle synchronization. At the end of diestrus, if an embryo is not present in the uterus to provide a pregnancy signal, the uterus releases prostaglandin that lyses the corpus luteum, resulting in a decline of progesterone and the cow returns to proestrus.

Bovine Pregnancy Diagnosis

Various methods of pregnancy diagnosis exist, but the most commonly employed is rectal palpation. An experienced person can diagnose pregnancy by 30 days' gestation. Ultrasonography is becoming more popular for pregnancy diagnosis. Machines have become more affordable, and accurate pregnancy diagnosis can be performed by 24 days or earlier in some cases. Fetal viability can be assessed and fetal sexing is possible between 55 and 70 days.

Technician Note

Various methods of pregnancy diagnosis exist, but the most commonly employed is rectal palpation.

Progesterone tests should not be regarded as pregnancy tests. Although a progesterone test can detect the presence of a corpus luteum, many scenarios exist where a corpus luteum is present and progesterone is high but the cow is not pregnant.

Breeding/Artificial Insemination

Most dairy cattle, and increasing numbers of beef cattle, are bred by artificial insemination. There are numerous advantages to artificial insemination, with rapid genetic improvement being the primary one. However, the need for estrus detection in order to time insemination is a major

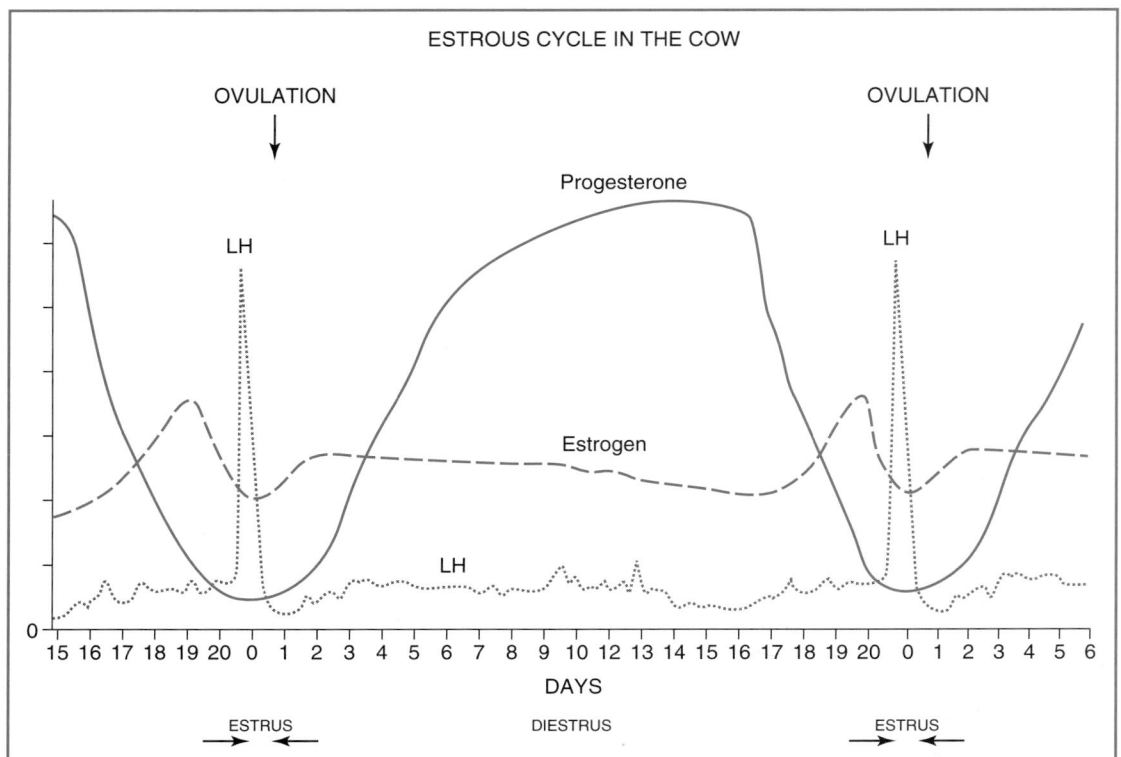

FIGURE 16-26. The bovine estrous cycle. Estrus is 24 hours long, and LH peaks during estrus. Diestrus lasts until about day 17, and progesterone is high throughout diestrus. If a pregnancy signal is not secreted by the early embryo by day 16 or 17, prostaglandin is released from the uterus, goes to the corpus luteum, and causes luteolysis (luteal death). The cycle then starts over.

drawback. Fortunately, cows, especially dairy cows, exhibit "standing heat" when in estrus and observation of this behavior is the best method of estrus detection. "Teaser" bulls, bulls that have been surgically altered to prevent vaginal penetration with the penis and have had vasectomies to render them sterile, can be used to help with estrus detection.

Estrus synchronization, through the use of hormones, also helps improve estrus detection. Many schemes have been devised using prostaglandin to lyse the corpus luteum. Other schemes use progestogen to mimic the luteal phase and suppress follicular growth. Currently, one of the most popular methods involves an injection of GnRH, followed by an injection of prostaglandin $F_{2\alpha}$ (PGF$_{2\alpha}$) 7 days later, followed by a second injection of GnRH 48 hours later and insemination 16 to 18 hours after that.

Abnormalities of the Estrous Cycle

Anestrus
The most common reason for failure of a cow to show estrus is pregnancy, whether as a result of poor record keeping or an unknown visit by a neighboring bull. For this reason it is always advisable to have a cow examined for pregnancy before attempting to "bring her into heat" with prostaglandin. After calving, a period of postpartum anestrus is common. This period is usually shorter for dairy cows (2 to 4 weeks depending on nutrition and environmental conditions) than for beef cows. Beef cows nursing calves have a longer period of postpartum anestrus, usually 45 to 90 days. The postpartum anestrus period in beef

cattle is prolonged if the cows are not in good body condition when they calve.

Pathologic reasons for anestrus include pyometra, luteal cysts, and follicular cystic degeneration. Pyometra may be caused by a number of factors, including trichomoniasis, bovine viral diarrhea (BVD) virus and postpartum uterine infection. It is characterized by a pus-filled uterus and a persistent corpus luteum. Treatment consists of simply administering prostaglandin, although two injections, 24 hours apart, may be needed to improve response.

Luteal cysts arise from follicles that fail to ovulate but do form luteal tissue. Progesterone is elevated, and a period of prolonged diestrus results. Treatment consists of prostaglandin injection. Follicular cysts result from follicles that fail to ovulate and do not form luteal tissue. Progesterone is low, and although some cows may exhibit persistent or frequent estrus, anestrus is much more common. Treatment consists of GnRH or hCG administration.

Abnormalities of Pregnancy

Uterine Prolapse
Uterine prolapse is easily recognized by the presence of the mucosal, or inner, surface of the uterus, with its characteristic caruncles, hanging from the vulva (Figure 16-27). It is more common in dairy than beef cattle. It occurs in the immediate postpartum period and is often associated with hypocalcemia or dystocia. Uterine prolapse should be considered an emergency, and the uterus should be replaced to its normal position as soon as possible. Uterine prolapse is not hereditary and is not considered to be likely to recur.

have calved yet so care will need to be taken to monitor her to reduce the chance of dystocia and mortality.

Dystocia

Dystocia is much more common in cattle than in mares. It is most commonly caused by fetal/maternal disproportion in size. Uterine torsion is also a fairly common cause of dystocia. As with mares, cleanliness and lubrication are essential for successful management of dystocia.

Milk Fever

Milk fever, or parturient hypocalcemia, most commonly occurs during the postpartum period although it may also occur during parturition. It is more common in dairy cattle than beef cattle. The incidence is increased when cattle are fed high levels of calcium prepartum. This condition should be viewed as an emergency and is treated by slow intravenous infusion of calcium gluconate. Milk fever is characterized by flaccid paralysis.

SWINE REPRODUCTION

Puberty

Gilts usually reach puberty at 4.5 to 6 months of age. Social environment and nutrition are important factors determining the onset of cyclicity in gilts. Onset of puberty is commonly seen in gilts weighing 82 kg or more. Direct contact between boars and gilts is very important in swine reproduction. Boars have pheromone-secreting salivary glands that sexually stimulate female pigs. This "boar effect" (stimulating or detecting estrus) is even more evident if mature, experienced boars are used. Daily exposure of 5- to 6-month-old gilts to a mature boar will hasten the onset of cyclicity. Season probably influences the onset of puberty, because gilts born in the fall start to cycle earlier than their spring-born counterparts. In addition, all factors that contribute to good management, such as number of gilts per pen, adequate physical space per gilt, ambient temperature, and health status (diseases, parasites) in general, will ensure that gilts reach puberty around 5 to 6 months of age.

Pharmacologic agents can also induce puberty. Fertile estrus and ovulation can be induced using exogenous gonadotropins. eCG in association with hCG is effective in inducing estrus in gilts. These two gonadotropins are marketed in a combination to induce estrus and ovulation. Estrogen administration is also effective but does not yield as reliable results as the eCG-hCG combination. GnRH is very effective, but it is expensive and needs to be delivered in a pulsatile fashion (every hour for 3 to 4 days), making this difficult to be done in a commercial unit.

Estrous Cycle

Domestic pigs are nonseasonal polyestrous animals. Female pigs exhibit estrus at 21-day intervals after they reach puberty. Longer estrous cycles, such as 26 days, have been associated with early embryonic mortality.

During proestrus, follicular development intensifies as the corpora lutea in the nonpregnant pig start to regress around day 15 of the estrous cycle. Initial behavioral signs of estrus are not always easily recognized. They include increased restlessness, reduced appetite, mounting other animals, homosexual behavior (malelike sexual activity), and lordosis. Lordosis occurs when pressure is applied on the pig's back by someone sitting on it and the female pig stands still, quiet, and passive, assuming a mating position. The vulva swells and becomes more pink and moist. A cloudy mucous discharge may be present during this phase.

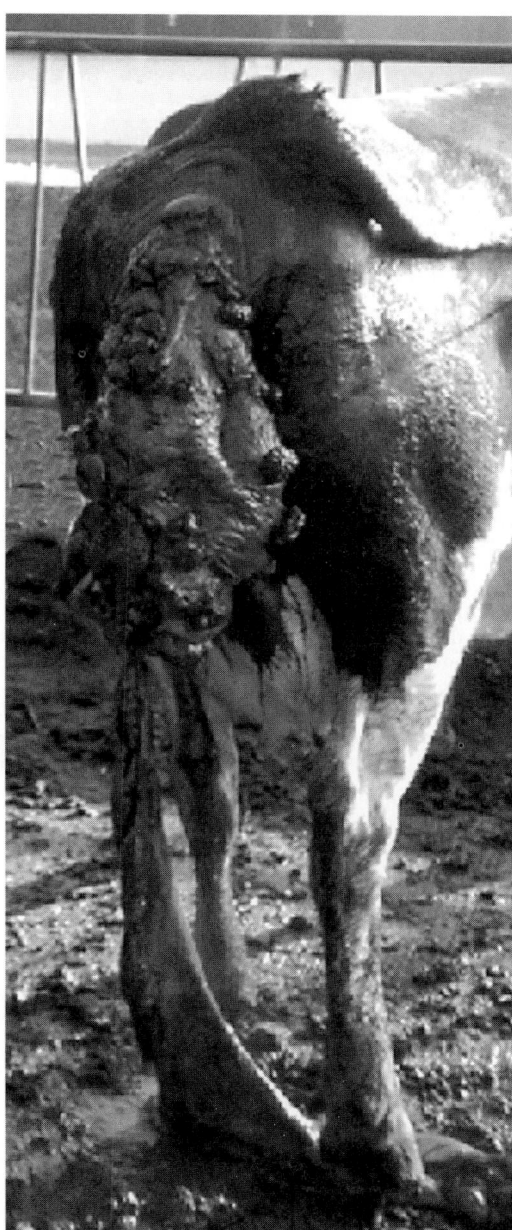

FIGURE 16-27. A bovine uterine prolapse. Note the caruncles on the exposed interior uterine surface.

Vaginal Prolapse

Although seemingly similar to uterine prolapse, vaginal prolapse is actually quite different. This is a hereditary problem. Therefore affected individuals should not be kept as breeding stock. It occurs under conditions associated with elevated estrogen, most commonly seen during late gestation, although it may also be associated with cystic follicular degeneration or ingestion of certain plants. Typically the affected animal will be a beef cow or heifer, in late gestation, and the vagina, and maybe also the cervix, will be protruding from the vulva. Various methods have been described to treat the condition, but all consist of cleaning the exposed tissue, replacing it, and preventing recurrence. It must be remembered that in most cases the cow will not

Estrus is the period when the female pig is responsive to the boar's approach. If male and female are put together during this stage, they start to show a precopulatory behavior (foreplay) that includes sniffing each other and head-to-head contact; the male starts to compulsively follow the female pig and initiate mounting attempts. Courtship culminates with the female pig standing still and allowing the boar to mount. The duration of estrus can be variable among individuals of different breeds or age or during different time of the year (longest in summer and shorter in winter). Estrus lasts on average 40 to 60 hours (2 to 3 days), but it can vary from 1 to 4 days. Ovulation usually takes place during the second day of estrus (36 to 44 hours after the onset of estrus), and mated females reportedly ovulate 4 hours before unmated female pigs. Follicular rupture of all follicles present in the ovary (10 to 20) may take 1 to 9 hours.

Diestrus is behaviorally characterized by a lack of sexual receptivity and lasts for 18 days if the female pig is not pregnant. Anestrus is mainly seen when sows are lactating.

Pregnancy

Deposition of semen in pigs is intracervical. The presence of cartilaginous rings in the sow's cervix in association with the fibroelastic spiral tip (corkscrew) of the boar's penis provides a natural and strong lock of the penis inside the cervix. Subsequently, during mating, strong contractions of the cervix are potentiated by oxytocin release in response to coitus. Several billion sperm cells are released during coitus in an average of 200 to 250 ml of semen. Uterine contractions allow a controlled number of sperm cells to reach the oviduct, where fertilization occurs. It seems that a minimum number of four embryos must be present in the uterus to cause appropriate maternal recognition of pregnancy. The average length of gestation is 114 days (3 months + 3 weeks + 3 days). Piglets are born weighing on average 1.4 to 1.6 kg. A tail-first presentation is not abnormal. Interval time between piglets averages 10 to 15 minutes. Intervals greater than 20 minutes are associated with an increasing number of stillbirths. All fetal membranes should be delivered in 4 to 6 hours.

Control of Farrowing

Farrowing can occur at any time of the day or night. Each sow may take several hours to deliver all the piglets and fetal membranes. It is important to assist sows during delivery because early detection and correction of potential problems during farrowing prevent piglet losses. Assistance during farrowing can be facilitated by pharmacologically inducing parturition. Accordingly, prostaglandin administration after day 112 of gestation will induce parturition in 20 to 30 hours. Combining prostaglandin with oxytocin or xylazine will help to improve the precision of response to prostaglandin administration.

Pharmacologic Control of the Estrous Cycle

Exogenous hormones can be used to alter or manipulate the estrous cycle in pigs. Estrus and ovulation can be induced by different means either in cycling pigs or in early pregnant pigs to synchronize estrus (Table 16-2).

PG 600 contains 400 IU of eCG and 200 units of hCG. It can be used to induce estrus in prepubertal gilts or in sows showing anestrus after weaning. It can also be used in cycling sows after day 16 of the estrous cycle. The administration of PG 600 will cause estrus and ovulation in 3 to 5 days following treatment. Estrus/ovulation can also be induced by administration of eCG and hCG 2 days apart. Prostaglandin can be used to terminate pregnancy or

diestrus only if given 12 days after ovulation. Before day 12, multiple injections (twice daily for 5 days) of prostaglandins are necessary to interrupt diestrus (short cycling) or to terminate pregnancy. Weaned sows usually show spontaneous signs of estrus in 11 to 12 days after weaning. Administration of PG 600 on the day of weaning will also induce estrus in 3 to 5 days. Sows that do not come into estrus in 2 weeks after weaning will show signs of estrus if PG 600 is administered.

Artificial Insemination

Artificial insemination with fresh or cooled semen is commonly performed in the swine industry. The boar is easily trained to mount a dummy and have semen manually collected. After collecting the sperm-rich portion of the ejaculate, semen is evaluated to determine its quality and how much extender to add. A sow should be inseminated with 3 to 4 billion sperm cells in a volume of 80 to 100 ml. The number of total insemination doses will depend on the frequency of collection, age of boar, breed, and some individual variation. Farrowing rates from sows artificially inseminated are comparable to those observed in sows naturally mated. Artificially inseminating twice, 12 to 24 hours apart, is likely to improve pregnancy rates. In a commercial unit, heterospermic insemination (mixing semen from two or more boars) is sometimes used and reportedly increases pregnancy rates.

Technician Note

Artificial insemination with fresh or cooled semen is commonly performed in the swine industry.

Pregnancy Diagnosis

Ultrasonography procedures are used to diagnose pregnancy in pigs. Doppler and amplitude-depth ultrasound were the first methods to be employed and are accurate between 30 and 90 days of gestation. Real-time (B-mode) ultrasound is being used with more frequency in the swine industry as equipment cost decreases. Accuracy is greater than 90% if used after 20 days of gestation.

Postpartum Complications and Diseases

Retained placenta is not a very common occurrence in pigs. Fetal membranes from all piglets are usually expelled after the last piglet is born. Manual examination of the birth

TABLE 16-2	HORMONES USED IN SWINE ESTROUS CYCLE	
Desired Effect	**Drug**	**Regimen**
Induction of puberty	PG 600 eCG/hCG	5 ml IM 400-1000 IU/ 200-1000 U IM
Estrus/ovulation	PG 600 eCG/hCG Regu-Mate	5 ml IM 500-1000 IU/ 500-1000 U IM 15 mg/gilt/day for 18 days orally
Abortion	PGF$_{2\alpha}$	10 mg Lutalyse or 500 µg Estrumate 12-45 days after breeding

eCG, Equine chorionic gonadotropin; *hCG*, human chorionic gonadotropin; *IM*, intramuscularly; *PG*, prostaglandin.

canal is warranted if the placenta is not passed out after sows apparently deliver their last piglet.

Obstetric problems are also not very common, and the great majority of sows and gilts deliver without any technical or veterinary assistance. Nevertheless, persistent and forceful abdominal contractions without delivery of a piglet for longer than 1 hour suggest potential complications. A problem will be even more evident if it is accompanied by vaginal discharge but not expulsion of a fetus. An increased time interval between deliveries is also suggestive of dystocia. The reason may be a primary absence of uterine contractions (primary inertia) or secondary to the presence of either an oversized, malpositioned, or malformed fetus. Oxytocin can be administered for primary uterine inertia. Removal of piglets is also helpful for stimulating progression of delivery. Occasionally, a cesarean delivery is needed to deliver the piglets.

Prolapse of the uterus can occur during parturition or after all piglets have been delivered. Excessive straining or a large pelvic inlet may predispose to uterine prolapse. Uterine prolapse is likely fatal. Vaginal prolapse generally happens a few days before parturition. It requires veterinary intervention to reposition it, and sows should be watched for any problems during labor.

Metritis and mastitis are the main diseases of the postpartum period and consequently lead to a disturbance in milk production. Hypogalactia (low milk production) and agalactia (absence of milk production) are often associated with mastitis and metritis. Any signs of abnormal, fetid vaginal discharge or abnormal enlargement of the udder warrant veterinary assistance. Oxytocin can be used to stimulate milk letdown during treatment.

Technician Note

Metritis and mastitis are the main diseases of the postpartum period and consequently lead to a disturbance in milk production.

OVINE AND CAPRINE REPRODUCTION

Seasonality

Sheep and goats are seasonally polyestrous, short-day breeders. Estrous cycles start to occur in the late summer and autumn. The photo period is the primary environmental cue controlling seasonal breeding in the ewe. Exposure of sheep and goats to increasing, or long, day length induces anestrus, whereas short or decreasing day length initiates estrous cycles. Perception of the day length by the eye is signaled to the pineal gland, which will cause melatonin release. Melatonin will induce the secretion of GnRH and LH, which initiates cyclicity. Low ambient temperature also cues small ruminants to start to cycle. Sheep and goats kept in tropical or subtropical areas do not display marked seasonality and can cycle almost year-round.

The geographic origin of a specific breed influences the length of the breeding season. For example, some breeds have a 2- to 4-month breeding season and some cycle all year long. Suffolk and Suffolk crosses average 6 months of breeding season. Dorset and Finn sheep have extended breeding seasons (8 months), whereas Merino ewes cycle almost all year-round.

Dairy goats (Saanen, Toggenburgh) cycle from August to February in the northern hemisphere. Most meat or crossbred-type goats have a more extended breeding season and undergo anestrus in late spring and summer.

Estrous Cycle

Ewes cycle regularly every 17 (range 14 to 19) days and does every 21 days (range 18 to 22 days) during the breeding season. During proestrus, ewes and does are not sexually receptive but attract the male's attention and courtship is initiated.

Estrus lasts 24 to 48 hours in ewes and 24 to 36 hours in does. Estrogen causes the vulva to be edematous and moist. Does show overt signs of estrus more often than ewes. Accordingly, does may exhibit homosexual behavior, but ewes do not. Estrus detection is efficiently achieved using males that have undergone vasectomy. Both species actively seek the male as they advance into estrus. Multiple copulations during the same estrus are correlated with higher pregnancy rates. A cloudy vaginal discharge may be seen at the end of estrus and should not be mistaken for infectious vaginal discharge. Ovulation occurs 24 to 30 hours after the onset of estrus in both species. Diestrus lasts 15 to17 days in ewes and 18 to 20 days in does.

Breeding Management

Puberty of ewes occurs at 6 to 9 months, but it can be as late as 1 to 2 years of age depending on breed, nutrition, and time of birth during the year (e.g., lambs and kids born in the fall come into puberty later than spring-born offspring). Pubertal ewes and does should be bred only if they have attained 65% of their mature body weight. The male/female ratio should be 1:50 in natural breeding situations or1:10 for synchronized breeding. Fresh or frozen semen can be used for artificial insemination. Deposition of semen can be intravaginal, intracervical, or intrauterine (Table 16-3). Laparoscopic procedures have become common practice in the sheep and goat industry.

Pregnancy

Gestation lasts approximately 150 days in both species. Ewes are dependent on luteal function only during the first 2 months of gestation. Because maintenance of pregnancy in ewes is accomplished by placental hormones after day 50 of gestation, administration of prostaglandin after 2 months of gestation does not induce abortion or

TABLE 16-3 ARTIFICIAL INSEMINATION (AI) BREEDING IN EWES			
Method	Semen	Semen Dose (Number of Spermatazoa)	Lambing Rate (%)
Laparoscopic IU	Fresh or frozen	$20\text{-}40 \times 10^6$	40-100
Transcervical IU	Fresh or frozen	$50\text{-}100 \times 10^6$	30-80
Cervical	Fresh only	200×10^6	40-80
Vaginal	Fresh only	400×10^6	20-60

*Modified from Youngquist RS, editor: *Current therapy in large animal theriogenology*, Philadelphia, 1997, WB Saunders.
IU, Intrauterine.

parturition. Does are dependent on luteal function throughout gestation, and prostaglandin administration interrupts pregnancy at any stage. Parturition can be safely induced by prostaglandin administration in goats after day 146 of gestation. Does come into labor on average 28 to 36 hours after prostaglandin administration. Dexamethasone induces parturition in ewes within 36 to 48 hours if administered after day 144 of gestation. Twinning is very common, and lambs and kids should be standing within 15 minutes and nursing within 1 hour after being born.

Ram/Buck Effect
Male pheromones produced under androgenic stimulation dramatically influence cyclicity in ewes and does. The introduction of a new, mature, odoriferous male during the transition from the anestrus season into the breeding season will induce estrus in most females. Ewes ovulate in 3 to 6 days, but the corpus luteum of this first cycle is short lived. After the second ovulation, regular cyclicity is established. The buck effect is more efficient in does inasmuch as cyclicity is regularly initiated with first ovulation.

Technician Note

Male pheromones produced under androgenic stimulation dramatically influence cyclicity in ewes and does.

Pharmacologic Control of the Estrous Cycle
Intravaginal sponges delivering progestogen are used to synchronize estrus in ewes and does. Controlled intravaginal drug-releasing devices (CIDRs) are widely used internationally but are not yet commercially available in the United States. Norgestomet implants (Synchro-Mate-B, Merial) can be implanted in the ear but are currently not available in the United States. Prostaglandin is also used to synchronize estrus alone or in combination with progestogen.

Pregnancy Diagnosis
Pregnancy diagnosis can be performed by checking for returning to estrus, ballottement (palpation) of the fetus in the abdomen, or ultrasonography. Return to estrus can be observed by using a marking harness and crayon on the male (Figure 16-28). Doppler ultrasonography is 90% accurate after 75 days of gestation. Real-time (B-mode) ultrasonography using a 5-MHz probe is 100% accurate after 60 days.

Periparturient Problems
Dystocia usually results from an abnormal fetal disposition or fetopelvic disproportion. It is important to recognize dystocia, because the cervix will close after 2 to 3 hours of nonproductive labor. A cesarean delivery is the treatment of choice. Ringwomb refers to the failure of the cervix to dilate during parturition.

Pregnancy toxemia is a common problem seen in ewes in the last 6 weeks of gestation. It is associated with multiple fetuses and inadequate nutrition. Hypoglycemia in these cases may lead to neurologic signs and incoordination. Vaginal prolapse usually occurs in late gestation (3 to 6 weeks before parturition), and dystocia is likely to result in a cesarean delivery.

Hypocalcemia is a condition of pregnant ewes and does leading to cool extremities, failure of the cervix to dilate, and generalized weakness. Treatment is intravenous calcium administration. The hypocalcemic female should be examined 3 hours after calcium treatment. If no progress in delivery is observed, a cesarean delivery is indicated.

Pseudopregnancy is a common condition in goats. It is characterized by a collection of fluid inside the uterus without pregnancy (hydrometra). If not treated with prostaglandin, the natural expulsion of the fluid is called *cloudburst*.

Infertility
The natural absence of horns in goats is associated with abnormal sexual development. This condition is called *polled (hornless) intersex*. The polled condition is determined by an autosomal-dominant gene that is the same or very closed linked to a recessive gene causing infertility. Homozygous polled genes cause sex reversal in the female. Affected animals may be genetically female but exhibit male, female, or mixed characteristics and sexual behavior.

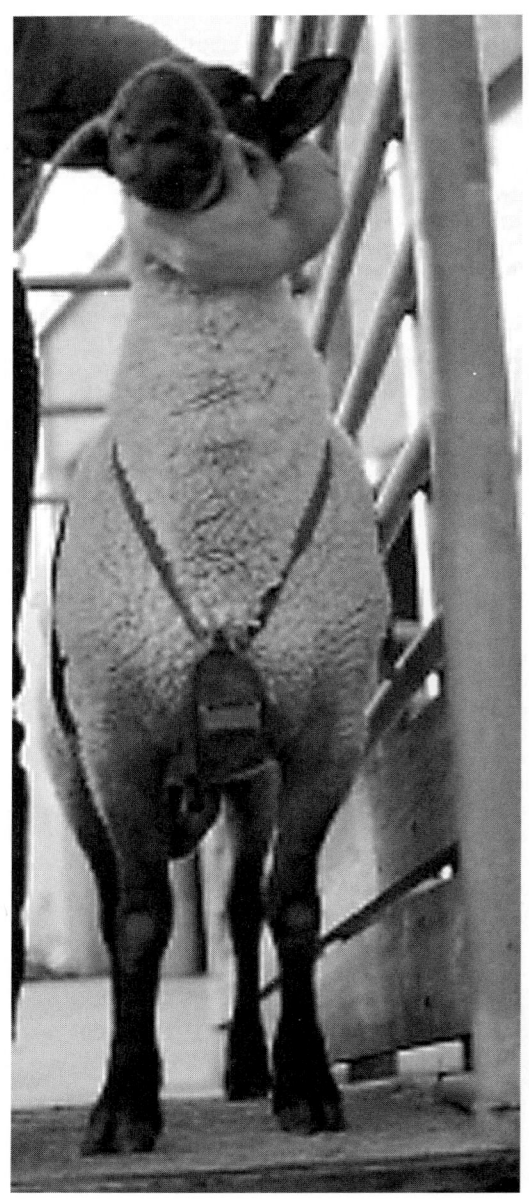

FIGURE 16-28. A ram fitted with a marking harness to detect estrus in ewes.

The polled gene is dominant, and the intersex condition is seen only in homozygous animals. Therefore this condition can be avoided by having at least one horned parent.

CAMELID REPRODUCTION

New world camelids include the llama, alpaca, vicuna, and guanaco. They developed from a common ancestry in South America before the arrival of Europeans. Many aspects of reproduction are similar, but there are differences that can be attributed to speciation.

Estrous Cycles

Puberty occurs at 10 to 12 months of age when the animal reaches approximately 60% of the adult body weight. Although llamas have peak fertility during the summer, they cycle year-round. Environmental and endocrinologic factors responsible for the onset and cessation of sexual activity are not yet clearly defined.

> ### Technician Note
>
> Camelids do not have regular estrous cycles. They are induced ovulators, similar to cats.

Camelids do not have regular estrous cycles. They are induced ovulators, similar to cats. Sexual receptivity can vary from 1 to 36 days. Coitus lasts 5 to 50 minutes with an average of 18 minutes. One mating is sufficient to induce ovulation, which occurs 1 to 3 days later. Delayed ovulation occurs in 30% and absence of ovulation in 10% of females after a single copulation. Treatment with hCG (500 to 700 IU) or GnRH (800 µg) is effective to induce ovulation. The use of a male that has had vasectomy is more effective to induce ovulation. The ovulatory follicle can be on either ovary, but the pregnancy is invariably in the left horn. Luteolysis is mediated by PGF. The CL remains functional throughout gestation. Prostaglandin can be used to induce parturition.

Gestation length averages 344 days (range 331 to 347 days). Parturition lasts 1 to 2 hours, and few complications occur. Approximately 90% of crias (baby camelids) are born between 7:00 AM and 1:00 PM.

GENERAL MALE REPRODUCTION

The development of the male reproductive tract occurs when an animal has an XY karyotype. The female tubular system regresses, and the male tubular system forms the vas deferens and epididymis.

The male differs greatly from the female in the production of gametes. Whereas in the female only one to ten oocytes ovulate during an estrous cycle, males are continually producing and excreting millions of sperm cells. Testicular anatomy differs significantly from ovarian anatomy. The testis is made up of many tubules, each of which connects to a central collecting duct. Between the tubules are the interstitial cells, which continually produce testosterone (Figure 16-29). Each tubule is lined by primordial

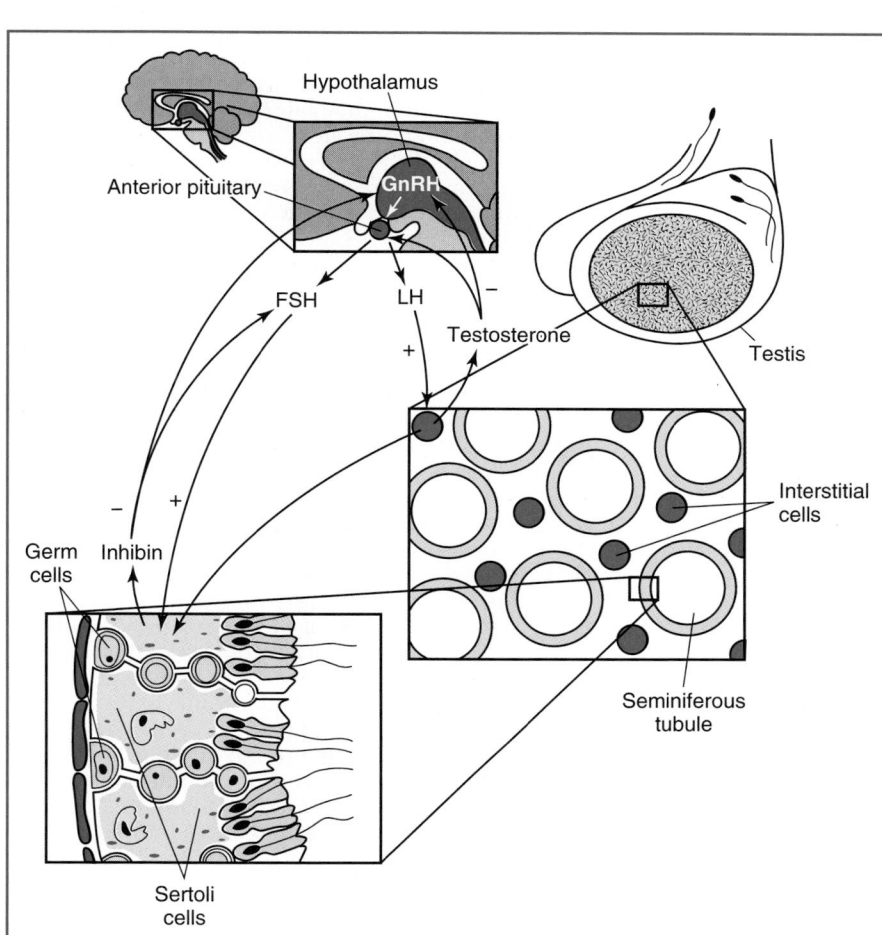

FIGURE 16-29. The general hormonal control of male reproduction. Pulsatile GnRH causes FSH to be released from the anterior pituitary. FSH causes increased sperm growth, maturation, and release. Inhibin from the Sertoli cells in the tubules feeds back on the anterior pituitary and causes less FSH to be released. GnRH secretion from the hypothalamus also results in LH release, which cause testoterone production by the interstitial cells of Leydig. The rise in testosterone causes less LH and GnRH to be released.

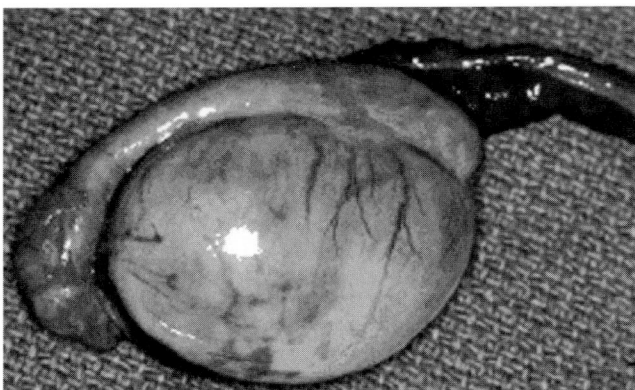

FIGURE 16-30. A canine testis showing the capsule surrounding the testicular tissue.

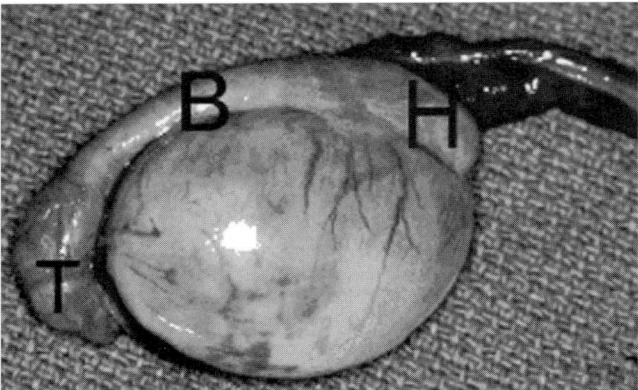

FIGURE 16-31. A canine testis and epididymis. The head (H), body (B), and tail (T) of the epididymis are marked.

germ cells (very immature sperm cell precursors) and Sertoli cells. The Sertoli cells surround all the developing sperm cells, leaving them with no other contact to the body. This is critical in that the developing sperm are recognized as a foreign substance to the male and would be destroyed by the immune system if they were not protected. As the sperm cells mature, they leave their attachment to the Sertoli cell and are moved through the tubules.

The entire testis is covered by a tight capsule, the tunica albuginea (Figure 16-30). The paired testes are contained within the scrotum. The scrotum maintains the testes at a lower body temperature than the rest of the body. If the testes are not kept at a lower temperature, sperm cell production will cease. However, even though sperm cell production ceases, the interstitial cells still produce testosterone. A common example of these consequences is in a cryptorchid animal. A cryptorchid animal has one or both of the testes retained in the abdomen. If the testes are in the abdomen, the animal is sterile but will still show masculine behavior.

Technician Note

If the testes are not kept at a lower temperature, sperm cell production will cease.

Although the anatomy of the testes differs from that of the ovary, the control of sperm cell production is quite similar to that of oocyte production; however, it is more continuous and does not occur in cycles. In the male, LH from the anterior pituitary causes an increase in testosterone production (see Figure 16-29). As testosterone production rises, it causes a decrease in GnRH and LH release. The decreased GnRH and LH release causes less testosterone to be produced. As less testosterone is produced, it follows that more GnRH and LH are produced, thus resulting in a balanced feedback mechanism and a relatively constant testosterone production. Testosterone is essential for the production of sperm cells. If testosterone is not present, sperm cells will not be produced. The concentration of testosterone within the testis is 10 times that in the systemic circulation. Administration of testosterone decreases endogenous testosterone production because of the negative feedback on the anterior pituitary and hypothalamus. This will result in lower testosterone concentrations within the testis. Because testosterone is needed for sperm

cell production, the exogenous testosterone will eventually decrease sperm cell production.

The other hormone involved in sperm cell production is FSH. Just as in the female, FSH release is triggered by GnRH from the hypothalamus. The FSH acts on the Sertoli cell to increase the division of primordial sperm cells and to release more sperm cells that are embedded in the Sertoli cells. As sperm cell production rises, the hormone inhibin feeds back on the hypothalamus and anterior pituitary to decrease GnRH and FSH, respectively. This causes fewer sperm cells to be produced. As fewer cells are produced, the FSH will increase to produce more sperm cells, thereby keeping sperm cell production relatively constant. In general, FSH causes production of the gamete (oocyte in the female and sperm cell in the male) and LH causes production of the dominant hormone (progesterone in the female and testosterone in the male).

After the sperm cells are released they move through the tubules and into the head of the epididymis. Within the epididymis, the sperm cells attain motility and the ability to fertilize. The movement through the epididymis to the tail of the epididymis is relatively constant and cannot be increased by increasing the number of breedings. The sperm cells are finally stored in the tail of the epididymis, where they are either ejaculated or voided in the urine if they are not ejaculated (Figure 16-31).

Ejaculation through the penis is the final process in sperm production and delivery. In most domestic species the penis comprises cavernous blood tissue surrounded by a firm covering, or tunic. An erection occurs when the male is sexually stimulated. During sexual stimulation, parasympathetic innervation causes blood flow increase into the cavernous portions of the penis. As blood flow increases to the penis, muscles around the proximal penis also contract to prevent blood outflow. Because the cavernous portions of the penis are contained within the tunic, the pressure increases, resulting in a penile erection. Any disruption of the cavernous tissue or the tunic can result in an erection failure.

During an erection the sperm cells in the tail of the epididymis are moved to the end of the ductus deferens, into the ampullae in the process called *emission*. Once the sperm cells are present in the ampullae, the stimulation to the penis during mating causes ejaculation. Ejaculation is the forceful expulsion of the semen through the penis. The force comes from sympathetic nerves causing smooth muscle contractions in the urethra. During ejaculation the sperm cells are mixed with fluid from the accessory sex glands. The accessory sex glands include the ampullae, prostate, vesicular glands, and bulbourethral glands. Each species has one or all of these glands, and different glands have different clinical problems in each species. When the sperm cells are mixed with the accessory sex gland fluid, the result is now termed *semen*. Secretions from the accessory sex glands fluid add various components to the ejaculate, increase the volume, and stabilize the sperm cell membrane. Once the sperm cells enter the female reproductive tract, the sperm cell membrane undergoes a physical and biochemical change called *capacitation*. Capacitation is required before the sperm cells are capable of fertilization. In the uterus, the sperm cells are quickly moved to the oviduct, where fertilization occurs. Sperm cells are moved to the oviduct by uterine contractions.

Technician Note

Once the sperm cells enter the female reproductive tract, the sperm cell membrane undergoes a physical and biochemical change called *capacitation*.

CLINICAL EXAMINATION OF THE MALE

Depending on the species, evaluation of the male as a sound potential breeder may employ different techniques to collect semen and evaluate sperm output. Although semen collection procedures may differ among species, analysis of the semen is quite similar.

SEMEN ANALYSIS

When evaluating semen it is important to have all equipment at 37° C. Sperm cells are very susceptible to cold shock and osmotic shock. Semen is best handled with a thin wooden stick, because the wood is thermoneutral and will not cold shock the sperm cells. The first step in semen analysis is to examine the motility. Motility will decline with time because of changes in the semen temperature and pH. Gross motility is examined by placing a drop of semen on a warm slide and examining it at 10×. The light on the microscope needs to be reduced greatly in order to see the cells. The sample is only evaluated for movement; however, the concentration can be estimated to help prepare other samples.

After the gross motility is evaluated, percent of progressively motile sperm is assessed. Individual motility slides are made by placing a drop of semen on the slide and then placing a coverslip over the sample. The sample should be evaluated at 40×. It is desirable to have approximately 10 cells per high power field. If there are more cells, the motility cannot be estimated accurately. Motility is estimated by determining the percent of cells that move progressively across the field. Cells that swim in tight circles are not progressively motile. If more than 10 cells are seen per high power field, the sample can be diluted. Dilution can be done by placing a drop of warm saline on a slide and then placing a small amount of semen into the saline (concentrated bull and ram semen usually only requires a quick touch of the saline with a wooden stick dipped into the semen). If the cells were alive on the gross motility examination but are dead on the individual motility examination, then the saline should be suspected of being hypertonic. As saline remains opened, the water evaporates and increases the

osmolarity of the solution. Replace the saline, and repeat the motility evaluation.

Sperm morphology is generally examined after staining with an eosin-nigrosin stain (Lane Manufacturing). Slides are made by painting a line of the stain across one end of the slide. A small amount of semen is placed in the stain. A second slide is then used to push the stain across the length of the slide. The objective of making the slide is to have a very dark background to highlight the cells. If there are lighter and darker areas on the slide, it may be easier to find a more suitable area to examine the cells. To examine the morphology slide, always use 100× magnification. Lower magnification will not allow adequate assessment of the sperm cells. A total of 100 cells are counted, and they are classified as normal or abnormal.

A spermiogram can be performed to differentiate the different types of sperm abnormalities, which include proximal droplets, distal droplets, kinked tails, coiled tails, acrosome abnormalities, midpiece abnormalities, and misshaped heads. Sperm concentration is also performed in situations where a physiologic ejaculate is obtained. In those species in which the sperm cell output is estimated using scrotal circumference (SC), a sperm count is not done. The concentration is calculated by diluting the sample 1:100 and then counting the diluted sample on a hemacytometer. The easiest way to make a 1:100 dilution is to prepare two tubes of 0.9-ml formal buffered saline. Add 0.1 ml of raw semen to the first tube, and mix. Take 0.1 ml of diluted semen from the first tube, and add it to the second tube. The second tube now has a 1:100 dilution. Place the 1:100 dilution on a hemacytometer, and count all the sperm cells in the middle big square surrounded by triple lines (it has 25 smaller squares). The total number of sperm cells counted and multiplied by 10^6 gives the concentration per milliliter. The volume of the sample multiplied by the concentration gives the total number of sperm cells in the ejaculate.

Bull, Ram, and Buck

The bull, ram, and buck have a fibroelastic penis that has a very low blood volume in the cavernous space, but it attains very high pressure. The stimulus for ejaculation in these species is temperature. When sensors on the penis encounter the correct temperature in the female vagina, the male ejaculates. It is important to note that even though there is no pain response on the penis, the temperature sensors may still be able to signal ejaculation. However, it is also difficult to ascertain whether the temperature sensors are functional. In order to obtain a physiologic ejaculate, an artificial vagina needs to be used to collect the semen. Most artificial vaginas consist of a hard shell with a rubber liner inserted. Warm water is placed between the rubber liner and the shell. The temperature of the water is critical in inducing ejaculation.

The animal is allowed to become sexually stimulated and mount an estrual female, restrained male, or immobile object; the collector then diverts the penis into the artificial vagina. Because this is not easy to do and most ruminants are not trained to breed an artificial vagina, most semen collections in the field are performed using an electroejaculator (Figure 16-32). An electroejaculator consists of a probe inserted into the rectum. On the ventral side of the probe are electrodes that stimulate the sympathetic and parasympathetic nerves. The probe is connected to a control box. The box controls how much stimulation the animal receives. The stimulation is very low at first and is gradually increased until the animal has an erection, protrudes the penis, and ejaculates. The ejaculate is then

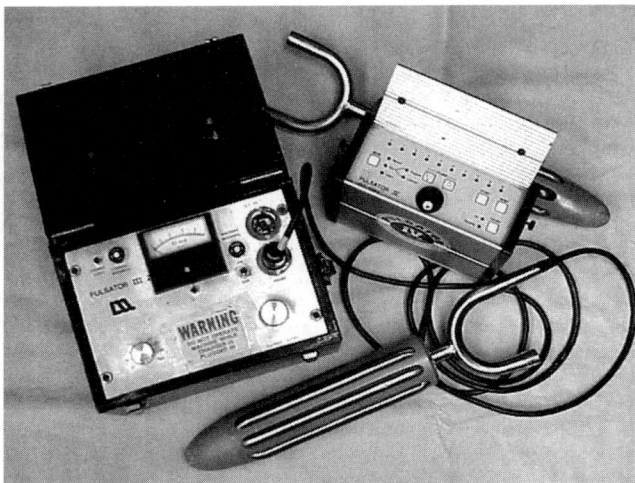

FIGURE 16-32. Two models of ruminant electroejaculators and two rectal probes.

collected into a receptacle. Some machines have an automatic progression of power settings, whereas other machines have to be stepped up manually to control the power.

Although commonly used, electroejaculation may be a painful process for the animal. As long as the power is applied, that animal will produce fluid (from the accessory sex glands), so the "ejaculate" is not truly physiologic. Because the ejaculate is not physiologic, other estimates must be used to estimate sperm output. Sperm output is generally estimated by measuring the scrotal circumference (SC). When measuring the SC, the testes and epididymides are also palpated for size and consistency. A normal bull testis has the consistency of a flexed human bicep. Standards have been set for the desired SC of different ruminant species of different ages.

Technician Note

When measuring the scrotal circumference (SC), the testes and epididymides are also palpated for size and consistency.

In the ram it is very important to palpate the epididymides carefully, because *Brucella ovis* causes infertility and epididymitis. In the bull a rectal examination is performed to evaluate the vesicular glands. Other body systems to evaluate are vision, teeth, and locomotion. The animal must be able to see, eat, and move around to be a successful breeder. Guidelines have been set by the Society for Theriogenology regarding the minimal criteria needed for an animal to be acceptable for breeding. Breeding soundness evaluation forms and criteria are available for veterinarians from the Society for Theriogenology (Figure 16-33).

Bulls commonly get seminal vesiculitis, and white cells will be seen in the semen. Other common problems in bulls are penile hematomas and preputial injuries (Figure 16-34). A penile hematoma usually occurs when a bull is breeding and the penis bends. This increases the pressure in the penis and causes a rupture of the penile tunic. The rupture almost always happens at the distal sigmoid flexure, and a blood clot forms. Preputial injuries are common

in *Bos indicus* bulls. These bulls have a very redundant prepuce that often is everted or hangs out. When the prepuce is damaged, it swells and the bull cannot retract it. Conservative therapy is common in these cases, but a reefing surgery or a circumcision may be needed.

Stallion

Semen is collected most commonly with an artificial vagina (AV) (Figure 16-35). The temperature and pressure of the artificial vagina are the criteria that contribute to the stallion ejaculating. A final temperature of 45° C is generally needed, and the pressure must be adequate. Some stallions prefer hotter and some colder; some prefer more pressure, and some prefer less pressure. Once the AV is prepared, the stallion is teased with an estrual mare until he attains an erection. If a mare is used for a mount, the stallion is led to the side of the mare and allowed to mount. The stallion will then position himself on the mare. As the stallion begins to thrust, the penis is diverted into the AV and the stallion allowed to thrust and ejaculate into the AV. As the stallion dismounts, the AV is held vertical to prevent semen from draining out the open end. Immediately after the dismount, the water in the AV should be drained out to prevent heat shock to the cells and to allow the semen to drain into the collection bottle.

Technician Note

Stallion semen often has a large gel fraction that must be removed before analysis can be performed.

Stallions can also be trained to mount dummies, or phantoms. A dummy allows collection of a stallion without an estrual mare present and is a safer way to collect semen. Stallion semen often has a large gel fraction that must be removed before analysis can be performed. This is usually done with an in-line filter attached to the collection bottle. Motility and morphology assessments are performed the same as in other species. Stallion semen may be diluted and counted manually or using a densimeter. A densimeter measures the amount of light that passes through the semen sample. The higher the concentration of cells, the less light passes through, the less the percent transmittance. Commercially available machines are calibrated to read out the sperm cell concentration based on internal calculations made from the percent transmittance (Figure 16-36).

The transport of cooled stallion semen is becoming more and more popular with certain breeds. Commercially available shipping containers cool the extended semen at a specific rate and keep it cool for up to 48 hours. Extenders are liquids added to the semen to help the longevity of shipped semen. Most extenders are made from skim milk and glucose and have some antibiotics added. When extending stallion semen, the final concentrations should be between 25 to 50 × 10^6 cells/ml; however, the final dilution ratio should be at least four parts of extender to one part of semen. If the semen cannot be extended to that concentration and ratio, the semen must be centrifuged and the resulting pellet resuspended to the desired 25 to 50 million/ml concentration. Many stallions, despite having semen that appears good, do not have semen that withstands even the best cooling and shipping procedures.

Stallions may have problems with decreased libido, hind limb lameness resulting in breeding difficulties, blood in the semen (hemospermia), or urine in the semen (urospermia). These may be challenging problems for the

Bull Breeding Soundness Evaluation

Guidelines Established by Society for Theriogenology
530 Church Street, Suite 700 • Nashville, TN 37219
Phone 615/244-3060 • FAX 615/254-7047 • www.therio.org

OWNER	CASE NO.	DATE
ADDRESS	BULL NAME	BREED
ZIP	I.D. NO.	Brand ☐ Tattoo ☐ Ear tag ☐
TELEPHONE ( )	BIRTH DATE	AGE (MO.)

HISTORY: Previous BSE

DATE	CASE NO.	CLASSIFICATION

PHYSICAL EXAMINATION

Body condition score _____ Thin ☐ Moderate ☐ Good ☐ Obese ☐
Beef 1, 2, 3, 4, 5, 6, 7, 8, 9   Pelvic Ht. _____ Width _____ Area _____
Dairy 1, 2, 3, 4, 5

Feet/legs	☐
Eyes	☐
Vesicular glands	☐
Ampullae/prostate	☐
Inguinal rings	☐
Penis/prepuce	☐
Testes/spermatic cord	☐
Epididymides	☐
Scrotum (shape)	☐

Other

SCROTAL CIRCUMFERENCE (CM) _____ . _____

This bull has been examined for physical soundness and quality of semen only. Unless otherwise noted, no diagnostic tests were undertaken for libido, mating ability or infectious disease status of this bull.

Remarks and interpretation (diagnosis, prognosis, recommendations)

SEMEN EXAMINATION

Collection method: EE ☐   AV ☐   Massage ☐

Response: Erection ☐   Protrusion ☐   Ejaculation ☐

Semen characterisitics	Ejaculate 1	Ejaculate 2
Motility — Gross (or) individual (%)		
% Normal cells		
% Primary abnormalities		
% Secondary abnormalities		
WBC, RBC, other		

CLASSIFICATION

Interpretation of data resulting from this examination would indicate that *on this date,* this bull is a:

☐ Satisfactory potential breeder

☐ Unsatisfactory potential breeder

☐ Classification deferred

Re-examination recommended on _____
DATE

Signed: _____
MEMBER—SOCIETY FOR THERIOGENOLOGY

Clinic:

FIGURE 16-33.   A bull breeding soundness examination form. These forms are copyrighted and available from the Society for Theriogenology.

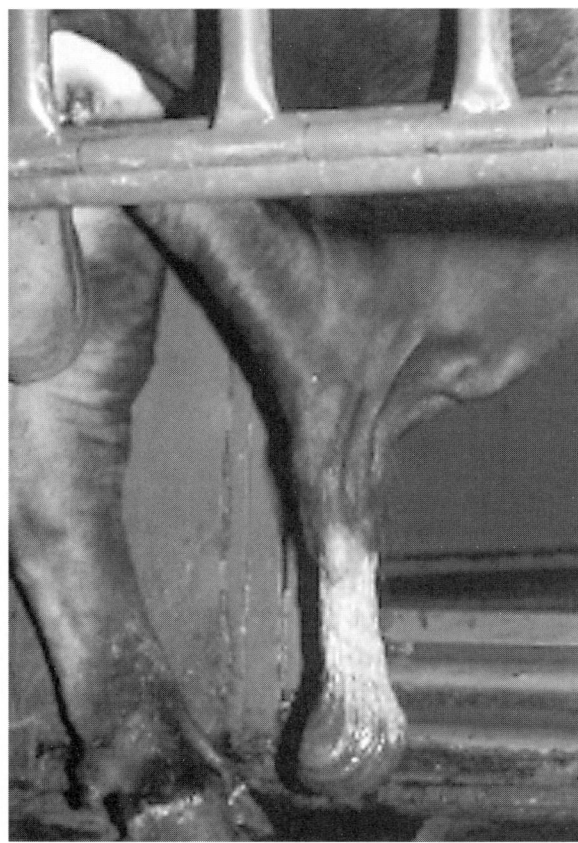

FIGURE 16-34. A *Bos indicus* bull with a preputial prolapse.

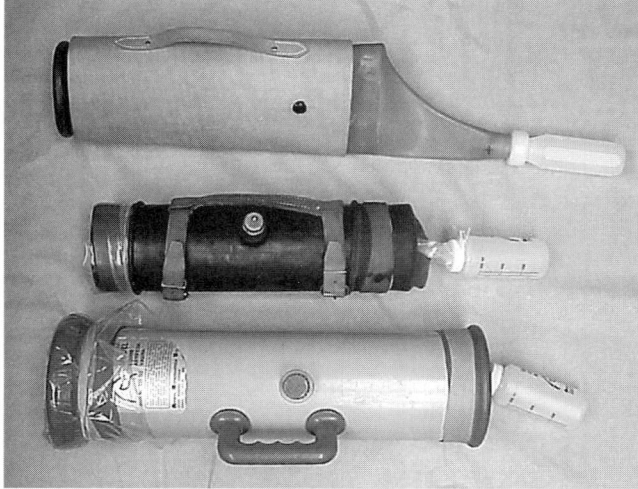

FIGURE 16-35. Three models of equine artificial vaginas. *From the top*, Missouri, Hannover ARS Colorado.

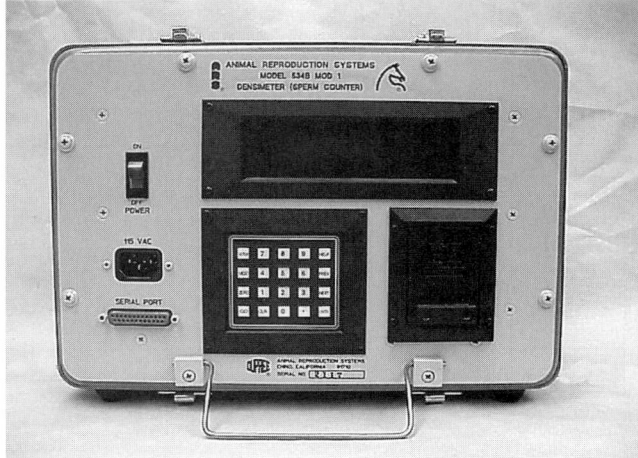

FIGURE 16-36. A densimeter used to measure the concentration of stallion semen.

kicked, the testes can swell and be damaged by both the heat from the inflammation and pressure necrosis of the testicular parenchyma swelling within the confined testicular tunic. Conservative therapy for these conditions includes hydrotherapy and antiinflammatories.

Canine

Canine semen evaluation is performed as in other species, which includes motility, morphology, and a semen count. The main difference is the way the semen is collected. Dog semen is collected by manual massage of the penis. It is best to have an estrual bitch present when the collection is attempted. Once the dog is somewhat aroused, the prepuce is pushed caudal to the bulbus glandis with a rubber or plastic cone. Circumferential manual pressure is then applied proximal to the bulbus glandis. Pressure is applied while the dog ejaculates. The initial portion of the ejaculate is clear, followed by the sperm-rich fraction. The final portion of the ejaculate is the clear prostatic portion. Normally, it is not necessary to collect the prostatic fraction. It is common for the dog to step over the collector's hand during the collection process. The criteria for a dog to be a good potential breeder have been published by the Society for Theriogenology. The most common reproductive disorder in the dog is prostatitis. A dog with prostatitis will have white blood cells in the ejaculate and possibly show pain during ejaculation.

 Technician Note

The most common reproductive disorder in the dog is prostatitis.

Tom

It is very uncommon to collect semen from the tom. However, semen can be collected using a small AV or an electroejaculator. A tom must be extensively trained to use an AV and must be anesthetized to use an electroejaculator. This is why semen evaluations are rarely performed in the tom. One option is to use a vaginal swab to detect the presence of sperm cells in a queen that has just been bred. The tom will also have retrograde ejaculation into the

veterinarian to diagnose and treat. The most common breeding injury in the stallion is when the mare kicks the penis or scrotum. The sequela to a kick on the penis is often a hematoma. This is a large blood clot on the outside of the penile tunic, which results in paraphimosis (the penis will not go back into the sheath). If the scrotum is bladder, so after breeding a cystocentesis can be performed in an attempt to find sperm cells as another option. The most common causes of infertility in the tom are poor teeth (because the tom bites the queen's neck during breeding) and hair rings around the penis.

Boar

Semen from the boar is collected by manual pressure of the distal penis. The boar is led to an estrual sow or can be trained to mount a dummy. As the boar mounts and extends the penis, the collector grasps the penis "back-hand" such that the tip of the penis is grasped mainly with the little finger. It is the manual pressure that elicits ejaculation in the boar. The tip of the penis is diverted to an open container. The bottle should be covered with gauze or cheesecloth to filter out the gel fraction of the ejaculate. The boar takes approximately 10 to 20 minutes to ejaculate and will continue to ejaculate as long as pressure is applied to the penile tip (the collector's hand usually tires before the boar). The most common breeding problems in boars are bite wounds to the penis and infections of the preputial diverticulum.

Camelids

Llamas and alpacas can have semen collected by electro-ejaculation or with an AV, or they can have semen recovered from the vagina of the female after natural mating. The AV is the best method to obtain a semen sample. The copulatory pattern of the llama is somewhat unique when compared with other domestic species. The female llama lies down, and the male llama will lie on top of the female during copulation. Copulation can take as long as 30 minutes, and the male may ejaculate several times. Semen is evaluated as with other species.

RECOMMENDED READING

Feldman EC, Nelson RW, editors: *Canine and feline endocrinology and reproduction*, ed 2, Philadelphia, 1987, WB Saunders.

Purswell BJ, Althouse GC, Root MV: Guidelines for using the canine breeding soundness form, *Proc Soc Therio*, p 174, 1992.

Younquist RS, editor: *Current therapy in theriogenology*, Philadelphia, 1997, WB Saunders.

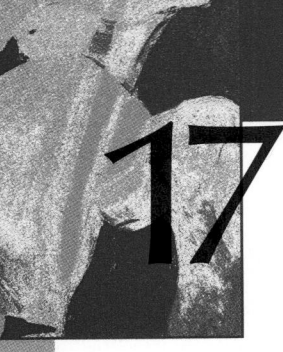

17

Birds, Reptiles, and Small Mammals

Thomas N. Tully, Jr.

The veterinary field of exotic or nondomestic pet medicine is growing as the popularity of these animals increases (Figure 17-1). Caged and aviary birds are now the third most common small animal pet. In a 1996 study, 4.6% of households in the United States owned a pet bird and 10.7% of the households owned pets other than a dog, cat, or pet bird (Wise, 1997). On the basis of the percentage of households with pet birds, the projected population of birds owned in 1996 was 12.6 million. This chapter discusses these species, with particular attention paid to the individual requirements of birds, reptiles, and small mammals. It is important to note that approximately 85% of the problems seen in exotic pet medicine result from lack of basic husbandry information among pet stores, pet owners, veterinarians, and veterinary technicians. With increased veterinary and public education, all species covered in this chapter will have a greater chance of living long and healthy lives.

Technician Note

Approximately 85% of the problems seen in exotic pet medicine result from lack of information on the part of pet stores, pet owners, veterinarians, and veterinary technicians.

BIRDS

The veterinary technician may, on occasion, be involved in telephone communication with clients. When clients call regarding avian patients, it is important to instruct owners in the following areas.

Ask the owners to bring the bird in its own cage if at all possible. They should not clean the cage, except to empty the water dish to prevent it from spilling during the trip. A good evaluation of the bird's environment is helpful to the veterinarian, and clean papers and a clean cage do not provide that information. All grit should be removed because some birds tend to gorge themselves on grit, particularly when ill. The cage should be covered with a towel or blanket to protect it from the weather, and the owner should be instructed to bring along any medication and vitamin supplements the bird is taking, as well as a sample of the food. Most avian telephone inquiries should be considered emergencies because of most owners' inability to note early signs of illness, the bird's inherent ability to mask clinical problems, and the rapid speed with which avian species succumb to disease.

Taking the Clinical History

The following is a suggested list of questions to ask the client regarding avian patients:

- Chief complaint
- Signalment (includes the species, gender, age, and breed) (Box 17-1)
- Origin: Where was the bird obtained? How long has it been owned?
- Environment: What is the construction and design of the cage? Is it painted? If so, what type of paint has been used? What types of water and food bowls, substrate (newspaper, wood shavings, corncob, etc.), and perches are used? Where is the bird kept (indoors or outdoors)? In what room of the house (e.g., kitchen or garage where potential toxins may be located)? Is it close to a window? Are insecticides, household cleaners, or other chemicals used around the house in the vicinity of the cage? Is the bird allowed out of the cage? If so, is it allowed to fly freely, and how well is it supervised?
- Diet: What is the bird being fed (e.g., seed, fruits, vegetables, grain)? How often is the animal fed? Are vitamins and minerals added to the food? How often is the water changed? How is the food prepared and stored?

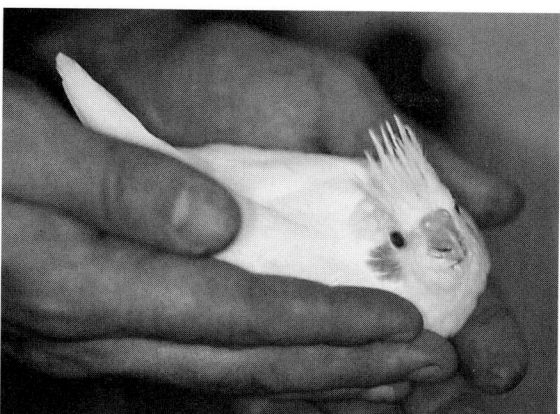

FIGURE 17-1. A bird is an attractive and popular companion.

FIGURE 17-2. Normal psittacine stool. Note the dark solid feces, white solid urates, and liquid urine.

Box 17-1	COMMON PET BIRDS
PSITTACINES	**PASSERINES**
Budgerigar	Canary
Cockatiel	Zebra finch
Amazon parrot	Java rice bird
Macaw	
Lovebird	
African gray parrot	

- Appetite: Notes should be made regarding the bird's overall appetite and daily food consumption.
- Feces: Questions regarding consistency, color, and number of droppings per day are all important. The client should be asked whether feces have been submitted for parasite evaluation previously.
- Cage mates: Are there other animals in the collection in the same cage or in the household? If so, how many, what species, and what degree of contact do they have with the patient? Does the owner maintain a quarantine policy?
- Molting cycle: When has the bird gone through its last general molt, and are there any abnormalities in the feather coat or feather growth?
- Overall attitude and behavior, including voice quality and changes in vocalization
- Previous medical history: Has the bird been ill before? Is there a history of disease in other pets in the house? If so, what illnesses have been diagnosed and treated in the past? Have they been to a veterinarian before?

Sample Collection and Diagnostic Procedures Commonly Used in Birds

Diagnostic plans in avian species are no different from the clinical approach to other domestic pets. Evaluation of the stool is an important first step. The technician should become familiar with normal stool to determine differences between polyuria (excessive urine output) and diarrhea (change in the fecal consistency and amount) (Figure 17-2). Fecal parasites may be detected on fresh smears with saline and a coverslip. This is the best method to check for

protozoa, such as *Giardia*. Fecal flotations will bring some parasite ova to the surface, such as ascarids and *Capillaria*. Fecal sedimentation is an important procedure for the diagnosis of flukes, which are common in imported cockatoos and raptors. Fecal specimens that are gram-stained are useful to determine the bacterial flora of the digestive tract. Most cage bird species have predominantly gram-positive organisms inhabiting the digestive system. Fecal Gram stains are only a preliminary diagnostic test and should be followed up with bacterial culture.

Technician Note

Most cage bird species have predominantly gram-positive organisms inhabiting the digestive system.

Cloacal Swab

A cloacal swab is often done on psittacine species to determine the bacterial flora of the lower gastrointestinal tract. A cotton swab is moistened, inserted into the cloaca, and gently rotated. Cloacal swabs are useful for cytologic evaluations, looking for inflammatory cells, such as heterophils. They may also be used for culture and sensitivity tests and *Chlamydia* or viral isolation.

Oral Examination and Crop Wash

The technician should become adept at assisting in the performance of oral examination and crop wash by the veterinarian. Good restraint technique is essential. An avian beak speculum is placed in the bird's mouth parallel to the commissure and then rotated to open the mouth (Figure 17-3). A choanal culture should be taken when birds are exhibiting upper respiratory signs. The Culturette is placed in the rostral area of the choana to prevent cross contamination with flora in the oral cavity (Figure 17-4).

Another important diagnostic technique is the crop wash. The crop wash permits examination of the upper gastrointestinal tract. A sterile or clean tube is passed through the mouth into the crop or into the esophagus in those birds that do not have a crop. A syringe of sterile saline is connected to the tube, and a simple flush is performed (Figure 17-5). Tubes may be made of plastic, rubber, or metal and have a ball tip (Figure 17-6). The crop

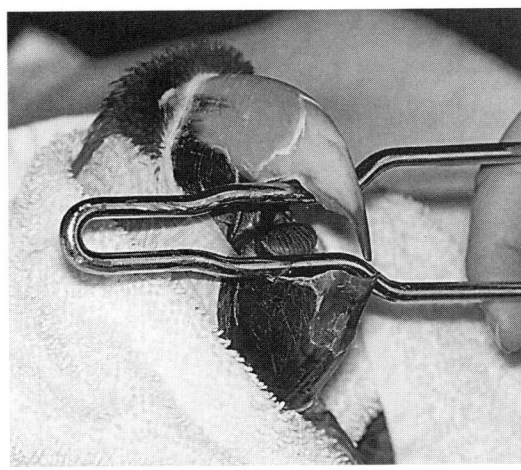

FIGURE 17-3. Oral examination demonstrating the use of a beak speculum on a macaw.

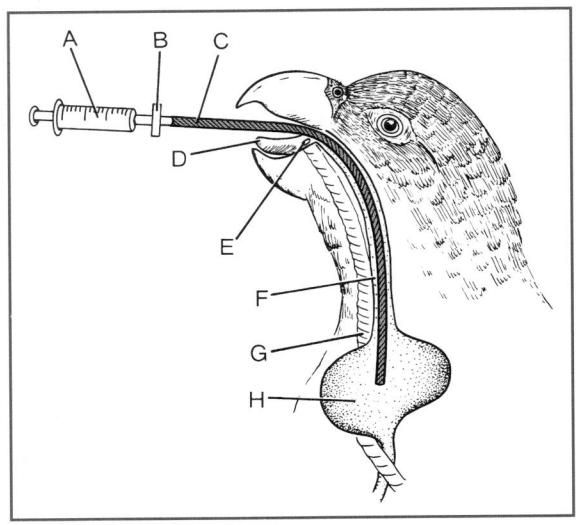

FIGURE 17-5. Proper tube placement for a crop wash or for tube feeding a bird. The bird's neck should be gently stretched. *A,* Syringe. *B,* Adapter if necessary. *C,* Tube. *D,* Tongue. *E,* Tracheal opening. *F,* Proximal esophagus. *G,* Trachea. *H,* Crop.

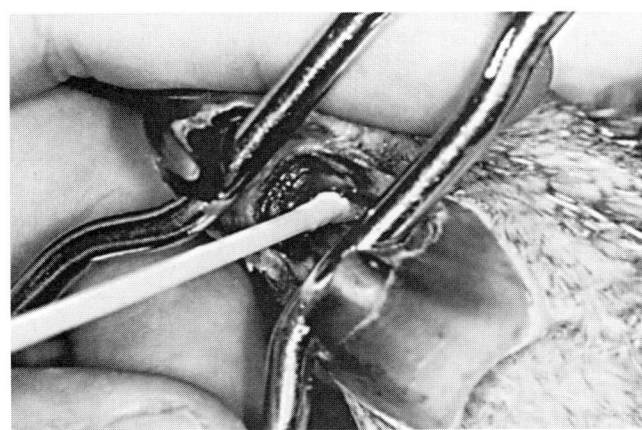

FIGURE 17-4. Culturette placement in the rostral aspect of the choana.

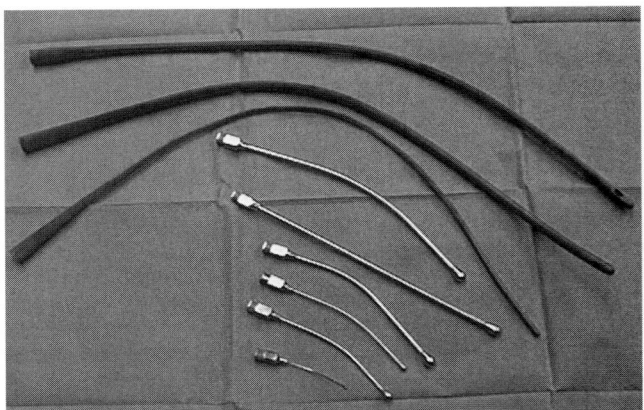

FIGURE 17-6. Various tubes used for tube feeding and crop washes.

wash is important for direct microscopic examination to check for protozoans, such as *Trichomonas* or yeast *(Candida albicans),* using a wet mount technique. Slides may be prepared for cytologic examinations with Diff-Quik stains or Wright's stain, looking for inflammatory cells, such as heterophils. A Gram stain is often done on crop wash samples from psittacine species, or the sample may be submitted for culture and sensitivity (see Plate I, in Chapter 5). A Culturette may be passed into a bird's crop for culture and sensitivity diagnostics. Care must be taken so that the patient does not bite the Culturette and swallow it. Young psittacine species readily accept Culturettes into the crop through normal feeding responses.

Passing a tube into the crop of the psittacine bird is an important technique to learn, because tube feeding is often necessary. Food that is administered using a feeding tube must have a lower temperature than the bird being fed. Most psittacine species have a body temperature of 102° F

to 104° F, so the food should be between 98° F and 101° F. The feeding formula must be thoroughly mixed before uptake into the syringe. Many baby birds develop thermal burns from hot feeding formula. This injury can be prevented by careful preparation of the food by the attending technician. The one rule of thumb to remember when using a tube for either feeding or a crop wash is to try to pick a tube with a diameter larger than the glottis. The glottis of the bird is located at the base of the tongue and is easy to visualize (Figure 17-5). The tube may be passed into the crop easily by positioning the tube in the side of the bird's mouth (Figure 17-5). The tube is easily palpated through the wall of the crop and the skin. While doing a crop wash or tube feeding, the handler should watch the back of the bird's mouth to ensure that food or water does not begin to accumulate. If the crop is overfilled, the bird may aspirate. If the crop overfills, put the bird down and let it attempt to clear its airway. The bird itself has a better chance of clearing its airway than does the technician or veterinarian using cotton-tipped applicators. Never handle a bird after placing oral medication into the crop or filling the crop unless the bird is experiencing respiratory difficulty.

Technician Note

The one rule of thumb to remember when using a tube for either feeding or a crop wash is to try to pick a tube with a diameter larger than the glottis.

Blood Work

Blood work is an important part of the diagnostic examination in avian species. Common venipuncture sites include the cutaneous ulnar vein, the right jugular vein, the medial metatarsal vein, and a toenail clipping, but other sites may be used depending on avian species and experience of the phlebotomist. Each has its own advantages and disadvantages, and the veterinarian and technician will tend to develop their own sites of preference, but the right jugular vein is the recommended site.

The right jugular vein is large and easily found in most birds on the right dorsolateral aspect of the neck. However, it is highly mobile and therefore difficult to stabilize. In most birds the right jugular vein is located in a featherless tract lateral to the trachea. With minimal practice and proper restraint, it becomes an easy procedure. An avian restraint board is recommended for blood collections from larger psittacine patients. Small psittacine and passerine patients can be hand held when blood is being drawn for diagnostic tests.

In general, the basilic vein is accessible but difficult to completely immobilize in the psittacine patient, because of the tremendous strength of the pectoral muscles (Figure 17-7).

The medial metatarsal vein is easy to immobilize and secure, even on an awake and fractious patient. However, if large volumes of blood are to be collected, the medial metatarsal vein may not be a good choice in psittacine patients (Figure 17-8).

A toenail clipping is available but is painful to the patient and often causes limping for several days following the procedure. It may result in a poor blood flow, low yield, and invalid results.

The blood may be collected in syringes, microhematocrit tubes, or blood collection tubes from the hub of the needle. A 3-ml syringe with a 26-gauge needle should be used in most avian patients. In extremely small psittacine and passerine patients a 1-ml syringe with a 30-gauge needle may be used. The technician should learn to proficiently perform a complete blood count (CBC) on avian blood.

Radiography

Radiography is an important diagnostic tool in avian patients. Typically, lateral and ventrodorsal views of the whole body or selected extremities may be taken (Figure 17-9). Technique charts must be developed based on the equipment available. Contrast films may be made with standard contrast agents, including iohexol and barium sulfate. Because good positioning and absence of motion are important to high-quality radiographs, it is generally recommended that all avian patients be sedated or anesthetized, except those who may be too ill (Figure 17-10). Proper positioning is important, and an avian restraint

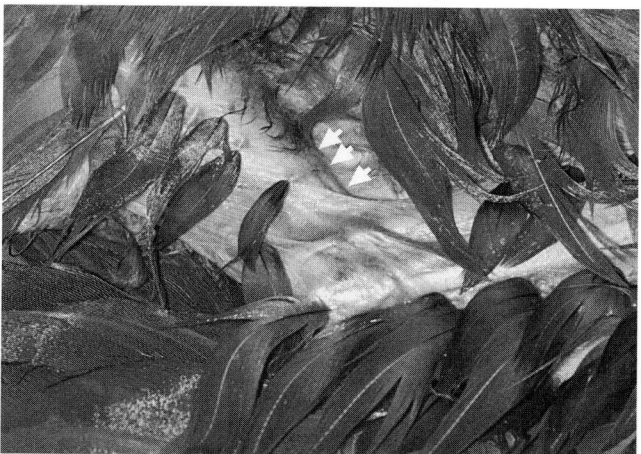

FIGURE 17-7. Location of the basilic vein *(white arrows)*. Ventral view of humerus, radius, and ulna.

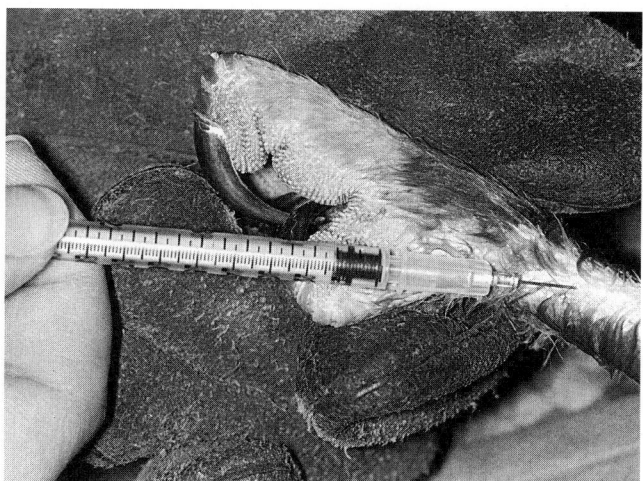

FIGURE 17-8. Intravenous injection using the medial metatarsal vein of a great horned owl.

board is essential. Other diagnostic procedures, such as laparoscopy, endoscopy, tracheal or air sac washes, biopsies, cytologic examinations, and bone marrow aspirates, may be performed on the patient. The technician's role may be to secure the animal with good restraint during these more sophisticated procedures.

Husbandry and Treatment in the Hospital

Generally speaking, drugs administered in the food or water will not reach adequate therapeutic levels. This is an unreliable way to administer medications because of the inconsistent intake of most birds. Direct oral absorption is inconsistent with tablets, but most liquid suspensions tend to work well. Injections of drugs into birds are best done in the large pectoral muscle mass. Drugs injected into the caudal half of the animal (e.g., the legs) may result in the drug's being absorbed into the bloodstream and shunted toward the kidneys by way of the renal portal system. Therefore potentially nephrotoxic drugs, such as aminoglycosides, should never be administered by injection into the legs except in ostriches, emus, and rheas.

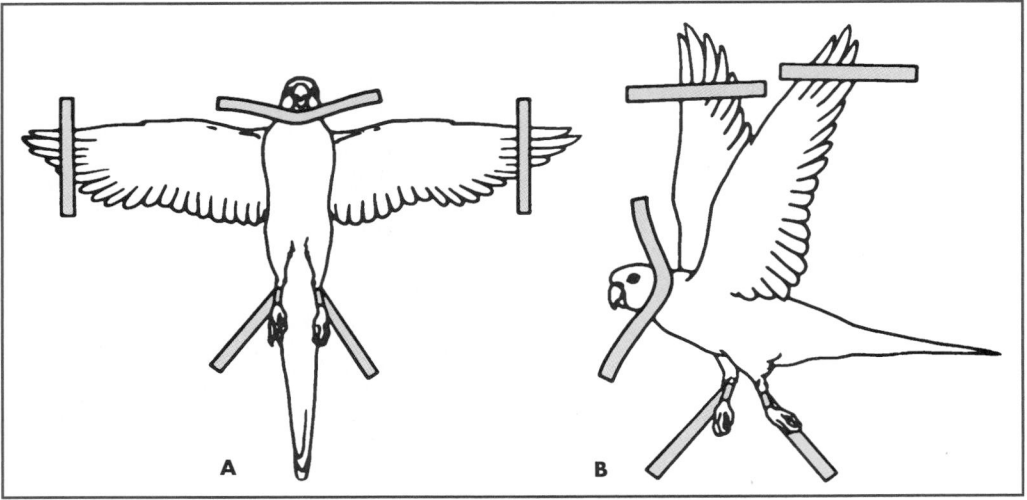

FIGURE 17-9.   Positioning of a budgerigar for radiographs using masking tape. **A,** Ventrodorsal and, **B,** lateral positions.

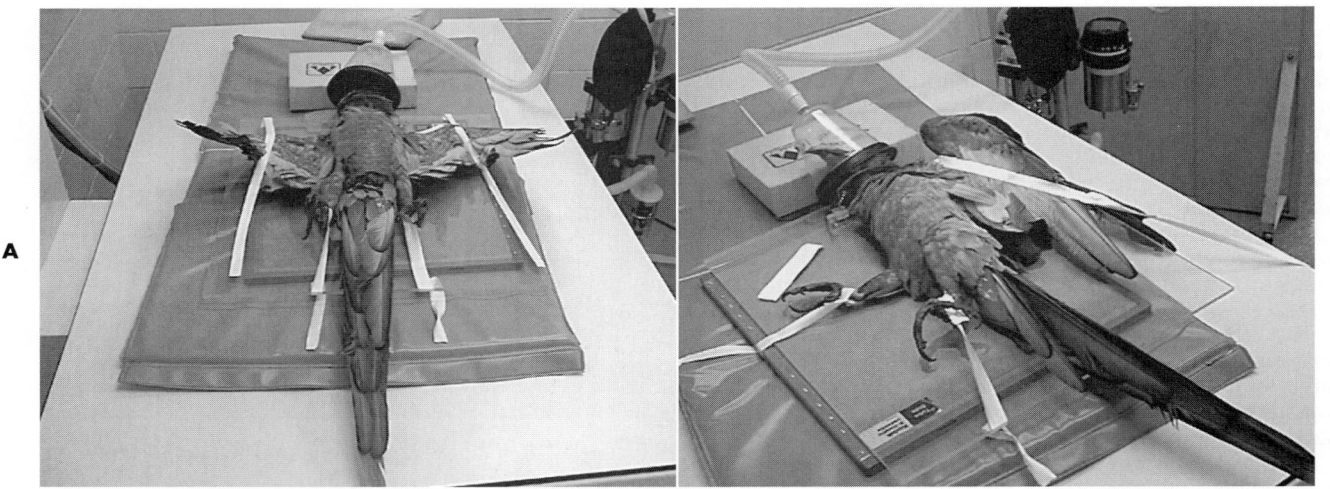

FIGURE 17-10.   **A,** Ventrodorsal and, **B,** lateral positioning of a macaw with the use of adhesive tape. The bird is on an avian Plexiglas restraint board for uniform positioning of patients. A face mask is used for the administration of inhalant isoflurane anesthesia.

Technician Note

Injections of drugs into birds are best done in the large pectoral muscle mass.

Common procedures that the veterinary technician often performs are nail trims and wing clips. Figure 17-11 illustrates one technique for clipping the flight feathers of pet birds. Both wings should be clipped for a symmetric effect, but there are many different feather clip variations that owners request. Typically the primary flight feathers are cut for heavier birds and both the primary and secondary feathers for lighter birds to achieve maximum flight restriction. If only one wing is clipped, the bird cannot control its flight and will be prone to injury. Wing clipping is flight restriction, not prevention. Find out what the owner wants to achieve through the wing clip and how the owner wants the wings to be clipped. No clipping technique will prevent the bird from flight. In the end, both the owner and technician or veterinarian have to be happy with the look and flight restriction of the trim.

Trimming nails in larger psittacines should be done with a Dremel Motor Tool (Dremel, Inc., Racine, Wis.). For small psittacines and passerines, human nail clippers should be used. Cautery units can be used on the nails of birds of all sizes but work especially well on the smaller species (Figure 17-12). Grinding the nails with a Dremel Motor Tool cauterizes as it reduces the length (Figure 17-13). Chemical cautery (as with silver nitrate sticks) should be ready for backup if bleeding occurs, especially in younger psittacines.

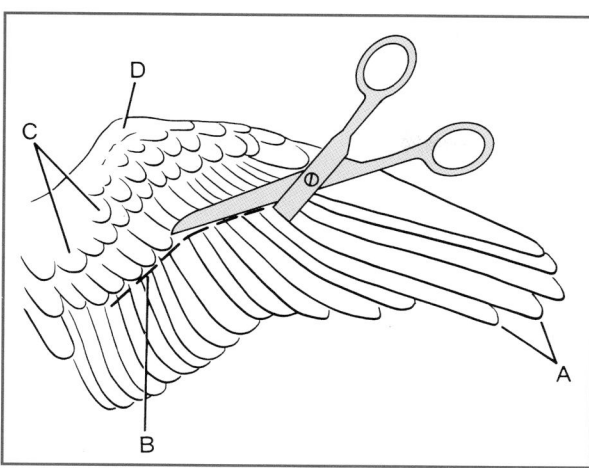

FIGURE 17-11.   Dorsal view of extended wing showing the proper technique for wing clipping. Leaving the first three or four primary or flight feathers intact *(A)*, the cutting line *(B)* should be underneath the overlying contour feathers *(C)* to maintain the appearance of the wing. The wing is grasped firmly at the carpal joint *(D)*.

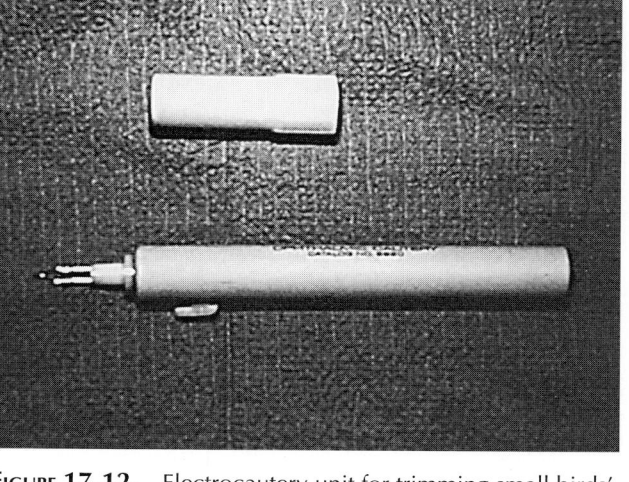

FIGURE 17-12.   Electrocautery unit for trimming small birds' nails.

Dietary management and nutritional support are particularly important in the compromised avian patient. Table 17-1 provides the basic feeding guidelines important in psittacine species and other seed eaters. It is important to remember to keep the cage as clean as possible. Food and water dishes should be cleaned at least daily and occasionally more often. Fresh fruits, vegetables, and meats should be left out only for short periods. Food consumption should be monitored closely. New foods should be introduced gradually, especially the pelleted avian diets. Some foods may provide the bird a source of activity during the ingestion process, such as peeling vegetables, fruits, and nuts. Tube feeding in psittacine birds is an important nursing procedure. Generally, a commercially available cereal-based baby avian formula is recommended for hand-raising young psittacine species. Tube feeding should begin with small amounts frequently, which are then slowly increased in volume and decreased in time interval. The bird should be weighed one or two times per day to chart weight gain. The crop should be monitored for prompt emptying, and the stools should be examined for consistency. The basal metabolic rate (BMR) may be calculated as a rough approximation of energy requirements. The normal BMR for a nonpasserine species, such as parrots, is approximately $79 \times$ body weight (in kilograms). This should be doubled for an ill bird. For passerine species, 130 times the body weight raised to the power of 0.7 should be used. For carnivorous birds, such as raptors, a high-quality canned cat food, such as Control Diet (Hill's Pet Products) may be used to meet their energy requirements.

Hospital facilities should be appropriate for the species being housed. Bird cages should be in a separate room if possible to minimize the stress of sounds and sights of other species. Isolation of birds also prevents contamination of potentially pathogenic bacteria. For example, most psittacine birds have a predominantly gram-positive gut flora. Housing these birds near animals with gram-negative gut flora, such as dogs, cats, reptiles, and carnivorous birds, could result in gram-negative enteric infections. A visual

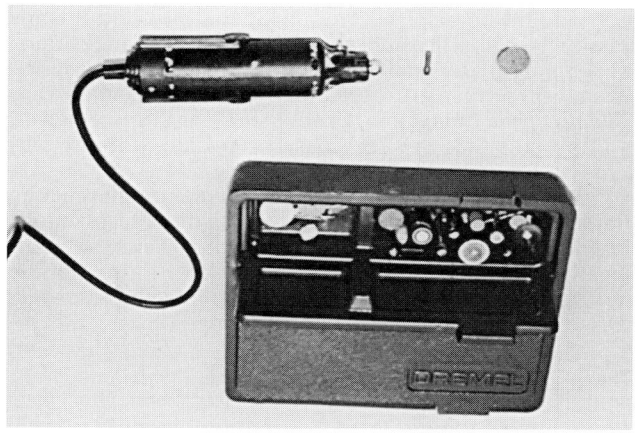

FIGURE 17-13.   Motor tool for grinding larger birds' nails and grooming beaks.

barrier should be provided for the bird, such as a cage cover or hide box in the cage. Large parrots may do well in standard dog or cat cages. Alternatively, Plexiglas custom cages work well and are easily cleaned. Perches should be disposable or easily disinfected and sized according to the individual patient. An isolation area should be available for psittacosis suspects. Again, cleanliness is one of the most important details in the hospital.

Temperature control is important, particularly with sick birds. In general, birds will tolerate cold better than heat. Sudden changes in temperature and drafts should always be avoided. Sick birds have difficulty maintaining and regulating their own body temperature, as do birds with poor feather coats, oil-damaged feathers, or plucked feathers. Therefore these birds should be kept warm but not hot. Temperatures between 80° F and 90° F are best. The bird should be observed for signs of heat stress or shivering. An environmentally controlled cage or unit should be available for the intensive care avian patients.

TABLE 17-1	RECOMMENDED PSITTACINE DIET	
Food Group	**What It Supplies**	**What It Lacks**
Cereals and grains, 45%-50% (commercial pellet diet)	Proteins, fats, B vitamins	Vitamins A, D, and K and calcium (high phosphorus)
Vegetables, 45%-50%	Vitamins A and K, fiber, carbohydrates ± calcium	Protein, fats, vitamin D₃
Fruit, approximately 5%	Sugars, simple carbohydrates	Proteins, vitamins, minerals
Meats (in combination with dairy products), about 5%	Proteins, fats, calcium	
Mineral supplements (e.g., cuttlebone, oyster shell, mineral blocks, or avian vitamins) may be added to the above diets.		

Zoonoses and Common Clinical Problems

Avian patients can present a wide range of clinical diseases; however, their clinical signs are relatively limited. Therefore a sick bird presented with signs of diarrhea, vomiting, or just not doing well should be considered as a potential source of *Chlamydophila psittaci* infections. Those that have recently been through quarantine or pet shops and exposed to high numbers of other birds are most suspect.

Psittacosis is a disease transmissible to humans, caused by the bacterium *Chlamydophila psittaci*. Those patients suspected of potentially being infected with *Chlamydophila* should be treated with appropriate techniques. The bird should be isolated, gloves and masks should be used, and feces should be disposed of quickly and promptly. Transmission is primarily through fecal contamination. Psittacosis is a potentially fatal disease in humans as well as birds when not properly treated. Many wild birds may carry *Chlamydophila* organisms without showing clinical signs. It is important that the veterinary technician working with birds become familiar with this disease.

Other clinical problems frequently encountered in a pet practice include lead poisoning, with signs of gastrointestinal disturbance such as vomiting and diarrhea; gram-negative enteric infections, which generally cause diarrhea and vomiting; and upper respiratory infections, usually caused by a gram-negative bacterium.

REPTILES

It is estimated that there are 7.3 million pet reptiles in the United States. Although the number of pet reptiles does not match dog and cat populations, this is a significant population of animals that require veterinary health services. The diversity of reptile species maintained in captivity requires owner education in health, nutritional, and environmental management (Box 17-2). With excellent owner care, most reptile species live long, healthy lives. In many cases, it is the responsibility of the technician to handle and collect diagnostic samples and educate the owner about their captive reptile.

Once a veterinary hospital decides to treat reptiles, there are a few pieces of specialized equipment needed to provide an adequate hospital environment and aid the technician and veterinarian. Required medical equipment includes an electronic gram scale, an incubating heating pad, tuberculin and microliter syringes, exotic animal formulary (see Recommended Reading), microhematocrit tubes, snake sexing probes, and metal feeding tubes. Common materials used on turtle shell repair include epoxy, resin, and fiberglass patches. Surgical equipment used for reptiles but available in most exotic animal practices includes a Dremel Moto Tool, stainless steel suture material, transparent surgical drapes, and a magnifying surgical headset.

Box 17-2	REPTILES COMMONLY MAINTAINED AS PETS

SNAKES
Boa constrictor (*Boa contrictor*)
Ball python (*Python regius*)
Corn snake (*Elaphe guttata*)
Burmese python (*Python molurus*)

CHELONIA
Box turtle (*Terrapene* spp.)
Red-eared slider (*Trachemys scripta elegans*)
Mud turtle (*Kinosternon* spp.)

LIZARDS
Bearded dragon (*Pogona vitticeps*)
Common tegu (*Tupinambis teguixin*)
Green iguana (*Iguana iguana*)
Green anole (*Anolis carolinensis*)
Jackson's chameleon (*Chamaeleo jacksoni*)
Panther chameleon (*Chamaeleo paradalis*)
Leopard gecko (*Eublepharis macularius*)
Tokay gecko (*Gekko gecko*)
Savannah monitor (*Varanus exanthematicus*)
Water dragon (*Physignathus lesueri*)

Reptile housing equipment must be adaptable to the different species that may be hospitalized. Examples of hospital caging and equipment include fluorescent light tubes (regular and full spectrum), humidifier, fiberglass cages, small aquaria with secure ventilated lids, a heated room, or heat lamps and pads. To aid in capture and restraint, a snake hook, tongs, Plexiglas tubes, and pole snare should be available. As with other exotic species, proper restraint reduces stress to the client, animal, and health care personnel. Once a practice is properly equipped and personnel are trained, interesting patients and cases will begin to receive quality health care.

Taking the Clinical History

The following is a list of questions to ask clients regarding reptile patients:

- Chief complaint: Why does the owner want the pet examined?
- Signalment (including the species as specifically as possible): What is the age and gender of the animal, and how long has he or she owned the animal?
- Origin: Where did the animal come from?
- Environment: Factors such as cage design, construction materials, substrates, perches, or branches are of critical importance in determining the health of these species. Temperature and humidity, as well as photo period and exposure to sunlight or full-spectrum artificial light,

may have a significant impact on the animal's health. The owner should be questioned as to where the cage is kept in the house, as well as the type of heat source used and the usual temperature gradient within the cage. For aquatic species, questions pertaining to water quality control, filter systems used, sources of water, and frequency of water change are important. It is also important to ask the owner about the types of cleaning agents and disinfectants being used and frequency.

- Food: How often is food offered? How much is consumed? What is the source of the food? How is the food stored, and how it is presented to the animal?
- Water: How often is the water cleaned or changed? How is it offered to the animal? If a water bowl is used, how large is it? For many species, it is important to offer water in a bowl large enough for the animal to completely submerge itself in.
- Feces: How often does the animal defecate in relation to feeding? What are the color and consistency of the stool? Has the owner submitted a fecal sample previously for parasite evaluation?
- Cage mates: Does the client have other animals in his or her collection or in the same cage? If so, what species are they, and where are they kept? Does the owner maintain a quarantine policy? If so, for how long?
- What are the current attitude and behavior of the patient, and have there been any recent changes?
- For lizards and snakes, how often does the animal shed? When was the last period of shedding or ecdysis?
- Previous medical history: Has the animal been ill previously? If it has, it is important to get the owner to describe its illness and any treatments that were done. It is often helpful to include the attending veterinarian's name. Have other animals in the collection ever been ill?

Sample Collection and Diagnostic Procedures

Diagnostic approaches in reptiles are often similar to those of other small animal species. As with any diagnostic procedure, ability through experience and confidence determines who will collect the sample needed from the patient. Any of the procedures listed in this section can be mastered by the technician who has the proper sampling equipment and desire.

Colonic Wash

Fecal samples may be collected and examined for gastrointestinal parasites. A fresh sample should be examined under a wet mount, and fecal flotation and sedimentation should also be done. If a fecal sample is not available at the time of the examination, specimens may be collected by performing a colonic wash; this is done by passing a lubricated tube or catheter through the cloaca into the colon. A syringe of sterile saline is attached, and a typical flush is performed (Figure 17-14). Samples may then be examined for parasites or parasite eggs or prepared for cytology or culture and sensitivity tests.

Bone Marrow

Large lizards, crocodilians, and some chelonians yield adequate bone marrow specimens from their femoral cavities (Frye, 1995). Bone marrow from turtles and tortoises may also be obtained by drilling a hole between the outer and inner layers of the bony shell and using a biopsy needle (Vim-Silverman, Becton-Dickinson Primary Care Diagnostics) to obtain the sample (Frye, 1995). The hole should be patched with epoxy or acrylic resin (Frye, 1995). Snake bone marrow specimens may be obtained from the marrow cavities in their ribs.

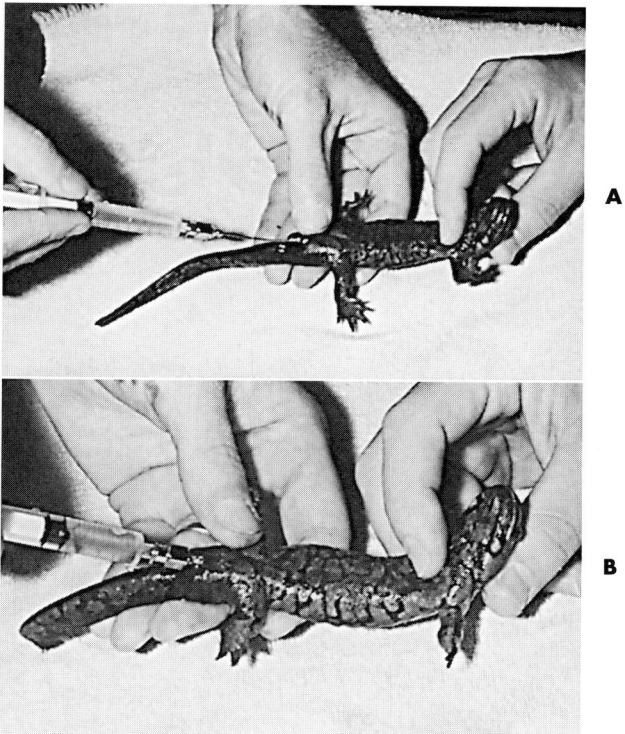

FIGURE 17-14. Colonic wash in a tiger salamander using a metal ball-tipped 18-gauge needle **(A)** and a syringe of warm sterile saline **(B)**.

Stomach Lavage

To examine the upper gastrointestinal tract, especially for identification of cryptosporidiosis, a stomach wash is often performed. This procedure is well tolerated by most reptiles and is a quick and easy procedure in the clinic. A lubricated soft rubber catheter is advanced through the mouth into the stomach after premeasuring alongside the animal. A syringe containing sterile isotonic saline is attached to the catheter, and a simple flush is performed after agitating the stomach with external palpation. Samples obtained are used for direct microscopic examination for parasites, to prepare slides for cytology, or to perform Gram stains or cultures and sensitivities.

Urine Samples

Urine samples may be collected from those species that produce a large volume of urine. Many turtles and lizards have urinary bladders. All reptiles have a cloaca into which the reproductive, gastrointestinal, and urinary tracts empty. A routine urinalysis may be performed on fresh urine samples. A cystocentesis may be performed on turtles by advancing a needle cranial to the hindlimb. Turtles will typically void when stressed; thus simply handling them may yield a urine sample. Green-stained solid urates when rehydrated with saline may reveal amoebic cysts or fluke ova when examined under a microscope.

Blood Samples

Blood collection in reptiles varies considerably, depending on the species. Do not withdraw more blood than is necessary. If you are not sure of the volume needed, contact your diagnostic laboratory. Direct cardiocentesis and venipuncture using the ventral and lateral caudal

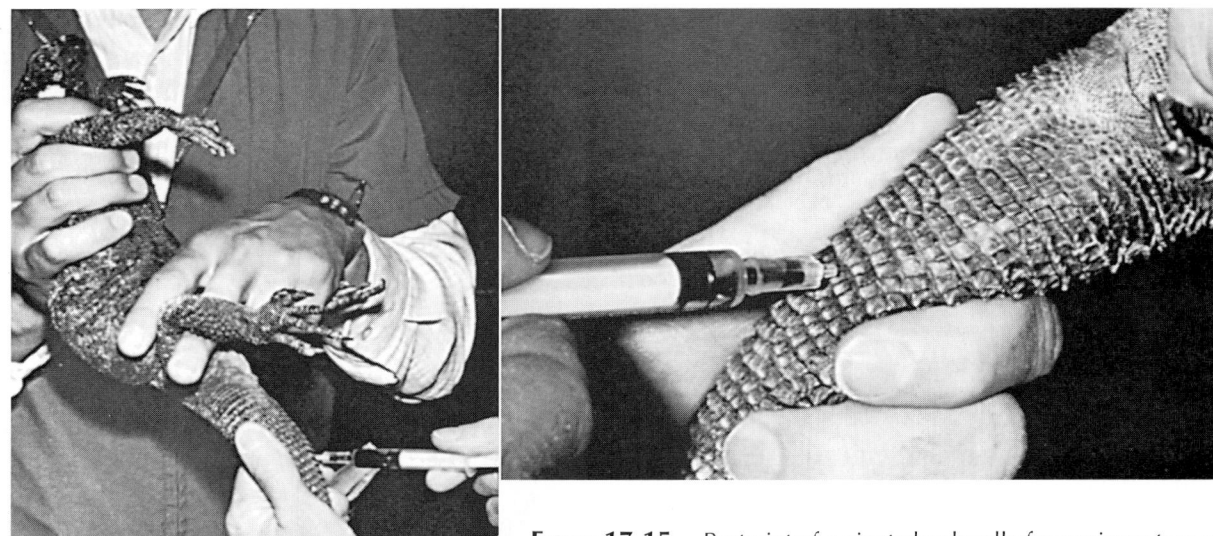

FIGURE 17-15.   Restraint of a giant chuckwalla for venipuncture using the tail vein.

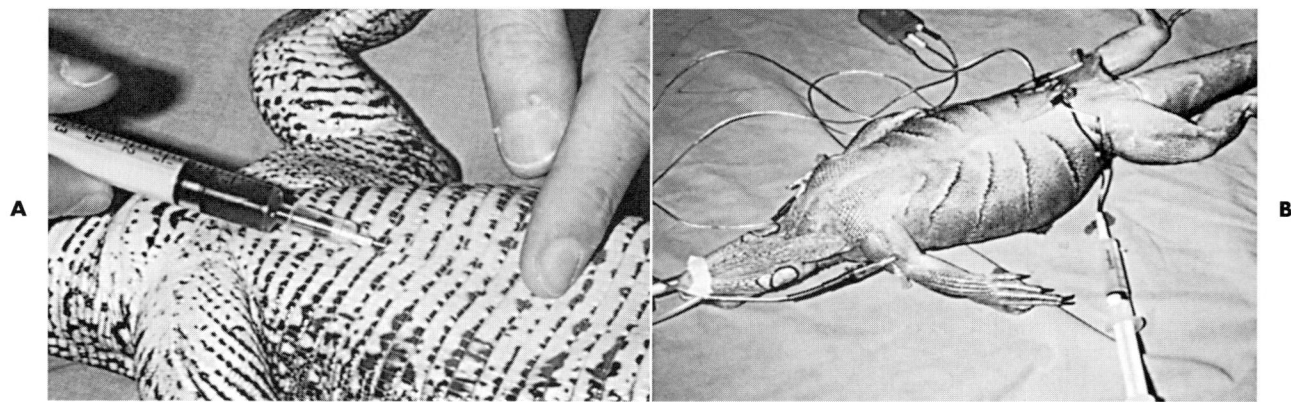

FIGURE 17-16.   **A,** Venipuncture from the ventral abdominal vein from an anesthetized tegu lizard. This is a blind technique. **B,** Intravenous catheter placed in ventral abdominal vein and electrocardiogram lead placement in an anesthetized common iguana.

veins, jugular, brachial, popliteal, periorbital, pterygopalatine, and dorsal postoccipital sinuses can be used depending on the species and size of the animal (Frye, 1995). Toenail clipping is not recommended for blood sample collection because of the inability to obtain reliable hematologic results from this site.

Venipuncture techniques in snakes depend on the experience of the handler. Sites that are often used include the caudal or coccygeal vein of the tail, cardiac puncture, and the ventral abdominal vein or palatine vessels. For any site, good restraint is necessary. For lizards, the caudal tail vein is often the most accessible; however, cardiac puncture and the ventral abdominal vein may also be used (Figures 17-15 and 17-16). In turtles, large jugular veins are present and are easily used for venipuncture sites (Figure 17-17).

In large crocodilians, turtles, and tortoises, the occipital sinus or the caudal vein of the tail may be used. The site chosen will depend on the veterinarian and the technician and their experience with that species. In small lizards, the peribulbar and retrobulbar plexi may be used for blood samples by inserting a heparinized microhematocrit tube between the eyelids and directing it to the inner edge of the

orbit. Rotating the tube will damage the plexus, yielding enough blood to fill the collection device.

Radiography
Radiography often is useful to aid in the diagnosis of reptile patients. For many species, radiographs may be taken on unsedated animals by restraining them in shallow boxes, acrylic tubes, or canvas bags. It is important to remember to take at least two views. With turtles, a third (frontal) view should also be taken. Contrast studies may be done, and barium sulfate is easily administered; however, gastrointestinal transit times are long, and it may take 1 week to complete a gastrointestinal barium study. Various other diagnostic procedures may be used, according to the preference of the veterinarian. The technician's knowledge of restraint and reptile behavior will aid in any immobilization process.

Husbandry in the Hospital
Reptiles require a controlled microenvironment in a hospital setting. It is important to remember that temperature and humidity are important because these animals are

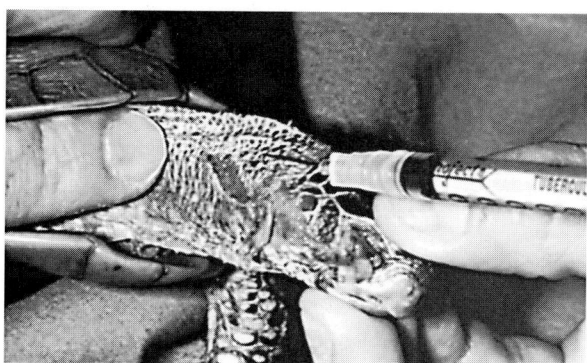

FIGURE 17-17. Jugular venipuncture in a box turtle. The jugular veins are located dorsally in the 10 o'clock and 2 o'clock positions.

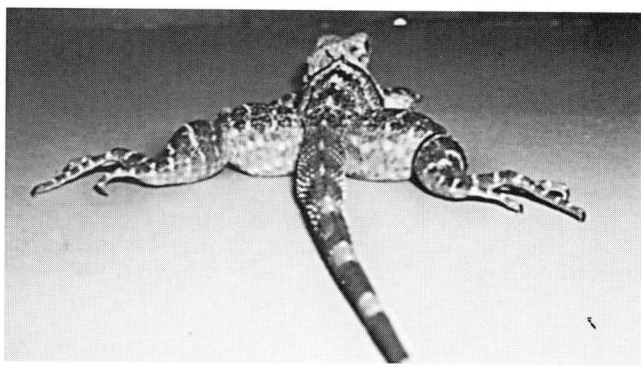

FIGURE 17-18. Metabolic bone disease in a lizard caused by an improper diet.

poikilothermic; that is, they depend on their environment to regulate their body temperature. A temperature gradient should be provided whenever possible by using a thermostat at each end of the cage, resulting in a cooler end and a warmer end. For most species, temperatures should not exceed 32° C (90° F) or dip below 24° C (75° F). It is important that hospitalized reptiles are maintained at the upper end of their temperature gradient during convalescence to aid in recovery. For many species, a variety of aquaria are sufficient for short-term hospitalization. Any substrate used should be one that is easily cleaned and disinfected or disposable, such as newspaper. It is important to house reptiles separately from psittacine birds, in particular, to avoid contamination of birds from the normal gram-negative flora of most reptiles. Cages should be provided with hide boxes or areas of seclusion, as well as perching for some species, such as iguanas and some snakes.

Technician Note

It is important that hospitalized reptiles are maintained at the upper end of their temperature gradient during convalescence to aid in recovery.

Tube feeding is an important technique for the veterinary technician to become adept at when handling reptiles. Tube feeding is easily accomplished, even by those without much experience with reptiles. A tube should be well lubricated and then passed the distance necessary to place it in the stomach. The glottis of reptiles is adjacent to the base of the tongue and is easily avoided. The glottis of snakes may actually be extended by the animal outside the mouth to accommodate large prey items. The tube is gently passed all the way to the stomach, and food is injected. Fluids may also be administered by this route. For patients that are anorectic, supplemental tube feeding may be accomplished by using a blended formula of food that is appropriate for the species being cared for. Dietary references for reptile species are listed in Recommended Reading. It is imperative that the technician become familiar with proper reptile diets to maintain healthy animals and supplement sick patients.

Injections in reptiles are usually performed on the cranial half of the animal's body. This is due to the renal portal system that routes blood from the caudal third of the body through a capillary network into the kidneys

before returning it to general circulation. It is important to remember not to give nephrotoxic drugs in the caudal third of the reptile's body. Injection sites are easily found in all reptile species, either in the forelimbs or in the epaxial musculature of the snake. Oral medications are easily given using a stomach tube. Liquids are preferred over tablets, which are not consistently absorbed.

Dietary requirements vary tremendously from species to species and may be an important factor in the disease of the patient. Dietary deficiencies are not commonly seen in snakes, which eat a whole-animal diet; however, a variety of dietary deficiencies are commonly seen in lizards, turtles, and crocodilians. One of the most common is metabolic bone disease. Metabolic bone disease is caused by inappropriately low calcium intake, low vitamin D_3 intake, or excessive phosphorous intake (Figure 17-18). This may be prevented by a suitable diet and exposing the animal to ultraviolet light, either naturally or artificially. It is essential that reptiles, especially lizards, have full-spectrum light available during normal daylight hours. Sunlight through glass is insufficient to prevent nutritional deficiencies. Animals with metabolic bone disease must be treated very gently because their bones are subject to pathologic fractures. Vitamin A deficiency is commonly seen in turtles and tortoises and usually manifests itself by overgrown beak, palpebral edema, and conjunctivitis. This underscores the importance of thoroughly researching the dietary history of the reptile patient.

Technician Note

It is essential that reptiles, especially lizards, have full-spectrum light available during normal daylight hours.

Skin

There are clinical dermatologic diseases noted in reptilian species as in other animals. Proper diagnostic techniques are needed to identify the problem to implement the appropriate treatment.

Skin specimens may be cultured for bacterial and fungal organisms. For fungal identification, DTM fungal growth medium or Sabouraud's culture media may be used. Bacterial organisms may be isolated on blood agar or subcultured in a thioglycollate-containing medium. Samples for skin culture may be taken using cotton-tipped Culturettes or by using pieces of the affected skin, scales, or dermal scutes.

Feces

Fecal material can be very useful in diagnosing parasite infestations, bacterial infections, pancreatic enzyme levels, and the presence of blood in the gastrointestinal tract. The fecal specimen should be as fresh as possible. If a fresh voided sample is not available, then fecal material may be removed from the terminal alimentary tract by gentle palpation or by the insertion of a fecal extractor or cotton-tipped applicator stick through the cloacal vent (Frye, 1995). The aid of a warm water enema may stimulate defecation in difficult cases.

Sputum

To obtain a sample of sputum, insert a cotton-tipped applicator into the discharge. Roll the sample applicator across a microscope slide, add a drop of coloring agent, apply a coverslip, and examine for parasite ova (Frye, 1995). Common parasites diagnosed in sputum samples are *Rhabdias* spp., *Entomelas* spp., and *Strongyloides stercoralis*. When handling diagnostic samples, proper hygiene is essential because of the zoonotic potential of many animal diseases and parasites.

Zoonoses and Common Clinical Problems

The technician should be aware of common zoonotic infections and clinical problems (see Chapter 18).

Most reptiles carry a variety of gram-negative enteric bacteria, including *Salmonella* spp., *Arizona* spp., *Klebsiella* spp., and *Providentia* spp. Many of these may cause infection in humans as well as in other animals. It is therefore important to keep the reptile separate and to maintain a high standard of sanitation when working with these animals. As with all animals, hands should be thoroughly washed after each time the patient is handled.

Bites from reptiles should be treated as potentially severe infections. Wounds should be thoroughly scrubbed out, and medical attention should be sought.

SMALL MAMMALS

FERRETS

Ferrets have been gaining in popularity over the past decade. Elective surgery (ovariohysterectomies, neutering) is common in these animals. Ferrets are seen with increasing frequency in veterinarians' offices; thus it is imperative that technicians become familiar with these pets.

When obtaining sample collections of blood, physical restraint alone is often inadequate. Chemical restraint therefore is commonly employed. Blood samples are drawn from either the jugular vein, the cranial vena cava, or the cephalic vein. To draw samples of blood from these sites, the animal's head must be securely restrained and grasped around the neck with thumb and fingers resting on the mandibles. To position an animal for jugular venipuncture, it is often best to stretch the animal out, using the other hand to grasp the hindlimbs. The ferret's thick skin and subcutaneous fat make blood collection from the jugular vein difficult. To draw adequate blood samples, the cranial vena cava therefore may be preferred (Figure 17-19). Ketamine hydrochloride or gas anesthetic agents such as halothane or isoflurane may be used for chemical restraint. When using gas anesthetics in ferrets, it is easiest to place them in an induction chamber, such as a Plexiglas box, to which the anesthetic machine is then attached. The animal may be removed from this chamber as soon as it loses the ability to right itself. Anesthesia may then be continued with the use of a face mask. Sample collection on the anesthetized animal is much easier, safer, and less

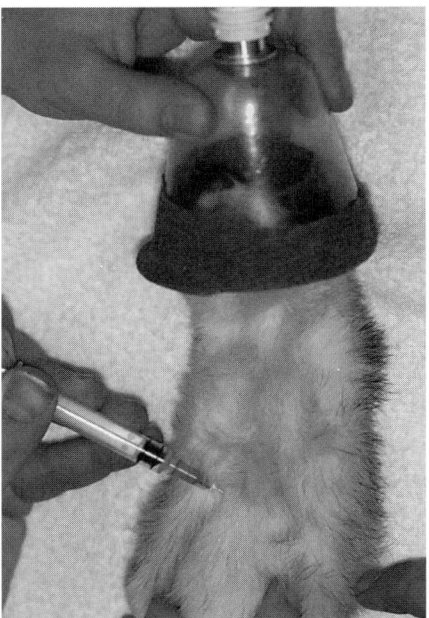

FIGURE 17-19. Cranial vena cava venipuncture of an anesthetized ferret with its head in an anesthetic mask to the right.

stressful to the animal. Urine may be obtained by cystocentesis because the bladder is easily palpated. If desired, for prolonged anesthesia, ferrets are easily intubated with small standard endotracheal tubes or Cole tubes.

Strategies for treating ferrets in the clinic revolve around the handler's ability to restrain the animal and perform the treatment in the most efficient and quickest manner possible. For giving drugs, Nutrical, dairy products, and sweets are useful in bribing animals and in hiding medications. Most ferrets will do almost anything for yogurt or ice cream. Liquid medications are much easier to administer than pills.

A potentially fatal common clinical problem of the ferret is estrogen toxicity in females as a result of prolonged estrus. Female ferrets are induced ovulators and occasionally will not cycle out of heat unless bred. These animals then become severely anemic and thrombocytopenic because of the toxic effects of estrogen on the bone marrow. Ferrets often present with signs of lethargy, dyspnea, petechial hemorrhages, vomiting, and diarrhea. This is best treated by prevention and client education. Female ferrets not intended for breeding should be spayed before their first heat.

Clinical signs similar to those of prolonged estrus include hair loss and swollen vulva, which may be caused by adrenal hyperplasia. Female ferrets that have been spayed at an early age are extremely susceptible to this clinical condition. An adrenal hyperplasia work-up should be performed on an older spayed female ferret exhibiting signs of vulvar swelling. Adrenal hyperplasia can be treated by a partial adrenalectomy and/or administration of therapeutic agents. Response to therapy and surgery has been varied.

Ferrets are susceptible to human influenza, and therefore clients should be counseled that when members of the family have influenza the ferret should not be handled. Human influenza in a ferret must be differentiated from canine distemper and bacterial pneumonia, to which ferrets are also susceptible. Both present with similar signs of respiratory disease: nasal and ocular discharges, coughing, and sneezing. The ferret with influenza will, in most cases, get over the infection on its own in 5 to 10 days. Topical antihistamines and decongestants may be of benefit. The nonvaccinated ferret will not survive a canine distemper infection, and signs usually progress to severe dyspnea, anorexia, and sometimes involvement of the central nervous system.

Technician Note

A potentially fatal common clinical problem of the ferret is estrogen toxicity in females caused by prolonged estrus.

Parasites are a problem that must be understood by the ferret owner. Heartworm prevention is required in animals that are maintained in an outdoor enclosure where they are exposed to mosquitos. Fleas commonly plague ferrets, even if maintained within a household setting. Feline flea control products are generally safe to use on flea-infested animals (see Chapter 7).

Ferrets are also fond of chewing on things, preferably soft rubbery objects, and, as such, should be watched closely for foreign body ingestion. A ferret that presents with signs of anorexia should be considered to have a potential gastrointestinal obstruction. There are also many reports of various neoplastic diseases in ferrets, including insulinomas, osteomas, lymphosarcomas, and fibrosarcomas. If a ferret presents depressed or moribund, a blood serum glucose test should be performed because of common hypoglycemia.

Ferrets should be vaccinated for canine distemper with a chick embryo cell line product. A distemper vaccine approved for ferrets is manufactured and recommended. Under no circumstances should a canine distemper vaccine of ferret cell origin be used. The animal should be revaccinated according to the schedule used for dogs (see Chapter 11). Ferrets are not susceptible to feline panleukopenia and therefore need not be vaccinated. Other preventive medicine measures regarding ferrets include good dental care and surveillance for gastrointestinal parasites. Ferrets are strict carnivores and therefore should be fed a strict carnivore diet. There are a number of commercially available ferret diets that will provide the proper nutrition for this unique animal. If these are not available, a high-quality cat food may be used. Although this may be slightly low in protein requirements for the pregnant or lactating ferret, few problems have been reported in ferrets eating high-quality cat food diets.

Technician Note

Ferrets should never be vaccinated against canine distemper using a vaccine of ferret cell origin.

The zoonotic disease of primary importance in ferrets is rabies. Although ferrets are potential carriers, their indoor lifestyle makes exposure very unlikely. Only one case of a rabid ferret that bit a human has been documented, and this was an animal that had escaped from its owner. Ferrets should be vaccinated for rabies, using only a vaccine approved for use in ferrets.

RABBITS

The rabbit is not a rodent but rather a lagomorph of the family Leporidae. Rabbits may be housed indoors or outdoors and may be fed one of many commercial pelleted feeds. Rabbits come in many sizes, ranging from the Flemish Giant (6 to 7.5 kg) to the Dutch and Polish breeds (1 to 2 kg). If proper husbandry practices are maintained, a pet rabbit should live a long, healthy life (5 to 6 years). Rabbits are sensitive to extreme hot and cold conditions.

Rabbits defend themselves by using their long incisors to bite and by kicking with the hind legs. To sex the rabbit, stretching the perineum while the animal is in dorsal recumbency will reveal the anogenital area. Males have a round urethral opening; females have a slit opening.

The rabbit that is a candidate for anesthesia should have food withheld for 8 to 12 hours and be free from respiratory disease. Some strains of rabbits have atropinesterase, which inactivates atropine. Atropine may be given subcutaneously as a preanesthetic to decrease salivation. If a rabbit has atropinesterase, it may be necessary to increase the dose of atropine. Rabbits are seldom intubated during anesthesia because they rarely regurgitate and are difficult to intubate. Recommended endotracheal tubes in rabbits have inside diameters of 2 to 4 mm. A medium laryngoscope will aid in passing the tube into the rabbit's glottis to near the thoracic inlet. Do not use topical anesthetic in rabbits to prevent laryngospasm.

Technician Note

Rabbits are seldom intubated during anesthesia because they rarely regurgitate and are difficult to intubate.

Injectable anesthetic agents used in rabbits include ketamine, xylazine, and acepromazine; isoflurane is the inhalation anesthetic of choice. The movement of the nictitating membrane over approximately one third of the cornea, a respiratory rate of 18 to 24 respirations per minute, abdominal musculature relaxation, and the loss of the ear, mouth, toe pinch, and palpebral reflexes indicate a suitable plane of surgical anesthesia in the rabbit.

By placing a rabbit in dorsal recumbency and gently stroking its ventrum, one causes hypnosis to occur. Hypnosis is a good restraint for injections and radiographic procedures.

To give intravenous injections to rabbits, the dorsal surface of the ear should be shaved to expose the marginal ear vein. Visibility of this vein will increase if alcohol is rubbed on the area. The central artery of the ear or the cephalic or lateral saphenous vein can also be used for bleeding. Cardiac puncture for blood collection should be used only under strict professional supervision and only as a last resort in the clinical setting. The lateral saphenous vein, which is located higher on the leg than in dogs, may be used to place an indwelling catheter.

Rabbits are affected by a number of infectious and parasitic organisms. A pet rabbit may be presented for hair loss caused by self-trauma, nutritional deficiencies, bacterial dermatitis (*Pasteurella multocida*, *Pseudomonas aeruginosa*, *Staphylococcus aureus*, and *Fusobacterium*), or parasites (ear mite *Psoroptes cuniculi* [Figures 17-20 and 17-21], fur mite *Cheyletiella parasitovorax*, and rabbit lice *Haemodipsus ventricosus*). Ulcerative lesions on the ventral surface of the rear hocks is usually due to poor husbandry or environmental pressures. Fungal organisms that have been noted to cause dermatopathies in rabbits are *Microsporum gypseum* and *Trichophyton mentagrophytes*.

An anorexic pet should be examined for malocclusion, hairballs, trauma, dietary change, stress, or poor feed. Heat stress (stroke) is common when adequate cooling is not provided in the summer. Diarrhea may be caused by

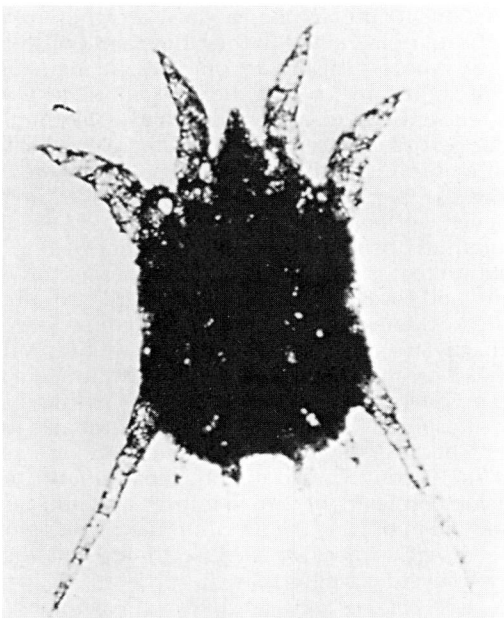

FIGURE 17-20. Microscopic view of *Psoroptes cuniculi,* the rabbit ear mite.

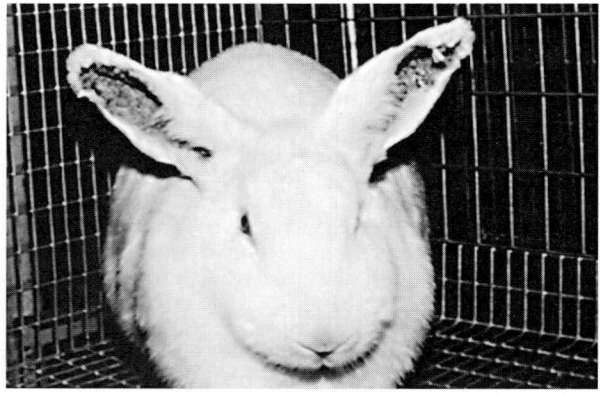

FIGURE 17-21. Rabbit exhibiting typical clinical signs of *Psoroptes cuniculi* infestation.

colibacillosis, rotavirus infections, *Clostridium* infections, mucoid enteropathy, antibiotic intake, or Tyzzer's disease *(Bacillus piliformis).* A high-fiber diet, which includes timothy hay, has been shown to improve digestive tract function and reduce the incidence of hairballs.

One of the main disease problems in rabbits is *Pasteurella multocida* infection (snuffles). Clinical signs include nasal discharge, torticollis, abscesses, conjunctivitis, and respiratory distress. Venereal spirochetosis should always be considered when rabbits are exhibiting infertility. *Eimeria stieda* is a hepatic coccidium that may affect attitude and eating habits.

Rabbits are territorial and fight when sexual maturity is reached or a male is placed in a female's cage for breeding. Neutering or ovariohysterectomy is recommended to prevent unwanted offspring.

RODENTS

Rodent species commonly presented to the veterinary hospital include guinea pigs, hamsters, gerbils, and, to a lesser extent, mice and rats. Although all these animals are rodents, each species has particular anatomic characteristics, dietary requirements, and diseases.

Antibiotics in Rodents

Care must be taken when prescribing antibiotics to rodents. Guinea pigs, rabbits, and hamsters are extremely sensitive to penicillin antibiotics, which may cause severe intestinal flora changes; penicillins, streptomycin, and dihydrostreptomycin are drugs that may cause this problem. Tetracyclines work well in cases that require antibiotic therapy. An exotic animal formulary is essential to an exotic animal practice to obtain specific information and dosage.

Technician Note
Guinea pigs, rabbits, and hamsters are extremely sensitive to penicillin antibiotics.

Anesthetics in Rodents

Ketamine hydrochloride, pentobarbital sodium, and thiamylal sodium are injectable anesthetics that may be used in rodents. Isoflurane is an acceptable gas anesthetic that provides quick induction and recovery while providing an adequate plane of anesthesia. Chapter 21 discusses anesthesiology.

Antiparasitic Agents in Rodents

Carbaryl powder, dichlorvos, and ivermectin can be used safely to treat ectoparasites. Dichlorvos, thiabendazole, and ivermectin are adequate to treat internal parasites. See Chapter 7 for additional information on parasitology.

Guinea Pig

The cavy, or guinea pig, is a rodent related to porcupines and chinchillas. Guinea pigs have a long gestation that leads to the birth of large, precocious young.

The most common guinea pig species kept as pets are the English or American, Abyssinian, and Peruvian long hair (Figures 17-22 and 17-23).

The guinea pig has open-rooted teeth that may become maloccluded. The overgrown teeth will irritate the gingiva, causing excessive salivation (Figure 17-24).

Although the female has only two vaginal mammary glands, it can successfully raise litters of three or more offspring.

A female that is bred past 7 or 8 months of age may have trouble separating the pubic symphysis. Fat pads may also occlude the pelvic canal, complicating parturition. These problems usually lead to dystocia or death. If the sow is experiencing dystocia, a cesarean retrieval of the young can often save the babies. Food preferences are established within a few days after birth for the young. Hand-rearing of the young requires regular stimulation of defecation and urination as with most neonatal mammals. Females usually allow foster nursing of other young.

Guinea pigs rarely become excited or bite when handled. Through their gentle nature, they become conditioned to their surroundings. However, if a group is contained in an enclosure, subordinate animals may be traumatized (as by hair loss and bite wounds) by dominant ones.

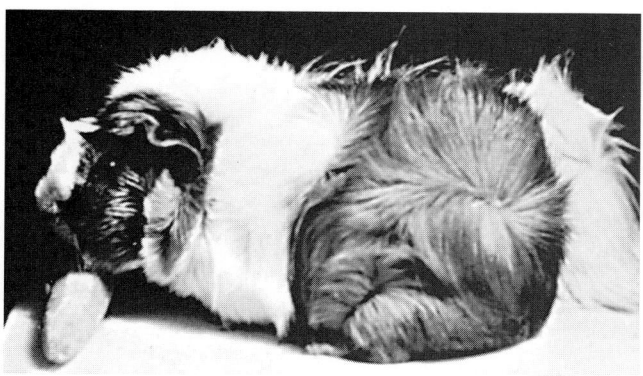

FIGURE 17-22. An Abyssinian guinea pig.

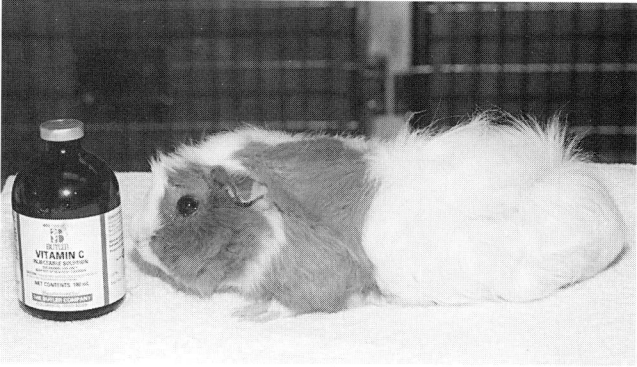

FIGURE 17-25. Vitamin C dietary supplementation is critical for maintenance of excellent health.

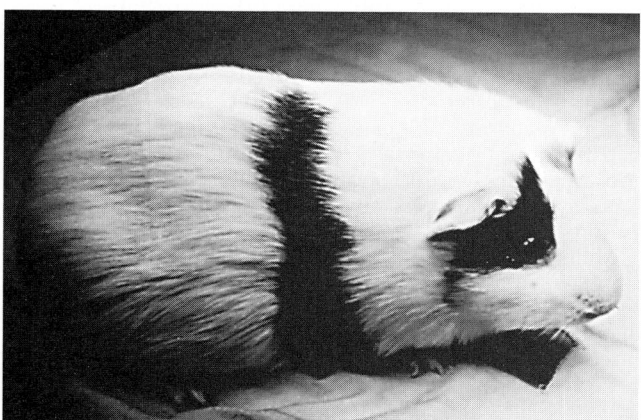

FIGURE 17-23. The English guinea pig, a common house pet.

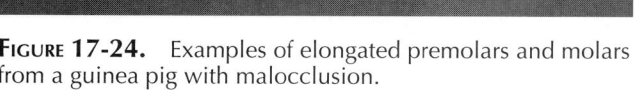

FIGURE 17-24. Examples of elongated premolars and molars from a guinea pig with malocclusion.

Foot pad dermatitis ulcers may develop on animals placed on wire. Metal, plastic, and glass make excellent habit cages. Substrate may be paper (shredded), wood shavings, or hay. Chewing their substrate is a vice commonly associated with an animal developing submandibular abscesses. Hard fibrous splinters penetrate the oral mucosa, inoculating the tissue with bacteria (usually *Streptococcus zooepidemicus*) that develop into abscesses. Changes in the substrate may be indicated to stop this problem, although it may be difficult to find an adequate alternative substrate, which must have absorptive qualities for the opaque, pale yellow, crystalline urine.

The feed and water are best placed in bowls that cannot be chewed (e.g., stainless steel or ceramic crocks). A vitamin C supplementation may be added to the water, such as Tang (General Foods Corp.). The food should be a freshly milled complete guinea pig ration. Storage in a freezer or refrigerator will extend the life of the food. All food and water containers should be placed above the substrate to prevent soiling.

Unlike other pet rodents, guinea pigs require dietary vitamin C supplementation. Vitamin C is highly unstable in the feed, especially when exposed to heat. Use of old feed is one of the primary reasons vitamin C deficiencies are seen (Figure 17-25).

 Technician Note

Unlike other pet rodents, guinea pigs require dietary vitamin C supplementation.

The cavy requires 0.5 mg/kg body weight dietary ascorbic acid per day because it lacks L-gulonolactone oxidase. Published doses of vitamin C for guinea pigs are 1 to 30 mg/kg intramuscularly twice daily or 200 to 400 mg/L in drinking water (freshly mixed daily). Guinea pigs *must* be fed species-specific food within 90 days of milling. Fruit and vegetable supplementation is discouraged because of the possibility of disturbing the normal gut bacterial flora.

To sex a guinea pig, the handler must observe the urethral orifice and anus. The male has no break in the ridge between the openings, whereas the female has a shallow U-shaped break.

One boar will service up to 10 sows beginning at 8 weeks of age. The sow becomes sexually mature around 5 to 6 weeks of age.

Gestation length is on average 63 to 68 days, with litter size ranging from one to six precocious offspring.

Hamster

The golden hamster is a native of Syria and comes in many different color varieties (Figure 17-26). Cheek pouches that

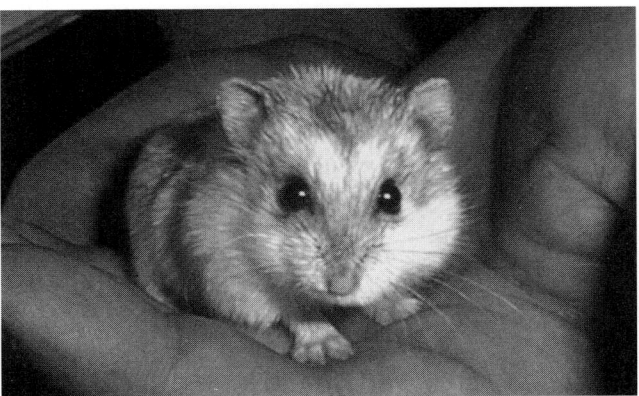

FIGURE 17-26. Siberian dwarf hamsters are popular pets.

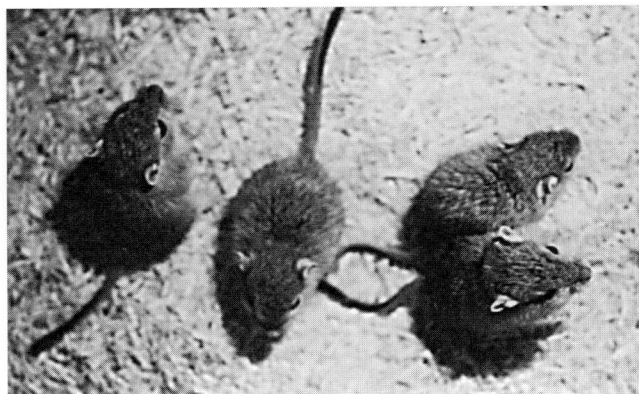

FIGURE 17-28. Young gerbils.

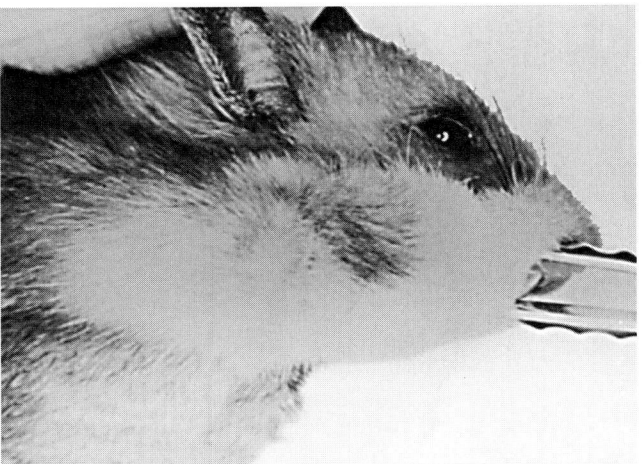

FIGURE 17-27. Hamster cheek pouches extended by forceps.

extend along the head and neck to the proximal dorsum of the back serve as a food transportation device (Figure 17-27). Along the caudal lateral abdominal region lie the flank glands. A dark brown patch of skin on each side delineates these sebaceous glands that are used to mark territory and in mating rituals.

Hamsters have a tendency to bite and are good at chewing through cage material. To accommodate the animal's physical nature, an exercise wheel should be placed in the cage.

Female hamsters often attack newly introduced males and females. Hamsters live, on the average, 18 to 24 months, have a gestation length of 16 days, and produce about five offspring on average. Offspring are weaned in 20 to 25 days. If disturbed, the female may cannibalize her litter or hide them in her cheek pouches. When the young are hidden in the cheek pouches, they may suffocate. Hamsters can be picked up by the nape skin at the base of the neck or by cupping the hands under the hindlimbs.

Technician Note

Hamsters live, on average, 18 to 24 months and have a gestation period of 16 days.

There are several commercially available hamster habitats. An aquarium with a mesh top may be used to house a hamster, with hardwood shavings being the choice substrate. Aromatic shavings such as cedar or pine may cause ocular and respiratory irritation, severe dermatitis, and allergic reactions. Sipper bottles are perfect for water dispensing, and nonchewable bowls should be used for food containers or the food should be placed on the floor. All food and water access should be made available to the young.

Males have a greater anogenital distance than females. Hamsters may be mated monogamously or in a harem situation. It is important that females with young are not disturbed so that cannibalism and abandonment of the litter do not occur.

Wet tail is a general term to describe diarrhea in the hamster. Bacterial infections, cestodiasis, and antibiotic administration are a few causes of diarrhea in these rodents.

Zoonotic Diseases

Lymphocytic choriomeningitis, salmonellosis, and hymenolepid tapeworm infections are diseases that may be transferred from hamsters to humans. Proper hygiene should be practiced after one has handled these animals.

Gerbil

The Mongolian gerbil is a popular pet native to Mongolia and northeastern China. It is an active burrowing animal adapted to desert environments. Gerbils have a midventral pad consisting of sebaceous glands used in territorial marking.

The gerbil has a life span of 3.5 years, with a gestation length of 25 days without lactation and 24 to 48 days with lactation. The litter sizes average five offspring that wean in approximately 25 days (Figure 17-28). Certain gerbil lines are prone to epileptiform seizure activity. Gerbils are friendly rodents that may be housed in hamster units (Figure 17-29). These animals are good at escaping; therefore the cage should be designed to prevent chewing.

The gerbil's diet may be similar to that of the hamster, and water can be supplied in a sipper bottle. Sexing is accomplished by measuring the urogenital distance. The male has a much longer distance than the female. Males aid in the care of the young.

Gerbils commonly present with a nasal dermatitis caused by a bacterial infection initiated by their burrowing activity. Topical antibiotic treatment is recommended for resolution of this infection.

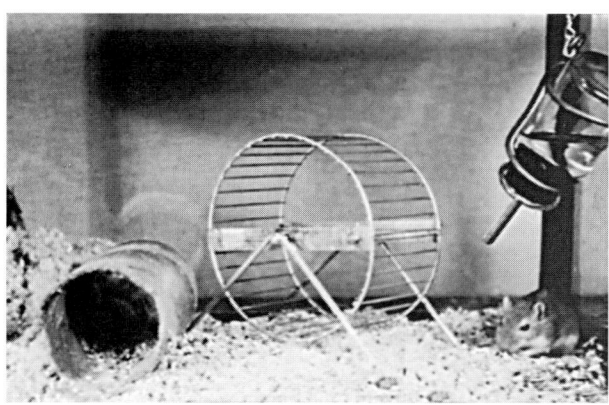

FIGURE 17-29. Typical small rodent cage containing gerbils.

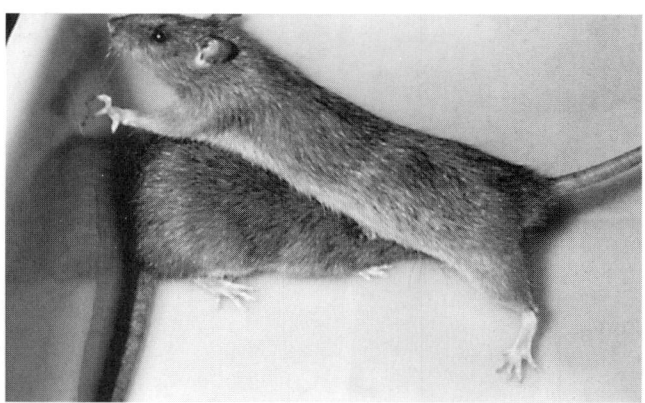

FIGURE 17-31. Rats make one of the best companion animals of all rodent species.

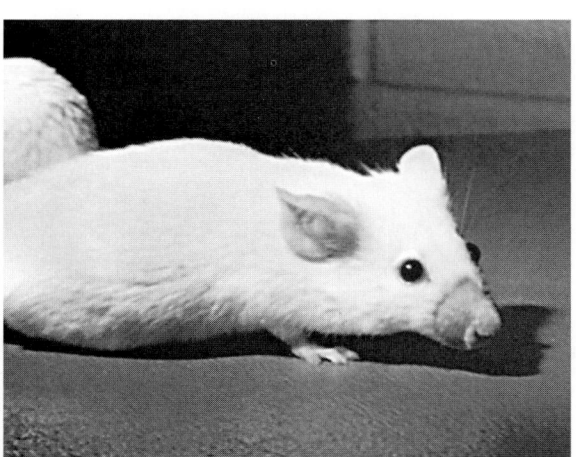

FIGURE 17-30. Trauma (cage mate–inflicted hair loss) on a mouse. This is commonly referred to as *barbering.*

Tyzzer's disease may be diagnosed in gerbils and is caused by *Bacillus piliformis.* Dietary change and colibacillosis also cause diarrhea in these animals.

Mouse

Mice are small rodents that are commonly used in the research setting but often are aggressive and bite. They are territorial animals and quickly develop a hierarchy when placed in groups (Figure 17-30). These small animals require small amounts of food and water but are escape prone and may develop an unpleasant odor.

Common clinical conditions affecting mice include ectoparasites, neoplasia, and trauma. Most mice have a life span of 2 years and are therefore prone to geriatric disease conditions within a relatively short time of ownership. One of the most common geriatric disease conditions is neoplasia. Tumors of various types have been identified in mice, making the education of owners particularly important to aid in early detection and treatment.

Housing should be similar to that of gerbils and hamsters. Hardwood shavings or chips are recommended in-

stead of the aromatic softwood chips (cedar and pine) because of potential liver damage and epithelial damage.

Housing should be cleaned regularly to prevent odor and health problems. Pelleted rodent feed and fresh water in sipper bottles should be supplied free choice.

Male mice have a greater urogenital distance than females. Female mice become sexually mature at 50 days of age and are best bred in the harem scheme, with one male combined with two to six females.

Rat

Rats are clean and unassuming and can be trained to be good pets (Figure 17-31). These animals may live up to 3 years or longer and become sexually mature at 1.5 to 2 months of age.

As with mice, rats are relatively short lived, predisposing them to geriatric diseases. Rats are also very susceptible to neoplasia, particularly mammary gland tumors. In addition, *Mycoplasma* spp. respiratory infections are commonly diagnosed and clinically may appear as dyspnea and nasal discharge. The nasal discharge is red because of the pigment of the harderian gland secretions. Enrofloxacin and tetracycline have been used to treat *Mycoplasma* spp. infections in rats.

> **Technician Note**
>
> Rats seldom bite, but caution must be used in a stressful situation.

Commercial rodent cages can be obtained for proper housing. Substrate should be similar to that of other rodents.

Males have a longer anogenital distance than females. The gestation length is 22 days, and nesting material should be provided before birth.

Although zoonotic diseases are rare in domestic rats, these animals can carry many diseases transmissible to humans. These diseases include rat bite fever, *Yersinia pestis,* leptospirosis, *Streptococcus* spp., cestodiasis, and Korean hemorrhagic fever.

Prairie Dogs

The black-tailed prairie dog *(Cynomys ludovicianus)* may present to a veterinary clinic even though it is illegal to keep wild North American species as pets. Wild prairie

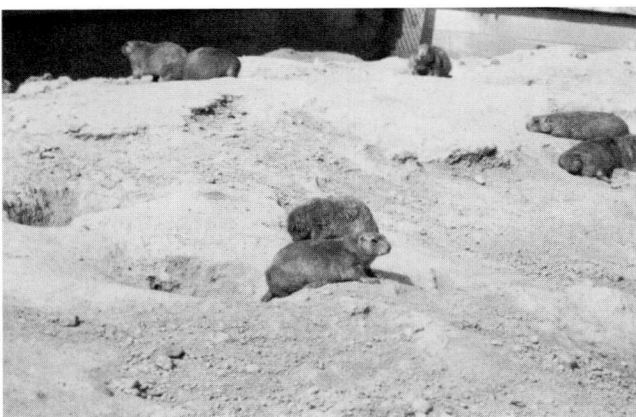

FIGURE 17-32.   Sociable prairie dogs may be a surprise patient to veterinary hospitals.

Box 17-3	RECOMMENDED DAILY DIET FOR HEDGEHOGS

- 3 teaspoons high-quality cat or kitten chow
- 1 teaspoon fruit/vegetable mix
- 4-8 small meal worms or 2-3 small crickets

dogs may carry *Hantavirus*, rabies, ectoparasites, *Salmonella* spp., the plague bacteria, and other bacterial agents. Some prairie dogs have been raised in captivity and are therefore less likely to carry dangerous zoonotic diseases. Nevertheless, it is recommended that all prairie dogs remain where they belong, in their natural habitat (Figure 17-32).

Prairie dogs may live up to 10 years and can survive on rodent chow and timothy grass hay. They are, however, susceptible to obesity, making it essential to monitor food intake, especially in adult animals. Digging and tunneling are important parts of their daily activity. The provision of deep bedding therefore enables this type of exercise and allows them to hide and feel secure. Prairie dogs can be managed much like rats in regard to their management and care. The scrotal sac is the identifying characteristic of male prairie dogs when sex determination is required. Venipuncture sites of choice include the lateral saphenous or cephalic vein. Jugular venipuncture or cranial vena cava collection should only be attempted when the patient is under general anesthesia.

Common disease problems identified in captive prairie dogs are obesity, respiratory disease, malocclusion, infectious pododermatitis, trauma, and neoplasia. The most difficult situation to overcome for most captively raised prairie dogs is the fat factor. Obesity usually complicates concurrent disease states, making it difficult at times to differentiate the primary disease problem from complications caused by obesity.

HEDGEHOGS

The African hedgehog *(Atelerix albiventris)* has become an increasingly popular pet in recent years. These nocturnal spiny animals are unique pets and may adapt best to captivity when left alone. Hedgehogs like to hide, like dark quiet areas, and will burrow to escape. Hedgehogs may be maintained much like rodents. For example, enclosures that are 20 gallons or larger and lined with an absorbable paper bedding make excellent habitats.

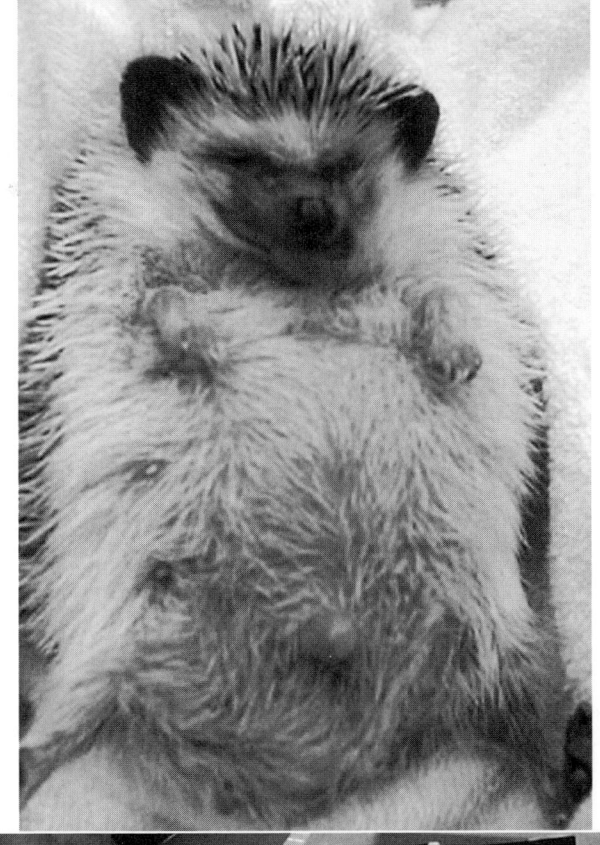

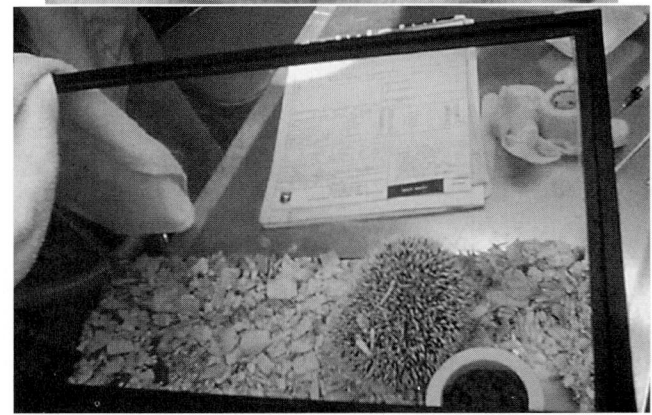

FIGURE 17-33.   **A,** The ventral surface of hedgehogs is devoid of spines. **B,** The dorsal aspect, as noted with this pet in its enclosure, is covered with sharp spines.

The life span of hedgehogs is 3 to 5 years. The most common disease conditions are neoplasia and external parasites. Yearly physical examinations are needed for teeth cleaning, nail trimming, and tumor checks. Hedgehogs are not rodents and rely on an insectivore/omnivore diet such as the one listed in Box 17-3.

One unique feature of hedgehog medicine is that hedgehog patients must be anesthetized simply to be examined. The spines are very sharp, so caution must be taken during handling and gloves are necessary, particularly before anesthesia (Figure 17-33).

Blood collection sites are cranial vena cava, jugular vein, cephalic vein, and lateral saphenous vein, with the

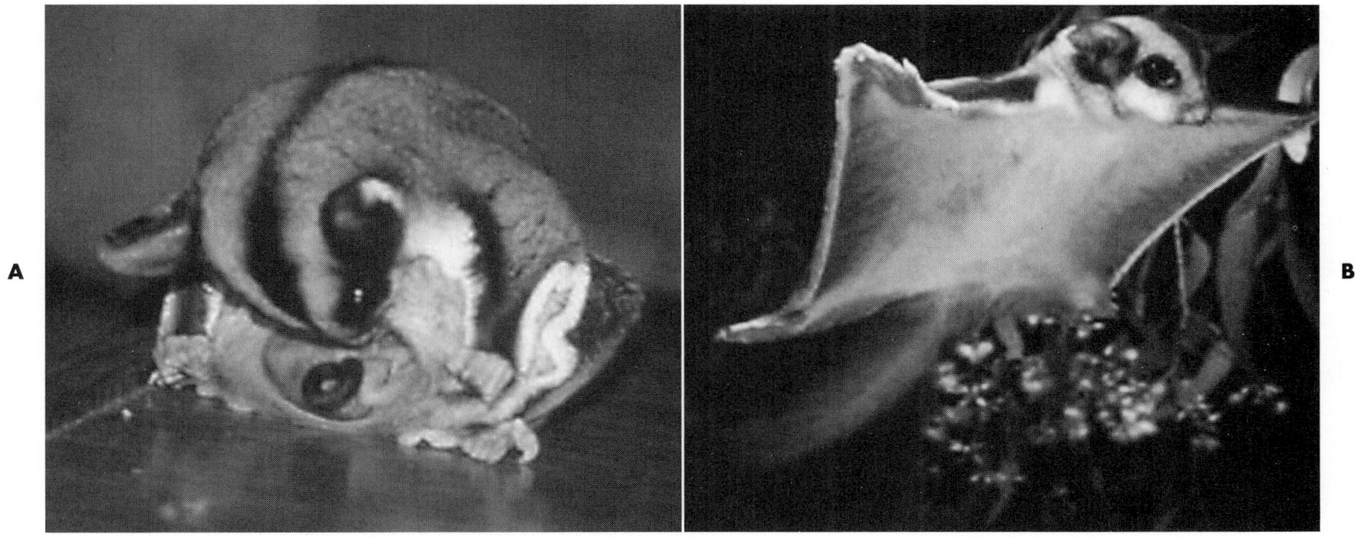

A

B

FIGURE 17-34. **A,** A sugar glider female with babies in her pouch. **B,** The skin stretched out, giving the sugar glider the ability to "fly" and also its name.

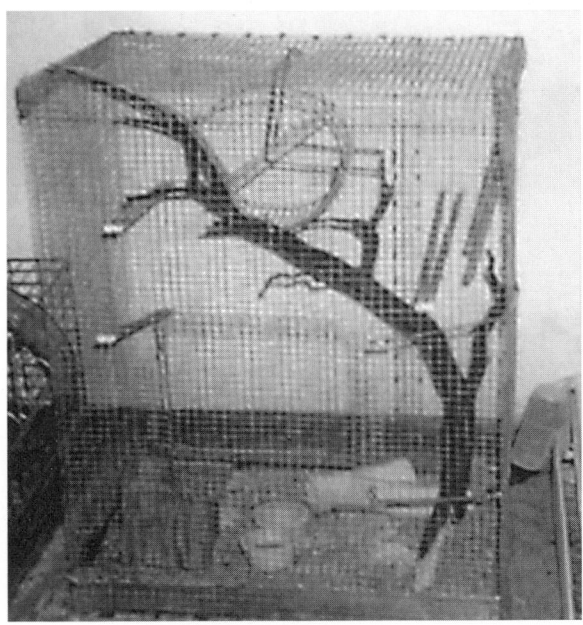

FIGURE 17-35. A typical sugar glider enclosure.

Box 17-4	DAILY SUGAR GLIDER DIET

- Zoo-formula insectivore diet
- Equal amounts:
  - Chopped apple
  - Grapes
  - Carrot
  - Sweet potato
  - Hard-cooked egg yolk
- 10-12 small meal worms
- Dust food and insects with vitamin mineral powder

cranial vena cava being the site of choice. Common diseases diagnosed in hedgehogs are neoplasia, obesity, otitis externa, dermatitis, external parasites, and respiratory disease.

SUGAR GLIDERS

Sugar gliders are nocturnal marsupials from Australia (Figure 17-34). As with hedgehogs, they are unusual pets with unique qualities that should be considered carefully by a potential owner before a purchase is made. They are very social animals. If maintained as a single pet, a glider will require additional attention from the owner to meet its psychologic needs. In addition, their nocturnal habits give rise to much activity throughout the night, which can be annoying to those who wish to sleep.

Housing needs to be a tall wire enclosure with fresh branches and places to hide, such as a bird box (Figure 17-35). The wire mesh should have spacing no more than 1-inch square to prevent escape. The bottom tray should be lined with shredded paper or pelleted paper products for easy cleaning and optimum absorption of urine, food, and water.

Malnutrition is one of the most common reasons for sugar gliders to present to the veterinarian. There are commercial pelleted glider diets available, but they are not actively marketed in most areas. One source of information worth exploring is the Internet. Web pages that focus on these animals can be found via search engines. An example of a complete sugar glider diet is listed in Box 17-4.

REFERENCES

Frye FL: *Reptile clinicians handbook,* Malabar, Fla, 1995, Krieger, pp 70-100.

Wise JK: *U.S. pet ownership and demographics sourcebook,* Schaumburg, Ill, 1997, American Veterinary Medicine Association, pp 1-58.

RECOMMENDED READING

Boyer TH: *A practitioner's guide to reptilian husbandry and care*, Lakewood, Colo, 1993, American Animal Hospital Association.

Campbell TW: *Avian hematology and cytology*, ed 2, Ames, 1995, Iowa State University Press.

Carpenter JW, Mashima TY, Rupiper DJ: *Exotic animal formulary*, Manhattan, Kan, 1996, Greystone Publications.

Fox JG: *Biology and diseases of the ferret*, Philadelphia, 1988, Lea & Febiger.

Fudge AM, editor: *Semin Avian Exotic Pet Med*, Philadelphia, WB Saunders (published quarterly).

Harkness JE, Wagner JE: *The biology and medicine of rabbits and rodents*, Philadelphia, 1995, Lea & Febiger.

Jacobson ER, Kollias GV Jr, editors: *Exotic Animals: contemporary issues in small animal practice*, New York, 1988, Churchill Livingstone.

Johnson CA, Harrison LR: *Guinea pigs: exotic companion medicine handbook for veterinarians*, Lake Worth, Fla, 1996, Wingers Publishing, pp 2-20.

J Avian Med Surg, Lawrence, Kan, Allen Press (published quarterly).

J Small Exotic Animal Med, Valley Village, Calif, Gray Publishing (published quarterly).

J Zoo Wildlife Med, Lawrence, Kan, American Association of Zoo Veterinarians, (published monthly).

Mader DR: *Reptile medicine and surgery*, Philadelphia, 1996, WB Saunders.

Mattison C: *The care of reptiles and amphibians in captivity*, New York, 1990, Sterling Publishing.

Ritchie BW, Harrison GJ, Harrison LR: *Avian medicine: principles and application*, Lake Worth, Fla, 1994, Wingers Publishing.

18

Zonoses and Public Health

Michael G. Groves • Kathleen Story Harrington

This chapter provides an overview of the major zoonotic diseases and other significant public health concerns that veterinary personnel are most likely to encounter in the course of their work. It is not the purpose of this chapter to present zoonoses, even important ones, that are unlikely to be transmitted to the veterinary technician in the course of his or her work. The focus is on the occupational exposure to these conditions, as opposed to exposure via other means. For example, some of the diseases discussed here, such as salmonellosis and brucellosis, also can be acquired by consuming contaminated food, water, or milk. Food-borne or waterborne transmission is mentioned but not described in detail; only those routes of infection that are specific to veterinary exposure are covered in depth. Likewise, outlined prevention strategies are oriented toward the veterinary profession rather than the public.

The animals listed as carriers or reservoirs of the various diseases are the ones most commonly implicated in transmission; no attempt has been made to list every host species that could possibly be associated with a given zoonosis. Absent also are those diseases that may affect both humans and animals (e.g., systemic mycoses such as blastomycosis or coccidiomycosis) but that are environmentally acquired rather than zoonotic. Finally, this chapter is not intended to be a comprehensive reference on zoonoses, but instead it presents a brief review of each disease or condition and provides suggestions for further reading. A summary of the major occupationally acquired zoonotic diseases is given in Table 18-1.

ANIMAL-ASSOCIATED INJURIES: BITE WOUNDS

There are many ways in which animals can adversely affect the health of humans, and for those who work with animals on a daily basis, the risk of sustaining an animal-associated injury is significantly higher than that of contracting a zoonotic disease. Large animals can inflict considerable damage with their feet if they kick or step on a person, and many orthopedic surgeons regard horses as the animal most likely to cause injury.

Technician Note

Animal-associated injuries most frequently sustained by veterinarians and animal care personnel are bite wounds from companion animals.

However, the animal-associated injuries most frequently sustained by veterinarians and animal care personnel are bite wounds from companion animals. A bite wound is defined as "any break in the skin caused by an animal's teeth, regardless of intention." In a recent survey of small animal practitioners, cat and dog bites accounted for more than two thirds of the injuries of veterinarians and their employees. A 3-year analysis of Workers' Compensation claims conducted for the American Veterinary Medical Association (AVMA) revealed that animal bites accounted for 49% of all reported incidents and accounted for more than $220,000 in payments to injured personnel each year.

Although cats are reported to inflict more bites in a veterinary setting than do dogs (54% vs. 45%, respectively), dogs are responsible for the most serious bites in both occupational and nonoccupational situations. Dog bites constitute a major public health problem. In the United States, more than 1 million dog bites are reported each year, which is equal to an annual incidence rate of 300 to 700 per 100,000 population. Probably fewer than half of all bites that occur are reported, however; and some reports estimate the true number is closer to 3 million per year. Annually, more than 585,000 bite wounds in the

TABLE 18-1   SUMMARY OF MAJOR OCCUPATIONALLY ACQUIRED ZOONOTIC DISEASES

	Agent	Source Animals*	Mode of Transmission	Type of Infection	Severity	Notes
BACTERIAL DISEASES						
Anthrax Cutaneous Inhalation	Bacillus anthracis	Cattle, sheep, horses, goats	Cutaneous inoculation Inhalation of agent in contaminated dust	Cutaneous lesion; may progress to septicemia Mild upper respiratory symptoms progressing to acute septicemia	Mild (cutaneous only) to fatal (septicemia) Usually fatal	Vaccine is available for people at high risk of exposure. Early treatment prevents progression to more severe disease.
Brucellosis	Brucella spp.	Cattle, sheep, goats, swine	Contact with placenta or birth fluids; inhalation; injection with strain 19 vaccine	Septicemia	Severe	Convalescence is prolonged; relapses frequently occur.
Campylobacteriosis	Campylobacter spp.	Dogs, cats, cattle	Fecal-oral	Gastroenteritis, diarrhea	Mild to severe	Most patients recover without treatment.
Capnocytophaga infection	Capnocytophaga canimorsus	Dogs, cats	Bite wound	Septicemia	Severe to fatal	Asplenic and other immunocompromised people are at increased risk.
Cat-scratch disease	Bartonella henselae	Cats	Bite, scratch, contact with broken skin	Influenza-like with regional lymphadenopathy	Usually mild, self-limiting	Most patients recover without treatment.
Erysipeloid	Erysipelothrix rhusiopathiae	Swine, turkeys	Cutaneous inoculation	Cutaneous lesion; rarely progresses to systemic disease	Usually mild	
Ornithosis (psittacosis)	Chlamydophila (Chlamydia) psittaci	Psittacine birds, turkeys	Inhalation of agent excreted in feces	Upper respiratory illness; pneumonia	Mild to severe	Early treatment shortens duration of illness.
Pasteurellosis	Pasteurella multocida	Cats, dogs	Bite wound	Cellulitis; progression to septicemia possible	Mild to severe	Septic arthritis may develop in persons with rheumatoid arthritis.
Q fever	Coxiella burnetii	Sheep, goats, cattle	Inhalation; contact with placenta or birth fluids	Systemic, influenza-like	Mild to severe	Usually mild; in rare cases chronic disease and endocarditis develop years after initial infection.

Disease	Agent	Animal reservoir	Transmission	Manifestation	Severity	Comments
Rat-bite fevers	*Streptobacillus moniliformis* and *Spirillum minus*	**Rodents**	Bite wound	Systemic, febrile, usually with polyarthritis	Mild to severe	Untreated infection may persist for weeks or months; fatalities have occurred.
Salmonellosis	*Salmonella* spp.	**Reptiles**, dogs, cats, chickens, ducks	Fecal-oral	Gastroenteritis	Mild to severe	Immunocompromised people at greater risk for severe illness
FUNGAL DISEASES						
Cryptococcosis	*Cryptococcus neoformans*	**Birds** (indirect)	Inhalation	Pneumonia; meningitis in HIV-positive people	Mild to severe	HIV-infected people at increased risk
Dermatophytosis (tinea)	*Microsporum canis, Trichophyton mentagrophytes, T. verrucosum*	Dogs, **cats**, sheep	Direct contact with infected animal or spores on hair or dander	Lesion affecting hair, skin, or nails	Usually mild	
PARASITIC DISEASES						
Cryptosporidiosis	*Cryptosporidium parvum*	**Cattle**	Fecal-oral	Gastroenteritis	Usually mild, self-limiting	May be life-threatening in HIV-infected people
Toxoplasmosis	*Toxoplasma gondii*	Cats	Fecal-oral	Systemic, mononucleosis-like; encephalitis	Usually subclinical in immunocompetent persons; can be life-threatening in HIV-infected people	Direct transmission from cats rare; primary infection during pregnancy can affect fetus
VIRAL DISEASES						
Contagious ecthyma (orf)	*Parapoxvirus*	**Sheep**, goats	Direct contact with infective material	Cutaneous lesion	Usually mild, self-limiting	
Herpesvirus simiae (B-virus) infection	*Herpesvirus simiae*	**Old World monkeys**	Bite wound or other cutaneous inoculation; possible aerosol transmission	Meningoencephalitis	Usually fatal	Survivors usually have permanent neurologic sequelae.
Newcastle disease	*Paramyxovirus*	**Poultry**	Direct contact of eyes with infective material; aerosols	Conjunctivitis; occasionally systemic, influenza-like	Usually mild, self-limiting	
Rabies	*Lyssavirus*	Dogs, cats, cattle, **skunks, raccoons, foxes, bats,** etc.	Bite wound or contact with saliva	Encephalomyelitis	Fatal	All animal care personnel should receive preexposure prophylaxis.

HIV, Human immunodeficiency virus.

*Boldface indicates most commonly implicated animals.

United States require medical attention, and dogs are responsible for 80% to 90% of those.

> ### Technician Note
>
> Zoonotic diseases that may be transmitted by dog bites include *Capnocytophaga canimorsus* infection, pasteurellosis, and rabies.

In the course of their work, veterinary personnel encounter many situations that may provoke a bite, even from a dog that is not normally aggressive. Some dogs resist being placed in submissive postures or situations, such as during restraint for examination, and will attempt to bite in response to this perceived insult. Other factors that may increase the risk of bites are the stresses that an already fearful dog experiences while in unfamiliar and often uncomfortable surroundings. The unintentional inflicting of pain in the course of restraining the animal, examining it, or administering medication also can provoke a bite.

If a bite occurs, there is a possibility of serious infection developing. At particular risk are persons who are immunocompromised, which includes people who are positive for the human immunodeficiency virus (HIV) or have acquired immune deficiency syndrome (AIDS). Other at-risk persons are pregnant women, people receiving long-term corticosteroid therapy, individuals who have had their spleen removed, and others who have weakened immune systems. All immunocompromised persons should take extra precautions to avoid exposure to infection. Zoonotic diseases that may be transmitted by dog bites include *Capnocytophaga canimorsus* infection, pasteurellosis, and rabies. (These diseases are detailed later in this chapter.) In addition, there is the possibility of permanent damage or disfigurement resulting from the wound.

Veterinary personnel should be alert to possible bite-provoking situations and take measures to ensure a dog does not have the opportunity to bite. In addition, people with immunosuppressive conditions should avoid handling animals that may bite.

If a bite does occur, regardless of the species of animal involved or the immune status of the person bitten, the wound should be washed immediately with soap and water and rinsed thoroughly with a strong stream of water. If the wound is severe, medical treatment should be sought as soon as possible. An immunocompromised person should consult a physician for even a minor wound because prophylactic antibiotics may be indicated. Normally healthy people with small wounds should seek medical advice if the wound penetrates a joint or the wound site becomes swollen, inflamed, or painful.

BACTERIAL ZOONOSES

Anthrax

Agent
Bacillus anthracis is a large, nonmotile, gram-positive rod that forms environmentally resistant endospores when exposed to air.

Reservoirs
Reservoirs for *Bacillus anthracis* are sheep, goats, cows, and other domestic and wild ruminants.

Occurrence
Incidence is worldwide except for the far north and some South Pacific islands, but it varies greatly by region. An-thrax in animals occurs sporadically in Eurasia, North America, and Australia but is endemic in Africa, the Middle East, India, Southeast Asia, Mexico, and parts of South America. Warm, humid areas tend to have anthrax "hot spots" because heat stress lowers animals' resistance and the climate encourages sporulation of shed organisms.

Estimates of human anthrax cases range from 20,000 to 100,000 per year, with most occurring in Africa, South America, Europe, the Middle East, and the former Soviet Union. In the United States, human anthrax is very rare, with only three cases reported between 1984 and 1993. Most cases of anthrax are occupationally acquired; people at greatest risk are veterinarians and animal care workers, abattoir workers, hide tanners, wool processors, and bone-meal producers.

Transmission
Infected animals shed the organism via hemorrhages that occur at death, thus contaminating soil with endospores that can remain viable for years. Other animals can become infected by grazing in the contaminated areas. Biting flies may be involved in mechanical transmission of the bacteria.

There are two forms of human anthrax that are occupationally associated: cutaneous and inhalation. Cutaneous anthrax is acquired when organisms enter broken skin, usually on the hands, arms, or face. Direct contact with tissues or body fluids of diseased animals and exposure to contaminated soil are the most common means of transmission. Inhalation anthrax results from inhaling viable spores that may be present in wool and processed hides of infected animals. A third form, gastrointestinal anthrax, results from eating contaminated undercooked meat and is not associated with any particular occupational exposure.

> ### Technician Note
>
> Inhalation anthrax results from inhaling viable spores that may be present in wool and processed hides of infected animals.

Disease in Animals
SIGNS.   Anthrax in animals manifests in three main forms: peracute, acute, and subacute to chronic. Peracute anthrax, which occurs in ruminants, is characterized by sudden death with few premonitory signs. The animal appears healthy until just before death, when there may be high fever, muscle tremors, dyspnea, and convulsions. A bloody discharge from various body orifices often occurs after death.

Both ruminants and horses can have anthrax in the acute form. In this form, signs appear up to 48 or more hours before death and may include a period of excitement followed by depression, lethargy, and anorexia. Fever, rapid respiration, and rapid heart rate occur, and mucous membranes become hemorrhagic or congested. The tongue, throat, sternum, perineum, and flanks may become edematous and swollen.

Swine, dogs, and cats that consume meat from diseased animals or other contaminated material can develop subacute to chronic anthrax. Organisms concentrate in lymph nodes in the pharyngeal region and cause swelling that obstructs the airways; death by suffocation follows. Bacteremia can also occur, and some animals may develop enteritis. Carnivores appear to be more resistant to anthrax and often recover.

DIAGNOSIS. The organism can be cultured from blood or tissues of affected animals. A necropsy should not be performed in cases of suspected anthrax to avoid exposing any *B. anthracis* organisms to air, thus causing sporulation and contamination of the site. Because blood does not clot following death from anthrax because of toxin produced by the organism, a sample can be collected from the jugular vein using a disposable syringe. Capped syringes should be refrigerated and submitted promptly to a laboratory for culture.

Disease in Humans

SIGNS AND SYMPTOMS. Cutaneous anthrax accounts for more than 95% of cases. Within 1 week of inoculation a small, painless, reddish, pruritic papule forms and develops into a fluid-filled vesicle. The area surrounding the lesion becomes edematous, and secondary vesicles may form around the initial site. The typical lesion of cutaneous anthrax is a black eschar that develops after a vesicle ruptures and ulcerates. Most patients recover within 10 days of onset, but in some cases cutaneous anthrax progresses to systemic disease. Disseminated anthrax is rapidly fatal if untreated.

Inhalation anthrax is almost always fatal. It begins with mild, nonspecific upper respiratory signs, but within 3 to 5 days the patient becomes acutely ill, with fever, shock, and rapidly progressing respiratory distress. Death occurs within 24 hours of onset of the acute phase.

DIAGNOSIS. Cutaneous anthrax is easily diagnosed if the disease is considered among the possibilities. Gram staining of the vesicular fluid often reveals large, gram-positive rods, and cultures of the fluid are usually positive for *B. anthracis* if specimens are collected before antibiotic therapy is begun.

The diagnosis of inhalation anthrax is much more difficult because early signs mimic a mild, influenza-like infection. Death usually occurs before the diagnosis is made.

Technician Note

A human vaccine for individuals at high risk of exposure to anthrax is presently available only to military personnel.

Treatment

Cutaneous anthrax responds well to antibiotic treatment. Inhalation anthrax, however, is often diagnosed too late in the course of the disease for even massive doses of antibiotics to be effective.

Prevention

Laws covering the prevention of anthrax are in force in most areas. Livestock vaccines are available and effective. When an outbreak occurs, affected animals should be treated with antibiotics and survivors quarantined for 21 days after the last death has occurred. As noted above, necropsy should not be performed on any animal suspected of having died from anthrax. Carcasses should be burned at the site, if possible, instead of buried because spores can survive for many years in soil. If an animal must be buried, there should be a deep burial, and the carcass should be covered with a layer of quick lime (anhydrous calcium oxide) before the dirt is replaced. Disposable material that must come in contact with infected animals should be burned or disinfected and buried. Contaminated surfaces and other nondisposable items should be cleaned with a disinfectant known to be effective against anthrax spores.

A human vaccine is available for personnel at high risk of exposure to anthrax, such as workers in wool or hide-processing plants, laboratory personnel working in anthrax research, and veterinarians and veterinary technicians working in highly endemic areas. Anyone coming into contact with an animal that may have anthrax should be particularly careful about hygiene and care of any wounds.

Reporting and Surveillance

Both human anthrax and animal anthrax are reportable diseases in the United States and other developed countries. In the United States, animal cases must be reported to the appropriate state animal health agency.

Avian Chlamydiosis (Ornithosis/Psittacosis)

Agent

Chlamydophila (Chlamydia) psittaci is an obligate, intracellular, gram-negative bacterium with a unique biphasic reproductive cycle, of which only one phase is infectious.

Reservoirs

Birds, especially psittacines (members of the parrot family), pigeons, and doves, and poultry, including ducks and turkeys, are reservoirs for chlamydiosis.

Occurrence

Incidence is worldwide; it is endemic in birds and sporadic in humans. Prevalence in avian species varies widely; active chlamydiosis in wild psittacines is about 1%, whereas 50% to 95% of some feral pigeon populations may carry the disease. Humans at risk are those who own exotic pet birds, bird breeders, pigeon fanciers, poultry farm or processing plant workers, veterinarians and their technicians who treat birds, zoo keepers, avian quarantine station employees, and others who come in contact with wild, pet, or domestic birds.

Transmission

Transmission occurs through inhalation of infective particles that have become aerosolized from dried feces, ocular or nasal secretions, dust from feathers, and so forth. Cleaning cages is a means of human exposure; sneezing and wing flapping by birds also spread infective material.

Disease in Animals

SIGNS. Birds may develop peracute, acute, or chronic disease; many are asymptomatic carriers. Clinical signs vary depending on species of host and virulence of the infecting strain, but most cases include depression, anorexia, yellowish or greenish diarrhea, conjunctivitis, nasal discharge, and respiratory difficulty. Morbidity and mortality also differ with strain virulence.

DIAGNOSIS. Diagnosis of avian chlamydiosis can be difficult. Clinical signs can suggest the disease, but there are no pathognomonic features. Microscopic examination of impression smears or fixed sections of spleen, liver, or air sac tissue of birds that have died from the disease sometimes reveals elementary bodies, the infectious phase of *C. psittaci*. Special staining techniques are required, however, and the absence of visible elementary bodies does not rule out chlamydiosis. Serologic tests, such as latex agglutination and enzyme-linked immunosorbent assay (ELISA), can be used to diagnose the disease in live birds, but results may be negative if testing is performed in the early stages of the infection. It is also possible to isolate *C. psittaci* from swabs taken from the palatine cleft, cloaca, or fresh feces, although a single negative culture should not be considered definitive because of intermittent shedding of the organism. Specimens submitted for culture attempts should be placed into a chlamydial transport medium and refrigerated until processed.

Disease in Humans

SIGNS AND SYMPTOMS. The incubation period for avian chlamydiosis in humans is 1 to 4 weeks. Onset can be either sudden or gradual; symptoms include fever, chills, headache, muscle aches, and upper and lower respiratory tract illness. Elderly people, particularly if not treated, may develop severe disease. Complications can include encephalitis, myocarditis, hepatitis, arthritis, and thrombophlebitis. Most cases, however, are mild or moderate, with recovery in 7 to 10 days in patients receiving appropriate treatment; the case-fatality rate among such patients is less than 1%.

DIAGNOSIS. A history of exposure to birds is suggestive. Serologic tests are the means of diagnosis most frequently used, with a fourfold rise in titer between paired sera collected 2 to 3 weeks apart being considered confirmatory. The agent can be isolated from sputum or blood, but if antibiotics have been administered, the chances of recovery of the organism are reduced.

Technician Note

Avian practitioners and others who work with birds should be aware of the possibility of chlamydiosis and take appropriate precautions.

TREATMENT. Avian chlamydiosis responds to various antibiotics, with tetracycline or doxycycline usually being the drug of choice.

Prevention

The aim of the 30-day quarantine period for imported birds mandated by law in the United States is to detect birds infected with Newcastle disease virus and does not ensure that birds entering the country are free from chlamydiosis; likewise, many domestically reared birds may be carriers. Infected birds can appear healthy and still shed the organism, particularly when stressed by crowding, shipping, or other adverse conditions. Therefore avian practitioners and others who work with birds should be aware of the possibility of chlamydiosis and take appropriate precautions. Rapid diagnosis and an effective treatment program for birds can help reduce human exposure.

If a bird is suspected of having chlamydiosis, it should be isolated, and all personnel caring for it should wear face masks and protective clothing. Cage papers should be wetted with a quaternary ammonium disinfectant before cage cleaning to minimize aerosolization of infective particles. Laboratory coats and other protective clothing should be removed and hands washed after contact with an infected bird. There is no vaccine for either birds or humans.

Reporting and Surveillance

In the United States and many other countries, avian chlamydiosis in humans must be reported to local health authorities.

Brucellosis

Agent

Brucella spp. are small, gram-negative coccobacilli. Humans are susceptible to infection by *B. abortus, B. melitensis, B. suis,* and *B. canis.*

Technician Note

More than 500,000 cases of human brucellosis are estimated to occur annually, with most in developing countries and most occurring as a result of contaminated milk.

Reservoirs

B. abortus is primarily carried by cattle, bison, Asian buffaloes, and North American elk; sheep, goats, horses, and other domestic livestock can maintain the infection within herds. Domestic goats and sheep are the major carriers of *B. melitensis;* cattle, camels, and dogs also are susceptible to infection with this species. *B. suis* is carried by swine, but European hares, reindeer, caribou, and some rodents are hosts for certain strains of this species. Canine species, both domestic and wild, are reservoirs for *B. canis.*

Occurrence

With a worldwide incidence, more than 500,000 cases of human brucellosis are estimated to occur annually, with most in developing nations and most occurring from contaminated milk. Countries bordering the Mediterranean and in the Middle East, India, central Asia, Mexico, and Central and South America have the highest incidence.

Human brucellosis has decreased radically in industrialized countries in which active programs to eliminate animal disease have been undertaken. In these countries, brucellosis primarily is an occupational disease among people who work with animals. In the United States, fewer than 200 cases are reported each year. Farm workers, abattoir workers, and especially veterinarians and their technicians are at the greatest risk.

Transmission

Among most animals, transmission occurs primarily through consumption of feed or other material contaminated with infected birth fluids. Although the organisms do not multiply outside a host, brucellae may survive in the environment for several months under moist, cool conditions, thus providing a source of infection for susceptible animals that may ingest contaminated material. *B. suis* and *B. canis* can be sexually transmitted.

As an occupational disease, human brucellosis is most often contracted by farmers and veterinarians via direct contact with aborted fetuses, placentae, or vaginal fluids from infected animals. The organism enters though broken skin. Accidental self-inoculation with strain 19 bovine vaccine is responsible for a small number of cases annually. Aerosol transmission is another important route of infection and can occur in farm, abattoir, and laboratory settings.

Disease in Animals

SIGNS. Abortion is the major sign of brucellosis, regardless of which species of animal is infected or which of the brucellae is the infective agent. *B. abortus* also can cause reduced milk production among infected cows and orchitis, seminal vesiculitis, and ampullitis among bulls; fertility of both genders is often adversely affected. *B. suis* infections of swine cause similar clinical signs, and arthritis also may occur. In sheep and goats, *B. melitensis* causes mastitis, orchitis, arthritis, and spondylitis. *B. canis* infection in dogs is characterized by bacteremia, lymphadenitis, and splenitis, in addition to reproductive tract lesions similar to those exhibited by livestock.

DIAGNOSIS. Isolation of organisms from infective material, such as aborted fetuses and blood, is definitive, but brucellae are slow growing, and standard laboratory culture procedures may not always be effective. A variety of serologic tests are available.

Disease in Humans

SIGNS AND SYMPTOMS. Human brucellosis is highly variable in presentation, with patients often having many vague, nonspecific symptoms. Onset may be sudden or insidious, with symptoms appearing gradually over 1 week or longer.

Most human cases are caused by *B. abortus* or *B. melitensis*. In acute systemic brucellosis caused by *B. abortus*, patients often have fever, nausea, vomiting, and other gastrointestinal complaints. In undulant fever caused by *B. melitensis*, cycles of waxing and waning fever occur. Each cycle lasts a few weeks and is followed by a brief afebrile period before another cycle begins. In both forms of the disease, osteoarticular involvement occurs in up to 60% of patients, and complications involving the male reproductive tract, such as epididymitis and orchitis, occur in up to 20% of cases. Endocarditis is a rare but significant complication and accounts for most of the fatalities associated with brucellosis (2% or fewer).

Infection with *B. suis* can produce similar clinical signs and also may result in chronic liver or splenic abscesses. *B. canis* infections are similar to those of *B. abortus* but tend to cause less severe illness and fewer complications. Some patients relapse repeatedly with febrile episodes even after successful treatment; chronic arthritis is often seen in these individuals.

DIAGNOSIS. Definitive diagnosis is possible only when the organism is recovered from a clinical specimen. However, unless brucellosis is suspected and the laboratory is notified, routine culture procedures may not allow sufficient incubation time for the slow-growing bacteria to become detectable. Serologic tests are available, but false-negative results are possible in many of these, and conventional testing does not detect antibodies to *B. canis*. Deoxyribonucleic acid (DNA) probes and polymerase chain reaction (PCR) techniques are new developments, but their practical application for clinical diagnosis has yet to be determined.

TREATMENT. Brucellosis responds best to combinations of antibiotics; treatment regimens using only one drug are not as successful. Relapses occur in some cases because of sequestered organisms; these patients require re-treatment with the original combination of antibiotics.

Prevention

Control of human brucellosis depends on the control of brucellosis in livestock. Reservoir animals should be eliminated through testing and slaughter of infected livestock. Farmers, slaughterhouse workers, and others who come into contact with potentially infected animals should be aware of the possibility of brucellosis and should take precautions to reduce risk. Laboratory personnel working with *Brucella* spp. should be aware of the potential for aerosol spread of the organisms and handle cultures or potentially infected tissues only within biologic safety cabinets.

Reporting and Surveillance

In most states and countries, both animal and human brucellosis cases must be reported to local health or veterinary authorities.

Campylobacteriosis

Agent

Campylobacter spp. are small, curved, gram-negative bacilli. *C. jejuni* and *C. coli* are responsible for most human clinical cases.

Reservoirs

Campylobacter organisms are carried, often asymptomatically, in the intestinal tracts of many birds and mammals. Chickens and other commercial poultry are the main reservoirs for *C. jejuni*. Cattle and swine also carry *C. jejuni* and *C. coli*, and kittens and puppies, particularly if feral or obtained from animal shelters or other large-scale pet suppliers, often are infected with the organism.

Occurrence

Campylobacteriosis occurs worldwide in all age-groups and is probably the most common cause of food or waterborne diarrhea in the world. In the United States, incidence is estimated to be 1000 cases per 100,000 population, with an annual total exceeding 2 million cases; other industrialized nations report similar incidence rates. In developing nations, the rate of infection may be much higher.

In animals, the rate among some commercial poultry flocks approaches 100%. Up to 40% of diarrheic puppies and 10% of adult dogs with diarrhea are infected with *C. jejuni* or *coli*. The rates vary widely for other farm and companion animals.

Transmission

Although ingestion of organisms in uncooked or undercooked food is the most common means of acquiring the infection, fecal-oral transmission in a farm or veterinary environment is also an efficient means of spread. Direct contact with infected diarrheic companion or farm animals can result in human infection if the bacteria are transferred from hands to mouth. The infective dose is very small, so even a small inoculum introduced into the mouth may cause disease. In one study, it was estimated that 6.3% of cases had been acquired through exposure to diarrheic animals, mostly dogs.

Campylobacter organisms are somewhat fragile and subject to desiccation and chemical disinfection but can survive for hours or days at room temperature in feces or other moist material.

Disease in Animals

SIGNS. Many animals and birds are asymptomatic carriers, shedding the organism in feces. Puppies and kittens may develop acute enterocolitis with diarrhea, vomiting, and fever. Infection in foals, calves, lambs, and kids is characterized by fever, mucoid or hemorrhagic diarrhea, depression, and dehydration.

DIAGNOSIS. The causative organism is isolated from feces. Specimens should be collected on sterile swabs and placed in a transport medium, preferably Cary-Blair, until laboratory processing. Special culture techniques, including selective media and reduced oxygen tension, are required for in vitro cultivation. Incubation at 42° C enhances the likelihood of recovery of the organism from clinical samples.

Disease in Humans

SIGNS AND SYMPTOMS. Campylobacteriosis ranges from asymptomatic infection to severe illness. The main symptoms are acute enterocolitis, with bloody, mucoid diarrhea, abdominal pain, nausea, vomiting, and general malaise. Although most people recover without specific treatment within 2 to 5 days, adults may experience prolonged illness, and relapses are possible. Rarely, extraintestinal infections may occur, or sequelae such as reactive arthritis, meningitis, or Guillain-Barré syndrome may follow the initial enteric infection.

DIAGNOSIS. Isolation of *Campylobacter* spp. as the sole pathogen from fecal samples is presumptive; isolation from blood culture is confirmatory. The specialized culture techniques mentioned above in the section on diagnosis of animal disease also apply here.

TREATMENT. Treatment is not usually necessary; in most cases, campylobacteriosis is self-limiting, and supportive care is sufficient. For prolonged or severe cases or those complicated by extraintestinal infection, erythromycin is the drug of choice.

PREVENTION. Strict attention to personal hygiene when handling or working around diarrheic animals or poultry can help reduce the risk of occupationally acquired campylobacteriosis.

Reporting and Surveillance

Many states require reporting of human cases to local health authorities, as do some countries. Animal infections are not reportable.

Cat-Scratch Disease
(*Bartonella henselae* Infection)
Agent

Bartonella (formerly *Rochalimaea*) *henselae* causes cat-scratch disease. This organism is a small, slightly curved, gram-negative bacillus.

Reservoirs

Domestic cats are the reservoirs for cat-scratch disease.

Occurrence

Cat-scratch disease occurs worldwide. As a clinical entity, cat-scratch disease affects only humans. In the United States, about 22,000 cases are reported each year. It occurs most frequently from July through January and affects all age-groups. Seropositivity rates in cats in the United States range from less than 15% in cool, dry areas to over 90% in the warmer, humid parts of the country; overall seroprevalence approaches 30%.

Transmission

B. henselae infection is transmitted both cat-to-cat and cat-to-human by fleas that have fed on infected cats. Cats infected with *B. henselae* often have persistent bacteremia in high levels. When a flea feeds on an infected cat, viable bacteria are ingested and excreted in the flea feces. When these infective flea feces contact a break in the skin, either on an uninfected cat or a human, the bacteria can enter and cause infection. It appears that a cat with both *B.*

henselae bacteremia and fleas is necessary for a human to become infected with cat-scratch disease. A cat scratch is not a requirement for development of the disease; any break in the skin that becomes contaminated with infective flea feces can serve as the inoculation site for *B. henselae.*

Disease in Animals

SIGNS. Cats infected with *B. henselae* usually do not exhibit obvious clinical signs, although at least one strain of *B. henselae* that is pathogenic for cats has been identified. Cats and kittens experimentally infected with this strain developed fever and lymphadenopathy and were lethargic and anorectic. Bacteremia persisted after clinical signs had resolved. Some studies have indicated that bacteremia may last for many months to several years despite the presence of a strong antibody response.

DIAGNOSIS. An immunofluorescent antibody (IFA) test can be used to detect *B. henselae* antibodies in serum, but this test cannot establish whether a cat has active bacteremia. Isolation of the organism from blood is definitive, but specialized culture techniques must be employed and several weeks are required for colony growth. In addition, experimental studies have shown that *B. henselae* is isolated intermittently from infected cats when they are monitored over time. It is unknown whether this is attributable to sporadic shedding of the organism from some internal focus of infection or whether it reflects a limitation of the microbiologic procedures.

If culture is requested, blood should be collected aseptically in a 1.5-ml Wampole Isolator microbial tube (Wampole Laboratories), an evacuated tube containing agents that lyse erythrocytes and prevent coagulation. If this is not available, a tube containing ethylenediaminetetraacetic acid (EDTA), such as a lavender-top Vacutainer tube (Becton-Dickinson Co.), may be substituted. It should be noted, however, that unless the red blood cells are lysed, chances of recovery of the organism are greatly reduced.

TREATMENT. Antibiotic therapy is not indicated for cats infected with *B. henselae.* Not only do infected cats show few or no clinical signs, but also efforts to eliminate bacteremia by administration of antibiotics have met with little success.

Disease in Humans

SIGNS AND SYMPTOMS. Most cases of cat-scratch disease are asymptomatic or so mild as to be unrecognized. When clinical disease does develop, it usually presents as a regional lymphadenopathy 3 to 14 days after dermal inoculation of the infectious agent. Low-grade fever, myalgia, and general malaise often occur, and a papular lesion sometimes develops at the site of inoculation. Lymph nodes affected usually are those proximal to the inoculation site; often they are very painful but rarely suppurate. In more than 90% of patients, cat-scratch disease follows a mild course and resolves spontaneously, although symptoms can persist for up to 2 months. Complications are rare, and the case-fatality rate is almost nonexistent.

B. henselae infection may be much more serious in immunocompromised people, however. In these patients, cat-scratch disease may progress to septicemia or disseminated disease affecting multiple organ systems. Very rarely, the infection may manifest as bacillary angiomatosis or bacillary peliosis instead of cat-scratch disease. Bacillary angiomatosis is characterized by a vasoproliferative tissue reaction that produces violaceous or colorless nodular lesions on the skin and in internal organs. In bacillary peliosis, blood-filled cysts develop in the parenchyma of the liver, spleen, and other reticuloendothelial structures. Both conditions are potentially life threatening and usually occur only in HIV-infected individuals.

DIAGNOSIS.   Although many physicians still diagnose cat-scratch disease solely on the basis of clinical signs and a history of cat exposure, a sensitive and specific IFA test to detect antibodies against *B. henselae* is now available. A titer of ≥1:64 is considered positive, and most patients show elevated antibody levels in the weeks following onset of lymphadenopathy. The organism also can be isolated from lymph node aspirates and blood, but, as in the cat, culture requires too much time to be useful as a diagnostic test.

TREATMENT.   Antibiotic therapy generally is not indicated for cat-scratch disease; in the typical patient it does not shorten the course of the disease or lessen the discomfort of the lymphadenopathy. Surgical excision of affected lymph nodes is not recommended, but needle aspiration can be used to relieve pressure and pain in severe cases. For most patients, rest, analgesics, and heat applied to swollen lymph nodes are adequate treatment. Systemic *B. henselae* infection in an immunocompromised person, however, does require immediate and aggressive antibiotic therapy.

Prevention

Aggressive flea control is essential for preventing the transmission of *B. henselae* infection to both cats and humans. Common sense and careful attention to hygiene are also helpful. Wash hands after handling cats. Avoid cat bites and scratches, and thoroughly wash with soap and water any scratches that do occur. Likewise, prevent cats from licking or coming in contact with any break in the skin; keep wounds covered until healed. Immunocompromised people should avoid handling cats with fleas and any kittens with clinical signs that suggest active *B. henselae* infection.

Reporting and Surveillance

Cat-scratch disease is not a reportable disease in the United States.

Capnocytophaga Infection

Agent

Capnocytophaga canimorsus, formerly known as CDC group dysgonic fermenter-2 (DF-2), is a slow-growing, fastidious gram-negative rod.

Reservoirs

Dogs and cats are the reservoirs for *Capnocytophaga*.

Occurrence

Incidence is probably worldwide. Human infections with *C. canimorsus* have been reported from North America, Europe, Africa, Australia, and New Zealand. Most cases have occurred in the summer and fall, and all age-groups are affected. Although only a comparatively few (fewer than 100) cases have been reported since the disease was first recognized, this is more likely attributable to the difficulty in isolating the organism from clinical specimens (making diagnoses difficult to establish) than to the true rarity of the infection.

Transmission

Dog bites or scratches are most often associated with *C. canimorsus* infection; about 65% of cases are attributable to dog-inflicted trauma. Nonbite exposure to dogs, cat bites or scratches, and other animal exposures also have been linked to *C. canimorsus* infection. Even small, apparently inconsequential, dog bites have, in some cases, led to fatal disease.

Disease in Animals

SIGNS.   There are no signs in animals. *C. canimorsus* is a commensal in the oral cavity of dogs and cats and can be isolated from the saliva of healthy animals of both species. Surveys indicate up to 24% of dogs and 17% of cats may harbor the organism.

DIAGNOSIS.   *C. canimorsus* can be isolated from gingivae, saliva, and nasal fluids. Samples should be collected using sterile cotton-tipped swabs, which should be placed in a holding medium until processed.

Disease in Humans

SIGNS AND SYMPTOMS.   *C. canimorsus* infections can be asymptomatic or self-limiting, even in immunocompromised patients. In most known cases, however, a life-threatening illness has developed. Usually presenting initially as a nonspecific febrile illness, *C. canimorsus* infection frequently progresses to an overwhelming septicemia. Disseminated intravascular coagulation, renal failure, endocarditis, cellulitis, and gangrene may occur. In these cases, mortality exceeds 30%.

Technician Note

All dog bites, no matter how small, should be vigorously cleansed first with soap and water followed by a povidone-iodine solution and then by thorough irrigation with water.

Many patients have some underlying medical condition that predisposes them to infection; splenectomy is most commonly reported. Other conditions associated with increased risk include age over 50 years, alcohol abuse, steroid therapy, and chronic neoplastic, hematologic, or pulmonary disease. It should be noted, however, that several otherwise healthy young people have developed fatal infections with this organism.

DIAGNOSIS.   *C. canimorsus* isolated from blood, cerebrospinal fluid, or tissues is definitive, but depending on the culture medium used, mature colonies may not develop for 1 week or longer after inoculation. In bacteremic patients, a rapid, presumptive test is a Gram stain of a blood smear or buffy coat. The organism appears as elongated, filamentous, gram-negative rods within polymorphonuclear cells.

TREATMENT.   Penicillin is the usual drug of choice for this infection.

Prevention

Animal care workers should be aware of the possibility of severe or life-threatening infection with this organism. All dog bites, no matter how small, should be vigorously cleansed with first soap and water followed by a povidone-iodine solution and then by thorough irrigation with water. Likewise, an existing wound that becomes contaminated with dog saliva should be thoroughly washed. Medical evaluation should be sought; surgical debridement may be indicated. Immediate medical treatment should be sought if fever or signs of cellulitis develop after an animal bite. Delay in treatment is a risk factor for development of severe infection.

Penicillin G as prophylaxis after a dog bite often is recommended for persons with underlying conditions associated with an increased risk of *C. canimorsus* infection. Asplenic individuals probably should never handle dogs or cats.

Reporting and Surveillance

No formal reports are required.

Erysipelothrix Infection

Agent

Erysipelothrix rhusiopathiae is a thin, non–spore-forming, gram-positive rod.

Reservoirs

Domestic swine are the principal reservoirs; up to 30% of healthy animals may harbor *E. rhusiopathiae* in their tonsils and continually excrete the organism in feces.

Occurrence

Incidence of swine erysipelas is worldwide and high in parts of Europe, Asia, North and South America, and Australia. Morbidity and mortality are variable, but in some areas intensive vaccination programs are required to allow profitable swine production. Many species of wild and domestic fowl, especially turkeys, also are frequently infected. Fish and shellfish are not known to develop clinical disease, but *Erysipelothrix* frequently is present in their exterior slime.

In humans, *E. rhusiopathiae* infection is related to occupation. Persons most often affected include veterinarians and animal care workers, butchers and other meat handlers, fishermen, fish and shellfish handlers, and microbiology laboratory personnel.

Transmission

Pigs and turkeys become infected through contamination of wounds or oral exposure. The organism is resistant to many environmental influences, including direct sunlight. It can survive for long periods in feces, sewage, carcasses, and water. In humans, most cases occur after occupational exposure to the organism, usually via scratches, abrasions, or puncture wounds to the hands or fingers caused by knives, bone splinters, and fish hooks.

Disease in Animals

SIGNS. Swine erysipelas can be acute, subacute, or chronic. The acute form of the disease is septicemia that may cause sudden death. Subacute erysipelas occurs in animals that survive the initial phase of the disease; this is characterized by the appearance of raised, reddish purple rhomboidal lesions (diamond skin disease) that subsequently become necrotic. Chronic erysipelas may affect the joints, causing arthritis and general unthriftiness, or the heart, resulting in endocarditis and death.

Turkey erysipelas mainly affects adult male birds. In the acute, septic form, birds are depressed and somnolent, with prostration and death occurring soon after onset. Subacute erysipelas is characterized by weakness, diarrhea, and cyanosis and swelling of the snood and dewlap. As in swine, chronic infection may cause arthritis or endocarditis.

DIAGNOSIS. The organism can be isolated from skin lesions and from blood and internal organs of animals with septicemia.

Disease in Humans

SIGNS AND SYMPTOMS. *Erysipelothrix* infection in humans has manifestations similar to those in animals. In humans, however, the localized cutaneous infection known as *erysipeloid* (to distinguish it from the human erysipelas caused by *Streptococcus* spp.) is the most frequently seen form. Erysipeloid is a cellulitis that usually develops on the fingers and hands after dermal inoculation with the organism; a raised, purplish lesion appears at the site and is accompanied by severe pain and swelling. Although erysipeloid is a self-limiting infection and usually resolves without treatment in 3 to 4 weeks, lesions may recur and last much longer in second attacks.

Systemic *Erysipelothrix* infections are uncommon and only rarely follow erysipeloid. Most patients with systemic disease develop subacute endocarditis; generalized cutaneous infection and septicemia also can occur.

DIAGNOSIS. The organism can be isolated from biopsy specimens taken from the edge of erysipeloid lesions. In cases of endocarditis or septicemia, routine blood cultures will allow isolation of the agent.

> **Technician Note**
>
> The chances of contracting human erysipeloid infection by those occupationally exposed can be lessened by frequent hand washing with disinfectant soaps or detergents.

TREATMENT. *Erysipelothrix* is susceptible to a variety of antibiotics. Some endocarditis patients may require valve replacement.

Prevention

For swine, vaccines and bacterins are available but do not always provide lasting immunity. Good management practices, especially those involving cleanliness and sanitation, must be used as well in areas where erysipelas is endemic.

The chances of contracting human erysipeloid by those occupationally exposed can be lessened by frequent hand washing with disinfectant soaps or detergents and prompt, appropriate treatment of any wounds. No vaccine is available.

Reporting and Surveillance

Erysipelothrix infection, whether in animals or humans, is not reportable in the United States.

Pasteurellosis

Agent

Of the various species of *Pasteurella*, *P. multocida* is most commonly encountered. *P. multocida* is a small, pleomorphic, nonmotile, gram-negative coccobacillus.

Reservoirs

Reservoirs for *Pasteurella* are domestic animals, especially cats and dogs. *Pasteurella* spp., which can infect bite wounds, are found in the oropharynx of 92% and 99% of healthy dogs and cats, respectively.

Occurrence

Incidence is worldwide. Carriage of *P. multocida* is common in domestic and wild animals and birds and affects a wide variety of species. In humans, pasteurellosis occurs most frequently as a cellulitis after a cat or dog bite. Respiratory infections acquired from exposure to farm and other domestic animals also occur.

Transmission

Pasteurella organisms are inhabitants of the upper respiratory tract of a variety of animals. Infection can be transmitted by both bites and aerosol routes. Among poultry, aerosol transmission is the predominant means of spread of the disease. Many people with respiratory infections caused by *Pasteurella* spp. have been exposed to cattle, fowl, or their products. Cats and dogs also may be a source of airborne infection, particularly for immunocompromised people.

Disease in Animals

Signs. Pigs, rats, rabbits, suckling mice, goats, and calves develop atrophic rhinitis after infection with certain toxin-producing strains of *P. multocida*. In sheep and swine, the infection can produce pneumonia or septicemia; in rabbits it causes coryza (snuffles). In Southeast Asia and Africa, certain serovars of the organism cause hemorrhagic septicemia among cattle and water buffalo. Avian pasteurellosis (fowl cholera) is an acute septicemic disease that affects all species of domestic poultry and causes high mortality. Although dogs and cats harbor the organism in their mouths and nasopharynges with no ill effects, abscesses caused by *P. multocida* often develop after bite wounds.

Diagnosis. *Pasteurella* spp. can be cultured from the blood or internal organs of animals or birds with septicemia. The organism also can be isolated from tracheal or bronchial washings or other respiratory specimens from animals with pneumonia and from purulent drainage from wound abscesses. The gums and teeth of many healthy cats and dogs yield *P. multocida*.

Specimens for culture should be collected on sterile swabs and placed in transport media; tissues obtained at necropsy should be placed in sterile containers and kept refrigerated until processing by a microbiologic laboratory.

Disease in Humans

Signs and Symptoms. *P. multocida* is the major cause of soft tissue infections of the hand after animal bites or scratches. The lower leg and face, especially in children, also may be involved. Risk factors for developing bite-associated pasteurellosis include age over 50 years, the hand being the site bitten, and puncture wounds, such as those inflicted by cats, that cannot be thoroughly cleansed. Acute inflammation, pain, swelling, serosanguineous or purulent drainage from the site, and lymphangitis develop, usually within 12 to 24 hours of the bite. In rare cases, the infection may spread into tendons, bones, or joints. In immunocompromised individuals, septicemia, endocarditis, meningoencephalitis, or other life-threatening disseminated infection may occur. *P. multocida* also can cause various respiratory infections, such as pneumonia, bronchitis, sinusitis, or tonsillitis.

Diagnosis. The acute onset of cellulitis after a cat or dog bite, as described above, is highly suggestive of pasteurellosis. Culture of the organism from the wound is definitive.

Treatment. Initial treatment should focus on immediate and thorough cleansing (preferably with a povidone-iodine solution) and rinsing of the wound, followed by professional medical evaluation. Debridement and high-pressure irrigation of the wound should be performed by a physician. As with any domestic animal bite, the rabies immunization status of the animal involved should be determined, and the patient's tetanus immunizations should be updated.

Hospitalization may be necessary if extensive cellulitis develops and there is proximal swelling of the involved limb. Most patients recover completely after treatment with topical, oral, and/or parenteral antibiotics.

Prevention

Hygienic management practices can help control pasteurellosis in animals. Bacterins and vaccines are available for some species.

Bite prevention is the single most important measure for humans. If a bite has already occurred, the major factors in development of bite-associated pasteurellosis are inadequate initial wound care and delay in seeking medical treatment. Debridement and irrigation of the wound are particularly important in preventing cellulitis. No vaccine is available for humans.

Reporting and Surveillance

Pasteurellosis is not a reportable disease in the United States.

Q Fever (Coxiellosis)

Agent

Coxiella burnetii is a small, obligately intracellular, gram-negative bacterium. Although in the past it was classified as a member of the Rickettsias, more recent studies have shown that *C. burnetii* is not closely related to other members of that group and therefore should not be considered a rickettsial organism.

Reservoirs

Cattle, sheep, and goats are the primary reservoirs; many other mammals, including companion animals and rodents, also may carry *C. burnetii*, as can birds, ticks, mites, and some insects.

Occurrence

Incidence is worldwide except New Zealand. All mammals and humans are susceptible to infection with *C. burnetii*; seroprevalence varies widely with geographic area. Humans at risk include ranchers, dairy farmers, abattoir and packing plant employees, veterinarians and animal care workers, and medical laboratory researchers who work with the organism.

Technician Note

The primary means of transmission of Q fever is inhalation of either aerosols from infected birth fluids and ruminant placentae or dust contaminated by birth fluids or urine.

Transmission

The primary means of transmission of Q fever is inhalation of either aerosols from infected birth fluids and ruminant placentae, which can contain up to 10^9 organisms per gram of tissue or dust contaminated by birth fluids or urine. The agent also may be present in high concentrations in wool or hides or in soil in areas in which livestock are kept. *C. burnetii* is resistant to high temperatures, sunlight, and many disinfectants. Cattle and other milk-producing animals that develop chronic infection in their mammary glands continually shed the organism in milk; thus consumption of unpasteurized milk from infected animals can lead to human infection.

Although farm animals are the most common sources of Q fever, household pets such as cats, dogs, and rabbits may also transmit the disease. Exposure to newborn or stillborn pet animals has been linked to Q fever among urban residents. *C. burnetii* is easily transmitted in a laboratory setting, with minimal exposures often resulting in disease.

Disease in Animals

SIGNS.   Most species have only asymptomatic infection, although coxiellosis in cattle, sheep, and goats sometimes causes abortion.

DIAGNOSIS.   Various serologic tests are used to diagnose coxiellosis in animals.

Disease in Humans

SIGNS AND SYMPTOMS.   Q fever usually manifests as an acute febrile disease, often with sudden onset of fever, chills, profuse sweating, intense retroorbital pain, and malaise 2 to 6 weeks after exposure. A maculopapular rash is common. Some patients develop atypical pneumonia and a mild cough; others may experience severe respiratory distress. Infections that occur during pregnancy may cause spontaneous abortion. Complications of acute infection may include meningoencephalitis and cardiac involvement. Most cases are mild and self-limiting; the case-fatality rate for untreated Q fever patients is less than 1% to 2.5%.

A few patients develop chronic infection, which gradually becomes apparent years after the initial illness and usually manifests as endocarditis. This form of Q fever occurs primarily in patients with a history of heart valve disease or other immunosuppressive conditions. Patients with this form of Q fever may develop hepatomegaly, splenomegaly, renal insufficiency, or stroke; progressive heart failure is common. Because of its insidious onset long after the primary episode of disease, medical care may not be sought until late in the course of the illness. Q fever endocarditis has a case-fatality rate of more than 60%.

DIAGNOSIS.   Diagnosis of Q fever is easy if a physician suspects the disease; serologic testing is effective in diagnosing both acute and chronic infection. Because the clinical picture of acute Q fever can mimic so many other infectious diseases, however, the illness may not be considered among differential diagnoses in areas in which Q fever does not often occur. A history of exposure to a reservoir is an important epidemiologic clue. Likewise, chronic Q fever has few obvious signs but should be suspected in a patient with valvular heart disease and an unexplained infectious or inflammatory process.

TREATMENT.   Antibiotics such as tetracycline or doxycycline are usually prescribed for both acute and chronic Q fever. The course of treatment for patients with acute disease is usually 15 to 21 days, whereas 3 or more years of antibiotic therapy may be required for cases of Q fever endocarditis.

Prevention

Avoid contact with possibly infected animals. A vaccine is available for people who work with reservoir animals.

Reporting and Surveillance

Q fever must be reported to local health authorities in the parts of the United States in which the disease is endemic. In many other countries, it is not a reportable disease.

Rat-Bite Fevers: Streptobacillosis and Spirillosis

Agents

Streptobacillus moniliformis is a pleomorphic, fastidious, gram-negative rod that causes streptobacillosis or streptobacillary fever. Spirillosis is caused by a spiral bacterium designated *Spirillum minus*, although it probably does not belong to that genus. Because *S. minus* cannot be cultured on artificial media, its true taxonomic position has not yet been determined.

Reservoirs

Primarily rats are carriers; mice, hamsters, gerbils, guinea pigs, squirrels, and other rodents may be occasional carriers. *S. moniliformis* is part of the normal oral and upper respiratory tract flora of both wild and domestic rats and is excreted in urine. *S. minus* is found on the teeth and in the blood and conjunctival secretions of rats and other rodents. This organism has been identified in up to 48% of rats, both wild and laboratory strains, and laboratory mice.

Occurrence

Both rat-bite fevers occur sporadically worldwide, mostly in poor urban areas and among laboratory or animal care personnel who handle rodents. Spirillosis is the more common rat-bite fever in Asia, particularly Japan, where it is known as *sodoku*.

Transmission

Rat bites are the most common means of transmission of both diseases. A form of streptobacillosis known as Haverhill fever is caused by ingestion of rodent-contaminated food or water.

Disease in Animals

SIGNS.   *S. moniliformis* generally does not cause disease in rats. However, mice, especially certain inbred laboratory strains, may be genetically more susceptible to infection. Epidemics of streptobacillosis have occurred among research colonies, causing polyarthritis and gangrene. Mortality and morbidity are high in these episodes. Streptobacillosis also may occur in turkeys that are bitten by rats. Clinical signs include purulent polyarthritis, foot-pad lesions, and sternal bursitis.

S. minus is not known to cause clinical disease in animals.

DIAGNOSIS.   *S. moniliformis* theoretically can be isolated from joint fluid or lesions of affected turkeys. Definitive diagnosis is difficult, however, because the organism has unusual growth requirements that routine microbiologic procedures may not provide.

Disease in Humans

SIGNS AND SYMPTOMS.   Streptobacillosis, or streptobacillary fever, usually develops within 10 days of a rat bite that has healed normally. The disease is characterized by sudden onset of headache, vomiting, malaise, fever, and chills, followed by a transient maculopapular or petechial rash that appears on the extremities. Severe pain and swelling develop in one or more joints. In untreated cases, complications can include endocarditis, myocarditis, meningitis, abscesses in various soft tissues or the brain, hepatitis, nephritis, and pneumonia; the case-fatality rate for untreated cases is about 13%. The clinical picture of Haverhill fever is similar, although there may be more gastrointestinal and upper respiratory signs.

Spirillosis often has a longer incubation period, with the

onset of symptoms 1 to 3 weeks or longer after exposure. The wound site heals during the incubation period but later becomes swollen, painful, and discolored and develops an indurated, encrusted ulcer. A cycle of relapsing fever begins, with episodes of elevated temperature that last 1 or 2 days and recur at 3- to 9-day intervals. An exanthematous or purplish rash appears, usually on the trunk, and may spread to other areas, especially joints. Muscle aches often occur. Some patients develop various neurologic symptoms, such as headache, nervousness, neuralgia, and weakness. Spirillosis can be complicated by meningoencephalitis, pneumonia, endocarditis, myocarditis, conjunctivitis, septic arthritis, and other lesions. About 10% of untreated cases are fatal, and fatalities have occurred despite antibiotic therapy.

Technician Note
Avoiding rat bites is the most effective means of prevention of either disease.

DIAGNOSIS. Streptobacillosis can be diagnosed on the basis of isolation of the etiologic agent from blood; as noted above, specialized media and processing are required.

Spirillosis is confirmed by microscopy. Either dark-field examinations or Wright's or Giemsa stains may be used to detect spiral organisms in wound exudates, lymph node aspirates, or, rarely, blood. Specimens also can be inoculated into guinea pigs or mice; spirilla can be microscopically detected in the peritoneal fluid and blood of these animals.

Both rat-bite fevers probably are underdiagnosed because the techniques required for identification of the etiologic agents are not among those usually performed in a standard clinical laboratory. Unless a physician suspects streptobacillosis or spirillosis and indicates this suspicion to the laboratory, ordinary microbiologic techniques and media may not be sufficient to identify either organism from clinical specimens.

TREATMENT. Both forms of rat-bite fever respond to antibiotic therapy.

Prevention
Avoiding rat bites is the most effective means of prevention of either disease. As with any animal bite, any wounds should be immediately and thoroughly cleansed, and medical advice should be sought.

Reporting and Surveillance
When streptobacillosis occurs epidemically in the United States, as in a food-borne or waterborne outbreak of Haverhill fever, it must be reported to health authorities. Single bite-associated cases are not reportable.

Salmonellosis
Agent
There are various serotypes of *Salmonella enteritidis*, a gram-negative rod of the family Enterobacteriaceae. These serotypes often are named for the place at which they were first isolated and are commonly referred to by genus and serotype name, such as *Salmonella arizonae*, instead of the more proper *S. enteritidis* subspecies *arizonae*. (Typhoid fever, caused by *Salmonella typhi*, has no

zoonotic occupational component and is not included in this discussion.)

Reservoirs
Salmonellae can infect a wide variety of warm- and cold-blooded animals, both domestic and wild. Reptiles, such as turtles, iguanas, and snakes, are particularly likely to be asymptomatic carriers of *Salmonella* spp.

Occurrence
Incidence is worldwide and common in both animals and humans. Human salmonellosis is mostly a food-borne or waterborne disease and a major cause of gastrointestinal illness and diarrhea. Incidence is highest among infants and young children; immunocompromised persons also are at increased risk. Occupational exposure to reptiles and other infected animals is a risk factor for veterinarians, animal care workers, zoo keepers, and pet shop employees.

Transmission
Consumption of contaminated food, particularly foods of animal origin such as poultry meat, eggs, and milk, is most often implicated in the transmission of salmonellosis. As an occupational disease, salmonellosis is transmitted via the fecal-oral route. Direct contact with infected animals, regardless of whether they show clinical signs of illness, can result in human infection if the bacteria are transferred from contaminated hands to mouth. In addition, indirect contact may be a source of infection; cages and food dishes used by infected animals may be contaminated with the bacteria, which can remain viable for months in dried feces.

Technician Note
Consumption of contaminated food, particularly foods of animal origin such as poultry meat, eggs, and milk, is most often implicated in the transmission of salmonellosis.

Disease in Animals
SIGNS. Infections may be clinical, subclinical, or inapparent. In clinically affected animals, regardless of species, most exhibit weakness, recumbency, fever, and diarrhea. Young animals are more likely to show clinical signs than are adults. Chronic carrier states are common in reptiles, birds, and other animals; in some reptiles, fecal carriage rates exceed 90%.

DIAGNOSIS. For clinically affected animals, isolation of the organism from blood or, at necropsy, from internal organs such as liver or spleen provides a definitive diagnosis. Carrier states can be detected by culturing *Salmonella* spp. from rectal or cloacal swabs or fecal samples.

Disease in Humans
SIGNS AND SYMPTOMS. Human salmonellosis usually manifests as an acute enterocolitis with sudden onset 12 to 36 hours after ingestion of the bacterium. Headache, abdominal pain, diarrhea, and nausea are common symptoms, and fever usually is present. Most cases are self-limiting and resolve in a few days. Salmonellosis is rarely fatal except in very young children, elderly persons, and debilitated or otherwise immunocompromised people. In these groups, there is an increased risk of severe

complications such as meningitis or septicemia. Asymptomatic infections can occur.

DIAGNOSIS.   Salmonellosis can be diagnosed in patients with enterocolitis by isolating the agent from fecal specimens; in most cases, fecal excretion persists for several days or weeks after symptoms have resolved. For patients with septicemia, *Salmonella* spp. can be cultured from blood as well as feces.

Isolates can be sent to reference laboratories for serotyping; knowledge of the causative serotype can provide an indication of the source of infection. For example, certain exotic serotypes are rarely isolated from animals other than reptiles. When the same unusual serotype is isolated from both the patient and a suspect reptile, it can be assumed that the reptile was the source of the person's illness.

 Technician Note

Working with reptiles is a specific risk factor for acquiring animal-borne salmonellosis.

TREATMENT.   Antimicrobial treatment is indicated only for those patients with severe or disseminated infections; chloramphenicol or fluoroquinolones are among the drugs of choice. Uncomplicated cases of gastrointestinal salmonellosis generally should not be treated with antibiotics because there seldom is any effect on the course of the disease and because their use can prolong fecal shedding of the organism.

Prevention

Working with reptiles is a specific risk factor for acquiring animal-borne salmonellosis because touching these animals or their surroundings can result in hands becoming contaminated with *Salmonella* spp. Wild fowl also frequently carry *Salmonella* spp., and diarrheic companion animals and livestock can also be sources of infection. Careful attention to personal hygiene, especially the use of gloves and frequent hand washing, can help reduce the risk of occupationally acquired salmonellosis.

Veterinarians and technicians should advise their clients who own reptiles, baby chicks, or ducklings that these animals increase the owners' risk of acquiring *Salmonella* infection and should stress the need for thorough hand washing after handling these animals or their cages. In addition, these pets should be kept out of food preparation areas. Kitchen sinks should never be used to bathe reptiles or to wash their dishes, cages, or aquariums. Likewise, sinks or tubs in which infants and children are bathed should never be used for such purposes. The U.S. Centers for Disease Control and Prevention recommend that people at increased risk for infection or serious complications of salmonellosis, including pregnant women, children under 5 years of age, and immunocompromised individuals, avoid all contact with reptiles. Reptiles may be inappropriate pets for households with young children because some cases have been reported in which there was no known contact, direct or indirect, between the child and the reptile.

Reporting and Surveillance

In the United States, confirmed cases of human salmonellosis must be reported to local health authorities.

MYCOTIC ZOONOSES

Systemic Infections: Cryptococcosis

Agent

Cryptococcus neoformans is an encapsulated yeast.

Reservoirs

Although a common saprophytic organism that can be isolated from many different environmental sources such as soil and plant materials, *C. neoformans* has a particular affinity for bird excrement, especially pigeon droppings. Sites contaminated with pigeon or chicken excreta often contain much higher concentrations of *C. neoformans* than do surrounding areas; it is thought that creatinine in the droppings enhances growth of the yeast. Viable cryptococci have been recovered from an aviary that had been unused for 10 years.

Occurrence

Incidence is worldwide and in all age-groups as sporadic cases, although adult males account for a majority of patients. Although many people have serologic evidence of exposure, clinical cases are relatively rare and usually occur in immunocompromised individuals. In the United States, 5% to 15% of patients with AIDS develop cryptococcosis; in this group, the infection is often life threatening.

Transmission

Transmission is by inhalation of the organism from environmental sources. Exposure to highly contaminated areas, such as aviaries or pigeon coops, can increase risk of disease.

 Technician Note

Exposure to highly contaminated areas such as aviaries or pigeon coops can increase the risk of cryptococcosis.

Disease in Animals

SIGNS.   There are no apparent signs in birds, although the organism can be recovered from the feces of many avian species. Most clinically affected mammals develop a disseminated infection that includes central nervous system signs; mortality is high. In cattle, the disease often manifests as mastitis and causes abnormalities of the udder and changes in milk.

DIAGNOSIS.   *Cryptococcus* can be detected through direct microscopic examination of various clinical specimens using an India ink preparation to reveal characteristic budding yeast cells. Culture and serologic testing can be used to confirm diagnoses.

Disease in Humans

SIGNS AND SYMPTOMS.   Most immunocompetent individuals develop only subclinical infection. Among patients with AIDS, meningitis is the most common presentation of cryptococcosis. It results from hematogenous dissemination of a primary pulmonary infection that can precede nervous system involvement by months or years. Pulmonary cryptococcosis is characterized by fever, chest pain, and coughing, with expectoration of blood-tinged sputum. When the infection spreads to the brain, headache, neck stiffness, and distorted vision occur. Confusion and other personality changes may follow. Even when treated aggressively, cryptococcal meningitis has a high mortality rate, and survivors often undergo relapses.

DIAGNOSIS. As described above, direct microscopic examination of India ink–stained cerebrospinal fluid, urine, or pus can reveal cells characteristic of *C. neoformans*. Serologic tests, culture, or histopathologic examination provides confirmation.

TREATMENT. Combinations of antifungal agents are used to treat human cryptococcosis.

Prevention

For normally healthy people, no special precautions are necessary. People with immunosuppressive conditions, such as HIV infection, diabetes, or Hodgkin's disease, or who are undergoing corticosteroid therapy should avoid exposure to accumulations of pigeon or other bird droppings. Contaminated sites may be disinfected with a 5% sodium hypochlorite solution.

Reporting and Surveillance

In the United States, cases should be reported to local health authorities. Because meningeal cryptococcosis is so strongly associated with AIDS, official reports are required in some areas.

Superficial Mycoses: Dermatophytoses

Agents

Dermatophytoses, or tinea, are opportunistic fungal infections of the hair, skin, or nails. *Microsporum canis*, *Trichophyton mentagrophytes*, and *T. verrucosum* are the zoophilic dermatophytes most important in human infection. *M. canis* causes tinea (ringworm) in both humans and animals; in humans, this species usually affects the scalp or body (tinea capitis or tinea corporis). *T. mentagrophytes* infection in humans may appear as tinea barbae (ringworm of the beard) or tinea corporis; *T. verrucosum* usually affects the face or upper body.

Reservoirs

M. canis is carried by dogs and cats. Wild mice and rats are primary reservoirs of *T. mentagrophytes*, but dogs, cats, horses, sheep, rabbits, guinea pigs, and other domestic and laboratory animals frequently are infected. *T. verrucosum* is carried by cattle, sheep, and other ruminants.

Occurrence

Incidence is worldwide in both humans and a variety of domestic and wild animals. People at greatest risk are those who work with animals or who live or work in areas that may be contaminated with hairs from infected animals.

Transmission

Transmission is by direct or indirect contact with infected animals or with hair from infected animals or humans.

Disease in Animals

SIGNS. For *M. canis*, about 90% of infected cats have no visible lesions; when present, lesions are usually on the face and paws and appear as 1- to 2-cm, hairless, scaly patches. Infected dogs usually have lesions similar to those in cats; they can appear on any part of the body. For *T. mentagrophytes*, most infected animals develop 1- to 2-cm, hairless, white, scaly lesions on the head or trunk. For *T. verrucosum*, young cattle are most frequently infected. Lesions can be small or extensive and begin as grayish white, scaly patches with hair loss. The skin later thickens and becomes scabby.

DIAGNOSIS. Examined microscopically in a wet mount of potassium hydroxide and ink, infected hairs from the inner edge of lesions of both *M. canis* and *Trichophyton* spp. may show an exterior cuff of arthrospores or mycelial elements within the hair shaft. Hairs infected with *M. canis* (but not *Trichophyton* spp.) also may fluoresce bright yellow-green when viewed under a Wood's lamp (365-nm filtered ultraviolet light), although this does not occur in all cases. Isolation of the organism from lesions is definitive. Scrapings or hairs from suspect lesions should be placed in a sterile container and submitted to a laboratory for culture.

Disease in Humans

SIGNS AND SYMPTOMS. For *M. canis*, tinea of the scalp produces scaly patches and temporary baldness because infected hairs are brittle and break easily. Infection of hairless parts of the body often causes formation of a *kerion*, a suppurative, boggy, raised lesion. For *T. mentagrophytes*, lesions are similar to those described for *M. canis* and usually occur on the face or upper body. Some individuals experience a highly inflammatory reaction to this infection. For *T. verrucosum*, lesions usually develop on the face, hands, arms, and upper body. The inflammatory response is severe, and kerions often form; scarring is a frequent result.

DIAGNOSIS. Diagnosis of dermatophytoses in humans is the same as in animals.

Technician Note

Both oral and topical antifungal agents, often in combination, are used to treat tinea infections in both humans and domestic animals.

TREATMENT. Both oral and topical antifungal agents, often in combination, are used to treat tinea infections in both humans and domestic animals. If kerions are present, a keriolytic cream may be prescribed. Antibiotics may be required if a secondary bacterial infection invades the lesions. Additional measures for tinea corporis include frequent and thorough bathing with soap and water and removal of scabs and crusts; for tinea capitis or barbae, daily washing of hair and scalp with a selenium sulfide shampoo is helpful.

Prevention

Vaccines to immunize animal populations against zoophilic dermatophytoses have been developed. If the infections can be controlled in animals, prevention of human infection will become much more feasible. Whenever possible, avoid direct contact with animals that show lesions suggestive of dermatophytoses.

Reporting and Surveillance

In the United States, reporting is required for epidemic outbreaks of any dermatophytosis but not for individual cases.

PARASITIC DISEASES

Cryptosporidiosis

Agent
Cryptosporidium parvum is a coccidian protozoan parasite.

Reservoirs
Reservoirs for *Cryptosporidium parvum* are humans, cattle, and other domestic animals.

Occurrence
Incidence is worldwide. In the United States and Europe, prevalence ranges from less than 1% to 4.5%; in developing nations, prevalence may be as high as 20% of the human population. People who come in contact with animals are at increased risk of contracting this infection.

Transmission
Transmission is fecal-oral, which includes human-to-human, animal-to-human, waterborne, and food-borne transmission. On reaching the intestine, the parasite infects epithelial cells and multiplies asexually via schizogony. After a sexual reproductive cycle, the organism produces infective oocysts that are passed in feces. These oocysts are resistant to many chemical disinfectants, including chlorination used in water treatment systems, and can survive in adverse environmental conditions.

Disease in Animals
SIGNS.   Cryptosporidiosis in animals often is subclinical, particularly in adults; younger animals, especially newborns, are more likely to develop clinical signs. Those affected usually develop diarrhea that can range from mild to severe. Calves are an important source of infection to humans and other animals because they develop profuse diarrhea, during which they shed massive quantities of oocysts into the environment. The mortality in livestock is low. Other animals that may develop clinical cryptosporidiosis are cats with underlying feline leukemia or feline immunodeficiency virus (FIV) infection or animals undergoing prolonged therapy with corticosteroid drugs.

DIAGNOSIS.   Oocysts can be detected in feces by direct microscopy of smears, sugar or zinc sulfate flotation, or special centrifugation techniques.

Disease in Humans
SIGNS AND SYMPTOMS.   Clinical cryptosporidiosis is characterized by profuse, watery diarrhea and cramping abdominal pain. Although symptoms may abate and recur for a time, in most otherwise healthy persons, the disease is self-limiting and resolves completely within 1 month. In immunocompromised individuals, however, the disease can be much more serious. Patients with AIDS and others who cannot clear the infection experience a severe and prolonged illness that can be fatal.

DIAGNOSIS.   Cryptosporidiosis can be difficult to diagnose unless suspected and sought. Direct identification of oocysts in fecal smears as detailed above can be successful. Likewise, various life-cycle stages can be detected by histopathologic examination of intestinal biopsy specimens, but *C. parvum* is very small and easily overlooked and can be mistaken for yeast cells if the proper stains are not used. An enzyme-linked immunosorbent assay (ELISA) and an immunofluorescence test have become available and are more accurate than direct microscopy.

TREATMENT.   There is no specific effective treatment. Supportive care, mainly in the form of rehydration, is effective for normally healthy people. Any immunosuppressive drugs the patient may be taking should be reduced or stopped if possible.

Prevention
People who are in contact with calves or other animals that have diarrhea should be especially careful about hand washing. Those with AIDS or other immunosuppressive conditions should avoid contact with diarrheic animals.

In areas in which water treatment facilities include filtration (which is standard for most cities in the United States), feces from infected animals can be discharged directly into sewers without prior disinfection. Areas contaminated with feces can be disinfected with a 10% formalin solution or 5% ammonia solution. Articles that withstand heat may be heated to 45° C for 5 to 20 minutes or to 60° C for 2 minutes.

Reporting and Surveillance
In the United States, cases of human cryptosporidiosis must be reported to local health authorities. Clusters of disease should be investigated epidemiologically to determine the source of infection.

Toxoplasmosis

> **Technician Note**
> The cat is the only known host of *Toxoplasma gondii*.

Agent
Toxoplasma gondii is an obligate intracellular sporozoan parasite.

Reservoirs
Cats are the only known definitive host (the animal in which the parasite completes its life cycle). Sheep, goats, swine, cattle, and chickens are intermediate hosts and can carry the infective stage encysted in muscle tissue.

Occurrence
Incidence is worldwide. Up to 70% of the human adult population is seropositive, indicating exposure and probable tissue infection. Cats frequently are infected; in some countries, up to 60% of cats have serologic evidence of exposure to the organism. The prevalence in livestock is related to the number of cats in pasture lands. Up to 43% of pigs and 35% of sheep have tissue cysts.

Transmission
After primary infection, cats shed oocysts in feces for only 1 to 2 weeks; subsequent intermittent shedding may occur, but this appears to be rare. *Toxoplasma* oocysts become infective 1 to 5 days after being passed; these are environmentally resistant and can survive for at least 1 year in soil in warm, humid environments. Other animals become infected when they consume soil or other material contaminated with sporulated oocysts.

In humans, toxoplasmosis may be primary or congenital. Primary toxoplasmosis is usually acquired through the ingestion of raw or undercooked meat, especially pork or mutton, in which the parasite has encysted. The mode that is of occupational importance, however, is the fecal-oral route (accidental ingestion of infective oocysts).

Congenital toxoplasmosis is acquired through transplacental infection. This occurs when a woman develops a primary infection during pregnancy; rapidly dividing tachyzoites circulate in the bloodstream and can infect the fetus. The risk of serious fetal disease is highest during the first and second trimesters.

Disease in Animals

SIGNS.   In most animals, toxoplasmosis produces only subclinical infection, with little morbidity or mortality. Toxoplasmosis in sheep, however, is an exception. In this species, the infection causes abortion or congenital disease that results in neonatal mortality; adults seldom are affected clinically. In some parts of the sheep-rearing world, economic losses from toxoplasmosis are significant. Swine are affected similarly, but the disease is not of economic importance in most areas. Outbreaks in cattle have been reported in which fever, dyspnea, and neurologic signs occur. Infection in horses is usually subclinical.

Most infected cats are asymptomatic, but kittens may develop diarrhea, hepatitis, pneumonia, encephalitis, and other signs. Dogs often are seropositive, but overt disease occurs mainly in puppies weakened by other conditions.

DIAGNOSIS.   Antemortem diagnosis is difficult. Oocysts can be detected in feline feces using various flotation techniques, although definitive identification requires considerable further laboratory testing (see Chapter 7). Serologic tests are available for many species but cannot be used to differentiate among active, recent, or past infections.

Disease in Humans

SIGNS AND SYMPTOMS.   Immunocompetent adults usually have only asymptomatic infection, although toxoplasmosis occasionally causes a self-limiting, mononucleosis-like illness. After the immune response causes the initial parasitemia to wane, *T. gondii* encysts in muscle tissue; these cysts can reactivate and cause disease if the person becomes immunocompromised at some later time.

Cerebral toxoplasmosis is a common opportunistic infection among patients with AIDS, with most cases resulting from activation of latent tissue infection as the immune system deteriorates. These patients often develop subacute meningoencephalitis, diffuse encephalopathy, or a space-occupying lesion in the brain. Lymphatics, lungs, heart, joints, or eyes also may be involved. Up to 40% of patients with AIDS develop cerebral toxoplasmosis, and at least 10% die. Other immunocompromised adults (chemotherapy patients, organ transplant recipients, people who have had a splenectomy) also are at increased risk of this form of toxoplasmosis.

Congenital toxoplasmosis results from primary maternal infection during gestation. When primary toxoplasmosis occurs during the first trimester of pregnancy, 17% of fetuses become infected, and 80% of those infections are severe. For second-trimester maternal infections, 25% of fetuses become infected, and 30% of that number have severe disease; abortion or premature birth often results. Infections acquired during the third trimester produce a higher fetal infection rate but fewer cases of severe disease. Neonatal central nervous system and ocular infections are the most frequent manifestations of congenital toxoplasmosis. Some babies develop encephalitis, hydrocephalus, or chorioretinitis; blindness, mental retardation, and seizures are possible sequelae.

DIAGNOSIS.   Diagnosis is based on clinical signs and results of serologic testing that support the presumption of toxoplasmosis. The organism also can be isolated from biopsy specimens or body fluids after intraperitoneal inoculation in mice; tachyzoites can be detected in mouse peritoneal fluid after 1 week, and cysts may be found in the brain after 6 weeks.

TREATMENT.   No specific treatment is indicated for otherwise healthy people, except for pregnant women with primary infections. In these patients, spiramycin is used to prevent fetal infection; if tests indicate fetal infection has already occurred, a combination of pyrimethamine and sulfadiazine can be used. Likewise, patients with severe symptomatic disease and infants born to mothers who had a primary infection during pregnancy are treated with a combination of antitoxoplasmal drugs and folic acid.

Prevention

Pet cats are seldom the source of human infection because of their fastidious nature. They bury their feces and clean themselves immediately, so feces do not remain on their fur long enough for oocysts to sporulate. In addition, oocyst shedding generally lasts only 1 or 2 weeks after the initial infection, and repeated exposure to the organism does not cause additional shedding. Oocysts can sporulate in litter boxes, so fecal material should be removed daily and disposed of in a toilet or by incineration. Wash hands thoroughly after handling litter boxes or cat feces.

Pregnant women and immunocompromised patients who work with animals should have serologic testing performed to determine whether they have a titer against toxoplasmosis. Those who are seronegative are at risk of developing primary toxoplasmosis and should avoid handling cat feces and changing litter boxes. Because most cases of toxoplasmosis are caused by consuming undercooked meat, those who are at risk also should avoid eating undercooked meat and handling raw meat, which are much more likely sources of infection than cat exposure.

Technician Note

Wash hands thoroughly after handling litter boxes or cat feces.

Cats should not be fed meat that may contain viable oocysts. Feed only commercial cat foods or thoroughly cook or freeze any meat that is to be fed to cats. (Freezing at −15° C for more than 3 days or −20° C for more than 2 days kills oocysts.) Because rodents and birds can be sources of infection, cats should be kept indoors when possible to prevent hunting.

Reporting and Surveillance

Reporting is not required in most areas, but it is in some states and countries in which epidemiologic studies are being conducted.

VIRAL DISEASES

Contagious Ecthyma (Orf)

Agent

Contagious ecthyma is caused by a DNA virus of the genus *Parapoxvirus*, family Poxviridae.

Reservoirs

Reservoirs are domestic and wild ungulates, including sheep, goats, domestic camels, deer, reindeer, and musk oxen. The virus is hardy and can persist for long periods in the environment and on the skin and hair of animals.

Occurrence

Incidence is uncommon but worldwide wherever sheep and goats are raised; many human cases occur in New Zealand. Contagious ecthyma (orf) is an occupational disease of sheep handlers, veterinarians, and abattoir workers.

Transmission

Humans contract orf through direct contact with lesions or mucous membranes of infected animals. In addition, contaminated knives, shears, or other objects can transfer the virus from animal to human. Preparation and administration of the crude live vaccine used in some endemic areas can also be a source of human infection.

Disease in Animals

SIGNS.   Most infections occur in young animals. Papules that progress into vesicles and pustules appear on the skin, eyelids, ears, lips, and nostrils. As lesions become confluent, they cause severe pain and often interfere with feeding. Females that nurse infected young may develop infection of teats and udders. Morbidity is often high, but mortality is low, usually resulting from secondary bacterial infection or infestation by fly larvae.

DIAGNOSIS.   Clinical signs alone often are sufficient to establish diagnosis; other diseases that produce similar lesions tend to have a different course.

Disease in Humans

SIGNS AND SYMPTOMS.   The most frequent presentation is the development of a single maculopapular or pustular lesion at the site of entry of the virus, usually on the hands, arms, or face. The papule is painful and progresses to become a firm, weeping nodule; secondary bacterial infection may cause pus formation. Most cases resolve completely in 2 to 4 weeks, but occasionally the infection is more serious. Reported complications include a widespread cutaneous eruption, ocular involvement with severe damage, and disseminated systemic disease.

DIAGNOSIS.   Demonstration of virus particles via electron microscopy of affected tissue and isolation of the virus in cell culture are definitive means of diagnosis. Serologic tests are available.

TREATMENT.   There is no specific treatment.

Prevention

Good personal hygiene, including thorough washing of skin that comes in contact with an infected animal, can help prevent human infection. Any broken skin should be kept covered, and gloves should be worn when examining or treating infected sheep.

Animal housing areas should be kept clean to reduce sources of infection for susceptible lambs. In some endemic areas, a crude live vaccine is made by pulverizing scabs from infected animals and suspending the material in a glycerinated solution. Lambs are vaccinated by applying the suspension to scarified skin in the axilla. However, the efficacy of this process is variable and, as mentioned above, can cause human infection. In addition, this practice can lead to perpetuation of the virus in the farm environment.

Reporting and Surveillance

Reporting of contagious ecthyma is not required.

Herpesvirus simiae Infection (B Virus)

Agent

Herpesvirus simiae is caused by a DNA virus of the genus *Herpesvirus*, family Herpesviridae; it is closely related to the human herpes simplex virus that causes fever blisters and mouth ulcers. It is also referred to as cercopithecine herpesvirus 1.

Reservoirs

Asian monkeys of the genus *Macaca*, especially the rhesus monkey, *M. mulatta*, are natural reservoirs; other primates in contact with infected *Macaca* spp. may acquire the virus.

Occurrence

Incidence is common in monkeys; 30% to 80% of rhesus monkeys are seropositive for this virus. In humans, B virus infection is a rare occupational disease that has been recorded in veterinarians, animal care workers, laboratory personnel, and others in contact with Old World monkeys or monkey cell cultures.

Transmission

H. simiae infection is transmitted between monkeys by direct contact, bites or scratches, and saliva-contaminated food or water. Infected monkeys may not show any clinical signs. Humans acquire the disease when bitten by a monkey that carries the virus, when saliva from an infected monkey comes in contact with broken skin, or by conjunctival, nasal, or pharyngeal exposure to aerosols that contain the virus.

Disease in Animals

SIGNS.   Primary B virus infection in macaque monkeys causes sores in or around the mouth that appear similar to fever blisters in humans. The small ulcers that form heal within 1 to 2 weeks. The condition is not serious in monkeys and is rarely noticed unless lesions appear on the lips, conjunctivae, or skin. After the initial outbreak of lesions, the virus becomes latent, and the monkey is then an asymptomatic carrier. In nonmacaque primates, the course of the disease is similar to that in humans and usually fatal.

DIAGNOSIS.   Serologic tests used to determine B virus infection include ELISA and radioimmunoassay. The virus can be grown in tissue culture, and identification is confirmed through the use of PCR, DNA restriction analysis, or other molecular methods.

Disease in Humans

SIGNS AND SYMPTOMS.   B virus in humans causes a severe and usually fatal meningoencephalitis. When infection follows a monkey bite or other cutaneous inoculation of the agent, the wound becomes reddened and painful; itching and numbness can occur. Vesicles appear at the site, and regional lymphadenopathy develops. After a few days to a few weeks, the disease becomes generalized, and there is sudden onset of fever, with headache, nausea, abdominal pain, and diarrhea. Various neurologic signs follow, including vertigo, diaphragmatic spasms, neck stiffness, and difficulty in swallowing. In late stages of the illness, the lower extremities develop flaccid paralysis; this spreads to the upper extremities and thorax. Respiratory failure and death usually occur within 5 to 28 days of onset of clinical symptoms. More than 70% of the known cases have been fatal, and most survivors have permanent and extensive neurologic damage, although recent improvements in diagnostic and therapeutic techniques offer hope for reducing fatalities and permanent sequelae.

DIAGNOSIS.   Serologic tests may be useful when a patient survives long enough to produce antibodies, but most cases are diagnosed post mortem through viral isolation from brain tissue.

TREATMENT.   Acyclovir has produced recovery in a few cases.

Prevention

Anyone who works with or comes into contact with Old World monkeys should take all precautions to prevent bites and aerosol exposure. Always wear gloves, masks, and protective clothing. Prompt treatment of any wound caused by a monkey (bite or scratch) or an object (cage or wires) that could be contaminated with monkey secretions is critical. Immediately and thoroughly scrub the wound with soap and water, and disinfect it with an iodine solution. Acyclovir may be an effective prophylaxis if administered promptly. If the wound becomes painful or numb or if itching or vesicular lesions appear at or near the wound site, seek immediate expert medical advice. No vaccine is available.

Technician Note

Anyone who works with or comes into contact with Old World monkeys should take all precautions to prevent bites and aerosol exposure.

Monkeys should be housed only in small groups, with a maximum of two per cage. Do not house rhesus monkeys with any other species. Quarantine all recently imported monkeys for at least 6 weeks; destroy any that have or develop lesions suggestive of *H. simiae*. Any animal responsible for a wound to a human should be observed for at least 2 weeks and tested to determine its B virus status.

Researchers who work with tissues or body fluids from macaques should follow biosafety level 2 (BSL 2) practices. If the material is known to contain *H. simiae*, BSL 3 facilities and precautions should be used.

Reporting and Surveillance
Report any human cases to local health authorities.

Newcastle Disease
Agent
This disease is caused by an RNA virus of the genus *Paramyxovirus*, family Paramyxoviridae.

Reservoirs
Chickens are the reservoir for Newcastle disease.

Occurrence
Incidence is worldwide. Newcastle disease occurs in wild birds and semidomestic and domestic fowl in both epizootic and enzootic forms; it is one of the most economically important diseases affecting the poultry industry. Human disease is rare and usually occurs among poultry slaughterhouse workers, poultry vaccinators using vaccines containing live viral strains, and laboratory personnel who work with the virus.

Transmission
Newcastle disease is spread from bird to bird mainly by aerosols, with the density of birds in commercial poultry farms facilitating transmission. The virus also is shed in feces. Humans become infected when the virus comes into contact with the eyes, as occurs with aerosolized vaccines.

Disease in Animals
SIGNS.   Numerous species of birds may be affected by ND, but chickens and turkeys are especially susceptible. Signs may be respiratory, nervous, or both and usually appear throughout a flock within 2 weeks of exposure. The strain of virus determines the severity of the outbreak; lentogenic strains are the least virulent, velogenic are the most, and mesogenic strains are intermediate. In birds with respiratory involvement, there is gasping and coughing; neurologic signs include drooping wings, twisted neck, depression, anorexia, and paralysis. Egg laying may cease. Some velogenic strains produce a viscerotropic syndrome, which is the most serious form of Newcastle disease. Affected birds have sudden onset of watery, greenish diarrhea, tracheal discharge, and edema of the face and wattles; small hemorrhages appear in the mucosa of the proventriculus, and the intestinal mucosa becomes necrotic. There is high mortality associated with this form of the disease.

DIAGNOSIS.   Newcastle disease virus can be isolated from tracheal exudate, lung, or spleen tissue taken early in the outbreak. Material taken for viral isolation attempts should be placed in a sterile container and transported to the laboratory. Various serologic tests also are useful.

Disease in Humans
SIGNS AND SYMPTOMS.   In humans, Newcastle disease usually causes a unilateral conjunctivitis, with excessive tear formation, pain, swelling of subconjunctival tissues, and inflammation of the lymph nodes in front of the ear. Generally, there is no systemic involvement, but some people exposed to aerosols of the virus develop an influenza-like illness that lasts 3 to 4 days. Recovery is complete in about 1 week. Subclinical infections also occur.

DIAGNOSIS.   Isolation of Newcastle disease virus is the only definitive means of diagnosis because many people do not develop a serologic response. The virus can be isolated from various body fluids, including conjunctival or nasal secretions, saliva, or urine. Inoculation of embryonated chicken eggs or tissue culture techniques can be used to isolate the virus.

TREATMENT.   Usually no treatment is necessary.

Prevention
Control of avian Newcastle disease depends on maintaining good hygiene on poultry farms. Poultry houses should be separated, and all birds in a flock should be vaccinated using a live lentogenic strain vaccine. People who administer the vaccine to poultry should wear masks; laboratory personnel should avoid creating aerosols when working with the virus.

Reporting and Surveillance
The United States requires that imported live birds of any species be quarantined and prohibits imports from countries in which Newcastle disease occurs.

Rabies

Agent

Rabies is caused by a ribonucleic acid (RNA) virus of the genus *Lyssavirus*, family Rhabdoviridae.

Reservoirs

Reservoirs for rabies are wild and domestic members of the Canidae family, including dogs, foxes, coyotes, and wolves; wild carnivores and omnivores, such as skunks, raccoons, and mongooses; and bats, including those that feed on blood (vampire bats), fruit eaters, and insectivores.

Occurrence

Incidence is almost worldwide in animal populations; the only exceptions are parts of the Pacific and far East, including Australia, New Zealand, Papua New Guinea, Japan, Taiwan, and most of Oceania; and some of Europe, including England, Scotland, Ireland, the Netherlands, Norway, Finland, Sweden, Spain, Portugal, and Greece. Rabies is present throughout most of the Americas except for a few Caribbean islands. In areas in which animal rabies occurs, the disease follows two cycles: urban and sylvatic. Urban rabies is transmitted by dogs and accounts for most human cases; sylvatic rabies circulates among wild carnivores and bats and causes some spillover infection of dogs, cats, and livestock. Rabies is responsible for an estimated 40,000 to 70,000 human deaths each year, most in developing countries.

Transmission

Rabies virus is abundant in saliva; thus most cases are attributable to a bite inflicted by an infected animal. Aerosol transmission is possible; a few cases have occurred among field biologists working in caves in which large populations of bats roosted.

> **Technician Note**
>
> Rabies virus is abundant in saliva; thus most cases are attributable to a bite inflicted by an infected animal.

Disease in Animals

Signs. Rabies in dogs may be either furious or paralytic ("dumb"). In the early stages of furious rabies, the animal becomes agitated, restless, and excitable. An aggressive phase follows, with the dog attempting to bite objects, other animals, humans, and itself. Salivation is profuse because throat muscles spasm and prevent swallowing; vocal cords become affected, and the bark changes to a hoarse howl. Convulsions and paralysis occur shortly before death. In paralytic rabies, the muscles of the head and neck initially are affected, and the animal has difficulty in swallowing. Paralysis spreads to the extremities and then becomes generalized; death follows.

Rabid cats usually manifest the furious variety, whereas in cattle, rabies generally is paralytic. Furious rabies is the more common form in wild animals, such as foxes, skunks, and raccoons.

Diagnosis. Behavioral changes and/or paralysis may suggest a presumptive diagnosis, particularly when rabies recently has been confirmed in the same species and geographic area. A positive direct immunofluorescence test on brain tissue is confirmatory. There are no tests available that produce satisfactory results on specimens from live animals.

Disease in Humans

Signs and Symptoms. The incubation period is variable; in most cases, onset of symptoms is within 3 to 8 weeks of exposure, but there are documented reports of disease occurring several years after a bite from a rabid animal. Rabies in humans usually begins with discomfort and irritation in the area of a previous animal bite. Vague sensory changes, apprehension, headache, low-grade fever, and malaise also may occur. As the disease progresses, salivation increases and eyes and ears become hypersensitive to light and sound. Paresis or paralysis develops, and spasmodic contractions of muscles used in swallowing cause the patient to develop an aversion to liquids (hydrophobia) and to stop swallowing his or her own saliva. Convulsions and various mental disturbances are terminal events. Death from respiratory failure usually occurs 2 to 8 days after onset of symptoms.

Diagnosis. A presumptive diagnosis sometimes can be made by immunofluorescence staining of skin sections taken from the back of the neck. As in animals, postmortem testing of brain tissue is necessary for confirmation.

Treatment. Rabies is always fatal. Once clinical disease has developed, there is no effective treatment.

Prevention

All pet dogs and cats should be vaccinated. Cattle and horses may be vaccinated in areas where skunk rabies is endemic or vampire bats are present.

Individuals at risk, such as laboratory workers, animal control personnel, veterinarians, technicians, field zoologists, and others who come into contact with wild or unvaccinated domestic animals, should receive preexposure prophylaxis. Human diploid cell vaccine (HDCV) is one of the best and most effective of available vaccines, but it is expensive and may only be available in developed countries.

Local laws may vary, but in general, a dog or cat that has bitten a person should be quarantined and observed for at least 10 days. If the animal develops any sign suggestive of rabies, the animal should be killed and its brain examined by fluorescent microscopy. Any wild animal that has bitten a person should be killed immediately and tested. Any unvaccinated animal that is bitten by a rabid animal should be destroyed.

The most effective means of preventing rabies in humans is to immediately and thoroughly cleanse any animal bite or scratch wound; if used quickly, soap and water are a good means of removing rabies virus. Flush the wound with a strong stream of water, wash with soap or detergent, and rinse well. Apply a disinfectant, such as alcohol, tincture of iodine, or a quaternary ammonium compound, and seek medical attention. Bite wounds should be left unsutured, if possible, so as not to interfere with bleeding and drainage.

> **Technician Note**
>
> All cases of animal and human rabies should be reported to health authorities.

For people who have not received preexposure immunization, postexposure prophylactic treatment consists of administering human rabies immune globulin (RIG) and rabies vaccine, preferably a 5-day course of HDCV or other approved vaccine. If the exposed person already has received a full course of vaccine before exposure, RIG is not considered necessary, and only two doses of vaccine are given.

Researchers who work with the virus should operate under strict biosafety level 2 (BSL 2) conditions; if aerosols are possible, BSL 3 precautions should be observed.

Reporting and Surveillance
All cases of animal and human rabies should be reported to health authorities.

RECOMMENDED READING

GENERAL
Beran GW: Zoonoses in practice, *Vet Clin North Am* 23: 1085, 1993.

Bottone EJ et al: *Cumitech 27, laboratory diagnosis of zoonotic infections: bacterial infections obtained from companion and laboratory animals,* Washington, DC, 1996, American Society for Microbiology.

ANTHRAX
Whitford HW, Hugh-Jones ME: Anthrax. In Beran GW, Steele JH, editors: *Handbook of zoonoses,* ed 2, Boca Raton, Fla, 1994, CRC Press.

AVIAN CHLAMYDIOSIS
Koschmann JR: Avian chlamydiosis. In Farris R et al, editors: *Health hazards in veterinary practice,* ed 3, Schaumburg, Ill, 1995, American Veterinary Medical Association.

BITE WOUNDS AND OTHER INJURIES
August JR: *Zoonosis updates,* ed 2, Schaumburg, Ill, 1995, American Veterinary Medical Association.

Beaver BV: Animal-related injuries. In Farris R et al, editors: *Health hazards in veterinary practice,* ed 3, Schaumburg, Ill, 1995, American Veterinary Medical Association.

Weber DJ, Hansen AR: Infections resulting from animal bites, *Infect Dis Clin North Am* 5:663, 1991.

BRUCELLOSIS
Metcalf HE, Luchsinger DW, Ray WC: Brucellosis. In Beran GW, Steele JH, editors: *Handbook of zoonoses,* ed 2, Boca Raton, Fla, 1994, CRC Press.

Radolf JD: Southwestern Medical Conference: brucellosis—don't let it get your goat! *Am J Med Sci* 307:64, 1994.

CAMPYLOBACTERIOSIS
Benenson AS: Campylobacter enteritis. In Benenson AS, editor: *Control of communicable diseases manual,* Washington, DC, 1995, American Public Health Association.

Saeed AM, Harris NV, DiGiacomo RF: The role of exposure to animals in the etiology of *Campylobacter jejuni/coli* enteritis, *Am J Epidemiol* 137:108, 1993.

CAPNOCYTOPHAGA CANIMORSUS INFECTION
Sasaki DM, Katz AR, Middleton CR: *Capnocytophaga* and related infections. In Beran GW, Steele JH, editors: *Handbook of zoonoses,* ed 2, Boca Raton, Fla, 1994, CRC Press.

CAT-SCRATCH DISEASE
Groves MG, Harrington KS: *Rochalimaea henselae* infections: newly recognized zoonoses transmitted by domestic cats, *J Am Vet Med Assoc* 204:267, 1994.

Zangwill KM et al: Cat scratch disease in Connecticut: epidemiology, risk factors, and evaluation of a new diagnostic test, *N Engl J Med* 329:8, 1993.

CONTAGIOUS ECTHYMA
Acha PN, Szyfres B: Contagious ecthyma. In *Zoonoses and communicable diseases common to man and animals,* ed 2, Washington, DC, 1987, Pan American Health Organization.

Benenson AS: Orf virus disease. In Benenson AS, editor: *Control of communicable diseases manual,* Washington, DC, 1995, American Public Health Association.

CRYPTOCOCCOSIS
Benenson AS: Cryptococcosis. In Benenson AS, editor: *Control of communicable diseases manual,* Washington, DC, 1995, American Public Health Association.

Levitz SM: The ecology of *Cryptococcus neoformans* and the epidemiology of cryptococcosis, *Rev Infect Dis* 13:1163, 1991.

CRYPTOSPORIDIOSIS
Benenson AS: Cryptosporidiosis. In Benenson AS, editor: *Control of communicable diseases manual,* Washington, DC, 1995, American Public Health Association.

Snowden KF: Cryptosporidiosis. In Farris R et al, editors: *Health hazards in veterinary practice,* ed 3, Schaumburg, Ill, 1995, American Veterinary Medical Association.

DERMATOPHYTOSES
Acha PN, Szyfres B: Dermatophytosis. In *Zoonoses and communicable diseases common to man and animals,* ed 2, Washington, DC, 1987, Pan American Health Organization.

Pier AC: Superficial mycoses (dermatophytoses). In Beran GW, Steele JH, editors: *Handbook of zoonoses,* ed 2, Boca Raton, Fla, 1994, CRC Press.

ERYSIPELOTHRIX INFECTIONS
Reboli AC, Farra WE: *Erysipelothrix rhusiopathiae:* an occupational pathogen, *Clin Microbiol Rev* 2:354, 1989.

Wood RL, Steele JH: *Erysipelothrix* infections. In Beran GW, Steele JH, editors: *Handbook of zoonoses,* ed 2, Boca Raton, Fla, 1994, CRC Press.

HERPESVIRUS SIMIAE INFECTION
Acha PN, Szyfres B: *Herpesvirus simiae.* In *Zoonoses and communicable diseases common to man and animals,* ed 2, Washington, DC, 1987, Pan American Health Organization.

Hilliard J, Lipper S: B virus. In Farris R et al, editors: *Health hazards in veterinary practice,* ed 3, Schaumburg, Ill, 1995, American Veterinary Medical Association.

NEWCASTLE DISEASE
Hugh-Jones ME, Hubbert WT, Hagstad HV: Newcastle disease. In *Zoonoses: recognition, control, and prevention,* Ames, 1995, Iowa State University Press.

PASTEURELLOSIS
Acha PN, Szyfres B: Pasteurellosis. In *Zoonoses and communicable diseases common to man and animals,* ed 2, Washington, DC, 1987, Pan American Health Organization.

Arons MS, Fernando L, Polayes IM: *Pasteurella multocida:* the major cause of hand infections following domestic animal bites, *J Hand Surg* 7:47, 1982.

Q FEVER
Raoult D, Marrie T: Q fever, *Clin Infect Dis* 20:489, 1995.

Williams JC, Sanchez V: Q fever and coxiellosis. In Beran GW, Steele JH, editors: *Handbook of zoonoses,* ed 2, Boca Raton, Fla, 1994, CRC Press.

RABIES

Benenson AS: Rabies. In Benenson AS, editor: *Control of communicable diseases manual*, Washington, DC, 1995, American Public Health Association.

Clark KA: Rabies. In Farris R et al, editors: *Health hazards in veterinary practice*, ed 3, Schaumburg, Ill, 1995, American Veterinary Medical Association.

RAT-BITE FEVERS

Will LA: Ratbite fever. In Beran GW, Steele JH, editors: *Handbook of zoonoses*, ed 2, Boca Raton, Fla, 1994, CRC Press.

Wullenberger M: *Streptobacillus moniliformis:* a zoonotic pathogen: taxonomic considerations, host species, diagnosis, therapy, geographical distribution, *Lab Anim* 29:1, 1995.

SALMONELLOSIS

Benenson AS: Salmonellosis. In Benenson AS, editor: *Control of communicable diseases manual*, Washington, DC, 1995, American Public Health Association.

U.S. Centers for Disease Control (CDC): Reptile-associated salmonellosis: selected states, 1994-1995, *MMWR Morb Mortal Wkly Rep* 44:347, 1995.

TOXOPLASMOSIS

Lappin MR: Toxoplasmosis. In Farris R et al, editors: *Health hazards in veterinary practice*, ed 3, Schaumburg, Ill, 1995, American Veterinary Medical Association.

19

Euthanasia

Joseph Taboada • Stephanie W. Johnson

Old Dog

 When the old dog had to die after long years full with love and honor,

 When the weight of time grew wearying and she was content to have it finished,

 I brought my old dog to our friend.

 Old dog lay soft against me, old eyes already closed, waiting.

 Our friend's hand was gentle on the weary body, with its ragged fur,

 So gentle to find the frail small vein where death could enter. DIFFICULT,

 Old blood runs sluggish, old veins slackly resisting.

 So patient, our friend, his knowing hands, all I can see through silent tears.

 I watch capable strong hands lightly coaxing, and at last a small red flower blooms briefly in the crystal before he eases the plunger in.

 Old dog only sighs very softly.

 The weary heart slows and stops as the joyful spirit leaps free.

 We wait a quiet minute, my tears dropping unheeded, into the soft fur.

 Our friend withdraws, his gentle hands leaving old dog's castoff body.

 My head bowed over the weathered white mask for a moment before I let her lie by herself and draw the blanket over her.

 I wish the old dog had made it easier for him.

 To bring even a kindly death brings sadness.

 He asked how many years she had, and I heard more than that in his voice.

 I wish I could thank him for keeping zest in her years, for making a good end of them, for his capable hands, for his gentle word, and caring heart.

 I took the old dog home, and laid her as if sleeping, wrapped in her worn blanket and sheltered deep in the kindly silent earth.

         Anonymous

Perhaps no single issue in veterinary medicine conjures up the range of emotion, ethical deliberation, and stress occasioned by euthanasia. Euthanasia was defined by the 1986 American Veterinary Medical Association (AVMA) Panel on Euthanasia as "the act of inducing painless

death," but the act is only one small aspect of the larger issue facing the profession.

The word euthanasia is derived from the Greek root *eu*, meaning good, and *thanatos*, referring to death. Few in the veterinary profession would argue that when used in the context of relieving suffering, the word runs counter to its Greek roots; however, as the word is currently defined, it also pertains to the killing of unwanted, abandoned, stray, or phenotypically undesired animals by veterinary professionals with problems in balancing conflicting interests. It is not always in the common interest of the patient, client, and veterinarian that euthanasia is performed. Euthanasia is an emotionally charged issue, with members of the profession varying significantly in their acceptance of the practice and in their views as to its utility. On the one hand, it might be viewed simply as "convenience killing," whereas on the other, it might be viewed as a means of furthering respect and love through the compassionate termination of hopeless suffering. No matter how one looks at it, the animal health professional may be caught in the middle, experiencing doubts, confusion, and moral questions over participation in the ending of an animal's life. It is an ethical dilemma that does not have an easy or even an absolutely right or wrong answer. It is an issue that all veterinary professionals must wrestle with, individually and collectively.

Technician Note

Euthanasia is an issue that all veterinary professionals must wrestle with, individually and collectively.

THE DECISION

The decision to perform euthanasia is one of the most difficult decisions that the owner of a companion animal will ever face. Some owners may make the decision quickly because of financial constraints or fear of what the illness may eventually cause, whereas others may never be able to make the decision, preferring to let their pet die naturally. The decision is often made more difficult by the fact that few pet owners have an adequate support group available that understands the bond that develops between an animal and the recipient of its unconditional love.

Most owners who elect to have euthanasia performed make the decision because they perceive that their pet's illness involves some degree of suffering. Suffering is difficult to define, and perceptions of animal suffering differ markedly between individuals and from case to case. The place the pet holds in the owner's family circle, how long the pet has been owned, the relationship between the pet and other loved ones, the financial resources available to the owner, and the disease process afflicting the pet are other factors that most owners take into consideration when trying to make the decision.

The veterinary team (veterinarian, veterinary technician, animal health care providers) can play an important role in the decision-making process. The veterinary staff often serves as a sounding board for the client who is trying to make the decision. Staff members can help with the decision by approaching the subject professionally with compassion and respect. The most important help that the team can give is to provide information. What the owner can expect from the disease process, what treatments are available, the prognosis with and without treatment, and what costs are involved are all questions that should be answered by the veterinarian. The veterinary technician can play a vital role as a client resource by answering questions about euthanasia. How euthanasia is performed, whether the animal will feel pain, how long the procedure will take, and what happens to the body afterward are all areas that a technician may be asked to address.

Technician Note

Veterinary technicians, as professionals, can help clients with euthanasia decisions by approaching the subject professionally with compassion and respect.

When interacting with an owner considering euthanasia, the veterinary professional should go to great lengths to lay out all options available while being careful not to make the decision for the client. Too many veterinary professionals make judgments as to the value of an animal (both monetary and personal) that only the owner can make. Questions such as "What would you do if he were your animal?" are difficult to address and perhaps best answered by urging the client to verbalize what he or she sees as the pros and cons of each choice. In doing this, it may become obvious that the client has already made the decision and is looking for support or validation. The client may feel guilt, anger, sadness, depression, pain, and helplessness during the decision-making process and after euthanasia has been performed (see Chapter 20). The veterinary professional can help by assuring owners that these feelings are normal, and indeed expected, and by assuring them that they are not alone in the pain they are feeling.

Once an informed decision has been made, it should be supported, even if it may not have been the decision that the veterinarian or veterinary staff would have made. Pet owners are sensitive to the actions of hospital personnel, and for this reason it is extremely important that persons interacting with the client or handling the animal in the presence of the owner be supportive, gentle, and empathetic.

AS THE END DRAWS NEAR: THE BEGINNING OF THE END

The death of a pet can be a devastating experience that can drastically affect the relationship between client and veterinarian. As many as 40% of clients change veterinarians after a pet has died. This number probably approaches 100% if euthanasia is handled in a manner that causes the client to perceive a lack of care, concern, or respect on the part of the veterinarian or other staff members. On the other hand, much can be done to foster a long-lasting relationship through the professional and compassionate handling of a euthanasia. It is often true that the client who loudly sings the praises of a veterinarian and staff is not the owner of an animal saved through long hours of hard work and outstanding medical care but rather the owner who was treated with compassion, care, and concern at and around the time of the loss of a pet.

Technician Note

Many clients change veterinarians after the death of a pet, especially if euthanasia is handled without the utmost care and respect.

Preparations for pet loss should begin as soon as it becomes apparent that death is a possibility. The veterinarian will often discuss euthanasia with a client early so that the client understands that it is an available option. However, it is important to discuss all other medical or surgical options first. Euthanasia should not be presented in such a manner that it is either completely discounted or viewed as the only reasonable course. Remember that the initial reaction of a client receiving bad news is often denial or feelings of numbness or shock. It is important to allow time for this initial reaction to fade and for the entire family to be given time to discuss the various options before allowing the client to make such a difficult and important decision.

While discussing options with the client, the veterinarian should use alternative jargon terms for euthanasia such as *put to sleep, put down, put away, humanely destroy, rock,* and *shoot* only when their meaning is understood by all individuals involved. Confusion will result from the use of a term such as *put to sleep* when talking to a companion animal owner who perceives the phrase to refer to anesthesia instead of euthanasia. Children are especially confused by the term *put to sleep* and may be afraid that they might die when going to sleep at night. Whatever term is used to describe the act of euthanasia, it is important that it be fully understood by all parties involved.

Once the decision has been made to have an animal undergo euthanasia, a client must make many decisions. When and where should the euthanasia take place? Should the client or other family members be present during the euthanasia? What is to happen to the body after euthanasia? Should a necropsy examination be allowed? What special method, if any, will the client use to memorialize the pet? It is best to discuss these concerns thoroughly in advance so that everyone understands precisely the wishes of the client.

The client, together with the veterinarian, should decide who will be present during the euthanasia. This is sometimes a difficult decision for both the client and the veterinarian. Some veterinarians do not offer this option to

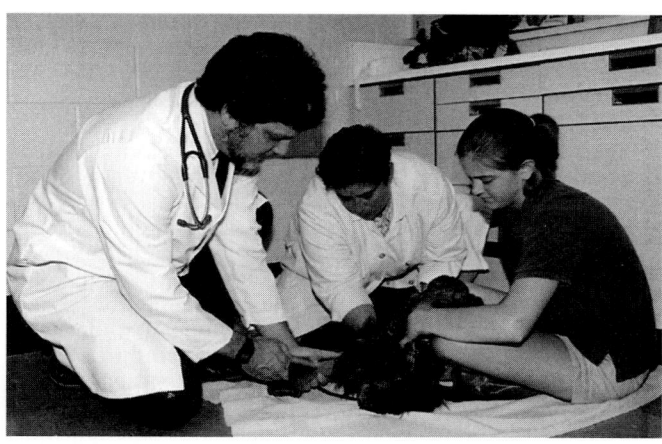

FIGURE 19-1. Being present during the euthanasia of the companion animal helps clients to say goodbye and complete the responsibilities of pet ownership. At times, clients will want to have euthanasia performed on a blanket on the floor or in a special place, making the event more personal and meaningful.

the client in the mistaken view that it will be too difficult for the client to watch. Contrary to this view, many clients will grieve more easily and accept more quickly the loss of their pet if they have had the opportunity to say goodbye in this most personal way (Figure 19-1). The chance to hold their pet and let it know that it is loved dearly while sharing its last moments is sometimes an important first step in the grief process. However, with the benefits to the client can come problems for the veterinarian and staff. Veterinary team members must realize that having the client present can increase their own stress level associated with euthanasia, and every attempt should be made to understand and minimize its effects.

Technician Note
Many clients will go through the grief process more easily if they are present at the euthanasia.

When the client or family members are to be present, euthanasia should be scheduled for a time of day when interruptions are unlikely, the waiting room is empty, and the potential for embarrassment by public exposure is minimized. Early mornings, evenings, or during the lunch hour may be suitable. It is best to schedule at least 30 minutes. The most important aspect of the euthanasia to consider is communication. The unexpected should be avoided at all costs, and before the procedure, the client should be given a detailed explanation of exactly what is about to happen to the pet and what he or she is about to see. Then the client should be talked through each step of the procedure. The euthanasia should proceed at a pace with which the client feels comfortable. Occasionally pets will urinate, defecate, vocalize, twitch, or gasp after they have become unconscious. Although these reflex acts can be minimized, they will still occasionally occur and will have a far less negative effect if they are expected and if the client is told that they are not a reflection of pain or suffering.

Technician Note
Communication is critical to a smooth euthanasia when owners are present.

Deciding where the euthanasia is to take place can be important. Using a hospital space that is less stark than the typical stainless steel hospital examination room is preferred. If the examination room is to be used, at least a blanket should be placed over the table and there should be a chair where the client can sit down. Some clients will request that the euthanasia be performed at home or at some special place. Many veterinarians will honor these requests or use the services of a house call practice for this need. Sometimes just being outside the "normal" environment of the veterinarian facility is a fair and acceptable compromise. A blanket on the floor, the lawn beside the clinic, and even the back seat of the family car might serve this purpose. One important consideration for the veterinarian in choosing the place is that many clients will feel uncomfortable coming back into the room where a pet previously underwent euthanasia. Indeed, many clients switch veterinarians because of a lack of sensitivity to this fact by the veterinary staff. To minimize this potential conflict in the future, it is best to choose a space that will not be routinely used for other client-related activities.

Clients who choose not to be present during euthanasia may still wish to see the body of the animal after it is dead. Seeing the animal dead conveys finality and also allows the client the opportunity to say goodbye. Many clients have a difficult time proceeding through the grief process if they have not been given this chance.

Technician Note
Clients who choose not be present for a euthanasia often still wish to see the body afterward.

Make arrangements in advance concerning how payment for services is to occur. Discuss with the client whether payment is going to be made in advance, at the time of services, or by a later bill. This can be an uncomfortable subject to broach after euthanasia has occurred.

AT THE END

Once all the preparations have been made, the euthanasia should be performed with skill and concern. Each member of the veterinary team should be well trained, know his or her responsibilities, and be available. The key, as already mentioned, is to expect and plan for the unexpected. Although many methods of euthanasia are deemed acceptable by the AVMA panel on euthanasia, only those that are aesthetically acceptable should be used when the client is going to be present.

Technician Note
Expect and plan for the unexpected.

If the examination room is to be used, the table should be covered with a cloth or blanket. Some owners will want to bring a favorite blanket for the pet to spend its last few moments on. It is important that they understand that it is possible, indeed likely, that the blanket will be soiled by feces or urine when euthanasia occurs. If the pet is likely to be aggressive or extremely apprehensive, tranquilizing it ahead of time should be considered. If the client is to be present, the animal should be taken away briefly so that a peripheral vein can be catheterized for smooth delivery of the euthanasia solution. It is advisable to put the catheter into a vein in a back leg; this will allow the client to hold the animal and pet its head without being in the way of the veterinarian while the injections are being given. Once the catheter has been placed, the client should be given the opportunity to be alone with the pet for a few moments.

Before administering the euthanasia solution, a saline solution should be injected into the catheter to ensure its patency. Next, the patient should be anesthetized with an ultra–short-acting barbiturate. This will decrease the incidence of excitement after the euthanasia solution is injected. Once the animal is anesthetized, the euthanasia solution can be injected. Sodium pentobarbital is the most commonly used euthanasia solution. It is a member of the barbiturate family of drugs that depress the entire central nervous system.* When large doses of this drug are administered, as for euthanasia, unconsciousness occurs first, and then breathing stops because of depression of the respiratory center. This is followed by cardiac arrest. The pentobarbital dose, concentration, and rate of administration determine the speed of action. When the drug is administered intravenously, animals die swiftly and quietly. Although intravenous administration is preferred, the drug is also effective when injected intrahepatically and, to a lesser extent, into the peritoneal cavity. Death following intraperitoneal injection may take as long as 15 minutes, however, because of relatively slow absorption. Pentobarbital for euthanasia is available alone or in combination with other drugs. The concentration of pentobarbital in most euthanasia solutions is approximately 20% by weight. The recommended dose is 2 ml for the first 4.5 kg of body weight and 1 ml for each additional 4.5 kg of body

weight. Sodium pentobarbital should be administered as rapidly as possible to provide the quietest and swiftest form of euthanasia. The veterinary team should be completely familiar with the use of the euthanasia solution chosen and the possible reactions that might be seen.

Because the cerebral cortex is affected by general anesthetic, predominant emotions may take over and the animal may show fear behavior, which is usually characterized by struggling and vocalization. Experimental studies indicate that the animal is not conscious of these feelings at the time. People who have undergone the "excitement" phase during general anesthesia do not remember that it took place. Although trained individuals may understand this excitement phase from the clinical standpoint, it is difficult for the owner to understand that struggling and vocalization are not due to pain or discomfort. Thus the owner's perception is that the animal is not experiencing a peaceful death. Clients who choose to be present should be warned that this phase may occur. The use of an ultra–short-acting barbiturate first will minimize the excitement phase.

THE END AS A BEGINNING . . . AFTER THE END

*A gentle touch,
barely audible she purrs,
goodbye, oh goodbye,
a final glimpse of life drifting away,
a lifeless stare;
. . . and then, I am alone.*

J. Taboada

Many veterinary professionals are good at the technical aspects of euthanasia but fall short in supplying what the client needs after euthanasia has been performed. The animal's death is often only the beginning of a long and difficult odyssey that the client is about to face. Some clients will feel a great sense of relief immediately after the pet's death, but most will soon feel empty, numb, or alone. They may question whether they did the right thing. Veterinary professionals can help them by again stressing that the pet's death was painless, assuring them that they did the right thing, and focusing on some positive things that the pet brought to their life. At the time of euthanasia, it is important that an environment be fostered that says, "It's all right to cry, it's all right to be emotional, it's all right to begin to grieve." Few of us have the gift of being able to say the right thing at the right time, so sometimes consolation can best be offered in a touch or an embrace. A touch on the arm or a simple embrace will often express best what the client needs to hear: "We care and you are not alone."

Technician Note
The pet's death is often only the beginning of a long and difficult odyssey.

Many clients, whether present for the euthanasia or not, need assurance that the animal is dead. Clients will feel more assured by the veterinarian who takes the time to listen to the animal's thorax with a stethoscope and shine a pen light into the animal's eyes before pronouncing the patient is dead. For those who choose not to be present,

---

*Note that all barbiturates are strictly controlled by federal regulations, and accurate accounting of the use of these agents is required. The Drug Enforcement Agency (DEA) of the U.S. Department of Justice is responsible for enforcement of laws governing the user of barbiturates. Sodium pentobarbital is a schedule II controlled substance and can be obtained only by a licensed medical practitioner, such as a physician, dentist, veterinarian, or approved institution. In addition to the DEA paperwork involved for procuring barbiturates such as sodium pentobarbital, careful handling of the drug is necessary after the drug is on the hospital premises. Thorough record keeping is required by law.

allowing them to view the animal's body can alleviate some of this fear. Before bringing the body to the client, it should be made as presentable as possible. It must always be treated with dignity and respect. Clean any blood from the fur, remove any catheters or bandages, place the tongue in the mouth, and close the eyes. Placing a drop of cyanoacrylate glue (Krazy Glue) in each eye will keep the eyelids closed. If time permits, bathe and brush the animal before laying it on a clean paper, blanket, or towel in a sturdy box. This will help to make the viewing as pleasant an experience as possible. This last, and often lasting, impression that the client takes away from the practice may go a long way toward determining whether he or she returns with another pet. If the animal's body is sealed in a box (commercially made boxes for home burial are available), let the client know how the body is wrapped and whether any signs of trauma or surgery are present. Even clients who assure the veterinarian that they will not open the box before burial or cremation often change their mind after leaving the office.

Technician Note

Always treat the pet's body with dignity and respect.

Having the client bring someone who will be able to drive him or her home will help ease the feeling of being alone and will also ensure a safe trip. It is nice to call clients after they have arrived home to check on them. Attempts should be made to call all clients who have lost a pet to answer any questions and to show concern. The veterinarian or a staff member may call. The show of concern is always appreciated, helps clients who are having difficulty dealing with grief, and assures clients that a relationship with the clinic fostered in life has not been ended by the death of their pet. Most clients will eventually choose to get another pet. A sympathy card or handwritten note is usually appreciated. Many beautiful sympathy cards designed for veterinary use are available (Figure 19-2).

One of the biggest concerns of clients who have just lost a pet is disposition of the body. When possible, all arrangements should be made in advance. The veterinary staff should be prepared with information to assist the client in making these arrangements. Know the laws concerning burial in the practice area. Make available names and telephone numbers of places that offer cremation and pet cemetery burial. If the client chooses to have the veterinarian handle the remains, it is best not to lie to the client concerning the disposal of the animal's body.

Technician Note

Memorializing the pet can be an important part of grieving for many clients.

Memorializing the pet is a step that many clients find comforting. It can be an important part of grieving for many clients. Offering the client a lock of hair and returning collars or leashes may facilitate these wishes. Having a memorial service, planting a special plant in memory of the pet, framing a photograph, keeping a lock of hair, writing a poem or special letter, offering a memorial scholarship at a veterinary school, or making a donation to organizations such as the American Veterinary Medical Association or a veterinary school foundation are actions that clients may use to memorialize their pet (Figure 19-3).

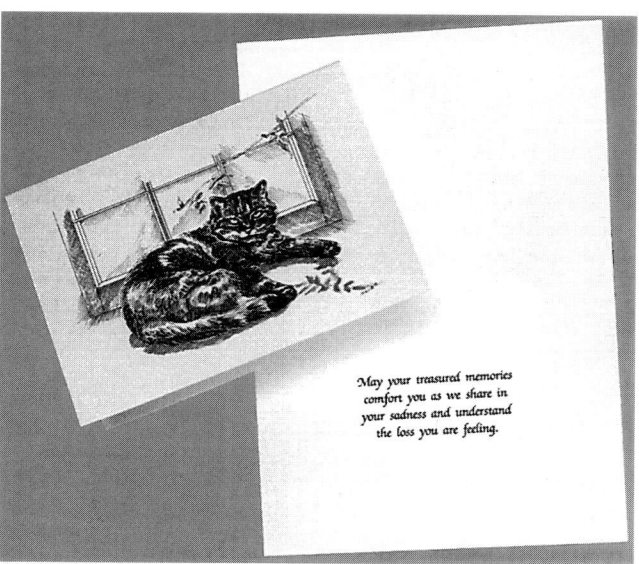

FIGURE 19-2. After a pet has died, a condolence card or letter from the veterinary practice is an appropriate symbol of support. Many clients will return to a practice that shows this type of caring gesture when they eventually invest in a new relationship with another pet.

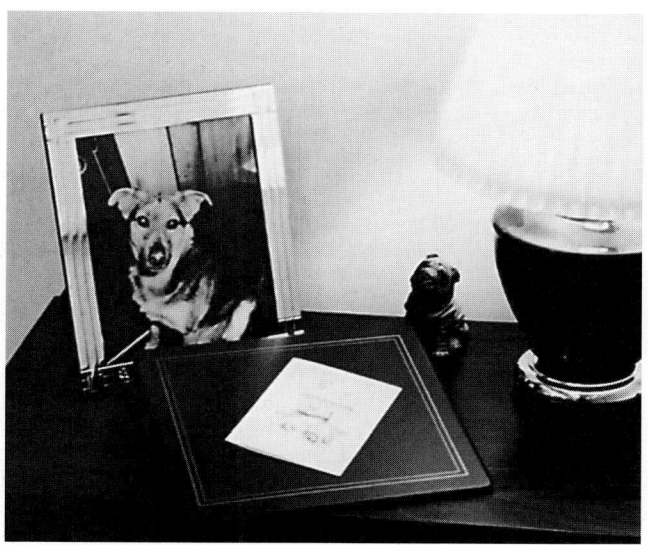

FIGURE 19-3. Memorializing a pet who has died can be an important part of grieving. A framed photo and a scrapbook are two effective ways to memorialize.

THE STRESS OF EUTHANASIA

Euthanasia is stressful not only to the client but also to the veterinarian and veterinary staff. Frequent performance of euthanasia is a primary cause of burnout within small animal practice (Box 19-1). It is at times even more stressful to the technical staff than it is to the veterinarian because staff members usually have little control over the situation. Euthanasias that go smoothly as well as difficult euthanasias will create stress. Difficult or inherently stressful euthanasias include euthanasia in which technical

Box 19-1	SIGNS AND SYMPTOMS OF BURNOUT
PHYSICAL SYMPTOMS	**PSYCHOLOGIC/BEHAVIORAL SYMPTOMS**
Ulcers	Withdrawal
Gastroenteritis	Overeating
Cardiac arrhythmia	Constant fatigue
Heartburn	Increased alcohol intake
Backache	Agitation
Nausea	Distraction
Skin disorders	Aggressive behavior
	Insomnia

problems arise, instances in which the animal reacts badly to the injections in the presence of the client, and the euthanasia of one's own pet, healthy animals, young animals, and animals for whom one has put a great deal of time and medical effort into fighting their disease. Euthanasia with the client present usually creates more stress on the veterinary staff than when the procedure is performed in the absence of the owner.

Each individual will have to decide in what type of euthanasia he or she is able to participate and one's personal tolerance for euthanasia. A technician may not be able to work effectively in a practice in which the veterinarian's views on euthanasia are vastly different from his or her own. Stress can become intense if these differences are not discussed and reconciled. Veterinarians differ markedly in their views on euthanasia. A survey of British veterinarians revealed that 74% would perform euthanasia on a healthy animal if the owner requested it. A similar survey in Japan revealed that 63% would not. There is room within the veterinary profession for this divergence of views; indeed, the diversity of opinions is one of the profession's strengths.

Technician Note

Euthanasia is stressful to both the owner and the veterinary staff.

One of the most important mechanisms of coping with the stress brought on by euthanasia is discussion with colleagues. Having sessions for the hospital staff in which people can openly express their feelings is a good outlet for emotions that, if unexpressed, can cause further stress and lead to burnout. This type of communication allows members of the veterinary team to understand their colleagues' feelings and tolerances for different situations. Members of the team may need to temporarily pass responsibility for euthanasia to their colleagues when they have reached the limit of their tolerance. Other mechanisms of managing stress include taking time off, making time for self, adopting recreational habits, helping clients deal with their grief, and finding strength in relationships formed with colleagues who experience the same stresses.

EUTHANASIA IN THE SHELTER AND RESEARCH FACILITY

Technicians in veterinary practice participate in an average of three to six euthanasias per week; however, shelter technicians and potentially research technicians experience much more death than this. Millions of animals must be euthanized each year because there are no homes for them or because of the needs of certain research protocols. These deaths are difficult to rationalize, making euthanasia a very stressful event for these technicians. The fact that there are different euthanasia methods employed depending on the species or facility is a complicating stressor. This factor brings up a wide range of both psychosocial and safety issues that need to be addressed (Table 19-1).

Staff members involved in these types of euthanasia often cope by shifting moral responsibility for killing animals away from themselves. Shelter technicians view their acts as a crusade for animals and against the ignorant public, whereas research technicians may view the euthanasia as necessary for the "greater good." To prevent burnout, they must see themselves as generators of medical knowledge beneficial to humans and animals, combatants of pet overpopulation, or providers of humane death. These technicians must remember their objectives in their work. Their objective, like every other technician's, is to prevent and release animals from suffering.

The same mechanisms for coping with the stress of euthanasia mentioned previously are very important for both shelter and research technicians. Perhaps one of the most important coping strategies is for the team to rotate euthanasia responsibilities. This rotation releases technicians from the moral stress of euthanasia and reschedules them to a more hopeful task, such as education or adoption responsibilities, or other important research missions; it is hoped that giving them a break will prevent burnout. Dark humor is also used to relieve stress. Such humor reduces tension by acknowledging death as part of the setting but also minimizing, for the moment, its tragedy and finality. Although this humor may appear callous and be misunderstood by those outside the shelter or research culture, it has been shown to be a very effective coping strategy. It is important to recognize this humor for what it is, a coping mechanism. These technicians care a tremendous amount but find themselves in an environment without much societal support.

Technician Note

Open discussion of issues surrounding euthanasia can help a hospital's staff deal with the stress.

EUTHANASIA OF LARGE ANIMALS

Euthanasia of large domestic animals presents specific hazards and problems not encountered in companion small animals. Safety must be a major consideration. The jugular vein should be used for injection whenever possible because this will place the person injecting the euthanasia solution in the safest position. On rare occasions, thrombosis of the jugular veins may have occurred from disease, and the cephalic vein must be used. However, this puts the individual under the animal's forequarters and in a dangerous position.

Euthanasia-strength pentobarbital can be administered with a large-gauge needle (14 to 16 gauge). The volume of solution is large, and even with a large-gauge needle, the time it takes to inject the solution is relatively long. The animal may go through the same excitement phase as that experienced by small animals, and it may come crashing to the ground on becoming unconscious. Generally, large animal euthanasia should be performed in an area with vehicle access to allow removal of the body. In some instances, the client may wish to bury a large animal. It should be remembered that all the same emotional con-

TABLE 19-1 SUMMARY OF AGENTS AND METHODS OF EUTHANASIA: CHARACTERISTICS AND MODES OF ACTION

Agent	Acceptability	Mode of Action	Ease of Performance	Safety for Personnel	Species Suitability	Efficacy and Comments
Barbiturates	Acceptable	Direct depression of cerebral cortex, subcortical structures and vital centers; direct depression of heart muscle	Animal must be restrained; personnel must be skilled to perform intravenous injection	Safe except human abuse potential; DEA-controlled substance	Most species	Highly effective when appropriately administered; acceptable intravenous and intrahepatic in small animals
Inhalant anesthetics	Acceptable	Direct depression of cerebral cortex, subcortical structures, and vital centers	Easily performed with closed container; can be administered to large animals by mask	Must be properly scavenged or vented to minimize exposure to personnel	Amphibians, birds, cats, dogs, fur-bearing animals, rabbits, reptiles, rodents and other small animals, zoo animals	Highly effective provided that subject is sufficiently exposed
Carbon dioxide	Acceptable	Direct depression of cerebral cortex, subcortical structures, and vital centers; direct depression of heart muscle	Used in closed container	Minimal hazard	Small laboratory animals, birds, cats, small dogs, mink, zoo animals, amphibians	Effective, but time required may be prolonged in immature and neonatal animals
Carbon monoxide (bottled gas only)	Acceptable	Combines with hemoglobin, preventing its combination with oxygen	Requires appropriately operated equipment for gas production	Extremely hazardous, toxic, and difficult to detect	Most small species, including dogs, cats, rodents, mink, chinchillas, birds, reptiles, amphibians, zoo animals	Effective; acceptable only when equipment is properly designed and operated
Microwave irradiation	Acceptable	Direct inactivation of brain enzymes by rapid heating of brain	Requires training and highly specialized equipment	Safe	Mice and rats	Highly effective for special needs
Tricane methanesulfonate	Acceptable	Depression of CNS	Easily used	Safe	Fish and amphibians	Effective but expensive
Benzocaine	Acceptable	Depression of CNS	Easily used	Safe	Fish and amphibians	Effective but expensive

Continued

Modified from Andrews EJ et al: *J Am Vet Med Assoc* 202(2), 1993.
DEA, U.S. Drug Enforcement Agency; *CNS,* central nervous system.

TABLE 19-1   SUMMARY OF AGENTS AND METHODS OF EUTHANASIA: CHARACTERISTICS AND MODES OF ACTION—CONT'D

Agent	Acceptability	Mode of Action	Ease of Performance	Safety for Personnel	Species Suitability	Efficacy and Comments
Cervical dislocation	Conditionally acceptable	Direct depression of brain	Requires training and skill	Safe	Poultry, birds, laboratory mice and rats less than 200 g, or rabbits less than 1 kg	Irreversible; violent muscle contractions can occur after cervical dislocation
Decapitation	Conditionally acceptable	Direct depression of brain	Requires training and skill	Guillotine poses potential employee injury hazard	Laboratory rodents, small rabbits, birds, fish, amphibians, reptiles	Irreversible; violent muscle contractions can occur after decapitation
Penetrating captive bolt	Conditionally acceptable	Direct concussion of brain tissue	Requires skill, adequate restraint, and proper placement of captive bolt	Safe	Ruminants, horses, swine, dogs, rabbits, zoo animals, reptiles	Instant unconsciousness but motor activity may continue
Gunshot	Conditionally acceptable	Direct concussion of brain tissue	Requires skill and appropriate firearm	May be dangerous	Large domestic and zoo animals, reptiles, wildlife	Instant unconsciousness but motor activity may continue
Electrocution	Conditionally acceptable	Direct depression of brain and cardiac fibrillation	Not easily performed in all instances	Hazardous to personnel	Used primarily in foxes, sheep, swine, mink	Violent muscle contractions occur at same time as unconsciousness
Pithing	Conditionally acceptable	Trauma of brain and spinal cord tissue	Easily performed but requires skill	Safe	Some poikilotherms	Effective but death not immediate unless double pithed
Nitrogen, argon	Conditionally acceptable	Reduced partial pressure of oxygen available to blood	Use closed chamber with rapid filling	Safe if used with ventilation	Cats, small dogs, birds, rodents, rabbits, other small species, mink, zoo animals	Effective except in young and neonates; an effective agent but other methods preferable; not acceptable in most animals less than 4 mo old

cerns encountered in small animal euthanasia pertain to large animals when a bond has formed between the owner and the animal.

CONCLUSION

Euthanasia is a skill that, like any other skill, must be well thought out and practiced. The entire veterinary team should be involved in a well-coordinated and professional manner. Euthanasia, if performed poorly, can be a disastrous experience for both the client and the veterinary practice. If performed with practiced care and gentle concern, it can be remembered positively for a long time.

RECOMMENDED READING

Arluke A: Coping with euthanasia: a case study of shelter culture, *J Am Vet Med Assoc* 198:1176, 1991.

AVMA Council on Research: Council report: report of the AVMA panel on euthanasia, *J Am Vet Med Assoc* 188:253, 1986.

Fogle B, Abrahamson D: Pet loss: attitudes and feelings of practicing veterinarians, *Anthrozoos* 3:143, 1990.

Grier RL, Schaffer CB: Evaluation of intraperitoneal and intrahepatic administration of a euthanasia agent in animal shelter cats, *J Am Vet Med Assoc* 197:1611, 1990.

Hart LA, Hart BL, Mader B: Humane euthanasia and companion animal death: caring for the animal, the client, and the veterinarian, *J Am Vet Med Assoc* 197:1292, 1990.

Kay WJ: Euthanasia, *Trends* 1:52, 1985.

Kogure N, Yamazaki K: Attitudes to animal euthanasia in Japan: a brief review of cultural influences, *Anthrozoos* 3:151, 1990.

Peters TG: Commander, *JAMA* 260:1460, 1988.

Randolph JW: Learning from your own pet's euthanasia, *J Am Vet Med Assoc* 205:544, 1994.

Tannenbaum J: *Veterinary ethics*, Baltimore, 1989, Williams & Wilkins, p 208.

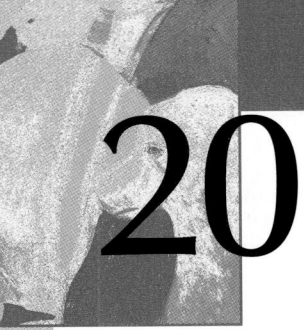

20

Client Bereavement and the Human-Animal Bond

Joseph Taboada • Stephanie W. Johnson • Katie M. Underwood

Today, with more than 58 million families owning one or more companion animals,* pets are considered part of the extended family network. Surveys and clinical experience indicate that many people consider their pets to be like children, partners, or best friends. Because of changing family structure and an increasing number of people who live alone, companion animals have taken on larger roles in people's support systems. With these changes have come added expectations of veterinary health care professionals. Members of the veterinary medical profession must realize that they are not treating just dogs, cats, birds, rabbits, or horses but important members of their clients' family and an important part of their clients' support system (Figure 20-1).

THE HUMAN-ANIMAL BOND

Today modern society is largely urban rather than rural. Through world urbanization, people tend to live in neighborhoods rather than on farms. Animals live with their owners in apartments or houses, thus increasing familiarity, dependency, and bonding.

Technician Note

Many people consider their pets to be like children.

Companion animals provide both parents and children with stability, constancy, and security. It is not unusual for families to change locales and residences several times within a 10-year period. As a result most people no longer live within a short distance of their extended families. The nuclear family is smaller, consisting of an average of less

than two children. The single-parent family is becoming common. Because an increasing number of U.S. women work outside the home, many school-age children return home to be greeted not by their mother but by the family pet. An increasing number of adults live alone and couples opt to remain childless. More and more people are filling these voids with pets, who provide a unique outlet for their owners' needs to nurture and be loved. As health and medical care improves, the number of people in the age-group older than 60 years has increased to nearly 25% of the population. Pets fulfill many needs for elderly people, including needs for interaction, exercise, companionship, protection, and motivation to remain active and independent.

It is becoming increasingly recognized that physically and mentally disabled individuals benefit from contact with animals. As society has realized the special talents of pets, new utilitarian functions have been found for them. Dogs are used with success to assist blind, hearing impaired, and physically challenged persons. These specially trained animals provide their owners with independence, companionship, social lubrication, protection, and love. Horses, cats, and dogs have been used successfully in animal-assisted therapy programs for people with all types of physical and mental disabilities. Animals facilitate interaction with people who may be reluctant to interact, and their presence reduces anxiety, lowers blood pressure, and decreases heart rate. Results of some studies indicate that animals may alleviate or prevent depression. Survival rates for cardiac patients who are pet owners are higher than for those who do not own pets. In fact, pet ownership is considered an important predictor of survival for patients with coronary artery disease.

In short, the relationships between people and animals have become physically closer, and the role of animals in the daily lives of their owners has become more emotional as society has changed. Of the more than 58 million families owning at least one pet, 87% describe their pets as

*1996 American Pet Products Manufacturers Association, National Pet Owners Survey.

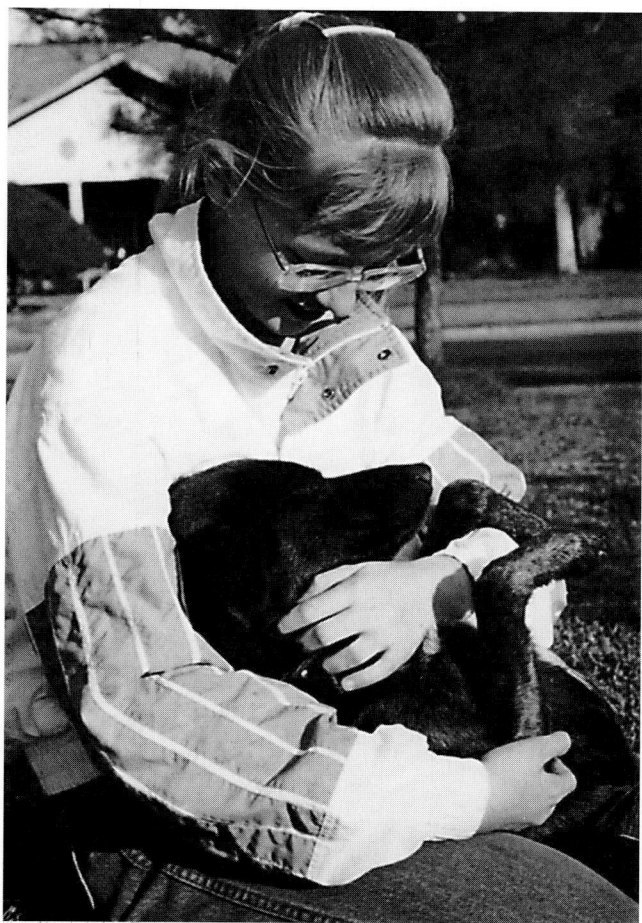

FIGURE 20-1. Pets have become important members of the extended family network. They provide tactile contact that can be important for young and old people alike.

family members and cite companionship, love, and friendship as the most important derivatives of the relationship. Further, it has been shown that 99% of pet owners talk to their pets; 65% buy them treats; 60% treat them as children; and 60% allow them to sleep on or near the family bed.

The Attachment Between Animals and Humans

Strong attachments can form between owners and any type of animal but are probably recognized most commonly in veterinary practice with dogs, cats, and horses. The degree of attachment varies greatly from the utilitarian attachment between a rancher and his or her cattle to the parent/child type of bonding that occurs between some people and their dog or cat. During the 1990s the cat supplanted the dog (59 million) as the most popular pet in the United States, with more than 75 million being owned.* It has recently been estimated that about 50% of these cat owners classify their attachment to their pet as strong. Of these "strong attachment" owners, about half see their cats as reflections of themselves or of their tastes who depend on the owner for love, affection, and care. The other half of the

_____

*2000 Pet Food Institute, Washington, D.C.

"strong attachment" owners report a reliance on their cats as an emotional crutch, supplying unconditional love and affection and sometimes acting as a substitute for family, friends, or children.

As pets are used to meet many of the changing psychosocial needs of modern society, the intensity of attachment has increased. When pet loss occurs, intensity and duration of attachment determine the significance of the loss and intensity of grief that follows. Attachment is more intense when the animal has functioned in many roles for the owner. The owner of an assistance dog may therefore suffer more intense bereavement than the owner of a dog used only for herding or hunting. Owners who have experienced previous significant losses, adjustments, or traumas and have been comforted by their pet's presence may also exhibit strong attachment and thus intense bereavement.

Benefits of Attachment

As reminders of both pleasant and traumatic events in people's lives, pets can take on symbolic meaning. There are several keys that are helpful in assessing the level of attachment between an owner and their animal or animals (Box 20-1). Even when the pet is simply another family member, grief can be intense. Grief is also very individual, and each family member may grieve in a unique way.

CASE EXAMPLE

Sneaky, a 12-year-old female domestic short hair cat, is brought into the clinic for lethargy and anorexia. After a work-up he is diagnosed as having cardiomyopathy. Even with appropriate treatment, the prognosis for a long lifetime is poor.

Sneaky is owned by a 73-year-old widow named Ruth. The cat was a gift from her husband, Ralph, who died of cancer 2 years earlier. During her husband's fight against the disease, Sneaky was his constant companion. Ruth can still vividly remember how Sneaky, as a kitten, used to make her husband laugh by hiding in his boots and jumping out at him when he leaned down to pick them up.

Sneaky was brought to the veterinarian for what was perceived to be a minor problem, but a severe, life-threatening disease was diagnosed. Ruth is likely to feel numb initially. The diagnosis is likely to be hard to accept. An important part of Ruth's attachment to Sneaky comes from her relationship with her late husband. Sneaky represents a tangible link between Ruth's life now and the many memories of her life with her husband. Not only is Sneaky's death going to be hard because of the loss of a faithful companion/family member, but it is also going to bring back many of the emotions that were associated with the death of her husband.

  Technician Note

If a pet is associated with an important person or significant life stage or event, it can take on added significance.

PET LOSS AND VETERINARY MEDICINE

Veterinarians and veterinary technicians are confronted daily with complex issues of attachment, loss, and grief in the course of their patients' illness and death. The diagnosis of life-threatening or terminal disease can be a difficult time for both the client and the veterinary professional (Figure 20-2). Considering all the emotional and utilitarian aspects of the human-animal relationship in modern society, it is not surprising that the breaking of the bond

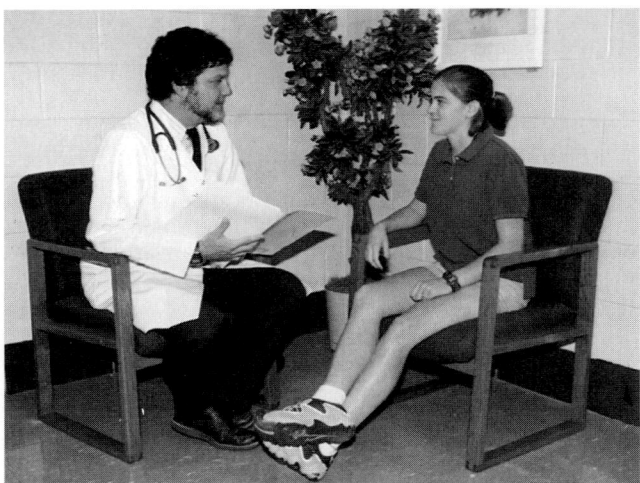

FIGURE 20-2. The diagnosis of a disease can be a difficult time for both clients and veterinary professionals.

BOX 20-1	KEYS TO ATTACHMENT

The levels of attachment are different for each pet and owner. Human-animal relationships may be perceived as stronger and more important when the following aspects are present:

- Owners believe they rescued their companion animals from death or near death.
- Owners believe that their companion animals got them through a difficult period in life.
- Owners spent their childhoods with their companion animals.
- Owners have relied on their companion animals as their most significant source of support.
- Owners anthropomorphize their companion animals.
- Owners have invested extensive time, effort, or financial resources into their companion animals' long-term medical care.
- Owners view their companion animals as symbolic links to significant people who are no longer part of their lives or to significant times in their lives.

---

because of the death of the pet is a significant event in the lives of many pet owners. The loss of the pet for many owners is made even more intense and personal in that the pet is often grieved by no one other than themselves. Daily routines are filled with reminders of activities once performed for or with the pet. The loss of a pet often means that a unique, irreplaceable member of the family is gone.

Technician Note

Veterinary technicians are confronted daily with complex issues of attachment, loss, and grief.

A person's support system is made up of people (and pets) that interact with one another on a daily basis, providing support, comfort, and social interaction. Support systems are especially important during times of loss. Unfortunately, many people who make up these support systems do not understand the full extent of attachment

between a pet owner and pet. This lack of understanding can present serious problems for the owner facing the odyssey of grief after the death of a pet. As a result, pet owners often turn to veterinary professionals as sources of support, comfort, and understanding at and around the time of their pet's death.

Technician Note

People tend to turn to the veterinary staff during grief over a pet because they feel the veterinary technician understands their attachment and loss.

The tendency for people to turn to the veterinary staff during the period of grieving the death of a pet places veterinary professionals in an awkward position, however. It demands that they have knowledge that is typically outside the boundaries of traditional veterinary medicine and requires that they find a comfort level in talking about death and the grief process. This is why the areas of attachment, animal behavior, human bereavement, and grief counseling are becoming increasingly relevant to veterinary medicine.

WHEN THE BOND IS BROKEN

In general people in U.S. society are uncomfortable talking about death. We know little about the experience of death, and we fear the unknown, yet veterinarians and their staff must frequently discuss death, participate in causing it, witness it, and deal with the emotions triggered by these experiences.

Although people in the midst of grief have a need and a right to understand what is happening to them, there are few places they can go to get helpful, supportive information about grief. This is particularly true when the loss they are grieving is that of a beloved pet. Like most of society, veterinarians and veterinary technicians rarely have formal training in this area. Despite this fact, veterinary professionals are still often the people clients instinctively turn to for support.

Making the job more difficult is the fact that grief and bereavement are emotional and often irrational areas of human interaction. Bereaved individuals may at times seem out of control or out of touch with reality. When this happens, those around the griever, including the veterinary professional, may feel uncomfortable; few veterinary professionals are taught how to support or deal with people who are irrational or emotional. Compassion is an important sensitivity to draw on when interacting with clients experiencing grief.

Grief is the companion to death. It is the mental anguish experienced by any human confronted with the loss of an object of attachment. Grief may ensue as an effect of any loss; the loss may be through death, divorce, loss of a job, or even moving or having friends move away. It can be intensely emotional and can affect mind, body, and spirit. When confronted with grief, the bereaved individual goes through a grief process. The term *grief process* implies that there is an intended end or result to be produced through grieving. Thus the grief process is the means of letting go of the object of attachment to feel better, reinvest, emotionally grow, and attach again.

The veterinary staff is in a unique position to assist clients going through the process of grief as it relates to the loss of a pet. By way of their unique role in the life of both the owner and pet, veterinary professionals are in a unique position to understand the bond that had developed. In addition, the veterinarian and the owner may have interacted uniquely in choosing the time of the pet's death (as occurs when euthanasia is performed). To assist clients during the difficult bereavement period, it is helpful to understand the normal grief process and the manifestations of it as applied to pet loss.

Pet Loss and the Grief Process

The death of a pet is all too often regarded as a trivial loss by society, perhaps in part because of the mistaken belief that pets can be easily replaced. There are no socially sanctioned rituals, such as funerals or memorial services, to help grieving pet owners gain support once the bonds between them and their animals have been broken. Further, people are rarely granted time off from their jobs to care for sick animals or to make arrangements for them after their deaths. Society also does not allow adequate time for mourning the death of a pet. Most people feel pressured to be "back to normal" within a few days of their pet's death to avoid being labeled as neurotic, hysteric, or overly attached. However, crying, taking time away from work, and wanting to memorialize a pet are healthy responses to the death of a pet. They should not be discouraged, nor should they be judged.

One of the most effective ways for veterinary professionals to assist grieving clients is to educate and reassure them that their feelings and behaviors are normal parts of the grief process. Other ways that veterinary professionals can help are listed in Box 20-2.

Technician Note

Veterinary professionals can assist clients by normalizing their feelings.

The Normal Grief Process

As stated earlier, the word *process* implies movement toward some end or result. In regard to grief, this movement is accomplished by passing through what have been termed *stages*, *phases*, or *tasks*. Although there are a few differences, the basic emotional process in pet loss is the same as in human loss.

Several models of the grief process can be modified to describe the emotional process that occurs during pet loss. the following discussion uses the classic model supplied by Elisabeth Kübler-Ross (see Recommended Reading).

Dr. Kübler-Ross was one of the first to work extensively with dying persons and their families during the late 1960s. She described the grief process as consisting of five stages: denial, bargaining, anger, depression, and resolution. She used the stages to describe the passage through grief, but it is helpful to remember that these stages are not a linear odyssey. Although people may travel through the grief process in a straight line, they more often fluctuate between stages, bounce back and forth, and feel the entire gamut of grief within minutes, days, or months.

Technician Note

The grief process consists of five stages: denial, bargaining, anger, depression, and resolution.

Denial and Bargaining

Denial is a normal defense mechanism that buffers humans from some unbearable news or reality. It is important to recognize the word "normal" here, because many individuals experiencing denial at the time a poor prognosis is given or during bereavement will seem to all observers to be out of touch with reality. The veterinary staff may wonder whether the client has even heard the veterinarian stating the seriousness of an animal's illness. A client in denial may listen attentively to a diagnosis of cancer with a poor prognosis but ask only if the toenails can be clipped or if their current flea shampoo is correct. A client informed of the death of his or her pet while it was hospitalized may chatter on about activities for the weekend. A simple form of denial is exemplified by the client who states repeatedly, "It can't be. I don't believe it."

It is tempting when presented with a client experiencing denial to insist that he or she recognize the seriousness of the situation. Many veterinarians and veterinary technicians worry that the client does not comprehend or has not heard correctly. There is no harm in repeating oneself to a client in denial (Figure 20-3). In fact, restating diagnoses, prognoses, treatment plans, and particulars is advisable. However, clients in denial will accept the unbearable reality of the situation only when they are ready internally; attempts to push them may backfire, resulting in frustration. Usually, a client will begin to ask appropriate questions about the time he or she arrives home and may telephone the veterinary office. Some may even seem to return to reality before your eyes while those toenails are being attended to. The veterinary professional must feel assured that the client has been told the basic information that needs to be given. Remember, however, that it may not have been fully understood; therefore always leave the door open for further communication.

Denial is reflected by the client's eyes and demeanor and by incongruous questions. The veterinary staff should not feel responsible to "break through" a client's denial. The client will move out of denial, accepting the reality of the situation, when he or she is ready. The veterinary staff's recognition of the client's denial can prevent impatience and frustration during the veterinary contact.

CASE STUDY

Captain, a 9-year-old boxer, is brought into the clinic for a check-up and vaccinations. His owner, Don, tells you that 1 year ago Captain was treated for lymphosarcoma. The cancer went into remission, and Captain has been doing fine ever since. However, it is obvious to you that Captain is not feeling very well.

The examination shows the cancer has returned. It takes Don some time to accept that fact. It is agreed that treatment should start up again immediately. After a lack of response to a rescue phase of chemotherapy, it is realized that Captain's death is imminent. When the news is given to Don he insists over and over again that the treatment should be continued. "If it worked before, it will work again just keep on trying." If the treatment really is not working, Don believes changing Captain's diet to one he read about on the Internet will have better results.

Don brought Captain in for a routine examination. It was immediately obvious to you that Captain was not feeling well. However, Don either could not recognize any of the symptoms or was denying that Captain was sick again. Despite the fact that Don went into the initial treatment protocol knowing relapse was eventually inevitable, he still exhibits signs of denial. It is also obvious he is not ready to accept Captain's impending death. It is important to realize Don's response is a normal part of the grief process. He will not be able to understand the seriousness of the situation until he is ready. Don also shows signs of bargaining when he wants other treatment options to be explored even though it is clear nothing can be done to save Captain at this point.

BOX 20-2   STAGES OF GRIEF: HOW VETERINARY PROFESSIONALS CAN HELP

DENIAL

What the client needs most is time, support, understanding, and permission to grieve.

Before Death

- Arrange to communicate with the client in person, if possible, where you both can sit down to talk without interruption or distraction. Recognize denial as a normal part of grief.
- Communicate clearly, and reiterate patiently. Phrase statements in words that are concrete and simple for the layperson. Avoid using medical jargon and lapsing into complicated medical explanations.
- Listen actively: maintain eye contact, use attentive body language, and paraphrase or clarify the client's statements as you respond. Give him or her permission to express feelings.
- Give the client time to think about and to grasp the reality of information that has been given. Some clients need only a slight pause in the conversation or a few minutes alone. Other clients may need more time to themselves before they comprehend the news of severe illness or actual death.
- Refrain from judging the client as "stupid" or "out of it."
- Remain nonjudgmental and unhurried toward the client, and state that you are available to talk about specifics or about his or her feelings whenever the time is right.
- *Never* attempt to force clients to "come to their senses" or to move out of denial. Clients will comprehend at their own pace.

After Death

- Encourage the client to view the body and say goodbye.
- Give permission to grieve.

BARGAINING

- Understand that bargaining is an attempt to control or reverse a dire situation. The client feels irrationally compelled to bargain during the grief process and does not mean to doubt the professionals involved.
- When the patient is terminally ill, do not become defensive or threatened when clients ask for other opinions or consider alternative treatments. Giving information, readings, and referral for second opinion will ameliorate bargaining attempts and facilitate commitment to treatment.
- After the death, be empathetic and educative about the stage of bargaining when clients confide their feelings and bargaining behaviors, such as prayers and dreams (or daydreams) of the pet still alive. Reassure them that the emotional basis for their behaviors and feelings is normal even though it may seem irrational.
- When clients inquire as to when to "replace" their pet, educating them about the role bargaining plays in shopping for a new pet can alleviate future disappointment. State that their dead pet was unique and cannot be replaced, but encourage them to obtain a new pet whenever all members of the family feel ready. Help them to find the type of animal they are looking for while gently steering toward one that is slightly dissimilar to the dead pet. Encourage them to choose a different breed, color, or gender, and a new name should be chosen.

ANGER

- Listen actively, and let the client know that you understand.
- Arrange for communication in a private room with no distractions. Sit at eye level, and use attentive body language. Take notes if the client is complaining or criticizing.
- Give the client permission to vent feelings. Listen actively using attentive body language, eye contact, nodding, and responses that paraphrase, clarify, and indicate your understanding of the client's feelings. (Example: "I can see that you're very angry. . . ." or "You feel that diagnosis could have been made sooner. . . .")
- If the client is directly angry at the veterinarian, technician, or clinic staff, take a mental step backward, and pause with either a deep breath or by counting to 10.
- *Do not become defensive or respond in like manner* to the client.
- Relieve guilt by assuring the client that he or she did the right thing and what he or she is feeling is a normal part of the grief process.

DEPRESSION

- Encourage depressed clients to talk about their feelings in regard to their pet. Follow up clients whose pets have died with a telephone call in a few days and then 2 weeks afterward.
- Listen actively.
- Attend to the client by positioning yourself at eye level, offering tissues or a drink of water, and leaning slightly toward the client. A nonthreatening yet compassionate touch on the forearm or on the shoulder communicates empathy and understanding.
- Offer a place to sit, a place to be out of the "public eye."
- Tell the client that it is all right, and even good, to cry. Listen supportively and actively, and touch the client gently on the shoulder or forearm. Some clients are known well enough to embrace, and this can be helpful as well.
- Validate the feelings of sadness by letting the client know that it is normal.
- Offer to call a family member or friend.
- Encourage and suggest means by which clients can memorialize their pet. Making scrapbooks, planting a tree, writing a letter to the pet, or writing the pet's life story all are cathartic activities that alleviate depression caused by grief.
- If a client expresses continued depression several weeks following the death of a pet, if his or her support system is poor, or if a client expresses a personal wish to die, referral to a compassionate professional counselor is necessary. Although referral may feel awkward, many clients appreciate the technician who states, "Grief as a result of pet loss is normal, but sometimes there can be no one to talk to, or the grief can be overwhelming. I know of a person who understands what you're going through. Would you like her (his) telephone number, or may I have her (him) call you?" Today, several schools of veterinary medicine employ counselors experienced in pet loss. Many communities have established support groups, and private counselors increasingly view pet loss as significant bereavement.*

RESOLUTION

- Acceptance is achieved once the above four stages have fallen into the background of the client's life. At this point, the bereaved person can channel emotional energy into a new relationship. The veterinary professional can help clients reach the resolution stage by offering insight into the grief process through his or her actions and by offering suggestions of reading material or seminars on the grief process.

---

*For a complete list of referral counselors or for a referral, write the Delta Society (Box 20-3).

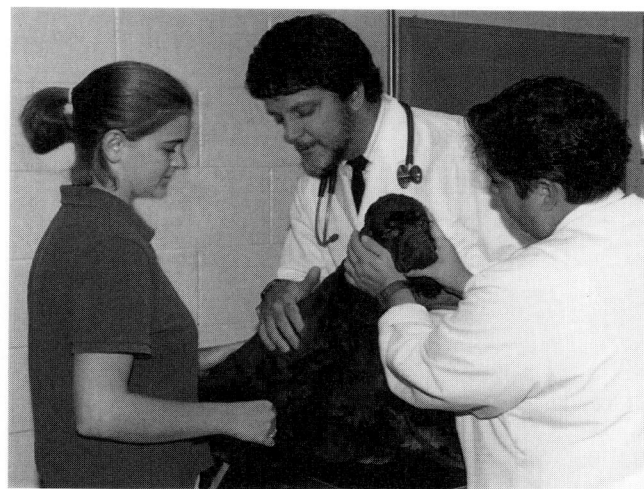

FIGURE 20-3. Even when dealing with attentive clients, veterinary professionals may be required to repeat themselves several times while clients decide on a course of treatment for their pet.

Technician Note

During denial the veterinary professional should repeat things without becoming frustrated or impatient.

Once the reality of death or impending death is realized, the client may show various impotent attempts to control or to reverse the reality. The client is grappling with the stage of the grief process that Dr. Kübler-Ross called *bargaining.* During this stage, the client maneuvers personally and privately, possibly praying and negotiating with God for miracles. The client might add various herbs and old family remedies to food. Children behave like little angels, hoping to be rewarded with a reversal of bad news. The veterinary staff may be subject to various inquiries by the client at this stage, relative to the latest "miracle cure" that the client has discovered on the Internet. It is while bargaining that a pet owner may also request permission to obtain a second (and sometimes third, fourth, or fifth) opinion. During this time be compassionate and when possible answer clients' questions. Help clients to understand that this stage of grief is normal.

Seeking to replace the lost animal without grieving at all is a form of bargaining. Many pet owners seek a new pet too soon, and they purchase the same species, the same color, and name them the same or a similar name.

It is important to recognize denial and bargaining as part of the normal grief process. Veterinary professionals who understand these stages will avoid frustration in their attempts to provide quality patient care and client service.

Anger

During the grief process, clients may move in and out of the stage called *anger.* Clients coping with this stage may exhibit anger in a wide variety of direct or indirect manners. The anger may be specific or nonspecific in the way that it is directed. Anger may also be exhibited in the form of guilt, which can be defined as anger turned inward.

Anger is a particularly difficult emotion to deal with when a client directs it toward the veterinary professional. Regardless of whether or not the client is justified in his or her stated cause for anger, staff members must use toler-ance and patience to avoid responding defensively. Bereaved clients may complain that the illness that resulted in death should have been discovered sooner, should have been treated differently, or should not have been allowed to happen. They may complain that their pet died while hospitalized because of neglect or inappropriate treatment rather than because of the tumor revealed by necropsy.

Anger may be apparent in the form of guilt. Clients feeling guilt use language with an abundance of "I should've" statements. They often seek the listening ear of the veterinary professional looking for absolution from guilt. They may ask whether the food they fed their pet could have contributed to the illness or death. They often ask whether it was the pesticide in their home or in the shampoo that caused a tumor or cardiac arrest. Clients may believe they allowed their pet to be too active or too fat; others may believe they caused the kidney failure in their cat by feeding an insufficient diet. These clients can direct anger at themselves, but frequently they cannot find a specific crime that they committed. When possible, the veterinary professional can assist the clients by assuaging their guilt. Reassuring clients that, in your opinion, they did everything possible for their pet, that they did only what they thought would benefit their pet, and that they made the right decisions for their pet will relieve much of the clients' guilt or anger and assist them in moving through the grief process.

Technician Note

Veterinary professionals can help by reassuring clients that they did everything possible and made the right decisions.

The client in this stage may be gruff or rude and generally hard to get along with. Stating that he or she is angry, the client may be at a loss to express the object of the anger. These clients may yell at the cashiers, the hospital manager, the receptionist, and the technicians, as well as the veterinarian. Giving the angry client an opportunity to express feelings (venting) is an effective way for the veterinary professional to help. At times, all that is needed is for the sensitive veterinary professional to explain that, considering the client's loss, anger is a normal feeling.

Anger is often exhibited by reluctance to pay the bill. On receiving an inquiry by telephone, the client implies that nonpayment is due to anger at treatment by the veterinarian or technician, the pet being neglected, the illness being mistreated, or the client being treated insensitively. Bereavement support can alleviate this client's anger. Listen attentively, state your apologies, if any, and follow up with this client. No admission of mistakes need be made, but the client needs to feel significant and understood.

Anger is difficult to work through, but it is guilt that may be hardest for the client to relinquish. In continuing to feel guilt and anger, the client avoids letting go of the beloved pet, and the grief process is stymied. Once the client is able to relinquish the guilt or anger, the grief process can continue.

The veterinary professional can assist the client with all types of exhibited anger by taking a mental step back and a deep breath, committing to a nondefensive attitude, and simply listening. Take notes if possible, and reassure the client of follow-up if anger is directed at veterinary staff. Assuage any guilt if the opportunity arises, and allow the client to vent. A few minutes on the telephone or in person may salvage a client relationship and go a long way in assisting the client through the grief process.

John brings Sparky, a 3-year-old Dalmatian, into the clinic. Sparky got out of the yard this afternoon because the gate was left open. He ran across the street and was hit by a car. His spine is fractured, and there is severe injury to his spinal cord. There is also a substantial amount of internal bleeding.

John is informed that Sparky has only a slim chance of surviving surgery. He elects for any measure to be taken regardless of cost. Unfortunately Sparky dies during the procedure. When you tell John, he immediately begins yelling at you, "How dare you let Sparky die? There must have been something else that could have been done!" He then refuses to pay the bill and storms out of the clinic.

The next day John calls and apologizes for his rude outburst. He lets you know that he realizes that every measure was taken to save Sparky. He also admits to feeling guilty for having left the gate open. Then he requests that the bill be mailed to him.

John is expressing his anger over Sparky's death, which should be recognized as a stage of grief. Although John initially expressed his anger at you, it should not be taken personally. It is not necessarily directed at you. You should not react defensively but instead listen politely and let John know that you empathize and understand. Realize that part of his anger may come from guilt that he left the gate open.

His call on the following day emphasizes that anger can be an uncomfortable but transient part of the grief process. He admits his anger was not really because of you. He attributes it to his feelings of guilt.

Depression

The stage of the grief process that is termed *depression* has also been called *grief*. Clients experiencing depression describe their mood as complete, overwhelming sadness. Intense grief can result in depression, which prohibits a client from functioning normally. Appetite is changed, energy level is lowered, the client withdraws from others, and sometimes the client is unable to go to work. More subtle symptoms of depression include irritability, sleep irregularity, restlessness, and inability to concentrate.

Technician Note

Depression has been described as complete, overwhelming sadness.

The veterinary professional has occasion to recognize depression as a result of pet loss when follow-up contacts are made with the client. Depression, when severe, usually sets in some time after the loss. Clients with poor social support systems, elderly clients, and clients with intense or symbolic attachment to the pet may experience worrisome depression. When contacts are made several days or weeks after bereavement and it is suspected that a client is depressed, referral can be made to a counselor or hotline specializing in pet loss (Box 20-3). Although referral sometimes is awkward, it might be gently phrased as, "I know a person experienced in counseling people who have lost their pets." Again, reassurance that grief is normal is beneficial.

Technician Note

If severe depression is suspected, referral can be made to a counselor or hotline.

Most clients experience the feeling of being overwhelmed by their emotions because of grief. They describe feeling as if their emotions are out of control. They may also state surprise and worry that they are reacting with such intensity to the death of an animal. They may be embarrassed. It comforts clients when veterinary professionals confide that most pet owners feel and act similarly on the loss of a pet. Assuring them of your knowledge of their pet's importance as well as your respect for their grief is valuable to them.

Grief must be worked through, not avoided; thus it is a process requiring some emotional catharsis. Many clients cry, and some are uninhibited about expressing anger and sadness. Becoming comfortable with one's own emotions facilitates comfort with others' emotions. It is human and necessary to feel empathy for grieving clients, but it can also be uncomfortable and painful. Separating your own feelings from theirs will allow you to transform empathy into sympathetic gestures that help the client.

Two weeks ago Micah brought her 10-year-old barrel racing horse, Lightning, to the clinic. Lightning had colic. Every possible remedy was explored; however, Lightning had to be euthanized. Micah was extremely distraught over the loss of Lightning, whom she described as "the other half of my soul."

You have a couple of free minutes so you decide to call and see how Micah is doing. Micah is still very upset about the loss of Lightning. She says that she has no desire to ever barrel race again and cannot even stand to go to the barn to visit the other horses. She also tells you that she has not been eating or sleeping well. Her parents and friends all think she is overreacting. At that Micah begins to cry and immediately apologizes. You respond, "It's okay. I know Lightning was very special to you. It is normal to still be grieving. I know of someone who specializes in pet loss counseling. Would you like her phone number?"

If you had not taken the time to call, Micah's depression might have gone unnoticed. Many times clients suffer through depression feeling alone. Depression may occur on and off during the entire grief process. Micah also explained to you that support was not available from her friends and family. It is important to follow up on clients who have poor support systems or who are very attached to their animals like Micah was. Referral to a professional counselor can be of great assistance in helping clients such as Micah in resolving the grief process.

Technician Note

Follow-up is important for those clients with poor support systems or unusual attachments.

Resolution or Acceptance

The stage of *resolution or acceptance* is the feeling that everything is okay, normal functioning is restored, and emotional energy is reinvested. This does not mean that the pet is forgotten but that it has been assigned to a special place in the bereaved individual's heart. New attachments can be made without regret and hesitation. Resolution may come easily for some and may be difficult for others. In general, children reach the stage of acceptance and resolution more quickly and more easily than do adults. (For more information on how to help children when a pet dies, see Box 20-4.) As stated previously, the grief process is not linear, and bits of this stage occur with more and more

Box 20-3 PLACES TO CONTACT FOR HELP OR REFERRAL SOURCES FOR CLIENTS NEEDING HELP WITH GRIEF

The Delta Society
ATTN: Librarian
289 Perimeter Road East
Renton, WA 98055-1329
Telephone: (206) 226-7357
(can be contacted for a list of referral sources in your area)
www.deltasociety.org

Veterinary Grief Counseling Hotlines
Companion Animal Association of Arizona, Inc.
Pet Grief Support Service
P.O. Box 5006
Scottsdale, AZ 85006
Telephone: (602) 995-5885

Pet Loss Support Hotline
Center for Animals in Society
School of Veterinary Medicine
University of California–Davis
Telephone: (530) 752-4200 or (800) 565-1526
(staffed by University of California–Davis veterinary students; weekdays, 6:30 PM to 9:30 PM PT)

The Chicago Veterinary Medical Association Pet Loss Support Hotline
Telephone: (630) 603-3994
(staffed by Chicago VMA veterinarians and staff; voice mail will be returned collect daily between 6 PM and 9 PM ET)

Pet Loss Support Hotline
College of Veterinary Medicine
Cornell University
Telephone: (607) 253-3932
(staffed by Cornell University veterinary students; voice mail messages will be returned within 24 hr)

Pet Loss Support Hotline
College of Veterinary Medicine
University of Florida
Telephone: (352) 392-4700; then dial 1 and 4080
(staffed by University of Florida veterinary students; weekdays, 7 PM to 9 PM ET)

Pet Loss Support Hotline
College of Veterinary Medicine
Michigan State University, G100
Telephone: (517) 432-2696
(staffed by Michigan State University veterinary students; Tuesday to Thursday, 6:30 PM to 9:30 PM ET)

Pet Loss Support Hotline
University of Illinois
College of Veterinary Medicine
Telephone: (217) 244-2273 or (877) 394-2273
(staffed by Illinois College of Veterinary students)

Pet Loss Support Hotline
Iowa State University
College of Veterinary Medicine
Telephone: (888) 478-7574
(staffed by Iowa State University veterinary students and community volunteers)

Pet Loss Support Hotline
Michigan State University
College of Veterinary Medicine
Telephone: (517) 432-2696
(staffed by Michigan State University veterinary students)

Pet Loss Support Hotline
Washington State University
College of Veterinary Medicine
Telephone: (509) 335-5704
(staffed by Washington State University veterinary students)

Pet Loss Support Hotline
College of Veterinary Medicine
The Ohio State University
Telephone: (614) 292-1823
(staffed by The Ohio State University veterinary students; Monday, Wednesday, and Friday, 6:30 PM to 9:30 PM ET)
E-mail: petloss@osu.edu

Virginia-Maryland Regional College of Veterinary Medicine
Virginia Tech
Telephone: (540) 231-8038
(staffed by Virginia-Maryland Regional College of Veterinary Medicine; Tuesday and Thursday, 6 PM to 9 PM ET)

School of Veterinary Medicine
Tufts University
Telephone: (508) 839-7966
(staffed by Tufts University veterinary students; Tuesday and Thursday 6 PM to 9 PM ET; voice mail messages will be returned collect daily)

Veterinary Schools and Colleges with Grief Counseling Programs
University of California
School of Veterinary Medicine
Center for Animals in Society
Davis, CA 95616
Telephone: (916) 752-4200

Colorado State University, Veterinary Teaching Hospital
CHANGES: The Support for People and Pets Program
300 West Drake Rd.
Fort Collins, CO 80523
Telephone: (970) 491-1242

Louisiana State University
School of Veterinary Medicine
The Best Friend Gone Project
Baton Rouge, LA 70809
Telephone: (225) 346-5710
E-mail: friendgone@vetmed.lsu.edu

University of Pennsylvania
School of Veterinary Medicine
3800 Spruce St.
Philadelphia, PA 19104-6044
Telephone: (215) 898-5438

Tufts University School of Veterinary Medicine
Center for Animals and Public Policy
200 Westboro Rd.
North Grafton, MA 01536
Telephone: (508) 839-7991

Washington State University
College of Veterinary Medicine
People-Pet Partnership
Pullman, WA 99164-7010
Telephone: (509) 335-4569

University of Wisconsin
School of Veterinary Medicine
Pet Loss Support Group
2015 Linden Dr.
Madison, WI 53706
Telephone: (608) 836-7297

BOX 20-4 | **HOW TO HELP CHILDREN WHEN A PET DIES**

When children's companion animals die, many parents follow their instincts to protect them from pain and grief. Some parents make decisions regarding the pet without discussing them with their children. Some may even lie to their children about the actual circumstances of the pet's "disappearance," preferring to tell them that a beloved pet ran away or was stolen rather than died. These tactics are not used maliciously by parents. They develop from a desire to spare children feelings of pain and from a belief that the parents, as parents, are inadequately prepared to discuss loss, death, and grief with their children.

Children, however, are tuned into their parents' emotions and, almost without exception, know that *something* is going on in the family. They don't know what that *something* is, but they do know that it upsets Mom and Dad. Consequently, children may feel anxious, confused, left out, and even guilty because, without honest explanations of a family crisis, children often believe that they are somehow responsible for the tension level in the home. At later ages, children may also feel betrayed by the parents they trusted when they discover the truth about their childhood pet's disappearance.

The knowledge, skills, and tools for dealing with loss and grief that are developed in childhood are the same ones used in adolescence and adulthood. It is of utmost importance, then, that children be given honest support and information about loss and death so their grief-coping strategies will be healthy, rather than unhealthy, ones.

HOW TECHNICIANS CAN HELP

Parents will often turn to veterinary professionals for assistance in telling their children about the death of a pet. Having books available for them to read and having information yourself to share can help ease an otherwise traumatic situation. Here are some suggestions:

- Always encourage parents to be honest with their children throughout a companion animal's illness, treatment, and death. Never agree to participate in a lie that the parents may want to tell their children to protect them. In the long run, lies create more problems for everyone involved and can be more damaging to children than the pet's death itself.

- Children under the age of 8 yr do not really understand that death is final. They may believe that a dead pet can return or that they will need food in their grave with them. Young children are also egocentric and believe quite strictly in the law of cause and effect. Thus they may develop the idea that they did something to cause the pet's death. Therefore they must be reassured repeatedly that the pet died because it had a disease or an accident or was very old.

- Straightforward explanations and concrete words such as *dead* and *died* should be used when talking to children about death. Young children do not understand euphemisms and can become upset when they hear terms such as *put to sleep*. Since they go to sleep every night and do not want to die like their pet did, attempts at softening the blow can actually make the situation more difficult and frightening for children.

- Children need to be held, reassured, and allowed to ask questions. Open communication about death is the desired atmosphere for keeping death anxiety manageable. Pets' names should be used in conversation whenever possible, and memories of them should be shared by the whole family. Older children should be included in the euthanasia process, the memorial ceremonies, and the goodbye rituals to whatever extent they wish to be and should be encouraged to demonstrate their sensitivity and compassion.

- It is always helpful to contact children's teachers, care providers, relatives, and other significant adults so they can help acknowledge the loss and grief process. Adults may observe children playing funeral or overhear them talking to friends about a pet's death. Although these activities may seem alarming and even morbid to adults, they are normal, healthy responses for children. Children deal with issues through play and experimentation. Unless they are in physical danger, their activities do not in most cases require interference.

- For adult information about helping children deal with pet loss, consult the following books:

Balk DE: *Children and the death of a pet*, Manhattan, 1990, Cooperative Extension Service, Kansas State University.

Jewett CL: *Helping children cope with separation and loss*, Boston, 1982, Harvard Common Press.

Nieburg HA, Fischer A: *Pet loss: a thoughtful guide for adults and children*, New York, 1982, Harper & Row.

Quackenbush J, Graveline D: *When your pet dies: how to cope with your feelings*, New York, 1985, Simon & Schuster.

Shirl-Potter JW, Koss GJ: *Death of a pet: answers to questions for children and animal lovers of all ages*, Stamford, Conn, 1991, Guideline Publications.

Stein S: *About dying: an open family book for adults and children*, New York, 1974, Walker & Co.

- The following children's books that may be helpful in explaining the loss of a pet to children:

Brackenridge SS: *Because of flowers and dancers*, Santa Barbara, Calif, 1994, Veterinary Practice Publishing.

Morehead D: *A special place for Charlie*, Broomfield, Col, 1996, Partners in Publishing LLC.

Rylant C: *Dog heaven*, New York, 1995, The Blue Sky Press.

Viorst J: *The tenth good thing about Barney*, New York, 1971, Aladdin Books.

---

frequency and with longer durations throughout the grief process. Eventually, the client who successfully resolves the grief process feels little, if any, of the first four stages.

There are many factors that may complicate the grief process (Box 20-5). These complicating factors may lengthen the time it takes to reach resolution or, in severe cases, may arrest progress through the grief process without allowing the individual to reach a resolution. Situations in which the grief process is complicated may not affect some individuals' ability to progress but may drastically affect

that of others. Few veterinary professionals are equipped to give the special kind of help that these complicated situations may require, but most have empathy and the ability to listen for signs that indicate someone may need help. Early recognition of factors that may complicate the grief process can be helpful when a person appears not to be progressing well through the process. Early recognition may also be important for timely referral in situations in which further assistance is required. Keeping on hand a list of professional alternatives for referral to someone who

Box 20-5   FACTORS THAT MAY COMPLICATE THE GRIEF PROCESS

- Multiple losses occurring within a related time frame
- Loss of a pet that was associated with a special person or event
- Loss of a pet on a day that is important, such as a birthday or holiday
- Loss of a pet because of factors that may have been preventable
- Feelings of guilt about the death of a pet
- An inability to afford expensive care that was offered
- Loss of a pet because of an illness or situation that previously caused the loss of another pet
- Sudden illness or trauma resulting in loss
- Witnessing the violent or unnecessary death of a pet

- Disappearance of a pet
- Lack of explanation as to why a pet died
- Situations in which the person experiencing loss has little or no support
- Insensitive comments from others who may not understand the bond between owner and pet
- Getting incorrect or bad information concerning the loss of a pet and/or the grieving process
- No previous experience with grief
- Not being present at the time the pet dies or not having the opportunity to view the body
- Not being able to say goodbye

can give the help that is needed is advised (see Box 20-3 for a short list of potential sources of help).

The question is often raised whether clients should get a new pet before they reach resolution of the grief process. The process itself is highly variable in length. It can be as short as a few weeks to as long as many years. Most pet owners are able to reinvest and reattach to a new pet at any time but only after they become aware that replacement of their unique loved one is impossible. If companionship, tactile closeness, and friendship are desired while grieving, these qualities can be obtained through a new pet. Cautioning and encouraging clients to choose animals somewhat dissimilar to their dead pet can be helpful. Having a new pet forced on the grieving individual who is not ready to reinvest in a new relationship will only end up furthering heartache in the bereaved and causing unhappiness in the new pet.

GRIEF AND THE VETERINARY PROFESSIONAL

Individuals in the veterinary profession deal with client grief on an almost daily basis. Rarely do they think about their own, however. The veterinary professional must realize the grief process that the client is struggling with is not taking place in an emotional vacuum. It is real and touches not only the bereaved person but also those around him or her, including the veterinary professional. It is common for veterinarians and veterinary technicians to cry with clients, to feel a lump in the throat, and to feel guilty or depressed or experience a sense of failure. The fact that veterinary professionals may go through a grief process each time a patient is lost must be recognized and accepted. Time should be spent thinking about these feelings and responses. Validation of the process within the profession, by way of staff meetings, discussions, and support sessions, can be important in recognizing and dealing with the stresses of "professional grief." Left unacknowledged, the grief process encountered by veterinary professionals can become destructive and lead to burnout.

Technician Note

Left unacknowledged, the grief process encountered by veterinary professionals can become destructive.

CASE STUDY

Two months later Micah (the client in the previous case study) calls back to let you know how she is doing. She expresses gratitude for your concern and compassion while she was grieving over losing Lightning. In his memory, she has decided to donate Lightning's winnings from last year to the Colic Research Foundation. She has also made a memorial plaque with Lightning's shoe on it to hang on his stall door. She would like for you and the veterinarian to come out to the farm to examine the soundness of a horse, Blaze, that she thinks has barrel potential. She is beginning to realize that Lightning would like for her to ride again.

Micah is doing well. She has gone through the process of grieving over Lightning. By memorializing Lightning with the plaque, she has a special way to remember him. Through the donation, she is able to feel like both she and Lightning have made an important contribution to equine medicine. Micah experienced a degree of personal growth through the process of grieving. Resolution and acceptance for Micah are symbolized by focusing her emotional energy into potentially developing a relationship with Blaze. It is important that Lightning is not forgotten.

CONCLUSION

Grief and the grief process are difficult to deal with. Despite this difficulty, veterinary professionals are asked to deal with it on a daily basis. Veterinary professionals are rarely trained in the area of bereavement and the grief process, yet they are still often the best qualified individuals when it comes to helping clients who have recently lost a beloved pet. Understanding what the client is going through by understanding the basics of the grief process will help the veterinary professional to empathize, maintain a balanced perspective, and be compassionate. The veterinary technician can play a vital role in helping bereaved clients by being available; listening; assuring clients that their feelings, emotions, and struggles are normal; and offering referral when clients think they need more help than their available support group is able to provide. This form of client help will strengthen the bond that develops between the client and the veterinary staff and will result in positive growth and added fulfillment for both the client and the veterinary professional.

The Feeling

. . . alone; the haunting thought of my old friend;
Alone; walking among those who could not possibly understand;
Alone; an unused bowl, an empty collar, a silent toy;
. . . the feeling is so strong;
How could I have let them do it?
What if there was something else that could have been done?
Sometimes I just want to yell;
Sometimes I just want to cry;
Sometimes I just want to die;
. . . the feeling is still so very strong;
I know that it was for the best;
My old friend was so sick, so frail;
We cried together on that day;
. . . the feeling was so strong;
I visited his grave today;
I could almost feel his kneading paws and hear his deep harsh purr;
Today I smiled . . . the feeling is so strong.

J. TABOADA

RECOMMENDED READING

Anderson M: *Coping with sorrow on the loss of your pet*, ed 2, Los Angeles, 1994, Peregrine Press.

Brackenridge SS, Elkins AD: Euthanasia and patient death: stressors in veterinary practice, *Vet Pract Staff* 4:1, 1992.

Church JA: *Joy in a wooly coat*, Tiburon, Calif, 1987, HJ Kramer.

Cohen SP, Fudin CE, editors: Animal illness and human emotions, *Prob Vet Med* 3:1, 1991.

Cusack O: *Pets and mental health*, New York, 1988, Haworth Press.

Fogle B, Abrahamson D: Pet loss: a survey of the attitudes and feelings of practicing veterinarians, *Anthrozoos* 3:143, 1990.

Harris JM: Nonconventional human/companion animal bonds. In Kay WJ, Nieburg HA, Kukscher AH, editors: *Pet loss and human bereavement*, Ames, 1984, Iowa State University Press.

Katcher A: Interactions between people and their pets: form and function. In Fogle B, editor: *Interrelations between people and pets*, Springfield, Ill, 1981, Charles C Thomas.

Kay WJ, Cohen SP, Nieburg HA, editors: *Euthanasia of the companion animal: the impact on pet owners, veterinarians, and society*, Baltimore, 1988, The Charles Press.

Kübler-Ross E: *On death and dying*, New York, 1969, Macmillan.

Lagoni L, Butler C, Hetts S: *The human animal bond and grief*, Philadelphia, 1994, WB Saunders.

Lawrence EA: Love for animals and the veterinary profession, *J Am Vet Med Assoc* 205:970, 1994.

Nieburg HA, Fischer A: *Pet loss: a thoughtful guide for adults and children*, New York, 1982, Harper & Row.

Quackenbush JE, Glickman L: Helping people adjust to the death of a pet, *Health Soc Work* 9:42, 1984.

Quackenbush JE, Graveline D: *When your pet dies: how to cope with your feelings*, New York, 1985, Simon & Schuster.

Rosenberg MA: Clinical aspects of grief associated with loss of a pet: a veterinarian's view. In Kay WJ, Nieburg HA, Kukscher AH, editors: *Pet loss and human bereavement*, Ames, 1984, Iowa State University Press.

Veevers JE: The social meanings of pets: alternative roles for companion animals. In Sussman MB, editor: Pets and the family, *Marriage Family Rev* 8:11, 1985.

Voith VL: Attachment of people to companion animals, *Vet Clin North Am Small Anim Pract* 15:289, 1985.

Walshaw SO: Role of the animal health technician in consoling bereaved clients. In Kay WJ, Nieburg HA, Kukscher AH, editors: *Pet loss and human bereavement*, Ames, 1984, Iowa State University Press.

Wilbur RH: Pets, pet ownership, and animal control: social and psychological attitudes. *Proceedings of the National Conference on Dog and Cat Control*, Chicago, 1976, American Veterinary Medicine Association.

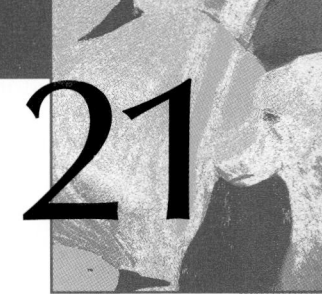

PART FOUR
Anesthesia and Pharmacology

21

Veterinary Anesthesia

Janyce L. Cornick-Seahorn

Anesthesia is a necessary part of veterinary medicine for restraint, elimination of pain sensation during surgical and medical procedures, control of seizure activity, and humane euthanasia. Anesthesia is an area in which veterinary technicians can contribute significantly to their employers and their patients.

Anesthesia is defined as total loss of sensation in a body part (local anesthesia) or in the entire body (general anesthesia), which results from administration of a drug (or drugs) that depresses the activity of part or all of the nervous system. The safe and effective use of anesthetic agents requires a general understanding of their pharmacologic actions and the refinement of several technical and interpretive skills for a variety of animal species. Anesthesia requires a thorough preanesthetic evaluation of the patient and a formulation of an anesthetic plan based on the patient, the surgical or medical procedure to be performed, drug availability, and the experience of the anesthetist. Careful patient monitoring is essential throughout the anesthetic period.

Five topics are discussed in this chapter: anesthetic pharmacology, anesthetic equipment, anesthetic monitoring and ventilatory support, anesthetic management of selected domestic species, and anesthetic emergencies.

PHARMACOLOGY OF ANESTHETIC AGENTS

Preanesthetic agents are an important part of safe patient management. Drugs most commonly used as preanesthetic agents in veterinary medicine include anticholinergic agents, tranquilizers, sedatives, opioids, and combinations of an opioid with a tranquilizer or sedative (neuroleptanalgesic combinations). These agents are used in the practice of anesthesia to aid in animal restraint; allay apprehension and minimize pain; decrease the amount of potentially more severe cardiopulmonary depressant drugs used to produce sedation, analgesia, or general anesthesia; produce a safe, smooth, and uncomplicated induction, maintenance, and recovery from general anesthesia; minimize the adverse and potentially toxic effects of concurrently administered drugs used for general anesthesia; and minimize autonomic reflex activity.

 Technician Note

Preanesthetic agents facilitate animal restraint, reduce patient anxiety, and smooth both induction and recovery.

Anticholinergic Agents

Anticholinergic agents are used to prevent bradycardia and excessive salivation and upper airway secretions. Atropine and glycopyrrolate are the two most commonly used drugs. Although atropine is more economical to use, glycopyrrolate offers some advantages, including a longer duration of action, less tendency to promote cardiac arrhythmias, and perhaps less suppression of intestinal motility. Glycopyrrolate appears to increase heart rate less than does atropine; this may be beneficial in animals with heart disease in which the increase in myocardial oxygen consumption associated with a profound increase in heart rate could be detrimental. Glycopyrrolate, unlike atropine, does not cross the placental barrier, thus having no effect on the fetus during cesarean delivery.

Although many veterinarians use anticholinergic agents as a routine part of a preanesthetic regimen, their use has become more selective and is based on the needs of the individual patient, the anticipated response to the anesthetic agents, and the tendency to develop bradycardia and excessive salivation. Procedures that may increase vagal tone include traction on abdominal organs and procedures involving the neck, throat, and eye. Anesthetic agents that promote bradycardia include opioids, alpha$_2$ agonists, barbiturates, and gas anesthetics. Dissociative agents, such as ketamine, may cause excessive salivation, which may be minimized by using an anticholinergic agent.

The use of anticholinergic agents is controversial in large animal species. They are never used routinely in horses because of the potential to cause ileus and colic, nor are they recommended for use in ruminants because the secretions become more viscid and difficult to clear from the respiratory tract. Anticholinergic agents may be used in swine in conjunction with drugs known to promote bradycardia or excessive salivation. Anticholinergic agents should be used in horses and ruminants only when life-threatening bradycardia develops (see Table 21-5 for normal ranges for heart rate).

Tranquilizers and Sedatives

These agents are used to depress the central nervous system (CNS), to aid in restraint, and to reduce anxiety and struggling. This action helps to minimize stress during both induction and recovery and to reduce the requirements for the more potent agents used for induction and maintenance of anesthesia.

Tranquilizers used in veterinary medicine include a phenothiazine commonly called PromAce (Fort Dodge) and benzodiazepines, such as diazepam, midazolam, and zolazepam. Acepromazine calms animals and decreases motor activity; however, animals may be readily aroused by external stimuli, especially animals that are highly excitable or apprehensive. Acepromazine does not provide analgesia but enhances the analgesic effects of concurrently used drugs. Acepromazine has a long duration of action and is dependent on metabolism by the liver; thus acepromazine should be avoided in patients with liver disease and in geriatric and pediatric patients. Other side effects and contraindications are listed in Table 21-1.

Benzodiazepine tranquilizers produce minimal tranquilization and may even increase excitability in dogs, cats, and horses. Benzodiazepines are rarely used alone but are useful for potentiating the effect of concurrently used premedications (e.g., opioids), for providing muscle relaxation in association with the dissociative drugs (e.g., ketamine), and for reducing the requirements for induction agents (e.g., barbiturates). Because of minimal cardiopulmonary effects, they are useful in geriatric and pediatric animals and animals with heart disease. Benzodiazepines have anticonvulsant activity and are useful in patients with a history of seizures or any neurologic disorder. Diazepam is usually used intravenously because its carrier, propylene glycol, causes pain when given intramuscularly. Midazolam is water soluble and may be used intramuscularly, subcutaneously, or intravenously.

Xylazine, detomidine (Dormosedan), and medetomidine (Domitor) are alpha$_2$ agonists that provide excellent sedation, muscle relaxation, and analgesia. Because of the profound cardiovascular effects (see Table 21-1), including bradycardia, conduction disturbances, and myocardial depression, alpha$_2$ agonists should be used only in healthy dogs and cats. Concurrent use of anticholinergic agents will help prevent bradycardia; however, this practice is controversial. Thermoregulation is impaired for several hours following xylazine administration, so extremes in environmental temperature must be avoided. Requirements for maintenance of anesthesia with inhalation agents are reduced by 50% or more when an alpha$_2$ agonist is used for premedication. Xylazine and detomidine are commonly used in horses. Xylazine is used in ruminants; however, both large and small ruminants are sensitive to xylazine, and low doses must be used (Table 21-2). Reversal agents, including yohimbine (Yobine), tolazoline (Tolazine), and atipamezole (Antisedan) are available for veterinary use.

Opioids

Opioids are used to provide analgesia and sedation. In horses and cats, they should be used in conjunction with a tranquilizer or sedative because excitement is likely when pure opioids, such as morphine or oxymorphone, are used. Opioids promote bradycardia, which is responsive to anticholinergic agents, but depression of cardiac contractility is minimal. Opioids produce respiratory depression; thus apnea and hypoventilation during general anesthesia are more likely to occur when opioids are used. Ventilatory support may be required to alleviate this effect, especially in animals with underlying respiratory abnormalities (e.g., pneumonia, diaphragmatic hernia).

> **Technician Note**
>
> An induction protocol should facilitate a smooth transition from consciousness to unconsciousness and provide adequate relaxation and immobilization for atraumatic endotracheal intubation.

Thermoregulation is impaired by opioids, which may delay the return of normothermia following anesthesia. External stimuli should be minimized before general anesthesia in animals that have received pure opioids because they are hyperresponsive, especially to noise. An advantage of opioids is the availability of opioid antagonists (e.g., naloxone) to reverse their effects (see Table 21-2).

Neuroleptanalgesia is defined as a state of profound CNS depression and analgesia produced by the combination of a tranquilizer or sedative with an opioid agent (see Table 21-2 and Box 21-1). Animals may become unconscious but remain responsive to external stimuli. These drug combinations provide more profound analgesia and calming than is the case when either agent is used alone and may provide adequate analgesia and restraint for procedures such as radiography, wound debridement, suturing of skin lacerations, and ear treatment. When a neuroleptanalgesic combination is used for premedication, dosage requirements of agents used for induction and maintenance are greatly reduced.

Dissociative Agents

Dissociative agents are usually used as part of an induction or maintenance protocol, but they may be used alone in cats as a premedication to produce immobilization for intravenous catheter placement and short noninvasive procedures and to facilitate induction of general anesthesia. They are discussed in more detail in the following paragraphs.

Induction and Maintenance

Induction agents are incorporated into an anesthetic plan to facilitate smooth and rapid transition from consciousness to unconsciousness for maintenance of general anesthesia. Agents most commonly used include the ultra–short-acting barbiturates, guaifenesin, dissociative agent combinations, propofol, and gas anesthetics via mask delivery. *Agents for maintenance* of anesthesia are most commonly the gas anesthetic agents. Effective anesthetic maintenance for short periods of anesthesia may be achieved using various combinations of those drugs used for induction.

Ultra–Short-Acting Barbiturates

The ultra–short-acting barbiturates include thiopental (thiobarbiturate) and methohexital (oxybarbiturate). They may be used without preanesthetic medication to produce rapid loss of consciousness; however, because of some undesirable cardiopulmonary effects (see Table 21-1), it is safer to use premedications to facilitate intravenous injection and to reduce the dosage required to achieve unconsciousness. The degree of respiratory depression associated with barbiturate administration is related to dosage and rate of administration. One should be prepared to intubate and provide ventilatory support if transient apnea occurs.

TABLE 21-1 EFFECTS OF ANESTHETIC DRUGS USED FOR PREMEDICATION AND INDUCTION

Drug	Cardiovascular	Pulmonary	Adverse Effects	Contraindications
PREMEDICATIONS				
Acepromazine	Hypotension Antiarrhythmic effect	Minimal	Penile paralysis (stallions) Lowers seizure threshold Promotes hypothermia	Liver disease History of seizures Dehydration Hypovolemia Shock Heart disease Geriatric patients Pediatric patients
Diazepam/ midazolam	Minimal	Minimal	Hypotension if injected too rapidly (diazepam) Burns when given IM (diazepam)	Should not use alone because excitement is possible
Xylazine/ detomidine/ medetomidine	Bradycardia Conduction disturbances Hypotension Arrhythmias with halothane anesthesia in dogs and cats	Respiratory depression	Impaired thermoregulation Hyperglycemia Profound muscle relaxation may exacerbate upper respiratory abnormalities	Heart disease Geriatric patients Pediatric patients Ruminants require low doses
Opioids	Minimal Bradycardia that is responsive to anticholinergic administration	Respiratory depression	Impaired thermo-regulation (panting in dogs) Hyperresponsive to external stimuli Excitement in cats and horses (pure agonists)	Use with tranquilizer or sedative in horses and cats
INDUCTION AGENTS				
Barbiturates	Myocardial depression Arrhythmias Hypotension	Respiratory depression (apnea)	Excessive salivation Laryngospasm Tissue necrosis with perivascular injection	Heart disease Liver disease Geriatric patients (low doses) Pediatric patients (low doses) Sight hounds (methohexital only) Obese animals (dose on lean weight)
Ketamine/ tiletamine	Increase in heart rate and blood pressure Some direct myocardial depression	Minimal Apneustic breathing May cause apnea when given IV	Profuse salivation Muscle rigidity when used alone Convulsions with high doses Poor visceral analgesia	Never use alone except in cats Must have good sedation before administration in horses (IV only) Animals with seizure history
Propofol	Myocardial depression Hypotension	Apnea	Heinz body formation with repeat administration (5-7 days) in cats	None
Guaifenesin	Minimal	Minimal	Tissue necrosis with perivascular injection	

IM, Intramuscular; *IV,* intravenous.

TABLE 21-2 Dosages* (mg/kg) of Commonly Used Anesthetic Agents for Premedication and Chemical Restraint

Agent	Dog	Cat	Horse	Cow	Goat/Sheep	Pig
ANTICHOLINERGICS						
Atropine	0.02-0.04	0.02-0.04	—	0.04 (max 20 mg)	0.04	0.04
Glycopyrrolate	0.011	0.011	—	—	—	0.003
TRANQUILIZERS						
Acepromazine	0.055-0.22	0.11-0.22	0.022-0.088	0.044-0.088	0.044-0.088	0.1-0.22
Diazepam	0.22	0.22	0.022-0.088	0.022-0.088	0.022-0.088	0.22-0.44
Midazolam	0.22	0.22	—	—	—	—
SEDATIVES						
Xylazine	0.44-1.1	0.44-1.1	0.44-1.1	0.022-0.11	0.022-0.066	1.1-2.2
Detomidine	—	—	0.01-0.02	—	—	—
Medetomidine	0.01-0.04	0.01-0.04	—	—	—	0.01-0.02
OPIOIDS						
Hydromorphone	0.1-0.2	0.1	—	—	—	—
Oxymorphone	0.01-0.05	0.055-0.011†	0.011-0.044†	—	—	—
Butorphanol	0.11-0.44	0.22-0.44	0.011-0.044	0.011-0.022	0.022-0.044	0.22-0.33
Morphine	0.44-1.1	0.11-0.22†	0.044-0.11†	—	—	0.44-0.88
Meperidine	0.44-1.1	0.22-0.44†	0.22-0.66†	—	—	0.44-1.1
Pentazocine	0.22-0.44	0.11	0.44-0.88	—	—	—
Buprenorphine	0.01-0.04	0.01-0.03	0.01-0.02	—	—	—
NEUROLEPTANALGESIC COMBINATIONS						
Acepromazine	0.1-0.22	0.1-0.22	—	—	—	—
Oxymorphone	0.11-0.22	0.055-0.11	—	—	—	—
Acepromazine	0.22	0.22	0.044	—	—	—
Butorphanol	0.22	0.22-0.44	0.022	—	—	—
Xylazine	0.22	0.22	0.66	0.022	0.022	—
Butorphanol	0.11-0.22	0.22-0.44	0.022-0.044	0.022-0.055	0.022	—
REVERSAL AGENTS						
Yohimbine‡ (alpha$_2$ antagonist)	0.11	0.11	0.11	0.11	0.11	0.11
Tolazoline (alpha$_2$ antagonist)	2.0-5.0	2.0	4.0	1.1	2.0	—
Atipamezole (alpha$_2$ antagonist)	0.2-0.35	0.2	—	—	—	—
Naloxone (opioid antagonist)	0.0066	0.0066	0.0055-0.022	—	—	0.0066

Modified from Muir WW: *Handbook of veterinary anesthesia*, St Louis, 1989, Mosby.
*Most agents may be used intravenously (IV) or intramuscularly (IM). As a general rule, use higher dose range IM and lower dose range IV.
†Use these opioids in these species *only* in conjunction with a tranquilizer or sedative.
‡Administer yohimbine "to effect" in large animal species. Calculate recommended dose and give in one-fourth increments until reversal of sedation is observed.

Box 21-1   SUGGESTED PROTOCOLS FOR CHEMICAL RESTRAINT AND GENERAL ANESTHESIA IN DOGS

NEUROLEPTANALGESIC COMBINATIONS
FOR CHEMICAL RESTRAINT

1. Acepromazine   0.22 mg/kg IV (max: 4 mg)
   Oxymorphone   0.22 mg/kg IV (max: 4 mg)
2. Acepromazine   0.22 mg/kg IV (max: 4 mg)
   Butorphanol   0.22-0.44 mg/kg IV
3. Atropine   0.044 mg/kg SC
   Xylazine or
      medetomidine   0.22 mg/kg xylazine or 0.01-0.02
                         mg/kg (medetomidine) IV or IM
                         followed by:
   Butorphanol   0.11-0.22 mg/kg IV

For animals in which acepromazine and xylazine should be
avoided:

4. Diazepam   0.22 mg/kg IV
   Oxymorphone   0.22 mg/kg IV (maximum: 4 mg)
5. Diazepam*   0.22 mg/kg IV
   Butorphanol   0.22-0.44 mg/kg IV

PROTOCOL FOR PHYSICAL STATUS I AND II ANIMALS

Premedication   Acepromazine: 0.11 mg/kg IM (max: 2 mg)
                   or
                   Acepromazine: 0.11 mg/kg IM (max: 2 mg)
                      plus
                   Butorphanol: 0.22-0.44 mg/kg IM
Induction   Thiopental
Maintenance   Halothane, isoflurane, or methoxyflurane

PROTOCOL FOR PHYSICAL STATUS ≥III ANIMALS

Premedication   Neuroleptanalgesic combination 4 or 5
                   listed above. Alternate administration of
                   one-quarter calculated dose of each drug
                   beginning with opioid until total dose has
                   been administered or until desired degree
                   of sedation is achieved.
Induction   Mask with isoflurane
                   or
                   Ketamine: 2.2-4.4 mg/kg IV "to effect"
                   or
                   Propofol: 2-4 mg/kg IV "to effect"
Maintenance   Isoflurane (if available). Halothane may
                   be used, but delivered concentrations
                   should be minimized.

INJECTABLE PROTOCOLS FOR SHORT-DURATION
ANESTHESIA†

1. Atropine   0.044 mg/kg SC
   Xylazine   0.66-1.1 mg/kg IV or IM
   Ketamine   6.0-12.0 mg/kg IV or IM
2. Diazepam   0.25 mg/kg Mix and inject IV
   Ketamine   5.0 mg/kg Provides 10-15 min of
                         anesthesia
3. Atropine   0.044 mg/kg SC
   Xylazine   0.44-0.88 mg/kg IV or IM
   Telazol   4.4-11.0 mg/kg IV or IM

IV, Intravenously; *IM*, intramuscularly; *SC*, subcutaneously.
*Midazolam may be used in place of diazepam at the same dose and may be administered IM, SC, or IV.
†Protocols 1 and 3 may be used IV or IM. Use higher dose range when administering IM. The IM route will be slower in
onset of effect and will give a longer duration of anesthesia and a longer recovery.

Detrimental cardiopulmonary effects are more likely to occur when large doses are administered rapidly and when higher concentrations are used. Although solutions up to 10% in strength are used in large animals, it is preferable to use a solution no stronger than 5% in small animals and safest to use a 2.0% or 2.5% solution. More dilute solutions will reduce the likelihood of adverse effects and cause less tissue necrosis with accidental perivascular injection. Should perivascular administration occur, 2% lidocaine diluted 1:9 with sterile saline should be infiltrated into the injection site. Barbiturates are metabolized by the liver and should be avoided in animals with liver disease. Recovery from thiopental anesthesia is due to redistribution to muscle. Repeated bolus doses to maintain anesthesia are not recommended because this practice will contribute to a rough and prolonged recovery.

Sight hounds (greyhounds, Irish wolfhounds, whippets) are unable to metabolize thiobarbiturates effectively, resulting in a prolonged recovery. An alternative induction method for sight hounds is with methohexital (6 to 11 mg/kg), which acts similar to thiopental but is effectively metabolized. Excitement during recovery may be more pronounced with methohexital induction, especially following short procedures, so preanesthetic tranquilization is recommended. With the introduction of propofol (see below), methohexital is not frequently utilized.

Propofol

Propofol (Rapinovet) is a nonbarbiturate, intravenously administered anesthetic agent that produces a rapid loss of consciousness for induction of anesthesia. The drug is noncumulative, being rapidly metabolized (even in the presence of liver dysfunction). Thus propofol provides a smooth and rapid recovery and may also be used for maintenance of anesthesia by infusion (0.4 mg/kg/min) or repeated bolus. The major side effects are transient apnea and cardiovascular depression. Both effects may be minimized by using adequate premedication to facilitate minimal dosage requirements and by titrating slowly to effect. Propofol is more expensive than thiopental but not prohibitive. The propofol formulation is a milky white emulsion containing soybean oil, egg lecithin, and glycerol. Although its milky appearance challenges the general rule of "do not administer any agent intravenously that is not clear," propofol is safe, effective, and versatile with negligible side effects when used conservatively following appropriate premedication. However, the carrier agents support bacterial growth; therefore, once opened or drawn from, the remainder should be refrigerated and discarded after 24 hours. This further increases the cost of the product.

Etomidate

Etomidate is a nonbarbiturate, noncumulative sedative-hypnotic administered intravenously for induction of anesthesia. Because of the expense, use in veterinary medicine is limited to high-risk patients. Etomidate's major advantage is that it does not depress cardiopulmonary function. Side effects, including pain on injection, myoclonus, vomiting, and excitement, are minimized by use of premedication.

Dissociative Agent Combinations

Dissociative agents produce immobilization and superficial analgesia. Swallowing and ocular reflexes remain intact, and muscle tone is increased. These agents may be administered intramuscularly or intravenously; however, intramuscular administration requires higher doses and results in a prolonged recovery. The intramuscular route is most commonly used in cats, dogs, small ruminants, and swine and is *never* used in horses.

Technician Note

Dissociative agents increase respiratory secretions and salivation, and some animals may require administration of an anticholinergic agent to ensure a patent airway.

Concurrent administration of an anticholinergic agent may be needed in some species (cats, dogs, swine) owing to excessive salivation. Although some direct depression of heart function occurs, an increase in sympathetic tone compensates for this effect by increasing heart rate and arterial blood pressure. This effect on heart rate and blood pressure offers an advantage over the thiobarbiturates for use in debilitated and septic patients or patients with heart disease. Because elimination of ketamine depends on both liver metabolism and renal excretion, high dosages should be avoided in animals with liver or kidney disease.

Ketamine combined with a benzodiazepine, along with propofol, offers an alternative method of induction for sight hounds. *Telazol* (A.H. Robins) is a commercial drug combination containing equal parts of zolazepam (benzodiazepine) and tiletamine (dissociative) that may be used for both induction and maintenance of anesthesia. Although approved only for intramuscular use, intravenous administration of very low doses provides an effective method for induction and for short-term anesthesia (Table 21-3).

Guaifenesin

Guaifenesin is an intravenously administered central-acting muscle relaxant that potentiates the effects of concurrently used preanesthetic and anesthetic agents, allowing for lower dosages of these agents to be used. Guaifenesin is used in large animals as part of both induction and maintenance protocols. Cardiopulmonary effects are minimal, and there is a wide margin of safety. Excessive dosages may result in paradoxic muscle rigidity of the forelimbs and neck and an apneustic breathing pattern, which is more likely to occur in young animals and can lead to respiratory arrest. Administration is best performed through an indwelling venous catheter because large volumes must be administered (usually as a 5% solution) and perivascular injection is caustic to tissues.

Epidural Analgesia/Anesthesia

Epidural drug administration provides a method of complete anesthesia (local anesthetics such as lidocaine and bupivacaine) or supplemental analgesia both intraoperatively and postoperatively (opioids). (See Chapter 22, discussion of pain management.) The site of injection is at the lumbosacral intervertebral space for small animals, small ruminants, and swine and at the first coccygeal space in horses and cattle.

Local anesthetics provide total analgesia and muscle relaxation to the caudal portion of the body, which will facilitate surgery of the hindlimbs, perineal region, and abdomen (lumbosacral administration). The cranial extent of the analgesia varies from patient to patient, and supplemental anesthesia may become necessary for some animals. This technique is good for cesarean delivery, because of minimal fetal effects, and for high-risk patients. Side effects may include hypotension as a result of vasodilation (which may be minimized by fluid loading before administration) and, in rare cases, respiratory arrest if excessive cranial migration occurs.

Animals receiving local anesthetics epidurally should never be placed in a head-down position. Dosage is approximately 1 ml/4.5 kg for both 2.0% lidocaine and 0.5% bupivacaine with a duration of action of 1.5 to 2 hours and 4 to 6 hours, respectively. Dosage should be reduced by 50% if cerebrospinal fluid is observed in the hub of the needle and by 10% to 20% in obese and pregnant animals.

TABLE 21-3	DRUGS (MG/KG)* COMMONLY USED FOR INDUCTION OR SHORT-DURATION ANESTHESIA					
Agent	**Dog**	**Cat**	**Horse**	**Cow**	**Goat/Sheep**	**Pig**
Thiopental	8.8-13	8.8-13	6.6-11	4.4-11	4.4-11	8.8-13
Propofol	2-6	2-6	1-3	—	—	—
Etomidate	0.5-2.0	—	—	—	—	—
Guaifenesin	44-88	—	66-132	66-132	66-132	44-88
Ketamine	—	2.2-18	—	—	2.2-6.6	2.2-6.6
Telazol	2.2-11†	2.2-11†	—	4.4-11	2.2-11	4.4-11†
Guaifenesin/thiopental	33-88	—	44-88	44-88	—	33-88
	2.2-6.6	—	2.2-6.6	2.2-6.6	—	2.2-6.6
Guaifenesin/ketamine	33-88	—	44-88	44-88	44-88	—
	1.1	—	1.1-1.5	0.6-1.1	0.6-1.1	—
Acepromazine/ketamine	0.11	0.22†	—	—	—	0.44†
	11.0	4.4-11†	—	—	—	2.2-6.6†
Xylazine/ketamine	0.66-1.1†	0.66-1.1†	1.1	0.044-0.088†	0.044†	2.2-4.4†
	2.2-11†	4.4-22†	2.2	2.2-6.6†	2.2-6.6	2.2-11†
Diazepam/ketamine	0.25	0.25	—	—	0.25-0.55	0.22-0.44
	5.0	5.0	—	—	4.4	4.4
Xylazine/telazol	0.44†	0.66†	1.1	0.022-0.11†	0.044-0.088†	0.66-1.1†
	6.6†	2.2-6.6†	1.1-2.2	2.2-6.6†	2.2-6.6†	4.4-6.6†
Xylazine/guaifenesin/ketamine	(See Boxes 21-1 to 21-5 giving specific species protocol.)					

Modified from Muir WW: *Handbook of veterinary anesthesia*, St Louis, 1989, Mosby.
*Dosage is for intravenous use unless otherwise designated.
†Indicates protocols that may be used intramuscularly in some species.

Morphine (0.1 mg/kg) is the most commonly used opioid for epidural injection because its duration of effect is 10 to 24 hours and it may be administered alone or in combination with a local anesthetic agent. The analgesic effects of epidural morphine may extend as far forward as the forelimbs. Morphine administered epiduralIly at the coccygeal space has been shown to be effective for managing pelvic limb and abdominal pain in horses and cattle. Contraindications for epidural injection include patients with sepsis, clotting abnormalities, or infected skin.

Inhalation Anesthetics

Inhalation agents used in veterinary medicine include isoflurane, halothane, sevoflurane, and methoxyflurane. Methoxyflurane use has greatly decreased since the introduction of isoflurane because of several undesirable effects, including significant hepatic metabolism and production of potentially toxic metabolites, prolonged recovery, and lack of availability that has resulted in an increased cost. Another inhalant agent, sevoflurane, which acts similarly to isoflurane, has recently been introduced for veterinary use. These agents produce general anesthesia, which includes unconsciousness and muscle relaxation, and are suitable for use in all species. Advantages include more rapid control of changes in depth of anesthesia and a more rapid recovery. However, these agents produce profound effects on cardiopulmonary function, and patients must be closely monitored throughout the anesthetic period. The use of gas anesthetics requires more complex and expensive equipment than is needed for injectable techniques, and an understanding of this equipment is necessary to use the agents safely and effectively.

Technician Note

Mask induction should be reserved for high-risk patients that are adequately sedated. This technique greatly increases waste gas contamination of the work environment.

Some properties of the gases (Table 21-4) must be reviewed to appreciate the anesthetic vaporizers used to deliver the gases and the speed at which the agents exert their anesthetic effect. *Vapor pressure* of a gas determines the maximum concentration that may be achieved in the carrier gas (oxygen) at any given temperature. For example, methoxyflurane, with a low vapor pressure (23 mm Hg), may only reach a maximum concentration of 3.5% at room temperature, whereas halothane and isoflurane, both with vapor pressures of approximately 240 mm Hg, may reach a maximum concentration of 32% at room

temperature. This means that a precision vaporizer (see discussion of equipment), which delivers a precise concentration of anesthetic gas according to settings on the vaporizer, is safer and helps to avoid potentially lethal concentrations of isoflurane and halothane. Although halothane, isoflurane, and sevoflurane have been reported to be used safely in nonprecision vaporizers, methoxyflurance is most commonly associated with this type of vaporizer.

Solubility determines the speed of induction and recovery of the anesthetic gas and is most frequently defined as its distribution between blood and gas phases. Methoxyflurane with a very high solubility is dissolved to a high degree in the blood. This delays the development of a tension (partial pressure) of anesthetic gas in the blood, which is essential for the gas to pass into the brain and render the patient unconscious. This high solubility of methoxyflurane is manifested clinically as a very slow induction of and recovery from general anesthesia, making it undesirable for use as an induction agent. The other agents listed in order of decreasing solubility are halothane > isoflurane > sevoflurane (see Table 21-4). All are effective for mask induction when indicated.

Minimum alveolar concentration (MAC) is a measure of anesthetic potency by which the gas anesthetic agents may be compared and is used as a guide to deliver adequate but not excessive concentrations for surgical procedures. MAC is defined as the minimum concentration of anesthetic in the alveoli at 1 ATM that prevents a response in 50% of patients exposed to a painful stimulus. The MAC values have been determined for the commonly used gas anesthetics for many animal species (see Table 21-4). For most surgical procedures in most species, 1.5 to 2.0 times MAC is adequate to maintain a surgical plane of anesthesia. Factors that may decrease the MAC requirement include age (older patients require less), hypothermia, administration of other depressant drugs (e.g., opioids, tranquilizers), anemia, and diseases such as septicemia.

The anesthetic gases cause dose-dependent depression of heart function, with isoflurane and sevoflurane having the least effect at clinically used concentrations. All anesthetic gases cause respiratory depression, and ventilation should be assisted (see Ventilatory Support) to minimize the development of hypercapnia and atelectasis. Halothane has the additional undesirable characteristic of sensitizing the heart to catecholamines, which can result in the development of arrhythmias. Methoxyflurane is less likely to induce arrhythmias, and isoflurane and sevoflurane do not have this effect. Isoflurane and sevoflurane, although more expensive than halothane, are the safest and most versatile anesthetic gases because they may be used in young, old, debilitated, and exotic patients with the fewest detrimental effects.

TABLE 21-4	CHARACTERISTICS OF COMMONLY USED INHALATION AGENTS IN VETERINARY MEDICINE									
Agent	Vapor Pressure (mm Hg)	Solubility Coefficient	MAC Values (%)				Induction (%)		Maintenance (%)	
			Dog	Cat	Horse	Pig	SA	LA	SA	LA
Isoflurane	240	1.4	1.5	1.6	1.3	1.47	2-4	4-5	1-3	2-3
Halothane	244	2.4	0.87	1.19	0.9	1.25	2-4	3-5	0.5-1.5	1-2
Methoxyflurane	23	13.0	0.23	0.16	0.3	*	2-3	†	0.2-1	†
Sevoflurane	157	0.68	2.38	2.58	2.31	—	—	—	—	—

LA, Large animal; *MAC,* maximum allowable concentration; *SA,* small animal.
*Value not available.
†Methoxyflurane is not used routinely in large animals.

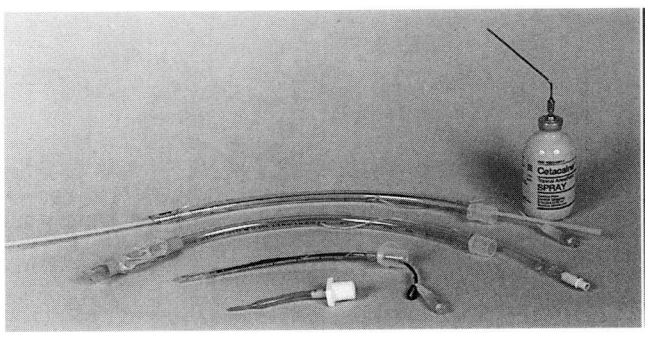
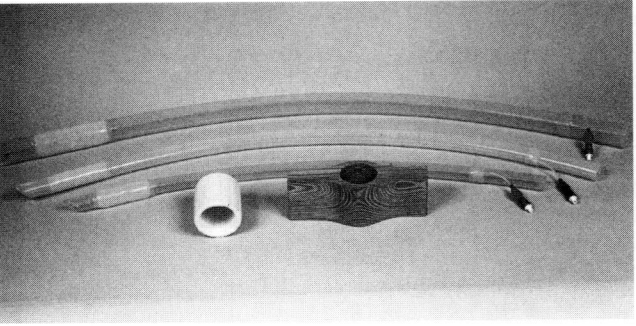

FIGURE 21-1. **A,** Representative sizes of cuffed endotracheal tubes appropriate for use in small animals, small ruminants, and swine. The top tube and the third tube from the top contain two types of stylets in place as they might be used clinically to facilitate intubation. A noncuffed Cole tube is also shown *(bottom)*. *Right,* Topical anesthetic spray (Cetacaine, Cetylite Industries Inc.) for desensitizing the larynx before intubation should not be used in cats. **B,** Cuffed tubes (Biovona) that are used for horses and cattle. Two types of oral specula for horses *(left)* and cattle *(right)* are also shown.

ANESTHETIC EQUIPMENT

Anesthetic equipment should be organized in a specific location in the hospital. This area should be quiet and away from mainstream hospital traffic. Once the technician knows what anesthetic drugs and equipment the veterinarian wants to have available, adequate supplies should be stocked and maintained.

Basic equipment and supplies that should be available to provide anesthesia include needles and syringes, intravenous catheters, tape for securing catheters, heparinized saline (2 units of heparin per milliliter of 0.9% saline), endotracheal tubes in a variety of sizes, laryngoscope, lubricant for the endotracheal tubes, ophthalmic lubricant, an oxygen source and method of delivery, an apparatus for manual ventilation (i.e., Ambu bag [see Figure 21-17] or anesthesia machine), and a selection of anesthetic agents. If gas anesthesia is used in the practice, an anesthesia machine, breathing systems, and a selection of rebreathing bags and face masks should be available. An emergency drug box (discussed under Anesthetic Emergencies) should also be accessible in this area.

Catheters

Intravenous administration equipment and catheters are covered in Chapter 3. As a general rule of anesthesia, dependable venous access, as with an intravenous catheter taped or glued securely in place, should be available in all anesthetized patients. An intravenous catheter provides a route of administration for polyionic fluids to maintain homeostasis; for additional drugs to maintain anesthesia, which is especially important when injectable techniques are used; and for emergency drug administration if cardiopulmonary arrest occurs.

Endotracheal Tubes

The endotracheal tube provides the connecting link between the patient's airway and the anesthetic equipment. Although it is not essential to place an endotracheal tube when injectable anesthesia is used, tubes must be available in rare instances when respiratory arrest dictates the need for assisted ventilation and delivery of oxygen or when the risk of regurgitation and aspiration is increased (as in patients who have not adequately fasted, who have a history of vomiting, or who are pregnant). Some veterinarians prefer to place an endotracheal tube routinely during injectable anesthesia as a precautionary measure. Cuffed tubes (Figure 21-1) are most commonly used and provide an effective seal within the airway to prevent aspiration and to facilitate effective ventilatory support. Cuffed tubes are available in a wide variety of sizes according to internal diameter (ID) in millimeters, with sizes 2.5 to 14 mm ID appropriate for dogs, cats, swine, and small ruminants and sizes 16 to 30 mm ID for large ruminants and horses. Noncuffed tubes (see Figure 21-1) are used in very small patients (e.g., newborn kittens and puppies, ferrets, birds) because they preserve a larger airway diameter.

> ### Technician Note
> All anesthetized animals should be intubated to ensure and protect the airway. Intubation, while not essential for short procedures that use injectable agents, should be performed on those animals with increased risk of regurgitation (not fasted, history of vomiting, pregnant).

Laryngoscopes

Laryngoscopes facilitate intubation in many species and are especially beneficial in small ruminants, swine, and cats. These instruments consist of a battery-containing handle with a detachable blade. Blades come in a variety of shapes and sizes. Two styles commonly used in veterinary anesthesia are shown in Figure 21-2.

Anesthetic Machines

The primary purposes of an inhalation anesthetic machine and breathing system are to deliver oxygen, to deliver a controlled amount of an inhalation anesthetic agent, and to provide a method of assisting ventilation. The variability of anesthetic machines, which are offered in a wide variety of types and sizes by numerous manufacturers, presents a challenge to the veterinary anesthetist; however, all machines have the same basic components (Figures 21-3 to 21-5).

The four basic components of an anesthetic machine are a *compressed gas source* (oxygen and sometimes nitrous oxide); the *pressure regulator,* which reduces and controls the pressure of gas leaving the compressed gas source to a lower pressure that will not damage the flowmeter; the *flowmeter,* which precisely controls the flow of gas entering

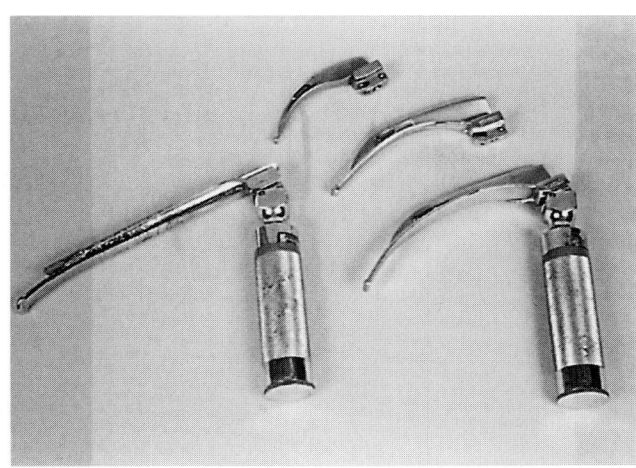

FIGURE 21-2. Laryngoscopes used in veterinary medicine. The three blades on the right are different-sized McIntosh blades. The blade on the left is a Miller blade, which is long enough to facilitate intubation of small ruminants and swine.

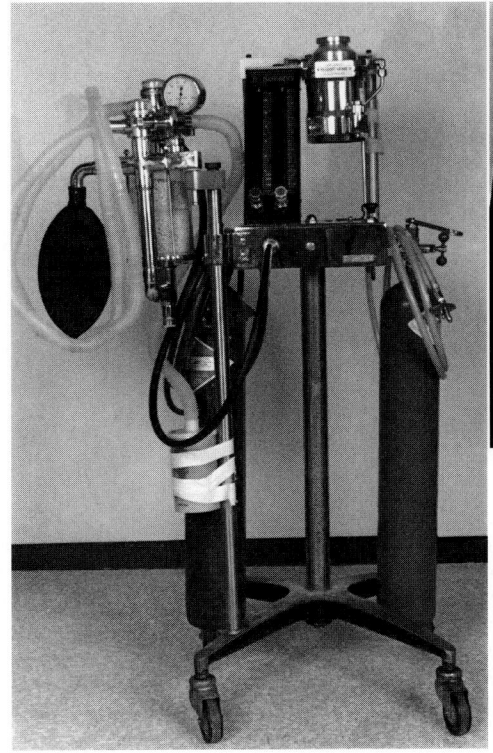

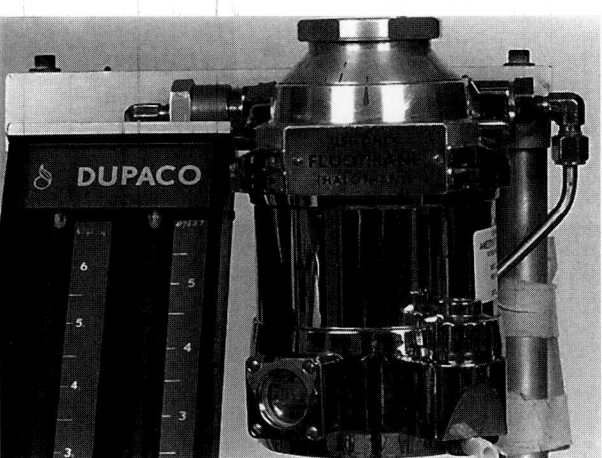

FIGURE 21-3. **A,** A basic veterinary anesthetic machine with a circle breathing system for use in animals weighing up to 135 kg. This machine may be connected to a central hospital gas pipeline system or to transportable "E" tanks of oxygen and nitrous oxide, which are mounted on the sides of the stand. **B,** A Fluothane Tec (Fluotec 3, Matrix Medical Inc.) vaporizer showing calibration of output in volume percent. The vaporizer is set at 0.5%. The small lever at the left of the vaporizer *(arrow)* is a locking mechanism that must be depressed to activate the control dial.

the patient's breathing system; and the *vaporizer,* which facilitates delivery of a controlled concentration of an inhalation anesthetic agent into the patient's breathing system.

Another feature is the pressure gauge, which reflects the amount of gas remaining in the compressed gas tank. Specifically, a full oxygen tank maintains a pressure of approximately 2200 psi, and that pressure decreases proportionately as the tank empties. An oxygen flush valve, which is included on most anesthetic machines, delivers oxygen directly and rapidly (35 to 75 L/min) to the common gas outlet of the machine, thus bypassing the vaporizer and quickly filling the breathing system with pure oxygen.

Older machines may flush through the vaporizer, which presents an inherent danger if the flush valve is engaged while the vaporizer is turned on. The flush valve may be used to quickly decrease the inhalation anesthetic concentration present in the breathed gases for a rapid decrease in anesthetic depth or to facilitate recovery from anesthesia. Use of the flush valve should be avoided as a method of filling the rebreathing bag unless a decrease in depth of anesthesia is desired. The oxygen flush valve should not be engaged when the pop-off valve is closed or when a nonrebreathing system is used because of the risk of delivering excessive pressure to the patient.

Vaporizers convert a volatile liquid inhalation anesthetic into a vapor for delivery into the patient's breathing

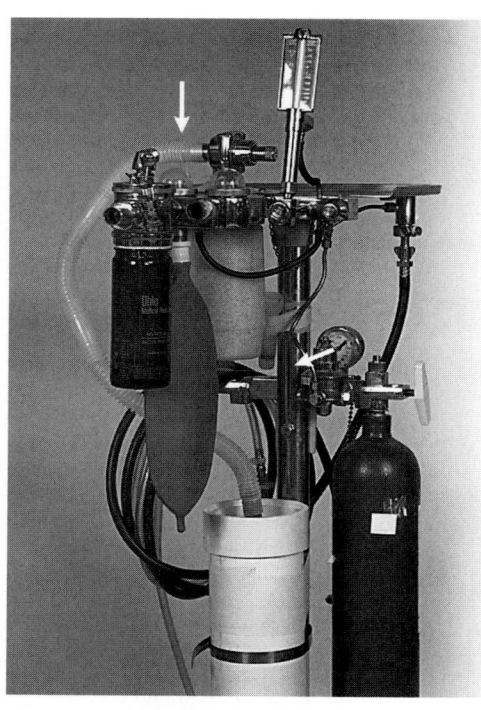

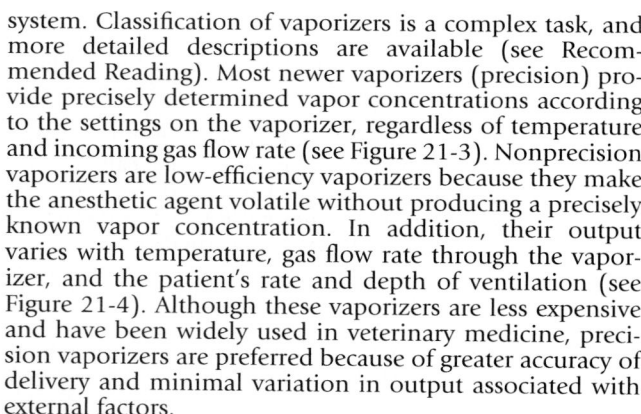

FIGURE 21-4. A basic veterinary anesthetic machine illustrating the position of the nonprecision vaporizer within the breathing circuit (the breathing tubes are *not* in place). Although this type of vaporizer has largely been replaced by the more accurate precision vaporizers, nonprecision vaporizers are still used in veterinary practice. Note the tubing *(arrow),* which connects the pop-off valve to the waste gas scavenging system.

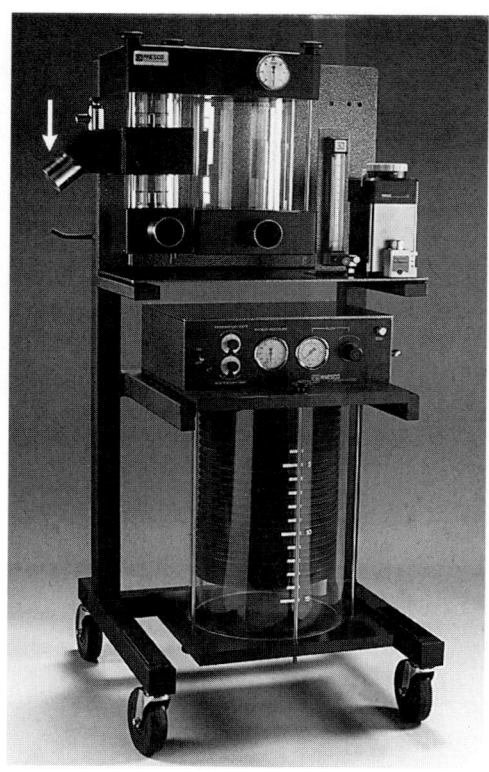

FIGURE 21-5. A large animal anesthetic machine with an isoflurane vaporizer and mechanical ventilator. The side connection *(arrow)* may be used for placement of a rebreathing bag for spontaneous ventilation or to connect the breathing circuit to the ventilator for controlled ventilation (IPPV). (Courtesy SurgiVet, Inc.)

system. Classification of vaporizers is a complex task, and more detailed descriptions are available (see Recommended Reading). Most newer vaporizers (precision) provide precisely determined vapor concentrations according to the settings on the vaporizer, regardless of temperature and incoming gas flow rate (see Figure 21-3). Nonprecision vaporizers are low-efficiency vaporizers because they make the anesthetic agent volatile without producing a precisely known vapor concentration. In addition, their output varies with temperature, gas flow rate through the vaporizer, and the patient's rate and depth of ventilation (see Figure 21-4). Although these vaporizers are less expensive and have been widely used in veterinary medicine, precision vaporizers are preferred because of greater accuracy of delivery and minimal variation in output associated with external factors.

Location of the vaporizer may be out of the breathing system (out-of-the-system precision) or in the breathing system (in-the-system nonprecision) as illustrated in Figure 21-6. There is an inherent danger in the use of an in-the-system (nonprecision) vaporizer. Whereas an out-of-system vaporizer can never deliver a concentration higher than what is set on the vaporizer dial (because fresh gas flow passes through the vaporizer one time only), an in-the-system vaporizer receives, in addition to fresh gas flow, a gas mixture containing anesthetic gas not taken up by the patient; therefore vapor concentration in the

breathed gas may increase over time. This increase is exacerbated by low fresh gas flows, which allow exhaled gases already containing anesthetic vapor to recirculate more times, and by ventilation, with greater ventilation resulting in increased vaporization. The latter effect theoretically provides a built-in safety factor *if* the animal is breathing spontaneously, because as anesthetic depth increases, ventilation becomes depressed, allowing anesthetic concentration in the breathed gases to decrease. Controlled ventilation is not safe to use with an in-the-system vaporizer.

Breathing Systems

The most commonly used breathing system is the circle rebreathing system, meaning that the patient rebreathes the gas mixture within the circle (see Figure 21-3). Three sizes are available, including pediatric (<7 kg), standard adult circle (7 to 135 kg), and large animal (>135 kg). These systems vary in internal volume owing to differences in diameter of the breathing tubes and the size of the rebreathing bags used.

Gases move in one direction because of the presence of one-way valves, and carbon dioxide produced by the animal is neutralized by soda lime or barium hydroxide lime contained in the absorbent canister (see Figures 21-3 and 21-4). Most absorbent granules contain an indicator dye, which becomes visible as a result of a color change as

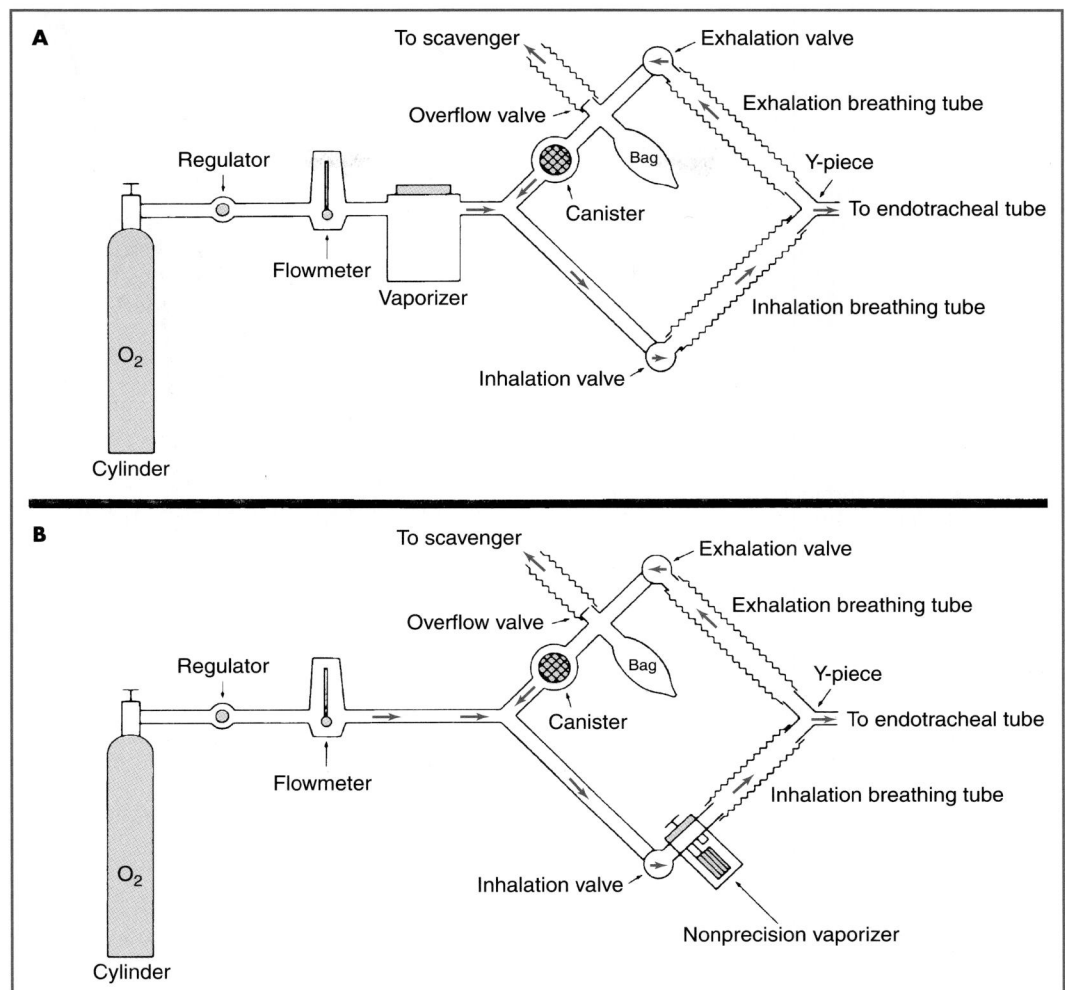

FIGURE 21-6. **A,** Diagram of the relationship of an out-of-the-system precision vaporizer to the various components of an anesthetic machine and a circle breathing system. **B,** Diagram of the relationship of an in-the-system nonprecision vaporizer to the various components of an anesthetic machine and a circle breathing system. (From Harstfield SM. In Short CE, editor: *Principles and practice of veterinary anesthesia,* Baltimore, 1987, Williams & Wilkins, p 403.)

the granules become exhausted. Although no set guidelines exist for when to change the absorbent granules, a general rule is that a strong color indicates the point of clinical exhaustion and the granules should be changed when the color shift is present in two thirds of the absorbent.

Rebreathing bag selection may be made by multiplying the patient's tidal volume (10 ml/kg) times six. Rebreathing bags available for animals less than 135 kg include 0.5-, 1-, 2-, 3-, 5-, and 6-L sizes, and for animals more than 135 kg, the bags include 15-, 20-, and 30-L sizes.

Fresh gas flow rates vary with personal preference. A setting that just meets the patient's metabolic oxygen needs (small animal = 4 to 10 ml/kg/min; large animal = 2 to 3 ml/kg/min) is termed a closed circle system, in which the pop-off valve is closed and flow rates are adjusted to maintain a constant volume in the rebreathing bag. Although this system is more economic, retains more heat and humidity, and causes less environmental pollution, hypoxia may develop if the patient is not closely monitored. The system must be flushed two to four times during

the first 15 minutes of anesthesia, and every 30 minutes thereafter, to prevent nitrogen (which is exhaled by the patient) from building up within the system. In a semi-closed circle system, defined by fresh gas flows of three times the patient's metabolic oxygen needs (small animal = 30 ml/kg/min; large animal = 6 to 10 ml/kg/min), the pop-off valve is open. Although these flow rates are less economic and result in more pollution, they ensure greater patient safety. Regardless of the flow rate used for maintenance, flow rates for mask induction and for a short period following intubation and connection to the breathing system (2 to 5 minutes) should be increased (except for in-the-system nonprecision vaporizers) to facilitate delivery of anesthetic gas to the patient and to aid in denitrogenation of the patient. A rate of two to three times the calculated maintenance flow rate will be adequate.

Nonrebreathing systems are also used in veterinary medicine for patients weighing less than 7 kg. Nonrebreathing (NRB) systems are simple to use and inexpensive, do not require carbon dioxide absorbent, and impart minimal

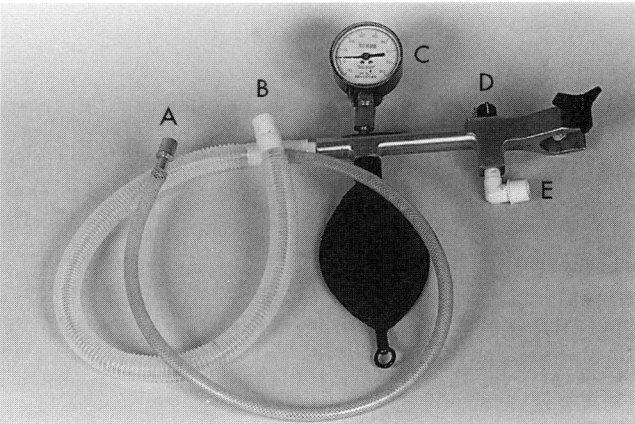

FIGURE 21-7. Bain circuit nonrebreathing system attaches to *(a)* the common gas outlet of the anesthetic machine. Patient connection end *(b)*. The system is also equipped with a pressure manometer *(c)*; a "pop-off" valve *(d)*, which remains open except during assisted ventilation; and an interface for connection to a waste gas scavenging system *(e)*.

resistance to breathing. Disadvantages include decreased economy and increased pollution because of the high flow rates required to remove carbon dioxide and a greater loss of heat and humidity. Flow rates vary according to the particular system used but are approximately 100 to 300 ml/kg/min with a minimum flow of 500 ml/min. A commonly used NRB system in veterinary medicine is the Bain coaxial system (Figure 21-7).

In veterinary hospitals in which inhalation anesthetics are used, it is important to minimize environmental exposure of attending personnel to waste gases (also see Chapter 35). Reduction of environmental pollution is facilitated by scavenging the waste gas exiting through the pop-off valve, checking equipment frequently for leaks (see Preparation of Equipment and Supplies), and practicing techniques that minimize environmental pollution. Although a cause-and-effect relationship has not been clearly demonstrated, studies of operating room personnel suggest that exposure to trace anesthetic gases may be a contributing factor in spontaneous abortion, congenital abnormalities, cancer, hepatic disease, renal disease, and neurologic disease. Scavenging systems include the gas-capturing device, the interface, and the disposal system, and detailed descriptions are available (see Recommended Reading). Considerations that help to minimize waste gas exposure include the following:

- Fill vaporizers at the end of the workday when fewer people are present, taking care to avoid spillage.
- Use low-flow techniques when possible.
- Have patients recover in well-ventilated areas, and leave the patient attached to the breathing system as long as possible so that expired gases can be scavenged.
- Do not turn on the vaporizer until the patient is connected to the machine.
- When disconnecting the patient from the machine, turn off the vaporizer and occlude the Y-piece until the patient is reconnected.
- Use mask or chamber inductions only when considered necessary for the safety of the patient or for unrestrainable patients.

> ### Technician Note
> Techniques to minimize waste anesthetic gas contamination of the work environment should be part of the daily anesthesia routine.

MONITORING

Intraoperative monitoring is essential to successful anesthesia because chemical restraint and general anesthesia impose a great stress on homeostasis in both normal and debilitated patients. Because irreversible brain and cellular changes occur in 3 to 5 minutes after the cessation of blood flow that occurs with cardiac arrest, vital signs should be assessed and recorded every 5 minutes. Life-threatening changes must be detected early so that action can be taken to avoid permanent damage to the patient.

The anesthetic record is a concise method for recording time of administration and doses (in milligrams) of anesthetic agents used and physiologic data measured throughout the anesthetic period. The record serves as a legal document, prompts the anesthetist to evaluate and record the patient's vital signs at regular intervals, permits recognition of trends in one or more of the recorded values that might signal an impending problem, and provides information for any subsequent anesthetic procedures in the same patient (Figure 21-8).

Monitoring includes both physical and technical methods. Physical methods parallel those skills involved in performing a physical examination plus assessment of muscle tone and eye reflexes. Technologic methods use sophisticated equipment to quantify various aspects of homeostasis. Monitoring should focus on the cardiovascular and pulmonary systems, the CNS, and body temperature because these are most affected by anesthetic drugs and surgical procedures. The preanesthetic physical status of the patient (see Preanesthetic Evaluation), the anesthetic protocol used, the procedure to be performed, and the anticipated duration of anesthesia help to determine the sophistication of the monitoring techniques used.

> ### Technician Note
> Vital signs should be monitored every 5 minutes on anesthetized animals and recorded in the anesthetic record.

Cardiovascular system monitoring involves integrated assessment of heart rate and rhythm, pulse quality, capillary refill time (CRT), and mucous membrane color. Heart rate and rhythm may be assessed by external auscultation or with an esophageal stethoscope in small animals (Figure 21-9). Palpation of a peripheral pulse may be easier to perform (vs. direct auscultation) during the surgical procedure and provides a way to count heart rate and assess pulse quality. Palpable peripheral pulses include the femoral, dorsal metatarsal, digital, and lingual arteries in dogs; the femoral artery in cats and swine; the facial, transverse facial, and lateral metatarsal arteries in horses; and the auricular, digital, coccygeal, and dorsal metatarsal arteries in ruminants. A continuous electrocardiogram (ECG) determines whether cardiac rate and rhythm are normal and aids in early detection of arrhythmias. Lead II is used in small animals, and a base-apex lead placement, recorded in lead II, is useful in large animals. Lead placement for a base-apex ECG (right arm over heart; left arm over jugular

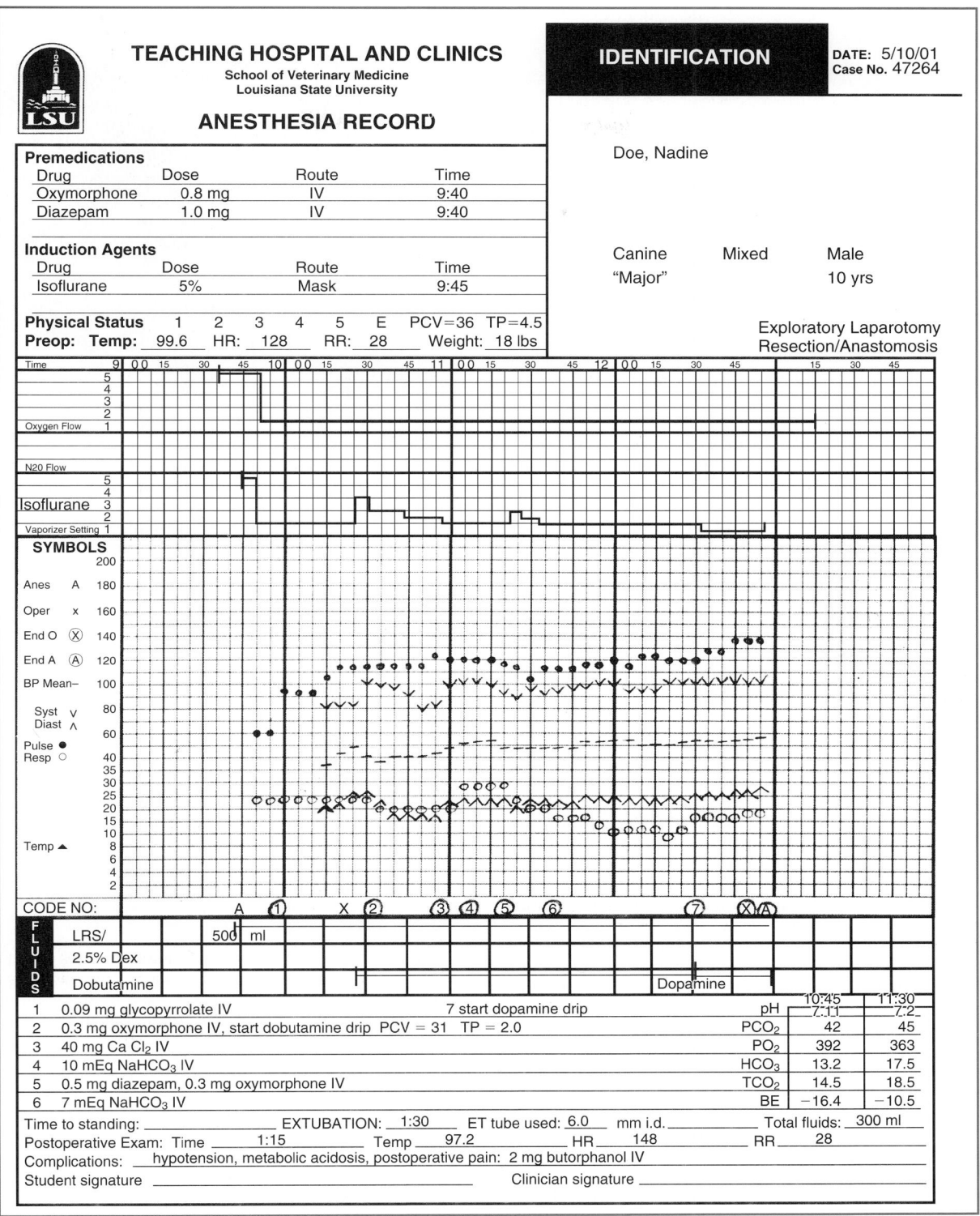

TEACHING HOSPITAL AND CLINICS
School of Veterinary Medicine
Louisiana State University
ANESTHESIA RECORD

IDENTIFICATION

DATE: 5/10/01
Case No. 47264

Doe, Nadine

Canine   Mixed   Male
"Major"   10 yrs

Exploratory Laparotomy
Resection/Anastomosis

Premedications

Drug	Dose	Route	Time
Oxymorphone	0.8 mg	IV	9:40
Diazepam	1.0 mg	IV	9:40

Induction Agents

Drug	Dose	Route	Time
Isoflurane	5%	Mask	9:45

Physical Status   1   2   3   4   5   E   PCV=36 TP=4.5
Preop: Temp: 99.6   HR: 128   RR: 28   Weight: 18 lbs

SYMBOLS

Anes   A
Oper   x
End O   (X)
End A   (A)
BP Mean–
Syst   v
Diast   ^
Pulse ●
Resp ○
Temp ▲

CODE NO: A ①   X ②   ③ ④ ⑤   ⑥   ⑦   (X)(A)

FLUIDS

LRS/	500 ml
2.5% Dex	
Dobutamine	Dopamine

1	0.09 mg glycopyrrolate IV	7 start dopamine drip
2	0.3 mg oxymorphone IV, start dobutamine drip PCV = 31 TP = 2.0
3	40 mg Ca Cl₂ IV
4	10 mEq NaHCO₃ IV
5	0.5 mg diazepam, 0.3 mg oxymorphone IV
6	7 mEq NaHCO₃ IV

	10:45	11:30
pH	7.11	7.2
PCO₂	42	45
PO₂	392	363
HCO₃	13.2	17.5
TCO₂	14.5	18.5
BE	–16.4	–10.5

Time to standing: _____   EXTUBATION: 1:30   ET tube used: 6.0 mm i.d. _____   Total fluids: 300 ml
Postoperative Exam: Time ___1:15___   Temp __97.2__   HR __148__   RR __28__
Complications: __hypotension, metabolic acidosis, postoperative pain: 2 mg butorphanol IV__
Student signature _____   Clinician signature _____

FIGURE 21-8. A sample anesthetic record that allows for sequential recording of heart rate, respiratory rate, and arterial blood pressures. Also included is a summary of the preanesthetic findings and the dose, route, and time of administration of drugs used.

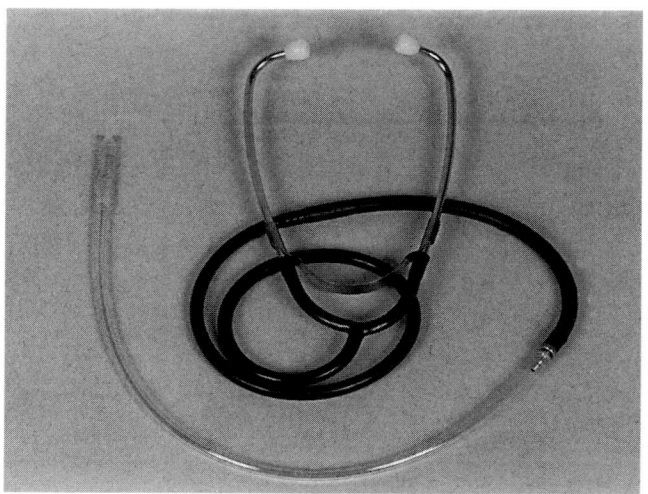

FIGURE 21-9. Esophageal stethoscope allows auscultation of heart sounds during the anesthetic monitoring period. The device may be coupled to a stethoscope earpiece (as shown) or an amplifier for transmission of audible sound.

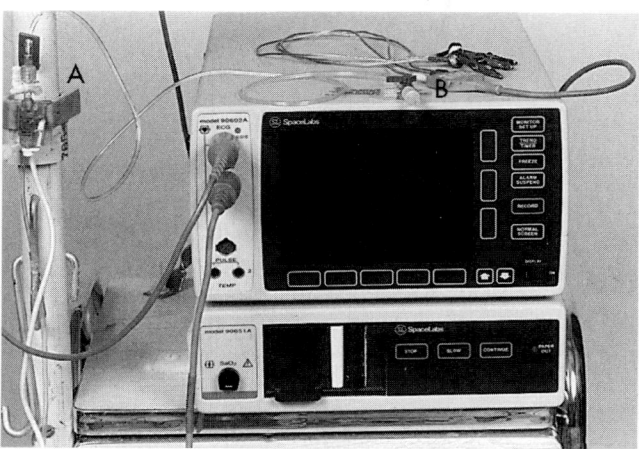

FIGURE 21-10. A computed electrocardiograph monitor for recording a continuous electrocardiogram. The monitor is also equipped with a pressure transducer *(a)*, which may be connected *(b)* to a catheter placed in a peripheral artery for direct measurement of systolic, diastolic, and mean arterial blood pressures. This machine can also record body temperature and hemogloblin oxygen saturation (pulse oximetry). (Courtesy Spacelabs, Inc.)

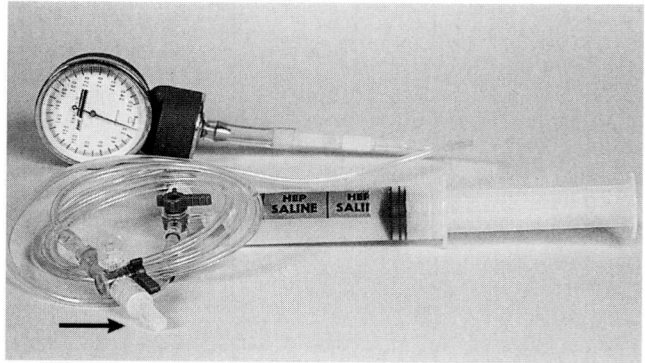

FIGURE 21-11. An aneroid manometer provides direct measurement of mean arterial blood pressure. The device is attached *(arrow)* to a catheter placed in a peripheral artery, and the air-water interface within the connecting tubing should be placed at the level of the patient's heart.

furrow; left leg over point of shoulder) will yield a large positive R wave. It is important to remember that a normal ECG only indicates normal electrical activity and yields no information regarding heart contractility or tissue perfusion.

Adequate perfusion is assessed by subjective evaluation of mucous membrane color, CRT (normal <2 seconds), and pulse quality.

Pulse oximetry is a noninvasive method of monitoring pulse rate and the amount of oxygen carried by hemoglobin in the arterial blood. Most pulse oximeters provide a pulse wave and a digital display of pulse rate and the percent oxygen saturation of hemoglobin (Sp_{O_2}). The Sp_{O_2} should be maintained above 95% in animals breathing 100% oxygen and above 90% in animals breathing room air. Values below 90% signal an arterial oxygen partial pressure (Pa_{O_2}) of less than 60 mm Hg, which defines hypoxemia.

Several sources of error can limit the usefulness of pulse oximetry, including hypotension, tachycardia, hypothermia, movement, and poor probe positioning. These potential sources of error should be considered when interpreting the values, and additional methods should be used in overall patient assessment. As a general rule, the closer the oximeter pulse rate is to the actual heart rate, the more accurate is the Sp_{O_2} value. Sites for probe placement in animals include the tongue, lip fold, toe web, ear, skinfolds, vulva, and nasal septum. A reflectance probe is also available, which may be used in the rectum or esophagus or laid flat against a mucous membrane.

Arterial blood pressure may be measured by either direct or indirect methods. Indirect methods, such as the oscillometric pulse monitor and the ultrasonic Doppler apparatus, require placement of an inflatable cuff on a peripheral artery. These methods are easy to use but are less accurate than direct methods.

For direct pressure monitoring, a catheter is placed in a peripheral artery and connected via heparinized saline-filled tubing to a pressure transducer (Figure 21-10) or aneroid manometer (Figure 21-11). Direct methods require more technical skill and knowledge of the equip-

ment. The aneroid manometer is relatively inexpensive and gives a continuous value for mean arterial pressure, whereas a pressure transducer records mean, systolic, and diastolic arterial pressures but requires relatively expensive equipment. Direct blood pressure monitoring is especially useful in equine patients during inhalation anesthesia to help assess anesthetic depth and to recognize and treat hypotension. The treatment of hypotension is important to minimize the risk of postanesthetic myopathy. Direct blood pressure monitoring is beneficial in high-risk patients of all species; a minimum of 60 mm Hg mean arterial pressure should ideally be maintained to ensure adequate tissue perfusion. Normal values for arterial blood pressure are listed in Table 21-5.

TABLE 21-5	REFERENCE INTERVALS FOR COMMONLY MEASURED CARDIOVASCULAR AND RESPIRATORY TESTS, BODY TEMPERATURE, AND LABORATORY VALUES IN COMMON DOMESTIC SPECIES					
Component	Dog	Cat	Horse	Cow	Goat/Sheep	Pig
Heart rate (beats/min)	70-180	145-200	30-45	60-80	60-90	60-90
Respiratory rate (breaths/min)	10-40	20-40	8-20	20-40	15-40	10-40
Temperature (°F)	101-104	101-104	99.5-101.5	100.5-102.5	101-104	101-103
Packed cell volume (%)	35-54	27-46	25-45	23-43	30-50	30-48
Total protein (g/dl)	5.7-7.8	6.3-8.3	6.0-8.5	6.7-8.6	6.3-7.1	6.0-7.5
Systolic arterial pressure* (mm Hg)	110-160	(Arterial blood pressure values tend to decrease during general anesthesia, especially with inhalation anesthetics and especially in debilitated patients, except in cattle, which tend to show an increase in blood pressure during general anesthesia. As a general rule, mean arterial blood pressure should be maintained above 60-70 mm Hg during general anesthesia in all species.)				
Diastolic arterial pressure* (mm Hg)	70-90					
Mean arterial pressure* (mm Hg)	80-110					
Arterial pH*	7.35-7.45					
$Paco_2$* (mm Hg)	35-45					
Pao_2 (mm Hg)	80-110	(as high as 500 when patient is breathing 100% oxygen)				
HCO_3^-* (mEq/L)	17-30	(mean = 24: higher values refer to horses and ruminants; lower values refer to dogs and cats)				
CO_2, total (mEq/L)	18-31					
Base excess* (mEq/L)	−4-+4					

HCO_3^-, bicarbonate; Pao_2, partial pressure of arterial oxygen; $Paco_2$, partial pressure of arterial carbon dioxide.
*Values are similar for all species; differences are explained in the table.

The *pulmonary system* is monitored by assessing breathing rate and rhythm. Although these assessments yield minimal information regarding adequacy of ventilation, sudden changes in the ventilatory pattern may signal an impending problem. For example, the onset of apnea during anesthesia may indicate excessive anesthetic depth. An increase in rate following initiation of surgery may indicate that the anesthesia is too light.

Respiratory apnea monitors sound an audible beep with each expiration and provide a method for monitoring breathing rate. The monitor is interfaced between the endotracheal tube and the breathing circuit. It is especially useful in small patients and birds whose respirations may be difficult to assess by either chest wall excursions or movement of the rebreathing bag. However, some apnea monitors may lack adequate sensitivity to detect expiratory flow of very small patients.

Most anesthetic agents are potent respiratory depressants, and apnea after anesthetic induction is not uncommon. Ventilation should be supported at this time (two to four breaths per minute) to ensure adequate delivery of oxygen and anesthetic gas until spontaneous ventilation returns (see Ventilatory Support).

The degree of collapse of the rebreathing bag provides a crude estimation of tidal volume. Arterial carbon dioxide ($Paco_2$) and oxygen (Pao_2) partial pressures provide the most accurate method of determining adequacy of ventilation; however, equipment for measuring blood gases is expensive and collection of arterial blood is required.

Capnometry provides a noninvasive method for monitoring breathing rate and adequacy of ventilation. The capnometer measures the partial pressure of carbon dioxide in expired gases and quantitates the end-tidal (end of expiration) carbon dioxide partial pressure (ET-Pco_2). The ET-Pco_2 is a close estimate of $Paco_2$ and should be maintained between 35 and 45 mm Hg. An increase indicates hypoventilation and the need for ventilatory assistance (see Ventilatory Support). The capnometer attaches to the patient's endotracheal tube and also provides a digital respiratory rate and an audible beep with each expiration. As a general rule, ET-Pco_2 tends to underestimate $Paco_2$ by 2 to 10 mm Hg.

Central nervous system evaluation yields information regarding depth of anesthesia and includes assessment of the position of the eye in the orbit and depression of eye reflexes (Table 21-6). Loss of the anal reflex is a crude indicator of excessive anesthetic depth. Degree of muscle relaxation (e.g., jaw tone) and absence of voluntary movement also aid in the evaluation of anesthetic depth. Muscle relaxation may be an unreliable indicator in animals given ketamine. Indicators of light anesthesia may include shivering and tensing of the neck and shoulder muscles.

Technician Note

Because anesthetized patients hypoventilate during anesthesia, ventilation should be periodically assisted or controlled to combat the development of hypercapnia and atelectasis, especially during prolonged procedures.

VENTILATORY SUPPORT

General anesthesia depresses respiration; therefore ventilatory support may often be necessary during general anesthesia. Special consideration must be given to high-risk patients, such as animals with pulmonary and pleural cavity disease, abdominal distention, diaphragmatic hernia, and obesity, and to animals undergoing open chest procedures. Although ventilatory assistance is not vital to the survival of most patients undergoing general anesthesia, ventilation should be periodically assisted to aid in the

Sign	Plane of Anesthesia		
	Too Light	Adequate	Too Deep
Corneal reflex	Brisk	Present	Absent
Palpebral reflex	Brisk	Slowed	Absent
Lateral nystagmus	Present	Absent or occasional	Absent
Unstimulated blinking	Present	Absent	Absent
Eyeball position	Centered	Rotated anteromedially	Centered
Tearing	Present	Absent or reduced	Absent

TABLE 21-6   EYE SIGNS* DURING MAINTENANCE OF ANESTHESIA

*Not useful after administration of dissociative anesthetics.
From Hubbell JAE: Monitoring. In Muir WW, Hubbell JAE, editors: *Equine anesthesia monitoring and emergency therapy,*
St Louis, 1991, Mosby,

maintenance of normal ventilation ($Paco_2$ = 35 to 45 mm Hg) and to minimize atelectasis, which tends to develop over time.

Assisted ventilation involves closing the pop-off valve and compressing the rebreathing bag. Many anesthesia machines are equipped with a pressure manometer, which measures the pressure inside the breathing system. A peak inspiratory pressure of 20 to 25 cm H_2O (small animals) and 25 to 30 cm H_2O (large animals) is sufficient to deliver an adequate tidal volume to most patients. Higher pressures may be needed in animals with open thoracic cavities or with primary lung disease. Ventilation should be assisted at least once every 2 or 3 minutes, and the animal should be "sighed" once every 5 to 10 minutes. The latter involves slightly higher peak inspiratory pressures to specifically combat atelectasis.

Many veterinary hospitals are equipped with mechanical ventilators and several types of ventilators are available that will enhance the quality of anesthesia during prolonged, complicated procedures (Figure 21-12). Indications for controlled ventilation (intermittent positive-pressure ventilation [IPPV]) include the following:

- Prolonged apnea
- Documentation of severe hypoventilation (increased $Paco_2$) on arterial blood gas analysis
- Intrathoracic surgery
- Intraoperative use of neuromuscular blocking agents
- Surgery duration longer than 90 minutes
- The need for hyperventilation in cases of head trauma
- To aid in the maintenance of a stable plane of surgical anesthesia by enhancing anesthetic agent delivery and uptake

Although IPPV does have a negative effect on cardiovascular performance, this may be minimized by ensuring adequate intravascular volume, using inotropes to enhance cardiovascular performance, and applying IPPV within the following recommended guidelines.

Tidal volume during IPPV is set above the actual tidal volume of the patient to allow for increases in breathing system and airway volume when positive pressure is delivered. The bellows volume is 15 to 20 ml/kg for small animals and 10 to 15 ml/kg for large animals.

Inspiratory time should be less than 1.5 seconds (up to 3 seconds in large animals), and the *I/E ratio* (inspiratory/expiratory ratio) should be less than 1:2 to minimize time spent in inspiration during the ventilatory cycle. Tidal volume and inspiratory time conjointly affect peak inspiratory pressure [PIP]. A value of 15 to 30 cm H_2O will expand the lungs of normal veterinary patients. Values on the high side of the range are needed for large animals, and for small animal patients, values of 12 to 20 cm H_2O are recommended.

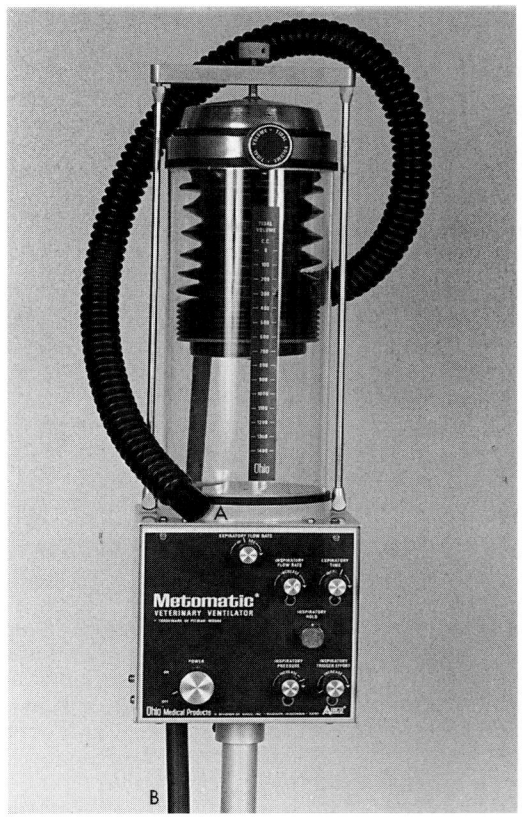

FIGURE 21-12. Metomatic veterinary ventilator for small animals. Tidal volume settings facilitate use in patients up to approximately 80 kg. The ventilator hose *(A)* is connected to the breathing system where the rebreathing bag is placed and the breathing system "pop-off" valve is closed. The waste gas scavenging system is then connected to the ventilator pop-off device *(B)*. (Courtesy Ohio Medical Products.)

The recommended *respiratory rate* during IPPV is 8 to 14 breaths/min for dogs and cats and 6 to 12 breaths/min for large animal species. When small tidal volumes must be used (i.e., animals with abdominal distention, diaphragmatic hernia), the rate should be increased accordingly.

ANESTHETIC MANAGEMENT

Several principles apply to the perianesthetic management of veterinary patients regardless of species. These are out-

TABLE 21-7	GUIDELINES FOR FASTING AND INTUBATION IN COMMON DOMESTIC SPECIES						
	Fasting* (hr)		Intubation				
Species	Food	Water	Technique	Desensitize Larynx	Laryngoscope Required	Regurgitation Possible	Comments
Dog	12	10	Visualization	No	No‡	Yes	—
Cat	12	10	Visualization	Yes	No‡	Yes	May need stylet
Horse	8-12	2	Blind	No	No	No	Oral or nasal
Cattle	36-48	12-24	Digital	No	No	Yes	Use guide tube
Sheep, goat, calves	18-24	2	Visualization	Yes	Yes†	Yes	Use guide tube
Swine	8-12	2-4	Visualization	Yes	Yes	Yes	Use guide tube

*Does not apply to neonates less than 1 mo of age.
†Incidence of regurgitation increases when animals are not adequately fasted, in animals with a history of vomiting, and in pregnant animals. Regurgitation may occur in horses presented for colic that have gastric distension.
‡A laryngoscope may be needed to visualize the larynx in some brachycephalic breeds and in dogs with pigmented mucosa. Although a laryngoscope is not essential for intubating cats, it may be necessary in some patients. Intubation may be performed blindly in small ruminants, but it is much more difficult and there is an increased risk of esophageal intubation, which may predispose to regurgitation and aspiration.

TABLE 21-8	PHYSICAL STATUS CLASSIFICATIONS AS DEFINED BY THE AMERICAN SOCIETY OF ANESTHESIOLOGISTS	
Classification	Definition	Example
I	Normal animal admitted for elective surgery	Elective castration
II	Animal with slight to moderate systemic disturbance	Obesity, dehydration
III	Animal with major systemic disturbance that limits activity but is not incapacitating	Heart disease, anemia, severe fracture
IV	Animal with very severe systemic disturbance that could lead to death if surgical or medical intervention is not applied	Frequent arrhythmias, ruptured bladder, internal hemorrhage, severe pneumothorax
V	Animal in a moribund state that will probably die despite surgical or medical intervention	Prolonged gastric dilation/volvulus, severe trauma with shock

lined and specific differences among species are noted in Table 21-7.

Preanesthetic Evaluation

The patient's history should be reviewed and a thorough physical examination performed, giving special attention to the cardiovascular and pulmonary system, before anesthesia (see Table 21-5). Minimal laboratory data include packed cell volume (PCV) and total protein concentration (see Table 21-5) in healthy animals. For high-risk patients, such as geriatric animals and animals with systemic diseases, a complete blood count (CBC), serum chemistry panel, electrolyte concentrations, and urinalysis should also be performed. An ECG should be recorded in traumatized and geriatric patients and in patients with evidence of cardiac arrhythmias or murmurs. Thoracic radiographs are indicated in patients with evidence of cardiac or pulmonary disease and those with a history of trauma. Abnormalities detected on physical examination and laboratory evaluation (e.g., anemia, respiratory distress, dehydration, electrolyte imbalance) should be corrected whenever possible before anesthetic induction.

Technician Note

Most animal species should fast before induction of general anesthesia to prevent regurgitation. Animals that have not fasted should only be anesthetized in an emergency situation.

On the basis of the foregoing information, the animal's physical status should be established (Table 21-8). The physical status indicates the risk for development of anesthetic complications in the individual patient and aids in the selection of an anesthetic protocol. The animal should *fast* before anesthesia; the duration varies among species (see Table 21-7). Neonates, birds, and patients under 2 kg should not be fasted because of limited glycogen stores and high metabolic rates.

Preparation of Equipment and Supplies

Selection of an anesthetic protocol is based on several factors, including the animal's temperament and physical status, the procedure to be performed, the available anesthetics, the familiarity of personnel with the drugs available, and the amount of assistance. Suggested protocols utilizing both inhalation and injectable techniques for the common domestic species are listed in Boxes 21-1 to 21-5.

Technician Note

Preparation of equipment and drugs is essential for successful anesthesia.

An anesthetic preparation checklist should be devised to optimize organization so that anesthetic induction and maintenance will be smooth and uncomplicated.

Box 21-2 SUGGESTED PROTOCOLS FOR CHEMICAL RESTRAINT AND GENERAL ANESTHESIA IN CATS

PROTOCOL FOR PHYSICAL STATUS I AND II ANIMALS

Premedication	Acepromazine: 0.06 mg/kg
	Ketamine: 15 mg/kg Mix and give IM.
	or
	Butorphanol: 0.44 mg/kg SC
Induction	Mask with halothane or isoflurane
	or
	Ketamine: 2.2-4.4 mg/kg IV "to effect"
	or
	Thiopental: 4.0-8.0 mg/kg IV
Maintenance	Halothane or isoflurane

PROTOCOL FOR PHYSICAL STATUS ≥III ANIMALS

Premedication (if needed)	Butorphanol: 0.44 mg/kg SC
Induction	Mask with isoflurane or sevoflurane
	or
	Diazepam: 0.25 mg/kg Mix and give IV "to effect."
	Ketamine: 5.0 mg/kg
	or
	Propofol 2-4 mg/kg IV "to effect."
Maintenance	Isoflurane or sevoflurane. Halothane may be used, but delivered concentrations should be minimized.

INJECTABLE PROTOCOLS

1. Butorphanol   0.44 mg/kg
   Telazol   6-11 mg/kg   Mix and give IM.
2. Butorphanol   0.44 mg/kg
   Xylazine   0.44 mg/kg
   Ketamine   15-22 mg/kg   Mix and give IM.
3. Diazepam and ketamine may be used as above to provide 10-15 min of anesthesia.
4. Acepromazine   0.1 mg/kg
   Butorphanol   0.44 mg/kg
   Ketamine   15-22 mg/kg   Mix and give IM.

IM, Intramuscular; IV, intravenous.

Preparations may be completed after the animal has been premedicated and should include the following:

I. Organize necessary supplies for intravenous catheterization, including appropriate catheters, tape, heparinized saline, and antiseptics for sterile preparation of the skin site.

II. Organize equipment for endotracheal intubation, including appropriately sized tubes that have been checked for cuff leaks, laryngoscope, stylet and topical anesthetic spray (if needed for the particular species), an oral speculum for cattle, gauze or tape to secure the tube in place, sterile lubricant to facilitate passage of the tube into the trachea, and a syringe to inflate the endotracheal tube cuff.

III. Prepare the anesthesia machine, and select a breathing system according to the animal's size (see selection criteria under Anesthesia Equipment):
   A. Fill vaporizer and check the oxygen supply.
   B. Evaluate soda lime absorbent, and refill if material is exhausted.
   C. Turn on flowmeter to check for free movement of indicator.

Box 21-3 SUGGESTED PROTOCOLS FOR CHEMICAL RESTRAINT AND GENERAL ANESTHESIA IN HORSES

STANDING CHEMICAL RESTRAINT

1. Xylazine   0.44-0.66 mg/kg IV
                   (Give xylazine first.)
   Butorphanol   0.022-0.044 mg/kg IV
2. Detomidine   0.022 mg/kg IV
3. Acepromazine   0.022-0.044 mg IV
                   (Give acepromazine 20 min before administration of other agents.)
   Xylazine   0.44 mg/kg IV
   Butorphanol   0.022 mg/kg IV

PROTOCOLS FOR INDUCTION OF ANESTHESIA BEFORE MAINTENANCE WITH AN INHALATION AGENT

1. Premedication   Xylazine: 1.1 mg/kg IV
                   (Give xylazine and wait 3-5 minutes before administering ketamine.)
   Induction   Ketamine: 2.2 mg/kg IV
2. Premedication   Xylazine: 0.44 mg/kg IV
                   or
                   Acepromazine: 0.044 mg/kg IV
   Induction   5% guaifenesin IV "to effect"
                   Thiopental bolus: 4.4-6.6 mg/kg IV
3. Premedication   Xylazine: 0.22-0.44 mg/kg IV
                   (This protocol works well in old, debilitated, and colic patients.)
   Induction   5% guaifenesin "to effect"
                   Ketamine: 1.5-1.8 mg/kg IV

INJECTABLE PROTOCOLS FOR INDUCTION AND MAINTENANCE OF GENERAL ANESTHESIA

Xylazine and ketamine as listed above provide 8-12 min of anesthesia. Duration of anesthesia may be extended by the following:

1. Administering butorphanol (0.022 mg/kg IV) or diazepam (0.055 mg/kg IV) before ketamine administration.
   or
2. Simultaneous administration of 50% of the original dose of xylazine and ketamine at 15- to 20-min intervals. Do not repeat more than two times.
   or
3. Administering a combination of 1 L of 5% guaifenesin containing 1 mg/ml of ketamine and 0.5 mg/ml of xylazine. The combination is administered at a constant drip (approximately 2.2 ml/kg/hr) until the procedure ends.

IV, Intravenously.

   D. Close pop-off valve, and pressurize the breathing system to 40 cm H_2O (on the pressure manometer) using the oxygen flush valve. This may be accomplished by placing your thumb over the patient connection. The system should maintain pressure if no leaks are present.
   E. Connect the breathing system (at the pop-off valve) to the waste gas scavenging system.
IV. Calculate the oxygen flow rate according to patient size and breathing system used.
V. Organize fluids for administration, and calculate the appropriate administration rate (see below).
VI. Calculate dosage for induction drugs. Withdraw drugs from bottles into labeled syringes.

BOX 21-4 SUGGESTED PROTOCOLS FOR CHEMICAL RESTRAINT AND GENERAL ANESTHESIA IN RUMINANTS

CATTLE

Premedication	Xylazine: 0.022-0.066 mg/kg IM (may not be required depending on animal's temperament and available restraint)
Induction	1 L of 5% guaifenesin plus 2-3 mg/ml of thiopental (give until animal assumes recumbency and can be intubated) *or* 1 L of 5% guaifensin plus 1.0-2.0 mg/ml of ketamine given "to effect"
Maintenance	Halothane or isoflurane

INJECTABLE PROTOCOLS FOR INDUCTION AND MAINTENANCE OF ANESTHESIA

1. 1 L 5% guaifenesin plus thiopental, 2 mg/ml, may be used for induction and maintenance: 1 L will provide induction and 30-45 min of anesthesia for a 500-kg animal. If a second bottle is required, thiopental, only 1 mg/ml, should be added to the guaifenesin.
2. 1 L 5% guaifenesin plus ketamine, 1 mg/ml, plus 0-50 mg of xylazine (total). Omit xylazine if the animal was premedicated with xylazine. This combination may be used for induction (2.2-4.4 ml/kg) and maintenance (2.2 ml/kg/hr), and one bottle may last 30-90 min, depending on the animal's size and type of procedure.

SHEEP AND GOATS

Premedication	Butorphanol: 0.05-0.1 mg/kg IV or IM Acepromazine: 0.055-0.11 mg/kg IV or IM Diazepam: 0.22-0.55 mg/kg IV (usually not required because animals are easy to restrain)
Induction	Thiopental: 11 mg/kg IV (Give "to effect" to facilitate intubation.) *or* Diazepam (0.25-0.5 mg/kg) plus ketamine (4.4 mg/kg): Mix and give IV "to effect" to facilitate intubation. (This combination is good for debilitated, old, or diseased animals.)
Maintenance	Halothane or isoflurane

INJECTABLE PROTOCOLS FOR INDUCTION AND MAINTENANCE OF ANESTHESIA

1. Xylazine: 0.11 mg/kg IM followed in 15 min by ketamine: 11.0 mg/kg IV (This combination provides 30-45 min of anesthesia. The recovery is prolonged but may be shortened by reversing the xylazine.)
2. Diazepam and ketamine as described above under induction provide 5-10 min of anesthesia.
3. Telazol: 2.2-6.6 mg/kg IV or IM provide 20-30 min of anesthesia.

IM, Intramuscular; *IV*, intravenously.

Endotracheal Intubation

Endotracheal intubation techniques in a variety of species are described in Table 21-7. Several principles should be remembered when performing intubation in any species:

- Inject air into cuff before use to check the cuff's ability to hold volume.
- Always have two or three tube sizes readily available for each patient in case the first selection is too small or too large.
- For cats, dogs, small ruminants, and swine, positioning the animal in sternal recumbency so that the head and neck are in a straight line offers the best visualization of the larynx for successful intubation. Some anesthetists prefer dorsal recumbency to perform intubation in swine. Horses and adult cattle are usually intubated while positioned in lateral recumbency with the head, neck, and back placed in a straight line to facilitate introduction of the tube into the larynx (Figures 21-13 and 21-14). Horses may also be intubated via the ventral meatus of the nasal cavity (a smaller tube must be used) with the head positioned as described above, and this position may be indicated for procedures involving the oral cavity. This method is especially applicable to foals and may be performed in the awake foal with minimal sedation to facilitate a rapid method of induction with inhalation anesthetics (Figure 21-15).
- A stylet with an atraumatic tip may be necessary in some situations. A rigid stylet will provide support for very flimsy tubes and will facilitate proper placement. In species such as small ruminants, swine, and sometimes cats, an atraumatic stylet such as a dog urinary catheter will facilitate introduction of the tube into the larynx. These species have a sensitive larynx, which is prone to

---

BOX 21-5 SUGGESTED PROTOCOLS FOR CHEMICAL RESTRAINT AND GENERAL ANESTHESIA IN SWINE

Premedication	Atropine: 0.044 mg/kg IM — Can mix and give as one injection Xylazine: 1.1-2.2 mg/kg IM *or* Medetomidine: 0.01-0.02 mg/kg IM Ketamine: 2.2-4.4 mg/kg IM *or* Atropine: 0.044 mg/kg IM — Can mix and give as one injection. Xylazine: 1.1 mg/kg IM Telazol: 6.0 mg/kg IM (decrease to 2.0-3.0 mg/kg for swine >50 kg)
Induction	Mask with halothane or isoflurane to facilitate intubation or maintain on mask
Maintenance	Halothane or isoflurane

INJECTABLE PROTOCOLS FOR MAINTENANCE OF ANESTHESIA

Premedication	See above protocols. These combinations will facilitate catheter placement in an ear vein.
Induction	1 L of 5% guaifenesin plus xylazine, 1 mg/ml, and ketamine, 1 mg/ml.
Maintenance	Drip at an approximate rate of 2.2 ml/kg/hr.

IM, Intramuscularly.

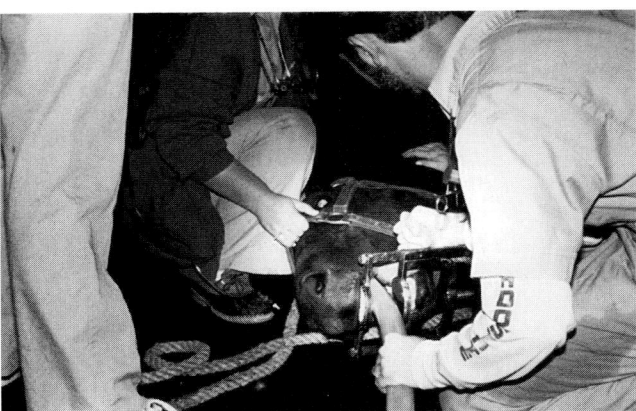

FIGURE 21-13. Positioning a horse to facilitate endotracheal intubation using the blind technique. An oral speculum is positioned between the incisor teeth to hold the mouth open, and the tongue is pulled out of the mouth.

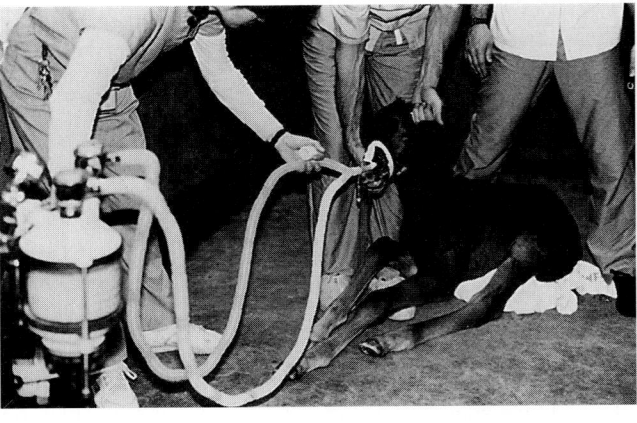

FIGURE 21-15. Newborn foal with an endotracheal tube introduced through the ventral meatus of the nasal cavity into the trachea for induction of anesthesia with isoflurane.

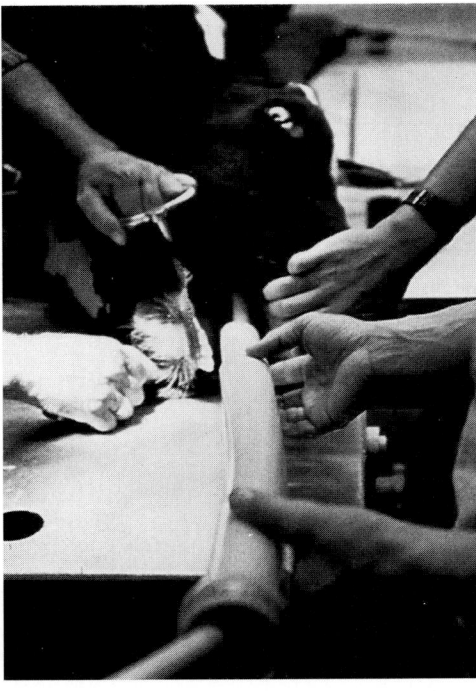

FIGURE 21-14. Endotracheal intubation of adult cattle requires placement of an oral speculum, digital palpation of the larynx, and introduction of a nasogastric tube into the trachea to guide the endotracheal tube into the trachea.

laryngospasm. Visualization is poor in small ruminants and swine because of their narrow oral cavity, and use of both a laryngoscope and a stylet is especially beneficial. In adult cattle, one can introduce a nasogastric tube into the trachea by digitally palpating the laryngeal opening. The endotracheal tube is then guided over the smaller and longer nasogastric tube and into the trachea. Use of a wire or any sharp instrument as a stylet is not advised; severe and even fatal tracheal trauma could result!

- Conservative use of a topical anesthetic agent in the laryngeal area (see Figure 21-1) specifically in cats, swine, and small ruminants, will facilitate intubation with minimal trauma. Laryngeal desensitization is effectively performed using 0.1 ml (cats) and 0.2 to 0.5 ml (other species) of 2% lidocaine delivered via syringe. Commercial topical benzocaine preparations (e.g., Cetacaine) should be avoided in cats because of reports of methemoglobinemia associated with its use.
- Adequate anesthetic depth and muscle relaxation are important for successful intubation. This will avoid unnecessary laryngeal trauma and excessive autonomic nervous system stimulation, which may give rise to cardiac arrhythmias.
- The endotracheal tube should be long enough to reach midway between the larynx and carina so that accidental dislodgment does not occur. It should not be too long because this can increase the risk of endobronchial intubation, and an excessive tube length that extends beyond the oral cavity constitutes dead space, which can contribute to hypercapnia.
- Proper tube placement may be assessed by (1) visualization of the tube passing between the arytenoid cartilages (not applicable in horses and cattle), (2) condensation of respiratory gases on the inside of the tube with expiration, (3) only one tubular structure (trachea) palpable in the neck region, (4) auscultation of lung sounds during assisted ventilation, and (5) absence of vocalization.
- The cuff should be inflated just enough to form an effective seal within the trachea. This can be assessed by closing the pop-off valve, assisting ventilation, and listening for air escaping around the cuff or checking for the smell of anesthetic gas.
- Secure the tube to the patient by tying gauze tightly around the tube and then securing it around the head (cats, brachycephalic breeds) or to the upper or lower jaw. This is usually not necessary in horses and adult cattle.

Fluid Administration During Anesthesia

Fluid administration is important to the maintenance of homeostasis during anesthesia and provides venous access for the delivery of agents used intraoperatively for supportive therapy (e.g., antibiotics, inotropic agents), for maintenance of anesthesia (injectable anesthetic agents), and for cardiopulmonary resuscitation. Imbalances may occur because of blood loss, drying of exposed tissues, removal of effusions, and the hypotensive effects of anesthetic agents. The following guidelines will keep fluid therapy during anesthesia simple and effective:

I. Fluids most commonly used are polyionic isotonic crystalloid solutions, such as lactated Ringer's or Normosol. For neonates (<1 month of age), very small patients, and birds, use 5% dextrose or supplement lactated Ringer's with 5 or 10 ml of 50% dextrose per 100 ml of Ringer's solution for a dextrose concentration of 2.5% or 5.0%, respectively.

II. For healthy animals during routine procedures the following fluid rates are suggested: small animals, 10 to 20 ml/kg/hr; large animals, 5 to 10 ml/kg/hr. The following exceptions to the foregoing fluid rates apply:
   A. Increasing the administration rate in animals with preexisting dehydration, excessive intraoperative blood loss, or hypotension and during cardiopulmonary resuscitation.
   B. Decreasing the administration rate in animals that have significant cardiac or renal disease or are hypoproteinemic. These situations make the animals more prone to the development of pulmonary edema because they are unable to handle the additional fluid load.

III. Blood lost during surgery should be replaced at a volume of three times the approximate loss in addition to the basic fluid rate during anesthesia. Ideally, when blood loss is significant, the PCV and total protein should be monitored to avoid excessive dilution. An acute fall in PCV below 20% should be treated with packed red cells or whole blood. Total protein should not fall below 3.5 g/dl because of the increased risk of developing pulmonary edema.

Induction and Maintenance

Guidelines for induction and maintenance are as follows:

- Turn on oxygen flow a few minutes before connection of the patient to the breathing system to fill the system with oxygen.
- Connect the endotracheal tube to the breathing system and turn on the vaporizer to the appropriate induction setting (see Table 21-4).
- Assess pulse rate and quality.
- Assess respiration. If the animal is apneic or the rate is slow, assist ventilation.
- Apply ophthalmic ointment.
- Reduce vaporizer settings to the appropriate maintenance concentration as indicated by the patient's anesthetic depth.
- Begin intravenous fluid administration.
- Begin monitoring and instrumentation with available monitoring equipment.
- Record all pertinent information in the anesthetic record, and begin recording vital signs every 5 minutes (see Figure 21-8).
- When using injectable techniques in horses and adult cattle, procedures should be limited to 1 hour. For procedures lasting longer than 1 hour, an oxygen source should be available to insufflate oxygen (10 to 15 L/min) into the nares to prevent the development of hypoxia as a result of hypoventilation and atelectasis.

The anesthetic period should also be limited to 1 hour in small animals when injectable protocols are used. For longer procedures, oxygen should be administered through an endotracheal tube or, preferably, inhalation anesthesia should be used.

Technician Note

Remember to check vaporizer liquid level periodically during the anesthetic period (especially during large animal anesthesia) to ensure the presence of adequate amounts of anesthetic.

Padding and Positioning of the Patient

Proper padding and positioning depend on the procedure to be performed and the particular species.

- Dogs, cats, neonates of all species, and all other small species should be placed on a covered heating pad, circulating water blanket, or forced air blanket heater when available to minimize hypothermia. *Never* place the animal directly on a heating pad or water blanket.
- When securing limbs to the surgery table, do not apply ties too tightly and do not apply excessive traction to the forelimbs. Both actions may result in neurologic damage, and the latter may impede ventilatory effort.
- Ensure that the head and neck are positioned to avoid kinking of the endotracheal tube or disconnection from the breathing system.
- Ensure that appropriate expansion of the thorax is not compromised.
- For horses and adult cattle, adequate padding, such as a thick foam pad, water-filled pad, or air dunnage bag, is essential to prevent the development of postoperative myositis and neuropathy. For procedures in the field, a grassy area offers the best padding. The down eye should be protected and the head padded if possible.
- For horses and cattle in lateral recumbency, the upper forelimbs and hindlimbs should be supported so that they are parallel to the table surface. The down forelimb should be pulled forward to avoid entrapment of the brachial plexus between the rib cage and humerus.
- Always remove the halter from horses during general anesthesia to avoid damage to cranial nerves by the metal connectors.
- Ruminants should be placed in right lateral recumbency *when possible* so that the rumen is on the up side. During lateral recumbency, the neck should be elevated with a soft pad so that the head angles downward to promote flow of saliva and regurgitation (if it occurs) out of the oral cavity.
- Because of the high incidence of regurgitation in mature ruminants, an endotracheal tube should be placed and the cuff inflated (even if injectable anesthetics are used) before positioning the animal (especially in dorsal recumbency).

Technician Note

Hypothermia is a significant problem during general anesthesia, especially in small animals, and can be life threatening. Precautions to minimize heat loss should always be part of anesthetic management.

Recovery

Guidelines for recovery from anesthesia vary according to species.

Dogs and Cats

1. Flush the breathing system with pure oxygen, and continue oxygen delivery for 5 to 10 minutes.
2. Deflate the cuff (*if* the animal is not at risk for regurgitation) and extubate only *after* swallowing is observed. Suction the oral cavity before extubation if excessive secretions have collected. Maintain the tube in place as long as possible in brachycephalic breeds, which are prone by conformation to upper airway obstruction following anesthesia.
3. Position the animal in sternal recumbency with the head extended if possible. This is especially important in brachycephalic breeds.
4. Most animals are hypothermic following general anesthesia, and an external heat source will hasten recovery and return to normothermia. Hot water bottles, heating pads, or a circulating water blanket may be used, but *never* place it directly on the patient's skin.
5. Changing the animal's position and rubbing the body will hasten recovery.
6. Use analgesics (e.g., opioids) postoperatively if the procedure was invasive (e.g., orthopedic surgery, thoracotomy, abdominal surgery).
7. Some patients may need continued intravenous fluid therapy (e.g., patients with renal disease, dehydration), and the suggested maintenance rate is 60 ml/kg/24 hr.
8. Check the animal frequently until it can maintain sternal recumbency and stand unassisted.

Horses

1. When inhalation anesthesia is used, the horse should be placed in a padded dark room and allowed to recover unassisted. Extubate with the cuff deflated when swallowing is observed. A safer method to ensure a patent airway throughout recovery is to extubate when anesthesia is discontinued and place a smaller noncuffed tube into the trachea via the nasal passage and secure it to the muzzle with tape. This tube may be left in place until the horse is standing.
2. If available, insufflate oxygen (10 to 15 L/min) via the recovery tube or nasal cavity for 15 to 30 minutes following the end of anesthesia.
3. For recoveries in the field, the halter should be replaced so that the animal can be assisted during recovery. The eye should be covered to minimize external stimulation.
4. Some horses have a rough recovery regardless of the technique used. Administration of a sedative such as xylazine or a tranquilizer such as acepromazine or diazepam in low doses will quiet the animal until it is ready to rise unassisted.

Ruminants

1. If inhalation anesthesia is used, 100% oxygen should be administered for 5 to 10 minutes after anesthetic delivery is discontinued.
2. Ruminants should be positioned in sternal recumbency as soon as possible to promote eructation and minimize the chance of regurgitation.
3. Extubation should be performed with the cuff *inflated* only after swallowing is observed.
4. A stomach tube should be passed to decompress the rumen if bloat has developed intraoperatively.

5. Ruminants generally recover smoothly from general anesthesia, and minimal assistance is required.

Swine

1. Continue oxygen for 5 to 10 minutes after anesthetic delivery has been discontinued when inhalation techniques have been used.
2. Extubate with the cuff deflated (unless there is evidence of regurgitation) when swallowing is observed.
3. Position the animal in sternal recumbency as soon as possible, and allow the animal to recover in a cool and quiet environment.

POSTOPERATIVE ANALGESIA

Any procedure considered to be painful to humans should be considered painful to animals; if there is any doubt whether an animal is in pain, it should be treated (see Table 22-2 for signs of pain in animals and an approach to evaluation). In large animals, nonsteroidal antiinflammatory agents, such as phenylbutazone or flunixin meglumine, are most commonly used. In small animals, systemic administration of opioids, such as oxymorphone, butorphanol, morphine, or buprenorphine, is excellent for postoperative pain management (see Table 21-2 for dosages). Buprenorphine offers the advantage of prolonged duration of effect (6 to 12 hours). Although butorphanol and buprenorphine are useful in cats, the pure opioid agonists (oxymorphone, morphine) may elicit an excitatory response and should be used in conjunction with a tranquilizer.

An alternative to systemic opioid administration is epidural administration, offering the advantages of longer duration of action and elimination of side effects such as respiratory depression and bradycardia. Epidural morphine (0.1 mg/kg) diluted in saline (1 ml/5 kg, not to exceed 6 ml) or with a local anesthetic provides a duration of action of 10 to 24 hours. Butorphanol (0.2 mg/kg), oxymorphone (0.1 mg/kg), and buprenorphine (0.003 to 0.005 mg/kg) may also be used epidurally, but they have a shorter duration than morphine. Systemic and epidural opioids are also useful for pain management in horses, ruminants, and swine (epidural dosages as listed above). Additional information concerning pain management may be found in Chapter 22.

ANESTHETIC EMERGENCIES

Anesthesia causes a stress to homeostasis, including respiratory and cardiac depression, which may increase the risk of cardiopulmonary arrest, especially in high-risk patients. Cardiopulmonary arrest is the sudden cessation of ventilation and effective circulation that requires rapid emergency intervention (cardiopulmonary resuscitation) to prevent death. Physical status categorization alerts the anesthetist to the likelihood that complications that may lead to arrest could occur in a particular patient and stresses the importance of careful monitoring throughout the anesthetic period. Complications may occur at any time during the anesthetic period, including induction, maintenance, and recovery.

Cardiopulmonary resuscitation (CPR) is subdivided into four phases: readiness and prevention, recognition and basic cardiac life support, advanced cardiac life support, and postresuscitative care.

Readiness and Prevention

Hospital personnel should be prepared to handle cardiopulmonary arrest by identifying an area in the hospital that

Box 21-6	READINESS CHECKLIST FOR CARDIOPULMONARY RESUSCITATION

- Well-lighted area with adequate workspace
- Clippers
- Emergency drugs (Table 21-10)
- Endotracheal tubes
- Tracheostomy tubes
- Face masks
- Method for artificial ventilation (anesthesia machine or Ambu bag)
- Oxygen source
- Gauze for securing endotracheal tube
- Needles and syringes
- Laryngoscope
- Aspiration device
- Intravenous catheters
- Electrocardiograph machine
- Defibrillator

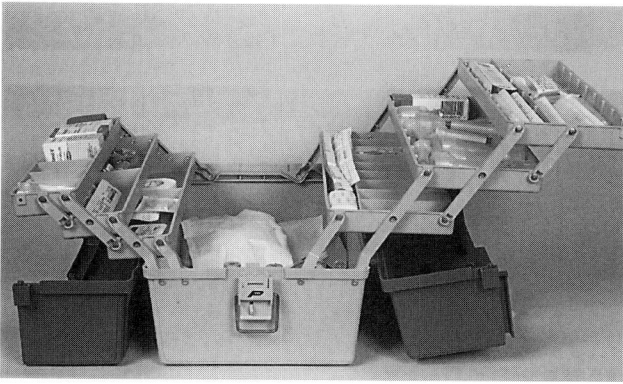

FIGURE 21-16. Example of a utility box used to organize emergency equipment and drugs for anesthetic emergencies.

is well lighted and stocked with emergency equipment and drugs (Box 21-6; Figures 21-16 and 21-17). Staff members involved in resuscitation should have an assigned role, which should be practiced periodically in mock drills to improve response time and the efficiency of intervention.

Prevention, as it applies to anesthetic-related cardiopulmonary arrest, involves recognition of high-risk patients and the application of appropriate and effective monitoring of all anesthetized patients. Clinical signs that may indicate an impending arrest include cyanosis; changes in respiration, such as apnea, tachypnea, dyspnea, or a marked abdominal effort associated with breathing; and changes associated with the cardiovascular system, such as bradycardia, tachycardia, weak, irregular or absent pulse, pale mucous membranes, and increased CRT. Hypothermia may increase the risk of arrest by contributing to the development of bradycardia and excessive anesthetic depth. A body temperature less than 30° C (86° F) predisposes to life-threatening ventricular arrhythmias. Recognition and correction of some potentially life-threatening problems are listed in Table 21-9.

Recognition and Basic Life Support

Early recognition of cardiopulmonary arrest is critical to successful resuscitation and is optimized by effective patient monitoring. The initial actions to be taken in the arrest of an anesthetized patient are to discontinue delivery of the anesthetic agent, flush the breathing system with pure oxygen, and increase the fluid administration rate. Reversal of anesthetic agents, such as opioids or alpha$_2$ agonists, may also be indicated in the anesthetized patient with cardiac arrest. The basic life support techniques should be initiated concurrently and include the following:

- *Airway.* If the animal is not already intubated, an endotracheal tube is placed. If the animal is already intubated, the tube should be checked for proper placement and patency. If an endotracheal tube cannot be placed or is not patent because of an obstruction, a tracheostomy should be performed or the tube changed, respectively.
- *Breathing.* Breathe for the patient using the anesthesia machine or an Ambu bag (see Figure 21-17), preferably with 100% oxygen, at a rate of 20 breaths/min performed simultaneously with every third to sixth chest compression, depending on the compression rate.

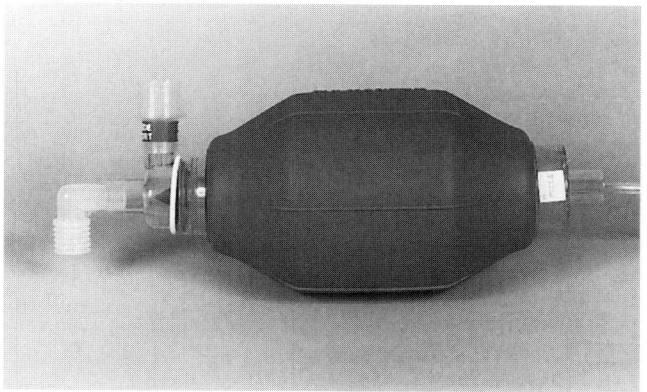

FIGURE 21-17. Ambu bag may be used to ventilate patients during cardiopulmonary arrest. The bag is attached to the endotracheal tube and squeezed to deliver a breath. Some Ambu bags are equipped with tubing for connection to an oxygen source.

- *Circulation.* If a pulse or heartbeat cannot be detected, external cardiac compressions should be initiated, with the goal of maintaining adequate blood flow to the brain and heart until normal heart rhythm can be restored. In most animals, compressions are performed at the level of the costochondral junction between the fourth and eighth ribs at a rate of 80 to 120/min, with the animal in lateral recumbency. In barrel-chested dogs, such as the brachycephalic breeds, compressions may be more effectively delivered in a ventrodorsal direction with the animal stabilized in dorsal recumbency. Abdominal wrapping or interposed rhythmic abdominal compressions may help to improve forward blood flow by increasing the intrathoracic pressure generated.

Advanced Life Support

Techniques for advanced life support include diagnosis of the type of arrest, the use of emergency drugs, defibrillation, and internal cardiac massage.

- *Drug/defibrillation.* Venous access is critical in the successful treatment of cardiac arrest. Drugs may be given

TABLE 21-9	DIFFERENTIAL DIAGNOSIS AND TREATMENT OF COMPLICATIONS THAT MAY OCCUR DURING ANESTHESIA	
Abnormality	**Potential Causes**	**Treatment**
Bradycardia	Excessive anesthetic depth	Correct underlying cause if possible
	Drugs: opioids, xylazine, gas anesthetics	Administer anticholinergic agent
	Hyperkalemia	Administer sympathomimetic agent
	Vagal reflex (intubation, oculocardiac reflex)	Dopamine: 2-10 µg/kg/min*
	Visceral manipulation	Dobutamine: 2-10 µg/kg/min*
	Hypothermia	Ephedrine: 0.05-0.5 mg/kg bolus*
	Terminal stages or hypoxia	Isoproterenol: 0.5-0.2 µg/kg/min*
	Exogenous and endogenous toxemias	
Tachycardia	Drugs: ketamine, thiobarbiturates, anticholinergics, sympathomimetics	Correct underlying cause if possible
	Hypokalemia	
	Hyperthermia	
	Inadequate anesthetic depth	
	Hypercapnia, hypoxemia	
	Anemia, hypovolemia	
	Hyperthyroidism, pheochromocytoma	
	Anaphylaxis	
Atrial and ventricular premature contractions	Light anesthesia	Correct underlying cause if possible
	Deep anesthesia	Evaluate anesthetic depth
	Hypoxia, hypercapnia	Check anesthetic machine and oxygen flow
	Hypovolemia	Assist ventilation
	Exogenous catecholamine therapy	If arrhythmia persists and meets one or more of the following criteria:
	Digitalis toxicity	• >20/min
	Hypokalemia	• Increasing in frequency
	Hyperkalemia	• Multifocal
	Hypercalcemia	• Occurring in runs
	Certain anesthetics (xylazine, halothane, thiobarbiturates)	• Causing significant effect on pulse
	Endocarditis or myocarditis	Treat arrhythmia as follows:
	Severe hypothermia	1. Turn off anesthetic gas
	End-stage visceral organ failure	2. Increase fluid administration rate
	Intracranial disorders	3. Administer lidocaine IV (max: 4 doses)
		Dog: 2.2 mg/kg
		Cat, horse: 0.5 mg/kg
Hypotension	Hypovolemia (i.e., blood loss)	Increase fluid administration rate
	Sepsis	Decrease anesthetic concentration
	Shock	Administer sympathomimetic agents
	Drugs (thiobarbiturates, inhalant)	Dopamine: 2-20 µg/kg/min*
		Dobutamine: 2-20 µg/kg/min*
		Ephedrine: 0.055-0.55 mg/kg bolus (small animals)*
		0.022 mg/kg bolus (horse)*
Tachypnea	Pain	Correct underlying cause if possible
	Hypoxia	
	Hypercapnia	
	Hyperthermia	
	Acidosis	
	Drugs (i.e., doxapram)	
Apnea	Hypothermia	Correct underlying cause if possible
	Hyperventilation with 100% O_2	Assist ventilation until spontaneous ventilation returns
	Drug effects (thiopental, ketamine)	
	Deep anesthesia	
	Aminoglycoside administration	

IV, Intravenously.
*These drugs may cause cardiac arrhythmias. Monitor electrocardiogram during administration.

by a peripheral venous catheter, if effective blood flow has been established by compression techniques. A fluid bolus should follow administration of every drug used. The tracheal route via the endotracheal tube is effective for epinephrine, atropine, and lidocaine administration. Dosages should be twice those given intravenously, the dose should be diluted in 3 to 10 ml of saline, and several rapidly applied ventilations should follow administration to ensure distribution to the pulmonary vasculature. The intraosseous route (via the tibial tuberosity, greater tubercle of the humerus, trochanteric fossa of the femur, wing of the ilium) may also be used for fluid and drug administration if venous access cannot be achieved. Table 21-10 lists some of the

TABLE 21-10 EMERGENCY DRUG DOSAGES AND DEFIBRILLATION SETTINGS USED FOR CARDIOPULMONARY RESUSCITATION

Drug		Concentration	Dosage	Indication	Comments
Epinephrine		1 mg/ml	0.02-0.2 mg/kg (SA)	Initiate heartbeat	Dose may be repeated every 5 min
			0.0011-0.0055 mg/kg (LA)	Increase heart rate	
				Increase contractility	
				Improve blood flow during CPR	
Atropine		0.5 mg/ml	0.044 mg/kg (SA)	Increase heart rate	
			0.011 mg/kg (LA)	Treat ventricular asystole	
Lidocaine		20 mg/ml	2.2 mg/kg (dogs)	Treat ventricular arrhythmias	
			0.5 mg/kg (cats)		
			0.5 mg/kg (LA)		
Prednisolone sodium succinate (Solu-Delta-Cortef)		10 mg/ml	22 mg/kg (SA)	Shock and ischemia	
		50 mg/ml	2.2 mg/kg (LA)	Stabilize cellular membranes	
or				Prevent cerebral edema	
Dexamethasone sodium phosphate		4 mg/ml	2.2-4.4 mg/kg		
Sodium bicarbonate		1 mEq/ml	0.5-1.0 mEq/kg per 5 min of arrest	Treat metabolic acidosis	Use after 10 min of arrest or with preexisting acidosis only
Calcium chloride		100 mg/ml	10 mg/kg (SA)	Prevent arrhythmias associated with hyperkalemia	Has been incriminated in reperfusion injury
			2.2 mg/kg (LA)	Treat hypocalcemia	
Hypertonic saline		70 mg/ml	4 ml/kg	Treat hypovolemic shock	Must be used with isotonic fluids
				Restore vascular volume	
Furosemide		50 mg/ml	1.1 mg/kg	Treat pulmonary and cerebral edema	Monitor hydration status
Mannitol		200 mg/ml	0.55-1.1 mg/kg	Treat cerebral edema	Monitor hydration status
				Protect brain against reperfusion injury	
Doxapram		20 mg/ml	1.1-4.4 mg/kg (SA)	Initiate breathing	
			0.22 mg/kg (LA)		
Direct current defibrillation	Body wt.	<8 kg	8-40 kg	>40 kg	Treatment of ventricular fibrillation	Better to treat underlying problem
	External	2 ws/kg	2-5 ws/kg	5-10 ws/kg		
	Internal	0.5-2.0 ws/kg				

CPR, Cardiopulmonary resuscitation; LA, large animal; SA, small animal; ws, watt-second (joules), which defines units of energy output produced by an electrical defibrillator.

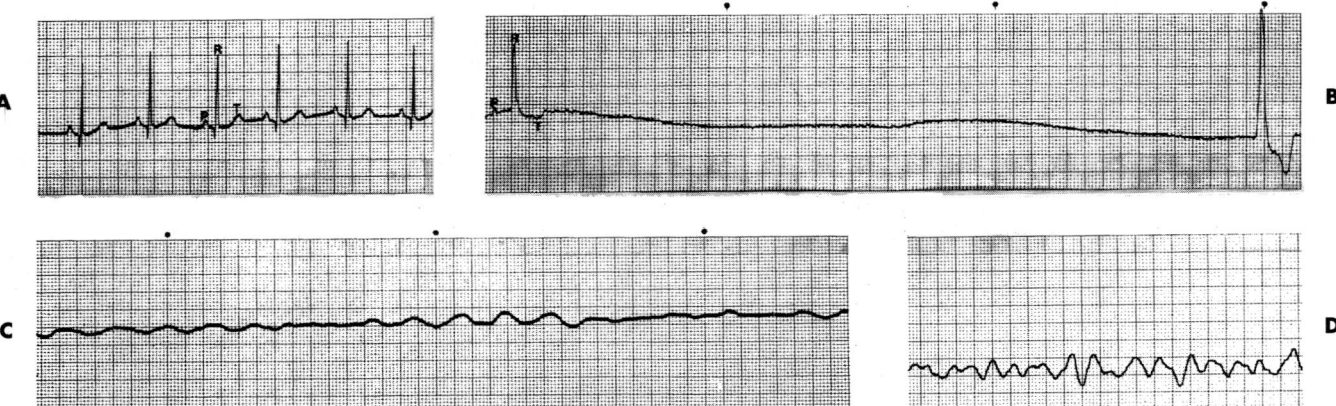

FIGURE 21-18. Representative electrocardiogram tracings of the different types of cardiac arrest. **A,** Electromechanical dissociation presents as a normal tracing, but no palpable pulse is associated with the electrical activity. **B,** Ventricular asystole presents as a flat tracing. Fine, **C,** and coarse, **D,** ventricular fibrillation present as wavy lines. It is important to distinguish between fine and coarse ventricular fibrillation because the latter is easier to convert to normal rhythm with defibrillation techniques. (From Tiley LP: *Essentials of canine and feline electrocardiography,* ed 3, Philadelphia, 1992, Lea & Febiger.)

TABLE 21-11	CLASSIFICATIONS OF CARDIAC ARREST AND SUGGESTED TREATMENT PROTOCOL	
Arrhythmia	**Treatment**	**Dosage**
Ventricular asystole	Epinephrine	0.02–0.2 mg/kg IV or IT*
	Atropine	0.044 mg/kg IV or IT
	Prednisolone sodium succinate (Solu-Delta-Cortef)	22 mg/kg IV
	Sodium bicarbonate (if >10–15 min)	1.0 mEq/kg IV
Ventricular fibrillation	Precordial thump (if defibrillator not available)	
	Epinephrine	0.2 mg/kg IV or IT
	Defibrillate	See Table 21-10
	Defibrillate	Double original dose
	Lidocaine	2.2 mg/kg IV or IT (cats: 0.5 mg/kg)
	Sodium bicarbonate (if >10–15 min)	1.0 mEq/kg IV
Electromechanical dissociation	Epinephrine	0.2 mg/kg IV or IT
	Prednisolone sodium succinate (Solu-Delta-Cortef)	22 mg/kg IV
	or	
	Dexamethasone sodium phosphate	2.2 mg/kg IV
	Sodium bicarbonate	1.0 mEq/kg IV

*IV, Intravenous administration; IT, intratracheal administration: double the recommended intravenous dose.

commonly used emergency drugs, indications for their use, and dosages.

- *Electrocardiogram.* An ECG should be recorded as soon as possible during the course of resuscitation to identify the type of arrest so that specific therapy for conversion to normal rhythm can be applied. The three types of cardiac arrest include ventricular asystole, ventricular fibrillation, and electromechanical dissociation. Figure 21-18 illustrates the three types of arrest, and Table 21-11 lists the specific treatment steps for each type of arrest.

- *Fluid therapy.* Cardiac arrest is a rapidly vasodilating process, and fluid therapy, most often with an isotonic polyionic solution is essential. Never use dextrose-containing fluids during resuscitative efforts because dextrose may exacerbate brain damage. It is recommended that fluids be given rapidly as calculated bo-

luses so that overhydration, which may predispose to pulmonary and cerebral edema, is avoided. For cats, boluses of 20 ml/kg are recommended, and for dogs and most other species, boluses of 40 ml/kg are recommended. These boluses may be repeated as needed throughout resuscitation to maintain an effective circulating volume. Three to seven percent hypertonic saline (4 ml/kg) has been shown to be beneficial in resuscitation efforts, in conjunction with isotonic fluid administration, to rapidly restore vascular volume and reduce the risk of development of pulmonary and cerebral edema.

- *Internal cardiac massage.* If external techniques and drug administration have not established effective circulation in 5 minutes or if the heart has not resumed normal rhythm in 10 minutes, a thoracotomy and internal massage should be performed at the left fourth or fifth intercostal space. This procedure should be performed immediately in very large or barrel-chested animals or in animals with fractured ribs or pneumothorax.

Postresuscitative Care

Patients may suffer arrest again following successful resuscitative efforts. Careful monitoring of the ECG, pulse quality, respiratory pattern, body temperature, and CNS (pupillary responses, mentation, seizure activity) is essential for several hours after the primary event. Neurologic damage may become evident 24 to 48 hours after the arrest, so serial neurologic examinations should be performed. Oxygen therapy should be administered for a period of time, depending on the condition of the patient.

Cardiopulmonary arrest in the anesthetized patient may be successfully treated only if the anesthetist recognizes the arrest early through careful monitoring and acts rapidly and correctly to reestablish normal cardiac rhythm before permanent organ damage occurs.

RECOMMENDED READING

Dorsch JA, Dorsch SE: *Understanding anesthesia equipment,* ed 4, Baltimore, 1999, Williams & Wilkins.

Muir WW, Hubbell JAE, editors: *Equine anesthesia monitoring and emergency therapy,* St Louis, 1991, Mosby.

Muir WW, Hubbell JAE, editors: *Handbook of veterinary anesthesia,* ed 3, St Louis, 2000, Mosby.

Seymour C, Gleed R, editors: *Manual of small animal anaesthesia and analgesia,* United Kingdom, 1999, British Small Animal Veterinary Association.

Short CE, editor: *Principles and practice of veterinary anesthesia,* Baltimore, 1987, Williams & Wilkins.

Thurmon JC, Tranquilli WJ, Benson GJ, editors: *Lumb & Jones' veterinary anesthesia,* ed 3, Baltimore, 1996, Williams & Wilkins.

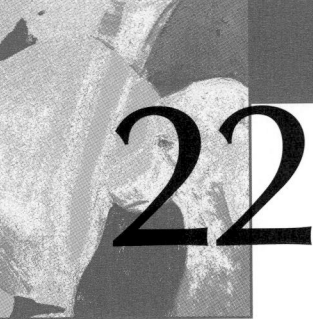

22

Pain Management

Jill E. Sackman

The veterinarian and veterinary technician together have an obligation to recognize and alleviate animal pain. This task is difficult, for only human patients can point to their specific source of discomfort and describe it. We must assume that veterinary patients experience pain under any circumstance in which humans would feel pain. There are, in fact, many similarities between animals and humans in the anatomic and chemical pathways of pain perception. Differences that do exist are generally attributed to alternative pathways for pain and not the absence of them. For many years there has been an erroneous but well-meaning belief that pain in animals is beneficial and that it provides a constant reminder to the patient to avoid movement that might cause further injury. This line of thought is illogical in that uncontrolled pain may lead to prolonged hospitalization, poor wound healing, and an increased rate of complications and mortality in both animals and humans. It has now become widely acknowledged that the recognition and alleviation of pain in animals is the essence of good patient care.

ORGANIZATION OF PAIN-CONDUCTING SYSTEMS

Peripheral Nervous System

The transmission of a painful sensation involves stimulation of receptors and peripheral nerves in the traumatized tissue with subsequent conduction through the spinal cord to multiple areas in the brain. When a painful stimulus occurs, a chain of events that lead to the sensation of pain is initiated. The degree of tissue sensitivity to pain is directly related to the density of pain receptors present. Pain receptors respond to traumatic stimuli by converting the chemical, mechanical, or thermal insult into nerve impulses. These impulses are conducted from the peripheral tissue to the spinal cord and brain. Tissues containing a high density of pain receptors include skin, periosteum, joint capsule, muscle, tendon, and arterial wall. The tissue of the brain is one of the most important pain-free regions in the body.

Technician Note

Tissues containing a high density of pain receptors include skin, periosteum, joint capsule, muscle, tendon, and arterial wall.

Peripheral nerves that transmit the sensation of pain to the central nervous system vary in size and in the speed with which they conduct sensation (Figure 22-1). Nerve fibers with a myelin sheath *(A delta fibers)* are larger and conduct pain much more rapidly than the smaller unmyelinated ones *(C fibers)*. Evidence indicates that A delta and C nerve fibers are capable of producing two distinct sensations of pain. Most painful events initially produce a sharp prickling pain followed by a dull burning sensation. The fast-conducting A delta fibers appear to be responsible for the rapid initial sharp sensation. The subsequent burning or throbbing pain involves conduction by the slower C fibers.

Some of the most intensely painful sensations result from chemical injury such as that associated with inflammation. Chemical substances such as prostaglandins, histamine, and proteolytic enzymes are made by the body during inflammation. These substances are so potent that they not only stimulate pain receptors but can actually damage them. One of the most important classes of chemical mediators of pain formed during inflammation is the metabolic products of arachidonic acid. This group of metabolites includes the prostaglandins and leukotrienes. Prostaglandin production from arachidonic acid is blocked by nonsteroidal antiinflammatory drugs (NSAIDs), of which aspirin is an example.

Technician Note

Some of the most intensely painful sensations result from chemical injury, such as that associated with inflammation.

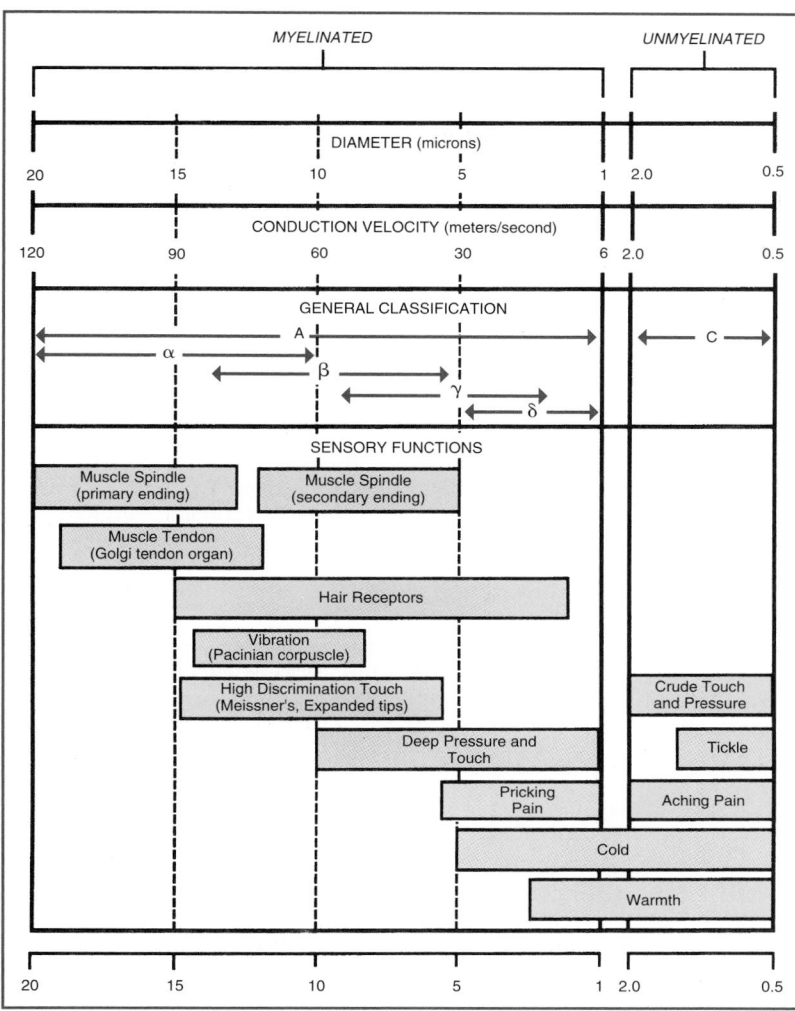

FIGURE 22-1. Physiologic classifications and functions of peripheral sensory nerve fibers.

Central Nervous System

The pathways for pain transmission in the central nervous system (CNS) are considerably more complex than those in the periphery. Nerve fibers transmitting pain impulses from the peripheral nerves enter the spinal cord through the dorsal nerve roots. Once the fibers have entered the spinal cord, they may associate with several types of neural hormones (e.g., substance P, somatostatin, cholecystokinin) that play a role in suppressing or augmenting the transmission and subsequent sensation of pain.

Once the impulse reaches the spinal cord, nerve fibers segregate into neural tracts, which carry specifically grouped fiber types (Figure 22-2). The spinothalamic tract is important in the transmission of pain impulses through the spinal cord and to the brain. The nerve fibers or axons, which travel in the *spinothalamic tract*, terminate in several areas of the thalamic area of the brain and brainstem. The fibers terminating in the thalamus are involved in the perception and conscious discriminatory aspects of pain, including location, nature, and intensity.

Pain Localization

The localization of pain to a particular area of the body is the responsibility of the CNS. Pain can be poorly localized because sensory nerve fibers may be present in low densities in the peripheral tissue or because pain pathways

frequently branch and converge, making it difficult for the brain to localize the sensation. For example, the pain resulting from gastroesophageal acid reflux in humans is felt as a diffuse burning sensation only vaguely localized to the sternum. A dull, poorly defined burning sensation is felt instead of well-localized pain, partly because of the poor sensory innervation that internal organs (viscera) have. Pain inflicted to tissues with a high density of pain receptors, such as the skin, is generally much more precisely localized than the pain associated with internal organs.

In clinical practice, pain associated with the viscera of the thorax and abdomen is often used to help diagnose disease. The sensation of pain experienced from visceral tissues is different from surface or somatic (e.g., skin) pain. Somatic pain from the skin is highly localized because of the large number of pain receptors present in this area. Visceral tissues, such as the bladder or intestinal tract, by contrast, are poorly innervated. Because of poor visceral innervation, abdominal and thoracic pain often occurs only following extensive, diffuse irritation. Common causes of visceral pain include leakage of damaging substances (e.g., bile, gastric acid) from the gastrointestinal tract leading to peritonitis or overdistention of the intestinal tract, which might occur with an obstruction or gastric torsion.

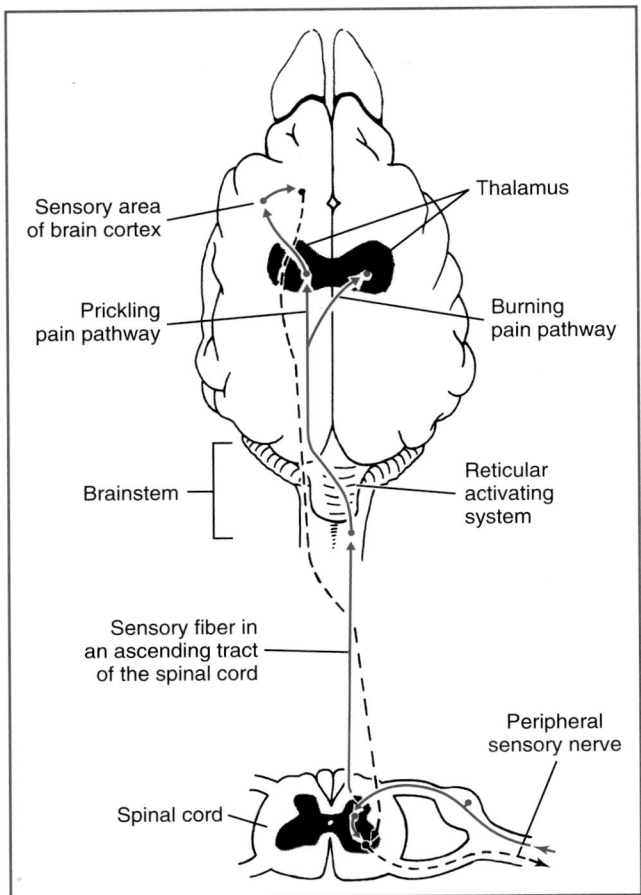

FIGURE 22-2. Transmission and segregation of nerve fibers carrying pain impulses within the central nervous system.

TABLE 22-1	COMMON CLINICAL SIGNS OF PAIN OR DISTRESS
System	**Signs**
Cardiovascular	Elevated heart rate and blood pressure, decreased peripheral circulation, prolonged capillary refill, cool extremities (ears, paws)
Respiratory	Rapid, shallow breaths; panting
Digestive	Weight loss, poor growth (young), vomiting, inappetence, constipation, diarrhea, salivation
Musculoskeletal	Unsteady gait, lameness, weakness, tremors, shivering
Urinary	Reluctance to urinate, loss of house training
Laboratory findings	Neutrophilia, lymphocytosis, hyperglycemia, polycythemia, elevated cortisol, elevated catecholamines

Technician Note

Recognizing pain and anxiety in animals is critical before appropriate analgesic selection and pain relief.

RECOGNIZING PAIN IN ANIMALS

Problems With Evaluation

Recognizing pain and anxiety in animals is critical before appropriate analgesic selection and pain relief. An animal confronted with a painful situation may exhibit specific behavior patterns, often secondary to stimulation of the autonomic nervous system. The typical nervous system response to pain and stress forms the basis of the classic fight-or-flight reaction. Autonomic nervous system stimulation results in the release of epinephrine and norepinephrine (catecholamines) from the adrenal glands, resulting in elevated heart rate, blood pressure, and respiratory rate and pupillary dilation (mydriasis). The fight-or-flight response, however, is not unique to painful situations; it may occur in purely stressful situations, such as the anxiety of being in the veterinarian's office. Because of its nonspecific nature, it is not possible to use autonomic stimulation as the sole criterion for pain evaluation. In addition to catecholamines, cortisol is released following pain and anxiety. Cortisol, like catecholamines, is released nonspecifically in response to stressful situations. Other nonspecific physiologic signs that animals may exhibit with pain and anxiety include neutrophilia and lymphocytosis (secondary to elevated epinephrine); hyperglycemia (especially in cats); and polycythemia (secondary to splenic contraction).

Signs of Pain and Distress: Animal Variability

Common physiologic responses to pain include increased heart rate and blood pressure, pupillary dilation, increased respiratory rate, and arousal (Table 22-1). It is essential for the veterinary staff to be aware of normal physiologic values, typical physical appearance, and behavior patterns for each species and breed seen in the practice. Behavioral responses to pain and anxiety vary not only by species involved but also between breeds and even among individuals. As an example, the behavioral response that a stoic hound might exhibit to postoperative pain will be considerably different from that of the nervous toy breeds. The veterinary staff is more likely to become aware of the pain and anxiety experienced by the toy breed than those experienced by the less vocal hound. Further, behavioral responses to pain may vary between individuals or even families within a breed, making generalizations about signs of discomfort extremely difficult.

Clinical Evaluation of Pain

In many cases, an animal initially reacts to a painful situation by retreating in an attempt to remove itself from the source of discomfort. If this reaction fails to bring relief, the animal may rely on other behavioral responses, such as vocalization, increased attempts to escape, pacing, guarding, sleeplessness, and aggression (Table 22-2). In horses, sweating, kicking, pawing, lip curling, and rolling are commonly exhibited with abdominal pain. Animals that are experiencing acute postoperative or traumatic pain may also respond by biting, licking, or scratching at the source of discomfort. Chronic, low-grade pain in animals is often associated with prolonged hospitalization, radiation, and chemotherapy; severe osteoarthritis may be manifested by failure to groom, lack of interest in surroundings, reluctance to move, anorexia, weight loss, constipation, and dysuria. Animals experiencing chronic pain may be withdrawn and quiet, unlike the seemingly "energized" state

Table 22-2	Postoperative Pain Evaluation		
Type of Surgery	**Signs of Pain**	**Suspected Pain Level**	**Duration**
Head, ear, oral, dental	Rubbing; shaking; salivating; reluctance to eat, swallow, or drink; irritability; vocalizing	Moderate to high	Intermittent
Ophthalmologic	Rubbing, vocalizing, reluctance to move	High	Intermittent to continual
Orthopedic	Guarding, aggression, abnormal gait, self-mutilation, reluctance to move, dysuria, constipation	Moderate	Intermittent
Abdominal	Guarding, splinting, abnormal posture, vomiting, inappetence	Mild to moderate	Intermittent
Cardiovascular/thoracic	Changes in respiratory rate and pattern, reluctance to move, vocalizing	Moderate to high	Continual
Perirectal	Licking, biting, scooting, self-mutilation, constipation	Moderate	Intermittent

From Johnson JM: *Compend Contin Educ Pract Vet* 13:804, 1991; Wright EM, Marcella KL, Woodson JF: *Lab Anim* 14:20, 1985; and author's clinical experience.

observed in animals experiencing acute pain. It is important to remember that not all signs of pain may be present at one time, and no single sign is a reliable indicator of the level of pain experienced.

Technician Note

Animals that are experiencing acute postoperative or traumatic pain may respond by biting, licking, or scratching at the site of discomfort.

CONTROL OF PAIN IN ANIMALS

Patient evaluation to identify the clinical signs of pain and distress is an area in which veterinary technicians can contribute significantly. The veterinary technician is often the one involved most closely with the minute-by-minute treatment and monitoring of postoperative surgical and intensive care patients. The observant technician can contribute a great deal to pain relief by learning to recognize the clinical signs of discomfort in patients.

Two main types of analgesics are often considered in the control of pain in companion animals: nonnarcotic antiinflammatory drugs (mild analgesics) and narcotics (strong analgesics). The clinical indications for each of these families of drugs are often very different. Likewise, their mechanism of action and adverse effects also differ significantly.

The first section below examines the indications and adverse effects of the narcotic (opioid) analgesics, which are the most commonly used analgesics in the postoperative patient. The antiinflammatory analgesics, covered later, are predominantly employed for mild to moderate chronic pain associated with the musculoskeletal system. Finally the use of tranquilizers along with analgesic drugs to treat the anxiety often associated with pain and distress in companion animals is discussed.

Environment and Nursing Care

Environmental factors often affect the emotional component of pain perception in both humans and animals. Keep the surroundings as familiar as possible to the animal, including providing toys or blankets from home or visits by owners in patients hospitalized for a long time. When possible, animals will often recover better at home from noncritical illnesses if owners are able to provide good nursing care. Recovery areas should be quiet and located away from busy areas with loud animal and human noise. Try to provide as stress free an environment as possible (Figure 22-3).

During patient recovery, interaction with humans may also help to relieve stress and anxiety. Talking to an animal, stroking, and petting can help to reduce restlessness, rapid breathing, increased heart rate, and other signs of discomfort. Also remember that an animal's pain may be greatly exacerbated by frequent moving, monitoring, or administration of medications. Prepare a dry, comfortable area for the patient, and schedule treatments and monitoring so that the animal is moved and disturbed a minimal amount.

ANALGESIC DRUGS: THE NARCOTICS

Narcotic drugs (opioids) are the oldest and most extensively studied analgesic drugs available. The analgesic effect of narcotics is due to their interaction at specific opioid receptors located within the CNS. Opioid receptors are present in both the brain and the spinal cord, making the alteration of pain sensation possible at multiple areas.

Five categories (mu, kappa, sigma, delta, epsilon) of receptors for opioid drugs have been described to date. Each receptor subtype produces a slightly different response following binding of an opioid drug (Table 22-3). For example, the mu receptor subtype will cause respiratory depression, sedation, euphoria, and addiction when a drug stimulates it. Another receptor subtype, the kappa receptor, produces analgesia and sedation without the drug addiction response.

Opioids referred to as *pure agonists* are substances that exert their effects by only stimulating opioid receptors. An example of a pure agonist is *morphine*. The subclass of drugs known as the opioid *antagonists* binds at opioid receptors but blocks or fails to elicit a response. The antagonists bind the opioid receptors and displace agonists, such as morphine. The antagonists are often referred to as *narcotic reversal agents* because of their ability to reverse the effects of the opioid agonists by displacing them at the receptor level. The classic opioid antagonist is *naloxone*.

The final category of opioid drugs is the *mixed agonist/ antagonist*. These substances have been synthesized to act like agonists at some of the opioid receptors and antago-

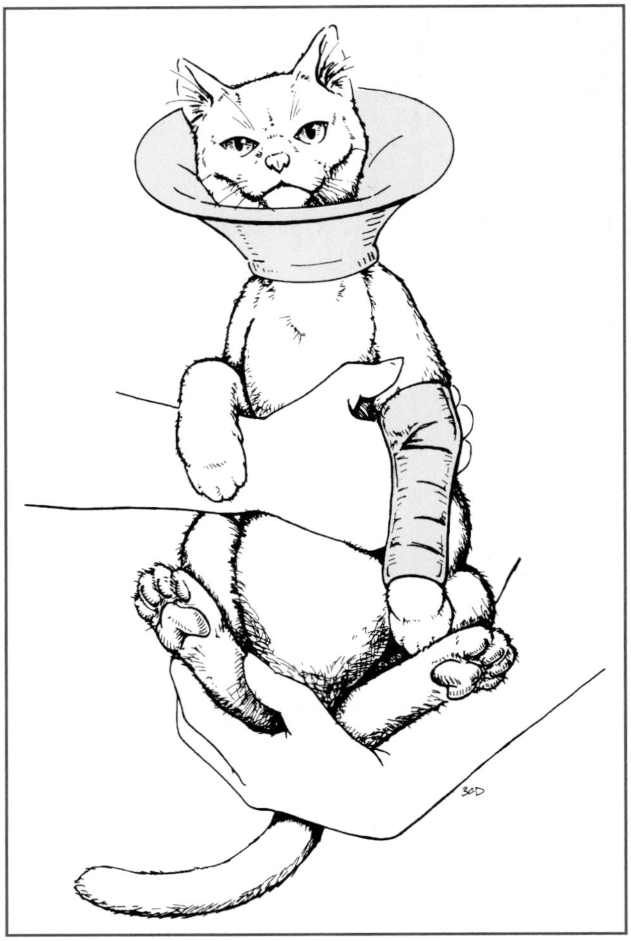

FIGURE 22-3. Good nursing care is critical to the management of patients experiencing pain and distress.

TABLE 22-3	RECEPTOR ACTIVITY OF OPIOID DRUGS		
	Receptor Activity		
Drug	**Mu**	**Kappa**	**Sigma**
Agonist opioids: fentanyl, morphine, meperidine, oxymorphone	Agonist	Agonist	Agonist
Butorphanol	Weak antagonist	Agonist	Antagonist
Pentazocine	Weak antagonist	Agonist	Antagonist
Buprenorphine	Weak agonist	Antagonist	Antagonist
Nalorphine	Weak agonist	Antagonist	Antagonist
Naloxone	Antagonist	Antagonist	Antagonist

nists at others. A good example of this class of drug is *butorphanol*. Butorphanol acts like naloxone at the mu receptor but binds like an agonist at the kappa receptor. This mixed effect allows butorphanol to be a good analgesic without having the addictive properties of morphine.

In general, the narcotic drugs produce minimal cardiovascular effects and are safe in patients with cardiac disease. They are known to produce bradycardia and can produce hypotension if they stimulate the release of histamine (morphine, meperidine). Their effects on the respiratory system include respiratory depression (decreased rate and tidal volume) and a decreased sensitivity of the respiratory center to increasing levels of carbon dioxide. Narcotics can also cause salivation, nausea, vomiting, and nonpropulsive

intestinal motility (segmental contractions). Along with their analgesic effects, these drugs will produce sedation and in some animals dysphoria (hallucinations).

The narcotic drugs are extensively metabolized by the liver and excreted in the urine. Animals with liver disease or neonates with poorly developed hepatic metabolism require reduced dosages of narcotics to avoid prolonged drug effects.

Morphine
Morphine is considered to be the prototypic narcotic analgesic (Figure 22-4). Two advantages of morphine are analgesia and sedation. The effects of morphine are reversed with narcotic antagonists, such as naloxone. Adverse

effects of morphine administration include depression of the respiratory and central nervous systems.

Technician Note

Morphine is considered to be the prototypic narcotic analgesic.

As with most of the narcotics, morphine is metabolized by the liver and excreted through the kidneys. Care should be taken when administering morphine to animals with renal or hepatic compromise, because drug elimination may be prolonged. At higher doses, morphine can be excitatory for cats, cattle, swine, and horses. Morphine given in lower doses or combined with a tranquilizer appears to reduce the undesirable effects in cats. Morphine is effective against moderate to severe pain. It has its greatest effect if given before the painful stimulus.

Fentanyl
Fentanyl (Sublimaze, Janssen) is a synthetic opioid with approximately 100 times the potency of morphine and 500 times the potency of meperidine. Fentanyl acts rapidly after intravenous or intramuscular injection. Profound analgesia and respiratory depression develop within 6 to 8 minutes after injection. Auditory sensitization and elevation of the thermoregulatory center leading to panting also frequently occur. Bradycardia is commonly produced, and therefore concurrent use of atropine or glycopyrrolate is recommended. Extreme caution should be used if fentanyl is administered concurrently with barbiturates (e.g., thiamylal, thiopental) because bradycardia, hypotension, and respiratory depression can be difficult to reverse.

Fentanyl has a short duration of action, with peak effects lasting for only 30 to 45 minutes. Although fentanyl is an excellent analgesic for moderate to severe pain, its use in veterinary medicine has largely been abandoned (with the exception of administration by continuous intravenous infusion) because of its short half-life. Fentanyl is most commonly available as a neuroleptanalgesic (narcotic and tranquilizer mix), for which purpose it is combined with the tranquilizer droperidol (Innovar, Pitman-Moore) (Figure 22-5).

FENTANYL PATCHES. Transdermal application of fentanyl has recently become popular in veterinary medicine. The transdermal patch (Duragesic, Janssen) is composed of a drug reservoir that is sandwiched between an impermeable backing and a permeable skin-contacting membrane. When patches are applied to cats or dogs, approximately 24 hours should be allowed for therapeutic concentrations to be reached. Patches are designed to provide about 72 hours of analgesia. Patches are available in 25, 50, 75, and 100 μg/hr concentrations. A patch with 2.5-mg fentanyl is designed to release 25 μg/hr. Some caution should be used with fentanyl patches, because therapeutic parameters have not been reliably established in cats and dogs. Patients should be evaluated for respiratory depression and sedation. Dosage guidelines are based on body weight: less than 3 kg, not recommended; 3 to 7 kg, 25 μg/hr; 8 to 18 kg, 50 μg/hr; 19 to 27 kg, 75 μg/hr; greater than 28 kg, 100 μg/hr. Patches should not be cut to reduce the concentration.

To place a transdermal drug patch, the hair over the lateral thorax or dorsal cervical region should be clipped without damaging the skin (avoid clipper burns). The site should not be cleaned with alcohol or surgical scrub. The

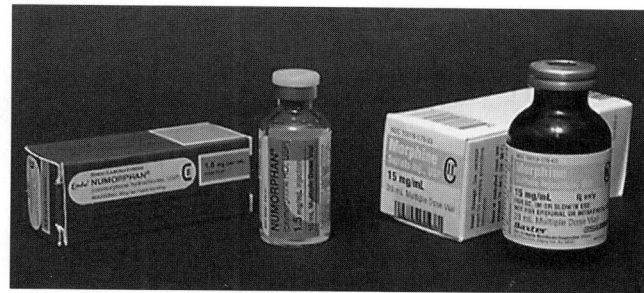
FIGURE 22-4. Narcotic agonists commonly used for pain control in small animal practice.

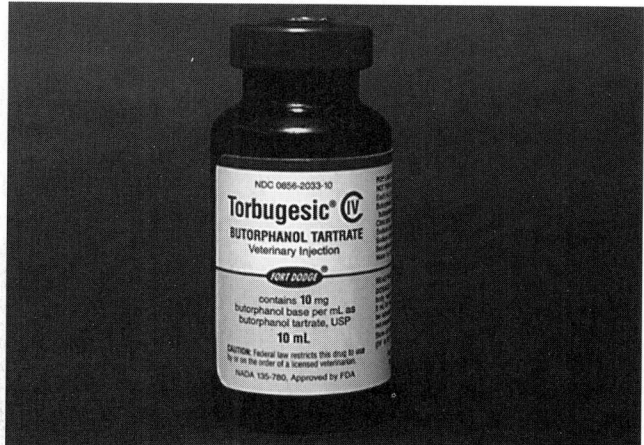
FIGURE 22-5. Butorphanol is a popular nonschedule, mixed agonist/antagonist analgesic. Fentanyl is combined with droperidol in the neuroleptanalgesic Innovar.

patch should be handled by the edges or with gloves and pressed firmly to the skin for at least 30 seconds. In dogs, the site should be bandaged. When removing the patch, use gloves. Fold the spent patch in half, and flush down the toilet. Patches are considered a controlled substance.

Oxymorphone
Oxymorphone (P/M Oxymorphone HCl, Pitman-Moore) is a semisynthetic narcotic analgesic that is approximately 10 times as potent an analgesic as morphine. It has a duration of action from 4 to 6 hours. Adverse effects are similar to those of morphine; however, it appears to cause less respiratory depression and gastrointestinal stimulation. Oxymorphone can cause significant auditory sensitization. Bradycardia is frequently observed if an anticholinergic (e.g., atropine, glycopyrrolate) is not administered concurrently. Elevation of the thermoregulatory center may lead to panting, as seen with other opioids. Oxymorphone is considered an excellent analgesic for moderate to intense pain because of its potency and duration of action.

Technician Note

Oxymorphone is considered an excellent analgesic for moderate to intense pain because of its potency and duration of action.

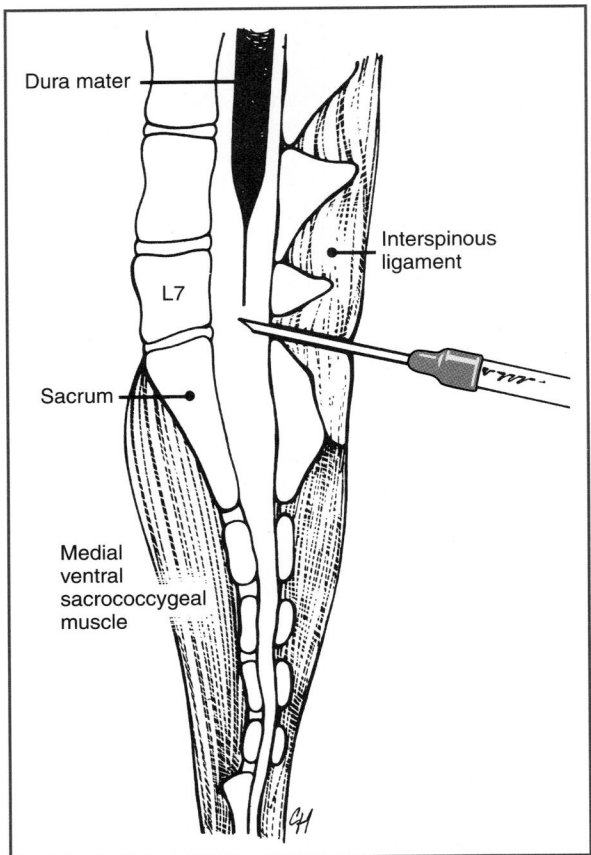

Dura mater

Interspinous
ligament

L7

Sacrum

Medial
ventral
sacrococcygeal
muscle

FIGURE 22-6. Epidural administration of an opioid drug has the advantage of providing analgesia for longer durations than systemic opioid use.

Epidural Use of Opioids

Because of significant success with the epidural use of opioid compounds in humans, much attention has been focused on their use in companion animals. Instead of being given systemically, epidural opioids are administered through spinal needles or catheters (Figure 22-6) on top of the outer meningeal covering of the spinal cord (dura mater). Because of the high density of opioid receptors in the spinal cord, epidural administration of opioids offers the advantage of prolonged analgesia (up to five times longer than intramuscular administration) without prolonged sedation and respiratory depression.

Opiates deposited epidurally enter the spinal cord by three pathways: (1) diffusion across the meninges, (2) along nerve roots, and (3) by uptake into the spinal arteries and epidural veins. The onset of action of epidural opioids varies markedly among drugs depending on their molecular weight, ionization, and lipid solubility. Lipid-soluble drugs such as fentanyl have a rapid onset of action and very short duration, whereas water-soluble morphine has a delayed onset and long duration.

For postoperative epidural analgesia in veterinary patients, morphine is used most commonly. Subarachnoid or epidural administration of preservative-free morphine (Duramorph PF, Elkins-Sinn; Astromorpho/PF, Astra Pharmaceutical Products) has been shown to be safe and efficacious. Epidural morphine is an excellent technique for providing postoperative analgesia after pelvic or hind-limb surgery. Administered at the lumbosacral space, it has been used after thoracic surgery, but it depends on cephalad migration of the drug within the cerebrospinal fluid (CSF). The dose of epidural morphine (preservative-free drug) commonly used in dogs and cats is 0.05 to 0.1 mg/kg of body weight. Epidural morphine should be administered 30 to 60 minutes before recovery from anesthesia. Duration of analgesia is 6 to 24 hours.

Mixed-Action Agonist/Antagonist Narcotic Analgesics

Butorphanol

Butorphanol (Torbugesic, Fort Dodge) belongs to a group of synthetic analgesics with combined agonist and antagonist properties. Butorphanol is considered to be a weak antagonist at the mu receptor but a strong agonist at the kappa receptor. Butorphanol is three to five times more potent an analgesic than morphine. The antagonist activity of butorphanol is nearly 50 times less than that of naloxone. The respiratory depression produced by butorphanol is similar to that of morphine; however, butorphanol reaches a ceiling effect beyond which higher doses fail to increase the depression. The ceiling on respiratory depression makes butorphanol a somewhat safer drug than morphine. Butorphanol is also a well-recognized antitussive and has been used as an antiemetic in cancer patients. Similar to other narcotics, butorphanol is metabolized by the liver and has a plasma half-life of 3 to 4 hours in dogs.

Butorphanol appears to have a relatively short duration of action and is a better analgesic for visceral pain than for somatic pain. Clinically, butorphanol appears to act as a good analgesic for mild to moderate pain in the dog, cat, and horse.

Butorphanol is effective for mild to moderate pain. Its short duration of action requires frequent redosing. Butorphanol is a Schedule IV controlled substance.

Buprenorphine

Buprenorphine (Buprenex, Norwich Eaton) is a mixed agonist/antagonist that has become popular in Europe as an analgesic and sedative drug. This drug differs from butorphanol in that its association and dissociation with the opioid receptors occur slowly. Because of its slow receptor association, it may take up to 30 minutes after intravenous injection for buprenorphine to take effect. Buprenorphine has a longer duration of action than butorphanol because of its tight binding to, and slow dissociation from, opioid receptors. Because it binds tightly to the opioid receptor, its effects can be difficult to reverse with naloxone. An important adverse effect following injection of buprenorphine is its delayed respiratory depression. It has been recommended that animals given buprenorphine be observed closely for at least 2 hours after administration. Buprenorphine is 300 times more potent than morphine and is effective for mild to moderate pain.

Narcotic Antagonists

Relatively minor structural changes to opioids can convert a drug with primary agonist activity to one with antagonist action. Narcotic antagonists allow for the quick reversal of a narcotic overdose and its associated respiratory depression, sedation, and analgesia.

Naloxone

Naloxone (P/M Naloxone HCl, Pitman-Moore) (Figure 22-7) is a pure antagonist with 50 times the reversal potential of butorphanol. Naloxone is regarded as a pure

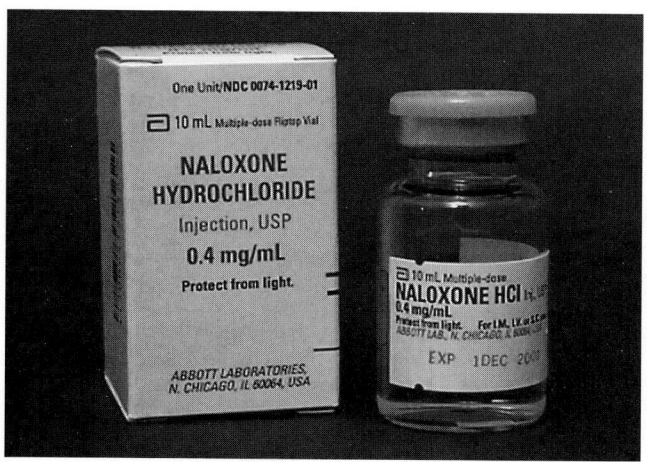

FIGURE 22-7. Naloxone is a pure opioid antagonist capable of reversing both the analgesic and untoward effects of opioid drugs.

competitive antagonist at all the opioid receptors and is not regulated by the Controlled Substances Act. Small doses of naloxone (0.4 to 0.8 mg), if administered intramuscularly or intravenously, rapidly reverse the effects of morphinelike opioids.

In patients with respiratory depression, an increase in respiratory rate occurs 1 to 2 minutes after naloxone administration. The sedative, cardiovascular, and analgesic effects of the opioids are also rapidly reversed. Antagonist effects will last for 1 to 4 hours, depending on the initial dose given. When naloxone is being used to reverse a pure agonist, readministration may be necessary, because many of the narcotics will last longer than naloxone. At low doses, naloxone has a high binding affinity for the mu receptor, which is responsible for respiratory depression and sedation; much higher doses are needed to antagonize the kappa receptor.

> **Technician Note**
>
> Naloxone rapidly reverses the effects of morphinelike opioids and is not regulated by the Controlled Substances Act.

Nalorphine

Nalorphine (Nalline, MSD-Agvet) is a morphine derivative that is classified as a partial agonist, but it reverses the effects of many opioids. Nalorphine is a Schedule III drug, which means that it is less addictive than a Schedule II drug, such as morphine. In the presence of narcotic agonists, nalorphine acts as a partial antagonist. Like butorphanol, nalorphine may be used alone for sedation and analgesia. The drug has the advantage of having less CNS and respiratory depression than the pure agonists.

MANAGEMENT OF CONTROLLED SUBSTANCES

Controlled substances, as defined by the Controlled Substances Act of 1970, include opioids (narcotics), barbiturates, hallucinogens (ketamine), amphetamines, and other addictive or habituating drugs. This act regulates the manufacturing, distribution, and dispensing of controlled substances. The licensed veterinarian wishing to prescribe or

maintain controlled drugs must register with the U.S. Drug Enforcement Agency (DEA).

Controlled substances must be kept in a locked cabinet or safe with attachment to a concrete floor. Strict inventory, including patient/client name and volume dispensed, is required by law.

Controlled drugs are listed in five different schedules (C-I, C-II, C-III, C-IV, C-V). *Schedule I* drugs have a high abuse potential and are not currently accepted in the United States for treatment. Examples include heroin, lysergic acid diethylamide (LSD), mescaline, and marijuana. *Schedule II* drugs have a high abuse potential and can produce severe psychic and physical dependence in humans. Examples include morphine, meperidine, oxymorphone, and pentobarbital. *Schedule III* drugs have less abuse potential than those in schedules I and II. Abuse of these drugs leads to moderate or low physical dependence. Examples include preparations with low levels of morphine as well as nalorphine, ketamine, and barbiturates. *Schedule IV* drugs are considered to have a low abuse potential and include phenobarbital and diazepam (Valium). Additional information on controlled substances may be found in Chapter 23.

NONSTEROIDAL ANTIINFLAMMATORY DRUGS (NSAIDs)

Inflammation

Nonnarcotic analgesics include the large family of drugs frequently referred to as nonsteroidal antiinflammatory drugs (NSAIDs). NSAIDs exert their analgesic effects in the peripheral tissues primarily by blocking the production of prostaglandins. Prostaglandins are normally produced in tissues during the process of inflammation.

Inflammation may be considered as a series of events (Figure 22-8) that are mediated by substances such as vasoactive amines (histamine, serotonin), leukocyte products (lymphokines, oxygen radicals, interleukins), and substances that are formed from the metabolism of arachidonic acid (prostaglandins, leukotrienes). Arachidonic acid, a phospholipid, is present in cell membranes, and when released, it can be metabolized to form prostaglandins and leukotrienes (Figure 22-9).

> **Technician Note**
>
> Nonnarcotic analgesics include the large family of drugs frequently referred to as nonsteroidal antiinflammatory drugs (NSAIDs).

Inflammation begins with local tissue injury. Vasoactive substances released from both blood cells (leukocytes, platelets) and cells in the peripheral tissue result in the production of pain, heat, and swelling. Fluid exudation from capillaries can cause swelling and pain secondary to the pressure exerted on local nerve endings. Along with the vascular changes, neutrophils and monocyte-macrophages migrate to the injured tissue to ingest and destroy foreign material. During this process, toxic oxygen radicals and enzymes are released into the local tissues, further exacerbating the inflammatory process.

NSAIDs control pain by inhibiting *cyclooxygenase*, a major enzyme in the arachidonic acid pathway leading to the production of prostaglandins. Cyclooxygenase also converts arachidonic acid to thromboxane (causes platelet aggregation) and prostacyclin (inhibits platelet aggregation). An important point to remember is that by blocking cyclooxygenase, NSAIDs inhibit the production of the

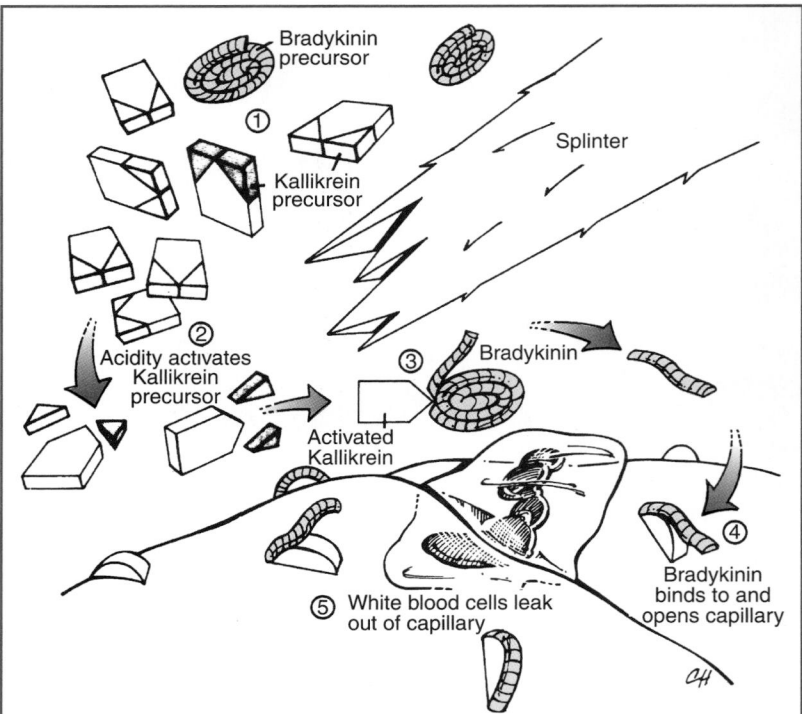

FIGURE 22-8. The inflammatory process involves the generation of many substances responsible for causing pain and swelling.

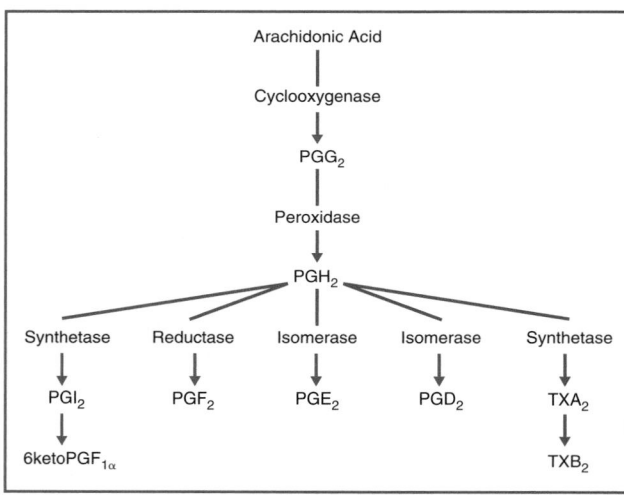

FIGURE 22-9. Many different prostaglandins are generated enzymatically after the release of arachidonic acid from cell membranes. *PG,* Prostaglandin; *TX,* thromboxane.

prostaglandins involved in inflammation as well as those involved in regulating such important functions as blood flow and gastric secretion.

Mechanism of Action

Recent research has shown why some NSAIDs produce more gastrointestinal adverse effects than others. There are two isoforms of cyclooxygenase (COX): COX-1, the constitutive gastroprotective form, and COX-2, the inducible form associated with inflammation. NSAIDs inhibit COX-1 and COX-2; dexamethasone inhibits only COX-2.

The current thought is that drugs with higher levels of COX-1 inhibition result in greater gastrointestinal injury. Pharmaceutical research has recently been directed toward developing COX-2 selective NSAIDs (Celebrex, Monsanto; Vioxx, Merck) that have fewer gastrointestinal complications.

Salicylate Analgesics

Salicylate analgesics were first introduced into clinical medicine in the late nineteenth century. Salicylates commonly used in veterinary practice include aspirin (Figure 22-10) and bismuth subsalicylate (Pepto-Bismol, Procter & Gamble). Salicylates are effective in relieving pain associated with peripheral inflammation, such as muscle and joint disease, but have virtually no effect on deep or visceral pain. Salicylates have antipyretic effects because of their ability to reduce the prostaglandin-induced fever response. Aspirin, like other NSAIDs, inhibits the generation of thromboxane and thus decreases platelet aggregation.

Salicylates are readily absorbed through the gastrointestinal tract and quickly enter synovial fluid, peritoneal fluid, milk, saliva, and placental membranes. These drugs are metabolized in the liver by the enzyme glucuronyl transferase. Once processed in the liver, metabolic byproducts are excreted through the kidney. The drug half-life of salicylates is higher in cats than in dogs because the cat has considerably lower levels of hepatic glucuronyl transferase and subsequently a decreased ability to metabolize the drug.

Clinical use of aspirin has centered around the management of inflammatory (e.g., rheumatoid arthritis) and degenerative joint diseases (Figure 22-11). Aspirin may be used in the cat as long as it is administered no more often than every 36 to 48 hours.

Clinical signs of toxicity associated with salicylates, as well as other more potent NSAIDs, include nausea and

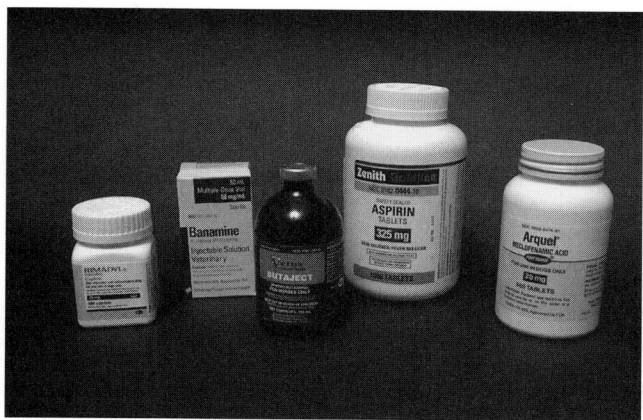

FIGURE 22-10.   Nonsteroidal antiinflammatory drugs commonly used in treating musculoskeletal pain in veterinary practice.

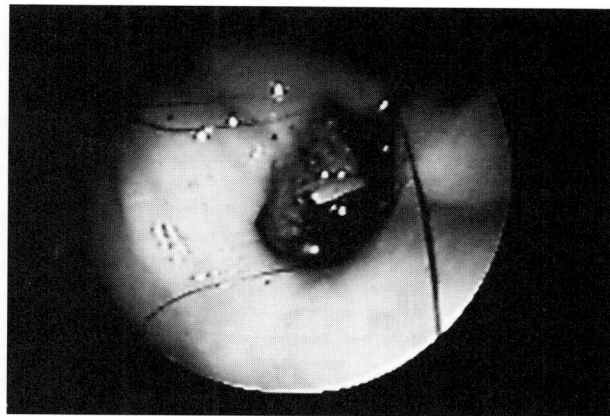

FIGURE 22-12.   Endoscopic view of deep gastric ulcer secondary to long-term nonsteroidal antiinflammatory drug use in a dog.

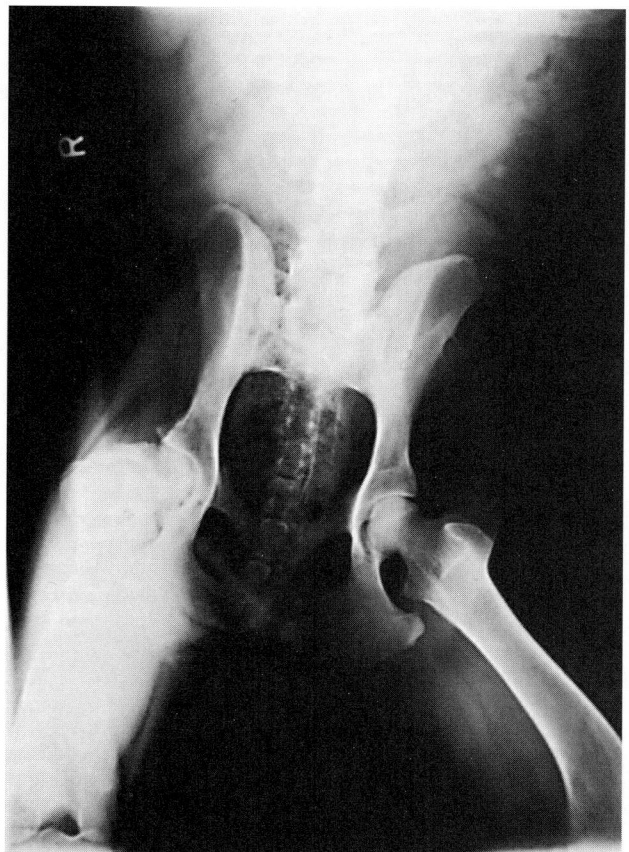

FIGURE 22-11.   Severe right coxofemoral osteoarthrosis amenable to treatment with nonsteroidal antiinflammatory drugs.

bloody vomitus (hematemesis) associated with gastric ulceration (Figure 22-12), renal disease, and bleeding tendencies secondary to platelet aggregation inhibition. Gastrointestinal ulceration is the most commonly encountered adverse reaction secondary to NSAID use in the dog and horse. Ulceration occurs secondary to direct irritation of the drug on the gastric mucosa and, importantly, secondary to prostaglandin inhibition. Prostaglandins produced by the gastric mucosa are normally involved in increasing gastric mucus and bicarbonate production, thus helping to coat the stomach lining, neutralize acid produced, and protect the mucosa from irritation. Prostaglandins are also involved in decreasing the volume and acidity of gastric secretion. By inhibiting prostaglandin production, NSAIDs contribute to decreased gastrointestinal protective mechanisms and predispose an individual to ulcer formation.

Propionic Acid Derivatives

Carprofen

Carprofen (Rimadyl, Pfizer Animal Health) is an NSAID recently approved in the United States for use in dogs with degenerative joint disease. The drug is a reversible inhibitor of COX-1 and COX-2. In dogs, carprofen is 90% absorbed after oral administration and has a mean half-life of approximately 8 hours after a single dose. Effective analgesic and antiinflammatory effects of carprofen have been established through subjective clinical trials, objective gait analysis, and force plate examinations. Carprofen is considerably more potent for management of signs of chronic pain than aspirin. Studies involving more than 450 dogs have been performed to evaluate the safety and efficacy of carprofen. The number of reports of adverse events has been minimal. The most common adverse events have been vomiting, lethargy, and anorexia. Recently, isolated drug-induced hepatotoxicity has been identified in dogs not previously showing signs of liver disease. Most animals recovered with supportive therapy after drug administration was discontinued. The Labrador retriever appears to be at increased risk. It has been recommended that evaluation of both renal and hepatic function be performed in dogs before administering carprofen.

Naproxen

There are a considerable number of propionic acid derivatives on the market, most of which act by inhibiting cyclooxygenase. Naproxen (Naprosyn, Synflex), an NSAID, has effective antiinflammatory, analgesic, and antipyretic properties and is an effective cyclooxygenase inhibitor. Naproxen has approximately 20 times the potency of the related drug ibuprofen. In humans, naproxen has been used successfully to treat degenerative joint disease as well as posttraumatic soft tissue injury.

The toxicity of naproxen is similar to that of other nonsteroidal drugs. Gastrointestinal ulceration leading to perforation and peritonitis has been reported. Because naproxen has a long duration of action in the dog, it can be administered once daily. Because of convenient single daily dosing, naproxen has gained some popularity in treating pain related to orthopedic conditions. The use of naproxen should be limited to dogs in which salicylates do not control pain. If clinical signs of gastric upset occur, administration should be discontinued immediately. In horses, naproxen is administered twice daily and is very effective for soft tissue inflammation.

Ibuprofen

Ibuprofen was the first phenylpropionate to be marketed in the United States and has been used successfully to treat rheumatoid arthritis and osteoarthritis in humans. In humans, ibuprofen is considered to have less of an analgesic effect than aspirin; however, it is preferred in many cases because it appears to be associated with a lower incidence of gastric bleeding.

The most common form of ibuprofen is available without prescription as 200-mg tablets under a wide variety of proprietary names (Advil, Whitehall; Medipren, McNeil; Midol, Upjohn; Motrin IB, Upjohn; Nuprin, Bristol-Myers).

Studies on ibuprofen use in the dog indicate that gastric irritation and repeated vomiting began after 2 to 4 days of administration and continued several days after the drug was discontinued. These studies indicate that dogs are more sensitive than humans to ibuprofen's gastric irritating effects. Ibuprofen offers no advantage over other NSAIDs, and because of significant gastrointestinal irritation, its use in the dog is not recommended.

> **Technician Note**
>
> Ibuprofen offers no advantage over other NSAIDs, and because of significant gastrointestinal irritation, its use in the dog is not recommended.

Ketoprofen

Ketoprofen (Ketofen, Fort Dodge) is a propionic acid NSAID approved for use in humans and horses. It is a strong cyclooxygenase inhibitor and is subsequently a powerful analgesic and antiinflammatory drug.

In a multicenter clinical trial, ketoprofen used intravenously at 2 mg/kg exhibited a potent analgesic effect in the management of pain in horses with colic. An excellent response was obtained in 89.5% of the horses, without any local or general side effects noted. Ketoprofen may be administered daily for up to 5 days in horses.

Fenamic Acids

Meclofenamic Acid

Meclofenamic acid (Arquel, Fort Dodge) inhibits cyclooxygenase and may also block cell surface receptors for prostaglandins. The drug has gained popularity for treating musculoskeletal pain that is refractory to aspirin. Toxic side effects have been observed in dogs and include diarrhea, vomiting, and gastrointestinal ulceration.

Meclofenamic acid is frequently used in dogs when aspirin therapy has failed to relieve pain associated with chronic degenerative joint diseases, such as elbow and hip dysplasia. In horses, meclofenamic acid is used for musculoskeletal pain.

Flunixin Meglumine

Flunixin meglumine (Banamine, Schering-Plough) is an NSAID with both analgesic and antipyretic activity. Like other NSAIDs, flunixin inhibits the enzyme cyclooxygenase, blocking the production of prostaglandins. Flunixin is considered to be one of the most potent cyclooxygenase enzyme inhibitors available. The analgesic potency of flunixin is greater than that of phenylbutazone, meperidine (narcotic), or codeine (narcotic).

Flunixin is recommended for relief of persistent, severe inflammation and pain associated with degenerative joint disease that is unresponsive to milder NSAIDs, such as aspirin. Because flunixin is a potent inhibitor of prostaglandin synthesis, it also frequently causes severe gastrointestinal ulceration and bleeding. Its use in the dog should not exceed 1 mg/kg once daily for 3 days. Flunixin is particularly useful for visceral analgesia in horses. Toxicity in horses is rare; it appears to have a wider margin of safety than phenylbutazone.

Pyrazolone Derivatives

Phenylbutazone

Phenylbutazone (Butazolidin, Coopers) has analgesic, antiinflammatory, and antipyretic properties similar to those common to the salicylate analgesics. As a member of the pyrazolone family, it has been associated with significant toxic effects in humans and, less commonly, in animals. Phenylbutazone in humans is known to cause fatal blood disorders (agranulocytosis). Prolonged use in the dog has also led to similar blood diseases.

Clinically, phenylbutazone has been used in the dog for treatment of painful arthritis and skeletal muscle disease and is considered to inhibit cyclooxygenase activity more effectively than aspirin but less effectively than meclofenamic acid and naproxen. Phenylbutazone is known to cause gastrointestinal ulceration, renal and hepatic disease, and, rarely, bone marrow suppression with prolonged use. Phenylbutazone is commonly used in horses for the control of musculoskeletal and visceral pain. The drug has a narrow margin of safety, and when compared to flunixin meglumine and ketoprofen, was found to cause a higher incidence of gastrointestinal ulceration. Certain pony breeds (Shetland and Welsh crosses) have been shown to exhibit acute toxicity to phenylbutazone. Lower daily doses (4.4 mg/kg once daily for 4 days and then every other day) have been recommended for ponies.

Treatment of Gastrointestinal Ulceration

Adverse drug reactions are common with the use of NSAIDs, especially when used long term and at high doses for musculoskeletal pain. Gastric ulceration, nausea, vomiting, and diarrhea commonly occur in dogs given NSAIDs. Gastric ulceration, weight loss, and inappetence occur in horses receiving NSAIDs long term. Several options have been suggested for the prophylaxis and treatment of ulcers associated with NSAID administration. Mucosal-adherent sucralfate (Carafate, Marion Merrill Dow) binds to mucosal defects, providing a barrier to gastric acid and may accelerate healing. The H_2 receptor antagonists cimetidine, ranitidine (Zantac, Glaxo), and famotidine (Pepcid, Merck) and the proton pump inhibitor omeprazole (Prilosec, Merck) are also commonly used. Misoprostol, a prostaglandin analog, has been shown to diminish gastric ulceration in dogs by providing the cytoprotective effects that NSAIDs reduce by blocking natural prostaglandins.

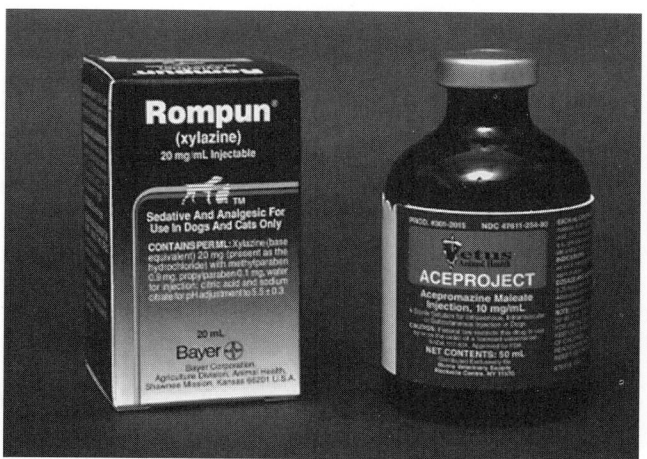

FIGURE 22-13. Tranquilizers, alpha$_2$ agonists, and steroids may have a role in the management of pain and distress in small animal patients.

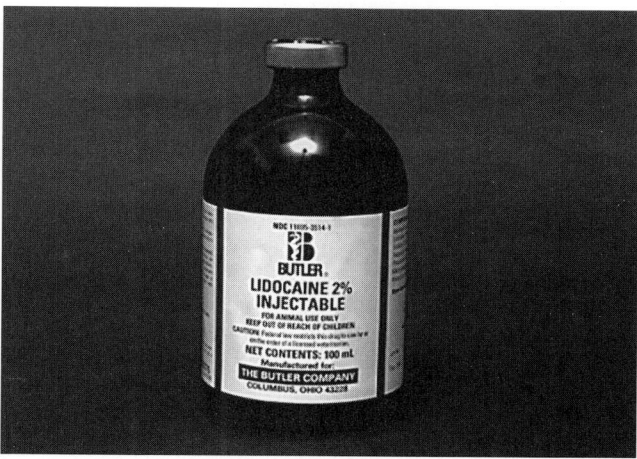

FIGURE 22-14. Local anesthetics may be used to provide regional analgesia.

PSYCHOTROPIC AGENTS

Tranquilizers

Animals experiencing pain and anxiety occasionally benefit from the effects of tranquilizers used in conjunction with analgesic drugs (Figure 22-13). Tranquilizers provide sedation, some muscle relaxation, and antianxiety effects. It is important to remember that tranquilizers provide minimal analgesia and that it is inappropriate to use these drugs alone for postoperative pain control. The phenothiazines (e.g., acetylpromazine, chlorpromazine, promazine) are used extensively for their sedative effects. Other useful tranquilizers include the benzodiazepine diazepam (Valium, Roche) and butyrophenones (droperidol, lenperone). The use of tranquilizers after surgery should be limited to providing sedation and relaxation to animals with pain-related distress and apprehension. Combining narcotics with low doses of tranquilizers often provides the most effective control of pain after surgery in anxious patients.

Alpha$_2$-Adrenergic Agonists

Xylazine

Xylazine (Rompun, Haver/Diamond Scientific) (see Figure 22-13) binds at alpha$_2$ receptors in the CNS, causing its sedative and analgesic effects. Many of the side effects of xylazine are secondary to its binding at peripheral alpha$_2$ receptors. Peripheral alpha$_2$-receptor stimulation causes vasoconstriction with an increase in arterial blood pressure. This increase in blood pressure is often followed by hypotension and arrhythmias (second-degree heart block). Xylazine can also cause smooth muscle relaxation and vomiting. One significant advantage of xylazine is that its effects may be reversed with the antagonists yohimbine, atipamezole, or idazoxan.

Xylazine hydrochloride is a potent visceral analgesic in the horse, but it is less effective for peripheral pain. In the dog and cat, xylazine provides 15 to 30 minutes of analgesia and is not generally considered to be very potent. Because of its short duration of analgesia and significant cardiovascular effects, xylazine is primarily used as an adjunct to other drugs to provide sedation in the dog and cat. Concurrent administration of atropine is recommended to counteract xylazine's cardiovascular side effects.

Detomidine

Detomidine (Dormosedan, Orion) is a sedative-analgesic originally developed for horses and cattle. Detomidine is more potent than xylazine and has a greater central alpha$_2$-adrenoreceptor specificity.

Detomidine has similar cardiovascular effects to xylazine when administered intravenously at 10 to 60 µg/kg. Sedation and analgesia are of a longer duration than xylazine. Administration of detomidine with opioids eliminates the excitation seen in horses given opioids alone. The combination of detomidine and butorphanol gives effective sedation and analgesia with few cardiovascular effects; detomidine (10 to 15 µg/kg intravenously) precedes butorphanol (20 to 30 µg/kg intravenously).

Corticosteroids

Corticosteroids principally act by dampening the fire of inflammation and not by eliminating the cause of it. Significant impairment of wound healing and masking of the underlying disease can occur with prolonged high doses of corticosteroids.

Useful corticosteroids for treatment of inflammation include the short-acting cortisone, hydrocortisone, prednisone, and prednisolone. The antiinflammatory effects of prednisolone and prednisone are approximately five times greater than those of cortisone. Corticosteroids are frequently used as short-term (3 to 5 days) antiinflammatory drugs in the treatment of acute exacerbations of chronic musculoskeletal pain (e.g., osteoarthritis of the elbow or hip). Corticosteroids should not be used with NSAIDs because of an increased risk of gastrointestinal ulceration.

Selective Nerve Blocks

The use of local anesthetics to selectively block peripheral nerves following surgery allows for the relief of pain without the significant side effects associated with other systemic analgesics, such as the opioids. Selective blocking of intercostal nerves before chest wall closure after thoracic surgery has been shown to provide analgesia equal to that of systemic morphine. The technique involves injecting 0.5% bupivacaine (Marcaine, Winthrop Pharmaceuticals) (Figure 22-14) into intercostal nerves as they pass behind the head of the ribs (Figure 22-15) for two to three rib spaces in front of and behind the thoracotomy incision.

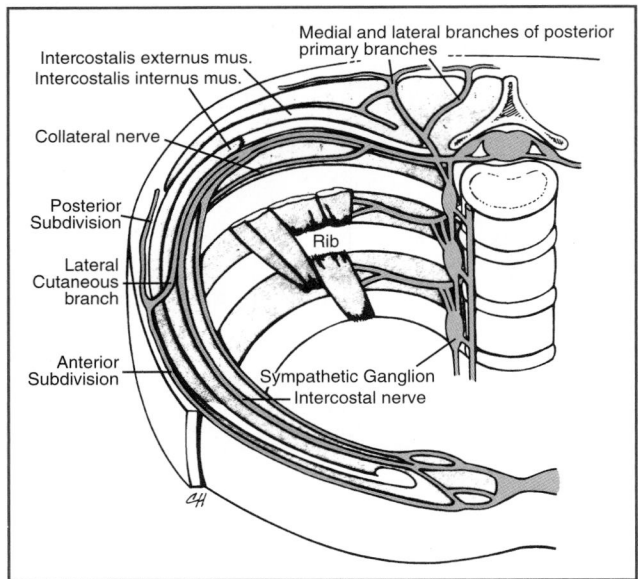

FIGURE 22-15. Intercostal nerve blocks may be used to provide regional analgesia after thoracic surgery.

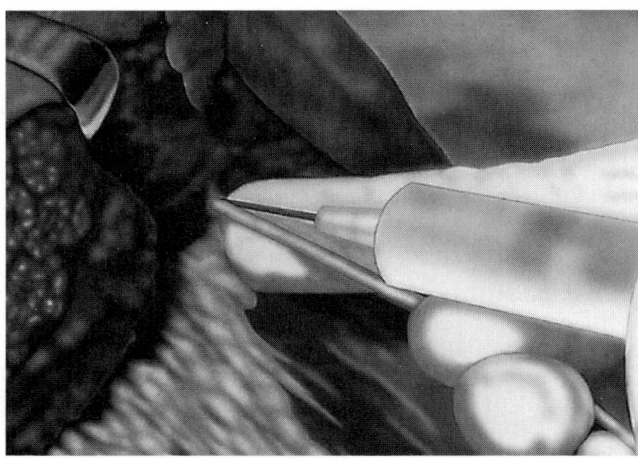

FIGURE 22-16. Bupivacaine injected into the severed sciatic nerve stump after rear limb amputation helps to provide regional analgesia.

A maximum total dose of 4 to 5 mg/kg in dogs and 2 to 3 mg/kg in cats should be used. Complete blocking of the intercostal nerves with bupivacaine will provide analgesia for 4 to 5 hours. Selective intercostal nerve blocks have a distinct advantage in not producing the respiratory depression associated with narcotic use.

Recently, analgesia in dogs for thoracotomy-associated pain has been achieved by instilling 0.5% bupivacaine, 1.5 mg/kg, through chest tubes placed during surgery. The analgesia provided is considered to be equal to either systemic morphine or intercostal nerve block. The technique involves instilling the appropriate dose of bupivacaine through the chest tube followed by flushing the tube with 5-ml sterile physiologic saline. The dog is then rolled on its back and slightly tilted to the incision side for

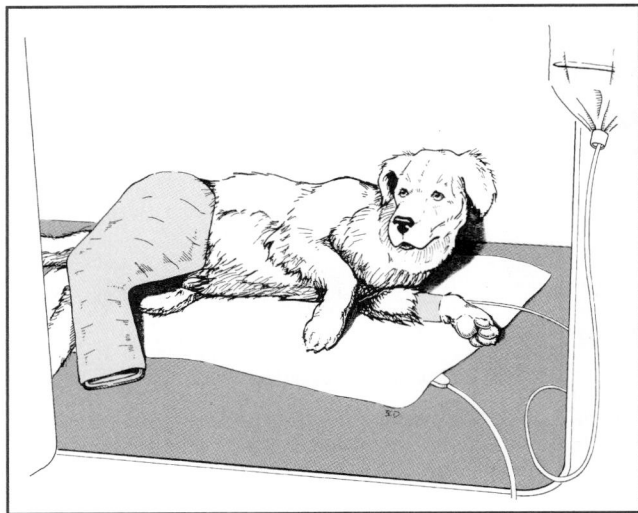

FIGURE 22-17. Avoid excessive movement in patients recovering from painful surgeries.

10 to 15 minutes. This technique allows the local anesthetic to block the nerve roots at the site of the incision.

Local nerve blocks are also used for injection of transected nerves following thoracic or pelvic limb amputation (Figure 22-16). Significant postoperative pain is often associated with cut nerve fibers following limb amputation. Analgesia may be provided by injecting 0.5% bupivacaine (0.5 ml per nerve, not to exceed 4 to 5 mg/kg in the dog) into the nerve stump before wound closure.

TREATMENT OF PAIN IN DOGS AND CATS

The first step in the management of pain in animals is recognizing the behavioral and physiologic signs associated with significant discomfort. Recognize that abnormal respiration, rapid heart rate, aggression, and changes in appetite and grooming behavior can all be associated with pain. It is critical to remember that no single sign is definitive in determining whether an animal is experiencing discomfort. It is helpful to remember, when clinical signs are confusing, that if the patient experienced a procedure that would be painful to a human, it is likely that it was painful to the animal.

Good nursing care is critical in the management of pain. Providing clean, dry, comfortable bedding in an area free from noise and confusion goes a long way in relieving the distress and anxiety associated with pain. Many patients will benefit from gentle human contact, such as talking and petting. Avoid excessive movement and treatments in patients recovering from a painful surgery (Figure 22-17).

 Technician Note

When administering any of the NSAIDs, always be aware that they can cause gastric upset, vomiting, and ulceration.

When one is selecting an analgesic drug for the treatment of pain (Tables 22-4 to 22-6 and Boxes 22-1 and 22-2), animals should be divided into at least two catego-

TABLE 22-4	NARCOTIC ANALGESICS USED IN DOGS			
Drug	Potency*	Dose	Analgesic Duration (hr)	Comments
Morphine	1	0.25-5.0 mg/kg IM, SC	4	Causes respiratory depression and vomiting; elevates intracranial and intraocular pressure; metabolized by liver
		Epidural: 0.1 mg/kg	10	
Oxymorphone	10	0.005-0.2 mg/kg IM, SC, IV; do not exceed 60-mg total dose	6	Causes respiratory depression, auditory hypersensitivity, and altered thermoregulation; metabolized by liver
		Epidural: 0.1 mg/kg	10	
Butorphanol	5	0.4-0.6 mg/kg IM, SC, IV	4	Agonist/antagonist; antitussive, antiemetic; ceiling on respiratory depression
Buprenorphine	25-50	0.006-0.01 mg/kg IM, SC, IV	6-8	Agonist/antagonist; prolonged (≥30 min) time from administration to onset of action; long duration; difficult to reverse with naloxone
Fentanyl	100	0.04-0.08 mg/kg IM, SC, IV	2	Causes respiratory depression, auditory sensitization, decreased cardiac output, bradycardia; metabolized by liver
Nalorphine	0.8	11-22 mg/kg IM, SC, IV	2-3	Agonist/antagonist
Naloxone		0.04 mg/kg IM, SQ, IV; may be repeated as necessary	2	Pure opiate antagonist; GABA-receptor antagonist

GABA, Gamma aminobutyric acid; IM, Intramuscularly; IV, intravenously; SC, subcutaneously.
*Morphine is used as a standard of potency.

TABLE 22-5	NARCOTIC ANALGESICS USED IN CATS			
Drug	Potency*	Dose	Analgesic Duration (hr)	Comments
Morphine	1	0.1 mg/kg IM, SC	4	Overdose causes excitation; causes respiratory depression, emesis; elevates intraocular pressure; metabolized by liver
Oxymorphone	10	0.1 mg/kg IM, SC, IV	6	May cause ataxia; *overdose* causes excitation; causes respiratory depression, auditory hypersensitivity, altered thermoregulation; metabolized by liver
Butorphanol	5	0.4-0.8 mg/kg IM, SC, IV	3-6	Analgesia for visceral pain lasts longer than for somatic pain
Buprenorphine	25-50	0.005-0.01 mg/kg IM, SC, IV	6-8	Agonist/antagonist; prolonged (>30 min) time from administration to onset of action; long duration; difficult to reverse with naloxone
Naloxone		0.04 mg/kg IM, IV; may be repeated as necessary	2	Pure opiate antagonist; GABA-receptor antagonist

GABA, Gamma aminobutyric acid; IM, Intramuscularly; IV, intravenously; SC, subcutaneously.
*Morphine is used as a standard of potency.

TABLE 22-6	ANTIINFLAMMATORY DRUGS USED IN DOGS		
Drug	Dose	Frequency (hr)	Comments
Aspirin	10-25 mg/kg PO	8	Induces gastric ulceration Decreases platelet aggregation
Phenylbutazone	10-25 mg/kg PO	8-12	May cause agranulocytosis Induces gastric ulceration
Carprofen	0.5 mg/kg PO	12	Gastric ulceration Hepatic toxicosis (idiosyncratic)
Flunixin meglumine	0.5-1.0 mg/kg IM, IV	24; 3-dose maximum	Induces gastric ulceration
Naproxen	3 mg/kg PO	24	Induces gastric ulceration
Meclofenamic acid	1.1 mg/kg PO	24	Induces gastric ulceration

IM, Intramuscularly; IV, intravenously; PO, orally.

| BOX 22-2 | SUGGESTED POSTOPERATIVE ANALGESICS FOR DOGS AND CATS |

ABDOMINAL SURGERY
Morphine
Butorphanol
Oxymorphone

Suggestions
- May add low doses of tranquilizers to opioids for additional sedation
- Opioids cause respiratory depression and are metabolized slowly in patients with liver disease

THORACIC SURGERY
Intercostal nerve block with bupivicaine
Intrapleural nerve block with bupivicaine
Morphine
Butorphanol
Oxymorphone

Suggestions
- Use low doses of opioids with local nerve blocks for additional pain control
- May add low doses of tranquilizers for additional sedation
- Opioids cause respiratory depression; use with caution in patients with respiratory disease

OPHTHALMIC SURGERY
Butorphanol
Oxymorphone

Suggestion
- May add low doses of tranquilizers for additional sedation

ORTHOPEDIC/NEUROSURGERY
Morphine
Butorphanol
Oxymorphone

Suggestions
- Butorphanol and morphine may not provide enough analgesia for severe postoperative pain
- May add low doses of tranquilizers for additional sedation
- By 24 hr after operation, NSAID may be tried in place of opioids; be alert for gastric ulceration

NSAID, Nonsteroidal antiinflammatory drug.

ries: those with acute pain resulting from surgery and those experiencing chronic, low-grade pain, frequently of musculoskeletal origin. Patients experiencing acute pain generally benefit the most from short-term opioid analgesics. When anxiety, as demonstrated by excessive vocalization, is involved with acute pain, low doses of tranquilizers may be added to opioid analgesics. Remember that tranquilizers alone have little or no analgesic effect. Patients with musculoskeletal pain often benefit from the use of one of the NSAIDs. In general, the most effective therapeutic approach is to begin with aspirin and then advance to one of the more potent NSAIDs, such as naproxen or meclofenamic acid, if aspirin is not effective. When administering any of the NSAIDs, always be aware that they can cause gastric upset, vomiting, and ulceration. Patients with existing kidney disease may also experience a worsening of their condition when given NSAIDs.

Principles of analgesia in the cat should follow the same basic guidelines as for the dog, with several exceptions. Of the nonsteroidal drugs, aspirin is the best choice. When using aspirin in the cat, remember that cats metabolize the drug slowly. Aspirin given orally every other day is generally effective. Narcotics are effective in controlling acute pain in cats. Doses of narcotics should generally be lower than for the dog to avoid the excitatory effects sometimes observed with high doses.

TREATMENT OF PAIN IN HORSES

The relief of pain in horses with gastrointestinal or musculoskeletal pain is important both for the comfort of the patient and to minimize injury to attending personnel. Technical staff must be aware that analgesics may mask many important clinical signs, including heart and respiratory rates, that are used for monitoring colic patients or lameness associated with musculoskeletal injury. In both cases, worsening of the condition may occur in the face of improving clinical signs. Analgesic therapy should be tailored to each case based on a thorough knowledge of the potency, mechanism of action, and drug side effects.

Analgesics in the Treatment of Colic

Colic produces many behavioral and cardiovascular changes that are frequently used to assess the severity and prognosis of the disease. Pain associated with gastrointestinal injury is most frequently related to abdominal visceral distention, obstruction, and torsion, along with the release of inflammatory mediators, such as histamine, serotonin, kinins, prostaglandins, and leukotrienes. Severe colic can cause such extreme pain that both the horse and attending technical staff may be at risk of injury. NSAIDs, narcotics, and tranquilizers are all used to control pain associated with colic (Table 22-7). In experimental equine models, xylazine was found to produce the most pronounced visceral analgesia for the longest period of time.

 Technician Note

In experimental equine models, xylazine was found to produce the most pronounced visceral analgesia for the longest period of time.

Visceral analgesia is immediate in onset after xylazine administration. Xylazine causes sedation characterized by lethargy, drooping and extension of the neck, and ataxia. Heart and respiratory rates are significantly depressed. Xylazine also depresses intestinal motility, which may contribute to postoperative ileus. Butorphanol produces visceral analgesia and is second to xylazine in potency. The combination of xylazine (1.1 mg/kg intravenously) followed by butorphanol (0.1 mg/kg intravenously) produces excellent analgesia. Morphine, meperidine, and oxymorphone produce visceral analgesia that is highly variable and often inferior to that of xylazine and butorphanol. Flunixin meglumine is also recommended for alleviation of colic pain and is widely considered the best NSAID for this purpose. Flunixin is also effective in preventing the clinical signs of endotoxemia.

TABLE 22-7   DRUGS THAT PROVIDE VISCERAL ANALGESIA IN HORSES

Drug	Recommended Intravenous Dose (mg/kg)
NARCOTIC AGONISTS	
Morphine	0.02-0.04
Meperidine	0.2-0.4
Oxymorphone	0.01-0.02
MIXED AGONIST/ANTAGONISTS	
Butorphanol	0.02-0.05
Pentazocine	0.4-0.8
NONSTEROIDAL ANTIINFLAMMATORIES	
Ketoprofen	2
Flunixin meglumine	0.6-1.1
ALPHA$_2$ AGONISTS	
Xylazine	0.3-0.5
Detomidine	0.005-0.02

TABLE 22-8   ANTIINFLAMMATORY DRUGS USED IN HORSES

Drug	Recommended Dose (mg/kg)
Aspirin	15-100 PO, every 12 hr
Flunixin meglumine	0.25-1.1 PO, IM, IV, every 8–24 hr
Meclofenamic acid	2.2 PO, every 24 hr
Naproxen	10 PO, every 12 hr
Phenylbutazone	2-4 PO, every 12-24 hr
Sodium hyaluronate	10-40 mg/joint intraarticularly every 7 days
Polysulfated glycosaminoglycans	250 mg/joint intraarticularly every 7 days 500 mg IM every 5 days

IM, Intramuscularly; *IV*, intravenously; *PO*, orally.

Analgesics for the Treatment of Musculoskeletal Pain

NSAIDs are extremely useful in the treatment of musculoskeletal pain in the horse (Table 22-8). This group of drugs provides analgesia when inflammation contributes significantly to pain. Examples include acute laminitis, joint sprains, severe muscle and tendon injuries, and chronic degenerative joint disease. The NSAID used most frequently in the horse is phenylbutazone. Drug actions and side effects for the nonsteroidal group in horses are similar to those described for the dog and cat.

Technician Note

The NSAID used most frequently in the horse to control musculoskeletal pain is phenylbutazone.

A miscellaneous group of agents used for modifying the disease process in degenerative joint disease includes sodium hyaluronate (Hylartin V, Pharmacia; Equron, Solvay; Hyalovet, Fort Dodge Laboratories) and polysulfated glycosaminoglycans (PS-GAGs; Adequan, Luitpold Pharmaceuticals). The mechanism of action of these drugs is variable, but all are aimed at returning the synovial joint to normal. Individual responses are variable and depend on the level of disease present. The intraarticular dose for hyaluronate is between 10 to 40 mg per joint. The dose may be repeated at weekly intervals. PS-GAGs are given at 250 mg per joint intraarticularly on a weekly basis. Alternatively, PS-GAGs may be given at 500 mg intramuscularly for 4 days for a total of seven treatments. The PS-GAGs have an advantage over hyaluronate in that they inhibit enzymes involved in cartilage degradation. Use of PS-GAGs is contraindicated in cases of infectious arthritis.

RECOMMENDED READING

Carroll GL: *Small animal pain management*, Lakewood, Col, 1998, AAHA Press.

MacPhail CM et al: Hepatocellular toxicosis associated with administration of carprofen in 21 dogs, *J Am Vet Med Assoc* 212:1895, 1998.

Sackman JE: Pain and its management, *Vet Clin North Am Small Anim Pract* 27:1487, 1997.

Scherk-Nixon M: A study of the use of a transdermal fentanyl patch in cats, *JAAHA* 32:19, 1996.

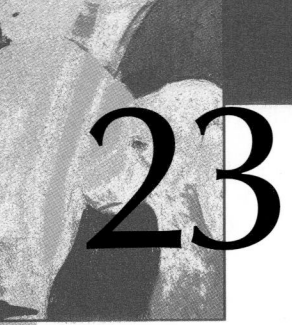

23

Pharmacology and Pharmacy

Marvene Augustus

In most practices, the technician shares the responsibility of administering drugs, which can range from the simplest chewable tablet to a gaseous anesthetic. As new drugs and strategies are applied to veterinary care, the role of the technician becomes increasingly sophisticated. The technician must have some knowledge regarding the mechanisms of drug actions and therapeutic uses and potential side effects. Verification that the drug and dosage are correct is a major responsibility of the technician. For this reason, the technician should be familiar with the dosage forms of drugs, able to recognize common medications, and able to translate drug dosages into the appropriate number of tablets or volume of drug for the individual patient.

This chapter is intended to provide the technician with a minimal basic knowledge of drugs, including the calculation of dosages; drug laws; and drug inventory control. Anesthetic agents and drugs used in the treatment of cancer are discussed in Chapters 10 and 21. Several good books written primarily for veterinary technicians are dedicated entirely to the subject of veterinary drugs and should prove helpful for those with greater interest in veterinary therapeutics.

GENERAL PRINCIPLES

Definitions

A *drug* is defined as any chemical agent that affects living processes; these agents may be used to prevent, diagnose, or treat diseases. *Pharmacology* is a broad term defined as the study of drugs. Aspects of pharmacology include the history and source of drugs *(pharmacognosy)*; physical and chemical properties of drugs and effects and actions of drugs on living organisms *(pharmacodynamics)*; characteristic ability of living organisms to absorb, distribute, metabolize, and excrete drugs *(pharmacokinetics)*; and therapeutic uses of drugs *(pharmacotherapeutics)*.

 Technician Note

Drugs do not create functions in tissues or organs; they can only modify or alter those that already exist.

Generally, use of the term *pharmacology* is limited to the study of the action of drugs on living systems to produce biologic effects. Drugs do not create functions in a tissue or organ but instead modify or alter existing ones.

PRINCIPLES RELATING TO DRUG ACTION

Pharmacokinetic factors of a drug (absorption, distribution, metabolism, excretion) will determine how the drug enters the body, reaches the site of action, and is removed from the body.

Drug Absorption

For drugs to exert an effect, they must reach their site of action *(target tissue)*. For some drugs, a simple topical application accomplishes this. Most drugs, however, must cross several barriers of cell membranes to produce the desired action. Cell membranes also must be crossed for the subsequent deactivation and elimination of the drug from the body. *Absorption* is defined as the uptake of substances into or across tissues.

Drugs with systemic actions that are administered orally must cross the gastrointestinal lining of the stomach or small intestine to be effective. Absorption of drugs from the gastrointestinal tract will be influenced by several factors. To pass through the membrane lining of the gastrointestinal tract, a drug must dissolve to some degree in oil *(lipid soluble)* because the membranes contain a high concentration of lipid (fat). Ionic *(charged)* forms of drugs do not easily pass through these membranes, whereas the nonionic forms of drugs pass more easily. Most drugs are weakly acidic or basic and have some lipid-soluble properties. The stomach is a highly acidic environment. The weakly basic drugs that are highly ionized (charged) in the acidic stomach will not be readily absorbed until they are farther down the digestive tract in the small intestine, because it is basic in nature. In the small intestine, the weakly basic drugs exist in an un-ionized form, which permits easier transport across the lipid membrane. Drugs that are weak acids are un-ionized in the acidic stomach and diffused more easily through the lipid membrane. They are rapidly absorbed from the stomach and therefore expected to exert their action more quickly than weakly basic drugs. Most drugs with poor lipid solubility cannot pass through cell membranes. Drugs such as the antimicrobial aminoglycosides (e.g., gentamicin) have poor lipid solubility and therefore are inadequately absorbed and ineffective after oral administration.

Stomach contents may inactivate or trap certain drugs. The volume of stomach contents also may delay absorption, thus delaying action. In ruminants, one is confronted not only with slow absorption from dilution but also with the effect of the action of the ruminal microorganisms on certain susceptible agents. Common drugs of plant origin, such as digoxin and atropine, are ineffective in the ruminant when administered orally because of digestive microorganisms.

Drugs that require injection *subcutaneously* or *intramuscularly* must be absorbed from the injection site to exert their action. The subcutaneous route is appropriate for small drug volumes (less than 1 ml) and drugs intended to be absorbed slowly. Because of limited blood flow, subcutaneous drug administration results in a more sporadic absorption compared with those drugs injected intramuscularly. Insulin and heparin are examples of drugs that are administered subcutaneously. In animals that are highly dehydrated, there is a restricted blood flow at body surfaces, so subcutaneous administration is not usually recommended.

Intramuscular injection is appropriate when a larger volume of drug must be administered. Absorption from the intramuscular site is faster than that from subcutaneous sites because muscles are better supplied with blood vessels than the skin. Procaine penicillin is an example of a drug to be injected in the muscle.

Absorption from the subcutaneous or intramuscular site can be hastened by applying heat or massage to the site to accelerate the blood flow. Conversely, absorption can be slowed by applying ice packs at the injection site to decrease blood flow.

Drugs that are introduced into the vascular system (*intravenous*) will not go through an absorption phase. These drugs are placed directly into the plasma compartment and take effect immediately.

Figure 23-1 depicts the distribution of drugs after administration. Drug concentration is a dynamic process that continually varies at different sites until it is virtually all excreted. Generally, another dose is administered before the complete removal of the previous dose, so the effective tissue levels (*site of action*) may be maintained. High lipid solubility and low protein binding are favorable characteristics indicative of the ability of a drug to diffuse through membranes. Drug transport into tissues involves passage through lipid-containing membranes. Diffusion is a difficult process for water-soluble compounds.

Most drugs in the bloodstream bind in varying degrees to plasma proteins such as albumin. Only the unbound drug (*free drug*), which may be as little as 10%, is available to diffuse into tissues and produce biologic effects. As a

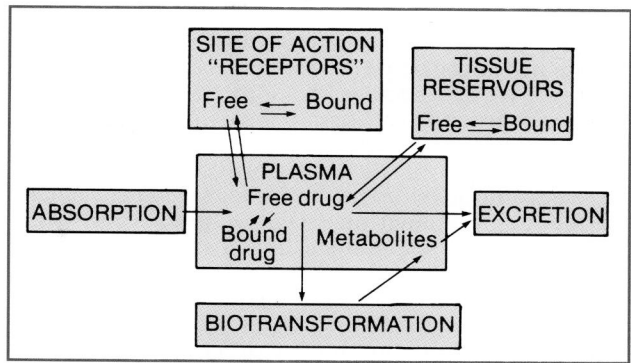

FIGURE 23-1. Schematic depicting fate of drug on administration.

rule, drugs bound to albumin or other proteins remain in the blood because these proteins do not diffuse through capillary walls. Drug binding to albumin is a reversible process. Protein binding serves as a reservoir site because the drug becomes available as the plasma concentration of the free drug is reduced. An equilibrium is maintained at all times between protein-bound and free drug in the blood. A common form of drug interaction occurs when a second drug has a stronger affinity for the plasma protein. The first drug is replaced and becomes free to exert its effects in a greater concentration at its site of action.

Accumulation of drugs may occur in various body compartments, such as fat, muscle, and liver, prolonging the effects of the drug as it is released from these storage sites. The potential of a drug to accumulate at these different sites will vary greatly among drugs, depending on their physiochemical properties. For example, a highly lipid-soluble drug, such as thiopental, will accumulate in body fat; this accounts for the slow recovery of obese dogs from barbiturate anesthetics compared with leaner dogs, such as the greyhound.

Although all the aforementioned distribution sites of a drug are important, the amount of drug reaching its site of action is of primary concern. The place at which a drug interacts with cellular components to exert its effect is called a *receptor*. There are numerous receptor sites throughout the body. Some sites are specific for certain drugs, whereas others are general and may respond or interact with several types of drugs.

The ability of a drug to bind to a specific receptor determines the biologic activity of the drug. The interaction of a drug with a specific receptor is similar to a lock-and-key fit (Figure 23-2). Only a certain critical portion of the drug is usually involved in binding with the receptor. Drugs that have similar critical portions but differ in other parts of the biologic molecule might be expected to have similar biologic activity.

A drug, in interacting with its receptor, may mimic the action of a natural body substance (*transmitter*). For example, acetylcholine is a natural transmitter that is secreted at terminal nerve endings, causing muscle contraction. A drug (bethanechol chloride) that is chemically similar to acetylcholine produces similar effects. Such drugs that directly produce the normal function of the receptor are termed *agonists*.

Drug Metabolism

For free drugs to be removed (*cleared*) from the blood, they must be excreted directly without change or metabolized *(biotransformed). Biotransformation* is the ability of a living organism to modify the chemical structure of drugs so that they are no longer active *(inactive metabolites)*. The liver is the principal organ responsible for biotransformation, but some of the activity may occur in the kidneys, brain, lungs, small intestine, and other organs.

Simple changes in the drug molecule, such as the removal or addition of certain atoms, may completely inactivate the drug. Through the mammalian enzyme system, potentially toxic compounds are changed into water-soluble compounds, which are more easily eliminated from the body by the kidneys. One means of removing many of the lipid-soluble drugs is through *conjugation*. This process involves the attachment of various endogenous substances to the drug. An example is the attachment of glucuronic acid to aspirin. After conjugation, the aspirin complex is much more water soluble, making it more readily excreted by the kidney. Cats are deficient in the enzymes required to conjugate drugs with glucuronic acid. This accounts for the relatively longer action of certain drugs in cats compared with most other mammalian species that do not have this deficiency.

Other common biotransformations of drugs by the liver include *hydroxylation* and *acetylation*. Biotransformation often inactivates drugs, but it does not always produce inactive products. Drugs such as codeine, diazepam, and amitriptyline are changed by the liver into metabolites that also exert a pharmacologic effect. These are called *active metabolites*.

In older animals or animals with hepatic disease, the ability of the liver to biotransform drugs may be impaired. Newborns less than 30 to 60 days of age are generally not capable of metabolizing many drugs because their liver enzyme system is not yet fully developed. To avoid drug toxicity, it might be necessary to reduce the drug dosage, increase the interval between doses, or switch to a drug that is not metabolized by the liver.

A few drugs are administered in an inactive form and do not become active until they are biotransformed by the liver; these are called *pro drugs*. For example, the angiotensin-converting enzyme (ACE) inhibitor enalapril must be converted by the liver to enalaprilat before it will exert any biologic activity.

Bacteria may carry out some biotransformation within the colon. This process may limit absorption of the drug from the bowel after oral administration, or it may help to eliminate drugs from the blood after parenteral administration.

Excretion

Most drugs or their metabolites are eliminated *(excreted)* by the kidney, although some drugs may be removed via the bowel or lungs or in some other minor way in limited amounts. The removal of drugs from the blood by the kidney is somewhat complex and will vary from drug to drug. One route of elimination involves the liver and kidney. Biotransformation of drugs by the liver tends to form more polar compounds, which can be more efficiently excreted by the kidneys. For example, the drug chloramphenicol is changed by the liver to chloramphenicol glucuronide. In this form, the drug cannot be reabsorbed via the kidney tubules from the urine back into the blood and therefore is excreted in the urine.

The pH of the urine will also influence excretion of drugs. Urine pH is normally basic, so drugs that are weakly acidic will exist in the ionized state and be more readily excreted. The weakly basic drugs will be in an un-ionized state and more apt to be reabsorbed back from the urine. For example, the elimination of aspirin, a weak acid, is enhanced in a more basic urine. The reverse is true of weak bases in an acidic urine. Ammonium chloride can be used to produce a more acidic urine, and sodium bicarbonate can be used to produce a basic urine.

Some drugs are not extensively metabolized by any organ in the body and are excreted unchanged in the urine. Some are excreted through passive diffusion into the glomerular fluid and are not reabsorbed to any significant degree and therefore enter the urine. Other drugs are actively secreted by specific systems in the renal tubules, which leads to more rapid drug elimination.

Drugs that are excreted by the kidney will accumulate in the body when there is a loss of kidney function. Creatinine (a natural waste product) levels in the blood are sometimes measured to determine the extent of renal damage so the dose of various drugs can be adjusted accordingly. Kidney function declines with age, even in the healthy animal. Elderly animals may show a reduced ability to excrete drugs in their urine. Certain drugs, such as the aminoglycosides, may directly damage the kidney *(nephrotoxicity)* and ultimately interfere with their own excretion.

Another route of drug excretion involves uptake by the

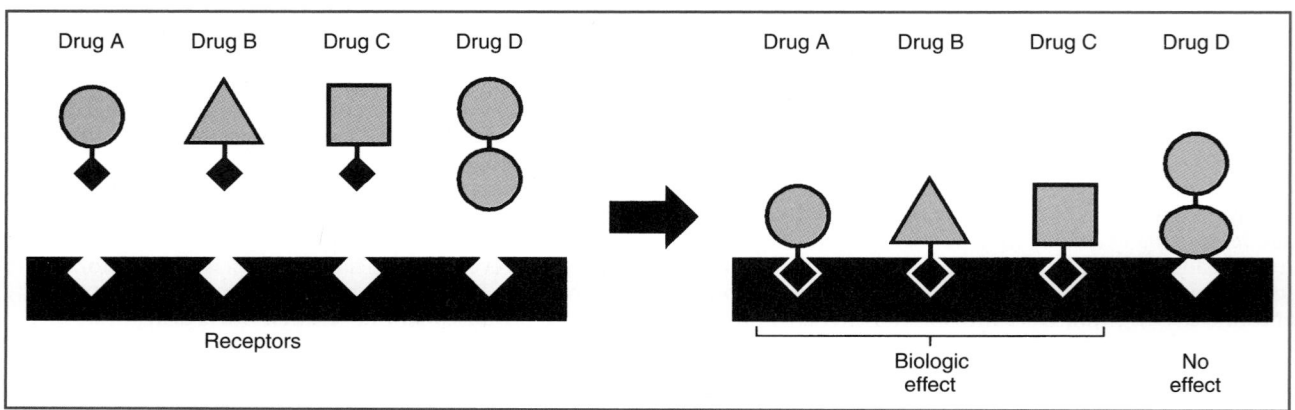

FIGURE 23-2. Lock-and-key fit between drugs and receptors through which they act. The drug and site, or receptor, must have definite shapes that conform to each other to bind and produce a biologic response.

liver, release into the bile, and elimination in the feces. Drugs in the bile enter the small intestine, in which they may be reabsorbed into the blood, returned to the liver, and secreted again into the bile. This process is called *enterohepatic circulation.* The drugs that are reabsorbed and resecreted will persist in the body much longer than the drugs that remain in the lumen of the intestine and pass out with the feces.

> ## Technician Note
>
> Pharmacokinetic factors include absorption (how the drug enters the body), distribution (how the drug reaches the target tissue organs), metabolism (how the drug is chemically altered), and excretion (how the drug is removed from the body).

ROUTES OF ADMINISTRATION

Several methods are available for administering drugs to animals. Each route of administration has advantages and disadvantages. The route selected will depend on a number of factors, including the patient's size, disease state, temperament, and unique species characteristics; the characteristics and commercial formulation of the drug; and the expertise *and* knowledge of the individual administering the drug. The cost of drugs should be a factor in the selection of a route of administration when all other clinical factors have been considered.

Oral Administration

Oral administration is one of the most convenient methods used by clients and animal health personnel for giving drugs. Tablets and capsules are fairly economic and provide accurate and uniform doses. Oral liquids offer some convenience, but the amount of active ingredient administered may vary from dose to dose, depending on measurement or the animal's acceptance. Administration of oral liquids by force in cats usually results in an undesirable salivary gag reflex episode. Oral paste forms for horses and food-producing animals have gained popularity because of their ease in administration. The acceptance of oral granules and powders, although variable among animals, offers convenience for dosing larger species. Drugs formulated for mixing in the animal's drinking water are least desirable because water consumption is highly variable and unpredictable. However, when dealing with large numbers of sick animals in flocks or herds, the use of water mixes may be the only economic and feasible method of treatment.

For small birds, medicated drinking water is sometimes used to avoid the stress that occurs with other methods.

> ## Technician Note
>
> Factors affecting routes of administration include physical characteristics and temperament of the animal, clinical state of the animal, characteristics and formulation of the drug, expertise in drug administration, and costs.

Absorption of drugs administered orally depends on a number of factors. Even when accurate doses are given, the actual amount of drug absorbed may vary, altering the expected therapeutic response. Most medications that can be administered orally can also be administered via feeding tube. It is preferred to give liquids by tube; however, some solid medications can be finely crushed and mixed with sufficient liquid to ensure complete passage of the drug into the stomach. Before administration of any drug via tube, make sure the tube is correctly placed.

Parenteral Administration

Parenteral administration of drugs is usually accomplished by subcutaneous, intramuscular, intradermal (Figure 23-3), or intravenous injections. Each requires sterile technique to reduce the possibility of introducing infection into the animal (see Chapter 3).

An *intradermal injection* is made just below the outer layer of skin *(epidermis).* This route of administration is used for allergy testing and giving local anesthetics. The volume of drug injected is small, usually less than 0.5 ml.

Subcutaneous injections are common in veterinary medicine because they are less painful to the animal and are easily administered. Some drugs cannot be given in this way because tissue irritation or sloughing may occur. Many vaccines are given subcutaneously, but some require intramuscular injection to produce the desired immune response.

Increased risks are inherent in the intramuscular administration of drugs. One must ensure the drug will not be injected into a vein or an artery by accident. The potential also exists for injecting the drug in or near a major nerve fiber, which could cause paralysis. One must have knowledge of the location of major nerves to avoid accidental damage.

When giving drugs subcutaneously or intramuscularly, only a limited amount can be administered at the injection site. Multiple sites may be used for some preparations, but the absorption may be more erratic.

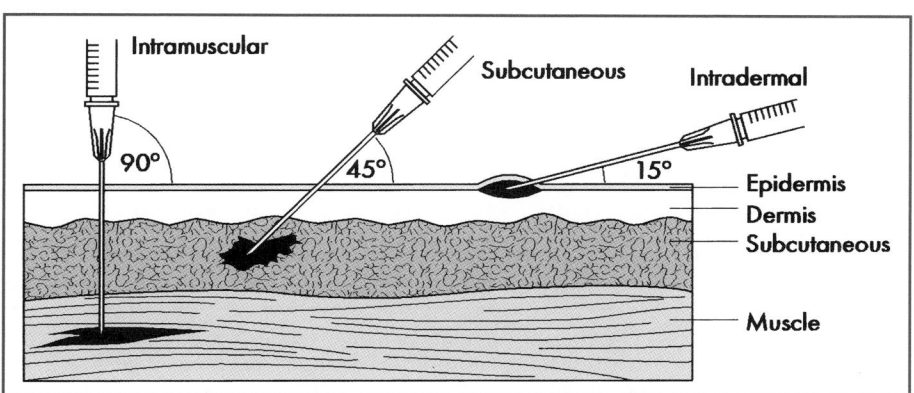

FIGURE 23-3. Comparison of angle of injection and location of medication deposit for intramuscular, subcutaneous, and intradermal injections.

The absorption from an intramuscular or a subcutaneous injection site is primarily through simple diffusion. A number of factors will influence the rate of diffusion from the site. Of primary importance is capillary circulation in the area. Because circulation is limited at subcutaneous sites, compared with intramuscular sites, one would expect slower absorption and longer action for drugs given subcutaneously.

Label directions should be followed regarding route of administration when administering drugs by injection. There may be a few exceptions for preparations with which sufficient experience exists for administration by routes other than those stated on the label. In most cases, however, there is a definite reason why the recommended route is stated. For example, antibiotics given by subcutaneous injection may not produce adequate blood levels to destroy microorganisms.

For intravenous administration, one must not only know the location of the larger veins that are used but also possess some skill in placement of the needle or catheter within these blood vessels. An immediate effect can be obtained from drugs administered intravenously without the delay of absorption encountered with other administrative routes. This route may also be used when larger volumes are required. Even certain irritating compounds can be given intravenously if they are given slowly, allowing adequate blood dilution.

Although intravenous administration has advantages, it also has risks. Highly irritating drugs, such as phenylbutazone, sodium thiopental, and triple sulfa, can severely damage blood vessels and surrounding tissue if injected outside the vein (perivascularly). Injecting certain drugs too rapidly may lead to untoward effects, including circulatory collapse and death.

Intravenous administration of drugs avoids the side effects caused by intramuscular or subcutaneous injection. Errors made with intravenous administration can be serious, even fatal, because the medications take effect quickly.

The technician should be aware there are several other important methods for introducing drugs into the body. Most, however, produce their effects locally at the site. Examples of other routes include topical (both skin and mucous membrane), intrathecal (into the spinal fluid), intraperitoneal, rectal, and inhalation.

DOSAGE FORMS

To administer drugs through the various routes, manufacturers have produced products in different formulations to accomplish the desired effect. For oral administration, there are not only traditional tablets and capsules but also chewable, flavored tablets to encourage animal acceptance and ease in owner administration. Oral liquids for human use may not be readily received by animals because of an undesirable flavor or high alcohol content. Liquids specifically flavored and designed for dogs and cats reduce stress for both client and patient during administration.

Many drugs cannot be administered orally to horses by their owners because of a disagreeable taste or odor. Some crushed tablets and powders can be mixed with molasses or other suitable compounds and then mixed with the animal's grain ration. Veterinary drug manufacturers have formulated granules and pellets for ease in oral administration. Oral paste forms, although somewhat more expensive, have gained popularity because of convenience to the owner and receptiveness of the animal.

Injectable drugs are frequently available in solutions or suspensions ready for use. Special buffers to maintain pH or absence of oxygen are required because of the instability of some components. Instability of some drugs may require a dry lyophilized powder be mixed with a diluent (reconstituted), such as sterile water or saline, just before use.

Some vials of drugs in solution are designed for single use only because the preparation may not have a preservative or the drug is highly susceptible to oxygen in the air. Certain vaccines or intravenous products may advise in their labeling that unused portions be discarded.

A variety of other dosage forms exist for use in veterinary medicine, such as ophthalmic ointments, solutions, or suspensions; topical sprays, creams, ointments, and lotions; and otic drops. Most are designed for a local effect, although occasionally there may be sufficient absorption from the application site to produce a systemic side effect. The transdermal patch is an example of a drug formulation designed for local application to produce systemic results.

Intrauterine administration of some antibacterials is not uncommon in mares, cows, and other breeding stock. Antibiotics are also formulated for intramammary infusion in milk-producing animals. Some of these products are used to prevent (prophylactic) infections at the end of the milking period only. These agents are designated for use in dry cows and usually have a longer duration of action. Other mastitis preparations are for use in lactating cows to treat an infection during the milking period. Milk must be discarded during the treatment period and for a time after the last treatment. The withdrawal time (usually 36 to 72 hours) will vary with the drug and formulation and is stated on the product label.

NEUROPHARMACOLOGY

Many different classes of drugs affect the nervous system, even though they are used for a variety of therapeutic uses. Some drugs will cause a direct effect, and others will alter functions of the nervous system as a side effect. The central nervous system includes the brain and spinal cord. Its function is to monitor, convey, and process signals from receptors throughout the body.

Neurons (nerve cells) relay information from the central nervous system to the rest of the body. They use neurotransmitters (NTs) to contact neurons and other cells. A neurotransmitter is a chemical substance released from the axon terminal of a presynaptic neuron or excitation (stimulation), which diffuses across the synaptic cleft to either excite or inhibit the target cell (receptor). Most neurons make only one kind of NT. The receptor recognizes only one specific NT and initiates a cellular response to it. The binding of the NT to its receptor is reversible. The stimulation of the cell is terminated when the NT is degraded or removed away from the receptor.

The nervous system is divided according to general function. The two primary divisions of the central nervous system are the autonomic nervous system or involuntary system and the somatic (motor) nervous system or voluntary system. The somatic system initiates muscle contraction by both conscious and unconscious control. The autonomic system innervates involuntary activities of the body. Although both systems have efferent fibers leading from the central nervous system, the focus of this discussion is on those of the autonomic nervous system.

AUTONOMIC NERVOUS SYSTEM

The role of the autonomic nervous system is to monitor and control internal body functions, such as digestive processes, blood volume, cardiac output, and kidney function. For impulse transmission to occur between nerves or

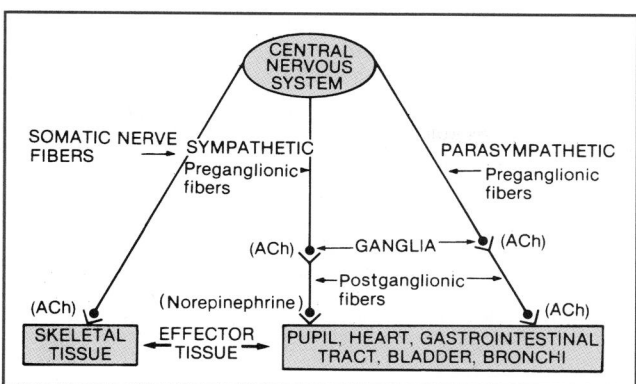

FIGURE 23-4.   Schematic of efferent fibers showing sites of neurohumoral transmitters.

TABLE 23-1	CHARACTERISTICS OF CHOLINERGIC (ACh) TRANSMISSION SITES	
Site	**Source of Stimulation**	**Response Blocked by**
Ganglionic (both sympathetic and parasympathetic)	ACh + nicotine	Hexamethonium, tetraethylammonium chloride
Postganglionic (parasympathetic primarily)	ACh + muscarine	Atropine and related belladonna alkaloids
Neuromuscular (somatic and skeletal muscle)	ACh + nicotine	d-Tubocurarine, gallamine

between nerves and effector sites (e.g., muscles, glands, organs), a small amount of an NT must be released by the efferent nerve (Figure 23-4). Two major NTs exist in mammals: *acetylcholine* (ACh) and *norepinephrine* (NE). ACh is released into the synapse. ACh that diffuses into opposing membranes is degraded into acetate and choline by the membrane-bound enzyme acetylcholinesterase. ACh that diffuses into the blood is degraded by nonspecific cholinesterases in the blood and tissues. NE is also deactivated by enzymes, but *reuptake* of NE by the nerve that released it occurs as well and the NT is again stored in the granules.

The autonomic nervous system is subdivided into the *sympathetic* and *parasympathetic* nervous systems. Both divisions commonly act on a given organ, but they produce opposite responses. NE is the predominant NT in the sympathetic system, and ACh is the principal NT of the parasympathetic system. ACh is also the transmitter substance found at the ganglia and at the neuromuscular junction in the somatic nervous system (Table 23-1).

Within the sympathetic nervous system, at least three different types of receptors exist (alpha, beta$_1$, beta$_2$), with others being postulated. All these receptors may be found within the same effector tissue, and response to the transmitter will therefore vary, depending in large part on the type of receptor that is predominant at the site as well as on the amount of transmitter substance present. The general responses of various effector tissues to normal sympathetic and parasympathetic stimulation are listed in Table 23-2. This antagonism allows full control of organ function according to body requirements. It should be noted that sympathetic response is a *fight-or-flight* response in that the animal's heart rate increases, bronchioles are dilated for better ventilation, and blood vessels to the heart and skeletal muscles dilate to increase blood supply. In the parasympathetic response the heart rate slows, bronchioles constrict to restrict airways, and blood vessels constrict in the heart and skeletal muscle.

Drugs affecting the autonomic nervous system may mimic or block all or selected effects of the NT, or they may alter the synthesis, storage, release or degradation, and

TABLE 23-2	PARTIAL LISTING OF GENERAL RESPONSES SEEN AT EFFECTOR SITES	
Effector Tissue	**Sympathetic Stimulation (Dominant Receptor Type)**	**Parasympathetic Stimulation**
Pupil	Dilated	Constricted
Glands		
Salivary	Scanty viscous secretion	Copious secretion (watery)
Gastrointestinal tract	—	Increased
Bronchioles	Dilated	Constricted
Heart		
Rate	Accelerated	Slowed
Contractile force	Increased	Decreased
Blood vessels		
Muscle (skeletal)	Dilated	—
Heart	Dilated	—
Skin	Constricted	Dilated
Gastrointestinal tract		
Muscle wall	↓ Peristalsis and tone	↑ Peristalsis and tone
Sphincter	↑ Tone	↓ Tone
Urinary bladder		
Wall	Relaxed	Contracted
Sphincter	Contracted	Relaxed

uptake of the transmitter. The classification of these drugs is difficult, not only because there are so many different types of action possible but also because most drugs possess more than one specific action. Drugs are generally classified based on their primary or predominant action.

Cholinomimetic (cholinergic or parasympathomimetic) *agents* are drugs that mimic the stimulatory effects of ACh. Cholinomimetic drugs can be further divided into muscarinic and nicotinic (see Table 23-1) agents. Receptor sites that are found to be postganglionic in the effector tissue may be stimulated by a naturally occurring alkaloid, *muscarine*. Most other ACh receptor sites, including end plates of muscle, may be stimulated by *nicotine*. *Anticholinergic* (cholinergic blocking or parasympatholytic) *agents* are those that are capable of blocking ACh effects. They can also be subdivided according to the site or sites blocked.

Sympathomimetic (adrenergic) *agents* and *sympatholytic* (adrenergic blocking) *agents* are those drugs that mimic or block, respectively, the effects of NE. These agents also are further classified by the particular receptor that they stimulate or block.

AUTONOMIC DRUGS

Cholinomimetic Agents

ACh is not effective systemically as a drug because it is rapidly *hydrolyzed* by the enzyme acetylcholinesterase at the receptor site. Only an ACh ophthalmic formulation is available for immediate constriction of the pupil during eye surgery.

Bethanechol is similar in structure to ACh and mimics much of its pharmacologic action. Bethanechol is sufficiently different from ACh in that it can resist hydrolysis by the cholinesterase enzymes; therefore it is a fairly long-acting drug. It is used as a smooth muscle stimulant. When given orally, indications for bethanechol use include gastric atony or stasis and urinary retention when there is no obstruction.

Adverse reactions to bethanechol in small animals are mild and may include vomiting, diarrhea, salivation, and anorexia. Arrhythmias, hypotension, and asthma are most likely to occur in overdosage.

Several drugs are able to bind with the cholinesterase enzyme, preventing it from breaking down ACh. This not only allows ACh to act longer but also creates increased concentrations, resulting in exaggerated effects. These agents are toxic (some related compounds were used as nerve gases in World War II), and their therapeutic usefulness is limited to a few unique medical problems. In veterinary medicine, the use of cholinesterase inhibitors is primarily for treatment of parasites—both internal and external. (These parasitic anticholinesterase compounds are discussed later in this chapter and in Chapter 7).

Cholinesterase inhibitors (anticholinesterases) are divided into three groups on the basis of reversibility: truly reversible (short acting, 5 minutes): edrophonium chloride; reversible (long acting, 30 minutes to 4 hours): physostigmine and neostigmine; and irreversible: organophosphates and ecothiophate iodide.

Edrophonium chloride is a drug used to diagnose myasthenia gravis, a disease of the nerves and muscles that is characterized by weakness and marked fatigue of skeletal muscles. Edrophonium chloride induces an immediate improvement, although it is of very short duration. The longer-acting agents *physostigmine, pyridostigmine,* and *neostigmine* are used to treat the disease in humans. Myasthenia gravis is a disease with a poor prognosis. It is a condition that is very expensive to treat; therefore treatment is rare in veterinary medicine.

A common veterinary use of injectable neostigmine is in the treatment of ruminal atony or gut stasis. Neostigmine is relatively short acting (2 to 4 hours), but its stimulatory effects may be beneficial in returning the rumen and gastrointestinal tract to normal peristaltic activity after surgery. This agent is sometimes employed to treat urinary retention because of its stimulatory effects on smooth muscle in the urinary bladder.

Neostigmine and physostigmine can also be used to treat atropine intoxication and to reverse the effects of certain neuromuscular blocking agents (e.g., tubocurarine, gallamine, pancuronium) used during surgery.

Technician Note
Neostigmine and physostigmine may be used to treat atropine intoxication and reverse the effects of some neuromuscular blocking agents.

Symptoms of overdose of the anticholinesterase agents include gastrointestinal effects (nausea, vomiting, diarrhea), salivation, sweating, respiratory effects (increased bronchial secretions, bronchospasms, pulmonary edema), ophthalmic effects (miosis, blurred vision, lacrimation), cardiovascular effects (bradycardia or tachycardia, hypotension, cardiac arrest), muscle cramps, and weakness.

Other cholinesterase inhibitors are available only as ophthalmic preparations to treat glaucoma. Glaucoma is a disease complex that is characterized chiefly by an increase in intraocular pressure that may lead to blindness if left untreated. The anticholinesterase agents reduce the intraocular pressure by lowering the resistance to outflow of the aqueous humor.

Anticholinergics

As mentioned previously, *nicotinic* receptors are predominant at the end plates of skeletal muscle and autonomic ganglia. *Muscarinic* receptors are predominant in smooth muscle, heart, and glands. Some drugs have the capability of stimulating both types of receptors to varying degrees, whereas other drugs are capable of blocking both sites in varying degrees. Further, some drugs may block the nicotinic effects at the skeletal muscle and not at the autonomic ganglia.

Drugs that inhibit the action of ACh at the muscarinic sites (antimuscarinic drugs) are used widely in veterinary medicine; the most popular drug in this class is *atropine*. Atropine is a belladonna alkaloid found in nature and commonly incriminated in plant poisoning. Other belladonna alkaloids, such as homatropine and scopolamine, are commercially available and have a slight difference in action.

Because these drugs exhibit their usefulness in inhibiting the action of ACh by competing at a number of sites, their potential for correcting a disorder or altering a response is significant. One can rarely choose a single site for therapeutic action without concomitant side effects occurring at other muscarinic sites. There have been numerous compounds synthesized in attempts to reduce certain unwanted actions and enhance desired effects. The success of such efforts has been limited, depending somewhat on the unique response of the individual patient.

The significant responses that are seen with therapeutic doses of atropine and related drugs are nearly the opposite of parasympathetic stimulation (see Table 23-2). The pharmacologic effects of atropine are dose related. Low doses will produce decreased salivation and bronchial secretions. Dilation of the pupil and increased intraocular pressure and heart rate are experienced with moderate systemic doses. High doses decrease motility and tone of the gastrointestinal and urinary tracts.

The antimuscarinic drugs are frequently used before and during surgery in small animals to reduce or prevent secretions of the respiratory tract and to reduce *bradycardia* (decreased heart rate). Atropine and its analogs have been used in combination with other drugs to treat diarrhea (see later discussion of antidiarrheal agents).

Technician Note

Anticholinergics increase intraocular pressure and are contraindicated in certain types of glaucoma.

Atropine is indicated in eye examinations and some ophthalmic surgery in which dilation of the pupil is desired. Atropine is long acting; therefore some of the shorter-acting *mydriatics* (dilating agents), such as tropicamide, are used. One of the most important uses of antimuscarinic drugs is to block spasms of the small ciliary eye muscles, thereby alleviating the associated pain.

Another significant use of atropine is as an antidote for organophosphates and other anticholinesterases found in many insecticides or parasiticides. Muscarine toxicity from poisonous mushrooms is also treated with atropine.

Atropine must be used with caution because of potential side effects, which are merely extensions of the pharmacologic effects. Some clinicians believe atropine is contraindicated in the horse except for life-threatening organophosphate toxicity because the decreased peristaltic activity in the lengthy gut of the horse leads to gas and toxin complications. Atropine can increase ocular pressure and is therefore *contraindicated* in the treatment of animals with certain types of glaucoma.

Neuromuscular Blockers

Neuromuscular blockers (NMBs) act at the junction of the nerve and skeletal muscle to paralyze skeletal muscle. These compounds are classified according to their onset and duration of action. Some of the more popular agents are d-*tubocurarine*, *succinylcholine*, *gallamine*, and *pancuronium*. Newer agents used in veterinary medicine are *vecuronium* and *atracurium*.

Some NMBs have been used in darts to capture animals, but they are dangerous because respiratory paralysis occurs. The main clinical use of NMBs is as an adjuvant in surgical anesthesia to obtain relaxation of skeletal muscle, particularly of the abdominal wall, and in orthopedic surgery. These agents are selectively used in veterinary medicine. *Guaifenesin*, another type of muscle relaxant, is commonly used in equine and bovine surgery. Symptoms of NMB overdose include increased risks of hypotension, histamine release, and prolonged muscle blockade.

Sympathomimetics

The *sympathetic nervous system* is extensively involved in regulating a number of body functions, including heart rate, blood pressure, bronchial airway tone, body temperature, carbohydrate and fatty acid metabolism, and appetite. Although NE is the primary transmitter substance, *epinephrine* is released from the adrenal gland when an animal is stressed through physical, psychologic, or other stimulatory means.

Because the NE molecule can be modified extensively and still possess some type of stimulatory properties, numerous agents are commercially available. Manufacturers seek a molecule that produces a desired response and eliminates or reduces all the other adrenergic effects. NE possesses only alpha effects and has limited therapeutic use in the treatment of certain hypotensive shock conditions.

Epinephrine has several therapeutic applications in veterinary medicine, although the actual frequency of use is limited. Clinical applications include the following:

- Allergic reactions (often lifesaving in the face of shock)
- Bronchospasm (provides rapid relief)
- Cardiac effects (sometimes used in specific heart disorders)
- Local hemostasis (may be used in dilute solutions [1:100,000 to 1:20,000] to control surgical bleeding in highly vascular tissue)
- Prolongation of the effects of local anesthetics, even though there may be undesirable systemic effects from epinephrine if overused

Isoproterenol, which has few alpha effects but powerful beta effects, is useful as a bronchodilator in respiratory disorders and as a cardiac stimulant in certain heart conditions.

A synthetic catecholamine gaining increased popularity in treatment of heart disorders involving depressed contractility is *dobutamine*. In therapeutic doses, the drug directly stimulates beta$_1$ receptors, resulting in cardiac stimulation with only a slight decrease in peripheral resistance, but it has little effect on beta$_2$ or alpha-adrenergic receptors.

Epinephrine and NE are not available in oral forms because both are destroyed by stomach acid. In addition, both drugs are relatively short acting when given by injection.

Isoproterenol is available in many preparations for humans that are designed for inhalation use or as tablets for under the tongue *(sublingual)*. Only the short-acting injectable form has application in veterinary medicine.

Epinephrine and *phenylephrine hydrochloride* are also commercially available as ophthalmic preparations. They cause the pupil to dilate, but unlike atropine, they directly stimulate those muscles of the eye controlled by sympathetic nerves. This mydriatic effect is useful in selected cases of glaucoma as well as in ophthalmic examinations.

Symptoms of toxicity include arrhythmias, pulmonary edema, dyspnea, vomiting, headache, and sharp rises in systolic, diastolic, and venous blood pressures.

Sympatholytics

Many chemicals interfere with the function of the sympathetic nervous system. Some agents act by interfering with the synthesis, storage, and release of the transmitter substance. Others interfere with the ability of receptors to interact effectively with NTs. Some blocking agents are specific in their action; for example, prazosin hydrochloride is specific in blocking the alpha receptors. Other agents (e.g., the phenothiazine tranquilizers, such as *acepromazine*) are more general in their action, blocking alpha and beta$_1$ receptors.

The alpha-adrenergic blocking agents cause vasodilation and are used mainly in animals for lowering blood pressure or improving blood flow in certain vascular diseases. An older, popular drug, *phenoxybenzamine hydrochloride*, which is used to dilate blood vessels and lower blood pressure, is being replaced by newer drugs, such as *prazosin*. Other hypotensive drugs, such as *hydralazine hydrochloride*, act directly on the vascular smooth muscle to cause relaxation.

Phentolamine, an expensive, injectable alpha blocker, is used to diagnose adrenal gland tumors and during surgery to control abnormally high blood pressure. Adverse effects seen with use of alpha$_1$-adrenergic blocking agents include first-dose syncope, transient lethargy and dizziness, nausea, vomiting, diarrhea, and constipation.

Beta-adrenergic blocking agents are therapeutically useful as antihypertensive agents and in the treatment of certain heart arrhythmias. *Propranolol* and *atenolol* are products used in humans that are gaining popularity in veterinary medicine.

Betaxolol and *timolol* are two beta-adrenergic blocking agents that are widely used in veterinary ophthalmology. After topical application to the eye, each reduces both elevated and normal intraocular pressure with or without glaucoma. Overuse of beta-adrenergic blocking agents results in symptoms of hypotension, bradycardia, bronchospasms, depressed consciousness to seizures, hypoglycemia, respiratory depression, and atrioventricular block.

Tranquilizers (Ataractics)

Tranquilizers are drugs that act on the central nervous system to produce a calmness of mind or detached serenity without loss of consciousness or marked depression. Their use in veterinary medicine is to modify the behavior of the animal to make it more manageable or less responsive to external stimulation.

Phenothiazines

Phenothiazine was originally used in veterinary medicine as an anthelmintic. Derivatives of the drug (chlorpromazine, acepromazine, promazine) have been synthesized to enhance the sedative effects of phenothiazine. Some of the derivatives are used as antihypertensive agents because they exhibit peripheral alpha-adrenergic blocking activity and cause vasodilation. The exact mechanism of action for sedation is unknown, but phenothiazines block postsynaptic dopamine receptors. These drugs have found usefulness as antihistamines, antiemetics, and anti-motion sickness agents.

The phenothiazine tranquilizers are used as preanesthetics by "taking the edge off the animal" and enhancing or prolonging the effects of certain anesthetics. Some side effects to be aware of when administering the phenothiazines include a drop in blood pressure, paralysis of the retractor penis muscle in horses, and lowering of the seizure threshold in dogs.

Alpha₂ Agonists

Although xylazine, detomidine, and medetomidine in the strictest sense may not be classified as tranquilizers, their sedative and analgesic properties are useful for chemical restraint, especially in the horse. Detomidine is approved for use only in the horse and has little application in other species. It appears to differ slightly from xylazine by producing greater analgesia and sedation. Although it is dose dependent, the duration of action of detomidine is longer than xylazine.

Both xylazine and detomidine are commonly used in combination with other sedatives, tranquilizers, and anesthetic agents. The effects of these drugs in combination are greatly potentiated and must be used with caution. Common side effects seen in the horse include muscle tremors, heart block, bradycardia, respiratory changes, sweating, and penile prolapse.

Xylazine is used widely in cattle, although it is not currently approved by the U.S. Food and Drug Administration (FDA) for use in food-producing animals. The popularity in ruminants results from its excellent anesthetic properties. Ruminants are sensitive to xylazine, requiring approximately one tenth the dose (based on body weight) used in horses. Adverse effects in cattle include ruminal atony, intestinal stasis, salivation, diarrhea, bloating, and regurgitation with aspiration pneumonia.

Technician Note

Yohimbine, an alpha₂-adrenergic antagonist, competitively blocks and antagonizes bradycardia and central nervous system and respiratory depression caused by xylazine.

Although xylazine is approved for the management of hyperexcitable behavior in the cat and dog, it is not widely used in these species. Vomiting is a common side effect seen in the cat, and xylazine is frequently used as an emetic when this effect is desired (e.g., emptying stomach before surgery).

Yohimbine is an alpha₂-adrenergic receptor antagonist that competitively blocks and antagonizes central nervous system depression or sedation and the bradycardia and respiratory depression caused by xylazine.

Antipamezole hydrochloride, which is a synthetic alpha₂-adrenergic antagonist, reverses the effects of medetomidine hydrochloride in dogs.

The use of *propofol* in veterinary medicine for induction in high-risk patients, such as those with compromised organ systems, is rapidly gaining popularity. It is used mainly for sedation/relaxation of 5 to 10 minutes in duration. Propofol is rapidly metabolized. Because propofol can cause respiratory depression its use should be restricted to situations where controlled intubation is available.

Anticonvulsants

Of the several different causes of *seizures* (convulsions) in dogs, only about two thirds can be controlled by the various anticonvulsant drugs. *Diazepam* may be the most popular injectable drug for use during seizures or in other emergency situations. This benzodiazepine agent depresses the subcortical levels of the central nervous system, thus exhibiting sedative, skeletal muscle relaxant, and anticonvulsant properties. Diazepam is relatively short acting (30 minutes to 2½ hours). *Phenobarbital sodium* is also available for injection when a longer effect (4 to 6 hours) is required.

Adverse effects seen with diazepam use include muscle fasciculations, weakness, and ataxia in the horse at sedative doses; irritability, possible development of hepatic failure, and aberrant demeanor in cats; and central nervous system excitement in the dog.

Phenobarbital is a barbiturate with central nervous system effects. The mechanism of action of this group of drugs is not quite understood, but they have been shown to inhibit the release of ACh, NE, and glutamate. Phenobarbital tends to depress motor activity without causing excessive sedation, which makes it a good anticonvulsant agent. One major side effect of this drug is dose-dependent respiratory depression.

An effective and inexpensive agent used to treat epilepsy (status epilepticus) and seizures caused by acute encephalitis or meningitis in dogs is *oral phenobarbital*. For some cases that are uncontrolled by phenobarbital, oral administration of potassium bromide has been effective. (Potassium bromide is not available in a commercial formulation. Authorization may be obtained from the FDA to compound preparations for treatment of refractory cases.)

Analgesics, Antipyretics, and Antiinflammatory Agents

Analgesics are agents that alleviate pain. Although local as well as general anesthetics inhibit the sensory perception of pain, analgesics are generally considered to increase the threshold of pain in the pain perception areas of the brain. Antiprostaglandins (e.g., aspirin, flunixin) inhibit the biosynthesis of these natural pain-producing substances and are also considered analgesics.

Opioid Analgesics

The naturally occurring narcotics (e.g., morphine, codeine) as well as synthetic narcotics (e.g., oxymorphone, hydrocodone, meperidine) are the most potent analgesics. These agents stimulate the *mu*-opioid receptor and are thought to have some activity at the *delta*-opioid receptor. Although these addictive agents are used for severe postsurgical or posttrauma pain in dogs and horses, their more common use is as an anesthetic or preanesthetic agent.

The pharmacologic effects differ somewhat among the various narcotics, but most will produce the following:

- Central nervous system depression in the dog, monkey, and human
- Central nervous system stimulation (excitement) in the cat and horse
- Cough sedation in the dog and human
- Respiratory depression (panting may initially be seen)
- Increased tone of intestinal smooth muscle, causing constipation

The effects of these drugs are reversed by narcotic antagonists, such as naloxone.

Unfortunately, the action of narcotic analgesics is fairly short in the dog and the horse (2 to 4 hours). Gut stasis in the horse is also a concern when considering opioid analgesics. Because the opioid analgesics have questionable efficacy in the ruminant, their use in veterinary medicine is limited.

The agonist activity of *butorphanol* is thought to be exerted at the *kappa* and *sigma* receptors. Butorphanol, a morphine congener, has shown promise in dogs as a longer-acting (4 to 8 hours) analgesic. Butorphanol is used in horses as an effective analgesic, although its stimulatory effects must be suppressed by the concurrent use of depressant drugs, such as xylazine. Butorphanol is also approved by the FDA as an antitussive in dogs. Adverse effects seen in the dog include sedation (occasionally) and anorexia or diarrhea (rarely). Transient ataxia and sedation may occur in the horse.

Gaining popularity in veterinary medicine for pain relating to surgery is *fentanyl*. Fentanyl shares the actions of the opioid agonists; the same precautions should apply. One advantage of using the transdermal patch system for pain management is that continual analgesia is provided for about 72 hours.

Hydrocodone bitartrate is a phenanthrene-derivative opioid agonist that is used in veterinary medicine mainly as an antitussive agent.

Opioid Antagonists

The opioid antagonists reverse the pharmacologic effects of the narcotics. Naloxone, which was discovered in 1960, appears to be the only true antagonist because it possesses no other apparent pharmacologic effect.

Although narcotic antagonists are used commonly in human addicts to reverse overdoses of self-administered narcotics, their principal use in veterinary medicine is to reverse the sedative and quieting effects of analgesics used for temporary restraint. Dogs receiving narcotic sedation for minor procedures (e.g., radiographs, suture removal) are easily "reversed" with naloxone; the animal is almost immediately alert. The duration of action of naloxone is shorter than that of most narcotics, and generally the effects of the unmetabolized analgesic are inadequate to cause the animal to return to its sedated state.

Corticosteroids

Corticosteroids are extremely active compounds that have numerous pharmacologic effects on all organ systems. They are valuable in the treatment of certain conditions; however, there are significant risks when one considers the potential adverse effects.

Because corticosteroids are naturally occurring body substances (cortisol is derived from the adrenal gland), one indication for the use of steroids would be replacement therapy to correct a deficiency. Such a deficiency is relatively rare. Most steroids used in veterinary medicine are given for their antiinflammatory effect; the mechanism for the antiinflammatory response is complex. They suppress the tissue swelling and pain that normally follow injury. Because inflammation is common in a variety of diseases, there is extensive use, perhaps overuse, of these agents.

Steroids also possess antiimmunologic effects, altering the immune response of the body. They are therefore used in certain allergic diseases because they reduce the hypersensitive and allergic reactions of the patient. Immunizations generally should not be given during corticosteroid therapy because of the potential for inadequate immune response.

 Technician Note

> Immunizations should not be given during corticosteroid therapy because of the potential for inadequate immune response.

Common side effects seen with the long-term use of steroids include gastrointestinal bleeding; increased susceptibility to infections or wounds that will not heal; potassium loss, causing irregular heartbeats, muscle cramps, and weaknesses; sodium and water retention (edema or ascites); muscle weakness resulting from protein breakdown; and behavioral changes.

Steroids are found in various dosage forms, including ophthalmic, otic, topical, injection, and oral. It should be noted that long-term use of these steroids as ophthalmic or topical agents may lead to some of the systemic toxic effects previously mentioned.

Dexamethasone is one of the most popular steroids used in veterinary medicine; it is fairly long acting (more than 48 hours). *Prednisone* is another very popular agent. These agents are commercially available in injectable, oral tablet, and liquid forms. *Prednisolone*, which is used interchangeably with prednisone, is available in tablet, ophthalmic, and injectable forms. *Triamcinolone* and *betamethasone* are also used extensively in veterinary medicine.

Nonsteroidal Antiinflammatory Drugs

To avoid side effects inherent to steroids, other agents possessing antiinflammatory action have been synthesized. *Phenylbutazone*, one of the original members of this group of compounds, remains one of the most widely used agents in equine medicine. Phenylbutazone is not frequently used in small animals, although there is a label claim for use in dogs. Dogs metabolize phenylbutazone rapidly, which makes it difficult to maintain therapeutic levels of the drug. Cats metabolize the drug slowly and thus become prone to its toxic effects.

Flunixin has gained popularity not only for its antiinflammatory effects but also for its ability to reduce gastrointestinal pain in horses and ruminants. Although not approved for food-producing animals, flunixin appears to be the best analgesic available for ruminants, providing relatively long, effective relief.

Technician Note

Phenylbutazone may be toxic to cats because of slow metabolism of the drug.

Ketoprofen is a propionic acid derivative structurally related to ibuprofen and naproxen. It has been approved for use in the horse to alleviate inflammation and pain associated with skeletal muscular disorders.

Oral administration of the nonsteroidal antiinflammatory drugs (NSAIDs) is apparently irritating to the gastrointestinal tract and may cause ulceration in the mouth, stomach, or intestine. *Carprofen* and *etodolac* are relatively new antiinflammatory drugs that have been approved for use in dogs. They cause less gastrointestinal distress than the older marketed drugs. Most NSAIDs used in human medicine are not used in small animal practice because dogs are prone to gastrointestinal tract side effects. Blood dyscrasia has been reported in several species receiving phenylbutazone. The drug has the potential for reducing the effects of other drugs metabolized by the liver because it increases the hepatic microsomal enzymes necessary to deactivate these drugs.

Diuretic and Cardiovascular Drugs

Fluid and electrolyte imbalances and their treatment are discussed in Chapter 27. The function of the kidney and its role in maintaining proper fluid volume and electrolyte concentration are also mentioned. Blood is initially filtered in the kidney, and most of the filtrate is reabsorbed from the kidney tubules back into the blood. Most diuretic drugs affect the reabsorption process, preventing the reabsorption of some sodium and water from the filtrate. As a result, urinary output and sodium excretion are increased.

Diuretics

Diuretic drugs are used primarily to relieve edema associated with diseases of the kidney, heart, or liver. Although there are numerous diuretic agents, *furosemide* appears to be the most routinely used diuretic in veterinary medicine. It is commercially available in convenient forms for oral and injectable administration in small and large animals. Besides being potent and effective in most cases, furosemide is rapid acting and usually produces diuresis within 5 minutes when given intravenously.

Furosemide can cause a "wasting" of potassium, so serum potassium levels should be monitored for animals that take furosemide. Potassium supplementation may be indicated during furosemide therapy.

Occasionally, when renal blood flow is inadequate because of trauma or shock, furosemide or similar diuretics are ineffective in altering tubular reabsorption. In such cases, an osmotic diuretic such as *mannitol*, which is poorly absorbed from the glomerular filtrate, is used to produce diuresis. Animals that have been hit by cars may be likely candidates to receive mannitol.

Cardiac Glycosides

Cardiac drugs are probably the most potent and hazardous group of drugs used in medicine because of their effects on such a vital organ. Any carelessness in calculations, administration, or observation of the patient may lead to death.

The dosage for these drugs should be individualized through frequent and careful monitoring to ensure the desired therapeutic response and avoid or minimize toxic effects.

The heart performs a relatively simple function (to circulate the blood), and it is essential to life. The heart consists primarily of muscle (myocardium), valves, and some specialized impulse-conducting nodes and fibers. Even though the heart has the ability to compensate for certain defects, disorders left untreated reduce the quality of life with severe disability, leading to premature death.

Significantly severe defects in the valves can only be treated surgically. Medical therapy is available for the treatment of a weakened myocardium and conductance disorders *(arrhythmias)*.

The normal healthy heart can increase its output readily when demands, such as increased exercise, are placed on it. This increased cardiac output is a result of either an increased heart rate or an increase in the volume of blood pumped per beat (stroke volume), but usually it is a combination of both. Heart muscle weakened with age does not contract as fully and therefore leads to reduced output. Because the body cannot tolerate much decrease in cardiac output, the heart rate will increase slightly and the heart will become enlarged because the myocardium will thicken in an attempt to improve contractility. *Congestive heart failure* is the condition of an enlarged heart with poor myocardium contractility.

Various glycosides found in the leaf of the plant digitalis have been found to be useful in the treatment of congestive heart failure. *Digitoxin* and *digoxin* are two of the glycosides that are commonly used in veterinary medicine, with the latter being more popular. The cardiac glycosides are unique in that they not only improve the contractility of the myocardium but also reduce the demand of the heart for energy and oxygen. These drugs also decrease the conduction of certain impulses within the heart and therefore decrease the heart rate. Glycosides are used for treatment of atrial fibrillation, an arrhythmic disorder of the heart.

Technician Note

Concomitant therapy of diuretics and cardiac glycosides may invoke low serum potassium levels, making animals more prone to digoxin toxicity.

Although the cardiac glycosides are effective by injection in horses and cattle, and to some extent orally in horses, it is not feasible to use these drugs to treat congestive heart failure because of the long-term nature of the disease. These drugs are commonly used in dogs and cats. There is adequate absorption of digoxin from the gastrointestinal tract in these species; however, it may differ somewhat among animals and can be influenced by feeding times.

Digoxin dosing is very critical. Toxic effects of the cardiac glycosides are seen at doses close to the therapeutic dose and therefore complicate its use. Owners should be aware of signs of toxicity, which include vomiting, diarrhea, loss of appetite, and depression. Associated with these symptoms are a decreased heart rate and drug-induced arrhythmias.

Animals that are concurrently using a diuretic may have low serum potassium levels and are more susceptible to digoxin toxicity.

Further complications to digoxin therapy are animals with reduced liver or kidney function, as is common to the older animal. Good client compliance and close monitoring are essential in digoxin therapy because of toxicity possibilities. The drug is available as oral tablet, oral liquid, and injection.

Antiarrhythmic Drugs

Arrhythmias of the heart fall into several categories and require skilled clinicians and electronic instrumentation for proper diagnosis and treatment. Some minor cardiac arrhythmias are likely to correct themselves and may be left untreated. The use of antiarrhythmic drugs in veterinary medicine is usually limited to treatment of those arrhythmias that are life threatening and require immediate attention.

Calcium channel blockers provide the veterinarian with an efficacious weapon in the treatment of certain cardiovascular disorders. This group of drugs has a low incidence of side effects. Of the numerous agents, *diltiazem* has surfaced as the most commonly used agent to treat supraventricular tachyarrhythmias in dogs and cats. It also is used in the treatment of hypertrophic cardiomyopathy in cats. Diltiazem acts as an antihypertensive agent through arteriolar dilation, but the benefit of this action is not fully known.

Three older commonly used antiarrhythmic drugs are *quinidine*, *procainamide*, and *lidocaine*. Only their more ordinary uses are mentioned because detailed discussion is beyond the scope of this chapter.

Quinidine is used in horses and large dogs for the treatment of supraventricular and ventricular arrhythmias. Other uses include treatment of atrial fibrillation and atrial flutters. Procainamide is related chemically to procaine, and it is used in the treatment of ventricular extrasystoles and tachycardia, atrial arrhythmias, ectopic contraction and tachycardia, flutter, and fibrillation. Lidocaine, although used primarily as a local anesthetic, has therapeutic application in the treatment of ventricular tachyarrhythmias. Clinical monitoring and electronic evaluations should accompany the use of these drugs.

All antiarrhythmic drugs are toxic to the heart and may produce their own serious arrhythmias. In addition, in the horse, quinidine can produce urticarial wheals, gastrointestinal disturbances (e.g., anorexia, colic, diarrhea), erythema, and edema of nasal mucosa with dyspnea and laminitis. Signs of quinidine toxicity in the dog include vomiting, depression, incoordination, and convulsions. Procainamide toxicities are exemplified in dogs by a loss of appetite, vomiting, and serious immunologic reactions with long-term use. A serious decrease in blood pressure may also occur when procainamide is given intravenously. Lidocaine is not effective orally and has brief action when given intravenously. In large doses, lidocaine can produce a drop in blood pressure.

Angiotensin-converting Enzyme Inhibitors

ACE inhibitors prevent the conversion of angiotensin I to angiotensin II (a potent vasoconstrictor). The drugs compete with angiotensin I for the active site of ACE. In veterinary medicine, this group of drugs is primarily used to treat canine congestive heart failure. *Captopril* was the first agent in this class to be commercially available. Treatment presented risks, such as renal failure. Other ACE inhibitors have been synthesized; they are *pro-drugs* because they require a functioning liver to convert them to the active metabolite. *Enalapril* is commercially available with label indication for use in veterinary medicine. Other ACE inhibitors that are in use, although experience is limited, are *benazepril hydrochloride* and *ramipril*.

The side effect profile of the second generation of ACE inhibitors has improved, and the dosing schedule is one or two times per day, which should improve client compliance.

AGENTS USED TO TREAT PARASITISM

Treatment of Internal Parasitism

Anthelmintics (wormers) are an extremely important group of drugs in veterinary medicine. The presence of internal parasites in an animal can shorten its life span or reduce the quality of life. It can contribute to considerable economic loss in food-producing animals. Although several different parasites are capable of infecting each species, most parasite infections can be effectively prevented or treated with proper care and medication. Current anthelmintics are much improved because they are more effective in eradicating the parasite and less toxic to the host. In addition, dosage forms such as pastes or chewable tablets are available. These formulations are much more easily administered, which reduces stress to the animal and client.

There are a vast number of anthelmintics currently available; however, this discussion is limited to a select, popular few. Parasite treatment summary charts and specific parasite information are given in Chapter 7.

Piperazine

Piperazine is an older, safe drug used for the eradication of roundworms (ascarids) in dogs, cats, horses, swine, and poultry. Because most of the newer anthelmintics are either more efficacious against ascarids than piperazine or have a broader spectrum of anthelmintic activity, piperazine has lost much of its popularity. Once commercially available as a single-ingredient product for large animal use, it is more frequently found in combination with other anthelmintics to broaden the spectrum or increase efficacy. Piperazine salts block neuromuscular transmission of the nematode, resulting in paralysis of the nematode in the gastrointestinal tract and passive removal from the body by peristalsis. Piperazine is considered to be a safe drug to use, even during pregnancy and concurrent gastroenteritis.

Benzimidazoles

Benzimidazoles are a large class of anthelmintics. They inhibit the enzyme fumarate reductase and thereby interfere with parasitic carbohydrate metabolism. *Thiabendazole, oxibendazole, mebendazole, albendazole, parbendazole, fenbendazole, cambendazole,* and *oxfendazole* are safe and effective agents against several gastrointestinal parasites. They are formulated primarily for large animals to eradicate strongyles, pinworms, and ascarids in the horse and roundworms as well as several other parasites in cattle, sheep, and goats. Albendazole is also active against liver flukes. Fenbendazole and mebendazole are available for use in small animals to eradicate roundworms, hookworms, whipworms, and some tapeworms, although neither is effective for the common *Dipylidium* tapeworm. Adverse effects are not usually seen at recommended doses of benzimidazoles.

Organophosphates

Trichlorfon, coumaphos, and *dichlorvos* are a group of agents that bind irreversibly to cholinesterase in the parasite, leading to ACh "poisoning" of the parasite. These drugs would also be toxic to the host, but they are selectively formulated to be poorly absorbed from the gastrointestinal tract of the animal. Precautions must be taken so animals dewormed with organophosphates are not exposed to other organophosphates, cholinesterase inhibitors, pesticides, or muscle relaxants, such as succinylcholine, until a few days after treatment. Organophosphates should be used only on the species indicated on the product label because the agents are toxic and specially formulated for the safety of each species. In addition, there is potential danger to humans in administration of these products.

Common toxic signs of organophosphate poisoning (e.g., widespread parasympathetic stimulation) include miosis, salivation, breathing difficulties, vomiting, defecation, and muscle fasciculation. *Atropine* is used as a specific treatment to block the muscarinic effects. *Pralidoxime* (2PAM) is an expensive product for humans and may be used in severe cases to reactivate the cholinesterase enzyme.

> ### Technician Note
> Atropine is the antidote for organophosphate poisoning. Pralidoxime (2PAM) is used to reactivate the cholinesterase enzyme.

The organophosphates are fairly effective in treatment of a number of principal parasites in horses, cattle, swine, sheep, dogs, and cats. With the potential toxicity of the organophosphates, many are being replaced with safer agents.

Tetrahydropyrimidines

Pyrantel and *morantel* are two drugs in the tetrahydropyrimidine class. These drugs act as cholinergic agonists and depolarize neuromuscular junctions. Morantel is a newer analog of pyrantel that is apparently safer and more effective in sheep and cattle than is pyrantel. Pyrantel is widely used in horses for the treatment of ascarids, strongyles, and pinworms. In dogs, pyrantel is used in the prevention and treatment of hookworms and ascarids. In general, the pyrantel products are safe and nontoxic to all species at the recommended therapeutic dose. There is no contraindication for use of these agents with other cholinergic drugs. Tetrahydropyrimidines are effective against the adult nematode but not active against larval forms.

Imidazothiazoles

Febantel is approved by the FDA for use in the horse to treat most of the common equine parasites except bots. Apparently, it is also effective against gastrointestinal parasites in a number of species, although it is not commonly used. This drug is reported to be safe and may be used in pregnant mares.

Levamisole has broad anthelmintic activity in a large number of hosts, including sheep, cattle, pigs, horses, chickens, dogs, and cats. Use and FDA approval are limited primarily to food-producing animals. Levamisole was used investigationally as a microfilaricide in heartworm infections of dogs when no other agents were commercially available. It causes neuromuscular depolarization. Although levamisole is relatively safe, some signs of toxicity occur similar to those of organophosphate poisoning. The toxic doses are only one or two times the therapeutic dose. Muzzle foam may be seen in ruminants after oral administration, but it usually disappears within a few hours. Transitory excitement has been seen in horses after treatment.

Milbemycins

The *milbemycins* are macrocyclic lactones that act by interfering with chloride-channel mediated neurotransmission in the parasite, thereby resulting in its paralysis and elimination.

Moxidectin is an oral dewormer and boticide for horses and ponies at least 4 months old. The label claims that one dose of the drug will suppress strongyle egg production through 84 days. *Doramectin* is an injectable drug marketed as a single dose for control of a wide range of roundworms and arthropod parasites in cattle and swine.

Ivermectins

The *ivermectins* enhance the release of gamma-aminobutyric acid (GABA), which paralyzes nematodes by blocking neurotransmission at excitatory motor neurons. Ivermectin has demonstrated effectiveness in a number of species against a wide variety of internal and external parasites. In cattle, swine, sheep, and goats, ivermectin is used to treat infestation by numerous gastrointestinal roundworms, lung worms, cattle grubs (cattle only), sucking lice, and mites.

The paste and oral liquid forms of ivermectin have been approved for treatment of infestations by large and small strongyles, pinworms, and bots, as well as for other equine parasite infestations. It is also approved for the treatment of ascaridiasis, although for some stages it may be less effective than desirable.

> ### Technician Note
> Most collie breeds are inherently sensitive to ivermectin toxicities.

Ivermectin has been approved for use in dogs only for heartworm prevention (see below); however, it has also been used at higher doses for treatment of other canine parasite infestations, including scabies. In certain dogs (most collie breeds) that are inherently sensitive to ivermectin, toxicities, sometimes fatal, have occurred with higher doses. Except for these unique toxicities, ivermectin has proved to be safe in other breeds and species when given at therapeutic doses.

AGENTS USED IN HEARTWORM TREATMENT AND PREVENTION

There is considerable risk involved in the treatment of heartworms; therefore the American Veterinary Medicine Association (AVMA) Council on Veterinary Service established guidelines suggesting that first adult heartworms and then the microfilariae be eliminated. Heartworm disease is primarily seen in dogs; however, cats may also become infected. Dogs subject to infestation or reinfestation must be found free of microfilariae and adult heartworms before being placed on a preventive heartworm regimen.

Melarsomine dihydrochloride (Immiticide, Merial Ltd.) is an organic agent used in treatment of heartworm disease caused by immature to adult infections. Dogs are at risk for posttreatment pulmonary thromboembolism; therefore they should be exercise restricted after treatment. The site of administration is critical for this drug, and it should be given only by deep intramuscular injection into the epaxial muscle. Adverse reactions observed with melarsomine dihydrochloride treatment include abdominal hemorrhage and pain, discolored urine, hematuria, tachypnea, disorientation, restlessness, and icterus. *Dimercaprol* (BAL) is an antidote for arsenic toxicity and may reduce signs of toxicity in overdoses. Coadministration of BAL may reduce the efficacy of melarsomine dihydrochloride.

Technician Note

Thiacetarsamide and melarsomine overdosages may show signs of arsenic toxicity. BAL is the antidote for arsenics.

Microfilariae ingested by mosquitoes from infected animals molt in the mosquitoes and are then introduced back into other dogs when another blood meal is taken. It is these reintroduced microfilariae that molt again into larvae and become adult heartworms. Drugs used for heartworm prevention, such as *diethylcarbamazine* (DEC), *ivermectin,* and *milbemycin,* act by killing the tissue-migrating larvae. To review the heartworm life cycle, see Chapter 6.

Milbemycin (Interceptor, Novartis) and ivermectin (Heartgard and Heartgard Plus, Merial Ltd.) are available as once-per-month heartworm preventatives. Milbemycin and Heartgard Plus have the added protection against adult hookworms caused by *Ancylostoma caninum.* Ivermectin toxicities (although rarely observed at the low-dose heartworm preventative level) unique to collies and collie-mix breeds are not seen with milbemycin.

DEC should be administered daily at the beginning of mosquito season and continued for 2 months after the season is over. If ivermectin or milbemycin is used, it should be given within 1 month of the initial exposure and then monthly. The final dose is given within 30 days of the last exposure. If more than 45 days elapse between doses, animals should be retested for heartworm before restoration of preventive therapy. In mild climates in which mosquitoes prevail year round, prophylactic treatment must be administered for the lifetime of the dog.

Although relatively nontoxic at the low dose used for heartworm prevention, DEC is somewhat irritating to the gastric mucosa. Oral administration is therefore recommended immediately after a meal to reduce nausea and vomiting. These adverse effects are usually seen only with the higher doses of DEC that are sometimes used to treat ascarids.

Anticestodal Drugs

Anticestodal drugs kill and/or facilitate expulsion of tapeworms. The original drugs used were agents that temporarily paralyzed the tapeworms, causing them to lose their attachment to the gastrointestinal tract. Even when these drugs contained purgative properties or were given with harsh laxatives, reattachment of a number of tapeworms was likely to occur. This treatment was stressful to the host because its ineffectiveness required repeated dosing. Newer drugs, although more expensive, kill the tapeworm.

When *praziquantel* (Droncit, Bayer) became commercially available for veterinary use, it soon replaced most other anticestodal drugs on the market because of its efficacy, limited toxicity, and wide margin of safety. It is quickly absorbed from the gastrointestinal tract after oral administration and can also be given by injection. Its distribution throughout the body makes praziquantel unique in that it is effective against various stages of tapeworm development, including the adult stage. In addition, it is nontoxic, with a wide margin of safety. The cost of praziquantel is the only factor discouraging the further development and expanded use of this drug in species other than dogs and cats.

Epsiprantel (Cestex, Pfizer Animal Health) has proven to be safe and effective. Unlike praziquantel, only trace levels of epsiprantel are absorbed after oral administration, and it remains at the site of action within the gastrointestinal tract. This drug exerts its action directly on the tapeworm.

Drugs Used to Treat Giardiasis

Giardia canis is a protozoan that may produce chronic diarrhea in dogs. Treatment with *metronidazole* is usually effective. In general, the toxicity is low, with few adverse effects reported during or after the 5-day treatment period.

Giardiasis is also found in cats, but clinically it is usually not a problem (its diarrhea-producing role is not known). For treatment in the cat, metronidazole is given in a dosage regimen similar to that used for dogs. The margin of safety in cats is much narrower, and overdosing must be avoided; several deaths have been reported.

Recent investigations show that *Giardia* with presenting diarrhea may be successfully treated with an alternating 7 days on/7 days off regimen of *fenbendazole.* The manufacturer of fenbendazole (Panacur, Hoechst) has not made label claim to this indication.

External Parasite Treatment
Chlorinated Hydrocarbons

Various *chlorinated hydrocarbon compounds* (e.g., *lindane, toxaphene, methoxychlor*) were once popular and marketed in several different formulations for a variety of uses in a number of species. Most compounds were effective and possess rapid knockdown capability, with some having residual effects for several days. The long-lasting residual properties posed a threat as environmental hazards, and as a result, many of these products have been banned. Other efficacious but less-endangering agents have been made available. Although the degree of toxicity will vary among the various chlorinated hydrocarbons, they should all be treated with caution and used as advised on the container label. Some diluted aqueous suspensions and powders may be applied directly to livestock. Signs of toxicity include vomiting, weakness, and other central nervous system effects, such as tremors, incoordination, convulsions, coma, and respiratory failure. Young, debilitated, or lean animals are more susceptible to the toxic effects. There is no specific antidote for chlorinated hydrocarbon toxicity. The animal should be removed from further exposure and given supportive treatment such as barbiturates to control seizures if necessary.

Organophosphates

Although *organophosphates* are the same class of drugs mentioned previously for treatment of intestinal parasites, these agents (*ronnel, coumaphos, trichlorfon, fenthion, malathion*) are formulated specifically for the treatment of external parasites. As with chlorinated hydrocarbons, a number of preparations exist, such as sprays, dips, foggers, pour-ons, and pest strips. These compounds have good insect-killing ability, but residual effects are related to the vehicle used to apply the agent. Topical application of these preparations permits significant absorption through the skin to produce signs of toxicity. Signs and treatment of toxicity are the same as those mentioned in the discussion on internal parasitism treatment. Persons applying these agents should avoid getting them in their eyes or on their skin. The use of disposable gloves and eye protection is recommended. Prolonged breathing of spray mists should also be avoided.

Pyrethrins

Pyrethrum flowers (chrysanthemums) have been used as insecticides for centuries, with the first powdered formulation being introduced in the United States in 1855. Before the advent of dichloro diphenyl trichlorethane (DDT), the annual importation of pyrethrins reached 18 million lb. Use dropped dramatically with the development of chlorinated hydrocarbons and organophosphates, but pyrethrins have gained in popularity. They are reported to be nontoxic to mammals as well as having little effect on the environment. Some toxicity has occurred in cats.

Pyrethrins are marketed in numerous formulations for convenient use. Most have chemicals, such as piperonyl butoxide, added to potentiate their killing power. Also, microencapsulation has significantly increased the residual activity of these compounds that were known initially for their quick "knockdown" effect.

Permethrin, a synthetic pyrethroid, is formulated and used similarly to the natural pyrethrins. Little can be found in the literature to compare the potency, toxicity, and environmental impact between the natural and synthetic agents.

Miscellaneous Agents

Several manufacturers have marketed new once-per-month flea control products. *Lufenuron* (Program, Novartis) is a benzoyl-phenyl-urea derivative classified as an insect development inhibitor. The product does not kill adult fleas but instead safely and effectively controls flea populations by breaking the life cycle at the egg stage. Preexisting flea populations may continue to develop and emerge after flea treatment, so noticeable control may not be seen for several weeks after dosing. Lufenuron is available in tablet formulation for dogs and oral liquid and injectable formulations for cats over 6 weeks of age.

Imidacloprid (Advantage, Bayer Animal Health) is a flea adulticide formulated for topical application. It is classified as a nitroguanidine and acts as an NT blocker in the insect. Imidacloprid will kill fleas within 1 day of treatment. The disadvantage with this product is that shampooing may shorten the duration of flea protection. The product is considered safe for dogs and cats over 4 months of age.

Fipronil (Frontline, Merial Ltd.) is classified as a phenylpyrazole and acts as a GABA inhibitor. It is a topical formulation for control of fleas by killing adult fleas. The manufacturer has also made product label claims for killing all stages of brown dog ticks, American dog ticks, lone star ticks, and deer ticks. After application, the animal can be handled immediately and shampooed the following day. Fipronil is safe for dogs and cats 8 weeks of age and older.

Milbemycin-lufenuron (Sentinel, Novartis) is an oral, once-per-month tablet that prevents heartworm disease and flea populations in dogs and puppies. The product also controls adult hookworms, roundworms, and whipworms. Sentinel should be administered immediately after or in conjunction with a normal meal.

Moxidectin (Cydectin, Fort Dodge Animal Health) is an endectocide of the milbemycin class used to treat infections caused by internal and external parasites in cattle.

Selamectin (Revolution, Pfizer Animal Health), a member of the avermectin class, is a once-per-month topical treatment for dogs and cats 6 weeks of age and older. Selamectin kills adult fleas and prevents flea eggs from hatching for 1 month. It is indicated for the prevention and control of flea infestations, prevention of heartworm disease, treatment and control of ear mite infestation, treatment and control of sarcoptic mange, control of tick infestation in dogs, and treatment of intestinal hookworm and roundworm infection in cats.

ANTIMICROBIAL AGENTS

Initially, *antibiotics* (antimicrobials) were defined as substances produced by microorganisms, which in low concentrations destroy or inhibit growth of other species of microorganisms. Many of these substances may be produced totally or in part through chemical synthesis. Because antibiotics have the potential to cure life-threatening infections, they are one of the most popular and useful groups of drugs in veterinary medicine.

It is important to know the characteristics and uses of the various antibiotics and have a proper understanding of the principles of antibiotic therapy *(chemotherapy)*. It is beyond the scope of this chapter to present a thorough discussion of chemotherapy; however, some basic principles are discussed. Not all microorganisms are harmful or disease producing *(pathogenic)*. Many bacteria normally found in the gastrointestinal tract, mucous membranes, and skin are helpful to their host. They compete with invading harmful pathogens and keep them from proliferating, thereby preventing progression to a disease state.

Each antibiotic is effective against specific groups of microorganisms. Some antibiotics are *bactericidal* (destroy bacteria), and some are *bacteriostatic* (inhibit growth); some may be both, depending on the concentration of the antibiotic (Box 23-1). The various species of bacteria that are affected by the antibiotic are known as the *spectrum*. *Broad-spectrum antibiotics* are those that are effective against a wide range of microorganisms.

For an antibiotic to be effective, it must be able to reach the site of infection in a sufficient concentration to exert its effect on the microorganism. In addition, the antibiotic concentration must be maintained or reached frequently over a period of time to completely destroy all bacteria or inhibit bacterial growth and provide time for the natural defense mechanisms of the body to eradicate the pathogen.

The length of antibiotic therapy may vary, depending on factors such as the site of infection, the microorganism, and the duration of infection. When antibiotics are prescribed, the treatment is usually for a minimum of 5 days. Although improvement may be seen with inadequate antibiotic therapy, it is an unwise practice. Microorganisms exposed to subtherapeutic antibiotic levels may develop

---

Box 23-1	ANTIBACTERIAL ACTION AT USUAL SERUM CONCENTRATIONS

BACTERIOSTATIC
Chloramphenicol
Tetracyclines
Erythromycin
Sulfonamides
Lincomycin

BACTERICIDAL
Pencillin
Aminoglycosides
Cephalosporins
Trimethoprim-sulfa combinations
Quinolones

resistance to that particular antibiotic, which will then be ineffective even when given at high doses. Bacteria not only can develop resistance to several antibiotics but also can pass resistance on to other species of bacteria. Multiple antibiotic-resistant bacteria are also a serious problem if resistance is developed in a hospital or clinic. *Nosocomial* (originating in hospitals) *infections* from resistant bacteria can be treated with only the most potent and expensive antibiotics. Nosocomial infections are discussed in Chapter 8.

The choice of antibiotic is obviously critical to successful therapy. The microorganism must be sensitive to the antibiotic chosen. A sample from the site of infection (blood, urine, or tissue) should be collected for culture and antibiotic sensitivity testing to determine the causative organism and the effective antibiotics (see Chapter 8). This is not always economically feasible, so a potentially effective antibiotic is frequently just chosen. Administered antibiotics that are not effective may actually worsen the disease by destroying nonpathogenic bacteria that are actively competing with the pathogen. Even when antibiotics are effective against the suspected pathogen, destruction of the nonharmful bacterial flora may allow a second pathogen to manifest and proliferate.

Ideally, it is desirable to choose an antibiotic that is effective only against the identified pathogen. Even the narrow-spectrum antibiotics are effective against a number of types of bacteria, both pathogenic and nonpathogenic. In selecting an antibiotic, one tries to choose an agent that is most likely to be effective against the pathogen and least likely to disturb normal, nonpathogenic bacteria. Indiscriminate use of broad-spectrum antibiotics eventually leads to resistant strains, ineffective antibiotic use, and expensive, perplexing therapeutic problems.

Penicillins

The discovery of penicillin in 1929 and its subsequent clinical use in 1940 represent one of the most significant advances in all of medical history. Penicillin dramatically changed the outcome of many life-threatening infections. Since its discovery, the basic penicillin molecule (Figure 23-5) has been continuously manipulated and changed to produce a number of improved penicillins with unique characteristics.

Penicillin G (benzylpenicillin), the first clinically used penicillin, is still used extensively in large animals in its procaine salt form. *Procaine penicillin G* is poorly soluble and is released slowly from its site of injection, providing adequate penicillin levels to allow once-daily dosing. However, twice-daily dosing is usually recommended. Penicillin G is effective when given orally, but high doses must be administered, because only approximately one fourth of it is absorbed from the gastrointestinal tract. Most of the antibiotic given orally is destroyed by stomach acid, so it should *not* be given directly after feeding, when stomach acid is greatest.

Penicillin acts by blocking bacterial cell wall synthesis in the final stages of replication. Without a cell wall, the bacteria swell and cannot function properly, and some *lysis* (rupturing) may occur. New infections in their high log growth phase are therefore most susceptible to penicillin. Penicillin has no direct effect on mammalian cells because they do not have cell walls.

One method of classification of bacteria is to determine their tendency to absorb dye (gentian violet) into their cell wall. Those absorbing stain are referred to as gram-positive (dark blue cell walls), and those that do not absorb the stain are known as gram-negative (light pink cell walls) (Box 23-2). Penicillin G is effective against most of the gram-positive microorganisms, including many of the streptococcal and staphylococcal species. Some staphylococcal species have the ability to produce penicillinase, an enzyme that hydrolyzes the lactam ring and thus renders the penicillin inactive. At high doses, penicillin G is effective against a few gram-negative species.

One alteration of the penicillin molecule was to make it more resistant to hydrolysis by stomach acid. Another improvement was to prepare penicillins that are resistant to the action of penicillinase. (*Clavamox* [Pfizer Animal Health] is a combination product containing amoxicillin and a specific beta-lactamase inhibitor, potassium clavulanate.) Table 23-3 provides some comparisons among various commercially available penicillins. From side-chain alterations of the molecule emerged penicillins that are effective against a wide variety of microorganisms. Some of the penicillins available for human use have a broad spectrum of activity and are the most important potent antibiotics for use against many gram-negative organisms that may be resistant to most other antibiotics. These penicillins are expensive and should be held in reserve and used when other agents are ineffective.

In general, the penicillins are safe. Allergic reactions, such as skin rashes, fever, urticaria, salivation, cutaneous edema, and other hypersensitivities, may occur and lead to justifiable concern.

Aminoglycosides

Aminoglycosides (*streptomycin, neomycin, kanamycin, amikacin, gentamicin*) have a fairly broad spectrum but are used primarily for their activity against gram-negative organ-

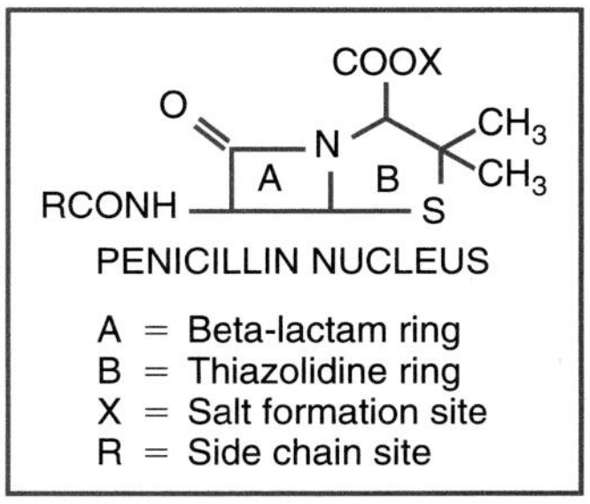

FIGURE 23-5. Penicillin nucleus.

BOX 23-2 COMMON ANIMAL PATHOGENS

GRAM-POSITIVE ORGANISMS
Streptococcus spp.
Staphylococcus spp.
Clostridium perfringens
Corynebacterium spp.

GRAM-NEGATIVE ORGANISMS
Escherichia coli
Proteus spp.
Pseudomonas spp.
Klebsiella spp.
Salmonella spp.
Brucella
Vibrio
Pasteurella spp.

TABLE 23-3	COMPARISON OF PENICILLIN PRODUCTS		
Penicillin	**Acid Stable**	**Resists Penicillinase Hydrolysis**	**Spectrum, Comments**
Penicillin G	No	No	Mostly gram-positive
Penicillin V	Yes	No	Mostly gram-positive, less effective than penicillin G against some species
Procaine penicillin G	NA*	No	Same as penicillin G
Dicloxacillin, oxacillin	Yes	Yes	Mostly gram-positive
Ampicillin, hetacillin	Yes	No	Mostly gram-positive plus *Escherichia coli, Proteus mirabilis,* and a few other gram-negative organisms
Amoxicillin	Yes	No	Spectrum similar to ampicillin, better absorbed
Carbenicillin	Yes†	No	Gram-positive plus several gram-negative, including *Pseudomonas aeruginosa* (oral form effective only in urinary tract infections)
Azlocillin, mezlocillin, piperacillin	NA	No	Broadest-spectrum penicillins effective against most gram-negative organisms, including *Klebsiella* spp.

*NA, Not applicable (no oral forms).
†Indanyl sodium salt for oral use

isms. Aminoglycosides are not adequately absorbed when administered orally, but they may be used orally for intestinal tract infections or "sterilization" of the gastrointestinal tract before surgery. Aminoglycosides exert their action by interfering with bacteria protein synthesis. Although toxicity may vary among agents, all are potentially *ototoxic* (affecting hearing balance) as well as *nephrotoxic* (renal toxicity). Neuromuscular blockage is also an adverse effect that is manifested by apnea and progressive paralysis of skeletal muscle. When aminoglycosides are administered to animals with preexisting renal damage, the patient must be closely monitored because the potential for toxicity is much greater.

Technician Note

All aminoglycosides are potentially ototoxic and nephrotoxic and cause neuromuscular blockade.

Resistance, toxicity, and expense are major considerations in the selection of these agents. Resistance demonstrated by organisms may be to a particular aminoglycoside or, commonly, to several within this class of drugs (cross resistance).

Dihydrostreptomycin, one of the first in this class to be discovered, is no longer commercially available even in the once popular combination with procaine penicillin. Most microorganisms were either resistant or readily developed a resistance to dihydrostreptomycin. Streptomycin is available as a product for humans and may be substituted as the agent of choice for some sensitive pathogens, such as *Bacteroides nodosus.*

Neomycin is nephrotoxic and therefore finds its use primarily in topical or ophthalmic preparations. Kanamycin, gentamicin, and amikacin are commercially available as veterinary products. Other aminoglycosides, although expensive products for humans, are finding use in veterinary medicine for highly resistant organisms that are not susceptible to other antibiotics.

Aminoglycosides are frequently used simultaneously with some of the newer penicillins or cephalosporins to treat stubborn gram-negative infections. Because the combinations are more effective than the use of either agent alone, the activity of the combination is called *synergism.* The use of aminoglycosides and chloramphenicol together is contraindicated because it is an *antagonistic* combination, resulting in decreased antibacterial action.

Cephalosporins

Cephalosporins *(cephalexin, cefadroxil, cephradine, cephapirin, ceftiofur)* are somewhat chemically similar (Figure 23-6) to the penicillins and share a similar mechanism of action and spectrum. Although some resistance exists to the cephalosporins, they are not destroyed by penicillinase-producing bacteria.

The cephalosporins are subclassified primarily by spectrum into first, second, and third generations. Only minor differences exist in the spectrum of the first generation; all are effective against most gram-positive bacteria and several gram-negative species. The second generation has a somewhat broader spectrum, displaying activity against most clostridial species. Although *Pseudomonas aeruginosa* is not susceptible to the first- or second-generation cephalosporins, it may be treated with the third-generation cephalosporins. Severe infections, such as *Pseudomonas* infection, are usually treated with a combination of antibiotics to ensure eradication and limit the possibility of developing resistance.

The cost of the cephalosporins limits their use in veterinary medicine. Even with the availability of veterinary cephalosporin and generic products for humans, cost remains a major concern when considering second- and third-generation cephalosporins. *Ceftiofur* (Naxcel, Pharmacia and Upjohn) is approved for use in cattle, horses, swine, dogs, and chickens. Ceftiofur under the trade name Excenel (Pharmacia and Upjohn) is approved for use in cattle only.

The cephalosporins have a low incidence of adverse effects. Long-term use of excessively large doses may lead to some complications similar to those of other antibiotics, including possible allergic reactions or overgrowth of nonsusceptible bacteria or fungi, leading to intestinal pain, bloating, and diarrhea.

FIGURE 23-6.   Cephalosporin nucleus.

Quinolones

Quinolones constitute a class of antibiotics finding extensive use in veterinary medicine for treatment of a wide variety of organisms, including *P. aeruginosa*. *Enrofloxacin* (Baytril, Bayer) is approved primarily for urinary, skin, and respiratory infections in dogs and cats, but it is also being used to treat bone and other infections in several additional species. It is a subcutaneous injection approved for cattle not intended for food to treat bovine respiratory disease (BRD) associated with *Pasteurella haemolytica*, *Pasteurella multocida*, and *Haemophilus somnus*.

Enrofloxacin seems to be well tolerated, and few side effects have been noted in animals. It is contraindicated in puppies during the rapid growth phase because it can induce abnormal cartilage formation, leading to weakness or lameness. This potential adverse effect discourages the use of enrofloxacin in other young animals as well as in adult horses. Although bacterial resistance to enrofloxacin is not yet common, indiscriminate use to treat routine infections is likely to produce resistant strains, making this very valuable drug worthless.

> **Technician Note**
>
> Quinolones should not be used in animals during rapid growth phases because they can induce abnormal cartilage formation, leading to weakness or lameness.

Second-generation quinolones encourage better compliance because of the once to twice daily dosing regimen recommended.

Chloramphenicol

Chloramphenicol use in humans is limited to a few specific infections because of a rare but potentially fatal occurrence of irreversible aplastic anemia. Even personnel who handle and administer chloramphenicol to animals should use care, avoiding direct contact with the drug. Although some blood dyscrasias have been seen in animals, particularly in neonates, the condition is usually reversible by withdrawal of the drug.

Chloramphenicol has been a popular, important antibiotic in veterinary medicine. To some extent, newer, safer, and more effective antibiotics have replaced it. Although chloramphenicol is bacteriostatic, it has a fairly broad spectrum of activity. It is rapidly distributed to most body compartments and tissues in adequate therapeutic concentrations. A small amount of chloramphenicol is excreted unchanged in the urine, but most undergoes biotransformation in the liver to the inactive glucuronide conjugate.

> **Technician Note**
>
> Chloramphenicol may cause blood dyscrasias. Personnel who handle and administer the drug should avoid direct contact.

Adverse effects include blood dyscrasias (as previously mentioned), anorexia, diarrhea, vomiting, and depression, as well as other rare but somewhat severe effects. Chloramphenicol in combination with other antibiotics is usually contraindicated. In addition, chloramphenicol interacts with several specific drugs or groups of drugs, including anticonvulsants, penicillins, phenylbutazone, and lincomycin.

Tetracyclines

Oxytetracycline and *tetracycline* are used practically interchangeably because of a similarity in spectrum and pharmacologic properties. One tetracycline available for human use, *doxycycline*, has gained acceptance for use in small animals. It requires less frequent dosing and penetrates the central nervous system better than other tetracyclines.

These bacteriostatic agents affect the vital protein synthesis of the microorganism. Although the tetracyclines possess a relatively broad spectrum of activity, the development of resistant organisms has been a factor limiting their use. Through more judicious use of these agents, less-resistant strains are being encountered.

The absorption of tetracyclines from the gastrointestinal tract is adequate but is decreased in the presence of food, milk, or antacids. Some injectable preparations use propylene glycol as a solvent and are not recommended for intramuscular use because they are painful. When given intravenously, the tetracycline must be injected slowly because the solvent and drug may exert a blocking effect on the heart, causing the animal to temporarily collapse. Other injectable preparations contain povidone or similar agents, which reduce intramuscular irritation and eliminate the cardiac problem. The intramuscular product formulated for extended action must not be given intravenously.

> **Technician Note**
>
> Tetracyclines form complexes with calcium in developing bones and teeth and should not be given to young animals. The absorption of tetracyclines is decreased in the presence of milk, food, and antacids. Out-of-date or improperly stored tetracyclines should never be administered because they form nephrotoxic products.

Tetracyclines are relatively inexpensive and widely used, especially in food animals. The tetracyclines are also commonly used at low levels as a livestock feed additive to increase weight gain and decrease liver abscesses. This practice promotes the development of resistant strains of bacteria, rendering the tetracycline useless for treatment even when given at therapeutic levels.

Although popular, the tetracyclines have toxicities. A common toxicity is the intestinal problems associated with disruption of the natural intestinal flora, including the possibility of superinfection by resistant organisms. Hypersensitivity reactions of rashes, fever, and liver damage may also occur with use of tetracyclines. The tetracyclines form complexes with calcium in developing bones and teeth; they should not be given to pregnant or young animals because tooth discoloration, increases in dental caries, and temporary suppression in bone growth may occur.

Although outdated products are never recommended, outdated or improperly stored tetracycline should never be used because the degradation products are actually toxic to the kidneys.

Miscellaneous Antibiotics

Erythromycin and *tylosin* are classified as macrolide antibiotics because of their high molecular weight. Their spectrum of activity is similar to that of penicillin; therefore they are commonly used instead of penicillin against penicillinase-producing microbes. Erythromycin does not alter intestinal flora extensively, but gastrointestinal effects such as vomiting and diarrhea have been observed.

Technician Note

Tilmicosin should be administered only by subcutaneous or intramuscular routes.

Tilmicosin is a macrolide used to treat bovine respiratory diseases, including those caused by *Mycoplasma*. A distinct advantage of tilmicosin is its long half-life, which allows a single-dose treatment. Tilmicosin must be administered only by subcutaneous or intramuscular routes because intravenously dosing has been fatal. Deaths have been reported after the use of tilmicosin in swine, horses, and nonhuman primates. The drug must be handled with extreme caution and administered in accordance with the detailed label instructions.

Lincomycin has a spectrum of activity similar to erythromycin and is particularly effective against *Staphylococcus* and *Streptococcus* spp. It has been useful when resistant strains or hypersensitivities to other antibiotics exist. Favorable results have been reported in the treatment of bone infections and various skin disorders (pyoderma) with lincomycin. The drug is concentrated and excreted in the bile. Lincomycin causes severe intestinal flora disturbances in horses, hamsters, and rabbits, so it should be avoided in these species.

Azithromycin is a long-acting macrolide administered orally that is used to treat *Chlamydia* infections of the eye.

Other Antimicrobial Agents

In addition to the antibiotics discussed, other chemical agents exist that are effective against certain strains of microorganisms. The *sulfa* drugs were the first antimicrobial agents to be used systemically in the treatment of bacterial infections.

Sulfonamides

Numerous sulfonamides *(sulfamethazine, sulfadiazine, sulfadimethoxine)* have been formulated, and many have been used clinically since their initial clinical use in 1932. Although their value and use have declined with the discovery of newer antibiotics, a few sulfonamides remain useful for certain conditions. These agents are relatively inexpensive, which makes them attractive for use in large animals for herd or flock treatment. The sulfonamides are particularly useful in the treatment of various infections of the respiratory system and urinary tract, bacterial diarrhea, foot rot, and coccidial infections. Unfortunately, bacterial resistance to the sulfonamides limits their effectiveness. A toxicity seen with the original sulfonamides was crystalluria, a condition in which the sulfa drug formed insoluble crystals in the urine, causing renal damage. Because the solubility of one sulfonamide is independent of other sulfonamides, the formulation of *triple sulfa* was developed to avert crystalluria. More soluble sulfonamides are also available, thereby further reducing concern. It is important that animals receiving sulfonamide have adequate water available.

The intravenous preparations of sulfonamides have a high (basic) pH and are therefore damaging to tissue when inadvertently given perivascularly. In addition, the intravenous preparations should be given slowly to avoid acute toxicity demonstrated by central nervous system effects, such as salivation, vomiting, diarrhea, weakness, ataxia, and convulsions.

Trimethoprim-Sulfonamide Combinations

A popular, effective antibacterial that is being used in veterinary medicine today is a combination product of one part *trimethoprim* and five parts *sulfadiazine* or *sulfamethoxazole. Ormetoprim with sulfadimethoxine* is a comparable combination with similar use and actions. These combinations block two essential sequential steps in the replication process of the bacteria, resulting in a synergistic antibacterial action. The combinations are effective against a wide range of organisms but not *Pseudomonas*.

Undesirable side effects seen with these combinations are infrequent. Although vomiting may occur, diarrhea is seldom seen. Animals that are deficient in folic acid may be prone to develop blood disorders, as has been reported in humans.

Nitrofurans

The nitrofurans *(nitrofurazone, nitrofurantoin, furazolidone)* have been replaced, to a great extent, by newer, more effective, and safer antibacterials. These synthetic agents have a fairly broad spectrum of activity, but they are not effective against *Pseudomonas*.

Although nitrofurazone and furazolidone are not absorbed from the gastrointestinal tract, they were once widely used orally in food animals to treat intestinal bacterial disorders. Except for topical application, their use in food animals is now strictly forbidden by the FDA because of their potential carcinogenicity.

Nitrofurantoin is sufficiently absorbed to have some use in small animals in the treatment of urinary tract infections. Nausea and vomiting, which are common adverse effects, can be reduced by administering nitrofurantoin with food or using the macrocrystal human preparations.

Antifungal Agents

Numerous agents are available to treat fungal infections of the skin *(dermatomycosis). Griseofulvin* is an antibiotic that is administered orally; it has no antibacterial activity but inhibits the growth of various skin fungi. It is an expensive product and is not usually the first-line choice unless the infection is widespread. Common topical agents found in creams, lotions, sprays, and other forms include miconazole, tolnaftate, undecylenic acid, iodine compound, nystatin, various dyes, and *phenolic compounds*.

The treatment of systemic fungal infections (e.g., cryptococcosis, blastomycosis, histoplasmosis) is usually expensive, requiring lengthy treatment with limited success. *Amphotericin B,* an antibiotic used for various fungal infections, is toxic, causing kidney and liver damage, central nervous system abnormalities, and so on. A newer formulation of amphotericin B in a lipid complex suspension (Abelcet, Liposome, Inc.) eliminates some toxic effects experienced with the original solution. *Nystatin*, another antibiotic, is relatively nontoxic but has a narrow spectrum of activity. *Ketoconazole*, an expensive antifungal agent, has proven to be effective against a variety of fungal infections. Ketoconazole causes *hepatotoxicity* (liver damage), so liver enzymes should be monitored during therapy. *Itraconazole* is a newer agent that is efficacious against a variety of fungal infections. It is less hepatotoxic than ketoconazole and more expensive.

Technician Note

Amphotericin B causes liver and kidney damage and central nervous system abnormalities.

HORMONES AND SYNTHETIC SUBSTITUTES

Hormones are substances that are produced and secreted by glands and carried by the blood, producing an effect on a target organ. A number of hormones are secreted by several different glands. This discussion is limited to the most clinically significant.

Thyroid Preparations

The thyroid gland is controlled primarily by the amount of *thyroid-stimulating hormone* released from the pituitary gland. When stimulated, the thyroid gland releases thyroid hormones consisting primarily of *thyroxin*. Because the thyroid hormones affect the metabolism of carbohydrates, protein, and fats, thyroid-deficient (hypothyroid) animals show signs of lethargy, reduced alertness, increased body weight, poor hair coat, and other related signs. Insufficient amounts of iodine in the diet can result in inadequate production of thyroid hormones. Such hormone deficiencies can be treated with desiccated thyroid because it is effective orally. *Sodium levothyroxine* (Synthroid, Knoll Pharmaceutical; Soloxine, Daniels Pharmaceuticals) may be the most popular agent for the treatment of hypothyroidism. *Sodium liothyronine* (Cytomel, SmithKline Beecham), the other active component of desiccated thyroid, is also available commercially.

Feline hyperthyroidism is treated with *methimazole* (Tapazole, JP Jones). It interferes with iodine incorporation into tyrosyl residues of thyroglobulin, thereby inhibiting the synthesis of thyroid hormones.

Insulin

Insulin is normally produced and released by islet cells of the pancreas. This hormone is necessary to facilitate the use of food by the body, especially sugar. Insulin enhances the absorption of glucose in most cells of the body. Animals with inadequate insulin will have abnormally high blood glucose levels (hyperglycemia) and other associated metabolic disorders. Insulin injection (regular Iletin) is a solution of dissolved insulin crystals, which accounts for its immediate action and short duration. There are other insulin preparations that are intermediate acting (approximately 24 hours) to long acting (approximately 36 hours). Isophane insulin suspension (NPH), an intermediate-acting insulin, tends to be the most widely used in small animal medicine.

With the emergence of recombinant products (e.g., Humulin, Lilly), it may be difficult to obtain insulin of animal origin. Animals that were originally administered insulin from animal sources may need to have dose adjustments if switched to recombinant products. Any change in insulin should be made cautiously and under the medical supervision of the veterinarian.

Overdoses of insulin produce hypoglycemia, which if severe can lead to coma and death. Treatment of hypoglycemia consists of administration of intravenous dextrose.

Oxytocin

Oxytocin is a hormone released at the end of pregnancy to stimulate uterine contractions during parturition and induce milk letdown. The synthetically produced oxytocin is beneficial during delayed parturition or for aiding milk letdown.

Prostaglandins

Although *prostaglandins* (PGs) were discovered in 1935, it has only been since the 1980s that these substances have been extensively studied and developed. PGs are found in many mammalian tissues and have been shown to have a wide variety of effects on a number of body systems, including the central nervous, cardiovascular, urinary, gastrointestinal, and reproductive systems. Commercially available PGs, such as *dinoprost* and *cloprostenol*, are used because of their effects on the reproductive system.

In cattle, PGs can be used to regulate the heat cycle so breeding and consequent calving times for a herd can be planned. PGs are also approved by the FDA to abort feedlot heifers. For certain conditions in mares, PGs can effectively restore the normal heat cycle so the animals can be bred.

Because these agents are abortifacients, they should not be handled by pregnant women. Bronchospasm is another serious adverse effect in animals and humans that may occur as a result of contact with the product. Consequently, PGs should not be handled by people with asthma or used on animals with respiratory diseases.

GASTROINTESTINAL DRUGS

Antiemetics

Certain species, such as horses, rabbits, and rodents, are unable to vomit, but protracted vomiting may become a problem in dogs, cats, and other species.

The vomiting reflex may be stimulated through at least four different pathways. For example, chemical substances in the blood (bacterial toxins or certain drugs) may mediate vomiting via the chemoreceptor trigger zone (CTZ) pathway (medulla of brain). Vomiting arising from movement of the head (motion sickness) is transmitted through another pathway (cortex of the brain). In selecting an antiemetic agent, it is desirable to know the underlying cause of vomiting and the pathway involved because some antiemetic drugs are specific in their site of action. Vomiting may be a symptom of a disease state, so initial attention should be directed to treatment of the primary disease.

Although independent of their antihistaminic activity, a few of the antihistamines (e.g., *dimenhydrinate, cyclizine, meclizine*) and *scopolamine* are effective in preventing vomiting induced by motion sickness. The principal side effect of antihistamines is drowsiness, which may be desirable in pets that are traveling.

A number of phenothiazine tranquilizers (e.g., *chlorpromazine, prochlorperazine, triflupromazine*) are classified as broad-spectrum antiemetics that control vomiting by blocking the CTZ at low doses and at the emetic center (in the medulla of the brain) at higher doses. Although these agents have the potential of producing a number of adverse effects, the risk of toxicity is low because of the low dose and short duration of therapy. Some potent broad-spectrum, human antiemetics (e.g., *haloperidol, metoclopramide*) are finding use in veterinary medicine.

Metoclopramide is a unique pharmacologic agent. Besides its potent antiemetic property, especially in drug-induced emesis (e.g., cancer chemotherapy), metoclopramide is a peristaltic stimulant that increases gut motility. It has been used for gastric stasis in a number of species, including horses and cattle. In addition, to facilitate radiologic examination of stomach or small intestine, metoclopramide may be used to stimulate gastric emptying and intestinal transit of barium in cases where delayed emptying interferes. Reflux esophagitis in dogs and cats has been treated with metoclopramide.

Cisapride (Propulsid, Janssen) is not classified as an emetic; however, its use is increasing as an equine gastrointestinal prokinetic agent (increases motility) in reflux conditions.

Emetics

Agents to induce vomiting are used clinically as a rapid means of eliminating certain poisons or to remove food from the stomach before induction of general anesthesia. A once common emetic used in veterinary medicine is *apomorphine*. Although still commercially available, it is extremely expensive and difficult to obtain. Apomorphine stimulates the CTZ and may be administered orally, intramuscularly, intravenously, or via the conjunctival sac of the eye. Because apomorphine depresses the emetic center, repeated dosing is not recommended when the initial dose is ineffective. Apomorphine should not be given to cats because it produces extreme excitement. *Xylazine*, a sedative analgesic, can be used as an emetic because of the routine vomiting it produces in the cat.

Ipecac, once used commonly in cats and occasionally in dogs, has the disadvantage of having to be administered via stomach tube because of taste. In addition, its effects may be somewhat sporadic. Some toxic effects, including death, may be induced with ipecac in cats. However, ipecac syrup remains a popular, convenient emetic for children for the removal of accidentally ingested noncorrosive poison.

Antidiarrheal Agents

Diarrhea, like vomiting, may be only a symptom of an underlying problem. Ideally, it is best to identify the specific problem and correct it. Current trends are not to slow the gut but to allow it to remain active to remove any present toxins or irritants. Most small animals with diarrhea recover regardless of therapy. Persistent diarrhea not only may be offensive to pet owners but also may require supportive treatment, such as electrolyte and fluid replacement. Anticholinergics, such as the various belladonna alkaloids (*atropine, homatropine, scopolamine*), have historically been used to treat diarrhea. Although *peristalsis* (propulsive intestinal contractions) is reduced, a minimal antidiarrheal effect results. The value of anticholinergic use is questionable because they have adverse effects, such as increased heart rate, dryness of mouth, and diarrhea from gut paralysis.

Technician Note

Atropine should never be used in horses except as an antidote to life-threatening organophosphate poisoning.

Opiates, including opium tincture, morphine, codeine, and similar derivatives, such as diphenoxylate, are unique in that they increase rhythmic segmentation contraction, which resists intestinal flow and decreases peristalsis. In addition, the opiates increase the tone of various sphincters and valves in the gastrointestinal tract, which further delays movement of the contents. The commercial product *diphenoxylate* (Lomotil, Searle), which is available with only a small amount of atropine, is effective in treating diarrhea in dogs.

The use of antidiarrheal opiates in cats is controversial because this species may react with excitatory behavior. Opiate antidiarrheals should be used with caution in patients with head injuries or increased intracranial pressures and acute abdominal conditions, such as colic, because the opiates may obscure diagnosis or clinical course of the condition. Opiate antidiarrheals should be used with extreme caution in patients with hepatic disease and central nervous system symptoms of hepatic encephalopathy because hepatic coma may result.

The use of opiates in animals with acute diarrhea that may be bacterially induced may enhance bacterial proliferation, delay the disappearance of the microbe from the feces, and prolong the febrile state. Acute overdoses of the opiate antidiarrheals could result in central nervous, cardiovascular, or respiratory system toxicity.

An over-the-counter combination suspension of *kaolin* and *pectin* is widely used in human medicine. Kaolin is thought to act as an adsorbent, binding toxins and bacteria and rendering them somewhat harmless. It also serves as a protectant because it coats the gastrointestinal tract. Pectin may also have some adsorbent and protectant properties. The kaolin-pectin mixtures are difficult to administer to animals because of poor palatability and the volume required per dose. Even though tablets are available, the number of tablets required to be effective makes treatment of large dogs expensive and cumbersome. Kaolin-pectin mixtures have been used to treat diarrhea in horses with varying results.

Another over-the-counter preparation that is extensively used in veterinary medicine is the human product *loperamide*. Loperamide is a synthetic piperidine derivative that slows intestinal motility through a direct effect on the nerve endings and/or intramural ganglia of the intestinal wall. In animals, loperamide does not have analgesic activity, even in extremely high doses. Loperamide is available in tablet, capsule, and oral liquid formulations.

Bismuth subsalicylate is thought to have weak antibacterial properties as well as being a protectant and antiendotoxin. Popular thought suggests the compound is cleaved in the small intestine into bismuth carbonate and salicylate. The bismuth carbonate is responsible for the protective, antiendotoxic, and weak antibacterial properties. The salicylate component has antiprostaglandin activity, which may contribute to its effectiveness and reduce symptoms associated with secretory diarrhea. In humans, the preparation is used for other gastrointestinal symptoms (e.g., indigestion, cramps, gas pain) and in the treatment and prophylaxis of traveler's diarrhea.

Cathartics (Laxatives)

There are relatively few clinical reasons to use cathartics in veterinary medicine. Occasionally, an older animal may have constipation, but usually alteration of the diet will correct the problem. Another indication might be for the treatment of hairballs in cats. After bowel or anal surgery, stool softeners may reduce stress at the surgery site until healing takes place. Cathartics as well as enemas may also be used before gastrointestinal tract radiographic examinations, proctoscopy, or elective surgery. One of the most legitimate uses of cathartics is in treating food animals and horses with overingestion of concentrated carbohydrates, such as grain. There are a few other unique circumstances in which the use of cathartics is appropriate; however, one is discouraged from overuse because it leads to dependence.

Cathartics increase the motility of the bowel by directly stimulating the smooth muscle or indirectly activating receptors through increased bulk. The irritant laxatives, which directly increase bowel motility, include *emodin*, found in cascara sagrada, aloe, and senna; *sodium ricinoleate*, a digestive end product of castor oil; and *danthron*, a synthetic compound. Bulk-producing cathartics include the following:

- Indigestible materials, such as psyllium seed (Metamucil, Searle), methyl cellulose, mineral oil, and white petrolatum, which not only increase bulk but also lubricate and soften the fecal mass
- Saline cathartics, such as magnesium sulfate, sodium sulfate, magnesium oxide, and phosphate salts, which draw water into the bowel
- Stool softeners, such as docusate sodium and dioctyl calcium sulfosuccinate (Surfak, Hoechst), which are surface-active agents like soap that increase bulk through water retention and lubricate and soften the fecal mass

The cathartics as a group are relatively safe for short-term use, although some may be harsh and cause cramping and diarrhea. Chronic use of the petrolatum-type cathartics may lead to deficiencies in fat-soluble vitamins because of absorption interference.

Ulcer Management Drugs

Gastric ulceration and subsequent blood loss appear to be related to acid damage commonly associated with high doses of corticosteroids or drugs NSAIDs as well as with certain medical disorders. Several methods are available for treatment and prevention.

Antacids were initially used, but they required round-the-clock administration every 2 to 3 hours to truly be effective. A major advancement in human medicine for ulcer management was the introduction of cimetidine, which is a histamine$_2$ receptor antagonist. Although these agents are not approved for veterinary use, cimetidine, ranitidine, and others are being used to block the acid-producing effects of histamine on the gastric parietal cells.

Sucralfate in an acid environment forms an ulcer-adherent complex providing a protective, BandAid-like barrier for the damaged mucosa. Sucralfate also inhibits pepsin activity.

Omeprazole is an agent that acts directly on the parietal cell, blocking acid secretion. It comes in an oral gel (Gastrogard, Merial Ltd.) and is oral indicated for treatment and prevention of recurrence of gastric ulcers in horses and foals 4 weeks of age and older. *Misoprostol* not only blocks gastric acid secretion but also appears to enhance natural gastromucosal defense mechanisms.

CALCULATIONS

The first step in solving any calculation problem is to express all quantities in the same system of units. If *strengths* (concentrations) of solution are given in percentages, they must be converted to grams per 100 ml.

Calculating the Strength of a Drug Solution

The following basic equation is used to calculate the concentration of a liquid dosage form:

$$\text{Concentration (g/ml)} = \text{Mass (g)} \div \text{Volume (ml)}$$

If you know any two of these quantities, the third can be found.

Example 1: What is the strength of a 1-L solution containing 50 g of drug?
You know:
1. Volume of solution (1 L = 1000 ml)
2. Mass of drug (50 g)

Solution:
Substitute all known quantities in the equation. Solve for the unknown:

$$\text{Concentration (g/ml)} = 50 \text{ g} \div 1000 \text{ ml} = 5 \text{ g} \div 100 \text{ ml}$$
$$\times \ 100\% = 5\% \text{ solution}$$

Manipulation of this equation is frequently used to find the quantity (mass) of a given volume of drug solution at a known concentration:

$$\text{Mass (g)} = \text{Volume (ml)} \times \text{Concentration (g/ml)}$$

Example 2: How much drug is needed to prepare 4 oz of a 2% solution?
You know:
1. Volume of solution (4 oz = 120 ml)
2. Concentration of solution (2% = 2 g/100 ml)

Solution:
Substitute all known quantities in the equation. Solve for the unknown:

$$\text{Mass (g)} = 120 \text{ ml} \times 2 \text{ g/100 ml} = 2.4 \text{ g}$$

The original equation is also used to find out the total volume of drug solution that can be prepared at a desired concentration with a given quantity of drug:

$$\text{Volume (ml)} = \text{Mass (g)} \div \text{Concentration (g/ml)}$$

Example 3: How much of a 10% solution can be prepared with 15 g of drug?
You know:
1. Concentration of desired solution (10% = 10 g/100 ml)
2. Mass of drug (15 g)

Solution:
Substitute all known quantities in the equation. Solve for the unknown:

$$\text{Volume (ml)} = 15 \text{ g} \div 10 \text{ g/100 ml} = 150 \text{ ml}$$

Calculating the Strength of Diluted Solutions

A basic equation can be used to solve problems for dilution stock (concentrated) solutions. (A more concentrated [stronger] solution can never be made from a diluted [weaker] solution without adding pure drug.)

$$\text{Concentration of desired solution} \times \text{Volume of desired}$$
$$\text{solution} = \text{Concentration of stock} \times \text{Volume of stock}$$

Knowing any three of these quantities, one can solve for the unknown.

Example 1: Prepare 2 qt of a 1:1000 solution from a 20% solution.
You know:
1. Concentration of desired solution (1:1000 = 1 g/1000 ml)

2. Volume of desired solution (2 qt = approximately 2000 ml)
3. Concentration of stock (20% = 20 g/100 ml)

Solution:
Substitute all known quantities in the equation. Solve for the unknown:

Volume of stock solution (ml) = 1 g/1000 ml × 2000 ml ÷ 20 g/100 ml = 10 ml

Example 2: How much of a 1% solution can be prepared from 6 ml of a 5% solution?
You know:
1. Concentration of desired solution (1% = 1 g/100 ml)
2. Volume of stock (6 ml)
3. Concentration of stock (5% = 5 g/100 ml)

Solution:
Substitute all known quantities in the equation. Solve for the unknown:

Volume of desired solution (ml) = 5 g/100 ml × 6 ml ÷ 1 g/100 ml = 30 ml

Calculating Drug Dosages

A drug dosage is expressed as units or mass of drug per body weight (BW) of the patient. The usual dosage for human drugs is based on the ideal BW of 140 lb (70 kg). There is no ideal BW in veterinary medicine because of the variety of species and breeds of animals. The usual drug dose for animals is based on BW expressed in pounds or kilograms.

The following equation is used for calculating the quantity of drug to be administered based on BW:

BW × Dosage ÷ Concentration of drug = Volume of drug (dose)

Example 1: An 88-lb dog is to receive a drug dosage of 25 mg/kg of BW. How many milliliters of the supplied drug at 50 mg/ml are required?
You know:
1. Drug dosage (25 mg/kg of BW)
2. Animal's body weight (88 lb = 40 kg)
3. Concentration of drug solution (50 mg/ml)

Solution:
Substitute all known quantities in the equation. Solve for the unknown:

Volume of drug = 40 kg × 25 mg/kg ÷ 50 mg/ml = 20 ml (dose)

The dosage of highly toxic drugs such as *antineoplastic* (anticancer) agents is calculated on the basis of body surface area (BSA). BSAs are difficult to calculate. Nomograms and charts (Table 23-4) have been constructed to help relate BW to BSA. BSA is expressed in *square meters.*

To determine dosage based on BSA, modification of the previous equation will enable this:

BSA (m²) × Drug dosage ÷ Concentration of drug = Volume of drug

Example 2: A 44-lb dog is to receive a dosage of 0.2 mg/m². What volume of a drug should be given at a concentration of 1 mg/ml?
You know:
1. BSA (44 lb = 20 kg = 0.74 m²)
2. Drug dosage (0.2 mg/m²)
3. Concentration of drug solution (1 mg/ml)

Table 23-4	Conversion Tables for Weight (kg) to Body Surface Area (m²)				
Dogs				**Cats**	
kg	m²	kg	m²	kg	m²
0.5	0.06	33	1.03	2.0	0.159
1	0.10	34	1.05	2.5	0.184
2	0.15	35	1.07	3.0	0.208
3	0.20	36	1.09	3.5	0.231
4	0.25	37	1.11	4.0	0.252
5	0.29	38	1.13	4.5	0.273
6	0.33	39	1.15	5.0	0.292
7	0.36	40	1.17	5.5	0.311
8	0.40	41	1.19	6.0	0.330
9	0.43	42	1.21	6.5	0.348
10	0.46	43	1.23	7.0	0.366
11	0.49	44	1.25	7.5	0.383
12	0.52	45	1.26	8.0	0.400
13	0.55	46	1.28	8.5	0.416
14	0.58	47	1.30	9.0	0.432
15	0.60	48	1.32	9.5	0.449
16	0.63	49	1.34	10	0.464
17	0.66	50	1.36		
18	0.69	52	1.41		
19	0.71	54	1.44		
20	0.74	56	1.48		
21	0.76	58	1.51		
22	0.78	60	1.55		
23	0.81	62	1.58		
24	0.83	64	1.62		
25	0.85	66	1.65		
26	0.88	68	1.68		
27	0.90	70	1.72		
28	0.92	72	1.75		
29	0.94	74	1.78		
30	0.96	76	1.81		
31	0.99	78	1.84		
32	1.01	80	1.88		

Solution:
Substitute all known quantities in the equation. Solve for the unknown:

Volume of drug solution = 0.74 m² × 0.2 mg/m² ÷ 1 mg/ml = 0.148 ml

Calculating Infusion Rates

Many drugs must be administered intravenously by slow infusion rather than as a rapid bolus injection. Large volumes of fluids are also given by intravenous infusion. Disposable intravenous sets and infusion pumps are used to deliver intravenous fluids at a steady rate over a period of time.

Calculations of infusion rates can be found by using the following equation:

Rate (drops/min) = drops/ml calibrated ÷ 60 min/hr × Total volume to be administered ÷ Total hr of infusion

Example 1: If 500 ml of a solution is to be infused over 6 hours, what is the correct infusion rate if the set delivers 10 drops/ml?
You know:
1. Drops/min calibration of intravenous set (10 drops/ml)

2.   Volume to be infused (500 ml)
3.   Infusion time (6 hours)

Solution:

Substitute all known quantities in the equation. Solve for the unknown:

$$\text{Rate (drops/min)} = 10 \text{ drops/ml} \div 60 \text{ min/hr} \times 500 \text{ ml} \div 6 \text{ hr} = 13.89 \text{ drops/min}$$

INVENTORY CONTROL

The maintenance of an active working inventory requires both planning and continuous monitoring. Failure to keep abreast of use and needs results in shortage, inefficient use of time, increased costs, and added stress. The time invested to sustain appropriate levels of stock is therefore beneficial to the overall operations of the practice.

Veterinary technicians who demonstrate interest in an active inventory may find themselves acquiring an increasing role in inventory control and maintenance. Assuming this additional responsibility not only increases employee value in the practice but also adds to job satisfaction.

Ideally, the quantities of each item stocked should be as small as possible without running out between reasonable ordering periods. Because it is worse to have a shortage of certain items than to have extra, most practices lean toward a higher inventory than actually required. Inventory turnover (the number of times per year an item is bought and sold) should be at least four to six times per year. Some items, such as pet food, may turn over 12 to 14 times per year. With the assistance of a computer, monitoring of daily usage, and keeping helpful records, the average turnover rate can usually be increased. The higher the turnover, the lower the investment in the item. Ordering of drugs can become a full-time duty if care is not given to organization and planning.

Inventory Maintenance

The primary disadvantage of having a large inventory is the expense of having working capital tied up in drugs and supplies. A large inventory makes switching to equivalent products difficult, even at a cheaper price. There is great potential for product outdates, breakage, spoilage, and obsolescence when the inventory is large. Some states have an inventory tax that provides added incentive for keeping working stock to a minimum.

Occasionally, there is some justification for increasing the purchase of certain products. The "savings" claimed through many of the deals offered by vendors should be approached with caution. Unless one can accurately predict the use of certain products, quantity buying is difficult to justify. To participate in most marketing promotions, a significant financial commitment is usually required. Before entering into these agreements, one should truly determine whether the products offered are desirable and will be used within a reasonable period and whether the savings really merit the capital commitment.

Processing small orders is costly because the time commitment required to process the order is not much different than that of a larger order with several items. One is justified in increasing quantities on these small orders, especially if the items are inexpensive, to reduce ordering frequency and cost of acquisition. Some vendors charge handling fees if the total order is below a minimal required dollar amount or volume.

Availability of replacement goods is a factor that will affect the inventory turnover. With some items, one may be able to accurately predict monthly use and maintain a few weeks' supply. Unfortunately, the use of most items cannot be readily anticipated, which results in larger inventory requirement, especially if delivery time cannot be predicted.

Procurement

Veterinary Suppliers

One may purchase supplies through veterinary wholesale suppliers (distributors) or directly from manufacturers. Distributors may specialize in one class of items, such as surgical supplies or bulk pharmaceuticals. Some wholesale suppliers may offer a complete line of products, ranging from buckets to gas machines.

One advantage in dealing with wholesalers is the ability to reduce the number of small orders that would be required in purchasing from several individual vendors. A few manufacturers only sell their products directly to veterinarians rather than distributors. *The Veterinary Pharmaceuticals and Biologicals* and the *Compendium of Veterinary Products* (see Recommended Reading) offer a fairly complete reference to veterinary pharmaceutical companies and their product lines.

Veterinary Clinics

It is an excellent idea to establish and maintain a good working relationship with another clinic in the area. In a crisis situation, you can borrow items from that clinic to see you through the emergency. Borrowing seldom-used items in an emergency is encouraged rather than stocking them. However, your practice is expected to order the item and return it. Thus inventory of seldom-used items is maintained elsewhere and record keeping is not necessary. Purchasing some items from another practice may be helpful, especially for expensive, short-dated items.

Several large buying groups have been established by some practices to increase their purchasing power and decrease costs.

Pharmacies and Drug Wholesalers

Using the services of a retail pharmacy is nearly essential to the practice of quality veterinary medicine. Veterinarians have need for various human products that are not obtainable through veterinary suppliers. Retail pharmacies may not stock many injectable products, but they can help with most ophthalmic and oral products and some topical preparations. In some locations, a human drug wholesaler may deal directly with the small, individual practitioner. Most, however, do not welcome these small accounts and will serve only as a distributor for hospitals and pharmacies. The veterinary practitioner must make arrangements with pharmacists to obtain human products for clinic or client use. Most pharmacists welcome this opportunity to serve the veterinarian.

Human Hospitals and Hospital Suppliers

A local human hospital may be a valuable resource for the veterinary clinic. Federal laws restrict hospitals with special buying privileges from selling to anyone outside their institution. As a result, it may be difficult for veterinarians and their clients to obtain some of the more potent, expensive, or rarely used medical supplies, except in an emergency. Human hospital contacts should be made to determine the local availability of drugs and supplies. The hospital's library and clinical laboratory may also provide some welcome assistance.

Local hospital suppliers will stock items such as syringes, needles, cotton balls, tongue depressors, and other disposable supplies. Although veterinarians do not routinely purchase from the local supplier, do not overlook them as an immediate source in times of shortages.

Other Sources of Suppliers

In addition to bulk chemicals, major chemical suppliers will stock glassware, balances, disposable beakers, brushes, carboys, and other laboratory and clinic supplies and equipment that would be useful in a veterinary practice. Most of these suppliers are located in metropolitan areas and have addresses and telephone numbers listed in the telephone directory.

Numerous mail order suppliers exist that provide not only pharmaceuticals but also a wide variety of veterinary products and equipment. The quality of products and service may vary greatly among these outlets. Of major concern are return policies for handling inferior or unacceptable items.

Feed stores and lay veterinary drug outlets can be used for an occasional urgently needed item. One may at times also want to take advantage of certain specials offered through these suppliers.

ORGANIZING THE PHARMACY

Whether planning a major hospital complex or rearranging a small portion of one hospital, a comprehensive list should be prepared of all activities conducted in the pharmacy. Activities related to the pharmacy include storage (refrigeration, security), ordering, receiving, clean-up, dispensing, withdrawal and administration of medication, compounding and manufacturing, product information, and so forth. In the design, the location of each activity must be determined, and each activity should be coordinated with other areas when required. Although most areas will be multifunctional, some activities may be unique and have their own special requirements.

A detailed list of functions pertaining specifically to the pharmacy inventory should include the following:

- *Ordering* requires a telephone, desk, file, and calculator.
- *Receiving* should be near an outside door and requires temporary counter or floor space.
- *Returns* require space for holding broken items, outdated, and damaged items.
- *Storage* areas must be adequate for working and backup (e.g., refrigeration for perishable items and security for volatile hazardous bulk materials).
- *Pricing* involves the use of a computer or price book, markup schemes, records, and a collection of material safety data sheets (MSDSs) for all products.

In addition, consideration should be given to the movement of items to areas of use or dispensing. Monitoring of inventory levels of all items is a much needed function to ensure an adequate supply at demand without shortages.

ARRANGEMENT OF INVENTORY

Working inventory should be placed on shelves in an organized fashion. One method is to arrange items by dosage form. Categories would include the following:

- Oral solids (tablets, capsules)
- Oral liquids
- Oral miscellaneous (boluses, powders, pastes)
- External liquids
- External miscellaneous (sprays, powders, ointments, creams)
- Ophthalmics (ointments, suspensions, solutions)
- Otics

- Small-volume injectables
- Large-volume injectables
- Mastitis preparations
- Miscellaneous, such as chemicals for compounding

Each section should be further arranged, perhaps by generic name, brand name, or the more common name used by individuals in the practice. One may wish to make exceptions for items that are popular, but they should be limited.

A different type of arrangement would be to group items by their most common therapeutic use. Classification would be similar to that in the discussion of drugs found in the first portion of this chapter:

- Anesthetics
- Tranquilizers
- Anticonvulsants
- Analgesics
- Antiinflammatories
- Cardiovascular drugs
- Fluids and electrolytes
- Diuretics
- Parasiticides
- Antibiotics
- Other antibacterials
- Antineoplastics
- Hormones and related substances
- Gastrointestinal drugs
- Vitamins

Each drug class could then be further divided into more specific uses, such as gastrointestinal drugs divided into antiemetics, emetics, and antidiarrheals. Some classes may have only two or three items. Disadvantages of using this system are the poor use of shelf space and the possibility of gallon jugs ending up next to ampules.

Another arrangement is to group items by company or vendor. This method may be acceptable for backup stock because it is helpful when preparing orders. In an active inventory, there may be poor use of shelf space. Perhaps the greatest disadvantage is trying to recall the last supplier for rarely used items. Another disadvantage is purchasing generic items from multiple vendors, which may lead to multiple locations of the same item and duplicate stock.

Pharmacy organization is desirable and has advantages, primarily by assisting each individual in locating items. The best method of organizing stock is probably a combination of the various arrangements above. Each practice should design its own method. In addition to the methods listed, placement of selected items in areas where they are frequently used should be considered.

DRUG LAWS

State Laws

Most state pharmacy laws are primarily concerned with the distribution of drugs within the state. These laws specify who is authorized to prescribe and dispense legend drugs, the licensing of outlets, records required, and certain processing standards.

Because state laws are unique to each state, it is the responsibility of those practicing veterinary medicine to know the laws that apply to them. State laws work in conjunction with federal laws. Sometimes state laws are more restrictive than federal laws; in such cases, one should comply with the stricter law.

Federal Laws

Although the Food, Drug and Cosmetic Act of 1938 has been amended numerous times, it is still the basic federal law governing drugs in the United States. This law assures the public that drugs have been prepared through approved manufacturing standards and are safe as well as effective for the claims made. The Durham-Humphrey Amendment (1951) restricted the availability of certain drugs to prescription through licensed practitioners. This class of drugs, referred to as prescription drugs or *legend drugs,* is deemed unsafe for lay medication, even with clear and precise label directions.

Veterinary labeled drugs bear the legend, "Caution: Federal law restricts this drug to use by or on the order of a licensed veterinarian." Human labeled prescription drugs bear the legend, "Caution: Federal law prohibits dispensing without a prescription." Commercial packaging may elect to utilize the "℞" symbol on the label copy to denote drug product status as a legend drug instead of the written legend.

The FDA has the responsibility for determining the marketing status of a drug, regardless of whether it is possible to prepare adequate directions for use under which a layperson can use the drug safely and effectively. Nonprescription or *over-the-counter* (OTC) drugs may be sold directly to clients but must bear extensive labeling, which includes warnings as well as instructions for proper use.

The American Veterinary Medical Association (AVMA) has approved the following guidelines regarding the use and distribution of veterinary drugs:

- A prescription drug can be dispensed only by or upon the lawful written order of a licensed veterinarian within the course of his or her professional practice where a valid veterinarian-client-patient relationship (VCPR) exists.
- All veterinary prescription drugs must be properly labeled when dispensed.

Technician Note

A prescription drug should be dispensed only where a valid VCPR exists.

Veterinarian-Client-Patient Relationship

A VCPR exists when all the following conditions have been met:

- The veterinarian has assumed the responsibility for making clinical judgments regarding the health of the animal and the need for medical treatment, and the client has agreed to follow the veterinarian's instructions.
- The veterinarian has sufficient knowledge of the animal to initiate at least a general or preliminary diagnosis of the medical condition of the animal.
- The veterinarian is readily available for follow-up evaluation or has arranged for emergency coverage in the event of adverse reactions or failure of the treatment regimen.

Label Requirements

Labeling requirements vary among states but may include name, address, and telephone number of the clinic; name of the client; animal identification; species of animal; date; prescribing veterinarian; name of medication; quantity of medication dispensed; adequate directions for proper administration of medication; number of refills authorized; and prescription transaction number (optional).

Auxiliary labels may also be required to caution or inform the client. Examples include "Shake well," "Keep refrigerated," "Do not use after [date]," "Poison," "External use only," and "For veterinary use only."

The ultimate responsibility for any medication dispensed through a veterinary practice lies with the authorizing veterinarian. In some states, the technician may be allowed to assist the veterinarian by typing labels, counting or pouring, attaching labels, and pricing. The technician *should not issue or refill medications without the veterinarian's approval.* For most medications, this would be in violation of federal law.

Readily retrievable dispensing records may be required by some states to safeguard public health. Accidental ingestion of prescription drugs by animals and small children is not uncommon. Proper records can provide attending physicians with the name and the amount of medication dispensed so appropriate treatment can be provided.

The federal Poison Prevention Packaging Act passed in 1970 requires pharmacists and physicians to dispense medications intended for oral human use in childproof containers. The AVMA recommends to companion animal owners that prescription drugs be placed in child-resistant containers. Certain states mandate the use of such. Veterinary clinics failing to use such a safeguard would be highly vulnerable to legal action in a case of accidental poisoning.

Material Safety Data Sheets

The U.S. Occupational Safety and Health Administration (OSHA) under the authorization of the U.S. Department of Labor set forth standards for current practice relations and requirements. The OSHA Act of 1970 was enacted to ensure the safe and healthful working conditions for working men and women. The law was based on the simple concept that every employee has the basic "right to know" the potential hazard of any substance in the workplace. Employees also need to know what protective measures are available to prevent adverse effects from occurring. Every drug and pharmaceutical aid has a material safety data sheet. A file of these fact sheets must be maintained in the veterinary practice and be accessible to every employee.

Technician Note

OSHA requires a file of MSDSs because every employee has a need and right to know the hazards and identities of the chemicals he or she is exposed to when working.

The essential parts of an MSDS are name, address, and telephone number of the manufacturer or supplier of the product; trade name and synonyms for the mixture or chemicals; hazardous ingredients, percentage, and toxicity; physical properties; fire and explosive hazard data; health hazard data; reactivity data; spill or leak properties; special protective information; and special precautions.

Technician Note

Each commercial container of a controlled substance shall have imprinted on the label the symbol designating the schedule in which such is listed (e.g., CII). The word *schedule* need not be used.

Controlled Substances

The Controlled Substances Act of 1970 was passed to reduce drug abuse by defining certain legal and illegal acts

CONTROLLED DRUG INVENTORY

Date	Dept. Rm No.	Vendor	Invoice No./ Control No.	Quantity Received	Quantity Issued	Balance on Hand	RPh	Date	Dept. Rm No.	Vendor	Invoice No./ Control No.	Quantity Received	Quantity Issued	Balance on Hand	RPh
			BEGINNING BALANCE → → →			20	MA								
1/2/01	SAICU		108221		1	19	MA								
1/7/01	SAICU		108236		1	18	MA								
1/9/01		M/D	9162710	25		43	MA								
1/10/01	63415		108376		1	42	MA								
1/13/01	64489		108389		1	41	MA								
1/15/01	64285		108401		1	42	MA								

FENTANYL TRANSDERMAL 75 MCG/HR (DURAGESIC)

FIGURE 23-7. Controlled drug inventory form. (Courtesy Veterinary Teaching Hospital, Louisiana State University, Baton Rouge, La.)

TABLE 23-5	SCHEDULE OF CONTROLLED SUBSTANCES				
Schedule	Abuse Potential	Dispensing Limits	Distribution Restrictions	Schedule Examples	Comments
I	High	Research use only	DEA form 222 required	LSD, heroin	No accepted medical use
II	High	Requires written prescription, no refills	DEA form 222 required	Oxymorphone, sodium pentobarbital injection	Abuse may lead to severe dependence
III	Less than I and II	Oral or written, refills up to five times within 6 mo	DEA registration number	Hycodan, Tylenol with codeine, anabolic steroids	Abuse may lead to moderate dependence
IV	Low	Oral or written, refills up to five times within 6 mo	DEA registration number	Diazepam, phenobarbital	Abuse may lead to limited dependence
V	Low	No DEA limits	DEA registration number	Lomotil, Robitussin AC	Lowest potential for abuse

regarding substances of high abuse potential. It is established and authorized by the Drug Enforcement Administration (DEA), which has the power to enforce this law. The law is designed to provide an approved means for proper manufacture, distribution, dispensing, and use of controlled substances through licensing of legitimate handlers of these drugs. This closed system has been effective in reducing widespread diversion of these drugs into the illicit market. Controlled substances are classified into five categories (schedules) according to their use or abuse potential (Table 23-5).

All veterinarians using these drugs in the course of their practice are required to have a DEA license number. Those who engage in administering or dispensing controlled substances in schedules II, III, IV, and V are required to keep records of such transactions for 2 years. Receiving records or reports of controlled substances received must also be kept for 2 years.

In addition, practitioners who handle controlled substances are required to take an initial inventory at the opening of business of all controlled substances. Biannual inventories are required after the initial inventory. Records for receipts and dispensing of schedule II substances must be kept separate from all other records. When schedule III, IV, and V drugs are incorporated with other drugs they should be identified with a red "C" in the lower right-hand corner of the record. All controlled substance records must be "readily retrievable."

Acquisition and distribution of controlled substances should be monitored by maintenance of a perpetual inventory (Figure 23-7) for each product stored in the clinic. A perpetual inventory is a "checkbook" balance system that provides an up-to-date balance of the drug. It is easier to reconcile inventory when this system is used.

It is best that those persons responsible for handling controlled substances be familiar not only with federal laws governing them but also with state laws, which may be more strict. Agencies such as the State Board of Pharmacy or the local DEA office are quite helpful in answering questions concerning compliance.

The law states that, "A practitioner who has controlled substances stored in his office or clinic must keep these drugs in a securely locked, substantially constructed cabinet or safe." A secure area is usually interpreted as a double-locked container that cannot be picked up and moved. Examples would be a locked metal box stored inside a floor safe or an attached locked wall cabinet. The responsibility for access to controlled substances should be restricted to only one or two persons in the practice. Practitioners experiencing theft or significant loss of controlled substances must report such loss to the DEA regional office and the local police department when the loss is discovered.

A government publication entitled the *Physician's Manual: An Information Outline on the Controlled Substances 1970* is an excellent guide for proper handling of controlled substances. This government manual may be obtained free by request from the following:

U.S. Department of Justice
Drug Enforcement Administration
1465 I Street, NW
Washington, DC 20537

RECOMMENDED READING

Adams HR, editor: *Veterinary pharmacology and therapeutics*, ed 7, Ames, 1995, Iowa State University Press.

Baumgartner K, Hoffman D, editors: *Controlled substances handbook*, Washington, DC, 1998, Government Information Services.

Bonagura JD, editor: *Current veterinary therapy XIII. Animal practice*, Philadelphia, 2000, WB Saunders.

Compendium of veterinary products, ed 5, Port Huron, Mich, 1999, North American Compendium.

Hardman JG et al: *The pharmacological basis of therapeutics*, ed 9, New York, 1996, McGraw-Hill.

Physician's desk reference, ed 54, Montvale, NJ, 2000, Medical Economics Co.

Plumb DC: *Veterinary drug handbook*, ed 3, White Bear Lake, Minn, 1995, PharmaVet Publishing.

USP DI: *Drug information for the health care professional*, ed 20, vol 1, Englewood, Col, 2000, Micromedex.

Veterinary pharmaceuticals and biologicals, ed 11, Lenexa, Kan, 1997, Veterinary Medicine Publishing.

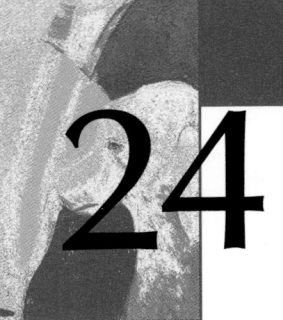

Surgical Instruments and Aseptic Technique

Jacqueline R. Davidson • *Daniel J. Burba*

The veterinary technician may need to assist the veterinarian with many aspects of surgery. The technician may need to prepare the patient for surgery, act as a circulating nurse in the operating room, and take responsibility for the care, cleaning, packing, and sterilization of the instruments. The technician is often responsible for ordering surgical instruments and implants, so familiarity with this equipment is essential. In addition, the principles of aseptic technique should be second nature. The technician may need to alert the veterinarian to potential problems with aseptic technique and may be required to "scrub in" to assist with surgical procedures. A surgical assistant can be of great value by anticipating which instruments the surgeon will need and by aiding in tissue retraction and hemostasis. The technician is an invaluable part of the surgical team and can greatly enhance the quality and efficiency of surgical procedures.

INSTRUMENTATION

Thousands of different surgical instruments are available, and new instruments are continually being designed to increase the efficiency and ease of performing surgery. The surgical technician must know the purpose of each instrument in order to anticipate when it will be used and must understand how to handle and care for it.

Technician Note

Each instrument is designed for a specific purpose, such as cutting, holding, clamping, or retracting.

General Surgery Instruments
Scalpel
The scalpel is the best instrument for incising tissues with minimal trauma. A variety of disposable blades are designed to fit several different scalpel handles (Figure 24-1).

The *Bard-Parker no. 3 handle* uses detachable blade nos. 10, 11, 12, and 15 and is the most useful for small animal surgery. The *Bard-Parker no. 4 handle* is larger and uses detachable blade nos. 20, 21, and 22. This handle is most commonly used for large animal surgery.

Electrosurgery
Electroscalpels can be used to cut or coagulate tissue and help to minimize bleeding. They work by passing a high-frequency alternating electrical current through the tissue (Figure 24-2). Cutting or coagulation can be performed through the same handpiece, and the surgeon can activate it by a switch on the sterile handpiece or by a foot switch. However, the power level must be adjusted by a nonsterile technician. In *monopolar electrosurgery*, current passes from the handpiece through the patient to a metal ground plate that is placed under the patient. Poor contact between the patient's skin and the ground plate can burn the patient at the site of the ground plate. In *bipolar electosurgery*, the current passes between two tips on the handpiece, which grasp the tissue. No ground plate is needed for bipolar electrosurgery.

Scissors
Specific scissors are designed to cut tissue, suture, wire, or bandage material. There are many types of dissecting scissors made for precise cutting and dissection of tissue. *Operating scissors* vary by the type of blades (straight or curved), the type of points (blunt-blunt, blunt-sharp, or sharp-sharp), and the cutting edge of the blades (plain or serrated) (Figure 24-3, *C*). *Mayo dissecting scissors* (Figure 24-3, *D*) are heavy scissors used for cutting tough tissue, such as heavy connective tissue. The blades may be straight or curved. *Metzenbaum dissecting scissors* (Figure 24-3, *E*) are fine, curved scissors used for cutting delicate tissue, such as fat or thin muscle. Metzenbaum scissors are preferred for most soft tissue dissection. They should never be used for cutting suture because this dulls their edges and causes the blades to separate and lose their effectiveness. Stitch scis-

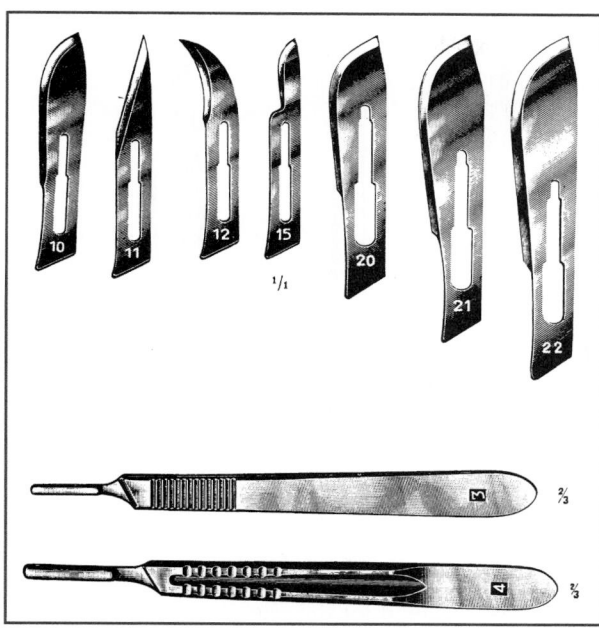

FIGURE 24-1. Scalpel handles and attachable surgical blades. Surgical blade nos. 10, 11, 12, and 15 fit the Bard-Parker no. 3 scalpel handle, and surgical blade nos. 20 to 22 fit the Bard-Parker no. 4 handle. The no. 3 handle and no. 10 blade are commonly used in small animal surgery. The no. 4 handle and no. 20 blade are commonly used in large animal surgery.

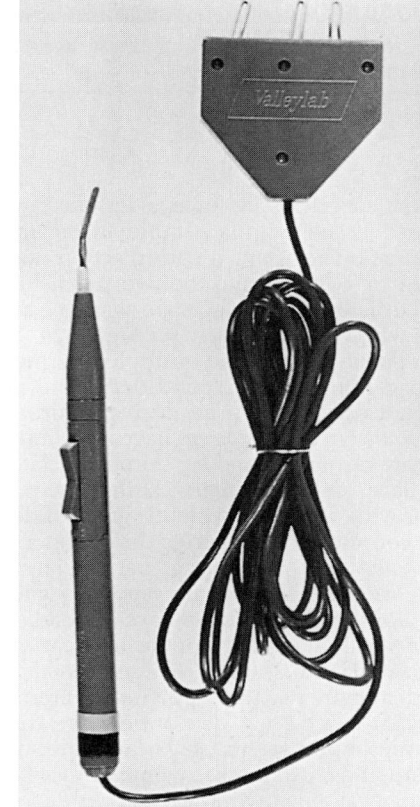

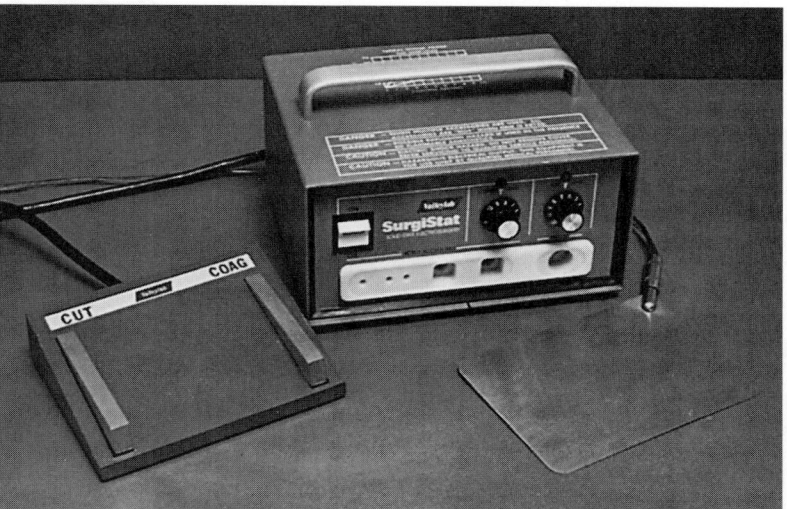

FIGURE 24-2. Electrosurgical equipment. **A,** Monopolar electrosurgery handpiece with a cutting/coagulation hand control. The handpiece is kept sterile. **B,** Electrosurgical foot switch, power source, and ground plate. The animal must have good contact with the ground plate for the electrosurgery unit to function correctly. These items are not sterilized.

FIGURE 24-3. **A,** Mayo-Hegar needle holder. **B,** Olsen-Hegar needle holder. **C,** Operating scissors: sharp-blunt, blunt-blunt, and sharp-sharp. **D,** Mayo dissecting scissors. **E,** Metzenbaum dissecting scissors.

sors or *Littauer suture removal scissors* (Figure 24-4, *A*) are used to cut all sutures except wire sutures. *Wire suture-cutting scissors* can cut wire suture (Figure 24-4, *B*). *Lister bandage scissors* are available to cut bandage material (Figure 24-4, *C*). One blade of the Lister scissors has a blunt end to facilitate sliding under a bandage without poking the skin. To prolong the life of any scissors, it should be used only for its intended purpose.

Technician Note

Scissors are specifically designed for many purposes, including tissue dissection and cutting suture or bandage materials.

Needle Holders

Needle holders are designed for holding curved suture needles during suturing and for performing instrument suture ties. *Mayo-Hegar* and *Olsen-Hegar* needle holders are two commonly used needle holders (see Figure 24-3, *A* and *B*). The Olsen-Hegar needle holder has a built-in suture scissors that negates the need for an assistant to cut suture. It allows the surgeon to work alone and cut suture without switching instruments. The potential disadvantage of this needle holder is that the suture may be accidentally cut during suture placement.

Needle holders consist of a set of jaws, a hinge or box lock, and handles with a ratcheted locking device (Figure 24-5). The size and design of these components vary greatly depending on their intended use. The jaws commonly have tungsten carbide inserts that provide excellent grip. The tungsten carbide insert is hard and resistant to wear and can be replaced when worn, thereby prolonging the life of the instrument. Worn inserts can result in improper closure of the jaws or sharp edges that inadvertently cut suture. Needle holders are available in different sizes, depending on the needle sizes they are designed to hold. Improper use of needle holders (e.g., using a needle

holder that is too small for the size of the needle or using the needle holder to bend or twist wire) may not only damage the jaws but also spring the box lock and ratchet.

Technician Note

Needle holders are designed for handling the suture needle and performing instrument suture ties.

Thumb Forceps

Thumb forceps are special tissue forceps designed to hold and easily release tissue with a simple finger motion (similar to tweezers). They have a spring action, and the jaws are opposed by compressing the two metal handles together. Several different jaw surfaces are available and are designed for use with various tissues (see Figure 24-4, *D* to *G*). *Brown-Adson thumb forceps* have multiple intermeshing teeth with a broad tip, providing good tissue and needle handling. They are commonly used during suturing and wound closure. *Rat tooth thumb forceps* have large interdigitating teeth and are primarily used for skin or fascia. *Adson thumb forceps* have delicate intermeshing teeth ("rat toothed") that provide a good, atraumatic grasp of delicate tissues. They are commonly used during dissection. *Cooley* and *DeBakey thumb forceps* have long, narrow jaws with multiple delicate sets of teeth that are especially good for vascular surgery. *Russian thumb forceps* have a broad curved surface good for needle handling but are traumatic when used to hold tissues (Figure 24-6, *A*). *Dressing thumb forceps* do not have teeth and are used for applying and removing dressings (Figure 24-6, *B*). They are not designed to grasp tissue and are undesirable for this use because the surgeon must squeeze hard and crush the tissue in order to grasp it. Thumb forceps are available in a variety of sizes depending on the intended surgery. For example, thoracic forceps have very long handles to enable the surgeon to reach tissues deep within the chest, but these same forceps would be too cumbersome and awkward to use on the skin.

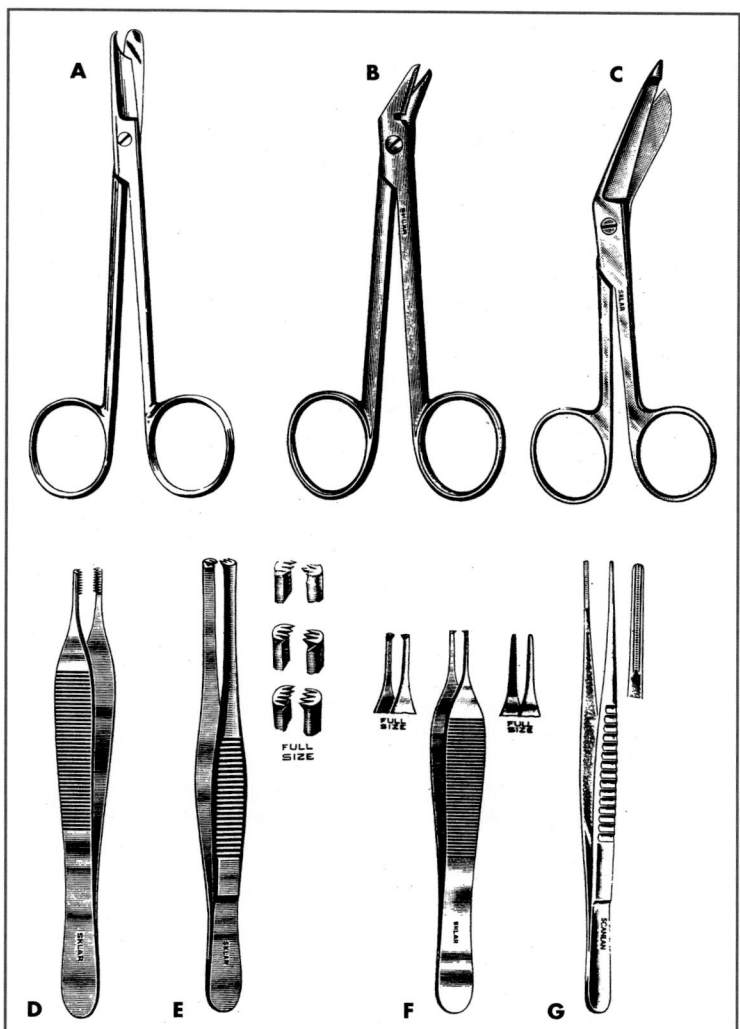

FIGURE 24-4. **A,** Littauer suture removal scissors. **B,** Wire suture cutting scissors. **C,** Lister bandage scissors. **D,** Brown-Adson thumb forceps. **E,** Rat tooth thumb forceps. **F,** Adson thumb forceps. **G,** DeBakey vascular thumb forceps.

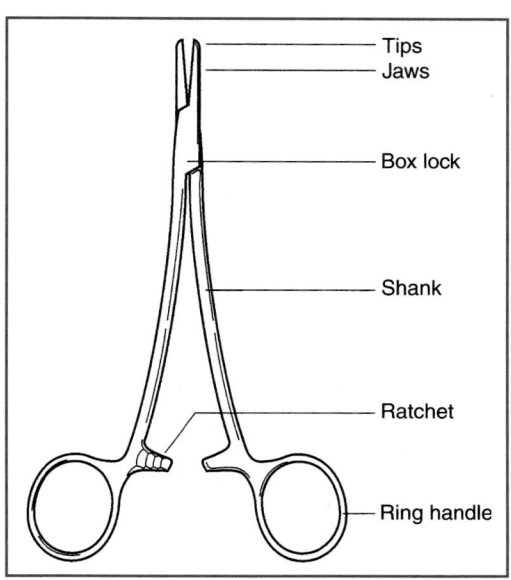

FIGURE 24-5. Basic components of a surgical instrument (Mayo-Hegar needle holder).

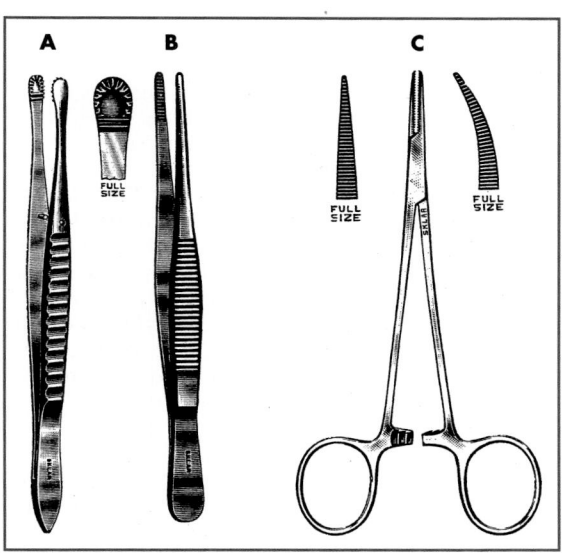

FIGURE 24-6. **A,** Russian thumb forceps. **B,** Dressing thumb forceps. **C,** Halsted mosquito hemostatic forceps.

Technician Note
Thumb forceps are commonly used in the surgeon's non-dominant hand to hold tissues while dissecting or suturing.

Tissue Forceps
Tissue forceps are locking instruments that clamp tissues. Different teeth patterns allow them to grip various types of tissues without slipping. *Allis tissue forceps* securely grasp tissue but also crush it (Figure 24-8, *C*). Therefore they are considered to be traumatic and should only be used on tissue that is being removed. *Babcock forceps* are shaped similarly to the Allis forceps but are less traumatic because they have a smoother grasping surface and less tip compression (Figure 24-8, *D*). The Doyen intestinal tissue forceps is a more delicate instrument used to occlude and hold intestine. The disadvantage of less traumatic tissue forceps is that they are less secure on the tissues.

Technician Note
Tissue forceps are used to clamp and hold tissues with a self-locking mechanism.

Towel clamps are forceps used to attach towels and drapes to the patient. These forceps have pointed tips that curve and join like ice tongs. *Backhaus towel clamps* and *Roeder towel clamps* are two common designs (Figure 24-8, *E* and *F*). The Roeder towel clamp has a metal bead or ball stop attached to the jaws that prevents deep tissue penetration and prevents the towel from slipping toward the box lock of the forceps.

Hemostatic Forceps
Hemostatic forceps are tissue forceps used to stop bleeding by crushing blood vessels. They are available in different sizes and may be straight or curved. Most hemostatic forceps have transverse grooves on the inside surface of the jaws to better grasp the tissue. *Halsted mosquito hemostats* are small and designed to occlude small vessels (Figure 24-6, *C*). When using hemostatic forceps, the tips of the forceps should be used to grasp only as much tissue as necessary. *Crile forceps* and *Kelly forceps* (Figure 24-7, *A* and *B*) are larger hemostatic forceps that are used on larger vessels. The jaws of the Crile forceps are transversely grooved for the entire length, but only the distal halves of the Kelly forceps are grooved. *Rochester-Pean forceps* are large, transversely grooved forceps that are used to clamp tissue bundles and large vessels (Figure 24-7, *C*). *Rochester-Ochsner forceps* are similar to the Rochester-Pean forceps but have interdigitating teeth at the tips (Figure 24-8, *A*) that aid in grasping the tissue. Rochester-Oschner forceps are used most commonly in orthopedic or large animal surgery. *Rochester-Carmalt forceps* are large crushing forceps with longitudinal grooves and cross grooves at the tip to provide more traction (Figure 24-8, *B*). These forceps are used for clamping across tissue containing vessels. The Rochester-Carmalt forceps are commonly used to crush the vessels of the ovarian pedicle or the body of the uterus during an ovariohysterectomy (spay) operation. When clamping across vessels, the forceps should be applied with the concave surface facing upward to facilitate tying the ligature.

Technician Note
Hemostatic forceps are used to clamp, crush, and hold blood vessels with a self-locking mechanism.

Retractors
Properly placed retractors do not interfere with the surgery yet provide good visibility of the surgical site and allow more room for the surgeon to work. Retractors may be hand-held or self-retaining. A surgical assistant is needed to maintain the position and tissue tension of a hand-held retractor. The *Army-Navy retractor* and the *Senn retractor* are double-ended, hand-held retractors commonly used to retract skin, fat, or muscle (Figure 24-9, *A* and *C*). The Army-Navy retractor is smooth bladed, whereas the Senn has one smooth blade and one blade with three sharp or blunt prongs (Figure 24-9, *C*). The *malleable retractor* is made of thin metal that is easily bent to the desired shape (Figure 24-9, *B*). It is commonly used to retract abdominal organs. The *Snook ovariohysterectomy hook* is a specialized type of hand-held retractor used to expose the horn of the uterus during an ovariohysterectomy (Figure 24-9, *D*). The *Hohmann retractor* consists of a single blade and a handle that are used to lever tissues out of the way for better visibility. It is used almost exclusively in orthopedic surgery and can provide good visibility in certain joint surgeries.

Technician Note
Retractors rather than hands are used to retract tissues and provide good visibility of the surgical site.

Self-retaining retractors are maintained in the desired position by some type of locking mechanism on the retractor handle. One advantage of the self-retaining retractors is that the surgeon and the assistant have their hands free for other tasks. The *Balfour retractor* provides increased exposure of the abdominal cavity (Figure 24-10, *A*). The two wirelike blades are used to distract the abdominal incision and the solid spoonlike blade is hooked onto the sternum to distract it cranially. The *Finochietto rib spreader* retracts the ribs to expose the surgical field within the thoracic cavity (Figure 24-10, *B*). The ratcheted part of the retractors is positioned at the dorsal aspect of the thoracic incision so it does not interfere with the surgeon. *Gelpi retractors* (Figure 24-11, *A*) and *Weitlaner retractors* (Figure 24-11, *B*) are self-retaining retractors commonly used for muscle retraction, especially in orthopedic and neurologic surgery.

Suction Tips
Several different suction tips are commonly used (Figure 24-12). The *Poole tip* is used primarily in the abdominal or thoracic cavity because it has an outer sleeve with small holes to prevent tissue, such as fat, from becoming entrapped in the tip. The *Frazier tip* is most commonly used in orthopedic and neurologic surgery. The *Yankauer tip* is a general-purpose suction tip. The suction tip is attached to a long, sterile suction tube. The other end of the suction tube is connected to a nonsterile suction canister.

Stapling Equipment
Several different surgical stapling devices are available for an array of purposes. There are many advantages to using

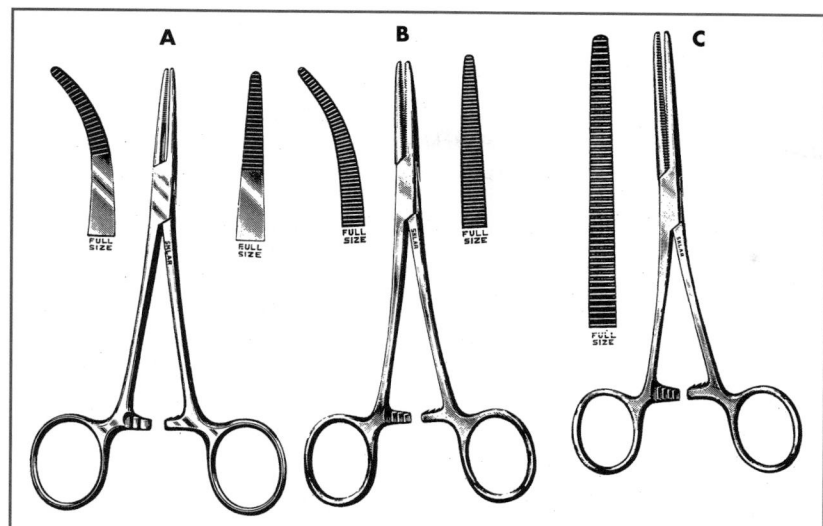

FIGURE 24-7. **A,** Kelly forceps. **B,** Crile forceps. **C,** Rochester-Pean forceps.

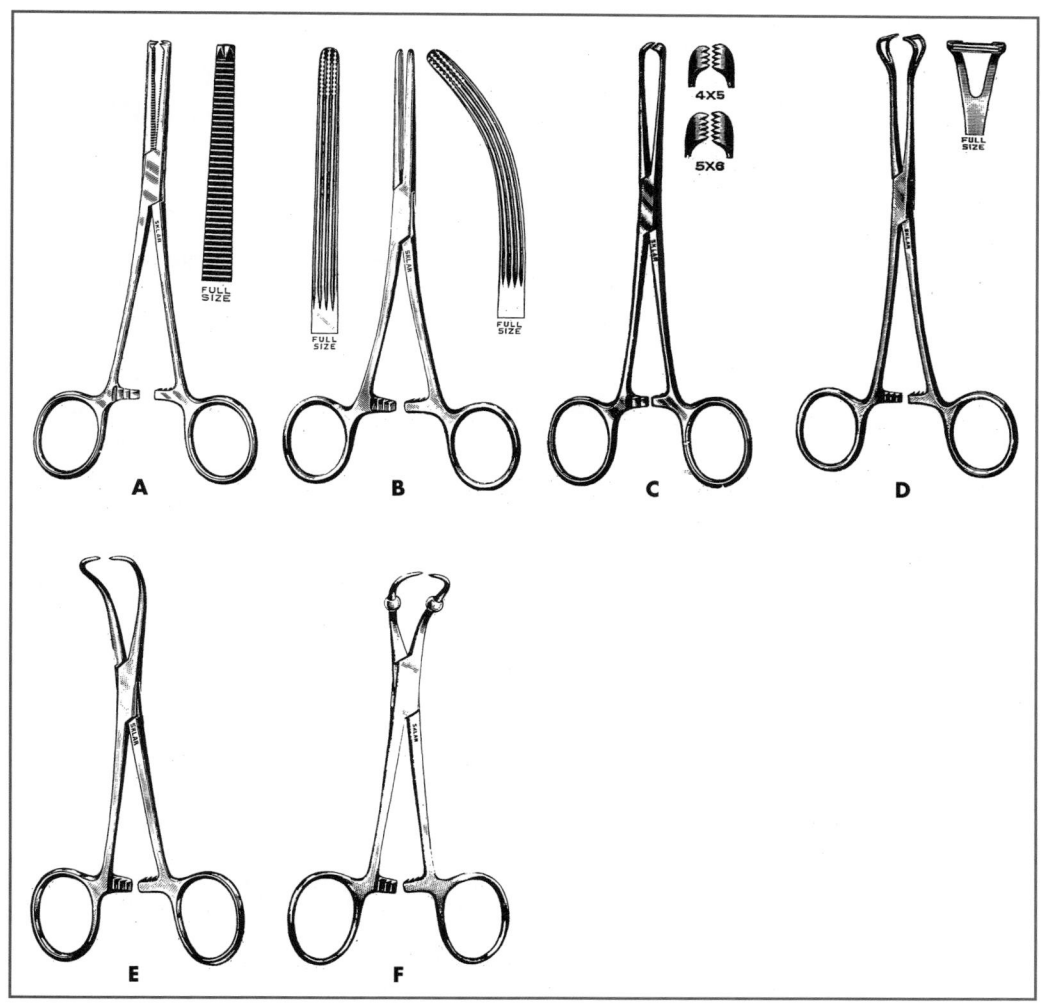

FIGURE 24-8. **A,** Rochester-Ochsner forceps. **B,** Rochester-Carmalt forceps. **C,** Allis tissue forceps. **D,** Babcock tissue forceps. **E,** Backhaus towel clamp. **F,** Roeder towel clamp.

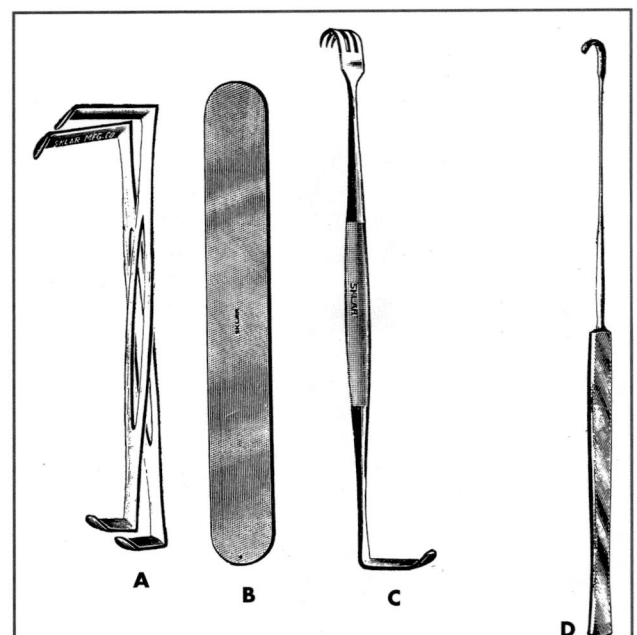

FIGURE 24-9. Hand-held retractors. **A,** Army-Navy retractor. **B,** Malleable retractor. **C,** Senn retractor. **D,** Snook ovariohysterectomy hook (spay hook).

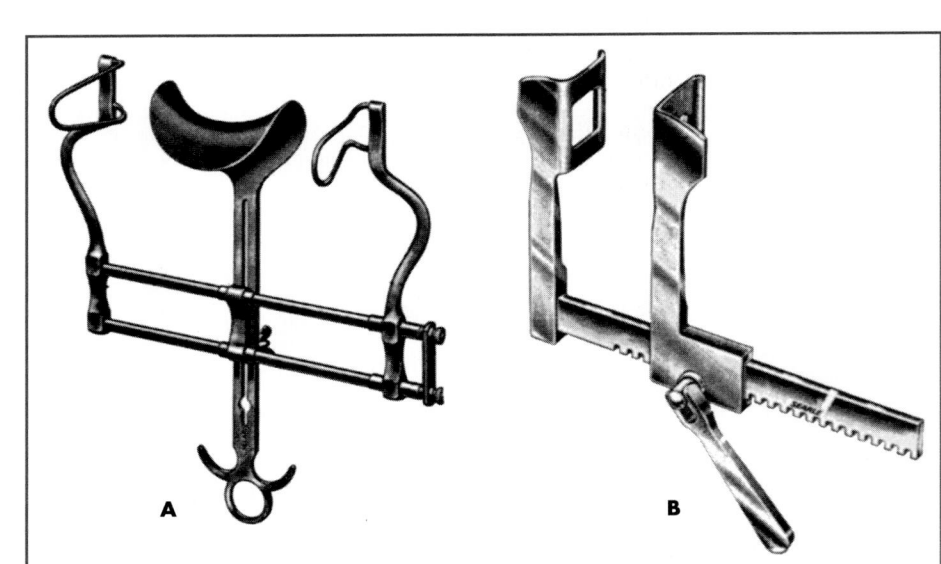

FIGURE 24-10. Self-retaining retractors. **A,** Balfour abdominal retractor. **B,** Finochietto rib retractor.

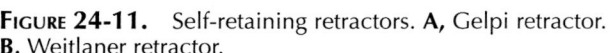
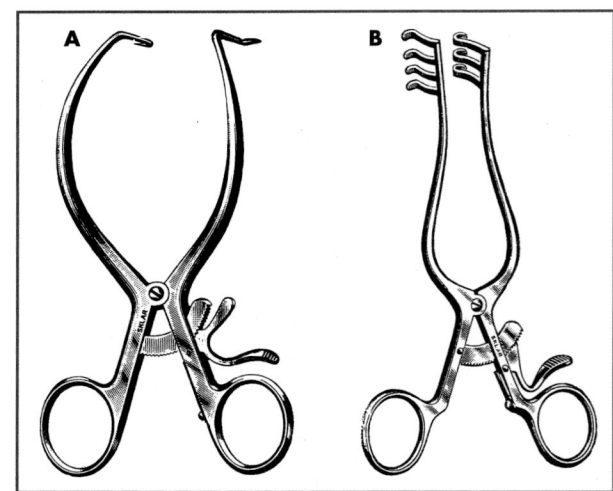

FIGURE 24-11. Self-retaining retractors. **A,** Gelpi retractor. **B,** Weitlaner retractor.

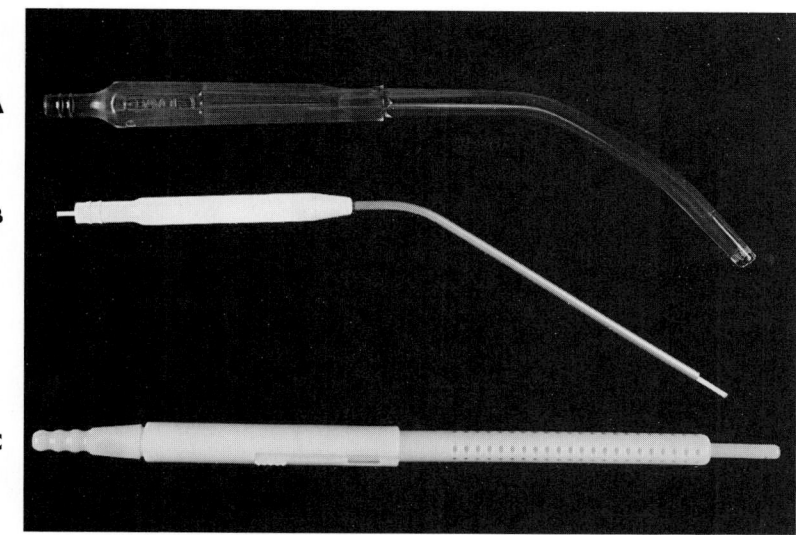

FIGURE 24-12.   Suction tips. **A,** Yankauer. **B,** Frazier. **C,** Poole.

TABLE 24-1	STAPLING EQUIPMENT		
Name	**Derivation of Name**	**Common Use**	**Comments**
TA	Thoracoabdominal	Lung resection	Places double or triple row of staples
GIA	Gastrointestinal anastomosis	Gastrointestinal resection and anastomosis	Places four rows of staples and cuts between the middle two rows
EEA	End-to-end anastomosis	Gastrointestinal anastomosis	Staples two intestinal segments together in a circular manner with a functional lumen
Skin and fascial stapler		Closes skin or fascia	Places a single staple
LDS	Ligate-and-divide stapler	Blood vessel ligation	Places two staples on a vessel and cuts between them

stapling devices in both large and small animal surgery. Stapling devices provide an easier and faster alternative to hand suturing. Some stapling devices also cut tissue after stapling. The staplers are named by an abbreviation of their designed function (Table 24-1). A number may be used after the name *TA* or *GIA* to indicate the length of the row of staples (e.g., a TA 30 places two rows of staples 30 mm long; Figure 24-13).

Michel Skin Clips

Drape material is often attached to the incised skin edge during surgical procedures to minimize contamination of the surgical field by the surrounding skin. The use of Michel skin clips is one method of attaching the drape to the wound edges (Figure 24-14). One end of the Michel clip applying-and-removing forceps grips the clip. When the handles are squeezed, the clip bends to pinch the edges of the drape and the skin together. The other end of the forceps has jaws that remove the clip by bending it backward and disengaging it from the incision edge. There are alternatives to Michel clips, including the use of suture, "scalp clips," towel clamps, and adhesive drapes.

Ophthalmic Instruments

Ophthalmic surgery requires the use of delicate instruments that must be handled carefully. Basic ophthalmic instruments include specialized scalpels, scissors, thumb forceps, needle holders, and retractors (Figure 24-15).

Orthopedic Instruments

Rongeurs

Rongeurs have sharp cupped tips that are used to cut small pieces of dense tissue, such as bone, cartilage, or fibrous tissue. Rongeurs have a double-action or single-action mechanism (Figure 24-16). Double-action rongeurs have a smooth cutting action and are mechanically stronger than single-action rongeurs, but they are also larger. Double-action rongeurs are preferred for removing large amounts of dense tissue. Single-action rongeurs are more commonly used in confined areas, as in removing bone to perform spinal surgery. Bone-cutting forceps are similar to rongeurs but have paired chisel-like tips. They are used for cutting bone and should not be mistaken for wire cutters.

Bone-Holding Forceps

Bone-holding forceps are designed to hold bone and bone fragments in alignment while orthopedic implants (screws, pins, wires, plates) are applied (Figure 24-17). Most bone-holding forceps are self-retaining. The *Kern bone-holding forceps* has a ratcheted handle that allows it to be clamped securely on the bone. The *self-retaining bone-holding forceps,* also known as "speed locks," has a nut that tightens against one handle to squeeze the handles together.

Curettes

Curettes are used to scrape hard tissue, such as bone or cartilage. Curettes are designed with a small cuplike struc-

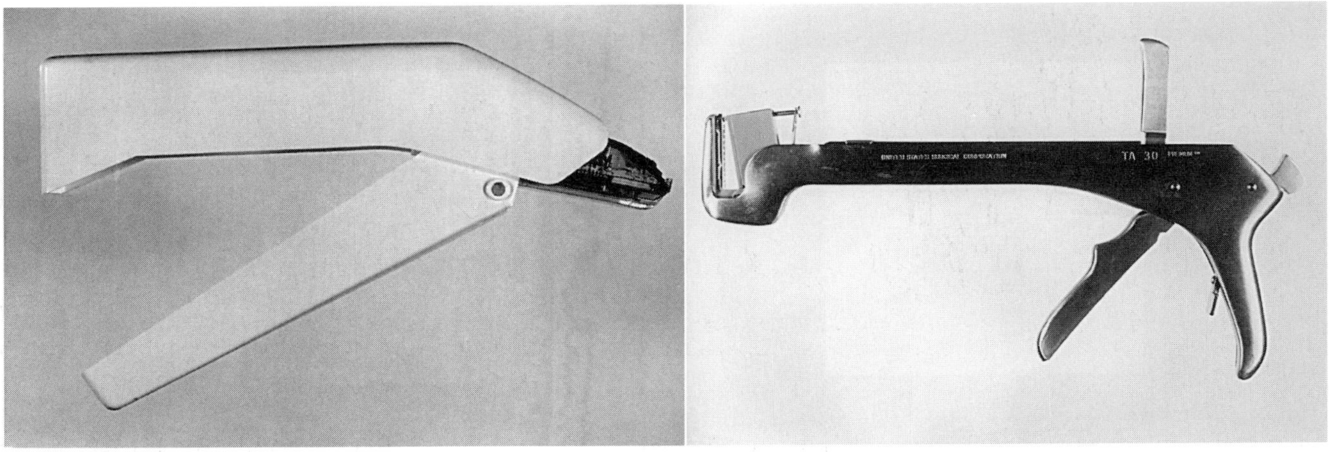

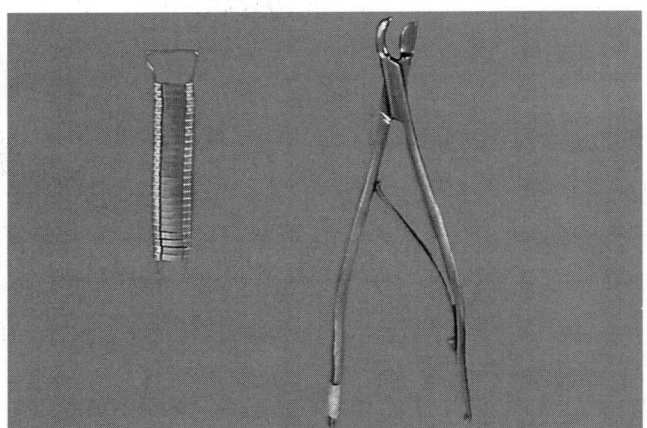

FIGURE 24-13. Surgical stapling equipment. **A,** Surgical skin stapler applies a single staple with each squeeze of the trigger (staple guns commonly hold 25 to 35 staples). **B,** Thoracoabdominal stapler (TA 30) applies two rows of staples simultaneously.

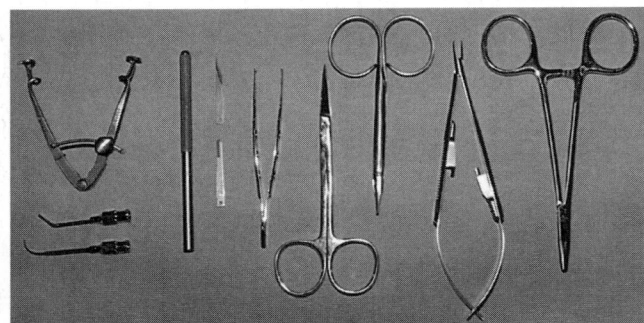

FIGURE 24-14. Michel skin clips and Michel clip forceps.

FIGURE 24-15. Common ophthalmic instruments. *Left to right,* Lid speculum *(above)* and lacrimal cannulas *(below),* Beaver blade handle with no. 64 and 65 surgical blades, Bishop-Harmon thumb forceps, iris scissors, tenotomy scissors, Castroviejo needle holder, and Derf needle holder.

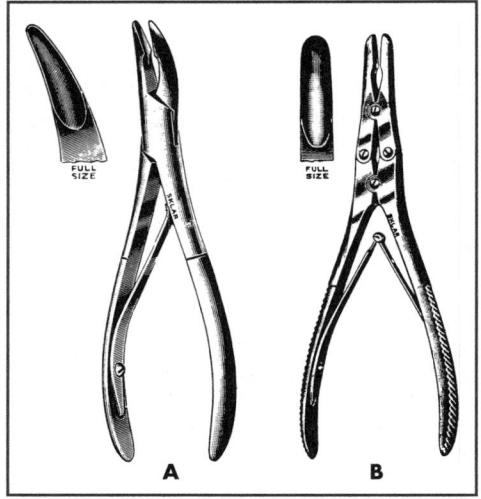

FIGURE 24-16. **A,** Single-action rongeur. **B,** Double-action rongeur.

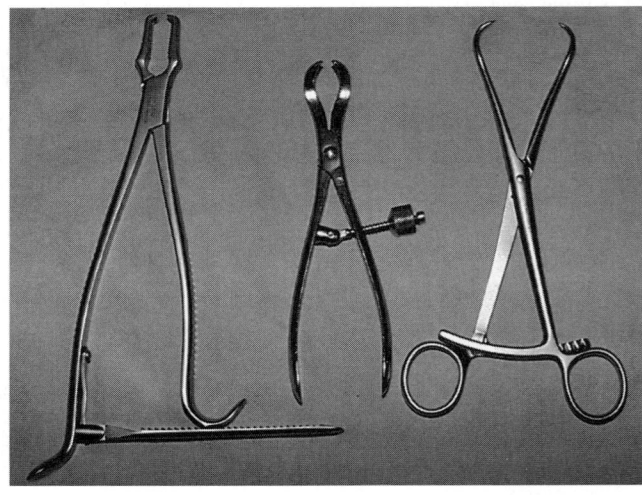

FIGURE 24-17. Bone-holding forceps. Kern forceps *(left),* speed lock forceps *(center),* and point-to-point forceps *(right).*

ture at one or both ends of a handle (similar to an ice cream scoop). The cup has a sharp cutting edge and is available in various sizes (Figure 24-18, *A*). A common use of bone curettes is to retrieve cancellous bone from the medullary cavity (tibia, humerus, ilium) for use as a bone graft. Cancellous bone grafts are often used during fracture repair.

Periosteal Elevators

Periosteal elevators are instruments that are used to pry periosteum or muscle from the bone surface. They have a bladelike structure at one or both ends of a handle. The blades have sharp or blunt edges and are available in various sizes (Figure 24-18, *B*).

Osteotomes and Chisels

Osteotomes and chisels are used to cut bone. The cutting edge of the osteotome is tapered on both sides, whereas the chisel is tapered only on one side (Figure 24-18, *C*). Osteotomes and chisels are used by pounding on the flared end of the handle with a mallet.

Gigli Wire

Gigli wire is used to cut bone by placing the wire around the bone and drawing it back and forth in a sawing fashion. T-shaped handles hook onto the wire to give the surgeon a firm grasp of the wire.

Trephines

Trephines are T-shaped tubular instruments with a cylindrical cutting blade (Figure 24-19). Trephines are usually used to remove a core of bone for biopsy.

Power Equipment

Some power equipment is commonly used in orthopedic and neurologic surgery. Although some drills are electric or battery powered (Figure 24-20, *C*), many orthopedic drills and saws are powered by nitrogen gas that is supplied via a sterile hose (Figure 24-20, *A* and *B*). A Hall air drill is a specialized high-speed burr that grinds away bone (Figure 24-21). It is most commonly used for spinal surgery.

Orthopedic Implants

Bone Pins

Bone pins vary in diameter, length, and the type of points. *Steinmann pins* are smooth, stainless steel pins ranging in diameter from one-sixteenth to one-fourth inch. Three different types of pin points are available: chisel, trocar, or threaded trocar (Figure 24-22). A power drill or a Jacobs hand chuck is required to insert the pin into bone, and a pin cutter is necessary to cut it to the proper length (Figure 24-23). Steinmann pins may be called *IM (intramedullary) pins* because they are often placed in the medullary cavity of long bones for fracture fixation. Kirschner wires (K-wires) are similar to Steinmann pins but smaller and can be used to pin small bone fragments. The available sizes are 0.035-inch, 0.045-inch, and 0.062 inch diameter.

Interlocking Nails

Interlocking nails are similar to intramedullary pins but have preplaced holes through the pin that allow screw placement. Interlocking nails have more rigid fixation than intramedullary pins. Equipment is similar to that required for pins, but specialized equipment is needed for screw placement.

Orthopedic Wire

Stainless steel orthopedic wire is supplied on spools. The common sizes used in small animal surgery are 22 gauge,

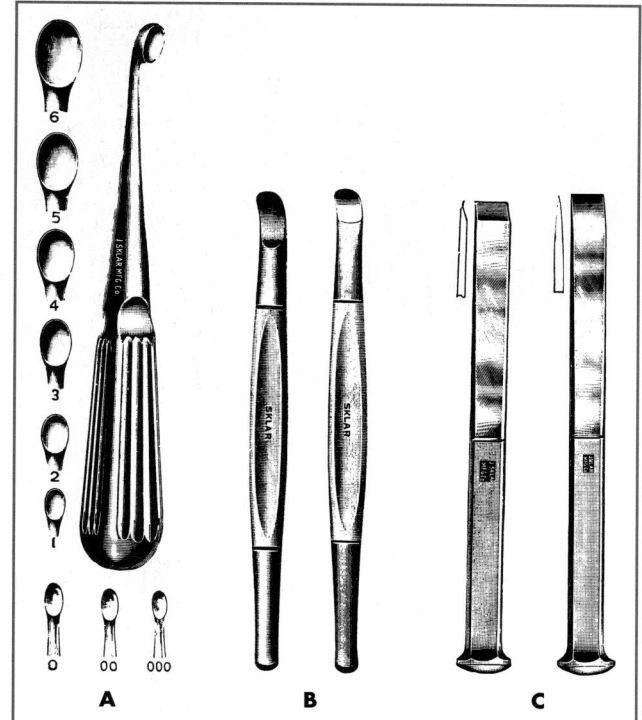

FIGURE 24-18.   A, Curettes. **B,** Periosteal elevators. **C,** Chisel *(left)* and osteotome *(right).*

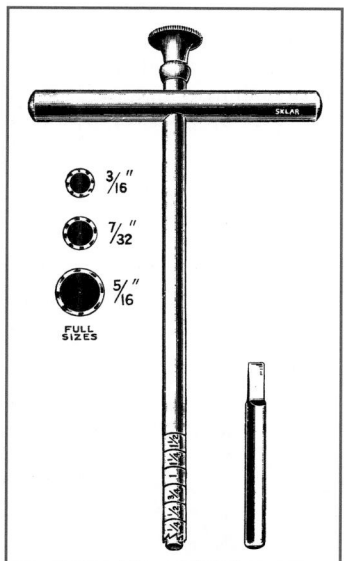

FIGURE 24-19.   Trephine.

20 gauge, and 18 gauge (Table 24-2). It is most commonly applied in a cerclage fashion by encircling the bone or bone fragments and twisting the ends in a "twist-tie" manner. Orthopedic wire is often used for fracture repair in combination with pins or bone plates.

External Fixators

External fixation is a means of stabilizing fractures using pins placed through the skin and bone. The pins are held rigid by a metal or acrylic connecting bar that is attached to

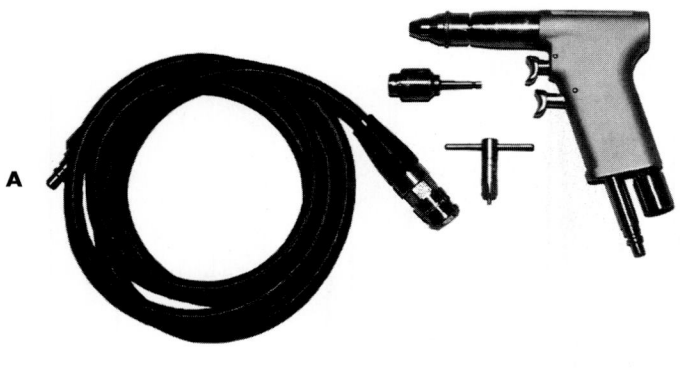

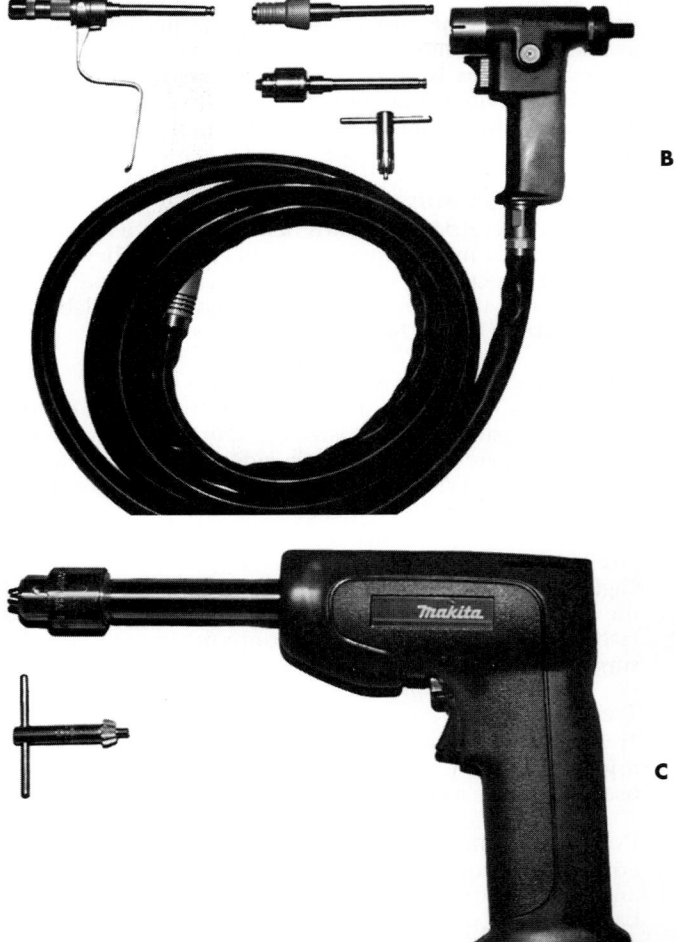

FIGURE 24-20.   Orthopedic drills. **A,** ASIF drill is powered by a tank of pressurized nitrogen gas. **B,** 3-M mini driver is also gas powered. It has an attachment for K-wires, and quick release or chuck attachments for drill bits. **C,** Makita drill is battery powered.

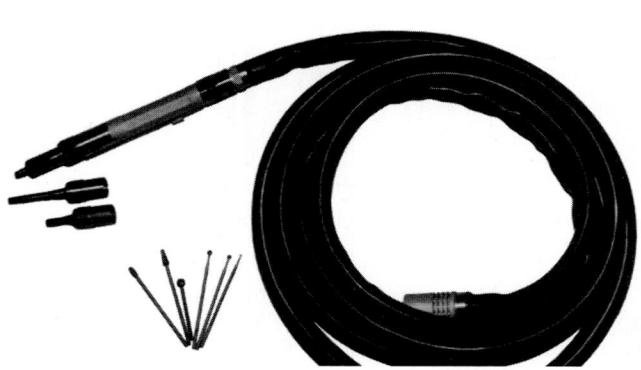

FIGURE 24-21.   Hall air drill with various burrs and two different-length burr guards.

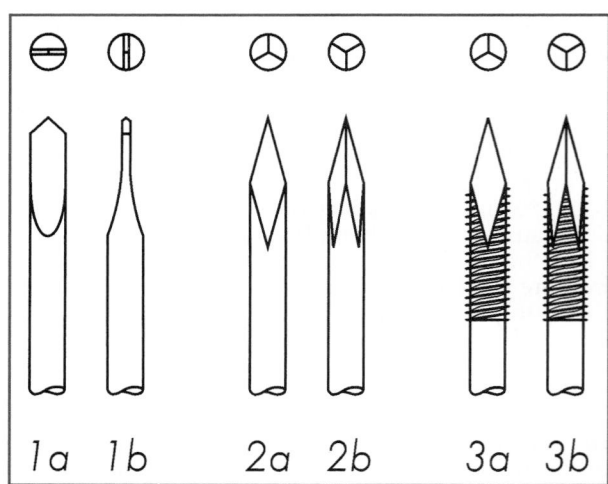

FIGURE 24-22.   Steinmann intramedullary pin points. *1a* and *1b,* Chisel tip is used to slide in the medullary cavity along the inner cortical surface. *2a* and *2b,* Trocar tip is a cutting tip. *3a* and *3b,* Threaded trocar tip can be used for better anchorage in bone.

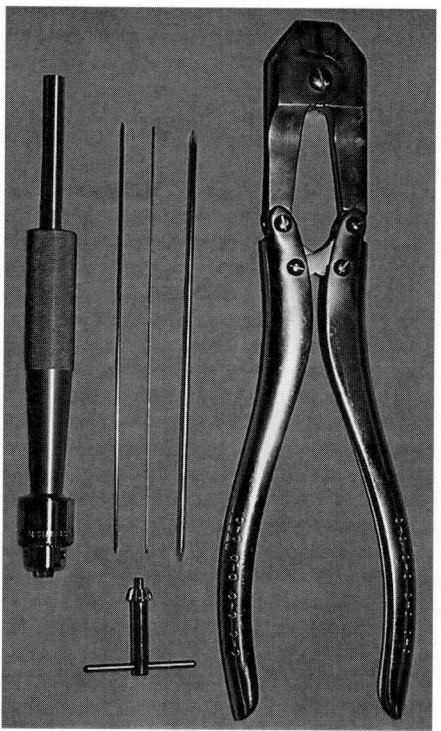

FIGURE 24-23. Jacobs hand chuck, key, various sizes of Steinmann pins, and pin cutter.

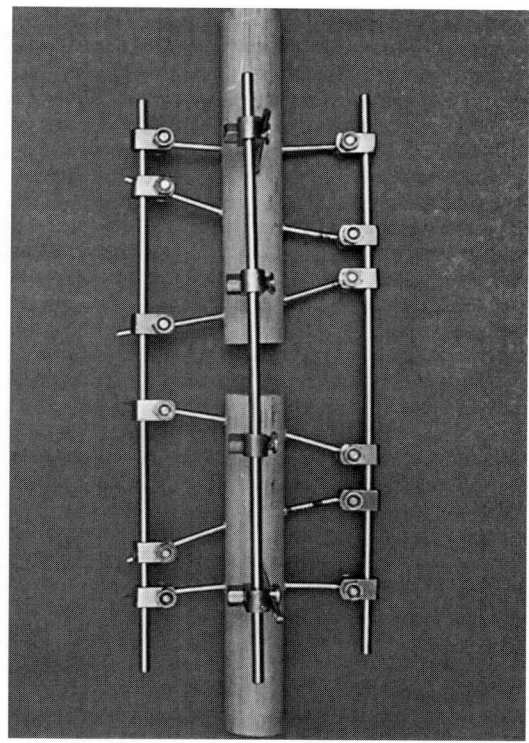

FIGURE 24-24. An external fixator placed on a wooden dowel fracture model.

TABLE 24-2	COMMONLY USED ORTHOPEDIC WIRE SIZES	
Gauge	**Inches**	**Millimeters**
22	0.025	0.64
20	0.032	0.81
18	0.040	1.02

the pins several centimeters from the skin (Figure 24-24). The Kirschner-Ehmer (K-E) apparatus uses special clamps to attach a metal connecting bar to the pins. Acrylic (methyl methacrylate) connecting bars are often made from dental acrylics or hoof wall repair acrylics because they are less expensive than surgical grades of acrylic. The acrylic connecting bar is more versatile and lighter than the metal K-E apparatus.

Bone Screws

The two basic screw types are cortical and cancellous screws. Cortical screws are fully threaded screws that are designed for dense (cortical) bone. Cancellous screws are either partially threaded or fully threaded and are made with wider threads in order to have better grip in the softer cancellous bone (Figure 24-25).

The general steps of screw placement include drilling a hole in the bone, measuring the hole with a depth gauge to determine the proper screw length, using a bone tap (a screwlike instrument with sharp threads) to cut a screw path in the bone, and inserting the screw with a specialized screwdriver. Bone screws may be used alone or in conjunction with a bone plate or interlocking nail.

Bone screws are named by both the screw length and

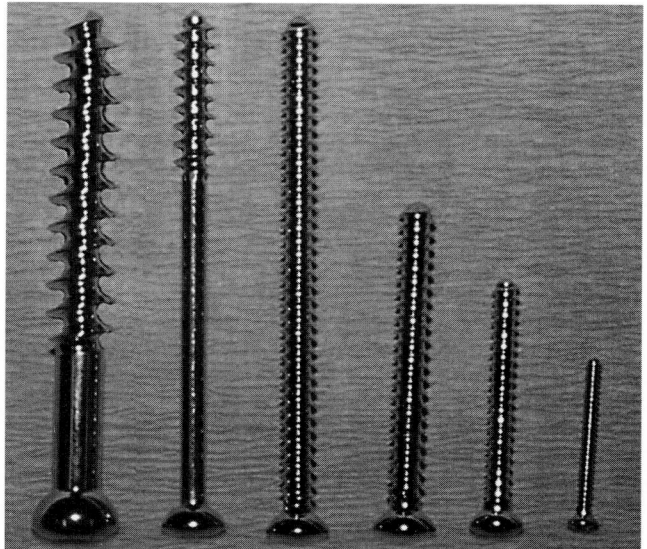

FIGURE 24-25. Partially threaded cancellous screws *(left)* and various sizes of fully threaded cortical screws *(right).*

thread diameter (in millimeters). Commonly used screws in small animal surgery are 2.7- and 3.5-mm diameter cortical screws and 4.0-mm diameter cancellous screws. All these screws have hexagonal heads and are driven by the same hexagonal screwdriver. Smaller screws (1.5- and 2.0-mm diameter) have cruciate heads and require a small,

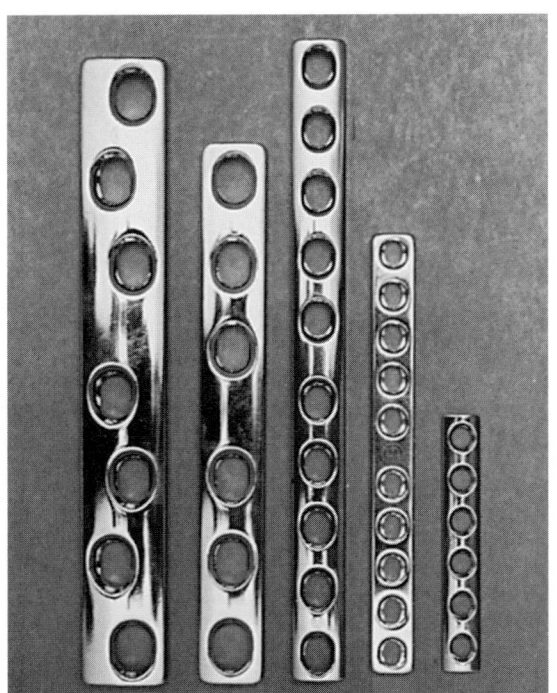

FIGURE 24-26.   Various sizes of bone plates.

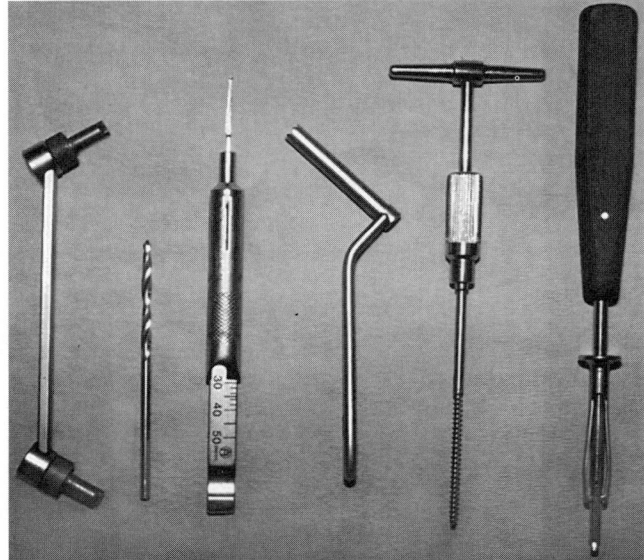

FIGURE 24-27.   Bone plating equipment. *Left to right,* Drill guide, drill bit, depth gauge, tap sleeve (to prevent soft tissues from being caught on the bone tap), bone tap, and screwdriver.

cruciate screwdriver. Larger screws (4.5-, 5.5-, and 6.5-mm diameter) are used in large animal surgery. These screws use a large hexagonal screwdriver.

Bone Plates

There are many different types of bone plates (Figure 24-26). Bone plates are named by the number of screw holes and by the screw diameter size that best fits the plate. For example, a seven-hole, 3.5-mm plate would use seven, 3.5-mm diameter screws. Bone plates must be bent to match the curve of the bone and fastened to it with bone screws. Instrumentation required to apply a bone plate is highly specialized and includes drills, drill bits, drill guides, depth gauges, bone taps, tap sleeves, screws, screwdrivers, and plate benders (Figure 24-27). Although bone plating is more complex than other types of orthopedic fixation, plate fixation is much more stable in most cases.

Arthroscopic Instruments and Equipment

The arthroscope is used as a diagnostic and surgical tool in veterinary surgery. It is used mostly to examine various joints of the horse, including the scapulohumeral, humeroradial, carpal, fetlock, distal interphalangeal, coxofemoral (foals only), stifle, and tarsocrural. It is also used to examine various joints in the dog. Arthroscopy is used primarily to remove osteochondral chip fragments and osteochondrotic lesions on the articular surface in joints of young horses and dogs. The arthroscope has been used to visualize intraarticular fractures for lag screw fixation, such as third carpal bone slab fractures in horses, as well as meniscal and cruciate injuries in dogs. The arthroscope has also been used to perform tenoscopy of the digital flexor tendon sheath and sinuscopy of the paranasal sinuses through trephined holes in the facial bones overlying the sinuses of horses. Most of the equipment used in veterinary arthroscopy has been adapted from human arthroscopy.

New technology is constantly being developed that will no doubt influence the veterinary field. This section is intended to allow the veterinary technician to become more familiar with the instruments and techniques of arthroscopy.

Arthroscope

There is a selection of different arthroscopes that have been developed with various diameters and viewing angles. For example, there is a 5-mm-OD (outer diameter) arthroscope with either a 10-, 25-, or 70-degree lens angle; a 4-mm OD with a 10-, 30-, 70-, or 110-degree lens angle; a 2.7-mm OD with a 5-, 30-, or 70-degree lens angle; and a 1.9-mm OD with a 5- or 30-degree lens angle. A 4-mm OD 25- or 30-degree angled lens scope is generally used by most equine surgeons (Figure 24-28), whereas a 2.7-mm-OD, 30-degree angled lens scope is commonly used for canine arthroscopy.

Ancillary Arthroscopic Equipment

Along with the arthroscope come various instruments used to introduce the scope into the joint and attachments for television viewing and fluid hookup. Stab incisions are made in the skin, over the joint space, through which the arthroscope and hand instruments will be inserted once the animal is positioned for surgery, and the site is surgically prepared (Figure 24-29).

SHARP TROCAR AND SLEEVE.   A pointed instrument called a sharp trocar is inserted inside a hollow, cannula-type instrument called the *sleeve* (Figure 24-30). The trocar and sleeve unit are used to penetrate the fibrous portion of the joint capsule through a stab incision (Figure 24-30).

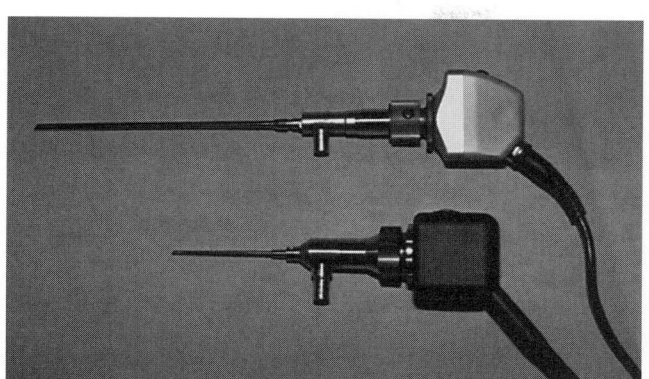

FIGURE 24-28. 4-mm–OD (outer diameter) and 2.7-mm–OD arthroscopes.

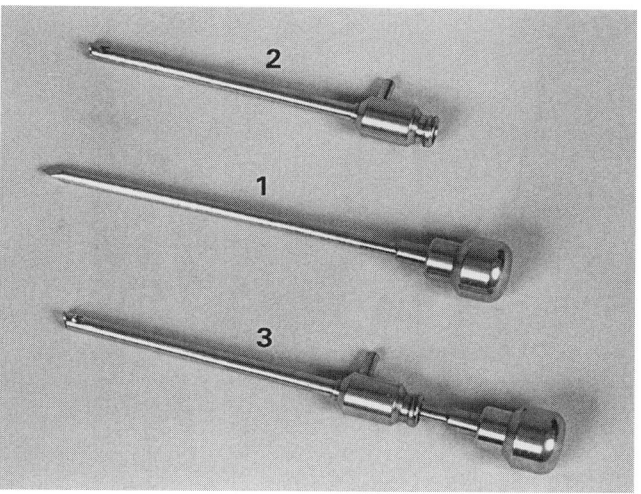

FIGURE 24-30. The sharp trocar *(1)* fits inside the arthroscope sleeve *(2)*. The unit *(3)* is used to penetrate the fibrous joint capsule through a stab incision in the skin.

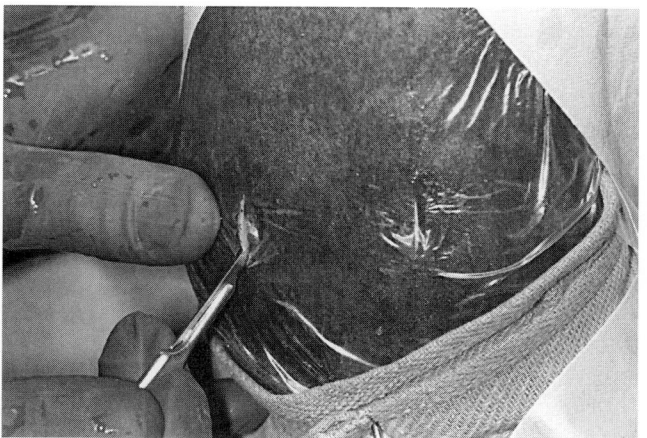

FIGURE 24-29. Stab incisions are made in the skin over the joint space, through which the arthroscope and hand instruments will be inserted.

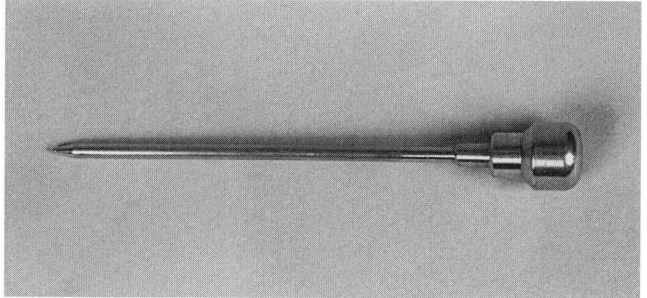

FIGURE 24-31. Conical (blunt) obturator.

BLUNT OBTURATOR. Once the sharp trocar has penetrated the fibrous joint capsule, the sharp trocar is replaced with a conical (blunt) obturator (Figure 24-31), which is used to penetrate the synovial membrane of the joint capsule and advance the sleeve into the joint space with less risk of damaging the articular cartilage (Figure 24-32). At this point the obturator is withdrawn from the sleeve. The joint space is distended with a sterile balanced electrolyte solution (fluids) before placement of the sleeve in the joint, so a rush of fluids through the barrel of the sleeve will occur as the obturator is being removed. The obturator is replaced with the arthroscope (Figure 24-33), which is designed to lock onto the sleeve once it is slid into position in the sleeve (Figure 24-34).

LIGHT CABLE, LIGHT PROJECTOR, AND TELEVISION CAMERA. Once the arthroscope is positioned in the joint a fiberoptic light cable (Figure 24-35) is attached directly to the optical light port on the arthroscope (Figure 24-36). A high-intensity light generated from a specially designed light projector is fed through the fiberoptic cable and through the arthroscope to illuminate the joint space (Figure 24-37). A television camera (Figure 24-38) then is attached to the eyepiece of the scope (Figure 24-39). Most arthroscopes today are coupled to a television camera, which allows the surgeon and surgical team to view the joint on a television monitor (Figure 24-40). A television monitor has the advantage of a larger image. This greatly improves visualization of the intraarticular space compared with direct viewing through the eyepiece of the arthroscope. This method also provides better aseptic technique, because the surgeon's face is not near the surgical field and an assistant can operate the camera-scope unit, allowing the surgeon more freedom. A monitor also allows several people to observe the procedure simultaneously, and a videotape record can be made for future replay.

Fluid Delivery Systems

Fluids, usually a balanced electrolyte solution, are infused into the joint under pressure to maintain distention of the

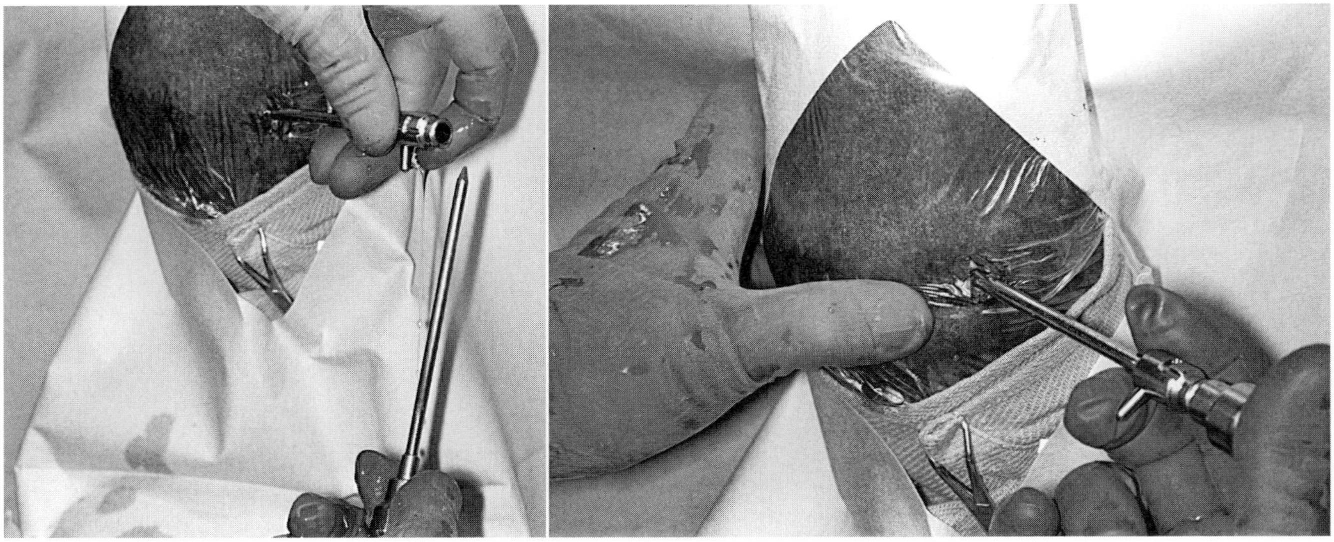

A

B

FIGURE 24-32.   The conical obturator replaces the sharp trocar in the sleeve and is used to penetrate the synovial membrane portion of the joint casule, **A,** and advance the sleeve further into the joint, **B.**

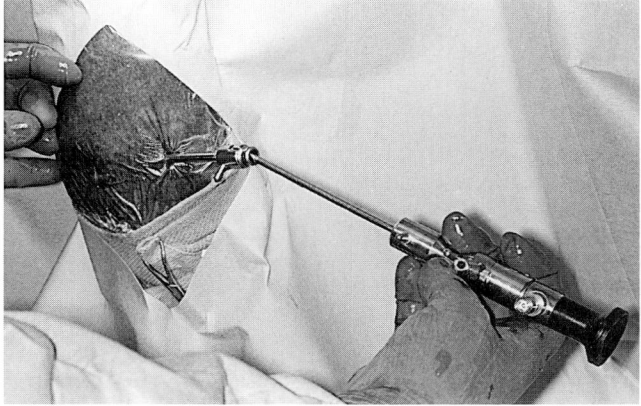

FIGURE 24-33.   Once the sleeve is in position in the joint, the obturator is removed and the arthroscope is placed into the sleeve.

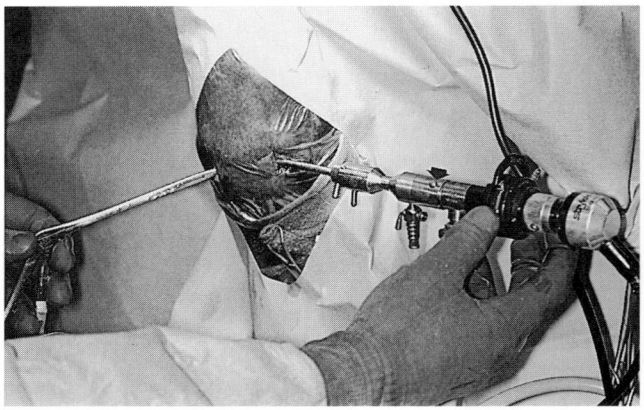

FIGURE 24-34.   The arthroscope is designed to lock *(arrow)* onto the sleeve to prevent dislodgement during surgery.

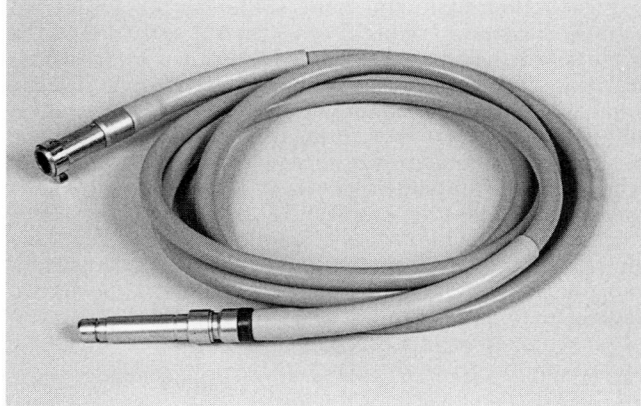

FIGURE 24-35.   Fiberoptic light cable. It should be handled very carefully to avoid damaging the optic fibers.

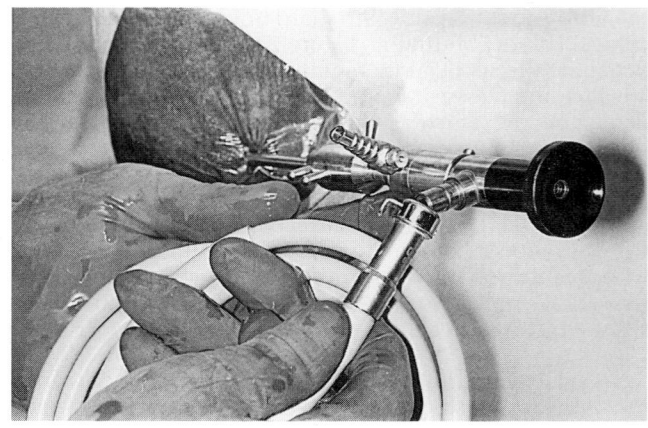

FIGURE 24-36.   The fiberoptic light cable attaches to the light port of the arthroscope.

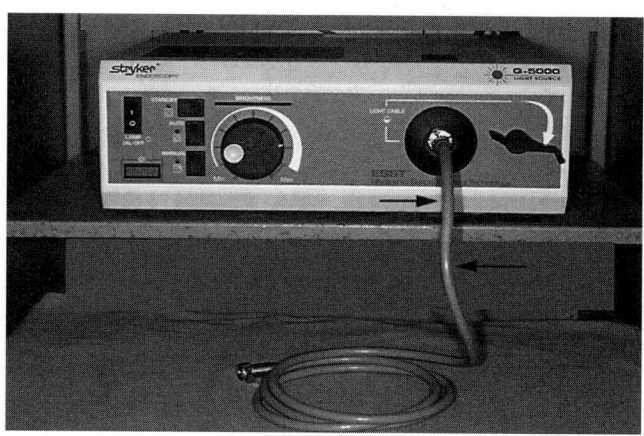

FIGURE 24-37. Light projector is designed to project light through a fiberoptic light cable *(arrow)* of the arthroscope.

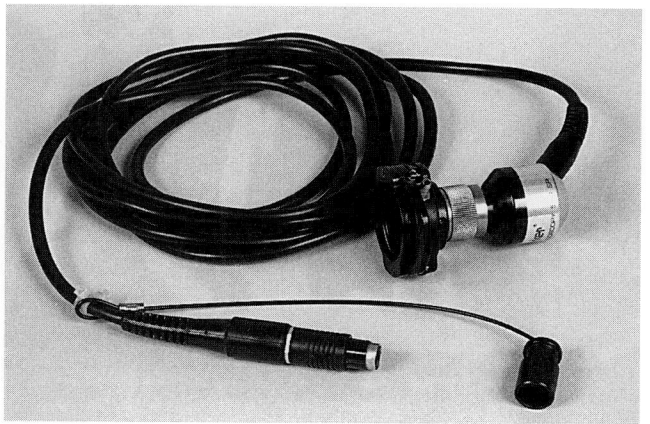

FIGURE 24-38. Television camera is designed for arthroscopic surgery.

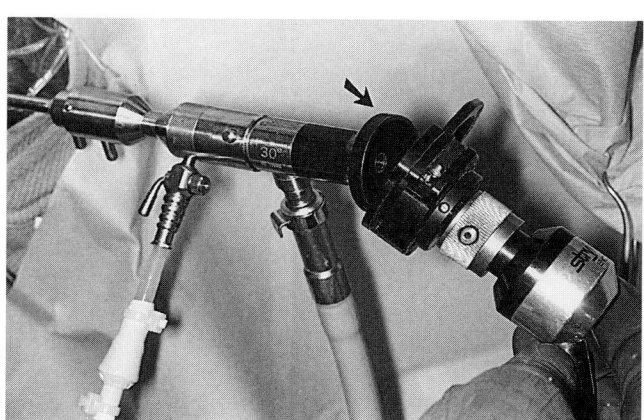

FIGURE 24-39. The television camera couples to the eyepiece *(arrow)* of the arthroscope.

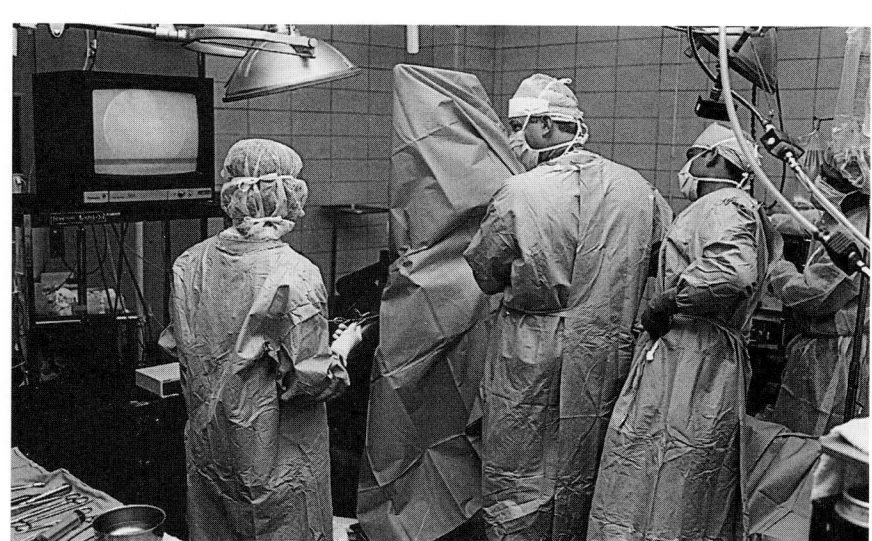

FIGURE 24-40. Most arthroscopic procedures are viewed on a television monitor.

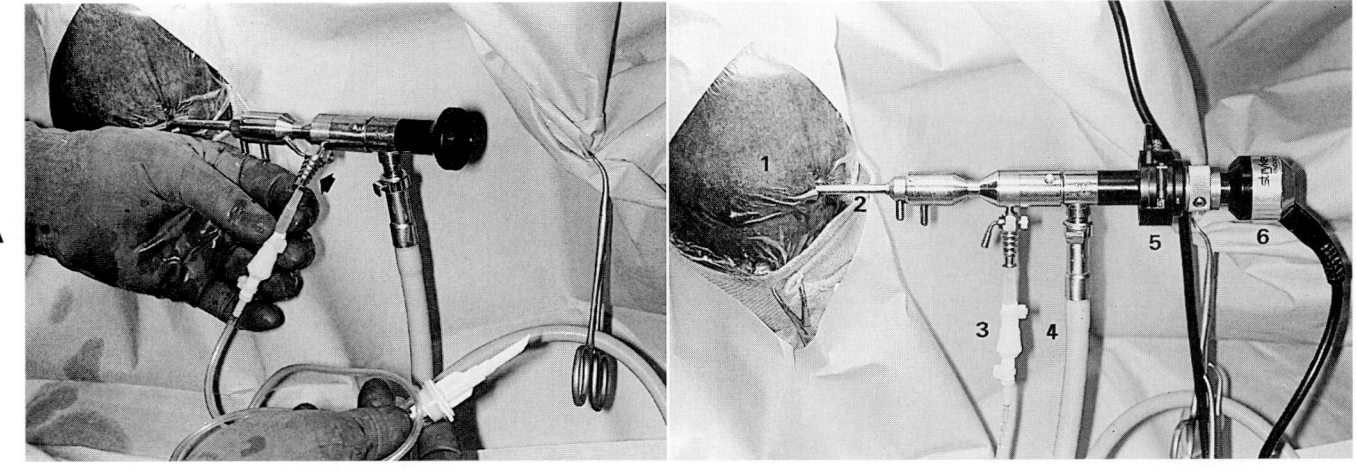

FIGURE 24-41.   **A,** The fluid line is connected to the stopcock of the arthroscope *(arrow).* **B,** Carpus of a horse *(1),* sleeve *(2),* fluid line *(3),* light cable *(4),* arthroscope *(5),* and camera *(6).*

joint capsule, which is essential for visualization of the intraarticular space. Gas insufflation, using carbon dioxide or nitrous oxide, has also been used as a method of distending the joint. However, a special system with a pressure-regulated device is required. One disadvantage of gas is that it does not allow for lavage of the joint space if osteochondral chip fragments become detached in the joint. The fluids are infused into the joint space through the sleeve, around the arthroscope. The sleeve has at least one stopcock that is used as an ingress port to connect a sterile fluid line (Figure 24-41).

PRESSURIZED BAG SYSTEM.   Various systems are available to deliver fluid to the joint. One system is a pressurized bag design. A pneumatic pressure cuff is slipped around a bag containing sterile fluids. The cuff is inflated with air, which squeezes the fluid bag, thus pressurizing the fluids (Figure 24-42). The amount of pressure is regulated by the amount of cuff inflation.

MOTORIZED PUMP SYSTEM.   Another type of system uses a motorized pump to regulate the fluid rate through the fluid lines connected to the arthroscope. One example of this type of system uses sterile silicone tubing that is threaded around the rollers of an infusion pump (Karl Storz Veterinary Endoscopy of America, Inc.) (Figure 24-43). The speed and fluid volume going into the joint are regulated by a foot pedal (Figure 24-43).

Automated pressure-sensitive pump systems are also available that incorporate a pressure feedback control. This allows the pump to maintain a preset pressure in the joint without the surgeon having to adjust the fluid pressure.

Hand Instruments for Arthroscopic Surgery

Numerous hand instruments of various types are available or have been adapted for arthroscopy. They are used to remove or retrieve osteochondral chip fragments, debride articular cartilage or subchondral bone, or probe cartilage or cartilage lesions. The instruments are inserted into the joint through a separate stab incision, and the arthroscopic operation is performed via a technique called *triangulation* (Figure 24-44). Only the most commonly used instruments are discussed here.

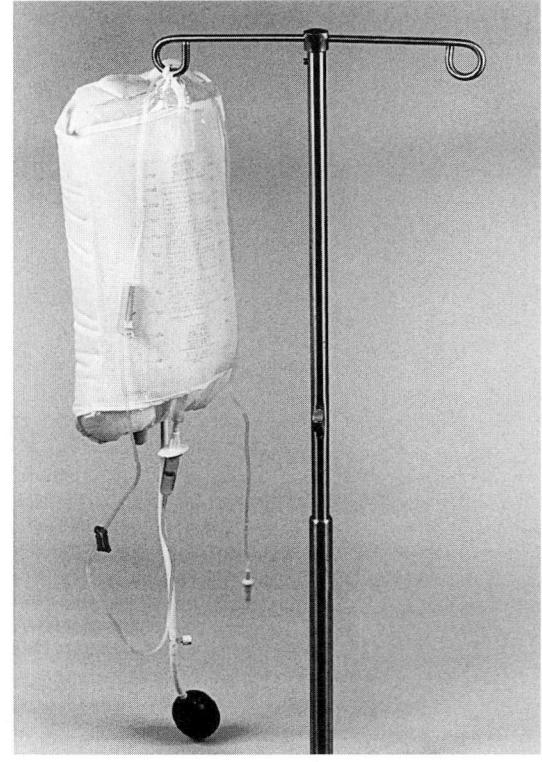

FIGURE 24-42.   Pressurized bag of fluids can be used to distend a joint during arthroscopy.

BLUNT PROBE.   The blunt probe is used to probe a site in the joint to determine such aspects as cartilage integrity or the extent of a cartilage lesion (Figure 24-45).

RONGEURS AND GRASPING FORCEPS.   Various types and sizes of rongeurs have been adapted for use in arthroscopy. These instruments have a beveled edge along the cupped jaws to cut the attachments of an osteochondral chip fragment as it is being removed (Figure 24-46). Forceps are

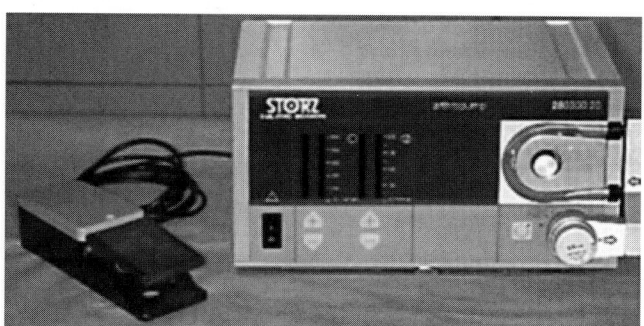

FIGURE 24-43. Infusion pump used to infuse sterile fluids into a joint during arthroscopy. The speed and amount of fluids going into the joint are regulated by a foot pedal.

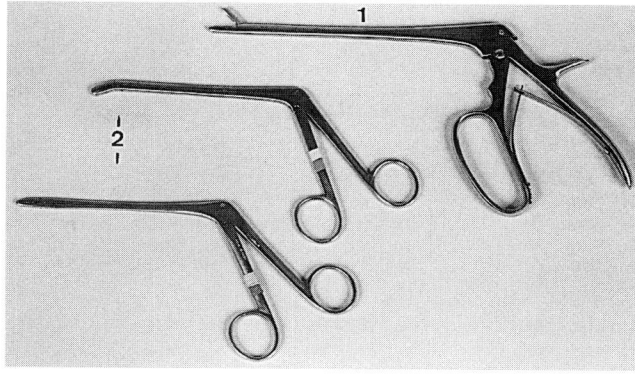

FIGURE 24-46. Rongeurs used in arthroscopy: Ferris Smith *(1)* and Love and Gruenwald *(2)*.

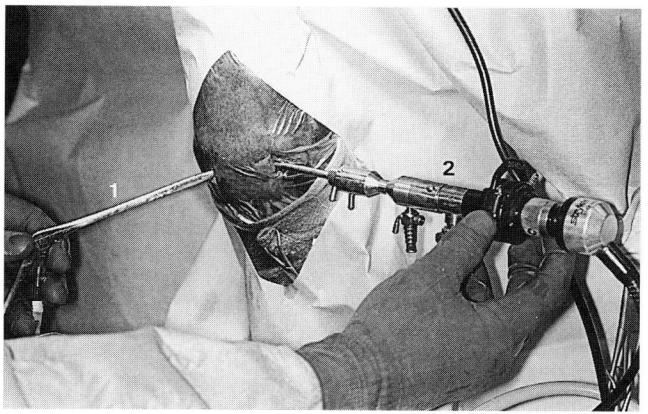

FIGURE 24-44. Arthroscopy is performed via triangulation of the hand instrument *(1)* and arthroscope *(2)* with the intraarticular lesion.

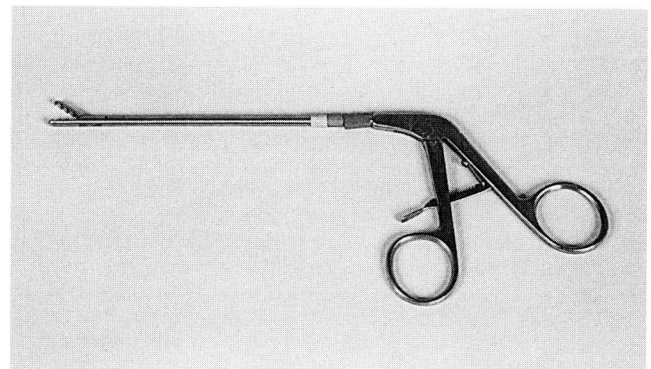

FIGURE 24-47. Forceps used in arthroscopy.

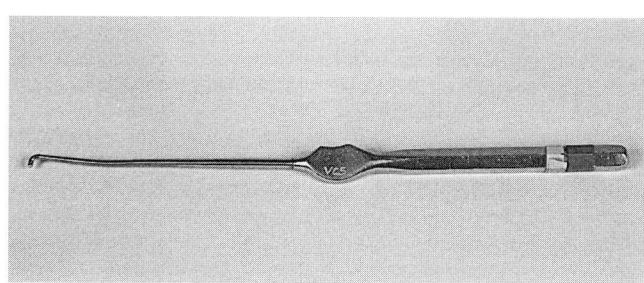

FIGURE 24-45. Blunt arthroscopy probe.

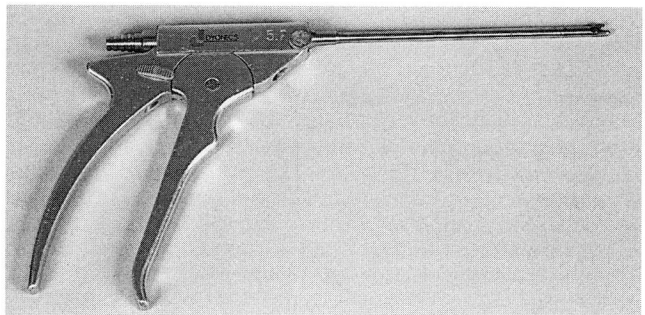

FIGURE 24-48. The Dyonics DynoVac suction forceps.

used primarily to retrieve loosely attached fragments (Figure 24-47). There are specially designed forceps that have a suction attachment to the hollow shaft of the instrument that allows evacuation of small fragments through the shaft as the surgeon grasps the fragments with the jaws of the instrument (Figure 24-48).

ELEVATORS AND OSTEOTOMES. These instruments have small beveled heads that are designed to cut or break down the attachments of an osteochondral chip fragment and

elevate it from the parent subchondral bone bed (Figure 24-49).

CURETTES. Curettes are inserted into the joint to debride a defect left in the articular cartilage or subchondral bone after removal of an osteochondral chip fragment or osteochondrotic lesion (Figure 24-50).

MOTORIZED BURRS. Motorized burrs are often referred to as a motorized arthroplasty system. The system consists of

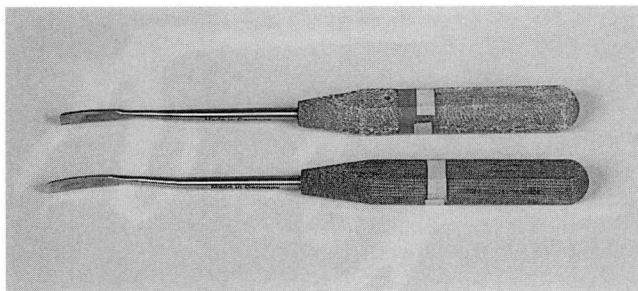

FIGURE 24-49. Elevator and osteotome used in arthroscopy.

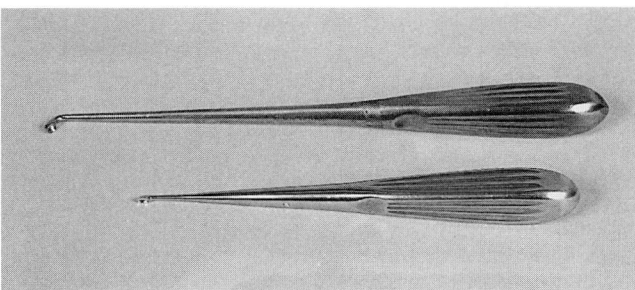

FIGURE 24-50. Small cupped bone curettes used in arthroscopy.

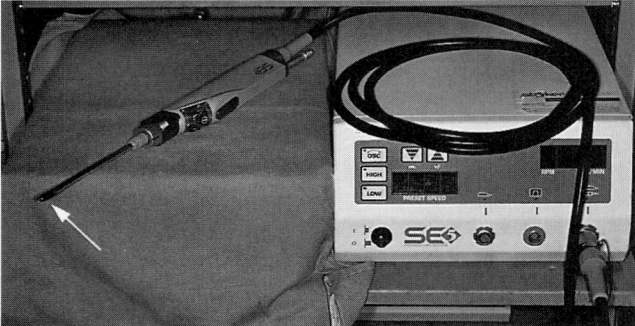

FIGURE 24-51. Motorized arthroplasty system with burr attachment *(arrow)*.

Box 24-1 SMALL ANIMAL INSTRUMENT PACKS

SOFT TISSUE/GENERAL PACK
No. 3 scalpel handle
Brown-Adson thumb forceps
Adson thumb forceps
Needle holder, Mayo-Hegar
Mayo scissors
Metzenbaum scissors
Wire suture scissors
Mosquito hemostats (4 curved, 4 straight)
Crile forceps (1 curved, 1 straight)
Carmalt forceps (2 curved)
Allis forceps (2)
Ovariohysterectomy hook (Snook hook)
Towel clamps (8)
Towels (6)
Stainless steel bowl
Sponges
Lap sponges (2)
Sterilization indicator

EMERGENCY PACK
No. 3 scalpel handle
Brown-Adson thumb forceps
Needle holder, Olsen-Hegar
Mayo scissors, curved
Mosquito hemostats (3 curved, 3 straight)
Crile or Kelly forceps (1 curved, 1 straight)
Allis forceps
Towel clamps (4)
Towels (4)
Sponges
Sterilization indicator

ORTHOPEDIC PACK
Army-Navy retractors
Senn retractors
Rongeurs
Large Kern bone-holding forceps
Small Kern bone-holding forceps
Bone curette
Periosteal elevator
Steinmann pins (5/64, 3/32, 7/64, 1/8, 9/64,
    5/32, 3/16, 1/4)
Kirschner wire (0.035, 0.045, 0.062)
Jacobs chuck and key
Roll 18-gauge stainless steel wire
Roll 20-gauge stainless steel wire
Roll 22-gauge stainless steel wire
Metal ruler
Michel clips and applicator
Sterilization indicator

a small rounded burr attached to a power-driven shaft. The burr and shaft are enclosed in a sleeve, with a portion of the burr protected to prevent inadvertent damage to surrounding articular cartilage (Figure 24-51). This instrument is also used to debride a defect left in the articular cartilage or subchondral bone after removal of an osteochondral chip fragment or osteochondrotic lesion. The speed of rotation of the burr can be adjusted, and the burr is usually operated at several thousand revolutions per minute. Most systems operate with an on/off foot pedal switch for the surgeon.

Instrument Packs

Most veterinary hospitals organize their surgical instruments into several different instrument packs based on the type of surgical procedure. Surgical pack organization depends on the type of practice and surgeries performed,

but some examples are as follows: general packs for soft tissue surgeries, bone packs for orthopedic surgeries, emergency packs for emergency and minor procedures, and neurologic packs for spinal surgeries (Boxes 24-1 and 24-2). A pack system helps to organize the instruments so the most commonly used instruments are readily available and infrequently used instruments are not contaminated and resterilized unnecessarily. For example, all commonly used instruments for spinal surgery are in one pack so it is opened, used, cleaned, sterilized, and repacked only when necessary. Infrequently used instruments are typically wrapped individually. Large and bulky instruments are also packed separately.

Box 24-2   LARGE ANIMAL STANDARD AND EMERGENCY PACKS

STANDARD PACK
No. 3 scalpel handle
No. 4 scalpel handle
Rat-tooth thumb forceps (3)
Adson thumb forceps (3)
Needle holders (2)
Mayo scissors (1 curved, 1 straight)
Operating scissors (sharp-sharp)
Metzenbaum scissors (1 curved, 1 straight)
Bandage scissors
Mosquito hemostats (4 straight, 4 curved)
Kelly or Crile forceps (2 straight, 2 curved)
Ochsner forceps, 15-cm (1 curved, 1 straight)
Allis tissue forceps (2)
Towel clamps (16)
Towels (4)
Saline bowl
Sponges
Sterilization indicator

EMERGENCY PACK
No. 3 scalpel handle
No. 4 scalpel handle
Rat-tooth thumb forceps
Brown-Adson thumb forceps
Needle holder
Mayo scissors (1 curved, 1 straight)
Mosquito hemostats (2 curved, 2 straight)
Allis tissue forceps (2)
Towel clamps (4)
Towel
Sponges
Sterilization indicator

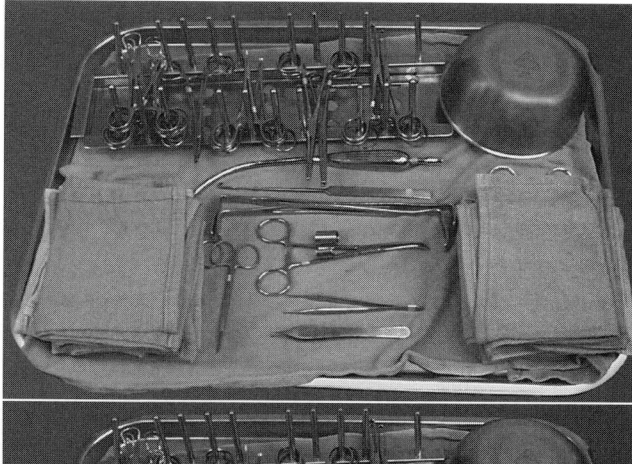
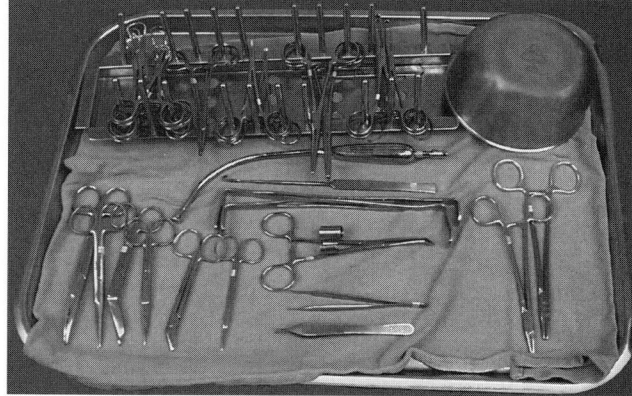

FIGURE 24-52. **A,** Properly organized instrument tray. **B,** Same tray but towels have been removed.

Each type of pack should be organized such that items are always placed in the same location on the tray (Figure 24-52). This makes it easier to inventory the instruments and facilitates finding the instruments quickly during surgery.

Instrument care

Most surgical instruments are made of stainless steel, which is rust resistant and retains a sharp edge. The two common instrument finishes are polished or satin. The polished finish is durable but tends to reflect light, which may impair the surgeon's vision. The satin or dull finish was developed to eliminate glare, but it is less resistant to spotting and discoloration.

Good-quality instruments are expensive but will last for years if treated properly. All instruments should be handled gently, and delicate instruments should be separated from the general instruments before cleaning. Multiple-component instruments should be disassembled before cleaning. Power equipment should be cleaned separately to ensure that water does not get inside the components.

Immediately after use, instruments should be rinsed with cold water to prevent blood and organic debris from drying in the serrations, hinges, box locks, or ratchets. Each instrument is scrubbed with a soft brush in warm water using a neutral pH instrument detergent. Abrasive cleaning agents should never be used on surgical instruments. Saline solutions are corrosive to stainless steel, so instruments should be rinsed with deionized or distilled water.

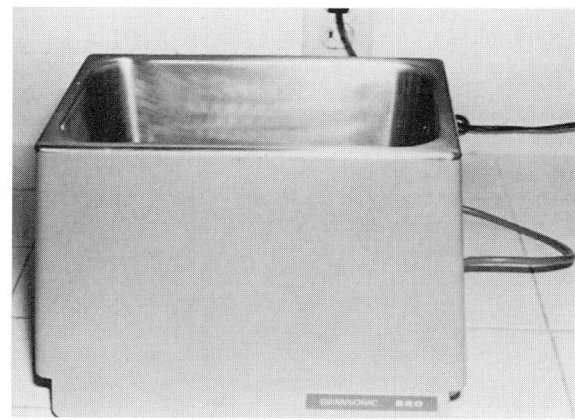

FIGURE 24-53. Ultrasonic cleaner. The instruments are placed in water inside the tub.

An ultrasonic (high-frequency sound) cleaner (Figure 24-53) is used after manual cleaning to remove tightly bound soil or clean areas that the brush cannot reach. Instruments should be thoroughly rinsed and dried before autoclaving to prevent rust spots.

Instruments with a working action, such as a hinge or box lock, should be treated with an instrument lubricant or instrument "milk" after each cleaning. The recommended lubricants are water soluble, so thorough cleaning will remove all the lubrication. Instrument lubricants are not oily or sticky, inhibit rust formation, and do not interfere with steam sterilization. Working components of power equipment should also be lubricated to maximize efficiency and to prolong the working lifetime of the equipment. Before instruments are repacked for sterilization they should be thoroughly inspected for cleanliness, stiff or "frozen" hinges, improper jaw alignment, and worn or broken parts.

Drapes and Gowns

Surgical drapes and gowns may be paper or cloth. Paper drapes and gowns are designed to be disposable and should be used only once. They are bought prepackaged and sterilized for individual use. Cloth drapes and gowns are designed for repeated use, but they require washing after each use. Immediately soaking the cloth in cold water will prevent blood and other fluids from setting. All cloth drapes and gowns should be washed in a mild detergent and thoroughly dried before sterilization.

> **Technician Note**
>
> Accordion folding of drape allows easy unfolding and placement on the patient.

Cloth gowns must always be folded and packed in the same manner (Figure 24-54). This technique allows the sterile gown to be unfolded and put on without contaminating it. Cloth drapes must also be folded and packed such that sterility can be maintained while they are unfolded and applied to the patient. Accordion folding allows easy unfolding and placement of the drape (Figure 24-55). Many specifically designed drapes are also available, including adhesive drapes, transparent drapes, fenestrated drapes, stockinettes, and compressive wraps. After the drapes and gowns have been properly folded, they are usually double-wrapped in paper or cloth before sterilization (Figure 24-56).

ASEPTIC TECHNIQUE

Asepsis is a condition of sterility in which no living organisms are present. Aseptic technique includes all steps taken to prevent contamination of the surgical site by infectious agents. A thorough understanding of aseptic technique is required to properly sterilize the surgical equipment and clean the operating room. Certain principles of aseptic technique must also be followed when scrubbing the surgical site and placing sterile drapes on the patient. The technician may need to act as a circulating nurse by getting the patient in the operating room and opening sterile equipment for the surgeon. In addition, the technician may be called on to "scrub in" as a scrub nurse or surgical assistant to organize and pass instruments to the surgeon or to assist with the surgical procedure. A working knowledge of aseptic technique is necessary to perform these tasks correctly and also to monitor for inadvertent breaks in sterile technique.

Microorganisms must be introduced into the surgical site for infection to develop. The sources of microorganisms include exogenous and endogenous routes. Exogenous sources of contamination include the air, the surgical instruments and supplies, the patient's skin, and the surgical team. Endogenous contamination arises from within the patient and reaches the wound through the blood-stream. Examples of endogenous sources are bacteria from gingivitis or dermatitis.

During every surgery, some bacterial contamination occurs at the surgical site. Whether the contamination progresses to an infection depends on many factors, including the general health of the patient, the degree of tissue damage in the wound, the virulence of the infectious agent, and the number of infectious agents. The factor over which the surgical team has the most control is the number of infectious agents that are introduced into the wound by an exogenous route. Strict adherence to the principles of aseptic technique will minimize exogenous wound contamination and prevent many infections from developing.

All procedures do not require the same degree of vigilance regarding aseptic technique. For example, the debridement of a cutaneous abscess is considered to be a contaminated or dirty surgery so aseptic technique would not be strictly followed. The wound would be scrubbed, but surgical instruments may be disinfected (cold sterilization) rather than sterilized (steam autoclave or gas sterilization), and the surgeon may wear sterile gloves but forgo complete sterile surgical attire. It may be preferable for such a patient to remain outside the operating room to prevent contaminating it. In contrast, total hip replacement surgery involves the implantation of synthetic material and infection can be devastating to the success of the surgery. In such cases, the surgical team adheres strictly to aseptic protocol. The surgeon will determine the degree to which the principles of asepsis are to be followed for each case.

STERILIZATION.   *Sterilization* is the destruction of all organisms and spores on an object. *Disinfection* is the destruction of the vegetative forms of bacteria but not the spores. Both sterilization and disinfection are used to prepare medical and surgical materials. The process used depends on the nature of the material and its intended use. Methods of sterilization and disinfection can be classified as either physical or chemical.

Physical Methods of Sterilization

The three general physical methods used for sterilization are filtration, radiation, and heat. Filtration and radiation are primarily used during the production and packaging of certain surgical products.

Filtration

Filtration is the use of a filter to separate particulate material from liquids or gases. Pharmaceuticals are commonly sterilized by filtration.

Radiation

Some materials that would be damaged by other methods of sterilization can be safely sterilized by radiation. Radiation destroys microorganisms without causing any significant temperature elevation. Gloves and some suture materials are sterilized by radiation during the manufacturing process.

Thermal Energy

The most common method used for sterilization is heat. The mechanism by which heat destroys microorganisms is not completely understood, but it is believed that death is the result of protein denaturation. This is probably a gradual process and may be reversible during the early stages of sterilization. The thermal susceptibility of micro-

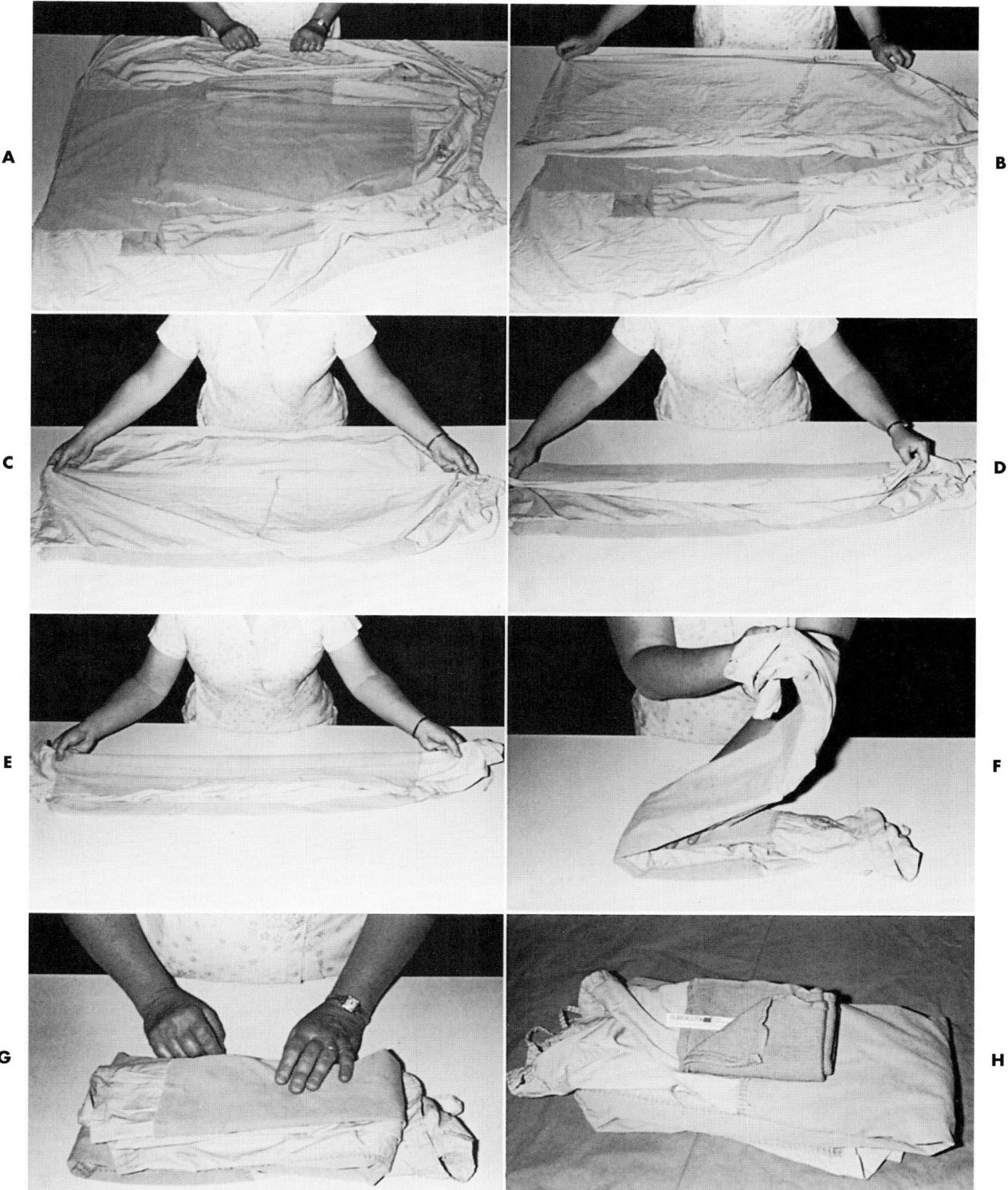

FIGURE 24-54. Method of folding a cloth surgical gown. **A,** The gown is spread on a countertop with the outside of the gown facing up. **B,** The near edge of the gown is folded to the center. **C,** Next, the far edge of the gown is folded toward the center to meet the near edge. **D,** The gown is folded in half. **E,** The gown is folded in half again. **F** and **G,** The gown is folded lengthwise in accordion fashion into thirds. **H,** A hand towel and sterilization indicator are placed on top, and the gown is ready for wrapping.

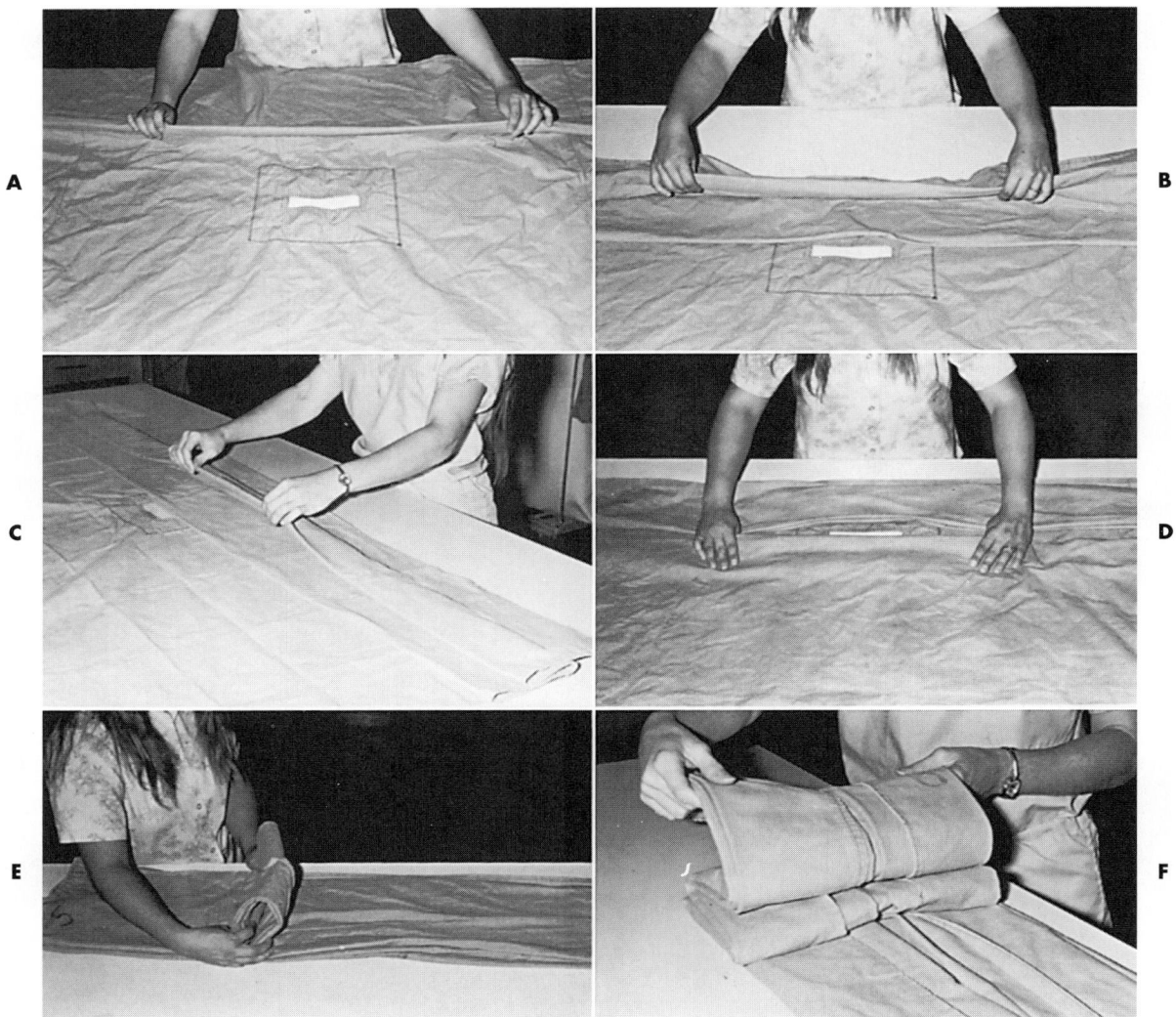

FIGURE 24-55.   Cloth drapes are folded in accordion fashion so that they are easily unfolded onto the patient. **A** to **C,** One side of the drape is folded to the center in accordion fashion. Each fold is approximately 15 cm wide. **D,** The opposite side is folded in a similar manner. **E** and **F,** Lengthwise, the drape is again folded to the center in accordion fashion. These folds are also approximately 15 cm in width.   *Continued*

organisms is influenced by several factors, including inherent resistance, individual variation, and age (young bacteria are more susceptible). There is no one temperature at which all microorganisms are killed instantly because death of bacteria and spores is a function of temperature and duration of heat.

The two basic types of heat sterilization are moist heat and dry heat. Dry heat is used to sterilize materials that cannot tolerate moist heat but can withstand high temperatures. Oils, powders, and petroleum products are most effectively sterilized by dry heat, whereas rubber, fabrics, and some metals may be damaged by the high temperatures. An advantage of dry heat is that it will not rust or corrode needles or sharp instruments. Dry heat is more difficult to control than moist heat, and the sterilization time is longer.

Both dry heat and moist heat destroy bacteria through protein denaturation; however, dry heat kills by protein oxidation whereas moist heat kills by coagulation of critical cellular proteins. Moisture facilitates the coagulation of proteins; thus moist heat kills bacteria and spores at lower temperatures and shorter exposures than dry heat.

Moist heat sterilization is accomplished either by boiling water or by steam under pressure. Boiling water at ambient pressures is not a reliable means of sterilization because of its relatively low temperature. The bactericidal effect of boiling water can be enhanced by alkalinization with sodium hydroxide (0.1 g/dl) or sodium carbonate (2 g/dl). The addition of these agents reduces instrument corrosion, but they cannot be used with glassware or rubber goods. Boiling water probably results in disinfection rather than sterilization and is rarely used.

The most common method of sterilization is saturated steam under pressure. Increased pressure causes steam to achieve a higher temperature. Materials to be sterilized in this manner must be penetrable by steam and not dam-

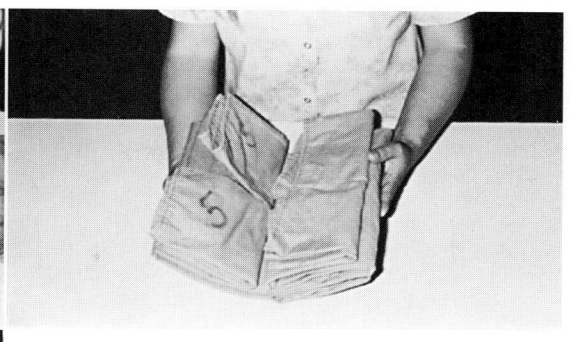

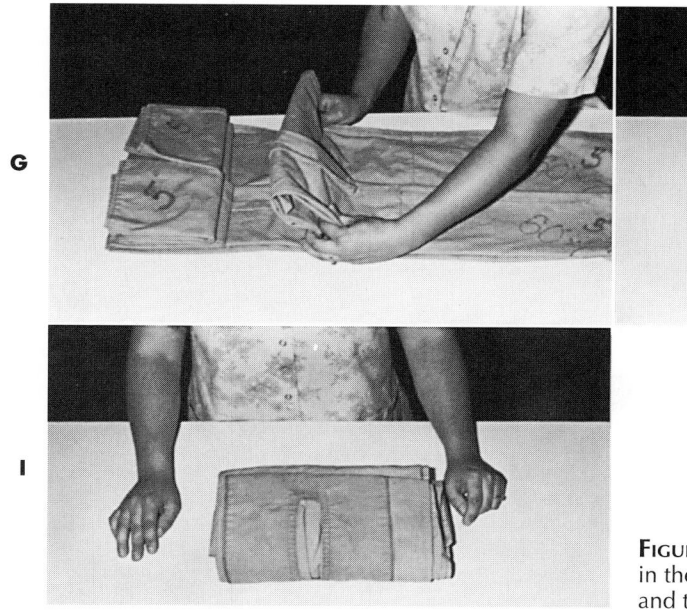

FIGURE 24-55, CONT'D. G, The opposite side is folded in the same manner. **H,** The two sides are folded together, and the drape is ready for wrapping, **I.**

aged by heat or moisture. Sterilizers that employ steam under pressure are called *autoclaves* (Figure 24-57).

AUTOCLAVE STERILIZATION. Autoclave sterilization is technique sensitive, so operating instructions accompanying the autoclave should be followed. An autoclave load is not sterile unless the steam has penetrated the packs completely so that all materials have been exposed to steam at the proper temperature and for the proper duration. Adequate steam penetration requires that the packs be properly prepared and loaded into the autoclave.

Proper pack preparation begins by checking that all materials are thoroughly clean and free from grease, oil, or protein residues. Packs must be properly wrapped with steam-permeable wrappers. Double-thickness muslin (thread count of 140 threads per 6.45 cm²) is a good wrapping material and will protect the surgical supplies following sterilization. Paper (crepe) can also be used as a wrapping material. Each pack must be labeled as to the pack contents, the person who prepared it, and the date it was sterilized.

Materials need to be packed as loosely as is practical to ensure good steam penetration. There should be 2.5 to 7.5 cm of space around each pack, and packs should be arranged to allow steam to flow readily from top to bottom. For example, a large pack should not be placed on top of several small ones because it will block the flow of steam down to the smaller packs. Steam flow may be facilitated by positioning packs vertically (on edge). It is recommended that packs be no larger than 30 cm × 30 cm × 50 cm and weigh no more than 5.4 kg, depending on the type of material being autoclaved. In many practices, the pack size is limited by the size of the autoclave.

A number of minimum time-temperature standards have been established for routine sterilization of surgical packs. Exposure to saturated steam at 121° C (250° F) for 13 minutes is considered to be a safe minimum standard. Five to ten minutes at 121° C will destroy most resistant microbes, and an additional 3 to 8 minutes provides a margin of safety. When the temperature in the exhaust line reaches the desired level the entire contents of the sterilizing chamber have been exposed to steam, so this is the beginning of exposure time. The time required to reach the sterilizing temperature is referred to as the heat-up time and is extremely short (about 1 minute) in prevacuum and pulsing-type sterilizers. Large linen packs require both a longer heat-up time and a longer exposure time. They should be saturated for 30 to 45 minutes at 121° C (250° F) in gravity displacement sterilizers and 4 minutes at 131° C (270° F) in prevacuum sterilizers.

Emergency sterilization, also called *flash sterilization,* is usually performed in prevacuum sterilizers. The recommended exposure time is 3 minutes at 131° C (270° F). The unwrapped instruments are placed in a perforated metal tray for sterilization and then carried to the operating room using detachable handles.

Technician Note

The safe minimal standard for autoclave sterilization is 121° C (250° F) for 13 minutes.

After sterilization, the autoclave door is unlocked and "cracked" open. If the autoclave door is opened wide, the cool outside air will condense the steam in the materials, making them soggy. About 10 minutes after cracking the door, the remaining moisture will have vaporized and escaped, leaving the contents thoroughly dry. Paper-wrapped products should not be left in the autoclave more than 15 to 20 minutes after cracking the door. If products are left too long, the heat will dry the paper, making it brittle and likely to crack and split when handled.

STERILIZATION QUALITY CONTROL. The only assurance that sterilization has been achieved is through proper technique and the use of dependable sterilization indicators. Indicators should always be checked before using the materials. There are four types of sterilization indicators used in autoclaves: (1) autoclave tape, (2) fusible melting

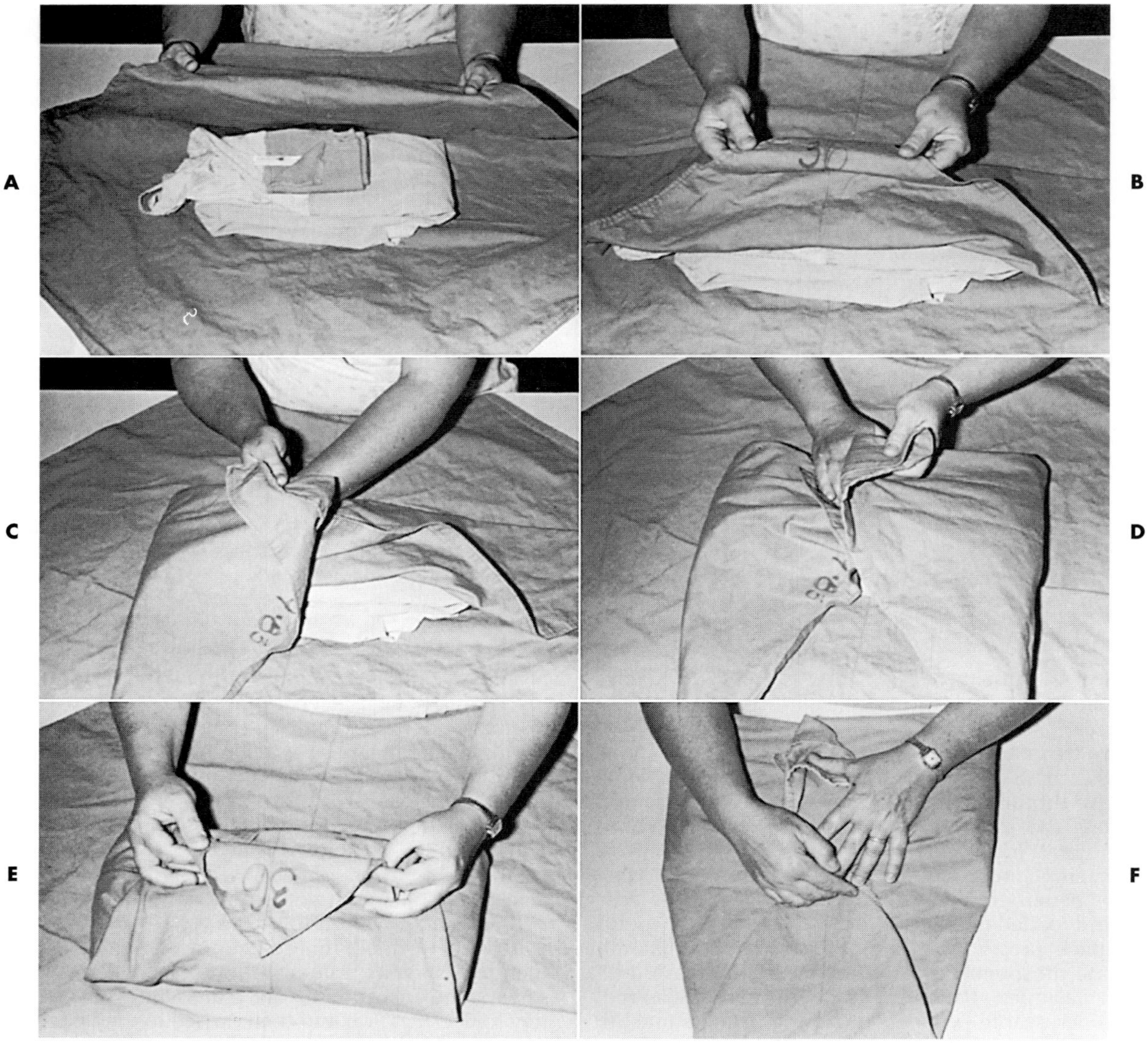

FIGURE 24-56. Wrapping a cloth drape or gown. **A,** The gown, along with a hand towel and sterilization indicator, is placed diagonally onto the drapes. **B** to **E,** The corners are folded over the gown. **F,** Three corners of the second drape are folded in a similar manner.

Continued

pellet glass type, (3) culture tests, and (4) chemical sterilization indicators. These indicators are meant to be used in combination because no one test alone can provide quality assurance of sterility.

Autoclave tape is useful for identifying packs and articles that have been exposed to steam, but it does not indicate whether the proper requirements of time, temperature, and steam have been met (Figure 24-58). The fusible melting pellet glass type indicates that a temperature of approximately 118° C (244° F) was reached but does not indicate whether proper time or steam saturation was achieved. Culture test indicators are strips that contain a controlled-count spore population of some particular strain of bacterium. This biologic challenge test is useful since it is the only test that proves microorganisms were killed. The disadvantages of this test are that the results are not immediately available and it does not assess steam penetration. Chemical sterilization indicators are available in

many types (Figure 24-59), and they undergo color changes when subjected to saturated steam for adequate periods of time. Most practices will use a combination of autoclave tape on the outside of the pack and a chemical sterilization indicator within the center of the pack to assess sterility.

Technician Note

The four types of sterilization indicators are autoclave tape, melting pellet glass, culture tests, and chemical sterilization indicators.

In the newer *prevacuum sterilizers,* an air removal test can be run daily to ensure that air is sufficiently removed from the autoclave. In *gravity displacement sterilizers,* temperature graphs can be kept as a record of autoclave performance.

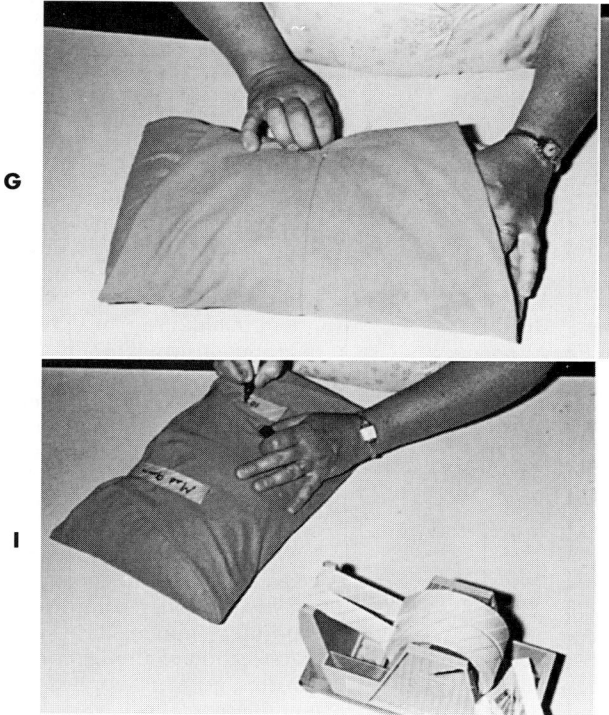

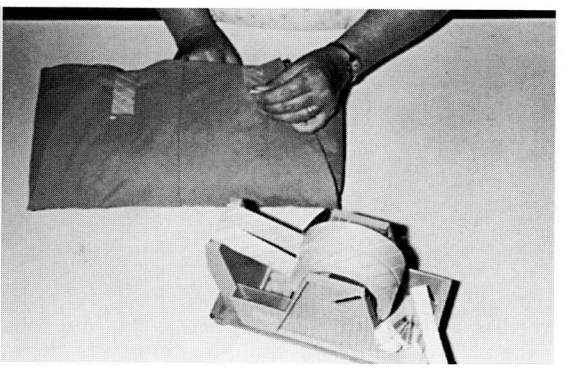

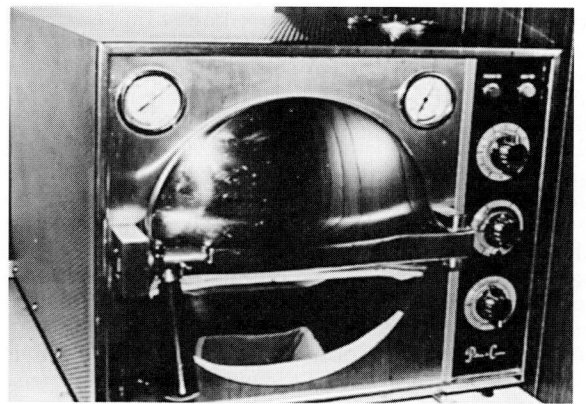

FIGURE 24-56, CONT'D.   G, The remaining corner is folded under and then folded over the top. **H,** The pack is secured with autoclave tape and is labeled with contents, date, and the initials of the individual preparing the pack **(I).**

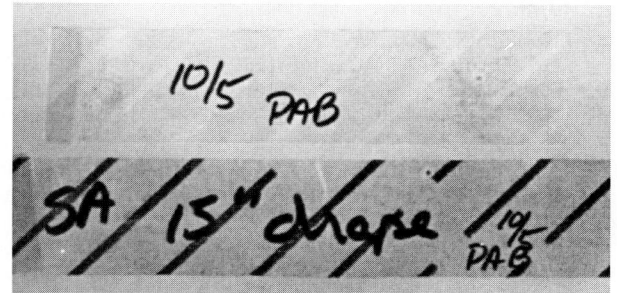

FIGURE 24-57.   Autoclave.

FIGURE 24-58.   Autoclave tape before *(above)* and after *(below)* sterilization. Note the appearance of the black line stripes.

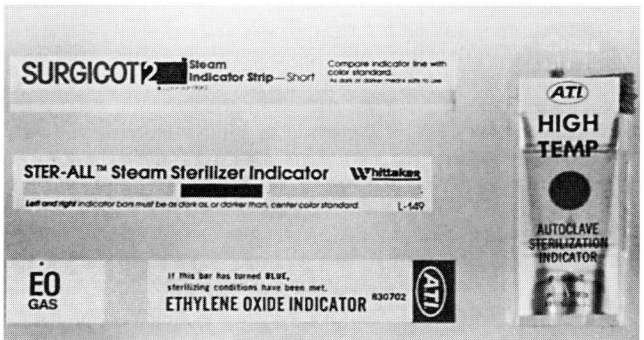

FIGURE 24-59.   Various sterilization indicator strips.

TABLE 24-3	SAFE STORAGE TIMES FOR STERILE PACKS	
Wrapper	**Closed Cabinet**	**Open Cabinet**
Single-wrapped muslin	1 wk	2 days
Double-wrapped muslin	7 wk	3 wk
Single-wrapped crepe paper	At least 8 wk	3 wk

Therefore quality assurance occurs at two levels, one to ensure that the pack runs through a sterilization cycle and another to ensure that the autoclave system is working properly. Quality control is essential for any surgical practice, because failure of proper sterilization can have far-reaching consequences.

CARE AND HANDLING OF STERILE PACKS.   Sterile packs should be stored in a dust-free, dry, and well-ventilated area away from contaminated equipment. Closed cabinets provide a cleaner storage area than open shelving. Safe pack storage times are listed in Table 24-3. If a pack is dropped, the tape sealing the pack is broken, or the pack wrap becomes wet, punctured, or torn, the pack should be considered contaminated. If there is any doubt as to the sterility of an item, consider it unsterile.

Technician Note

Ethylene oxide is the most commonly used type of chemical sterilization, and good ventilation is critical.

Chemical Methods of Sterilization

Chemical sterilization is performed with certain liquids or gases. Liquid chemicals can be used for instrument sterilization. The most common agent used for liquid sterilization is glutaraldehyde. Gas sterilization is used for items that cannot tolerate the high temperatures or steam associated with autoclaving (some power equipment or plastic products). The most common agent used for gas sterilization is ethylene oxide.

Ethylene Oxide

Ethylene oxide is a colorless gas at room temperature. It is flammable, explosive, toxic, irritating to skin and mucous membranes, and therefore a potential health hazard. Ethylene oxide penetrates paper and plastic film packaging. The item to be gas sterilized is wrapped in plastic packaging (polyethylene, polypropylene, or polyvinyl chloride) and heat sealed before sterilization.

Ethylene oxide destroys metabolic pathways within the cells by alkylation, and it is capable of killing all microorganisms. Effective sterilization with ethylene oxide depends on the concentration of gas, exposure time, temperature, and relative humidity. Ethylene oxide activity is enhanced by increasing the temperature or the gas concentration. Ethylene oxide sterilizers usually operate at temperatures between 21° C and 60° C (70° F and 140° F). The activity of ethylene oxide approximately doubles with each 10° C increase in temperature. Doubling the ethylene oxide concentration decreases the sterilization time by approximately one half. Moisture is necessary for the lethal action of ethylene oxide, and optimal relative humidity for sterilization with ethylene oxide is 40%. Exposure time

TABLE 24-4	GLOSSARY OF KEY TERMS
Term	**Definition**
Antiseptic	An agent capable of preventing infection by inhibiting the growth of infectious agents; term generally applied to living tissues
Autoclave	Sterilizer that uses saturated steam under pressure to achieve high temperatures for sterilization; minimal exposure to saturated steam: 13 min at 121° C (250° F)
Disinfectant	An agent that destroys or inhibits microorganisms; typically refers to inanimate objects
Ethylene oxide	A gas chemical sterilization agent used to sterilize objects that cannot withstand heat; a good exhaust system must be used
Flash sterilization	Emergency sterilization in which object (instrument) is placed unwrapped in an autoclave and taken directly to the surgery following sterilization; recommended exposure: 3 min at 131° C (270° F)
Sterilization	The destruction of all microorganisms; generally applied to inanimate objects

varies from 48 minutes to several hours, but 12 hours of exposure is commonly used when sterilizing at room temperature.

After ethylene oxide sterilization, materials should be quarantined in a well-ventilated area for a minimum of 24 hours. Color-coded chemical sterilization indicators are commonly placed within the packs when using ethylene oxide sterilization (see Figure 24-59). Biologic indicators are available for ethylene oxide sterilization and are the only truly reliable test for sterility. Because results are unavailable for several days, biologic indicators are most commonly used to evaluate the sterilization system and not individual packs.

Gas plasma sterilization is quickly replacing ethylene oxide because it is safer for the environment and personnel. Many hospitals have converted to this system. The chlorofluorocarbon component (CFC-12) of 12/88 ethylene oxide systems was banned by the U.S. Food and Drug Administration (FDA) in 1996 and is no longer manufactured. Therefore many hospitals had to recalibrate their ethylene oxide system or convert to a gas plasma system.

Chemical Disinfection

A *disinfectant* is an agent that destroys bacteria or inactivates viruses. Disinfectants are chemical agents that are applied to inanimate objects to destroy the vegetative form of bacteria but not necessarily the spore forms. Disinfectants that are capable of destroying vegetative bacteria plus spores, tubercle bacilli, and viruses may be used as chemical sterilizers.

Disinfection time is the time required for a particular agent to produce its maximum effect. It is influenced by many factors, including the nature of the material being disinfected, the degree of soil and microbial contamination, and the concentration and germicidal potency of the disinfectant.

TABLE 24-5   COMMON ANTISEPTIC AND DISINFECTANT AGENTS

Agent	Examples	Common Uses	Spectrum of Activity	Residual Activity
Povidone-iodine detergent	Betadine scrub (Purdue-Frederick) (brown sudsy solution)	Preoperative scrubs	Bacteria, viruses, fungi, protozoa, yeast	4-6 hr, but inactivated by organic debris and alcohol
Povidone-iodine solution	Betadine solution (Purdue-Frederick) (brown solution)	Preoperative antiseptic application; wound lavage when diluted 1:100	Bacteria, viruses, fungi, protozoa, yeast	4-6 hr, but inactivated by organic debris and alcohol
Chlorhexidine detergent	Nolvasan scrub (Fort Dodge Laboratories) (blue solution), Hibiclens scrub (Stuart Pharmaceuticals) (pink solution)	Preoperative scrubs	Bacteria, viruses, fungi, yeast	2 days; not inhibited by organic matter or alcohol; less skin irritation
Chlorhexidine solution	Nolvasan solution (Fort Dodge Laboratories) (nonsudsy, blue solution)	Preoperative antiseptic application; wound lavage when diluted 1:40	Bacteria, viruses, fungi, yeast	2 days; bactericidal but not cytotoxic in open wounds at diluted concentrations
Alcohol: isopropyl and ethanol	Many manufacturers	Surgical preparations; disinfection antisepsis; do not use in open wounds	Bacteria, some fungi	None
Phenol: hexachlorophene	pHisoHex scrub (Sanofi; Winthrop) (white)	Preoperative hand scrub	Bacteria (more effective against gram-positive than gram-negative species)	Up to 2 days
Phenol: glutaraldehyde		Cold sterilization; not intended for living tissues	Bacteria, viruses, fungi, yeast, spores	None; causes skin irritation

Antisepsis is the prevention of infection by inhibiting the growth of infectious agents. Antiseptic agents, such as iodine or chlorhexidine, are substances used on living tissue to effect antisepsis. A glossary of key terms used in describing aseptic technique is given in Table 24-4.

Antiseptic and Disinfectant Compounds

IODINE.   Iodine compounds are effective antimicrobial agents but have limited activity against bacterial spores. Iodine solutions are used for surgical preparation, topical wound therapy, and joint and body cavity lavage (Table 24-5). Iodine compounds are available as aqueous solutions, tinctures, and iodophors. *Aqueous solutions* contain higher levels of free iodine than iodophors and therefore have greater bactericidal activity. However, aqueous solutions are also cytotoxic and cannot be used in living tissue unless they are greatly diluted. Aqueous iodine also stains materials and is corrosive to instruments.

Tincture of iodine is a solution of 2% iodine in 50% ethyl alcohol and is intended for use on intact skin. It is not commonly used in veterinary practices.

Iodophors contain iodine complexed with surfactants or polymers, so free iodine is slowly released. The adverse properties of staining and irritation are reduced, and delivery of iodine to the tissues is enhanced. *Povidone-iodine* is the most commonly used iodophor and is available as scrubs or solutions. Dilution of stock solutions (common dilutions include 1:10, 1:50, and 1:100) increases the

bactericidal activity and decreases the cytotoxicity. The residual bactericidal activity (i.e., continued action when left on the skin) of povidone-iodine is 4 to 6 hours, but this greatly diminished in the presence of organic matter.

Povidone-iodine is one of the most common surgical scrubs used in veterinary hospitals. Although it is a relatively safe skin preparation there are several considerations regarding its use. Alcohol, lavage solutions, or organic debris such as blood will destroy residual bactericidal activity. Povidone-iodine can cause skin irritation or acute contact dermatitis in up to 50% of canine patients, and it may be a problem for some hospital staff. Rarely, individuals who have repeated contact with iodine scrub solutions may develop systemic iodine toxicity, resulting in metabolic acidosis and thyroid dysfunction.

Technician Note

The two most commonly used antiseptic agents are povidone-iodine and chlorhexidine.

CHLORHEXIDINE.   Chlorhexidine is an antiseptic agent that is available in aqueous, tincture, and detergent formulations. It is an effective antimicrobial agent with activity against bacteria, molds, yeasts, and viruses. Chlorhexidine has a rapid onset and a long residual activity that is not affected by alcohol, lavage solutions, or organic debris. It has become a popular surgical scrub because of its effectiveness and because it is nonirritating to the skin. In several human studies, chlorhexidine has been found to be superior to povidone-iodine as a surgical hand scrub. The effectiveness of povidone-iodine and chlorhexidine is similar when used as surgical scrubs for canine surgery.

As a lavage solution for open wounds, chlorhexidine must be diluted 1:40 with sterile water or saline to produce a 0.05% solution. At this concentration, chlorhexidine has significant antibacterial activity with no cytotoxicity and is superior to povidone-iodine, saline, and other antiseptics. Higher concentrations can cause inflammation and cytotoxicity, so they are not recommended in open wounds. When chlorhexidine is mixed with electrolyte solutions (e.g., lactated Ringer's solution), it will precipitate, but this does not affect antimicrobial activity and the solution can still be used for wound lavage.

Technician Note

Chlorhexidine is an effective antimicrobial agent with rapid onset and long residual activity.

ALCOHOLS.   Alcohols are used as disinfectant and antiseptic agents. They are organic solvents that evaporate rapidly and leave no residue. Alcohols are bactericidal but ineffective against spores and fungi. They have no residual effects and are inhibited by organic debris. Ethyl and isopropyl alcohols are more effective than methyl alcohol as disinfecting agents. Alcohols should never be used in open wounds because they are both painful and cytotoxic.

PHENOLS.   Phenols (carbolic acid) have been used historically as both antiseptics and disinfectants, but phenols have been routinely replaced by newer, safer, and more effective agents. Hexachlorophene, a skin preparation, was one of the most popular phenols, but it has been replaced by povidone-iodine and chlorhexidine.

QUATERNARY AMMONIUM.   Quaternary ammonium compounds are synthetic cationic detergents that act on cell membranes and are effective against bacteria but not spores or some viruses. Very bland and nontoxic, these agents are quite popular. Benzalkonium chloride is the most commonly used quaternary ammonium compound and is used as a disinfectant.

CHLORIDE.   Chloride compounds were among the first agents to be used as medical disinfectants and found popularity for wound treatment in World War I as Dakin's solution. Antimicrobial chlorine compounds, specifically the hypochlorites, have broad bactericidal and virucidal activity but can be cytotoxic when improperly used on living tissues. Presently, sodium hypochlorite (bleach) is commonly used as a disinfectant in many hospitals.

ALDEHYDE.   Formaldehyde and glutaraldehyde are the most commonly used aldehydes in veterinary medicine. They are both toxic and irritating, which restricts them from use on living tissues. They are very effective antimicrobial agents but may require several hours of exposure time. Formaldehyde is commonly used in the preservation of tissue specimens. Glutaraldehyde is commonly used for chemical sterilization in cold trays and for endoscopy equipment.

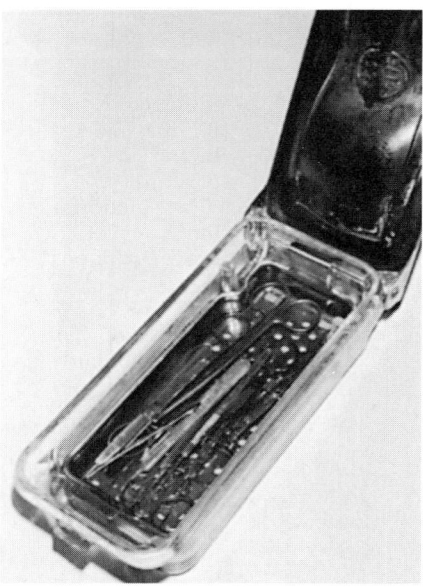

FIGURE 24-60.   Cold sterilization tray. Instruments are kept submerged in disinfectant and retrieved by lifting the rack.

Cold Sterilization

Cold sterilization refers to soaking instruments in disinfecting solutions, such as chlorhexidine or glutaraldehyde. Metal trays used to soak instruments in disinfectant are called *cold trays* (Figure 24-60). Because sterility cannot be guaranteed, cold-sterilized instruments should be used only for minor procedures (superficial lacerations, dental procedures) or for equipment that cannot tolerate other forms of sterilization, such as endoscopic equipment. Exposure times should exceed 3 hours, and the equipment must be rinsed thoroughly before use.

Technician Note

The arthroscope, fiberoptic light cable, and camera should never be steam sterilized.

Sterilization of Arthroscopic Equipment

Most hand instruments and ancillary equipment can be steam sterilized. They can also be gas sterilized with ethylene oxide or cold sterilized using a glutaraldehyde-based solution (Cidexplus, Johnson & Johnson Medical Inc.) (Figure 24-61). Cold sterilization affords the ability to use the equipment more than once in a single day, unlike steam and gas sterilization in most situations. The arthroscope, light cable, and camera can be gas sterilized or cold sterilized but *not* steam sterilized.

With cold sterilization, the instruments are soaked for a minimum of 20 minutes in the Cidexplus just before surgery. The electrical plug of the camera cable is not submerged in the cold sterilization solution, which would damage it. The end is draped out over the top of the container with the Cidexplus (Figure 24-62). The surgeon or assistant double-gloves and removes the instruments from the solution. The instruments are then placed in a sterile autoclave tray containing sterile water (Figure 24-63). Once the instruments have been submerged in the water, each piece is gently agitated, individually removed

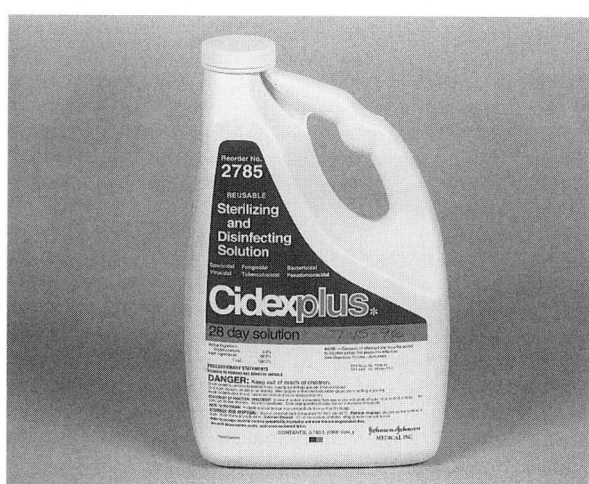

FIGURE 24-61. Cold sterilization solution (Cidexplus, Johnson & Johnson Medical Inc.).

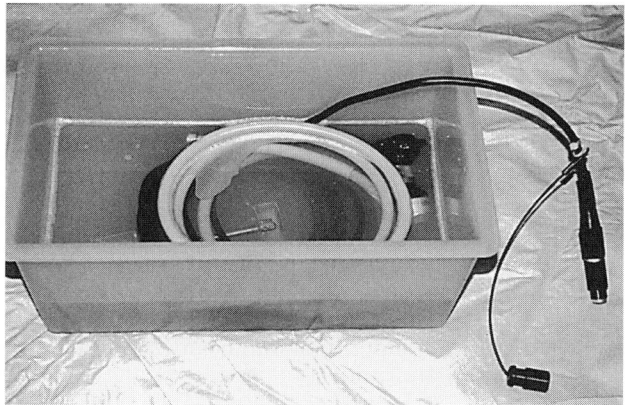

FIGURE 24-62. The electrical plug of the camera cable is draped over the top of the cold sterilization container to prevent it from being submerged, which could damage it.

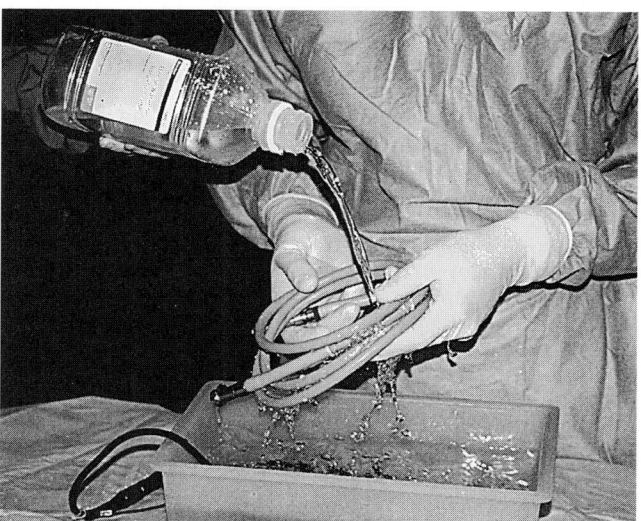

FIGURE 24-63. Once the arthroscopic equipment has been cold soaked, it is rinsed and transferred aseptically to a sterile tray that contains sterile water.

from the tray, rinsed with sterile water by a scrub nurse or other assistant, and transferred to the instrument table. The surgeon or assistant removes his or her outer gloves and dries the instruments. It is important that the Cidexplus be thoroughly rinsed from the instruments. Glutaraldehyde can cause a chemical synovitis and is injurious to chondrocytes. A double rinse further reduces the amount of glutaraldehyde residue remaining on the instruments.

> **Technician Note**
>
> Glutaraldehyde causes a chemical synovitis and is injurious to chondrocytes.

Operating Room Preparation

Operating room design is important for ease of cleaning. The operating room should be simple and uncluttered.

Commonly used equipment and materials should be readily available, but excess stock should not be stored in the operating room. When additional equipment is needed it is brought to the operating room by the circulating nurse.

Operating room cleanliness is essential for proper aseptic technique. A routine daily and weekly cleaning schedule should be established to keep the operating room clean and dust free. The surgery table should be cleaned and disinfected, and soiled areas of the floor should be cleaned and disinfected by damp mopping immediately after each surgery. It is preferable to perform thorough daily cleaning at the end of each day because cleaning creates airborne dust that takes several hours to settle. Buckets should be emptied and cleaned. The operating table and all equipment should be cleaned and wiped with a disinfectant solution. (The operating room is never dry mopped or dusted because this produces excessive airborne dust.) The casters on equipment should be cleaned, and the entire floor should be mopped.

Once each week, the operating room should undergo a thorough cleaning in which movable equipment is removed and cleaned with a disinfectant solution. Permanent structures, such as walls, air vents, window sills, light fixtures, and the surgical table, should also be wiped clean. Cabinets should be emptied, washed, and restocked. The operating room floor should be scrubbed and disinfected. Disinfectant can be applied with a mop, although this may actually spread dirt and microorganisms throughout the room. To avoid this, the mop head should be laundered daily and not stored in used disinfectant solution. The wet-vacuum method in which the clean floor is flooded with disinfectant solution and then vacuumed is superior to mopping. Cleaning equipment used in the operating room should be kept separate from all other cleaning equipment.

Daily cleaning of the surgical preparation room is also important because this room is subject to continual contamination. Sinks and plumbing fixtures should be scrubbed. Buckets and vacuum canisters should be emptied. Furniture and cabinets should be wiped clean and the floor scrubbed. If there are holding cages in the preparation room, they should be cleaned and disinfected. All surgical preparation solutions and supplies should be replenished.

Patient Preparation

Surgical Clip

The surgical site is usually prepared after the animal is anesthetized. The hair is first clipped in the same direction as the hair growth. Then it is clipped against the direction of growth to achieve the closest shave possible (using a no. 40 clipper blade). A wide region of skin is clipped around the proposed surgical incision. A general rule is to shave at least 2 to 4 cm in every direction from the proposed incision, depending on the size of the animal and location of the incision. For abdominal procedures, the clip should extend several centimeters cranial to the xyphoid, caudal to the pubis, and lateral to the nipples. For orthopedic procedures, the entire circumference of the limb is clipped from the foot up onto the body. Long hair growing near the periphery of the clipped area should be cut short enough that it cannot hang over the clipped area. Sterile, water-soluble lubricant may be placed in open wounds before clipping around them. The lubricant will collect hair, allowing it to be rinsed away before the surgical scrub. Areas that appear to be infected should be clipped last so the clippers do not spread infected material. After clipping, a vacuum cleaner may be used to eliminate loose hairs on the skin. The surgical clip should be thorough but gentle. Unnecessary roughness will result in inflamed or traumatized skin, which can cause greater postoperative complications.

Surgical Scrub

Initial skin preparation is done in the preparation room to remove gross contamination. The surgical scrub is usually performed by alternating between an antiseptic scrub (e.g., povidone-iodine or chlorhexidine scrub) and alcohol. (Remember not to use alcohols or detergents in open wounds, eyes, or mucous membranes.) The surgical site is scrubbed a minimum of three separate times or until the sponges do not pick up dirt. Scrubbing should begin over the proposed incision site and extend outward in a spiraling pattern, never going back toward the center with the same gauze sponge (Figure 24-64). An antiseptic solution may be applied to the surgical site via a spray bottle or sterile sponge after the final surgical scrub. If contamination occurs when moving the animal to the operating table, the area is rescrubbed. Many veterinarians routinely have the surgical site rescrubbed after the animal is positioned on the operating table.

> ### Technician Note
>
> It is generally recommended that the surgical site be scrubbed and rinsed three times. An antiseptic solution is often applied to the skin following the scrubs.

There are many modifications to the surgical preparation technique. For example, in preparation for feline orchiectomy (castration) the scrotal hair is plucked rather than clipped. Feline onychectomy (declawing) and tail docking and dewclaw removal of neonatal puppies are commonly performed without clipping the hair. The surgical site is soaked or gently scrubbed with detergent and swabbed with alcohol or antiseptic solution. Bovine and porcine castrations are performed without clipping the hair, and an

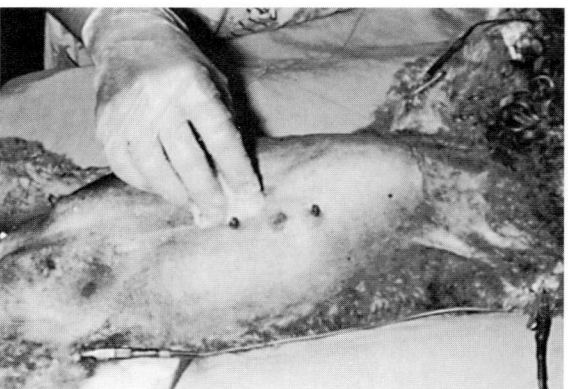

FIGURE 24-64.   The surgical preparation should begin at the proposed incision site and should progress outward, never returning to the proposed incision line with the same gauze sponge. Examination gloves worn during the preparation decrease contamination from human hands.

alcohol or antiseptic wash is usually used. Equine castrations may be prepared with three thorough washes using dilute chlorhexidine or povidone-iodine solution.

Patient Positioning

There are several common positions in which to place an animal for surgery. The position of the animal is described by the region of the body that contacts the table. For example, right lateral recumbency means the animal is lying on its right side, dorsal recumbency means the animal is on its back, and sternal recumbency means the animal is on its belly. Maintaining patient positioning is facilitated by the use of adjustable surgical tables, portable table-top V troughs, sandbags, or vacuum-activated "beanbags."

In orthopedic surgery the affected leg is often suspended from an overhead support or intravenous stand during skin preparation and initial surgical draping. The advantage of hanging the leg is that it allows aseptic preparation of the entire circumference of the limb, so the surgeon can manipulate it during surgery. To hang the leg, the distal limb is wrapped (using gauze or an examination glove covered with tape) to cover any unclipped areas and strips of tape ("stirrups") are extended from the end of the foot. The leg is suspended by these stirrups (Figure 24-65). The entire limb circumference is clipped and scrubbed from the foot to the level of the inguinal or axillary region. The skin preparation usually extends to the dorsal and ventral midlines of the body. The surgeon places sterile drapes on the body, around the base of the limb, and then covers and holds the foot with a sterile wrap while the circulating nurse cuts the stirrups. A cotton stockinette or adhesive drape may be used to cover the entire leg. The stockinette-covered limb is passed through a hole in a large sterile drape that covers the entire animal. After making the skin incision, the cut edge of the adhesive drape or stockinette is sutured or clipped to the skin edges.

> ### Technician Note
>
> The dorsal recumbent position is commonly used for abdominal surgical procedures.

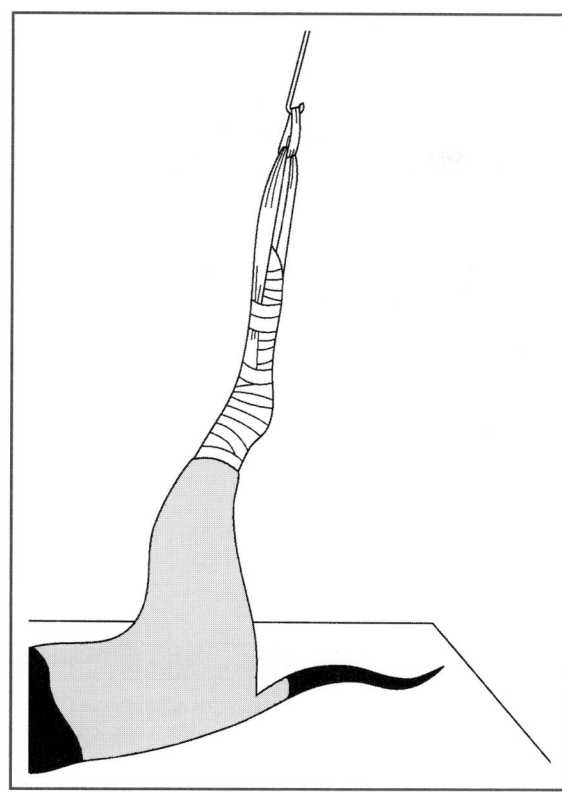

FIGURE 24-65.   Hanging leg surgical preparation. This is commonly used for orthopedic surgeries of legs including the shoulder and hip. The operated limb is suspended by tape stirrups that cover all distal leg hair. The surgical scrubs are started at the highest aspect of the clipped leg and worked downward with gravity in a circular fashion. At surgery, the taped foot is wrapped in a sterile towel, and the stirrups are cut.

A   **B**   **C**

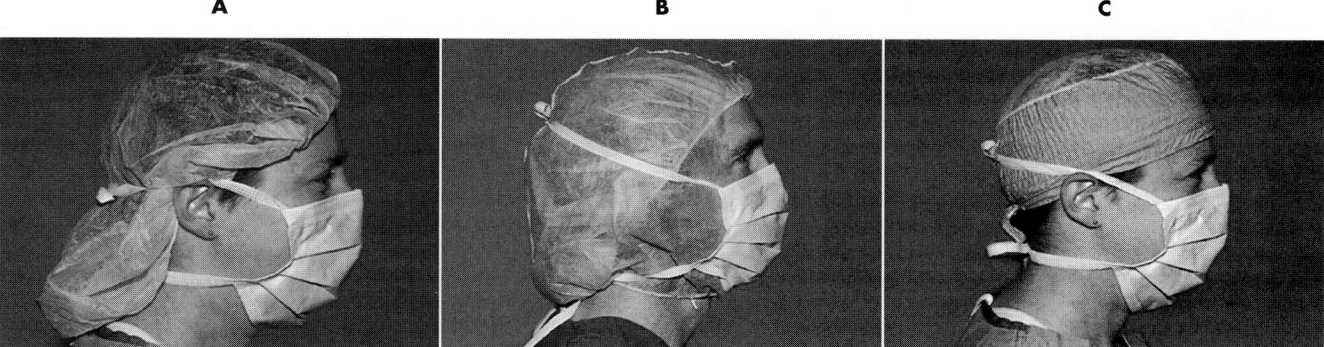

FIGURE 24-66.   Surgical caps and masks. **A,** Bouffant head cover is used to cover long or short hair. **B,** Hoods are available for individuals with sideburns or a beard. **C,** A cap may be suitable to cover very short hair.

Surgical Team Preparation
Attire
Proper surgical attire and proper scrubbing, gowning, and gloving procedures are important aspects of aseptic technique. Street clothing, especially shoes, are a major source of contamination and should not be worn into the operating room. Ideally, each person should have a pair of shoes designated for use only in the operating room. Also, disposable shoe covers may be worn in the operating room and discarded on leaving the room. Cotton scrub suits should be worn in the operating room. The shirt should be tucked into the pants to reduce the amount of skin debris dispersed into the room. Outside the operating room, scrubs suits should be protected by a laboratory coat.

Surgical caps and masks are worn during surgery. The surgical cap covers the hair and prevents airborne contamination. Different types of surgical head covers are available to cover short hair, long hair, or beards (Figure 24-66). The mask filters air exhaled from the nose and mouth. Masks are effective for relatively short periods and should be changed between operations.

Hand Scrub
The purpose of scrubbing the hands and arms is to remove dirt and decrease the concentration of bacterial flora. The surgical cap and mask must be donned and all jewelry removed from hands and arms before beginning the sterile hand scrub. Once the scrubbing has begun, the hands and arms should not touch unsterile objects. If this occurs the scrub is started over.

The hands and arms are lathered for about 1 minute without a brush and then rinsed in running water. While

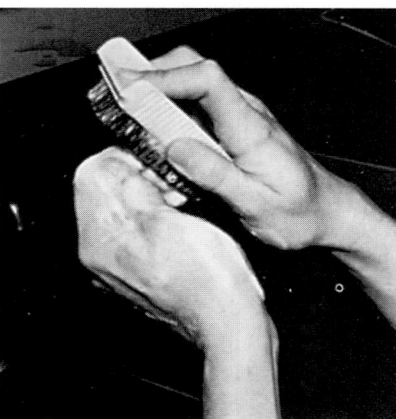

FIGURE 24-67.   Surgical hand scrub. Thoroughly scrub all surfaces of each finger, hand, and forearm.

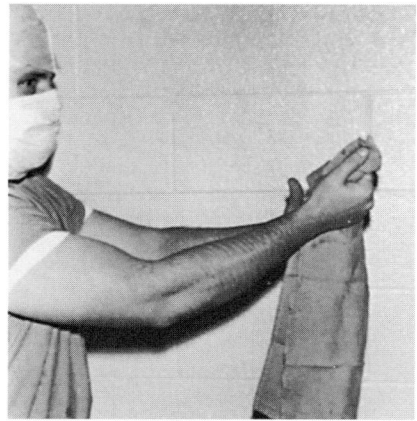

FIGURE 24-69.   One hand is dried first, then the arm, using half the towel. The other hand and arm are dried, using the other half of the towel. The towel should be held away from the body so it does not brush against anything.

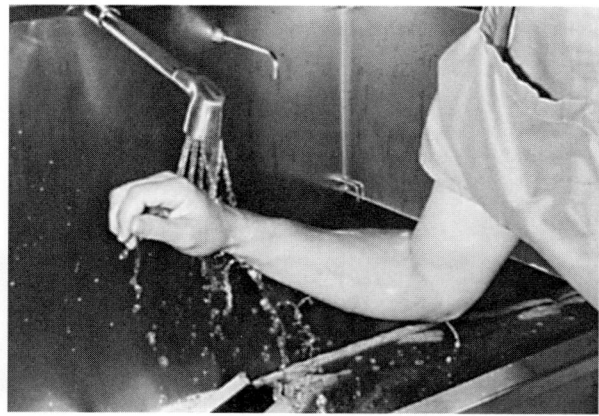

FIGURE 24-68.   Rinse hands, forearms, and brush after each scrub, always keeping the hands above the elbows.

personnel are scrubbing, the hands are always held above the level of the elbows so the water drains off the elbows. Soap is applied to a sterile brush, and a systematic scrub is begun. Scrub all four sides of each finger, with special attention to the fingernails (Figure 24-67). The back, both sides, and the palm of the hand are scrubbed. Next, the wrist and forearm are scrubbed, working toward the elbow. After both hands and arms have been scrubbed, they are rinsed in running water (Figure 24-68). The entire scrub process is then repeated.

The two basic types of surgical scrubs are anatomic and timed. The anatomic scrub is performed by counting the number of brush strokes used on each skin surface. Ten brush strokes are made on each surface of the hands and arms before rinsing. This is performed four times. The more commonly used timed scrub is performed by repeated scrubs over a set period of time. The initial scrub of the day should last about 10 minutes. For subsequent scrubs between surgeries, 5 minutes is adequate unless gross contamination has occurred.

Technician Note

The surgical hand scrub requires that all surfaces of the fingers, hand, and forearm be scrubbed. Skin-soap contact time should last 10 minutes.

Gowning and Gloving

The hands and arms are thoroughly dried (Figure 24-69) before gowning and gloving. The sterile gown is picked up and held by inside shoulder seams, allowing it to unfold. Sometimes it is necessary to gently shake the gown to completely unfold it. Hands are at chest level, and the gown is held out away from the body. The sleeve openings are located, and the arms are slid into the sleeves but not extended through the cuff openings (Figure 24-70). The gown is secured at the neck and waist by a nonsterile assistant.

The two methods for gloving are *closed gloving* and *open gloving.* The risk of contamination is minimized with closed gloving (Figure 24-71) since the outside of the gloves never contacts skin. There is a much higher risk of contamination during open gloving (Figure 24-72), and it is generally reserved for minor procedures when a gown is not worn. If it is necessary to replace gloves during surgery, it is preferable to have a nonsterile assistant remove the old gloves and simultaneously pull the gown sleeve so the hands remain inside the sleeves. If the old gloves are removed in this manner, new gloves can be put on by the closed gloving method.

The Sterile Field

It is important for the entire surgical team to be aware of the sterile field even if they are not "scrubbed in." Nonsterile personnel should only touch nonsterile items or areas. They should not lean over or reach across a sterile field. Sterile packs are touched only on the outside of the wraps and are opened away from the body.

Sterile personnel should only touch sterile items or areas. To maintain sterility of an item while removing it from its wrap, it should be grasped by a gloved hand or

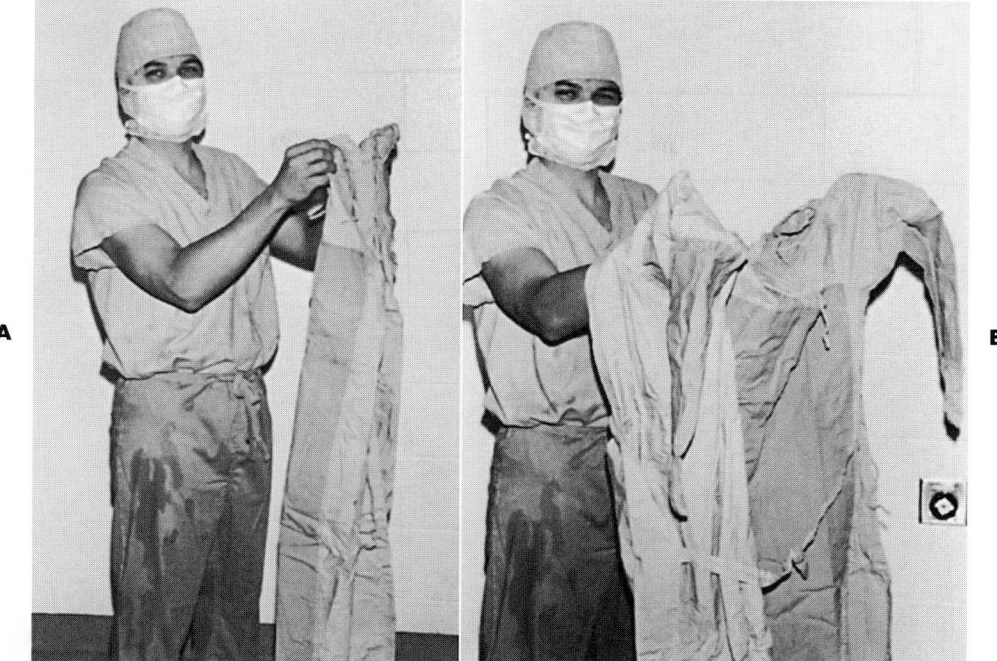

FIGURE 24-70. **A,** The gown is held by the inside shoulder seams. The gown is held away from the body at shoulder height and allowed to unfold. **B,** The arms are slid into the sleeves.

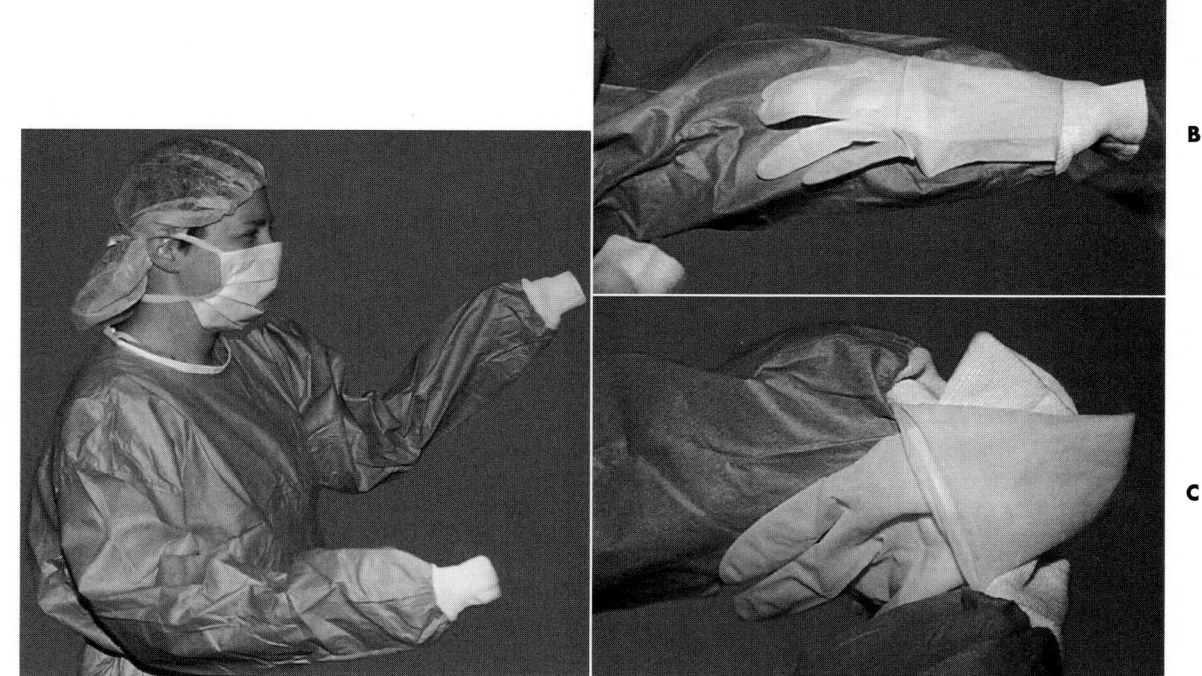

FIGURE 24-71.   Closed gloving. **A,** When performing closed gloving, the hands are kept inside the sleeves while gloving takes place. **B,** The palm side of the glove is grasped at the cuff through the sleeve. **C,** The opposite side of the cuff is grasped in the other hand.   *Continued*

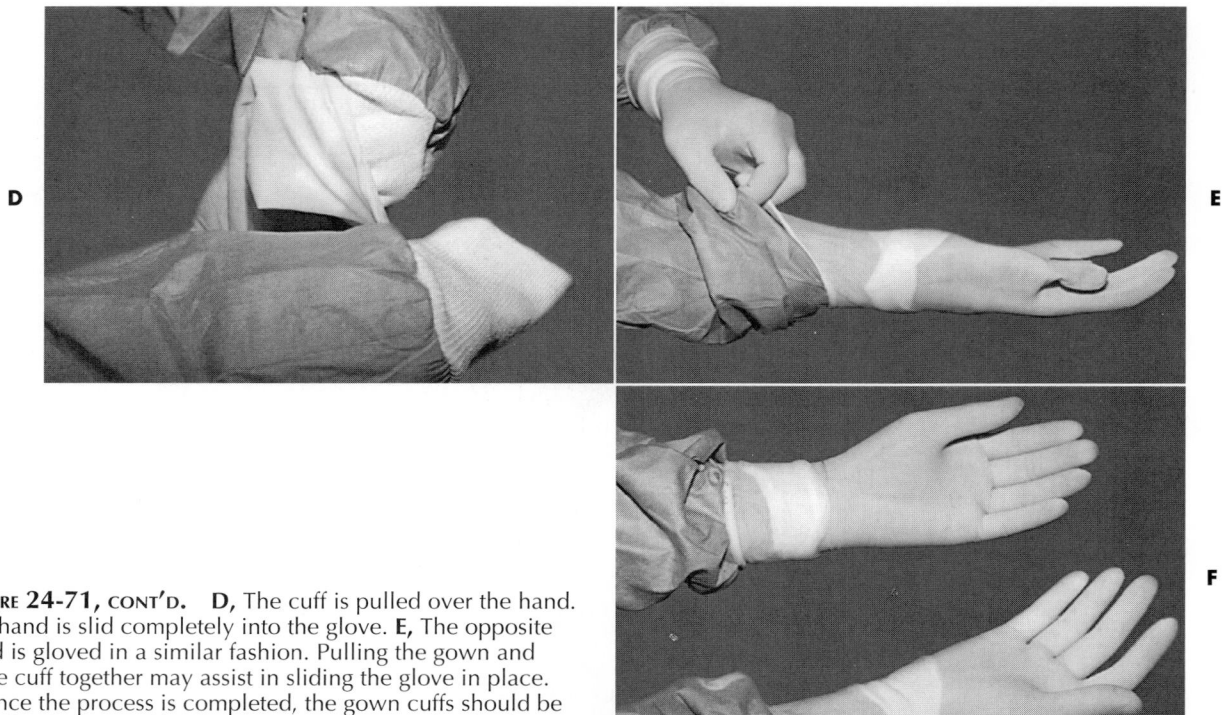

FIGURE 24-71, CONT'D. D, The cuff is pulled over the hand. The hand is slid completely into the glove. **E,** The opposite hand is gloved in a similar fashion. Pulling the gown and glove cuff together may assist in sliding the glove in place. **F,** Once the process is completed, the gown cuffs should be completely covered by the gloves. At no time should skin be visible while performing closed gloving.

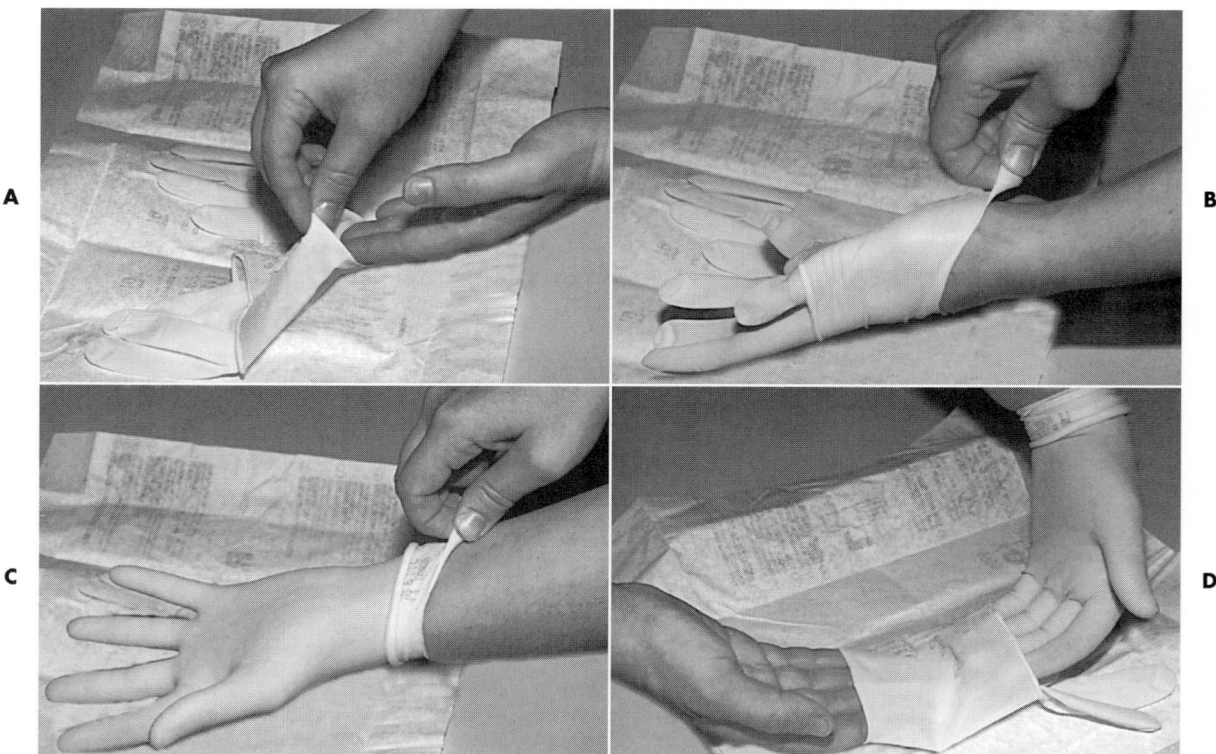

FIGURE 24-72. Open gloving. **A,** Open gloving is usually done for procedures where a gown is not required. The glove pack is opened near the edge of a table. The left hand is inserted into the glove opening, taking care not to touch the outside of the glove. The inside of the glove will not be sterile, so the cuff may be touched. **B,** The glove is pulled on by grasping the cuff fold with the other hand. **C,** The left glove should be on well enough to allow use of the hand. Minor adjustments in fit can be made once both gloves are on. **D,** The left hand can now touch the outside portion of the right glove, so it is placed between the cuff and the palm of the right glove to assist gloving the right hand.

Continued

FIGURE 24-72, CONT'D. E, The left hand should only touch the sterile areas of the right glove. **F,** Once both gloves are on, adjustments can be made to both gloves, taking care to touch only the outside portions of the gloves.

sterile instrument and lifted up and out. The edges of a sterile container are considered to be contaminated so items should not be dragged over the edge of the container. The gown is considered to be sterile on the front of the sleeves and from the waist to shoulder level in front only. The back of a gowned person is considered to be nonsterile and should not be turned toward the sterile field. Draped tables are considered to be sterile only at the table level, so if a sterile item extends below the table it is considered to be contaminated and should no longer be touched by sterile personnel.

Technician Note

The two methods of gloving are *closed gloving* and *open gloving.*

RECOMMENDED READING

Berg RJ. Sterilization. In Slatter DH: *Textbook of small animal surgery*, ed 2, Philadelphia, 1993, WB Saunders.

Fries CL. In Slatter DH: Assessment and preparation of the surgical patient. *Textbook of small animal surgery*, ed 2, Philadelphia, 1993, WB Saunders.

Hobson HP. In Slatter DH: Surgical facilities and equipment. *Textbook of small animal surgery*, ed 2, Philadelphia, 1993, WB Saunders.

Hurov L: *Handbook of veterinary surgical instruments and glossary of surgical terms*, Philadelphia, 1978, WB Saunders.

Knecht CD et al: *Fundamental techniques in veterinary surgery*, ed 3, Philadelphia, 1987, WB Saunders.

Lemarie RJ, Hosgood G: Antiseptics and disinfectants in small animal practice, *Compend Cont Ed Pract Vet* 17: 1339, 1996.

McCurnin DM, Jones RL. In Slatter DH: Principles of surgical asepsis. *Textbook of small animal surgery*, ed 2, Philadelphia, 1993, WB Saunders.

McIlwraith CW: *Diagnostic and surgical arthroscopy in the horse*, ed 2, Philadelphia, 1990, Lea & Febiger.

Nieves MA et al. In Slatter DH: Surgical instruments. *Textbook of small animal surgery*, ed 2, Philadelphia, 1993, WB Saunders.

Pavletic MM: Surgical stapling, *Vet Clin North Am* 24:225, 1994.

Tracy DL: *Small animal surgical nursing*, St Louis, 2000, Mosby.

Wagner SD. In Slatter DH: Preparation of the surgical team. *Textbook of small animal surgery*, ed 2, Philadelphia, 1993, WB Saunders.

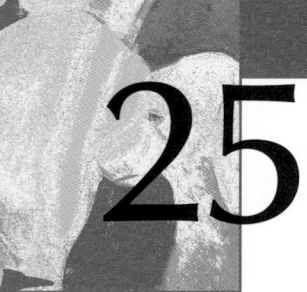

25

Surgical Assistance and Suture Material

Erick L. Egger • Susan Kretzmer

ROLE OF THE VETERINARY TECHNICIAN IN SURGICAL ASSISTANCE

The purpose of surgery in veterinary medicine is primarily that of service. In cases of clinical disease or injury, surgery is used to relieve suffering and improve the quality of life for the animal patient and consequently the owner. Veterinary surgery is also performed to maintain or increase the economic value of animals that are used for food, breeding, show, or competitive purposes. The veterinary technician's role is to assist in providing this specialized service to the animal and owner. The technician accomplishes this by both helping the surgeon and protecting the patient. Surgical assistance includes improving the surgeon's visualization by providing retraction and hemostasis in the surgical field, being familiar with the objectives of the technique, and manipulating the instrumentation and tissues into position for completion of the surgical task. The second charge of the technician is to protect the patient from hazards of surgery, such as infection, by maintaining an aseptic surgical field and expediting surgical completion by anticipating needs for proper instruments and suture readiness. Because the surgeon is often concentrating on the surgical procedure, the technician must also be constantly aware of the patient's anesthetic and cardiovascular status while assisting.

PROPER TISSUE-HANDLING TECHNIQUES

Each of the various body tissue systems has specific attributes that require consideration when being surgically approached. If the technician understands the general surgical principles of each system, the appropriate actions and measures to be taken in each specific case will be apparent.

Skin

The preparation of the patient's skin for surgery has been described in Chapter 24. One must remember that preparation results in an *aseptic* but not *sterile* skin. This means that the number of bacteria has been reduced below the number required to overwhelm the body's defense mechanism. However, with a depressed immune system or prolonged surgery, these resident bacteria can start to multiply and result in infection. Therefore the surgeon and assistant should avoid unnecessary direct handling of the skin with the gloves or instruments that will be used in the deeper incision. These items could then carry organisms into the deeper tissues. For lengthy or complicated procedures, a sterile plastic drape (Barrier, Johnson & Johnson) that directly adheres to the skin surface may be used (Figure 25-1). A spray adhesive may be applied to the skin to augment the plastic's ability to remain in place throughout the surgery. The incision is made directly through the plastic drape. Alternatively, sterile towels or drapes may be applied to the margins of the skin incision to protect the deeper incision (Figure 25-2). These towels may be attached with additional towel clamps spaced every 5 to 10 cm along the incision (Figure 25-3) or by suturing the rolled edge of the towel or drape to the subcutaneous tissue with a simple continuous pattern of a strong, inexpensive suture material. For orthopedic surgery, the limb is often enclosed in a sterile stockinette to allow movement and manipulation and to limit exposed skin. The edges of the incised stockinette are, likewise, often attached to the surgical incision. This can be accomplished by suturing as

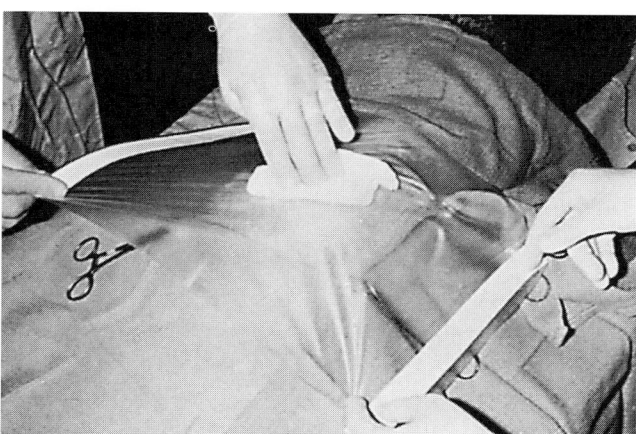

FIGURE 25-1. Application of a sterile plastic drape that adheres directly to the skin and minimizes potential contamination.

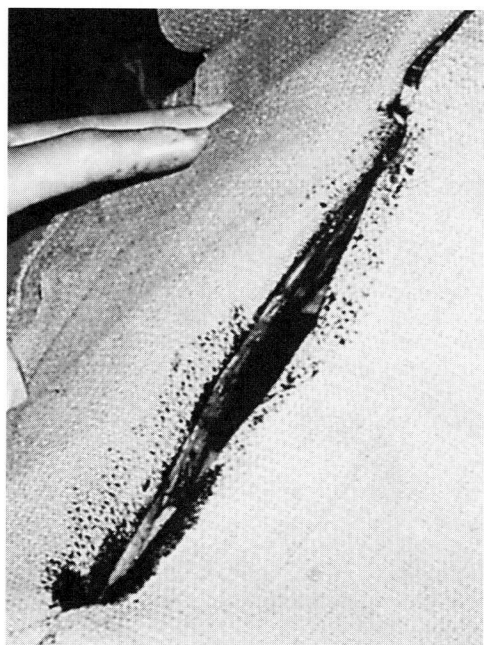

FIGURE 25-2. Application of sterile towels to skin margins to protect the deeper incision.

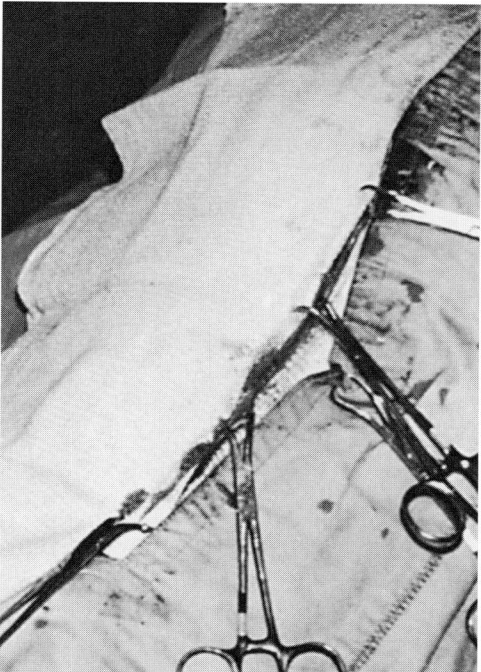

FIGURE 25-3. Use of towel clamps to attach towels to the incision margins.

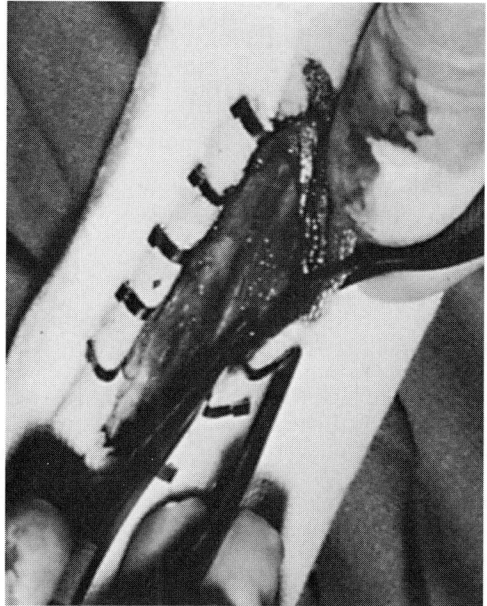

FIGURE 25-4. Use of Michel clips to attach the edge of the stockinette to the skin incision margins.

previously described or by the use of Michel clips (Figure 25-4). The cut edge of the stockinette should be rolled under so that cut fragments of the stockinette material will not fall into the incision. The rolled-under stockinette is usually pulled over the skin edge and attached to the subcutaneous tissue to completely cover the cut skin edge. This will also control much of the minor hemorrhage that occurs following skin incision.

Technician Note

Surgical preparation of the skin results in aseptic, not sterile, skin.

Technician Note

The skin incision should be performed with a sharp scalpel blade.

The skin incision itself should be performed with a sharp scalpel blade. A scissors will crush and shear skin as it

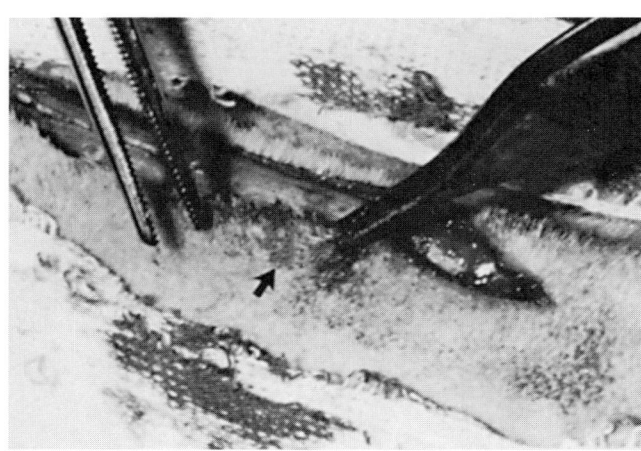

FIGURE 25-5. Smooth-jawed instruments hold tissue by pressure and can damage it by crushing *(arrow)*.

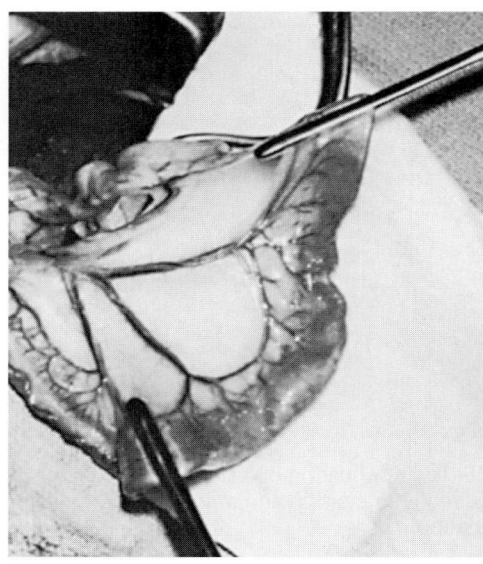

FIGURE 25-6. Use of Doyen intestinal forceps to prevent luminal content leakage during an enterotomy or a resection.

cuts. Skin is generally sensitive to this form of injury and will commonly react with severe swelling and scar formation. The skin is relatively thick and elastic; therefore it will also tend to force or "spring" the blades of the scissors apart, damaging the instrument. A sharp incision with a scalpel blade results in the most rapid healing and the least amount of scar formation. Skin incision with an electro-scalpel somewhat delays healing and generally results in a larger scar. The principles and use of the electroscalpel are discussed later under Electrosurgery.

Any instrument used to hold or manipulate skin should grip the tissue with teeth or hooks. Instruments that have smooth tips hold the tissue by pressure, which tends to crush skin and damage it in much the same way as scissors do (Figure 25-5).

Hollow Organ Surgery

Surgery of the hollow organs (i.e., stomach, intestines, bladder, esophagus) requires both complete control of luminal contents to avoid contamination and careful handling to avoid damage to these delicate tissues. Whenever possible, the surgical site is isolated from the body cavity with saline-moistened laparotomy sponges. Specific intestinal forceps (Doyen) have been developed and can be used to prevent luminal content leakage when performing enterotomies or intestinal resections (Figure 25-6). However, even these specialized clamps can damage tissues if tightened excessively or left in place too long (Figure 25-7). Consequently, many surgeons prefer the assistant to occlude the intestinal lumen by using moistened gloved fingers (Figure 25-8). Large, hollow organs, such as the stomach or urinary bladder, often cannot be exteriorized. Consequently, the incision is made into the most elevated portion of the viscus to avoid leakage into the body cavity. This is usually accomplished by placing *stay sutures* at four points around the incision. Stay sutures are simple loops of suture that pass through the outer layers of the viscus and are held together at their ends with a clamp (Figure 25-9). The surgical assistant supplies traction to the clamps to keep the incision in the desired location and elevated to avoid content leakage (Figure 25-10).

Musculoskeletal Surgery

Surgery of the musculoskeletal system often requires surgical assistance. Although muscle itself is highly vascular and has great healing ability, bone has a limited blood supply and heals slowly. Consequently, as the assistant retracts and manipulates fractures, all efforts should be made to preserve soft tissue attachment to bone. The assistant must also be cognizant of adjacent structures and protect them from damage by bony fragments or the surgeon. The most significant endangered structures are nerves. Specifically, the radial, ulnar, and ischiatic nerves course very closely to commonly occurring fractures and their surgical exposures. The surgical assistant must be familiar with the anatomic location of these structures.

Retraction Techniques

Retraction of tissues is often used to increase visibility and ease of manipulation in the incision. This can be accomplished with hand-held retractors by which the assistant provides traction in one direction with one retractor and countertraction in the opposite direction with a second retractor (Figure 25-11). Retractors are available with various tips and blades to be used on different tissues. Care should be taken that retractors do not slide around or pull out of the incision, because this causes significant tissue trauma. Consequently, sharp-tipped retractors that maintain a grip on the tissue (without crushing) are often preferable to blunt-tipped retractors, particularly for muscle and skin retraction. Self-retaining retractors are also often used to free the assistant for other duties (Figure 25-12). Excessive retraction for prolonged periods must be avoided with self-retaining instruments.

Technician Note

The surgical assistant must be familiar with vital structures to avoid injury during retraction of tissues during surgery.

Manual traction on adjacent tissues is often used to increase visibility or expose organs. Deep structures of the

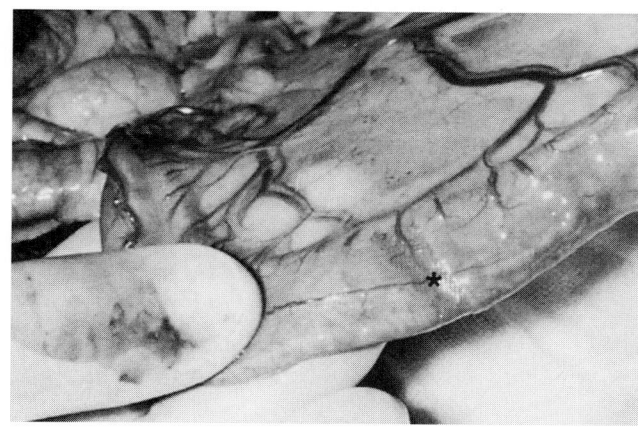

FIGURE 25-7. Area of intestinal damage *(asterisk)* from excessive tightening of a Doyen intestinal clamp.

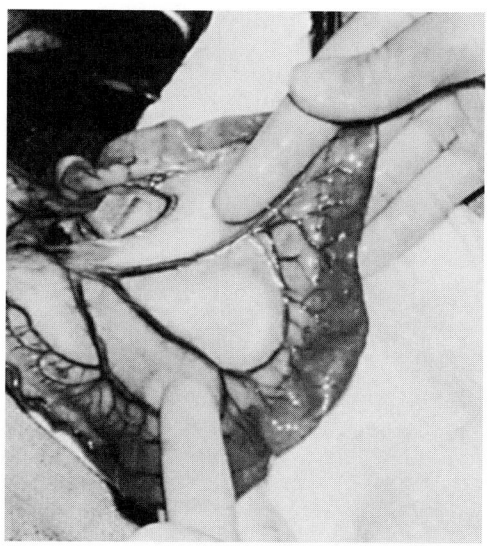

FIGURE 25-8. Use of moistened gloved fingers to occlude the intestinal lumen.

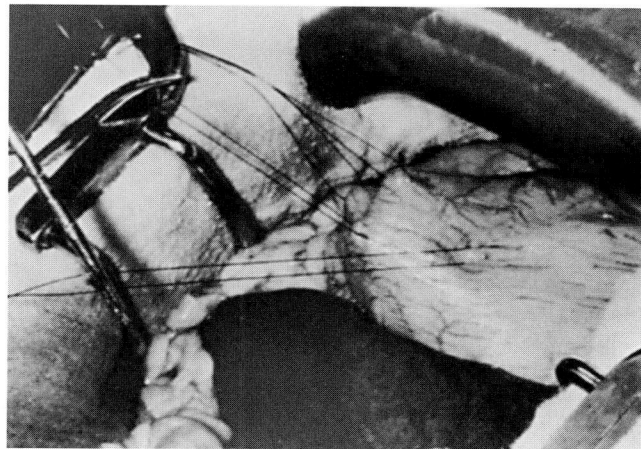

FIGURE 25-9. Stay sutures are passed through the outer layers of hollow organs. Both ends are held with a clamp.

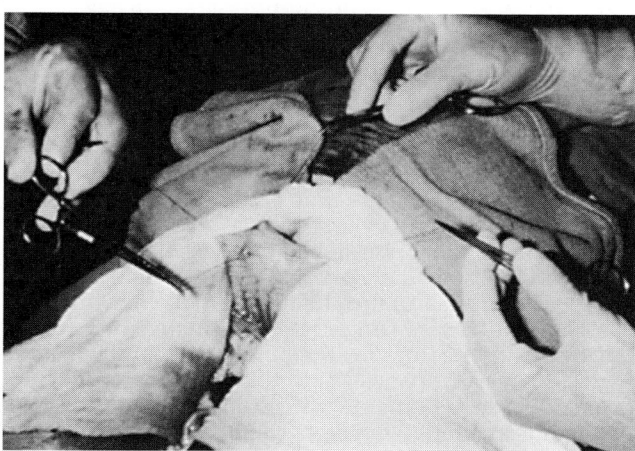

FIGURE 25-10. The assistant elevates the area of incision by applying traction to the stay sutures.

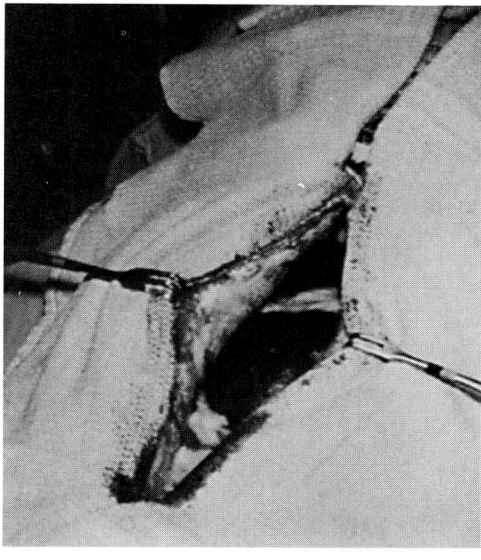

FIGURE 25-11. Exposure in the incision can be increased with hand retractors by the application of traction in one direction and countertraction in the opposite direction.

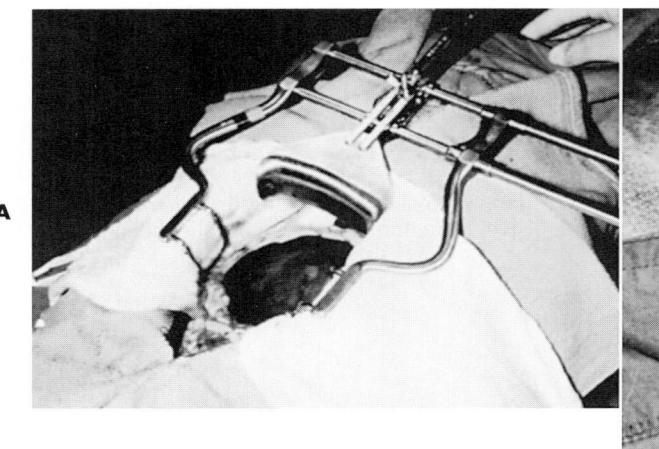
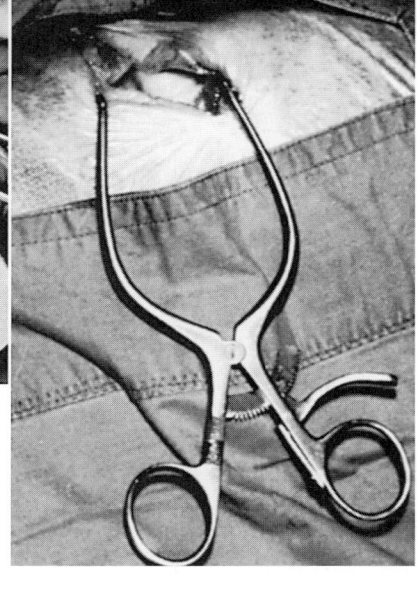

FIGURE 25-12.   **A,** Use of a blunt-tipped, self-retaining retractor (Balfour) in an abdominal incision during an exploratory laparotomy. **B,** Use of a sharp-tipped, self-retaining retractor (Gelpi) between muscles during an arthrotomy.

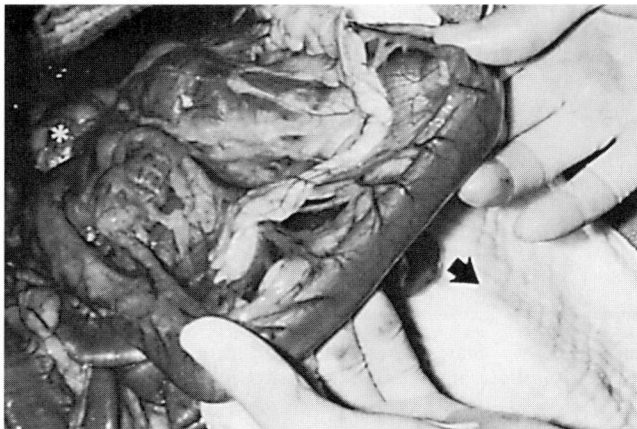

FIGURE 25-13.   Retraction of the proximal duodenum to the left *(arrow)* exposes the right kidney *(asterisk).*

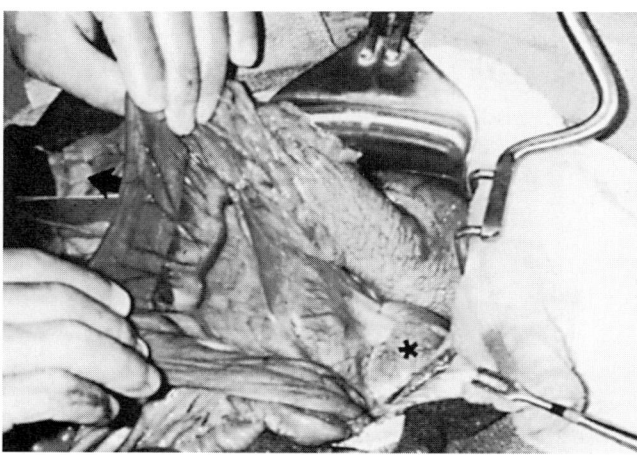

FIGURE 25-14.   Retraction of the descending colon to the right *(arrow)* exposes the left kidney *(asterisk).*

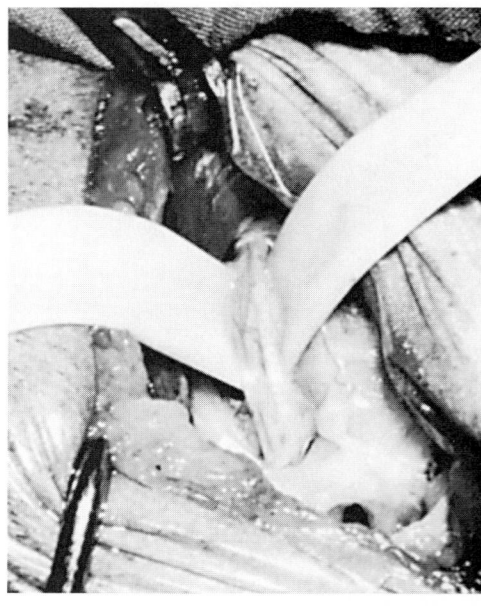

FIGURE 25-15.   A Penrose drain is passed behind a nerve and used as a retractor.

right half of the canine or feline abdominal cavity may be visualized by retracting the proximal duodenum, which holds the abdominal viscera behind the mesentery, to the left, thus exposing the right kidney and ureter (Figure 25-13). The left half of the abdominal cavity may likewise be visualized by retracting the abdominal viscera to the right, behind the mesocolon of the descending colon (Figure 25-14). The pancreas is best exposed by traction on the adjacent duodenum. As when using fingers for occluding the intestinal lumen, gloves should be moistened and excessive pressure should be avoided.

Nerves or large blood vessels are often retracted to improve visualization or to avoid potential damage. Careful blunt dissection is used to free the nerve or vessel from surrounding tissue. A broad, flat band, such as a Penrose

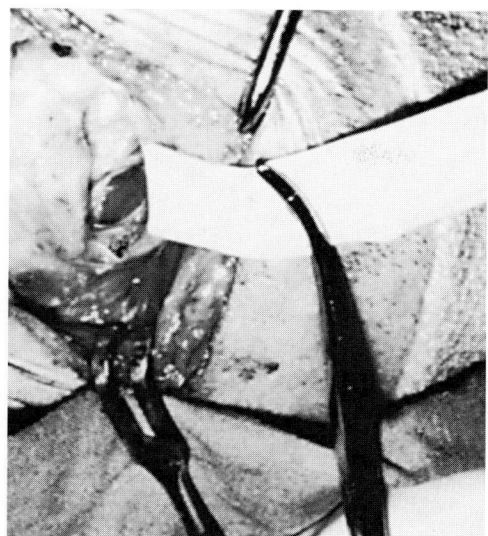

FIGURE 25-16. The ends of the drain are clamped together, and the nerve is pulled to one side to avoid damage.

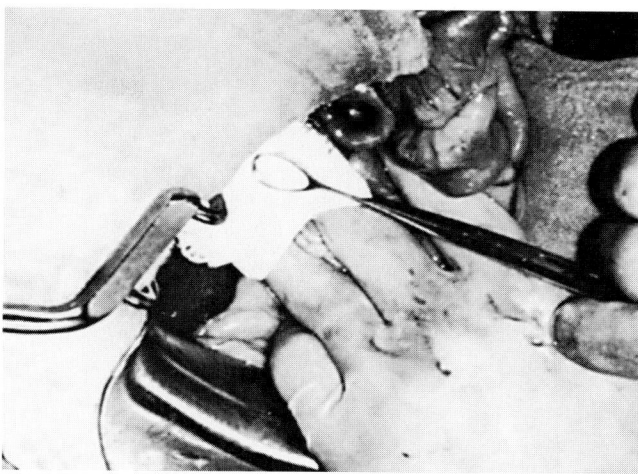

FIGURE 25-17. Gauze sponge held in a sponge forceps.

drain or moistened umbilical tape, is passed around the structure (Figure 25-15), and the ends are clamped together much like a stay suture. The assistant can gently retract the nerve or vessel to one side, carefully avoiding entanglement with other instruments or equipment (Figure 25-16).

HEMOSTASIS

The surgical assistant is often responsible for maintaining hemostasis during surgery. Hemostasis is needed both to limit the volume of blood loss and to obtain optimal visibility in the incision. Hemostasis can be obtained by a variety of methods with which the surgical assistant should be familiar.

Sponge Hemostasis

Gauze sponge is often used to remove existing hemorrhage from incised tissues. Because any dry material is damaging to body tissues, many assistants slightly moisten sponges with saline before using them in the incision. The sponge should be applied with a blotting type of motion. A wiping motion will irritate tissue and will often renew bleeding by pulling the forming blood clots out of incised capillaries. Sustained pressure through gauze sponges can be used to control bleeding from small vessels. The pressure apparently stops hemorrhage by collapsing the vessels until clotting can occur. With persistent hemorrhage, pressure may need to be sustained for up to 5 minutes to allow adequate coagulation.

Sponge Complications

Gauze sponges are extremely irritating and will cause severe tissue reaction, adhesions, and drainage if they are left in a closed incision. The abdominal and thoracic cavities are particularly hazardous locations for sponges to become lost. Consequently, many surgical assistants count sponges in such areas to make sure all sponges have been removed. Before surgery begins, sterile sponges are counted out in piles on the Mayo stand. Usually, two or three piles of 10 sponges are used to start. The total number is recorded, and all other sponges (e.g., those used for skin preparation) are

removed from the area. If additional sponges are required during surgery, they are supplied in packs of 10, and their number is added to the total. The used sponges are saved in a separate pile and are counted at the termination of the procedure before the incision is closed. The number of used sponges plus the remaining clean sponges must equal the total amount to account for all sponges.

> **Technician Note**
> The surgical assistant should always count sponges in and out of the large body cavities (thorax or abdomen).

For particularly deep incisions, sponges may be held in a sponge forceps (Figure 25-17) or tied with a long piece of umbilical tape (Figure 25-18). The end of the tape (called the tail) is left extending out of the incision as the sponge is used (Figure 25-19). The sponge can then be easily removed by pulling the tail.

Hemostatic Forceps

Hemorrhage from larger vessels can be occluded by clamping with a hemostatic forceps. The clamp should be applied perpendicular to the tissue surface and the bleeding vessel, with a minimal amount of adjacent tissue being grasped in the tips of the clamp (Figure 25-20).

Suture Ligation

A bleeding vessel that has been clamped can be ligated to achieve permanent hemostasis. After the suture material is passed around the vessel, the assistant lowers the handles of the clamp, which raises the tips (Figure 25-21). This causes the ligation loop to form around the vessel and not the instrument. As the first throw of the knot is pulled tight, the assistant releases the clamp. This allows the vessel to totally collapse, thus occluding the lumen. However, the assistant should return the vessel to its origin before releasing the clamp so the knot is not snapped off the cut end of the vessel. After the surgeon finishes the knot, the assistant cuts off excessive suture, using the tips of the scissors (Figure 25-22). Care must be taken not to pull

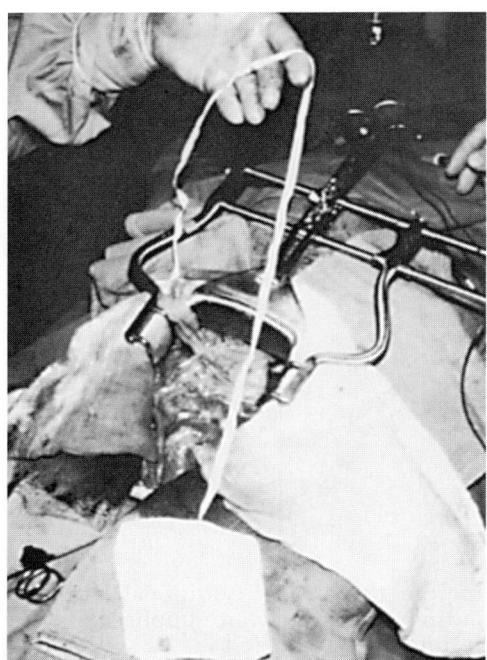

FIGURE 25-18.   Gauze sponge tied to a long piece of umbilical tape.

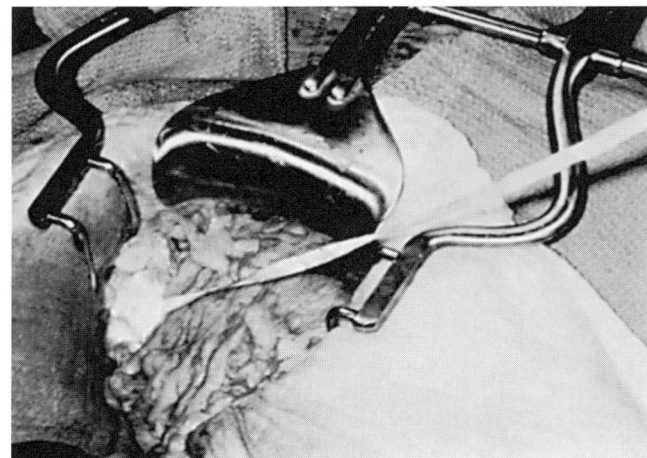

FIGURE 25-19.   The tail is left extending out of the incision, allowing easy retrieval.

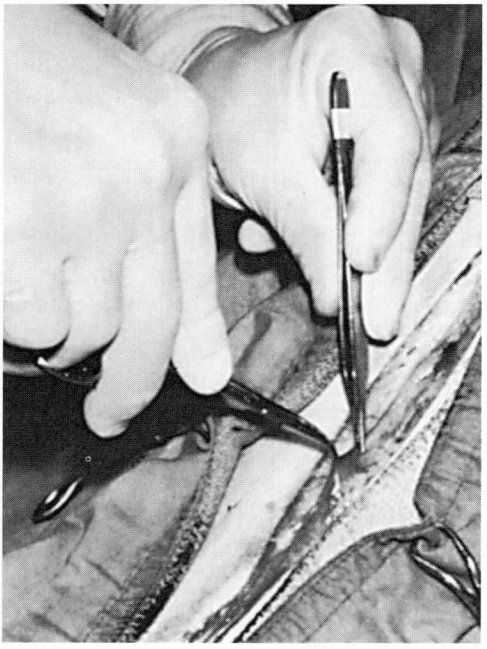

FIGURE 25-20.   A hemostatic forceps is perpendicularly applied to the bleeding vessel with a minimal amount of adjacent tissue included.

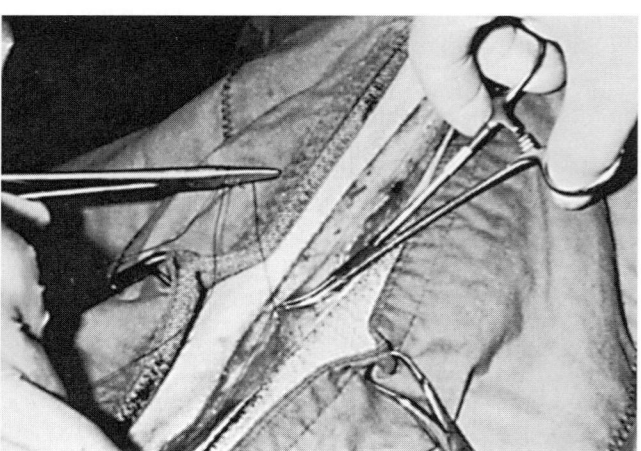

FIGURE 25-21.   Lowering the handles of the hemostatic forceps raises the tips, forcing the ligation loop to form around the vessel.

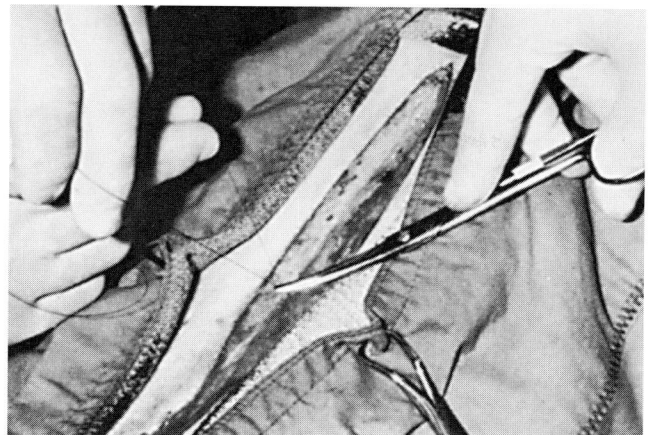

FIGURE 25-22. The tips of the scissors are used to cut off excess suture.

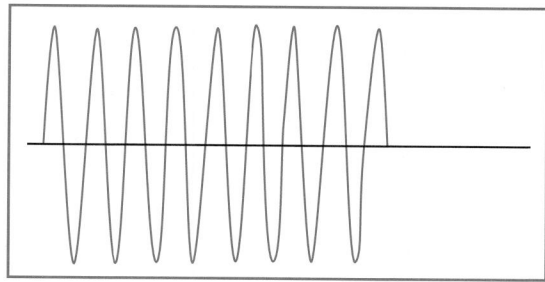

FIGURE 25-24. Diagram of the undamped sine wave current, which "cuts" tissues.

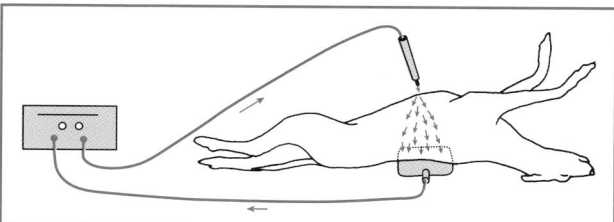

FIGURE 25-23. Diagram of electrical current passing from the handpiece, dispersing in the body, and returning to the generator via the ground plate.

the ligature off the end of the vessel. Only enough material to secure the knot should be left. Arteries are commonly ligated twice, particularly if they are more than 2 mm in diameter.

Electrosurgery

Electrosurgery offers a means of stopping hemorrhage after a vessel has been cut, either with electrocoagulation or by using an electroscalpel that coagulates as it cuts. Either coagulation or incision can be obtained by passing an electrical current from a unipolar handpiece to a small contact area on the patient. The current then spreads out through the body and returns to the current generator via a ground plate that is necessary to complete the electrical circuit (Figure 25-23).

Electroscalpel

Electrocutting occurs when the current generated is an undamped sine wave (Figure 25-24). It causes microcoagulation of the tissue proteins at a small point of contact. A slow, steady motion of the handpiece is used to create an incision. As the protein coagulation occurs, carbon tends to build up on the active tip of the handpiece (Figure 25-25). This carbon tends to insulate the current and should be periodically removed by the assistant, who scrapes it with a hard metallic edge, such as a scalpel handle.

Electrocoagulation

Electrocoagulation uses a damped electrical wave (Figure 25-26) to produce protein coagulation of the blood elements within the blood vessel wall. Electrocoagulation

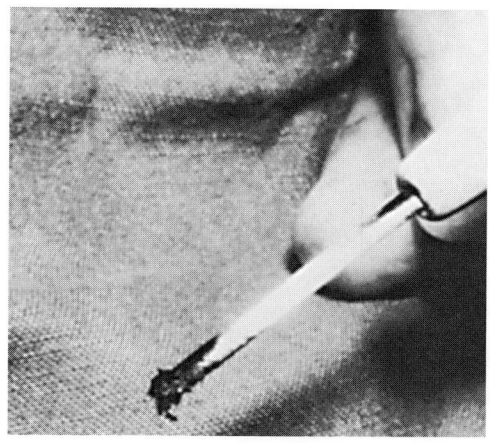

FIGURE 25-25. Buildup of protein on the handpiece tip, which prevents passage of current.

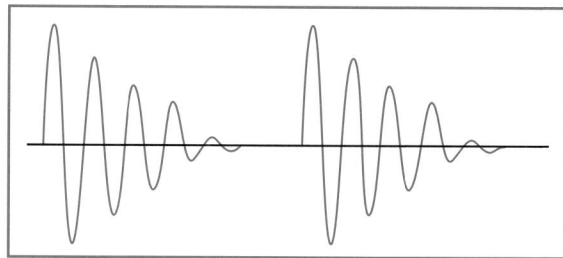

FIGURE 25-26. Diagram of the damped sine wave current, which causes coagulation.

should be used only on vessels smaller than 1.5 mm. Larger vessels should be ligated. The current can be applied through a hemostatic forceps clamped on the vessel (Figure 25-27). Current can be directly applied to the vessel from the handpiece tip only if all blood and fluid, which would dissipate the current, have been blotted away. Most modern electrosurgical generators allow the blending of cutting and coagulation currents to achieve a truly bloodless incision (Figure 25-28).

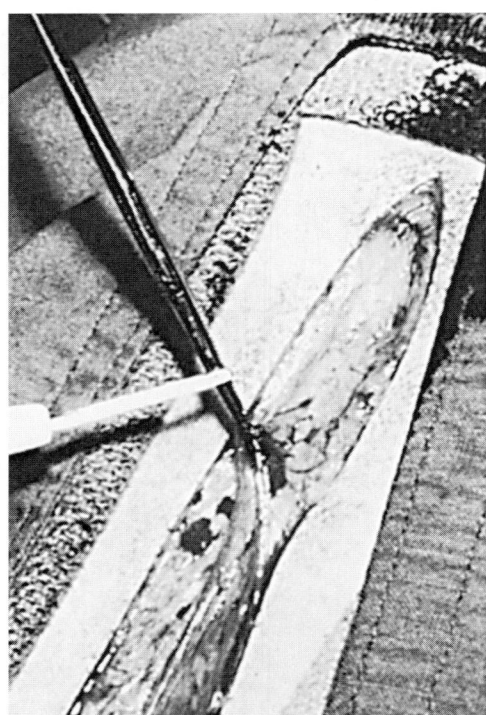

FIGURE 25-27. Application of current to a bleeding vessel by touching the handpiece to the hemostatic forceps.

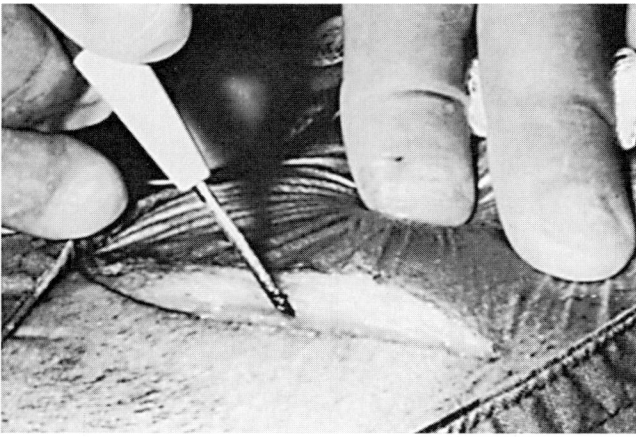

FIGURE 25-28. A bloodless incision can be obtained by blending cutting and coagulating currents.

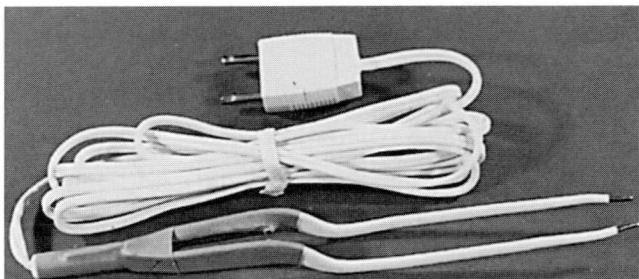

FIGURE 25-29. The thumb forceps-like handpiece used for bipolar cautery.

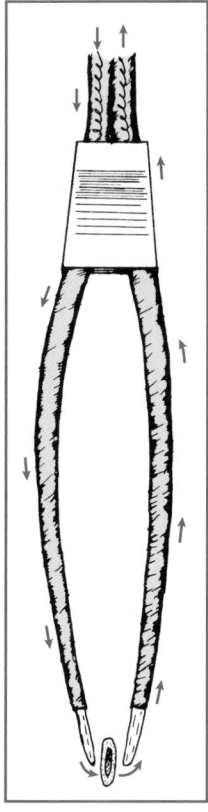

FIGURE 25-30. Diagram of the bipolar coagulation current as it passes from one tip of the handpiece to the other.

Bipolar Electrocautery

Bipolar electrocautery utilizes a thumb forceps-like handpiece (Figure 25-29). The vessel to be cauterized is grasped between the blades of the forceps, and the coagulating current runs from one blade to the other, not through the body (Figure 25-30). This form of electrocoagulation is particularly useful in neurosurgery in which unipolar currents can stimulate unwanted muscle contractions and injure the central nervous system.

Safety With Electrosurgery

Electrosurgery will result in spark formation, and therefore it should *not* be used when explosive anesthetics, such as ether and cyclopropane, are present. Likewise, some antiseptic preparation materials (alcohol based) and adhesive agents are volatile and should be avoided or allowed to dry thoroughly before using electrosurgery. The patient must have good electrical contact, using a conductive gel or fluid to a large area of the ground plate to avoid a burn at the point of current grounding (Figure 25-31). An electrical shock to hands holding the clamp or electrosurgical handpiece is usually caused by a hole in the glove. Regloving should alleviate the problem. Continued shocking reflects poor grounding or an equipment malfunction that should be checked by a qualified service representative.

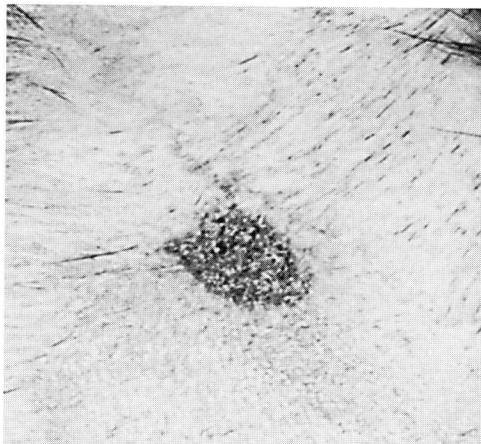

FIGURE 25-31. Cautery burn caused by inadequate conductive contact to the grounding plate.

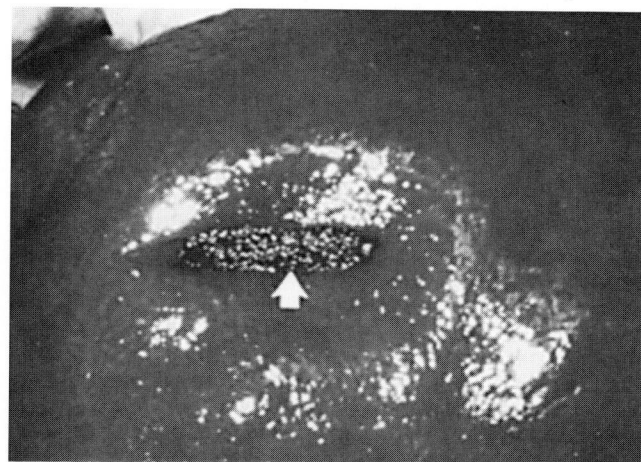

FIGURE 25-33. Cellulose sponge packed into a bleeding crevice *(arrow)* in a liver.

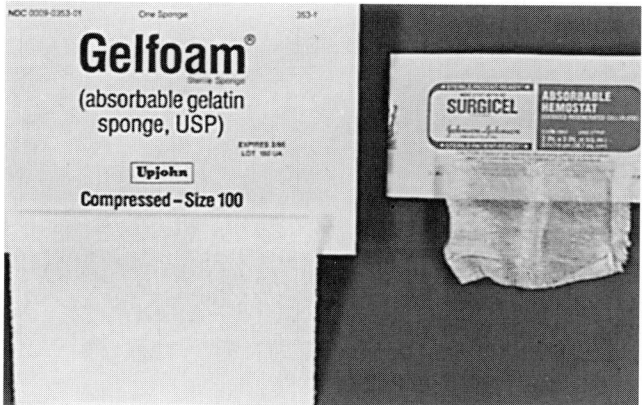

FIGURE 25-32. Biologic hemostatic agents, such as gelatin foam or cellulose sponge, promote coagulation and clot adherence.

Technician Note

Electrosurgery should not be used in the presence of explosive anesthetics (ether) or alcohol-based antiseptic materials.

Tissue healing following the use of the electroscalpel has been shown to be significantly delayed. Likewise, the incidence of incisional infection is somewhat increased. Therefore techniques of asepsis and atraumatic tissue handling must be strictly adhered to when using electrosurgery.

Biologic Coagulants

Biologic agents, such as gelatin sponge (Gelfoam, Upjohn) or cellulose gauze (Surgicel, Johnson & Johnson) (Figure 25-32), can be used to achieve hemostasis on tissues that tend to continually ooze or to pack small bleeding cavities (Figure 25-33). These agents promote coagulation and provide a lattice for the forming clot to adhere to. They are normally absorbed in 2 to 6 weeks, depending on the area of implantation and the specific material.

Chemical Cauterization

Chemical cauterization by agents such as phenol and silver nitrate will achieve hemostasis by denaturing the proteins of the tissues they contact, thus sealing small blood vessels. However, these agents are difficult to apply without contacting and damaging adjacent soft tissues. This usually precludes their use in general surgery.

Metal Clips

Metal clips made of noncorrosive materials (Hemoclip, Versaclip) and the specialized forceps to apply them are available in a variety of sizes and designs (Figure 25-34). They are very effective and can be applied quickly. Their use in veterinary surgery is becoming more widespread as their expense relative to convenience decreases. Vascular stapling devices that automatically occlude both sides of a vessel with small metallic staples, as well as divide it, are available (LDS, U.S. Surgical Corp.) and are commonly used in human surgery. Although the staple cartridges are expensive, the supplying company will often lease the application device.

INCISION IRRIGATION AND SUCTION

Incision irrigation and suction (lavage) serve four main purposes. The first is to physically dilute and remove bacteria carried into the incision from the skin or the air or from spillage from incising a contaminated or infected structure, such as the intestine. The body has a tremendous ability to resist infection from low numbers of bacteria. Consequently, lavaging the site after the initial skin incision, and periodically throughout the procedure to decrease bacterial numbers, will dramatically reduce the incidence of infection. Second, irrigation and suction are used to remove hemorrhage, increasing visibility at the surgical site. This makes both hemostasis and surgical manipulations easier to accomplish. Third, lavage keeps the tissues moist, particularly during longer procedures. If the tissues desiccate (dry out), cell damage and death occur. This decreases the rate of healing and increases the incidence of infection by devitalizing the natural cellular defense mechanisms. There is an old surgical saying that "moist tissues are happy tissues." Finally, lavage is used to dilute and remove irritating and degenerative material, such as urine, bile, or bony fragments. Although these materials will not cause infection, they can cause undesirable biologic reactions and should be removed.

Lavage Fluid

Many different fluids are used for lavage, but they all have common characteristics. The fluid should be a physiologically neutral, isotonic solution (i.e., buffered normal saline or lactated Ringer's solution), meaning it has the same pH (acidity) and osmolality (mineral concentration) as serum. Excessively acid or basic fluids can promote bacterial growth and cause cell damage. Hypotonic (less concentrated) solutions, such as distilled water, will be imbibed by the tissues, resulting in significant edema. Hypertonic (more concentrated) solutions will pull water out of tissues and result in dehydration. This reaction is occasionally used to reduce preexisting edema.

Antiseptic and antibiotic agents are commonly added to the irrigation solution. Povidone-iodine (Betadine, Purdue-Frederick) is used to make a 10% (10 ml of Betadine in 100 ml of normal saline) solution with saline. The addition of 10 ml of chlorhexidine hydrochloride (Nolvasan solution, Fort Dodge Laboratories) per 1 L of saline also makes a useful lavage solution. Care should be taken not to use scrub materials for lavage solutions, since they contain detergents that are highly irritating to tissues. Aminoglycoside antibiotics (e.g., gentamicin) should not be used in lavage of the abdominal and thoracic cavities, because they may be rapidly absorbed and may cause a neuromuscular respiratory paralysis. Antibiotic solutions in general should not be used with cancellous bone grafts, because the antibiotic will diminish the graft's biologic activity.

Technician Note

Scrub solutions should not be used for lavage irrigation solutions because they contain detergents that are irritating to delicate tissues.

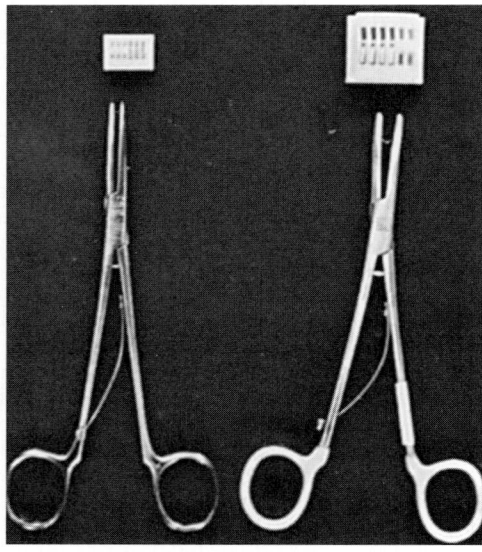

FIGURE 25-34. Metallic hemostatic clips are available in several sizes.

Lavage Technique

Irrigation solutions can be applied with a bulb syringe or a large syringe to obtain a hydraulic cleansing effect. They should be warmed to body temperature to avoid causing hypothermia. This is particularly important in very small or debilitated patients. Cloth drapes should not become excessively damp during surgery, since this will allow capillary movement of bacteria from the underlying nonsterile area. Alternatively, waterproof draping materials, such as baby crib sheets, may be used.

Suction of the surgical incision requires a suction tip, tubing, and a suction bottle. The suction tip may have a single orifice or multiple fenestrations. The single-orifice tip is most useful in orthopedic surgery, neurosurgery, and general surgery, in which the exposure is limited and relatively small amounts of liquid must be removed from very precise areas (Figure 25-35). The multiple-fenestrated tips are used in thoracic and abdominal procedures in which large volumes of fluid are removed (Figure 25-36).

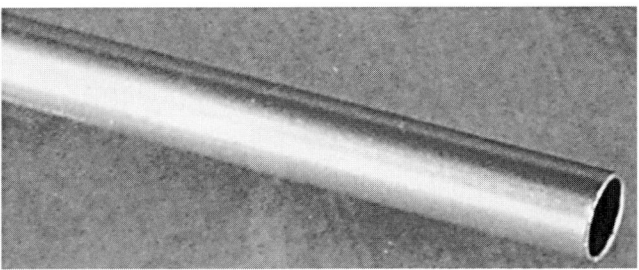

FIGURE 25-35. The single-orifice suction tip is used for precise control.

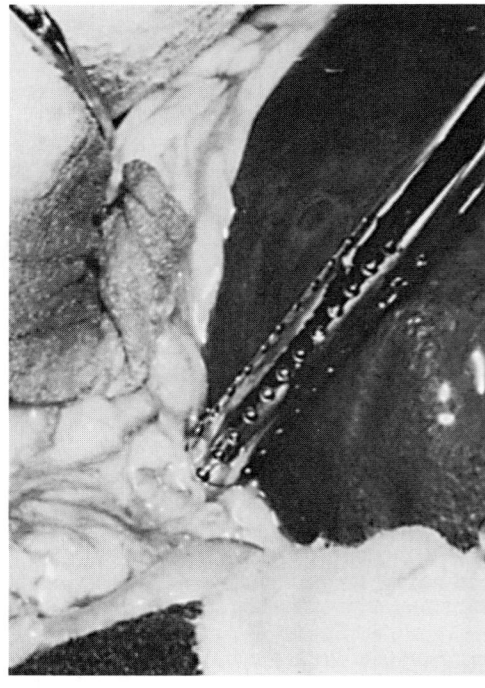

FIGURE 25-36. The multiple-fenestrated suction tip is used to remove large volumes of fluids and avoid omental occlusion.

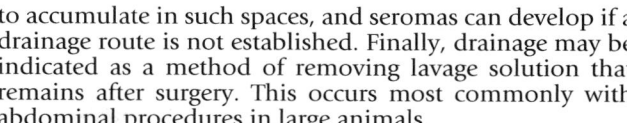

Fenestrated tips also reduce the incidence of plugging with movable soft tissue, such as omentum and mesentery. The surgical assistant controls the strength of suction by occluding the vent hole in the handle of the suction tip. If the tip becomes plugged, it can be cleared by passing a stylet made of slightly smaller stainless steel wire. Periodic suction of clean irrigation solution during the surgical procedure will reduce the incidence of suction tube plugging and make cleaning of the tube much easier.

SURGICAL DRAINS

Postoperative drainage of the surgical area may be indicated for several different reasons. Any incision that is thought to be infected should be allowed to discharge. This can be accomplished by leaving the wound open or by inserting a drain. A drain is also indicated when soft tissues cannot be opposed to obliterate dead space. Serum tends

to accumulate in such spaces, and seromas can develop if a drainage route is not established. Finally, drainage may be indicated as a method of removing lavage solution that remains after surgery. This occurs most commonly with abdominal procedures in large animals.

Two types of drains are commonly used in veterinary surgery. *Penrose drains* are thin-walled, collapsible, latex rubber tubes. Discharge escapes by moving along the *outside* of the drain (Figure 25-37). Therefore the holes in the tissues through which the drain runs must be kept spread open and clean for the drain to work properly. Cleanliness is particularly important, because the hole and drain can act as an avenue for retrograde infections. *Suction drains* are thick-walled tubes of rubber or Silastic. Suction is applied to the outside end of the drain, and discharges are pulled through the lumen of the tube. Multiple openings are created in the wall of the tube on the implanted end (Figure 25-38). This decreases the problem of soft tissues obstructing the drainage. A fenestrated Penrose drain can be placed over the end to further maintain flow, particularly in the abdominal cavity in which the omentum tends to isolate the drain (Figure 25-39). Suction must be maintained for this type of drain to work. Spring-activated devices are commercially available (HemoVac) (Figure 25-40). A homemade device can be made from a large injection syringe and a hypodermic needle (Figure 25-41).

Technician Note

Surgical drains are used to provide an open site of discharge in infected tissues, evacuate dead space, and remove lavage solutions.

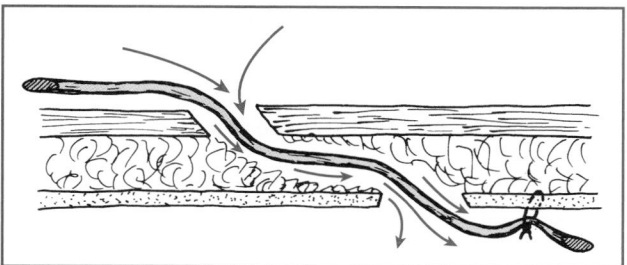

FIGURE 25-37.   Diagram of discharge escaping around the outside of a Penrose drain.

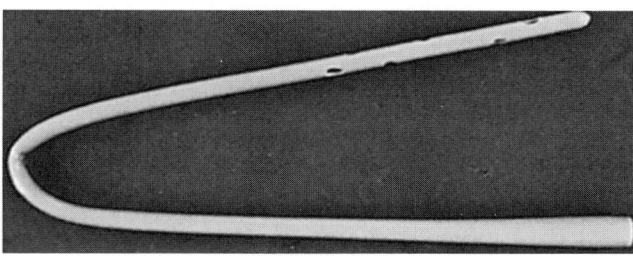

FIGURE 25-38.   Multiple openings on the implanted end of a suction drain.

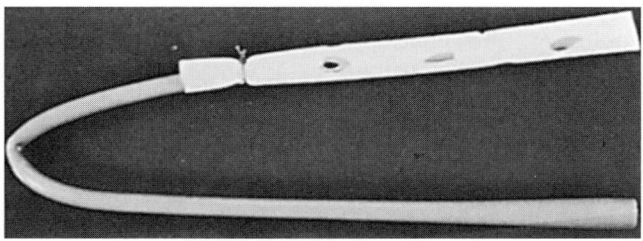

FIGURE 25-39.   Placing a fenestrated Penrose drain over the end of a suction drain decreases occlusion from the omentum.

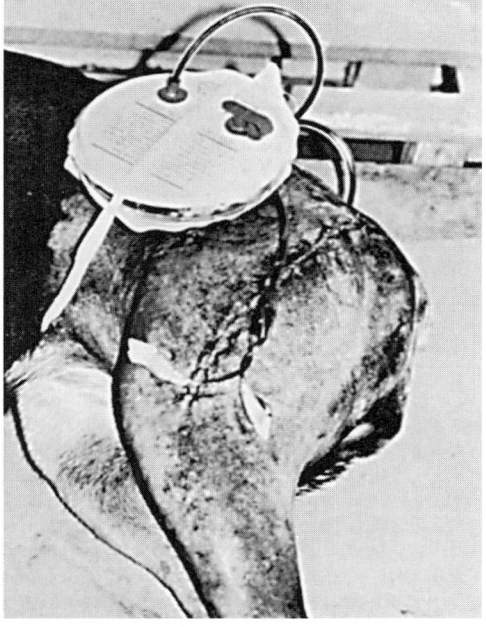

FIGURE 25-40.   A commercially available spring-activated, constant-suction device.

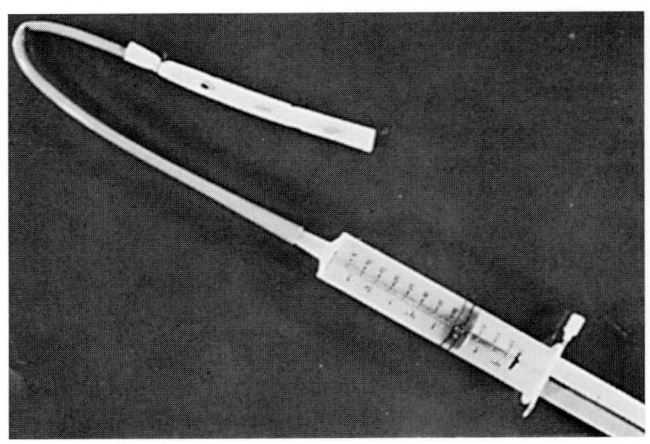

FIGURE 25-41. A homemade constant-suction device constructed from a large syringe and hypodermic needle.

SURGEON: Dr. McCurnin	**PROCEDURE:** Anterior Cruciate Repair
GLOVE SIZE: 7½	**POSITION OF PATIENT:** VD, leg hung
SKIN PREP: Standard	**DRAPES:** 25 cm fenestrated drape 17.5 cm × 15 cm back table drape
SUTURES AND NEEDLES	**INSTRUMENTS AND EQUIPMENT**

TIES:
 	
PERITONEUM:
 	
FASCIA:
 	
SUB-CU: 2-0 chromic gut, cutting
 	
SKIN: 2-0 nylon, cutting
 	
RETENTION:
 	
OTHER: joint capsule: 0 Prolene, Taper
	BASIC:
	        Standard set
	        Bone set
	        Suction hose
	        Large Frazier tip
	        Cautery
	        Stockinette
	
	EXTRA INSTRUMENTS:
	        Stryker saw
	        *Chronic: Round file
	                        Small rongeur

DRESSINGS:	

FIGURE 25-42. A technique card that is used to detail the necessary equipment for each surgical procedure.

SURGICAL THEATER CONDUCT

The principles of aseptic technique and proper preparation are discussed in Chapter 24. The surgical assistant should review these concepts and be constantly cognizant of them during surgery. The assistant must monitor not only his or her own activity but also the surgeon's and that of anyone else in the surgical theater. Ignoring a break in aseptic technique, regardless of the origin, results in contamination and leads to infection. This may destroy an otherwise perfectly performed surgical procedure unless the break is recognized and proper steps are taken to rectify it. Unnecessary traffic and visitors in the surgery suite should be avoided, not only during the procedure but at all times, to help control dust and aerial contamination of the facility.

To be truly efficient and effective as a surgical assistant, the veterinary technician must be familiar with the procedure being performed. This allows readiness of proper instruments and supplies and minimizes the time spent explaining positioning and retraction. This may require

maintenance of a card file detailing necessary equipment and a brief review of the operative technique for each procedure (Figure 25-42).

The surgical assistant is responsible for organizing the instrument set and passing instruments to the surgeon. Although no specific organizational scheme is universally used because of the variation in instruments and specialty equipment, the surgical assistant should be consistent in the general arrangement of the instrument stand. This will save time and effort for the assistant and speed up the procedure. In general, the most-used instruments are placed in the front of the tray, and specialty instruments are placed toward the back (Figure 25-43). A specific region should be reserved for the saline bowl, suture, and sponges. The saline bowl should be placed either inside a sterile tray or on waterproof drapings to prevent wicking from underlying nonsterile surfaces (Figure 25-44). Technicians should follow the progress of the procedure closely to anticipate the surgeon's needs. When passing instruments, the assistant should firmly "snap" the handle or

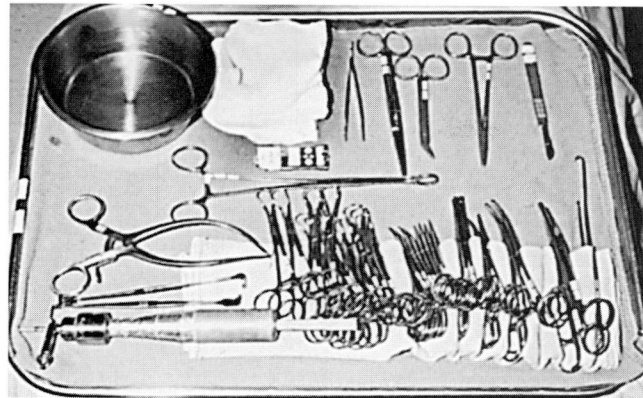

FIGURE 25-43. Example of a typical instrument arrangement on the Mayo stand.

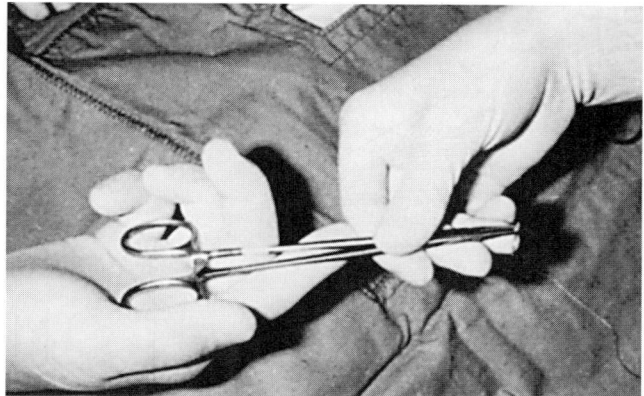

FIGURE 25-45. Instruments are passed, ready for use, into the open hand of the surgeon.

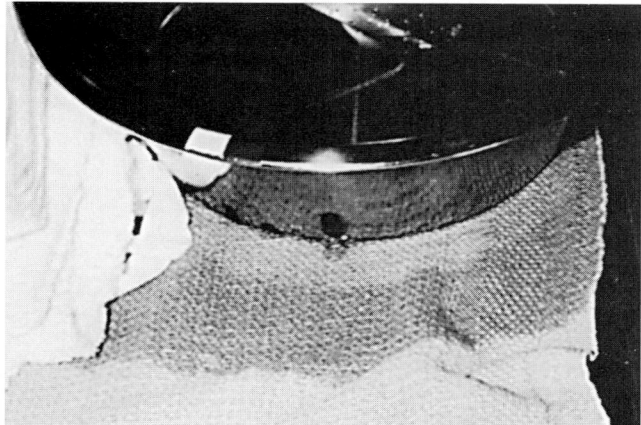

FIGURE 25-44. The saline bowl is placed inside a sterile tray to avoid wick contamination after spillage.

handles into the open hand of the surgeon (Figure 25-45). This keeps the instrument firmly under control and in position for use. When the surgeon has finished with an instrument, it should be quickly wiped clean of blood and tissue and returned to its position on the instrument stand. Prolonged soaking of instruments in water (particularly saline) should be avoided because this ultimately causes corrosive damage to sharp cutting edges and hinges.

SUTURE MATERIAL

Suture is any material that holds tissues together until they heal. The use of suture has been documented since the first century AD. However, it was not until the advent of sterilization and aseptic technique that suture became commonly used. During the late 1800s and early 1900s, suture materials were derived mainly from natural sources. Synthetic suture materials first became available in the 1930s and are still being developed.

Some uses of suture include the following:

- Apposing the edges of an incision or wound
- Obliterating open space in which serum would tend to accumulate

- Tightening and stabilizing joints that have sustained ligament injury or have luxated
- Strengthening or replacing weakened tissues, as in hernias
- Ligating blood vessels or tissues that will be removed

Qualities of the Ideal Suture Material

The ideal suture material would have the following qualities:

- Able to be used for any procedure with the same characteristics in all tissues
- Easily handled and tied by the surgeon
- Causes minimal tissue reaction and does not support, spread, or sequester bacterial growth
- High tensile strength in a small diameter, yet not cut through tissues
- Knots securely with a minimum number of throws and small knot size
- Easy and economical to produce and sterilize
- Does not induce allergic, electrolytic, or neoplastic changes
- Holds tissues until healing occurs, then resorbs with minimum tissue reaction

Obviously, no such suture material exists or probably ever will since several of these attributes are contradictory. Consequently, veterinary personnel must be aware of the advantages and disadvantages of all available sutures and choose the one most appropriate for the use at hand. The technician will need to become familiar with all sutures used by the surgeon.

Suture Nomenclature

Suture material can be classified by a number of characteristics. *Absorbable suture* is broken down and resorbed by the body, resulting in a loss of tensile strength within 60 days. Consequently, it should be used in tissues that heal rapidly to adequate strength. *Nonabsorbable suture* does not significantly weaken with time. It is used in areas that heal slowly and are subject to disruptive stresses. *Multifilament* or *braided suture* material is made up of a number of very small elements that are braided or twisted together to form the desired diameter (Figure 25-46). Multifilament suture tends to be relatively strong, handles well, and has good knot-holding abilities. However, many braided sutures induce significant tissue reaction and can harbor bacteria,

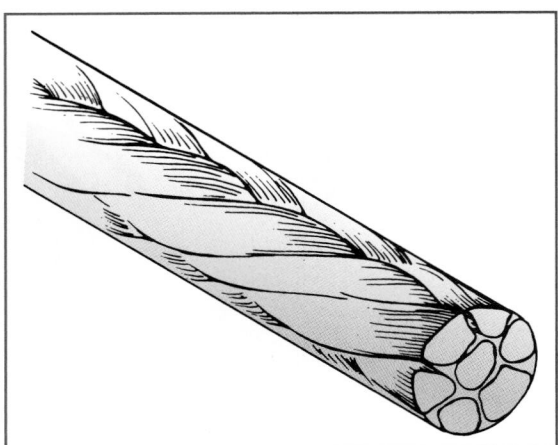

FIGURE 25-46. Constructed multifilament suture. (From Meeker MH, Rothrock JC: *Alexander's care of the patient in surgery,* ed 11, St Louis, 1999, Mosby.)

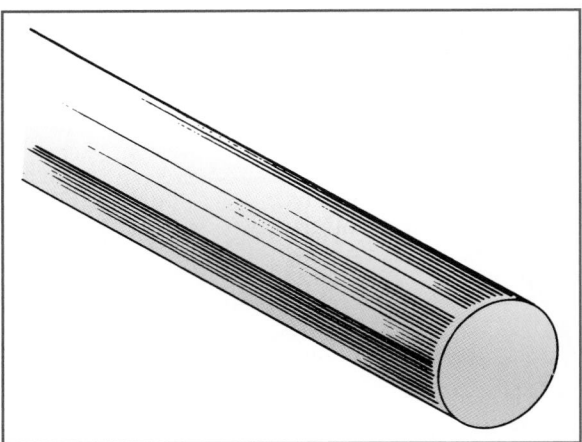

FIGURE 25-47. Monofilament suture. (From Meeker MH, Rothrock JC: *Alexander's care of the patient in surgery,* ed 11, St Louis, 1999, Mosby.)

leading to intractable suture tract infections if they become contaminated. Moreover, most braided suture will exhibit capillary or "wicking" characteristics in which fluids travel along the length of the suture between the filaments. Therefore multifilament suture should not be used in hollow organs or in the skin when part of the suture is exposed to a contaminated environment and the wicking fluid can carry bacteria into the body. *Monofilament suture* (Figure 25-47) avoids the capillary problem and consequently has a lower incidence of infection. It also has a low coefficient of surface friction, making it easy to generally pull through tissues. However, the low surface friction results in poor knot security, necessitating many throws on each knot. Some monofilament suture also has a tendency to return to its original shape (called *memory*), resulting in poor handling characteristics (Figure 25-48).

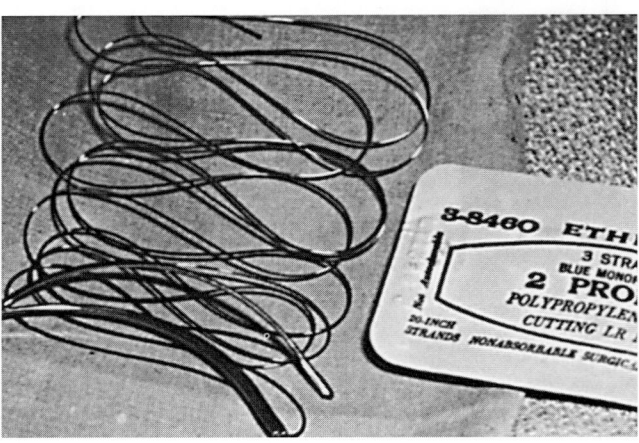

FIGURE 25-48. Memory is the tendency of suture to return to its package shape.

Technician Note

Suture material can be classified as absorbable or nonabsorbable and monofilament or multifilament.

Absorbable Suture Material

Surgical gut is collagenous protein obtained from the submucosal layer of sheep small intestine. It was originally known as kit gut (meaning fiddle string, because the material was used for stringed instruments). Over the years, the term *kit* was mistakenly changed to *cat*, resulting in the common misnomer *catgut.* When implanted in tissues, surgical gut incites an inflammatory reaction that ultimately resorbs the suture by phagocytosis. The severity of reaction, and consequently the rate at which the gut loses strength, can be decreased by tanning the material with chromic salts. Surgical gut has been classified into four groups: *plain, mild, medium,* and *extra chromic* treated with resorption times of 10, 20, 30, and 40 days, respectively. Because surgical gut is broken down by phagocytosis, implantation in inflamed, highly vascular, or biologically active tissue will result in a faster rate of resorption. Medium chromic gut is relatively inexpensive and has predictable handling and knotting characteristics, and therefore it is still one of the most popular absorbable sutures for ligations in veterinary practice. However, its

variability in rate of tensile strength loss, particularly in response to an inflammatory environment, should be considered and has led most surgeons away from its use for closure of support layers.

Other absorbable suture materials, such as collagen, kangaroo tendon, and fascia lata, have been developed but have shown few distinct advantages over surgical gut.

Synthetic Absorbable Suture Material

Synthetic absorbable sutures have been developed to avoid the variation of resorptive rates in inflammatory environments. Polyglycolic acid (Dexon, Davis-Geck) is a synthetic polyester polymerized from hydroxyacetic acid. It is produced in fine filaments that are braided into sutures of various sizes. Consequently, it has excellent handling and knot-holding characteristics. Dexon is broken down in the body by enzymatic hydrolysis, which does *not* induce a significant inflammatory reaction. Further, the rate of absorption is not affected by placement in an inflamed or infected environment. Dexon loses about 33% of its tensile strength in 7 days and 80% of this strength within 2 weeks. Some studies have shown that Dexon absorbs more rapidly in the presence of urine. Overall, it has a superior initial strength, but it loses its strength more rapidly than surgical gut.

Polyglactin 910 (Vicryl, Ethicon) is a copolymer of lactic and glycolic acids. Its production and resorption processes are similar to those of Dexon. Vicryl also has a high initial strength that declines rapidly when implanted. Likewise, it has good handling qualities and knot security.

Poliglecaprone (Monocryl, Ethicon), polydioxanone (PDS, Ethicon), and polyglyconate (Maxon, Davis-Geck) are newer synthetic polyester materials that are pliable enough to be produced and used in monofilament form. Consequently, they have significantly less tissue drag in placement. However, they do possess some memory characteristics and must have multiple throws to knot securely. The process of resorption is similar to that of the other synthetic absorbable materials. Monocryl absorbs at a rate similar to medium chromic gut. Its predictability has led to its replacing gut for many applications. PDS and Maxon are significantly stronger, retaining 74% strength at 2 weeks, 58% strength at 4 weeks, and 41% of their original strength at 6 weeks after implantation. Consequently, they are particularly useful in slow-healing tissues. The major disadvantage of these sutures is their expense, which is approximately twice that of surgical gut and one and one-half times that of Vicryl or Dexon in comparable sizes.

Technician Note

Absorbable sutures retain their tensile strength in tissues for several weeks, whereas nonabsorbable sutures last 60 days or more.

Nonabsorbable Suture Material

Nonabsorbable suture retains its tensile strength for more than 60 days. It can be natural fiber, metallic, or synthetic and will be described according to origin.

Silk is one of the first and still most commonly used nonabsorbable materials. It is obtained from the cocoon of the silkworm and is braided or twisted into multifilament strands. It has excellent handling and knotting qualities. However, it can induce a severe soft tissue reaction, allow capillary migration of contamination (wicking), and serve as a nidus for infection. Despite its nonabsorbable classification, the inflammatory reaction usually results in complete loss of tensile strength within 6 months.

Cotton and linen are natural fibers that are also used to make suture. They both increase slightly in strength when wet but otherwise behave very much like silk. They have seen limited use in veterinary surgery.

Metallic sutures have been used since the fourteenth century, when the biologically nonreactive nature of gold was first described. Stainless steel is the major metallic suture in use today. It is biologically inert and will not support bacterial growth. Also, steel retains its high tensile strength when implanted. Consequently, it is particularly useful in infected wounds or tissues that are expected to be stressed while healing slowly. Stainless steel suture is available in monofilament and multifilament forms. The major disadvantage of steel is its poor handling quality and its tendency to kink. Silver, aluminum, and tantalum sutures have some limited use in human surgery.

Synthetic Nonabsorbable Suture Material

Polyamide (nylon) is a polymerized plastic that is available as suture in both monofilament and braided forms. It does not cause tissue reaction when implanted, but it gradually loses its tensile strength over several years. It is somewhat stiff and slippery, and it has significant memory, making handling and knot security exacting.

Polypropylene (Prolene, Ethicon) is a synthetic plastic that is similar to nylon. However, polypropylene does not weaken with time, making it useful when permanent suture support is needed.

Polybutester (Novafil, Davis-Geck) is a similar synthetic suture that is much more elastic. This means it can stretch and return to its original length without breaking, making it useful for repairing ligaments and other structures that must stretch under weighted motion.

Polyester fibers (Mersiline, Ethicon; Dacron, Davis-Geck) are braided to form a strong noncapillary suture. Handling quality is good, but five or six throws are required for good knot security. It also has significant tissue drag and induces just slightly less tissue reaction than silk. Some manufacturers coat the polyester fibers with Teflon (Tevdek and Polydek, Deknatel) or silicone (Ticron, Davis-Geck) to reduce drag and reaction. However, chronic infection and draining fistulae remain common complications of polyester use.

Polymerized caprolactum (Vetafil, B. Braun Melsungen AG) is made of synthetic fibers coated with a smooth plastic-like material. It has high tensile strength and does not induce a significant tissue reaction. Vetafil is usually provided on a large spool in a multiple-use cassette that may become contaminated. Therefore it must be steam sterilized if implanted beneath the cutaneous layer.

Suture Size and Strength

Technician Note

Oversized sutures do not strengthen a wound and may lead to overtightening and strangulation of tissues.

The size or diameter of suture has been classified by the U.S. Pharmacopeia. Table 25-1 lists the established limits of surgical gut from 7-0 (pronounced "seven ott" or "seven zero") to no. 3. Other suture materials use the same sizing limits and have extended down to an 11-0 nylon for microvascular anastomosis and up to no. 7 stainless steel for orthopedic use. The appropriate-sized suture for each procedure needs to be no stronger than the tissue on which it is used. Oversized sutures do not strengthen a wound and may lead to overtightening and strangulation of tissues. In addition to suture tensile strength, knot security should be considered when selecting suture size. Because the knot is the strength-limiting area of most suture, and the relative knot security decreases as suture size increases; smaller suture offers a mechanical advantage. This is particularly true of the synthetic monofilament sutures, which have a low coefficient of friction (slippery). Besides untying, knotting decreases a suture's strength by converting the longitudinal tensile force into a shearing force that collects at the base of the knot, at which point strands cross and angle. The process of tying the knot also weakens suture by abrading its surface as strands cross. This is particularly true of surgical gut sutures and braided sutures. Excessive suture material should be cut off, leaving the ends just long enough to secure the knot on buried sutures. Of course, this length varies with surface friction and knot security. In general, multifilament and metallic sutures can be cut off quite close to the knot (about 2 mm). Monofilament sutures with memory and polyesters need to have 3 to 4

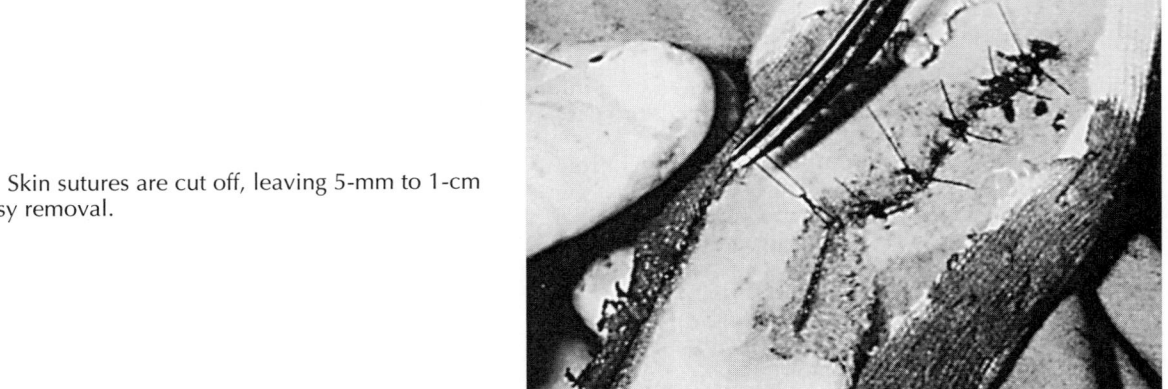

FIGURE 25-49. Skin sutures are cut off, leaving 5-mm to 1-cm tails to allow easy removal.

TABLE 25-1	LIMITS ON SUTURE DIAMETER				
		Millimeters		**Limits on Knot-Pull Tensile Strength**	
Size		**Minimum**	**Maximum**	**kg**	**lb**
7-0		0.025	0.064	0.06	0.125
6-0		0.064	0.113	0.16	0.35
5-0		0.113	0.179	0.32	0.7
4-0		0.179	0.241	0.68	1.5
3-0		0.241	0.318	1.13	2.5
2-0		0.318	0.406	1.18	4.0
1-0		0.406	0.495	2.50	5.5
1		0.495	0.584	3.40	7.5
2		0.584	0.673	4.80	9.0
3		0.673	0.762	5.22	11.5

From US Pharmacopeial Convention: *United States pharmacopeia,* ed 16, Rockville, Md, 1960, The Convention.

mm left to prevent knot untying. Skin sutures usually have about 0.5- to 1.0-cm tails to aid in easy removal (Figure 25-49).

Suture Reaction

As previously noted, some suture materials induce more tissue reaction than others. In descending order of reactiveness, surgical gut is most reactive, followed by multifilament natural fiber, synthetic multifilament suture, synthetic monofilament suture, and finally metallic suture. Recognizing a suture's reactivity becomes particularly important when suture reaction might affect function of the tissue, as in neurosurgery or cardiovascular surgery.

Tissue reaction also impedes healing of normal tissue. The presence of infection or contamination has a much greater effect on the more reactive sutures. For example, the inflammatory process associated with infection will often phagocytose surgical gut at an increased rate, leading to resorption before healing and wound dehiscence. Likewise, the presence of silk has been shown to increase the incidence of infection 10,000-fold in contaminated incisions. Finally, nonabsorbable suture, such as silk or polyester, may cause ulceration of the gastrointestinal tract or serve as the nidus for stone formation in the urinary bladder or gallbladder if it penetrates the lumen of those hollow organs.

Preparation of Suture Material

Several methods are used by suture producers to sterilize various suture materials. Many prepackaged sutures are sterilized by gamma irradiation. Ethylene oxide is used on those products that will not tolerate irradiation. Prepackaged suture material has a sterile shelf life that varies as denoted by the expiration date printed on the package. Consequently, expiration dates should be periodically checked and stock rotated when new supplies arrive. Steam sterilization (autoclaving) can be used on some materials, with variable damaging effects. The following describes the effects of autoclaving:

I. Severe damage, destroys tensile strength
  A. Surgical gut
  B. Polyglycolic acid (PDS)
  C. Polyglactin (Vicryl)
II. Mild damage, reduces tensile strength
  A. Silk
  B. Linen
  C. Cotton
III. Tolerates at least three autoclavings without loss of tensile strength
  A. Polyester
  B. Nylon
  C. Polypropylene
  D. Metallics

Sutures that can be steam sterilized are often bought in bulk and are sterilized in the practice. When preparing such suture, an appropriate number of strand lengths (usually 30 to 60 cm) should be cut and coiled or loosely wound around a card or sponge (Figure 25-50). This will avoid repeated autoclaving, which will damage even the most steam-tolerant material.

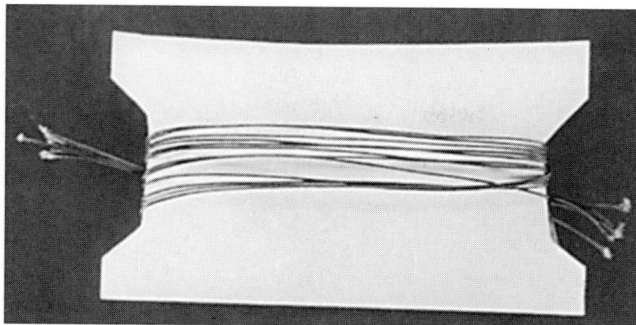

FIGURE 25-50.   Precut strands of suture loosely wrapped around a card.

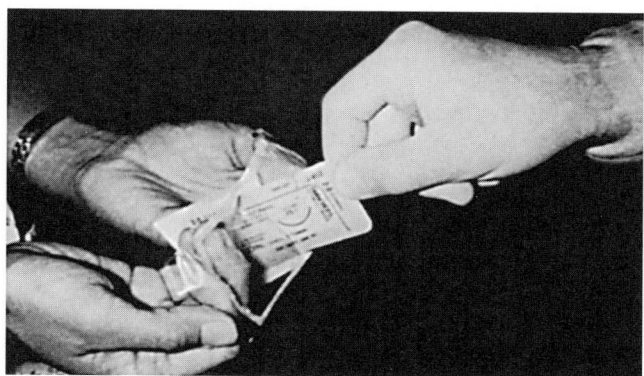

FIGURE 25-51.   Peeling back the outer covering of a prepackaged suture material.

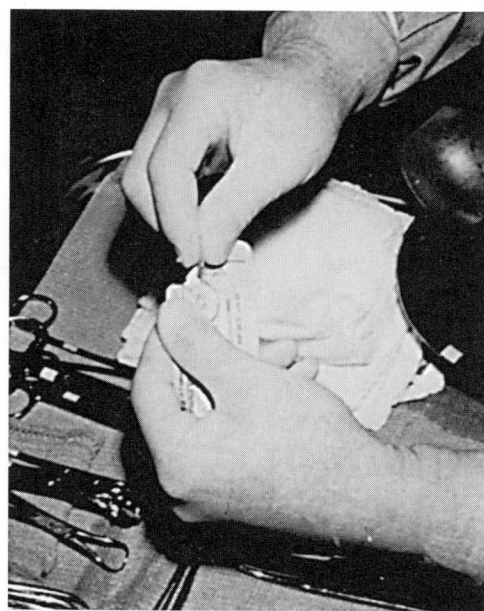

FIGURE 25-52.   Tearing off the end of the inner suture package.

Prepackaged suture material is opened (by a nonsterile assistant) onto the instrument tray by peeling back the outer packaging (Figure 25-51). The surgical assistant opens the inner pack by tearing off one end and grasping the suture end or swaged needle with needle holders as directed on the package (Figure 25-52). Before use, the suture should be stretched slightly to overcome memory but not snapped because this commonly leads to contami-

nation of the suture end. Any excessive preserving fluid should be wiped off. The tissue drag of many sutures (particularly the synthetic multifilaments) can be reduced by moistening with sterile saline. However, this will reduce the tensile strength of silk, and surgical gut will imbibe water to swell and soften. Multifilament suture strands tend to accumulate blood as they pass through tissue and should be wiped off with a moistened sponge between use.

Suture Needles

Suture needles vary considerably in shape, point design, method of attachment to the suture (eye), and size. The size and shape of the needle are determined by the thickness of tissue being sutured and the depth of the incision (Figure 25-53, *A*).

Technician Note

Cutting-edged needles should not be used when an airtight or watertight suture line is required (lung, urinary bladder, intestine, etc.).

The point design varies with the toughness of tissue being sutured (Figure 25-53, *B*). Skin, eye tissues, and some facial tissues are sutured with a *cutting-edged needle*. *Reverse-cutting needles* (K needles) are preferred by some surgeons for their increased needle shank strength. Cutting-edged needles actually incise a slightly larger hole than the size of the needle shank. Although this makes passage of the needle and suture easier, a true incision that can leak is created. Therefore cutting-edged needles should not be used when an air-tight or watertight suture line is required. *Taper needles* do not actually cut tissue but spread it open around the needle and following suture. This spreading effect avoids hemorrhage and results in a sealed

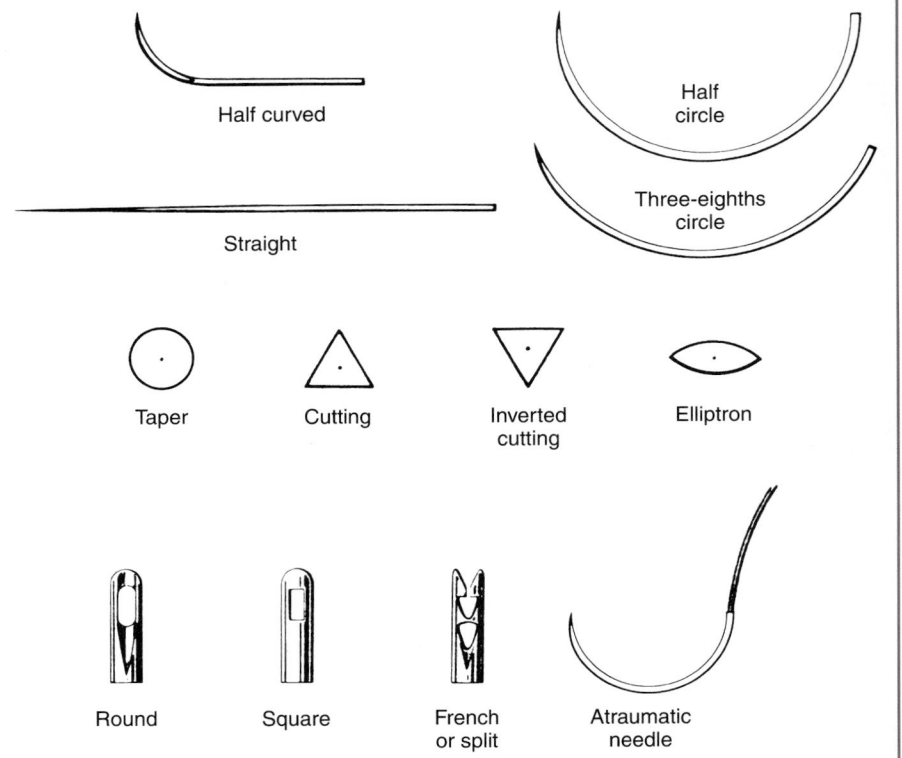

FIGURE 25-53. **A,** The size and shape of the needle are chosen according to the thickness of the tissue. **B,** The needle point design is determined according to the toughness of the tissue on which it is used. **C,** The needle is attached to the suture either by threading through an eye or being swaged. (Courtesy Sherwood Davis & Geck, Milford, N.J.)

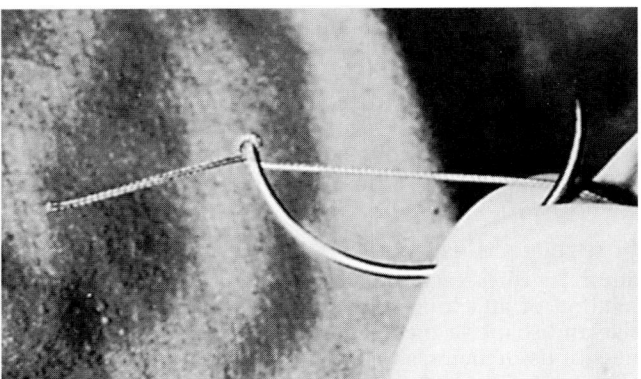

FIGURE 25-54. Double threading should be avoided because it results in a large bulk of suture that causes severe tissue drag.

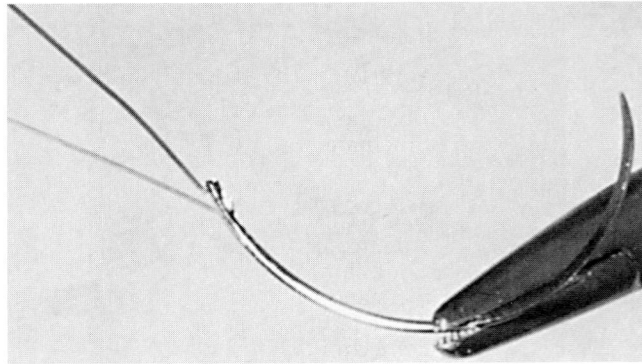

FIGURE 25-55. Threading of a French eye needle by passing the suture through the complete eye and pulling it down through the spring eye.

suture line. Taper needles and reverse-cutting needles are used in suturing most hollow organs.

The needle can be attached to the suture by three different methods (Figure 25-53, *C*). Single-eyed needles have one hole in the head of the needle. The eye should be single threaded, since double threading leaves a large bulk of suture around the shank (Figure 25-54), which will cause excessive tissue drag and damage as the needle is passed. A curved needle is threaded from within the curve so that the short end of the suture falls away from the outside curve. About 10 cm of suture should be pulled through the eye. These steps will help to prevent the suture from pulling out of the eye during suturing. Spring or French-eyed needles have a complete eye and an incomplete "spring" eye. Suture is threaded through the complete eye and is then forced back through the spring eye, which grips the suture end (Figure 25-55). Eyeless or swaged needles are attached directly to the end of the suture by the factory. The surgeon draws a single strand through the tissue and uses a new sharp needle with every strand. Therefore swaged needles are the most atraumatic and are the most popular surgical needle.

RECOMMENDED READING

Evans HE, Christenson GC: *Miller's anatomy of the dog,* ed 3, Philadelphia, 1993, WB Saunders.

Slatter D: *Textbook of small animal surgery,* ed 2, Philadelphia, 1993, WB Saunders.

26

Small Animal Surgical Nursing

Matt G. Oakes

GENERAL PRINCIPLES OF SURGICAL NURSING

The role of the veterinary technician in veterinary surgery can best be discussed by dividing the duties into preoperative, operative, and postoperative considerations. Before surgical intervention, the patient must be properly evaluated, prepared, and monitored. The veterinary technician is responsible for the adequate restraint of the patient before anesthetic induction (see Chapters 1 and 21) and for knowing proper anesthetic techniques and monitoring (see Chapter 21). In addition, the veterinary technician must have a solid understanding of surgical instrumentation and aseptic technique (see Chapter 24) and positioning requirements. These techniques are discussed in detail in this text and should be reviewed before operative assistance techniques.

Many operative procedures require the assistance of a veterinary technician. A working knowledge of common surgical procedures will help to make the veterinary technician proficient at surgical assistance. Procedures that often require such assistance include orthopedic surgery (retraction, reduction, traction, countertraction), open chest procedures (artificial ventilation, retraction), and complicated abdominal procedures (diaphragmatic hernia repair, renal surgery, tumor resection). An understanding of aseptic technique, a familiarity with surgical instrumentation, and a working knowledge of the specific surgical procedure are prerequisites for proper intraoperative assistance. Surgical assistance is discussed in Chapter 25.

Small animal surgical nursing includes many aspects of the primary care of the veterinary surgical patient. This chapter deals primarily with the postoperative care and evaluation of patients by the veterinary technician. In addition, the more commonly performed small animal surgical procedures are discussed, with emphasis on the role of the veterinary technician.

Patient Monitoring

Postoperative care can be divided into immediate and delayed categories. The veterinary technician should continue patient monitoring in the immediate postsurgical period in a fashion similar to preoperative and intraoperative monitoring (e.g., respiratory rate, heart rate, reflex changes). The postoperative phase is a critical transition period and must be monitored continuously until the patient is safely extubated, normothermic, and in sternal recumbency.

As the patient becomes more conscious and aware of its surroundings, evaluation of discomfort at the surgical site should be made.

Technician Note

If the patient is having an unusually "stormy" recovery that can be related to surgical pain, the veterinarian should be alerted, and a proper analgesic should be prescribed. When in doubt, it should be assumed that the patient is having some degree of postoperative pain.

In the daily evaluation of any postsurgical patient, the technician should be aware of several important indicators. First, the patient should be evaluated for its general appearance, attitude, and appetite. A general examination should include temperature, pulse, and respiration. Abnormalities in these can often be the first changes to occur in significant postoperative complications. Second, a visual and palpable inspection of the surgical wound should be made.

Common abnormalities in the early postoperative period (1 to 3 days) include redness, swelling, drainage, excessive licking, and dehiscence (wound breakdown).

Incision Evaluation

An incision should be evaluated with respect to the type of surgical procedure performed on the patient. Elective operations, such as ovariohysterectomy and castration, can be expected to produce mild redness and swelling with no drainage from the incision site. However, if the wound was contaminated (e.g., laceration, perianal wound) or if the surgical exposure was extensive, the incision can be expected to be somewhat swollen, reddened, and warm to the touch and have mild to moderate drainage in the first 24 to 48 hours postoperatively. Swelling secondary to surgical trauma can be expected to resolve in several days. However, *seromas* (serum pockets) and *hematomas* (pockets of hemorrhage) may persist and should be treated early. They are recognized by localized areas of fluctuant, fluid-filled swellings and are treated by drainage, warm compresses, and bandaging. If the swelling occurs 4 to 6 days postoperatively, is warm to the touch, and is associated with an elevated body temperature, the possibility of an abscess or cellulitis (infection along tissue planes) must be considered. These conditions must be treated by drainage, warm compresses, and systemic antibiotics.

Wound dehiscence is defined as the separation of all layers of an incision or wound. Early recognition is imperative in any wound but especially in abdominal and thoracic incisions. Critical evaluation of surgical wounds is of paramount importance for the ultimate welfare of the patient.

> ### Technician Note
>
> Dehiscence of an abdominal wound may result in evisceration of the abdominal organs, with subsequent contamination and infection. Dehiscence of a thoracic wound will result in a severe open *pneumothorax* (air within the chest causing collapse of the lungs), a problem that may result in sudden death.

During the first 12 to 24 hours after surgery, it will become apparent which patients will aggressively lick at their suture line. It is important to recognize these patients early to prevent subsequent wound dehiscence and infection.

Patient Restraint

Several methods can be used effectively to prevent postoperative self-trauma. They are divided into two groups: chemical restraint agents and mechanical restraint devices.

The most commonly used chemical restraint agents are tranquilizers and noxious-tasting agents. Tranquilizers must be used with some caution, since they are often insufficient when used alone and may have undesirable side effects. In combination with other devices (e.g., Elizabethan collar, side bar), however, they can be useful. Acepromazine (Ayerst) is the most commonly used tranquilizer in veterinary medicine.

Noxious-tasting agents must also be used with discretion. Some commonly used substances include Bandguard Cream (Schering-Plough), bitter apple, Tabasco, and various thumb-sucking preparations. The agent can be impregnated into bandage material, and some can be placed directly on the skin around the incision. It should not, however, be placed directly on the incision because it could be irritating. Alternating various substances helps to

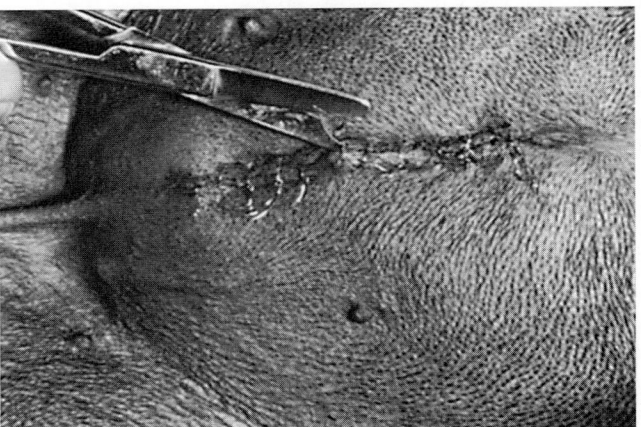

FIGURE 26-1. Proper instrumentation and technique for removal of sutures.

prevent the patient from becoming accustomed to the taste of one. The combined use of mechanical restraint devices and chemical restraint agents has been helpful in controlling intractable patients.

Mechanical restraint devices include the Elizabethan collar, the body brace, the side bar, hobbles, and various bandages. The assembly, materials necessary, specific indications, contraindications, and complications have been adequately described elsewhere (see Recommended Reading) and are beyond the scope of this chapter. A properly selected, constructed, and applied device will be well tolerated by the patient and effective for its desired purpose.

Suture Removal

Suture removal is commonly performed by the technician. Most sutures are removed 10 to 14 days after surgery. Incision healing should be evaluated before suture removal. Suture scissors allow removal with minimal discomfort to the patient (Figure 26-1).

COMMON SURGICAL PROCEDURES

The veterinary technician must have a working knowledge of common surgical procedures in order to properly prepare the patient preoperatively, act as an efficient surgical assistant, and manage the immediate and long-term postoperative care. The remainder of this chapter reviews the most commonly performed small animal surgical procedures in a veterinary practice. A brief description of the procedure, with emphasis on the role of the veterinary technician, will be given.

Elective Surgery Versus Nonelective Surgery

It is ideal to perform surgery on a healthy patient, thus allowing the surgeon to choose the best time to operate. This is known as an *elective* surgical procedure. Occasionally, a patient will be admitted to the hospital requiring immediate surgery. The patient is often compromised. This is not the ideal time to perform the operation, but it must be done as a lifesaving measure. This is known as *nonelective* or emergency surgery.

Tail Docking on Puppies

DEFINITION. Tail docking refers to partial amputation of the tail. Tails are docked to conform with standards set for certain breeds. The American Kennel Club has a recom-

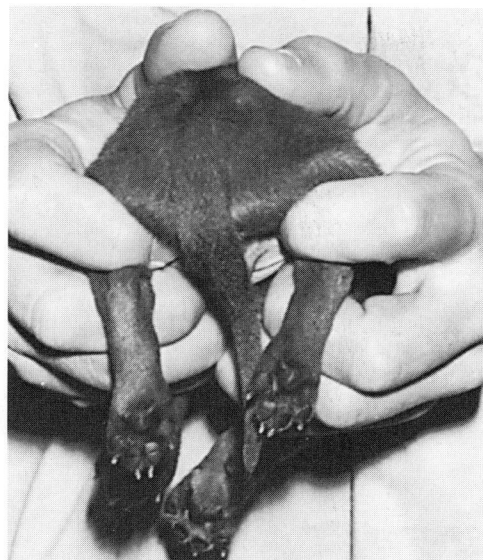

FIGURE 26-2.   Patient properly restrained and positioned for tail-docking procedure.

mended tail length for each breed. This standard should be followed carefully unless the owner or breeder specifies otherwise. Tail docking should be performed at an early age (3 to 5 days). This allows the procedure to be performed without general anesthesia.

TECHNIQUE.   The pup should be cradled in the palms of both hands, with the hindlegs held between the index and middle fingers and the tail directed toward the surgeon (Figure 26-2). The surgical site is prepared in the usual manner. The desired length of remaining tail is marked, and the skin of the tail is retracted craniad. The tail is amputated with a pair of scissors, bleeding is controlled with electrocautery or pressure, and the skin is released, allowing it to retract over exposed bone. One simple interrupted absorbable suture is placed to appose the skin edges.

AFTERCARE.   The pups should be returned to the mother. The procedure is relatively atraumatic to the pups, and they will begin to nurse minutes after surgery. The suture remains until it is absorbed or licked out by the mother.

Dewclaw Removal on Puppies

DEFINITION.   The claws located on the medial aspect of the forelegs and hindlegs are known as *dewclaws*. Dewclaws are commonly removed from the forefeet and hindfeet of purebred dogs for show purposes and from hunting dogs because they may be torn as the dog runs over densely shrubbed terrain. It should be remembered that in certain breeds (e.g., Great Pyrenees, Newfoundland) the presence of dewclaws is necessary for proper show quality. Dewclaws should be removed at an early age (3 to 5 days). Removal is generally performed at the same time as tail docking.

TECHNIQUE.   The surgical site is prepared in the usual manner. The pup is cradled in the palm of one hand, and the extremity is extended with the other hand. Scissors are used to clip the dewclaws off. Hemorrhage is controlled with electrocautery or pressure. The skin edges may be left unsutured or apposed with one absorbable suture.

AFTERCARE.   The pups are returned to the mother immediately.

Tail Docking and Dewclaw Removal in the Adult

Tail docking and dewclaw removal should ideally be done within the first week of life. In some instances, adult dogs are presented for one or both procedures.

TECHNIQUE FOR DEWCLAW REMOVAL.   The patient must be placed under general anesthesia. The surgical site is clipped and prepared in the usual manner, and an elliptical incision is made at the base of the dewclaw. The dewclaw is dissected and is transected at the carpometacarpal joint in the front paw or the tarsometatarsal joint in the hindpaw. Hemorrhage is controlled with electrocautery and pressure. The skin edges are apposed with a subcuticular suture pattern. A foot bandage is used to prevent swelling and self-trauma. An Elizabethan collar should be used if needed.

TECHNIQUE FOR TAIL AMPUTATION.   The tail should be clipped and hung from an intravenous stand, the skin should be prepared in the usual manner, and the end of the tail should be covered with a sterile stockinette. A tourniquet is placed at the base of the tail, and the tail is amputated at the desired location by skin incision and transection of the coccygeal vertebra at the appropriate site. Blood vessels are identified and ligated. The skin edges are sutured over the remaining vertebrae, and the tourniquet is removed. The tail can be bandaged or left unbandaged. In any case, an Elizabethan collar should be placed on the patient postoperatively. The patient should be examined frequently during the first 6 to 8 hours to be certain that the tail cannot be traumatized.

Feline Onychectomy

DEFINITION.   Onychectomy (declawing) involves removal of the claw and its associated third phalanx. The third phalanx must be removed to ensure adequate excision of germinal epithelium. If this is not accomplished, regrowth of the claw may occur.

INDICATIONS.   Onychectomy is an elective procedure to prevent furniture mutilation by the cat. Most veterinarians recommend declawing the front feet only. This does not significantly impair the cat's ability to climb trees or defend itself from intruders. Onychectomy is often performed at the same time as castration or ovariohysterectomy, but young cats (8 to 16 weeks) tend to have less hemorrhage and postoperative pain.

TECHNIQUE.   The feet are surgically scrubbed but need not be clipped unless the patient is a long-haired breed. A tourniquet is placed above the elbow. A Rescoe nail trimmer is positioned snugly onto the dorsal surface of the toe between the second phalanx and third phalanx. During positioning of the nail trimmer, the claw should be pulled cranially. As little skin as possible should be excised. The cutting edge of the Rescoe nail trimmer is positioned at the cranial edge of the foot pad. As the cutting edge is advanced, the pad is moved caudally while rotating the nail dorsally and caudally. The third phalanx is then excised by the Rescoe nail trimmer (Figure 26-3). Care is taken to avoid cutting the foot pad or leaving any portion of the third phalanx. Each nail is amputated in a similar fashion.

The paws are bandaged snugly with strips of tape and a gauze sponge. The sponge is placed over the excised digits.

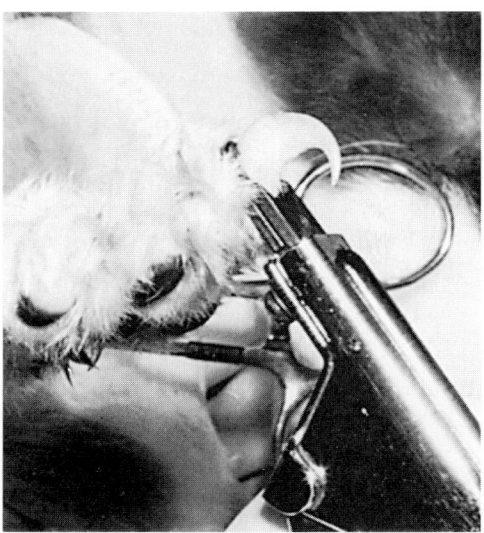

FIGURE 26-3. Proper placement of claw and third phalanx in the cutting edge of the Rescoe nail trimmer for an onychectomy.

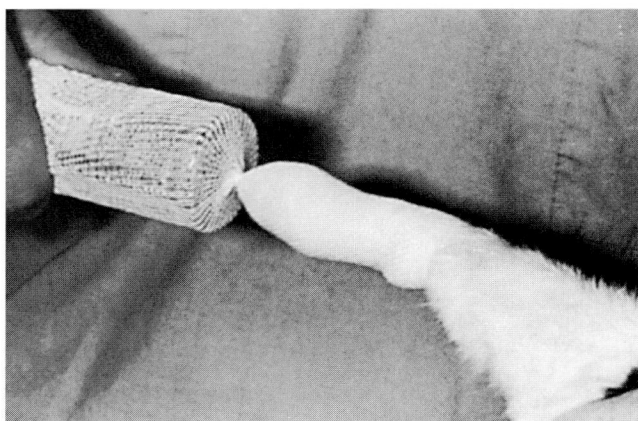

FIGURE 26-5. Tube gauze used to bandage paws after onychectomy.

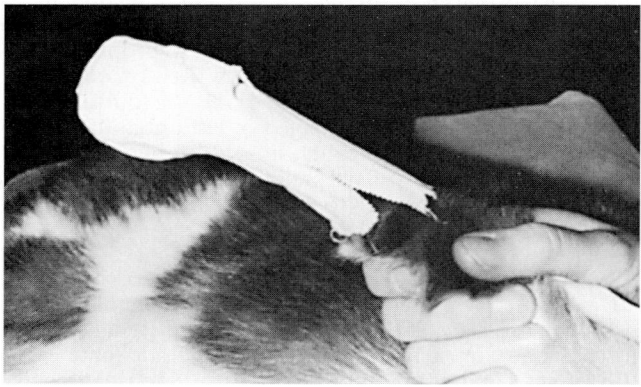

FIGURE 26-4. Tape and gauze used to bandage paws after onychectomy.

Strips of tape are placed longitudinally along the leg and distally around the paw (Figure 26-4). Tape is then placed circumferentially around the paw up to the elbow. Care is taken to lay tape on the leg and not to pull too tightly. Tube gauze (Figure 26-5) can also be used, but its expense precludes its use in most practices. The tourniquets are removed as soon as bandaging is complete. The bandages should not be left on longer than 24 hours.

Technician Note

The bandage from an onychectomy should be removed within 24 hours.

The patient generally remains in the hospital until the bandages are removed. Most cats allow removal of the bandages by carefully cutting the bandage apart longitudinally and gently peeling it off the leg. If the patient is intractable, the bandage may be cut and the cat returned to its cage. The patient will then remove the bandage on its own. In severely intractable patients, a light dose of intravenous ketamine may be necessary to remove the bandages safely. Patients are generally kept for observation for 12 hours after bandage removal. If no signs of hemorrhage occur, the patient can be discharged.

When patients are discharged, it is important to inform owners that the litter must be changed to shredded paper for the first 5 to 7 days at home. This prevents contamination of the paw with litter and subsequent infection.

COMPLICATIONS. Onychectomy complications can be divided into those that occur in the early postoperative period and those that occur in the late postoperative period. Early complications include loose bandages and postoperative bleeding. Onychectomy patients should be checked frequently for evidence of loose, bloody bandages or complete bandage removal and severe hemorrhage. In the event of hemorrhage, the paws should be rebandaged snugly. Late complications include regrowth of the claws, chronic lameness, or both. Claw regrowth requires reoperation and removal of remaining germinal epithelium. Chronic lameness without evidence of regrowth may be seen with incomplete removal of the phalanx or cut foot pads. For this reason, it is essential that the pads be preserved during the operative procedure.

Variations of the above-described technique have been used to successfully declaw the cat. Included are blade excision of the third phalanx, CO_2 laser excision, suturing the defect after claw excision, and the use of cyanoacrylic tissue adhesive to close the wound. The most acceptable technique is that with which the veterinarian is most familiar.

Celiotomy

DEFINITION. *Celiotomy* (laparotomy) is a surgical incision into the abdominal cavity. There are several locations in which the incision can be made: ventral midline, paramedian, paracostal, parapreputial, and flank (Figure 26-6). The most commonly used incision site is ventral midline.

INDICATIONS. A celiotomy incision can be performed in an elective procedure or in a nonelective procedure. Some

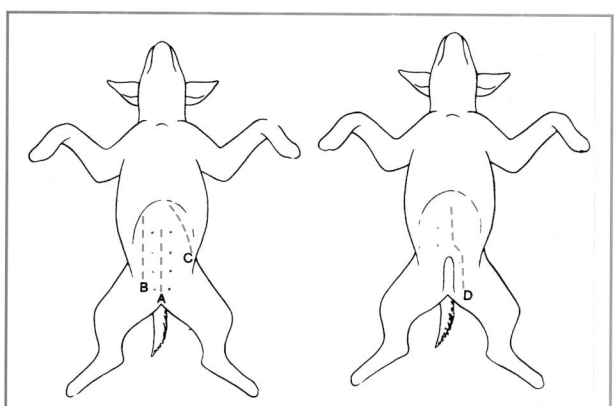

FIGURE 26-6.   Locations for celiotomy incisions. *A,* Ventral midline. *B,* Paramedian. *C,* Paracostal. *D,* Parapreputial.

of the common elective procedures include ovariohysterectomy, cystotomy, cesarean delivery, intestinal surgery, gastric surgery, and retained abdominal testicles. Some common nonelective procedures include gastric dilation and volvulus (bloated, twisted stomach), intussusception, gastrointestinal foreign bodies, ruptured spleen, penetrating foreign bodies (e.g., knife wound, arrow wound, bullet wound), severe abdominal bleeding, and diaphragmatic hernia. In some instances, the patient is presented for an unknown abdominal problem. These patients may need elective or nonelective celiotomy, referred to as an *exploratory celiotomy.* Exploratory celiotomy is often performed for abdominal masses of unknown origin and is used as a diagnostic tool.

TECHNIQUE.   The patient is placed in dorsal recumbency. Larger dogs should be placed in a V trough to support their shoulders. Smaller dogs and cats can be placed on moldable beanbags or sandbags. All patients should be placed on a circulating water heater, but this is especially important for smaller dogs and all cats. The abdomen is widely clipped from 2 cm craniad to the xiphoid cartilage to 2 cm caudad to the pubis. The skin is aseptically prepared in the usual fashion (see Chapter 24).

The various incisions (paramedian, paracostal, etc.) are all slight variations of the ventral midline incision (see Figure 26-6). For this reason, emphasis will be given to the ventral midline incision.

The line of the incision is from the xiphoid process to the pubis. The length used varies with the type of procedure (see specific procedures). The incision is made with a scalpel blade or electrocautery in the cutting mode. The incision is carried through the subcutaneous tissue to the level of the linea alba, which is elevated with forceps to pull it away from the underlying abdominal viscera. This will prevent the inadvertent puncture of abdominal organs when entering the peritoneal cavity. A scalpel blade is used to nick through the linea alba into the peritoneal cavity. The incision is extended the desired length with scissors. Moistened laparotomy pads (sponges) are used to protect the incision edges. A Balfour self-retaining abdominal retractor can be introduced, if necessary, into the incision to facilitate visualization of abdominal structures (explor-

atory celiotomy). It is important to remember that minimal manipulation of abdominal viscera is the rule. Whenever retraction or manipulation of structures is necessary, atraumatic technique is mandatory. Retract viscera with moistened laparotomy pads, manipulate viscera with moistened gloves, blot any excess hemorrhage with moistened sponges (do not wipe surfaces with sponges), and when using suction be careful not to suck the walls of visceral structures against the suction orifice. The postoperative sponge count should be made before closing the abdomen.

> ### Technician Note
>
> A thorough inspection of the abdomen should be made before closure to avoid leaving instruments or sponges in the abdominal cavity. A preoperative and postoperative sponge count is recommended.

The abdomen is sutured closed in three layers. The linea alba is the layer of strength and must be securely closed. The subcutaneous tissues are then sutured to decrease the amount of dead space. This helps reduce the frequency of postoperative hematoma or seroma formation. The skin is then sutured to complete the celiotomy closure. (For additional information about sutures, see Chapter 25.)

POSTOPERATIVE CONSIDERATIONS.   During the first 24 hours, the skin incision should be examined carefully for evidence of self-trauma. If problems arise, an Elizabethan collar should be considered. If there is evidence of dehiscence, the veterinary technician should notify the veterinarian immediately. Emergency closure may be necessary.

Ovariohysterectomy in the Dog and Cat

DEFINITION.   An ovariohysterectomy involves the surgical removal of the uterus and ovaries. The uterus is removed with the ovaries to prevent subsequent development of uterine disease. If any ovarian tissue is inadvertently missed, the animal will continue to have heat cycles.

INDICATIONS.   In the normal female the principal objective is prevention of estrus and the accompanying problems associated with bloody discharge, attraction of male dogs or cats, accidental matings, pregnancy, and unwanted puppies or kittens.

Other indications for ovariohysterectomy include endocrine imbalances, infections, injuries, cysts, tumors, and congenital abnormalities. Endocrine disturbances are associated with varied clinical manifestations, such as sterility, skin lesions, mammary tumors, pseudocyesis (false pregnancy), and nymphomania. Among the uterine diseases that may require ovariohysterectomy are metritis, pyometra, endometrial hyperplasia, neoplasia, injury, neglected dystocia, and congenital abnormalities.

Although the operation can be done at almost any age and at any phase of the reproductive cycle, it is best performed either before puberty or during anestrus. About 6 months of age is generally considered best. At this age, the animal can be anesthetized with relative safety. The female cat may be spayed any time after 5 months of age.

>
> ### Technician Note
>
> The incidence of mammary neoplasia can be greatly reduced in the dog by spaying before the first heat.

The surgery is most hazardous during estrus and pregnancy and in old, obese females. The blood supply to the reproductive tract and the risk of intraoperative hemorrhage are increased during estrus and pregnancy. The most favorable time to spay a mature bitch is 3 to 4 months after estrus. Female cats may be spayed during heat with minimal increased risk. After whelping, the operation should be done as soon as the puppies or kittens have been weaned and lactation has ceased, about 6 to 8 weeks following parturition. Gestation does not alter the usual 6- to 8-month estrus cycle in the canine.

TECHNIQUE.   The patient is clipped and aseptically prepared for a routine ventral midline celiotomy. The skin incision is made from the umbilicus caudally 3 to 6 cm in a dog and from 2 cm caudad to the umbilicus caudally 3 to 4 cm in length in a cat. When the abdominal cavity is entered, the uterine horns are located and exteriorized from the abdomen. The ovarian arteries (pedicles) are ligated with the appropriate-sized absorbable suture material. The uterine body is then exteriorized and ligated. The abdominal cavity is carefully examined for hemorrhage. The celiotomy incision is closed in a routine fashion.

COMPLICATIONS.   The most common postoperative complication of ovariohysterectomy is abdominal hemorrhage. The patient should be carefully monitored during the first 3 to 6 hours postoperatively. Temperature, pulse, respiration, and character of mucous membranes should be examined periodically.

When monitoring the patient's body temperature, it should be appreciated that all postoperative patients experience hypothermia. It is considered a good sign if periodic readings show a trend toward an increasing body temperature. If the temperature remains low or continues to fall, it may be an indication of potential problems. Attempts should be made to maintain the patient at normal body temperature during recovery.

The pulse should be evaluated with respect to rate and character. If it becomes rapid and weak, it may be a sign of hemorrhage, developing shock, or both. Frequent evaluation to determine the trend of the pulse rate and its character is necessary to properly evaluate the patient.

Respiratory rate may help to determine the patient's postoperative condition. If the patient is experiencing significant blood loss, the respiratory rate may increase significantly.

The mucous membranes should be examined frequently. They should be evaluated with respect to color and capillary refill time. Normal mucous membranes should be pink and have a capillary refill time of less than 2 seconds.

Technician Note

If the mucous membranes become pale and the refill time is greater than 2 seconds, the patient may be experiencing significant blood loss.

One abnormal sign at one given time is not enough to diagnose a significant problem. All indicators (temperature, pulse, respiration, mucous membranes) should be evaluated serially to determine a trend in the patient's condition. It is this trend that will determine the severity of the postoperative problem and dictate the appropriate treatment. A detailed description of shock is given in Chapter 28.

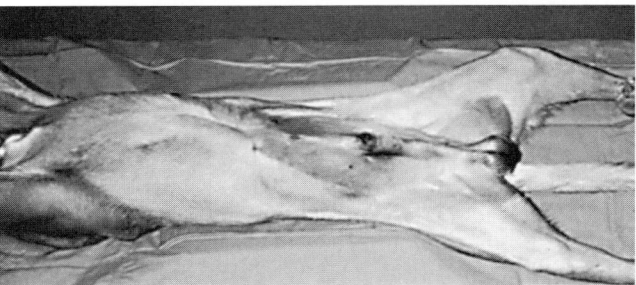

FIGURE 26-7.   Proper positioning and preparation for canine castration.

In severely hemorrhaging patients, the veterinary technician may observe weakness, abdominal enlargement, bleeding from the incision, or a combination of these. They generally occur late and denote a prolonged episode of hemorrhage.

When the patient is suspected of having significant internal bleeding, a packed cell volume (PCV), a total protein determination, and paracentesis (abdominal tap) should be performed to confirm the diagnosis. Reoperation in the severely bleeding patient may be necessary to save the life.

Body weight gain may occur as a late sequela to ovariohysterectomy in the bitch. The reasons for this excessive weight gain are poorly understood but may be partially caused by ovarian endocrine deficiency. In most instances, obesity can be controlled by proper diet and exercise.

Canine Castration

DEFINITION.   Canine castration involves the removal of both testicles.

INDICATIONS.   There are numerous indications for canine castration, the most common being an elective procedure in the young male dog to help prevent roaming, aggressiveness, unwanted breeding, or a combination of these. The optimal age for elective castration is 6 to 9 months. Several medical problems may also be treated by castration, including prostate disorders, anal and perianal tumors, perineal hernias, and testicular tumors. Preanesthetic evaluation should include palpation of both testicles to detect retained testicles before surgery.

TECHNIQUE.   The abdomen is clipped from the tip of the prepuce to the margin of abdominal skin and scrotal skin (Figure 26-7). The clipped area should extend widely into the inguinal region. Ideally, the scrotum itself should not be clipped. The scrotum has very delicate, thin skin that is easily subject to clipper burn and laceration. If, however, there are long scrotal hairs protruding into the surgical field, they can and should be clipped. Care should be taken, however, not to touch the clippers to the scrotal skin.

The animal is secured in dorsal recumbency, and a standard surgical preparation of the prescrotal skin (craniad to the scrotum) is performed. Again, when scrubbing the scrotal skin, care should be taken not to be as aggressive as on the abdominal skin.

A midline incision is made in the prescrotal skin. With gentle pressure, one of the testicles is pushed craniad into the incision. The testicle is then exteriorized through the incision by carefully incising over the common tunic (tissue that encases the testicle). The major vessels are then easily identified and ligated with two absorbable sutures. The remaining scrotal ligament is gently dissected from the testicle. The opposite testicle is handled in a similar fashion. The incision is closed with a continuous subcuticular suture pattern.

COMPLICATIONS. Several postoperative complications can occur. The veterinary technician is most commonly the first person to observe early postoperative complications.

If the presurgical preparation is not done carefully so as to preclude scrotal dermatitis (clipper burn, excessive scrubbing), the patient will lick aggressively at the scrotum and the incision. This often results in severe inflammation and swelling of the scrotal and prescrotal skin. If this problem is not detected early, the results can be suture removal and wound dehiscence. The best treatment is prevention. If scrotal dermatitis does occur, the patient should be immediately placed in an Elizabethan collar. The scrotum and incision are then treated with an antiinflammatory and antimicrobial ointment combination.

 Technician Note

The most common complications associated with canine castration are secondary to self-trauma.

Another less common complication is hemorrhage. When the testicles are removed from the scrotal sac, a significant amount of free space remains in the scrotum. If there is any hemorrhage, either from the subcutaneous tissue or common tunic, the space will fill with a considerable amount of blood before there is enough pressure to create hemostasis, resulting in a large hematoma within the scrotum. If a hematoma is detected early, before the scrotum is full, cold compresses can be applied with slight pressure to the scrotal area to encourage hemostasis. If the scrotum is full, its surgical removal may be necessary.

Feline Castration

DEFINITION. Feline castration involves the removal of both testicles.

INDICATIONS. The major indications for feline castration are to prevent fighting, roaming, and urine spraying and to decrease urine odor. Castration in the cat may provide a rapid response (2 to 4 weeks) to these objectionable characteristics. Preanesthetic evaluation should include palpation of both testicles to confirm the gender of the cat and to detect retained testicles before surgery.

TECHNIQUE. There are several acceptable techniques for feline castration. The patient is generally placed in dorsal recumbency with the legs tied craniad (Figure 26-8). The scrotal hairs are gently plucked from the scrotum with the thumb and finger. This is easily accomplished by grasping the base of the scrotum by the thumb and index finger of one hand and gently pushing the testicles into the scrotum. With the other hand, the thumb and finger are used to gently strip the hair from the scrotal skin. Unlike the dog, the cat is not susceptible to severe scrotal dermatitis. The scrotum is then scrubbed and draped in an aseptic manner.

An incision is made directly through the scrotum. The testicle is protruded through the incision by gentle pressure with the thumb and index finger. The testicle and its spermatic cord (vessels) are exteriorized and then may be ligated with suture, ligated with metal clips, or tied in a

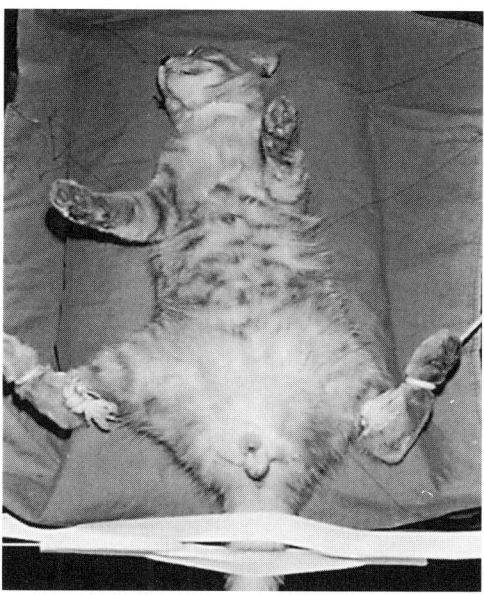

FIGURE 26-8. Proper positioning and preparation for feline castration.

knot on itself, or the vessels can be separated from the vas deferens and tied in a square knot. The scrotum is left unsutured.

COMPLICATIONS. Scrotal swelling and bleeding are the two most common complications of feline castration. Scrotal swelling is due primarily to traumatic surgical preparation and hair plucking. An Elizabethan collar may be necessary to control licking. Hemorrhage from a scrotal vessel may be detected immediately postoperatively. Cold compresses on the scrotum for 5 to 7 minutes will help to encourage hemostasis.

When the patient is sent home, the owner should be informed to change the litter from gravel type to shredded or pelleted newspaper for the first 5 to 7 days. This will prevent pieces of litter from contaminating the surgical site.

Cesarean Delivery

DEFINITION. *Dystocia* (Greek: *dys*, difficult + *tokos*, birth) literally translated means difficult birth. Cesarean delivery derived its name from Caesar, allegedly the first to be born by such a technique. The procedure involves making an incision into the abdominal cavity and then into the uterus to deliver the newborn.

INDICATIONS. Cesarean delivery is indicated when a bitch or queen cannot deliver the pups or kits through the birth canal by normal uterine contractions, because of either maternal or fetal abnormalities. Some of the common causes of dystocia are seen in Figure 26-9. Normal stages of parturition are discussed in Chapter 16.

PREOPERATIVE CONSIDERATIONS. The aim of treatment should be the successful delivery of live and undamaged pups or kits without harm to the dam. Before medical therapy can be instituted, a diagnosis of the cause of dystocia must be made. Medical therapy may do more harm than good when used in the wrong type of dystocia. An example would be giving a drug (oxytocin) that would

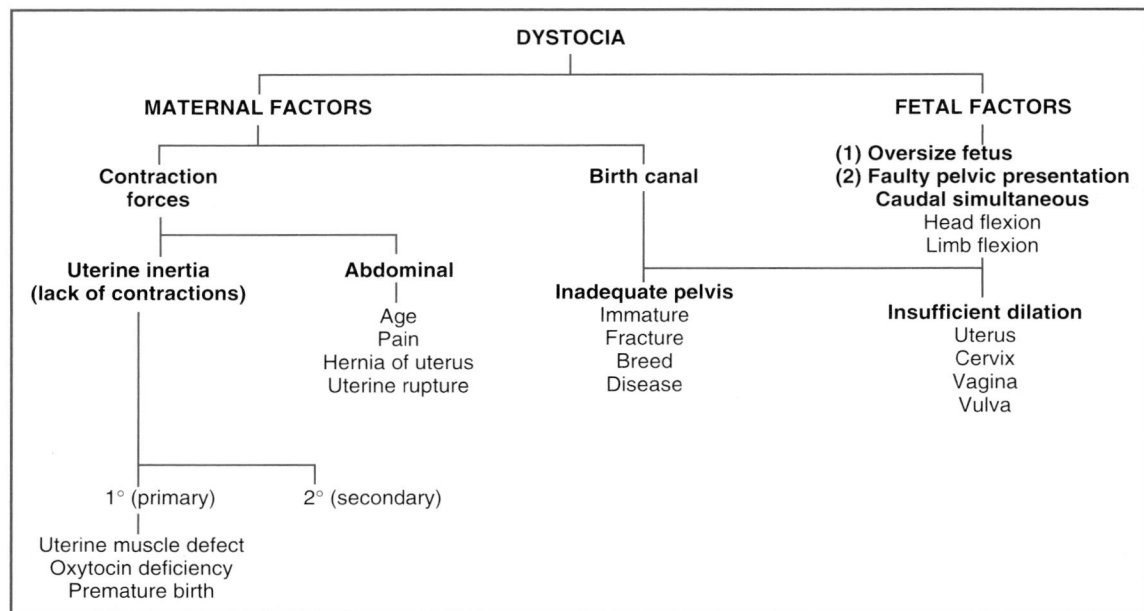

FIGURE 26-9.   Common causes of dystocia.

increase uterine muscular contraction in a bitch that has a malpositioned pup. When proper diagnosis of the type of dystocia is made, and medical therapy is either contraindicated or not effective, the dam should be prepared for surgery.

The anesthetic regimen is of prime importance when considering cesarean delivery. In order to get strong, healthy pups or kits, the agents used should have minimal effects on the newborn. A detailed discussion of anesthetic regimens for the dystocia patient is given in Chapter 21.

TECHNIQUE.   The patient is clipped *before* anesthesia. After anesthetic induction and maintenance, the patient is placed in dorsal recumbency. It is important to remember that the increased weight of the pups or kits on the diaphragm may compromise the normal breathing capacity of the dam.

Technician Note

It is important to do as much preoperative preparation in lateral recumbency as possible and then place the patient in dorsal recumbency just before the surgical preparation.

A ventral midline celiotomy is performed (see Figure 26-6, *A*). The uterus is exteriorized and isolated with surgical towels. Uterine isolation helps prevent the uterine contents from entering the abdominal cavity. An incision is made into the dorsal aspect of the uterine body. Care is taken not to cut the fetus. The fetus and fetal membranes are advanced through the uterine incision by applying gentle pressure to the uterine wall. On presentation, the fetal membranes are removed, the umbilicus is clamped or ligated, and the newborn is handed to the assistant. Each successive newborn is handled in a similar fashion until all pups or kits are delivered. The uterine incision is closed in two layers. The celiotomy incision is closed in a routine

fashion. The skin can be closed with stainless steel sutures in an interrupted pattern or with a synthetic nonabsorbable suture in a *continuous* pattern. This will discourage the pups or kits from removing the sutures when they are nursing.

IMMEDIATE CARE OF THE NEWBORN.   The assistant should be ready to grasp the pup or kit from the surgeon and immediately place it in a dry towel. The assistant can then massage the animal gently to stimulate respiration, dry any secretions around the mouth and nose, and dry the remainder of the body to decrease the chance of hypothermia. The mouth should be inspected for evidence of mucus that may be plugging the airway. At the same time, a quick examination for the presence of cleft palate is made. If the mouth and nostrils are clogged with mucus, the pup or kit should be cradled in the palm of the right hand with the left hand stabilizing the animal; it is then swung smartly downward in an arc, which removes any fluid by centrifugal force (Figure 26-10). Weak newborns or those with faint respirations may be stimulated by injecting doxapram (a respiratory stimulant) in the umbilical vein or under the tongue, using a 25-gauge needle and a tuberculin syringe. A thorough examination for congenital defects is made, and the pup or kit is placed in an incubator or warm, padded area.

The animals can be safely returned to the dam as soon as she has recovered from anesthesia. Care should be taken not to return them so early that the dam may unknowingly harm them by stepping or lying on them. The dam should be returned to her home environment as soon as possible so that she can begin caring for her newborn pups or kits.

Cystotomy

DEFINITION.   Cystotomy involves incising through the urinary bladder wall to expose the lumen (inside of the bladder).

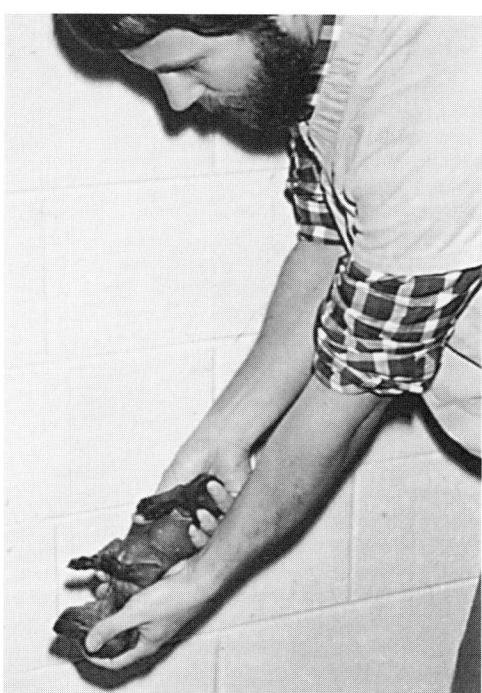

FIGURE 26-10. Removal of mucus and fluid from nostrils and mouth of the newborn pup can be accomplished safely by cradling the pup in the hand and swinging it smartly downward in an arc.

INDICATIONS. The most common indication for cystotomy in small animals is cystic calculi (bladder stones). A cystotomy is also indicated when tumors, mucosal outpouchings, congenital defects, or traumatic rupture occurs.

TECHNIQUE. The abdomen is widely clipped from the xiphoid to the pubis. In male dogs, care is taken to clip the hair from the prepuce. The preputial orifice and penis are then gently flushed with a 1% povidone-iodine (Betadine) solution. A stiff polyethylene male urinary catheter is aseptically passed from the tip of the penis into the urinary bladder. This will allow flushing of any urethral calculi back into the bladder for easy removal. Although it is more common for urinary stones to lodge in the urethra of the male, a urethral catheter should also be passed in the female, because urethral calculi have been reported.

The animal is placed in dorsal recumbency and prepared for surgery with a standard skin preparation. In male patients, the abdominal skin incision will curve laterally to avoid the prepuce (see Figure 26-6, *D*). Care should be taken to thoroughly prepare this area aseptically.

In the female, a standard caudal midline celiotomy is performed (see Figure 26-6, *A*). In the male, a caudal midline skin incision is made from the umbilicus to the sheath of the penis and is then extended lateral to the sheath. Major vessels lateral to the prepuce are encountered—the caudal superficial epigastric artery and vein—which are ligated and transected. The sheath is retracted laterally, and a ventral midline celiotomy is performed. The bladder is exteriorized and packed off with laparotomy pads to preclude urine spillage into the celiotomy incision. An incision is made on the ventral aspect of the bladder, in a relatively avascular area, between preplaced stay sutures. A urine culture is immediately taken, the cystic calculi are removed and submitted for stone

analysis, and the entire tract (bladder to urethra) is flushed with sterile physiologic saline solution until all calculi have been removed. The bladder wall is inspected for abnormalities and is then closed with a simple interrupted or inverting suture pattern. The laparotomy pads are removed, the abdomen is lavaged with sterile physiologic saline solution, and the incision is closed in a routine fashion.

POSTOPERATIVE CONSIDERATIONS. The immediate postoperative care of the cystotomy patient includes monitoring the patient's urination. During the first 48 to 72 hours postoperatively, a mild hematuria (bloody urine) with or without blood clots can be expected. Owners should be informed of this if the patient is released during this time.

> ### Technician Note
> During the first 48 to 72 hours following a cystotomy, a mild hematuria with or without blood clots can be expected.

Following surgical removal of cystic calculi, the major treatment regimen begins—calculi prophylaxis. The stone must be analyzed, the culture and sensitivity must be evaluated, and the client must be informed about recurrence of cystic calculi. Some stones have a specific treatment and dietary regimen that must be strictly followed to prevent the re-formation of calculi. The prompt treatment of urinary tract infections with the appropriate antibiotics is also very important in preventing stone formation.

Prescription Diet (S/D Hills) has been developed as a nutritional aid for the dissolution of struvite uroliths. This diet increases the solubility of struvite crystals by maintaining an acid urine.

Feline Perineal Urethrostomy

DEFINITION. Perineal urethrostomy is performed in male cats with recurrent urethral obstruction to provide a larger-diameter opening in the penis that will allow passage of urine crystals and mucus.

INDICATIONS. The most common indication for a perineal urethrostomy is multiple episodes of feline urologic syndrome. Other less common indications include rupture of the penile urethra secondary to traumatic catheterization or rupture secondary to blunt trauma (e.g., hit by car, abdominal kick).

PREOPERATIVE CONSIDERATIONS. A cat with feline urologic syndrome can present for examination with an array of clinical findings. The presentation often depends on the duration and completeness of the urinary obstruction. If the patient is brought for examination early, there is little chance that other organ systems are affected. If the patient is presented 12 to 24 hours after a complete obstruction, severe electrolyte abnormalities, cardiac arrhythmias, kidney dysfunction, and shock can be present. These patients must have the obstruction removed and become stabilized, and normal renal function must be restored before surgery. This is a *true* emergency situation.

TECHNIQUE. The hair on the perineum and external genitalia is clipped. The patient is placed in a perineal position (ventral recumbency with the perineum elevated approximately 30 degrees). The tail is extended directly over the dorsal midline and immobilized with tape. A purse-string suture is placed in the anus to eliminate fecal

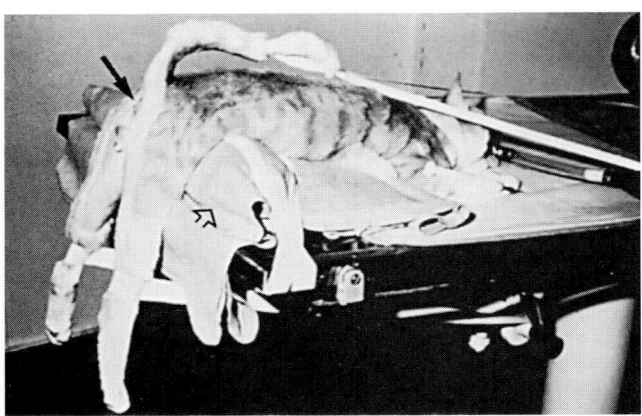

FIGURE 26-11. The perineal position can be used in the dog or cat. *Open arrow,* Padding in front of the legs. This cat is positioned for a perineal urethrostomy. *Arrow,* Purse-string suture in the anus.

contamination of the surgical field. Standard skin preparation is performed (Figure 26-11).

If the cat is intact, he is first castrated (see Feline Castration). An elliptical skin incision around the scrotum and prepuce is made. The urethra is dissected free from its pelvic attachments. A catheter is placed in the urethra, and a longitudinal incision is made through the penile urethra extending craniad to the level of the pelvic urethra. The diameter of the pelvic urethra is approximately two times that of the penile urethra. This allows normal urination in the face of crystalluria (sandlike material in the urine) and mucous plugs. The urethral mucosa is sutured to the skin. This results in a new, permanent opening that will easily accommodate the excess mucus and crystals.

POSTOPERATIVE CONSIDERATIONS. The purse-string suture is removed. Immediate postoperative care includes placement of an Elizabethan collar and examination of the surgical site for evidence of hemorrhage. The Elizabethan collar is essential to keep the patient from licking the sutures. Occasionally, especially in intact male cats, postoperative hemorrhage may be a problem. In such instances, cold compresses can be gently applied to the surgical site to control hemorrhage. Rarely is the bleeding severe enough to require additional surgery or transfusion.

During the first 2 to 3 days postoperatively, the bladder should be gently expressed to determine that a normal flow of urine exists. Postoperative catheters are *discouraged* because of the increased incidence of strictures. The perineal urethrostomy site should be manipulated as little as possible. Ointments and warm cleansings are also discouraged. This may delay healing or aggravate hemorrhage. When the patient is dismissed from the hospital, the use of shredded paper in the litterbox is recommended for the first 7 to 10 days at home.

The most common late postoperative complication is stricture. This is generally manifested by chronic stranguria (straining to urinate). Stricture requires reoperation.

Hernias

The strict definition of *hernia* is protrusion of an organ from its normal cavity (generally the abdominal cavity) through a congenital or acquired defect in the wall of that cavity. The most common hernias in the dog and cat are umbilical hernias, inguinal hernias, and diaphragmatic hernias.

Umbilical Hernia

DEFINITION. An umbilical hernia is one in which bowel or, more commonly, omentum protrudes through a defect in the abdominal wall under the skin at the umbilicus. This hernia is most commonly congenital, and it is recognized on physical examination by the presence of a swelling at the umbilicus. Very small hernias in young dogs (2 to 4 months of age) are often self-limiting. Larger hernias in older dogs (6 to 9 months of age) generally require surgical repair. The most common complication of larger umbilical hernias is strangulation of the intestine. Some of the smaller umbilical hernias are repaired during ovariohysterectomy.

TECHNIQUE. The abdomen is widely clipped from xiphoid to pubis. The patient is placed in dorsal recumbency, and a standard skin preparation is performed. An elliptical skin incision is made around the hernia. The skin is dissected away from the hernial sac; the contents are then exposed and are either replaced into the abdominal cavity (intestine) or excised (falciform or omental fat). The edges of the hernial ring are trimmed to ensure healing of the defect. The abdomen is closed in a routine fashion as for the celiotomy incision.

POSTOPERATIVE CONSIDERATIONS. Postoperative care is similar to that given for any celiotomy incision.

Inguinal Hernia

DEFINITION. An inguinal hernia is one in which intestine, uterus, broad ligament, or another abdominal organ protrudes through the inguinal canal. This is more common in the bitch than in the male dog. An inguinal hernia is diagnosed on physical examination by the presence of a soft, doughy, nonpainful mass in the inguinal region. It does not spontaneously regress and should be surgically repaired when diagnosed, because the abdominal contents may become entrapped within the hernial sac.

TECHNIQUE. The abdomen is widely clipped from the umbilicus to and including the inguinal area. The patient is placed in dorsal recumbency, and a standard skin preparation is performed. A midline incision is made in the caudal abdominal region just across from the inguinal hernia. The inguinal ring is exposed with its hernial sac and external pudendal vessels. The hernial sac is emptied of its contents and is excised and sutured along with the margin of the inguinal ring. Care is taken during closure to avoid the external pudendal vessels that exit from the caudal medial aspect of the ring. The skin incision is then closed as for a celiotomy closure.

POSTOPERATIVE CONSIDERATIONS. The incision is monitored as for any abdominal incision.

Diaphragmatic Hernia

DEFINITION. A diaphragmatic hernia exists when abdominal organs protrude through an opening in the diaphragm into the thoracic cavity. Diaphragmatic hernias may be congenital or traumatic. Any patient with a history of trauma or suspected trauma should be examined for a diaphragmatic hernia. Diaphragmatic hernias may be life threatening. They may be insidious and difficult to identify. Signs may be masked by other problems.

An animal with a massive hernia will have a diminished

intrathoracic space as a result of migration of abdominal contents into the thoracic cavity, resulting in a reduction of lung volume. Presumptive diagnosis is based on a thorough physical examination. The classic signs of diaphragmatic hernia are a "tucked-up" abdomen, intestinal sounds in the chest, muffled heart and lung sounds, and dyspnea. The diagnosis is confirmed by chest radiograph.

Once the diagnosis of diaphragmatic hernia has been made, the patient should be stabilized before anesthesia. This includes *minimal* stress, oxygen cage confinement to allow maximal oxygenation of available lung capacity, and constant monitoring for respiratory insufficiency or arrest. Rarely is diaphragmatic hernia repair an emergency. Only in cases of massive hernia or severe gas distention of a herniated viscus (stomach, intestine) is immediate operation necessary.

> ### Technician Note
>
> Diaphragmatic hernia patients should have oxygen cage confinement to allow maximal oxygenation, minimal stress, and constant monitoring for respiratory insufficiency before surgery.

TECHNIQUE.　The most critical time for the diaphragmatic hernia patient is at anesthetic induction. It is very important to be thoroughly familiar with induction procedures as well as resuscitative techniques in the event of respiratory or cardiac arrest (see Chapter 28).

The skin is widely clipped from just ahead of the xiphoid process to the pubis. The patient is placed in dorsal recumbency on an incline, with the head slightly higher than the hindquarters. This will allow any easily movable viscera to "slide" from the thorax back into the abdominal cavity, allowing an increase in lung capacity and easier breathing.

A ventral midline celiotomy from xiphoid to umbilicus is performed. The edges of the incision are protected with laparotomy pads, and a Balfour self-retaining abdominal retractor is placed to enhance visualization. The diaphragmatic defect is inspected, and any herniated viscera are gently reduced into the abdominal cavity. A thorough inspection of abdominal and thoracic viscera is made to rule out organ rupture or vascular compromise.

Diaphragmatic hernia repair requires working in a deep cavity. Gentle retraction of viscera to expose the defect is necessary throughout the procedure to preclude damage to abdominal organs. The diaphragmatic defect is sutured with a nonabsorbable suture material in a simple continuous suture pattern. This will effect an airtight and watertight seal. The completed suture line is inspected for leaks by filling the abdominal cavity with warm, sterile physiologic saline solution. The lungs are then inflated, and the incision is inspected for bubbles. Air is evacuated from the chest by thoracocentesis through the diaphragm. The celiotomy is closed in a routine fashion.

POSTOPERATIVE CONSIDERATIONS.　The patient should be monitored carefully for signs of respiratory distress. If dyspnea occurs, the chest should be evacuated with a hypodermic needle, three-way stopcock, and a large syringe. A rapid return to normal negative thoracic pressure and normal lung capacity should occur.

In some patients, an indwelling chest tube is placed for the first 1 to 2 days postoperatively. In these cases, periodic aspiration using positional changes (right lateral recumbency, left lateral recumbency, standing on hindlegs, standing on front legs) will afford maximal removal of air and fluid. During the drain management period, it is of utmost importance to keep the patient from chewing a hole in the drain or removing it from the chest cavity. Removal can result in acute death. It is also imperative to keep all connections on the chest drain airtight. Leaks will result in a pneumothorax, respiratory difficulty, and possibly death. Proper management of a chest drain requires full-time patient monitoring.

A chart quantitating the amount of air and fluid removed during a given period of time (12 to 24 hours) will help to determine when the drain should be removed. Generally, the drain can safely be removed as the amount of air and fluid decreases toward zero.

Mammary Neoplasia

Mammary cancer is the most frequently occurring neoplasm in the female dog, and mammary gland neoplasms are the third most frequently found tumors in the female cat.

In dogs there is a significantly higher incidence of mammary gland tumors in nonspayed females or females that are spayed at an age older than 2.5 years. Spaying before the first estrus cycle provides a definite protective factor.

In the initial stages, the tumor will usually appear as a hard lump in any of the glands of the mammary chain. Long-standing or fast-growing tumors may present a sizeable mass with ulceration and drainage. Early diagnosis and therapy will give the best possible prognosis for mammary gland cancer.

Before surgery can be considered, an examination for possible metastasis (spread) of the tumor is done. Malignant tumors will generally metastasize to the lymph nodes and lungs. Biopsy of regional lymph nodes and chest radiographs may detect metastases. About 50% of mammary tumors in dogs are malignant, and about 80% to 90% of mammary tumors in cats are malignant.

Surgery is currently considered the most effective therapy. Early surgery can cure up to 50% of canine mammary gland cancer. The primary objective of surgical treatment is complete removal of the tumor tissue.

TECHNIQUE.　The skin is clipped widely to include all affected mammary glands. The patient is placed in dorsal recumbency, and a standard skin preparation is performed. An elliptical incision is made, attempting to include a 1-cm margin around the tumor. The skin, mammary gland, and tumor are gently undermined and removed. The skin incision is often gaping after tumor excision, requiring a meticulous subcutaneous closure. Subcutaneous tissues are closed with a simple interrupted pattern using absorbable suture material. The skin is closed in a routine fashion. The excised mammary masses are placed in formalin and sent to a laboratory for histopathologic evaluation.

POSTOPERATIVE CONSIDERATIONS.　Major complications that can occur postoperatively are generally related to the tension placed on the skin to adequately close the wound. Dehiscence is not common, but the incision should be examined daily for evidence of separation. Bruising along the incision edges is common and is no cause for alarm. Immediate postoperative hemorrhage can occur. In the event of oozing blood, an abdominal bandage should be applied with gentle pressure. This will help ensure hemostasis and is also comfortable for the patient. The incisions are often very long and must be kept clean and dry at all times. Dogs that prefer to lie on the incision should be well padded or bandaged. If the patient irritates the incision by licking, an Elizabethan collar should be applied until suture removal.

NEUROLOGIC PATIENT CARE

The most common neurologic disorder in the dog is spontaneous intervertebral disk disease. Disks are normally found between vertebral bodies in the spine and act as shock absorbers during spinal movements. With time, the disks can undergo degeneration and calcification. When this occurs, the normal shock absorber-like effect is impaired, and extrusion (rupture) of the disk material into the spinal canal can occur. This puts pressure on the spinal cord and can cause an array of neurologic deficits or pain.

One neurosurgical procedure occasionally performed in small animal practice is *intervertebral disk fenestration*. In this procedure, each disk that is calcified or that may become calcified is removed (scraped) from the intervertebral space. This procedure is performed to *prevent* rupture of the disk material into the spinal canal. Dogs may develop spontaneous intervertebral disk extrusions in the cervical spine (neck) or the thoracolumbar spine (lower back). If the disk has already ruptured, a "decompressive" procedure must be performed. The most common decompressive procedures are the ventral slot (for cervical disk rupture) and hemilaminectomy or dorsal laminectomy (for thoracolumbar disk rupture). The most commonly affected breed is the dachshund, but the beagle, Pekinese, poodle, and terrier breeds also frequently experience disk herniation.

The preoperative and postoperative care of neurologic patients depends on their neurologic status. Patients that have the ability to walk (ambulatory status) on presentation can be managed much like any other animal in the hospital, except that they must be handled with care so as not to exacerbate their cervical or thoracolumbar disk herniation. Patients that have motor weakness (inability to walk normally) or paralysis (inability to walk) on presentation demand frequent attention and careful preoperative and postoperative care.

SURGICAL TECHNIQUE.   When a patient with a herniated cervical or thoracolumbar disk is anesthetized, the normal protective abilities of muscle support and conscious perception of pain are removed. It then becomes the responsibility of the veterinary technician, anesthesiologist, and surgeon to protect the patient from further neurologic deficits by handling the spine with extreme care. It is important to keep the neck and back as straight as possible when moving the patient from one location to another. This needed support can be achieved in various ways. The patient can be taped to a rigid, flat surface or can be cradled in the arm, being careful to completely support the affected area (Figure 26-12). The means of transportation may

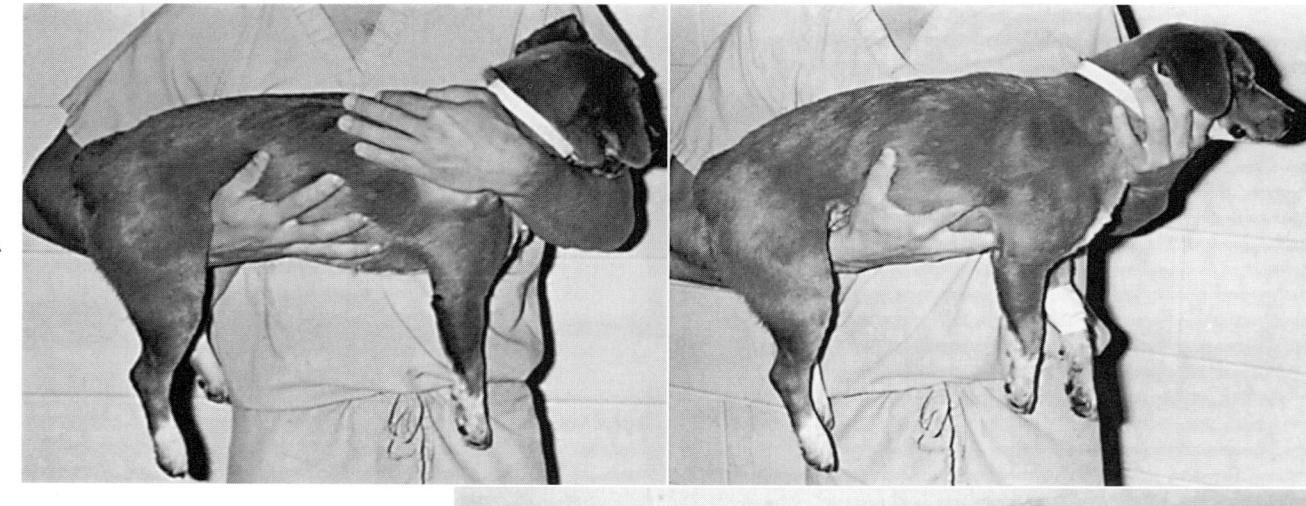

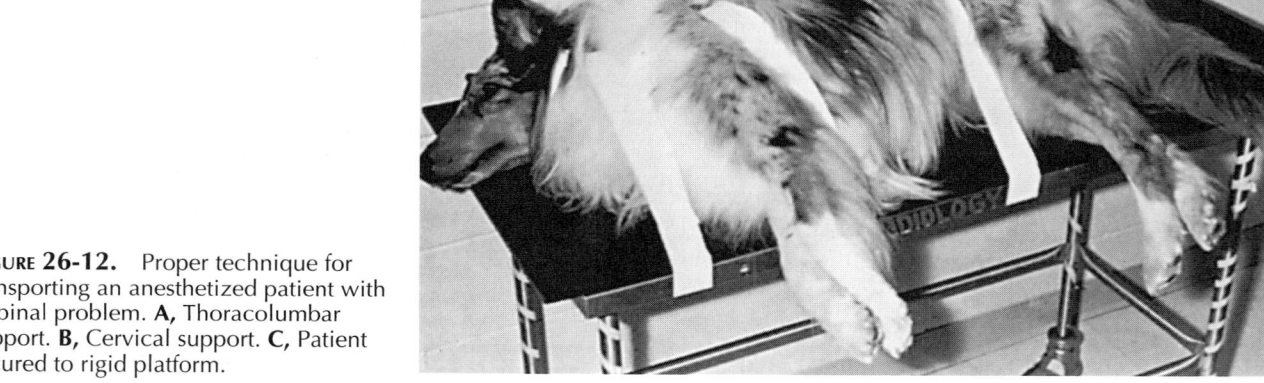

FIGURE 26-12.   Proper technique for transporting an anesthetized patient with a spinal problem. **A,** Thoracolumbar support. **B,** Cervical support. **C,** Patient secured to rigid platform.

often be dictated by the size of the patient, but, generally speaking, a rigid, flat surface is the preferred method.

Patients undergoing cervical disk surgery are placed in dorsal recumbency with the head and neck in slight extension (Figure 26-13). The ventral aspect of the neck is widely clipped from the manubrium sterni to the cranial aspect of the larynx. A standard skin preparation is performed. A ventral midline incision is made through the skin and muscles to expose the intervertebral spaces. A dental tartar scraper, curved needle, fenestration hook, or curette can be used to remove the disk material from the interspace. The fenestration technique is carried out from the C2 to C3 disk space to the C6 to C7 disk space. If decompression is needed, an oblong slot is made through the vertebral bodies into the spinal canal using a pneumatic or electric-powered burr. The disk material is then carefully removed from the spinal canal. The surgical wound is closed in layers with a continuous suture pattern using an absorbable suture. The skin is closed in a routine fashion.

Patients undergoing thoracolumbar disk surgery are placed in ventral recumbency (Figure 26-14). The back is widely clipped from the midthoracic region to the pelvis. A standard skin preparation is performed. A skin incision is made from T11 to L6. Careful dissection between epaxial muscles (muscles of the back) allows palpation and limited visualization of the disk spaces. Each space between T10 and L5 is curetted with a technique similar to that described for cervical disk fenestration. If decompression is needed, a portion of the bony lamina covering the spinal cord is removed with a pneumatic or electric-powered burr or bone rongeurs. The ruptured disk material is then carefully removed from the spinal canal. The muscles, subcutaneous tissue, and skin are closed in a routine fashion.

POSTOPERATIVE CONSIDERATIONS. Postoperative management for the nonambulatory patient is demanding. These patients are subject to decubital ulcers (bed sores or pressure sores), urinary bladder infections, joint stiffness, muscle atrophy (muscle wasting), pneumonia, and gastrointestinal ulceration. Preventing these conditions from occurring is the main objective of proper postoperative management and should include the following:

• Passive range-of-motion exercises and whirlpool baths to encourage joint motion and muscular activity
• Urinary bladder expression four or five times per day

to keep the urinary bladder empty, thus lowering the incidence of infections secondary to large residual volumes
• Turning the patient frequently to reduce the incidence of pneumonia
• Keeping the patient well padded to prevent the formation of decubital sores
• Using an elevated, perforated, rubber-coated rack to keep the patient from urinating and defecating on itself (Figure 26-15)
• Observation of the stool for evidence of fresh blood (bright red on feces) or digested blood (dark, tarry feces), which may be an indicator of colonic or gastric ulceration, respectively; this may be observed following cortisone therapy

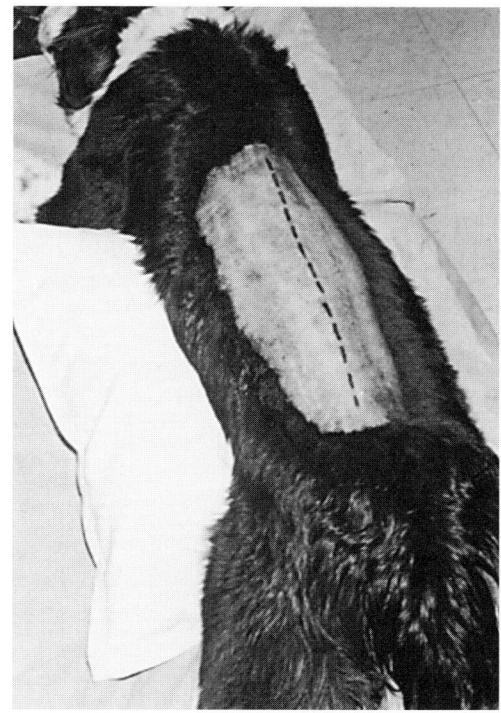

FIGURE 26-14.   Proper positioning for thoracolumbar disk surgery.

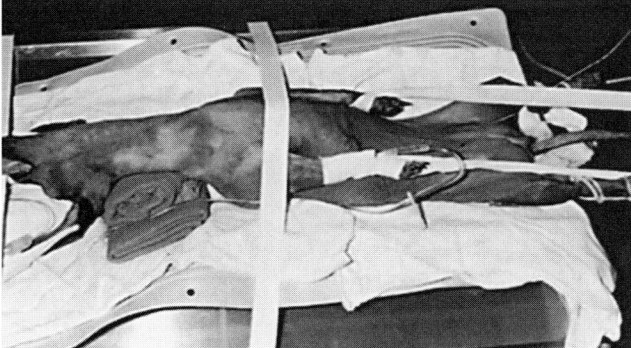

FIGURE 26-13.   Proper positioning for cervical disk surgery.

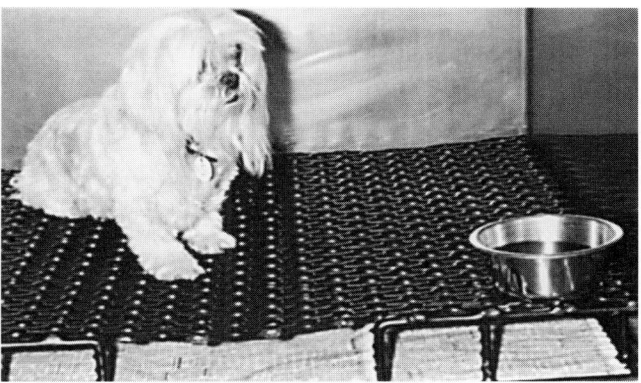

FIGURE 26-15.   Spinal trauma patient on an elevated rack. The rack protects the patient from being soiled with urine and feces and helps prevent decubital sores.

- Observation for vomiting, especially if the vomitus contains coffee grounds-like material, indicative of gastric bleeding

As can be seen from the preceding list, the veterinary technician and veterinarian must work diligently and continually to properly manage the nonambulatory neurologic patient back to health.

ORTHOPEDIC SURGERY

Long Bone Fractures

PREOPERATIVE CONSIDERATIONS.   When a patient is brought to the veterinary hospital with a fracture, several steps must be taken to ready the patient for a permanent repair. First, the patient must be stabilized with respect to all other body systems (treated for shock, chest injuries, abdominal injuries). Second, any open wounds associated with the fracture should be managed, and, third, the fracture must be immobilized by means of a bandage, cast, or sling. Once these three things have been achieved, fracture repair can be safely considered. Most long bone fractures are not life threatening and do not require emergency surgery.

 Technician Note

Most long bone fractures are not life threatening and do not require emergency surgery.

OPERATIVE CONSIDERATIONS.   An extensive clip is required on all limb preparations. The surgeon and assistant will manipulate the limb during reduction and repair. For this reason, the limb is clipped from the level of the metacarpus or metatarsus to the scapula or pelvis, respectively, including the medial and lateral aspects of the extremity. This may vary slightly, depending on the particular bone that is fractured, but the general rule should be a wide and thorough clip. The remaining hair at the tip of the paw is covered with a rubber glove that is taped to the clipped skin (Figure 26-16).

POSITIONING.   Patient positioning depends on the specific bone that is fractured. Generally, the following positions are recommended for each fracture:

- Femur: lateral recumbency, affected side up
- Tibia-fibula: lateral recumbency, affected leg down
- Humerus: lateral recumbency, affected leg up
- Radius-ulna: dorsal recumbency, affected leg craniad
- Pelvis: lateral recumbency, affected leg up

With so much skin exposed, skin preparation is time consuming, but it must be meticulous. The surgeon eventually covers the extremity with a sterile stockinette, but this should not preclude an adequate skin preparation.

SURGICAL ASSISTANCE.   Orthopedic procedures are often very difficult and time consuming and may demand the help of an assistant. Often, the veterinary technician is called on to participate as a surgical assistant and therefore should have a general understanding of orthopedic tissue handling.

Several basic maneuvers commonly needed by the surgeon are often performed by the veterinary technician. They include retraction, muscle fatigue, alignment and reduction, and suction of the field. Proper techniques for each are discussed separately.

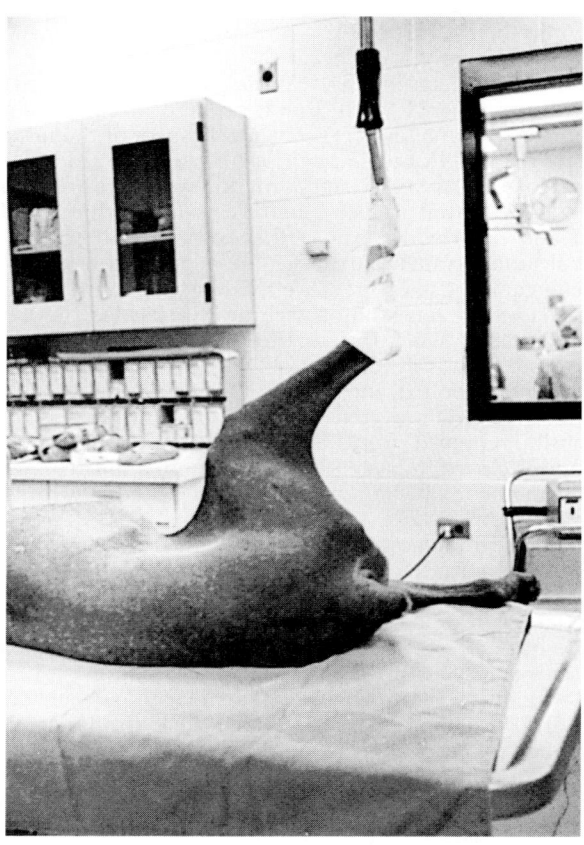

FIGURE 26-16.   Properly prepared extremity must include a thorough clip of the medial and lateral aspects and proper covering of the paw.

Retraction.   Care should be taken to preserve the soft tissues in the operative field. It will be necessary to have functional muscle groups remaining when the bone is repaired. Retraction should be firm but not so traumatic as to bruise or tear the muscle.

Muscle Fatigue.   Large-breed dogs or fractures that are 3 to 5 days old may be difficult to reduce because of heavy muscle mass or severe muscle contraction, respectively. In such cases, constant steady traction on the muscle groups will cause them to fatigue and relax, thus facilitating reduction.

Alignment and Reduction.   In order to repair fractured bones, the ends must be reduced and aligned. It is often necessary for an assistant to hold reduction during the fixation of the fracture. For rapid bone healing to occur, the fractured bone must be held in rigid fixation. Pins, wires, screws, and plates of stainless steel may be used to achieve the necessary fixation.

Suction.   Whenever a fracture occurs, bleeding into the fracture site can be massive. Some continuous oozing occurs during fixation. A clean surgical field is of the utmost importance in facilitating early and accurate reduction and fixation.

POSTOPERATIVE CONSIDERATIONS.   Some postoperative orthopedic patients may require external coaptation. The patients should be managed as described in Chapter 4. Other patients may require range-of-motion exercises, but the majority require limited activity. It is important to

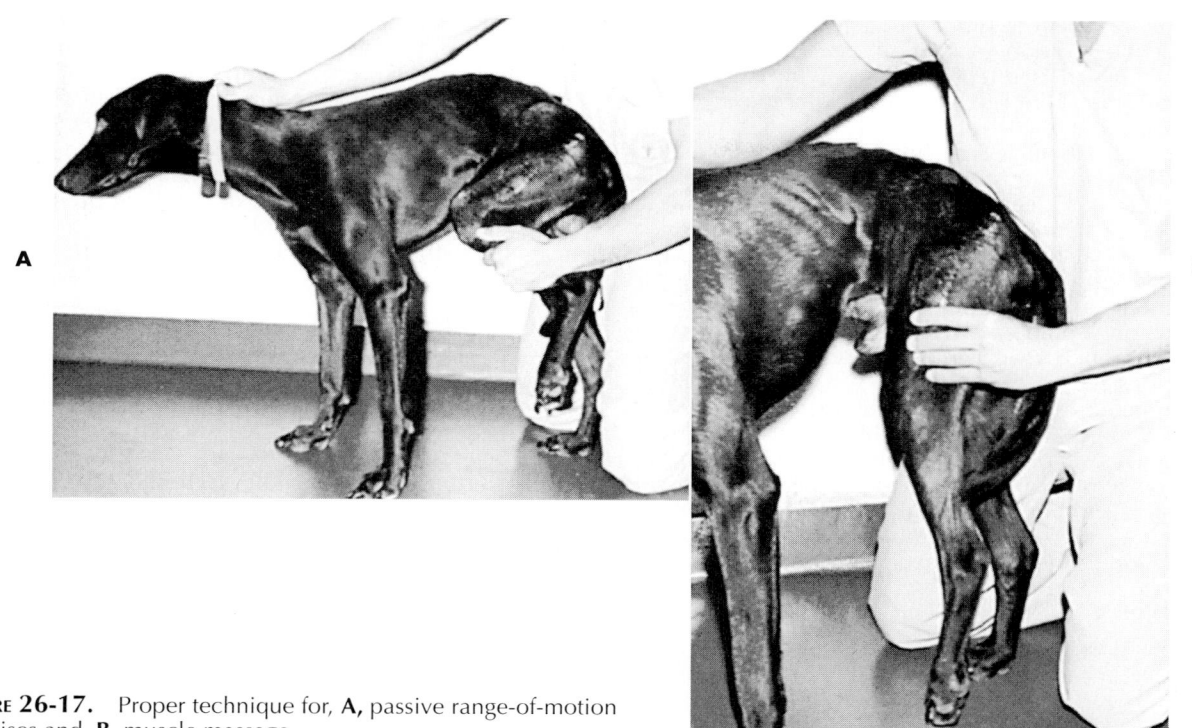

FIGURE 26-17.   Proper technique for, **A,** passive range-of-motion exercises and, **B,** muscle massage.

realize the relatively unsure gait of a three-legged dog or cat, and, when exercising it, one must be certain to avoid slippery surfaces (vinyl or wet floors). Cement, grass, gravel, or dirt provides a much more sure-footed environment. Physical therapy should become part of most fracture patients' rehabilitation therapy. Flexing and extending the affected limb along with muscle massage will improve blood flow and muscle tone as well as reduce muscle contraction (Figure 26-17). Therapy should be done for a period of 5 minutes each time, repeated two to three times per day. A demonstration by the technician of the proper technique will aid the client in understanding the therapy.

Joints

PREOPERATIVE CONSIDERATIONS.   The majority of orthopedic procedures involving the joints are elective and rarely need emergency care. The preoperative management includes limiting the patient's activity. External coaptation is rarely necessary. The indications for joint surgery involve dislocations, ligament ruptures, infections, fractures involving the joint surfaces, joint capsule biopsy, and osteochondrosis (lytic lesions of the articular cartilage).

OPERATIVE CONSIDERATIONS.   An extensive clip, as for fractures, should also be done for joint surgery. Positions will vary depending on the joint involved. Generally, the following positions are recommended for each joint:

- Hip: lateral recumbency, affected leg up
- Stifle: lateral recumbency, affected leg up, or dorsal recumbency (can be used for unilateral or bilateral stifle surgery surgeon's preference)
- Shoulder: lateral recumbency, affected leg up
- Tarsus: lateral recumbency, affected leg up
- Elbow: lateral recumbency, affected leg up
- Carpus: lateral recumbency, affected leg up

Intraoperative assistance in joint surgery is similar to that necessary in fracture repair. Some special precautions should be taken while joints are exposed.

Retraction.   Care should be taken *not* to place retractors in direct contact with the articular cartilage. Cartilage has a relatively poor response to trauma. When exposure of the joint is necessary, sharp retraction of the joint capsule will decrease trauma.

Technician Note

Care should be taken *not* to place retractors in direct contact with the articular cartilage. Cartilage has a relatively poor response to trauma.

Flush.   The cartilage should be frequently flushed with saline to keep it from drying out during the procedure. This is true of all tissues, but especially the articular cartilage because of its poor regenerative ability.

POSTOPERATIVE CONSIDERATIONS.   Postoperative care of patients undergoing joint surgery can be variable, depending on the surgical procedure, the joint involved, and the surgeon's preference. Generally, the joint is immobilized for 1 to 2 weeks, is gradually exercised with passive range-of-motion exercises for 7 to 10 days, and then is gradually (1 to 2 weeks) worked back to normal activity.

CLIENT EDUCATION

When a patient is discharged from the professional care available in a veterinary hospital, it becomes the responsibility of the hospital staff to instruct the client to provide the same type of care at home. This requires that time be spent with the client and the pet to educate the client on appropriate treatment techniques. There are several methods of client education in surgical cases, the degree of difficulty of which is often associated with the type of surgical procedure performed (e.g., ovariohysterectomy vs. disk fenestration).

Whenever a patient is sent home with a sutured skin incision, the client must be instructed to observe the incision daily for evidence of swelling, redness, or drainage and to feel the incision for heat. The client should also watch the animal for aggressive licking, removal of skin sutures, or both.

If a patient is sent home with a bandage, a written discharge form should be given to the client describing in detail the proper management necessary to prevent complications.

In orthopedic cases, as well as in many elective soft tissue surgery cases, the owner should be instructed specifically on what kind of limited activity should be enforced. If passive range-of-motion exercises are expected, the client should be given both oral and written instruction in providing the correct care. A demonstration by the technician of the correct method of therapy is helpful.

In many instances, such as complicated orthopedic and neurologic discharges, a handout explaining in detail the care necessary is very informative and gives a handy reference for the client to refer to if a problem arises.

The use of visual aids, such as a skeleton or overlay books that illustrate anatomy, can be effective in helping the client understand the scope of the problem. Clients are generally willing and capable of handling the postoperative patient, and with a little help from the veterinary hospital staff, a predictably successful result can be expected.

RECOMMENDED READING
Pascoe PJ: Patient aftercare. In Slatter D, editor: *Textbook of small animal surgery*, ed 2, Philadelphia, 1993, WB Saunders.

Seim HB III, Creed JF: Restraint techniques for prevention of self-trauma. In Bojrab MJ, editor: *Current techniques in small animal surgery*, ed 3, Philadelphia, 1990, Lea & Febiger.

27

Small Animal Medical Nursing

T. Mark Neer

Small animal medical nursing consists of attending to the total needs of a medical illness. The nursing process can be viewed as a traditional exercise in problem solving. Problem solving can be divided into several components: data collection, data interpretation, implementation of a plan, and evaluation of the response to the plan. The veterinary technician should apply each of these steps to small animal medical nursing.

The cornerstone of data collection for the technician is *observation*. Effective observation requires an understanding that many clinical problems are dynamic processes that are capable of rapid change. If change is to be recognized, careful, detailed, and systematic observation is required. The precise system and nature of patient monitoring will vary depending on the specific clinical situation; however, the evaluation of all patients should take place according to a regular and reliable schedule. An important part of any system of observation is to establish an accurate baseline for whatever parameters are being serially monitored.

Observations by the veterinary technician are invaluable in providing optimal medical care for the ill animal. In many instances, the technician has observed the patient for longer periods of time than has the veterinarian. Thus the technician may be able to recognize changes that are not readily apparent to the veterinarian during routine daily physical examination. Also, the manifestations of certain significant medical problems, such as pain, can be subtle. Dogs may manifest pain by being restless or uneasy without displaying any other sign of discomfort.

Technician Note

An integral aspect of any system of observation is the technician's ability to establish an accurate baseline for the parameter to be serially monitored.

Data interpretation by the veterinary technician consists of recognizing and correctly interpreting the observations that have been made. Stated differently, the technician must recognize and define clinical problems. A clinical problem is anything that interferes with the well-being of the animal patient or anything that requires treatment or further diagnostic evaluation. Examples of clinical problems that might be recognized by the technician include diarrhea, vomiting, anorexia, and respiratory distress.

It is important to document that a problem exists before implementing a diagnostic or therapeutic plan. For example, the technician may suspect increased water consumption, but before an extensive evaluation is initiated it may be wise to accurately measure the water consumed over a 24-hour period. In certain instances, documentation of a problem may simply consist of repeating a clinical determination or measurement.

Formulation, organization, and implementation of a diagnostic or therapeutic plan constitute the next step in the total nursing process. Usually, this occurs after consultation with the attending veterinarian. For nursing to be optimally effective, a mechanism should exist for the ready exchange of information between technician and veterinarian. A team approach to animal health care is the ultimate goal, with veterinarian and technician each contributing their unique skills and abilities to the task of returning the patient to health.

The need for thorough observation does not end once the diagnostic or therapeutic plan has been initiated. Frequently, the plan is modified because of a changing clinical situation or because of the response to the specific plan.

When implementing any diagnostic or therapeutic plan, it is important to remember that the quantity and nature of nursing care should always be individualized. One patient may readily accept a specific procedure, whereas another will resist to the point that the intended benefit is lost. Although excessive intervention may be detrimental to certain animals, this should not be construed as an excuse for medical neglect. The fundamental principle is that if a patient is not meeting a requirement for survival, the technician must promptly intervene. Certain animals require tremendous amounts of attention and affection from the technician simply to maintain the will to live during periods of separation from the owner.

Each technician and the head of every animal hospital should establish and maintain consistent standards of nursing care. Veterinary technicians have a professional and moral obligation to every animal patient to provide the following basic necessities:

- A clean, comfortable environment, as free of stress as possible
- Food and water at all times unless restricted for medical reasons
- Adequate exercise and grooming care unless restricted for medical reasons
- Prompt and humane relief of suffering
- Humane treatment of every patient with dignity at all times

GENERAL CARE

Grooming and bathing are aspects of the general care of the animal patient that are important for several reasons. First, a clean and well-groomed animal has an enhanced sense of well-being and potentially will recover from an illness more rapidly. Second, a clean animal is much less likely to develop severe contact dermatitis from urine scalding and fecal soiling of the skin, which, if it does occur, becomes another clinical problem to manage. Third, grooming and medicated baths are recommended for the prevention or treatment of many dermatologic problems. Bathing with shampoo that contains an insecticide is a useful adjunct in the control of ectoparasites. Finally, the cleanliness of the patient at the time of discharge is an indication to the owner of the overall quality of the health care provided.

Every animal hospital should have an adequate collection of grooming and bathing equipment and supplies, that is, combs, brushes, scissors, towels for drying, electrical dryers, and a selection of shampoos appropriate for different situations. Care must be taken to prevent the spread of infectious problems, such as dermatomycosis, from one animal to another via grooming instruments. These instruments should be thoroughly cleansed in an appropriate disinfectant solution after each use.

When clipping or removing hair from an animal for medical reasons, it is important to obtain the owner's permission, whenever possible. This is particularly important in animals used for show purposes. In certain breeds, such as the Afghan hound, regrowth of hair is extremely slow.

Bathing

The basic technique for bathing dogs and cats is self-evident; however, the following points warrant emphasis. The eyes should be protected from chemical injury by instilling a drop of mineral oil or a small amount of boric acid ophthalmic ointment before the bath. Care should be exercised to prevent water from entering the external ear canal; this can be accomplished by placing a small piece of cotton in each ear. Remember to remove the cotton when the bath has been completed. Thermal injury from excessively hot water can be prevented by constantly monitoring the water temperature. Thorough rinsing with clean water prevents irritation of the skin from residual shampoo. The axillary and scrotal regions of long-haired dogs are particularly vulnerable to residual shampoo irritation. If a cage dryer is used, caution must be exercised to prevent overheating (hyperthermia). Shampoos containing insecticides should be used only with the approval of the attending veterinarian because of the possibility of cumulative toxicity or drug interactions. If insecticidal dips are used, correct dilutions are necessary to avoid toxic reactions. If a complete immersion bath is contraindicated, localized soiling of the animal may be handled with a sponge bath.

Exercise

Moderate exercise is beneficial for the general care of the animal patient. Exercise should take place in a secure, controlled, and safe environment so that injury or loss of the animal does not occur. Contraindications to exercise include many, but not all, respiratory, cardiovascular, and musculoskeletal problems. The decision whether to restrict exercise should be made after consultation with the attending veterinarian. Moderate exercise can be considered the simplest and most basic form of physical therapy and can be a useful means of reducing peripheral edema and improving muscle tone and strength.

Feeding

The animal health technician plays a particularly pivotal role in ensuring that each patient remains in a positive energy balance, in which caloric intake exceeds metabolic requirements. As stated earlier, the technician is in an excellent position to observe complete or partial anorexia (loss of appetite) and to take appropriate action to rectify the situation. In certain instances, merely substituting a more palatable food will solve the problem. Familiarity with the home feeding regimen will aid in the selection of palatable alternative diets. In certain instances, it may even be advisable for the owner to prepare food at home and bring it to the hospital. It is helpful to stock a variety of types of food, such as canned, semimoist, and dry, in a variety of flavors to satisfy even the most discriminating patient. Although not suitable for long-term nutritional maintenance, meat-flavored baby food may be used to stimulate an animal's appetite. In other instances, personalized attention at the time of feeding will increase food intake. Hand feeding will usually be sufficient, but forced feeding may be required in selected cases. Forced feeding consists of manually placing boluses of food in the caudal pharynx to stimulate the swallowing reflex. High-calorie density supplements, such as Nutrical (Evsco), may facilitate meeting the caloric requirements of the patient but by no means will meet the animal's daily requirements by themselves. In many animals requiring forced feeding for an extended period, gastric gavage is preferred because it is less stressful (both to the patient and to the veterinary technician). The technique for gastric gavage (stomach tubing) is discussed in Chapter 3. Other methods of enteral nutrition are being used with increased frequency; these include feeding by way of nasopharyngeal, pharyngostomy, gastrostomy, and jejunostomy tubes. Specially tailored complete diets may be administered through these routes to ensure adequate nutrition in a variety of disease states, such as hepatic lipidosis in cats and renal failure. One such complete diet, which can be forced through a 60-ml syringe, is Prescription Diet A/D (Hills).

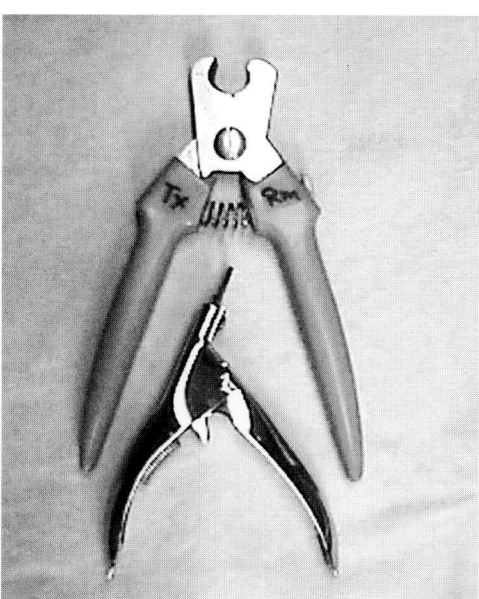

FIGURE 27-1. The two common types of nail trimmers, Whites *(top)* and Resco *(bottom)*. The Whites nail trimmer is useful for very long nails that have curled back toward the foot pad.

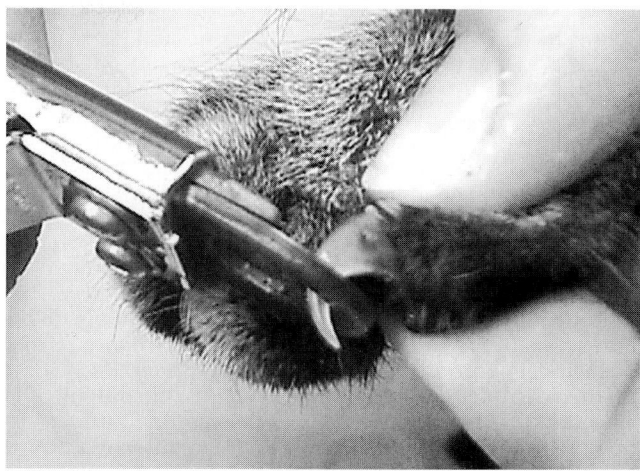

FIGURE 27-2. To trim the nails in cats, extend the claw by compressing the caudal part of the nail just in front of the foot pad with the thumb and forefinger. At this point, one can visualize the vein or "quick" (pink area in claw) and the nail trimmer can be placed in front of the vein for trimming.

Nail Trimming

Nail trimming (pedicure) is an important general care technique. Excessive nail length results in altered gait and the potential accentuation of lameness problems. Excessively long nails are more likely to be traumatically avulsed. Finally, untrimmed nails can become ingrown (usually into the foot pads), resulting in cellulitis or abscess formation.

A sturdy, durable nail trimmer is required for this procedure. Two common types are available (Resco and Whites; Figure 27-1). To avoid cutting pigmented (black) nails too short in the dog, the cutting surface of the nail trimmer should be held parallel to the palmar (plantar) surface of the digital foot pads, and the nail is cut in this plane. In cats, the nails can be exposed by grasping the paw between the thumb and index finger and sliding the skin on the dorsum of the paw away from the nails (Figure 27-2). Once exposed, the nails can be trimmed as described for the dog. It should be noted that nails that have not been trimmed for an extended period of time have a "quick" or nail vein that extends further into the claw than that of regularly trimmed nails. In this instance, one should be conservative with regard to how much nail is trimmed. The center of the nail takes on a fleshy, shining appearance in the region next to the quick (Figure 27-3. This is an indicator to trim no further. Because certain animals vehemently resent handling of their feet for nail trimming, it is a good practice to routinely give a pedicure to any animal anesthetized or tranquilized for any procedure. If the blood vessel in the nail is inadvertently severed ("the quick is cut"), silver nitrate sticks can be used to stop the hemorrhage by means of chemical cautery. Other products available for chemical cautery include styptic powder and blood-stop powder, which are available from numerous companies. If the owner is receptive, it is desir-

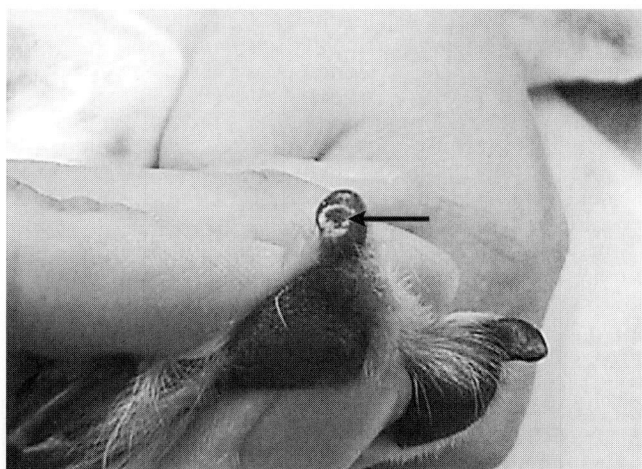

FIGURE 27-3. When trimming black nails, always trim a small amount at a time. Once you get close to the "quick," you will note that the center of the nail begins to have a shiny, fleshy appearance *(arrow)*. Once you see this, no further trimming is necessary.

able to provide instructions in the proper technique of nail trimming so this routine task can be accomplished at home.

Ear Cleaning

The external ear canal may accumulate cerumen, exudate, or cellular debris as a sequela to otitis externa or a foreign body (e.g., grass awn), which then requires cleaning. Certain breeds, notably poodles, Bedlington terriers and

Kerry blue terriers, may also accumulate excessive hair in the external ear canal. The initial and essential step in the treatment of any external ear problem is complete and thorough cleaning of the entire ear canal. Frequently, satisfactory cleaning requires the administration of a short-acting general anesthetic or heavy tranquilization. The first step is to remove any hair that is present, and, if excessive wax is present, a ceruminolytic agent (i.e., dioctyl sodium succinate [Cerusol, Burns-Biotech Labs]) can be instilled to soften the wax. Caution should be used when instilling ceruminolytics into an ear canal when the integrity of the tympanum is not known. If this is the situation, one may elect to use normal saline as the initial cleansing agent. Excessive wax and debris can then be removed by using a soft rubber bulb syringe and a dilute disinfectant solution to lavage the external ear canal. Balls of cotton and cotton applicator sticks can be used to gently wipe the wax from the external ear canal. It is important to remove only debris that is visible in the vertical canal so that debris is not pushed deep into the horizontal canal (Figure 27-4). Some of this debris should be suspended in mineral oil and smeared on a microscope slide to be examined under low power for the presence of *Otodectes* (ear mites). Cleaning the horizontal ear canal should be done gently and with extreme caution to prevent damage to the tympanic membrane or the packing of debris deep into the horizontal canal (Figure 27-4). If the ear canal contains purulent debris, a sample should be obtained for cytologic evaluation (smear) and bacterial culture before instrumentation and cleaning. If bacterial growth is observed, antibiotic sensitivity should be evaluated in vitro (see Chapter 8). If the cytologic preparation reveals the presence of yeast *(Malassezia)*, appropriate therapy should be initiated. Some practitioners advocate the use of pulsating streams of water from a dental hygiene apparatus (Water Pik, Teledyne Inc.) to clean the external ear canal. Approximately 5 ml of povidone-iodine (Betadine, Purdue-Frederick) or Nolvasan solution (Fort Dodge Laboratories) is added to approximately 236 to 384 ml of warm water. The stream of water should be applied in a rotating motion and directed parallel to the external ear canal. The excess water and debris can be caught in an ear irrigation basin or similar vessel. An inexpensive alternative is the use of a rubber bulb syringe to manually loosen debris and aid in flushing the ear canal. This technique is not recommended if the tympanic membrane is not intact.

Technician Note

Ceruminolytics and disinfecting solutions should be used with caution if the integrity of the tympanic membrane is not known. Cleansing with warm normal saline should be attempted first.

Regardless of the technique employed to clean the external ear canal, a second otoscopic examination should be performed to evaluate the completeness of the ear cleaning. Once the ear canal is sufficiently clean, the canal should be carefully dried with clean cotton swabs, and the initial dose of prescribed otic preparation instilled.

Anal Sacs

The anal sacs are reservoirs for the secretions produced by the anal glands. The anal glands line the walls of the anal sacs and produce a foul-smelling fluid that varies from serous to pasty in consistency and is brown to off-white. The anal sacs are paired structures, approximately 1 cm in

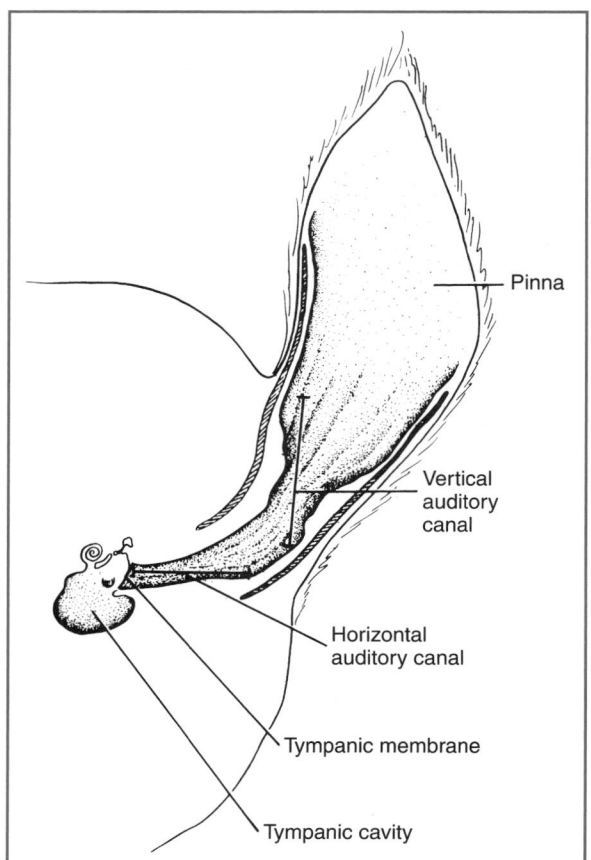

FIGURE 27-4. Schematic diagram of the anatomy of the canine ear.

diameter, that lie between the internal and external anal sphincter muscles on either side of the anal canal. Each sac opens into the lateral margin of the anus by a single duct, at approximately the four and eight o'clock positions of the anus.

Clinical signs associated with impacted anal sacs include excessive licking of the perineum; "scooting," or dragging the perineum on the floor; abnormal carriage of the tail; and vague indications of pain or discomfort in the perineal region.

The anal sacs are best expressed by inserting a lubricated, gloved forefinger into the rectum. The distended sacs are immobilized between the forefinger and the thumb, which remains external to the anus. The sacs are generally found in a ventrolateral location. Gentle pressure is applied until the secretions are forced through the ducts. Because the ducts as well as the sac are occasionally compressed with this technique, if the sac cannot be expressed with gentle pressure, the finger and thumb are repositioned and pressure is reapplied. Paper toweling or cotton placed over the anus can be used to prevent the extremely unpleasant liquid from soiling the patient, environment, or technician.

Bedding

The optimal means of keeping an ambulatory dog clean is by the appropriate use of bedding and exercise runs. Several types of bedding are routinely used in small animal practice; they include newspaper, other types of paper products, blankets, and towels. It is important that the bedding material selected be either disposable or readily and effectively cleaned between uses. Because occasionally dogs will ingest their bedding, it is also important that the material be safe and nontoxic. Most dogs are extremely reluctant to urinate or defecate in their cage; therefore keeping the cage and patient clean is facilitated by the regular use of exercise runs. Specifically, dogs should be placed in the runs several times daily for an adequate period of time.

Generally, cats are easier to keep clean than dogs during periods of hospitalization. Cats will use litter pans and groom and clean themselves unless they are seriously ill. Litter should be changed daily, and pans or trays should be either disposable or constructed of materials that will allow thorough cleaning and disinfection between uses. It is unnecessary to place cats in exercise runs unless the hospital stay is unusually long.

Decubital Sores

Keeping the nonambulatory patient clean and free of associated problems is far more challenging. Prevention and management of *decubital sores* (bedsores) and urine scald are extremely important aspects of the care of recumbent patients. Animals with various neurologic or orthopedic problems can be recumbent for prolonged periods and require special care. Urine and fecal soiling can cause serious problems that can complicate recovery from the underlying condition. Scalding from urine or diarrhea can be prevented by a light topical application of a protective compound, such as Aquaphor (Beiersdorf, Inc.) or petrolatum (e.g., Vaseline) to susceptible perineal or inguinal areas.

Decubital sores not only complicate recovery but also can be a source of sepsis, which can lead to the demise of the patient. The best treatment for decubital sores is *prevention*. Decubital sores develop over bony prominences as the result of continuous pressure and damage to the overlying skin. Various types of bedding have been advocated to reduce the frequency and severity of decubital sores; they include the use of air or water mattresses, foam padding, synthetic fleeces, grids or grates, and straw. The material should either be disposable or have an impermeable surface that does not retain moisture or microorganisms and can be thoroughly cleaned. A potential problem with impermeable surfaces is that urine and moisture tend to remain in contact with the skin and can exacerbate the problem. Therefore care should be taken to keep the skin surface as dry as possible. This is why, for long-term management, straw is beneficial since adequate cushioning is available for the animal and urine drains through the straw away from the patient.

Other routine measures that help to prevent decubital sores include frequent turning of the patient from side to side, intermittent use of slings or carts to prevent continuous pressure over the bony prominences, and frequent baths to keep the skin clean.

Once decubital sores have developed, they should be thoroughly cleaned with a surgical scrub. Surgical debridement of necrotic tissue may be necessary. After cleaning, the area should be completely dried. Soaking the affected area two to four times daily with a mild astringent will aid in keeping the decubital sore dry. A 1:40 astringent solution of aluminum acetate (Burow's solution) may be made by dissolving one packet (Domeboro solution, Dome Laboratories) per pint of warm water. Ideally, the area of the decubital sore should be padded to prevent further pressure injury; however, the sore itself should remain exposed to the air to prevent retention of moisture. One way of accomplishing this is to fashion a "donut" from foam rubber and to fix this to the skin by means of adhesive tape. Unfortunately, it is difficult to maintain these pads in the proper location for long periods of time.

Topical antimicrobial agents should be applied judiciously because many contain ointment or cream bases that form an occlusive dressing that will retain moisture. Further, it is questionable how beneficial they are in controlling an infected decubital sore.

Geriatric Nursing

With improved veterinary care, pets are enjoying an increased life span; consequently, the number of geriatric patients seen in small animal practices is increasing. The geriatric patient can be presented with a number of problems that directly influence the nursing process. These problems are generally related to or are secondary to degenerative diseases and other geriatric changes, such as arthritis, deafness, and blindness.

Dogs with arthritis or other degenerative diseases of the musculoskeletal system may be suffering from chronic pain. These animals are likely to react aggressively when an affected body part is touched or manipulated. Dogs suffering from central nervous system disorders (e.g., a brain tumor or cerebral infarction) may also display aggressive behavior.

Deafness is another disorder that frequently accompanies old age. It is easy to surprise or startle a deaf, older dog, and certain dogs will instinctively respond by biting. When approaching a deaf dog, it is important that the patient is able to see you before you attempt to handle it or perform a procedure.

Blindness can occur in older dogs from cataracts, retinal degeneration, glaucoma, and other diseases. As is the case with deaf dogs, blind dogs should be approached cautiously. It is best to move slowly and speak while approaching the dog. Generally, elderly dogs and cats show less response to external stimuli. They appear to be less interested in their surroundings and frequently remain inactive for prolonged periods. In fact, they tend to resent any interference and react aggressively when disturbed. Some dogs forget previous training and may fail to respond to basic commands. Finally, the geriatric dog or cat is resistant to changes in daily routine. The stress of hospitalization alone can sometimes cause rapid deterioration. Obviously, it is impossible to correct or reverse many of the changes associated with aging; however, a willingness to provide gentle, compassionate nursing care is of paramount importance.

Pediatric Nursing

The clinical situation that best illustrates the skills required in pediatric nursing is the hand rearing of orphaned puppies or kittens. The first step is to determine the caloric requirements of the puppy or kitten. During the first week of life, these requirements are approximately 27 calories/kg/day, 32 to 36 calories/kg/day during the second week, 36 to 41 calories/kg/day during the third week; and 41 to 45 calories/kg/day during the fourth week. A number of artificial milk replacers (Esbilac, Pet-Ag; Just Burn, Farnham) are available for use in puppies. KMR (Pet-Ag) is an artificial replacement for queen's milk (see Table 27-1 for formula dosage). The following formula can be used as a short-term emergency supplement in puppies: 8 oz of cow's milk mixed with two egg yolks and 1 tsp of corn oil. For an emergency formula in kittens, 4 oz of cow's milk can be mixed with two egg yolks and one drop of

TABLE 27-1	ORPHAN FORMULA DOSAGE FOR PUPPIES AND KITTENS	
Age (wk)	**Dosage* (ml/100 g body weight/day)**	
1	13	
2	17	
3†	20	
4	22	

*Divide and feed four times daily.
†Begin to feed solid food.

multivitamins. Once the total daily requirement has been calculated, this amount can be divided into four equal feedings. Frequent feedings are necessary to prevent over-distention of the stomach and subsequent emesis and aspiration pneumonia. Generally, it is faster and easier to use gavage via an orogastric tube than to bottle feed.

The technique for gavage is to use a soft rubber feeding tube (Fr. 8 to 16). The tube is marked with a marking pen or tape at a point equal to the distance between the tip of the nose and the eighth rib. The tube is advanced into the pharynx and down the esophagus to the level of the midthorax. A syringe can be used to inject the artificial milk replacer slowly. The stomach capacity of puppies and kittens can be calculated by using the following formula: body weight in grams times 5% equals the capacity of the stomach in milliliters. This milliliter amount should not be in a single feeding.

If the puppies or kittens are vigorous nursers, an alternative technique would be to use Pet Nursettes (Peg-Ag) or human premature baby bottle nipples. This technique is slower but may satisfy the pups and kittens more, so the incidence of litter mates nursing on each other will be reduced.

The neonatal puppy is essentially poikilothermic (body temperature varies with ambient temperature); therefore it is imperative that the ambient temperature of the whelping box be maintained between 30° C and 33° C. If hypothermia occurs, it will reduce feeding by the neonate and may enhance the pathogenicity of certain viruses, such as canine herpes. To detect hypothermia in neonates, it is desirable to use a low-reading clinical rectal thermometer.

A highly effective monitoring technique during the neonatal period is to weigh the neonates frequently. Newborn puppies and kittens should be weighed daily. Puppies should gain approximately 10% to 20% of their birth weight daily for the first week of life. Postage or food scales should be used to weigh each animal two or three times daily, especially during the first 2 weeks of life. Weight loss or failure to gain weight each day may be the first sign of illness.

PRACTICAL NURSING PROCEDURES

In many veterinary practices, it is the responsibility of the veterinary technician to monitor the patient's vital signs (i.e., temperature, pulse, respirations).

Temperature

One routine method for determining the body temperature of a small animal is to use a standard mercury-in-glass clinical rectal thermometer. Veterinary thermometers differ from those used in humans in that the storage reservoir for the mercury is short and spherical rather than elongated. Human thermometers can be used in dogs and cats with-

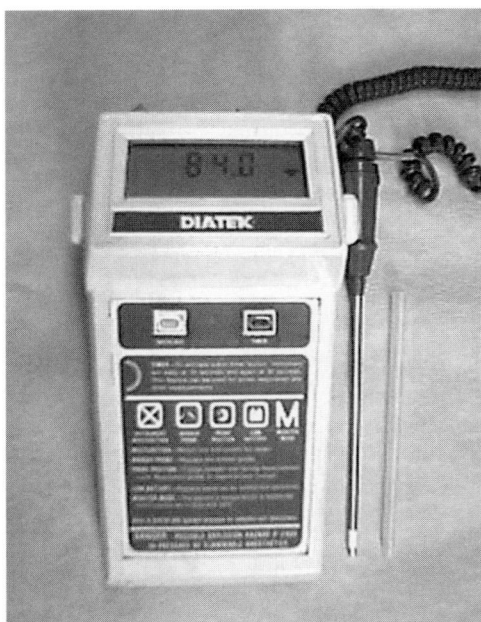

FIGURE 27-5.   Digital electronic thermometer by Doatek with removable and disposable plastic sheaths. These are very accurate and quick for the measurement of rectal temperature.

out difficulty. Thermometers can be calibrated in Fahrenheit or Celsius degrees. A Fahrenheit reading can be converted to Celsius by using the following formula: degrees C = (degrees F − 32) × 5/9.

When taking the patient's temperature, one should first shake the thermometer so that the mercury is below the constriction in the glass tube. The thermometer is well lubricated with petrolatum, mineral oil, or a mild soap and inserted into the rectum with a gentle twisting motion. The thermometer is advanced into the rectum beyond the bulb and is held in place for the minimum period of time stated on the thermometer. The patient is restrained to prevent the thermometer from being broken. The thermometer is withdrawn, and the bulb and stem are wiped clean with an alcohol-soaked cotton swab. The thermometer is held horizontally and rotated until the magnified scale is clearly visible. Because of the constriction in the glass tube, the level of the mercury does not fall until it is shaken down. Finally, the thermometer should be stored in an antiseptic solution (e.g., benzalkonium chloride). Hot water should not be used for cleaning thermometers.

The more common and quicker method of obtaining a body temperature is with the use of digital thermometers (Figure 27-5). There are many brands available, and with most an auditory "beep" alerts the technicians when the reading is final.

Certain diseases that produce fever display a diurnal pattern (i.e., the temperature fluctuates) during the day. If the patient's temperature is taken just once per day, the periods of fever may not be recognized. If this situation is suspected, a temperature chart may be kept by taking and recording the temperature at regular intervals, for example, every 4 hours.

The normal rectal temperature in the dog is 38.9° C. The normal rectal temperature in the cat is 38.6° C. Excitement or activity can elevate the temperature above these limits.

In rare clinical situations (i.e., rectal laceration, rectal prolapse), it may not be possible to measure the rectal temperature. In these situations, the temperature may be taken in either the axilla or external ear canal. The temperature recorded in these sites will be significantly lower than the simultaneous rectal temperature. In general, 2° C can be added to an axillary or ear canal temperature to approximate rectal temperature. These alternative techniques for determining the body temperature are useful when the same site is used serially in an individual patient, and the results are compared. The temperature is taken by placing the bulb of the thermometer deep in the axilla or ear canal for several minutes.

Recently, infrared thermometers have been developed that record accurate body core temperatures by focusing the infrared beam on the tympanic membrane. This thermometer is helpful in those patients with very low rectal temperatures or in those for which taking a rectal temperature is contraindicated (Ototemp Veterinary, Exergen Corp.).

Pulse

The rate and character of the pulse are valuable means of assessing the cardiovascular status of the patient. The pulse can be palpated in any artery located close to the body surface. The pulse is most commonly felt in the femoral artery. The femoral artery is usually palpated on the medial aspect of the thigh, proximal to the stifle. Palpation of the femoral pulse requires practice and can be difficult in a trembling patient or in a patient with short, heavily muscled legs. Alternative sites for taking the pulse are the palmar aspect of the carpus and the ventral aspect of the base of the tail. The *normal pulse rate* in adult dogs is 60 to 160 beats/min, up to 180 beats/min in toy breeds and 220 beats/min for puppies. The maximum rate in cats is 240 beats/min.

The heart rate can be counted by palpation or auscultation at the point of maximal intensity of the heartbeat. The point of maximal intensity is located at the costochondral junction between the left fourth and sixth intercostal spaces. If the pulse rate is taken at the same time as the heart rate and the pulse rate is less, this is called a *pulse deficit*. A pulse deficit generally indicates an abnormal heart rhythm.

The dog can have heart and pulse rates that are "regularly irregular." Characteristically, the heart and pulse rates increase with inspiration and decrease with expiration. This normal variation is called *sinus arrhythmia*.

In addition to taking the pulse rate, it is beneficial to evaluate the pulse pressure and character of the pulse. Decreased pulse pressure may indicate systemic hypotension (drop in blood pressure) secondary to a process such as hypovolemic shock. Instrumentation has been developed for the noninvasive measurement of blood pressure in the dog and cat (Dinamap 8300, Critikon; Figure 27-6).

Respiration

The respiratory rate should be counted when the animal is at rest but not sleeping. Respiration involves both an inspiratory and expiratory phase. When counting the respiratory rate, it is necessary to count either inspirations or expirations but not both. The normal rate in the dog is between 15 and 30 breaths/min. Smaller breeds tend to have a more rapid rate of respiration than larger breeds. The rate in cats is between 20 and 30 breaths/min. In addition to determining the rate, it is important to characterize the respiratory status of the patient by inspection.

Several terms are used to describe respiratory function.

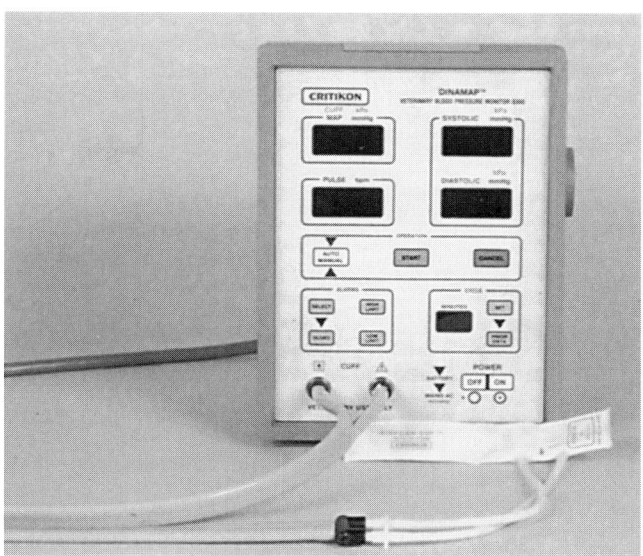

FIGURE 27-6.   Dinamap 8300 (Critikon) instrument for noninvasive measurement of blood pressure.

Tachypnea refers to very rapid breathing. *Hyperpnea* indicates a condition in which the respiration is deeper and more rapid than normal. *Depth of respiration* indicates the volume of air inspired with each breath. Increased depth of respiration indicates a greater demand for oxygen. Shallow respiration can be caused by either metabolic derangement (e.g., acidosis) or mechanical injuries (e.g., fractured ribs). *Dyspnea* is a term used to indicate the subjective impression of increased difficulty or distress in breathing.

All hospitalized patients should have their vital signs monitored at least once per day. Depending on the underlying problem and the status of the patient, it may be necessary to monitor the patient more frequently. The temperature, pulse, and respiration rate should be recorded in the medical record every time they are taken. This will facilitate recognition of abnormalities as early as possible. Further, serial observations will permit recognition of clinical trends.

Administration of Medications

It is important for the animal health technician to be familiar with several basic principles of clinical pharmacology. These principles are important when considering the route of administration of various drugs. Drugs can be administered parenterally (e.g., by injection), orally, or topically. The parenteral techniques routinely used in veterinary medicine include the intravenous, intramuscular, and subcutaneous routes. The specific techniques used to administer drugs by these various routes are discussed in Chapter 23. The discussion in this chapter is concerned with the selection of an appropriate route in various clinical situations.

In choosing the route of administration, a variety of factors must be considered. First, the pharmacologic properties of the drug should be considered. Certain drugs are not adequately absorbed when given by a certain route (e.g., gentamicin is poorly absorbed from the gastrointestinal tract). Similarly, insulin must be given by injection because it is destroyed in the gastrointestinal tract. Other drugs cannot be given by a certain route because they produce severe tissue reactions (e.g., thiamylal sodium causes sloughing of the skin if it is given subcutaneously). Another pharmacologic factor to consider is the rate of absorption. If an animal is critically ill, the route of administration that will provide the earliest onset of action is preferred. For example, an animal with a severe, overwhelming infection should receive an antibiotic intravenously rather than orally.

It is also important to consider the patient when considering the route of administration. For example, it is generally inadvisable to administer oral medications to a vomiting patient or to an animal with severe respiratory embarrassment. The temperament of the patient should also be considered. In a fractious animal, it may be impossible to administer drugs topically, orally, or intravenously. Subcutaneous or intramuscular injections may be the only feasible routes of administration. Finally, convenience and compliance of the client will influence therapeutic decision. Obviously, the topical and oral routes are preferred for treatment at home.

The principal advantages of the oral route are convenience and reduced risk of infection or abscess caused by faulty injection technique. Disadvantages of the oral route include the potential for inhalation of liquid medications and the potential for animals to spit out the medication so the prescribed dose is not absorbed.

Advantages of parenteral injections include, in general, more rapid absorption and greater assurance that the prescribed dose is accurately delivered.

The major advantage to topical medication is that systemic effects are reduced and safety is thus increased. The major disadvantage is that most systemic illnesses do not respond to topical medication alone.

Whenever any drug is administered, it is essential to record the treatment (drug, dose, time) and route of administration completely and accurately in the medical record. The notation should be made immediately after administering the medication. If this procedure is consistently followed, patient care will improve because it is less likely that treatments will be omitted or inadvertently repeated. In addition to improving the level of patient care, it should be remembered that this policy is important because the medical record is a legal document, and every treatment should be recorded in case of subsequent litigation.

It is also of utmost importance that all medications, either those used in the hospital or those dispensed for use at home, be labeled correctly. The dispensing label information should include the complete name of the drug, size or concentration of the drug, number of tablets or capsules or milliliters of drug dispensed, dose and frequency of administration, name of the client, and name of the hospital. If potentially toxic drugs are dispensed, child-proof containers should be used, as determined by state and federal regulations.

Fluid Therapy

The veterinary technician generally will not be called on to formulate a fluid order in a hospitalized patient without supervision of the attending veterinarian. However, familiarity with certain fundamental points will allow the technician to participate actively in this essential process.

The total volume of fluid required to treat an animal can be approximated by considering the volume of fluid needed to rehydrate the patient, volume of fluid needed for maintenance requirements, and volume of fluid needed to correct ongoing losses:

- Dehydration deficit—estimate as percentage from chart in Table 27-2

TABLE 27-2	DIAGNOSIS OF DEHYDRATION: PHYSICAL EXAMINATION FINDINGS
Dehydration (%)	**Clinical Signs**
<5	Undetectable
5-6	Skin slightly doughy, inelastic consistency
6-8	Skin definitely inelastic; eyes very slightly sunken in orbits
10-12	Increased skin turgor; eyes sunken in orbits, prolonged refill time, dry mucous membranes
12-15	Shock and imminent death

- Maintenance requirement—60 ml/kg of body weight per day for the adult and 100 ml/kg/day for young (less than 5 months of age) animals
- Contemporary (ongoing losses)—estimated volume lost in diarrhea or vomitus in milliliters

Sensible losses are roughly equivalent to urine output. *Insensible losses* represent the fluid lost in the feces and during respiration. These losses are considered as part of the daily maintenance requirements. *Contemporary losses* are due to ongoing problems (i.e., vomiting, diarrhea).

The hydration status, and thus the rehydration requirement, can be assessed by the following physical examination criteria: skin turgor, dryness of the mucous membranes, capillary refill time, and degree of sinkage of the eyes into the bony orbit. Several laboratory criteria are beneficial, particularly if they are followed serially; these include the hematocrit, total protein determination, and urine specific gravity (SG). Finally, serial body weights can be valuable in determining changes in hydration status. One pound of body weight is equivalent to 1 pint or 480 ml of fluid.

By using the physical examination findings mentioned, the degree of dehydration is estimated as a percentage of body weight (see Table 27-2). Thus an animal that shows only a slight alteration in skin turgor is approximately 5% to 6% dehydrated. Skin turgor is evaluated by pinching a fold of the skin and subjectively assessing the rate at which it returns to its normal position. An animal that is 10% to 12% dehydrated will display pronounced changes in skin turgor; dry, tacky mucous membranes; prolonged capillary refill time; and eyes that are sunken into the orbits. The physical alterations associated with dehydration are a continuum so an animal that is 8% dehydrated should have abnormalities midway between the end points described. It should be stressed that physical examination findings are at best very crude indicators of the degree of dehydration. The quantitative value of these parameters is improved if they are carefully and critically assessed over time.

The laboratory criteria used to assess the degree of dehydration evaluate the extent of hemoconcentration. Thus the higher the hematocrit and the total protein determination, the more hemoconcentrated and thus dehydrated is the patient. These laboratory tests are useful in detecting relative changes and do not necessarily measure the absolute hydration status of the patient. If the concentrating ability of the kidneys is normal, a urine SG of more than 1.035 in the dog and 1.040 in the cat provides further evidence that the patient may be dehydrated.

Because changes in body weight over short periods are caused by changes in fluid balance rather than by the loss or gain of body mass, an accurate daily weight can also be helpful in assessing changes in the hydration status of the patient.

The most reliable means of establishing the degree of dehydration is to make a collective judgment based on as many of the criteria mentioned as possible.

Once the degree of dehydration has been estimated, it can be used in calculating the volume of fluids needed to rehydrate the patient. The percent dehydration is multiplied by the body weight in kilograms and then by 1000. This is the number of milliliters needed to rehydrate the patient.

Generally, the volume required to rehydrate the animal is not replaced immediately. One procedure is to administer approximately 80% of this volume over the first 24 hours and the remaining 20% over the next 24 hours. In addition to the volume required for rehydration, the maintenance requirement must be incorporated in the calculation of the daily fluid order. The maintenance requirement consists of estimates of both sensible and insensible losses.

As mentioned, sensible losses refer to the urine output. Insensible losses represent the fluid lost from the body via the gastrointestinal and respiratory tracts. Although sensible and insensible losses will vary somewhat depending on the clinical setting, a useful clinical approximation is 60 ml/kg/day. If the animal is not taking any liquids by mouth, a volume equivalent to the sensible and insensible losses (e.g., the maintenance requirement) should be included in the daily fluid order.

Most animals with problems that require fluid therapy do not have these problems resolve immediately on initiation of fluid therapy. Therefore contemporary or ongoing losses must also be considered in determining the daily fluid order. For example, if a patient has gastroenteritis, the volume of fluid lost with each episode of vomiting and diarrhea should be estimated and added to the rehydration and maintenance volumes. The volume of diarrhea and vomitus is frequently underestimated; therefore it has been recommended that the visual estimate be *doubled* to more accurately reflect the actual volume lost.

Routes of Fluid Administration

Oral fluid administration is the preferred method because of reduced expense, ease of administration, and safety. Contraindications to oral fluid administration include vomiting and severe, life-threatening fluid imbalances that require immediate correction.

Many conditions respond well to subcutaneous administration of fluids. Fluids given subcutaneously should be warmed to body temperature and must be isotonic with extracellular fluid. Isotonic fluids have an osmotic pressure approximately equal to that of extracellular fluid. Never give subcutaneously dextrose solutions with a concentration of more than 2.5%; sloughing of skin and abscess formation are common sequelae. The volume and rate of subcutaneous fluids that can be given will vary from patient to patient. A rough guideline for total daily volume is approximately 60 ml/kg. Absorption of subcutaneous fluids will occur over 6 to 8 hours; therefore this total daily dose can be divided and given every 6 to 8 hours. It is necessary and desirable to administer this divided dose in as many sites as possible. Subcutaneous fluid administration is safe and easy; however, it is not the recommended route of administration when prompt correction of severe deficits is required.

The intraperitoneal route is not a routine method of fluid administration because peritonitis and intraabdominal abscess formation may result from this form of fluid therapy. The rate of absorption of intraperitoneal fluids is roughly equivalent to the rate of absorption of subcutaneous fluids and therefore the intraperitoneal route is not adequate when prompt correction is needed. The exception to this is the use of intraperitoneal fluid administration in the neonate and wildlife neonate, where this route may be very effective.

Signs of volume overload include restlessness, hyperpnea (increased respiratory rate), serous (watery) nasal discharge, chemosis (edema of the ocular conjunctiva), and pitting edema. Volume overload can be caused by either an excessive total volume or an excessive rate of fluid administration. Decreased cardiac function or decreased plasma protein can predispose to a volume overload state. If volume overload is suspected, the lungs should be auscultated for evidence of pulmonary edema, and the central venous pressure should be determined. Before the development of pulmonary edema or elevated central venous pressure, weight gain may be seen. Therefore it is advisable to weigh the animal three times daily while intravenous fluid therapy is being used, especially in those patients who are less able to handle a fluid load (e.g., patients with cardiac or renal disease).

Fluid therapy is a dynamic process that must be reassessed at frequent intervals and adjusted to obtain the maximum results. The technician's role in clinically assessing the patient is important in making appropriate adjustments.

Central Venous Pressure

The measurement of central venous pressure is a useful aid in evaluating the fluid status of a patient. When used and interpreted properly, it can substantially reduce the likelihood of excessive fluid administration. Measurement of the central venous pressure is a simple technique that can be performed in all veterinary practices.

To measure the central venous pressure, an indwelling intravenous catheter is placed in the cranial vena cava via the external jugular vein. It is very important that the catheter tip be located in the cranial vena cava. If the intravenous catheter is properly placed, a 2- to 5-mm fluctuation in central venous pressure will be noted with each respiration.

Next, a sterile three-way stopcock is attached to the intravenous catheter. The open line of the three-way stopcock is connected to the intravenous fluid source. The intravenous fluids are used to prime the manometer; that is, the manometer is filled to overflowing with the intravenous fluids. With the patient in lateral recumbency, the zero point of the manometer is positioned at the level of the sternum (Figure 27-7). The central venous pressure is equal to the level of intravenous fluid in the manometer once equilibrium has been established. To improve accuracy, this determination should be repeated a total of three times. If the pressure is high, prevent blood from entering the manometer because a blood clot may alter the measurements.

The following points are important considerations when measuring and interpreting central venous pressure measurements. Serial measurements should be performed with the same zero point and the patient in the same position. If the catheter is obstructed because of blood clots or kinking, the central venous pressure will be falsely elevated. Obstruction should be suspected if the level of the manometer does not fluctuate with respiration. Because continuous recording is not possible, pressure measurements are made intermittently. If intravenous fluids are not being administered between central venous pressure measurements, the catheter should be flushed with heparinized saline. Heparinized saline is prepared by adding 5 U of heparin per milliliter of saline. When evaluating the central venous

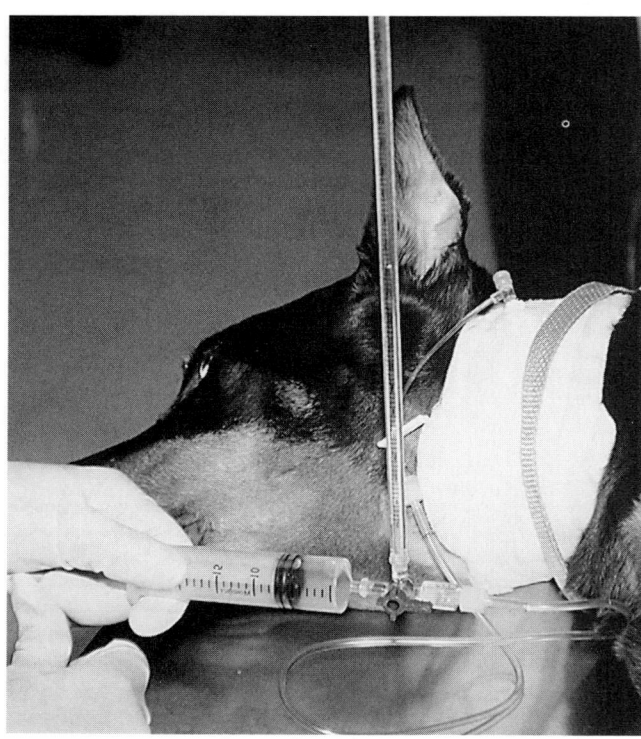

FIGURE 27-7. Use of a manometer to measure central venous pressure in a dog.

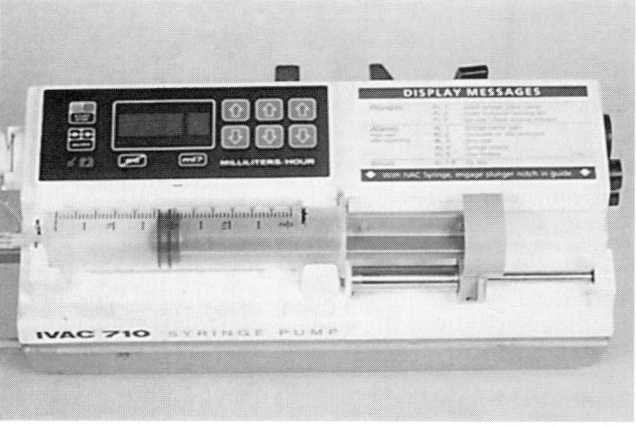

FIGURE 27-8. IVAC 710 Syringe Pump fluid pump used for the administration of small volumes and slow rates of fluid to the cat and small dog.

pressure, it is better to evaluate trends rather than single measurements. Usually, changes of less than 3 cm of water are not significant. Using the sternum as the zero point, normal central venous pressure in the dog and cat varies between 0 and 5 cm of intravenous fluid. If the central venous pressure is consistently more than 8 to 10 cm of intravenous fluid, volume overload is suspected and fluid administration should be slowed or stopped.

Technician Note

Heparinized saline can be prepared by adding 5 units of heparin per milliliter of saline. For example, add 500 units of heparin to a 100-ml bag of saline.

The chance of inadvertent fluid overload can be reduced by using indwelling intravenous catheters and administering fluids over prolonged periods of time rather than using rapid bolus techniques. In addition, Minidrip (Travenol Laboratories, Inc.) and Buretrol (Travenol Laboratories, Inc.) administration sets can be used in cats and small dogs. Also, syringe pumps are useful in administering fluids to cats and very small dogs (IVAC 710 Syringe Pump; Figure 27-8).

Several basic types of fluid are routinely used in small animal practice. They include physiologic (0.9%) saline, 5% dextrose in water, and extracellular fluid replacement solutions such as lactated Ringer's solution or Ringer's solution. Combinations of these basic fluid types are also used. These basic parenteral fluid types can be supplemented with concentrated solutions of electrolytes and dextrose to produce the desired fluid composition appropriate for the specific clinical situation (Table 27-3).

Frequently, antimicrobials are added to intravenous fluids for administration. A number of the commonly used antimicrobials are incompatible with certain fluids (Table 27-4). The physical incompatibilities include precipitation of the drug out of solution and chemical inactivation. In addition to these incompatibilities, it has been noted that when certain drugs are mixed in infusion solutions, inactivation occurs. For example, when carbenicillin is added to a solution containing gentamicin, the gentamicin is inactivated. As a general rule, it is undesirable to mix multiple drugs in a syringe or intravenous fluids. Frequently, the interaction is visible on mixing, but other times it will not be observed before administration.

Blood Transfusion

Blood transfusion is an effective method of fluid replacement but a potentially hazardous form of treatment. Clear indications for its use must be present. The effectiveness of transfusion is temporary. Consequently, every effort must be made to identify and correct underlying problems.

Severe blood loss is an indication for transfusion therapy. Massive hemorrhage can occur after trauma or surgery. Measurement of the packed cell volume (PCV) can be misleading immediately after acute blood loss because of compensatory vasoconstriction and splenic contraction. The PCV may remain normal for as long as 6 hours after an acute bleeding episode, but the total protein will decrease soon after the bleeding episode and therefore can be used as an early indicator of blood loss. As the intravascular volume is restored by the redistribution of body fluids, the PCV will drop. Collectively, the following clinical parameters are better indicators of acute hemorrhage than the PCV: total protein, pulse pressure, depth and rate of respiration, mucous membrane color, capillary refill time, urine production, central venous pressure, and arterial blood gases.

In the treatment of chronic anemia, blood is used primarily for its oxygen-carrying capabilities and should not be considered definitive therapy. The decision to transfuse should be based on clinical signs (e.g., respiratory distress, weakness) rather than an arbitrarily determined PCV or hemoglobin concentration. Some animals with chronic anemia have been shown to be able to increase oxygen delivery at the tissue level by means of biochemical changes within the red cells. Thus one dog with a PCV of

TABLE 27-3	BASIC FLUIDS						
	Fluid Composition per Liter						
Fluid Type	Na$^+$	Cl$^-$	K$^+$	Ca^{2+}	Lactate	Kcal
Lactated Ringer's solution	130	109	4	3	28	9
Ringer's solution	147	156	4	5	0	0
0.9% Saline	154	154	0	0	0	0
2.5% Dextrose in ½ normal saline	77	77	0	0	0	85
5% Dextrose in lactated Ringer's solution	130	109	4	3	28	179
5% Dextrose in water	0	0	0	0	0	179
Normosol-R	140	98	5	0	0	18

TABLE 27-4	PHYSICAL INCOMPATIBILITIES OF ANTIMICROBIALS IN INTRAVENOUS SOLUTIONS
Antimicrobial	**Incompatible with:**
Amphotericin B	Normal saline
Cephalothin sodium	Lactated Ringer's solution, calcium gluconate, calcium chloride
Chloramphenicol sodium succinate	Vitamin B complex with vitamin C
Chlortetracycline hydrochloride, oxytetracycline hydrochloride, tetracycline hydrochloride	Lactated Ringer's solution, sodium bicarbonate, calcium chloride
Penicillins	Dextrose-containing solutions with pH >8 (i.e., added sodium bicarbonate)
Penicillin G potassium	Vitamin B complex with vitamin C

12 may be well compensated, whereas another with the same PCV will be severely compromised and will require a transfusion.

Transfusions may be indicated to stop or prevent bleeding resulting from decreased number of platelets or abnormal platelet function, but large quantities of blood are needed to significantly raise the platelet count; therefore platelet-rich plasma is the preferred method to replace platelets. Because platelets survive for less than 12 hours in stored blood, freshly drawn blood should be used. Transfusion therapy is also useful in the treatment of hereditary or acquired bleeding disorders, such as hemophilia or disseminated intravascular coagulation (DIC). As with platelets, some coagulation factors are labile, so transfused blood should be less than 12 hours old. The basis for this use is to provide adequate concentrations of the deficient coagulation factor at the bleeding site.

Transfusion of blood is indicated in autoimmune hemolytic anemia only in life-threatening situations. Transfusion of a patient with autoimmune hemolytic anemia can initiate or accelerate a hemolytic crisis and increase production of antibodies directed against red blood cells (RBCs). If transfusion is necessary as a life-saving measure, only the absolute minimum number of RBCs should be administered. An initial replacement volume of not more than 12 ml/kg of body weight would be acceptable in this situation.

Transfusions to correct leukopenia (low white blood cell [WBC] count) or hypoproteinemia (low serum protein) are of equivocal long-term benefit and require such large volumes to effect a significant rise in these parameters that they are impractical for this use.

There are eight canine blood groups. Blood groups are designated by the presence of specific *canine erythrocyte antigens* (e.g., CEA-1, CEA-2, CEA-3). Any of these erythrocyte antigens can stimulate antibody production if it is transfused into a recipient that is negative for that particular antigen. CEA-1 is the most powerful stimulus for such antibody production. Reactions to CEA-2 are less pronounced; however, they can still be of clinical significance. Reactions to the other canine erythrocyte antigens are generally clinically insignificant. Antibodies directed against CEA-1 and CEA-2 do not occur naturally; consequently, clinically significant adverse reactions do not occur on initial transfusion.

Because 60% of dogs have either CEA-1 or CEA-2 antigens, transfusion with blood from a random donor (i.e., untyped donor) has a 24% chance of stimulating CEA-1 or CEA-2 antibody production. On subsequent repeated random transfusions, the incidence of transfusion reactions is about 15%. Besides the possibility of transfusion reactions, other problems associated with the transfusion of untyped blood include decreased survival of transfused cells in the recipient and hemolytic disease of newborn pups born to dams sensitized by transfusion.

Unfortunately, blood typing sera are not readily available. Therefore in many veterinary practices it is necessary to use untyped blood. If multiple blood transfusions are required, cross-matching should be performed to detect donor-recipient incompatibility. A major cross-match is performed by combining two drops of a 4% suspension of the donor's RBCs suspended in the donor's serum with two drops of the recipient's serum and incubated in a test tube at room temperature for 15 minutes. The tube is centrifuged at 1000 revolutions per minute (rpm) for 1 minute, and the contents are examined for hemolysis. If hemolysis is present, the transfusion is incompatible, and that donor blood should not be used.

Although blood groups have been reported in the cat, most cats appear to belong to the same blood group. Transfusion reactions caused by blood group incompatibility are rarely observed in practice.

Blood Donors

Canine blood donors should not have CEA-1 or CEA-2 and should be negative for heartworms, *Ehrlichia canis*, and *Babesia canis*. Donor cats are not routinely typed; however, they should not have feline leukemia virus, feline immunodeficiency virus, or *Haemobartonella*. In large blood donor programs, each animal should be permanently identified and have a permanent medical record.

Routine periodic laboratory evaluation, that is, a complete blood count (CBC), biochemistry panel, urinalysis, and fecal flotation, will help to assess the health status of donors. Routine immunizations should be performed as required. The donors should be fed a good commercial diet and receive a hematinic (vitamin and iron supplement).

The ideal canine donor is an 18- to 27-kg, medium-build dog in good health and of good temperament. Approximately 10 to 20 ml of blood per kilogram of body weight may be drawn every 3 weeks without excessively stressing the canine donor. In the cat, approximately 60 ml can be drawn every 3 weeks without excessive stress to the donor.

Blood Collection

The actual method of collection will vary, depending on the specific situation. The donor that is to be sacrificed at the end of the collection is first anesthetized, and a surgical preparation of the collection site is performed. Possible collection sites in the dog include the jugular vein, heart, or femoral artery. In the cat, the jugular vein and heart are possible sites. In permanent donors, the jugular vein is the preferred site. Blood collection should be performed rapidly and without interruption, using a single site to avoid excessive activation of the clotting cascade and damage to the RBCs. If acid citrate dextrose (ACD Evacuated Blood Collection Bottle, Diamond Laboratories, Inc.) is being used, a separate collection set should be used. If citrate phosphate dextrose (CPD) plastic blood pack units (with Integral Donor Tube, Fenwall Laboratories, Inc.) are used, the attached needle should be used. If the vacuum bottles are used, care should be taken not to lose the vacuum at the time of venipuncture.

In the cat, a 19-gauge butterfly needle (Travenol Laboratories) and a large syringe containing the desired anticoagulant can be used.

Several anticoagulants are available for routine collection of blood. Blood drawn in heparin must be used within 24 to 48 hours because of the marked increase in pH and the subsequent decrease in red cell adenosine triphosphate observed when heparin is used as an anticoagulant. These chemical changes result in rigid red cells that do not deform and thus are rapidly removed from the recipient's circulation.

If blood is to be stored for longer than 48 hours, either acid citrate dextrose (ACD Evacuated Blood Collection Bottle) or citrate phosphate dextrose (CPD Blood Pack Units with Integral Donor Tube) must be used as the anticoagulant and the blood stored at 1° C to 6° C. The temperature cannot vary by more than 2° C, and if the blood is out of refrigeration long enough to warm to 10° C (approximately 30 minutes), it must be used immediately. During storage, the blood should be gently mixed periodically. When collected and stored as described, blood drawn in ACD has an effective storage life of approximately 14 days, and blood drawn in CPD has an effective storage life of approximately 21 days. Blood stored beyond these limits will have reduced posttransfusion survival.

Blood should be gradually warmed to approximately 37° C before administration. Refrigerated blood can be warmed by passing it through a coiled tube in a 40° C water bath or by other appropriate means. Care should be exercised to prevent excessive warming (more than 50° C). Excessive warming will cause hemolysis.

It is essential that strict asepsis be maintained during collection, storage, and administration of blood and blood products. Once a blood storage container has been entered, the stored blood should be used within 24 hours.

Blood should be administered through a sterile blood administration kit (Blood Administration Set, Diamond Laboratories, Inc.). A micropore filter is suggested to reduce the transfusion of microemboli found in stored blood. Administration of blood and blood products can be given by the intravenous (the most common route), intraperitoneal, or interosseous routes. The intraperitoneal and intraosseous (into the bone marrow) routes are used more in the neonate.

If the practice has a frequent demand for transfusion therapy, it is desirable to make optimal use of the available donors by separating blood into its components and administering only the needed component. Packed red cells can be produced by either centrifugation or by sedimentation of whole blood. Sedimented packed red cells are separated from plasma by gravity. The recovery of plasma is less efficient by this method; however, a centrifuge is not necessary. If collected in glass vacuum bottles, approximately 25% to 30% of the blood volume separates into plasma by 7 to 9 days, and 45% of the blood volume is available as plasma after 14 to 16 days. Plasma is harvested from the glass collection bottles with a sterile 17.5-cm needle and a sterile syringe. Blood in plastic packs separates more rapidly than blood in glass bottles. Plasma can be collected from plastic packs by means of either a sterile needle and syringe or a plasma transfer pack (Plasma Transfer Sets, Fenwall Laboratories) and a plasma extractor (Plasma Extractor, Fenwall Laboratories). The plasma transfer packs have attached tubing and adaptors as well as sealable entry ports. Thus the plasma can be collected in a closed, sterile system. If the plasma is to be stored at refrigerator temperatures (1° C to 6° C) for longer than 24 hours, a closed system is essential. Plasma frozen at less than –20° C has a storage life of longer than 1 year. If frozen plasma is to be used to treat bleeding disorders, it should be frozen within a few hours of collection.

If the major indication for transfusion is decreased oxygen-carrying capability, the patient should receive packed red cells. Packed red cells can be administered rapidly with less risk of creating volume overload in a patient with compromised cardiovascular function. The use of packed red cells will also reduce the frequency of transfusion reactions caused by plasma protein incompatibility.

Plasma transfusions are used primarily to expand the extracellular fluid volume. Plasma is also used for its transient benefit in the management of hypoproteinemia. Fresh frozen plasma is a source of coagulation factors V and VIII.

Transfusion Reactions

Complications of blood transfusion can be both immunologic and nonimmunologic in origin. Immunologic reactions can result from the transfusion of incompatible blood. Incompatible RBCs in a previously unsensitized recipient will be destroyed 7 to 10 days after transfusion. If the recipient is subsequently exposed to incompatible blood, a more acute hemolytic reaction may occur. Clinical consequences of hemolytic transfusion reactions include the rapid development of tachycardia, hypotension, vomiting, salivation, and muscle tremors. Laboratory changes associated with significant acute hemolysis include hemoglobinemia, hemoglobinuria, and possible acquired coagulation disorders.

Delayed hemolytic reactions will sometimes occur following multiple transfusions. Delayed hemolysis should be suspected if the PCV drops unexpectedly 2 to 21 days after transfusion. The clinical and laboratory signs of acute hemolysis mentioned may not be detected in delayed hemolytic reactions. Transfusion reactions may also be caused by immunologic reactions caused by leukocyte, platelet, or plasma protein incompatibilities. Reactions between antigens and antibodies may activate the complement system and thus release vasoactive substances that may be responsible for trembling, vomiting, and urticaria (hives). Prior transfusion is not required for these reactions to occur. Some authors have advocated the use of antihistamines (diphenhydramine hydrochloride) approximately 30 minutes before transfusion to reduce these reactions.

Transfusion-induced fever is due to the response of the donor to foreign proteins. The initial step in controlling transfusion-induced fever is to slow the rate of transfusion. If no response is noted when the rate is reduced, antipyretics, such as aspirin, should be administered. Bacterial contamination of the transfused blood will also produce fever.

Nonimmunologic transfusion reactions are principally due to vascular overload. Signs of vascular overload include a dry cough, respiratory distress, and vomiting. If there is evidence of preexisting cardiac dysfunction, the rate of administration of blood should be reduced to approximately 1 ml/kg/hr. Because vomiting is a potential adverse reaction to transfusion, food and water should be withheld from the patient during the transfusion.

Technician Note

Since vomiting is a potential adverse reaction to transfusions, if the situation allows, the patient should be fasted and have water withheld during the transfusion.

Physical Therapy

Physical therapy can be defined as the use of cold, heat, water, electrical impulses, and therapeutic exercise to treat an injury or disease. When used appropriately, these techniques can either prevent permanent dysfunction or hasten the return of normal function. Physical therapy is especially useful in treating diseases of the musculoskeletal and neuromuscular systems.

Physical therapy can be of tremendous value in reducing muscle spasm, relieving pain, resolving peripheral edema, improving blood supply to a specific site, improving muscle tone, and increasing the range of motion of a joint.

In veterinary practice basically five treatment modalities are employed: superficial heat, cold, massage, active exercise, and electrical stimulation. All these forms of treatment will influence blood supply and edema.

Superficial heat increases the temperature of local tissues, which results in increased metabolism, improved blood supply, and mild analgesia. In contrast, deep heat (e.g., *diathermy*) can potentially increase peripheral edema by increasing capillary hydrostatic pressure. Superficial heat can be applied by means of whirlpool baths, hot packs, or infrared radiation. Moist heat is preferred to dry heat because of its greater action in reducing pain and muscle spasms. Use of a whirlpool bath provides superficial heat as well as buoyancy to support the affected body part. The jet streams of warm water can also stimulate

peripheral nerves and cleanse soiled areas. The technique for applying hot packs is to soak a towel or cloth in water as hot as the technician can comfortably stand, wring lightly, and apply to the affected part. As the temperature of the towel decreases, the towel can be rinsed with hot water and reapplied. Twenty minutes is an adequate period of time for this form of heat treatment.

In most traumatic injuries, *early* application of cold will reduce swelling and muscle spasm. Towels or cloths soaked in either cold water or ice water and wrung lightly are a means of applying cold to an animal patient. Alternatively, commercial cold packs or ice packs can be used; however, they should be used with caution in order to prevent cold-induced injury. Fifteen to twenty minutes are usually required for treatment.

If peripheral edema is present, massage may be beneficial. The technique for therapeutic massage consists of gentle stroking and light kneading of the involved area. An attempt should be made to direct the peripheral edema from the involved area toward the heart. This will enhance venous return of the edematous fluid.

Active movement should be encouraged as soon as it can be accomplished safely and without pain. Active movement can be accomplished by swimming the patient in a whirlpool or bathtub. Most animals will swim with encouragement and then actively exercise a body part that otherwise would not be exercised. A towel or sling can be used for support and to keep the animal upright. When appropriate, therapeutic exercise can occur on any nonslippery surface. If the patient is not able to ambulate without assistance, a towel or sling can provide the necessary support. Active therapeutic exercise is of greater benefit than passive exercise.

Although not widely used in veterinary practice, electrical stimulation is beneficial in the treatment of some neuromuscular diseases and neurogenic atrophy.

Owners of animals that would benefit from physical therapy are usually willing to perform physical therapy at home. However, the owner must be carefully instructed on how to perform the treatment and why it will be beneficial to the patient. The technician is usually the best person in the practice to demonstrate the proper technique.

Oxygen Therapy

The primary indication for oxygen therapy is *hypoxia*, which refers to a deficiency of oxygen at the tissue level. Tissue hypoxia may be caused by a reduction in perfusion (reduced blood flow) or a reduction in oxygen content of the blood. Hypoxia is probably more common than is recognized in veterinary medicine since a caged animal at rest will not show signs until the oxygen content of the blood is severely reduced.

Hypoxia can be manifested in a variety of ways, and the veterinary technician must be alert to identify these changes. Abnormalities that may be noted in the cardiovascular system include tachycardia or arrhythmias. An increased respiratory rate, open-mouthed breathing, and dyspnea may also be noted. *Dyspnea* is the term used to indicate subjective difficulty or distress in breathing. With severe hypoxia, central nervous system changes may be noted and include drowsiness, altered motor abilities, or increased excitability. Finally, cold extremities may indicate an inadequate supply of oxygen at the tissue level. *Cyanosis* is not a reliable indicator of hypoxia, especially if the animal is anemic. Cyanosis refers to dark bluish or purplish discoloration of the skin and mucous membranes.

Although the basic defect in hypoxia is decreased oxygen

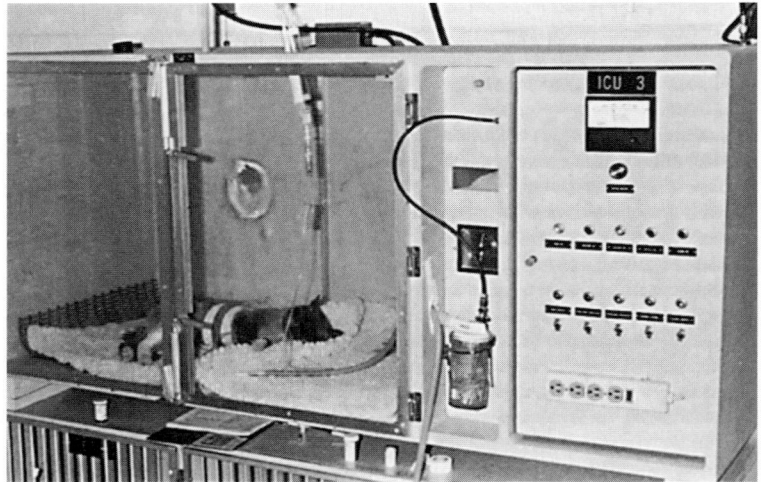

FIGURE 27-9. Small animal oxygen cage.

availability at the tissue level, it can occur by a variety of mechanisms. For example, it can result from lung disease, decreased cardiac output, or severe anemia.

In small animal practice, oxygen therapy is used primarily in the following clinical situations: pulmonary edema, severe bronchopneumonia, upper airway disease in brachycephalic breeds such as English bulldog and Boston terrier, pulmonary trauma, collapse of lung lobes, and shock.

Methods of oxygen therapy include oxygen cages, human pediatric incubators, masks, nasal catheters, endotracheal tubes, and intratracheal catheters.

Oxygen Cage

Oxygen cages for veterinary use are sold commercially. These cages permit control of not only the oxygen concentration but also temperature and humidity (Figure 27-9). These cages are useful in animals able to ventilate without assistance. However, they are expensive and consume large amounts of oxygen. Surplus human pediatric incubators are a less expensive means of providing similar therapy to small dogs, cats, or exotic animals. Oxygen cages and incubators should be flushed (filled) with oxygen after they have been opened. Some units are equipped with entry ports that allow access to the patient without excessive loss of oxygen.

An inspired oxygen concentration of 30% to 40% is adequate for animals requiring oxygen therapy. Excessively high oxygen concentrations can result in oxygen toxicity. Neonatal kittens appear to be particularly susceptible to retinal changes induced by oxygen toxicity.

Mask Induction

In certain circumstances, masks can be used to administer oxygen. Masks are available in a variety of sizes and shapes suitable for use in dogs and cats. If an oxygen mask is used, it is important to provide a high oxygen flow rate to prevent excessive accumulation of carbon dioxide. Administration of oxygen via a mask is suitable for short periods of time only and only in selected patients. Some patients will resist the use of an oxygen mask, and the resultant stress will negate any beneficial effect of the oxygen.

Intratracheal Catheter Induction

An alternative means of oxygen administration that is both inexpensive and effective is the intratracheal catheter. This technique is reserved for critically ill patients. The skin is aseptically prepared, and a local anesthetic is administered over the trachea in the midcervical area. An intravenous catheter (14, 16, or 18 gauge) is introduced into the trachea and advanced to a point craniad to the bifurcation of the trachea. The delivered oxygen should be humidified and administered at a flow rate of 0.5 to 4 L/min. The flow rate should be adjusted, depending on the size of the animal.

Nasal Catheter Induction

Nasal catheters can also be used to administer oxygen for brief periods to severely depressed animals. In this technique, a small (5 to 8 Fr.) soft rubber feeding tube or urinary catheter is inserted through the external nares to the level of the caudal nasopharynx. The catheter can be coated with a topical anesthetic cream, or topical anesthetic drops can be instilled in the nostril to facilitate passage. Adhesive tape is attached to the catheter, and the tape is sutured to the forehead. An Elizabethan collar should be used to prevent the patient from dislodging the catheter.

Respiratory Physical Therapy

Physical therapy of the respiratory system is a valuable adjunct to other forms of therapy for diseases of the lungs and airways. Appropriate physical therapy is also useful as a preventive measure in patients at high risk for the development of pulmonary disease. Secondary bronchopneumonia is a common complication in patients with lung lobe collapse. Stimulation of the cough reflex by compressing the trachea will expand the lungs maximally and help prevent lung collapse. Regular turning of recumbent patients will enhance drainage and circulation and thus prevent hypostatic congestion.

Percussion (coupage), also known as *tapping* or *clapping,* is a technique of striking the animal's chest to loosen bronchial secretion and thus facilitate drainage. The chest is struck with the hand held slightly cupped with fingers and thumb closed so a cushion of air is trapped between the technician's hand and the chest wall. Best results come from using both hands alternately in rapid sequence for several seconds, moving from ventral to dorsal on the lung fields. When done properly, this is a noisy procedure; however, it is not painful to the patient. An electric hand vibrator can be used to set up fine vibrations that will also aid the drainage of secretions. If the animal is ambulatory, a brief walk after coupage will aid in mobilization of respiratory secretions.

Whenever possible, animals with pulmonary problems should be maintained in an upright position (i.e., sternal recumbency). If necessary, slings or supports should be used to maintain this posture. This position will decrease the amount of hypostatic congestion that develops.

Topical Therapy

Topical therapy plays an important role in the treatment of dermatologic disease. It can be used to treat a specific disease, such as sarcoptic mange. More frequently, however, topical therapy is used either in conjunction with systemic medications or as a form of symptomatic therapy when the diagnosis is unknown.

Plain tap water is one of the most effective topical agents. Depending on how water is used, it can either hydrate or dehydrate the skin. Frequent wetting of the skin will stimulate evaporation from the skin and thus cause dehydration. This approach can be useful in managing any acute moist dermatitis ("hot spot"). In contrast, if a film of oil (e.g., Alpha Keri, Westwood Pharmaceuticals, Inc.) is applied immediately after soaking with water, evaporation is slowed or stopped, and the skin remains moist.

Soaks

Soaks are an effective means of handling localized acute eruptions. Soaks can be applied with moist towels or by placing the animal in a water-filled basin or tub. Soaks for local acute dermatosis should be applied for 10 to 15 minutes three or more times daily. The involved area should be kept constantly moist, and the warm temperature of the soak should be maintained by adding hot water as needed. Some of the solutions commonly used for soaks in veterinary medicine include water, aluminum acetate (Burow's solution, Domeboro solution, Dome Laboratories), and magnesium sulfate or Epsom salts (1:65 solution in water, 1 tablespoonful per 1000 ml of water).

Astringents

Astringents precipitate proteins on the surface of an area of acute damage and form a beneficial covering. These agents do not penetrate deeply. Aluminum acetate is an excellent mild astringent. Another effective astringent is tannic acid. Tannic acid is combined with salicylic acid and alcohol in several products to form a potent astringent. These combination products are especially useful as part of the management of localized acute moist dermatitis; however, astringents should be applied only once to an involved area.

Baths

Cleansing baths are an important part of topical dermatologic therapy. Baths aid in the removal of dirt, debris, and scale. A variety of effective mild cleansing soaps or detergents are available. Mild dishwashing detergents or soaps (e.g., Joy, Palmolive Liquid) are effective and inexpensive. If a milder, less irritating product is desired, a balanced pH soap, such as Johnson's Baby Shampoo (Johnson & Johnson), can be used. If an even milder product is needed, vegetable oil soaps (coconut oil) are the most bland. Regardless of how mild the soap or detergent, it should always be thoroughly rinsed out of the coat with copious volumes of clean water.

A medicated bath can be applied as a shampoo or as a rinse applied to the animal after a routine cleansing bath. Medicated baths contain ingredients that enhance the actions of routine cleansing shampoos. Medicated shampoos should be lathered into the coat for 10 to 15 minutes.

This allows the medicated component of the shampoo time for effect or limited absorption. Types of medicated baths used in small animal practice include colloidal oatmeal, tar-sulfur, sulfur-salicylic, and benzoyl peroxide products. Colloidal oatmeal (Aveeno, Cooper Care, Inc.; Epi-Soothe cream rinse, Allerderm, Inc.) baths are used for their soothing and antipruritic properties. Tar-sulfur shampoos (Lytar, Dermatologics for Veterinary Medicine, Inc.; Allerseb-T, Allerderm, Inc.) are used in the management of oily, flaky seborrheic conditions. Sulfur and salicylic shampoos (Sebalyte, Dermatologics for Veterinary Medicine, Inc.; Sebolux, Allerderm, Inc.) are used in the management of dry, flaky seborrheic conditions, and benzoyl peroxide shampoos (Oxydex, Dermatologics for Veterinary Medicine, Inc.; Pyoben, Allerderm, Inc.) are useful in the treatment of superficial pyoderma (bacterial skin infection), excessive crusting and debris problems, and oily seborrheic conditions. The underlying condition and the individual response to the medicated bath determine the required frequency of application.

Dips and Rinses

Dips or rinses use water as a means of delivering various antifungal or antiparasitic agents to the skin. Although applied to the skin, some of these agents have the potential to cause systemic toxicities. Clipping the hair and using cleansing baths help to obtain greater penetration in animals with excessive scale or crust. Dips that are useful in the treatment of dermatophytosis (ringworm) include dilute sodium hypochlorite solution, dilute Nolvasan solution (Fort Dodge Laboratories), dilute iodine solutions, or lime-sulfur solutions. Antiparasitic products used as dips or rinses include chlorpyrifos (Dursban), pyrethrins, pyrethroids, organophosphates (malathion), and carbamates. Amitraz (Mitaban, Upjohn Co.) is useful in the treatment of generalized demodectic mange.

Before using any topical agent the label should be checked to be sure it is safe to use in dogs, cats, puppies, and kittens. The age of young animals should be noted because some products are not recommended in the very young.

Powders

Powders are occasionally used in veterinary medicine as drying agents and vehicles for parasiticides and to reduce friction and irritation. When used as a drying agent, powders may be in the form of true powders, shake lotions, or pastes. Components that improve the drying action of various powdered products include talc, zinc oxide, cornstarch, and tannic acid. Carbaryl powders are a valuable part of flea control programs in the dog and cat. Labels should be checked carefully to be certain that the specific product is safe for dogs and cats. The powder must be worked down into the hair coat to increase the parasiticidal effect. This can be accomplished by rubbing the hair coat against the grain as the powder is applied. The powder should be applied to the entire body, excluding the face. Fractious or frightened cats can be treated by wrapping them in a thick bath towel and medicating small sections until the entire animal has been covered. Flea sprays can be used similarly.

Creams and Ointments

Creams and ointments are also used in the topical treatment of dermatologic problems. The area of treatment should be clipped, if not hairless, and protected from immediate removal by licking. For practical and economic reasons, the area to be treated should be relatively small.

Ointments are thicker than creams and leave a greasy feeling when applied to the skin. Ointments and creams soften, lubricate, and protect the skin and aid in the removal of scale and crusts. Ointments and creams form an occlusive covering and therefore are not indicated for moist or oozing skin lesions.

Topical creams and ointments can be used to treat localized dermatophytosis (ringworm). They can be used as the sole type of therapy or as an adjunct to oral therapy or topical rinses. Creams and ointments must be restricted to small lesions because of expense and convenience. Effective topical fungicidal products used in veterinary medicine contain miconazole and thiabendazole. Because the use of ointments and creams alone is often insufficient to clear the infection or prevent reinfection, rinses or dips are important.

Otic Preparations

Most topical otic preparations contain various combinations of antibiotic, antiinflammatory, fungicidal, and parasiticidal agents. Topical antimicrobial agents are indicated whenever infection is present. Chloramphenicol, neomycin, polymyxin, and gentamicin are the commonly used antibiotics in these combination otic preparations. Neomycin and gentamicin have been reported to cause ototoxicity when used for prolonged periods in dogs with ruptured eardrums. (Gentamicin is inactivated by pus; therefore the ears must be thoroughly cleaned before use.)

Corticosteroids are used in these combination products because they decrease inflammation and the buildup of discharge and, consequently, decrease self-trauma by the animal. The antifungals are useful in treating dermatophytes and yeast organisms such as *Malassezia pachydermatis (Pityrosporon)*. Thiabendazole and miconazole are effective topical antifungal agents.

Certain drugs owe their efficacy to their ability to alter the pH in the ear canal. Acetic acid (dilute vinegar solution) and Domeboro Otic (Dome Laboratories) are specific examples.

Products that contain rotenone in oil or thiabendazole are used to treat ear mites. It is essential that treatment for ear mites be continued for at least 3 weeks and that all animals in the household be treated. Otic instillation of ivermectin, as a one-time application (on occasion, two to four treatments may be needed), has also been shown to be effective in the treatment of ear mites.

INFECTIOUS DISEASES

This section will discuss a number of common medical problems of dogs and cats. It is not intended to be a comprehensive review of internal medicine; rather, several specific problems have been selected that illustrate or emphasize important aspects of medical nursing.

Canine Respiratory Disease Complex

Synonyms for canine upper respiratory disease complex include kennel cough and infectious tracheobronchitis. This complex is composed of a number of different disease processes. Causative factors include viral and bacterial agents as well as predisposing environmental factors. These factors may occur singly or in combination. The diagnosis of this complex is usually based on historical and physical examination findings rather than on laboratory tests. This problem is most often self-limiting, and the duration of signs generally is no more than 2 weeks.

Treatment involves nursing care and the correction of any environmental factors that may have predisposed to the illness. The dog should be kept in a warm space that is well ventilated and free of drafts and should be fed a highly palatable diet. Appetite will be enhanced if eyes and nose are kept free of accumulated discharge. If anorectic, the patient should be hand or force fed. Intravenous or subcutaneous fluid therapy is occasionally necessary. Steam or vaporizer therapy may provide symptomatic relief. Steam therapy can be performed by placing the dog in a steam-filled bathroom several times per day. Alternatively, cold mist vaporizers can be used several times daily.

The decision to use antitussive (cough suppressant) therapy should be based on the frequency of coughing and how prolonged the episodes are. If codeine-derivative cough suppressants are used to excess, depression and anorexia will result.

Treatment with antibiotics usually is not indicated unless there is evidence of lower respiratory or systemic involvement, for example, fever. If antibiotic therapy is instituted, a complete regimen of 10 to 14 days at full therapeutic doses should be completed. The selection of an antibiotic would ideally be based on the results of culture and sensitivity testing of a transtracheal wash. If these are not available, chloramphenicol, trimethoprim-sulfonamide combination, or tetracyclines are usually effective. The use of systemic products containing both antibiotics and corticosteroids is not indicated. Likewise, the intratracheal injection of any product is inappropriate therapy.

Because of the highly contagious nature of the causative organisms, an infected dog should be isolated from other hospitalized patients. If possible, hospitalization should be avoided. Once an outbreak occurs in a kennel or veterinary hospital, control is difficult. Ideally, the area should be kept vacant for approximately 2 weeks, and appropriate preventive measures should be instituted, consisting of the implementation of an effective vaccination protocol for every hospitalized patient. All dogs should preferably be vaccinated at least 10 days before exposure. Yearly revaccination of all patients should be a consistent hospital policy. Although parenteral immunization is widely used, studies suggest that intranasal vaccines are more efficacious in preventing infection. Vaccination is recommended more often than yearly for animals at high risk of exposure to the causative agents (e.g., frequent boarding or dog shows). The commonly used disinfectants, such as chlorhexidine (Novalsan) and benzalkonium (Roccal), effectively kill the causative bacteria and viruses.

Feline Respiratory Disease Complex

The principal components of the feline respiratory disease complex are feline viral rhinotracheitis and feline calicivirus. Less frequently incriminated agents include feline reovirus, feline pneumonitis (*Chlamydia psittaci*), *Mycoplasma*, and *Bordetella bronchiseptica*.

Clinical signs of this complex include fever, cough, paroxysms of sneezing, and hypersalivation. As the infection progresses, mucopurulent ocular and nasal discharge, lacrimation, and open-mouthed breathing can be seen. Ulceration of the tongue, hard palate, and nasal pad has been reported with feline calicivirus. The severity of signs and the mortality are greatest in young (less than 1 year of age), nonvaccinated cats and kittens. The severity of the clinical signs will vary widely from patient to patient. The variability results from a number of interacting factors, which include the virulence of the virus, infecting dose of virus, and general health and immune status of the infected cat.

Diagnosis is based primarily on history and clinical signs rather than on laboratory findings. Occasionally, laboratory confirmation of the diagnosis by means of virus isolation or the demonstration of serum antibodies is indicated. The additional expense of laboratory confirmation is justified only when dealing with groups of cats having a chronic history of feline respiratory disease complex.

Treatment will vary, depending on the severity of signs. Some cats will show only mild, transient signs, and they require no treatment. Secondary bacterial infection will occasionally be a sequela to the feline respiratory disease complex, and therefore a broad-spectrum antibiotic may be indicated in the very young kitten (<12 weeks of age).

General nursing care is of much greater importance than antibiotics in typical cases. Whenever possible, infected cats should be treated at home rather than in the hospital.

A vital part of nursing care is to gently clean away accumulated ocular or nasal discharge. If the nostrils are kept patent, the cat is more likely to continue eating. To ensure that this happens, the owner should indulge the pet and provide highly palatable foods. Strongly flavored or odorous foods are more likely to stimulate the appetite of an anorectic cat. Steam therapy is frequently useful and can be achieved by placing the cat in a steam-filled bathroom or by using a vaporizer.

In cats that become completely anorectic, subcutaneous or intravenous fluids may be required until the appetite returns to normal. Force feeding or repeated syringe feedings may be attempted; however, in certain cats, the associated stress may negate any beneficial effect. Alternatives that appear to be better tolerated include nasoesophageal or pharyngostomy tubes. These procedures should be reserved for severely cachectic cats.

The virus is usually transmitted through direct contact with an infected cat. Sneezing with subsequent aerosolization of the virus will spread the virus a distance of approximately 15 to 20 cm. Fomite transmission via hands, clothing, litterboxes, and food and water dishes is a more significant means of transmission than aerosolization in veterinary hospitals. The agents responsible for the feline respiratory disease complex are sensitive to hypochlorite disinfection.

The best way to prevent outbreaks of feline respiratory disease complex in hospitalized cats is to have an effective immunization protocol. Adequate ventilation will reduce the likelihood that infection will spread within the hospital. The humidity should be maintained between 30% and 50%. Disposable food trays and litter pans and autoclavable water dishes should be used. Cats should not be moved from one cage to another unless absolutely necessary during an outbreak. Cages should be thoroughly cleansed with a dilute hypochlorite solution. Finally, because the infection can be spread via hands and clothing, meticulous hygiene on the part of all hospital personnel is essential. It is important to understand that up to 80% of the cats that develop this respiratory complex remain lifelong carriers of the organism or organisms. They can pose a risk to other cats or can experience a recrudescence of the complex in stressful situations.

Canine Distemper

Canine distemper is an important viral disease of dogs because of the ubiquitous nature of the virus and the mortality associated with infection. The severity of signs will vary from a transient, subclinical infection to a severe fatal disease that involves several different organ systems.

This variability is due to the differing virulence of various virus strains and differences in host immunity.

The initial phase of the infection is associated with fever, transient anorexia, lethargy, and a mild serous ocular discharge after an approximate 9- to 14-day incubation period. Obviously, these signs are not specific for canine distemper. Later, as the virus spreads to the respiratory and gastrointestinal systems, mucopurulent ocular and nasal discharge, coughing, diarrhea, and, occasionally, vomiting are noted. Many dogs are anorectic at this point and become severely dehydrated. Involvement of the central nervous system may occur and can be the only signs manifested by some dogs. These dogs may develop seizures or other evidence of neurologic disease. Some dogs will seemingly recover from the severe respiratory and gastrointestinal signs, but weeks or months later they develop neurologic signs that either are fatal or require euthanasia because of their severity.

Although the virus may survive in the environment for weeks at near-freezing temperatures (0° C to 4° C), it is susceptible to heat, drying, and ultraviolet light. Routine disinfection is usually effective in destroying the virus in a hospital or kennel.

Feline Panleukopenia

Feline panleukopenia is a potentially severe, highly contagious parvoviral disease of cats. Synonyms are feline distemper and infectious enteritis.

The typical clinical signs associated with feline panleukopenia include lethargy, anorexia, vomiting, and diarrhea after a 7-day incubation period. Characteristically, the feces are yellowish and semiformed to fluid in consistency; they may be blood tinged. Severe dehydration may be present. Cats will occasionally hang their heads over water bowls but will not drink. The temperature may be elevated or subnormal. Feline panleukopenia can be an acute disease. Rarely, development of signs is so rapid that the owner may suspect malicious poisoning. Kittens and young cats appear to be more severely affected.

Diagnosis of feline panleukopenia is based on the presence of the clinical signs described above in the presence of a low total leukocyte count (less than 2000 WBCs/mm^3). The low total count is primarily due to low numbers of neutrophils. The diagnosis of feline panleukopenia can be confirmed by virus isolation and serologic and histopathologic characteristics.

Treatment is primarily supportive because specific antiviral drugs are not available. The cornerstone of successful therapy is the correction of fluid and electrolyte imbalances and prevention of sepsis by the use of broad-spectrum antibiotics. Symptomatic control of vomiting and diarrhea is usually indicated. Another complication the technician should be alert to is the development of hypoglycemia (low blood glucose). This may be manifested by the development of extreme weakness, seizure activity, or both.

The prognosis for recovery is good if the cat survives the initial 3 to 6 days of severe clinical signs. The prognosis for kittens and young cats is guarded. A rising WBC count indicates a more favorable prognosis. During the recovery phase, the WBC count may exceed 50,000/mm^3 and reveal a significant leftward shift. This should not be confused with the development of another infection, because this can be a normal response.

If the queen is infected during pregnancy, fetal death or congenital defects in the kitten may result. The fetus is susceptible to the virus because most tissues have high cell-proliferation rates. If the fetus is infected just before or immediately after birth, the development of the cerebellum may be affected. These kittens show balance and coordination problems beginning at about 3 to 4 weeks of age.

Fortunately, because of the availability of excellent vaccines, feline panleukopenia is currently an infrequent clinical problem.

Feline Leukemia Virus and Feline Immunodeficiency Virus Infection

These two distinct retroviral infections in cats may cause similar clinical signs. Feline leukemia virus (FeLV) has been recognized for many years and may cause immunosuppression, neoplasia, or both. Lymphosarcoma and bone marrow disorders are the more common disorders associated with FeLV. The virus is transmitted between cats by direct contact through grooming, sharing food dishes, and fighting. The virus is easily killed in the environment, and isolation of an infected cat is adequate to prevent transmission to susceptible cats. Although most cats that are exposed to the virus successfully eliminate the infection, 1% to 3% of cats in single-cat households and up to 30% of cats in multiple-cat households will become persistently infected with the virus. These infected cats are then at risk for the development of the plethora of FeLV-related diseases. FeLV infection can be identified by an in-hospital test. There are many such in-hospital tests on the market and available to the practicing veterinarian. There are several vaccines available for the prevention of FeLV, and as many as 70% of cats will be protected with a successful immunization program.

Feline immunodeficiency virus (FIV), also called T-lymphotrophic T cell lentivirus (FTLV), is another virus that causes immunosuppression in the cat. Common clinical signs of infection with this virus include gingivitis, chronic diarrhea, generalized lymphadenopathy, fever, conjunctivitis, rhinitis, and dermatitis. It is notable that all these signs may be seen in cats infected with FeLV. FIV is found nationwide and, indeed, worldwide. Most cats infected with this virus will not become immune, which differs from FeLV infection. The disease is spread by inoculation of the virus through cat bites. Transmission of the virus by direct contact through grooming, sharing of food dishes, and close contact is less than that seen with FeLV. No treatment or vaccine is available for this disease. Commercial kits detecting antibodies to this virus are available for in-hospital testing.

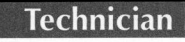

Technician Note

FeLV infection is spread by direct and repeated close contact such as grooming or sharing of food and water dishes, whereas FIV infection is transmitted by inoculation of the virus through cat bites.

Routine Immunization Program for Dogs and Cats

One of the greatest areas of advancement in veterinary medicine in the past 50 years is in the prevention of infectious diseases. The purpose of any vaccination program is to prevent clinical disease by preventing or limiting infection. The vaccination program can also be the foundation of a complete well-animal health maintenance program. At the time of vaccination, owners should be counseled regarding nutrition, parasite control, and matters regarding reproduction. Chapter 11 provides a complete overview of canine and feline preventive health programs and vaccination recommendations.

A physical examination by the veterinarian at the time of vaccination is extremely important because a number of conditions will potentially influence the immunization procedure, such as pregnancy, debilitation, and fever.

Numerous factors influence the patient's ability to respond to vaccination. Factors that are of practical significance include colostral antibodies, vaccine type, route of administration, age of the patient, nutritional status of the patient, and concurrent infection or drug therapy.

Colostral Antibodies

In puppies and kittens, approximately 95% of the circulating immunoglobulins come from absorption of *colostrum* (first milk) shortly after birth. These circulating immunoglobulins provide essential temporary protection, but they also have the ability to interfere with more permanent protection. Interference occurs because the vaccine does not reach the appropriate cells to stimulate the active immunity process. Consequently, it is necessary for the level of circulating immunoglobulins derived from the colostrum to be reduced before successful vaccination is possible. In puppies born to bitches that have received vaccinations against canine distemper and infectious canine hepatitis, this period of uncertain response to vaccination may extend to 14 weeks of age. Thus the last dose of vaccine should be administered at 14 to 16 weeks of age to optimize the success of the vaccination program. Colostral immunoglobulins to canine parvovirus may persist for at least 16 weeks in puppies; therefore the last dose of vaccine for parvovirus should be given no earlier than 16 weeks of age. In the Rottweiler and Doberman breeds, it is suggested that the last dose of parvovirus vaccine be given at 18 weeks of age.

An alternative technique to prevent or reduce the blocking effect of colostral antibodies on canine distemper vaccination is to use measles virus vaccine. Approximately 50% of puppies at 6 weeks of age will not respond to canine distemper virus vaccination, whereas the vast majority will respond to measles virus vaccine. The measles virus stimulates resistance against canine distemper in puppies regardless of circulating antibodies that the pup has acquired from the colostrum. Measles virus vaccine prevents clinical disease but does not prevent infection. Measles virus vaccine should be considered a temporary method of preventing canine distemper until the dog can respond to the canine distemper vaccine. There is no reason to use vaccines containing measles virus in dogs older than 16 weeks of age. There are no known public health dangers associated with the use of measles virus–containing vaccines. Measles virus vaccine does not provide protection against infectious canine hepatitis.

Methods of overcoming the effects of colostral (maternal) antibodies are not absolute. Therefore research is continuing in this area. Although colostral antibodies interfere with the immunization process, colostrum is extremely important for the protection of the neonate against a number of potentially harmful microorganisms. Puppies and kittens should never be deliberately deprived of colostrum.

Type of Vaccine

The type of vaccine is very important in formulating a successful vaccination program. Viral vaccines can be either *inactivated* or *modified live* virus vaccines. Because live virus vaccines depend on viral replication in the recipient animal to provide protection, the vaccine must be handled strictly according to the instructions supplied by the manufacturer. Inactivated vaccines are less labile; however, in general they must be administered several times to get an adequate protective response. It is impossible to state that one type of vaccine is categorically better than another; in the future, both inactivated and modified live virus types of vaccine will continue to be used.

To achieve the optimal response, the entire dose of vaccine should be given as recommended; the dose should not be split and given to more than one animal. Different vaccine products should not be mixed in the same syringe before administration. Frequently, vaccines contain preservatives that will interfere with another vaccine.

Route of Administration

The route of administration specified in the manufacturer's instructions should be followed. With certain viruses, significant differences in response occur, depending on the route of administration. For example, with measles virus and some rabies virus vaccines, the intramuscular route is much more effective than the subcutaneous route. The manufacturer's recommendations must be understood and followed for all vaccines.

With certain viruses (e.g., feline viral rhinotracheitis, calicivirus, feline infectious peritonitis) vaccines that produce local immunity have been developed. These vaccines are given by the intranasal and intraocular routes. An example of a bacterial disease for which an intranasal vaccine has been developed is *Bordetella bronchiseptica*. The basis for this approach is the concept that if the vaccine is administered by the same route that natural infection takes, greater protection will be achieved. Unfortunately, these vaccines can produce mild clinical disease.

Because of the concern of development of feline sarcomas secondary to vaccination procedures, specific guidelines have been developed for vaccinating cats. Sarcomas have been associated more with rabies and feline leukemia virus vaccines than others. The suspected incidence of vaccine-induced sarcomas is approximately 1 in 1000 to 10,000 cases per year.

The suggested route of administration of rabies and feline leukemia vaccines is to give the rabies in the right rear leg (over the tibia) and the feline leukemia vaccine over the left tibia by the subcutaneous route. In this way, if a sarcoma does develop, amputation of the limb can be done to save the cat's life.

Age of Patient

The age of the animal is important, not only because of the persistence of colostral antibodies but also because of the relative immaturity of the immune response in the puppy and kitten during the first 2 weeks of life. This phenomenon is at least partially due to the hypothermia that exists during this period. Optimal functioning of the cells of the immune system depends on a normal body temperature.

Orphaned pups should not be vaccinated during the first 2 weeks of life. Instead of being vaccinated, pups and kittens should be given *immune serum*, either by parenteral injection or by mouth. The immune serum can be mixed with artificial milk replacer.

Age of vaccination is also important in older patients. It has been shown that certain older dogs (more than 7 years of age) do not respond as well to vaccination as do younger animals. Thus, annual revaccination is important in these patients to ensure adequate protection.

Nutritional Status

An animal in poor nutritional condition may not respond adequately to vaccination. Generally, caution should be exercised in giving modified live virus vaccines to debilitated animals. However, a debilitated animal should be vaccinated if it is to be hospitalized. Although there is a chance the animal may not respond to the vaccination, it is also possible that the animal will be protected from infection with a virulent organism. If a debilitated dog or cat is vaccinated, vaccination should be repeated when the patient's nutritional status has improved so that immunity is more certain. Every veterinary hospital should establish a specific vaccination policy and protocol and adhere to it at all times. This will prevent errors of omission that could result if the vaccination policy is not clearly defined.

Concurrent Disease or Therapy

Occasionally, dogs and cats presented for vaccination are incubating an infectious disease. A detailed history of possible exposure to infected animals as well as a complete physical examination may suggest this situation. However, it is impossible to definitively diagnose most infections in the incubation stage. If there is a history of exposure to an infected animal, the owner should be informed that there is a risk of their animal developing disease despite vaccination.

Certain infections and diseases may be associated with alteration of the immune system and may interfere with successful response to vaccination; examples include dogs infected with demodectic mange and cats infected with feline leukemia virus or feline immunodeficiency virus.

It has been suggested that certain virus vaccines may increase the susceptibility of the recipient animal to the development of the disease for which one is vaccinating against, if the animal is incubating or infected with another virus simultaneously. For example, dogs infected with the canine parvovirus that are subsequently vaccinated with a modified live distemper vaccine may be prone to develop distemper encephalitis because of infection with the parvovirus.

Modified live virus vaccines are not recommended in dogs and cats receiving immunosuppressive agents. Drugs that suppress the immune system are frequently given to animals with cancer or autoimmune diseases, such as immune-mediated hemolytic anemia. Commonly used immunosuppressive agents include cyclophosphamide, azathioprine, methotrexate, and corticosteroids. When corticosteroids are used at antiinflammatory dose levels (less than 2 mg/kg of body weight), the response to virus vaccines is not altered.

Program Guidelines

When all the clinical factors discussed are considered, along with economic factors, it is safe to conclude that there is no single perfect vaccination program. Nonetheless, certain general guidelines are possible. Usually, the first vaccination should be administered when the animal is between 6 and 8 weeks of age. Animals should be revaccinated at 10, 12, and 16 to 18 weeks of age. Revaccination should occur annually for the entire life of the animal. Although annual revaccination is probably unnecessary for certain viral diseases, for others it is of critical importance.

Currently, there has been much debate concerning the frequency of vaccination procedures and whether yearly vaccines are needed. More study is required to effectively answer this question (see Chapter 11 for more discussion).

Pet-Associated Zoonoses

A zoonosis is a disease of animals that is transmissible to humans under natural conditions. The technician is frequently questioned by clients about the public health significance of animal diseases. Hospitalized animals may represent potential sources of zoonotic infection; thus these infections may be considered occupational diseases.

It is beyond the scope of this section to discuss all the pet-associated zoonoses, but several of the more important infections are described. It is important to stress that when questions about human medical care arise, a physician should be consulted.

Canine brucellosis rarely occurs in humans. Transmission from an infected dog to a human can occur by contact with blood, urine, semen, milk, and infected tissues. Vaginal discharges, aborted fetuses, and placental material after abortion contain large numbers of bacteria. Infection in humans can be an insidious, chronic disease that resembles infection with other strains of *Brucella*, or it can result in relatively mild flulike symptoms.

Toxoplasmosis can be acquired by human exposure to cat feces containing infective oocysts. Cats are an obligate host in the life cycle of *Toxoplasma*. *Toxoplasma* oocysts can remain viable in the environment for as long as 6 months under ideal conditions. The following recommendations to reduce the exposure hazard from toxoplasmosis-infected cats should be followed. Plastic gloves should be worn when cleaning litter pans or handling potentially contaminated soil. Children's sandboxes should be covered, and basic principles of sanitation should be followed. Immunodeficient people and women of child-bearing age should exercise extreme caution to reduce the risk of exposure. Women contemplating pregnancy should have their antibody status determined by a physician. Those with a significant titer against toxoplasmosis are probably protected from reinfection. Antibody titers in cats are of little value because they do not indicate which cats are actively shedding infective oocysts. An enzyme-linked immunosorbent assay (ELISA), currently available through the University of Georgia and Colorado State University veterinary schools, identifies immunoglobulin M (IgM) and immunoglobulin G (IgG) antibodies in a cat's serum and may provide evidence for an acute or a recent infection in a cat. It should be stressed to the concerned client that eating raw or improperly cooked meat probably is the most common source of human toxoplasmosis.

Campylobacter and *Salmonella* are bacteria that can produce pet-associated zoonoses. Pets appear to be relatively infrequent sources of *Campylobacter*. When pets are incriminated, it is usually a stray or recently adopted puppy or kitten that has had recent diarrhea. The incidence of *Salmonella* infection acquired from pets is unknown. Animals can be asymptomatic shedders of this organism for an average of 6 weeks. Because the route of transmission is the fecal-oral route, good sanitation is important.

Reports of human leptospirosis attributed to vaccinated pets have appeared in medical literature. The *Leptospira* bacteria that are used for routine immunization may not protect against subclinical infection and shedding of the organisms in the urine. Because transmission is via infected urine, good sanitation is essential.

Visceral larva migrans and cutaneous larva migrans are caused by the migration of animal parasite larvae in human hosts. The technician plays an important role in prevention by educating clients about the risks posed by pets infected with intestinal parasites. Treatment of infected animals and reducing environmental contamination will reduce the incidence of these problems.

Plague is an infectious disease of animals that is transmitted to humans by the bite of an infected ectoparasite, usually the flea. Although the majority of cases in humans result from exposure to infected wild rodents, domestic cats have been associated with a number of infections in humans. Infections have been reported in persons employed in veterinary hospitals. Cats with suppurative lymphadenitis (infected draining lymph nodes) should be considered plague suspects, and caution should be exercised by the veterinary technician when handling exudates or treating draining wounds.

Cat-scratch disease is a disease of humans that usually is associated with cat scratches or close contact with cats. Rarely, exposure to cats has not occurred and other injuries are incriminated, such as splinters, thorns, or dog scratches. The causative agent is *Bartonella henselae*. It is presumed that cats simply act as vectors for the disease because they are not ill. Multiple cases in the same household have occurred over a period of months or even years. In immunocompromised patients (e.g., humans infected with the human immunodeficiency virus), the disease can cause severe problems and therefore may pose a significant risk to these individuals. Usually, the disease in humans is a mild, self-limiting problem.

Rabies is an acute, fatal viral disease of the central nervous system that affects all mammals. Rabies is transmitted by infected secretions, usually saliva. In the United States, the skunk and bat are the most important sources of human exposure. However, raccoons, foxes, and unimmunized dogs and cats may also represent a hazard. In most areas of the world, the dog is the most important vector of rabies.

If human exposure to rabies is suspected, a physician or public health official should be consulted immediately. Technicians should be familiar with local laws governing the handling of animals who have bitten humans.

Animal bites can cause serious infectious complications, including cellulitis, lymphangitis, soft tissue abscesses, osteomyelitis, meningitis, and bacteremia. Humans who have undergone splenectomy are at particular risk of bacteremia and possibly death if the organism known as DF-2, isolated from the nasal and oral secretions of healthy dogs, is inoculated into tissues by a bite.

More information regarding zoonoses and public health is found in Chapter 18.

OPHTHALMOLOGY

Glaucoma

Glaucoma is defined as an increase in intraocular pressure. Glaucoma may cause blindness, and there are certain breeds predisposed to primary glaucoma (Box 27-1).

The signs in early glaucoma are often subtle and can be variable. Acute glaucoma is a painful process; signs include tearing, sensitivity to bright light, and pawing at the eye. Inspection of the eye may reveal congested episcleral blood vessels, a dilated nonresponsive pupil, and a cloudy cornea. In chronic glaucoma, the major finding is an enlarged globe.

The diagnosis is made by documenting an increased intraocular pressure. Several methods are used to measure intraocular pressure. Tonometers are the most accurate, but some are expensive. The Schiötz tonometer is useful and costs approximately $300 to $400, which is well within the means of most veterinary practices (Figure 27-10).

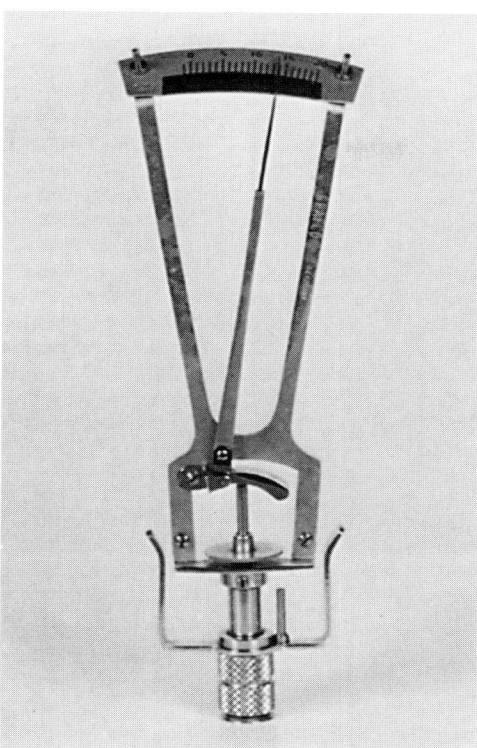

FIGURE 27-10. Tonometer (Schiötz Tonometer) used for measurement of intraocular pressure. The tonometer is placed on the cornea to obtain the pressure reading.

Box 27-1	BREEDS PREDISPOSED TO DEVELOPMENT OF GLAUCOMA

Afghan
American cocker spaniel
Basset hound
Beagle
Bedlington terrier
Brittany spaniel
Dachshund
Dalmatian
English cocker spaniel
English springer spaniel
Fox terriers
Great Dane
Malamute
Norwegian elkhound
Saluki
Samoyed
Sealyham terrier
Siberian husky
Toy and miniature poodles

Glaucoma is considered a medical emergency because delay in treatment may result in permanent damage to the eye. Several drugs are available to treat glaucoma, all of which work by either reducing aqueous production or increasing the opening at the drainage angle.

Cataracts

A cataract is a focal or diffuse opacity within the lens and its capsule. Cataracts may be hereditary or nonhereditary. They should be differentiated from nuclear sclerosis, which is a normal aging change that decreases the clarity of the nucleus of the lens.

Inherited cataracts occur in many breeds and may be associated with other eye abnormalities. Different modes of inheritance have been reported in different breeds. Breeds reported to have inherited cataracts include the beagle, German shepherd, golden retriever, Labrador retriever, Afghan hound, American cocker spaniel, Boston terrier, poodle, and miniature schnauzer. Inherited cataracts have not been reported in the cat.

Cataracts can be the result of metabolic abnormalities, such as diabetes mellitus, inflammation, or trauma. Inflammatory diseases associated with cataracts include feline infectious peritonitis, feline leukemia virus, leptospirosis, and systemic mycoses.

There is no successful medical treatment for cataracts, but any associated inflammation should be treated. Medications that dilate the pupil may be helpful in improving vision in cases of immature or hypermature cataracts. Currently, the only effective therapy for cataracts is surgical removal of the lens.

Corneal Ulcers

Superficial corneal ulcers may result from trauma, decreased tear production (keratoconjunctivitis sicca), aberrant eyelashes (distichiasis, districhiasis), inward rolling of the eyelid (entropion), and inability to blink. Animals with superficial corneal ulcers experience a significant amount of pain. This pain is manifested as excessive tearing, sensitivity to bright light, and squinting (blepharospasm). Corneal ulcers are diagnosed by using fluorescein dye. Fluorescein is a water-soluble dye that will not stain the epithelial layer but stains the underlying layers if the superficial epithelial layer is damaged.

Treatment should be directed first toward correcting the underlying cause. Once this has been accomplished, epithelialization of the ulcerated area is rapid and usually uncomplicated. Broad-spectrum antibiotics are generally used to eliminate infection. It has been shown that ointments may retard healing more than solutions; however, the difference in healing may not be clinically significant. One advantage to solutions is that the dose can be more easily controlled. Systemic medications usually are not necessary with corneal ulcers. Occasionally, a surgical flap over the cornea is necessary until epithelialization is complete.

DERMATOLOGY

Veterinary dermatology is an important part of small animal practice. Veterinary dermatology is a challenging discipline; although there are many causes of skin disease, there are only a limited number of ways in which the skin can react. Consequently, in many cases a specific etiologic diagnosis can be difficult to make.

It is beyond the scope of this chapter to consider all the common dermatologic diseases of dogs and cats. Instead, emphasis is placed on several diagnostic procedures that are commonly performed by veterinary technicians.

Skin Scraping

Skin scraping is one of the most frequently used tests in veterinary dermatology. It should be part of the minimum data base whenever the diagnosis has not been established. The skin scraping is used to identify microscopic ectoparasites such as *Demodex* and *Sarcoptes* as well as dermatophytes. The material and equipment needed to identify ectoparasites include mineral oil, scalpel blade, microscope slide, coverslip, and microscope. The material and equipment used to identify a dermatophyte include saline, scalpel blade, microscope slide, coverslip, potassium hydroxide solution, a heat source (e.g., Bunsen burner), and a microscope.

A representative area should be selected for the skin scraping. In general, an area that has not been disturbed or medicated should be selected. If a dermatophyte is suspected, an area near the margin of the lesion should be selected. If *Demodex* is suspected, a fold of skin should be gently pinched and the skin scraped until there is a slight ooze of blood. When scraping for ectoparasites, a drop of mineral oil should be placed on the scalpel blade so it is possible to transfer the material to a microscope slide. When scraping for dermatophytes, saline or water is used to wet the blade to facilitate the transfer of the specimen to the microscope slide.

Once the accumulated material and mineral oil have been transferred, one or two drops of mineral oil are added, and the mixture is spread evenly with an application stick. A coverslip is added, and the specimen is carefully examined under the microscope. If parasites are not found, demodectic mange is generally eliminated as a diagnostic possibility; however, as many as eight to ten sites should be evaluated and found to be negative before eliminating sarcoptic mange as a possibility.

If a dermatophyte is suspected, a potassium hydroxide preparation should be examined. The material is collected, using the technique described, and placed on a microscope slide. Several drops of 10% potassium hydroxide are placed on the sample, a coverslip is added, and the slide is gently heated for 15 to 20 seconds. Alternatively, the preparation can be placed on the microscope stage and heated by the microscope light source for 15 to 20 minutes. Interpretation of the specimens obtained requires patience and experience. Identification of dermatophytosis can be made by finding branching mycelia. The mycelial filaments are uniform in diameter (2 to 6 μm), are divided into compartments, and vary in length and degree of branching. Hair shafts should be carefully examined for spores. The dermatophytes that infect animals generally have ectothrix spores, which form a prominent sheath on the outside of the hair shaft, in addition to growing inside the hair shaft.

If there is any doubt about the interpretation of the potassium hydroxide digestion, a fungal culture should be performed. A culture is considered the most reliable means of identifying dermatophytes.

The equipment needed for culture includes culture media, a sterile scalpel blade, sterile forceps, and alcohol swab. Appropriate culture media include Sabouraud's media and dermatophyte test media (DTM).

Before a specimen is obtained, the area is cleansed with 70% alcohol to reduce bacterial contamination. A small scraping of superficial debris and hair should be obtained, using the sterile scalpel blade and forceps. Alternatively, a small tuft of hair can be plucked from the margin of a lesion, using mosquito hemostats. The hair sample should be deposited partially beneath the surface of the culture medium. The culture medium bottle cap should be left open one-fourth turn to provide aerobic conditions, and the specimen should be incubated at room temperature. Care should be taken not to inoculate the medium with too large a specimen because this may confuse interpretation of the results. A number of commercial media containing agents that inhibit the growth of bacteria and indicator dyes that help to differentiate pathogens from saprophytes are available (e.g., Fungassay, Pitman-Moore).

Another commonly used diagnostic technique in veterinary dermatology is bacterial culture of suspected pyodermal lesions. The technique used to obtain the specimen is extremely important because skin contaminants are usually present. A representative site should be selected, and an unopened lesion should be gently prepared with a surgical scrub. The lesion should be opened with sterile instruments, and a sterile swab should be inserted deep into the cavity or tract. Alternatively, after the area has been scrubbed, a sterile needle is introduced into the unopened lesion, and the purulent material is aspirated into a syringe. Inoculation of the culture medium should be made immediately. Direct smears should also be made immediately and stained with Gram's stain.

CARDIOLOGY

Congestive Heart Failure

Congestive heart failure is a clinical term used to describe the state when the heart is unable to maintain adequate cardiac output. Because of decreased cardiac output, the body's tissues do not receive sufficient blood supply for normal function. The decreased cardiac output and the resultant increase in pressures within the vessels entering the heart stimulate complex compensatory mechanisms that contribute to the clinical signs of congestive heart failure. The term *congestive heart failure* does not indicate a specific etiology.

Tachycardia and cardiomegaly (heart enlargement) are general signs associated with congestive heart failure. However, depending on the principal site of involvement, signs of left-sided or right-sided heart failure will predominate.

Left-sided heart failure results from dysfunction of the left atrioventricular valve (mitral valve), ventricle, or both. Clinical signs associated with left-sided heart failure include cough, exertional dyspnea, orthopnea, and, at times, syncope. Characteristically, early in left-sided heart failure the cough occurs in paroxysms and at night or in the early morning. The cough in left-sided heart failure is usually secondary to the development of pulmonary edema or occurs because the left atrium has enlarged and compressed the left main-stem bronchus. Exertional dyspnea refers to labored breathing associated with increased activity. This may be manifested as decreased exercise tolerance or reluctance to exercise. *Orthopnea* means difficult or labored breathing in the recumbent position. Pulmonary edema refers to the accumulation of abnormal fluid in the interstitial spaces and alveoli of the lungs. It can be detected by auscultating rales (crackles) in the lungs or by observing the characteristic pattern on chest radiographs. Syncope, or fainting, results from decreased cardiac output to the brain.

Right-sided heart failure results from a pathologic condition of the right atrioventricular valve (tricuspid valve), right ventricle, or both. Clinical signs associated with right-sided heart failure include hepatic enlargement, ascites, pleural effusion, and subcutaneous edema. Increased pressure in the abdominal veins results in congestion and enlargement of the liver. Increased hydrostatic pressure in capillaries results in leakage of fluid and the subsequent development of ascites, pleural effusion, and subcutaneous edema. Subcutaneous edema is a relatively rare sign in the

Box 27-2	CLINICAL SIGNS OF LEFT- AND RIGHT-SIDED HEART FAILURE

LEFT CONGESTIVE SIGNS

Pulmonary congestion and edema resulting in cough, tachypnea, dyspnea, orthopnea, pulmonary crackles, tiring, hemoptysis, cyanosis

Secondary right-sided heart failure

Cardiac arrhythmias

RIGHT CONGESTIVE SIGNS

Systemic venous congestion: high CVP (central venous pressure), jugular vein distension

Liver and spleen enlargement

Fluid in chest cavity (pleural effusion) causing dyspnea, orthopnea, and cyanosis

Fluid in abdominal cavity (ascites)

Subcutaneous edema

Fluid in pericardial sac (pericardial effusion)

---

dog and is seen late in the course of the condition. (Box 27-2 provides a list of signs seen with left- and right-sided heart failure.)

Certain cardiovascular problems result in both left-sided and right-sided heart failure. Obviously, the signs described are not specific for heart disease. Consequently, when evaluating a patient for cough or ascites, the conditions to rule out should include noncardiac problems.

Mitral Insufficiency

Mitral insufficiency resulting from chronic mitral (left atrioventricular) valvular fibrosis is the most frequently diagnosed form of heart disease in the dog. It is followed in prevalence by chronic tricuspid (right atrioventricular) valvular fibrosis, which causes tricuspid insufficiency. *Valvular insufficiency* is a term used to indicate functional incompetence (leakage) of the valve with subsequent regurgitation (backward flow) of blood from the ventricle into the atrium during ventricular systole.

The signs associated with chronic mitral insufficiency are those of left-sided heart failure (e.g., cough, exertional dyspnea, pulmonary edema). The specific cause of mitral valvular fibrosis is unknown; however, it appears to be associated with aging. Certain breeds appear to be predisposed, the majority of these being small breeds of dogs (e.g., miniature poodles). Mitral insufficiency as a cause of left-sided heart failure is much less common in the cat. The diagnosis of chronic mitral insufficiency is based on the clinical history, auscultation of the heart and lungs, thoracic radiography, and electrocardiography. Although the traditional treatment for this condition has included the use of cardiac glycosides (e.g., digoxin), recent evidence indicates that cardiac contractility is normal to increased in the majority of these dogs, and therefore digoxin is not indicated until late in the course of the failure state.

Initially, the use of diuretics such as furosemide (Lasix), a sodium-restricted diet, and exercise restriction are the primary mode of therapy. Treatment with vasodilators such as hydralazine (Apresoline), captopril (Capoten), and enalapril (Enacard) is also beneficial. These drugs work by decreasing the resistance against which the heart has to pump. As more long-term data are accumulated, we may find in dogs, as in people, that vasodilators may help to prolong survival of dogs with heart failure if they are begun earlier in the disease state.

Heartworm Disease

Heartworm disease, caused by *Dirofilaria immitis*, is characterized principally by the presence of right-sided heart failure. The adult parasites lodge in the right atrium, right ventricle, right ventricular outflow tract, pulmonary arteries, and venae cavae. The major effect of heartworm disease is to produce pulmonary hypertension (increased blood pressure in pulmonary arteries), which results in right-sided heart failure.

Heartworm disease has a geographic distribution. The highest incidences of infection occur along the southeastern Atlantic and Gulf coasts. Gradually, heartworm disease has spread to most of the eastern and midwestern United States. Small endemic areas have also been reported in the western United States. With the increased travel of dogs from one region to another, heartworm disease is possible anywhere.

Mosquitoes are an intermediate host for the parasite. The disease is spread by mosquitoes ingesting microfilariae (immature parasites, the L$_1$ larvae) from the blood of an infected dog. The microfilariae undergo maturation within the mosquito to become an infective larva. Infective larvae (L$_3$ stage) enter the dog through the skin puncture wound produced by the mosquito and migrate to subcutaneous tissue, muscle, or fat. Two more molts occur within the dog's body, and the young adult heartworm arrives in the heart approximately 110 days after infection. The adult female heartworms begin producing circulating microfilariae 6 to 7 months after infection.

The most practical method to detect heartworm disease is to observe the presence of circulating microfilariae in the peripheral blood. The microfilariae of a nonpathogenic filarial worm, *Dipetalonema reconditum*, must be differentiated from those of *Dirofilaria immitis*. The most useful diagnostic characteristics of the microfilariae of *D. reconditum* are the blunt shape of the head and the serpentine progressive movement demonstrated in direct blood smears. There are three basic tests used to detect microfilariae. They include the direct smear, modified Knott test, and filter tests. Each test has its advantages and disadvantages; however, if cost, sensitivity, and ease of species identification are considered, the modified Knott test is preferred. During the past few years, serologic testing for heartworm disease has become the preferred method of documenting heartworm infection. There are multiple kits available to detect heartworm antigens in dog serum, and these can be easily performed in practice.

It has been estimated that as many as 25% to 65% of dogs with heartworm disease have no circulating microfilariae. This is referred to as *occult heartworm disease*. If heartworm disease is suspected based on history, physical examination, radiography, and electrocardiography, yet circulating microfilariae are not present, a serologic test for detection of adult heartworm antigens should be performed.

The treatment of heartworm disease can be divided into three phases. The first phase is to kill the adult heartworms (adulticidal therapy) that are present in the heart and blood vessels. The next phase is to eradicate the circulating microfilariae (microfilaricidal therapy). Finally, preventive medication (prophylactic therapy) is administered to those dogs at risk of developing heartworm disease. This would include any dog residing in or traveling to an endemic area.

Adulticide therapy consists of administering thiacetarsamide sodium (Caparsolate, Abbott Laboratories) intravenously. The recommended regimen is to administer the drug twice per day for 2 days. An adulticide (melarsomine dihydrochloride, Merial) is available for intramuscular administration. It is an arsenical compound given by intramuscular injection into the epaxial muscles in the lumbar region. Two treatments are given 24 hours apart. If needed, a second treatment can be given 4 months later.

The adult heartworms will die slowly over a 2- to 3-week period. Fever, coughing, and, in more severe cases, dyspnea and hemoptysis (coughing up blood) are the signs observed as the worms die and pass to the lungs (pulmonary thromboembolism). Prednisone therapy (1 mg/kg) is the accepted therapy for pulmonary thromboembolism. Administration of aspirin therapy (5 mg/kg once daily) is recommended in dogs with moderate to severe heartworm disease to reduce thromboembolism. It may be started 1 week before treatment and continued for 4 to 6 weeks after treatment.

To minimize the development of clinical pulmonary thromboembolism, it is important to restrict exercise for 3 to 4 weeks after completion of adulticide therapy. If the signs associated with pulmonary thromboembolism are severe, hospitalization and the administration of bronchodilators, antiinflammatory drugs, and antibiotics are recommended. DIC may occur in dogs with severe clinical signs. Treatment of advanced DIC is usually unsuccessful.

Microfilaricide therapy is begun 3 weeks after adulticide therapy. Ivermectin (Ivomec), 50 µg/kg orally once, is the current accepted method of treatment for microfilaria, even though it is not approved by the U.S. Food and Drug Administration (FDA) for this function.

Heartworm disease may be prevented with the use of one of several products. Some of these also have protective activity against some endoparasites. Table 27-5 lists the products currently available for heartworm prevention in the dog.

Cardiomyopathy

Cardiomyopathy is a general term that merely indicates that the basic pathologic lesion involves the heart muscle. Cardiomyopathies can be primary or secondary. Primary cardiomyopathies indicate that the myocardial disease is not due to any recurrent or preexisting cardiovascular or systemic disease. Primary cardiomyopathies in cats are further subdivided into hypertrophic, dilated, and restrictive forms. Secondary cardiomyopathies in dogs and cats are less frequent and are the result of diseases such as infection, metabolic disorders (e.g., uremia), endocrine problems (e.g., hyperthyroidism), and infiltrative processes (e.g., neoplasia).

Hypertrophic cardiomyopathy is characterized by increased thickness of the myocardium and a small left ventricular lumen. Clinical signs are seen in middle-age cats of all breeds. The most prominent sign is the sudden development of respiratory distress secondary to pulmonary edema. Hindlimb paresis (weakness) and severe pain may also be present. These hindlimb signs are caused by aortic thromboembolism (blood clots) disrupting the blood supply to the hindlimbs. This problem can usually be diagnosed easily if femoral pulses are found to be poor or absent. Diagnosis of cardiomyopathy is based on history, physical examination, radiography, electrocardiography, and echocardiography. If echocardiography is not available, nonselective angiocardiography may be necessary for diagnosis. The basic initial therapeutic approach may include diuretics (e.g., Lasix, Hoeschst-Roussel Pharmaceuticals), cage rest, oxygen therapy, beta-adrenergic blockers such as propranolol (Inderal, Ayerst Laboratories), and calcium channel blockers such as diltiazem hydrochloride (Cardizem, Marion Merrell Dow). Long-

TABLE 27-5	CURRENTLY AVAILABLE HEARTWORM PREVENTIVES			
	Trade Name	Ingredient(s)	Company	Antiparasitic Activity
	Multiples	Diethylcarbamazine	Multiple	Roundworms Heartworm prevention
	Filaribits	Diethylcarbamazine	Pfizer	Roundworms Heartworm prevention
	Filaribits-Plus	Diethylcarbamazine Oxibendazole	Pfizer	Hookworms Roundworms Whipworms Heartworm prevention
	Heartgard	Ivermectin	Merial	Heartworm prevention
	Heartgard-30 Plus	Ivermectin Pyrantel pamoate	Merial	Heartworm prevention Roundworms Hookworms
	Heartgard for cats	Ivermectin	Merial	Heartworm prevention Hookworms
	Interceptor	Milbemycin oxime	Novartis	Heartworm prevention Hookworms Whipworms Roundworms
	Sentinel	Milbemycin oxime Lufenuron	Novartis	Heartworms Fleas Whipworms Roundworms Hookworms
	Revolution	Selamectin (topical)	Pfizer	Fleas Heartworms *Otodectes cynotis* Ticks Hookworms Roundworms

term management consists of diuretics, beta blockers, calcium channel blockers, a sodium-restricted diet (feline H/D, Hill's), aspirin, and restricted activity. Aspirin is used to reduce the likelihood of aortic thromboembolism.

Dilated cardiomyopathy is characterized by extreme ventricular dilation and moderate atrial enlargement. This results in impaired pump function of the ventricle. This type of cardiomyopathy is also known as *congestive cardiomyopathy*. Signs of right-sided heart failure usually predominate. In addition, cats may show a gradual onset of lethargy and anorexia and at times may be brought in dehydrated, hypothermic, and in cardiovascular shock. Respiratory distress secondary to pleural effusion and aortic thromboembolism resulting in hindlimb paresis is also occasionally seen. The basic therapeutic approach is to mechanically remove as much fluid as possible from the pleural cavity (thoracocentesis), administer digitalis (digoxin therapy), and administer diuretics. Aspirin is used as a preventive measure against aortic thromboembolism. Vasodilators, such as nitroglycerin ointment (Nitrol ointment, Kremers-Urban Co.), may have a role in the management of dilated cardiomyopathy.

Some cats with dilated cardiomyopathy have low plasma taurine levels, and cardiac function will increase with oral taurine supplementation of 250 to 500 mg daily. Cardiac function usually improves over a period of months, and if cats are placed on a diet containing ample taurine, cardiac drugs and taurine supplementation may eventually be discontinued. It should be stated that because this association of low taurine levels and cardiomyopathy in the cat has been made, almost all commercial and prescription diets have adequate levels of taurine, so low-taurine dilated cardiomyopathy is much less common than it used to be.

Restrictive cardiomyopathy is the least common form of primary feline cardiomyopathy. A synonym is endomyocardial fibrosis. Respiratory distress is the most common clinical sign. Diagnosis is similar to the other forms of primary cardiomyopathy. Response to therapy is generally poor.

Primary cardiomyopathies in the dog are categorized as dilated (congestive), boxer cardiomyopathy, Doberman pinscher cardiomyopathy, and hypertrophic cardiomyopathy.

Dilated cardiomyopathy is most common in large and giant breed male dogs aged 4 to 6 years; however, English and American cocker spaniels are smaller-breed dogs that may be affected. Presenting signs often include weakness, lethargy, respiratory distress, cough, anorexia, weight loss, and possibly ascites, and syncope. The left ventricle and atrium are dilated with decreased contractility. Diagnosis is confirmed by physical examination, radiography, electrocardiography, and echocardiography. Treatment consists of diuretics, a low sodium diet, arteriolar dilators, and positive inotropes, such as cardiac glycosides. The long-term prognosis is guarded in that most dogs with the dilated form of cardiomyopathy have an average life span of 6 to 8 months after the diagnosis has been made.

Technician Note

Dilated cardiomyopathy is primarily a disease of large and giant purebred dogs, although medium-sized breeds, such as English and American cocker spaniels, are being diagnosed with increasing frequency with this acquired heart disease.

A specific cardiomyopathy occurs in boxers. These dogs may be asymptomatic or present with syncope and episodic weakness. Arrhythmias are common and may

cause sudden death. Diagnosis is confirmed by the same methods as those used in dogs with dilated cardiomyopathy. Treatment with diuretics and antiarrhythmics, such as propranolol, may be useful; however, prognosis is still poor.

Doberman pinschers may present with a primary cardiomyopathy that is similar to congestive or dilated cardiomyopathy. Ventricular contractility is often severely compromised, and atrial arrhythmias are common. These dogs are often in fulminant congestive heart failure and require supportive care with oxygen, diuretics, positive inotropes, and vasodilators. Prognosis is poor.

Hypertrophic cardiomyopathy is the most uncommon primary cardiomyopathy. It is most often seen in German shepherd dogs and other large breeds. Presenting signs are referable to cardiac disease, and sudden death may occur. Treatment with diuretics and propranolol may improve cardiac output and clinical signs.

ENDOCRINOLOGY

Canine hyperadrenocorticism (Cushing's syndrome) is a disorder that results from the excessive production of cortisol by the adrenal cortex. The clinical signs of canine hyperadrenocorticism include polyuria, polydipsia, abdominal distention, polyphagia, muscular weakness, dermatologic changes, and reproductive problems (anestrus, testicular atrophy). Cushing's syndrome can result from excessive production of adrenocorticotropic hormone (ACTH) by the pituitary gland (pituitary-dependent hyperadrenocorticism) or from a functional tumor of the adrenal cortex. Pituitary-dependent hyperadrenocorticism is by far the most common, comprising approximately 80% of the cases. Diagnosis is based on measurements of the plasma cortisol levels after stimulation with ACTH or suppression with dexamethasone. Treatment is different for these two conditions. If a functional adrenal tumor is present, the recommended treatment is surgical removal. The drug used to treat Cushing's syndrome caused by excessive ACTH production is mitotane (Lysodren, Bristol Laboratories). Side effects associated with the use of mitotane include anorexia, lethargy, vomiting, and depression.

Canine hypoadrenocorticism (Addison's disease) is caused by a lack of absent glucocorticoid and/or mineralocorticoid levels and activity. It is generally seen in the middle-aged female, and the most common signs are gastrointestinal (vomiting, anorexia), weakness, depression, and collapse. These signs may have a waxing-waning course.

In an acute crisis these patients may present in acute collapse and in hypovolemic shock. The classic laboratory abnormalities are a low serum sodium (Na^+) level and a high serum potassium (K^+) level, resulting in a low Na^+/K^+ ratio (usually less than 25:1). These patients may also be azotemic and have a low urine specific gravity, which could be confused with renal failure.

The most accurate means of diagnosis is to perform an ACTH stimulation test and show that the patient has a very poor response to this drug, because cortisol levels will not increase following ACTH administration.

The treatment consists of aggressive fluid therapy and supplementation with glucocorticoid and mineralocorticoid therapy. Prednisolone sodium succinate and desoxycorticosterone are the glucocorticoid and mineralocorticoid used to treat this disease.

Hypoglycemia

Canine hypoglycemia is a clinical problem associated with a variety of diseases rather than a specific diagnosis itself.

The signs associated with hypoglycemia include weakness of the rear legs, generalized weakness, focal or diffuse muscle twitching, incoordination, blindness, generalized seizures, and behavioral changes. These behavioral changes include aggressive behavior and anxiety as evidenced by incessant running, barking, and loss of bowel and bladder control. These signs tend to be episodic, regardless of the cause of hypoglycemia. Hypoglycemia should be considered a differential diagnosis in any dog that is having seizures or is comatose.

The first step in evaluating a patient with suspected hypoglycemia is to verify or document that hypoglycemia exists. Improper handling of blood samples may result in falsely low blood glucose levels. The blood glucose level can be lowered if the serum is not removed from the clot or if the specimen is stored at room temperature for a prolonged period. It is preferable to remove serum from the clot within 10 to 15 minutes of drawing the blood sample. If this cannot be done, use of sodium fluoride tubes may be helpful.

Once hypoglycemia has been verified, the signalment, history, clinical findings, and further laboratory tests may be needed to reduce the long and rather diverse list of conditions that may cause hypoglycemia. Functional beta-cell tumors (insulinomas of the pancreas), nonpancreatic tumors, hypoglycemia-ketonemia in pregnant bitches, glycogen storage diseases, septic shock, juvenile and neonatal hypoglycemia, canine parvoviral diarrhea, and excessive insulin administration in diabetic patients are all examples of diseases that can cause hypoglycemia.

Hypothyroidism and Hyperthyroidism

Hypothyroidism is one of the most common endocrine disorders in the dog, but it is rare in the cat. Some of the common clinical signs include oily seborrhea, alopecia, thickened skin, weight gain, lethargy, and cold intolerance. There are some breeds with an apparent increased incidence of hypothyroidism (Box 27-3). The thyroid-stimulating hormone (TSH) stimulation used to be the most accurate diagnostic test. TSH is no longer readily available; therefore a combination of three tests (total T_4, free T_4, and TSH levels) is used to diagnose the routine hypothyroid patient. Treatment of hypothyroidism consists of supplementation with thyroxine (T_4).

Hyperthyroidism is the most common endocrinopathy affecting cats older than 8 years of age, but it is rare in the dog. The most common clinical signs of hyperthyroidism are weight loss despite a good appetite, restlessness, hyperactivity, and diarrhea. In many cases, a thyroid nodule can be palpated in the ventrocervical region of the neck. The diagnosis can usually be confirmed by documenting an elevated serum T_4 level. Treatment may consist of medical therapy with methimazole (Tapazole, Eli Lilly and Co.), surgical removal of the thyroid nodule, and/or radioactive iodine (^{131}I).

Diabetes Mellitus

Diabetes mellitus is seen in the older dog and cat, and it is more common in the female dog and the male cat. Common clinical signs include excessive water intake (polydipsia), large volumes of urine (polyuria), weight loss in spite of a good appetite, and rapidly developing lens opacities (cataracts) in the dog. If the dog or cat is ketoacidotic, then weakness, vomiting, depression, and, possibly, coma may develop. The diagnosis of diabetes mellitus is made by documenting hyperglycemia, glucosuria, and, if the animal is ketoacidotic, ketonuria or ketonemia.

BOX 27-3	BREEDS WITH AN APPARENT INCREASED INCIDENCE OF HYPOTHYROIDISM

Afghan hound
Airedale
Beagle
Boxer
Brittany spaniel
Chow chow
Cocker spaniel
Dachshund
Doberman pinscher
English bulldog
Golden retriever
Great Dane
Irish setter
Irish wolfhound
Malamute
Miniature schnauzer
Newfoundland
Pomeranian
Poodle
Shetland sheepdog

The technician's role in the treatment of patients with this endocrinopathy is twofold: (1) management of the ill ketoacidotic diabetic animal in the hospital and (2) education of clients concerning home management and treatment of their pets.

The ketoacidotic diabetic patient represents a true challenge for the veterinarian and technician alike, and it is important that they work in unison so optimal patient care is achieved. The technician's role involves close monitoring of vital signs, ensuring fluids are given at the proper rate, frequent blood glucose determinations, and administering short-acting (regular/crystalline) insulin. Because the ketoacidotic patient requires such close monitoring, the technician plays a major role in the minute-to-minute and hour-to-hour evaluation of the patient, so minor changes in the patient's condition can be recognized early and the veterinarian be informed. Because of the complexity of the ketoacidotic diabetic patient, all these functions should be done under the direct supervision of a veterinarian.

The second aspect of diabetic management involves the instruction of the client concerning home management of the pet. This can be a time-consuming function, and the technician who has a good understanding of diabetes management can be a tremendous asset to the veterinarian. Examples of areas in which the client should be instructed and/or shown include how to mix the insulin, read the syringes, draw up the insulin into the syringe, give the subcutaneous injection, and read urine test strips for urine glucose measurement. In addition, the client needs to be instructed (1) about the type of diet to be fed and how much and when to feed, (2) *not* to give the insulin if the pet does not eat in the morning, and (3) if the pet has a seizure, to give the animal Karo syrup orally and call the hospital immediately. All these items can be compiled into a handout that the technician can develop with the aid of the veterinarian. This handout can then be given to the client, who can refer to it as needed at home.

THERIOGENOLOGY

Postpartum Disorders in the Bitch

The postpartum bitch may be brought to an animal hospital for a variety of serious problems after whelping. These problems include mastitis, metritis, and eclampsia. *Mastitis* refers to inflammation of one or more mammary glands. In severe cases, affected glands are hot and painful, and the patient is systemically ill. Bitches with septic mastitis are depressed, anorectic, and reluctant to care for the puppies. In less severe cases, the bitch may not be symptomatic; however, the puppies may fail to gain weight or may show signs of septicemia. Systemic antibiotics are used to treat mastitis. Because the affected glands produce abnormal milk, and the antibiotics excreted in the milk may be harmful to the puppies, it is recommended that the puppies be hand reared.

Severe mastitis may progress to abscess formation or gangrenous mastitis. Surgical drainage and treatment may be required in these cases.

Stasis of milk in the mammary glands can occasionally result in enlarged, painful mammary glands. Galactostasis may be observed during pseudopregnancy or at the time of weaning when the body is attempting to resorb milk. Unlike mastitis, dogs with galactostasis are not systemically ill. Treatment consists of application of cool towels and compresses to decrease inflammation. Care should be taken not to massage the glands because this can stimulate additional milk letdown.

Metritis is a uterine disease of the immediate postpartum period. Signs usually develop within the first week of whelping. Metritis is associated with retained placentae, retained fetuses, and dystocia. Clinical signs suggestive of metritis include fever, depression, and reduced interest in the puppies. A foul-smelling, brown or reddish-brown vaginal discharge may be present; the normal discharge after whelping is nonodorous and greenish. The diagnosis is based on history, clinical findings, and laboratory results. Laboratory tests that are useful include vaginal cytologic studies, CBCs, and bacterial cultures.

Initial therapy consists of replacing fluid deficits, treating shock, if present, and initiating antibiotic therapy after cultures have been obtained. Medical drainage of the uterus can be attempted in valuable breeding bitches. In severe cases, ovariohysterectomy may be indicated to save the bitch's life.

Hypocalcemia (eclampsia) usually occurs 2 to 3 weeks postpartum in small bitches with large litters but occasionally can occur before birth. Presenting signs include weakness and trembling and may proceed to tonic convulsions. The temperature is usually elevated during convulsions.

Diagnosis is based on clinical signs in a lactating female. Treatment includes removing the young for 12 to 24 hours, treating the dam with intravenous 10% calcium gluconate, and ensuring the dam receives oral calcium lactate or calcium gluconate and vitamin D at home. If the condition recurs, the young should be weaned.

Canine Brucellosis

Canine brucellosis is primarily an infection of the reproductive tract, although other organ systems may be involved. *Brucella canis* also has been isolated from dogs with discospondylitis and chronic recurrent fever. Brucellosis is a frequent cause of infertility and other reproductive problems in both males and females.

Definitive diagnosis requires demonstration of the organism by a culture of blood or body fluids. Serologic tests can be diagnostic as well. The rapid slide agglutination test is an easy, readily available test; however, false-positive results occur. The rapid slide agglutination can be used as a screen, with positive tests being confirmed using an alternative technique (e.g., agar gel immunodiffusion).

The mode of transmission is venereal. However, infection can also result from the ingestion of infected material, for example, aborted fetuses, placentae, and vaginal discharge. Because of these means of spread, brucellosis can quickly become a kennel-wide problem.

Although a variety of antibiotic combinations have been recommended, therapeutic success cannot be guaranteed. After antibiotic therapy, some dogs will continue to harbor the organism and represent a risk to other dogs. Canine brucellosis is considered a possible zoonotic disease. For these reasons, some experts advocate removal of all infected dogs from the premises. Other experts feel that this position is extreme and instead recommend castration or ovariohysterectomy and antibiotic therapy for infected pet dogs.

Because treatment is not always successful, prevention is emphasized. All dogs should be tested before breeding or before introduction into a kennel.

Pyometritis

Pyometritis is a uterine disease that occurs during the luteal (approximately 1 month after estrus) phase of the reproductive cycle. It occurs in both bitches and queens. Pyometritis may be part of a complex that initially starts with cystic changes in the endometrium and endometrial hyperplasia. Prior estrogen therapy may predispose to pyometritis (see also Chapter 16).

Clinical signs are variable. A vaginal discharge may or may not be present, but, if present, the color of the discharge can be green, yellow, or reddish brown. Bitches with pyometritis frequently will be polydipsic and polyuric. Affected animals can be severely depressed and septic or clinically normal.

An enlarged uterus on radiographs and leukocytosis with a left shift are considered diagnostic. Fluid therapy to correct fluid and electrolyte deficits followed by ovariohysterectomy is the treatment of choice in nonbreeding animals. In valuable breeding bitches, medical treatment with prostaglandin $F_{2\alpha}$ has been advocated to preserve the breeding life of the patient. Treatment with prostaglandin $F_{2\alpha}$ is expensive and potentially dangerous; therefore it should be strictly reserved for dogs of significant breeding value.

Canine Prostatic Disease

Prostatic disease is occasionally seen in older intact male dogs. Clinical signs include straining to urinate (stranguria), painful urination (dysuria), blood in the urine (hematuria), and/or difficulty in defecation. The conditions that affect the prostate include benign prostatic hypertrophy, bacterial prostatitis, prostatic abscess, prostatic cyst, and prostatic neoplasia.

The following noninvasive techniques are used to evaluate the prostate: rectal palpation, routine radiology, sonography (ultrasound), urethrography, cytologic studies, and bacterial cultures of prostatic washes or the prostatic fraction of the ejaculate. Frequently it is difficult to differentiate neoplasia, infection, and hypertrophy with these noninvasive techniques. Consequently, surgical exploration and biopsy may be required to establish a definitive diagnosis.

Treatment varies, depending on the specific process.

Dogs with benign prostatic hypertrophy respond to castration. Although estrogen therapy reduces the size of the prostate in benign prostatic hypertrophy, it is not recommended because of possible adverse reactions. Recently, finasteride (Proscar, Merck & Co., Inc., West Point, Pa) has been shown to be an effective medical treatment for reduction of prostatomegaly secondary to benign prostatic hypertrophy. Prostatic abscesses and cysts require surgical drainage. Bacterial prostatitis and prostatic abscesses are treated with antibiotics. Prostatic neoplasia is generally highly malignant, and treatment is directed toward palliation rather than cure. Some dogs with prostatic cancer may benefit from castration because the tumors possess testosterone receptors.

GASTROENTEROLOGY

Acute Gastroenteritis

Acute gastroenteritis is one of the more common problems seen in canine practice. Some examples of conditions that may cause this problem include dietary indiscretion, viral gastroenteritis, bacterial gastroenteritis, gastrointestinal foreign bodies, gastrointestinal parasites, intussusception, ingestion of toxins, acute pancreatitis, and hypoadrenocorticism. The clinical history, signalment, and physical examination may suggest the diagnosis. Frequently, response to symptomatic therapy is used to assess whether further diagnostic study is warranted. The intensity and degree of symptomatic and supportive care are determined by the severity of clinical signs.

The fundamental decision of whether to hospitalize the patient is based on a number of factors; they include the hydration status of the dog, severity and frequency of vomiting and diarrhea, presence or absence of blood in the vomitus or stool, and presence of fever or profound lethargy. Non–patient-related factors to be considered include the client's ability to provide adequate care for the patient at home and ability of the client to pay for hospitalized care.

Clinical management of outpatients consists primarily of dietary restriction, administration of locally acting gastrointestinal medications, and use of fluid therapy when indicated. Dietary restriction is the most important aspect of the symptomatic care of acute gastroenteritis. The objective is to rest the gastrointestinal tract. This is accomplished by withholding all food for 12 to 24 hours, depending on the details of the case. If vomiting is severe, water is also withheld. If diarrhea is present and vomiting has not occurred, warm electrolyte-containing solutions can be given by mouth. During this period of symptomatic therapy, it is imperative that the patient be observed closely to prevent ingestion of foreign material and detect any worsening of clinical signs.

After food has been withheld for the prescribed period, small, frequent, bland meals should be offered. These meals should be low in fat, low in fiber, and easily digested and absorbed. These criteria are met by prescription diets, such as Prescription Diet I-D (Hill's), and by homemade diets, such as cottage cheese and boiled rice. These diets should be warmed before feeding. These frequent, small, bland meals should be continued for 2 to 3 days. If the patient is doing well, the regular diet and feeding schedule can be gradually reintroduced over the next 3 to 5 days. If clinical signs recur during this process, the dog should be reevaluated. Further diagnosis, evaluation, and more intensive supportive therapy may be warranted.

Although a vast number of locally acting preparations are available for the treatment of acute gastroenteritis, most have not been proved effective in controlled clinical trials. An over-the-counter preparation containing bismuth subsalicylate (Pepto-Bismol) has been shown to shorten the duration of symptoms in humans with experimental viral enteritis. It is theorized that the beneficial response is not due to the coating action of the product but rather to the salicylate inhibiting prostaglandin synthesis. Prostaglandins play a role in diarrhea by affecting both motility and secretory activity of the gastrointestinal tract. The technician should be aware that Pepto-Bismol may cause the stool to be dark to black, giving the false impression that melena is present when it is not.

Technician Note

Pepto-Bismol causes the stool to be colored black and therefore should not be confused with melena.

In animals that are slightly to mildly dehydrated, some form of fluid therapy is appropriate. Fluids can be administered by mouth if the patient is not vomiting. Commercial water and electrolyte solutions, such as Gatorade, can be used to restore hydration and correct electrolyte imbalances. Alternatively, a homemade solution can be prepared inexpensively. One formula that has been recommended consists of 3.5 g of sodium chloride, 2.5 g of sodium bicarbonate, 1.5 g of potassium chloride, and 20 g of glucose added to 1 L of water. Approximately 13.6 ml/kg/day of this solution will meet the maintenance requirements of the patient.

If the dog is mildly to moderately dehydrated or is vomiting, subcutaneous fluids are indicated. Lactated Ringer's solution or Normosol are the fluid of choice. If signs have been prolonged, the lactated Ringer's solution can be supplemented with potassium chloride. Generally, the dose of subcutaneous fluids is 4.5 to 9.0 ml/kg of body weight administered at multiple sites. This can be repeated if necessary.

Client education is an essential part of the symptomatic care for acute gastroenteritis. The client should be informed that a definitive diagnosis has not been established and that merely the symptoms are being treated. If the animal is getting worse or if the signs persist longer than 36 to 48 hours, the animal should be reevaluated. The technician should have a concerned, caring attitude during the outpatient visit so if signs persist, the client will not hesitate to return or call for additional help. In many practices, it is standard procedure to telephone the client to receive follow-up progress reports. This ensures close client contact and thus improves the chances of successful management of the problem.

If initial clinical signs are severe or there is no response to symptomatic therapy, hospitalization is necessary. A major indication for hospitalization is the need for intravenous fluid therapy. Details about intravenous fluid therapy have been discussed earlier.

Medications that alter the motility of the gastrointestinal tract may be indicated in cases of severe gastroenteritis. Improved understanding of the pathophysiology of intestinal motility has resulted in the more rational use of medications that are used to symptomatically treat vomiting and diarrhea. Anticholinergics decrease the resistance to intestinal flow and thus are of questionable efficacy in treating diarrhea. Antispasmodics are of minimal benefit as well.

Narcotics and narcotic-like drugs increase the rhythmic

segmental contractions of the bowel, slow the passage of ingesta, and thus help to control diarrhea. These drugs should be used cautiously because of potential problems. Generally, they are reserved for more chronic or severe cases that are unresponsive to conservative therapy. A major disadvantage of the narcotic derivatives is that they can cause central nervous system depression. The decreased ingesta flow rate may result in increased absorption of toxins and altered bacterial flora in the gut. These compounds are contraindicated in the presence of intestinal obstruction.

Drugs used for the treatment of acute vomiting can be divided into several categories (Box 27-4).

Drugs that have been used to decrease gastric acidity include anticholinergics. Anticholinergics probably have no effect on acid secretion. Antacids do not decrease the secretion of acid; however, they neutralize the acid that is produced. Antacids must be given frequently because their duration of action is brief. Paradoxically, if antacids are not given frequently, total daily acid secretion increases. Antacids administered according to a schedule of two or three times per day are probably of no value and may, in fact, be harmful. In most practices, more frequent administration is not practical. Drugs that block H_2 (histamine) receptors inhibit secretion of gastric acid. Cimetidine (Tagamet, SK&F Lab Co.) works by this mechanism. Phenothiazine-derivative tranquilizers, such as chlorpromazine, work on the vomiting center of the central nervous system. These drugs are effective at controlling vomiting at much lower doses than the usual tranquilizer doses. These agents should be used with caution in dehydrated patients because of their blood pressure–lowering effects. Other antihistamines act by inhibiting a neural center involved in vomiting called the *chemoreceptor trigger zone*. Vomiting induced by certain drugs, such as digoxin, is mediated by this center. Vomiting caused by motion sickness or vertigo may also respond to drugs in this group.

When the patient has improved, oral fluids and frequent, small, bland meals can be instituted. After discharge from the hospital, the dog can be treated as already described under outpatient management.

Canine Viral Enteritis

The two most important causes of viral enteritis in the dog are canine coronavirus and canine parvovirus. Other viral agents can occasionally produce gastroenteritis; they include canine distemper and canine rotavirus.

Clinical signs vary from subtle lethargy and anorexia to severe, rapidly fatal hemorrhagic gastroenteritis. Dogs of any age can be affected; however, the more severe cases typically occur between 6 and 20 weeks of age. On physical examination, the pups are usually febrile, depressed, and dehydrated. Vomiting or diarrhea may be observed. The stool may be watery, watery with flecks of blood, or severely hemorrhagic. Occasionally, infected dogs will display abdominal tenderness or pain. The presence of fever is more commonly associated with parvovirus than with coronavirus. A history of vaccination does not rule out viral enteritis because maternal antibodies may have prevented a protective immune response to the vaccination. It should be noted that the gastroenteritis and clinical disease secondary to coronavirus infection are much less severe than those seen with parvovirus infection.

Hemograms are usually normal with coronavirus enteritis but may be abnormal with parvovirus enteritis. Transient leukopenia is present in roughly one third to one half

---

Box 27-4 COMMONLY USED DRUGS FOR ACUTE GASTROENTERITIS

NARCOTICS
Lomotil (diphenoxylate, atropine)
Donnagel-PG (opium, atropine, hyoscyamine, kaolin, pectin)
Imodium (loperamide)
Diban (opium, atropine)
Parapectolin (paregoric, pectin, kaolin)

TRANQUILIZERS
Thorazine (chlorpromazine)
Darbazine (prochlorperazine, isopropamide)
Tigan (trimethobenzamide)

ANTICHOLINERGICS
Atropine
Scopolamine
Methscopolamine
Robinul-V (glycopyrrolate)
Centrine (aminopentamide hydrogen sulfate)
Diathal (diphemanil methylsulfate, penicillin, dihydrostreptomycin, chlorpheniramine maleate)
Darbazine (prochlorperazine, isopropamide)
Biosol-M (methscopolamine, neomycin)
Amoforal (kanamycin, aminopeptamide hydrogen sulfate, pectin)
Sulkamycin tablets (phthalylsulfacetamide, neomycin, belladonna alkaloids, pectin)

LOCALLY ACTIVE AGENTS
Kaopectate (kaolin, pectin)
Kao-forte (kaolin, pectin)
Pepto-Bismol (bismuth subsalicylate)

SMOOTH MUSCLE RELAXANTS (ANTISPASMODICS)
Oct-Vet (isometheptene)
Novin (dipyrone)
Jenotone (aminopropazine)
Myoquin-65V, Neopavin (ethaverine)

ANTIHISTAMINES
Dramamine (dimenhydrinate)
Bonine (meclizine)
H_2 Blocker
Tagamet (cimetidine)

---

of dogs with parvovirus infections. Severely leukopenic patients may develop secondary infections because of a compromised immune system.

Plain abdominal radiographs do not reveal specific changes. Gastrointestinal contrast study changes may mimic small bowel obstruction. Abnormalities include dilated loops of bowel, tremendously prolonged passage time, and gas-capped fluid lines.

Definitive diagnosis is possible by several techniques. The viruses may be detected in the stool by electron microscopy. An ELISA performed on the feces can detect parvoviral antigen and can be used to demonstrate the virus in the feces during the period of active viral shedding. This period corresponds to the clinical illness. An easy-to-perform in-house test is available to check for parvovirus antigen in the stool (Probe-Canine Parvovirus Antigen test kit, Idexx Labs).

It should be stressed that the treatment of canine viral gastroenteritis is supportive because there are no effective antiviral agents. Treatment includes aggressive intravenous fluid therapy, antibiotics, injectable antiemetics, and keeping the animal clean and comfortable. One other complication seen with parvovirus infection, to which the technician should be alert, is the development of hypoglycemia. If profound weakness and/or seizures develop, a blood glucose level should be determined.

A myocardial form of canine parvovirus has been described in young pups. This form of the disease is characterized by sudden death in otherwise healthy pups; however, it is becoming less common. This may be because most pups have maternal antibodies at the critical period when they are susceptible to the myocardial form.

Both canine parvovirus and coronavirus are highly contagious. The major route of the infection is fecal-oral. Dogs showing clinical signs will shed large numbers of viral particles for 1 to 2 weeks. The canine parvovirus is hardy; therefore once the environment is contaminated, infective virus will survive for prolonged periods. The virus has been shown to remain infectious in dog feces held at room temperature for longer than 6 months.

Good sanitation will reduce the numbers of infective virus in the hospital environment. Dilute hypochlorite (chlorine bleach and water, diluted to a ratio of 1:32) solutions have significant viricidal properties. Because the virus is ubiquitous, however, the best means of prevention is an appropriate immunization program.

NEPHROLOGY AND UROLOGY

Canine Uroliths

A *urolith* is a pathologic stone formed from mineral salts found in the urinary tract. Clinical signs depend on location, number, size, shape, and whether there is concurrent urinary tract infection. Urolith classification is generally based on the predominant mineral component, such as phosphate or urate. In the dog, more than 90% of uroliths are located in the bladder and urethra and fewer than 10% are located in the kidneys. Although uroliths can occur in any breed, some breeds suspected to be at greater risk include the miniature schnauzer, Dalmatian, dachshund, pug, English bulldog, Welsh corgi, basset hound, Pekinese, and Scottish terrier.

If the urolith is located in the bladder, there may be no clinical signs, but more commonly stranguria, increased frequency of urination (pollakiuria), and hematuria will be seen. If the urolith is in the urethra, there may be frequent attempts to urinate and dribbling of urine. If the urethra is completely obstructed by the stone or stones, abdominal distention, pain, anorexia, depression, and vomiting will be observed.

Laboratory findings generally are not specific for uroliths. Radiology, including contrast studies such as cystograms and pneumocystograms or ultrasound, may be necessary to establish the diagnosis. Generally speaking, uroliths are managed surgically. A prescription diet (S/D, Hill's) has been advocated as a means of medically treating phosphate uroliths. The diet is high in sodium and low in protein and phosphorus and has an acidifying effect on urine. Dissolution of the uroliths occurs over a period of weeks. Unfortunately, this medical approach has several important limitations. A prescription S/D diet is effective in the dissolution of only phosphate calculi and is not recommended as a long-term maintenance diet.

The overall recurrence rate for bladder stones is high, approximately 25%. Therefore efforts to reduce the chance of recurrence are very important. The first step is to analyze the mineral composition of the stone because different stone types are managed differently. It is also important to determine whether infection is present and, if so, which antibiotics are most likely to be effective.

Several preventive measures are appropriate regardless of the stone type. These include elimination of any infection and stimulation of increased urine output. The urine output can be increased by salting the diet and thereby increasing water intake.

Depending on the specific stone type, it may also be desirable to initiate dietary therapy and modify the urine pH. Ammonium chloride is commonly used to acidify the urine, and sodium bicarbonate is used to alkalinize it.

Because the recurrence rate for uroliths is high, client education is extremely important. First, long-term therapeutic compliance will be achieved only if the importance of these measures is stressed to the client. Second, the owner should be aware of signs that indicate recurrence of the problem.

Feline Lower Urinary Tract Disease

Feline lower urinary tract disease (FLUTD) is the term used to describe a condition of unknown etiology in cats characterized by dysuria, hematuria, pollakiuria, urinating in uncommon places, and occasionally urethral obstruction. Urethral obstruction, if it occurs, is potentially fatal because of the associated severe metabolic derangements. The emergency treatment of feline urethral obstruction is covered in Chapter 28.

Because recurrence of the urethral obstruction is frequent, some clinicians prefer to routinely use indwelling urethral catheters for a brief period of time after relief of the obstruction. The justification for the use of indwelling catheters is to maintain urine flow without the trauma associated with recatheterization and manual compression of the bladder. Indwelling urethral catheters should be used judiciously because of the risk of ascending urinary tract infection and catheter-induced injury to the bladder or urethra. Complications associated with the use of indwelling catheters can be minimized if an appropriate catheter is selected. Commercially manufactured polypropylene catheters (Sovereign tomcat catheters and open-end tomcat catheters, Sherwood Medical Industries) can be either too short or too long. Therefore care should be taken to select a catheter with an appropriate length. Soft, flexible polyvinyl catheters, such as the Sovereign sterile disposable feeding tube and urethral catheter, are preferred because of decreased damage to the urethral and bladder mucosa. To pass these catheters, they are kept frozen until immediately before use. This will make the catheter sufficiently rigid to allow passage in a male cat. The catheter should be well lubricated before passage.

Indwelling urethral catheters are generally secured by suturing the catheter to the prepuce. Adhesive tape is attached longitudinally and transversely to the end of the catheter. If the catheter is wet when the tape is applied, it may not stick. Two simple interrupted sutures on either side of the prepuce penetrate the tape and thus prevent movement of the catheter. If analgesia is required to place the sutures, the prepuce can be numbed by applying an ice cube for 1 or 2 minutes. When the catheter is sutured in place, it should be done in such a way that there is no chance of kinking. An Elizabethan collar can be used to prevent the cat from removing the indwelling catheter.

To prevent ascending urinary tract infection, sterile technique is required when placing and maintaining the indwelling catheter. The collection apparatus should be a closed, sterile system. The entire system—catheter, plastic tubing, and collection bottle—must be sterile initially and must be kept sealed to prevent bacterial contamination. Povidone-iodine ointment should be applied several times daily at the point at which the catheter exits the urethra.

Indwelling urethral catheters should be used for as brief a time as possible. The prophylactic use of antimicrobials does not reduce infection. If infection does develop, it is frequently caused by an organism resistant to the prophylactic antimicrobial.

Because the recurrence rate for feline urologic syndrome is high, preventive measures are an important aspect of its medical management. Unfortunately, because the etiology of feline urologic syndrome is unknown, preventive measures are largely empirical. The most frequently recommended preventive measures include providing an ample supply of fresh, potable water, cleaning the litter pan frequently, and lightly salting the food to increase water intake and thus urine volume. Exclusive feeding of diets that contain 20 mg of magnesium per 100 Kcal or less and that maintain a urine pH of 6.4 or less is the most important preventive measure. Certain diets, such as C/D or Feline Maintenance (Hill's), meet this requirement. Although urinary acidification with ammonium chloride has been recommended, it should be emphasized that some diets, such as the ones mentioned above, cause urinary acidification, and additional acidifiers are contraindicated. The basis of acidifying the urine is to increase the solubility of this crystalline material, which is incriminated as the cause of feline urologic syndrome.

If ammonium chloride is used with a nonacidifying diet, it should be thoroughly mixed with the food to improve palatability. It should also be administered with every meal. Any change in diet or introduction of a food additive, such as ammonium chloride or salt, should be done gradually over several days. This will reduce the chances of the cat's rejecting the new or altered food. Enteric-coated ammonium chloride tablets are not effective in the cat.

In recent years, calcium oxalate bladder stones have become recognized in the cat as a new cause of FLUTD. Calcium oxalate stores are more likely to form in an acid urine, and therefore cats that eat an acidifying diet may be at risk for the formation of calcium oxalate stones.

In addition, some cats with FLUTD have no definable cause but may benefit from drugs such as amitriptyline (Elavil) or glycosaminoglycans (Adequan).

Chronic Renal Failure

Animals in renal failure should be fed diets containing reduced quantities of high-quality protein and adequate nonprotein calories. This can be accomplished by using prescription diets such as K/D (Hill's). K/D is a moderate protein-restricted diet available for dogs in canned, semimoist, and dry forms. Feline K/D is a canned product suitable for use in uremic cats.

If desired, homemade diets can be used. The following is a recipe for a moderately low-protein diet for dogs:

¼ lb regular ground beef
1 hard-boiled egg, finely chopped
2 C cooked rice without salt
3 slices white bread, crumbled
1 tsp calcium carbonate
Balanced vitamin and mineral supplement

The meat should be braised, retaining the fat, and thoroughly mixed with the other ingredients. This recipe will meet the daily requirements of a 13.5-kg dog.

The following is an example of a homemade protein-restricted diet for cats:

¼ lb liver
2 large hard-boiled eggs

2 C cooked rice without salt
1 tbs vegetable oil
1 tsp calcium carbonate
Balanced vitamin and mineral supplement

Dice and braise the liver, retaining fat. This recipe provides a total of 635 Kcal/lb.

Many animals with renal failure are anorectic because of nausea and vomiting. Small, frequent meals are recommended to reduce the nausea. If the animal can tolerate food orally but is not eating, feeding by means of an orogastric tube is recommended. The diets described can be administered through a stomach tube if the ingredients are thoroughly mixed with water in a kitchen blender.

Supportive therapy for chronic renal failure includes the use of phosphorous binders, anabolic steroids, sodium bicarbonate, sodium chloride, calcium, and vitamin D metabolites. The use of these treatments should be based on documented abnormalities because the inappropriate or incorrect use of these agents can do more harm than good.

ORTHOPEDICS

Canine Hip Dysplasia

Hip dysplasia refers to a developmental problem of the canine coxofemoral joint. Subluxation of the femoral head leads to abnormal wear and eventual degenerative joint disease. The acetabulum is more shallow than normal, and the femoral head is flattened.

The etiology of hip dysplasia is multifactorial. Genetics and environmental factors such as nutrition appear to be important. Hip dysplasia is seen in most large breeds and is inherited by a polygenic mode of inheritance. This means that many genes are responsible for its development. It is also quantitative in its expression. In other words, affected dogs can show slight or severe changes. As is characteristic for traits with a polygenic mode of inheritance, hip dysplasia is modified by environmental factors. For example, it has been suggested that dogs fed a high-calorie diet during growth have an increased incidence, whereas dogs fed a low-calorie diet have a decreased incidence.

The Orthopedic Foundation of America in Columbia, Mo., is an organization established to evaluate the hip radiographs of potential breeding dogs. Radiologists identify those dogs with radiographically normal hip joints. Unfortunately, because of the factors mentioned, breeding two radiographically normal dogs does not ensure normal progeny. It is better to evaluate entire families (siblings and progeny) when selecting dogs to be included in a breeding program to decrease the incidence of hip dysplasia. It is also important to recognize that good hip joints should not be the sole criterion for selection. Other traits, such as disposition, working ability, and conformation, should also be considered.

The clinical signs of hip dysplasia vary tremendously from occasional slight discomfort to a severe disabling disease. It should be remembered that the clinical signs of hip dysplasia do not always correlate with the severity of hip dysplasia detected radiographically.

Dogs with hip dysplasia will respond differently to varying levels of exercise. Some dogs are most comfortable with minimal activity, yet others do best with a regular regimen of moderate exercise. Swimming is an excellent form of exercise, since muscle tone is increased with the hip joints in a non-weight-bearing position. Any exercise program should be instituted gradually. Forced sudden activity such as ball playing or rough play should be discouraged. Severely affected dogs should be treated symptomatically with analgesics and antiinflammatory drugs.

Several surgical procedures have been advocated for the treatment of hip dysplasia. They include procedures such as pectineal myotomy, pelvic osteotomy, excision arthroplasty, and total hip prosthesis. A discussion of these surgical procedures is beyond the scope of this chapter.

Intervertebral Disk Disease

Intervertebral disk disease is a relatively common problem affecting the spinal cord of chondrodystrophoid and other breeds. Breeds commonly affected include dachshunds, Pekingese, cocker spaniels, poodles, pugs, and beagles. The chondrodystrophoid breeds tend to develop signs at an earlier age than the nonchondrodystrophoid breeds.

The intervertebral disks are structures located between the vertebrae and function as a shock-absorbing system. The disk itself is composed of two parts: the firm fibrous outer annulus and the softer inner nucleus. In intervertebral disk disease, the annulus undergoes degeneration, and the nuclear material protrudes or is completely extruded. The result is compression of the spinal cord with the subsequent development of neurologic signs. These signs vary from simple pain to complete paralysis.

Intervertebral disk disease can be managed either conservatively with cage confinement and antiinflammatory drugs or more aggressively with neurosurgery. Management decisions are based on the history, neurologic signs, and wishes of the owner.

If conservative therapy is elected, the technician plays a vital role. Extreme care should be taken in handling the patient because movement may result in the extrusion of additional disk material and worsening of signs. To reduce handling, these patients should be placed in lower cages whenever possible. Because these patients are frequently in severe pain, gentle, compassionate care is essential. Many cases will benefit from some of the physical therapy techniques described earlier.

Dogs with intervertebral disk disease receiving antiinflammatory drugs, such as dexamethasone, may develop secondary problems, such as gastrointestinal hemorrhage or acute pancreatitis. Consequently, these patients should be observed closely for fever, anorexia, abdominal pain, hemorrhagic vomiting, and diarrhea.

Additional information regarding orthopedics is found in Chapter 26.

RECOMMENDED READING

Feldman EC, Nelson RW: *Canine and feline endocrinology and reproduction,* ed 2, Philadelphia, 1996, WB Saunders.

Ford RB, Schultz RD. In Bonagura JD: *Kirk's current veterinary therapy XIII,* Philadelphia, 2000, WB Saunders.

Hand MS et al: *Small animal clinical nutrition,* ed 4, Marceline, Mo, 2000, Walsworth Publishing.

28

Emergency Nursing

Lee Ann Eddleman • Steven L. Marks

The field of veterinary medicine is dynamic and continues to evolve. The quality of veterinary care continues to improve as technologic advancements become available. The specialty of emergency and critical care medicine has greatly contributed to the evolution of veterinary medicine. The critically ill patient has unique requirements and presents a challenge to the veterinary clinician. These challenges have helped highlight the important role of the veterinary technician.

In 1994, a group of technicians and veterinarians in the emergency and critical care field created a body that would recognize veterinary technicians in this field as a specialty. This organization would provide continuing education and evaluate the competency of veterinary technicians who work in the area of emergency and critical care. In January 1996, the North American Veterinary Technician Association (NAVTA) recognized the Academy of Veterinary Emergency and Critical Care Technicians as a specialty in veterinary technology.

Successful management of the emergency patient depends on the training and skills of the personnel and the quality and readiness of the hospital. The implementation of a team approach through the use of established policies, protocols, and procedures reduces stress, builds camaraderie, and provides a coordinated resuscitative effort. By understanding the principles of triage and the basic principles for assessment and treatment of shock and trauma the technician is able to perform efficient and effective evaluation and monitoring of critically ill patients. The veterinary technician must have a basic understanding of anatomy, physiology, pathophysiology, and pharmacology to fulfill this indispensable role. The technician must also have a clear understanding of his or her role in cardiopulmonary resuscitation (CPR) and of the general principles of fluid and drug therapy. It is through clinical experience and understanding of the pathophysiology of disease that the veterinary technician is able to excel in this profession.

ELEMENTS OF EMERGENCY CARE

Personnel

Survival of the emergency patient depends on the collaborative effort of the veterinarian and technician. Technicians and veterinarians should work together to evaluate, resuscitate, stabilize, diagnose, and treat the emergency patient. The emergency patient requires prompt attention and rapid stabilization, which makes teamwork essential. A collaborative environment exists when there is mutual respect and understanding of the unique contributions each individual makes to the care of the patient. Improved patient care is the result of careful planning and anticipation by the veterinarian and technicians to identify problems and address them in a logical, prioritized manner.

Technician Note

The emergency patient requires prompt attention to ensure rapid stabilization.

Success of the clinical team depends not only on the knowledge base and technical skills of each member but also on the consistent performance of the team. The predetermined assignment of specific nursing tasks in the emergency setting, such as allowing the technician to initiate basic CPR, fosters the efficient utilization of talents and manpower, reduces stress, and builds camaraderie. Most importantly, this decreases the time between onset of the precipitating event responsible for the emergency and the delivery of definitive care.

The technician should be competent at phlebotomy, placement of intravenous (IV) catheters, administration of medications utilizing various routes (IV, subcutaneous [SC], intramuscular [IM]), performance of basic CPR, administration of anesthesia, and assistance of the veterinarian in advanced CPR and surgery if required. The

Box 28-1	RECOMMENDED SKILLS FOR THE VETERINARY TECHNICIAN PROVIDING EMERGENCY CARE

BASIC SKILLS
Triage skills
Physical examination and interpretation skills
Recognition of life-threatening conditions and clinical signs
Venipuncture of various veins
Ability to perform various stat. blood work as well as interpret results: packed cell volume (PCV), blood glucose, total solids (TS), activated clotting time (ACT), buccal mucosal bleeding time, blood gases, electrolytes
Catheterization of peripheral veins
Nasal oxygen catheter placement
Endotracheal intubation
Basic first aid techniques, such as hemostasis and CPR

MORE ADVANCED SKILLS FOR THE VETERINARY TECHNICIAN
Arterial blood sampling and arterial catheter placement
Nasoesophageal, nasotracheal, and nasogastric tube placement
Central vein catheter placement (jugular and saphenous)
Cricothyroid and tracheal oxygen delivery catheter placement
Mechanical ventilatory assistance to include appropriate ventilator settings, trouble shooting, and patient care
Calculation and preparation of continuous-rate infusion drugs, such as lidocaine, dobutamine, and dopamine
Knowledge of how to perform radiographic and advanced imaging techniques, such as ultrasound

technician should be able to provide effective patient monitoring and understand basic monitoring equipment. Knowledge of basic emergency laboratory testing and interpretation is also essential for the veterinary technician (Box 28-1).

Facility Capabilities

The receiving area of the veterinary clinic or hospital should have wide corridors with good lighting and be arranged to facilitate the rapid transport of injured animals to the emergency or centralized treatment area of the building. Stretchers and gurneys should be easily accessible for transporting nonambulatory patients. Long boards and various sizes of plastic sheets are also recommended to be available for transport of nonambulatory patients. Duct tape may be useful to secure and immobilize dogs in lateral recumbency during transport. Blankets, towels, and bubble wrap can also be used to provide insulation and protection.

Emergency equipment and drugs required for resuscitation should be organized and readily available for use in the emergency area (Box 28-2). A portable cart should be used to store instruments and equipment if shared by other areas of the hospital. A portable fishing tackle box may be a useful portable container for emergency drugs. The anesthesia induction area is often chosen as the emergency area because key pieces of equipment, such as oxygen and endotracheal (ET) tubes, are readily accessible. The proximity of the operating room can also be advantageous because some patients may require immediate surgical intervention once stabilized.

Box 28-2	RECOMMENDED EMERGENCY EQUIPMENT

OXYGEN DELIVERY DEVICES
Portable oxygen tank or wall oxygen
Rebreathing bags (assorted sizes)
Face masks of various sizes, oxygen canopy, nasal catheters, oxygen tubing, Ambu bag

RESUSCITATION CART AIRWAY DRAWER
Endotracheal tubes (assorted sizes)
Laryngoscope (large and small blades)
Tracheostomy pack
Chest tap device: 19- or 21-gauge butterfly catheter or needle, three-way stopcock, 35- to 60-ml syringe

DRUG DRAWER
Epinephrine, lidocaine, and atropine
Syringes of assorted sizes with needles

CATHETER DRAWER
IV and IO catheters of various sizes
Spinal needle
Butterfly catheters of various sizes
Central catheters
Surgical scrub
Tape
Heparin flush

MISCELLANEOUS
Scissors
Scalpel blades
Sterile gloves
Bandage materials
Sponge forceps

FLUIDS
Fluid pressure infuser
Fluid administration sets
Infusion pumps
Isotonic crystalloids and synthetic colloids
Hemoglobin-based oxygen carriers

SUCTION APPARATUS
Suction reservoir
Suction tubing
Suction cannulas

BLOOD PRESSURE MONITORING
Doppler unit or oscillometric blood pressure unit
Various-size cuffs
Sphygmomanometer
Conduction gel

ELECTROCARDIOGRAPHY
ECG unit
Electrode paste

DEFIBRILLATOR
Internal and external paddles
Conduction gel

ADDITIONAL EQUIPMENT
Chest tube pack
Thoracotomy pack

IO, Intraosseous; IV, intravenous.

The mobile resuscitation cart or "crash" cart remains in the emergency area and has several drawers for storage. Essential equipment such as an electrocardiograph (ECG), blood pressure monitor, and suction device should be visible and easily accessible. The drawers can be organized into different sections, such as an airway management drawer, an emergency drug drawer, and a catheter drawer (Figure 28-1). A CPR log is kept within the resuscitation cart for recording vital information, such as the cause and time of arrest, drug dosage, and route of administration (Figure 28-2).

The airway drawer should contain different sizes of ET tubes with a syringe for inflating the cuff and at least one laryngoscope with different-sized tongue blades. Forrester sponge forceps for retrieval of airway foreign bodies and tracheostomy tubes are kept in this drawer as well. A butterfly catheter or 20-gauge, 1.25-inch needle attached to an IV extension set with a three-way stopcock and syringe is set up for immediate thoracentesis (Figure 28-3). A sterile chest tube pack (Box 28-3) should be available to expedite chest drain placement. The drug drawer should contain atropine, epinephrine (containing preservative and not requiring refrigeration), and lidocaine with different sizes of syringes that are preloaded with needles. Urinary catheters should be available for intratracheal drug administration. Other drugs, including antibiotics, glucocorticoids, dopamine, or dobutamine, are kept in the crash cart or on a nearby shelf. Emergency drug and defibrillation dosages should be available, and a wall chart that is centrally posted can provide quick reference during CPR.

The catheter drawer should include all materials required for the placement of IV and intraosseous (IO) catheters. An additional drawer is stocked with bandage material, sterile gloves, and hair clippers with long extension cords. This equipment is useful for treating bleeding and open wounds and for placement of chest drains.

For cardiac monitoring, an ECG with alligator clips is necessary for easy attachment. A defibrillator with internal and external paddles is also kept on the cart ready for use in patients with ventricular fibrillation.

A suction device with different suction tips should be available. Large rigid dental suction tips work well for suctioning pharyngeal fluid, and small flexible suction tips will allow suction of ET or tracheostomy tubes. Hand-powered suction units should be available if there is no electrical suction system present.

Basic laboratory tests used in the emergency setting include packed cell volume (PCV), total solids (TS), blood glucose (Accu-Chek), blood urea nitrogen (BUN; Azostix), serum electrolytes, activated clotting time (ACT), urinalysis (Multistix), and urine specific gravity. Blood collection tubes, microcentrifuge tubes, a centrifuge, laboratory test strips, and a timer are part of the basic emergency laboratory equipment located in the emergency area.

To guarantee constant preparedness, each technician starting a shift reviews a checklist of all contents of the emergency cart. The instruments should be tested for proper function (e.g., light bulb on the laryngoscope), and emergency drugs are checked for quantity, proper location, and expiration date. By reviewing the checklist, the techni-

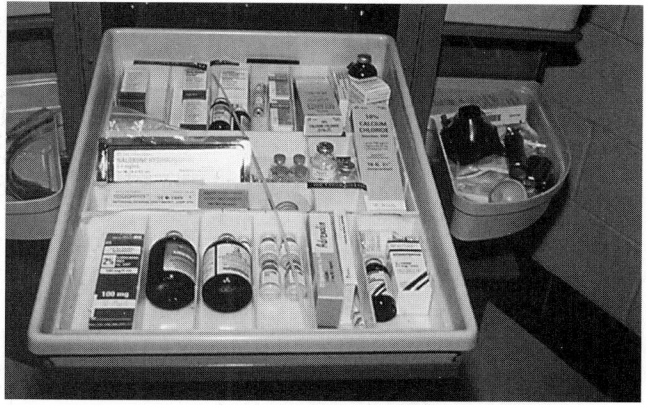

FIGURE 28-1. The use of predetermined slots in the crash cart facilitates identification of essential equipment that is missing or has been misplaced.

cian and veterinarian become familiar with the supplies and their location.

Policies and Procedural Protocols

Algorithms, procedural protocols, and guidelines provide consistency and efficiency within the emergency room. Algorithms and procedural protocols mandate how to do things in a step-by-step fashion to minimize stress and errors during an emergency. Established policies and protocols can also be used to ensure consistency of care. All team members should be familiar with the protocols, which should be discussed and reviewed at staff meetings (Box 28-4).

KEY ASPECTS OF EMERGENCY NURSING

Initial Contact and First Aid

The receptionist or technician usually makes initial contact with the owner on the telephone. The person who provides the first contact with the caller is termed a *first responder*. It is recommended that specific protocols be established on exactly what information or advice the first responder is to give the caller. The first responder should have some medical knowledge to properly assist the client in first aid, transport, and recognition of catastrophic emergencies (airway obstruction, respiratory arrest, cardiopulmonary arrest). Appropriate first aid can prevent further injury at the scene or during transport. The client should be given precise instructions for the easiest route to the hospital. The telephone number for a poison control center should be readily available for reference in cases of suspected toxin ingestion.

Telephone Contact, Handling, First Aid at the Scene, and Transport

It is important that during initial telephone contact, vital information be recorded, such as client name and telephone number; patient species, age, and gender; presenting complaint; patient's current condition; and expected

LOUISIANA STATE UNIVERSITY SCHOOL OF VETERINARY MEDICINE

INTENSIVE CARE

Date______, 20___

Primary Clinician____________

Time of Arrest_____AM/PM Hospital

Patient ID Card

Location at Time of Arrest____________

Type of Arrest: Respiratory____ Cardiopulmonary_____

Time CPR Instituted_____AM/PM

IV Catheter____Y/N Location of Catheter__________

Problems Before Arrest:

1.______________________________
2.______________________________
3.______________________________
4.______________________________
5.______________________________
6.______________________________

Basic Cardiac Life Support

Dorsal Recumbency____ Lateral Recumbency____

Ventilation only____

1:1 Simultaneous Compression/Ventilation_____ 5:1 Compression/Ventilation_____

Chest Compression Rate____/Min Interposed Abdominal Compression_____

Jen Chung: Y/N Successful? Y/N

Emergency Thoracotomy: Y/N

Advanced Cardiac Life Support

ECG Diagnosis at Time of Arrest____

Drugs

Time	Medication	Volume	Route	Defib	ECG Before	ECG After
Outcome						

CPR Team Members:_______________________________________

Time of Death:____AM/PM Owners Notified? Y/N CPR Clinician__________________________

FIGURE 28-2. A cardiopulmonary resuscitation (CPR) log can be useful for recording all vital information when cardiopulmonary arrest occurs.

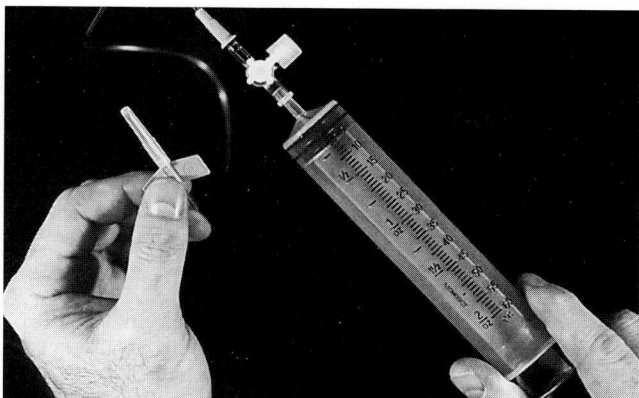

FIGURE 28-3. Thoracentesis can be performed by using a 60-ml syringe, butterfly catheter, or fluid extension set and 20-gauge needle and three-way stopcock.

Box 28-3	EMERGENCY CHEST DRAIN PLACEMENT PACK CONTENTS

Large curved Carmalt forceps
Scalpel handle
Scalpel blade
Sharp-to-sharp scissors
4 × 4 gauze sponges
Metzenbaum scissors
Surgical towels for draping
Towel clamps

Box 28-4	THORACENTESIS PROTOCOL

Gather supplies:
Thoracentesis setup (60-ml syringe, three-way stopcock, IV extension set, 20-gauge needle)
Surgical scrub
Sterile gloves
Vacutainer tubes
Clippers
Position pet in sternal or lateral recumbency.
Give sedation if needed.
Shave hemithorax on side or sides to be tapped (fifth to twelfth intercostal spaces).
Aseptically prepare area.
Introduce needle into pleural space at seventh to ninth intercostal space, staying close to the cranial edge of the rib. Initially start at level of the costochondral junction.
Adjust three-way stopcock so line is open to patient and aspirate with minimal pressure (5 ml).

IF NEGATIVE TAP:
Redirect needle in a cranial, caudal, dorsal, and ventral direction.
Enter different intercostal space.

IF POSITIVE TAP*:
Air+: remove until negative pressure.
Fluid: remove as much as possible or until clinical signs improve. Submit for fluid analysis.

*If frequent productive taps, chest drain placement should be considered.
+, Always quantitate fluid and air removed.

Box 28-5	COMMON HISTORIC OR OBSERVED PROBLEMS THAT WARRANT IMMEDIATE MEDICAL ATTENTION

Arterial bleeding
Respiratory distress
Near drowning
Heat prostration
Shock
Dystocia
Gastric dilation volvulus (GDV)
History of poisoning (especially ethylene glycol)
History of decreased urine output
Burns
Seizures
Prolapse of organs
Potential snake bites
Open wounds with exposure of extensive soft tissue or bones
Penetrating thoracic or abdominal wounds

time of arrival. When answering a call, an immediate assessment must be made and the clinical problems prioritized. This phone triage enables the first responder to determine whether a life-threatening condition exists and to instruct the client on the next step to take (Box 28-5). If first aid advice is required, guidance should be offered according to protocols approved by the hospital administration.

Technician Note

Advise the owner to remain calm and cautiously handle the injured pet.

Owners and good Samaritans may provide important medical assistance at the scene of the injury. The first concern must be for the handler's safety. Advise the handler to take a quiet, gentle approach while handling the injured pet. Warn handlers to watch for signs of aggression or any clues that they may have difficulty safely handling the animal.

When a dog is in pain or acting aggressively, a muzzle may be required. A blanket or towel may help provide the rescuer with adequate protection while attempting to handle an aggressive cat. Callers should always be cautioned that despite these preventive measures, they might be injured while assisting the animal.

It is possible to gain control of an aggressive pet by placing a heavy blanket over the animal while an assistant restrains the head behind the ears away from the mouth. A muzzle can be beneficial but should not be placed by anyone inexperienced because of the risk to both handler and animal. Muzzles that hold the mouth closed may be contraindicated if the animal is bleeding from the nose, the nasal passages appear to be occluded, or any type of respiratory distress is present. Cats should be picked up slowly, with one hand supporting the chest while transporting the animal in a firm, secure manner under the arm. The front legs should be held with one hand, and the head and neck held with the other. Placing the cat into a cardboard box or pillowcase is an alternative means of immobilization and transport.

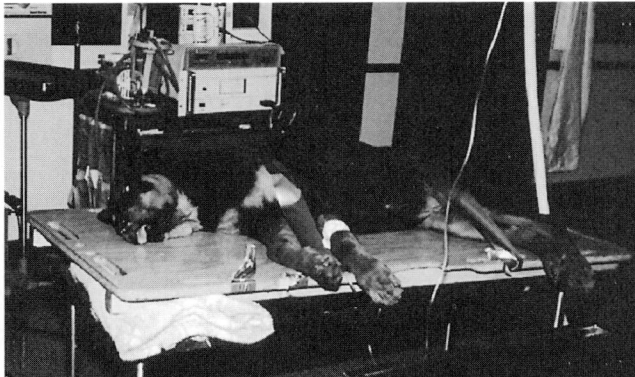

FIGURE 28-4. Unconscious animals should be transported from the accident site and in the veterinary facility on a firm surface such as a plastic, fiberglass, or wood board or a gurney until head and spinal injuries are ruled out.

BOX 28-6	**EMETIC AGENTS**

HOUSEHOLD EMETIC
Hydrogen peroxide (3%), 1 tsp/10 lb body weight; can repeat up to three times every 15 minutes

IN-HOSPITAL EMETICS
Hydrogen peroxide (3%)
Apomorphine

Unconscious or stuporous animals are at risk for developing injuries and vomiting with aspiration that may lead to life-threatening complications. These animals should be transported in a sternal or lateral position to avoid placing pressure on the neck or chest, which may lead to vagally mediated bradycardia, hypotension, and cardiac arrest (Figure 28-4).

If the injured animal is uncoordinated, unconscious, or nonambulatory, a spinal or head injury should be suspected. These animals should be immobilized in lateral recumbency for transportation to the hospital. When possible, animals sustaining trauma to one side of the chest should be transported with the injured side down to allow full expansion of the normal or less injured lung on the opposite side. Tape can be used to restrain the patient on a flat rigid carrier, such as a board. This will allow for safe transportation as well as immobilization during initial diagnostic procedures. Immobilization is important to prevent exacerbation of orthopedic, thoracic, abdominal, and spinal injuries. When sliding the animal onto a board, make certain the body remains parallel to the surface of the board to prevent excessive manipulation of the head or spine. Do not elevate the head if at all possible in order to maintain cerebral blood flow. If the animal will not lie down and becomes agitated, respiratory injury should be suspected and excessive restraint may be life threatening.

Fractures of the long bones below the elbow, hock, or stifle with significant displacement have potential for nerve, muscle, and skin penetration and should be supported during transport. The owner can fashion a splint from a rolled newspaper or magazine. The splint should include the joint above and below the fracture, which is then secured in place with tape or a piece of fabric such as a necktie or scarf.

If there is a large volume of blood or pulsating bleeding from a wound (arterial bleeding), direct pressure should be applied to the site. A pressure bandage may be made using a nonshedding material over the site and then wrapping an over material snugly around the site. Tourniquets are avoided because they may disrupt blood flow to and from the affected limb.

In the case of toxin ingestion, induction of emesis before transport to the hospital may be indicated. Hospital policy for induction of emesis should be followed (Box 28-6). The pet owner should be instructed to bring the label or packaging of the toxin ingested for further information. Poison control center telephone numbers should be available at the veterinary hospital for possible consultation on uncommon toxicities.

If after speaking with a pet owner, the technician feels the condition is not an emergency, an appropriate appointment should be made to evaluate the pet during normal hospital hours and the content of the conversation recorded in a telephone log.

The Veterinary Technician: Rendering First Aid

When the critically ill patient arrives at the veterinary facility, first aid is the initial care provided to a pet that has been injured or is acutely ill. Knowledge of how to triage and stabilize the pet will improve the overall chances of survival.

Triage

The word *triage* is a French term meaning *to sort* and was originally used by French wool traders. In the medical context, triage has been used to describe the objective clinical evaluation of multiple casualties in order to prioritize therapy. Triage systems were developed for use in battlefield conditions. In veterinary medicine, triage describes a medical decision-making process that is used in several clinical settings. In the emergency medical field, triage is used to screen patients into categories on the basis of severity of illness to determine their relative priority for treatment. In many cases, triage is used to prioritize the presenting problems in a given clinical case and helps to provide a systematic approach to the critically ill patient. When used correctly, the principles of triage guide the veterinary team in the efficient delivery of medical and patient care.

> **Technician Note**
>
> *Triage* means *to sort* and was adapted from the battlefield to assist in prioritizing problems and treatment provided.

The person performing triage must possess excellent assessment as well as interpersonal skills. He or she must be able to convey concern and empathy while gathering objective information from the pet owner. Establishing trust and rapport is fundamental to providing emotional support during this time.

During triage, a brief history is obtained from the owner that includes the nature of the emergency, the time it occurred, and any previous medical conditions or therapy. Further information can be obtained after initial assessment.

In some cases, the severity of disease may be readily recognizable for patients with life-threatening disorders or those with low-priority, nonurgent complaints. The triage nurse or technician must make decisions regarding the

TABLE 28-1	TRIAGE PARAMETERS		
Parameter		**Normal Value**	**Abnormal Value**
Heart rate (beats/min)			
Cat		150-210	<150; bradycardia
			>250; tachycardia
Dog			
	>25 kg	70-100	<70; bradycardia
			>140; tachycardia
	<25 kg	90-160	<70; bradypnea
			>160; tachypnea
Respirations (breaths/min)			
Cat		8-30	<8; bradypnea
			>40; tachypnea
Dog		8-20	<8; bradypnea
			>30; tachypnea
Mucous membrane		Pink	Pale, brown, yellow
Capillary refill time (sec)		1-2	<1 or >2
Temperature (° C [° F])		38-39 (100-102)	<37 (99); hypothermia
			>40 (>103); hyperthermia
Blood pressure (mm Hg)			
	Systolic	100-150	>160; hypertension
	Diastolic	60-110	<60; hypotension
	Mean arterial	80-120	<60; hypotension
Urine output (ml/kg/hr)		1-2	<1

life-threatening nature of the situation based on chief complaint, general appearance, vital signs, past history, current medications, and patient age (Table 28-1).

Although the purpose of triage is not to diagnose, experienced technicians are able to recognize clinical syndromes and use this knowledge when deciding on the severity of disease. When it is determined that immediate assessment or intervention is required, the animal is moved to the ready area, and the owner is assured that someone will be with them immediately. To accelerate treatment, permission for initial intervention (IV catheter placement, fluid administration, oxygen supplementation) should be obtained from the owner at this time.

Triage of multiple critically ill patients involves the identification of conditions that require immediate treatment and then performing treatments that make the most efficient use of the available work force and skills. Patients with potential for compromised airway, breathing, or circulation (ABCs) are given first priority for immediate treatment. The assessment examination should follow a systematic approach, and several triage systems are available. The acronym *A CRASH PLAN* is easy to remember and simple to follow (Box 28-7).

Before patient triage, observing the owner and the animal for anything that may indicate risk can help assess the situation. This includes an animal that is growling and not well controlled. Obvious fractious dogs should not be approached until the handler has a muzzle on the dog. Any signs of respiratory distress or possible airway obstruction, such as hemorrhage from the nose or mouth, should dictate the use of fenestrated plastic or wire cage muzzle to avoid further respiratory compromise (Figure 28-5). If blood is observed on the pet, gloves should be worn and possibly protective eye wear if blood or other chemicals could be sprayed. Animals with an unusual neurologic history in rabies-endemic areas should be considered rabies suspects, and gloves and eye wear should be worn.

Box 28-7	THE TRIAGE SYSTEM
A	Airway
C	Circulation
R	Respiratory
A	Abdomen
S	Spine
H	Head
P	Pelvis
L	Limbs
A	Arteries and veins
N	Nerves

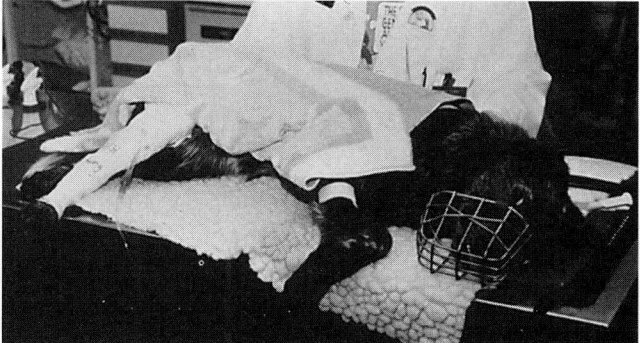

FIGURE 28-5. A wire cage muzzle can restrain the pet without impairment of breathing.

Hand washing after the handling of each emergency patient is required. Animals having difficulty breathing should receive oxygen by face mask (Figure 28-6) before handling. The feline patient in respiratory distress presents a high-risk case, and oxygen should be provided before any

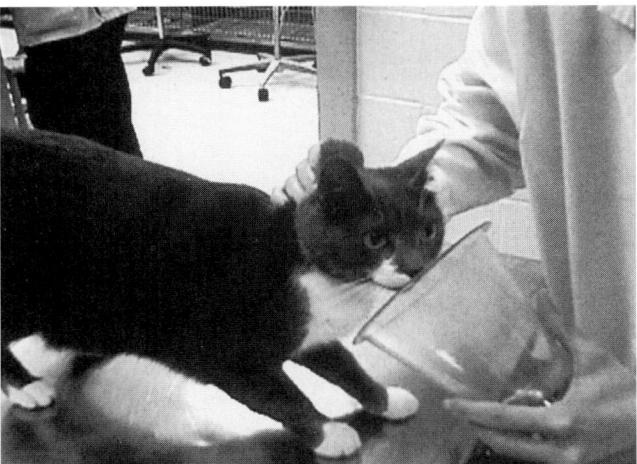

FIGURE 28-6. Oxygen supplementation can easily be provided via face mask.

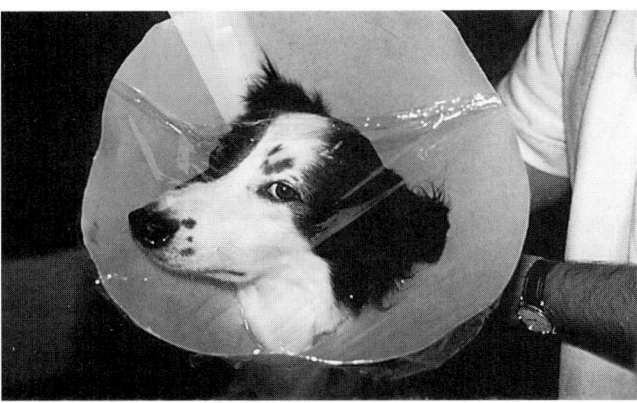

FIGURE 28-7. An oxygen canopy or hood can be made with an Elizabethan collar and cellophane wrap.

intervention is considered. Oxygen supplementation can also be provided by oxygen canopy made using an Elizabethan collar and a clear plastic bag or cellophane (Saran) wrap (Figure 28-7).

Technician Note

Patients in respiratory difficulty should receive oxygen before they are handled extensively.

History

On arrival, after a capsule history is obtained, it is recommended that the owner be given a history form to complete. This helps save time, determines the owner's ability to read and follow directions, and provides a thorough case review. It also gives owners something to do while waiting and makes them feel they are helping. When reviewing the history with the pet owner it is important to ask specific questions to obtain as much detailed information as possible.

Examination

To help prevent problems and body systems from being overlooked during the examination, the following mne-

monic has been used to triage emergency cases: *A CRASH PLAN. A* represents airway and breathing (nose, mouth, trachea, thoracic inlet, all lung fields); *C,* cardiovascular system (mucous membrane color, capillary refill time, peripheral pulses, heart sounds); *R,* respiratory system (breathing effort, chest and abdominal movement, thoracic percussion); *A,* abdomen (palpation, wounds, bruises, inguinal and retroperitoneal region; auscultation, abdominocentesis); *S,* spine (palpate entire spine; ambulation, wounds, bruises, pain); *H,* head, eyes, ears, nose, and throat (face, skull, jaw, teeth, tongue, pharynx); *P,* pelvis (palpate ilial wings, tuber ischii, greater trochanters, rectal area, genitalia); *L,* limbs (distal to proximal: check movement, pain perception, function, joints); *A,* arteries and veins (clip neck and examine jugular vein filling, check pulses); and *N,* nerves (assess level of consciousness, cranial nerves, spinal function, peripheral nerves) (Box 28-7).

VITAL SIGNS: PATHOPHYSIOLOGY, ASSESSMENT, AND INTERVENTION

Evaluation of the patient through physical findings is the most objective way of determining patient status. Obtaining and assessing parameters constitute a dynamic process, with the initial and successive values acting as continued points of comparison. It is important to know normal values for each patient so abnormal values can be recognized. It is important that all abnormal values are noted in the medical record. This allows consistent monitoring, especially when several technicians and clinicians are managing the case. It is also important to inform personnel of anticipated problems, especially during personnel or shift changes. If there are changing trends, the technician should inform the clinician, and more frequent monitoring or reassessment may be required. Identifying trends or changes can be much more useful than documenting one-time values. The parameters should always be interpreted in the context of the clinical case.

Respiration and Respiratory Patterns
Pathophysiology
Respiration is the exchange of oxygen and carbon dioxide between the air and tissues. The lung, with its network of capillaries and alveoli, is the primary site of gas exchange with the blood. In addition to the lungs, the airways, larynx, pharynx, and nasal passages comprise the respiratory tract. Other functions of the respiratory tract include control of acid-base balance, defense against inhalation of foreign particles, and filtration of the circulation. The brain and respiratory muscles control the respiratory rate and pattern. Normally, the diaphragm is responsible for 80% to 90% of the work of breathing when the animal is resting. When increased work of breathing occurs, as might happen with pneumonia, the intercostal muscles are also utilized.

The rate and effort of breathing can be affected by pathology of the respiratory tract, central nervous system, or respiratory muscles. Trauma to the thoracic wall and associated structures (e.g., diaphragmatic hernia, pressure on the diaphragm, rib fractures, intercostal muscle damage) can affect respiration by making it painful for the animal to breathe and disrupting the normal mechanics of breathing. Metabolic changes leading to acid-base abnormalities and pain are other causes for abnormal breathing patterns.

When blood carbon dioxide increases or bicarbonate decreases, the brain responds by increasing pulmonary

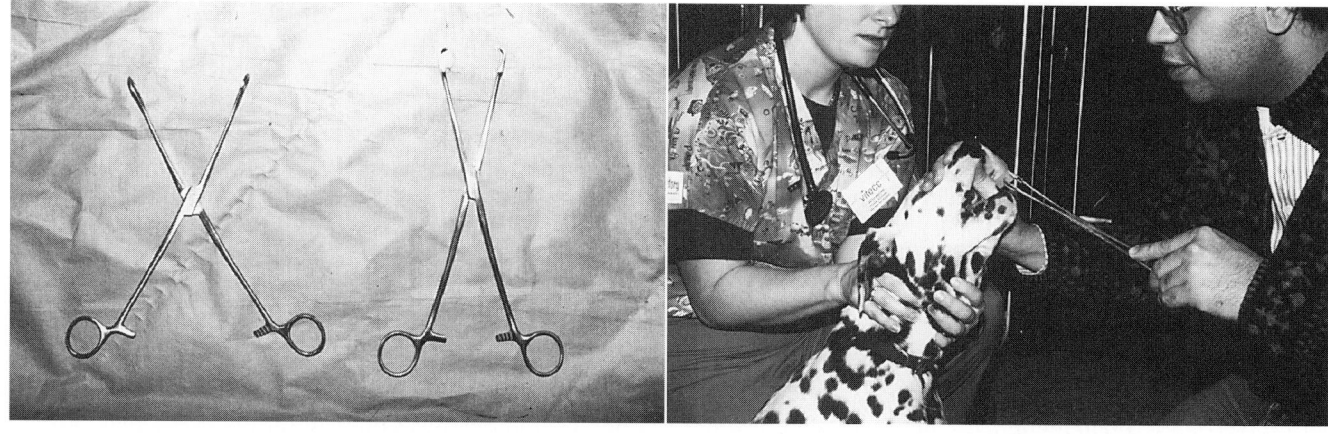

FIGURE 28-8. **A,** Forceps, such as the Laufe polyp forceps (commonly known as sponge forceps *[left]*) and the vulsellum forceps *(right),* aid in the removal of foreign bodies from the oropharyngeal area. **B,** Use of forceps in the removal of oropharyngeal foreign body.

ventilation in an effort to exhale carbon dioxide and normalize blood pH. Chemoreceptors in the carotid bodies detect increased carbon dioxide levels and stimulate the respiratory center. When carbon dioxide levels decrease, the stimulus for ventilation is removed. In addition, a decrease in blood oxygen content or pH is detected by carotid chemoreceptors and stimulates ventilation through the respiratory center.

Assessment

Clinical signs of respiratory distress change as the disease progresses. The first subtle sign of respiratory distress is an increase in respiratory rate. This is followed by a change in respiratory pattern, which may indicate the site of the pathologic finding. As the distress progresses, the animal may assume postural positions of relief, followed by open mouth and labored breathing. Cyanosis is a very late sign (P_{AO_2} <60 mm Hg) that carries a guarded prognosis.

Respiratory patterns guide the veterinary team to help localize the anatomic site of disease for life-saving intervention. Loud breathing or stridor (heard without the aid of a stethoscope) indicates large airway disease (nasal passages, larynx/pharynx, trachea). Inspiratory stridor directs investigation of the extrathoracic airways, especially the larynx. Expiratory stridor is usually due to intrathoracic tracheal changes. Rapid, shallow breathing is suggestive of pleural space disease (e.g., accumulation of air or fluid). Labored breathing on both inspiration and expiration is most typical of lung parenchymal disease. Distress on expiration, with a short inspiratory phase, directs attention to the small airways.

Auscultation can help distinguish pleural disease from lung disease. Moist lung sounds suggest fluid in the lung tissues. Dry, coarse sounds on inspiration and expiration suggest fibrosis of the lung. The absence of lung sounds indicates that air, fluid, or tissue in the pleural space is dampening airway sounds. Thoracic percussion may aid in distinguishing between the presence of air or fluid in the pleural space.

As the work of breathing increases, the animal will assume a posture to assist the efforts. Cats often sit crouched with their sternum elevated from the surface whereas dogs extend their neck, abduct their elbows, and arch their back.

Respiratory rates below 8 breaths/min or above 30 breaths/min are considered abnormal (Table 28-1). Low respiratory rates can be caused by trauma to the brain or spinal cord, diseases that affect respiratory drive (chronic obstructive pulmonary disease, low blood carbon dioxide level), and drugs (sedatives). Increased respiratory rates can be caused by fever, pain, anxiety, trauma to the brain or chest, metabolic alterations (alkalosis), pulmonary diseases (pneumonia or pulmonary edema), and drugs (oxymorphone).

Intervention

Any change in breathing pattern or effort warrants immediate notification of the veterinarian. The veterinary technician should administer oxygen until a complete assessment can be made. If an upper airway foreign body is suspected, the technician can examine the mouth and retrieve the foreign body with a pair of sponge forceps (Figure 28-8) or by performing the Heimlich maneuver. When the breathing pattern suggests pleural space disease, the technician should prepare for thoracentesis and possibly chest tube placement by the veterinary team.

Technician Note

Any change in breathing pattern or effort warrants immediate notification of the veterinarian.

When respiratory distress is severe, ET tubes and a laryngoscope should be placed in close proximity to the cage. The veterinarian may need to rapidly sedate or anesthetize the animal in order to intubate. In some cases, a tracheostomy is performed to gain control of the airway, minimize the work of breathing, and provide oxygenation and ventilation. In the event that the animal stops breathing, the technician should rapidly intubate and ventilate with 100% oxygen and have equipment available for thoracentesis, chest tube placement, or tracheostomy as directed by the veterinarian.

Heart Rate and Rhythm
Pathophysiology

RATE. The function of the heart is to pump blood to the tissues. The amount of blood pumped by the heart is termed *cardiac output* and is dependent on the heart rate and the volume of the left ventricle (stroke volume). The force of contraction results from stretch of the myocardium from ventricular filling. The amount of blood returned to the heart (venous return) determines ventricular filling, also called *preload*. Heart rate and contractility are affected by both the sympathetic and parasympathetic nervous system. Decreased venous return as a result of hemorrhage or intravascular fluid loss (volume depletion such as dehydration) initiates a reflex increase in heart rate (tachycardia) and strength of contraction (inotropism) mediated by the sympathetic nervous system. However, sympathetically induced tachycardia can also occur with stress, pain, elevated temperature, and drugs.

An increase in heart rate (Table 28-1) and contractility will attempt to increase blood pressure and improve tissue perfusion. Sinus tachycardia can be normal or associated with shock, stress, excitement, fever, and hyperthyroidism. However, when the heart rate increases above a critical level, energy demands increase, ventricular filling is impaired, and coronary perfusion decreases, causing myocardial hypoxia. Cardiac arrhythmias and myocardial failure can result, leading to systemic hypoxia and multiple organ failure.

A decreased heart rate (bradycardia) can lead to decreased cardiac output. Extracardiac causes of bradycardia include hypothermia, metabolic disorders (hyperkalemia, hypoglycemia, hypothyroidism), and parasympathetic (vagal) stimulation. Parasympathetic stimulation can occur with brain, pulmonary, and gastrointestinal diseases. Bradycardia can also occur with the administration of drugs that either stimulate the parasympathetic nervous system (parasympathomimetics) or decrease the sympathetic system (sympatholytics). Heart rates that fall below a critical level can lead to tissue hypoxia, organ failure, and death.

RHYTHM.   The conduction system supplies the electrical pathway coordinating the contraction of the heart. The rhythm of contractions depends on the route of electrical impulse through the nerve pathways in the heart. A normal impulse starts at the sinoatrial (SA) node in the right atrium and travels through the atria to the atrioventricular (AV) node at the junction of the atria and ventricles. From this location the impulse proceeds to the bundle of His and ventricular Purkinje fibers. This pathway provides the normal sinus rhythm detected on thoracic auscultation and the ECG recording.

An arrhythmia or dysrhythmia is defined as an irregularity of the heart rhythm that may be detected on physical examination by simultaneously auscultating the heart and palpating a peripheral pulse. When the ventricular contraction has not been successful in forcefully propelling blood to the periphery, a pulse deficit is detected. An arrhythmia can also be defined as a heartbeat that is abnormally fast or slow. An abnormal conduction system or diseased heart muscle (cardiomyopathy) can cause an arrhythmia.

Not all arrhythmias are pathologic. Basic ECG interpretation is a valuable skill for the emergency and critical care veterinary technician. Normal sinus rhythm is defined by a regular rhythm and the presence of characteristic P-QRST complexes on the ECG. Sinus arrhythmia can be mistaken on examination as pathologic but is a normal fluctuation in the heart rate with respiration decreasing with expiration and increasing with inspiration. The presence of P waves and upright and narrow QRS complexes characterizes supraventricular rhythms. Ventricular arrhythmias lack P waves and have wide and bizarre QRS complexes. Supraventricular and ventricular arrhythmias can be subdivided according to rate into normal rate, bradyarrhythmic (be-

low normal rates), or tachyarrhythmic (faster than normal rates).

Assessment
The technician should listen to the heart by placing the stethoscope over the left and right sides of the thorax at the third to fifth intercostal space while palpating the pulse. Pericardial fluid, pleural air or fluid, severe hypovolemia, or herniated abdominal organs may cause muffled heart sounds. Tachycardia, bradycardia, muffled heart sounds, and pulse deficits require immediate attention by the veterinary team.

Intervention
When an arrhythmia is suspected during physical examination, the veterinarian is alerted, and an ECG is performed. Thoracic radiographs and echocardiography may also be required to better define the cause of muffled heart sounds.

Continuous ECG and blood pressure measurements may be necessary to detect changes in rate and rhythm. All vomiting animals require close monitoring because collapse may occur as a result of severe bradycardia from increased vagal tone during emesis. Treatment of an arrhythmia is warranted if it is associated with impaired perfusion. Oxygen supplementation is indicated while the veterinary team is treating the arrhythmia.

Perfusion Parameters
Pulse strength and quality, jugular distention, mucous membrane color, capillary refill time, and body temperature are parameters that help evaluate how well the animal is perfusing peripheral tissues.

Pathophysiology
PULSE.   Blood pumped into the aorta during ventricular contraction creates a fluid wave that travels from the heart to the peripheral arteries; this wave is called a *pulse*. The character of the pulse depends on stroke volume, heart rate, and force of ejection as well as vascular tone. Evaluation of the pulse strength is based on the difference between the systolic and diastolic pressures (pulse pressure). A normal pulse pressure makes the pulse easily palpated and strong. When the difference is wide, the pulse will be bounding (hyperkinetic). Causes of hyperkinetic pulses include fever, hyperthyroidism, patent ductus arteriosus, and hyperdynamic phases of shock.

When the difference is small or the time to maximal systolic pressure is prolonged, the pulse feels weak (hypokinetic). Causes of hypokinetic pulses include any disease conditions that have a decreased cardiac output, such as septic shock, heart failure, and severe arrhythmia.

Assessment
Pulses are palpated by lightly placing the index and middle fingers on the part of the body where an artery crosses over bone or firm tissue. The most common pulse points assessed are the femoral and dorsal pedal arteries. In dogs and cats, both femoral pulses should be assessed simultaneously to determine symmetry and to evaluate for obstruction, as seen with saddle thrombus.

Intervention
Any changes in pulse quality should be reported to the veterinarian. Bounding pulses may reflect pain, fever, or early shock and will require intervention with pain medication or fluid replacement by the veterinary team. Weak pulses are cause for immediate concern and warrant aggressive measures to improve cardiac output (IV fluids for

shock and appropriate cardiac medications for heart failure).

Hemorrhage

Catastrophic hemorrhage is life threatening because of the massive volume of blood that may be lost. Internal bleeding into areas that surround vital organs such as the heart and brain can create increased pressure that compromises vital organ function. Internal hemorrhage can occur in other areas, such as the chest, abdomen, and osseous compartments (e.g., pelvis, humerus, femur).

Bleeding into the thorax and abdomen requires the assessment and management skills of a veterinarian. Clinical signs associated with abdominal hemorrhage include red circular discoloration with its center at the umbilicus (caused by an accumulation of red cells under the skin) and abdominal distention from blood accumulation. Abdominal distention usually requires a blood loss of approximately 40 ml/kg or more. Bleeding along fascial planes is generally due to blunt trauma and may be accompanied by lacerations, bruising, and swelling.

When hemorrhage is recognized, attempts should be made to stop or slow bleeding and restore volume to prevent vascular collapse (decreased volume of blood in veins and arteries). Shock in these patients is a result of circulatory collapse and hypoxia. Restoration of volume to these patients becomes a major priority. These patients require rapid IV infusion of fluids consisting of crystalloids, colloids, and transfusions with blood components such as whole blood or packed red cells. Rapid restoration of blood volume is needed to maintain sufficient pressure to perfuse vital organs such as the heart, brain, and kidneys and to restore red cells to serve as oxygen-carrying vehicles.

Jugular Vein Distention

Pathophysiology

Jugular pulse waves are related to atrial contraction and filling. Observed jugular pulses indicate right-sided heart disease or arrhythmia. Persistent jugular vein distention occurs with right-sided congestive heart failure secondary to high right filling pressures, external compression of the cranial vena cava (as occurs with pericardial effusion/tamponade, tension pneumomediastinum, tension pneumothorax, or right-sided heart mass), jugular vein thrombosis, and other causes of increased central venous pressure (see section on central venous pressure).

Assessment

Jugular pulses may be normal in lateral recumbency; therefore the patient should be observed when sternal. The presence of jugular pulsations higher than one third of the way up the neck is abnormal.

Mucous Membrane Color and Capillary Refill Time

Pathophysiology

The normal pink color of nonpigmented membranes depends on an appropriate blood hemoglobin concentration, tissue oxygen tension, and peripheral capillary blood flow. The capillary refill time (CRT) is a result of blood flow to the capillary beds of the membranes. This flow depends on cardiac output and vascular tone.

Assessment

Pressing on oral or gingival mucous membranes is the most common means of assessing mucous membrane color and CRT. The conjunctiva of the eye and membranes of the vulva and penis can also be used. To obtain a CRT, pressure is applied by the index finger to a nonpigmented area of the mucous membrane and then released. The time for color to return to the blanched area is recorded as the CRT. Normal values are 1 to 2 seconds. A prolonged CRT (more than 2 seconds) suggests poor peripheral perfusion (as found in the late stage of shock, severe vasodilation or vasoconstriction, pericardial effusion, heart failure). A rapid CRT (less than 1 second) can be due to anxiety, compensatory shock, fever, and pain.

> ### Technician Note
> A CRT of more than 2 seconds suggests poor peripheral perfusion.

Intervention

Abnormal mucous membrane color or CRT should be immediately brought to the attention of the veterinarian. Pale or cyanotic mucous membranes with prolonged CRT necessitates oxygen administration and a rapid search for the underlying cause. The veterinary technician should be prepared to measure the blood pressure and central venous pressure, perform an ECG, or determine the PCV while recording the data. Aggressive fluid resuscitation might be required, and the technician should be prepared for rapid intervention.

Level of Consciousness

Pathophysiology

A deteriorating level of consciousness is suggestive of a progressive brain pathologic condition and worsening prognosis. The levels (in declining order) are alert and responsive, depressed, uncontrolled hyperexcitability, stupor, and coma. A mentally depressed animal is conscious but slow to respond to stimuli. An unconscious patient that responds to noxious (painful) stimuli is in a stupor. The patient that is unconscious and does not respond to any stimuli is in a coma. Coma carries the worst prognosis.

An animal can be conscious but have abnormal mental abilities. These mentation changes can include slow but appropriate responses to stimuli (severe depression), inappropriate responses to situations or stimuli (dementia), bizarre behavior (aggression, fly biting), and slow response with the animal unaware of the stimuli (mental dullness).

Etiologies for changes in level of consciousness or mentation include metabolic problems (liver failure or shunts, hyperglycemia or hypoglycemia, hypernatremia or hyponatremia), hypoxia, hypotension, trauma, toxins (ethylene glycol), intracranial disease (tumors, infectious disease, inflammation), and drugs (sedatives, anesthetics). Any pathologic condition can lead to brain edema or hemorrhage and result in increased intracranial pressure. When this occurs, the brain tissue is compressed. This is a medical emergency, and rapid deterioration of neurologic status or death may occur.

Stupor and coma result from injury to the brainstem, midbrain, and cerebral cortex. Localization of the lesion to the cerebral cortex or midbrain-brainstem area is important to determine prognosis and detect deterioration in clinical status. A diffuse cortical pathologic condition generally carries a better prognosis than one involving the midbrain or brainstem.

Assessment

The veterinary technician must monitor the animal's mentation and level of consciousness. Changes in the animal's behavior, response to stimuli, or posture may be significant. Any decline in the level of consciousness suggests a worsening pathologic condition and warrants immediate neurologic examination and medical or surgical intervention.

In the conscious animal with altered mentation, the cerebral cortex and diencephalon are the sites of pathologic findings. The animal can show behavioral changes, dementia, circling to the side of the lesion, seizures, stupor, or coma. Animals may also have mild weakness in their limbs.

The neurologic evaluation of the unconscious animal should be used to localize the lesion and determine the progression of the pathologic condition. Pupillary size and response to light are noted. Normal, responsive pupils or equal, miotic pupils are associated with disease within the cerebral cortex or subcortical structures. Dilated or midrange fixed pupils are most commonly caused by midbrain pathologic problems and represent a grave sign. Eye position is noted, with ventral lateral strabismus (lateral gazing) indicating a midbrain pathologic condition. Nystagmus may be vertical, horizontal, or rotary. This suggests central or peripheral vestibular disease. Disease affecting the vestibular system can be located within either the ear or the brainstem. If there are changes in the patient's level of consciousness along with nystagmus, the cause is more likely central vestibular disease (involving the brain) versus peripheral vestibular disease (lesion involving the ear or vestibular nerve). Vertical nystagmus generally indicates a central lesion, whereas horizontal or rotary nystagmus may be found with peripheral or central vestibular disease. The ability to demonstrate changes in nystagmus suggests a central lesion, and conscious proprioceptive deficits also indicate a central lesion. Changes in posture, with the forelimbs and neck in extensor rigidity in the unconscious patient (decerebrate rigidity), are a grave neurologic sign, indicating a severe midbrain lesion (Figure 28-9).

Respiratory changes in the unconscious patient imply serious pathologic findings. Rhythmic waxing and waning of respirations (Cheyne-Stokes respirations) are caused by diffuse, severe cortical pathologic conditions. Apneustic breathing (nonrhythmic waxing and waning of breathing) and uncontrolled hyperventilation may result from a brainstem lesion.

Intervention

Any change in level of consciousness or mentation requires immediate intervention. Frequent neurologic evaluation is recommended for at-risk patients. Animals with uncontrolled hyperexcitability may require sedation or anesthesia and a well-padded, quiet enclosure to avoid injury. Bowls and toys are removed from the environment to prevent injury.

Efforts are required to lower intracranial pressure in the unconscious patient. The head and neck should be in a level position with the body level or slightly elevated to 20 degrees. The airway is secured in patients that cannot swallow (ET tube) because salivary secretions, regurgitation, or vomiting can cause airway obstruction or aspiration pneumonia. The carbon dioxide level should be maintained between 30 and 35 mm Hg for optimal cerebral blood flow and to prevent or manage cerebral edema; this may require intubation and ventilation. The arterial oxygen must be maintained above 60 mm Hg. Oxygen supplementation may be required. Nasal oxygen should be used with caution because stimulation of a sneeze during nasal catheter placement could abruptly elevate intracra-

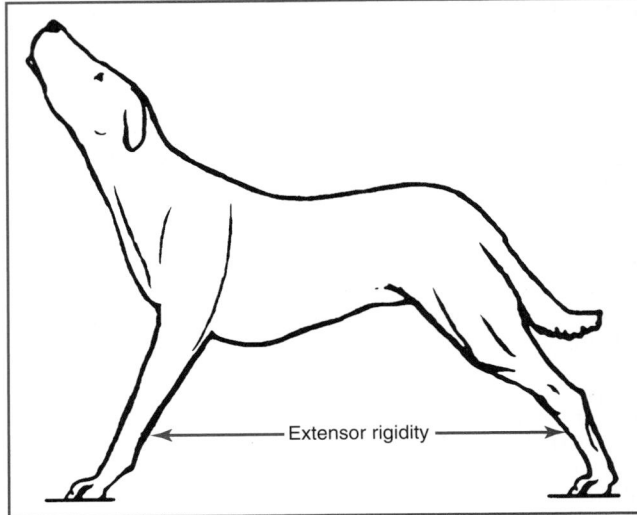

FIGURE 28-9.   Decerebrate rigidity carries a poor prognosis.

nial pressure. An oxygen face mask and canopy must be used with care to prevent increased levels of carbon dioxide.

The tongue is kept moist with water and the eyes lubricated with an ophthalmic ointment. No pressure should be placed on the jugular veins, and jugular venipuncture is avoided. Usually, urinary catheter placement is recommended to keep the bedding and patient clean and dry. Frequent and gentle physical therapy and turning are recommended to avoid pressure sores. The unconscious patient has higher metabolic demands, and appropriate nutritional support must be provided.

Temperature
Pathophysiology
The body maintains temperature homeostasis by balancing heat production with heat loss through a thermostatic feedback mechanism in the hypothalamus. This mechanism may be altered by systemic disease or neurologic injury. Chemical substances released in the disease state can reset the thermoregulatory center causing an increase in metabolic rate and other physiologic processes resulting in elevated body temperature. These chemicals may be pyrogens secreted by bacteria or cytokines associated with inflammation. Primary brain disease (cerebral edema, brain trauma, tumors) can reset the thermostat to a higher level. In cases where the thermoregulatory center has been reset, the term *pyrexia* or *true fever* is used. Other conditions, such as heat stroke, are better termed *primary hyperthermia*.

All causes of elevated body temperature create increased tissue oxygen requirements. The body responds by increasing ventilation and vasodilation to release body heat. Should the P_{CO_2} decrease to a low level, cerebral vasoconstriction and brain hypoxia can result. Cardiac workload and oxygen demands are also increased. Damage to vascular cells can lead to disseminated intravascular coagulation (DIC), sloughing of gastrointestinal mucosa, bacterial translocation, and significant intravascular volume deficits.

Hypothermia results in a reduced metabolic rate and enzyme functions. There is a decrease in oxygen consumption and a decrease in the ability of hemoglobin to release oxygen to tissues. Hypothermia affects the cardiovascular system by causing peripheral vasoconstriction, decreased heart rate, and hypotension. Gastrointestinal motility is also decreased, and ileus may occur.

Assessment

Emergency patients should have their temperature monitored several times daily. Patients with inflammatory disease, excessive panting, or hyperactivity and postoperative patients should have their temperature checked more frequently. Ideally, temperatures are monitored from the same site, usually rectally. Other sites of monitoring include the ear canal, the axilla, and the inguinal region. These areas usually are 1° to 2° F lower than rectal temperature. Ear canal temperatures can also be obtained using an ear canal thermometer. Serial temperatures taken from the same area provide more information than single readings.

Intervention

Any abnormal temperature must be reported to the veterinarian, who will determine what methods are required to cool hyperthermic patients and warm hypothermic patients. External cooling may benefit some hyperthermic patients. Some commonly used measures include cooling with a fan or placing cool compresses, such as towels soaked in cool water. Cold or ice water should be avoided because this may lead to peripheral vasoconstriction and inhibition of heat dissipation. Active cooling techniques include IV fluid therapy with cool fluids and cool water enemas. Cooling measures should cease when the rectal temperature reaches 40° C (104° F) to prevent overcooling. All patients with long-term elevation of body temperatures should be placed on IV fluid therapy.

Hypothermic patients can be treated by covering them with a warm blanket and water bottles filled with warm water. The patient can be placed under a heating lamp, but strict monitoring is essential to prevent burns. Circulating warm water blankets are preferred over heating blankets and lamps because there is less chance of accidental thermal injury. An innovative warming system that is now available in some practices is the Bair Hugger, which is a forced warm air heating system. No surface heat should be provided without volume replacement because vasodilation from the heat may exacerbate the condition. Severe or prolonged hypothermia may require more aggressive approaches, such as active core warming with warmed IV fluids, warm peritoneal lavage, or intracolonic lavage with warm isotonic fluids. The recumbent patient should be turned every 2 to 4 hours to avoid thermal injury. Heating should be discontinued after the rectal temperature is low normal (38° C [100° F]).

PHYSIOLOGIC PARAMETERS ASSESSED IN THE EMERGENCY PATIENT

Hydration Status

Hydration status is evaluated by combining clinical history with physical examination. Parameters to assess the hydration status of the emergency patient can be defined as qualitative or quantitative. The qualitative assessment includes skin turgor, moist quality of the mucous membranes, position of the eye within the socket, and thoracic auscultation. Quantitative parameters include body weight, packed cell volume, plasma protein, urine specific gravity, and central venous pressure. No single parameter should be used as the sole indicator of hydration status. The combined assessment of multiple parameters remains the best indicator of dehydration or overhydration.

By definition, dehydration is a loss of fluid volume. This loss can be detected in peripheral tissues. In overhydrated patients tissues become swollen (edematous) with excess fluid. Lifting the skin between the shoulder blades assesses skin turgor. These tissues are elastic and rapidly return to normal position in a well-hydrated animal. Prolonged skin tent may occur in geriatric patients because of decreased skin elasticity. In general, decreased skin turgor correlates well with a state of dehydration. Skin turgor in overweight patients may appear normal even in the event of dehydration because of fat deposition in the subcutaneous tissues.

Mucous membranes are normally glossy and moist. Dehydrated small animals will have membranes with a tacky texture. However, this may be undetected if the patient has concurrent hypersalivation as a result of oral disease, dental disease, nausea, or vomiting. The conjunctival mucous membranes are another important site to evaluate for hydration. In dehydration, the eyes will appear sunken as these tissues lose moisture. With overhydration, chemosis characterized by swollen and puffy conjunctiva may occur. In the event of overhydration harsh lung sounds may be auscultated, and a serous nasal discharge may be noted.

Acute changes in body weight are directly attributable to changes in fluid volume. Serial body weight measurements are invaluable in monitoring the ability to achieve and maintain adequate hydration status. An initial body weight is important for later comparison; however, there is less immediate value unless there is prior data for comparison.

Packed cell volume and plasma protein will reflect hydration status. The ratio of fluid to packed cells and protein is decreased in dehydration, resulting in increased packed cell and plasma protein (hemoconcentration). The ratio of fluid to packed cells and plasma protein is increased in overhydration, resulting in a decreased packed cell volume and plasma protein. These parameters also reflect anemia, hypoproteinemia, hyperproteinemia, and polycythemia. If any of these are present, hydration status based on these parameters is difficult to assess without serial measurements and a more complete assessment.

Urine Output
Pathophysiology

The main function of the kidneys is to excrete metabolic wastes and reabsorb vital electrolytes and water. The volume and contents of urine are a result of the net function of individual nephrons. Each nephron, the functional unit of the kidney, comprises a glomerulus and renal tubules. The volume of urine produced depends on the glomerular filtration rate (GFR) and the ability of the renal tubules to reabsorb sodium and water. Factors governing the GFR are the size of the glomerular capillary bed, permeability of the capillaries, and hydrostatic and oncotic pressure gradients across the capillary walls. Variations in these factors have predictable results. For example, if the mean arterial blood pressure falls below 60 mm Hg, the hydrostatic pressure gradient declines across the glomerular capillary beds and glomerular filtration decreases.

Procedure

Accurate and frequent measurement of urine output requires bladder catheterization. A sterile soft red rubber or other soft feeding tube is used in the male dog, and a Foley catheter is used in the female dog. A 3.5 Fr. soft red rubber catheter or other feeding tube is used in cats. Soft and pliable catheters or tubes are preferred to reduce irritation to the urethra. The use of aseptic technique while placing the catheter minimizes iatrogenic urinary tract infection.

The catheter is lubricated and advanced slowly through the urethra into the neck of the urinary bladder and sutured in place to the vulva or prepuce. A closed urinary collection system with a sterile collection bag is attached to the catheter. Collection systems should be maintained below the level of the catheter. The bladder is immediately emptied, and the time is recorded as time zero (start of collection). The frequency of measuring urine output is determined by the animal's clinical condition. In general, urine output is measured every 4 to 6 hours. Daily examination of urine sediment is performed to monitor for infection. Urinary catheters should be flushed with sterile saline and inspected for kinks and clots in the line if there is a sudden decline in collected urine.

Indirect methods of estimating urine output are occasionally used. Absorptive pads or towels are placed in the patient's cage to collect the urine. The bedding must be weighed before and after placement in the cage. The weight of the dry material is subtracted from the weight of the urine-soaked material. Each 1-g increase in weight equals 1 ml of urine. An alternate method is to place the animal on a grate elevated off the cage floor or a special cage called a *metabolic cage.* Urine is then collected and measured after each voiding.

In the medical record, enteral and parenteral fluid intake and urine output are recorded. Quantities of fluid lost through vomiting and diarrhea are estimated and recorded. A good rule of thumb to used when estimating volume of vomitus or diarrhea is to double your initial estimate.

Technician Note

Normal urine output is 1 to 2 ml/kg/hr.

Assessment

Normal urine output is 1 to 2 ml/kg/hr. Oliguria (low urine production) is defined as less than 1 ml/kg/hr. Anuria (no urine output) is defined as less than 0.08 ml/kg/hr. Oliguria can result from prerenal, renal, or postrenal causes. Prerenal conditions such as hypovolemia, cardiac failure, hypotension, or excessive vasoconstriction lead to oliguria by reducing GFR. Dehydration and hypotension will decrease urine output until adequate intravascular volume has been restored. Renal diseases that affect the glomeruli or tubular cell function, including sepsis, trauma, toxins (aminoglycosides, ethylene glycol, amphotericin), radiocontrast agents, and infections (pyelonephritis), may manifest as oliguria or anuria. Postrenal problems cause interruption of the flow of urine through the ureters, bladder, or urethra and include renal calculi, blood clots, neoplasia, or trauma.

True oliguria in an animal receiving IV fluid will result in a decreased PCV and TS as a result of hemodilution. The central venous pressure (CVP) will increase, and harsh or wet lung sounds may develop. The body weight will increase as overhydration occurs. Increasing serum levels of urea nitrogen, creatinine, and potassium suggest renal failure or postrenal obstruction and warrant immediate veterinary intervention.

Excessive urine production is called *polyuria* and can be caused by IV fluid overload or impaired renal tubular absorption of sodium and water. Other conditions, such as renal medullary washout, postobstructive diuresis, and sepsis, can cause polyuria and require large volumes of replacement fluids.

Intervention

The technician must evaluate the urine output in relation to the hematocrit, TS, CVP, blood pressure, heart rate, and body weight. Any decrease in urine output in an adequately hydrated and perfused animal warrants immediate notification of the veterinarian. Initially the urinary collection system is examined for postrenal causes of urine outflow obstruction. If the origin of the condition is determined to be renal, and the animal is well hydrated, the veterinarian may administer vasoactive agents, such as mannitol or dopamine. Dopamine may be used in conjunction with furosemide, and these agents may work synergistically to improve urine output.

Blood Pressure
Pathophysiology

Arterial blood pressure is a product of cardiac output (heart rate and stroke volume) and peripheral vascular resistance. Systolic pressure is the pressure exerted by the blood as a result of contraction of the left ventricle. Diastolic pressure is the pressure exerted by the blood within the vessel when the ventricle is at rest. The difference between diastolic and systolic pressures is called the *pulse pressure.* Mean arterial pressure (MAP) is the diastolic pressure plus one third of the pulse pressure. Any factor that alters cardiac output or peripheral vascular resistance will alter the blood pressure.

Procedure

Blood pressure can be measured directly or indirectly. Direct (invasive) blood pressure measurement requires the insertion of a catheter into an artery (e.g., femoral or dorsal pedal artery) and connecting a transducer linked to a monitor. The direct arterial pressure is demonstrated in a waveform on an oscilloscope with the high point being the systolic pressure and the low point being the diastolic pressure. Although direct measurement provides the most accurate pressure values, expensive and sophisticated monitoring equipment is required.

Indirect (noninvasive) blood pressure measurements, although less accurate, are more easily obtained with affordable equipment. Blood pressure cuffs can be placed around the distal portion of a leg or around the tail. The two most common methods used for indirect blood pressure measurements in veterinary medicine are oscillometry and Doppler.

Oscillometric blood pressure measurement involves the use of a microprocessor and cuff that determines systolic and diastolic pressures from oscillations detected from the blood vessel as the cuff is automatically inflated and deflated. The optimal width of the cuff bladder is 40% to 60% of the circumference of the extremity to which it is applied. It is important when using an automated oscillometric unit to obtain five consecutive readings; discard the lowest and highest values and average the remaining three (Figure 28-10). Shivering, trembling, struggling, vasoconstriction, and inappropriate cuff size are common causes of erroneous measurements when using the oscillometric method.

The Doppler flow probe emits ultrasonic signals and detects these signals as they are reflected from the moving column of blood in the vessel. The reflected wave is shifted slightly from the transmitted wave, and the difference is converted into an audible signal. The frequency varies directly with blood velocity. The flow probe is lubricated with ultrasonic gel and secured to the shaved skin over an artery (e.g., the digital or dorsal metatarsal artery). The flow probe is attached to an amplifier that produces the pulsatile sound of blood moving through the vessel.

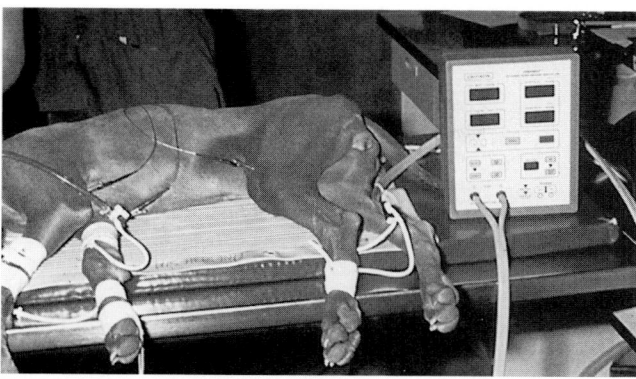

FIGURE 28-10. The inflatable cuff in place for oscillometric blood pressure measurement.

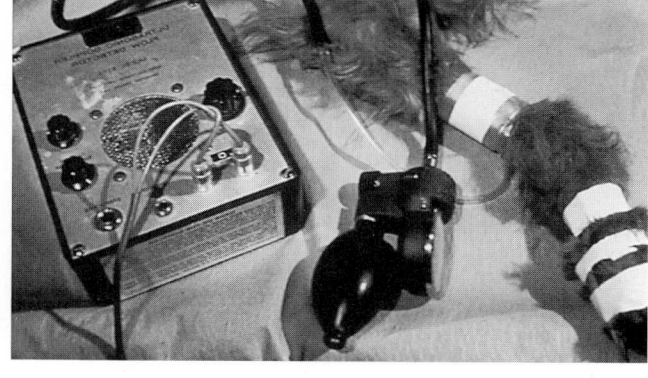

FIGURE 28-11. The Doppler technique can be utilized for indirect blood pressure measurement.

A blood pressure cuff with sphygmomanometer is secured to the limb proximal to the probe. The optimal width of the cuff bladder is 40% to 60% of the circumference of the extremity to which it is applied (Figure 28-11). The cuff is inflated until the pulse sound is not heard. The valve on the manometer is gradually opened to slowly allow the cuff to deflate. The point at which the pulse sound is first heard again is the systolic pressure. The point at which the swishing sound changes from its short pulsatile character to a more continuous swishing, longer-lasting sound is the approximate diastolic pressure. Determination of diastolic pressure is less reliable than systolic pressure with this technique. Erroneous results can occur with the Doppler method because of malpositioning of the transducer, inappropriate cuff size, poor contact with coupling gel, and flexion of the limb.

Assessment

The normal blood pressure in the dog and cat averages 120 mm Hg systolic and 80 mm Hg diastolic. The mean arterial pressure is normally 80 to 90 mm Hg. Systolic pressure should be above 100 mm Hg. Systolic pressure below 80 mm Hg is significant, and pressure below 60 mm Hg may be associated with poor renal perfusion and oliguria. Cerebral circulation is compromised when systolic pressure falls below 50 mm Hg, with brain ischemia occurring when systolic pressures are below 30 to 35 mm Hg for 2 hours. Coronary perfusion is best maintained when systolic pressures are higher than 70 mm Hg. Decreases in blood pressure can be caused by cardiac failure, hypovolemic shock, and drugs (e.g., sedatives, opioids, anesthetics). Blood pressure should be evaluated together with the animal's perfusion parameters, urine output, and disease state. As with any monitoring technique, repeated measurements are needed to detect a trend or change. Renal perfusion over the short term is considered adequate if systolic blood pressure is maintained above 60 mm Hg.

Increases in blood pressure can be caused by any condition that increases cardiac output, such as fever, exercise, and septic shock. Increases in total peripheral resistance will also lead to increases in blood pressure. Hypertension with systolic pressures above 200 mm Hg can be associated with a hyperdynamic stage of shock, excessive endogenous production of renin, chronic renal failure, hyperthyroidism, hyperadrenocorticism, pheochromocytoma, and excessive sympathetic stimulation.

Intervention

Any blood pressure outside the normal value must be reported to the veterinarian. Intervention by the veterinary team is performed after complete patient assessment, including level of consciousness, CVP, perfusion, and urine output. Addressing the underlying cause, such as hemorrhage, may treat hypotension. Volume expansion with crystalloid or colloid infusion is often the first line of therapy for hypotension. Pharmacologic intervention with positive inotropic or vasopressor agents may also be indicated. The two most common agents are dobutamine and dopamine. Addressing the underlying disease, such as renal failure or hyperthyroidism, often treats hypertension. Other causes of hypertension, such as pain, can also be managed. Sustained or life-threatening hypertension may be treated with diuretics, vasodilators, or calcium channel blockers.

Central Venous Pressure
Pathophysiology

CVP is a function of four independent forces: volume and flow of blood in the vena cava, distensibility and contractility of the right heart chambers during filling, venomotor activity in the vena cava, and intrathoracic pressure. When right-sided heart function and intrathoracic pressure are normal, CVP can be used as a reflection of intravascular volume. Changes in blood volume will result in pressure changes in the vena cava and are reflected by the CVP.

Procedure for Central Venous Pressure
Monitoring Setup

CVP measurement requires placement of a central catheter into the cranial vena cava (through the jugular vein), with the tip lying near the base of the heart (right atrium). The catheter is attached to IV extension tubing, which is connected at right angles to a water manometer by a three-way stopcock (Figure 28-12). Across from the IV extension tubing on the stopcock is an IV line and fluids or a syringe filled with isotonic fluid. The zero on the water manometer should be at the level of the right atrium. A horizontal line drawn between the thoracic inlet and the manometer establishes the zero reference level.

The stopcock is off to the manometer when the patient is receiving IV fluids. To measure CVP, the manometer is filled with fluid from the IV bag and the stopcock is turned off to the bag, leaving a column of fluid within the manometer. The stopcock is then opened toward the patient, allowing a continuous fluid column from the

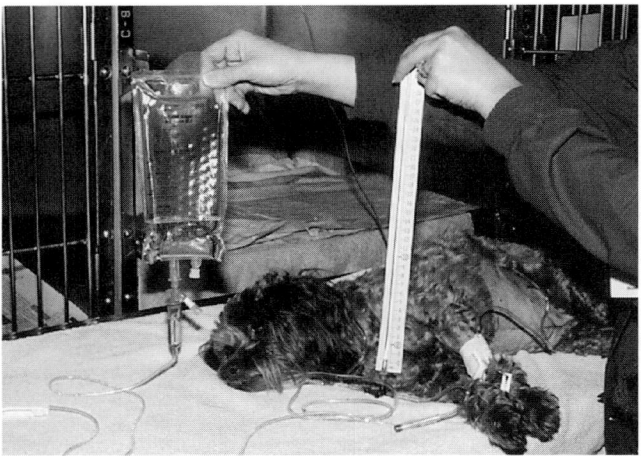

FIGURE 28-12. Central venous pressure can be measured to help assess hydration and monitor fluid therapy.

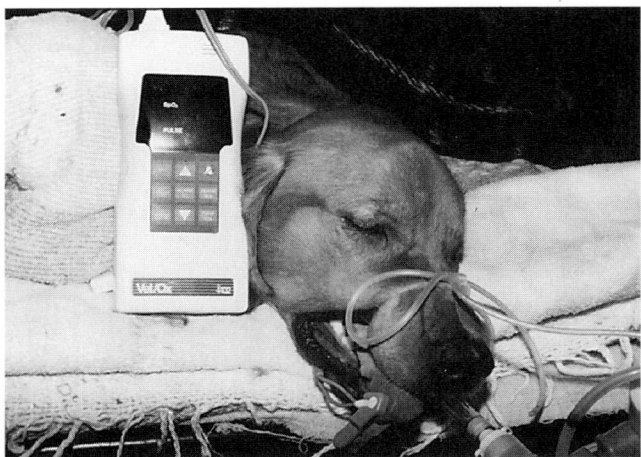

FIGURE 28-13. Pulse oximetry is used to noninvasively measure arterial oxygen saturation and is routinely used to monitor patients during and after surgery.

manometer to the patient. The fluid level in the manometer is allowed to equilibrate with the pressure in the jugular vein. The fluid level may oscillate a few millimeters with each respiration. Three values or readings are obtained to ensure consistent readings.

Assessment

Normal CVP measurements are reported as 0 to 5 cm H_2O. However, animals in critical condition are resuscitated to supranormal values, and the CVP is optimally maintained between 5 and 8 cm H_2O. Values of less than 5 cm H_2O are suggestive of insufficient intravascular volume. Values of more than 12 cm H_2O are of concern for right-sided heart failure or significant volume overload. Factors unrelated to right-sided heart function and volume overload (e.g., pleural, pericardial, or mediastinal pressure and pulmonary hypertension) can also raise the CVP.

The CVP can be performed in lateral or sternal recumbency but should be consistent. If readings do not fluctuate with respiration, the readings are inaccurate. Always obtain three or five consecutive readings at a time. Each reading should be approximately close in measurement. Huge discrepancies in readings should alert the technician to troubleshoot the CVP setup for kinks, obstructions, or problems with catheter or patient position.

Intervention

The CVP can be used to guide aggressive intravenous fluid resuscitation. When the CVP is low in a hypotensive animal, crystalloids and colloids are rapidly administered until the CVP is between 5 and 8 cm H_2O. At that time, if hypotension persists, vasopressor or positive inotropic agents may be required.

Elevated CVP measurements warrant examination of the system for occlusion of the catheter. If the system is patent, then fluid overload or right-sided heart disease should be suspected. Fluid overload should lead to other signs, such as change in PCV/total protein and changes in body weight. If overhydration or right-sided heart disease is suspected, the fluid rate is lowered, and the veterinarian may choose to administer diuretics or drugs specific for the cardiac condition. Any CVP measurements outside the target values set by the veterinary team should be reported to the attending veterinarian.

Pulse Oximetry
Pathophysiology

Pulse oximetry is a quick and reliable noninvasive method of measuring arterial oxygen saturation (S_{AO_2}) (Figure 28-13). S_{AO_2} is the percentage of hemoglobin sites that are chemically combined with oxygen. S_{AO_2} and pulse rate are determined by passing two wavelengths of light, one red and one infrared, through body tissue to a photodetector. The signal strength resulting from each light source determines the S_{AO_2}. Pulse oximetry can be affected by the color and thickness of body tissues, probe placement, intensity of the light source, and absorption of arterial and venous blood in the body tissue.

> ### Technician Note
>
> The use of pulse oximetry can provide an early warning of pulmonary or cardiovascular deterioration.

Procedure

Several types of probes can be placed. Probes that are clamps can be placed on the tongue or on a shaved, nonpigmented skin surface. The rectal probe is placed against the rectal mucosa, which has been cleared of feces. The oximeter is turned on, and S_{AO_2} and pulse rate are digitally reported.

Assessment

Animals requiring oxygen therapy or under anesthesia should have their S_{AO_2} monitored as well as physical signs of hypoxia (e.g., decreased level of consciousness, tachycardia, arrhythmias, restlessness, altered blood pressure, increased respiratory rate, changes in mucous membrane color). The use of pulse oximetry for monitoring S_{AO_2} and pulse rate can provide early warning of pulmonary or cardiovascular deterioration before it is clinically apparent. Normal S_{AO_2} is 98%. Values below 90% are correlated with P_{AO_2} of less than 60 mm Hg, a hypoxemic patient, and eminent cyanosis. Limitations of pulse oximetry include its inability to differentiate carboxyhemoglobin (seen with carbon monoxide poisoning) from hemoglobin. In addition, the pulse oximeter cannot distinguish a declining

P_{AO_2} that is above 100 mm Hg (e.g., a fall from 330 to 100 mm Hg will still generate a report of an S_{AO_2} of 100%) or the presence of methemoglobin. Results can be erroneous in animals with poor peripheral perfusion, heavily pigmented skin, hypothermia, icterus, and anemia.

Intervention

Any sudden decrease in S_{AO_2} with proper probe placement requires immediate notification of the veterinarian and rapid assessment of the animal's cardiopulmonary function. The oxygen concentration may need to be increased or the method of ventilation improved.

SHOCK: PATHOPHYSIOLOGY, CLINICAL SIGNS, AND THERAPY

Shock may accompany many emergency situations, and an understanding of its pathophysiology, assessment, and therapy is essential for those providing emergency care. Shock can be defined as ineffective circulation and failure to provide adequate oxygen-rich blood to organs throughout the body. Shock is usually caused by a failure of the patient's circulatory system to function properly, leading to inadequate tissue perfusion.

Circulation depends on a proper balance of the following: adequate blood volume, efficient cardiac output, and healthy vascular bed (vascular resistance). The vascular bed maintains the peripheral resistance necessary to distribute blood and maintain venous return. The vascular bed is composed of a network of arteries, veins, and capillaries or microcirculation (composed of arterioles and venules). All these anatomic structures normally work together in a state of dynamic equilibrium. However, the heart, arteries, and veins function somewhat independent of the microcirculation. Impulses from the sinoatrial node induce myocardial contraction. The heart, arteries, and veins are also subject to direct stimulation of the sympathetic nervous system.

The microcirculation is primarily responsive to local tissue needs. It delivers body fluids and solutes, such as nutrients, electrolytes, and oxygen, to the tissue cells and removes waste. It also helps regulate total blood volume and adjust and direct blood flow by constricting and relaxing precapillary sphincters. The ability of some vessels in the capillary network to dilate and constrict permits the microcirculation to selectively supply undernourished tissue while temporarily bypassing tissues with no immediate need. The microcirculation includes more than 90% of the body's blood vessels, and at any given time only 6% to 7% of capillary vessels are perfused with blood. If a disproportionate number of capillary bed vessels dilate and fill with blood, the remainder of the circulatory system becomes depleted, and blood pressure drops precipitously.

At the Cellular Level

Shock can be a result of various causes, but the end result of cellular damage or death is the same regardless of the precipitating factor. Shock is a progressive process, with an initial systemic compensatory reaction, but if adequate intervention is not instituted at this time, decompensation and an irreversible stage of shock will ensue. Regardless of the type or cause, shock produces circulatory insufficiency that reduces blood flow through the microcirculation.

Inside the cell, the mitochondria are responsible for producing the energy supply of the cells. By oxidizing glucose and other nutrients, the mitochondria manufacture adenosine triphosphate (ATP), the fuel for all cellular activity. The mitochondria use 90% of all oxygen entering the cell to make ATP; this process is called *aerobic metabolism*.

During shock, cells supplied by the microcirculation become so deprived of oxygen that they can no longer maintain aerobic metabolism and other normal activities. Consequently the cell mitochondria adopt an anaerobic metabolism (metabolism without oxygen). This process permits the cell to continue manufacturing ATP but far less efficiently. As a result, the cell uses up ATP faster than it can replenish the supply and eventually runs out of fuel for other cell functions, such as membrane maintenance.

Anaerobic metabolism also produces lactic acid. Normally, only muscle tissue produces lactic acid, which is then metabolized by the heart and liver. However, in shock, lactic acid pours out through the debilitated cell membranes of hypoxic cells in other tissues. The liver and heart cannot accommodate this excess, which then accumulates in the blood, resulting in a metabolic acidosis.

Alterations in the cellular metabolism and oxidative energy production of ATP eventually lead to failure of the sodium-potassium pump, causing redistribution of cellular ions and fluid shifts. The cell membrane, by means of passive and active transport, moves oxygen and nutrients into the cells and moves out waste products. Active transport requires energy expenditure by the cell. This transport mechanism handles molecules and particles (glucose, potassium, sodium) that cannot easily pass through the pores of the cell. Hypoxia, which is a key finding that accompanies shock, debilitates the cell membrane, causing this transport mechanism to malfunction.

Increased amounts of sodium and fluid enter the cell, causing cell swelling and death. Potassium exits from the intracellular compartment into the extracellular spaces, leading to hyperkalemia. Lysosomes (cytoplasmic organelles containing proteolytic enzymes) deteriorate and release enzymes into the cytoplasm of the cell. Cellular acidosis enhances their activity, and they begin to digest the cytoplasm.

If the cycle is not interrupted, cellular hypoxia leads to cell and tissue death, the final stage in the progression of shock. As more cells are compromised or destroyed, the tissues and organs begin to fail. In most instances, oxygen restoration within several minutes can return cell function and energy production to normal.

Finally, decompensatory stages of shock ensue as a result of unequal tissue oxygen supply compared with oxygen demand at the cellular level, resulting in an oxygen debt. In shock, the cellular oxygen debt, along with cellular damage and poor removal of waste products, occurs as a result of inadequate perfusion or inadequate oxygen delivery to tissue structures.

Clinical Characteristics of Shock

Clinical signs of shock develop in a specific order. Patients in shock will demonstrate different clinical signs depending on the stage of shock they are experiencing at the time of the assessment. Also see Chapter 28.

Decompensatory Stage of Shock

Clinical signs include cyanotic, pale mucous membranes; cold skin; decreased rectal temperature; absent or weak femoral pulses; oliguria (from arterial blood pressure less than 60 mm Hg), prolonged or absent CRT; and unconsciousness, stupor, or semiconsciousness. During substantial hemorrhage, the animal may have seizures because of low blood pressure.

Mild Stage of Shock

Clinical signs include pale or ashen mucous membranes, cool skin, low rectal temperature, weak femoral pulses, tachycardia, decreased urine output, prolonged CRT, and altered mental status (depression, seizures, uncontrolled hyperexcitability). Hemorrhage may be active or a slow bleed.

Compensatory Stage of Shock

Clinical signs include slightly rapid or labored breathing or normal respiration, red or pale mucous membranes, normal skin and rectal temperature, normal or bounding pulses, tachycardia, normal urinary output, and CRT less than 1 second or normal. The animal is mentally alert and conscious (aware of surroundings, mildly depressed to excited). Hemorrhage may be slight to absent.

Early Compensatory Shock

Patients in early compensatory shock are less serious, but the condition is still pressing and requires action within 24 hours. Clinical signs consist of a breathing pattern that is outwardly normal, normal perfusion or signs of early compensatory shock, red or pink mucous membranes, normal skin and rectal temperature, normal or bounding pulses, normal or rapid heart rate, normal urinary output, normal or rapid CRT, and normal or excited mental state.

Technician Note

The major goal of shock therapy is to restore and maintain tissue perfusion by expanding intravascular volume.

Therapy in Shock

The main goal of therapy is to restore and maintain tissue perfusion and correct the underlying physiologic abnormality. This is accomplished by replacing intravascular volume with a combination of crystalloids (lactated Ringer's, Plasmalyte, Normosol-R), colloids (albumin, dextran, hetastarch), and blood. Initially, the lost volume is replaced quickly through more than one peripheral catheter until the state of shock is corrected, as demonstrated by normalization of heart rate, arterial blood pressure, CVP, and urine output.

Crystalloid solutions are used most commonly as the primary fluid for acute intravascular volume expansion. Care must be taken to titrate the total amount of fluid volume needed to reach the physiologic end point to avoid the development of pulmonary edema. A concern with the use of isotonic fluids is the large volume often required for resuscitation. Only about 25% of the volume administered remains in the vascular space 1 hour after administration. The suggested shock volume of crystalloid for a dog is 90 ml/kg/hr. A convenient way of administering this fluid is to divide the total dose into four equal volumes or one-fourth shock doses. A quick rule of thumb is to take the dog's body weight in pounds and add a zero. This volume is the one-fourth shock dose. For example, a 40-lb dog would have a one-fourth shock dose of 400 ml of crystalloid. This dose of fluid is given over one fourth of the time frame, or 15 minutes. The patient is then reassessed, and if more fluid is required, another one-fourth dose is administered. In 1 hour 1600 ml would be given (4 × 400). Using the standard formula of 90 ml/kg/hr the dose of fluid would have been 1800 ml (20 kg × 90 ml). So the quick rule is very close to the calculated volume.

A similar formula can be used for shock doses of fluids in the cat. Most cats are 10 lb, or 5 kg. The shock dose of fluids for the cat is 45 ml/kg/hr. This means that taking the body weight of the cat in kilograms and adding a zero gives the one-fourth shock dose. For example, a 5-kg cat would receive 50 ml as the one-fourth shock dose over 15 minutes. Four doses of 50 ml will equal 200 ml in 1 hour. Using the formula of 45 ml/kg/hr the fluid volume would be 225 ml (45 × 5). Again, this quick rule is very close to the calculated amount of fluid required.

IV colloid solutions are composed of larger molecules that provide oncotic pressure and remain in the vascular space for a prolonged period of time compared with crystalloids. Commonly used synthetic colloids include hetastarch and dextrans. These products are administered at a rate of 20 ml/kg/24 hr but can be administered to effect during shock therapy.

After an acute massive blood loss, red blood cell transfusions are indicated for restoration of the oxygen-carrying capacity of the blood. The development of blood component therapy has made it possible to reduce the number of whole blood transfusions. Component therapy consists of fractionation of whole blood at the time of collection into red blood cells (packed red blood cell unit), platelets (platelet-rich plasma), and plasma.

Autotransfusion, which is the collection of the patient's blood from a body cavity (abdomen or thorax) and its readministration, is an accepted resuscitative measure in trauma and emergency patients. Hemoglobin-based oxygen carriers, such as Oxyglobin, are also useful for fluid resuscitation.

Pharmacologic agents such as vasoactive drugs are frequently required because of either myocardial depression or persistent hypotension after fluid resuscitation efforts. Dobutamine is a $beta_1/beta_2$-adrenergic agent that has inotropic and vasodilatory properties and is used to augment cardiac output when persistent evidence of hypotension exists. Dopamine administered at low dosages improves renal blood flow in patients with reduced urine output. At higher dosages, dopamine improves contractility and increases cardiac output and peripheral vascular resistance, causing renal and mesenteric arterial vasoconstriction.

CARDIOPULMONARY RESUSCITATION (CPR)

Chaos often surrounds initial attempts at CPR. A prompt and well-directed resuscitative effort is critical to achieve adequate cardiopulmonary function. Many authors now refer to CPR as CPCR, which is cardiopulmonary cerebral resuscitation. Resuscitative equipment should be close at hand; there should be established protocols and a predetermined team. One person must be in charge of the resuscitation team. This person should integrate all pertinent information and establish priorities for response. The team leader should monitor the ECG, order therapeutics, and direct the actions of the team members but not be distracted from the leadership role by performing procedures.

Advance Directives

Advance directives refer to discussions with the pet owner before a medical catastrophe. This is a venue for discussing what life-saving procedures should be performed in the event of a medical emergency. In other words, does the pet owner want CPR performed on the pet if cardiopulmonary arrest occurs. The reason this is so important is that some patients may have irreversible underlying disease or disease that carries a poor prognosis. These pets are generally not good candidates for resuscitation. With the still extremely low rates of resuscitation in dogs and cats (<10%), these factors should be discussed with the pet owner before a medical emergency if at all possible. The veterinary technician often is involved in these discussions. The goal of these discussions is to provide the pet owner with the most accurate and current information concerning the disease, the prognosis, and the emergency procedures that may be required. The pet owner can then make an educated and well-informed decision.

ABCs of Basic Cardiac Life Support

The main purpose of basic cardiac life support is to maintain organ function by promoting perfusion of the two major organs: the brain and heart. Cerebral perfusion and coronary artery perfusion are the priority during resuscitation.

Several conditions are considered life threatening, but three in particular require immediate attention: respiratory arrest, circulatory failure, and severe bleeding. Respiratory arrest or circulatory failure can set off a chain of events that will lead to death. Severe uncontrolled bleeding can lead to an irreversible state of shock in which death is inevitable. Thus first aid priorities that demand rapid and accurate assessment can be grouped as those that restrict airway, breathing, and circulation (cardiovascular to include bleeding)—after which other injuries may be addressed. The *ABCs* refer to the following:

Airway
Breathing
Circulation

> ### Technician Note
>
> The first priority in resuscitation is to maintain a patent airway.

Airway

Any interference with breathing produces oxygen depletion (hypoxia) throughout the body. Therefore the first priority is to ensure there is a patent airway and maintain its patency. The technician must be able to objectively assess the airway during examination of the patient. A partial obstruction can become a complete airway obstruction, resulting in unconsciousness and respiratory arrest. Total or partial airway obstruction may occur because of a foreign body (bone, meat chunk, ball, stick), large blood clots, vomitus, thick saliva, or direct trauma to the larynx or trachea causing hemorrhage or spasm. During the summer months, some dogs may develop laryngeal edema from overexertion and heat-induced illness.

Signs that indicate a partially obstructed airway are difficulty breathing on inspiration, exaggerated airway sounds (usually by this time 75% of the airway is compromised), accessory muscles of the face and neck being used, and eventually cyanosis.

First aid measures in the animal with a partially obstructed airway consist of removal of any visible object from the mouth that may be causing the obstruction. Precautions should be taken to avoid being bitten by the animal. Remember partial obstructions can turn into total obstructions. As the animal struggles for more air, it becomes more distressed and may be nonresponsive to commands, even from the owner. If the type of material causing the obstruction is known or suspected, the rescuer can attempt to dislodge the object via abdominal thrust compressions similar to those used in the Heimlich maneuver in humans. It is important that these patients be

taken to the closest veterinarian immediately. Clinical signs observed in animals with total airway obstruction include lack of airway sounds, loss of consciousness, cyanosis, and no movement of the chest wall. First aid measures to consider in these patients, especially the unconscious patients, include the following:

1. Maintain the animal in a horizontal position. Elevation of the head in a hypotensive animal may decrease blood flow to the brain and can precipitate cardiopulmonary arrest.
2. Open the animal's mouth, pull the tongue forward, and extend the neck. If an obstruction is suspected, perform a finger sweep (insert index finger down the side of the cheeks and into the back of the throat to the base of the tongue; then "sweep" across the back of the throat in a hooking action to dislodge the obstruction). If the airway is thought to be clear, attempts should be made to perform rescue breathing by performing mouth-to-mouth and mouth-to-nose breathing or using a mask with an Ambu bag or anesthetic machine with a rebreathing bag. If air can be forced into the lungs, the rescue breathing should continue until tracheal intubation can be performed. If one is unable to inflate the lungs, the head, neck, and tongue should be repositioned and another attempt made to ventilate the patient. If ventilation still cannot be accomplished, a laryngeal examination and tracheal intubation should be performed. Mechanical or manual suction may be needed to clear blood, saliva, or vomitus from the airway. If a foreign body is observed, it should be removed either by a finger sweep or with the use of instruments (see Figure 28-8). If instruments are not available and the foreign body cannot be removed using the finger sweep, perform 5 to 10 abdominal (subdiaphragmatic) thrusts to aid in moving forward the object.
3. Once the object has been removed, the rescuer may have to provide artificial breathing. If the animal regains consciousness, it may still be necessary to provide artificial breathing because of secondary neurologic dysfunction or pulmonary edema that can occur as a result of hypoxemia. The patient should be observed closely for secondary consequences of severe airway obstruction. A veterinarian should assess the patient to determine whether any conditions developed because of hypoxia or an injury occurred secondary to the laryngeal obstruction (e.g., lacerations or swelling from the foreign body).

Breathing

Breathing consists of two separate acts: inhalation, in which the chest cavity is expanded so air flows into the lungs, and exhalation, in which the size of the chest cavity is decreased so air is driven out. The diaphragm provides most of the energy for the mechanics of inspiration, and exhalation is normally passive.

PROVIDING ARTIFICIAL VENTILATION (RESCUE BREATHING).   An animal can stop breathing for many reasons, including electrical shock injury, drowning, airway obstruction, head trauma, congestive heart failure, severe hypovolemic shock, various toxicities, pulmonary thromboembolism, and other lung diseases.

When there is absence of respiration, the rescuer should begin artificial ventilation. If at all possible having two or three people to help resuscitation is ideal. If outside of the hospital environment, the technician can start mouth-to-

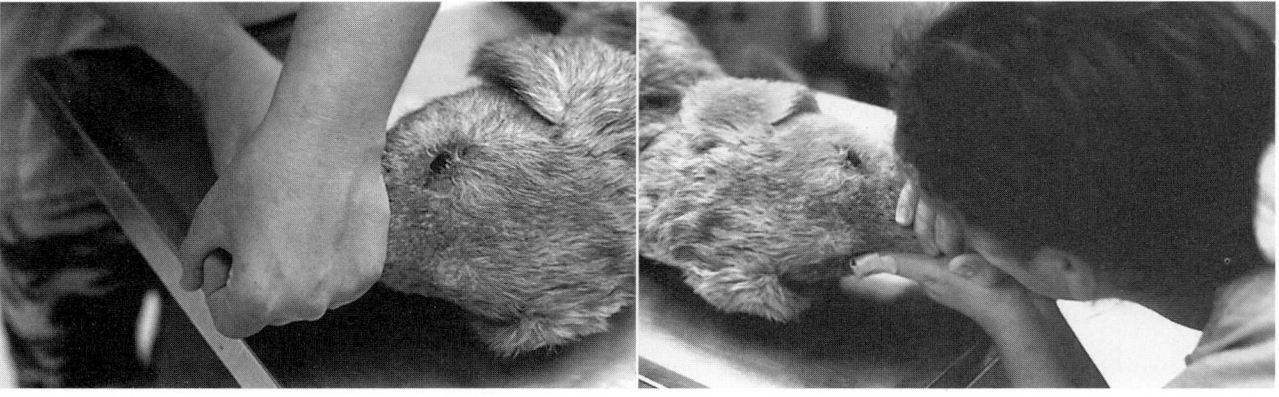

FIGURE 28-14. The hand can be used to form a seal when performing mouth-to-mouth or mouth-to-mouth and nose resuscitation.

mouth or mouth-to-nose rescue breathing. This can be accomplished by extending the animal's neck, pulling the tongue out, and closing the mouth to allow the incisors to hold the tongue and not allow it to move back into the mouth and obstruct the airway. Breathing is started by placing the mouth over the animal's nose or nose and mouth and blowing in air (Figure 28-14). Provide the animal with two breaths while watching for the animal's chest to rise and fall and see if spontaneous breathing begins. If there is no response then continue breathing at a rate of 12 to 20 breaths/min.

In a hospital setting, if an animal is found in respiratory arrest, the airway should be checked for patency as discussed previously, and if clear the animal should be immediately intubated with an endotracheal tube. Breathing can then be accomplished by Ambu bag (Figure 28-15) or anesthesia machine and rebreathing bag. In some cases of respiratory arrest, the use of acupuncture to stimulate respiration has been suggested. The Jen Chung (GV26) maneuver may be used by using a 25-gauge needle at the nasal philtrum (Figure 28-16).

 Technician Note

The use of clear plastic endotracheal tubes allows visualization of fluid or exudate from the trachea or lungs.

It is recommended to use clear plastic ET tubes with inflatable cuffs that are high volume and low pressure. A clear tube allows visualization of any fluid or exudate from the trachea or lungs. A high-volume, low-pressure cuff helps reduce the incidence of pressure necrosis of the trachea when the tube is maintained for extended periods.

During assessment of breathing the technician must evaluate for the presence of a pulse or heartbeat. The lack of pulse or heartbeat suggests cardiopulmonary arrest, and the technician must move on to "C," or circulation.

If the arrest is of pulmonary origin and the heart is still beating but at a very slow rate, initial ventilations may be sufficient to reestablish breathing and increase heart rate. If the patient continues to breath on its own, supplemental oxygen should be provided via nasal cannula, via oxygen canopy, or transtracheally. It is very important to observe the patient's respiratory pattern. If it is unusually slow, shallow, or unstable, continued ventilatory support may be required.

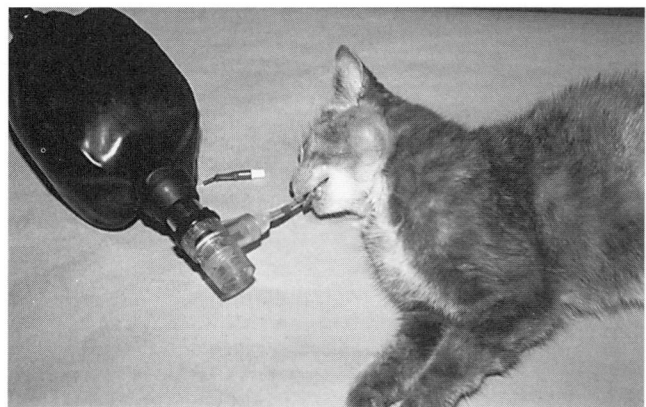

FIGURE 28-15. Ambu bag ventilation allows the operator to evaluate airway inflation resistance and lung compliance.

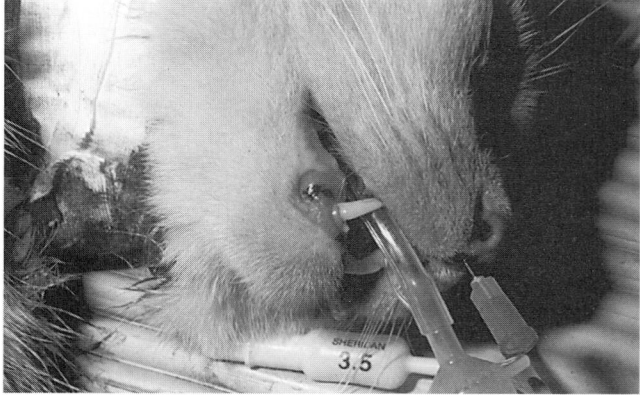

FIGURE 28-16. The Jen Chung acupuncture point can be used during respiratory arrest.

Patients with respiratory arrest should be intubated in lateral or dorsal recumbency to avoid manipulation of the head or neck in cases of hypotension or cervical/head trauma. Using 100% oxygen, ventilate and ensure the lungs expand well. Use a stethoscope to listen for bilateral lung sounds while the patient is being ventilated. Failure to hear lung sounds bilaterally can indicate ET tube placement in one side of the main pulmonary tree or unilateral pleural space disease. If a manometer is available, ventilation should achieve inspiratory pressures of 20 cm H_2O in the dog and 10 to 15 cm H_2O in the cat. Patients with suspected pleural space or lung parenchymal disease will require greater inspiratory pressures. Overzealous inflation of the lungs may interfere with venous return and cause damage to the pulmonary tree, leading to pneumothorax. In the absence of a manometer, provide sufficient inspiratory pressure so that movement of the chest wall can be visualized. When attempts to ventilate are met with increasing resistance, one should suspect pneumothorax, and thoracentesis should be performed. In the majority of cases in veterinary medicine, respiratory arrest is the principal inciting factor that leads to cardiac arrest. One exception may be the Doberman pinscher, which has been observed to have sudden onsets of ventricular fibrillation before respiratory arrest. Another exception is an animal that undergoes a vasovagal reflex with sudden cardiac arrest caused by vagus nerve stimulation. This is most commonly observed in animals after or in conjunction with micturition, defecation, vomiting, or another manipulation that can stimulate parasympathetic nerve discharge in the face of ongoing sympathetic responses, such as that seen postoperatively or posttraumatically. The vasovagal reflex is more likely to occur in animals that are hypoxemic and acidemic. In debilitated and older animals, a vasovagally induced arrest may also occur with insertion of the rectal thermometer or laryngeal manipulation during endotracheal intubation.

The patient with a total upper airway obstruction should have a tracheostomy performed to allow effective ventilation. In the patient with a partial airway obstruction, emergency aid can be delivered by insufflation of oxygen via a large-bore needle or catheter puncture at the cricothyroid membrane, providing adequate oxygenation until a more definitive airway is established. During CPR, ventilation should normalize arterial pH and provide adequate oxygenation. The cornerstone of pH correction is adequate ventilation, not sodium bicarbonate administration. Venous blood gases can be used to assess the effectiveness of the compressions. High Pco_2 is seen with poor blood flow generation. End-tidal CO_2 monitoring can also be used to determine effectiveness. A value of more than 12 mm Hg has been associated with increased brain survival in experimental studies. Clinical studies in humans seem to substantiate this.

Circulation/Cardiac Compression

Cardiopulmonary arrest can be defined as the cessation of functional ventilation (breathing) and effective circulation. For example, during shock, as the victim's condition progressively worsens, the brain and heart begin to decompensate. Reduced blood flow to the heart muscle (coronary blood flow) leads to damage of the heart muscle, resulting in heart failure (myocardial failure). The resulting reduced blood flow to the brain causes depression of respiratory and cardiovascular centers that control heart rate and respiratory rate. During this stage, the blood vessels dilate in the muscles, skin, and abdominal organs, causing blood to pool in these tissues. All these alterations feed a vicious cycle of changes that eventually precipitate cardiopulmonary arrest.

Signs observed in the cardiopulmonary arrest patient are absence of an auscultated or a palpable heartbeat, lack of palpable pulses (from arterial hypotension), apnea (cessation of breathing) or agonal breathing (ineffective breaths taken before death), absence of bleeding even in the

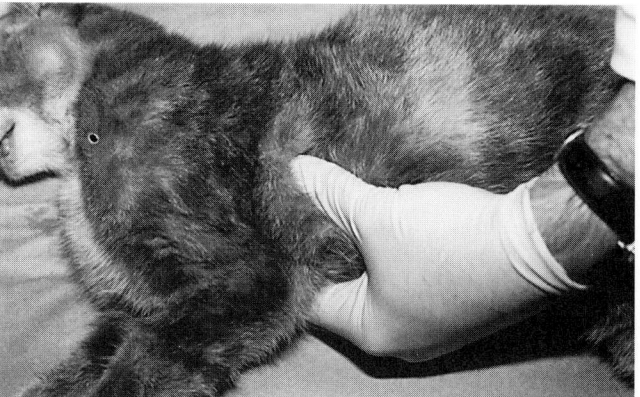

FIGURE 28-17. The cardiac pump mechanism being performed during cardiopulmonary resuscitation (CPR).

presence of a wound or laceration of considerable size (this will occur with blood loss of more than 40% to 55% blood volume), loss of consciousness (10 to 15 seconds after arrest), and pupillary dilation (30 to 45 seconds after arrest).

If the animal has not responded to artificial ventilation and an apex heartbeat or pulse is not detectable, chest compressions must be started in an attempt to improve circulation. Ventilation and compression rates depend on the size of the animal and number of personnel available. One-person CPR is very difficult and often ineffective. If only one person is available, two breaths should be administered and followed by 15 chest compressions. When multiple staff members are available for resuscitation the outcome may be better.

Blood flow during CPR is theorized to occur via two mechanisms: the cardiac pump and thoracic pump. The cardiac pump theory proposes that chest compressions generate positive intraventricular pressure, stimulating cardiac muscles to contract and making the heart valves function to achieve forward blood flow with each compression. The cardiac pump mechanism is utilized by performing chest compression directly over the heart. This can be done one handed or two handed (Figure 28-17) with the animal in lateral recumbency. Unfortunately, in animals weighing more than 7 kg, direct compression of the heart is not very effective because of the large size of the chest and the space taken up by the lung. The thoracic pump theory proposes that the heart serves as a passive conduit for blood flow. Chest compressions create positive intrathoracic pressure, and this pressure is reflected on the giant vessels, leading to coronary and cerebral artery perfusion.

The thoracic pump mechanism is utilized in dogs with body weights more than 7 kg. With this technique, compression of the chest wall is performed with two hands placed on the widest portion of the chest with the animal in right lateral recumbency (Figure 28-18). The chest should be compressed about 30% with each compression.

Ideally this technique requires two people. The second person ventilates the pet via the endotracheal tube at either a 1:1 rate with chest compressions or ventilates with every other compression. This technique is referred to as *simultaneous ventilation compression.* Compressing the thorax against an inflated lung contributes to the increase in intrathoracic pressure.

Binding of the caudal abdomen and rear limbs using bandage materials, towels, or commercially produced MAST (military antishock trousers) was once thought to be

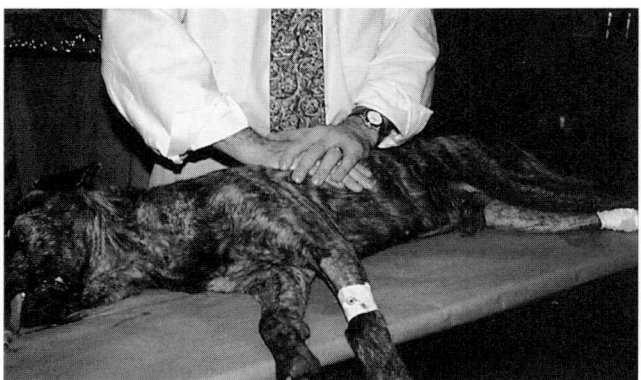

FIGURE 28-18. The thoracic pump mechanism being performed during cardiopulmonary resuscitation (CPR).

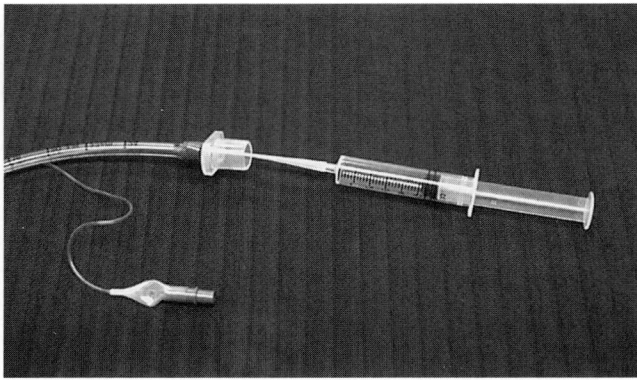

FIGURE 28-19. Intratracheal administration of emergency drugs is performed using a urinary catheter.

beneficial by increasing blood supply to the cranial portion of the body. These procedures are not currently suggested. However, interposed abdominal compressions are currently advocated.

Closed-chest CPR may not be effective, especially in large animals, or it may be precluded because of underlying disease, such as severe chest trauma; thus the emergency team must be prepared to perform an emergency thoracotomy. CPR should continue until one of the following occurs:

- Spontaneous cardiac function returns; a pulse or heartbeat is palpable or auscultated. In the majority of cases, artificial ventilation will be required for a period of time, even though heart function has returned. This is due to the nervous system depression secondary to the arrest.
- The pet owner requests no further resuscitation.
- The primary clinician requests no further resuscitation.

ADVANCED CARDIAC LIFE SUPPORT

The goal of advanced cardiac life support is to intervene with appropriate pharmacologic agents, restore an ECG rhythm, achieve adequate acid-base balance, and diminish neurologic impairment. Advanced cardiac life support begins where basic cardiac life support stops. Where basic cardiac life support has the components A, B, C, advanced cardiac life support has the components D, E, F:

Drugs
ECG
Fibrillation control
Fluid resuscitation

Ideally, four or five individuals should be involved with advanced cardiac life support procedures. It is imperative that participants have predetermined assignments to make the emergency situation less stressful. The team leader makes the decisions and may be involved with invasive techniques such as thoracotomy or vascular access. In animals with circulatory collapse, venous access is often achieved by cut-down or placement of an IO catheter. A second person performs ventilation while a third team member performs thoracic compressions. A fourth person can perform interposed abdominal compressions, and a fifth team member (if available) is there for drug acquisi-

tion and administration as well as to act as a scribe to document all activities during an arrest. CPR log sheets are useful for documentation of CPR protocol (see Figure 28-2).

Drug Administration

The goal of administration of emergency drugs during CPR is to deliver the agent to the myocardium via the coronary vessels as quickly as possible. Oxygen is the first and most important therapeutic agent provided during CPR and should have been addressed during management of the airway and breathing. Cardiopulmonary arrest patients should be intubated and ventilated using a system such as an Ambu bag that is capable of delivering 100% oxygen. In the majority of cases treated for cardiopulmonary arrest, the drugs epinephrine and atropine will be used. It is important to understand how these agents work. All dosages should be checked by at least two team members, at least one being a veterinarian, before administration.

Most cardiopulmonary arrest cases will have an ET tube placed to establish an airway. Specific drugs, including *l*idocaine, *e*pinephrine, *a*tropine, and *n*aloxone, can be administered via an ET tube directly to the pulmonary tree, where they are rapidly absorbed into the circulation. The acronym *LEAN* can be used to remember which agents can be administered through the endotracheal tube. An important point to remember is that the dose of these drugs that would be delivered intravenously should be doubled for endotracheal administration. If there is insufficient volume, the dosage can be diluted with saline. It is easiest to deliver these agents using a syringe and urinary catheter (Figure 28-19).

Other routes of administration during CPR include central IV catheter, IO catheter, and intralingual and peripheral IV catheter. If a central IV catheter is in place before cardiopulmonary arrest, this is the route of choice. In most cases ET tube administration is the primary route used. If underlying disease such as pulmonary edema or pulmonary hemorrhage is present, intratracheal administration is contraindicated. In these cases IO and intralingual routes should be considered. The small volume that can be delivered limits the use of the intralingual route. Peripheral catheters are the least effective route of administration. Intracardiac administration of emergency drugs should not be used because of serious complications that may occur unless open chest CPR is being performed.

Electrocardiography

The ECG allows characterization of any existing arrhythmia and determination of the presence of ventricular fibrillation. The major arrhythmias associated with cardiac arrest include ventricular asystole, ventricular fibrillation, electromechanical dissociation, ventricular tachycardia, and sinus bradycardia. It is important for the veterinary technician to be able to recognize different arrhythmias and have an understanding of what emergency drugs may be utilized. It is also imperative to understand that the ECG is only providing information about electrical activity and not cardiac function.

Ventricular Asystole

Ventricular asystole rhythm is defined as the complete absence of electrical activity and is seen as a flat line on the ECG. The presence of this disturbance suggests significant myocardial ischemia, and the prognosis for resuscitation is poor. Underlying problems, such as hyperkalemia and metabolic acidosis, should be corrected when possible. This is a nonperfusing rhythm, and CPR should be performed and epinephrine and atropine administered.

Ventricular Fibrillation

Ventricular fibrillation rhythm implies disorderly depolarization of the ventricular muscle or myocardium. It may sometimes look like asystole if the amplitude of depolarizations is small. Immediate electrical defibrillation is the treatment of choice for this life-threatening arrhythmia. This arrhythmia is also time dependent. The longer the rhythm persists, the less likely resuscitation will be successful.

Electromechanical Dissociation

Electromechanical dissociation is an arrhythmia characterized by the inability to detect pulsatile activity in response to coordinated ECG complexes. This emphasizes the point that the ECG does not reflect cardiac function. The ECG demonstrates electrical activity but is uncoupled from mechanical contractions of the myocardium. The presence of this arrhythmia indicates a grave prognosis. Treatment includes epinephrine, atropine, and possibly naloxone.

Fibrillation Control or Defibrillation

It is uncommon for most veterinary practices to have an electrical defibrillator. However, this may change with the new incentives in human medicine to increase public access to automated electrical defibrillators. If a defibrillator is present in the hospital it should be used with extreme care and should only be used by the veterinarian unless training on its use has been provided. Doses for defibrillation are published and based on body weight. Only one person should use the defibrillator during CPR. The operator should have dry hands, apply conductive gel to the paddles, and give the command "clear" before delivering the shock. It is the responsibility of the defibrillator operator to make sure all team members are safe before delivering the shock. This means no one can be in contact with the table or patient, including the operator.

Fluid Therapy

Fluid therapy during resuscitation is somewhat controversial. Large volumes of IV fluids should only be administered if the suspected predisposing disease would have required this therapy. During the arrest, fluids should be given to effect based on the clinical response of the patient. The use of crystalloids, colloids, blood products, and hemoglobin-based oxygen carriers (Oxyglobin) may be indicated.

PROLONGED CARDIAC LIFE SUPPORT OR POSTRESUSCITATIVE CARE

Once resuscitation has been successful, it is important to maintain diligent monitoring and continued supportive care. Mechanical ventilation is often required if effective spontaneous ventilation is not present. Treatment for alterations in intracranial pressure may be addressed using mannitol and furosemide. Mannitol is also considered an oxygen free radical scavenger and may be useful in management of reperfusion injury. The value of free radical scavenger therapy in this situation is not completely understood. Other long-term considerations should include nutritional support via enteral tube feeding or total parenteral nutrition until the animal recovers and is able to eat by mouth.

Continued monitoring should include but is not limited to serial measurement of pulse, respiration, body temperature, CRT, arterial blood pressure, CVP, body weight, arterial blood gas, venous blood gas, electrocardiography, serum chemistry analysis (especially electrolytes, BUN, and creatinine), urine output, and neurologic status.

Special Procedures

Although the veterinary technician will not be performing an emergency thoracotomy or aortic compression to increase blood flow to the heart and brain during CPR, it is recommended that these procedures still be understood. In many veterinary emergency centers, technicians are part of the team performing open-chest and aortic compression or cross clamping. They also are expected to be able to assist in the procedure and perform cardiac compressions.

SUMMARY

Emergency nursing is a vital component of veterinary emergency care. The quality of care provided and the monitoring of patients often depend on the quality of nursing care. The veterinary technician is a part of a team where each member's knowledge and skill become synergistic with the other team members. This is the prime example where the team functions more effectively than any given team member. Veterinary medicine in general and emergency medicine specifically rely on the training and the dedication of the technician to keep patients pain free and to save lives.

RECOMMENDED READING

Battaglia AM: *Small animal emergency and critical care: a manual for the veterinary technician*, Philadelphia, 2001, WB Saunders.

Bistner SI, Ford RB: *Kirk and Bistner's handbook of veterinary procedures and emergency treatment*, Philadelphia, 1995, WB Saunders.

Crow SE, Walshaw SO: *Manual of clinical procedures in the dog, cat and rabbit*, Philadelphia, 1997, Lippincott Raven.

Kirby R: *Small animal emergency and critical care medicine*, Ames, 1998, Iowa State University Press.

Mathews KA: *Veterinary emergency and critical care manual*, Ontario, Canada, 1996, Lifelearn.

Murtaugh RJ, Kaplan PM: *Veterinary emergency and critical care medicine*, St Louis, 1992, Mosby.

Plunkett SJ: *Emergency procedures for the small animal veterinarian*, Philadelphia, 2001, WB Saunders.

Wingfield WE: *Veterinary emergency medicine secrets*, Philadelphia, 2001, Hanley & Belfus.

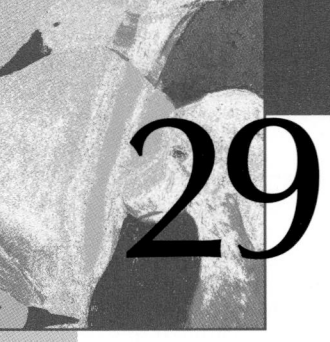

29

Veterinary Dentistry

Ashley B. Oakes

Every pet with teeth will need dental care at some point in its lifetime. Whether the pet mouse, snake, or horse will receive the quality of care dogs and cats now receive remains to be seen. As dental home care products continue to improve, clients have more options available to provide dental care for their pets. It is not uncommon to find photographs in veterinary and dental literature of exotic animals such as killer whales, dolphins, and sea lions opening wide for dental care. Preventive dentistry (tooth brushing, dental cleanings) is important to maintain good health and quality of life in pets just as it is for humans. Most family veterinary offices provide routine professional dental cleanings for their patients. Some practices also provide advanced dental care, such as endodontics, exodontics, and periodontal treatments. Dental radiography has a place in every veterinary practice that examines and cleans teeth. Veterinary technicians play an important role in providing these dental services to the client's pets. It is important that the dental technician or veterinary dental assistant have a good understanding of the different dental problems and treatment options available for these problems.

This chapter provides a detailed discussion of periodontal disease and its prevention with proper diet, routine professional dental cleanings, and dental home care. Because veterinary technicians often perform dental scaling and polishing procedures, it is important to have a good understanding of the necessary equipment and its proper use and care. Dental radiology is extremely beneficial in veterinary medicine because patients often do not show obvious signs of dental pain. Veterinary personnel must examine the teeth closely and radiograph teeth with abnormalities or use periodic survey films. The procedures for taking diagnostic dental radiographs are covered. The remainder of the chapter addresses the specialty branches endodontics, exodontics, orthodontics, and restorative dentistry.

ETHICAL AND LEGAL ASPECTS

The level of dental care a veterinary technician can provide varies from state to state, and the rules for the particular state in which a person is working need to be reviewed before providing dental care. The American Veterinary Dental College (AVDC) published a position statement in the *Journal of the American Veterinary Medical Association* (vol. 213, no. 5, September 1, 1998) regarding veterinary dental heath care providers. The purpose of this statement was to develop a means to safeguard veterinary dental patients and ensure the qualifications of persons performing veterinary dental procedures. The AVDC considers it appropriate for the veterinarian to delegate maintenance dental care and certain dental tasks to veterinary technicians.

Tasks appropriately performed by veterinary technicians include dental prophylaxis and certain procedures that do not result in alterations in the shape, structure, or positional location of teeth in the dental arch. A veterinarian may direct a technician to perform these tasks providing the veterinarian is physically present and supervising the treatment and providing the technician has received appropriate training.

The AVDC supports advanced training of veterinary technicians to perform additional ancillary dental services (e.g., taking impressions, making models, charting veterinary dental lesions, taking and developing dental radiographs, performing nonsurgical subgingival root scaling and debridement) providing that they do not alter the structure of the tooth.

The AVDC supports appropriate training of veterinary assistants (not registered, certified, or licensed) to perform the following dental services: supragingival scaling and polishing, taking and developing dental radiographs, taking impressions, and making models.

The American Society for Veterinary Dental Technicians (ASVDT) was established in 1994. This organization currently has 900 to 1000 members who have taken and passed a self-taught home study video and workbook course. All veterinary staff personnel are eligible to take the examination (i.e., veterinary technicians, veterinary assistants, veterinarians, receptionists, kennel workers). The purpose of the course is to improve the individual's dental knowledge to better serve clients and their pets. To find out more about the ASVDT contact Mr. Gerry Selin at (800) 613-3647.

PERIODONTICS AND PERIODONTAL DISEASE

Periodontics is the branch of dentistry concerned with the study and treatment of the periodontium. The periodontium is composed of the supporting structures of the tooth. These supporting structures are the *gingiva*, periodontal ligament, alveolar and supporting bone (tooth socket), and the cementum of the tooth root (Figure 29-1). Healthy *gingiva* has a sharp, tapered edge (margin) that lies closely against the crown of the tooth (Figure 29-2). The free gingiva forms a moat around the tooth called the *gingival sulcus*. The epithelial attachment of the gingiva to the cementum of the tooth root forms the bottom extent of the gingival sulcus. The depth of this sulcus ranges from 1 to 3 mm in a healthy mouth of a dog and is up to 1 mm deep in the cat.

Periodontitis means inflammation of the structures around the tooth (Greek *peri*, around + *odous*, tooth + *it is*, inflammation). It is the most common disease of animals and humans and is caused by plaque. Approximately 80% of dogs and 70% of cats have some form of periodontal disease by 3 years of age.

Plaque is a white, slippery film that collects around the gingival sulcus of the tooth. It is composed of bacteria, food debris, exfoliated cells, and salivary glycoproteins. Over time, plaque will mineralize on the teeth to form dental calculus, a brown or yellow deposit (Figure 29-3). As the plaque collects around the tooth, it damages the gingival tissues by releasing bacterial endotoxins. The animal's immune system further damages these tissues through the release of harmful byproducts from white blood cells as they attempt to destroy the bacteria. In the

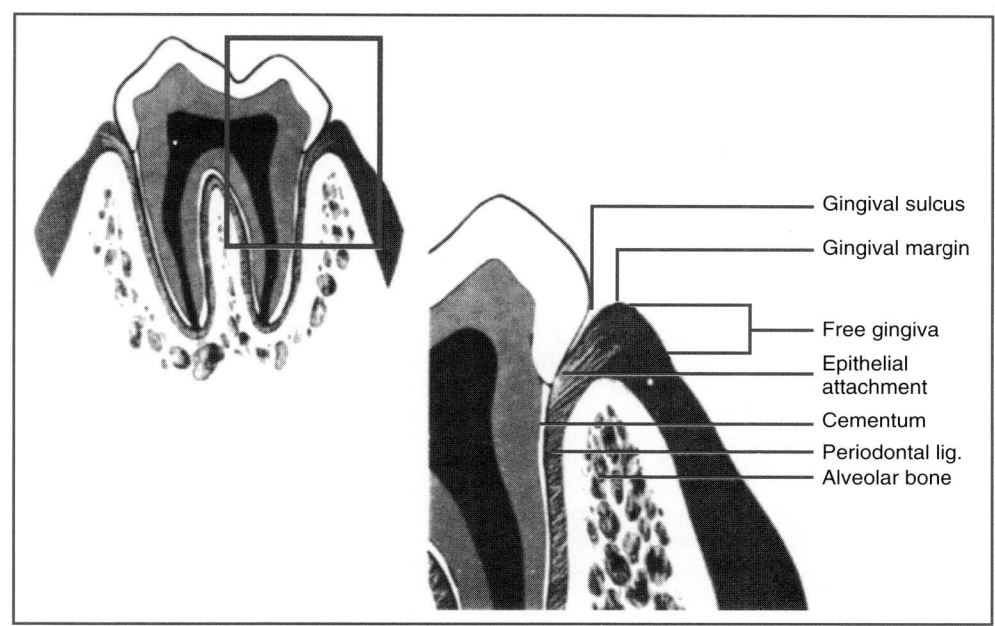

Gingival sulcus
Gingival margin
Free gingiva
Epithelial attachment
Cementum
Periodontal lig.
Alveolar bone

FIGURE 29-1. Structures collectively referred to as the periodontium. The tooth is suspended in the socket by the periodontal ligament. (From Bojrab MJ, Tholen M: *Small animal oral medicine and surgery,* Philadelphia, 1990, Lea & Febiger.)

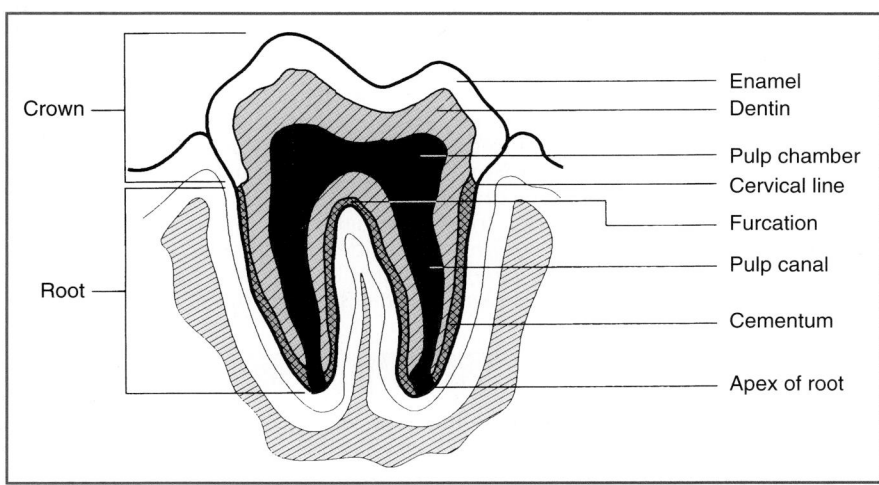

Crown

Root

Enamel
Dentin
Pulp chamber
Cervical line
Furcation
Pulp canal
Cementum
Apex of root

FIGURE 29-2. Typical external and internal gross anatomy of a tooth. The model is a premolar. (From Bojrab MJ, Tholen M: *Small animal oral medicine and surgery,* Philadelphia, 1990, Lea & Febiger.)

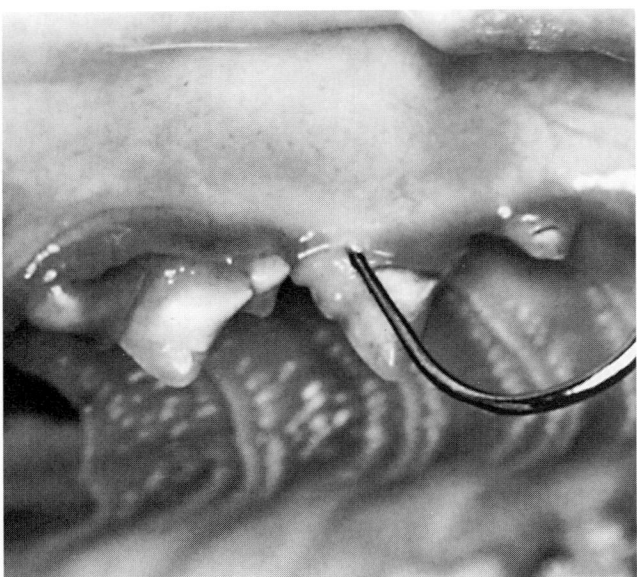

FIGURE 29-3. The calculus and plaque deposits on these teeth have caused the gingiva to become inflamed (gingivitis). A dental explorer is used to detect subgingival (under the gingiva) calculus or dental abnormalities.

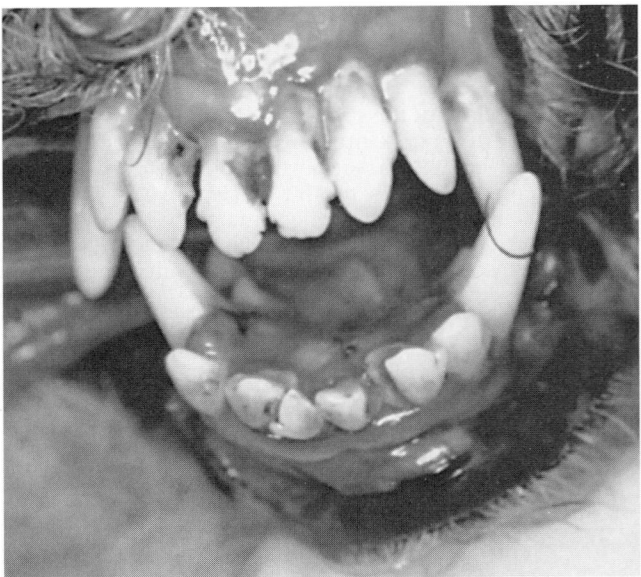

FIGURE 29-4. Periodontal disease has destroyed a significant portion of the alveolar bone and periodontal ligament of these incisor teeth. The gingiva has receded from the crowns of these teeth, and the tooth roots are now exposed.

early stages, the *gingiva* becomes inflamed and bleeds easily. This stage is called *gingivitis* (Figure 29-3). As the disease progresses and destruction of the periodontium begins to occur (e.g., loss of alveolar bone, periodontal ligament, and gingiva), an irreversible stage of disease begins that is termed *periodontitis* (Figure 29-4).

 Technician Note

The key to prevention of periodontal disease is to minimize plaque accumulation by means of proper diet, routine professional dental scaling and polishing, and daily teeth brushing or mouth rinsing.

Periodontal disease is difficult to control once it has developed. For this reason, great emphasis must be placed on its prevention. Many diseases can contribute to the severity of periodontal disease, but the bacteria in plaque are believed to be the primary cause.

When periodontitis is already present, destruction of the periodontal tissues has begun and will continue if not treated. Once the periodontal ligaments are destroyed, they are extremely difficult to replace. As the tooth begins to lose its periodontal tissue, it becomes more susceptible to plaque accumulation in the deep periodontal pockets that form around the tooth root or roots. When the tooth loses a significant portion of its periodontium, it becomes mobile (loose) and will eventually fall out. This is nature's way of clearing the infection from the body. The infection, however, is usually present for months to years before the tooth is eventually lost. During this time, the bacteria can gain entrance to the animal's bloodstream and become systemic, spreading to numerous organs such as the liver, kidney, heart, and lungs.

For patients with periodontal disease, the treatment goal is to remove the plaque and calculus from the teeth and to minimize plaque reattachment. Treatments to minimize plaque accumulation include those listed for prevention of periodontal disease, as well as periodontal surgery when deep periodontal pockets have formed around tooth roots.

Root planing and subgingival curettage are important procedures in periodontal treatment. *Root planing* is the removal of calculus and necrotic cementum from the diseased tooth roots (Figure 29-5). The root surface must be thoroughly cleaned before healing can occur. Curettes are used to clean the root surface using multiple overlapping strokes in vertical, horizontal, and oblique directions until the root surface is as smooth as glass. Pressure created with each stroke ranges from firm to light as the tooth root is cleaned. Care must be taken not to gouge the root surface. The gingiva covering these roots must be cleaned of foreign debris and granulation tissue as well. This procedure is called *subgingival curettage*, and curettes are used for this procedure too. The blade of the curette is directed toward the pocket lining, and digital pressure is placed on the gingival tissue to support it while the tissue is debrided.

Subgingival curettage and root planing can be done without incising and elevating the gingival tissue as long as there is sufficient access to the roots and gingival pocket epithelium to thoroughly debride the area. This process is called *closed root planing*. If the gingiva impedes proper cleaning of the tooth roots, the gingiva should be incised and reflected to allow visualization and instrumentation of the roots for proper debridement. This technique is termed *open root planing* and must be performed by a veterinarian or dentist under the direct supervision of a veterinarian.

Technician Note

If the gingiva impedes proper cleaning of the tooth roots, the gingiva should be incised and reflected to allow visualization and instrumentation of the roots for proper debridement. This technique is termed *open root planing*.

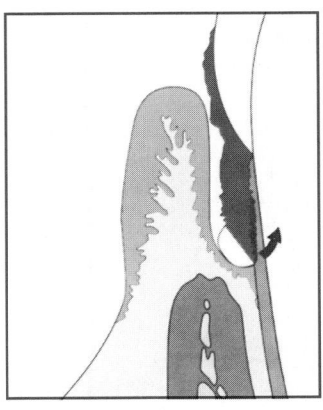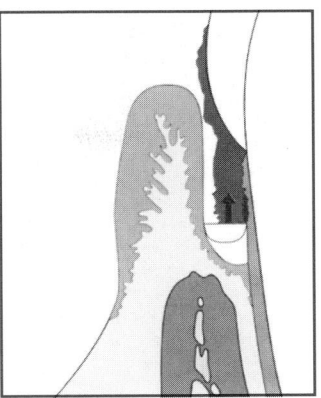

FIGURE 29-5. Root planing. *Left,* The curette is inserted into the pocket with its curved back against the epithelium. It is turned to engage the cutting edge into the necrotic cementum and debris. *Right,* The curette is withdrawn, removing the subgingival debris and necrotic cementum and scraping the pocket epithelium. (From Emily P, Penman S: *Handbook of small animal dentistry,* ed 2, Oxford, England, 1994, Pergamon Press Ltd.)

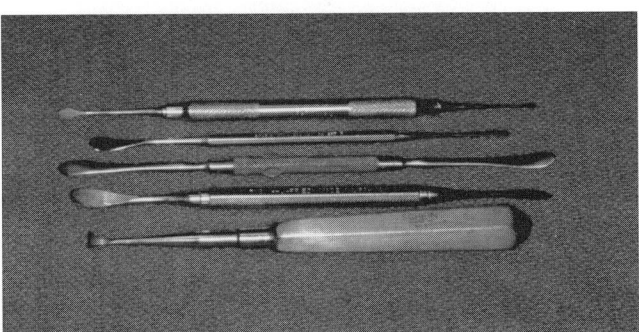

FIGURE 29-6. Periosteal elevators. *Top to bottom,* Cislak Ex-9, Schein no. 7, Freer, Molt no. 9, Schein ST 7.

Several types of gingival flap procedures are used to expose the diseased tooth roots. The instruments required to create the gingival flaps are a scalpel blade (no. 11 or 15) and handle as well as a periosteal elevator. Small elevators, such as the Cislak EX-9, are commonly used for single teeth or small surgery sites. Larger periosteal elevators, such as the Schein ST 7 or Molt 9, are used for larger teeth and/or surgery sites (Figure 29-6). Once the roots and pocket lining are exposed and debrided with an ultrasonic scaler and curette the surgery site is lavaged with 0.2% chlorhexidine followed by sterile saline. The tissue is reapposed with 4-0 absorbable suture material placed interdentally in a simple interrupted pattern and digital pressure is applied to the gingiva for 60 seconds. The patient should be placed on a soft food diet for 1 week and have the mouth rinsed daily with a 0.2% chlorhexidine solution for 2 weeks. The owner should start brushing the teeth 1 week postoperatively and be very gentle around the surgery site.

A grading system is helpful to categorize periodontal disease and determine appropriate treatment. Grade I periodontal disease is a reversible gingivitis and requires routine dental cleaning. Grade II periodontal disease is an early form of periodontitis. There is some attachment loss (approximately 1 to 2 mm), and root planing or subgingival curettage may be required. Grade III periodontal disease is considered a moderate degree of periodontitis; attachment loss is in the range of 3 to 6 mm and root planing, subgingival curettage, and periodontal surgery are often required. These teeth have a fair to guarded prognosis. Grade IV periodontal disease is severe periodontitis; attachment loss is greater than 6 mm, and the tooth has a poor prognosis. Many of these teeth are extracted. Efforts to save these teeth require root planing, subgingival curettage,

periodontal surgery, and possibly periodontal splinting. (The attachment losses mentioned above apply to dogs, not cats.)

Loose teeth can be stabilized by splinting them to adjacent teeth to prevent their loss while the periodontium is healing. A thorough dental cleaning with radiographs, root planing, and subgingival curettage must be performed before splinting the loose teeth. Splinting is performed only if the pet owner is willing to provide dental home care and have the teeth professionally cleaned as needed. If the owner does not properly clean the splints and teeth, the splints will retain foreign debris and worsen the condition. Pets with advanced periodontal disease may require professional dental cleaning every 3 to 4 months.

Proper Diet

The semimoist and canned pet foods are tacky and tend to stick to the teeth. This accelerates plaque accumulation.

> **Technician Note**
>
> Dry pet food is the diet of choice for minimizing the rate of plaque accumulation on the dentition. Hill's t/d is a prescription diet specifically developed to remove dental calculus.

Tartar control pet products have entered the marketplace. The active ingredients are sodium hexametaphosphate (HMP) and sodium tripolyphosphate. The tartar control products work by sequestering the calcium in plaque fluids to reduce calculus formation. Research studies on dogs and cats have shown that these products can reduce calculus up to 46% in dogs and 30% in cats.

Hill's Pet Nutrition has produced a pet food called t/d that is nutritionally balanced and designed to help minimize calculus buildup. The t/d biscuit fibers are longer than traditional fibers and are primarily oriented in one direction to keep the biscuit from crumbling readily when the dog or cat bites into it. This design allows the biscuit to mechanically scrape the sides of the teeth clean as the teeth penetrate the biscuit.

Proper chew toys should be encouraged. Rawhide bones and chews are excellent for exercising the teeth and periodontium to help maintain a healthy mouth. Some pets have a desire to chew on hard objects such as rocks. Hard objects can damage the teeth and should be removed from the pet's environment when possible. Any chew toy has the potential to cause damage so the owner should monitor the pet while using these items.

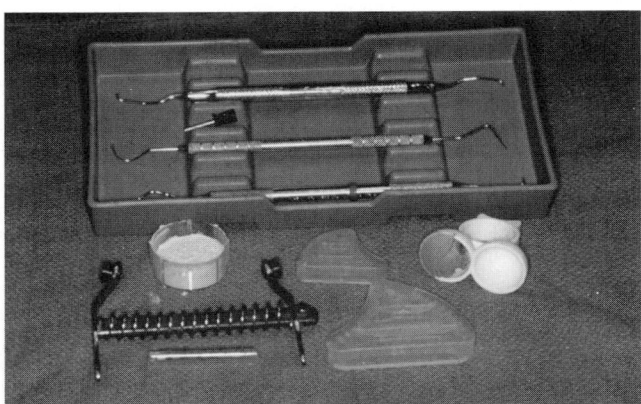

FIGURE 29-7. Dental cleaning tray (subgingival curette, explorer and periodontal probe, supragingival curette, prophy cup), prophy paste in ring, variety of mouth gags, flour pumice.

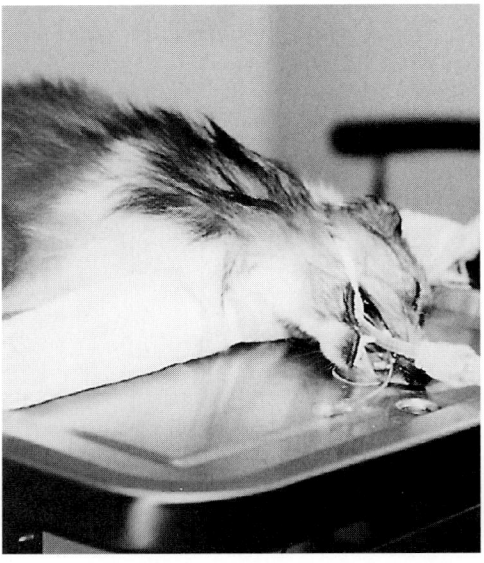

FIGURE 29-8. Proper patient positioning for dental scaling and polishing. Note that the head is placed in a downward position.

Dental Scaling and Polishing

Before beginning the dental cleaning procedure, the dental treatment area should be prepared. The proper instruments should be out for easy access, and they should be clean and sharp (Figure 29-7). The patient should be examined by the veterinarian before anesthesia for bacterial infection of the periodontium. When oral infection is present, preoperative antibiotics should be given to help prevent the systemic spread of oral bacteria to internal organs. Patients with moderate or advanced periodontal disease should begin antibiotic treatment at least 3 days before the dental cleaning procedure.

The patient is anesthetized, and a cuffed endotracheal tube is used to prevent water and foreign debris from entering the trachea. Care should be taken not to overinflate the endotracheal tube cuff, which could damage the trachea. In 1994 the American Veterinary Medical Association Professional Liability Insurance Trust received 18 claims on pets (all cats) diagnosed with subcutaneous emphysema following an anesthetic procedure. All cases were intubated, and 16 patients were under anesthesia for dentistries. The cause of the subcutaneous emphysema was not confirmed in every case, but tracheal tears were found in some of the cases. To avoid injury to the trachea, disconnect the animals from the anesthesia circuit when repositioning them, minimize movement of the endotracheal tube, and inflate the cuff just enough to stop the leak of anesthetic gases.

 Technician Note

To avoid injury to the trachea, disconnect the patient from the anesthesia circuit when repositioning is needed, minimize movement of the endotracheal tube, and inflate the cuff just enough to stop the leak of anesthetic gases.

The patient's head should be placed on a slight incline (nose downward) if possible. This can be done by tilting a surgery table or placing a rolled towel under the animal's neck to ensure that the pharynx is higher than the nose (Figure 29-8). This allows water and debris to run out of the mouth while mechanical scalers are being used.

Once the anesthetized patient is prepared, the technician should don the proper attire and begin the dental cleaning. Proper attire consists of a mask, gloves, eye protection (glasses or a shield), cap, and laboratory coat. It is important to wear these protective coverings because large numbers of bacteria are aerosolized during the mechanical scaling procedure, and these could be inhaled or could saturate clothing, leading to contamination of other areas in the hospital.

The dental cleaning begins with a thorough examination of the oral cavity. The mouth is propped open, and the cheeks and tongue are lifted to evaluate all areas of the mouth thoroughly. Do not forget to examine the tongue, tonsils, and pharynx as well. Just before beginning the oral examination a chlorhexidine rinse can be given to the oral cavity to decrease the bacterial load substantially. This increases safety for the pet and dental care provider. Clinical findings should be recorded at either the beginning or the end of the procedure. Important findings to include are areas of ulceration, missing teeth, loose teeth, periodontal pockets, receded gingiva, degree of periodontal disease, and fractured teeth (Figure 29-9). Box 29-1 defines and illustrates dental terminology that is useful for describing specific locations in the mouth.

The teeth can be referred to by numbers. Unfortunately there are several numbering systems in existence, which can cause confusion. Most people who do a large volume of dentistry will adapt a numbering system because it is easier to discuss and record teeth by numbers such as 208 as opposed to "the left upper fourth premolar." The most commonly used system is the Modified Triadan System. Teeth in the maxillary right quadrant are assigned the 100 series, left maxillary quadrant 200 series, left mandibular quadrant 300 series, and right mandibular quadrant 400 series. Each tooth within the quadrant has a two-digit number starting at the anterior midline and moving along the dental arch in a caudal direction. The right maxillary

Tampa Bay Veterinary Dentistry
1501A Belcher Road South, Suite 1A
Largo, Florida 33771
Phone: (727) 535-3500
Fax: (727) 539-7865

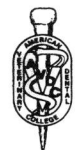

Ashley B. Oakes, DVM,
Diplomate American Veterinary Dental College

Date:_____

Canine Dental Record

Patient:_____

Reason for Visit:_____

History:_____

_____

_____NPO_____

Right Upper Quadrant   **Left Upper Quadrant**

Buccal   Buccal

Occlusal   Occlusal

Palatal   Palatal

110	109	108	107	106	105	104	103	102	101	201	202	203	204	205	206	207	208	209	210
G																			G
411	410	409	408	407	406	405	404	403	402	401	301	302	303	304	305	306	307	308	309	310	311

Lingual   Lingual

Occlusal   Occlusal

Buccal   Buccal

A

Right Lower Quadrant   **Left Lower Quadrant**

KEY

CE – Cervical Erosion	F1 - Grade 1 Furcation	GH - Ging. Hyperplasia	M1 - Grade 1 Mobility	ONF - Oronasal Fistula
D - Discolored Tooth	F2 - Grade 2 Furcation	GR - Gingival Recession	M2 - Grade 2 Mobility	PE - Pulp Exposure
E - Enamel Defect	F3 - Grade 3 Furcation	HX - Hemisection	M3 - Grade 3 Mobility	PH - Pulp Hemorrhage
ERR – External Root Resorption	F4 - Grade 4 Furcation	IRR – Internal Root Resorption	M4 - Grade 4 Mobility	PN - Pulp Necrosis
	FX - Fractured Tooth		O - Missing Tooth	RD - Retained Deciduous Tooth

RR - Retained Root   - Rotated Tooth
RSP – Root Resorption
SN - Supernumerary Tooth   - Crowding
T - Twinning
W - Worn Tooth   ↓ or ↑ - Super-erupted Tooth

Calculus	**Gingivitis**	**Periodontitis**
None	None	None
Slight (s	Mild (1)	Early (P1)
Moderate (m)	Moderate (2)	Moderate (P2)
Heavy (h)	Severe (3)	Advanced (P3)

Diagnosis:_____

_____

_____

_____

_____

_____

_____

Plan:_____

_____

_____

_____

_____

FIGURE 29-9.   A, Canine dental record: note each tooth has a 3-digit number.

Continued

Tampa Bay Veterinary Dentistry
1501A Belcher Road South
Largo, Florida 33771
Phone: (813) 535-3500
Fax: (813) 539-7865

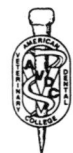

Ashley B. Oakes, DVM,
Diplomate American Veterinary Dental College

Date:_____

Feline Dental Record

Patient:_____

Reason for Visit:_____

History:_____
_____
_____NPO_____

Right Upper Quadrant   Left Upper Quadrant

Buccal   Buccal
Occlusal   Occlusal
Palatal   Palatal
         109 108 107 106   104 103 102 101 201 202 203 204   206 207 208 209

    G   G

         409 408 407   404 403 402 401 301 302 303 304   307 308 309
Lingual   Lingual
Occlusal   Occlusal
Buccal   Buccal

Right Lower Quadrant   Left Lower Quadrant

KEY

CE - Cervical Erosion	E - Enamel Defect	FX - Fractured Tooth	M1 - Grade 1 Mobility	ONF - Oronasal Fistula
CR - Crown Reduction	F1 - Grade 1 Furcation	GH - Ging. Hyperplasia	M2 - Grade 2 Mobility	PC - Pulp Capping
CT - Contour Tooth	F2 - Grade 2 Furcation	GP - Gingivoplasty	M3 - Grade 3 Mobility	PE - Pulp Exposure
D - Discolored Tooth	F3 - Grade 3 Furcation	GR - Gingival Recession	M4 - Grade 4 Mobility	PH - Pulp Hemorrhage
DB - Dentinal Bonding	F4 - Grade 4 Furcation	HX - Hemisection	O - Missing Tooth	RC - Root Canal

RD - Retained Deciduous Tooth   W - Worn Tooth
RS - Root Planing/Subging. Curettage   X - Extraction
RR - Retained Root   ↻ - Rotated Tooth
SN - Supernumerary Tooth   ↔ - Crowding
T - Twinning   ↑or↓ - Super-erupted Tooth

Calculus	**Gingivitis**	**Periodontitis**
None	None	None
Slight (c/s)	Mild (I)	Early (PI)
Moderate (c/m)	Moderate (II)	Moderate (PII)
Heavy (c/h)	Severe (III)	Advanced (PIII)

Diagnosis:_____
_____
_____
_____
_____
_____

Plan:_____
_____
_____
_____
_____
_____
_____

FIGURE 29-9, CONT'D. B, Feline dental record.

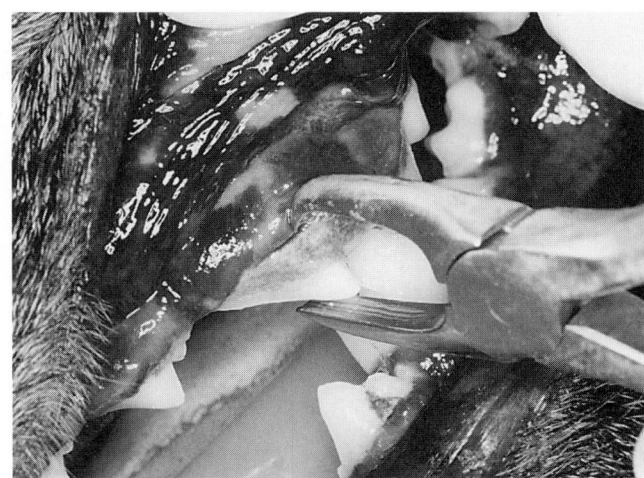

FIGURE 29-10. Large pieces of calculus can be quickly removed with forceps. Care should be taken not to place excessive pressure on the tooth, especially cusp tips, to avoid fracturing the tooth.

first incisor is 101, right maxillary second incisor is 102, right maxillary third incisor 103, right maxillary canine 104, and so on. The left maxillary canine is 204; left mandibular canine is 304 and right mandibular canine 404 (see Figure 29-9). Deciduous teeth are assigned the 500 series for right maxillary quadrant, 600 series for left maxillary quadrant, 700 series for left mandibular quadrant, and 800 series for right mandibular quadrant.

Felines have fewer teeth than canines (dogs) so the system is modified in felines to keep numbers consistent. In other words, no. 108 should refer to the upper fourth right premolar whether discussing a dog, hyena, cat, or lion. Since the cat has three maxillary premolars instead of four like the dog the 105 number is skipped and the first tooth behind 104 (maxillary right canine) is 106 (see Figure 29-9). The feline mandible has only two premolars, so 305, 306, 405, and 406 are skipped and the numbering starts with 307 and 407. Keeping these numbers consistent among species allows veterinary personnel to quickly learn the tooth by one specific number. When someone says tooth 208 is fractured, one should think of the left maxillary fourth premolar (carnassial tooth) since its anatomic shape is very similar for all mammalian carnivores.

Large pieces of calculus can often be easily removed with calculus-removing forceps (Figure 29-10). If the patient has minimal amounts of calculus present, the calculus can be removed with hand scaling instruments alone. Electric and air-driven mechanical scalers can be used on patients with significant amounts of calculus present (most patients!) because they remove calculus rapidly (Figure 29-11). Since the mechanical vibrations of the tips of these scalers dislodge the calculus, minimal pressure is used when operating these instruments. Most of these instruments generate heat owing to the rapid vibrations, so it is imperative to use irrigation to cool the working tips of these instruments so that the pulp tissue does not receive thermal damage.

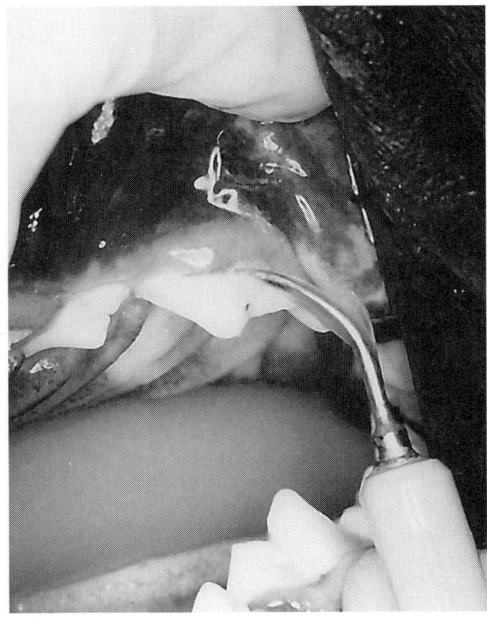

FIGURE 29-11. An ultrasonic scaler is used to clean the tooth of calculus and plaque deposits. The water helps cool the instrument tip and flush debris off the tooth and gingiva.

If the scaling of a tooth is not completed in 10 to 15 seconds, the adjacent tooth can be scaled while the first tooth cools. Once cool, the first tooth can be scaled again.

Most dental cleaning procedures require the use of mechanical and hand scalers. Hand scalers can be used to reach those areas that are inaccessible to the mechanical scaler.

There are a large number of different types of dental scalers and curettes on the market. It is important to understand the different components of these instruments so they can be used properly and aid the technician's decision on which instruments to purchase. Scalers and

Technician Note

When using mechanical scalers, the instrument must be kept moving on the tooth surface and should not be on the tooth for more than 10 to 15 seconds to avoid heat buildup.

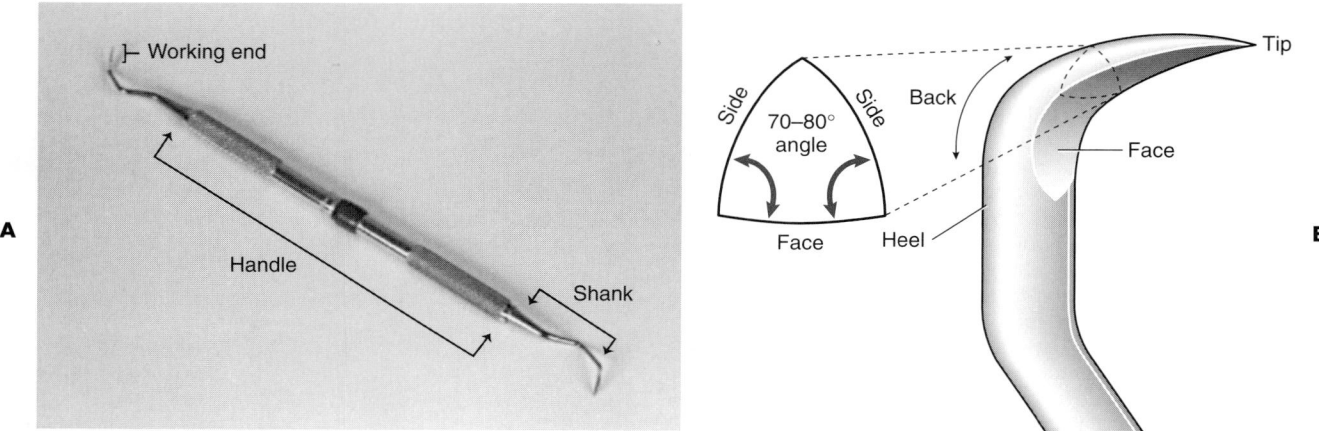

FIGURE 29-12.   A, Supragingival scalers are used to scale the crowns of the teeth. A Jacquette scaler is shown here. **B,** Drawing of the working end. The face of the instrument joins the sides to create a blade edge of 70 to 80 degrees.

curettes are designed with three main components: the handle, shank, and working end (Figure 29-12). The handles can be purchased in slim to wide diameters and be hollow or solid, based on personal preference. The shank attaches the handle to the working end and allows adaptation of the working end to the tooth surfaces. The shank is the most variable part of the curette. A relatively straight shank is good for working in the anterior segment of the mouth and in deep periodontal pockets. An angled shank improves instrumentation in the distal segment of the mouth where space is minimal.

The working end of the instrument has several components: the blade or cutting edge, back, face, heel, and toe or tip. The blade is the portion that cleans the tooth and gingival pocket epithelium. The face of the working end is the flat surface, which creates one of the edges of each blade. The back is the rounded bottom of the working end. These instruments can be purchased as single or double ended depending on whether they have a working end at one or both ends of the handle. Double-ended scalers are designed so that one end adapts to the anterior surface of the tooth and the other end adapts to the distal surface. The term *scaler* includes supragingival (above the gingival margin) and subgingival (below the gingival margin) scalers. All curettes can be used subgingivally because they have a round toe and back to help prevent damage to the gingival tissue (Figure 29-13). They may be used supragingivally as well. Supragingival scalers are not to be used subgingivally because they have a pointed tip that could damage the gingival sulcus (Figure 29-12, *B*). Supragingival scalers are often referred to as *scalers* and subgingival scalers as *curettes*.

Dental scalers should be held in a modified pen grasp (Figure 29-14). The thumb and index finger hold the handle close to the shank. The middle finger is placed just in front of the index finger to further support the instrument. The ring finger is placed on a stable surface (e.g., the tooth or gingiva) to act as a fulcrum and support the hand. The strokes of the scaler should be made through the wrist and not the fingers to avoid operator hand fatigue.

To remove subgingival calculus from the gingival sulcus, the curette is placed to the bottom of the gingival sulcus with its curved smooth back toward the gingival epithelium. Once it is seated at the bottom of the sulcus, the cutting edge is turned to engage the calculus on the tooth root. The curette is then pulled toward the crown to dislodge the calculus and remove it from the sulcus, as illustrated for root planing (see Figure 29-5). This pull stroke is repeated until all the calculus has been removed from the tooth. Proper instrument positioning takes practice and concentration. It is important to master this technique to ensure that the instruments do not damage the gingival tissue and the subgingival calculus is completely removed.

After the teeth have been properly scaled, they must be polished. This step is performed to smooth the microscopic pits and scratches on the tooth surface created by the scaling procedure and routine chewing. If this step is skipped, the plaque will rapidly return because of increased surface area created by the scratches. Polishing is achieved using a slow-speed handpiece with a prophy cup attached and filled with prophy paste. Enough pressure should be applied to just flare the edge of the prophy cup. Flaring the edge will allow it to be gently inserted into the gingival sulcus to polish subgingivally (see Figure 29-15).

All surfaces of the tooth crown should be polished. The rotational speed should be kept slow (4000 rpm or less), and the polisher should be constantly moved on the tooth surface to prevent thermal damage to the tooth and gingiva. The tooth should not be polished for more than 5 seconds, or thermal damage could result. If the polishing is not completed in 5 seconds, another tooth should be polished, and the unfinished tooth can be polished once it has been given time to cool.

Technician Note

All surfaces of the tooth crown should be polished. The rotational speed should be kept slow and the polisher should be constantly moved on the tooth surface to prevent thermal damage to the tooth and gingiva.

Ample prophy paste should be kept in the prophy cup to help prevent excessive heat generation and to smooth the tooth surface. Several polishing pastes are available. For routine dental cleanings, the fluoride-containing pastes are preferred. Fluoride strengthens enamel, decreases tooth

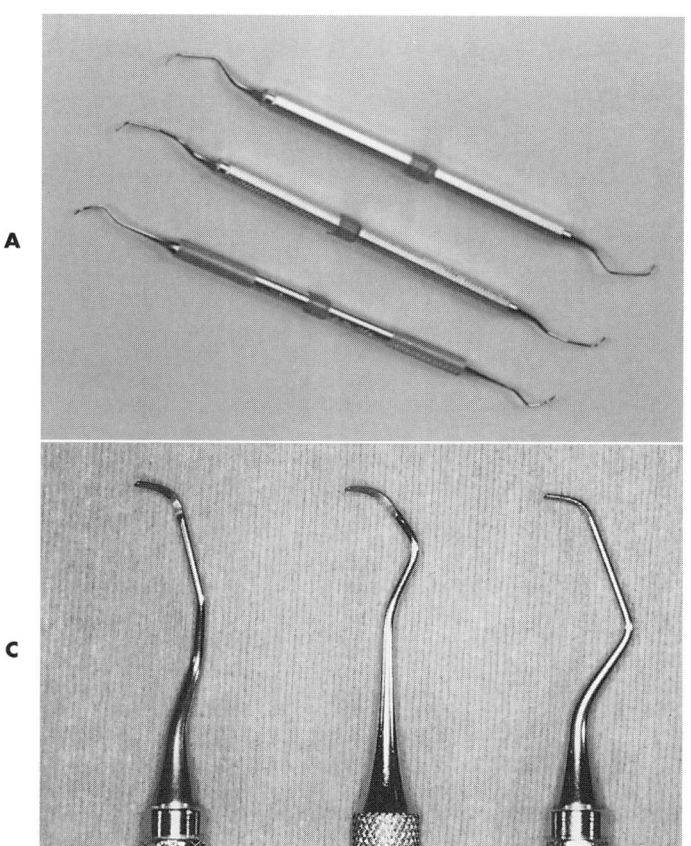

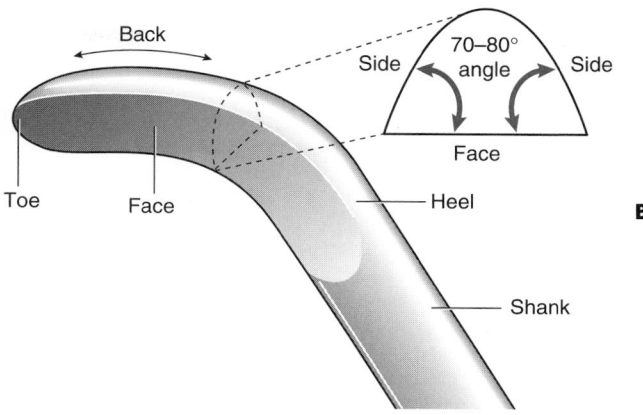

FIGURE 29-13. Curettes can be used subgingivally (below the gingival margin) to scale tooth roots and debride the gingival sulcus. Note the rounded toe and curvature of the instrument. Curettes are available with different angles to the shank to improve access to the tooth roots. **A,** Double-ended curettes. **B,** Drawing of the working end. **C,** Shank and working end of curettes.

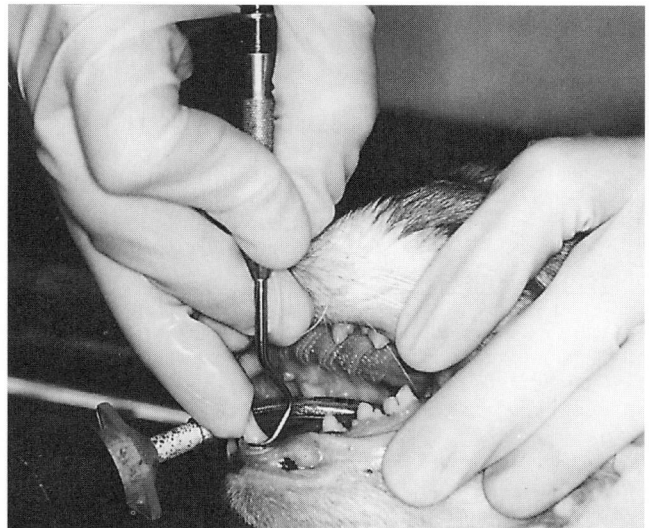

FIGURE 29-14. The scaler is held in a modified pen grasp.

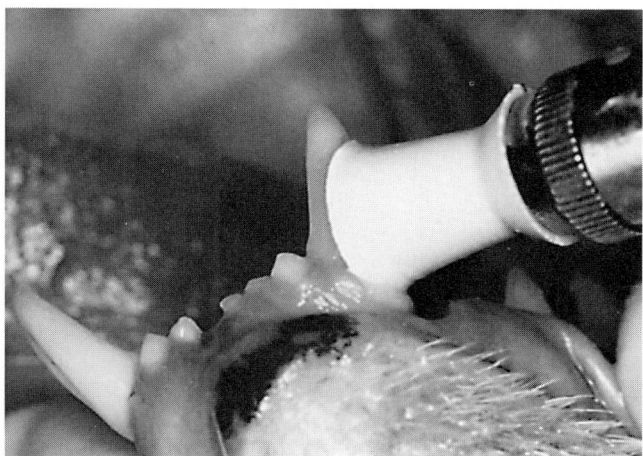

FIGURE 29-15. Polishing the teeth after scaling is extremely important to prevent rapid plaque accumulation following dental cleaning. The flared edge of the prophy cup can be placed into the gingival sulcus to polish the subgingival enamel.

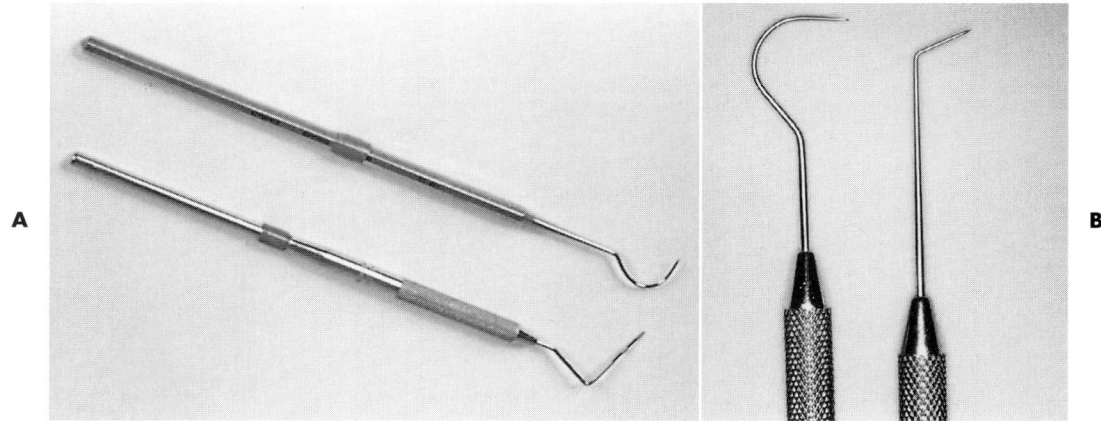

FIGURE 29-16. A, Dental explorer *(top)* and periodontal probe *(bottom)*. The periodontal probe is marked in millimeter increments to measure periodontal pocket depth. The dental explorer has a fine tip and is used to detect subgingival calculus and tooth abnormalities. **B,** Shepherd's hook explorer *(left)* and no. 6 explorer *(right)*.

sensitivity, has antimicrobial properties, and decreases the rate of plaque reattachment. The zirconium silicate pastes (sodium or potassium aluminum silicates) are very effective polishing pastes and will not abrade the tooth enamel.

The oral cavity is rinsed of prophy paste and calculus after all surfaces of the teeth have been polished. The gingival sulcus should be irrigated to remove debris if present. Irrigating systems or syringes can be purchased, or a blunt needle on a syringe can be used. A dilute 0.1% chlorhexidine solution is an excellent irrigation agent because of its antibacterial property, but other solutions can be used, such as physiologic saline, 3% hydrogen peroxide, or zinc ascorbate.

The teeth are checked for any abnormalities and remaining plaque after they have been scaled and polished. Plaque disclosing solutions, such as Reveal (Henry Schein Inc.), are available to enhance visualization of areas of plaque retention. Drying the teeth with air will further enhance visualization of any remaining plaque and calculus.

A dental explorer is used to check for subgingival pathologic changes, such as root caries or erosion, calculus, and tooth root furcation exposure. Explorers come in a variety of shapes to aid exploration of the periodontal pockets in the different areas of the mouth (see Figures 29-3 and 29-16). Commonly used explorers are the shepherd's hook for dogs and the no. 6 for cats. The tip of the explorer has a sharp delicate point that gives good tactile sensation to the operator's hand when exploring the subgingival area.

A periodontal probe (see Figure 29-16, *A*) must be used to check the level of epithelial attachment in the gingival sulcus of each tooth. The probe is placed parallel to the long axis of the tooth root, and multiple sites along each tooth should be checked (see Figure 29-17). The clinical probing depth of any periodontal pocket should be recorded on the pet's dental chart and is a measurement taken from the gingival margin to the epithelial attachment level (base of the pocket).

Periodontal probes come in a wide variety of calibrations, which are either color coded or notched and measure pocket depths up to 10, 11, or 12 mm. The probes are either round or flat. It is useful to have a variety of probes, but the most popular probe is a color-coded probe that measures 3-, 6-, 9-, and 12-mm increments. Factors that affect the probing depth of a periodontal pocket are

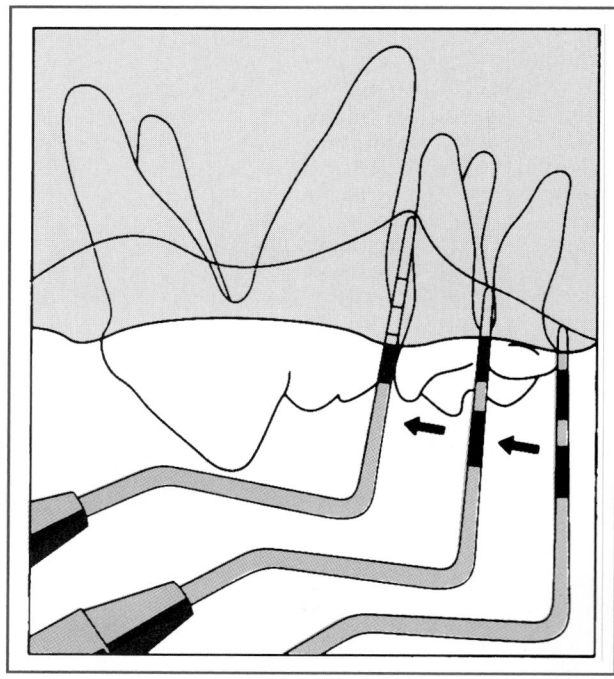

FIGURE 29-17.   Multiple sites on a tooth should be probed to detect any deep pockets present. (From Emily P, Penman S: *Handbook of small animal dentistry,* ed 2, Oxford, England, 1994, Pergamon Press Ltd.)

epithelial attachment level, alveolar bone loss, gingival margin swelling (reversible), and gingival recession. Gingival recession should be measured with the periodontal probe from the level of the cementoenamel junction (CEJ) of the tooth to the gingival margin and recorded on the dental record. This value plus the clinical probing depth will equal the amount of attachment loss for that particular tooth (attachment loss = clinical probing depth + gingival recession) (see Figure 29-9). Any problems noted during the dental cleaning should be brought to the attention of the veterinarian, and dental radiographs should be taken if

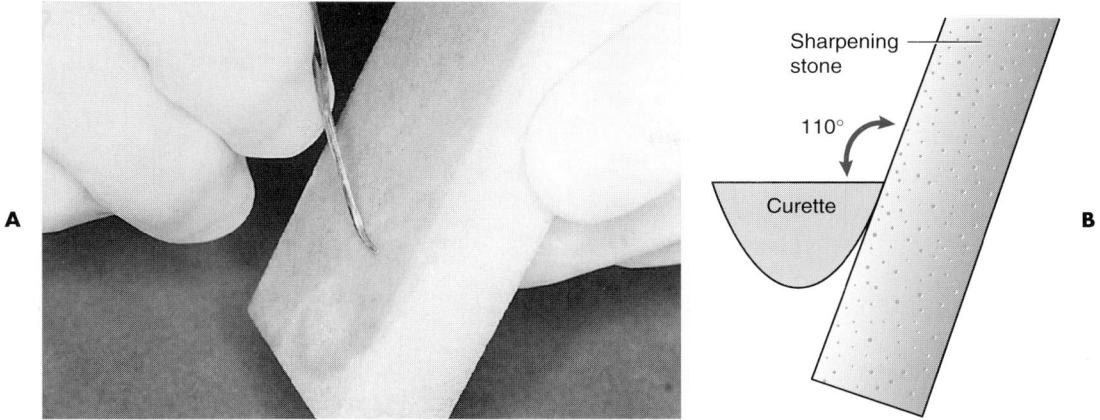

FIGURE 29-18.   A, The sharpening stone should be kept at an angle of 100 to 110 degrees to the scaler face to maintain the proper shape of the instrument. **B,** Curette face in cross section to sharpening stone showing the 100- to 110-degree angle.

indicated. After scaling, polishing, and sulcus irrigation have been performed and all problems have been addressed, the animal can recover from anesthesia.

Dental Home Care

The final stage of dental cleaning is client education on dental home care treatment along with the dispensing of dental home care products. Many products are available to encourage good compliance and meet individual needs.

When the owner comes to pick up the pet, he or she should be taken into an examination room, where the technician can demonstrate the proper brushing technique on a dental model. The owner should be instructed to start slowly with the pet and to use ample praise. The owner should then be asked to repeat the brushing procedure on a dental model to ensure correct technique. The pet can then be brought in to the owner. The owner should be shown how to properly grasp the muzzle so that the pet is not injured when brushing the teeth. Daily dental home care is the best way to prevent the accumulation of plaque. For owners with busy schedules, however, a home care session on alternate days or three times per week will still provide benefits to the pet.

Technician Note

The key to success with dental home care is finding a product that works well for the owner and is acceptable to the pet. With patience, praise, and guidance, the owner should be able to find a dental home care treatment that will work for his or her pet.

The owner should be informed of any dental problems the pet might have as well as the date on which the pet's next dental cleaning will be due. As a general rule, pets with healthy mouths or mild to moderate gingivitis will benefit from annual dental cleanings. Those with early periodontitis will probably require a dental cleaning every 6 to 8 months, and those with moderate to severe periodontitis may require a dental cleaning every 3 to 4 months.

The key to success with dental home care is finding a product that works well for the owner and is acceptable to the pet. There are many different types of toothbrushes available. Dog and cat toothbrushes can be purchased, or the owner can buy a child's soft-bristled toothbrush. Some pets will not tolerate a toothbrush and may respond better if the owner uses a sponge-type swab or a gauze pad wrapped around the owner's finger. If this is unacceptable to the pet, or if the owner risks being bitten, a mouth rinse or spray can be used.

Pet toothpaste formulas are well tolerated by most pets because they like the malt, poultry, or beef flavoring that has been added. Human toothpaste should not be used on pets. The flavors of the veterinary chlorhexidine and zinc ascorbate oral rinses and spray products are not as well liked by pets. However, they are excellent for keeping oral bacterial levels under control and for healing damaged gingival tissue. They can be applied more quickly than pastes and are easier to use on animals that will not tolerate much handling.

Another product is a bioadhesive pellet (Stomadhex, Virbac) that releases chlorhexidine diacetate and niacinamide into the oral cavity as it is slowly dissolved. The tablet is placed on the labial mucosa once daily for the desired length of treatment. This may be beneficial for pets that do not tolerate tooth brushing well or that are too tender to be brushed after periodontal therapy. With patience, praise, and guidance, the owner should be able to find a dental home care treatment that will work for his or her pet.

Sharpening Dental Scalers

Dental scalers must be kept sharp to work properly. Dull instruments burnish calculus into the tooth rather than remove it and can cause operator hand fatigue. There are several different methods to sharpen scalers. A helpful instructional textbook is *Smarten Up, Sharpen Up* by Hu-Friedy, which is available through most dental supply companies. An oiled sharpening stone should be used to sharpen dental scalers. The finer grades of sharpening stones (e.g., the Arkansas stone) maintain a smoother cutting edge, remove less metal, and as long as instruments are sharpened frequently the sharp edge is rapidly restored. A thin layer of oil should be placed on the surface of the stone before sharpening. The instruments should be cleaned before sharpening, and sharpening should be performed in a well-lit area.

A simple sharpening method is the moving flat stone, stationary instrument technique. The flat stone is held at an angle of 100 to 110 degrees to the face of the curette or sickle scaler (Figure 29-18). This angle will maintain the 70- to 80-degree bevel of the cutting edge (see Figures

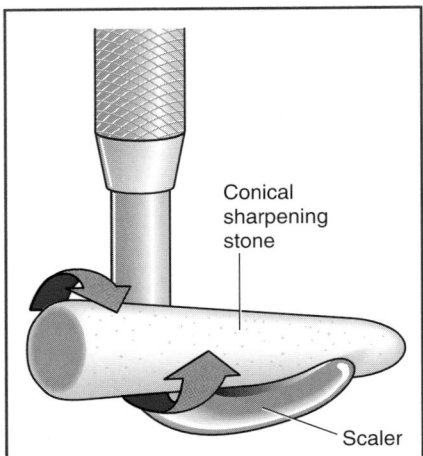

FIGURE 29-19.   The conical sharpening stone is rolled across the face of the scaler to remove wire edges.

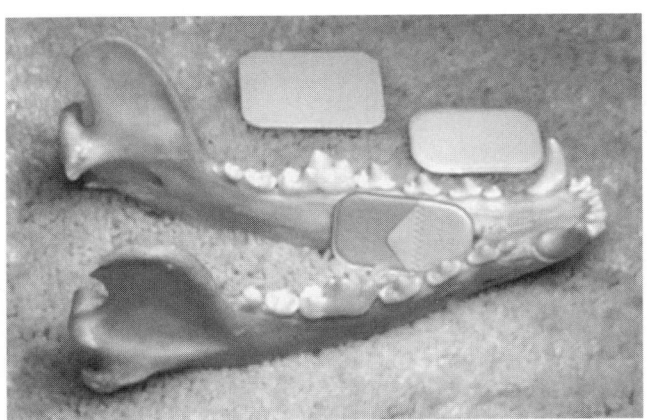

FIGURE 29-20.   Intraoral dental film size 2 and size 0.

29-12, *B*, and 29-13, *B*). Begin sharpening with short up and down strokes starting at the heel of the instrument and working toward the toe or tip of the instrument. The technician's dominant hand should hold the stone, and the other hand should hold the instrument with the face up and parallel to the floor. The instrument hand should be braced on a stable surface, such as a counter or tabletop. Sharpening always finishes on a down stroke, and greater pressure is placed on the down strokes than on the up strokes. Once the stone reaches the tip of the supragingival scaler the stone is removed on completion of the down stroke. The rounded toe must be maintained on curettes to avoid soft tissue trauma. As the stone approaches the toe, the sharpening is continued, maintaining the same angle around the toe to finish on the down stroke.

The instruments should be checked for sharpness on an acrylic stick. A sharp instrument easily engages the acrylic and shaves thin strips off with little effort. The sharpening procedure is repeated until the instrument is properly sharpened. The wire edges are then removed from the face of the instrument by rolling a round stone over the face a few times (Figure 29-19). Finally, the instrument is cleaned of oil and metal debris and sterilized.

Instruments need to be sharpened based on use. If a scaler is used very little it may be able to go through three or four procedures without dulling. If a dental case requires extensive hand scaling the scaler may require sharpening after that case. A good rule of thumb is to check scalers frequently with an acrylic stick to identify the dull instruments.

DENTAL RADIOGRAPHY

Dental radiography is an important tool in the diagnostic and prognostic evaluation of oral disorders in veterinary medicine. As advances have been made in veterinary dentistry, there has been a demand for high-quality dental radiographs to evaluate teeth and oral structures more accurately. The use of dental radiograph machines and intraoral dental film in veterinary medicine has increased dramatically during this time.

Traditionally, radiographs of the teeth, mandible, and maxilla were taken to evaluate disorders such as oral masses, fractured jaws and teeth, and facial pain and swelling. Many veterinarians are now using this diagnostic aid to assess problems such as discolored teeth, feline odontoclastic resorptive lesions, and periodontal disease and to aid in the treatment of endodontically compromised teeth, dental restorations, and difficult extractions.

Dental radiographs can be taken with the film placed in the mouth (intraoral technique) or outside the mouth (extraoral technique). Intraoral dental film is a non-screened flexible film (Figure 29-20). Regular screened or nonscreened x-ray film can be used for extraoral radiographic views (see Chapter 9) and a limited number of intraoral views. Nonscreened x-ray films provide greater detail than the screened films but require increased exposure times.

There are several advantages of the intraoral radiographic technique over the extraoral technique. Perhaps the greatest advantage of the intraoral technique is the ability to minimize the superimposition of teeth and surrounding structures on the area of study. Intraoral dental film can be purchased in sizes small enough to fit in the mouth next to the tooth or teeth to be studied. The closer the x-ray film is to the subject of interest (the tooth), the better the detail. The aiming cylinder of the dental radiograph machine can be moved and angled to radiograph the tooth of interest and be placed close enough to the tooth to eliminate the opposite dental arch.

When using the extraoral technique, there is usually some degree of superimposition of teeth from the contralateral arches that are in the path of the primary beam (Figure 29-21). The teeth in the opposite arch may obstruct the view of the teeth of interest, and dental abnormalities could be missed.

The film focal distance (FFD) for the dental radiograph machine is 16 inches or less, in contrast to the standard radiograph machines for which an FFD of 36 to 40 inches is commonly used. The shorter FFD of the dental radiograph machine allows closer placement of the anode to the tooth, eliminating the opposite dental arch, surrounding soft tissue, and/or bone from the path of the primary beam. The shorter FFD also minimizes harmful scatter radiation, as does the small cone size and lead lining, which many of the dental radiograph cones contain.

The extraoral views require the patient to be placed in many different positions so that the skull is angled in order for the primary beam to avoid the surrounding oral structures. This proper positioning takes time and skill. Intra-

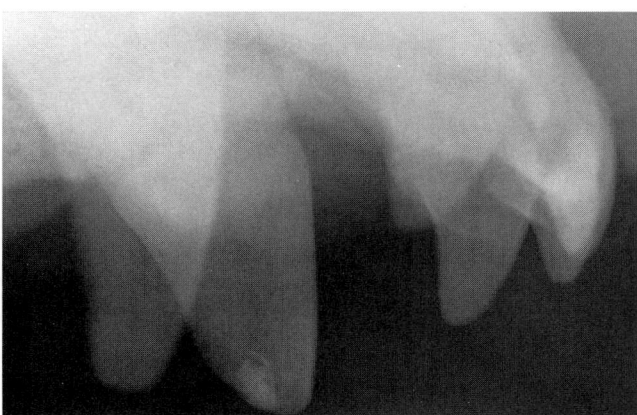

FIGURE 29-21. Superimposition caused by placing the film extraorally. The teeth in the contralateral arch are interfering with the image of the area of interest.

oral dental film can be placed in the mouth, and the tube head of the x-ray machine can be moved instead of the patient. The patient is placed in dorsal recumbency to radiograph the mandible and in ventral recumbency to radiograph the maxilla. A complete evaluation of all four oral quadrants requires at least six to eight views.

Intraoral dental film can be processed by hand or "piggybacked" to a regular film with electrical tape and automatically processed. Extraoral nonscreened x-ray film may not be compatible with the automatic processor's developer and might require hand developing. The extraoral nonscreened x-ray film is considerably more expensive than the smaller intraoral dental film. If rapid developer and fixative are used, intraoral dental film can be hand developed in approximately 2 minutes, which is helpful in minimizing anesthesia time.

To use the intraoral radiographic technique, one must master the bisecting angle technique. The bisecting angle technique was developed to minimize image distortion caused by the inability to place the dental film parallel to the central axis of the tooth. Placing the film parallel to the teeth in the maxillary arch and anterior mandible is particularly difficult because of the flat palate and impeding soft tissue structures of the mandibular symphysis. To utilize the bisecting angle technique, the film is placed as close to the tooth as possible. The primary x-ray beam is then aimed perpendicular to the plane that bisects the angle created by the plane of the central axis of the tooth to the plane of the dental film. The bisecting angle (or bisector angle) is the imaginary plane that divides this angle created between the tooth and film into two equal parts (Figure 29-22). Distortion of the tooth is minimized but is still present because the film is closer to the crown of the tooth than it is to the root apex.

> ### Technician Note
>
> To use the intraoral radiographic technique, one must master the bisecting angle technique. The bisecting angle technique was developed to minimize image distortion caused by the inability to place the dental film parallel to the central axis of the tooth.

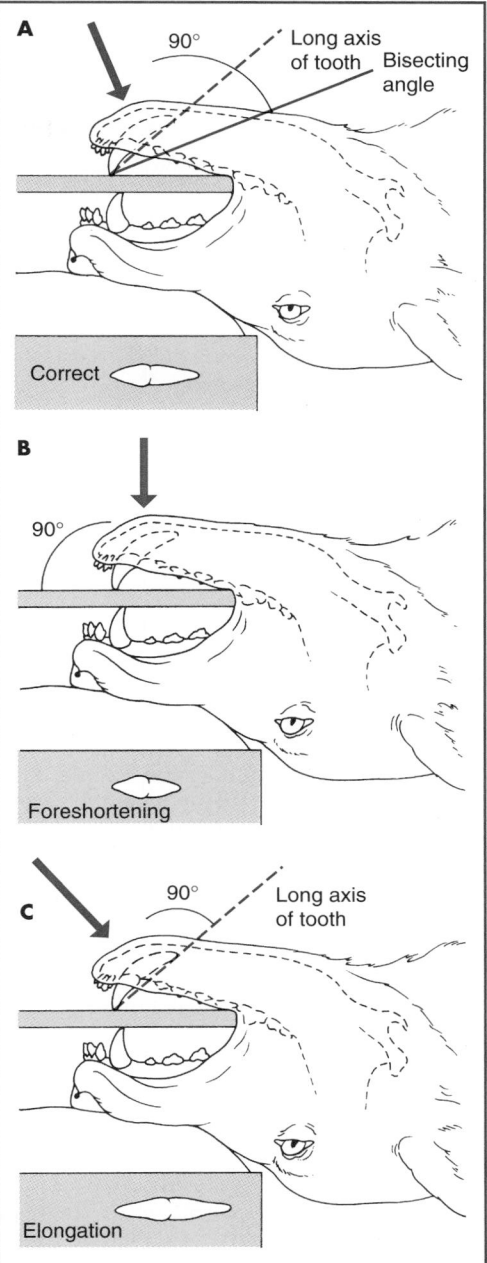

FIGURE 29-22. **A,** Bisection angle technique produces an accurate image of the tooth. **B,** Direction of the x-ray beam at right angles to the film shortens the tooth's image. **C,** Direction of the x-ray beam at right angles to the long axis of the tooth elongates the tooth's image. (From Emily P, Penman S: *Handbook of small animal dentistry,* ed 2, Oxford, England, 1994, Pergamon Press Ltd.)

The buccal object rule (tube shift technique or Clark's rule) is useful for object localization as well as isolating structures for better visualization. Objects that are lingual to a reference point will move in the same direction as the change in position of the tube head (either rostrally or distally); and objects buccal to the reference point move opposite the direction of the tube head. For example, a cat presents for epistaxis and a wound on the face below the

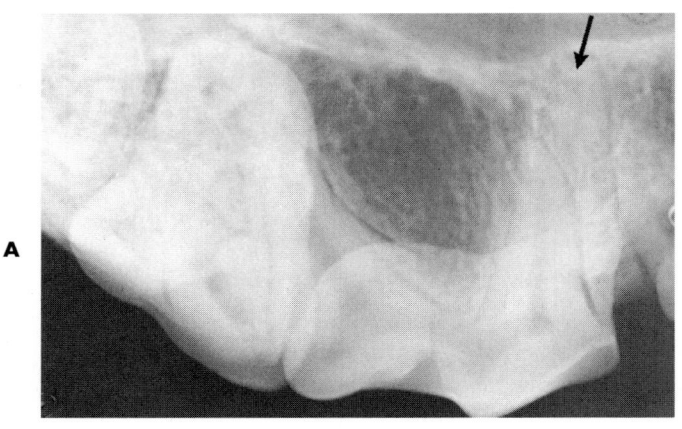

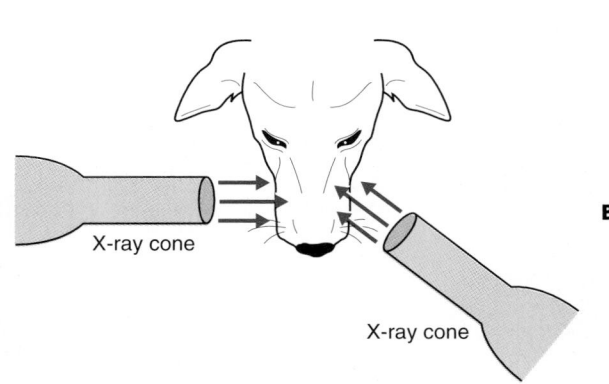

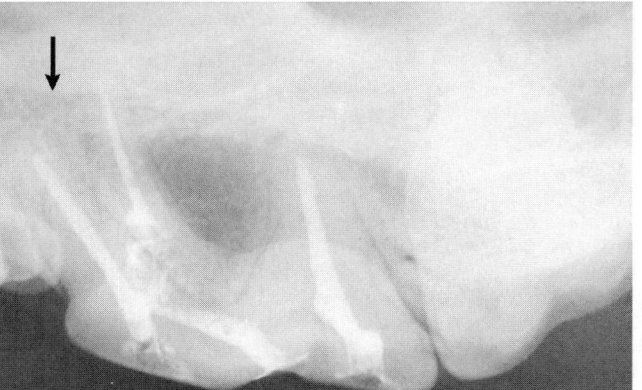

FIGURE 29-23.   A, Rostrocaudal oblique view of the upper fourth premolar tooth *(arrow)* of the anterior roots. The most mesial root is the palatal root. **B,** This diagram illustrates how the position-indicating device (PID) is positioned to take an oblique view. **C,** Caudorostral oblique view of the upper fourth premolar. The most mesial root is the buccal root *(arrow).* Note the nice separation.

eye. A lateral skull survey radiograph reveals a bullet in the maxilla by the upper fourth premolar tooth roots. Veterinary personnel need to determine if the bullet is lodged lingual to the premolar and in the maxillary sinus or if it is buccal to the tooth. An intraoral x-ray can be taken with the tube head positioned rostral to the upper fourth premolar. The x-ray is taken in a rostrocaudal oblique projection, and the bullet will be rostral to the premolar tooth roots on the x-ray film if the bullet sits in the sinus. An acronym to help remember this rule is SLOB, which stands for same-lingual, opposite-buccal.

This technique is used frequently in veterinary dentistry to isolate the palatal (lingual) and buccal roots of the maxillary fourth premolars. For example, if the tube head is moved rostrally, the palatal (lingual) root of the upper fourth premolar will be the most rostral root on the radiograph and the anterior buccal root will be distal to the palatal root (Figure 29-23, *A*). To change the position of the tube head, the perpendicular angle to the bisecting angle is maintained, and the tube head is simply angled obliquely at the object either in a slightly more anterior oblique view or posterior oblique view (Figure 29-23, *B*).

Intraoral Radiography in the Dog and Cat

Intraoral radiographs of the mandibular premolars and molars are obtained by using standard radiographic technique. The film is placed on the lingual side of the teeth and parallel to the central axis of the teeth. The dental x-ray beam is then aimed perpendicular to the film (Figure 29-24). This is the only area in the oral cavity of the dog and cat where the standard technique can be used.

The mandibular incisors can usually be radiographed on one dental film. The animal is placed in dorsal or lateral recumbency with the dental film as close to the incisors as possible on the lingual side. The position-indicating device (PID) is then centered over the first incisors pointing in a caudal direction with the x-ray beam aimed perpendicular to the bisecting angle. The apices of both mandibular canines can be obtained in this view if the dental film extends far enough caudally. The frenulum of the tongue may prevent proper placement of the intraoral film in some pets, particularly cats. If this becomes a problem, the tongue can be placed between the teeth and the film (Figure 29-25).

To obtain a radiograph of the mandibular first, second, and third premolars in a dog and third premolars in the cat where the symphysis prevents proper parallel placement of the film, place the animal in dorsal recumbency. Position the film on the lingual side of the teeth as close to the teeth and ventral border of the mandible as possible. Direct the PID at the teeth from a lateral position, and aim the x-ray beam at the bisecting angle (Figure 29-26).

Radiographs of the maxillary dentition are commonly taken with the bisecting angle because the flat palate makes it difficult to place the film parallel and in close apposition to the tooth roots. The maxillary incisors are radiographed with the same technique as is used for the mandibular incisors except the animal is placed in sternal or lateral recumbency (Figure 29-27). The apices of the maxillary canines are usually superimposed over the first and second premolars in this view. The maxillary canines should be radiographed from a lateral or rostrocaudal oblique view using the bisecting angle technique (Figures 29-23, *B*, and 29-28).

To radiograph the maxillary premolars and molars the

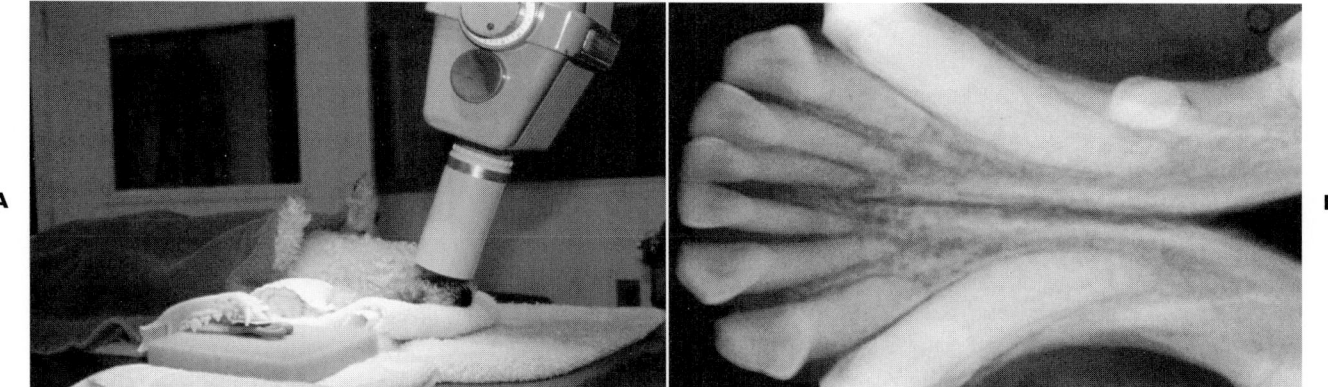

FIGURE 29-24.   A, Proper positioning for a radiograph of the mandibular premolars and molars. **B,** Radiograph of teeth 408, 409, and 410. The area of interest in this study was 409.

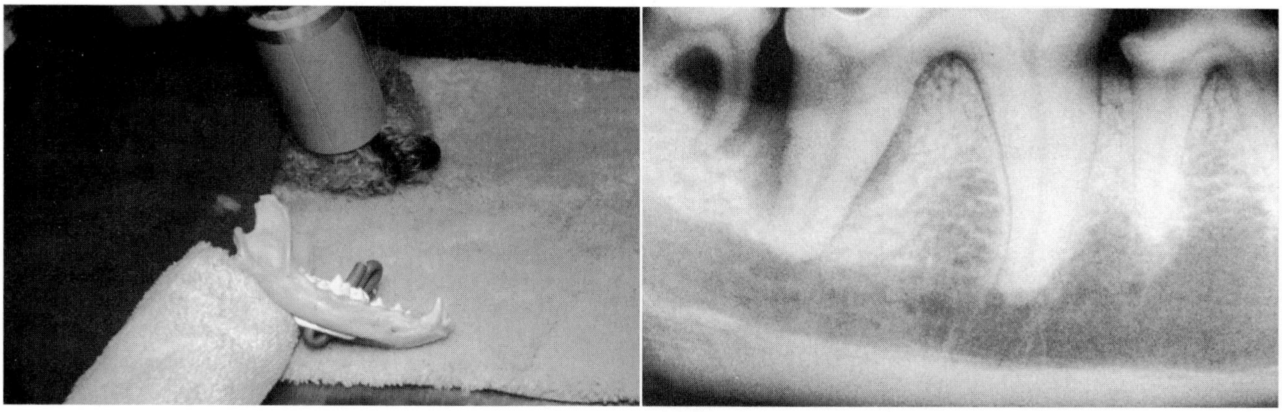

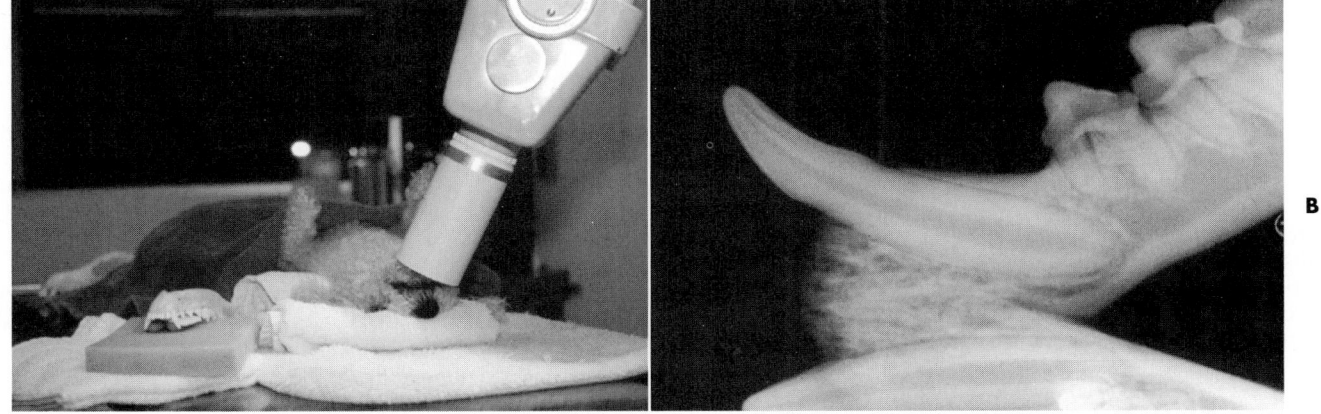

FIGURE 29-25.   A, Positioning for a study of the mandibular incisors and canines. **B,** Radiograph of the mandibular incisors and canines.

FIGURE 29-26.   A, Positioning for a study of the rostral mandibular premolars. This can also be used to obtain a lateral view of the incisors and canine tooth. **B,** Radiograph of 304, 307, and 308 in a cat. Note the incisor teeth are missing.

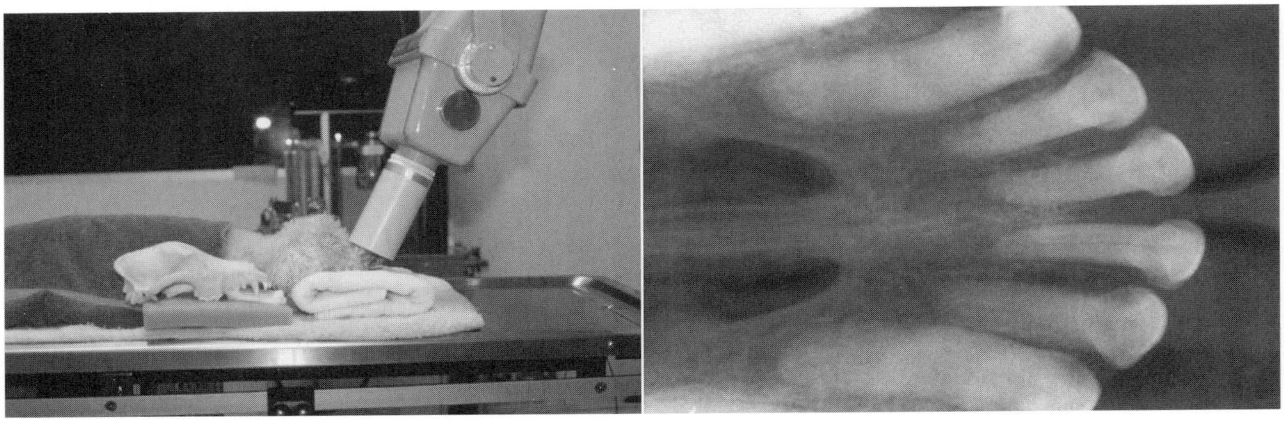

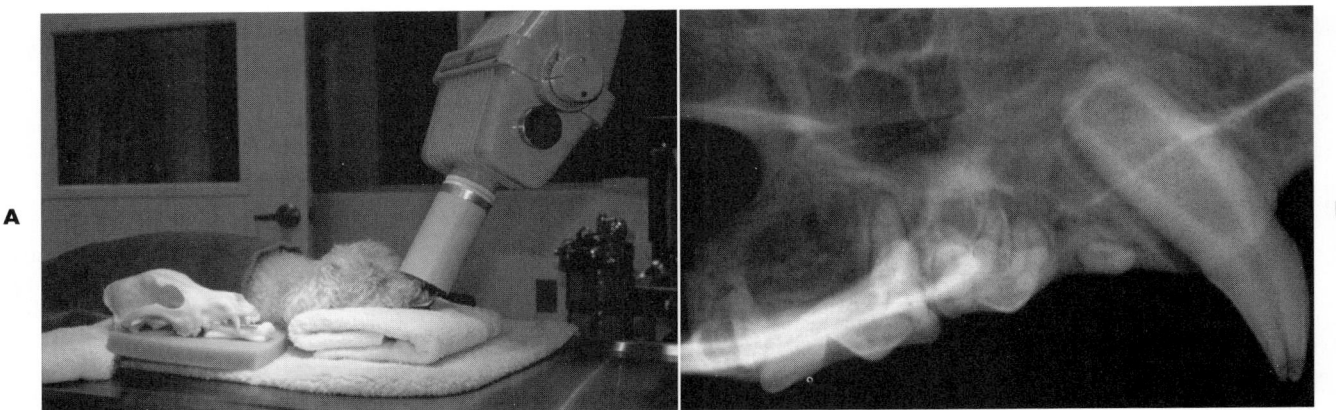

FIGURE 29-27.   **A,** Positioning for a study of the maxillary incisors. **B,** Radiograph of the maxillary incisors.

FIGURE 29-28.   **A,** Positioning for a study of the maxillary premolars. This can also be used to obtain a lateral view of the maxillary incisors and canine tooth. **B,** Radiograph of 204, 206, 207, 208, and 209 in a cat.

animal is placed in sternal or lateral recumbency. The film is placed as close to the tooth as possible on the lingual side of the dentition. Maxillary premolars one through three can be viewed with the tube head placed lateral to the teeth (see Figure 29-28). If the animal has crowding or rotation of these teeth, additional views in a rostrocaudal oblique position may be required to improve visualization of tooth roots.

Rostrocaudal or caudorostral oblique views are needed to isolate the different tooth roots of the maxillary fourth premolar and first and second molar teeth. A rostrocaudal view of premolar four provides an isolated view of the anterior tooth roots, but the distal root may be superimposed over the first molar. An additional view of the tooth from the caudorostral oblique projection will isolate the distal root, but the anterior roots may now be superimposed over the third premolar. The crowns of the molar teeth will superimpose their roots so the technique may need to be adjusted to penetrate the additional structures.

In cats and in brachycephalic dogs, the zygomatic arch may be superimposed over the maxillary premolar tooth roots. If the PID is placed in a rostrocaudal oblique position, the zygomatic arch can be shifted off the area of interest.

When one is learning the positioning techniques for

intraoral dental radiographs, it is easiest to place the dog or cat in sternal recumbency for views of the maxillary dentition, in dorsal recumbency for views of the anterior mandible, and in lateral recumbency for views of the mandibular premolars and molars. As one masters the technique, the animal can be left in lateral recumbency (since many veterinarians perform dental procedures with the animal in this position) and the views taken following the same principles. Film holders are often needed for many of these views to keep the film from moving once it is placed in proper position. Gauze squares and Flexi-film holders (Dr. Shipp's Laboratories) are useful for this purpose (see Figures 29-24, *A,* and 29-25, *A*). Box 29-2 is a technique chart to serve as a reference for taking intraoral radiographs with a dental x-ray machine and intraoral film.

Technician Note

When one is learning the positioning techniques for intraoral dental radiographs, it is easiest to place the dog or cat in sternal recumbency for views of the maxillary dentition, in dorsal recumbency for views of the anterior mandible, and in lateral recumbency for views of the mandibular premolars and molars.

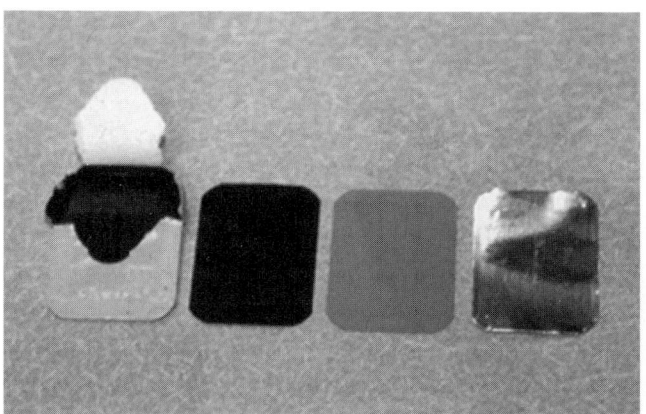

FIGURE 29-29. Components of intraoral dental film. *Left to right,* Outer water-resistant wrapper, black paper, dental film, lead foil.

BOX 29-2	EXPOSURE TIME (SEC) USING D SPEED INTRAORAL DENTAL FILM

Cats: 0.1-0.3
Dogs: 0.2-0.5
Dental machine: 70 kVp, 15 mA, FFD 12 inches

FFD, Focal-film distance; *kVp,* kilovolts peak; *mA,* milliamperes.

An intraoral dental film packet has four main components (Figure 29-29). The film itself is wrapped in black paper to protect it from light exposure. The back of the film contains lead foil to shield the film from back-scatter radiation that could cause film fog. These components are then wrapped in a paper or plastic outer wrap that is moisture resistant. Intraoral dental film is available in D and E speeds. The exposure time of E speed film is 50% less than D speed, but there is less sharpness and more film fogging with E speed film. Either film is acceptable for use.

Intraoral dental film comes in three sizes: periapical, bite-wing, and occlusal. The composition of the film does not vary in the different film sizes. In veterinary medicine the periapical and occlusal sizes are used primarily. Periapical films are used to evaluate the crown, root, and periapical region and come in the following three sizes: size 0 ($^7/_8$ inch × 1$^3/_8$ inches), size 1 ($^{15}/_{16}$ inch × 1$^9/_{16}$, and size 2 (1¼ inches × 1$^5/_8$ inches). Size 0 is used commonly in cats and small-breed dogs. Size 2 is used for medium to large-breed dogs and for single tooth studies, such as an endodontic case.

Occlusal film is size no. 4 film and is used to evaluate a larger area of the mandible or maxilla than would be seen on a single periapical film. It is commonly used for full mouth dental radiographic studies in medium to large breed dogs to get more teeth per film with each radiation exposure. The dimensions of no. 4 film are 2¼ inches × 3 inches.

ENDODONTICS

Endodontics deals with the study and treatment of the inside of the tooth (pulp) and periapical tissues. The periapical tissue is located around the tip (apex) of the tooth root. The tooth pulp consists of nerves, blood

vessels, lymphatics, and connective tissue. The pulp tissue is found in the pulp chamber (crown) and pulp canal (root) of the tooth and enters the tooth through numerous small openings in the apex of the tooth root called the *apical delta.*

The dental pulp is important to the development of the tooth in a young animal. It supplies the nutrients needed by the odontoblasts to deposit dentin. This makes the walls of the root and crown thicker, so the tooth is stronger. Once the dog or cat is past 10 to 18 months of age, the majority of the dentin has been deposited, the tooth walls are fairly thick, and the root apex should be closed. As the animal continues to age, the pulp chamber and canal will become smaller because the odontoblasts will continue to deposit dentin (Figure 29-30).

The treatment options for teeth with endodontic disease will depend on the age of the animal, duration of endodontic disease, and anatomy of the tooth. Conventional root canal therapy is usually performed on dogs and cats 12 months of age and older with endodontic disease. Treatment involves removing the dead or dying pulp tissue from the tooth with small files or reamers, disinfecting and shaping the root canal, and filling the canal (obturation) with an appropriate material to seal the apex from the periapical tissues. Radiographs are necessary to ensure that a proper apical seal has been achieved. A detailed discussion of this procedure will follow below.

Among the most common causes of endodontic disease in dogs and cats are pulp exposures from fractured teeth as well as dental abrasion (wear from a foreign object) and attrition (wear from tooth on tooth). Many dogs will cause severe abrasion of their teeth by chewing on hard objects such as rocks or fences. The teeth most commonly fractured are the canines and the maxillary fourth premolars (carnassial) (Figure 29-31). Attrition and abrasion usually occur on the incisors and canines but can be seen on the premolars and molars as well. If the dental wear occurs slowly, the odontoblasts will deposit tertiary dentin over the pulp tissue to prevent pulp exposure as enamel and dentin are lost. The pulp tissue may be visualized through the tertiary dentin as a brown or red dot (Figure 29-32). A dental explorer should be run over the tooth surface to make sure the pulp tissue is not exposed. When the pulp tissue is exposed, the tip of the dental explorer will drop down into the pulp chamber as it crosses the surface of the tooth.

In fresh fractures the tooth may bleed from the center. If the tooth is treated within the first 48 hours, a vital pulpotomy procedure can usually be performed. This involves removing the coronal pulp tissue (the pulp tissue in the tooth root remains), covering the pulp tissue with calcium hydroxide, and sealing the coronal exposure site with appropriate dental restorative materials.

All teeth with exposed pulp tissue should be treated either by endodontic treatment (conventional root canal, pulpotomy) or by extraction. If left untreated, infection from the exposure site will spread to the periapical tissues, and a periapical abscess may develop. This condition is seen fairly frequently in dogs with maxillary carnassial tooth abscesses. The owner will notice swelling or a draining tract just below the dog's eye, and treatment is usually sought (Figure 29-33). Surprisingly, only about 20% of periapical abscesses will form a fistula to the skin, which means that unless the teeth of these pets are being examined for endodontic disease, many abscesses go untreated. These abscesses can be very painful and are a source of infection, which can spread to other teeth and the bloodstream.

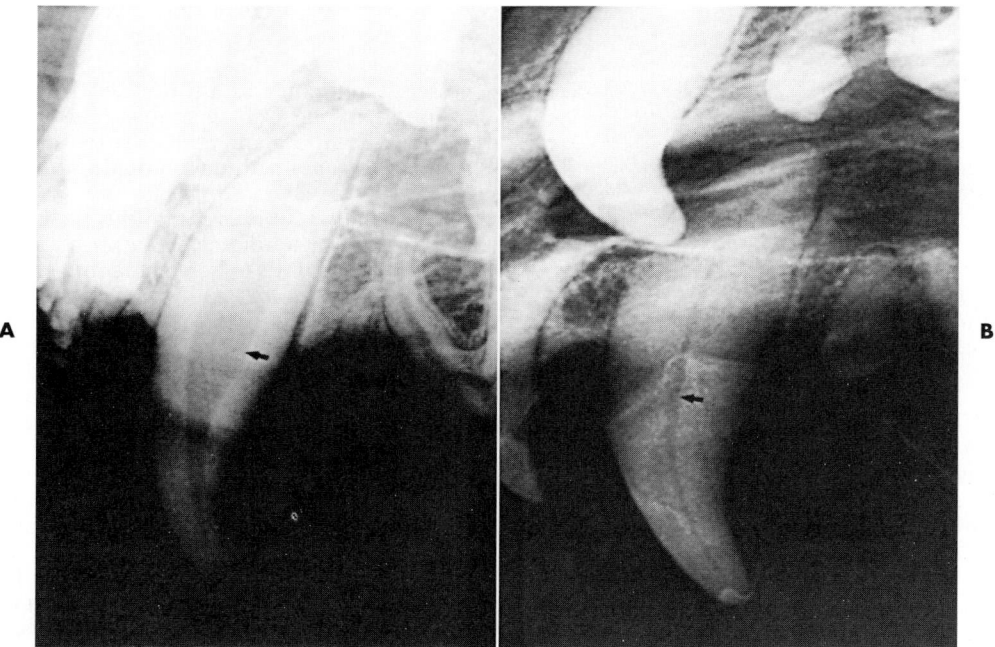

FIGURE 29-30. **A,** Large pulp chamber and canal in a young cougar's canine tooth *(arrow)*. **B,** As animals age, dentin is deposited, and the pulp chambers and canals narrow *(arrow)*.

FIGURE 29-31. Slab fractures of the maxillary fourth premolar teeth are a common problem in dogs. This fracture extends subgingivally, and the pulp tissue has been exposed *(arrow)*.

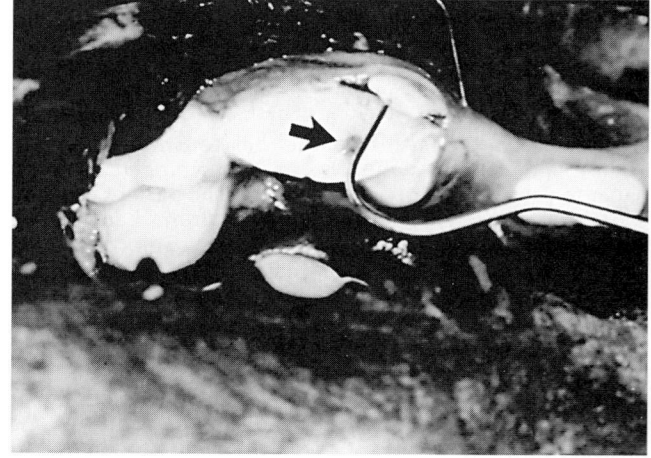

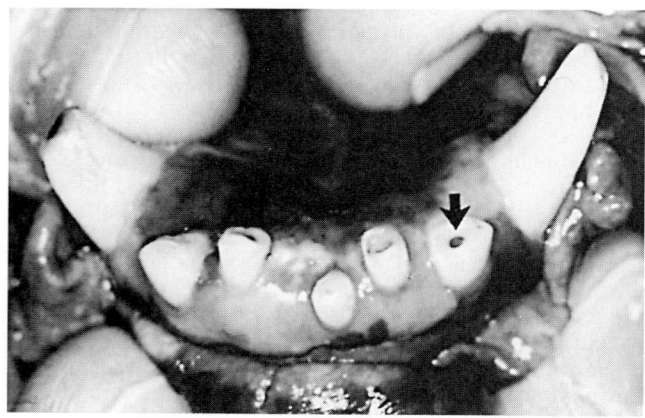

FIGURE 29-32. Severe abrasion of the incisors and canine teeth. The brown or red dots *(arrow)* in the center of these teeth are the pulp tissues below the less opaque tertiary dentin.

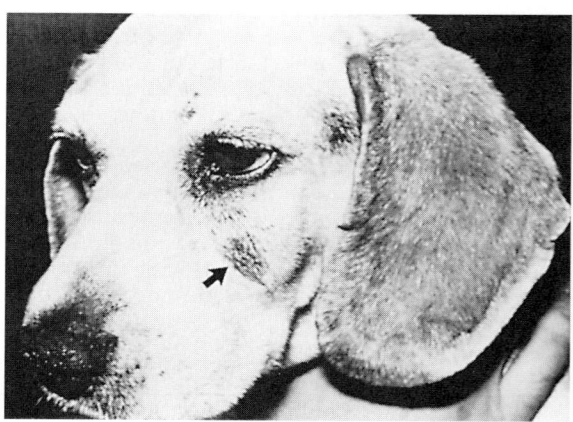

FIGURE 29-33. Patient with a maxillary tooth abscess with a draining tract fistula *(arrow)*.

Other signs of endodontic disease include discolored teeth and painful teeth. Diagnosing a painful tooth in an animal can be difficult, but when there is a question, a dental radiograph can be taken to assess the periapical area for signs of disease.

Conventional Root Canal Therapy

Box 29-3 lists equipment and supplies needed for conventional root canal therapy . These items should be ready for use before the root canal treatment is started.

A preoperative radiograph is taken to evaluate the tooth root and periapical region. The veterinarian will make the appropriate access to the root canal through the crown of the tooth with a dental bur of proper size determined by the size of the crown being treated. The canal may have pulp present that will require removal with a barbed broach (Figure 29-34). The broach is placed in the canal and rotated to ensnare the pulp. The broach and pulp tissue are removed from the canal. This step is repeated until all pulp has been removed. Many teeth will not have any visible pulp tissue remaining (necrotic pulp), and the barbed broaches will not be needed.

The next step is to begin filing the root canal in order to clean and shape the canal for proper obturation. Obturation means to fill the canal. There are several types and sizes of files. Hedstrom and K files are the most commonly used files (Figure 29-35). Hedstrom files have a sharper edge and can remove dentin faster than K files. They are used in a push/pull motion. They are more susceptible to file fracture than K files, however. K files are used in a push quarter clockwise turn/pull motion. Their edges are not as sharp so dentin removal is less efficient than with Hedstrom files but they are structurally sounder and less

---

likely to fracture in the canal. The files are available in a number of different lengths and diameters. The smallest diameter file is a no. 6. They increase in diameter by even number increments from 6 to 10 and then they increase by increments of 5. For instance, the following diameters exist: 6, 8, 10, 15, 20, 25, 30, 35, 40, and so on until file 60, at which point the diameter increases by 10. The largest diameter file is a 140. The length is 21 mm, 25 mm, 30 mm, or 31 mm. Special veterinary files are available for canine teeth that are 40 mm, 60 mm, or, most recently, 120 mm (see Figure 29-35). This variation in length is necessary so that the tip of the tooth root can be reached in very long teeth (canines). The variation in diameter is necessary so that the narrow canals of old and/or small animals as well as the large canals of young or big animals (lions, horses) can be properly filed.

Files should be removed from the package and placed in an organized manner. In our practice we place the files in a piece of foam in increasing diameter from 6 to 40 or 45, and all the files in this group should be a standard length (e.g., 21 mm). The files in the foam can be autoclaved, and when the veterinarian is ready to perform the root canal

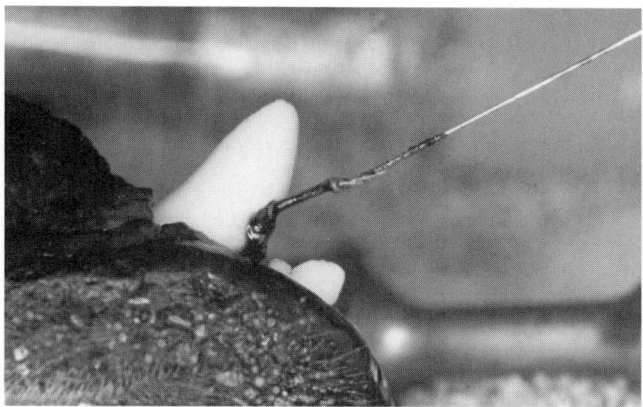

FIGURE 29-34. A barbed broach is used to remove pulp tissue from the tooth.

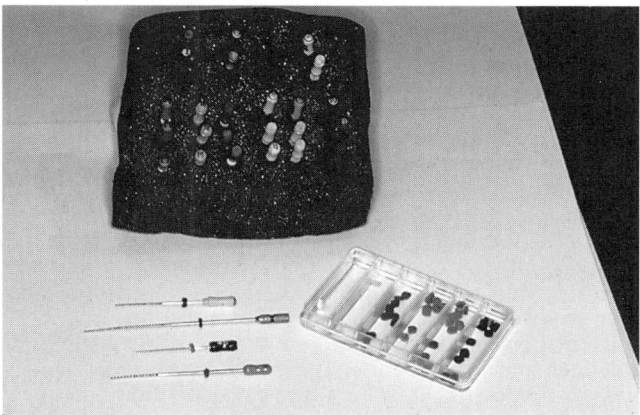

FIGURE 29-35. A sterile sponge and sterile endodontic files are organized and ready for use. Endodontic stops are in the container on the right. Different file lengths and types are displayed below the sponge. *Top to bottom,* 30-mm size 20 H file, 60-mm size 25 H file, 25-mm size 40 K file, and 40-mm size 35 K file.

Box 29-3	ROOT CANAL INSTRUMENTS AND MATERIALS

- A dental cleaning tray (supragingival scaler and small blade subgingival curette, dental explorer and probe, new prophy cup, flour pumice) (see Figure 29-7)
- Several dental films, dental film positioner, dental machine turned on and set to the proper technique for the patient
- Barbed broaches, endodontic files with endodontic stops, measuring gauges
- Canal irrigants, endodontic irrigation needles, canal lubricant, dental dam
- Engine-driven endodontic files (rotary files) and corresponding handpiece
- Tongue depressors, gauze squares
- Round (½, 1, or 2) or pear (330) carbide or diamond burs
- Gutta-percha cones, cannulas, and syringes; machinery used to heat gutta-percha should be turned on and filled with gutta-percha if extended heating times are required (i.e., Ultrafil and Successfil products)
- Glass bead sterilizer should be turned on
- Endodontic cement and mixing pack, spreaders and pluggers, sterile paper points
- Restorative materials and dentinal bonding agent

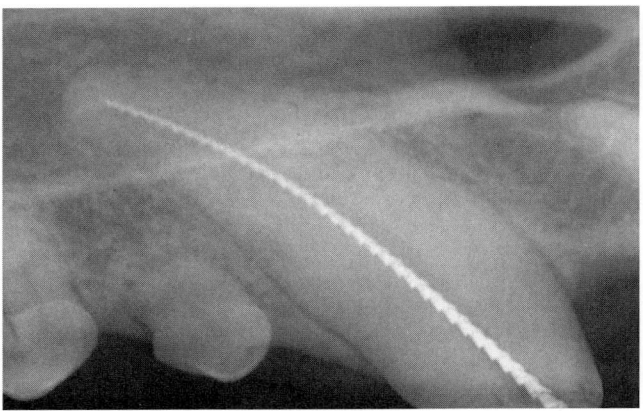

FIGURE 29-36. This radiograph verifies that the file is at the proper working length because the file tip goes all the way to the apex of the root canal.

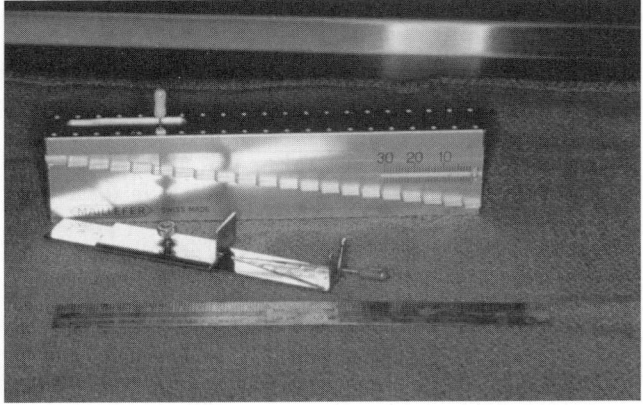

FIGURE 29-37. Measuring gauges used to measure the working length of the root canal. The two gauges at the top are used to quickly slide the endodontic stop to the correct length.

the foam of files will be sterile and in an organized manner. Several files of each diameter should be included. For instance, we put three of each size from 6 to 25. Two of these three files are K files, and the other one is a Hedstrom file. The files are organized with the 2 K files in front and the Hedstrom file in back (see Figure 29-35). This attention to detail is helpful in minimizing anesthesia time because root canals can take 1 to 2 hours depending on the tooth and degree of skill.

Endodontic stops are small pieces of rubber that go around the file to mark a specific length (see Figure 29-35). The file is placed in the root canal, and a radiograph is taken to make sure the file goes all the way to the apical extent of the root canal system (Figure 29-36). The distance from the endodontic stop (placed at a convenient location on the crown of the tooth) to the file tip is called the *working length*. The rest of the files are set to this length to ensure the root canal is filed to the proper depth. Measuring gauges are available that allow quick adjustment of the endodontic stop to the proper working length (Figure 29-37).

If rotary files are used they can be placed in a sterile sponge in order from smallest diameter to largest as well. The handpiece that attaches to these files should be set up. It will either be attached to the low-speed handpiece of the air-driven dental unit or have an electrical connection. The rotary engine-driven files may have two different file types available. The first type is a shorter file with a greater diameter increase along the taper. These files are referred to as orifice shapers, and they are used to open the coronal third of the root canal. The other set of files will be longer and should reach the apex of the tooth. The diameter of these files does not increase as rapidly along the taper.

Canal lubricants are sold that are used to soften the dentinal walls to ease filing and help prevent file breakage. One of these lubricants should be on hand. An irrigant is used in between file sizes to rinse the canal of dentinal shavings and other debris. The most common irrigant is sodium hypochlorite (i.e., Clorox bleach) because of its excellent disinfecting properties and ability to break down organic debris (pulp). Endodontic irrigation needles are placed on the syringe that contains the irrigant. These needles have a blunt end with a side opening to prevent forcing noxious irrigant periapically (Figure 29-38).

After the canal has been properly cleaned and shaped by

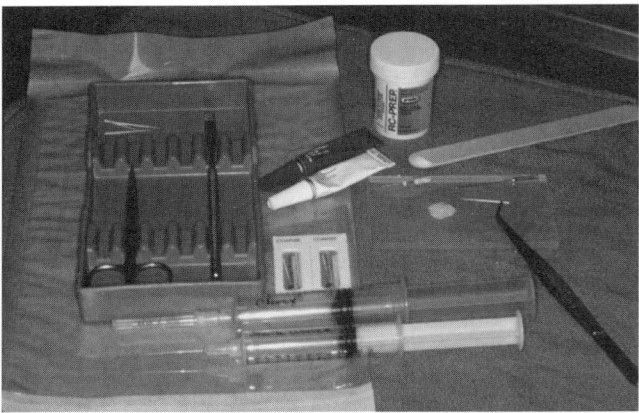

FIGURE 29-38. Root canal irrigants *(bottom),* paper points, and sterile glass slab with endodontic cement. The small jar contains a canal lubricant. Some of the lubricant has been placed on a tongue depressor. The files can be coated with lubricant without contaminating the stock bottle. The pink tray is autoclaved with the glass slab, cotton forceps, spatula, and iris scissors. The cement is mixed with the spatula on the glass slab.

the files, it is then ready for obturation. This simply means filling the canal with a material that will seal it from the periapical area. The canal should have a final rinse of sterile water then it is dried with sterile paper points. Successive paper points are inserted and removed until the points come out of the canal dry. An endodontic sealer is then applied to the canal walls. Sealer application can be done with a sterile paper point, K file, or spiral paste filler on a slow-speed handpiece (see Figure 29-38).

Gutta-percha is used to provide the bulk of the filling agent. It is a radiopaque viscoelastic material that can be vertically and laterally condensed to adapt to the shape of the root canal. The material can be heated to allow it to flow into the canal and adapt to the canal shape easier. Ultrafil cannulas are heated in a specially designed heater. When the heater indicates that the cannula is ready (flashing light) it is attached to a syringe and injected into the

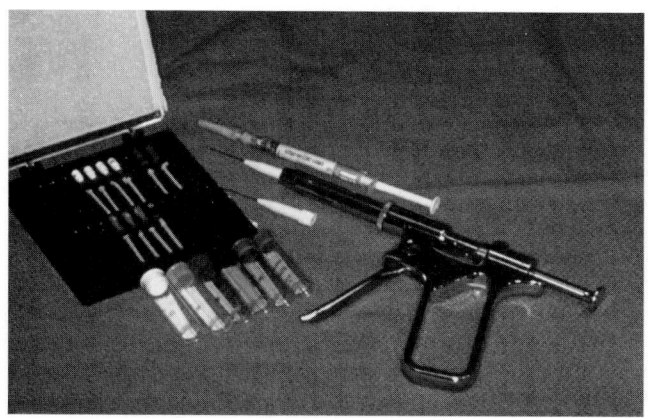

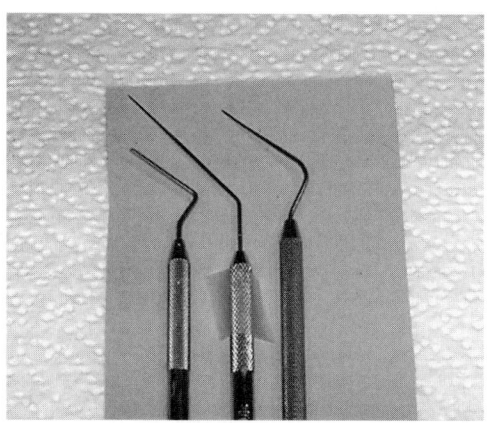

FIGURE 29-39.   Gutta-percha products. The TB syringe contains gutta-percha (Successfil), the white cannulas go in the silver gun to inject gutta-percha (Ultrafil), and the gutta-percha–coated files in the black box are inserted into the canals and the handle is removed. These three techniques require heating of the gutta-percha beforeplacement. The gutta-percha points in the vials are color coded to indicate size. These are placed in the canal without heating but can be heated once in the canal if desired.

FIGURE 29-40.   An endodontic plugger *(left)* and endodontic spreaders *(middle* and *right)*. The spreaders have a pointed end, and the pluggers have a flat end.

canal. The Thermafil system has gutta-percha coated on a file. The appropriate size gutta-percha–coated files are selected based on the size of the canal and with the aid of a size verifier file. The correct size verifier file will fit passively in the root canal to the appropriate working length. The corresponding gutta-percha–coated file is then placed in the Thermafil system's oven and heated for the amount of time indicated on the oven button for that size file. When the oven beeps the file is removed from the oven and placed in the root canal. The file handle is removed, and the rest of the file remains in the canal (Figure 29-39). Vertical and lateral condensation is performed with pluggers and spreaders, and additional gutta-percha is added if needed. Pluggers have a blunt end that pushes the gutta-percha vertically in an apical direction. Spreaders have a pointed tip and push the gutta-percha laterally to create room for more gutta-percha for a solid fill. Spreaders and pluggers come in a variety of lengths and sizes (Figure 29-40). Extra long veterinary length spreaders and pluggers are available as well.

Once obturation of the canal has been accomplished, the restorative filling material is placed. This can be done with a single filling material or in two layers with an intermediate and final filling material used. Composite fillings cannot be placed next to eugenol because eugenol can interfere with the set of the composite. Gutta-percha

does contain a large amount of eugenol. Glass ionomers are a commonly used intermediate or final filling material. If used as an intermediate filling material, a composite final filling material is then used for optimal esthetics.

Teeth that have undergone pulp death do become more brittle over time because of the lack of hydration that was originally provided by the pulp tissue. A good history should always be taken to try to determine how the pet fractured the tooth. If inappropriate chew toys are in the environment these should be removed when possible. A metal cap may be desired to help prevent fracture of the tooth in the future.

EXODONTICS

Some people feel that tooth extraction is equivalent to failure for a dentist. Although it is fantastic to be able to save teeth for pets, it is not always in the pet's best interest to save a very diseased tooth. A good history from the owner is necessary to determine his or her level of commitment to the pet's oral health. If owners do not feel they can brush their pet's teeth daily or at least 3 times per week and are not likely to bring the pet back for professional dental care as necessary, then tooth extraction may be the best option for the pet. It can be very disheartening to have a pet go through advanced periodontal therapy only to see that the owner is not following through with the dental care at home and the pet returns to the office with an infected mouth and oral pain. The veterinary practice's ultimate goal is to provide the pet with a healthy and comfortable mouth.

Sometimes owners are willing to provide all the treatment necessary but the tooth is too damaged to have successful results. In either scenario tooth extraction will be necessary. Very loose teeth can be easy to extract and sometimes fall out on their own when the technician is cleaning the teeth. These teeth should be set aside for the veterinarian to examine to make sure no portion of the root remains in the mouth, and they should be recorded on the dental record. Teeth with a healthy periodontium can be very difficult to extract, especially if they are multi-rooted. Tooth extraction techniques will be discussed so that the technician can have the appropriate equipment on hand for the veterinarian. In many instances a preoperative radiograph of the tooth will be taken to evaluate the roots and surrounding bone so that risk factors are minimized.

A no. 11 or 15 scalpel blade is used to sever the epithelial attachment of the gingiva around the cervical region of the tooth (neck). If the tooth is multirooted a periosteal

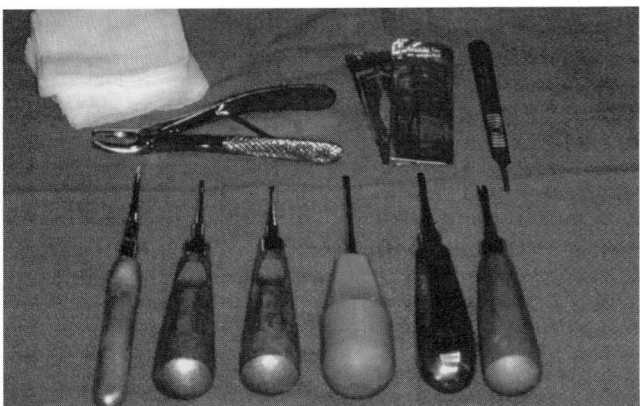

FIGURE 29-41.   An assortment of dental elevators is necessary. Elevators with a small narrow blade are used initially, and as the periodontal ligament breaks down, larger-bladed elevators can be used. Small breed extraction forceps, scalpel blades and handle, and gauze sponges are on hand as well. Dental elevators *(left to right):* Cislak 100c, Cislak EX5, Cislak 301MX, luxator, Cryer 34S, E34.

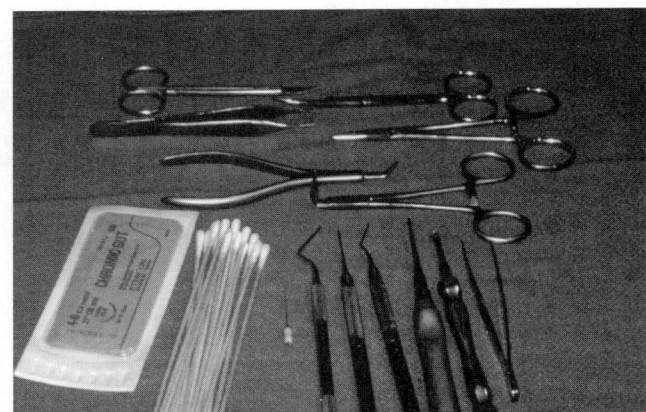

FIGURE 29-42.   Small root tip picks are necessary to retrieve broken roots or to extract teeth in very small animals. Dental elevators *(left to right):* Schein ST11, Cislak WA1, Cislak WA2, Cislak 100C, and a Farenkrug. A small tip tissue forcep or an endodontic file can also work well to retrieve loose root tips. Small root tip forceps and suturing instruments should be on hand.

elevator (Cislak Ex-9, Schein ST 7, Molt 9) (see Figure 29-6) can be used to lift the gingiva off the buccal or lingual bone to visualize the furcation. Vertical releasing incisions may be needed to allow further elevation of the gingiva to expose alveolar bone for removal over the tooth roots or to create a mucogingival flap to close the extraction site. Next, small dental elevators are used to place in the periodontal ligament space and are rotated to put pressure on the tooth root (Figure 29-41). Pressure is held for 5 to 10 seconds, and then the elevator is advanced apically and rotated against the root in the opposite direction to create pressure and hold again. The goal is to fatigue the periodontal ligament and avoid tooth root fracture. Larger elevators are used as the periodontal ligament breaks down and allows more room to place a larger instrument (see Figure 29-41). The veterinarian will therefore need a surgery pack of small to large dental elevators, a periosteal elevator, scalpel handle and blade, gauze squares, extraction forceps, suture, needle holders, thumb forceps, and scissors (dissection and suture).

Sometimes a root will fracture, and additional instruments will be needed to retrieve the retained tooth root. Small dental elevators called *root tip picks* are helpful for root tip retrieval as are very small-tipped extraction forceps called *root tip forceps* (Figure 29-42). Cotton tip applicators are helpful to bloat hemorrhage in the alveolar socket to visualize the root tip. Once all tooth root material has been extracted, the socket should be debrided of any calculus and excessive granulation tissue with a spoon curette (Figure 29-43). If the site is to be closed with a mucogingival flap, tetracycline powder can be placed in the socket before closing the site if the animal is mature. The pet should be given soft food for 7 to 14 days following treatment and be given antibiotics and pain medications as deemed necessary by the veterinarian. Regional nerve blocks are very helpful with pain management and can be given at the time of surgery (see Chapter 22). The owner can resume tooth brushing in 3 to 14 days but may wish to avoid the extraction site until the pet no longer seems tender.

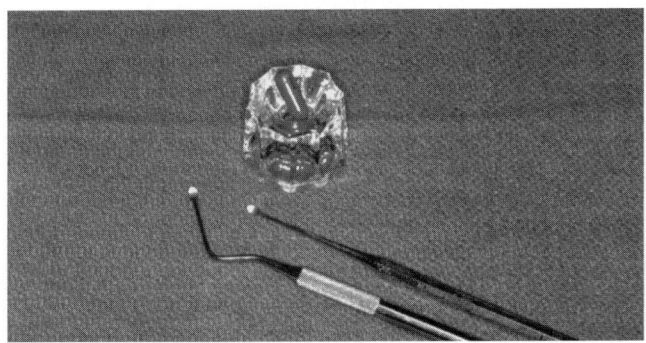

FIGURE 29-43.   Bone curettes (Lucas 75, Schein ST10) and a tetracycline capsule in a dental dappen dish. The tetracycline powder can be poured into the dappen dish and placed into the alveolar socket with the bone curette.

Tooth extraction is considered a surgical procedure in most instances, and serious complications can arise that the owner should be made aware of before admitting the pet for the procedure. Complications to address with the owner are those associated with anesthesia as well as the possibility of hemorrhage; eye trauma if working on teeth in the mid to caudal maxilla; and jaw fracture. Iatrogenic jaw fracture can easily occur when extracting diseased mandibular first molars or canine teeth in cats or small breed dogs if care is not taken.

Technician Note

Tooth extraction is considered a surgical procedure in most instances, and serious complications can arise that the owner should be made aware of before admitting the pet for the procedure.

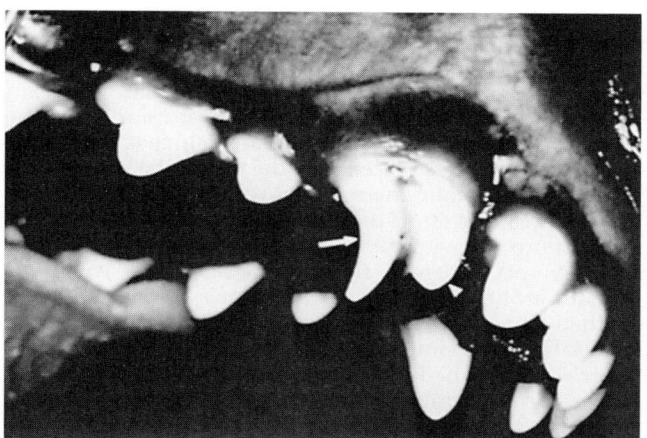

FIGURE 29-44.   A retained deciduous maxillary canine tooth *(arrow)* has displaced the permanent canine tooth mesially (toward the nose) *(arrowhead)*. The abnormal tooth alignment can lead to periodontal disease and interfere with other teeth or oral soft tissues.

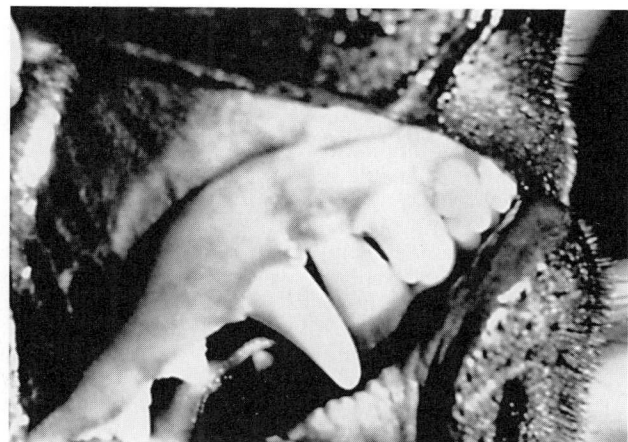

FIGURE 29-45.   Lingually displaced mandibular canine tooth. The mandibular canine is displaced toward the tongue and is striking the gingival tissue.

ORTHODONTICS

Orthodontics is concerned with the correction and prevention of irregularities and malocclusion of the teeth. The primary reason for performing orthodontic correction of malaligned teeth in veterinary medicine is to alleviate a painful malocclusion or a malocclusion that will lead to endodontic or periodontal disease. When genetic malocclusions are suspected, the owner should be counseled on the problem in order to prevent breeding of these animals and the propagation of inferior genes.

Interceptive orthodontics involves the extraction of retained deciduous teeth that will usually cause displacement of the permanent dentition (Figure 29-44). This treatment can be extremely beneficial, and many abnormally erupting permanent teeth will correct spontaneously after extraction of the retained deciduous teeth. The most important factor determining success with this treatment is early detection of the problem. Many companion animals have completed their vaccination series by the time they reach this mixed dentition stage and will not be seen again until 6 months of age if the owner has elected to neuter the pet. To prevent this condition from going undetected, the owner should be instructed to monitor the dentition closely to ensure that the deciduous tooth is shed before the emergence of the permanent tooth. Dental models can be used to show the owner the difference between deciduous teeth and permanent teeth. Dental examinations can be scheduled so that a dental problem does not go undetected.

Some of the most common dental malocclusions seen are lingually displaced mandibular canine teeth (Figure 29-45), mesially displaced maxillary canine teeth (Figure 29-46), and even or level bites. These malocclusions can be corrected by orthodontics in most cases, but the owner must be willing to invest the time to clean the oral appliance and return for rechecks as needed. Orthodontic treatment generally costs more than tooth extraction and involves more anesthetic procedures, but it is less invasive than extraction. Orthodontics can be an important treatment option when considering alternatives to extraction of large teeth such as the canines, or multiple teeth, such as the six incisors in a dog with an even bite. Many cases that

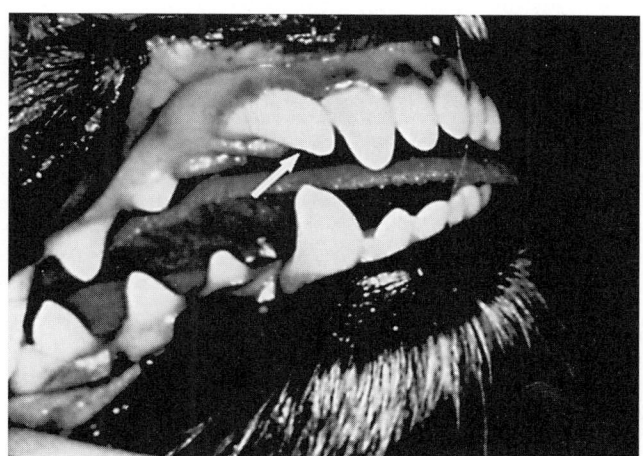

FIGURE 29-46.   Mesially displaced maxillary canine tooth. The maxillary canine tooth is displaced mesially *(arrow)* and is striking the mandibular canine tooth when the mouth is closed.

present with the malocclusions listed above can be corrected rapidly with orthodontic treatment.

Crown height reduction with or without a vital pulpotomy is another option for animals with malocclusions, particularly severe malocclusions. This procedure entails shortening the tooth to remove the interference it is causing with another tooth or surrounding soft tissue. This method is less invasive than extraction, removes the animal's source of discomfort, and achieves results more quickly than does orthodontics. However, it does permanently alter the appearance of the tooth (Figure 29-47). The pulp chamber is often exposed when the crown is reduced sufficiently. When this occurs, a vital pulpotomy will be necessary to protect the pulp tissue.

Impressions and Models

Veterinary technicians and dental assistants can be given the task of taking an impression and pouring a stone model if an orthodontic study model is needed. These stone dental models will aid treatment and serve as a record for treatment progress. The orthodontic appliances are often constructed from these models as well.

Alginate is the material that records the imprint of the teeth. The teeth should be cleaned before the impression is made. The appropriate size dental impression tray is selected for the patient. The area of interest must fit into the tray without touching the sides, and the tray must completely cover these teeth. Impression trays made for dogs and cats can be purchased. These trays are designed for the anterior portion of the mouth from about the level of the third premolar forward. This is where most of the treated orthodontic problems occur in dogs. Cats are rarely treated by orthodontic means because of poor patient acceptance.

The jar of alginate should be agitated (fluffed) with the top on before use and should be allowed to sit for at least 5 minutes after agitation so the dust will settle. Level scoops of alginate are placed in a rubber mixing bowl. The scoop comes in the jar of alginate. A proper scoop of alginate will be level on the surface and will not contain filling voids. Gently tap the scoop of alginate to eliminate any voids, and then level the surface with the blade of the alginate spatula (Figure 29-48).

Alginate spatulas have a wide blade that is used to blend the alginate powder with the water. A cylinder comes with the alginate to measure out the proper amount of water. The cylinder is clear plastic with three lines on it. Water is filled to the first line if one scoop of alginate is used, the second line if two scoops of alginate are used, and so on. The amount of alginate used is based on the size of the impression tray. The water is added to the alginate all at once, and the spatula is used in a stirring action to wet the powder. Once the powder is wet, the wide blade is used to

start spatulating. This term means to spread and smear the alginate from one side of the bowl to the other in a back and forth motion. The bowl is held in the palm of the hand while the dominant hand works the spatula. Once the alginate is mixed, it is loaded into the impression tray with the spatula. The lips of the animal are held away from the teeth, and the tray is placed over the teeth. The tray should be held steady while the material sets. This takes about 5 minutes from the start of the mix. Cold water and room temperature will increase the set time, and warm water and room temperature will shorten the set time. The extra alginate around the rim of the impression tray can be touched periodically to determine when it is set. Once the material sets it is similar to rubber and will not stick to the finger when touched. The impression tray and alginate are then removed from the teeth in one quick pulling motion in the direction of the long axis of the teeth.

Once removed from the teeth, the impression should be inspected to be sure the area of interest was adequately recorded (Figure 29-49). The material should then be rinsed off and a moist paper towel placed on it until the

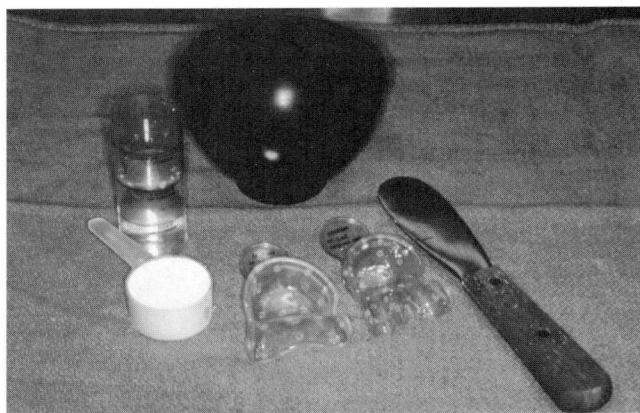

FIGURE 29-48.   Materials used to take an alginate impression: rubber mixing bowl, alginate spatula, impression trays (mandibular and maxillary), alginate scoop, and water measuring cylinder.

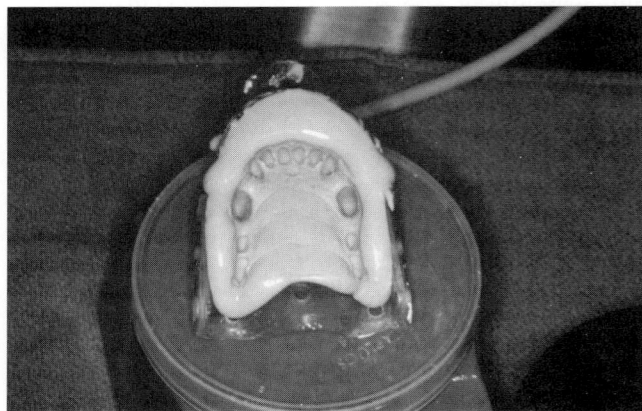

FIGURE 29-49.   Alginate impression of the rostral maxillary dentition.

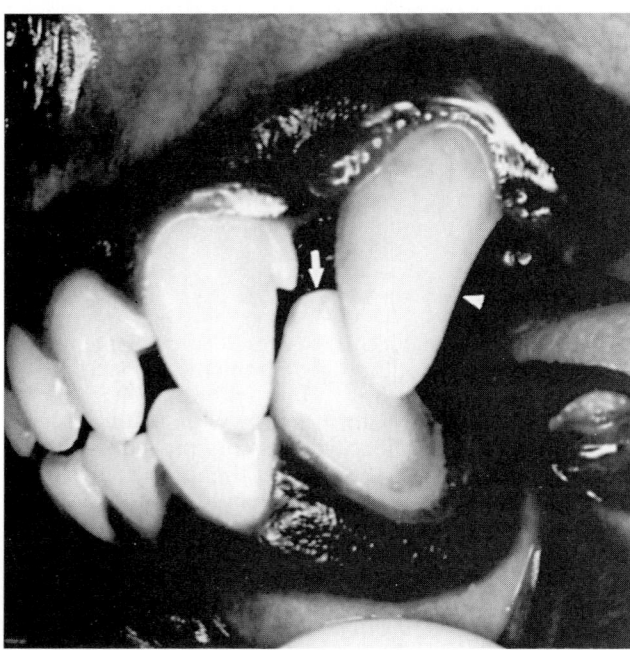

FIGURE 29-47.   The mandibular canine tooth *(arrow)* has been shortened to prevent it from impinging on the palate. The maxillary canine tooth *(arrowhead)* is displaced mesially, preventing the mandibular canine tooth from returning to its normal position.

stone can be poured into it. The sooner the stone is poured the more accurate the impression will be since alginate is susceptible to desiccation and overhydration. Most technicians pour the stone as soon as the animal is recovered from anesthesia or sooner when safely possible.

Dental stone is used to make the positive image of the mouth. The stone comes in a powder form and is mixed with water. The powder can be weighed out and mixed with a specified volume of water. Experienced technicians can determine the approximate amount of water and stone powder by the thickness of the mix. A good mix will slowly run off the mixing blade when held above the bowl. The rubber mixing bowls and a narrow blade spatula are used for the stone (Figure 29-50).

Once the stone is mixed, the alginate impression should be cleared of excess water by gently tapping or shaking it. The impression is then held on a laboratory vibrator while small amounts of stone are placed on the impression and allowed to run into the teeth. This step is critical because if an air bubble gets trapped in the teeth the impression will be missing part of the tooth. The vibrator serves two purposes. First, it helps to remove bubbles from the stone, and second, it causes the stone to flow into the teeth. Once the teeth have been filled with stone, the rest of the stone can be added at a faster rate since this step is less critical. The stone mix can then be made thicker by adding more powder. This portion can be placed on the top of the model to give it a strong base. The vibrator is not used for this step. Optimal working time for the stone is about 10 minutes. Complete set of the stone takes about 1 to 2 hours.

The model should be removed from the alginate impression after the stone has had at least 45 minutes to set. Do not wait several hours because the alginate will dry and stick to the stone model. The model should be carefully pulled from the alginate and inspected to make sure all teeth are adequately recorded. If a portion of a tooth is missing this could be a result of an air bubble or the tooth could have broken off and still remain in the impression. The canine teeth are particularly susceptible to fracture because of their long curved anatomy. If the stone tooth breaks, it can be glued back on the model. The model should then be labeled with the pet's name and the date.

Technician Note

The impression is then held on a laboratory vibrator while small amounts of stone are placed on the impression and allowed to run into the teeth. This step is critical because if an air bubble gets trapped in the teeth the impression will be missing part of the tooth.

RESTORATIVE DENTISTRY

The goal of restorative dentistry is to restore a tooth as closely as possible to its natural structure and function. No restorative material is as strong as the original tooth structure, so an attempt is always made to preserve as much of the original tooth as possible. Indications for restorative dentistry include teeth with dental caries (cavities), fractured teeth, and endodontically treated teeth.

Dental caries rarely occurs in the dog and cat. When present, the carious tooth structure must be completely removed and the defect restored. If left untreated, the caries will dissolve the enamel and dentin and gain access to the pulp tissue. The tooth will eventually be destroyed.

A common problem of feline dentition is the development of idiopathic feline odontoclastic resorptive lesions (Figure 29-51). It is estimated that 20% of cats are affected by this problem. The lesions are usually found at the neck of the tooth (the junction of the enamel of the crown and the cementum of the tooth root), which is often hidden by the gingiva. Cats must be examined closely for these lesions. Often the gingival tissue over these lesions is inflamed. A dental explorer must be used to check for

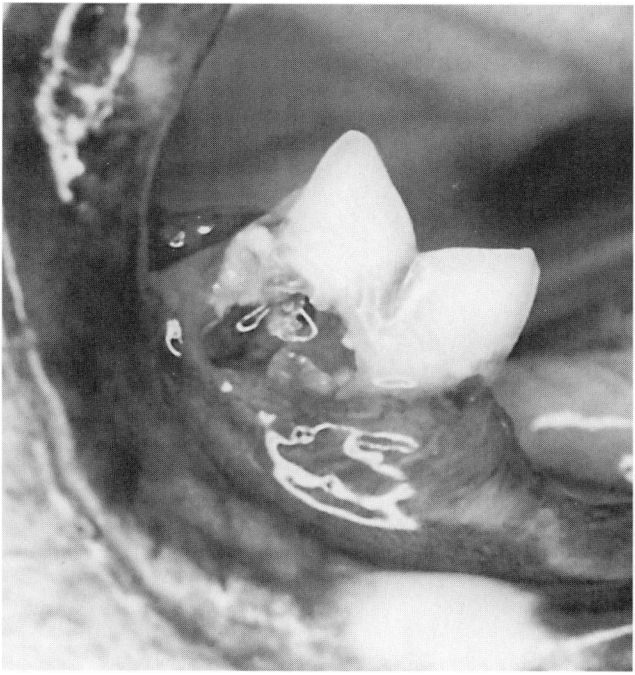
FIGURE 29-51. Feline odontoclastic resorptive lesion. The large erosion on this tooth involves the distal root and cervical portion of the tooth crown. A dental radiograph is necessary to evaluate the tooth roots.

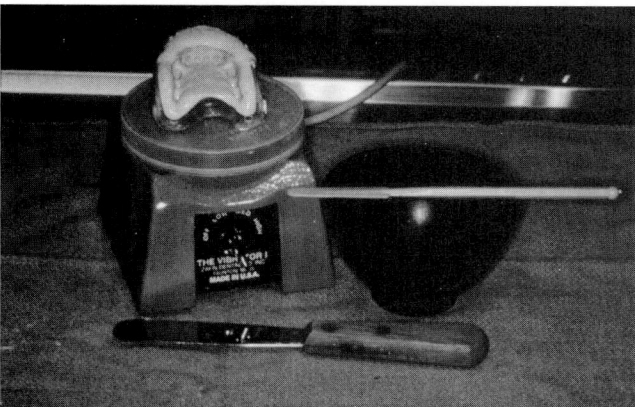
FIGURE 29-50. Materials used to pour a stone dental model: rubber mixing bowl, small blade spatula, narrow blade spatula, laboratory vibrator, and alginate impression.

irregularities below the gingiva. Early detection and restoration of these lesions may prevent the continued resorption of the tooth. Many of these teeth are identified in the advanced stages of the disease with pulp exposure and root resorption. When the resorption has progressed this far, the tooth cannot be saved and should be extracted. Dental radiographs of these teeth are necessary to evaluate the severity of resorption.

Fractured teeth are frequently restored to return function and maintain periodontal health. The cheek teeth (premolars and molars) have a natural design called the *cervical bulge* that deflects food away from the gingival sulcus. When the teeth lose this proper contour they can become predisposed to periodontal disease. Fractured teeth can be restored with restorative materials alone or in combination with retention pins or posts or both. Pins and posts do not add strength to the restoration but aid in retaining the restoration. Restoration of the bulge on the upper fourth premolar is usually best achieved with a metal crown because of the powerful shearing forces this area receives.

Caps or prosthetic crowns are placed on teeth with fractured crowns to protect the tooth, to improve function, and sometimes to improve esthetics. The silver-colored metal caps, which are made of nonprecious metals, are the most common type used because of their greater strength and lower cost when compared with gold or porcelain caps. The teeth most commonly capped in dogs are the canines and maxillary fourth premolars (Figure 29-52). In the cat, the canine is the most commonly capped tooth.

Veterinary dentistry is a specialty field in veterinary medicine. Advanced procedures require strong background knowledge of the materials used, the anatomy and physiology of the teeth and periodontium, and the principles applied to each procedure. It is important for the general practitioner and veterinary technician to be able to identify dental abnormalities and to be able to recommend treatment alternatives to the owner. The pet can then be

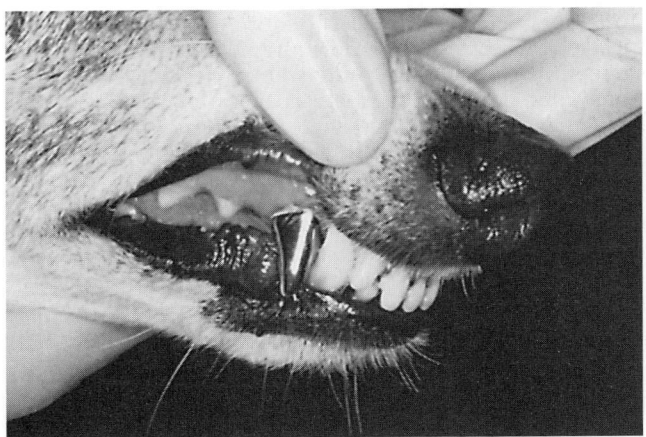

FIGURE 29-52. A non–precious metal crown has been cemented to the maxillary canine tooth after the tooth was traumatically fractured and received endodontic treatment.

referred for advanced dental procedures if the owner wishes to pursue treatment.

RECOMMENDED READING

DeForge DH, Colmery BH: *An atlas of veterinary dental radiology,* Ames, 2000, Iowa State University Press.

Holmstrom SE, Frost P, Eisner ER: *Veterinary dental techniques,* ed 2, Philadelphia, 1998, WB Saunders.

Torres HO et al: *Modern dental assisting,* ed 5, Philadelphia, 1995, WB Saunders.

Wiggs RB, Lobprise HB: *Veterinary dentistry principles and practice,* Philadelphia, 1997, Lippincott-Raven.

30

Equine Medical and Surgical Nursing

Rustin M. Moore • Lais R.R. Costa

The role of the veterinary technician in equine practice is to be a team member with a goal of providing efficient, quality health and nursing care for horses. A skilled, observant veterinary technician with equine-specific training is an invaluable resource in an equine hospital. Technicians are expected to provide patient monitoring, treatment, surgical assistance, nursing care, and client education. Providing veterinary care for horses is particularly cumbersome because they are large, fractious, and fragile animals. Skilled technical support with expertise in patient handling and restraint, specialized instrumentation, and equine-specific disease is crucial for the equine veterinarian to provide quality intensive care or perform advanced techniques. Familiarity with equine behavior will allow the veterinary technician to recognize abnormal behavior, permitting the early recognition of colic, pain, neurologic disease, and respiratory distress during patient monitoring, for example. The technician is often the first to identify a change in patient status and may save valuable time at a crucial turning point for therapeutic intervention. Familiarity with equine-specific surgical equipment will reduce surgical time and improve patient prognosis. Recognition of the unique layperson's language in equine medicine and surgery will help the technician recognize the significance of the patient's historical data and physical examination findings and improves client communication. Equine technical support imparts a tangible contribution to the quality and efficiency of patient care in a hospital setting.

PHYSICAL EXAMINATION OF THE EQUINE PATIENT

A thorough physical examination is an integral part of the diagnostic assessment and monitoring of ill horses. Because veterinary technicians play an important role in the day-to-day monitoring of hospitalized patients, learning to perform a thorough and complete physical examination is vital (see Chapter 2). A knowledgeable veterinary techni-

cian should ensure the safety of the handler, the examiner, and the patient when performing a physical examination. Handling the ill horse is inherently dangerous because most horses are more difficult to control when in pain or under stress. It is crucial to record all observations and findings of the physical examination in the medical record. The medical record provides the only record of the patient's progress or deterioration, and moreover it is a legal and scientific document (see Chapter 33).

Technician Note

The veterinary technician plays a pivotal role in the day-to-day monitoring of and caring for hospitalized patients; therefore the ability to be observant and to perform a thorough and complete physical examination is vital.

Physical examination should begin with observation of the equine patient from a distance and overall inspection of the animal and its surroundings, followed by a detailed assessment of each body system. The observation of the patient from a distance provides a more accurate assessment of the animal's mental status and attitude (the animal's interaction with its environment and other animals and response to external stimuli; thus the animal may appear bright and alert, depressed, obtunded, demented, responsive or unresponsive, excitable, etc.). Observation from a distance also allows assessment of the horse's breathing pattern and respiratory effort. Young horses and foals are likely to have increased respiratory rate and shallow breathing when approached. The horse's general body condition should be noted. The ribs should not be visible but should be easily palpated in a horse in ideal body condition. The horse's use and the physiologic demands, such as intense training, pregnancy, and lactation, should be considered when assessing body condition. Moreover, horses with mild depression or mild abdominal pain are more likely to demonstrate their true behavior when observed from a distance, whereas they may appear relatively normal when approached and examined. Several signs can indicate the horse is experiencing mild abdominal discomfort or pain. Those signs include pawing the ground with the front feet; kicking at the abdomen with the rear feet; looking at the flank or abdomen; curling the lip; posturing or straining to urinate or defecate; playing in the water bucket; lying down in sternal, lateral, or dorsal recumbency; and rolling on the ground.

Inspection of the horse's environment can also provide important information. Evidence of disrupted stall bedding could be an indicator of the horse being cast (unable to stand because the horse lies down too close to the wall) or could be an indication that the horse has experienced discomfort such as colic (abdominal pain). Exposed bare stall floor often indicates pawing of bedding. The amount of hay, feed, and water in the stall can be an important indicator of the horse's appetite and water intake. The amount, character, and quantity of feces in the stall and observation of the horse's drinking, urination, and defecation can also yield important information.

Close inspection of the horse should include evaluation of the head for swelling, wounds, and asymmetries; the nostrils for the presence and character of nasal discharge and for flared nostrils; and the eyes for ocular discharge (epiphora), the character of ocular discharge, and "squinting" (blepharospasm). Serous nasal discharge is often present in horses with viral respiratory disease, whereas horses with an infection of the frontal or maxillary sinuses or guttural pouches or horses with pneumonia often have a mucopurulent nasal discharge. Horses may have evidence of blood at the nostrils (epistaxis) as a result of guttural pouch mycosis, ethmoid hematomas, or exercise-induced pulmonary hemorrhage. Epiphora may be associated with a primary ocular disease or occlusion of the nasolacrimal duct system, or it may manifest secondary to a viral respiratory disease. Blepharospasm is usually a sign of ocular pain and is commonly observed in horses with corneal ulceration and uveitis. Coughing is generally a sign of lower respiratory tract disease (pneumonia, chronic obstructive pulmonary disease [COPD]) and can be productive or nonproductive. The presence of inspiratory or expiratory noise usually reflects an obstructive disease of the upper respiratory tract (nostrils to trachea). Dyspnea (difficult breathing) is characterized by flared nostrils, rapid and shallow thoracic excursions, and, if very severe, cyanotic mucous membranes; this should be brought to the attention of the attending veterinary clinician immediately. Flared nostrils (Figure 30-1) combined with the presence of prominent external abdominal oblique musculature ("heave line") extending anywhere from the tuber coxae toward the elbow (Figure 30-2) and a forced expiration usually signifies a horse with obstructive pulmonary disease.

Evaluation of the manner in which the horse ambulates in the stall can provide important information regarding the musculoskeletal and neurologic systems. Horses with laminitis (founder) often stand with their rear limbs camped underneath their torso and their front limbs extended in front of their torso in order to take weight off the toe and have an arched and tense back (see Figure 30-10). These horses may ambulate in the stall, but it is particularly painful when they are forced to turn. Horses with navicular disease may stand with the heels of the front feet elevated. Horses with severe unilateral limb lameness may stand with all their weight on the unaffected limb and may hold the affected limb in a slightly flexed position.

Evidence of ataxia (incoordination), generalized weakness, head tilted to one side, involuntary muscle tremors, and circling are suggestive of neurologic disease. Horses spending long periods in sternal or lateral recumbency because of painful musculoskeletal ailments (e.g., laminitis, rhabdomyolysis or "tying up," botulism) or neurologic diseases (hepatic encephalopathy, severe spinal cord disease) may often develop decubital ulcers (see Figure 30-25).

Monitoring of vital signs, including rectal temperature, respiratory rate, heart rate, and character of the pulse, is very important. One must be careful when taking a horse's rectal temperature and take appropriate safety precautions to prevent self-injury. Some horses resent having their rectal temperature taken and will kick. The horse should be approached from the left side, standing as close to its body as possible. The handler should also be located on the left side of the horse. One should slowly work toward the rear of the horse, carefully raise the tail, and slowly insert a lubricated thermometer into the rectum. Some horses will clamp down their tail. Do not stand directly behind the horse when taking the temperature because a kick could cause serious injury or death. The thermometer should be attached to a string or piece of rubber tubing and an alligator clip so that it can be attached to the tail hairs,

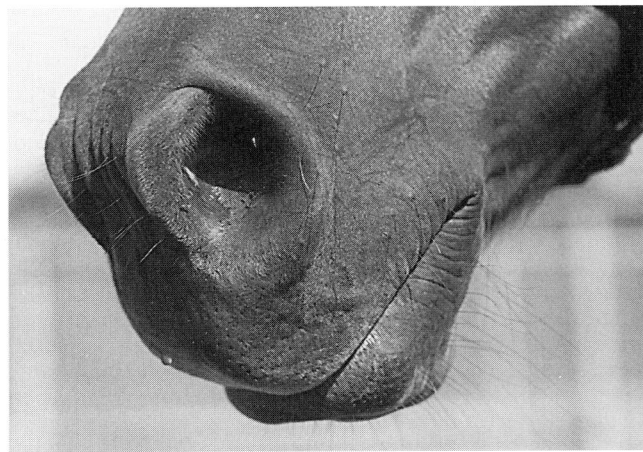

FIGURE 30-1.   Flared nostrils on a horse with chronic obstructive pulmonary disease.

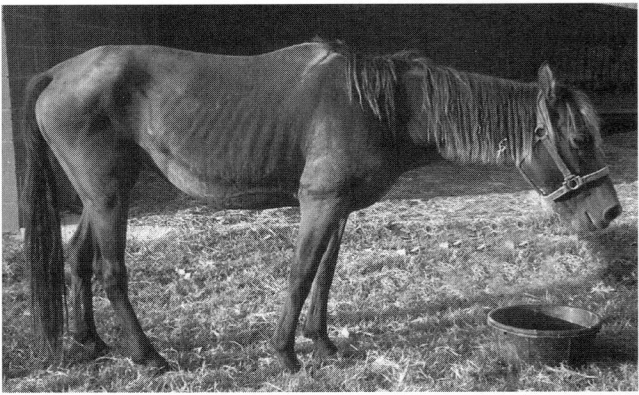

FIGURE 30-2.   Horse with increased expiratory effort and heave line caused by obstructive pulmonary disease.

which will prevent it from dropping to the floor during defecation. The normal rectal temperature of adult horses is approximately 37° C to 38.5° C (99° C to 101.5° F). An increased rectal temperature usually indicates an inflammatory or an infectious process somewhere in the body, but hyperthermia can occur after exercise and secondary to environmental conditions (hot, humid, poor ventilation), especially in anhidrotic (unable to sweat) horses. Hypothermia can occur regardless of the environmental temperature, particularly in foals and also in old and debilitated horses. The heart rate of adult horses should range from 25 to 50 beats/min and is generally 30 to 40 beats/min. The respiratory rate is generally 8 to 20 breaths/min. The heart rate can be determined by auscultating the heart or by obtaining the pulse from the linguofacial or transverse facial arteries (Figure 30-3).

The heart rhythm should also be assessed during auscultation of the heart; second-degree atrioventricular block is a common arrhythmia in adult horses and usually is alleviated by exercise. Atrial fibrillation is characterized by an irregular cardiac rhythm and can be confirmed on an electrocardiogram by a rapid and irregular rate and absent P waves. Auscultation and percussion of the thoracic cavity are important to assess the status of the lower respiratory tract and thoracic cavity. Both lung fields should be auscultated carefully (Figure 30-4). Frequently a rebreathing bag is used during auscultation of the lungs in adult horses to increase the depth of breathing by increasing the inspiratory and expiratory volumes and thus exacerbating adventitious sounds (Figure 30-5). Abnormal lung sounds, such as crackles and wheezes, can be auscultated in horses with pneumonia. End-expiratory wheezes can often be heard in horses with COPD. The heart and lungs sounds can be muffled in horses with pleural effusion; frequently a fluid line can be identified by auscultation and percussion of the thorax.

Oral mucous membranes should be assessed for color, moistness, capillary refill time after blanching, icterus, and

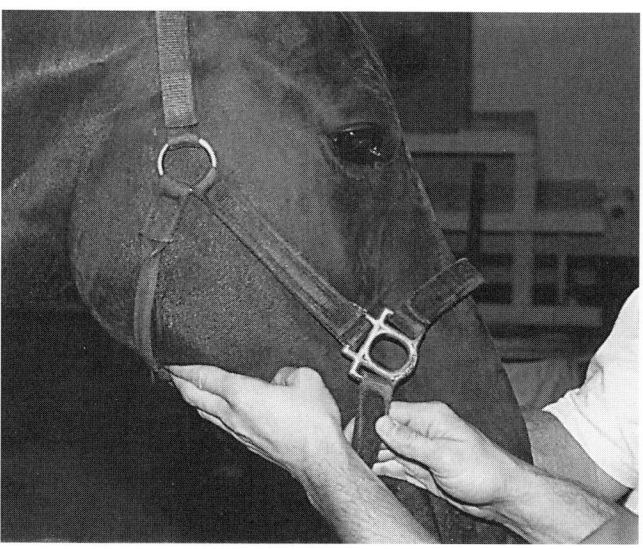

FIGURE 30-3. Determination of pulse rate and arterial pulse pressure through palpation of the facial artery.

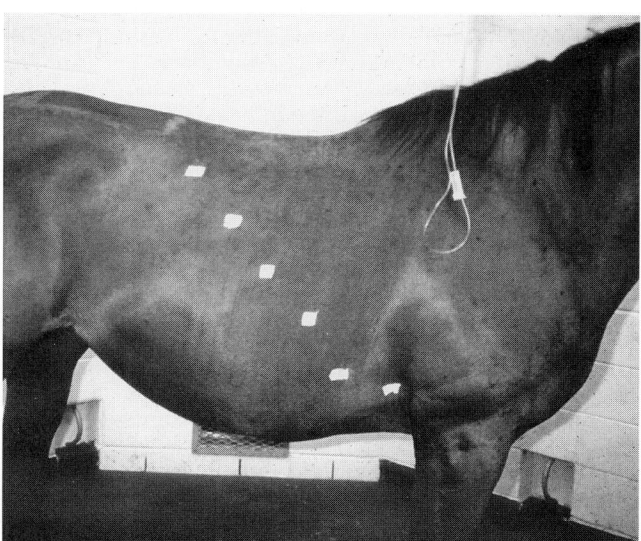

FIGURE 30-4. Outline of the lung fields in the horse.

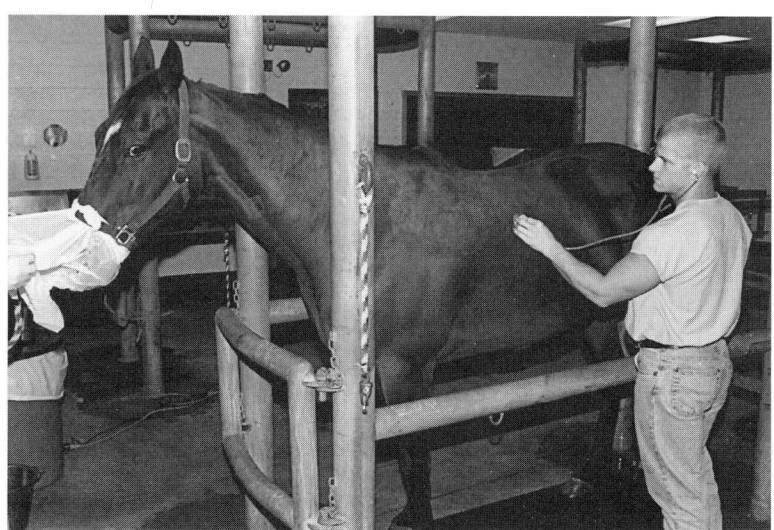

FIGURE 30-5. Use of a rebreathing bag to stimulate the horse to breathe more deeply to accentuate both normal and abnormal lung sounds during thoracic auscultation.

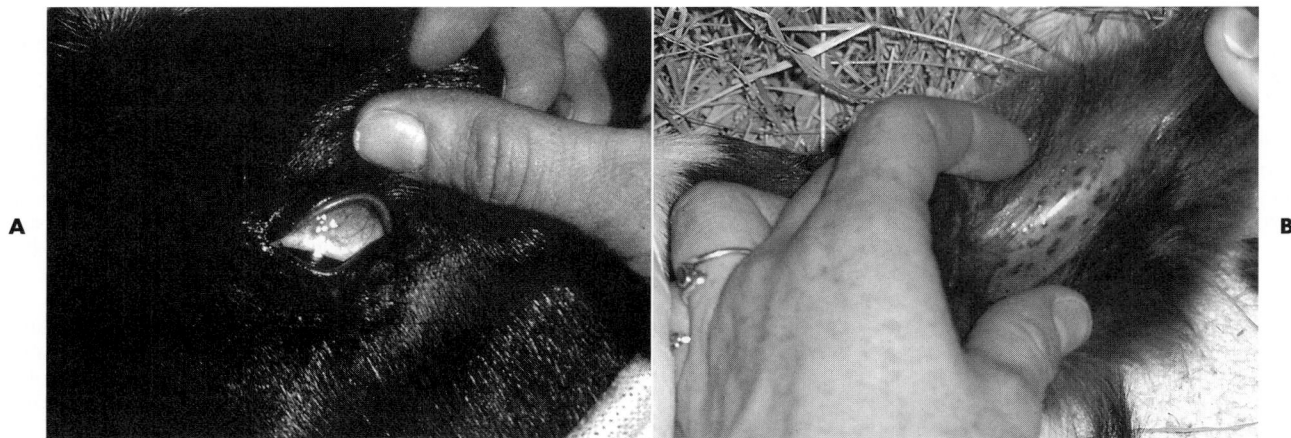

FIGURE 30-6. **A,** Scleral injection in a neonatal foal is suggestive of sepsis. **B,** Petechial hemorrhages in the pinna are also suggestive of sepsis.

petechiae. The oral mucous membranes should typically be light pink in color and moist to the touch. The capillary refill time should be less than 2 seconds. Cyanotic (whitish blue) mucous membranes often indicate severe hypoxemia (insufficient quantity of oxygen present in the blood) and are often observed in horses with respiratory disease. Dark pink to bright red mucous membranes are often observed in horses with endotoxemia. Dry, tacky mucous membranes often reflect volume depletion and are frequently observed in horses that are dehydrated or in shock. The sclera should also be examined for injection and icterus; this is particularly important in neonatal foals (Figure 30-6, *A*).

Auscultation and percussion of the abdominal cavity (Figure 30-7) should be performed carefully and thoroughly, especially in horses with gastrointestinal tract diseases (colic, diarrhea). The abdominal cavity is generally arbitrarily divided into right and left dorsal and ventral quadrants for purposes of auscultation and percussion. In addition, the degree of abdominal distention should be assessed and monitored. This can be performed by subjective visual observation or can be assessed more objectively by measuring abdominal circumference at a consistent site. Monitoring of abdominal distention is especially useful in colicky foals. Last, rectal examination is important in the evaluation of adult horses with conditions involving the abdominal cavity, and it is often considered an extension of the physical examination of horses with colic, diarrhea, or weight loss. Rectal examination should only be performed by a veterinarian in horses that are properly restrained (Figure 30-8). Rectal trauma can be sustained during a rectal examination and can lead to a tear or perforation that is fatal. Likewise, digital rectal palpation of a young foal suspected to have a meconium impaction should be carefully performed by a veterinarian.

Technician Note

Horses are unable to evacuate their stomach by vomiting; therefore it is important that the veterinary technician become knowledgeable and proficient in nasogastric intubation to prevent a catastrophic rupture of the stomach.

Because ill horses are predisposed to develop laminitis, the digital pulse and hoof heat should be evaluated often.

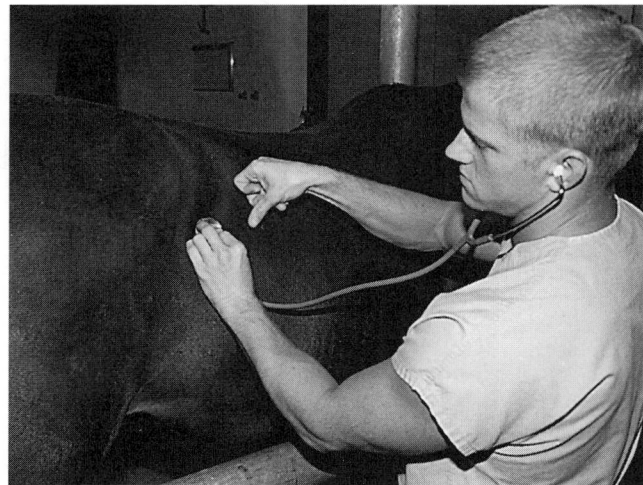

FIGURE 30-7. Auscultation and percussion of the abdominal cavity.

The digital pulse can be palpated at the level of the fetlock over the abaxial surface of the sesamoid bones (Figure 30-9). Normally the pulse can be palpated, but it should not be bounding. Although subjective, evaluation of hoof heat can be useful, particularly if there is a unilateral disease process. Hoof heat increases secondary to laminitis, sole abscess formation, and other infectious or inflammatory conditions of the foot. The digital pulse can increase subsequent to any disorder of the foot, but an increase occurs commonly with laminitis, sole abscess, and third phalanx fractures. Laminitic horses are reluctant to move, particularly when turning or stepping on a hard surface (Figure 30-10). Proper management measures and therapy for acute laminitis should be instituted as soon as possible.

Passage of a nasogastric tube is an essential part of the examination and treatment of horses with colic. Because horses are unable to evacuate their stomach by vomiting, it is important that the technician becomes knowledgeable and proficient in nasogastric intubation to prevent a catastrophic rupture of the stomach. The nasogastric tube can be passed by standing on the horse's left side and placing the right hand on the bridge of the nose to control

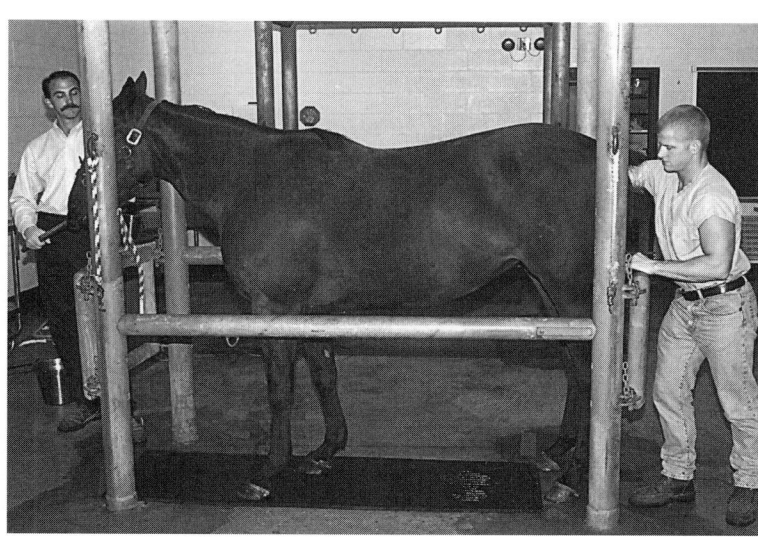

FIGURE 30-8. Rectal examination of a horse that is physically restrained with the use of stocks and a twitch.

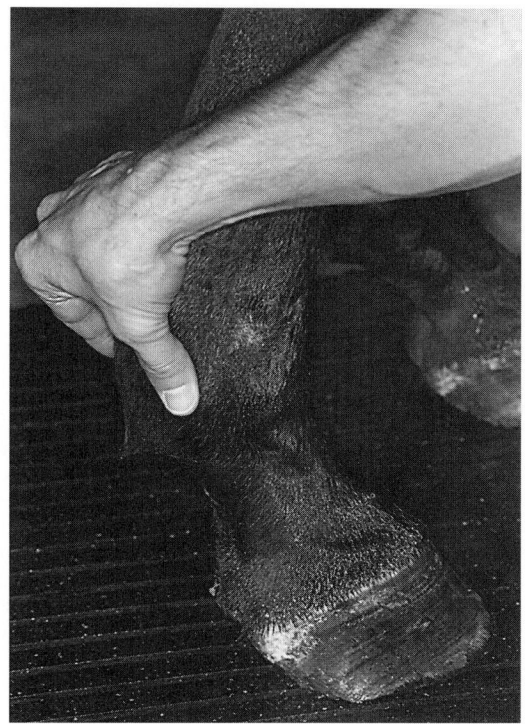

FIGURE 30-9. Location for palpation of digital pulse in a horse.

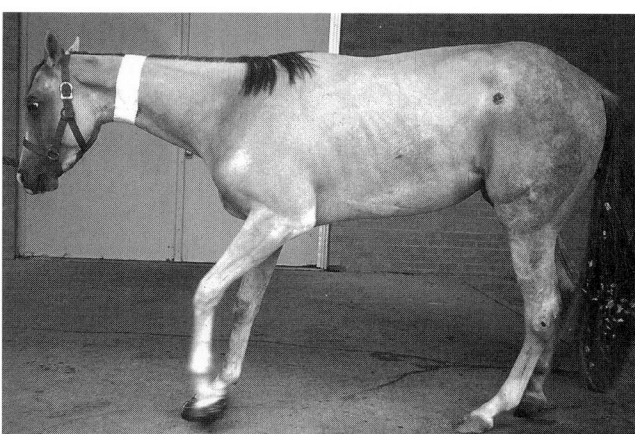

FIGURE 30-10. Typical posture of a horse with laminitis walking or turning on a hard surface.

movement of the horse's head (Figure 30-11). The end of the nasogastric tube to be passed into the stomach should be held in the left hand, and the opposite end of the tube should either be held in the mouth or draped around the neck of the person passing the tube. Lubrication of the end of the tube with warm water or a water-soluble jelly may facilitate the passage through the nasal canal. The thumb of the right hand is used to push the tube into the ventral meatus of the nasal passages. The tube should be advanced slowly through the nasal passages because if the tube briskly contacts the ethmoid turbinates, profuse bleeding can occur. As the nasogastric tube is advanced through the

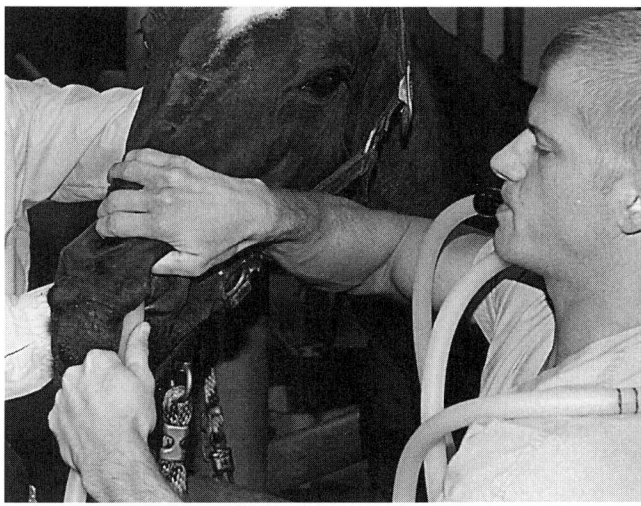

FIGURE 30-11. Nasogastric intubation in an adult horse.

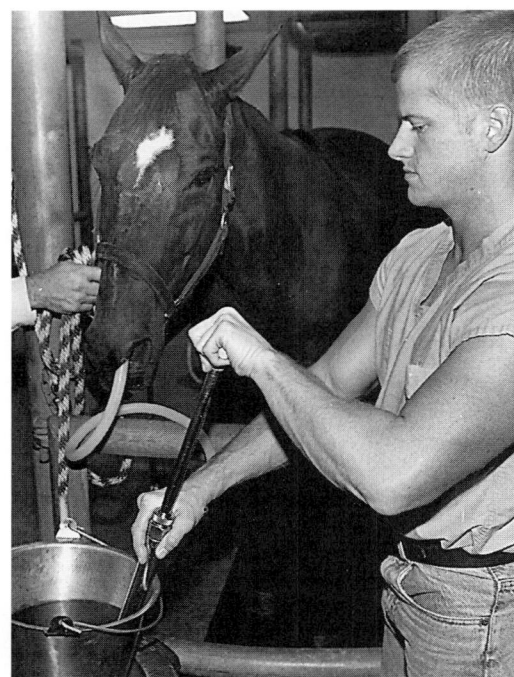

FIGURE 30-12. Once the nasogastric tube is confirmed to be within the stomach, the tube should be primed with water to initiate a siphon effect. This can be achieved by filling the tube with water through the use of either a pump or gravity flow with a funnel.

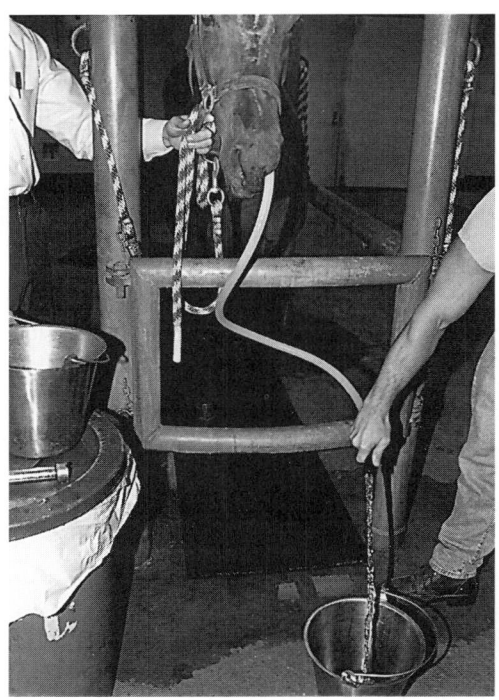

FIGURE 30-13. Evacuation of fluid from the stomach of a horse through a nasogastric tube.

nasopharynx the neck should be flexed to facilitate swallowing of the tube and avoid the placement of the tube into the trachea. Once the horse swallows the tube, the nasogastric tube should be advanced. The person passing the nasogastric tube should confirm that the tube is within the esophagus by obtaining negative pressure when sucking back on the tube or by visually observing or manually palpating the tube within the esophagus on the left side of the neck above the jugular groove. Adult horses often cough vigorously when the nasogastric tube is accidentally passed into the trachea; however, severely depressed and sedated horses may not cough at all. After it has been confirmed that the tube is within the esophagus, air can be blown through the tube to dilate the esophagus as the tube is being advanced into the stomach.

Special care should be taken when intubating the stomach of a neonatal foal. Neonatal foals often do not have a normal swallow reflex, and they rarely cough when the tube is located in the trachea. Avoid blowing into the nasogastric tube because accidental rupture of the foal's stomach can occur.

Once the tube is within the stomach it should be primed with water to obtain a siphon effect. The tube can be primed by pumping water or allowing water to flow by gravity through a funnel (Figure 30-12). Once the tube is primed, the end of the tube should be lowered to allow stomach contents to flow; sometimes it is helpful to pull the tube out in small movements until flow becomes steady (Figure 30-13). It is helpful to use a tube of as large a diameter as possible to facilitate removal of feed material from the stomach. It is also helpful to have several fenestra-

tions along the end of the tube to encourage drainage if the end of the tube or some fenestrations become occluded with feed material. The quantity of fluid that is placed within the tube and stomach for priming should be subtracted from the total amount of fluid obtained to determine the net amount of reflux, which should be recorded in the medical record. This provides a monitoring tool for determining the magnitude of the intestinal obstruction, determining whether ileus (abnormal intestinal motility) is improving, and monitoring fluid therapy. Moreover, the character of the gastric fluid (e.g., hemorrhagic, yellow, fermented grain, putrid smell) and the pH of the fluid will provide important information.

If no net reflux is obtained, then fluids or medications such as mineral oil (intestinal lubricant), magnesium sulfate (osmotic cathartic), dioctyl sodium succinate (surface-acting agent), psyllium hydrophilic mucilloid (bulk laxative), and bismuth subsalicylate (intestinal protectant) may be administered through the nasogastric tube. The total capacity of the stomach of adult horses is not very large, and no more than 6 to 8 L should be administered at one time. In horses being administered oral fluids, 6 to 8 L can be administered every 2 to 4 hours. In situations where net reflux is obtained or when fluids are being administered via nasogastric tube, the tube can be secured in place with adhesive tape and tied to the halter (Figure 30-14). If the tube is kept in place because the horse is continuously refluxing, the external end of the tube may be left unplugged to allow spontaneous drainage. Alternatively, the horse with voluminous continuous reflux may be checked hourly and the amount of reflux quantified. Indwelling

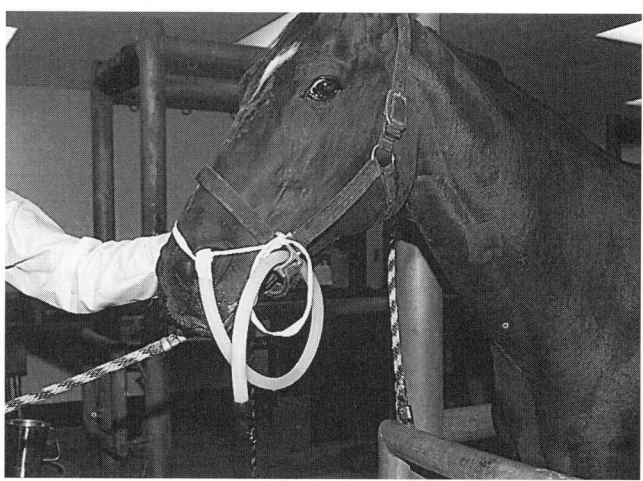

FIGURE 30-14. Technique for securing a nasogastric tube in the proper position. Adhesive tape can be applied to the tube and then tied to a securely fitting halter. This will help prevent dislodgment of the tube.

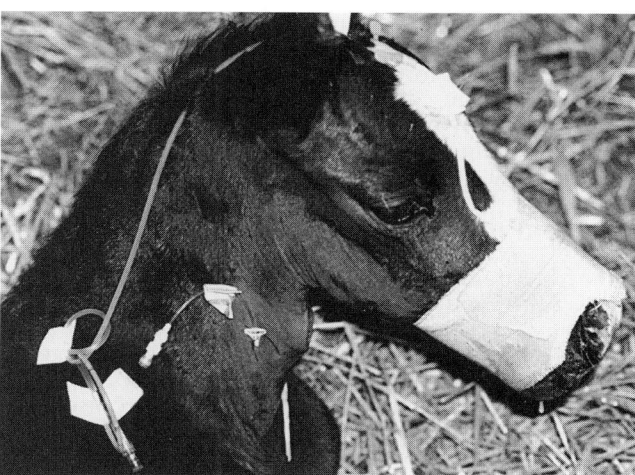

FIGURE 30-16. Alternative technique for securing a nasogastric feeding tube in a foal. The tube is sutured to the nostril and secured to the maxilla with adhesive tape (Elasticon) placed circumferentially around the foal's muzzle.

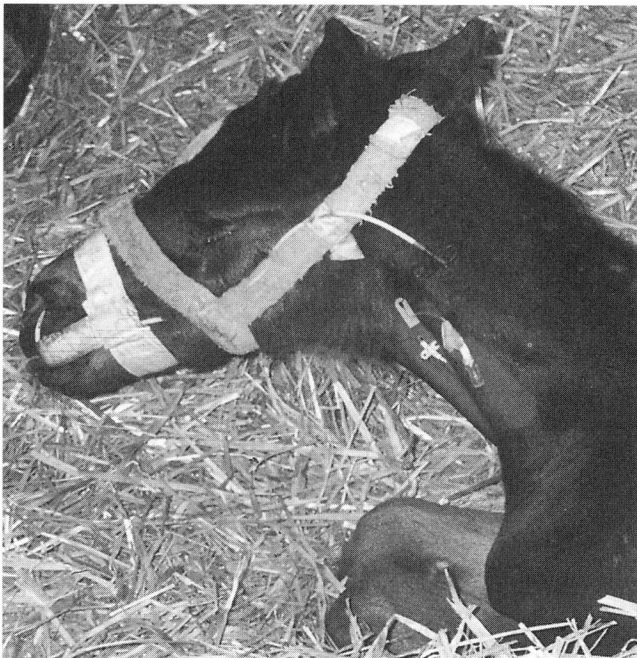

FIGURE 30-15. Nontraumatic technique for securing a nasogastric feeding tube in a foal. A tongue depressor is taped to the nasogastric tube and then taped to the foal's maxilla with adhesive tape placed circumferentially around the foal's muzzle. (Courtesy Dr. J. Palmer.)

nasogastric tubes are not benign; horses with tubes that are kept in place for long periods can develop inflammation and ulceration of the pharynx and esophagus. Therefore horses that salivate or chew excessively should be closely monitored because these horses are prone to develop esophageal ulceration or perforation. Nasogastric tubes can become fragmented, and the tube fragments could potentially cause gastrointestinal tract obstruction.

A similar method is used for nasogastric intubation in foals, but a smaller diameter, more pliable tube should be used. Indwelling tubes are often used for feeding sick foals; the end of the tube should be placed in the middle or distal esophagus rather than the stomach. When priming the tube with water or administering medication via a nasogastric tube in foals, the fluid should be administered with a funnel via gravity flow. It is often helpful to secure the tube to the foal's nostril with a tongue depressor attached to the tube and taped to the foal's head (Figure 30-15). Alternatively, the tube can be secured with a tape butterfly and suture to an elastic tape around the foal's head (Elasticon, Johnson & Johnson) placed over the bridge of the nose (Figure 30-16).

The technician should be familiar with the normal range of vital signs in foals and the differences among adult horses. Temperature should range from 37.3° C to 38.8° C (99° F to 101.8° F). The heart rate varies considerably in foals within the first week of life; it is usually 40 to 80 beats/min in the immediate postpartum period, increases to 120 to 150 beats per minute during the next several hours, and then stabilizes at approximately 80 to 100 beats/min during the first week of life. The respiratory rate in the neonatal foal is approximately 60 to 80 breaths/min in the immediate neonatal period and decreases to approximately 30 breaths/min within 1 hour of birth. Thoracic auscultation is not a reliable indicator of lower respiratory disease in the foal; often only subtle abnormalities are detectable on auscultation, even in the presence of severe pulmonary disease.

Physical examination of foals is similar to that of adult horses; however, there are several areas that need to be more closely evaluated in foals than in adult horses. The sclera, mucous membranes, and pinna should be evaluated for the presence of icterus and petechiae (see Figure 30-6). Icterus and petechiae are often associated with neonatal sepsis and hemolysis. The umbilicus should be observed and palpated for heat, pain, swelling, and moisture which is an indicator of umbilical remnant disease; ultrasonography may help in further evaluation of umbilical remnant disease. All joints of foals should be evaluated and palpated on a daily basis; effusion (joint swelling) or periarticular swelling and heat are indicators of joint infection. See Neonatal Care for more information.

RESTRAINT OF THE EQUINE PATIENT

Proper restraint of the equine patient is important to protect the handler, examiner, and patient from injury or death (see Chapter 1). Both physical and chemical methods can be used to achieve proper restraint (see Chapter 1). The handler should always stand on the same side of the horse as the examiner. This is important because if the horse is anxious or fractious and is moving, the handler can turn the horse's front end toward the examiner so that the rear limbs of the horse go away from the examiner. This will prevent injury from occurring secondary to the horse kicking the examiner. The handler should always lead the horse from its left side. The snap of the lead shank should be attached to the ring of the halter on the chin strap. A cotton or nylon lead shank can be used with or without a chain attached. The chain is useful when handling fractious or difficult horses. The chain portion of the shank can be placed over the bridge of the nose, under the chin, or over the gums to provide more secure control of some horses. This may be particularly necessary in stallions. The chain should be placed through the rings of the halter on the chin strap and on both sides of the halter, and then the snap should be attached to the ring on the chin strap. Care must be taken when using the chain in this manner because many horses are not accustomed to this and may rear or resist handling.

Technician Note

Horses can be dangerous; therefore proper handling and restraint of the equine patient are critical to protect the handler, examiner, and patient from injury or death.

Technicians are often involved in conducting lameness or neurologic examinations of equine patients. When walking or jogging a horse, the handler should walk or jog along on the horse's left side and allow approximately 1 foot of shank between the right hand and the horse's head. This allows the horse to have some movement of its head, which can be important when conducting a lameness examination. This also enables the handler to stay far enough away from the horse to prevent getting stepped on. The handler should not look back at the horse when walking or jogging because this often causes the horse to resist forward movement. The surface where the horse is being walked or jogged is important. A hard surface, such as concrete or asphalt, allows one to better hear and sometimes better observe a subtle lameness, but this kind of surface can cause damage to unshod hooves and can be slippery, particularly if wet. Therefore caution must be taken when handling horses on this type of surface.

In a hospital setting, horses can be placed in stocks for performing many necessary procedures. Although this helps control the horse's movement, it is not the best method of restraining some horses. Some very anxious or fractious horses can actually cause more injury to themselves if placed in stocks. Therefore the horse's tempera-

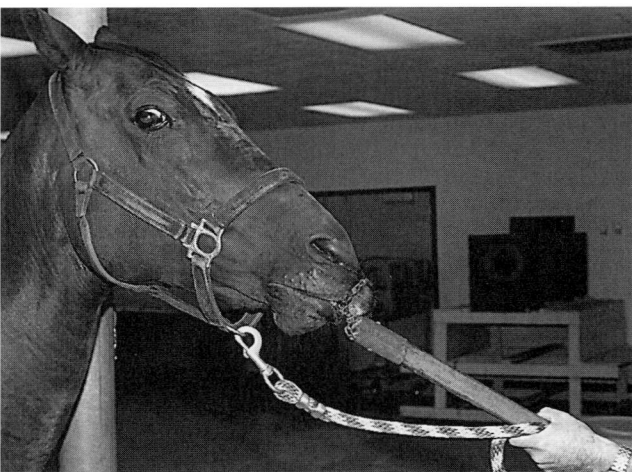

FIGURE 30-17. Technique for restraining a horse with a nose twitch.

ment and level of training should be taken into consideration when contemplating the use of stocks for restraint. When placing a horse in stocks, both the front and rear gates should be opened and the handler should walk through from rear to front and allow the horse to follow. An assistant should close the gate behind the horse and secure it before the handler closes the gate at the front of the stocks. This will prevent the horse from suddenly backing out of the stocks before the rear gate can be closed. Many stocks have a set of cross ties at the front. Many horses can be secured with cross ties, but they should not be used on fractious horses. Rather, the handler should remain at the horse's head. Horses should never be left unattended in stocks because they can easily become frightened or anxious and attempt escape. This can lead to severe injury, sometimes necessitating humane destruction.

A twitch can be used as the sole method of physical restraint or can be used in combination with other forms of physical or chemical restraint (Figure 30-17). A chain or rope twitch can be placed over the horse's upper lip and tightened by rolling it toward the horse's poll. This should help prevent it from coming off the lip. The twitch should be placed on the nose from the side where the handler is standing. The restraining effects of a twitch have a limited period of effectiveness; therefore the twitch should not be placed on the lip until immediately before it is needed. Some horses resist twitching, particularly if they have had it performed several times in the past. Other horses will tolerate it at first but then start resisting it. If the procedure is lengthy, then taking the twitch off for a period may prevent the horse from becoming very anxious. It may be better to use chemical restraint in certain horses in which lengthy procedures are being performed. Other forms of physical restraint, such as twitching an ear or the skin in front of the scapula, will provide variable degrees of restraint and are not widely accepted by many people (Figure 30-18). When restraining horses for certain procedures, such as nerve blocks during a lameness evaluation, one of the horse's limbs can be picked up and held off the ground by an assistant. This often helps prevent the horse from lifting the limb that is being worked on.

Chemical restraint (sedation or tranquilization) is prob-

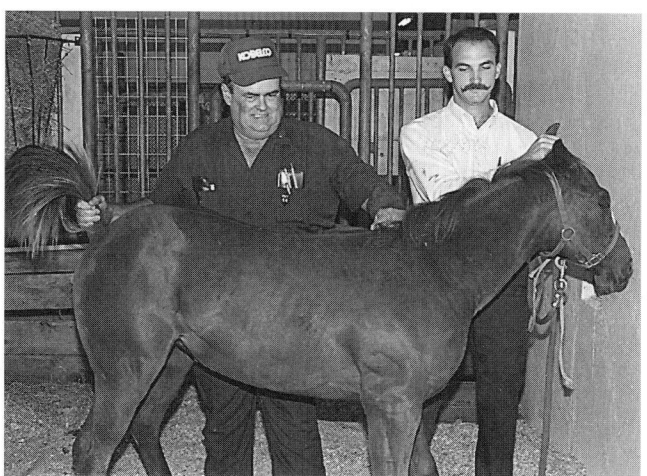

FIGURE 30-18.   Technique for restraining a foal or weanling that is not halter broken.

ably the most effective and safest form of restraint, but it can sometimes interfere with certain procedures. For example, sedation can alter the gait of horses and interfere with interpretation of a lameness or neurologic examination. Some sedatives also have analgesic properties that could possibly alleviate or alter lameness. Sedation can also interfere with interpretation of an upper airway endoscopic examination. Because some sedatives have muscle-relaxing properties they can alter abduction and adduction of the arytenoid cartilages and can alter function of the epiglottis and soft palate. Therefore, if sedation is required during an endoscopic examination of the upper airway, this should be taken into consideration when interpreting the endoscopic findings.

The most commonly used drugs for chemical restraint include alpha$_2$ agonists (e.g., xylazine, detomidine), narcotic agonist/antagonists (e.g., butorphanol), and phenothiazines (e.g., acepromazine). These can be administered alone or in different combinations; they can be administered intravenously or intramuscularly. Xylazine and detomidine are potent sedatives that have muscle-relaxing and analgesic properties. They provide marked visceral analgesia, which makes them effective in controlling pain associated with colic. The duration of effect depends on the dose and the route of administration; xylazine lasts 20 to 30 minutes when administered intravenously. Detomidine is more potent and has a greater duration of effect; this can be beneficial in some instances but can also cause problems because it can mask pain for an extended period. Moreover, detomidine has more cardiovascular side effects than xylazine. Butorphanol is a narcotic, and it is best used in combination with one of the alpha$_2$ agonists or acepromazine. Acepromazine provides tranquilization but no muscle relaxation or analgesia. It is frequently used in combination with other drugs. It can lead to marked hypotension and therefore should not be used in horses that are dehydrated or in shock. It can also cause permanent penile paralysis (paraphimosis) in stallions.

Foals are restrained differently from adult horses. Many foals have not been trained to be led by a halter; attempts at leading foals with a halter can lead to injury. Many times the foal can be moved by walking the mare to the desired location and allowing the foal to follow. This also works

well when attempting to evaluate the foal's gait. It is probably best to have at least two and preferably three people when working on a foal. One person should handle the mare, one should restrain the foal, and the other should examine or treat the foal. Foals are probably best restrained by holding one arm around the lower portion of the foal's neck and grasping the tail at its base with the opposite hand. Some foals tend to sink in the rear end if the handler tries to support them by holding too much tension on their tail. Therefore the tail should be used as a handle to help control the foal's movement rather than as a method to support the foal's hindquarters. Foals should not be placed in stocks because the stocks are too large for their body size and foals are generally not trained to stand. Horse trainers have many other effective methods of walking and restraining foals. Foals can be chemically restrained with tranquilizers or sedatives as with adult horses; the dose must be adjusted to body weight.

CARE OF HOSPITALIZED PATIENTS

In the equine hospital setting, veterinary technicians are often responsible for primary patient monitoring, administration of medications, general daily care of horses, and supervision of lay technical support. This section provides an overview of daily management of equine patients in the hospital setting.

Patient Monitoring

The level of patient monitoring required for a hospitalized horse will depend on the severity and nature of its disease. Horses hospitalized for elective surgery (castration, bone chip removal) require a thorough physical examination at presentation to ensure they are healthy surgical candidates. During hospitalization, elective patients usually require twice daily monitoring of heart rate, temperature, respiratory rate, appetite, and fecal output. Horses with infectious disease or extensive traumatic injuries require antibiotic administration and patient monitoring every 6 hours. Neonates; horses with colic (medical or surgical), diarrhea, renal failure, or respiratory distress; and any critically ill patients need constant intravenous fluid administration and intensive care monitoring. Most will be monitored continuously or hourly for signs of discomfort, abdominal pain, respiratory distress, shock, laminitis, gastrointestinal motility, heart rate, respiratory rate, hydration and capillary refill time. Recumbent foals are particularly fragile and labile. A 24-hour attendant is required to maintain an esophageal feeding tube, intravenous fluids, oxygen therapy, and sternal recumbent positioning. In addition, the attendant will administer medications and monitor heart rate, temperature, character and rate of respiration, mental status, abdominal distention, and urinary output.

Patient monitoring forms are designed to identify trends in physical signs, and patient treatment forms are designed to coordinate treatment periods when several individuals may be responsible for administering medications. Treatment sheets and monitoring forms may be combined for low-maintenance, elective patients (Figure 30-19). However, for intensive care patients, monitoring should be more detailed and indicated appropriately in a flow sheet. Considering the diversity of conditions of intensive care patients, the flow sheet should outline the parameters to be evaluated, such that the evaluation of a horse with colic (Figure 30-20) or a horse with diarrhea (Figure 30-21) would differ from the evaluation of a neonate (Figure 30-22) or any other intensive care patient (Figure 30-23).

Text continued on p. 721

Date	T	P	R	Treatment	7AM	1PM	3PM	7PM	11PM	1AM

EQUINE TREATMENT SHEET
SID, BID, TID, and QID

Person Administering Treatment Should Initial Box Under the Appropriate Time

FIGURE 30-19.   Elective patient flow sheet for monitoring of patient's progress and treatments.

COLIC FLOW SHEET

Clinician: _____
Student: _____
Date: _____
Page: _____ of _____

Date: _____	AM/PM	AM/PM	AM/PM	AM/PM	AM/PM	AM/PM	AM/PM	AM/PM	AM/PM	AM/PM	AM/PM	AM/PM
Attitude												
Temperature												
Heart rate												
Resp. rate												
Refill/color												
Est hydration												
GI sounds RD/RV												
LD/LV												
Feces												
Urine												
Digital pulse												
PCV _____ % / TP _____ g/dl												
N-G reflux vol												
Rectal exam												
Abdominal centesis												
Lab submitted												
Fluid type												
Fluid rate												
Drugs (record doses, routes, rates on the treatment sheet)												
Signature:												

Instructions: _____
_____
_____

Heart rate more than _____
PCV more than _____ less than _____
TP more than _____ less than _____
Respiratory rate _____ __ temp _____
Signs of colic

COLIC FLOW SHEET

FIGURE 30-20.   Colic flow sheet for intensive care unit patients to identify monitoring, treatments, and administration schedule.

DIARRHEA/ISOLATION FLOW SHEET

Clinician: _____
Student: _____
Date: _____
Page: _____ of _____

Date: _____	AM/PM	AM/PM	AM/PM	AM/PM	AM/PM	AM/PM	AM/PM	AM/PM	AM/PM	AM/PM	AM/PM	AM/PM
Attitude												
Temperature												
Heart rate												
Resp. rate												
CRT/MM color												
Est hydration												
GI sounds RD/RV												
LD/LV												
Feces output consistency												
Fecal culture												
Urine vol./ua												
PCV _____ % TP _____ g/dl												
Digital pulse												
Water consumption electrolyte water*												
Feeding/appetite												
Evaluate catheter site												
Fluid therapy rate Fluid therapy vol												
Lab submitted												
TX: drugs/dose												
Initials:												

Instructions: _____
_____
_____

- **Measure and refill water buckets (plain and electrolyte water)**

DIARRHEA/ISOLATION FLOW SHEET

FIGURE 30-21.   Diarrhea flow sheet for quarantine intensive care unit patients to identify monitoring, treatments, and administration schedule.

NEONATOLOGY/ICU FLOW SHEET

Clinician: _____
Student: _____
Date: _____
Page: _____ of _____

Date: _____	AM/PM	AM/PM	AM/PM	AM/PM	AM/PM	AM/PM	AM/PM	AM/PM	AM/PM	AM/PM	AM/PM	AM/PM
Attitude												
Temperature												
Heart rate												
Resp. rate												
CRT/MM color												
Est hydration												
GI sounds RD/RV												
LD/LV												
O2 suppl.												
Feces output consistency												
Urine vol./ua												
Blood glucose												
PCV _____ % TP _____ g/dl												
DIP/CK umbilicus												
Feeding nursing												
Milk from mare												
Fluid therapy rate Fluid therapy vol												
Lab submitted												
TX: drugs/dose												
Initials:												

Instructions: _____
_____
_____

If recumbent, turn foal q2 hours

NEONATOLOGY/ICU FLOW SHEET

FIGURE 30-22.   Neonatal flow sheet to identify monitoring, treatments, and administration schedule for critically ill newborn foals.

ICU FLOW SHEET

Clinician: _____
Student: _____
Date: _____
Page: _____ of _____

Date: _____	AM/PM	AM/PM	AM/PM	AM/PM	AM/PM	AM/PM	AM/PM	AM/PM	AM/PM	AM/PM	AM/PM	AM/PM
Attitude												
Temperature												
Heart rate												
Resp. rate												
Refill/color												
Est hydration												
GI sounds RD												
RV												
LD												
LV												
Feces out put consistency												
Urine vol./ua												
Digital pulse												
PCV _____ % TP _____ g/dl												
Drugs (record doses, routes, rates on the treatment sheet)												
Signature:												

Instructions: _____
_____
_____

Heart rate more than _____
PCV more than _____ less than _____
TP more than _____ less than _____
Respiratory rate _____ __ temp _____
Signs of colic

ICU FLOW SHEET

FIGURE 30-23.   Intensive care unit flow sheet to identify monitoring, treatments, and administration schedule for critically ill patients. This helps readily identify trends that may indicate a deterioration in the patient's condition.

A separate treatment sheet should be used to outline the detailed medication schedule, the route, the dose of the drug per body weight, the strength, and the total amount given to the patient (Figure 30-24). The intensive care unit (ICU) flow sheets for all patients in the hospital may be assembled in a central area to allow one technician to easily identify treatment periods and thus coordinate efforts. It is important to recognize that monitoring and treatment forms are a permanent part of the medical record, which represents a legal document to record all events during hospitalization.

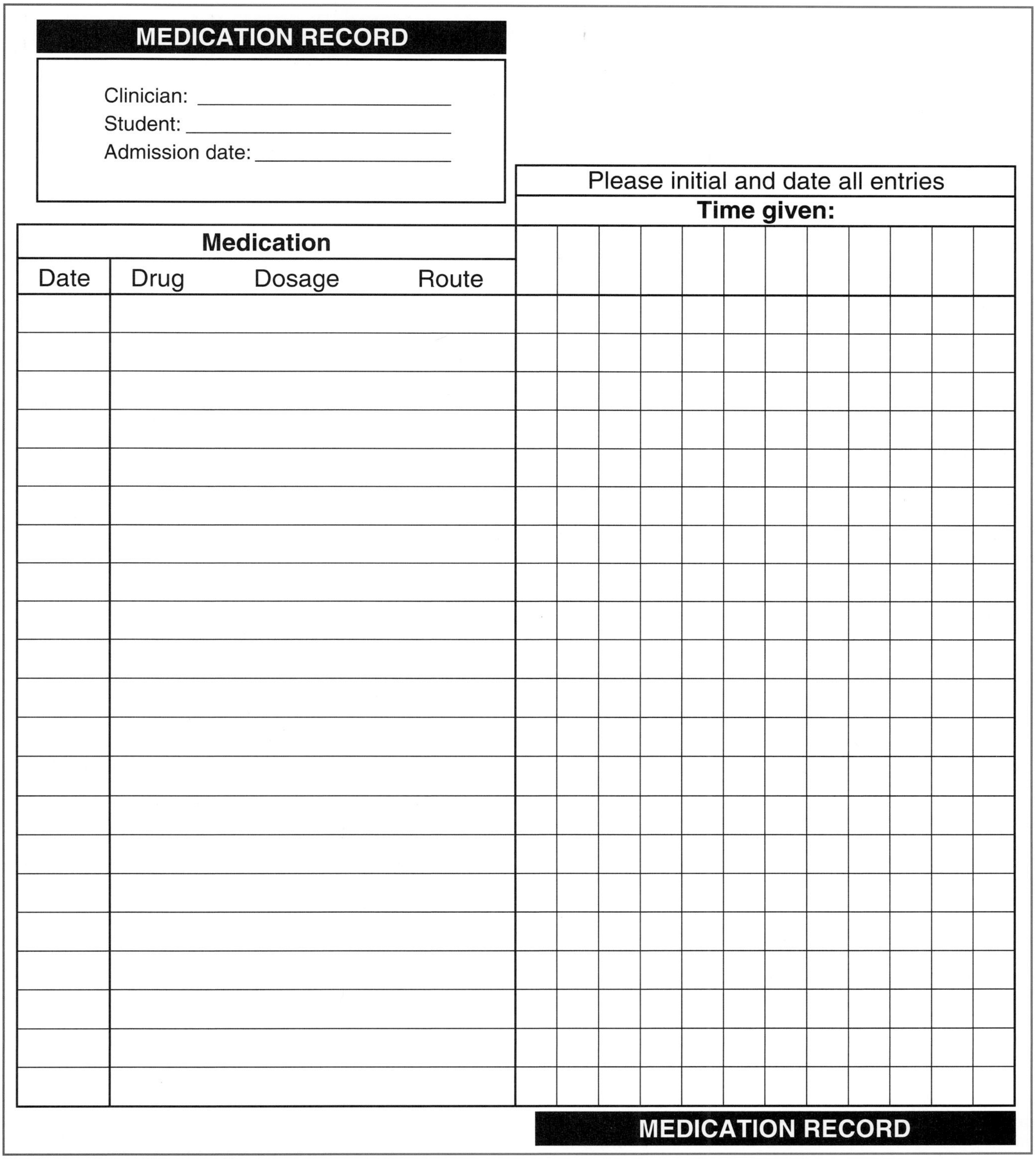

MEDICATION RECORD			

Clinician: _____
Student: _____
Admission date: _____

Please initial and date all entries
Time given:

Medication					
Date	Drug	Dosage	Route		

MEDICATION RECORD

FIGURE 30-24. A treatment sheet should list all the medications, the drugs' concentration, the dose per body weight, the total amount, the appropriate route, and the times to be administered. Following administration, the treatment must be recorded promptly.

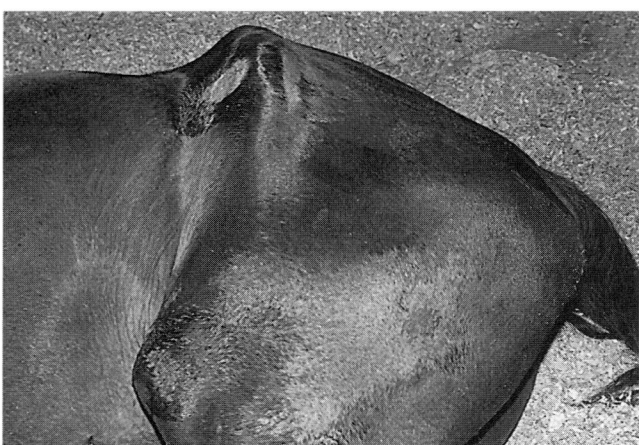

FIGURE 30-25. Pressure sores on a horse with chronic laminitis secondary to prolonged recumbency.

Horses with infectious, contagious diseases should be hospitalized in isolation facilities. The most common infectious diseases that require an isolation protocol are colitis (salmonellosis) and strangles *(Streptococcus equi)*. Personnel should be supplied with disposable gloves, boots, and body suits to wear while attending to isolation cases; a disinfectant foot dip should be used when entering and exiting each stall and the protective boots, gloves, and suits should be discarded when exiting the isolation area. Horses in isolation should not be walked in areas where other horses are grazing, and waste from the stall should be disposed of in an inaccessible area. If possible, personnel attending to isolation cases should not attend to foals or immunocompromised patients.

Recumbent horses are a particular challenge to manage effectively in a hospital setting. Neurologic and musculoskeletal diseases are the most common problems resulting in recumbency in horses. Horses and foals that are recumbent will quickly develop pressure sores over the point of their hip (tuber coxae), elbows, and head (Figure 30-25). Pressure sores rapidly become deep and may infect underlying bony structures. In addition, recumbent horses may have decreased intestinal motility and failure to void urine, and they are predisposed to developing colic, urinary bladder distention, and even rupture. Therefore laxatives and soft laxative feeds, such as fresh grass and bran mash, should be offered to recumbent horses to facilitate evacuation and prevent impaction. Horses unable to defecate should have feces manually removed twice daily. Placement of an indwelling urinary catheter or periodic catheterization of the urinary bladder is necessary when managing recumbent patients. Recumbent horses should be deeply bedded on straw, placed on a padded mat, or placed on a waterbed to prevent development of pressure sores. Their position should be changed every 4 hours; multiple attendants are required to move an adult recumbent horse. A sling can only be used in horses that can support their own weight but are too uncoordinated to remain standing (Figure 30-26). The sling acts as a safety net to catch them when they stumble. Horses cannot be supported solely by the sling because of constriction of breathing and sling-induced pressure sores. Rarely can recumbent adult horses be managed for more than 1 or 2 weeks without development of life-threatening complications (pneumonia, urinary tract infection, colic, pressure sores).

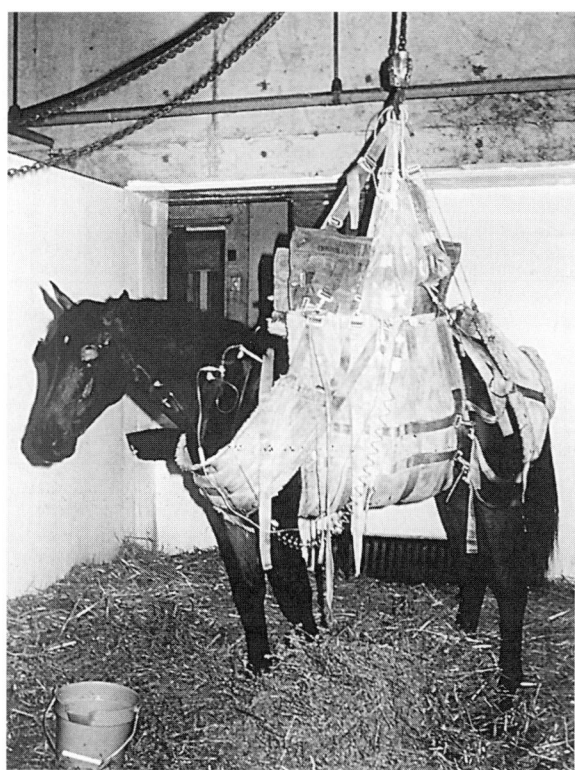

FIGURE 30-26. Use of a sling and hoist to provide some balance and support to an ataxic or weak horse.

Feeding

Whenever possible, hospitalized patients should be offered feed similar to what they are fed at home. Sudden changes in diet can predispose horses to colic or diarrhea. In some instances, feeding must be specialized to accommodate the patient's disease. Horses with diarrhea should not be offered rich, calorie-dense feeds, such as corn, barley, or alfalfa, that may exacerbate colitis. Grass hay, bran mash, and oats are the most appropriate feeds for horses with diarrhea. After colic surgery or medical resolution of colic, horses should be offered soft, laxative feeds, such as bran mash, fresh grass, and small amounts of good-quality hay. Feed should be offered frequently in small quantities to horses with gastrointestinal tract disease rather than offering two large daily meals. Horses with allergic airway disease (heaves, COPD) should be offered water-soaked hay and dust-free complete pelleted diet. Horses with inappetence owing to infectious disease should be offered highly palatable, calorie-dense feeds to increase energy intake (see Chapter 15).

Therapeutics

Medication in tablet form is best administered to horses by crushing the pills with a mortar and pestle and mixing the powder with corn syrup, molasses, or applesauce. The resultant solution is sticky and palatable and can be placed directly in the horse's mouth with a syringe. Alternatively, the prepared medication may be placed over feed, but the attendant must observe closely to ensure medication placed over feed is completely ingested.

Oral medications may also be administered via nasogastric intubation. The nasogastric tube is passed through the nasal passages into the esophagus and stomach. Proper

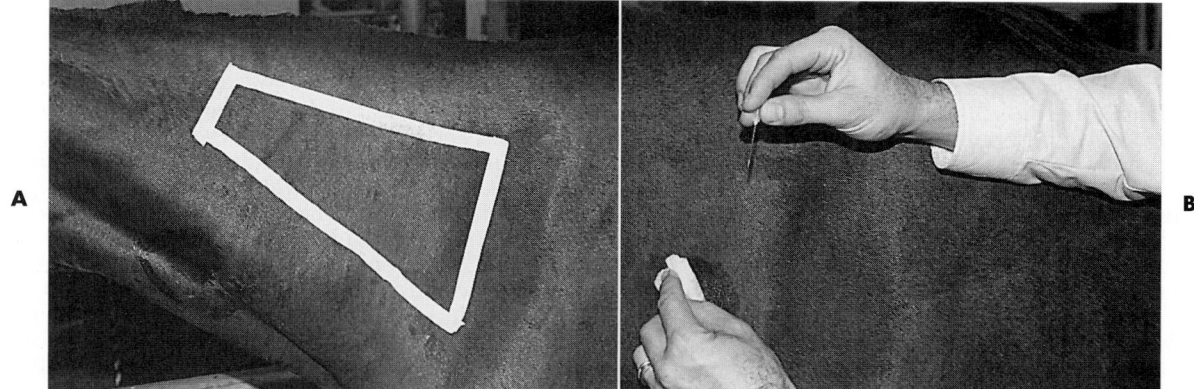

FIGURE 30-27.   **A,** Location considered safe in the cervical region of horses for the administration of intramuscular injections. **B,** Technique for administering intramuscular injections; the skin should be cleansed and then swabbed with an alcohol-soaked gauze pad before insertion of the needle. The needle (1.5-inch) should be extend into its hub to deposit the medication deep within the muscle.

placement of the nasogastric tube should be confirmed before administration of medications. The tube should be visualized as it passes through the cervical portion of the esophagus, negative pressure should be obtained when the examiner aspirates on the tube, and the aroma of stomach contents may be noted as gas escapes from the tube. Inadvertent administration of medication into the lung using an improperly placed nasogastric tube (in the trachea) can result in death of the horse.

Nonirritating, sterile solutions can be administered intramuscularly in horses. The volume of medication to be injected at a single intramuscular site should not exceed 20 ml. Sites for intramuscular injection include the semimembranosus or semitendinosus muscle and the musculature of the neck. The appropriate region for injection in the neck is above the cervical spine, cranial to the scapula, and below the nuchal ligament (Figure 30-27, A). Because of excessive postinjection swelling, the pectoral muscles are not recommended for intramuscular injection. The gluteal muscles are not recommended for intramuscular injection, because this region cannot effectively drain if an abscess forms at the injection site. In rare instances, postinjection abscesses in the gluteal muscles may drain into the abdominal cavity. Irritating medications, such as phenylbutazone, tetracycline, and thiamylal, should never be administered intramuscularly.

Intravenous medications may be administered directly into the jugular vein, using an 18-gauge, 1.5-inch needle. The jugular vein is most superficial and most distant from the carotid artery in the proximal one third of the neck. The needle should be seated in the jugular vein to the hub without the syringe attached to ensure the needle has not been accidentally placed in the carotid artery. Blood flows continuously and slowly from an 18-gauge needle in the jugular vein, whereas blood spurts in a pulsatile manner from a needle placed in the carotid artery. Inadvertent intracarotid injection may result in seizure, coma, permanent neurologic deficits, or death.

An intravenous catheter can be placed for repeated administration of medications or continuous fluid infusion. Intravenous catheters may be placed in the jugular, cephalic, and lateral thoracic (spur) veins in horses. Catheters should be placed aseptically and secured appropriately to prevent their dislodgment (Figure 30-28). Teflon

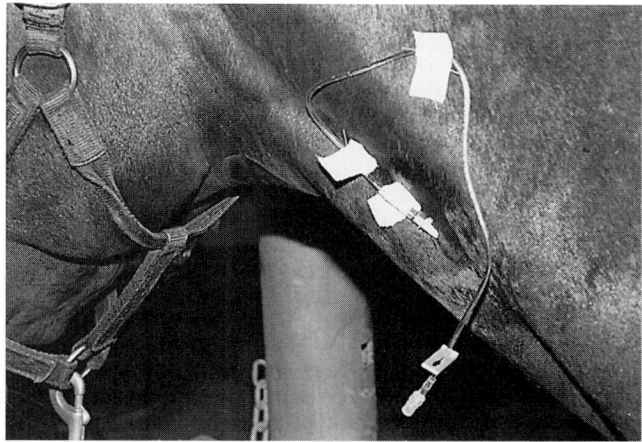

FIGURE 30-28.   Technique for securing a catheter in the jugular vein of a horse.

catheters are relatively irritating and should be replaced every 3 days. Silastic catheters can remain in the vein as long they are patent and show no signs of infection. Central venous catheterization using a wire-guided polyurethane catheter often used in critically ill patients. Intravenous catheters should be flushed with heparinized saline flush (2-10 µ/ml) every 4 to 8 hours, and monitored twice daily for heat, swelling, pain, and positioning. Infection at the catheter site may occur in the subcutaneous tissue or within the vein (septic thrombophlebitis). Septic thrombophlebitis can be life threatening in horses.

The ideal antibiotic is effective against a wide range of bacterial organisms (broad-spectrum), easy to administer, and nontoxic (see Chapter 23). Penicillin has good efficacy against common gram-positive pathogens in the horse *(Streptococcus zooepidemicus, S. equi)* and is relatively safe. It is frequently administered intramuscularly (procaine penicillin) and intravenously (potassium penicillin). Procaine penicillin should never be administered intravenously. Life-threatening anaphylactoid reactions are reported with procaine penicillin administration and should be treated with epinephrine. Aminoglycoside antibiotics (gentamicin, amikacin sulfate) are efficacious against gram-negative pathogens and can be administered intramuscularly or intravenously. These antibiotics are nephrotoxic, and renal function should be monitored during the period of administration. Trimethoprim-sulfa antimicrobials have a moderate gram-positive and gram-negative spectrum, are administered orally, and are used for treatment of mild to moderate infection. Ceftiofur sodium has a good gram-positive and gram-negative spectrum, may be administered intramuscularly or intravenously, and is used for moderate to severe infection. Metronidazole is administered orally or per rectum to treat anaerobic bacterial infections. There are specific indications for administration of tetracycline, erythromycin, and rifampin in horses, but these antibiotics are not widely used because of the risk of antibiotic-induced colitis. Chloramphenicol is used sparingly in horses because of the human health risk of idiosyncratic, fatal aplastic anemia after exposure during administration.

There are many analgesic medications available for horses. Phenylbutazone, ketoprofen, and flunixin meglumine are nonsteroidal antiinflammatory drugs (NSAIDs) that provide mild to moderate pain relief without sedation or immunosuppression. The NSAIDs also reduce fever (antipyretic) and inflammation. Phenylbutazone is the most widely administered analgesic of horses and is most effective for treatment of musculoskeletal pain. Ketoprofen, meclofenamic acid, and naproxen are less commonly used drugs that provide mild to moderate analgesia for musculoskeletal pain. Flunixin meglumine is more effective for soft tissue and visceral pain. In addition, flunixin meglumine may combat the effects of endotoxemia in horses with gastrointestinal tract disease. Xylazine and detomidine are alpha$_2$-agonist sedative analgesic medications that provide immediate relief of moderate to marked pain with moderate to profound sedation. Xylazine provides 20 to 30 minutes of sedation and analgesia, whereas detomidine provides up to 1 hour of sedation and analgesia. Butorphanol is a narcotic agonist/antagonist that provides up to 1 hour of sedation and analgesia for moderate to severe pain. Acepromazine has no analgesic properties, and it only provides moderate tranquilization. Acepromazine causes hypotension, and it can lead to the development of persistent paraphimosis in stallions.

Corticosteroids have potent antiinflammatory properties and are administered for allergic airway disease, allergic skin conditions, immune-mediated disease, and joint inflammation. Corticosteroids are administered topically, orally, parenterally (intravenously or intramuscularly), and intraarticularly. Adverse effects of corticosteroid administration include immunosuppression, polyuria or polydypsia, poor hair coat, muscle wasting, poor wound healing, laminitis, and progression of degenerative joint disease. Therefore corticosteroids are administered with caution in instances with specific indications for their use.

Dimethyl sulfoxide (DMSO) is a common antiinflammatory drug used in horses to relieve swelling and edema associated with central nervous system trauma, traumatic musculoskeletal injuries, laminitis, and myositis. DMSO may be administered topically, orally, or intravenously (diluted in crystalloid fluids as a 10% to 20% solution). The technician should wear gloves while handling the product. Rapid intravenous administration may result in hemolysis, hematuria, and sweating in horses.

ENDOSCOPY

Fiberoptic endoscopes of different lengths allow evaluation of the upper respiratory tract (nasal passages, sinuses, ethmoid turbinates, nasopharynx, guttural pouches, trachea, bronchi), proximal gastrointestinal tract (esophagus, stomach, duodenum), distal gastrointestinal tract (rectum), and urogenital tract (uterus, urethra, urinary bladder). The endoscope is frequently used for evaluating athletic horses with poor performance and those making respiratory noise. The endoscope can be used with horses standing (Figure 30-29) or with horses exercising on a high-speed treadmill. The latter enables the upper respiratory tract to be evaluated dynamically. The most common abnormalities detected in the upper respiratory tract include left laryngeal hemiplegia, dorsal displacement of the soft palate, epiglottic entrapment, arytenoid chondritis, and subepiglottic cysts. The endoscope can also be used to determine the source of mucopurulent nasal discharge or epistaxis. The most common source of mucopurulent nasal discharge is the lower airway; endoscopy would enable observation of this material in the trachea and bronchi. Other possible sources of discharge could be guttural pouch empyema or sinusitis. Horses with maxillary sinusitis often have mucopurulent discharge exiting the nasomaxillary opening into the nasal passages. Potential sources of epistaxis include ethmoid hematoma, guttural pouch mycosis, and exercise-induced pulmonary hemor-

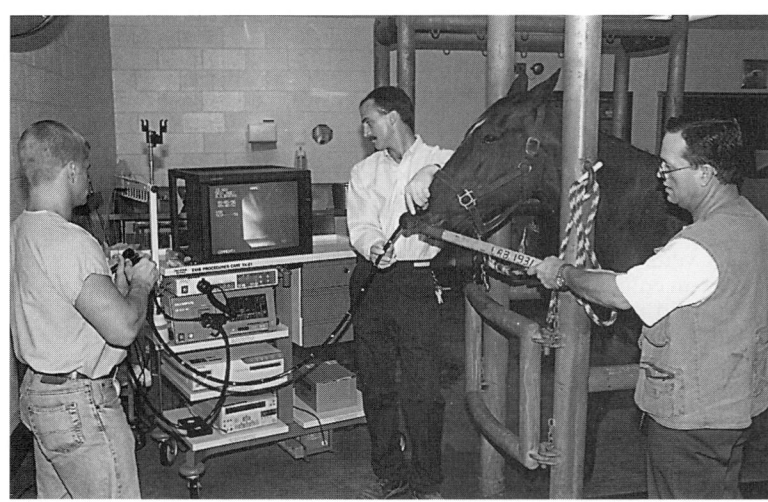

FIGURE 30-29. Use of endoscopy to evaluate the upper airway of a horse.

rhage. The endoscope is also used to obtain a tracheal wash or bronchoalveolar lavage sample in horses with inflammatory or allergic lung disease.

The endoscope is useful for evaluating horses with esophageal obstruction (choke) to determine the location and cause of the obstruction. It is also useful for evaluating the integrity of the esophagus after resolution of the choke to determine if the mucosa is ulcerated, which could predispose the esophagus to form a diverticulum or stricture. Development of the long endoscope (3 m) has allowed examination of the stomach and duodenum in foals and adult horses for gastric and duodenal ulceration. Endoscopy has revealed that the incidence of gastric ulceration in adult performance horses is greater than previously suspected. This enables the clinician to document the presence and severity of ulceration and monitor the response to treatment.

The endoscope is often used to assess the integrity of the urethra and urinary bladder in horses with hematuria (blood in the urine), stranguria (slow and difficult urination), and pollakiuria (frequent urination in small amounts) . It may reveal erosive or neoplastic lesions in the urethra. Urinary bladder abnormalities that can be identified endoscopically include inflammatory and neoplastic diseases and cystic calculi. The endoscope has been used to assess the uterine lining for cysts and other pathologic conditions.

The technician is integrally involved in the care, use, and maintenance of the endoscope and associated equipment. There are specific instructions on the proper methods for cleaning and disinfecting the endoscope. It is important that the proper methods be followed to ensure that infectious agents are not transmitted from one patient to another and to prevent damage to the endoscope.

IMAGING TECHNIQUES

The veterinary technician in equine practice often participates in diagnostic imaging techniques. In some instances, the technician may be solely responsible for obtaining radiographic or scintigraphic images for interpretation by the veterinarian. The technician must recognize good-quality images on the basis of technique and positioning and understand indications for special radiographic studies. Additional information on imaging techniques may be found in Chapter 9.

Plain Film Radiography

Plain film radiography is used to identify disruption of bony structures, such as fracture, osteochondrosis, osteomyelitis (bone infection), malalignment (luxation, subluxation), or degenerative joint disease (arthritis). If it is necessary to be near the horse when the x-ray examination is performed, lead aprons and gloves should be worn. Long-scale (low milliamperage [mAs], high kilovolt peak [kVp]) techniques are used for plain film radiographic technique to preserve resolution of soft tissues and bone. Portable radiograph machines are typically used to image the carpus, hock, skull, and distal limbs in adult horses. The standard focal spot-to-film distance using portable radiographic units is 85 cm. To obtain detailed radiographs of the coffin and navicular bone, the horse's shoes should be removed and the frog should be packed with Play-doh. Portable radiograph units may also be used to image the thorax, abdomen, and cervical spine in neonatal and weanling foals. Large overhead radiograph units (1000 mA, 150 kV) are required to image the spine, thorax, elbow, shoulder, stifle, and hip in adult horses. The standard focal spot-to-film distance using overhead radiographic units is 100 cm. Radiographs of the thorax, cervical and thoracic spine, elbow, and stifle may be obtained in standing, sedated horses. However, high-quality radiographic imaging of the lumbar spine, shoulder, and hip usually requires general anesthesia. It is important to label the radiographs correctly with the name of the patient, the date of examination, the affected limb, and the radiographic marker used for orientation. Radiographic markers are generally used when performing radiographs of the limbs; the markers are placed externally on the radiographic cassette in a location that will either be lateral or dorsal to the limb.

Technician Note

In some instances, the technician may be solely responsible for obtaining radiographic or scintigraphic images for interpretation by the veterinarian.

Contrast Radiography

Special radiographic techniques use a contrast agent to better define or outline lesions suspected clinically or radiographically but not visualized on survey (plain film) radiographs. Positive-contrast agents are most commonly used in equine radiography for investigation of puncture wounds or draining tracts (fistulogram), joints (arthrogram), bladder (cystogram), spinal cord (myelogram), and esophagus (barium swallow). Short-scale (high mAs, low kVp) techniques are used to highlight visualization of the contrast agent. Triiodinated, water-soluble contrast materials are used for the fistulogram, arthrogram, and cystogram. Nonionic, water-soluble benzoic acid derivatives are used for myelographic examination, and oil-based barium solutions are used for evaluation of the gastrointestinal tract. The fistulogram is most commonly used to outline foreign bodies or a sequestrum (dead bone) or to define the extent of a penetrating wound. A fistulogram can easily outline involvement or penetration of a synovial structure, such as a joint or tendon sheath. Arthrograms allow a complete evaluation of articular cartilage integrity, synovial membrane proliferation, and joint capsule integrity. A surgical skin preparation is required before injection of sterile contrast agent into a joint. Positive-contrast cystography can only be performed in foals and is used to identify a tear in the bladder wall or persistent urachal remnants. Myelography is used to diagnose cervical stenotic myelopathy (wobbler's syndrome) wherein the cervical spine is malformed and narrowed, which compresses the spinal cord. Attenuation or obliteration of the contrast column is identified at vertebral sites where the cervical vertebrae are compressing the spinal cord. A barium swallow may be useful for investigating dysphagia, esophageal motility, esophageal integrity, gastric emptying and duodenal structures (foals only).

Ultrasound

Ultrasound examination is useful for investigating soft tissue structures and body cavities. The ultrasonic image is formed by ultrasound waves reflecting from tissue interfaces. The reflection of ultrasound waves is caused by the difference in acoustic impedance between tissues. Ultrasound can be used to investigate any soft tissue structure, solid organ, or swelling but is most commonly used in horses to examine tendon, lung, heart, pleural space, abdominal organs, and reproductive tract. It is important

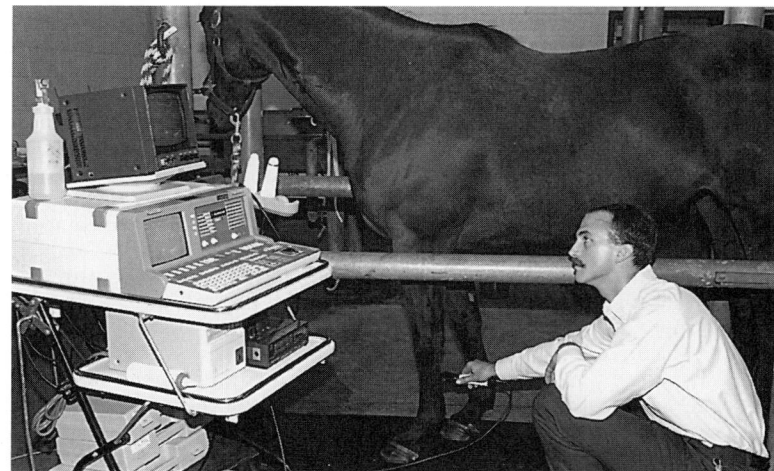

FIGURE 30-30. Use of ultrasonography to evaluate tendon injury in a horse with suspected flexor tendinitis.

to recognize that air impedes ultrasound penetration; therefore investigation of gas-filled intestines and air-filled lung is unrewarding. Tendon ultrasound allows the examiner to identify and monitor core lesions, tears, and fibrosis of the tendons during the healing process (Figure 30-30). Ultrasound examination of the heart is termed *echocardiography* and is used to identify congenital defects, valvular disease, and congestive heart failure. Ultrasound examination of the thorax is particularly useful in horses with pleuropneumonia to identify the location, depth, and character of pleural fluid. Identification of free gas, fibrin, or highly cellular fluid within the pleural space using ultrasound examination is a poor prognostic indicator in horses with pleuropneumonia. Pulmonary abscesses can only be identified if they communicate with the pleural space; deep pulmonary abscesses cannot be visualized because air in the lungs impedes ultrasound penetration. Abdominal ultrasound in foals is used to identify peritoneal effusion resulting from ruptured bladder, enlarged umbilical structures, and gastrointestinal dilatation and intestinal intussusception (telescoping of the bowel). In adult horses, abdominal ultrasound is used predominately to investigate solid visceral organs, such as the liver, kidney, and spleen. Reproductive ultrasound examination is used to identify the appropriate time for breeding, follicular development, early pregnancy diagnosis (15 days), twins, and metritis (dense fluid accumulation in the uterus).

Nuclear Scintigraphy

Nuclear scintigraphy (bone scan) is performed by injecting a radioactive isotope intravenously and monitoring its distribution in the bones and soft tissue of the limbs. Technetium-99m is the most commonly used radioactive isotope. Technetium is combined with phosphate compounds that localize within bone after intravenous administration. Localization of phosphate-labeled technetium is identified using a gamma camera. Bony uptake of phosphate-labeled technetium is greater in regions of high bone turnover or increased blood flow. Areas of increased uptake are termed *hot spots* and usually indicate an abnormality or disease process. Nuclear scintigraphy is indicated in horses with obscure, unlocalized lameness (using local anesthesia) and localized lameness with normal radiographic examination. Hot spots may identify nondisplaced fractures or stressed or damaged bone. Nuclear scintigraphic examination is quickly performed on an entire limb or multiple limbs, whereas radiographic examination of an entire limb is cost and time prohibitive. In instances of unlocalized lameness, a plain film radiographic examination should be performed after nuclear scintigraphy to identify bony abnormalities. Serial nuclear scintigraphic imaging should be performed in horses with normal plain film radiographic examination to monitor progression and healing of the injury.

A white blood cell scan can be performed to identify occult infection. In this procedure, the patient's white blood cells are isolated from a blood sample (60 ml) and labeled with technetium 99m. These technetium-labeled white blood cells are injected back into the patient and the patient is scanned with a gamma camera. The white blood cells travel to a focus of infection and create a hot spot detectable with the gamma camera. This technique may be used to identify a tooth root abscess, osteomyelitis (infected bone), or an intraabdominal abscess.

CLINICAL PATHOLOGY

Clinicopathologic testing provides important information for the veterinarian to identify functional impairment of an organ system, confirm a clinical diagnosis, assess response to therapy, and formulate a prognosis. The normal values of many clinicopathologic tests vary among species. In addition, there are species-specific characteristics associated with diseases and significance of abnormal findings. This section concentrates solely on equine-specific alterations in clinicopathologic values in health and disease (also see Chapter 6).

Serum Chemistry

A serum chemistry panel provides specific information pertaining to the liver, kidney, muscle, and serum electrolyte concentrations. The serum sample should be drawn into a tube without anticoagulant (red-top tube) and submitted to the laboratory. Some laboratories can perform chemistry profiles in heparinized blood samples (green top). If there will be more than a 1-hour delay in submission, the tube should be centrifuged, serum or plasma removed and stored in the refrigerator. Delayed sample submission without centrifuging produces artificially low serum glucose and high serum potassium concentrations. Horses have high serum bilirubin compared to other species, and serum bilirubin concentrations will increase dramatically if feed is withheld for more than

24 hours. Fasting hyperbilirubinemia in horses is a normal physiologic response and is not indicative of liver disease. Most species develop low serum albumin with chronic liver disease because of decreased production; however, horses maintain production of albumin even with marked impairment of liver function. Reliable indicators of liver dysfunction in horses are high serum gamma glutamyltransferase (GGT) activity, high serum sorbitol dehydrogenase (SDH) activity, high serum bile acid concentrations, and low blood urea nitrogen (BUN) concentrations.

In most species, renal failure produces low serum calcium and high serum phosphorus concentrations. Horses are obligate calcium excretors, and chronic renal failure often produces a marked increase in serum calcium concentration. Reliable indicators of renal failure in horses include high serum creatinine and BUN and electrolyte abnormalities, including low sodium and chloride and high potassium and calcium. The large colon of horses exchanges a vast amount of electrolytes and fluids on a daily basis. Horses with colonic inflammation may develop marked electrolyte abnormalities before development of diarrhea. Low serum sodium, chloride, and potassium in horses with abdominal pain or depression often indicate loss of electrolytes into the lumen of the colon and impending diarrhea.

Serum creatine phosphokinase (CK) is an indicator of muscle damage in all species. Horses have large muscle masses in comparison to ruminants and small animals. Moderate increases in serum CK (two to four times normal) readily occur in horses following prolonged transport, prolonged recumbency, exercise in an unconditioned horse, or rolling owing to abdominal pain. Moderate increases do not usually indicate primary muscle disease. Horses with primary muscle disease, such as exertional rhabdomyolysis (tying up, azoturia, Monday morning sickness), have increases in serum CK activity of up to 200 times normal values.

Hematology

A complete blood count (CBC) provides information pertaining to the red blood cell (RBC) count, RBC morphology, total white blood cell (WBC) count, differential WBC (including neutrophils, lymphocytes, eosinophils, monocytes), WBC morphology, and fibrinogen concentration. Samples for CBC should be submitted in a tube with ethylenediaminetetraacetic acid (EDTA) anticoagulant (purple-top tube). The RBCs are most easily estimated, using the packed cell volume (PCV); low PCV is indicative of anemia. Horses have a large muscular spleen that normally contains up to one third of the circulating RBC volume. With excitement and exercise, PCV in horses can increase by as much as 50% secondary to splenic contraction. Therefore the resting PCV is highly variable and must be serially evaluated in excitable patients. In addition, the response of the spleen to massive hemorrhage precludes use of the PCV to estimate the magnitude of blood loss for at least 24 hours. The normal range of PCV depends on the breed. Hot-blooded breeds (thoroughbreds, Arabians, quarter horses) have higher resting RBC counts, compared with cold-blooded breeds (ponies, draft horses).

Evaluation of the total and differential WBC count is important to identify the presence of infection. In most instances, bacterial infection will manifest as an increase in WBC count (leukocytosis) characterized by an increase in the number of mature neutrophils (mature neutrophilia). Fibrinogen is a coagulation factor and an acute-phase reactant in horses. The liver produces fibrinogen in response to bacterial infection and inflammation within 72 hours, and fibrinogen concentrations remain increased until the infection is resolved.

Horses are particularly sensitive to circulating endotoxin released from the cell wall of gram-negative bacteria. Endotoxin causes margination and sequestration of WBCs. Therefore a profoundly low WBC count (leukopenia) characterized by low neutrophil count (neutropenia) and immature band neutrophils (left shift) is indicative of either gram-negative septicemia or gastrointestinal disease with mucosal absorption of gram-negative bacteria. High eosinophil counts (eosinophilia) are indicative of massive parasite infestation or possibly allergic diseases, and low lymphocyte counts (lymphopenia) are observed in horses with early viral infections.

Urinalysis

Urinalysis is essential for evaluation of primary renal disease. Urine can be collected as a voided sample or after catheterization of the bladder. Normal horse urine is usually alkaline (pH 7 to 9) and contains many calcium carbonate crystals. Alkaline urine usually produces a false-positive reaction for protein on urine dipsticks. Horses have a large number of mucous glands located within the renal pelvis; therefore normal horse urine may appear very thick and mucoid. Normal horse urine may appear red or bloody in the snow, which often alarms novice horse owners. Truly red urine is abnormal and results from the presence of frank blood (primary urinary tract disease), hemoglobin (hemolytic anemia), or myoglobin (myositis). Differentiation of these sources of red urine requires special testing of urine and serum samples. Urine specific gravity and urinary electrolyte excretion ratios should be obtained to investigate primary renal function. Urine specific gravity indicates the ability of the kidney to concentrate urine, and normal values in resting horses should be 1.020 to 1.035. Urinary electrolyte excretion ratios indicate the ability of the kidney to conserve electrolytes. Identification of WBCs and bacteria indicates a urinary tract infection.

Evaluation of Body Fluids

Evaluation of cerebrospinal, synovial (joint), and abdominal cavity fluid provides important information pertaining to inflammation, infection, or neoplasia within that particular body cavity. These body fluids are analyzed for total protein, total cell count, differential cell count, and bacterial culture.

Any form of neurologic disease in horses constitutes an indication for cerebrospinal fluid (CSF) analysis. CSF is collected in standing, sedated horses with spinal cord disease from the lumbosacral space using a 6-inch, 18-gauge spinal needle. In horses with brain and brainstem disease, CSF is collected in anesthetized horses from the atlantooccipital space using a 3-inch, 18-gauge spinal needle. Normal nucleated cell counts are less than five cells per microliter (predominately lymphocytes), and normal total protein concentration is variable depending on the laboratory but is usually less than 80 mg/dl (higher than in other species). Abnormalities in protein and cell counts can identify an inflammatory, infectious, or neoplastic process, but results of CSF analysis are often nonspecific. Antibody to the causative agents of several equine neurologic diseases (rabies, protozoal myelitis, herpes myeloencephalopathy, equine encephalomyelitis) can be detected in CSF, which provides specific information regarding the cause of neurologic signs. Complications associated with CSF tap include iatrogenic (operator-induced) spinal cord trauma and introduction of bacteria into the central nervous system.

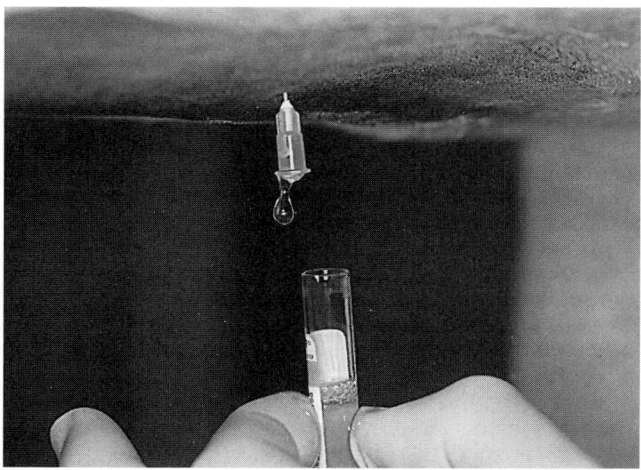

FIGURE 30-31. Technique for performing abdominocentesis in a horse.

Joint effusion, pain, or heat is an indication for arthrocentesis (joint tap) in horses. Synovial fluid is obtained by needle aspiration of almost any joint on the limbs of horses. Before needle aspiration, the hair must be clipped and a sterile preparation must be performed over the joint. Normal synovial fluid is highly viscous and will string 2 to 3 cm between your fingers before breaking. Normal synovial fluid is clear yellow in color and does not clot. Normal total protein is less than 2 g/dl and the normal cell count is less than 300/µl (less than 10% neutrophils). Analysis of synovial fluid can differentiate between synovial inflammation and infection. Bacterial culture of synovial fluid can identify the offending bacteria in horses with septic arthritis. Complications associated with arthrocentesis include iatrogenic septic arthritis and trauma to joint structures.

Abdominal pain, abnormal rectal examination, abdominal distension, and fever of unknown origin are indications for abdominocentesis in horses. Abdominal fluid is obtained by placing an 18-gauge, 1.5-inch needle into the peritoneal space of the ventral abdomen (Figure 30-31). The needle should be placed one hand's breadth behind the sternum, off the midline to the right of the horse (to avoid the spleen). If a 1.5-inch needle is insufficient to reach the peritoneal cavity, a teat cannula or female dog urinary catheter may be used. The use of a teat cannula is more invasive and increases the risk of traumatic bowel rupture. Normal abdominal fluid total protein is less than 2.5 mg/dl, and normal total nucleated cell count is less than 5000/µl (50% neutrophils). Analysis of abdominal fluid can identify devitalized bowel in horses with acute abdominal pain (colic); abdominal abscess; tumor in horses with a mass in the abdomen identified via rectal palpation; and ruptured bladder in foals with abdominal distention. Complications of abdominocentesis include traumatic bowel rupture, intraabdominal hemorrhage from trauma to the spleen, and iatrogenic septic peritonitis.

Bacterial Culture and Susceptibility Testing

The veterinary technician often plays an important role in bacteriologic testing of specimens collected from patients with infectious diseases (see Chapter 8). Specimens (blood, joint fluid, abdominal fluid, urine, wound exudate, infected bone, etc.) are frequently collected from horses with infectious diseases for culture. Following the proper procedures during collection and transport of these specimens to the laboratory for culture and susceptibility testing improves the chances of growing the causative organism. There are specific guidelines that should be followed for collection and transport of different types of specimens. For example, blood is usually placed in a special enhancement medium immediately after collection for transport to the laboratory. Likewise, there are special methods for collection and transport of samples submitted for aerobic and anaerobic culture. Identifying the causative agent in an infectious process and determining its in vitro susceptibility pattern to antibiotics are often critical in choosing the appropriate antibiotic regimen. Therefore the technician contributes greatly to the successful outcome of equine patients with infectious diseases. Fecal samples are often submitted for *Salmonella* spp. or *Clostridium* spp. cultures from horses with diarrhea. Fecal samples for *Salmonella* culture should be submitted daily for 5 consecutive days. If no salmonellae are isolated from these five samples, then one can be reasonably confident that the horses are not shedding *Salmonella* organisms. Fecal samples may be submitted to other diagnostic tests as ELISA for rota virus and clostridial toxin.

PREVENTIVE HEALTH CARE

The equine veterinary technician may be a valuable resource for client education in areas of general horse care, vaccination programs, deworming protocols, and interstate shipment guidelines. Specific information in these areas will depend on geographic location. The technician and veterinarian should prepare standard recommendations that are appropriate for their region and clientele.

Vaccination

Vaccination plays a crucial role in equine management programs in preventing and controlling infectious disease within a herd. Appropriate vaccination protocols will differ among horses depending on geographic location, age, use, and reproductive status. All horses must be vaccinated against tetanus and eastern and western encephalitis; and vaccinations against influenza, rhinopneumonitis, and rabies are highly recommended (see Chapter 11). The frequency of vaccination for these five diseases depends on age and reproductive status. Geographic and epidemiologic circumstances dictate indications for administering vaccines to protect horses from botulism, strangles, equine viral arteritis, rotavirus, and Potomac horse fever. Initial vaccination schedules for naive horses should be administered according to manufacturer recommendations.

 Technician Note

The equine veterinary technician may be a valuable resource for client education in areas of general horse care, vaccination programs, deworming protocols, and interstate shipment guidelines.

Vaccinations are administered either subcutaneously or intramuscularly, depending on manufacturer instructions. Vaccinations are frequently given in the neck musculature; however, local inflammatory reactions may make the horse reluctant to lower or raise its head. The impact of local reactions can be reduced by administering vaccines deep in the semimembranous and semitendinosus muscles.

Administration of vaccines into the pectoral or gluteal muscles is not recommended in horses.

Tetanus is a highly fatal neurologic disease in horses. It is characterized by a stiff, stilted gait, hyperexcitability, seizure, and coma. The causative organism is ubiquitous in the environment. The most common portals of entry for disease in horses include a subsolar abscess, penetrating wound, and infected intramuscular injection site. Tetanus toxoid (inactivated) is a safe and efficacious vaccine for preventing clinical disease. Healthy horses without risk factors should be vaccinated for tetanus annually. Horses that acquire penetrating wounds or subsolar abscesses or require surgery (colic, castration) should receive a booster vaccine if the most recent vaccination was administered more than 3 months before this incident. Unvaccinated horses at high risk of development of tetanus (wounds, subsolar abscess, surgery) should receive tetanus antitoxin in addition to tetanus toxoid to provide immediate protection against disease. Tetanus antitoxin is associated with fatal serum hepatitis, and administration should be limited to cases at high risk of disease.

There are three main types of viral equine encephalitis: eastern, western, and Venezuelan. The viral equine encephalitides produce rapidly progressive, highly fatal neurologic disease in horses. Mosquitoes transmit the infection to horses; therefore disease incidence is seasonal in most geographic regions. Vaccines for eastern and western equine encephalitis are highly efficacious. Clinical disease in vaccinated horses is rare. All horses in the United States should be vaccinated against eastern and western equine encephalomyelitis virus before the mosquito season, which is generally in the spring. Horses that live in southern states with a year-round mosquito season should be vaccinated in the fall and summer in addition to the spring vaccination. Brood mares should receive a booster of their vaccination in the tenth month of gestation (use only killed vaccines in pregnant animals) to ensure adequate colostral antibody protection for the foal. Vaccination against Venezuelan equine encephalomyelitis is not routinely recommended because the disease has not been reported recently in the United States and does not currently pose a threat to the U.S. horse population except those near the Mexican border.

Influenza is a highly contagious respiratory disease in horses and is characterized by fever, cough, and depression. The intramuscular influenza vaccines do not provide consistent protection from influenza virus challenge, but vaccination programs do reduce the incidence of disease within the herd and the severity and duration of disease in individual horses. On the other hand, intranasal influenza vaccine closely resembles the protective immunity achieved with natural infection. Sedentary adult horses, not exposed to other horses, are at low risk of contracting influenza and should be vaccinated once or twice per year. Young horses and horses engaged in performance activities (racing, showing, training) are at high risk of contracting influenza because of their exposure to other horses and should be vaccinated every 3 to 4 months or 3 to 4 weeks before exposure to other horses. Brood mares should be vaccinated with the injectable vaccine against influenza in the tenth month of pregnancy to ensure adequate colostral transfer of antibody against influenza for the foal. Some horses may suffer a transient systemic reaction characterized by fever, inappetence, and depression several days after influenza vaccination.

Equine herpesvirus (the causative agent of rhinopneumonitis) is a highly contagious virus that produces respiratory disease, abortion, neonatal and neurologic disease in horses. Protection against respiratory disease following equine herpesvirus vaccination is inconsistent and relatively short lived. Sedentary adult horses, not exposed to other horses, should be vaccinated once or twice per year, whereas young horses and horses engaged in performance activities should be vaccinated every 3 to 4 months. Inactivated univalent vaccines should be administered to brood mares during the third, fifth, seventh, and ninth months of pregnancy to prevent abortion. Although 100% protection against abortion is not achieved, the incidence of equine herpesvirus abortion is significantly reduced by institution of this vaccination program. None of the current vaccines claims to provide protection against the neurologic form of herpesvirus in horses.

Rabies is a rapidly progressive, fatal neurologic disease in horses. Although the incidence of rabies is low, equine infection does represent a human health hazard. The most likely source of infection in horses is the bite of a rabid wild animal. Skunks, foxes, raccoons, and bats are the most common reservoirs in North America. Horses should be vaccinated against rabies on an annual basis. Vaccinated horses that have been exposed to a rabid animal should be revaccinated promptly and observed for 90 days. Unvaccinated horses with a known rabies exposure should be observed for 6 months and should not be vaccinated.

Botulism is a rapidly progressive, fatal neurologic disease in horses characterized by profound weakness, muscle fasciculations, and dysphagia (inability to swallow). The causal organism produces a neurotoxin that may gain entry to the body by colonizing the intestinal tract (foals), infected wounds, or contaminating feedstuffs. Colonization of the intestinal tract in foals occurs in particular geographic regions of the United States, especially Pennsylvania, Ohio, and Kentucky. Foals in endemic regions may be protected by vaccination of mares with botulism toxoid before foaling.

Strangles is a highly contagious respiratory disease of horses caused by *Streptococcus equi*. Although strangles is common in young horses, vaccination is not routinely recommended. The injectable vaccine induces incomplete, short-term immunity against infection, whereas natural disease provides protection against infection for up to 10 years. In addition, injectable vaccines are commonly associated with swelling and abscess formation at the injection site and immune-mediated reactions (purpura hemorrhagica). Therefore routine vaccination should be limited to herds with endemic clinical disease and rapid turnover of horses. The recently developed modified-live intranasal vaccine induces mucosal immunity, providing better protection and fewer side effects, but it should not be given to pregnant mares and young foals.

Equine viral arteritis is a contagious viral disease that produces limb swelling, abortion, and respiratory disease in horses. Stallions can develop a persistent infection in their reproductive tract, which they readily transmit to mares during breeding. The vaccine for equine viral arteritis is approved for use in stallions and nonpregnant mares under the supervision of the U.S. Department of Agriculture (USDA). Pregnant mares should not be vaccinated for equine viral arteritis. Vaccination induces seropositivity and may interfere with testing requirements for export.

Potomac horse fever is caused by *Ehrlichia risticii* and produces diarrhea, fever, abortion, and laminitis. The mode of transmission is not completely elucidated, but it is suspected to involve an insect vector. Geographically, clinical disease is observed predominantly in states east of the Mississippi. Two inactivated bacterins are commercially available and should be administered to horses living in or traveling to endemic regions of the United States. Vaccination should precede the months of peak disease incidence (March through October).

Systemic reactions may occasionally occur after vaccine administration. Anaphylaxis is a life-threatening systemic reaction that produces cardiovascular shock and respiratory distress. Anaphylaxis should be treated immediately with epinephrine. Local reactions characterized by swelling, heat, and pain are more common and are generally self-limiting. Administration of NSAIDs may speed recovery of local swellings, fever, and pain associated with vaccination. Fatal local reactions are rare and are associated with infection of the injection site with clostridial organisms (malignant edema).

Deworming

Internal parasite control is an essential part of an effective preventive medicine program for all horses and is especially beneficial in young horses (see Chapter 7). Effective internal parasite control will allow young horses to grow to their full potential and will reduce the incidence of colic in horses of any age. An effective internal parasite control program should be directed at control of ascarids (large roundworms), small strongyles, large strongyles, and bots. Adult ascarids predominately affect young horses, live within the lumen of the intestinal tract, and may produce colic. Ascarid larvae migrate through the lungs and may produce parasitic pneumonia. The larvae of large strongyles migrate through the vascular system of the intestinal tract and may reduce blood flow and cause colic. Bot larvae attach to the stomach wall, creating inflammation, irritation, and potentially obstruction. Small strongyles encyst into the intestinal wall, which impairs nutrient absorption and creates inflammation. Small strongyles are particularly difficult to control because they have developed resistance to many of the commercially available anthelmintics.

The frequency of anthelmintic administration depends on geographic location. In the northern United States, a seasonal deworming program can be used wherein dewormer is administered from March through November at 8- to 12-week intervals. A boticide should be administered after the first frost in the northern United States and Canada. In the southern United States, dewormer should be administered year-round at 8- to 12-week intervals. Foals should be dewormed beginning at 8 weeks of age. Properly administered paste dewormers have an efficacy equal to tube deworming. Daily administration of pyrantel tartrate is effective in controlling small strongyles, large strongyles, and ascarids. This product is added to the feed daily and kills larvae before their migration. A boticide (ivermectin) must be administered in the fall of the year in addition to daily administration of pyrantel tartrate. Daily deworming is more expensive than interval deworming. Larvacidal deworming effective against encysted small strongyles includes single-dose moxidectin and five consecutive days of fenbendazole at twice the regular dose. The only reliably effective anthelmintic against equine tapeworms is a double dose of pyrantel pamoate.

Dental Care

Dental care is an important but frequently neglected part of health maintenance programs for horses. Regardless of age, the teeth of all horses should be examined annually. Dental problems may interfere with mastication, contribute to systemic infection, and cause chronic weight loss. Abnormal eating habits, such as dropping grain, excessive salivation, dropping feed boluses (quidding), or tilting of the head during mastication, are indications of dental problems. Thorough examination of the oral cavity often requires sedation, a flashlight, and a mouth speculum (gag). The frequency of routine dental care depends on the age and occlusal anatomy of the individual horse. Normal horses have three pairs of incisors, three pairs of premolars (second, third, and fourth premolars), and three pairs of molars on each arcade. Males usually have canine teeth, whereas females usually do not. Some horses will have "wolf teeth," which are remnants of the upper first premolar. Wolf teeth are small, round teeth adjacent to the second premolar (first cheek tooth). They often interfere with the bit and require removal between 12 and 18 months of age. Wolf teeth can be removed in standing, sedated horses.

Horses have a hippsodontic dentition, meaning their teeth continue to elongate and wear throughout their lives. Therefore dental surfaces that are not opposed by the adjacent arcade because of abnormal anatomy, malalignment, or malocclusion develop sharp, protruding enamel surfaces called *points* and *hooks*. The upper arcade of normal horses is wider than the lower arcade; therefore points develop on the buccal (cheek) surface of the upper arcade and the lingual (tongue) surface of the lower arcade. Often the upper arcade is shifted rostrally (with respect to the lower arcade) and hooks will develop on the rostral surface of the first cheek tooth on the upper arcade and the caudal surface of the last molar on the lower arcade. Dental hooks and points can cause erosion and ulceration of the tongue and cheek, dropping feed, and weight loss. Most hooks and points can be removed by floating (rasping) the teeth with dental floats (Figure 30-32). Large hooks may be removed using molar cutters. Many of the severe, often untreatable malocclusions and wear abnormalities seen in older horses can be prevented by regular dental care.

The most common malocclusive disorder in horses is parrot mouth, or prognathism, and there is likely a heritable component to this disorder. Prognathism is characterized as an unsoundness in horses and results in difficult prehension of food and dental hooks on the first cheek tooth (upper) and last molar (lower). Dental examination should be performed every 6 months in horses with prognathism.

Horses with an infected tooth root typically present with malodorous nasal discharge. The tooth roots of the last four teeth on the upper arcade are located within the maxillary sinus; therefore infected teeth result in secondary sinusitis. The affected tooth can be identified by skull radiographs, and the fourth premolar and first molar are most commonly involved. Removal of the affected tooth is the only effective treatment approach. Teeth generally cannot be removed from the oral cavity. Rather, teeth are repelled from their roots via an incision into the maxillary sinus or trephination in the maxilla or mandible (with the horse under general anesthesia) and driven into the oral cavity for removal.

Young horses (2 to 3 years) may retain deciduous caps after eruption of the permanent teeth. Retained caps can produce ulcerations on the cheeks, inadequate mastication, and dropping of feed and should be removed if retained for more than a few months. Retained caps can be removed in standing, sedated horses.

Equine Infectious Anemia

Equine infectious anemia (EIA) is a viral disease of horses that results in anemia, fever, and weight loss. The virus is transmitted from infected horses by large biting flies, tabanides. Once infected, horses become permanently

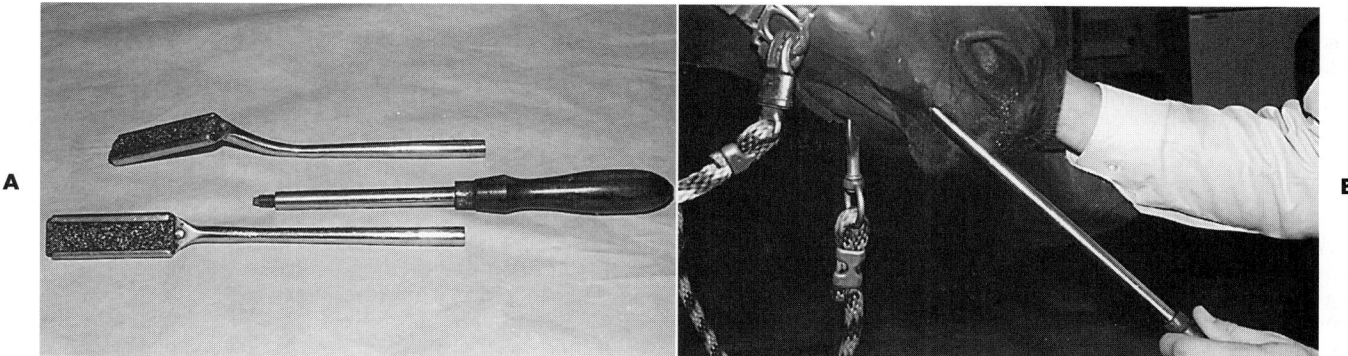

FIGURE 30-32. **A,** Tooth floats used to file off the enamel points of the upper and lower cheek teeth of horses. **B,** Technique for floating teeth in a horse.

infected and therefore are carriers of the virus. Horses must have a negative (Coggins') test for EIA within 1 year for issuance of health certificates for interstate travel, international travel, show, and sale. A USDA-accredited veterinarian must draw blood for testing and provide a detailed description of the horse on specified forms. The health certificate for interstate travel cannot be issued until the negative test is returned from a state or federally recognized laboratory. Horses that are not traveling or sold should still be tested on a yearly basis. If a positive test is obtained, the entire herd is quarantined until all horses on the premises are tested (usually 60 days). Only the state veterinarian can release the quarantine. Because horses that test positive for EIA are persistent carriers, they serve as a reservoir of the virus. Therefore infected horses must be quarantined for life (greater than 200 yards from other horses) or euthanized. The veterinary technician may be involved in collection of blood, completing submission forms, and sending samples for EIA testing under the direct supervision of the attending veterinarian.

SELECTED MEDICAL DISEASES

Equine Respiratory Diseases

Strangles is a common, highly contagious respiratory disease of horses caused by the bacterial pathogen *Streptococcus equi*. Strangles typically produces swelling and abscesses of the submandibular and retropharyngeal lymph nodes. Affected horses have fever, depression, poor appetite, and painful swellings under the mandible. The abscesses under the mandible enlarge, rupture, and drain a large volume of purulent exudate. Horses may develop abscesses within the guttural pouch, thorax, abdomen, and central nervous system. Development of abscess in abnormal locations is termed *bastard strangles*. These cases are particularly difficult to treat successfully. Horses with complicated cases of strangles should be treated with antibiotics, and *S. equi* is typically sensitive to penicillin. Horses with strangles should be maintained under strict isolation protocol. Recovered horses remain contagious and represent a threat to susceptible horses for approximately 6 weeks after recovering from clinical disease. Immunization against *S. equi* is controversial (see Vaccination).

Influenza is a highly contagious viral respiratory disease in horses characterized by an increased body temperature of 40° C (104° F), cough, and depression. The incubation period is short (2 to 3 days), and horses remain ill for 3 to 4 days. Equine influenza virus is transmitted through a herd via aerosolization of virus during coughing. The virus damages the clearance mechanisms in the lung and predisposes horses to bacterial pneumonia. Horses should be rested for a minimum of 3 weeks after recovery from viral respiratory disease. Immunization against influenza is recommended (see Vaccination).

Equine herpesvirus is a very contagious virus that produces respiratory disease, abortion, and neonatal and neurologic disease (ascending paralysis) in horses. The clinical signs of respiratory disease caused by equine herpesvirus are milder but hardly distinguishable from equine influenza. The incubation period is longer (2 to 10 days), and horses may remain ill for 4 to 5 days. Equine herpesvirus is transmitted through the herd by aerosol transmission, respiratory secretions, and fomite transmission. Protection against respiratory disease following equine herpesvirus vaccination is inconsistent and relatively short lived. Abortion secondary to equine herpesvirus occurs in the seventh to eleventh month of gestation, and the mare does not appear sick at the time of abortion. Vaccination is recommended for performance horses and brood mares. Neurologic disease caused by equine herpesvirus is not common. Affected horses demonstrate signs of incoordination, inability to urinate, and poor tail tone. Recovery from neurologic diseases is prolonged (2 to 3 months), and horses may not return to completely normal neurologic function. None of the currently available vaccines claims to provide protection against the neurologic form of herpesvirus in horses.

Equine viral arteritis is a contagious viral disease that produces limb swelling, conjunctivitis, abortion, and respiratory disease in horses. Limb swelling is painful and results from vasculitis (inflammation of blood vessels). Stallions infected after puberty develop a persistent infection in their accessory sex glands (ampullae) and transmit the viral infection to mares during breeding. Abortion can occur at any point during gestation and results from viral damage to the blood vessels of the placenta. The vaccine for equine viral arteritis is approved for use in stallions and nonpregnant mares under the supervision of the USDA. Pregnant mares should not be vaccinated against equine viral arteritis.

Chronic obstructive pulmonary disease (COPD, heaves) is an allergic airway disease that produces narrowing of small airways (bronchoconstriction) and excessive mucous production. The clinical signs of COPD are cough, nasal discharge, flared nostrils, increased respiratory rate, and increased expiratory effort. The severity of clinical signs may range from exercise intolerance to severe respiratory distress (dyspnea) at rest. Most affected horses are allergic to the molds present in hay and straw. Ideally, horses should be maintained at pasture and hay should be removed as the source of roughage in the diet. A similar form of this disease is observed in horses during the summer months in the southern United States. Summer pasture–associated obstructive pulmonary disease (SPAOPD) usually occurs from May to November, and it is thought to result from exposure to mold spores present on the pasture. Horses cannot be "cured" of COPD or SPAOPD, but the diseases can often be controlled with appropriate management practices. Changing the environment to remove offending allergens is the single most important principle in the treatment of COPD and SPAOPD. Medical therapy of horses with COPD or SPAOPD may be intermittently necessary in moderate to severely affected horses and consists of corticosteroids to reduce inflammation and bronchodilator therapy to relax small airways.

The guttural pouches are two large symmetric dilations of the eustachian tube that are present in all Equidae. They are located just above the pharynx and larynx and can be accessed during endoscopic examination through small openings in the dorsal lateral nasopharynx. The internal and external carotid arteries and several cranial nerves travel superficially under the surface of the guttural pouch lining and are vulnerable to damage from pathologic conditions. The purpose of the guttural pouches may be to lower the temperature of the blood that is traveling to the brain (internal and external carotid arteries) during exercise. Bacterial infection of the guttural pouch is termed *guttural pouch empyema* and is often associated with strangles. Fungal infection of the guttural pouch is termed guttural pouch mycosis, and the causative agent is often *Aspergillus* sp. The fungal plaque usually forms over the internal carotid artery, adjacent to nerves that control swallowing. Horses may have life-threatening blood loss from rupture of the internal carotid artery or dysphagia from damage to the nerves. Accumulation of air in the guttural pouches (guttural pouch tympany) occurs in foals and weanlings and is usually associated with an abnormality of the opening to the pouches. It can occur unilaterally or bilaterally and is characterized by a fluctuant, nonpainful swelling in the throat-latch region. Guttural pouch empyema is characterized by accumulation of mucopurulent material in the pouches, which is often secondary to retropharyngeal lymph node abscess formation from a streptococcal infection.

Gastrointestinal Disease

"Choke" refers to obstruction of the esophagus. Chronic dental disease and retained deciduous caps are common predisposing conditions for development of choke. The esophagus is usually obstructed by grain or hay, and most horses will continue to attempt to eat despite their inability to swallow. Clinical signs include anxiety, gagging, excessive salivation, and feed and saliva coming from the nostrils. The obstruction can be visualized via endoscopic examination and in most instances can be relieved by manipulation and hydropulsion using a nasogastric tube. Horses must be heavily sedated to lower their head during manipulation of the nasogastric tube to prevent water and feed from entering the trachea. Aspiration pneumonia is a significant complication and must be addressed in all cases. Esophageal stricture or rupture is a less common complication and occurs in horses with circumferential damage to the esophageal mucosa.

Young horses are particularly prone to development of gastric ulceration. Stress, a high-grain diet, musculoskeletal pain, and administration of NSAIDs are common predisposing factors. Clinical signs of gastric ulceration are bruxism (grinding teeth), hypersalivation, and abdominal pain after eating. Foals with gastric ulceration will often lie still in dorsal recumbency with their forelimbs over their head or extended out straight. Human antiulcer medications, such as histamine H_2 blockers, intestinal protectants, and hydrogen ion pump blockers, are used to treat gastric ulceration in horses. Most equine facilities administer prophylactic antiulcer therapy to hospitalized foals because of the stressful environment.

Colitis in horses can result in rapid, life-threatening fluid loss (hypovolemia), shock, endotoxemia, electrolyte loss, and acid-base imbalance as a result of diarrhea. Some horses may develop hypovolemic shock and electrolyte imbalance before the appearance of diarrhea. In addition to diarrhea, clinical signs of colitis include depression, inappetence, abdominal pain, tachycardia (increased heart rate), injected (brick red) mucous membranes, and prolonged capillary refill time. Etiologic agents that produce life-threatening diarrhea in horses include *Salmonella, Clostridium,* and *Ehrlichia risticii.* Horses with diarrhea should be considered contagious and maintained under isolation protocol. Intravenous fluid therapy is crucial to support the cardiovascular system, replace fluid losses, and correct electrolyte and acid-base imbalance. Complications of colitis include laminitis (founder), cardiovascular collapse, cardiac arrhythmias, and thrombophlebitis.

Phenylbutazone toxicosis in horses can produce renal insufficiency and oral, gastric, and colonic ulceration in horses. The colonic ulcers occur in the right dorsal colon and are the most difficult aspect of phenylbutazone toxicity to treat. Colonic ulcers secondary to phenylbutazone toxicity can produce abdominal pain, marked protein loss, melena (blood in manure), peritonitis, colonic stricture, or colonic rupture. Dehydration and excessive dosages are the most important predisposing factors for development of phenylbutazone toxicosis.

Neurologic Disease

The five most common disorders of the spinal cord are cervical vertebral myelopathy caused by stenotic or dynamic compression of the spinal cord (wobbles), equine protozoal myelitis, equine herpesvirus myeloencephalopathy (rhinopneumonitis), equine degenerative myeloencephalopathy, and vertebral fracture. Damage to the spinal cord produces spinal ataxia (incoordination of the limbs without abnormalities of the brain and brainstem). Diagnostic aids to differentiate these diseases include neurologic examination, cervical radiographic examination, myelographic examination, and CSF analysis. CSF can be obtained at the lumbosacral space in standing, sedated horses, and at the atlantooccipital space in anesthetized horses. CSF travels from the cranial area in a caudal direction. Therefore CSF should be obtained at the lumbosacral space in horses with spinal cord disease and at the atlantooccipital space in horses with brain and brainstem disease.

Cervical vertebral myelopathy is a manifestation of developmental orthopedic disease characterized by compression of the cervical spinal cord by malformed or unstable cervical vertebrae. Males are affected four times more frequently than females, and thoroughbreds appear to be predisposed. Clinical signs of symmetric incoordination usually begin between 6 months and 3 years of age. The hindlimbs are usually more severely affected than the forelimbs. Likelihood of disease is determined by plain film cervical radiographs, and the diagnosis is confirmed by myelographic examination. Surgical stabilization improves the neurologic status of some patients.

Equine protozoal myelitis (EPM) is the most common cause of spinal ataxia in the United States. Horses are dead-end, aberrant hosts of the protozoan parasites. *Sarcocystis neurona* is the most common of the protozoan parasites that cause spinal cord disease in horses; opossums are the primary hosts of this parasite, and horses are likely infected via fecal-oral transmission. Birds are the secondary hosts, and do not appear to be infectious for horses. The clinical signs of EPM are directly referable to the location of the organism in the central nervous system. Therefore EPM should be considered in any horse demonstrating neurologic signs. Most horses with EPM (85%) demonstrate signs referable to spinal cord damage. Diagnosis is confirmed by identification of antibody to the organism in CSF. Treatment consists of administration of two antibiotics that inhibit folic acid metabolism: sulfadiazine and pyrimethamine. The average treatment period is approximately 120 days, and the prognosis for return to normal neurologic function is 60%. Folic acid should be administered to prevent development of anemia during treatment.

Equine herpesvirus can produce respiratory disease, abortion, and neonatal and neurologic disease in horses. The neurologic form is characterized by ascending paralysis with the hindlimbs more severely affected than the forelimbs. Horses often demonstrate urinary incontinence, poor tail tone, and penile prolapse. Diagnosis is confirmed by cytologic analysis of CSF. Administration of corticosteroids may improve recovery if administered early in the disease process. Prognosis for return to normal neurologic function is approximately 80%.

Equine degenerative myelopathy results in symmetric spinal ataxia with both the forelimbs and hindlimbs equally affected. Clinical signs appear between 6 months and 2 years of age, and the disease appears to be familial in some breeds. There is no definitive antemortem diagnostic test, and diagnosis is usually made on the basis of the neurologic examination, CSF analysis, cervical radiographs, and myelographic examination. Dietary supplementation with vitamin E may prevent progression of disease and may result in improvement in clinical signs in some instances. The prognosis for return to normal neurologic function is poor.

The most consistent clinical sign associated with vertebral fracture is pain. The cervical vertebrae, caudal thoracic vertebrae, and thoracolumbar junction are the most common sites of vertebral fracture. Cervical vertebral fracture results in tetraparesis (weakness of all four limbs), whereas fracture of the thoracic and lumbar vertebrae produces paraparesis (weakness of hindlimbs) or paraplegia (paralysis of hindlimbs). Diagnosis is confirmed by plain film radiography. If the fracture is nondisplaced, nuclear scintigraphy may aid in identification of the fracture site. Surgical correction may be attempted for fractures of the cervical vertebrae, but repair of thoracic or lumbar vertebrae is not attempted.

The four most common disorders of the brain and brainstem in horses are rabies, equine viral encephalitis (eastern, western, Venezuelan), leukoencephalomalacia (moldy corn toxicity), and head trauma. Damage to the cerebrum may produce altered mentation, altered states of consciousness, head pressing, and seizure. Damage to the brainstem may potentially damage the cranial nerves, which control the muscles of facial expression, facial sensation, mastication, swallowing, balance, vision, taste, and ocular position. Brainstem lesions also produce incoordination of the limbs and altered breathing patterns. Diagnostic aids for evaluation of horses with cerebral or brainstem dysfunction include CSF analysis and skull radiographs.

Rabies is a zoonotic infection (infectious to humans) and is universally fatal (see Chapter 18). Horses usually acquire the infection by a bite wound from a rabid skunk, fox, or bat. Clinical signs are highly variable but often begin as fever, hindlimb ataxia, and hyperesthesia (hyperresponsiveness to touch). Neurologic signs rapidly progress to involve the brain and brainstem. The duration of neurologic signs before death varies from 3 to 10 days. Diagnosis is confirmed by fluorescent antibody stain of brain tissue. Humans handling potentially rabid horses should avoid contact with saliva, wear gloves, and avoid contact with CSF. Individuals with occupational exposure to livestock and wildlife should undergo a prophylactic rabies vaccination series. Postexposure rabies vaccination should be administered to humans in contact with rabid animals.

The equine viral encephalitides (eastern, western, Venezuelan) are transmitted to horses by mosquitoes. Clinical signs include profound depression, fever, and multiple cranial nerve abnormalities, and mortality is extremely high. Treatment consists of supportive care to provide fluids, nutrition, and a clean, dry environment. The prognosis is poor with eastern equine encephalitis and guarded with western and Venezuelan encephalitides. Diagnosis is confirmed by mouse inoculation. The viral encephalitides can be prevented by vaccination 1 month before mosquito season. In southern regions of the United States, vaccinations should be administered two or three times per year.

Equine leukoencephalomalacia (moldy corn toxicity) is caused by ingestion of a fungal toxin produced by *Fusarium moniliform*. This mold has a predilection for moldy corn, and affected kernels are usually pink to brown. The fungal toxin produces liquefactive necrosis of the cerebral cortex, and clinical signs include profound depression, head pressing, altered states of consciousness, incoordination, and aimless wandering. Treatment consists of supportive care, and the prognosis for recovery is poor. Horses often die within 24 hours of manifesting neurologic signs.

Horses acquire two types of skull fractures depending on the nature of their traumatic injury. Horses that suffer frontal impact with a solid object develop depression fractures of the frontal and parietal bones. The common neurologic signs observed in horses with this type of fracture are referable to cerebral damage and include depression, seizure, stupor, and aimless wandering. Horses that flip over backward develop fractures of the petrous temporal bone and the junction of the basisphenoid and basioccipital bone. Neurologic signs associated with these fractures include abnormalities of balance, incoordination of limbs, nystagmus (rhythmic eye movement), abnormal respiratory patterns, and coma. Diagnosis is confirmed by radiographic examination of the skull. Treatment consists of supportive care and antiinflammatory therapy (corticosteroids, DMSO). Surgical decompression of frontal and parietal fractures may improve the neurologic status of some horses.

Dermatologic Disease

Equine dermatophytosis (ringworm) is a fungal infection of the superficial layer of skin. The fungi commonly involved are *Trichophyton* and *Microsporum* spp.

Transmission of the fungal infection is by direct contact between affected animals, and younger animals (less than 4 years old) are more likely to be affected. Infected areas of skin have a bull's-eye appearance with circular patches of hair loss with a circle of inflammation at the periphery of the lesion. Diagnosis is confirmed by fungal culture on commercially available dermatophyte culture medium. Although the infection is usually self-limiting, application of topical antifungal drugs will speed recovery.

Dermatophilosis (rain scald, rain rot) is a common bacterial infection caused by *Dermatophilus congolense* that produces crusting lesions. The crusts can be pulled out with a tuft of hair, and the remaining lesion is a glistening yellow crater. The organisms readily colonize wet, macerated skin, and therefore the disease is common in the winter and spring. An impression smear of the tuft should be stained with Wright's stain, and organisms are identified as a double chain of cocci with a "railroad track" appearance. The organisms are usually easily cultured and form an applesauce-like colony on specialized growth medium. Affected horses should be bathed with an iodine-based or chlorohexidine shampoo and placed in a dry environment. Administration of penicillin will speed recovery in severely affected horses.

Culicoides hypersensitivity is a syndrome characterized by mane and tail rubbing whereby affected horses develop an allergic pruritic skin condition secondary to the bite of *Culicoides* flies. The classic body regions affected include face, ears, mane, withers, rump, base of the tail, and ventral abdomen. The dermatitis usually begins as a seasonal condition, but its severity and duration increase as the horse ages. Pruritus usually is noted during the fly season but will vary in length depending on geographic location. The condition is diagnosed by correlating the historical findings of seasonal pruritus with physical evidence of self-mutilation, especially in the mane and tail areas. Intradermal skin testing can be useful in confirming the diagnosis. Treatment involves reducing insect exposure and concomitant use of antiinflammatory medication. Because *Culicoides* breeds in stagnant waters, affected horses should be moved from proximity to ponds, lakes, or irrigation canals. Water troughs and barrels should be cleaned frequently and the water kept fresh to prevent use as breeding sites by the flies. Because *Culicoides* feeds primarily at dusk, night, and dawn, horses should be kept stabled during these times. Stabling is most effective if the doors and windows can be closed and if the stall is lined with a fine-mesh screen. Frequent application of insecticide to the screen may also be useful. Ceiling fans help reduce exposure because *Culicoides* cannot fly well in brisk breezes. Application of insecticides and repellents is a necessary part of disease control. The most effective products are those containing pyrethrins with synergists and repellents. Frequent bathing not only decreases scale and crust but also seems to decrease pruritus. Corticosteroid therapy may be required in some horses to control the pruritus.

Equine sarcoid is a benign, locally invasive tumor of skin and is the most common tumor in horses. These tumors produce either raised, hairless lesions with a corrugated surface that often bleed when traumatized, known as *fibroblastic sarcoids*, or a flattened form known as *verrucous sarcoids*. The cause of sarcoid is unknown, but a viral agent is suspected. Surgical resection, cryotherapy (freezing), laser therapy, immunotherapy (intralesional mycobacterial cell wall extract), radiotherapy (iridium 191), and chemotherapy (intralesional cisplatin) are accepted treatment modalities with variable success. It is difficult to predict response to a given treatment modality, and combination therapy is often necessary.

Melanomas are relatively common skin tumors that develop particularly in gray horses. They occur most commonly in the perineal region but can occur on other areas of the body. Melanomas appear as darkly pigmented nodules in the skin. They are usually benign but tend to progress and can cause mechanical problems, such as interfering with defecation. Most clinicians believe it is better not to attempt surgical removal unless they are located in an area that interferes with tack or they are so large that they interfere with normal body functions. These tumors often become more aggressive following unsuccessful attempts at complete surgical removal. Administration of cimetidine has been reported to be effective in some horses in causing reduction in size or resolution of melanomas, but it does not seem to be effective in all horses. Once the cimetidine is discontinued, the tumors usually enlarge.

Ophthalmologic Disease

Recurrent uveitis (moon blindness, periodic ophthalmia) is the most common cause of blindness in horses. Affected horses experience episodes of intraocular inflammation characterized by blepharospasm, corneal edema, and hypopyon (inflammatory cellular exudate in the anterior chamber). Over time, the episodes become more frequent and severe and produce permanent ocular lesions, including retinal degeneration, cataracts, synechiae (adhesions of the iris to either the lens or the anterior chamber), and low ocular pressure. The disease may be unilateral or bilateral. Recurrent uveitis is classified as an unsoundness in horses, which constitutes failure during prepurchase and insurance examinations. Recurrent uveitis cannot be cured but can be controlled in some instances with long-term antiinflammatory therapy (aspirin). Acute episodes are treated with ophthalmic preparations containing atropine and corticosteroids; systemic antiinflammatory therapy may be beneficial, including flunixin meglumine, phenylbutazone, or aspirin. It is an immue-mediated condition, and many factors have been implicated (heredity, parasites, leptospirosis), the inciting cause of uveitis is unknown. Horses with end-stage uveitis are blind and have very small, collapsed, ocular globes (phthisis bulbi).

Corneal ulceration commonly results from ocular trauma. Corneal ulceration can be detected by application of fluorescein dye to the surface of the eye. Defects in the corneal surface will stain an apple-green color. Corneal ulceration in most horses responds readily without complications to administration of ophthalmic antibacterial ointment (bacitracin, neomycin, polymyxin B). In some instances, the ulcer will be colonized by *Pseudomonas* or *Aspergillus* spp. These organisms produce collagenase, which destroys the cornea and creates a "melting" corneal ulcer. These ulcers are rapidly progressive and prone to uveal prolapse or ocular rupture. Frequent antibiotic dosage regimens may require placement of a subpalpebral lavage system, wherein polyethylene tubing is placed into the eyelid and exits the conjunctiva dorsal to the globe (Figure 30-33). The port of the tubing can be braided into the horse's mane, which facilitates frequent dosing for a painful eye. Aggressive topical antibacterial therapy may be successful, but suturing a conjunctival pedicle flap to provide blood supply to the affected area may be necessary to save the globe in some instances. Deep, melting corneal ulcers often heal with a fibrous scar that may impair vision in the future.

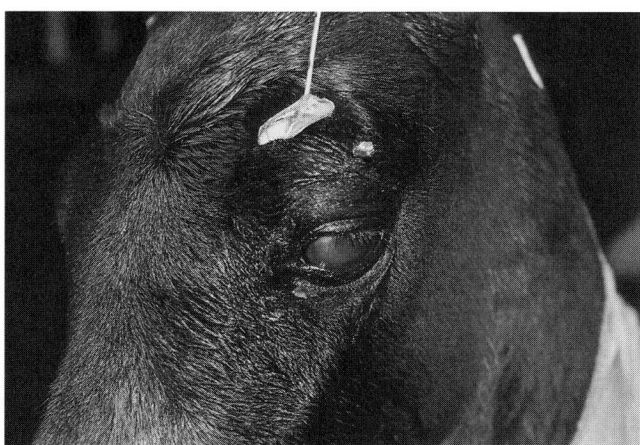

FIGURE 30-33. Subpalpebral eye lavage system for administration of ophthalmic medication without touching the affected eye.

Neonatal Care

The normal gestation period of mares varies considerably, ranging from 320 to 360 days. As a mare approaches parturition, the udder begins to enlarge ("bagging up") and may leak small amounts of colostrum that dry over the ends of the teats ("waxing"). Increasing calcium and magnesium concentrations in milk correspond to impending (less than 24 hours) parturition and can be detected using commercially available foal predictor kits. In mares with placentitis, parturition cannot be predicted by the increase in milk calcium. Parturition occurs in three stages. Stage 1 is under voluntary control of the mare and is characterized by repositioning of the fetus to a dorsosacral position and initial uterine contractions; it generally lasts a few hours, although it can be interrupted for hours to days. External signs of stage 1 labor include restlessness, sweating, pacing, inappetence, and raising the tail. The onset of stage 2 labor is signaled by rupture of the chorioallantoic membrane and release of allantoic fluid (breaking water). Delivery of the foal should be complete within 20 to 40 minutes of the onset of stage 2 labor. The third stage of labor begins after expulsion of the foal and is defined by expulsion of the fetoplacental membranes. Fetoplacental membranes should be passed within 1 hour of expulsion of the foal. Retained placenta (failure to pass fetal membranes within 3 hours of delivery) is an emergency in mares and may result in toxic metritis and laminitis. After parturition, the umbilicus is dipped in a chlorhexidine or an iodine solution, foals are examined for developmental anomalies and traumatic injury, the mare's reproductive tract is examined for traumatic injury, and the placenta is inspected for completeness and evidence of thickening or infection (also see Chapter 16 for additional information on reproduction).

Normal foals should stand within 1 hour, suckle within 2 hours, and pass meconium within 3 hours of parturition. It is important for the foal to ingest the colostrum ("first milk") produced by the mare. Colostrum contains immunoglobulins and other factors and provides protection against infection. Foals are born without immunoglobulin in their blood, and the immunoglobulin in colostrum represents the only form of immune protection (passive transfer of immunity). The immunoglobulin in colostrum is absorbed intact by the intestinal tract for the first 18 hours of life. After that time, the intestinal tract will no longer absorb the large immunoglobulin proteins (gut closure). Foals that do not receive adequate colostral maternal immunoglobulins shortly after birth are said to experience *failure of passive transfer*. Failure of passive transfer can occur with failure or delay to suckle, premature gut closure, failure of the dam to produce good-quality colostrum, and leakage of colostrum before parturition and is the single most important predisposing factor for development of life-threatening neonatal infections.

Adequate transfer of immunity should be assessed at 18 to 24 hours of life, using one of the several commercially available immunoglobulin G (IgG) test kit, that provide a semiquantitative measurement of IgG concentration in serum, plasma, or whole blood. This test is frequently performed by the veterinary technician. Early assessment of passive transfer is often indicated in high risk pregnancies and can be performed at 12 hours of age; although blood IgG levels may increase some, most of the absorption occurs in the first 8 to 12 hours. If the foal has not received adequate colostrum, it should be supplemented by intravenous plasma transfusion, using either commercial hyperimmune plasma or plasma collected from an appropriate donor as soon as possible. Moreover, if signs of sepsis are present blood cultures should be collected using sterile technique and broad-spectrum antibiotic therapy instituted immediately. The antibiotic therapy should be modified appropriately in accordance with the organism cultured. Bactericidal antibiotics with a broad spectrum, particularly activity against gram-negative organisms, may also be recommended to prevent bacterial infection in neonatal foals.

Normal foals suckle every 30 to 40 minutes and are very active. Foals are particularly fragile, and failure to suckle is the first sign of disease. Neonatal septicemia is the most common life-threatening disease of foals and results from entry of bacteria via the gastrointestinal tract, respiratory tract, and umbilicus (navel ill). Clinical signs include depression, fever, tachycardia, injected mucous membranes, icterus and petechiae seen on the mucous membranes and pinna (see Figure 30-6), recumbency, respiratory distress, shock, hypothermia, and coma. If untreated, neonatal septicemia usually results in death of the foal. Septic arthritis (joint ill) and osteomyelitis are common sequelae to neonatal septicemia that are difficult to cure and may produce permanent damage.

Hypoxic-ischemic (HI) syndrome is a result of prolonged birth asphyxia associated with insufficient placentation, difficult labor (dystocia), premature placental separation known as red bag (Figure 30-34), and premature cord rupture and failure to rupture placental membranes. The organs most susceptible to the HI injury include the central nervous system, the gastrointestinal tract, kidneys, and liver, respectively. Neonatal maladjustment syndrome (dummy foal) is a manifestation of HI encephalopathy. Foals may show neurologic abnormalities since birth or may develop those abnormalities within 24 hours after birth. The range of neurologic abnormalities includes failure to suckle, hyperresponsiveness, depression, bizarre vocalization (barkers), failure to recognize the dam, stupor, seizures, and coma. The neurologic signs result from neuronal damage associated with the hypoxia and ischemia in the brain and brainstem; edema and hemorrhage are commonly seen. Less commonly, the HI injury affects the other organs mentioned above, resulting in necrotizing enterocolitis and renal and liver insufficiencies.

Other causes of neonatal distress include constipation (meconium impaction), abnormal intestinal distention resulting from enterocolitis, uroperitoneum resulting from ruptured urinary bladder, profound anemia because of

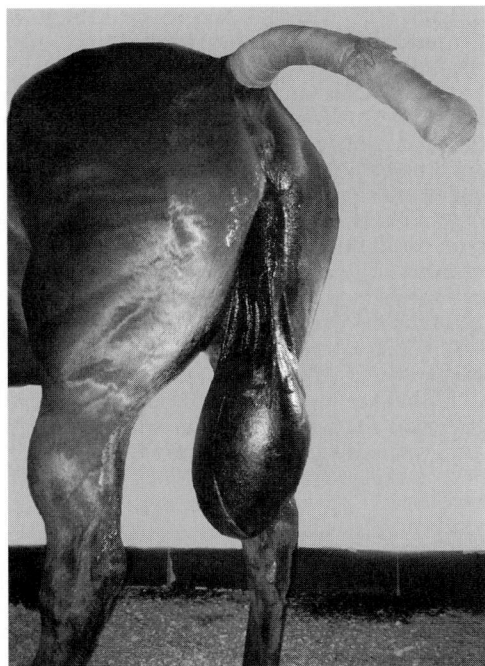

FIGURE 30-34. Mare with premature placental separation (red bag), which is often associated with prolonged birth asphyxia.

neonatal hemolysis resulting from incompatible blood type with mare (neonatal isoerythrolysis), and pulmonary insufficiency as a result of prematurity (failure to produce surfactant). Foals readily develop gastric ulceration under conditions of stress. Signs of abdominal discomfort, bruxism, and salivation are indicative of gastrointestinal ulceration, and therefore prophylactic antiulcer medication may be administered to all foals in intensive care.

> ### Technician Note
>
> Regardless of the primary disease process, neonatal intensive care is a daunting task. The veterinary technician attending to the recumbent foal must be diligent, thorough, aseptic, and observant.

Normal foals suckle approximately 30 times per day, ingest 15% to 20% of their body weight in milk, and gain 1.0 to 2.5 kg (2.2 to 5.5 lb) per day. Adequate nutritional support is of paramount importance in neonatal care. Nutritional support can be provided by feeding the mare's milk using a small nasoesophageal feeding tube. The mare should be hand milked every 2 hours, but, if the mare does not produce sufficient milk to meet the nutritional requirements of the foal, equine milk replacers may be used. Nonevaporated goat's milk may be used as a substitute; cow's milk should only be used as a last option, and it should be modified by the addition of lime water; calf milk replacers should be avoided. Total parenteral nutrition (TPN) is an intravenous nutritional support that may be necessary in foals with poor gastrointestinal motility and primary gastrointestinal disease. Parenteral nutrition requires a dedicated intravenous catheter and a constant infusion pump. Moreover, TPN may predispose or exacerbate septicemia; therefore appropriate handling and strict sterile technique are required when giving parenteral nutrition. Intravenous fluid therapy is often necessary to support the cardiovascular system, correct electrolyte abnormalities, and maintain acid-base balance.

Recumbent neonatal foals require intensive supportive care consisting of a 24-hour attendant, constant intravenous infusion system, nutritional supplementation, oxygen supplementation, and accessible blood gas and electrolyte analyzers. Recumbent foals are sometimes placed on a foal bed, which is designed to allow the attendant to care for the foal from one side and the mare to access the foal from the other. Foals should be maintained in sternal recumbency to prevent collapse of the down lung, allowing maximal ventilation. Foals must be kept clean and dry, and their position should be changed every 2 hours. Recumbent foals are prone to corneal ulceration; therefore triple antibiotic ointment or artificial tears should be placed in their eyes every 4 hours. Heart rate, respiratory rate and character, temperature, mucous membrane character, capillary refill time, abdominal distention, and gastrointestinal motility should be monitored every 2 hours. Urinary and fecal output should be recorded. Arterial blood gas, PCV, total protein, serum electrolyte, and serum glucose concentrations should be determined every 4 to 12 hours depending on the severity of the disease. Palpation of the umbilicus and joints should be performed at least daily.

Most recumbent foals demonstrate some degree of respiratory insufficiency. Oxygen can be supplemented to the foal using nasal insufflation with humidified 100% oxygen at 4 to 8 L/min. If nasal insufflation is inadequate, the foal may require mechanical ventilation to ensure adequate oxygenation. Mechanical ventilation requires nasotracheal or endotracheal intubation and positive pressure ventilation. Pulmonary function can be monitored using serial arterial blood gas evaluation obtained from the greater metatarsal artery. Pulse oximetry is a noninvasive alternative for monitoring arterial oxygen saturation.

Regardless of the primary disease process, neonatal intensive care is a daunting task. The veterinary technician attending to the recumbent foal must be diligent, thorough, aseptic, and observant. Deterioration in patient status occurs rapidly and without warning. Meticulous patient care and monitoring will allow rapid correction of the therapeutic plan, which often determines the final outcome for neonatal foals. Additional information on neonatal care of the foal is found in Chapter 12.

Dystocia

Dystocia means difficult birth and is relatively uncommon in horses compared with cattle. However, when dystocia occurs in mares it is usually a serious problem. Because parturition is rapid in horses and the expulsive efforts of the mare are violent, veterinary obstetric manipulations are difficult and exhausting. Care must be taken at all times to avoid injuring the reproductive tract of the mare. There are many causes of dystocia in the mare; the most frequent ones include premature placental separation and abnormal presentation of the fetus, especially when either the head or limbs or both are deviated. Because the neck of the foal is relatively long, it can easily become twisted. Sometimes the foal may come hindfeet first (rare), or if the hindfeet are retained, the tail comes first. This latter situation is true breech position. Transverse presentation is also rare in mares. Other occasional causes of dystocia include an excessively large fetus or fetal monsters (e.g., hydrocephalus). An anatomic or physiologic abnormality in the mare herself may cause dystocia. For example, a mare that has sustained a pelvic fracture can develop callus formation, which impairs the shape and size of the birth canal. Another cause of dystocia is torsion of the uterus. This may occur during gestation, particularly during the last trimester.

Dystocia in mares is corrected using a variety of methods, depending on the cause of the dystocia, the status of the foal, and the condition of the mare. Sometimes the dystocia can be corrected by manipulating fetal position or presentation with the mare standing, with or without the use of sedation or an epidural anesthetic. Placement of a nasotracheal tube will prevent the mare from exerting an abdominal press and will relieve straining. Sometimes a short-acting anesthetic protocol combined with rolling the mare on her back or hoisting her hindlimbs is enough to relieve the dystocia and provide the veterinarian with sufficient relaxation in the mare to deliver the fetus. Fetotomy is sometimes performed to relieve dystocia, particularly if the fetus is dead. Fetotomy is a process in which a dead foal is cut into pieces while within the uterus and removed. Caution must be taken while performing a fetotomy to prevent serious injury to the reproductive tract of the mare.

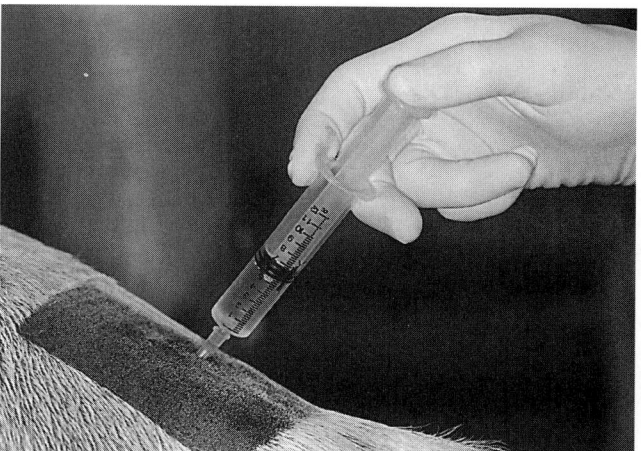

FIGURE 30-35. Technique for injecting a caudal epidural anesthetic between the first and second coccygeal vertebrae in a horse with an 18-gauge, 1.5-inch needle.

Technician Note

Most cesarean deliveries are performed in the mare with general anesthesia. Generally, time is critical for saving the foal and for the overall health and well-being of the mare. The technician must be prepared for the surgery and have the necessary equipment, personnel, and drugs ready for reviving the foal if necessary.

Most cesarean deliveries are performed in the mare with general anesthesia. Generally a cesarean delivery is performed though a caudal ventral midline or flank incision in mares. Time is usually critical for saving the foal and for the overall health and well-being of the mare. The technician must be prepared for the surgery and have necessary equipment, personnel, and drugs ready for reviving the foal if necessary. The same instruments that are used for colic surgery are often used for cesarean delivery, but additional instruments may be necessary. If the foal is alive, the technician or other personnel need to be prepared and equipped to revive it. The foal will usually be depressed from the effects of general anesthesia and may need vigorous rubbing and drying. Oxygen should be available, as well as heat lamps and a nasotracheal tube and Ambu bag to ventilate the foal. Forceps to clamp the umbilicus should be readily available if excessive bleeding occurs. A suction device to remove mucus and stomach contents from the airway should be attended to by the technician or other personnel. The technician should be cognizant and attentive to the needs of the surgeon during this time even though the foal is requiring assistance.

A piece of straw inserted in the nostril is one of the most practical methods of initiating respiratory movements in a newborn foal. The foal's neck should be extended to help ensure a patent airway. The foal should be vigorously dried because fluid will conduct heat away from the animal, resulting in hypothermia and a weak foal. The foal can be resuscitated with the self-inflating nonrebreathing Ambu bag. Air can be delivered through a cone-shaped face mask similar to the one used to induce anesthesia in small animals. The mask must fit tightly over the nostrils and mouth. Mouth-to-nose ventilation may be performed and is done by covering one nostril, closing the mouth, and blowing in the opposite nostril. A few short breaths are

all that is usually required. Overinflation can obviously cause permanent damage to the lungs. Frequently the veterinarian may order intravenous fluids, respiratory stimulants, and drugs to support the cardiovascular system. The foal should be kept warm (not hot) with heat lamps, circulating warm water pads, and blankets. The next important thing is to ensure that the foal consumes or is administered an adequate amount of colostrum to provide passive immunity to infectious agents during the first few weeks of life (see Neonatal Care). Enteral feeding of foal that underwent severe asphyxia may be contraindicated, as it may contribute to the development of neonatal necrotizing enterocolitis.

Surgery of the Female Caudal Reproductive Tract

Perineal surgery is relatively common in equine practice. Primiparous mares develop rectovaginal and cervical lacerations during foaling. Abnormal perineal conformation can lead to reproductive unsoundness. Mares with abnormal conformation can develop pneumovagina or pneumouterus secondary to aspirating air into the reproductive tract. They also can develop vesicovaginal reflux in which urine pools in the cranial vaginal cavity; this can drain into the uterus during estrus when the cervix is opened, leading to endometrial inflammation. Most surgical procedures to correct these caudal reproductive tract abnormalities are performed in standing mares that have been sedated, and a caudal epidural anesthesia is used.

A caudal epidural anesthesia is performed after clipping the hair over the tail head and aseptically preparing the skin. An 18-gauge, 1.5-inch needle is inserted through the skin between the last sacral and first coccygeal vertebrae or between the first and second coccygeal vertebrae and advanced (Figure 30-35). The correct location can be confirmed by checking to see if local anesthetic placed in the hub of the needle is drawn into the epidural space. Once the correct location has been identified, the local anesthetic is injected. The most commonly used agents for horses are lidocaine, mepivacaine, or xylazine. A caudal epidural anesthetic will desensitize the perineal region. Because horses will also become incoordinated in their rear limbs following the procedure, care should be taken when moving them until the effects of the anesthetic dissipate.

There are several surgical procedures for correcting caudal reproductive tract abnormalities. The most important factor in the eventual success of repairing a rectovaginal tear is that the mare's feces be made soft (cow patty consistency) and kept soft for at least 30 days after surgery. This decreases the straining and tension placed on the repaired rectal shelf. The most effective method for getting the feces soft is to remove hay and other coarse roughage from the diet and feed the mare on lush pasture or a complete pelleted feed. Administration of mineral oil or magnesium sulfate to the diet also helps soften the feces.

The most commonly formed perineal surgery is Caslick's operation. This is performed in many fillies on the racetrack and in mares with poor vulvar conformation to prevent pneumovagina and fecal contamination of the vagina, respectively. This procedure is usually performed with sedation and local anesthetic infiltration of the edge of the vulva. The edges of the dorsal vulvar labia are incised and then sutured using a continuous suture pattern. The closure is extended down to the level of the pelvic floor. The suture should not be any lower than this because it may interfere with urination and contribute to urine pooling.

Urogenital Tract Surgery

Urinary calculi occur infrequently in horses. Urinary calculi in horses are usually composed of calcium carbonate and have a spicular appearance. These calculi may develop in the kidney or urinary bladder. Small-diameter calculi can be passed during normal urination and go unnoticed. Clinical signs of urinary calculi include stranguria (slow and difficult urination or straining to urinate), pollakiuria (frequent urination), and hematuria (bloody urine). Horses that develop renal calculi will develop signs of abdominal discomfort when the stones become lodged in the ureter. In addition, cystic (urinary bladder) calculi that become lodged in the urethra in male horses cause an inability to urinate and subsequent abdominal pain. Urinary calculi can be diagnosed based on clinical signs, urinalysis, palpation of the urinary bladder per rectum, and endoscopic evaluation of the urethra and urinary bladder. Occasionally a calculus can be palpated in the proximal urethra of male horses at the level of the ischial arch. There are several techniques and certain instruments available for removing urinary tract calculi.

Foals commonly develop diseases of the umbilical remnants, including infection (navel ill) in the umbilical arteries, veins, and urachus. These foals often become depressed, inappetent, and febrile. Many foals also develop secondary septicemia and septic arthritis. Umbilical remnant infection may be diagnosed based on clinical signs of swelling, heat, or drainage in the umbilical area. However, foals can have infection within these structures and be normal on palpation. Transabdominal ultrasonography is also helpful in diagnosing diseases of the umbilical structures. Foals with umbilical remnant infection require treatment with broad-spectrum antibiotics; many of these foals require surgical removal of the affected structures. Surgery for umbilical remnant disease involves a similar approach and instrumentation as for repairing an umbilical hernia. It is necessary to proceed with caution and have suction available and ready while dissecting the umbilical structures to prevent contamination of the abdominal cavity.

Patent urachus is a condition wherein foals dribble urine from the umbilicus because a patent canal between the urachus and urinary bladder is present at birth or develops in the postnatal period. Because those that develop in the postnatal period often occur secondary to an infectious process, it is imperative to rule out umbilical remnant infection and systemic infectious disease. Foals with a patent urachus may be treated nonsurgically by applying an irritant, such as iodine solution, or using silver nitrate sticks on the external surface of the urachus to promote scarification and closure. This is probably most effective in those foals that have a patent urachus at birth. Foals that do not respond to this treatment or those that have an infectious process occurring in the umbilical remnants should have an umbilical remnant resection.

Castration is one of the most commonly performed surgeries in horses. It is usually performed in the field and does not require extensive surgical facilities or instrumentation. Although under most circumstances castration is performed under short-acting intravenous general anesthesia, it can be performed in the standing horse with heavy sedation and infiltration of a local anesthetic into the scrotum and spermatic cord. The most common drugs for castration with the horse under intravenous anesthesia include xylazine/ketamine or xylazine/thiobarbiturate; both combinations can be used with or without guaifenesin. It is important to document that both testicles have descended into the scrotum before commencing with castration in the field. One needs to be prepared for a more extensive surgery requiring entrance into the abdominal cavity (as in a retained testicle); this needs to be planned for because it often takes more time than a routine castration. If both testicles cannot be palpated in the scrotum, then the testicle may be located intraabdominally, in the inguinal canal, or immediately outside the external inguinal ring. A horse with a testicle located outside the abdominal cavity, but not within the scrotum, is referred to as a "high flanker." If the testicle cannot be palpated in the scrotum, then sedation may relax the horse and the cremaster muscle and allow the examiner to palpate the testicle or a portion of it. If the testicle still cannot be palpated after sedation, then a rectal examination with or without ultrasonography may help confirm the location of the testicle. Involvement of the veterinary technician for castration includes general restraint, handling, administering and monitoring anesthesia, preparation of the surgical site, and preparation of instruments.

Castration is usually performed with the horse in lateral recumbency with the upper rear limb pulled forward and tied around the horse's neck. Castration involves making an incision over each testicle parallel to the median raphe through the skin and subcutaneous tissue. The testicles are removed by crushing and cutting the spermatic cord proximal to the testicle and epididymis using emasculators (Figure 30-36). The emasculators should be placed on the spermatic cord so the cord is crushed on the side toward the body wall and cut on the side toward the scrotum (Figure 30-37). There are numerous types of emasculators, and each surgeon may have an individual preference. The entire spermatic cord may be crushed and cut simultaneously within the tunic (closed castration) or the tunica albuginea may be opened and the emasculators can be applied to the vascular structures separately (open castration); this is often done in aged stallions that have an excessively large-diameter spermatic cord. The spermatic cord should be examined after the emasculator is removed to make sure there is no bleeding. The skin incisions are stretched manually to promote drainage.

Postoperative care usually includes strict stall confinement for 24 hours and then controlled exercise (hand walking) once or twice daily for 1 to 2 weeks to promote drainage, prevent excessive swelling, and prevent or reduce stiffness and soreness. The horse should be monitored

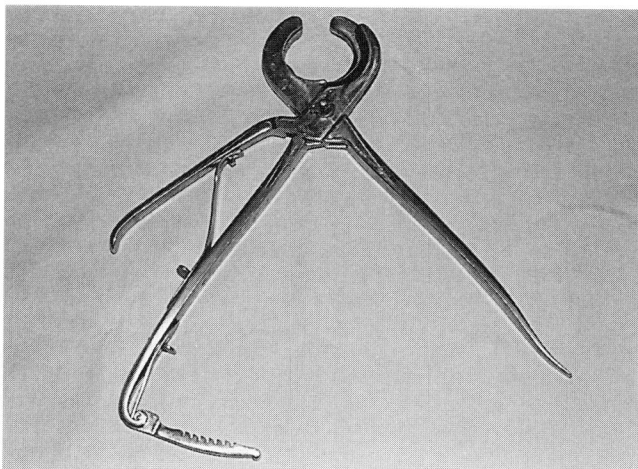

FIGURE 30-36. Emasculators used to crush and cut the spermatic cord of horses during castration.

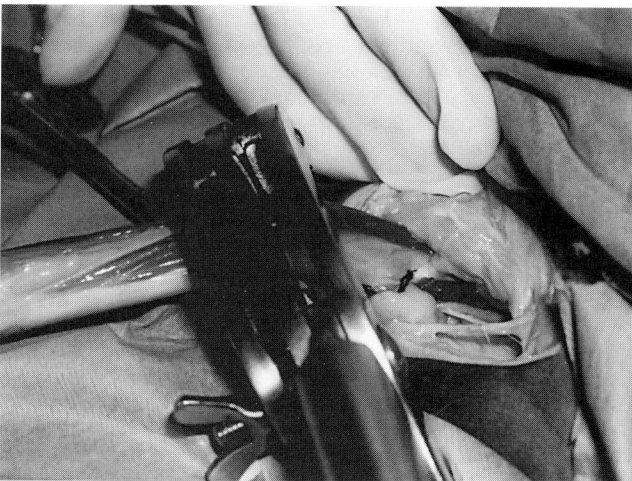

FIGURE 30-37. Use of emasculators during castration of a horse. The emasculators are placed around the spermatic cord so that the nut on the emasculators is located toward the testicle; this will ensure that the spermatic cord is crushed toward the body side and the cord is cut toward the testicle side.

closely during the first day after surgery for signs of excessive hemorrhage, evisceration of intestine or omentum (herniation), or excessive swelling.

If the testicle has not descended (cryptorchidism), then surgery is more involved and requires anesthesia of longer duration. Cryptorchidectomy (removal of a cryptorchid testicle) also requires the surgeon to use a different surgical technique than for routine castration. The testicle can be approached through various incisions, but an approach through the inguinal ring is most often used. A sponge forceps is used to grasp the structures that lead to the scrotum (gubernaculum), and the testicle is extracted from the inguinal canal. In some horses the testicle cannot be retrieved in this manner and the surgeon must manually explore the inguinal canal or caudal abdominal cavity. Once the testicle is retrieved, it is removed using a similar

technique as described for routine castration. Following removal of the retained testicle, the other one is removed in a routine manner. Occasionally horses have both testicles retained.

It is believed that cryptorchid horses are more at risk for evisceration after surgery. To prevent this, some surgeons may elect to temporarily pack a length of gauze soaked in sterile saline or an antiseptic into the subcutaneous areas of the inguinal canal. The gauze packing is held in place with large sutures in the skin and is usually removed in 24 to 72 hours. Other surgeons place interrupted absorbable sutures in the external inguinal ring.

Ovariectomy is performed in mares with diseased ovaries, in mares with normal reproductive tracts for use as teaser mares, and in some mares used as performance horses that have unacceptable behavior associated with estrus. An ovariectomy can be performed unilaterally or bilaterally depending on the reason for the procedure. Diseased ovaries are usually enlarged and require removal through an incision in the ventral body wall (caudal midline or diagonal paramedian) or the flank. The most common cause of ovarian disease necessitating removal is neoplasia; the most common types of ovarian neoplasia include granulosa theca cell tumors and teratomas. Mares with granulosa theca cell tumors often display abnormal behavior, such as anestrus, persistent estrus or nymphomania, or stallion-like behavior. Ovarian tumors and other diseases are diagnosed by clinical signs, palpation findings per rectum, and transrectal ultrasonography. Nondiseased ovaries of normal size can usually be removed through a flank incision or via an incision in the vaginal wall (colpotomy) in standing sedated mares with either local anesthetic infiltration in the body wall or a caudal epidural anesthetic. Hemostasis of the ovarian pedicle is provided either by transfixing with multiple sutures, application of an automatic stapling device, or crushing with a chain ecraseur. Complications include hemorrhage, abdominal pain, myositis, and other problems related to anesthesia and abdominal surgery.

Hernia Repair

Herniation of omentum or abdominal viscera through the abdominal wall can occur with an umbilical hernia, inguinal (scrotal) hernia, or incisional hernia. Umbilical hernias are usually congenital and are relatively common in foals. Small hernias may close spontaneously as the foal grows, whereas others require surgical intervention. Umbilical hernias can be repaired using several different methods. Generally the body wall is closed with either interrupted or continuous absorbable suture. Some surgeons open the peritoneum (open herniorrhaphy) and others leave the peritoneum intact (closed herniorrhaphy). If an umbilical hernia is large or it has not closed by several months of age, then it should probably be surgically repaired. The owner should be instructed to manually reduce hernial contents at least daily; if at any time the hernia cannot be reduced, then it should be evaluated immediately by a veterinarian. If intestine becomes incarcerated in the hernia, then vascular compromise can occur leading to ischemic injury.

Inguinal or scrotal hernias can occur in horses of any age, but newborn foals and adult breeding stallions are probably the most commonly affected. Frequently the herniated contents do not become incarcerated and can be easily reduced. The hernia should be reduced at least daily in foals because intestine could become incarcerated, which would necessitate emergency surgery. Sometimes, these hernias will spontaneously resolve in foals, but many foals require surgical repair. Because the tissues are friable

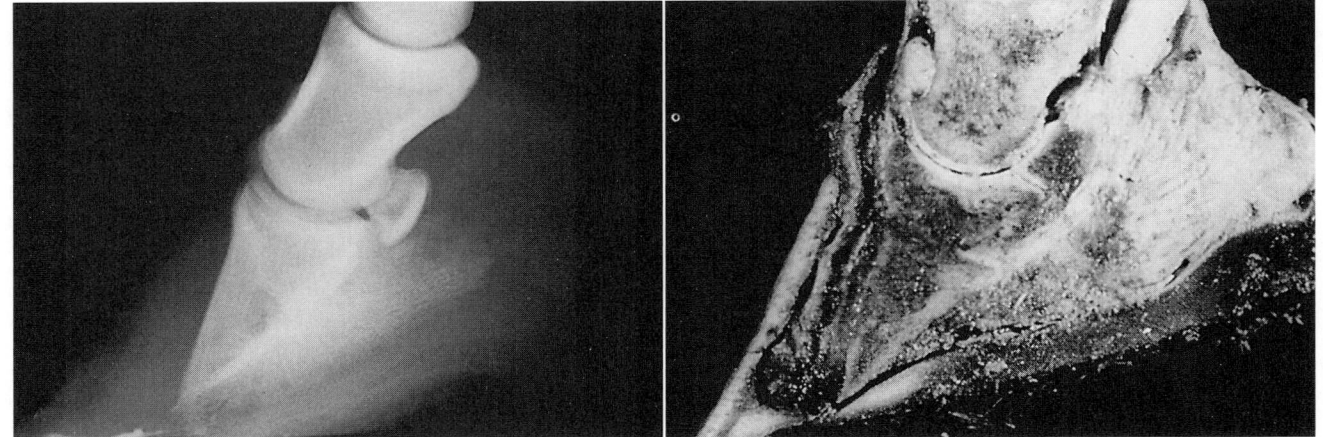

FIGURE 30-38. **A,** Lateral radiograph of the front foot of a horse with laminitis that has evidence of coffin bone rotation. **B,** Gross pathologic photograph of a sagittal section of the front foot of a horse with laminitis that has undergone coffin bone rotation.

in foals, successful surgical repair can be difficult. Scrotal hernias in adult horses most commonly occur in stallions shortly after breeding. In most instances, the herniated structure or structures become incarcerated (not reducible), which necessitates immediate surgery. Incarceration of intestine within the scrotum will result in a large, firm, and cold scrotum on the affected side secondary to compromised testicular blood flow. The blood supply to the intestine also becomes compromised, resulting in ischemic injury. Generally the testicle on the affected side is removed and the affected segment of intestine often requires resection. This necessitates preparation of the horse for inguinal and ventral midline surgery.

Acquired body wall herniation occurs in horses subsequent to trauma and following surgery. Blunt trauma such as a kick can lead to disruption of the body wall musculature. Body wall hernias occur secondary to abdominal incisions; these occur more frequently in horses that develop incisional infection or other complicating factors. Small body wall hernias can be repaired primarily by suturing. Larger body wall defects require the use of mesh implants. It is critical that there be no residual incisional infection present at the time of mesh herniorrhaphy and that aseptic technique be followed during placement of the mesh.

Musculoskeletal Diseases

Laminitis (founder) is a serious, often life-threatening disease of horses. It involves ischemic necrosis and inflammation of the sensitive laminae of the feet. It often involves both front feet or all four feet. However, it can occur in only one fore or rear foot if there is a severe lameness in the opposite limb. The cause of laminitis is unknown, but horses with serious infectious or inflammatory diseases resulting in endotoxemia, such as ischemic or inflammatory bowel disease, pleuropneumonia, septic metritis, and grain overload, are predisposed. Certain medications, such as corticosteroids, have also been incriminated as a potential cause of laminitis. Laminitis occurs almost exclusively in adult horses; it rarely occurs in horses less than 1 year of age.

Acute laminitis occurs in the initial stages of the disease, resulting in extreme pain and reluctance to move. Horses often have increased heat in the hooves and have a pronounced or bounding digital pulse. They are reluctant to walk, turn, or allow their feet to be picked up. They stand with a characteristic stance with their rear legs camped underneath their torso and their front feet camped out in front (see Figure 30-10). Chronic laminitis occurs when, because of degeneration of the sensitive laminae on the coffin bone (distal phalanx), the dorsal laminar attachments to the insensitive laminae of the hoof detach and the coffin bone rotates. In severe chronic laminitis, the rotated coffin bone may protrude through the sole of the foot. A lateral radiograph of the foot is usually required to determine whether coffin bone rotation has occurred (Figure 30-38). In more severe cases, all laminar attachments may become detached and the coffin bone is displaced distally within the hoof wall. Horses that have distal displacement of the coffin bone develop a characteristic depression at the coronary band and are termed *sinkers*. Horses with chronic laminitis develop characteristic concentric rings on the hooves as well as an abnormal shape of the hooves.

The main focus of treatment of horses with laminitis involves reducing inflammation and providing analgesia with antiinflammatory drugs (phenylbutazone), promoting digital blood flow with vasodilator drugs (acepromazine, isoxsuprine, topical glyceryl trinitrate), and mechanically supporting the distal phalanx by providing frog support (frog pads or heart bar shoes). Nursing care is also an important component of the therapeutic regimen, particularly in chronic laminitis. Because laminitis is extremely painful, horses often spend long periods of time lying down. This necessitates care of decubital ulcers. In addition, they often develop subsolar abscesses that require daily soaking and bandaging. The prognosis for return of the horse to athletic competition depends on the occurrence and severity of rotation or sinkage of the coffin bone. Most horses that have appreciable rotation do not return to athletic function. The prognosis for horses that develop distal displacement of the coffin bone is poor.

Rhabdomyolysis (myositis, tying up, azoturia, Monday morning sickness) is an acute inflammatory disease of muscle. It can be initiated by exertion or by a change in either the diet or the amount of exercise. It is characterized by a stiff, stilted gait with firm or hard muscles. The most commonly affected muscles are those of the hindlimb and back. Severely affected horses may be reluctant to move, and some may become recumbent and be unable to rise. Affected horses are often anxious, sweat excessively, and have elevated heart and respiratory rates and body temperature. Horses often have dark, discolored urine secondary to myoglobinuria. Confirmation of this disease is often based on increased serum muscle enzyme (creatine phosphokinase, aspartate aminotransferase) concentrations. Treatment involves exercise restriction, diet modification, intravenous fluid therapy, NSAIDs (phenylbutazone, flunixin meglumine), muscle relaxants, and tranquilization.

Bog spavin is a term used to describe the accumulation of synovial fluid (effusion) in the tarsocrural joint of the hock. Fluid can accumulate secondary to osteochondrosis, synovitis, and arthritis. Degenerative joint disease (arthritis) is a common performance-limiting condition of horses and can affect numerous joints. Bone spavin refers to arthritis in the distal intertarsal and tarsometatarsal joints of the hock. High ring-bone and low ring-bone refer to arthritis in the proximal interphalangeal (pastern) and distal interphalangeal (coffin) joints, respectively. Osselet is a term used to describe arthritis in the metacarpophalangeal or metatarsophalangeal (fetlock) joint.

Tendinitis (bowed tendons) is an injury involving primarily the superficial digital flexor tendon and occasionally the deep digital flexor tendon of the front limbs. This injury is usually sustained secondary to racing or other strenuous activity. There are different degrees of tendinitis ranging from mild edema and inflammation, to tendon fiber separation, to tendon fiber tearing or disruption. When tendon fibers tear the result is hemorrhage and inflammatory debris accumulating in a cavity within the tendon, which is known as a *core lesion*. Treatment of tendinitis includes hydrotherapy, NSAIDs, support bandages, topical antiinflammatory agents (sweats, poultices), and exercise restriction or controlled exercise. Several surgical procedures have been used to either treat tendinitis or prevent its recurrence. The most commonly performed surgery is tendon splitting, which evacuates the core lesion and allows more rapid vascularization and healing of the area. The prognosis for return to athletic function depend on the severity of the injury; some horses with severe core lesions can return to athletic function if given appropriate treatment and time for convalescence.

Osteochondrosis is a form of developmental orthopedic disease in which the articular cartilage and underlying subchondral bone do not develop appropriately. This can result in the formation of osteochondritis dissecans (cartilage flaps), osteochondral fragments, cartilage erosion, and subchondral bone cysts. These abnormalities often manifest as joint effusion and lameness when young horses are first put into strenuous exercise. Many of these lesions are amenable to treatment via arthroscopy, resulting in the horse returning to athletic function.

Subsolar abscess is a common cause of severe lameness. Horses usually will not bear weight on the limb. There is palpable heat in the hoof and a bounding digital pulse similar to that in a horse with laminitis. However, the difference is that subsolar abscesses usually occur only in one foot. Pain can be localized by applying focal pressure to the sole with hoof testers. Occasionally, purulent debris will accumulate and migrate, and an area breaks open at the coronary band and drains (gravel). Treatment involves paring out the sole until the abscess is located to provide drainage. The foot should be kept bandaged to keep it dry

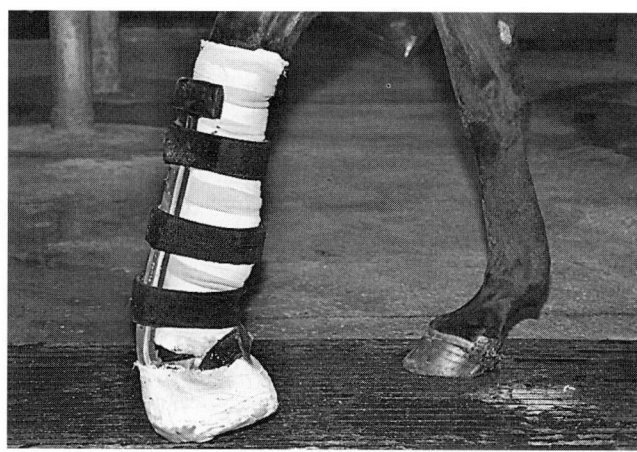

FIGURE 30-39. Use of Kimsey splint to stabilize fractures or joint subluxations in the lower limb of horses.

and clean. The affected foot can be soaked daily in a solution of povidone-iodine (Betadine) and magnesium sulfate (Epsom salts) and then rebandaged. The horse should be given analgesics (phenylbutazone) for a few days. Appropriate tetanus prophylaxis should be administered. The foot needs to be protected from dirt and debris until the area fills in with granulation tissue and is covered with cornified tissue.

Septic arthritis is a common occurrence in adult horses secondary to iatrogenic inoculation of joints during arthrocentesis or joint surgery or subsequent to traumatic joint injuries. It occurs commonly in foals subsequent to hematogenous spread from a focus of infection, such as the umbilicus (navel ill), lungs (pneumonia), or intestinal tract (enteritis). The cornerstone of treatment of septic arthritis includes broad-spectrum antibiotics administered systemically, intraarticular antibiotics, NSAIDs, and joint drainage and lavage.

Horses frequently sustain severe musculoskeletal injuries, such as long bone fractures or disruption of tendons or ligaments. These injuries often require stabilization with the use of bandages, splints, or casts before transport to a referral hospital. Successful stabilization of these injuries and safety of transport are important considerations in the outcome of these cases. Most severe injuries should be bandaged and splinted or casted to a level at least one joint above the injury. A heavy Robert Jones bandage should be applied and then rigid splints placed on the lateral and either the dorsal or palmar aspects of the limb to provide appropriate support. Splints can be made out of rigid materials, such as wood, steel, or aluminum. The splints should not be excessively heavy or bulky but must provide appropriate support. Horses with phalangeal fractures can be casted with their distal limb in flexion or can be placed in a commercially available device such as a Kimsey splint (Figure 30-39). Horses with limb injuries should be hauled in a trailer with partitions to provide some support for them to balance themselves. The head should be tied loosely enough to enable the horse to use the head and neck for balance. Horses with front limb injuries should be transported with their head toward the rear of the trailer, and those with rear limb injuries should be transported with their head toward the front of the trailer.

SURGERY OF THE EQUINE PATIENT

Preoperative Preparation of the Equine Patient

Numerous procedures are required in preparation of the equine patient for anesthesia and surgery. Many if not all of these procedures involve the veterinary technician. It is probably wise that a checklist be developed that the technician can use to make sure all procedures are performed. This is particularly helpful in a hospital where more than one technician is working on the same case. Because of the dense hair coat of horses, thorough grooming is necessary. This may include simply brushing or currying the horse's coat, or it may require that the horse be bathed. The aim of grooming is to remove as much loose hair, dander, and dirt from the horse's body as possible, thereby keeping such material out of the operating room. If the horse is shod, the shoes are generally removed before surgery to prevent injury to the horse during recovery from anesthesia or damaging the recovery stall flooring. The horse's feet need to be picked out and cleaned. One of the main responsibilities of the technician will be to clip a wide area of hair in the vicinity of the surgery site before anesthetic induction. If the surgery will be performed on a limb, then the hair can be clipped the day before surgery and the limb can be cleaned and a bandage placed to keep the site clean. The final aseptic preparation is performed once the horse is under anesthesia. Clipping the hair and cleaning the surgery site before anesthetic induction will reduce anesthesia time.

Technician Note

A checklist should be developed to ensure that the technician performs all procedures required for preparation of the equine patient for anesthesia and surgery.

It is important that the technician consult the clinician as to the exact site that should be clipped. Areas of the mane and tail should be clipped only under special circumstances. Most owners are adamant that these areas should not be clipped for cosmetic purposes. The hair of the mane and tail takes months to years to grow out, and unnecessarily clipping these areas may cause needless delay in a show horse's convalescence. The location of the skin incision and the appropriate part of the horse to clip before surgery can usually be found in equine surgical textbooks. However, because of variation among surgeons, the technician should always consult the surgeon before clipping the patient.

Unlike ruminants and small animals, horses do not regurgitate or vomit. Adult horses are generally held off feed for approximately 12 hours to allow time for emptying of the stomach, which may allow the horse to ventilate more easily. Horses are generally provided water during this time. Young foals that are still nursing are generally not held off feed before anesthesia, but, if they are, it is usually only for 1 to 2 hours. A complete physical examination should be performed, including auscultation of the heart and lungs. In adult horses, a rebreathing bag may need to be used to increase the respiratory effort sufficiently to hear air moving through the lung fields. An electrocardiogram should be performed if there is any evidence of an abnormal heart rhythm detected during auscultation. Preoperative blood work usually includes a complete blood count (CBC) and fibrinogen determination. Some clinicians also perform a chemistry profile depending on the age and health of the horse.

Before general anesthesia, an intravenous catheter is placed in one of the jugular veins. The anesthetic agents for induction are administered through the catheter. Some anesthetic agents (thiobarbiturates) and perioperative medications (phenylbutazone) are irritating if injected perivascularly. Therefore it is imperative that the catheter be placed into the vein and appropriately secured. Catheter placement can be performed by the clinician or by the technician under the supervision of the clinician. Perioperative medications such as antibiotics and NSAIDs are usually administered before anesthetic induction. However, if an infectious process is suspected, then the surgeon may opt to start antibiotics after a sample has been obtained at surgery for culture and susceptibility testing. In this case, the medication can be administered during anesthesia or after recovery; this will depend on the medication and the condition of the patient while under anesthesia. Because horses are generally intubated with an endotracheal tube through the oral cavity, it is important that the mouth be thoroughly washed out before anesthetic induction; this will reduce the chance that feed material will be carried into the airway during intubation. Once the horse is intubated, the cuff should be inflated to prevent saliva and other materials from draining into the lower airway and leading to aspiration pneumonia.

Intraoperative Nursing

The technician should consult the surgeon regarding which instruments will be required. In a hospital where there is more than one technician and several surgeons, a card system that has the necessary instruments listed for each surgical procedure should be used. This will allow the technician to know the different requirements of individual surgeons. One common difference among surgeons is the type of suture material chosen to close wounds. The technician must learn to adapt to these individual preferences. It is recommended that the technician have all the available instruments close to the surgery. Even if the instrument is used infrequently, it is better to have it nearby rather than waste time looking for it once it is needed. Time-wasting activities lead to prolonged anesthetic time, which could lead to increased morbidity or mortality. Correctly labeled radiographs are essential for most limb surgery. The radiographs should be placed on a radiographic view box in the operating room. The technician should have available gloves, gowns, and drapes and all other supplies that are anticipated to be used. In some lower limb surgeries, an Esmarch bandage (Latex Rubber Bandage/Tourner Wrap, Smiths & Nephew Richards) and tourniquet are used to assist with hemostasis during surgery (Figure 30-40). An Esmarch bandage is a flat, gum-rubber elastic bandage that is wrapped around the limb in a spiral fashion from distal to proximal to a point above the surgical site. At this point, an inflatable tourniquet is applied and secured. The aim of the Esmarch bandage is to force blood out of the limb while the tourniquet prevents blood from entering into the site. The Esmarch bandage is removed after the tourniquet is fully inflated. The use of an Esmarch bandage and tourniquet enables the surgeon to operate in a bloodless field and results in a shorter surgery time. Following surgery, a pressure bandage is applied and the tourniquet is released.

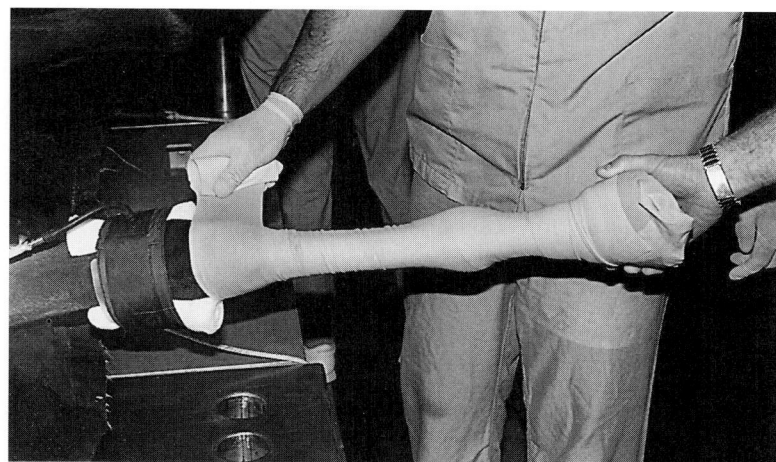

FIGURE 30-40.   Application of an Esmarch bandage and tourniquet on the limb of a horse. The uninflated tourniquet is placed around the limb just proximal to the carpus. An Esmarch bandage is placed tightly around the limb beginning at the foot and extended to the level of the tourniquet. The tourniquet is then inflated, and the Esmarch bandage is removed.

Technician Note

In a hospital where there is more than one technician and several surgeons, a card system that has the necessary instruments listed for each surgical procedure should be used.

The technician must help ensure that the patient is properly padded. Because of their body weight, horses are prone to myositis (muscle damage) that can be life threatening. The pressure of the horse's body and the hypotension that can occur during anesthesia can result in hypoperfusion of the muscles. If this condition is prolonged, the muscles can undergo metabolic change, resulting in extreme soreness and pain. In severe cases, muscle pigment (myoglobin) is released into the bloodstream and excreted in the urine (coffee-colored urine); the pigment can lead to kidney damage. The first sign that muscle damage has occurred during anesthesia is manifested during recovery. Usually the front or rear limb, or both, on the side the horse is lying on will be affected. However, the uppermost limb or any limb in a horse in dorsal recumbency can be involved. The horse may be unable to bear weight on the limb. If a forelimb is involved, the horse will drag the limb in a flexed position and will be unable to bear weight; this is associated with triceps damage. If the hindlimb is involved, the horse may knuckle in the lower joints and walk on the dorsal aspect of the fetlock, and the limb will collapse as the horse tries to bear weight. Most horses show some improvement over the first few days, but some horses are unable to rise. Management of a postoperative recumbent patient presents a number of problems to clinicians and technicians. Appropriate padding materials are an inflatable waterbed, semiinflated tire inner tubes under the shoulder and hip, dunnage bags, or foam rubber pads.

The patient and the surgery site must be positioned so it is comfortable to the surgeon and safe for the patient. This will help ensure that the surgeon does not become fatigued or frustrated and a subsequent compromise in technique does not occur. It is not wise to overextend, overflex, abduct, or adduct the limbs because of potential complications of myopathy and neuropathy.

Aseptic preparation of the surgery site, surgical instruments, and the surgeon is imperative to a successful and uncomplicated surgery. It is the responsibility of all personnel involved to maintain asepsis, but the technician or technicians should assume primary responsibility for ensuring that the surgical site is properly prepared and the instruments are properly sterilized and packaged. The technician must be cognizant of all activities in preparation for surgery and during the surgical procedure. If a technician observes a break in aseptic technique it should be brought to the attention of the surgeon so the problem can be remedied. The techniques involved in sterilization of surgical instruments and supplies and aseptic preparation of the surgery site are covered in Chapter 24.

Postoperative Nursing

Technicians play a vital role in the postoperative care of the equine patient. Although veterinarians are responsible for the patients' care, technicians are often primarily involved with postoperative monitoring, administering medications, changing bandages, grooming, and other tasks required on postoperative patients. Monitoring the postoperative patient is similar to previously discussed patient monitoring. Although all body systems should be evaluated, the important things to consider in the postoperative patient are the presence and magnitude of postoperative pain, whether the patient is febrile, and whether there are any signs of infection (swelling, erythema, heat, pain) at the incision site. The postoperative patient should be examined for any complications such as pneumonia, diarrhea, jugular vein thrombophlebitis, or laminitis.

Technician Note

Although veterinarians are responsible for the patients' care, technicians are often primarily involved with postoperative monitoring, administering medications, changing bandages, grooming, and other tasks required on postoperative patients.

Technicians are generally responsible for administering medications postoperatively. This may involve giving antibiotics or NSAIDs orally, intravenously, or intramuscularly. Many horses that undergo surgery have an intravenous catheter that is used in the postoperative period to administer perioperative antibiotics. The duration of antibiotic therapy depends on clinician preference and the type and severity of the underlying disease process. Many horses are administered NSAIDs in the postoperative period for their antiinflammatory and analgesic properties.

Horses undergoing limb surgery generally have a bandage placed on the limb at the conclusion of surgery before recovery from anesthesia. The limbs are often kept bandaged until the skin sutures are removed 10 to 14 days postoperatively. The bandages should probably be changed every 2 to 3 days initially or more frequently if they become wet or soiled from the outside or if wound drainage soaks through from the inside. There are several types of materials used for limb bandages in horses and several methods of application (see Chapter 4). In general, a sterile nonadherent material is usually placed directly against the incision and held in place with sterile, soft roll gauze (Kling, Johnson & Johnson). The next layer of the bandage is usually a sterile, soft combine that covers the circumference of the limb for the entire distance of the bandage, which is also held in place with soft roll gauze. This layer can be skipped if the outer bandage that is placed is a thick, sterile combine material. Next, a thick layer of rolled cotton, sheet cottons, or combine material is placed on the limb and secured with soft roll gauze. An Ace bandage, Elasticon (Johnson & Johnson), or Vetwrap (Animal Care Products/3M) can be used as the final layer of the bandage. Elasticon is useful for securing the top of the bandage to the skin above it and the bottom of the bandage to the foot below. This helps seal the bandage and prevent debris from getting between the skin and the bandage. All layers of the bandage should be applied in the same direction (dorsal to palmar or plantar) and with even tension; this should help prevent constriction of the tendons in the metacarpal or metatarsal area and subsequent tendinitis (bandage bow). When the bandages are changed postoperatively the incision should be examined for swelling, heat, exudate, and pain on palpation. The exudate should be removed, the wound gently cleaned, and the bandage reapplied. If there has been an appreciable change in the horse's gait or in the incision from the last bandage change, this should be brought to the immediate attention of the veterinarian.

Colic

Colic is a general term used to describe abdominal pain; many diseases can result in abdominal pain or signs that mimic abdominal pain. Diseases of the gastrointestinal tract are the most common causes of abdominal pain in horses. Because of the anatomy and physiology of the gastrointestinal tract and the fact that horses experience varying degrees of parasitic infestations (e.g., *Strongylus vulgaris*), they are more predisposed to colic than are most other animals. It is one of the most common and important diseases of horses and is one in which the veterinary technician plays a vital role in assisting in the diagnosis and both medical and surgical treatment. The technician is also intimately involved in the daily monitoring and treatment of horses with colic.

The typical cause of colic in horses is an obstruction to flow of ingesta and gas in the gastrointestinal tract, causing intestinal distention, stretching of the intestinal wall, and tension on the mesentery, all of which lead to pain that is manifested in a variety of behavioral signs. Not all signs of abdominal pain are attributable to intestinal obstruction. For example, a mare that is near parturition will show similar signs owing to uterine contractions. A horse with an obstruction of the urinary tract (urethral calculus) may also show signs of abdominal pain. Although it is important that the veterinary technician recognize signs of colic, the diagnosis of the actual cause of colic is the responsibility of the veterinarian. Various signs of abdominal pain are displayed by horses with different types and magnitudes of colic; however, certain signs are common to most. Mild signs of colic include inappetence, stretching more frequently than normal, yawning, and looking at the flank. Other signs include playing with water or frequent urination. More obvious signs of colic include pawing the ground, stamping the feet, walking the stall, kicking the abdomen, and violent rolling. Some horses will actually sit like a dog or roll into dorsal recumbency to relieve the pain. Horses with colic often sweat profusely, have increased heart and respiratory rates, and have congested mucous membranes.

The causes of gastrointestinal tract–related colic include volvulus (twisting of the intestine), intestinal incarceration, impactions of feed material or foreign bodies, obstruction caused by enteroliths (stones that form in the intestinal tract), parasitic infections, displacement of the intestine, tympany (primary gas distention), and inflammatory bowel disease (anterior enteritis, enterocolitis). Volvulus (twisting) can occur in numerous portions of the intestinal tract, but it most commonly occurs in the small intestine and large colon. The small intestine frequently becomes incarcerated (entrapped) in numerous sites, such as the inguinal ring, epiploic foramen, mesenteric rent, and a diaphragmatic hernia. Intestinal incarceration and volvulus result in obstruction of the intestinal lumen and occlusion of the intestinal blood vessels resulting in intestinal distention and ischemic necrosis of the bowel wall. Therefore these horses display severe abdominal pain and usually develop signs of shock owing to absorption of endotoxin through devitalized bowel. These horses require emergency abdominal exploration with correction of the volvulus or reduction of the incarceration; depending on the duration and magnitude of the disease, the affected segment of intestine often requires resection. Because of the anatomy of the gastrointestinal tract, horses are predisposed to large intestinal displacement. Large colon displacement results in luminal obstruction but no vascular occlusion. Therefore these horses develop mild to severe abdominal pain depending on the magnitude of the luminal distention but do not develop intestinal ischemia. Treatment usually involves surgical correction. However, one particular type of large colon displacement (entrapment of the large colon in the nephrosplenic space) is sometimes correctable by rolling the horse under general anesthesia.

Horses develop impactions in the ileum, cecum, and large and small colon. Many of these horses can be treated medically with intravenous or oral fluids, lubricants (mineral oil), cathartics (magnesium sulfate), and analgesics. Other horses with intestinal impactions require surgery to evacuate the intestinal contents to prevent rupture. Intestinal contents are usually evacuated through an incision in the bowel wall (enterotomy), and the lumen is lavaged to remove as much of the contents as possible. The enterotomy incision is then sutured. Intestinal obstruction can occur secondary to an enterolith (stone) lodging in a segment of the large intestine that has a reduced diameter (pelvic flexure, transverse colon, small colon). Enterolithiasis results from mineral deposition that forms around a nidus within the intestinal tract. Sometimes horses pass numerous small-diameter stones in the feces, whereas larger-diameter stones may develop and obstruct the lumen; these larger-diameter stones frequently cause abdominal pain secondary to luminal distention and require removal through an enterotomy. Horses can develop intestinal obstruction secondary to ingestion of foreign bodies; young curious horses are most commonly affected, and the most common type of foreign bodies is fibrous (nylon rope or string, hay netting, feed sacks, rubber fencing, hair). Occasionally a horse will be able to pass these fibrous foreign bodies, but often surgery is required to remove the foreign body and relieve the intestinal obstruction.

Although parasite-related causes of colic are less common now than in the past because of the development of effective anthelmintic drugs and management strategies, they still represent a possible cause of colic, especially on farms with poor preventive medicine programs. Larvae of *Strongylus vulgaris* (blood-sucking worms) migrate through the mesenteric arteries causing arteritis; this can lead to thromboembolic colic wherein segments of the intestine become infarcted. Ascarids *(Parascaris equorum)* usually cause a problem in young horses. The problem usually arises after deworming a heavily infested foal when a large number of adult ascarids die and obstruct the intestinal lumen (ascarid impaction). The best way to prevent this is to begin effective deworming programs early in the foal's life or to use a dewormer that is not especially effective in a heavily infested foal. Once the ascarid impaction occurs, the most effective treatment is evacuation of the worms via an enterotomy. Tapeworm *(Anoplocephala perfoliata)* infestation has been anecdotally related to cecocolic and ileocecal intussusception and to development of cecal impactions. These parasites are frequently identified in the cecal lumen in horses with these conditions, but no cause-and-effect relationship has been confirmed. The most effective treatment regimen for tapeworms is twice the recommended dose of pyrantel pamoate. Small strongyles are probably the most important intestinal parasite in horses because of their resistance to benzimidazole anthelmintics. Infestation with small strongyles can cause poor doeing, weight loss, diarrhea, and colic (see Chapter 7).

Horses with inflammatory bowel disease often have signs of abdominal pain, fever, increased heart and respiratory rates, congested mucous membranes, diarrhea, and nasogastric reflux. These horses are usually best treated with intravenous fluids, gastric decompression, and administration of intestinal protectants, antibiotics, analgesics, and antiinflammatory drugs.

The prognosis for horses with colic depends on the type of abnormality and its magnitude and duration. In general, horses with simple obstruction (no compromise in blood flow) of the intestinal tract (impaction, enterolith, displacement, tympany) have a good prognosis for survival with appropriate medical or surgical treatment. Horses with strangulating obstruction (compromised blood flow) of the intestinal tract (volvulus, incarceration, intussusception) have a more guarded prognosis, but some of these horses will survive and be functional if treated early and appropriately. The prognosis for horses with parasitic and inflammatory bowel diseases depends on the severity and duration before treatment and the development of life-threatening complications, such as laminitis.

The veterinarian will conduct a thorough examination and perform several diagnostic procedures in an attempt to arrive at an accurate diagnosis of the cause of colic. Most of these procedures will either directly or indirectly involve the veterinary technician. Such procedures include a rectal examination, nasogastric intubation, abdominocentesis and abdominal fluid analysis, collection of blood for CBC and chemistry profile, transabdominal ultrasonography, urinalysis, fecal flotation for intestinal parasites, and fecal cultures for *Salmonella*. The technician may be involved in organizing the instruments and supplies for performing these procedures or actually participating in the procedures.

The veterinary technician will be intricately involved in both medical and surgical treatment of horses with colic. Medical treatment is usually appropriate for impactions, tympany, and spasmodic colic, whereas surgical treatment is necessary for intestinal volvulus and incarceration, enterolithiasis, fibrous foreign body obstruction, and intestinal displacements. Fortunately, most horses with colic respond to conservative treatment, such as analgesic, antiinflammatory, or antispasmodic drugs; intestinal lubricants or cathartics; intravenous or oral fluids; restriction of feed; and controlled exercise. Only a small percentage of horses with colic require surgery. Sometimes surgery is necessary to arrive at an accurate diagnosis. Abdominal surgery is a major undertaking and requires a full team to perform it in an effective and efficient manner.

Abdominal Surgery

Adult horses and foals frequently undergo abdominal surgery for gastrointestinal and urogenital tract disease. Although a flank incision in a standing, sedated horse is sometimes used for horses with colic or other abdominal disease, the most common approach to the abdominal cavity is through a ventral midline incision with the horse under general anesthesia and positioned in dorsal recumbency (Figure 30-41). Because most horses with colic requiring surgery will be operated on with the patient under general anesthesia, the veterinary technician will be involved in the preparation of the horse for surgery. This will include placing a catheter, administering perioperative medications, passage of a nasogastric tube, washing out the mouth, clipping the hair, preparing the anesthetics, aseptically preparing the incision site, and opening surgical packs at the time of surgery. Most colic patients can be clipped before anesthesia, but if the horse is in severe pain it may be done after anesthetic induction for the safety of the horse and personnel. The hair should be clipped from rostral to the xiphoid area to the udder or preputial area and to the flank folds on either side; clipped hair and other debris can be removed with a vacuum. The incision site (ventral midline) may be shaved to remove the hair remaining after clipping, and the clipped area is then aseptically prepared. The incision is draped with four small drapes or towels and then a large, water-impermeable drape is placed that covers the entire horse. The incision is usually made from the umbilicus rostrally toward the xiphoid until the necessary exposure is achieved, but the incision can be extended caudal to the umbilicus. This is particularly necessary for urogenital tract surgery, such as a cystotomy for removal of cystic calculi. Once the incision is made, a thorough exploration is usually performed depending on the reason for surgery. Once the abnormality is identified it is corrected. Suction is often necessary to decompress gas from the gastrointestinal tract or aspirate fluid such as urine from the bladder during a cystotomy.

There are numerous surgical techniques and manipulations that the veterinarian may perform at the time of abdominal surgery. They are too numerous to describe here, and the veterinary technician will become familiar with them through instruction and experience. Many specialized instruments are required for abdominal surgery (see Chapter 24). One group of instruments that has become increasingly popular with veterinary surgeons for use in equine abdominal surgery is gastrointestinal stapling equipment. The technician must become familiar

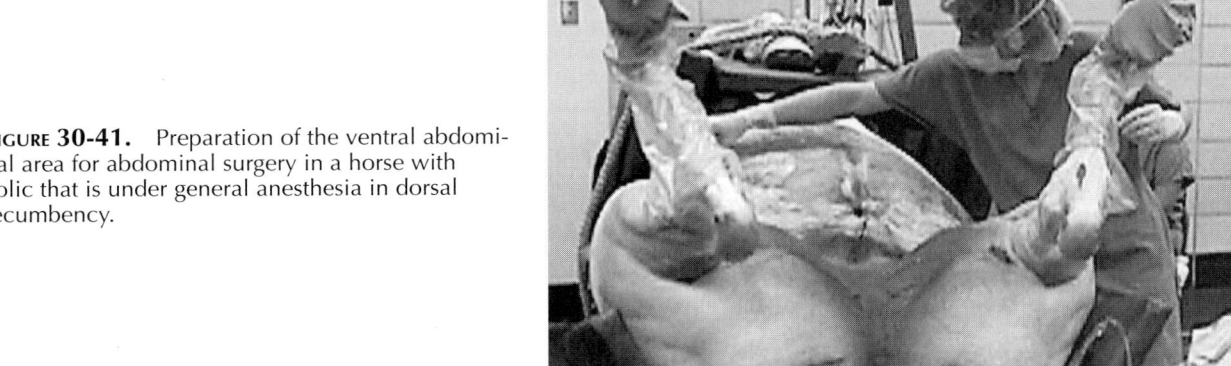

FIGURE 30-41. Preparation of the ventral abdominal area for abdominal surgery in a horse with colic that is under general anesthesia in dorsal recumbency.

with the different instruments and cartridges. Intestinal resection and anastomosis often require specialized instruments and supplies.

Once the cause of colic or other abdominal problem has been corrected and the horse has recovered from anesthesia, the veterinary technician becomes even more closely involved with patient management. Horses usually require administration of intravenous fluids, antibiotics, antiinflammatory drugs, and other medications in the postoperative period. The veterinary technician usually administers or oversees administration of these medications. The technician may also be involved in nasogastric intubation, blood collection, intravenous catheterization, and changing bandages. In addition, the technician will often be responsible for feeding and watering, exercising, grooming, and monitoring the horse.

Arthroscopic Surgery

Arthroscopy is commonly performed for the diagnosis and treatment of joint disease. It is commonly performed for removing osteochondral chip fractures, treating cartilaginous and bony abnormalities associated with osteochondrosis, treating septic arthritis, and evaluating causes of joint lameness that have no definitive radiographic abnormalities. Depending on the joint being evaluated and the type and location of the lesion, the horse may be positioned in dorsal or lateral recumbency. It is necessary to have the radiographs on a view box in the operating room so the surgeon can evaluate them intraoperatively. During arthroscopy the technique of triangulation is used whereby the lesion forms one corner of the triangle and the arthroscope and surgical instruments serve as the other two corners of the triangle. Generally the arthroscope is placed in the joint on the side opposite the lesion and the surgical instrument is placed in the joint on the same side as the lesion. The portal for placement of the arthroscope is usually made by making a small (1-cm) incision in the skin and subcutaneous tissue and then using a sharp trocar to advance the arthroscopic cannula through the fibrous joint capsule and synovial lining. Once the cannula has penetrated the joint cavity, the sharp trocar is replaced with a blunt obturator to pass the cannula across the joint; this prevents iatrogenic damage to the cartilage. The skin incisions are usually made before joint distention in the carpus but after joint distention in other joints. The joint is distended with sterile polyionic fluid to facilitate place-

ment of the arthroscope. Once the arthroscope is in place the joint is evaluated; once the lesion is identified the most appropriate location for the instrument portal is determined by using a needle to triangulate the lesion with the arthroscope. Once the appropriate location for the instrument portal is identified, the instrument portal is made with a scalpel blade (no. 11 or 15). The appropriate instrument is placed into the joint. The instruments commonly used in arthroscopy include a blunt probe for palpating intraarticular structures, rongeurs for removing osteochondral fragments, and curettes for debriding diseased cartilage and bone. A fenestrated cannula is often used at the end of surgery to facilitate removal of cartilage and bone debris via lavage. Motorized equipment is available and is sometimes necessary for debridement of large areas of diseased bone.

The surgeon uses specific instruments for arthroscopy, and these may vary depending on the joint involved and the individual surgeon's preference. Generally there will be a standardized set of arthroscopy instruments that are packaged together. Instruments are steam sterilized, but if they are to be used on more than one case per day, they are sterilized with a cold sterilization solution before each use. Following sterilization, the instruments are packed in a sterile stainless steel pan that is later used to rinse disinfecting solution off the arthroscopy instruments. One of the most important and most expensive instruments is the arthroscope; it should be handled carefully to prevent damage. Additional items necessary are a sterile needle (usually 18-gauge) and syringe, which are used for distending the joint. During arthroscopic surgery, the joint is kept distended with sterile physiologic solution; this solution is usually delivered with a pump through a sterile intravenous set.

Many hospitals perform arthroscopy using a video camera so that the entire procedure can be viewed on a television screen (Figure 30-42). This causes less strain on the surgeon's eye, makes the procedure more educational for surgery assistants and technical staff, provides an opportunity to videotape the procedure, and probably allows the procedure to be performed with fewer breaks in aseptic technique. To provide the intense light required to illuminate the inside of the joint, a fiberoptic light source and light cable are required. It is essential that the technician be familiar with the assembly and function of the arthroscopic equipment and the proper care, cleaning, and

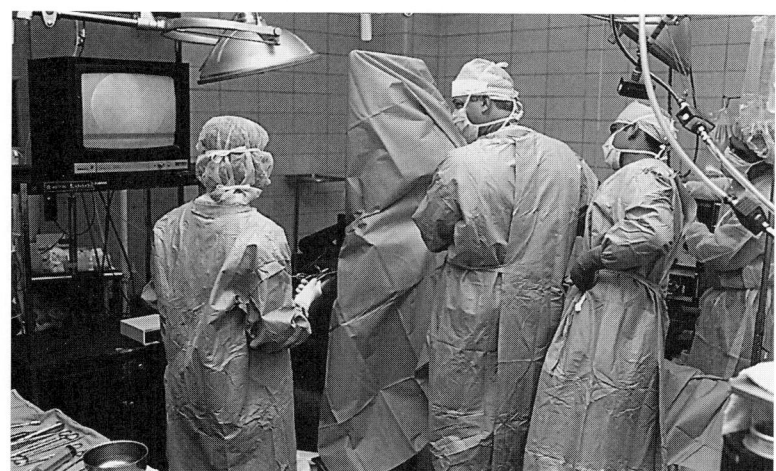

FIGURE 30-42. Use of arthroscopy for evaluating joint disease in horses. The arthroscope is inserted into the joint and attached to a camera that projects the image on a television screen for easy viewing by the surgeon and other personnel.

disinfecting of the instruments. The arthroscopy instruments are disinfected using a cold sterilization solution such as activated dialdehyde (Cidex, Surgikos); the instruments, arthroscope, and light cables are soaked for a minimum of 10 minutes. One should read the manufacturer's recommendations regarding the time required for disinfecting. To avoid delays, the instruments can be placed in the sterilizing solution at the start of anesthesia. This will also ensure adequate sterilization time. Before using the instruments, they are transferred sterilely into an empty sterile tray. The instruments are then rinsed with sterile saline to remove the sterilization solution.

After the surgical site has been aseptically prepared and draped and the instruments removed from the sterilizing solution, the technician will be responsible for attaching the fiberoptic cable to its light source. The system that delivers the fluid to distend the joint must also be connected to the appropriate fluid source. Once the system is connected to the fluid source, the surgeon must run fluid through the system to flush all air bubbles out of the tubing so they do not enter the joint. Electric fluid pumps are generally used to maintain joint distention; these may be manually or pressure controlled.

Following surgery, all specialized arthroscopy equipment and instruments need to be cleaned. The arthroscope lens should be examined for scratches and the video camera dried carefully. If several arthroscopy surgeries are scheduled for the day, then the instruments are placed in the cold sterilization solution in preparation for the next surgery.

Orthopedic Surgery

Orthopedic surgery has become more common in horses. Athletic horses develop numerous orthopedic conditions that are amenable to surgical correction. Historically, fractures of long bones in adult horses were considered irreparable. However, with advanced techniques and more rigid surgical implants many of these injuries are potentially correctable. Certain bony fractures are amenable to surgical correction using bone screws that are placed in lag fashion to stabilize the fracture by creating compression of the bone fragments (Figure 30-43). Although developing an understanding of the principles of lag screw fixation and the instrumentation involved will help the equine technician in preparing instruments and assisting with surgery, this area is beyond the scope of this book. Major fractures of long bones in horses are best repaired with screws and

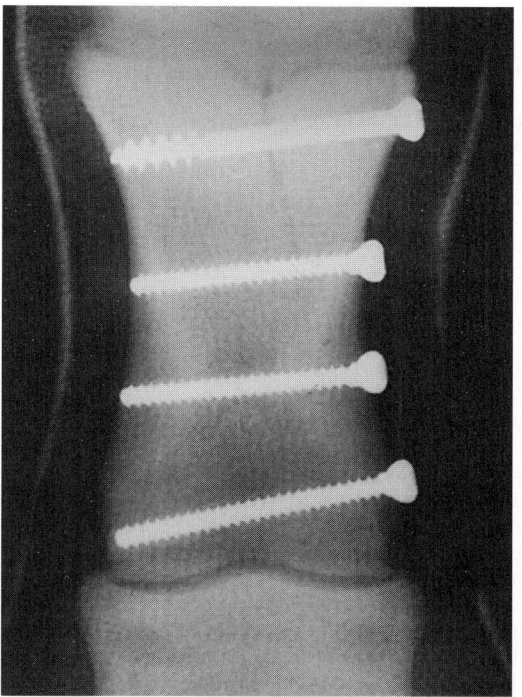

FIGURE 30-43. A proximal phalanx fracture in a horse repaired with cortical bone screws placed in lag fashion to compress the fracture line.

bone plates to prevent movement at the fracture site while the bone heals under rigid fixation. Although aseptic technique is imperative for all surgical procedures, it is especially crucial to the overall success of orthopedic surgery in horses. If bony infection develops, it can lead to instability of the implants and fixation failure, which often necessitates euthanasia. It is the responsibility of all personnel to follow aseptic protocol. The technician should strive to maintain asepsis by monitoring the activities of all personnel involved in surgery. Orthopedic surgery requires the use of several specialized instruments and implants; because many of these surgeries are performed on an emergency basis, it is imperative that the technician make sure instruments are available and ready for use. Many orthopedic injuries that are surgically repaired require the use of external coaptation (cast) for anesthetic recovery or for longer periods postoperatively (see Chapter 4). Therefore the technician should anticipate this need and have the appropriate materials available at the conclusion of surgery. The technician may also be needed to assist with anesthetic recovery of the orthopedic equine patient.

Postoperative monitoring of the orthopedic patient is vital for early detection of potential problems. It is particularly important to observe how the horse is using the affected limb in the stall; any dramatic change in use of the limb may signal an impending problem (infection or cast sores). The cast should also be monitored for heat, odor, or exudate, which would indicate the development of cast sores. The most common locations for sores to develop in association with a half-limb cast are at the proximal, dorsal aspect of the metacarpus or metatarsus, at the palmar or plantar aspect of the fetlock over the sesamoid bones, and over the heel bulbs. Bandages need to be changed frequently, and the incision sites should be monitored for swelling, erythema, and discharge. Drains are commonly used in orthopedic surgery following repair of a long bone. Drains can be useful in preventing seroma formation, but they can serve as potential routes for inoculation of the surgery site. Therefore it is important to maintain these drains sterile by keeping a clean, sterile bandage on the leg. This may require changing the bandage more frequently than once daily.

Upper Respiratory Tract Surgery

Abnormalities of the upper respiratory tract can be performance limiting to athletic horses and, if severe, can also be life threatening. Many obstructive diseases of the upper respiratory tract are amenable to surgical correction. The most common of these are left laryngeal hemiplegia, epiglottic entrapment, dorsal displacement of the soft palate, and arytenoid chondritis. Others are subepiglottic cysts, guttural pouch empyema, guttural pouch tympany, and guttural pouch mycosis.

Left laryngeal hemiplegia ("roarer") is a condition resulting in paralysis of the left arytenoid cartilage, which prevents it from being abducted during inspiration. This results in the arytenoid collapsing and being pulled into the airway secondary to the negative pressure that is generated during inspiration. The cause of this condition is unknown, but it results in a recurrent laryngeal neuropathy. Because this nerve normally provides innervation to the major abductor muscle of the arytenoid cartilage, the cricoarytenoideus dorsalis, a neuropathy results in muscle atrophy and an inability to abduct the arytenoid. As the name implies, this condition occurs almost exclusively on the left side (95%); it is believed that this is related to the longer length of the nerve on the left side and the fact it may become damaged from the vibrations as it courses around the aortic arch. This condition is diagnosed using endoscopy at rest or during exercise on a high-speed treadmill; the left arytenoid cartilage is not fully abducted during inspiration and in severe cases actually collapses into the airway. Horses with this condition make a characteristic inspiratory noise (roaring) and develop exercise intolerance. Surgical treatment is a prosthetic laryngoplasty, which involves placing a suture between the cricoid cartilage and the muscular process of the arytenoid cartilage to mimic the action of the cricoarytenoideus dorsalis and abduct the arytenoid cartilage (tieback). The laryngeal ventricles (saccules) are also everted and resected (ventriculectomy or sacculectomy) through either a ventral laryn-

gotomy or by use of an endoscopically guided laser. Approximately 70% of horses treated with a prosthetic laryngoplasty and sacculectomy return to athletic function. Most horses will continue to make some noise, and in some the noise may not improve. The laryngotomy incision is usually left open to heal by second intention. This requires daily cleaning with gauze sponges with saline or water followed by application of petrolatum to the skin around the incision and on the mandible and neck to prevent skin scald from the drainage. It usually takes approximately 3 weeks for the incision to heal. Some clinicians partially close the incision, which reportedly shortens the time required to heal.

Epiglottic entrapment is a condition where the aryepiglottic membrane that extends from the arytenoid cartilage to the ventral surface of the epiglottis hypertrophies and rolls upward to envelope the rostral and abaxial portions of the epiglottis. Normally the epiglottis should have a serrated edge and a distinct vascular pattern present on the dorsal surface. When the epiglottis becomes entrapped, the serrated edge and vascular pattern can no longer be seen. The shape or outline of the epiglottis can still be observed (unlike that seen with a dorsal displacement of the soft palate), but the tip appears more rounded and the abaxial surface is smooth rather than serrated. In more chronic cases, the tip of the epiglottis may become ulcerated. The cause of epiglottic entrapment is unknown, but it is believed these horses have an instability between the caudal edge of the soft palate and the epiglottis and that the aryepiglottic membrane hypertrophies and makes the epiglottis more rigid. Epiglottic entrapment can be intermittent or permanent. Some horses can continue to perform athletically with an entrapped epiglottis, but it does appear to affect performance in most horses. Treatment of epiglottic entrapment includes transecting the aryepiglottic membrane to release the epiglottis. This can be done using several techniques. First, it can be performed with a hooked bistoury placed through the nasal passages in a standing sedated horse with or without endoscopic guidance; care must be taken to prevent trauma to other structures and to prevent laceration of the soft palate. Second, it can be performed in an anesthetized horse with a mouth speculum by manually guiding a hooked bistoury and transecting the membrane on midline. Third, it can be performed using an endoscopically guided laser in a standing sedated horse. Finally, in more severe or chronic recurring cases the aryepiglottic membrane can be resected through a ventral laryngotomy. The prognosis for return to athletic performance is good, but entrapment can recur. Some of these horses may develop dorsal displacement of the soft palate after the entrapment is released. Horses that have the entrapment released using the hooked bistoury or laser can generally resume training in a few days, whereas those treated via resection through a laryngotomy require approximately 3 weeks before resuming training.

Dorsal displacement of the soft palate (DDSP) is generally a dynamic obstructive disease of the upper respiratory tract that occurs during exercise. Normally the soft palate remains ventral to the epiglottis. However, if the epiglottis is small or flaccid or the caudal edge of the soft palate is flaccid, the soft palate can become displaced dorsal to the epiglottis during strenuous exercise. The cause of this condition is unknown, but it is believed the factors listed above predispose the palate to become displaced during inspiration when negative pressure is generated in the upper airway. This condition usually is intermittent, occurring during strenuous exercise and dissipating once exercise has stopped and the horse swallows. Because horses are obligate nasal breathers, dorsal displacement of the soft palate interferes with the horse's breathing. Horses with DDSP usually make a characteristic gurgling or snoring type of noise, which will dissipate as soon as they swallow and replace the palate into its normal position.

Treatment options for a horse with DDSP include placing a cloth or leather tie on the horse's tongue and pulling the tongue rostrad and tying the tongue to the mandible in the interdental space. The epiglottis, tongue, and sternothyrohyoideus muscles are attached to the hyoid apparatus. Because the tongue is attached at the rostral aspect of the hyoid apparatus and the sternothyrohyoideus muscles are attached at its caudal aspect, a tongue tie prevents caudal retraction of the hyoid apparatus, including the epiglottis. This seems to help approximately 50% of horses with DDSP because it prevents caudal retraction of the epiglottis and maintains normal epiglottic-palate alignment. Because of its noninvasive nature, the tongue tie is generally the first thing attempted in horses with DDSP. If this does not work, a section of the sternothyrohyoideus muscles can be resected in the midcervical region; this also prevents caudal retraction of the hyoid apparatus. This myectomy procedure helps in approximately 50% of horses with DDSP that fail to respond to a tongue tie. If this procedure does not work, then the caudal margin of the soft palate can be resected (staphylectomy). There are two theories as to why this may help prevent DDSP. First, it is believed the caudal edge of the palate becomes more fibrous as it heals with scar tissue; this makes the caudal edge more rigid and therefore more resistant to displacement. The other theory is that, if the palate does displace, then it enables the palate to be replaced more easily. Regardless of the mechanism it seems that it helps prevent DDSP in approximately half of the horses that do not respond to the tongue tie or myectomy.

Arytenoid chondritis is an inflammatory, degenerative condition of the arytenoid cartilages resulting in a proliferative mass on one or both arytenoids. This usually results in an obstructive disease of the upper airway with signs similar to the conditions described earlier. These cartilages are usually enlarged and more fibrous than normal, which prevents them from being effectively treated with a tieback. The treatment of choice is to remove the affected arytenoid cartilage through a ventral laryngotomy. Because of the time required for dissection in the laryngeal region during an arytenoidectomy, a tracheotomy is usually performed in the middle or proximal trachea to provide a mechanism for ventilation during anesthesia. The tracheotomy can be performed either before anesthetic induction or once the horse is anesthetized. These horses are prone to upper airway obstruction postoperatively and need to be closely monitored. The tracheotomy tube is usually left in place, at least for a couple of days, until it is believed the horse has an airway of adequate diameter for breathing. It is imperative that these horses be monitored closely while the tracheotomy tube is in place to make sure it does not become dislodged or obstructed with mucus or other discharge. The laryngotomy and tracheotomy sites require daily cleaning and application of petrolatum on the skin around the incisions. Both these incisions will heal by second intention in approximately 3 weeks.

Bacterial infection of the guttural pouch (empyema) usually is a sequela to strangles or retropharyngeal lymph node abscesses. Clinical signs include swelling in the throat-latch region and a bilateral mucopurulent nasal discharge. Horses with guttural pouch empyema can be treated conservatively with antibiotics and guttural pouch lavage; this may be effective in many horses that are treated early in the course of the disease. However, in more chronic cases the mucopurulent material becomes inspissated and forms gelatinous concretions (chondroids) that lie in the floor of the guttural pouches. Resolution of empyema requires removal of the chondroids, and long-term effective drainage can usually only be achieved with surgical drainage. Several approaches are reported for surgical drainage of the guttural pouches, but the most common surgical approach for guttural pouch empyema is the modified Whitehouse technique; the incision is made in the skin on the ventrum of the throat region just axial to the linguofacial vein and is followed by blunt dissection into the pouch. The guttural pouch is lavaged intraoperatively. Indwelling catheters can be placed into the guttural pouches in standing sedated horses under endoscopic guidance; these catheters enable frequent lavage of the pouches. The guttural pouches should not be lavaged with irritating solutions because of the proximity of blood vessels and nerves coursing through the area. The incision is managed similarly to a laryngotomy or tracheotomy incision.

Guttural pouch tympany is an accumulation of air in the guttural pouches; this occurs in foals and weanlings and is usually associated with an abnormality of the opening to the pouches. It can occur on one or both sides and is characterized by a fluctuant nonpainful swelling in the throat-latch region. If unilateral guttural pouch tympany is present, then it is usually treated by surgically creating an opening in the septum between the left and right pouches; this is usually approached through an incision in Viborg's triangle on the affected side. If bilateral tympany is present, then creating an opening in the septum will not effectively drain the two sides. Therefore the opening to one or both of the guttural pouches is surgically revised through a Viborg's triangle approach. Surgical revision of the guttural pouch opening may be performed on only one side with creation of an opening in the septum to enable both pouches to evacuate the air through one opening.

Guttural pouch mycosis can be life threatening. Fungal plaques form in the lining of the guttural pouches; if the plaques involve vascular structures such as the internal carotid artery, then severe fatal hemorrhage can occur. Fatal hemorrhage is often preceded by several episodes of substantial epistaxis. However, once the diagnosis is made, surgery should not be delayed. The most accepted method of surgical treatment involves either direct ligation or use of a balloon-tipped catheter to occlude either the internal carotid artery, external carotid artery, or both depending on which vessels are affected. Both the internal and external carotid arteries can be ligated unilaterally with no untoward effects. The major potential complication of external carotid artery occlusion is blindness. Once the affected vessels are ligated, the fungal infection is treated by lavage of the guttural pouches and instillation of antifungal medication into the pouch via indwelling catheters or via the endoscope.

Surgical Musculoskeletal Diseases

Flexural and angular limb deformities (crooked legs) are abnormalities of the limbs that arise from abnormal development of bones and musculotendinous structures in the limbs. Flexural limb deformities result in overflexion of certain joints. There are three main manifestations of flexural limb deformities in horses. These can be present at birth or develop during the first few months or years of life. Carpal flexural deformities result in the front limbs being flexed or buckled forward at the carpus. This may range from mild deformity to a severe deformity that prevents

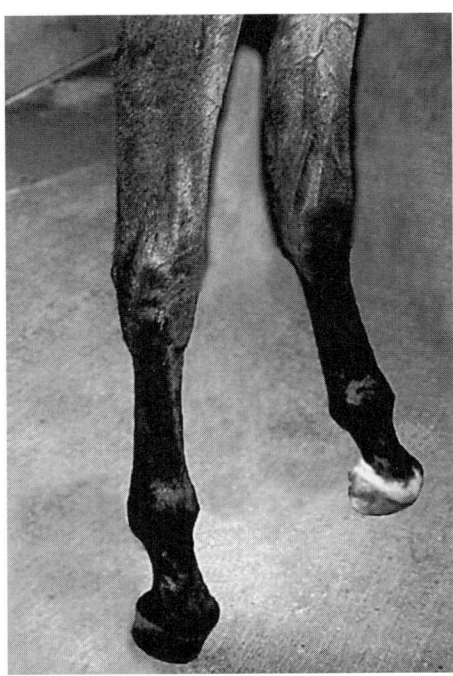

FIGURE 30-44. Severe flexural deformity of the distal interphalangeal (coffin) joint of both front limbs in a weanling horse.

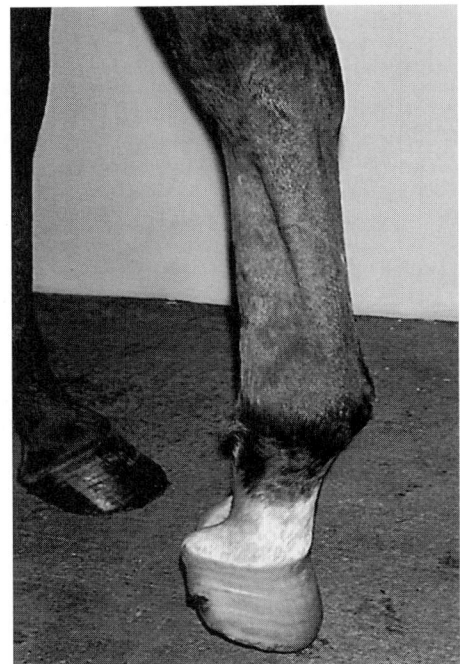

FIGURE 30-45. A flexural deformity of the metacarpophalangeal (fetlock) joint of a yearling horse.

the foal from standing. Mild to moderate cases are often amenable to treatment with controlled exercise combined with application of bandages and splints that extend from the ground to the elbow or tube casts that extend from just above the fetlock to the middle portion of the antebrachium. Intravenous administration of oxytetracycline may be beneficial to help relax the musculotendinous structures.

The second type involves flexural deformity of the distal interphalangeal (coffin) joint, which results in a characteristic clubfoot-shaped hoof (Figure 30-44). This often is first noticed when the foal is a few months of age and can progress to the point that the foal walks on the toe or the dorsum of the hoof wall. Mild to moderate cases (those in which the foot has not passed the vertical plane) often respond to corrective trimming (lower heel) and application of an extended toe shoe, which helps to stretch out the deep digital flexor tendon. More advanced cases usually require surgical transection of the inferior check ligament, which lengthens the deep digital flexor musculotendinous unit.

The third type of flexural deformity involves the metacarpophalangeal joint and is characterized by an increased steepness to the pastern and fetlock (Figure 30-45). This usually begins to develop around 1 year of age but may occur as late as 2 years. It can progress until the horse knuckles over at the fetlock. This condition commonly occurs in rapidly growing heavily muscled horses such as 1- to 2-year-old quarter horses. Conservative treatment involves controlled exercise, dietary management (balanced minerals, low energy and protein), management of pain (arising from osteochondrosis or physitis) with

NSAIDs, and application of bandages and splints that extend from the ground to the elbow. More severely affected horses or those that do not respond to conservative treatment may be successfully treated surgically by performing a superior check or inferior check ligament desmotomy or both, depending on whether the superficial digital flexor or deep digital flexor tendons or both are involved.

Angular limb deformities are deformities that develop in the appendicular skeleton in a medial-to-lateral direction. These deviations can be present at birth or develop during the first few months of life. Mild deformities may self-correct, others may persist but not worsen, and still others may become more severe with time. These deformities are named in reference to the joint involved and the direction of the deviation. The most common deviation is carpal valgus, where the limb distal to the carpus deviates laterally (Figure 30-46). Other common deviations include fetlock varus, where the limb distal to the fetlock deviates medially (Figure 30-47), and tarsal valgus. These deviations can occur because of disproportionate growth of bone on either side of the growth plate, incompletely ossified cuboidal bones in the carpus and tarsus, or ligamentous laxity. The deviations in foals with incompletely ossified cuboidal bones or ligamentous laxity can usually be manually straightened, whereas those with disproportionate growth at the physis cannot.

Treatment of mild to moderate angular deviations may include stall rest with controlled exercise, depending on the age of the foal. Successful surgical procedures have been developed to treat moderate to severe deformities. Transection and elevation of the periosteum near the

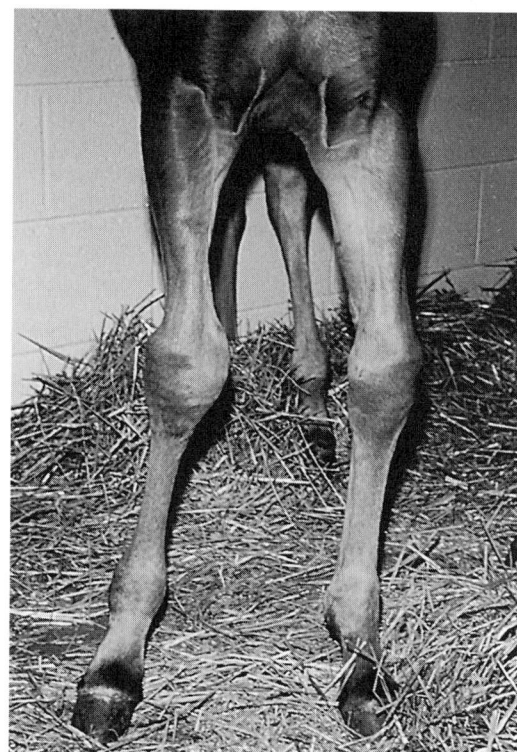

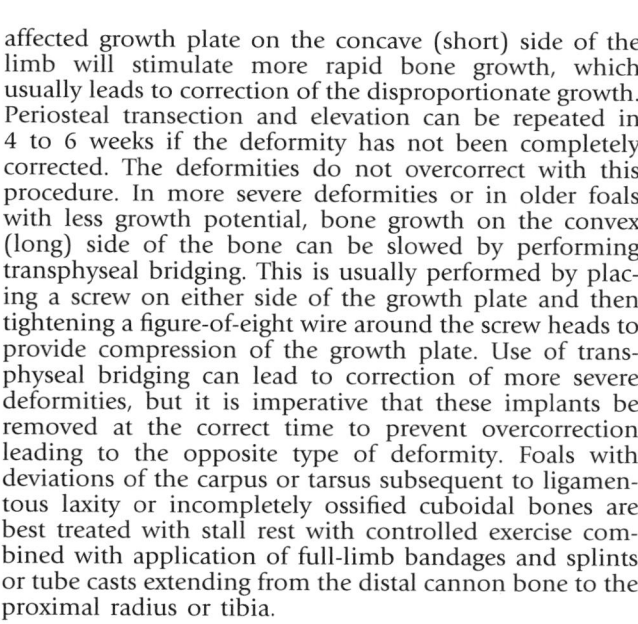

FIGURE 30-46.   A valgus deformity of the right carpus and a varus deformity of the left carpus in a foal.

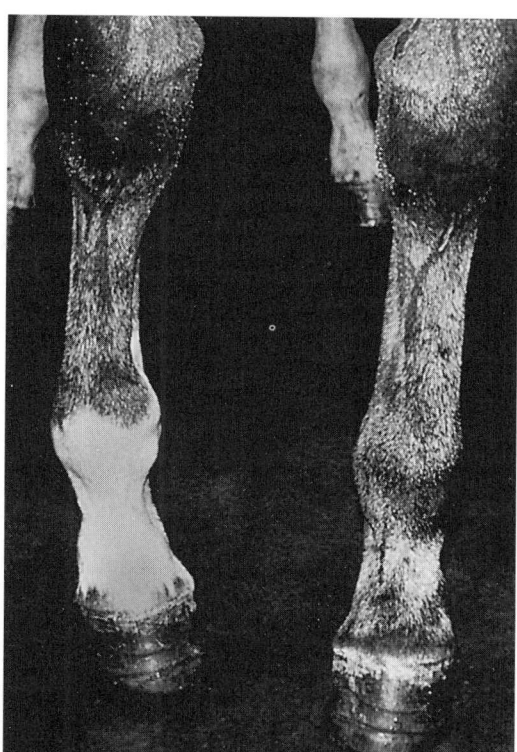

FIGURE 30-47.   A varus deformity of the right front fetlock in a foal.

affected growth plate on the concave (short) side of the limb will stimulate more rapid bone growth, which usually leads to correction of the disproportionate growth. Periosteal transection and elevation can be repeated in 4 to 6 weeks if the deformity has not been completely corrected. The deformities do not overcorrect with this procedure. In more severe deformities or in older foals with less growth potential, bone growth on the convex (long) side of the bone can be slowed by performing transphyseal bridging. This is usually performed by placing a screw on either side of the growth plate and then tightening a figure-of-eight wire around the screw heads to provide compression of the growth plate. Use of transphyseal bridging can lead to correction of more severe deformities, but it is imperative that these implants be removed at the correct time to prevent overcorrection leading to the opposite type of deformity. Foals with deviations of the carpus or tarsus subsequent to ligamentous laxity or incompletely ossified cuboidal bones are best treated with stall rest with controlled exercise combined with application of full-limb bandages and splints or tube casts extending from the distal cannon bone to the proximal radius or tibia.

EMERGENCY SITUATIONS AND PROCEDURES

Several emergency situations can arise that necessitate immediate action on the part of a technician or clinician to prevent death of a horse. One of the most common emergency situations is the development of upper airway obstruction leading to dyspnea. Obstructive diseases involving the nasal passages, nasopharynx, and larynx can be alleviated by a tracheotomy. A tracheotomy is generally performed at the junction of the middle and proximal thirds of the neck on the ventral midline. An incision is made on the ventral cervical midline through the skin, subcutaneous tissue, and cutaneous colli muscle parallel to the trachea. The paired sternothyrohyoideus muscles are then split on midline to expose the tracheal rings. The membrane between two adjacent rings is then cut with a scalpel on the ventral surface for a distance of approximately one half the circumference of the tracheal rings. Care should be taken not to cut the tracheal rings and not to cut vital structures adjacent to the trachea (carotid artery, recurrent laryngeal nerve, jugular vein). Many times the tracheotomy must be performed on an extremely anxious horse or after the horse has collapsed from insufficient oxygen. Therefore one should be careful not to get into a situation where injury occurs.

Technician Note

One of the most common emergency situations is the development of upper airway obstruction leading to dyspnea.

Veterinary technicians should become familiar and comfortable with the dosages and indications for drugs commonly used in emergency situations. A list of drugs and doses along with the drugs and syringes should be kept readily available in several locations throughout the hospital. These can be prepared in small emergency packs.

Technician Note

Veterinary technicians should become familiar and comfortable with the dosages and indications for drugs commonly used in emergency situations. A list of drugs and doses along with the drugs and syringes should be kept readily available in several locations throughout the hospital.

Occasionally horses develop reactions to certain drugs. These may be anaphylactic reactions resulting in shock or death or allergic-type reactions resulting in skin wheals. Horses may develop a reaction to procaine penicillin, which usually results in an anaphylactoid reaction. These horses usually require treatment with corticosteroids and epinephrine. They may recover or die subsequent to pulmonary edema. Horses often develop skin wheals in response to drugs or environmental allergens. The drugs that most commonly cause these wheals in horses are NSAIDs and trimethoprim-sulfa antibiotics.

Intracarotid injection of drugs can cause seizurelike activity. This can be life threatening to the horse and is potentially injurious to the handler and other personnel in the vicinity. The chance for this can be minimized by using an 18-gauge needle that is unattached from the syringe and directed down the jugular vein. Normally, if the needle is in the jugular vein, blood will slowly ooze out of the needle hub only if the jugular vein is occluded. If the carotid artery is inadvertently entered with the needle, then blood will exit in a pulsatile manner. If this occurs, do not inject the medication. The needle should be removed, and compression should be applied to decrease hematoma formation. The needle should be reinserted into a different location using the same technique.

ANESTHESIA FOR THE EQUINE PATIENT

Technician Note

Frequently the technician is primarily responsible for all aspects of anesthesia, including selection of induction and maintenance anesthetic agents, instrumentation, monitoring, and recovery of patients.

The veterinary technician may be directly or indirectly involved in anesthesia of horses. Frequently the technician is primarily responsible for all aspects of anesthesia, including selection of induction and maintenance anesthetic agents, instrumentation, monitoring, and recovery of patients. It is important that the technician be familiar with the properties and recommended doses of the anesthetic agents being administered and the equipment (ventilator, blood pressure monitor, anesthetic machine, etc.) being used (see Chapter 21). Numerous complications can arise, and it is important that the technician be familiar with the methods of treating these complications, including the correct drugs and doses for treating hypotension and cardiac arrhythmias. Because it is important to maintain mean arterial blood pressure at 70 mm Hg or greater to help prevent myopathies and neuropathies, blood pressure should be monitored via an indirect or direct method. Hypotension is usually treated by reducing the depth of anesthesia and increasing the rate of administration of intravenous fluids and vasoactive drugs, such as dobutamine, dopamine, or phenylephrine. It is important to monitor how well the horse is being oxygenated and ventilated during anesthesia; this can be done most effectively by monitoring arterial blood gases. The technician should monitor recovery from anesthesia and be prepared for any potential complications.

RECOMMENDED READING

Auer JA, Stick JA, editors: *Equine surgery*, Philadelphia, 1999, WB Saunders.

Koterba AM, Drummond WH, Kosch PC, editors: *Equine clinical neonatology*, Philadelphia, 1990, Lea & Febiger.

Robinson NE, editor: *Current therapy in equine medicine*, ed 2, Philadelphia, 1987, Saunders.

Robinson NE, editor: *Current therapy in equine medicine*, ed 3, Philadelphia, 1991, WB Saunders.

White NA, Moore JN, editors: *Current practice of equine surgery*, Philadelphia, 1990, Lippincott.

White NA, Moore JN, editors: *Current techniques in equine surgery and lameness*, Philadelphia, 1998, WB Saunders.

31

Food Animal Medicine and Surgery

Margaret L. Cebra • Christopher K. Cebra

The food animal industry encompasses a wide variety of animal species and economic functions. Domestic food animal species include cattle, sheep, goats, llamas, alpacas, and pigs. The major functions of food animals include food and fiber production and providing genetic stock. Although the trend in the food animal industry has shifted from small farms toward intensively managed, large production systems and treatment decisions are often based on economics, a knowledge of the medical and surgical problems of individual food animals is the basis of effective herd health and production management.

Veterinary technicians play a vital role in food animal practice. They work closely with veterinarians to restrain and handle animals for examination, collect samples for diagnostic testing, and treat sick animals. Other functions of veterinary technicians include preparing equipment and animals for surgical or diagnostic procedures, assisting the veterinarian in performing diagnostic and surgical procedures, and preparing animal health and production records, written reports, and financial statements for the animal producer. In addition, the technician is responsible for stocking equipment, pharmaceuticals, biologics, and supplies used by the veterinarian. A technician who is well trained, competent, and efficient can enhance the success and efficiency of the veterinary service provided to the food animal producer. The more knowledgeable the veterinary technician is about the diseases and procedures performed, the better he or she can anticipate the needs of the veterinarian.

The purpose of this chapter is to acquaint the veterinary technician with common medical and surgical problems of food animals. The chapter has been organized by organ system using a problem-oriented approach. Because the principles of surgery and medicine are the same for all species, the various food animal species are discussed together, unless a unique feature of a specific animal warrants special mention. Emphasis has been placed on those diseases and procedures that are commonly encoun-

tered in food animal practice and with which the veterinary technician should be familiar.

HEAD PROBLEMS

Infectious keratoconjunctivitis (pinkeye) is caused by *Moraxella bovis* in cattle and *Mycoplasma* spp. or *Chlamydia* in small ruminants. Bacteria may be spread by flies or through direct contact. In cattle, the lesion often starts as a central corneal opacity, which helps differentiate this lesion from viral conjunctivitis (Figure 31-1). In small ruminants, the lesion starts as conjunctivitis and spreads to the cornea. Photophobia, ocular reddening, and discharge are commonly seen. Systemic or subconjunctival antibiotics are used to treat affected animals, and fly control is important to prevent new cases.

Oral and nasal vesicular or ulcerative lesions are common in ruminants and swine with a variety of viral diseases. Some of these are accompanied by conjunctivitis, diarrhea, abortion, and coronary band lesions and should be investigated because of the significant effect on a herd. Sore mouth (orf) is a less severe (but zoonotic) disease that is common and transient in small ruminant neonates (Figure 31-2). Morbidity is due to the pain caused by the mouth lesions and teat lesions on the dams. Basic supportive care is essential for animals that cannot eat.

Facial swelling is a common complaint because of its visibility. To determine the cause, careful palpation of the swollen area is necessary. Hard masses suggest that bony structures are affected, whereas softer, moveable masses suggest that the lesion is primarily within the soft tissue. The causes of bony swelling include displaced or healing fractures, osteomyelitis (lumpy jaw, actinomycosis [most common in cattle]), tooth root abscesses (most common in camelids and pigs), and bony tumors (rare in all species) (Figure 31-3). Causes of soft tissue swelling include snake or insect bite, cellulitis or lymphadenitis (actinobacillosis in cattle or corynebacterial caseous lymphadenitis in small

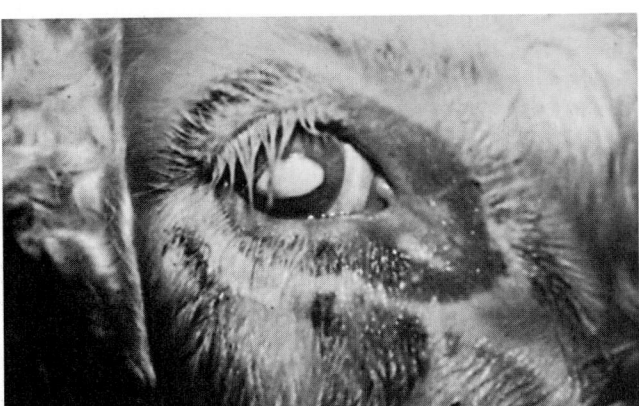

FIGURE 31-1. Cow with infectious bovine keratoconjunctivitis (pinkeye) with a large central corneal opacity.

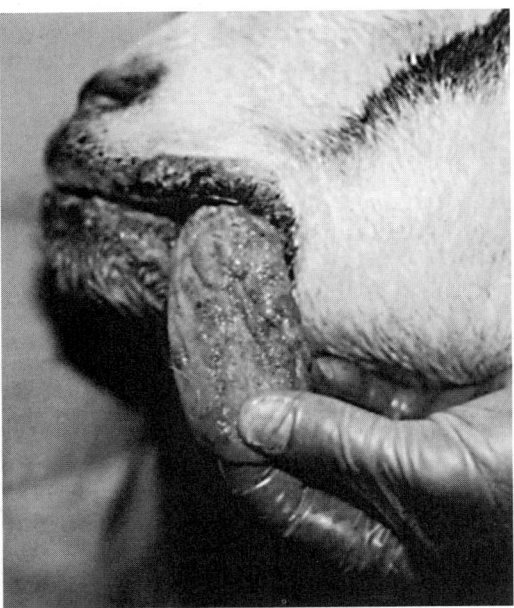

FIGURE 31-2. Goat with contagious ecthyma (orf, sore mouth) with ulcerative and proliferative lesions on the lips and tongue.

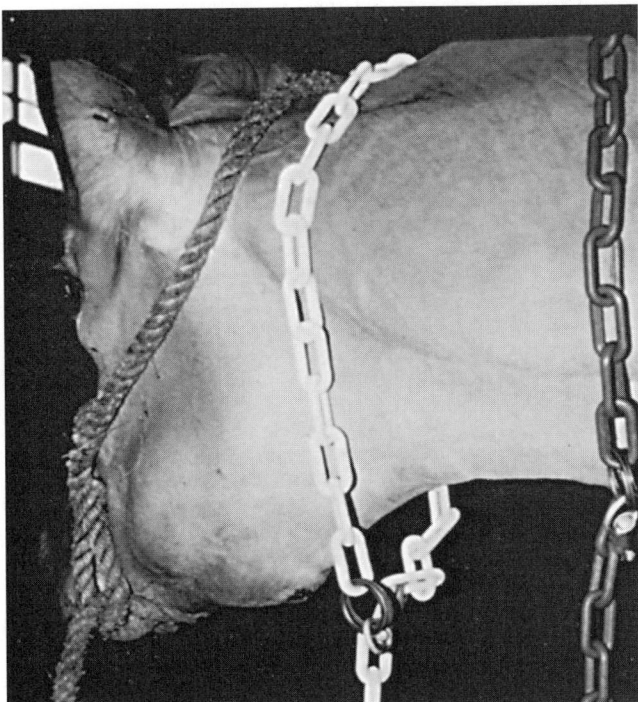

FIGURE 31-3. A bony mass on the mandible of a cow with actinomycosis (lumpy jaw).

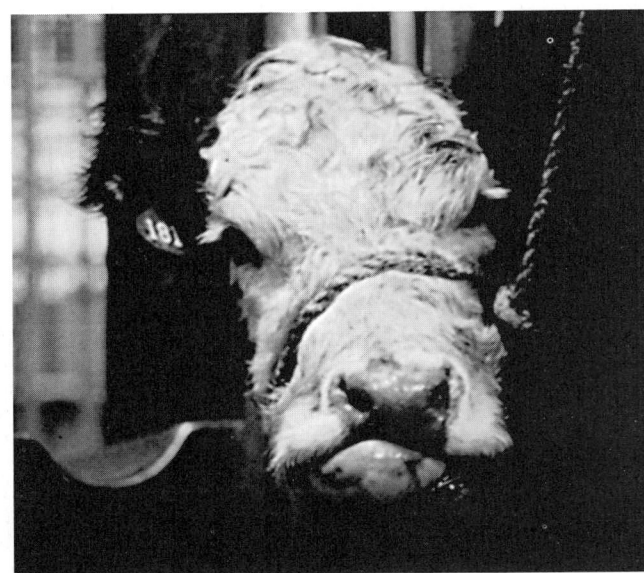

FIGURE 31-4. Calf with actinobacillosis (wooden tongue). The enlarged tongue protrudes from the calf's mouth.

ruminants), foreign body reactions, lymphoma or other soft tissue tumors, or salivary mucocele (Figure 31-4). Bony lesions also may lead to inflammation and draining tracts in the adjacent soft tissue.

Other clinical information may aid in arriving at a diagnosis. A fracture or tooth root abscess frequently causes the animal pain on mastication. Dysphagia, quidding (dropping food out of the animal's mouth), or weight loss may be seen, although camelids with a tooth root abscess rarely show evidence of oral pain. Malalignment of teeth secondary to osteomyelitis or a tumor also may cause painful trauma to soft tissue. Radiographs are helpful in differentiating the causes of bony swelling but are not always practical. They are especially useful in differentiating osteomyelitis from a tooth root abscess. Gram stains or cultures of discharges or aspirates may help determine a

bacterial etiology. Biopsy is necessary to definitively diagnose a tumor.

There usually is a surgical and medical option to treat all facial swellings. Fractures may be repaired surgically, whereas infected bone may be curetted, abscessed teeth removed, tumors debulked, and abscesses drained. Because of the size of most food animals, surgical repair of mandibular fractures is uncommon. Curettage of osteomyelitis also is uncommon, because surgery does not significantly improve the prognosis, and fractures may result. Repulsion of abscessed teeth is facilitated through a sinus flap or trephine hole. Drainage from abscesses may be facilitated by lancing. This is best achieved by clipping and surgically preparing a site over the softest, most ventral part of the swelling, using a hypodermic needle to establish the purulent nature of the material within the mass and then opening a large hole with a scalpel blade into the center of the mass.

Medical treatment also can be very effective. Mandibular osteomyelitis in cattle may be treated successfully with a 1-month course of antibiotics if the lesion is not too extensive. Camelids with tooth root abscesses appear to respond satisfactorily to a similar regimen of antibiotics without surgery. Because bacteremia with metastasis of infection may occur in cattle with tooth root abscesses, medical treatment of this lesion may be inferior to removal of the tooth. Lymphadenitis and cellulitis may be treated with a combination of antibiotics and sodium or potassium iodide; the iodide salt reduces inflammation, which allows better penetration of the antibiotic into the lesion. Prognosis is poor for caseous lymphadenitis in small ruminants because internal abscesses often are present.

Simple management changes may be necessary. If multiple animals in a herd are affected by bony or soft tissue infection of the mouth, the feed should be checked for grass awns or foxtails. If quidding is noted, providing the animal with soft feed will help it maintain weight. This is especially useful for healing fractures.

Tooth Trimming

Male llamas and pigs may develop prominent canine teeth that can cause injury to others. Annual trimming of these teeth is recommended. This may be accomplished with the animal under heavy sedation or general anesthesia. A piece of obstetric wire is placed around the tooth above the gum line, and the tooth is sawed off.

Dehorning

Except for polled breeds, most ruminants of either gender will develop horns. Horn buds can be palpated toward the back of the skull within the first weeks of life. Although favored by some people for their appearance, horns can be dangerous weapons. Removal or destruction of the horn buds early in life is easier and less traumatic than the removal of a fully developed horn (Figure 31-5).

Sensation to the horn comes from the cornual nerve in cattle. This may be blocked by infiltrating the area midway between the horn base and the lateral canthus of the eye with a local anesthetic agent. Goats and older cattle have additional innervation and may require a ring block around the base of each horn. Horn buds may be burned with a hot iron or removed with a scoop or gouge (Figure 31-6). Burning is best done on animals less than 1 month old, whereas the scoop or gouge may be used on any horn that fits within its lumen. In adult animals, a skin incision may be made around the horn base, and the horn is then cut off with a wire or hand saw. Regardless of the technique, it is important to remember that the horn is produced by the germinal epithelium around the horn base, and this tissue must be destroyed or removed to prevent regrowth. Extreme care must be taken when dehorning small ruminants because their poorly developed frontal sinus often leaves the brain cavity in direct contact with the horn base.

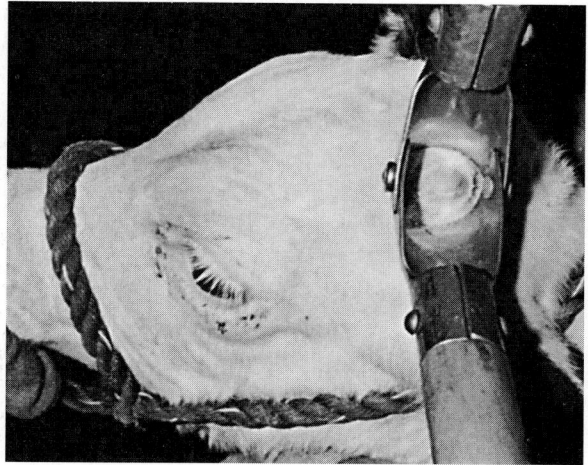

FIGURE 31-5.   Dehorning a calf with a Barnes scoop dehorner.

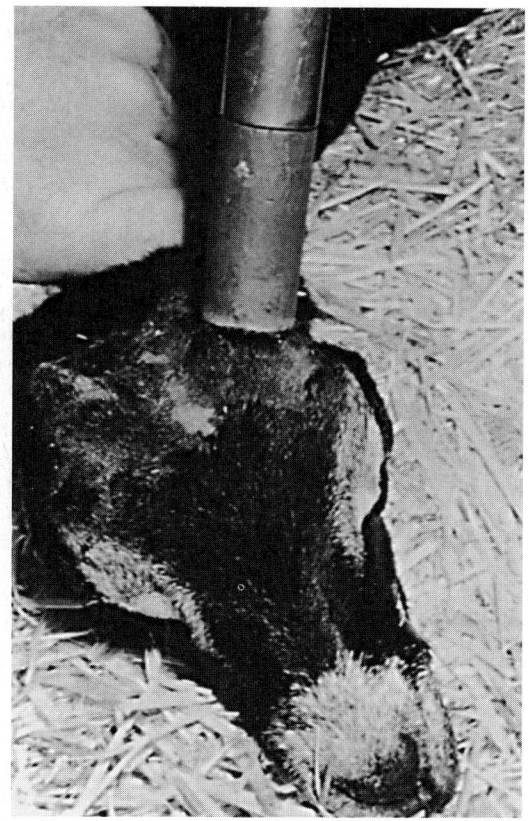

FIGURE 31-6.   Disbudding a kid by burning with an electric dehorning iron.

RESPIRATORY DISEASE

Respiratory problems in food animals are commonly infectious and can be divided into upper and lower respiratory tract disorders depending on whether the pharynx, larynx, or trachea (upper) or lungs (lower) are involved. Assessment of the respiratory system involves auscultation and percussion of the thorax as well as ancillary tests, such as transtracheal wash and bronchoalveolar lavage.

Transtracheal Wash

Both percutaneous and endoscope-guided sampling may be done. In both cases, the animal should be adequately restrained, preferably standing with the head and neck extended. For endoscope-guided sampling, a double-sheathed catheter should be used. The trachea can be visualized with the endoscope and positioned with the tip of the endoscope near a pocket of fluid if present. The catheter or tubing is passed into the trachea, and 20 ml of sterile saline is flushed into the trachea and followed by rapid aspiration. For percutaneous sampling, the ventral midcervical area is clipped, surgically prepared, and infiltrated with local anesthetic. One sterile hand is used to grasp the trachea while a 1-cm longitudinal scalpel incision is made through the skin over the trachea. Tracheal rings should be palpated and an area between rings identified. A stab incision is made into the lumen of the trachea between rings with a 9-gauge bleeding trocar (bevel directed down) while continuing to stabilize the trachea with the other hand. Sterile, polypropylene tubing (90 cm) is passed into the trachea at least 15 cm. Once the tubing is within the trachea, the trocar is removed, leaving the tubing in place. Sterile physiologic saline (30 ml for a cow) is injected via a 15-gauge needle that is placed in the end of the tubing. Immediately afterward, the saline wash is aspirated using the same or a different sterile syringe. From 5 to 10 ml of saline wash is sufficient for analysis. The sample is placed in a tube with ethylenediamine tetraacetic acid (EDTA) for cytology or transported in the syringe or onto transport medium for culture.

Upper Respiratory Disease

Causes of upper respiratory tract infections include viral and bacterial agents. Common viral infections include infectious bovine rhinotracheitis (IBR), bovine virus diarrhea (BVD), and malignant catarrhal fever (MCF) for cattle; border disease in sheep; and influenza (paramyxovirus) in swine. Common clinical signs include fever (often up to 41° C [105.8° F] with MCF), conjunctivitis, rhinitis, tracheitis, oral and nasal erosions and ulcers, listlessness, coughing, and dyspnea (Figures 31-7 and 31-8). BVD and border disease are also associated with reproductive and gastrointestinal diseases, whereas MCF often causes corneal opacification. Typically, the viruses facilitate bacterial invasion of the lungs by damaging the respiratory defense mechanisms. Recovery from acute viral infection is often rapid if not complicated by bronchopneumonia. Diagnosis for all viral respiratory diseases consists of viral isolation from nasal swabs (IBR, influenza) or white blood cells (BVD, border disease, MCF) or serologic testing. Treatment consists of supportive care and prophylactic antibiotics. Control is based on vaccination for IBR, BVD, and swine influenza (see Chapter 11).

Probably one of the most common causes of bacterial upper airway disease in cattle between 3 to 18 months old is necrotic laryngitis (calf diphtheria). It is an acute-to-chronic infection of the laryngeal mucosa and cartilage. Damaged mucosa allows invasion by *Fusobacterium necrophorum*. Signs include acute onset of moist, painful cough, inspiratory dyspnea with loud stridor and open-mouthed breathing, hypersalivation, anorexia, depression, fever, bilateral nasal discharge, fetid breath, ill-thrift, and death. Mild pressure to the larynx causes cough, pain, marked dyspnea, and stridor. Aspiration pneumonia may develop. Diagnosis can be confirmed by endoscopy or laryngos-

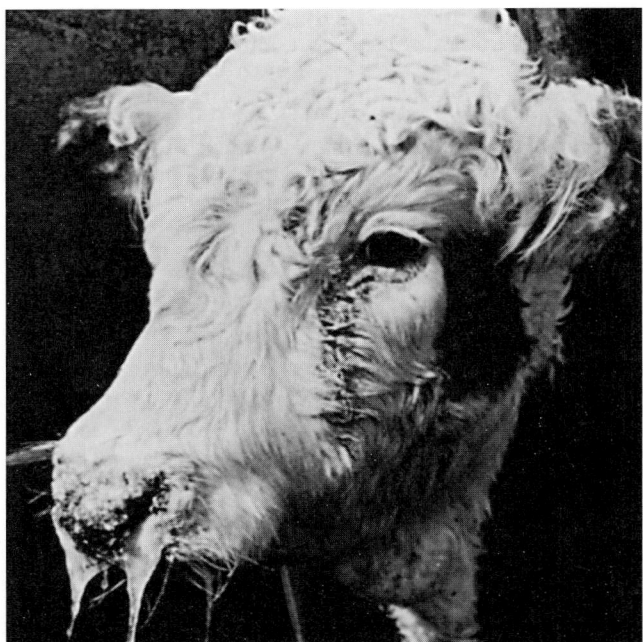

FIGURE 31-7. Mucopurulent oculonasal discharge in a calf with respiratory disease.

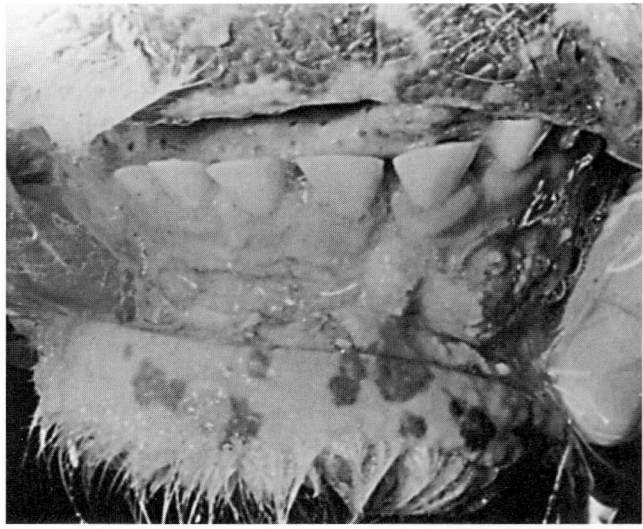

FIGURE 31-8. Calf with ulcers and erosions of the gums associated with bovine virus diarrhea (BVD).

copy. Treatment consists of long-term antibiotic administration, antiinflammatory agents, or surgical removal of the diseased arytenoids through a ventral approach.

Atrophic rhinitis is a multifactorial disease complex in pigs caused by toxigenic *Bordetella bronchiseptica* and *Pasteurella multocida*. The disease is characterized by turbinate atrophy and nasal deviation. Treatment includes antimicrobial therapy of sows, piglets, and weaners. Poor environmental conditions contribute to increased incidence and severity of atrophic rhinitis (e.g., poor ventilation, overcrowding, temperature extremes).

Lower Respiratory Disease

Two of the common viral causes of pneumonia in cattle are parainfluenza 3 (PI-3) and bovine respiratory syncytial virus (BRSV). PI-3 also causes pneumonia in sheep. Uncomplicated PI-3 infection is usually mild, often asymptomatic. BRSV infection occurs in calves less than 6 months of age, causing pneumonic signs and subcutaneous emphysema. Animals affected with either virus often succumb to secondary bacterial pneumonia caused by impaired clearance of organisms from the lungs. Diagnosis is confirmed by viral isolation from nasal mucosa (PI-3) or tracheal or bronchial secretions (BRSV) collected early in the disease process or by serologic testing. Prevention is through vaccination, which reduces the severity of disease but does not prevent infection. Immunity to natural infection with BRSV does not prevent reinfection.

In small ruminants, there are three retroviral causes of pneumonia: two nononcogenic retroviruses, ovine progressive pneumonia (OPP) and caprine arthritis and encephalitis virus (CAE), and pulmonary carcinoma or adenomatosis. OPP causes chronic pneumonia in sheep and can also cause disease in goats, whereas CAE causes interstitial pneumonia in goats only. Both OPP and CAE have long incubation periods and insidious, progressive clinical disease courses. Small ruminants rarely show signs before 2 years of age. Several syndromes can occur for both OPP and CAE, of which respiratory disease is only one. Clinical signs include weight loss; listlessness, with progression to exercise intolerance; dyspnea, often without pyrexia; and death within 18 months. Routes of transmission for OPP and CAE include lactogenic (through nursing) and transplacental (rarely). Diagnosis is by serology, clinical signs, and histopathology. Control measures are directed at identification of infected animals with serologic testing and depopulation. Newborn lambs and kids should be separated from seropositive ewes and does immediately after birth before colostral ingestion. The lambs and kids should be fed pooled seronegative or pasteurized colostrum.

Pulmonary carcinoma is a contagious neoplastic disease (possibly caused by OPP) of adult sheep characterized by insidious, progressive weakness, dyspnea, nasal discharge, and death. Transmission is by inhalation. Diagnosis is based on typical signs and histopathologic lesions. There is no specific treatment for any of these viral infections, but antibiotics and antiinflammatory agents may temporarily improve the quality of life.

Coronavirus has been identified as a cause of pneumonia in cows and pigs. The virus is antigenically related to the organism associated with gastrointestinal disease in both species but causes bronchointerstitial pneumonia in naive animals. Pseudorabies virus (PRV) causes pneumonia or upper respiratory tract infection in grower-finisher pigs. Signs are nonspecific and referable to the respiratory system. Morbidity is usually high, but mortality is low, with recovery often within 10 days. PRV persists in infected swine and is actively shed during periods of stress. Transmission may occur during mating, transplacentally, or through aerosol. Pseudorabies virus also causes rabieslike signs in other species, including cows, sheep, dogs, and cats. Efforts to eradicate the disease are currently underway in the United States.

Porcine respiratory and reproductive syndrome (PRRS) is associated with respiratory distress in sows. Pigs have increased susceptibility to bacterial causes of pneumonia. Nursing pigs develop rapid abdominal breathing and a characteristic "thumping" sound on auscultation. Mortality may be as high as 50% in some litters. Infected finishing pigs may exhibit rapid breathing, dyspnea, rough hair coat, and poor growth. Reproductive problems have also been associated with PRRS.

The primary bacterium responsible for producing acute fibrinous bronchopneumonia in ruminants is *Mannheimia* (*Pasteurella*) *haemolytica*, whereas chronic pneumonia in ruminants and pigs is often caused by *Pasteurella multocida*. *M. haemolytica* is part of the normal nasal flora but present in the lungs only when causing pneumonia. Management, environmental, and infectious stressors may facilitate infections. *M. haemolytica* can cause pneumonia independent of viral or other bacterial agents; however, viral agents and bacteria such as *Mycoplasma bovis* increase susceptibility to challenge with *M. haemolytica*. *Haemophilus somnus* and *Haemophilus parasuis* can cause conjunctivitis, tracheitis, pleuritis, suppurative bronchopneumonia, pericarditis, arthritis, and meningoencephalitis in cattle and pigs, respectively. The respiratory form is seen in feedlot calves and nursing, nursery, and finishing pigs. The route of transmission is unknown. Mycoplasma are small bacteria lacking a cell wall. *M. bovis* causes pneumonia. *Mycoplasma dispar* and *Ureaplasma* spp. are probably associated with respiratory disease in calves. Transmission occurs through direct contact, exposure to droplets or fomites, discharge from nose or eyes, and aerosolization. Diagnosis of bacterial pneumonia is by culture of tracheal or bronchial secretions. Treatment consists of antibiotics and antiinflammatory agents. Vaccines are available for most of the bacterial agents; however, efficacy is not completely satisfactory.

Many simple pneumonias in calves, pigs, and adult cattle are syndromes involving one or more infectious agents, environmental and management stressors, and a susceptible host. Enzootic pneumonia of calves is commonly diagnosed in housed calves from 2 to 6 months of age. The syndrome in pigs often occurs during the growing and finishing stages. Adult cattle with respiratory disease complex (shipping fever) often manifest clinical signs within 2 weeks of arrival at a feedlot. Several different pathogens have been implicated in all three syndromes with combinations of organisms common. Viral agents often associated with enzootic pneumonia of calves include PI-3, BRSV, BVD virus, IBR, and several adenoviruses. For adult shipping fever, IBR, BVD, PI-3, coronavirus, and BRSV are often implicated. *M. haemolytica* is the most significant cause of shipping fever, although *P. multocida* and *H. somnus* are sometimes involved. For enzootic pneumonia of calves, common bacterial agents include the same three agents in addition to *Mycoplasma* spp., *Actinomyces pyogenes*, and *Salmonella* spp. Common agents for enzootic pneumonia of swine include *Mycoplasma hyopneumoniae* (primarily) and *P. multocida*.

Clinical signs for all three syndromes range from subclinical to acute and fulminating to chronic. Signs include ill-thrift with poor weight gain, prolonged recumbency, listlessness, persistent and dry hacking cough, intermittent fever, dehydration, and a history of recurrent episodes of mild pneumonia that tend to become refractory to therapy. Auscultation may reveal wheezes and crackles. Radiographs often show evidence of atelectasis and consolidation of cranioventral lung lobes.

Diagnosis for all three syndromes can best be achieved by a postmortem examination, premortem serologic testing, and culture of lung or tracheal secretions from the most severely affected animals. Treatment is largely supportive, consisting of appropriate antibiotics for bacterial pathogens, fluids, antiinflammatory agents, and oxygen as needed. The most successful cases will be those that are recognized and treated early before irreversible damage to the lung and growth potential of the animal occurs.

Management considerations for avoidance of these syndromes emphasize colostral management for calves, nutritional support for pigs and older cattle, good-quality housing facilities (air quality, ventilation, low population density), preconditioning for older cattle (processing before marketing), and appropriate vaccination programs.

Acute bovine pulmonary emphysema and edema is a nonfebrile, noninfectious respiratory distress syndrome of adult beef cattle that usually occurs in the fall. It occurs in cattle grazing on alfalfa, rape, kale, or turnip tops. Clinical signs include dyspnea and crackles and wheezes on auscultation. Mortality of affected cattle may approach 50%. Treatment is primarily supportive in addition to removal of the animals from affected pastures. Prevention involves gradual introduction to lush pasture, ionophores such as monensin and lasalocid, and prophylactic oral antibiotics.

Parasites such as *Ascaris suum, Dictyocaulus viviparus, Dictyocaulus filaria, Protostrongylus rufescens,* and *Muellerius capillaris* can cause inflammation in the lungs with resultant eosinophilic or granulomatous pulmonary infiltrates in food animals. All except *A. suum* primarily invade the pulmonary system, whereas larvae from *A. suum* migrate through the lungs, causing inflammation and impaired resistance to secondary infectious pathogens. Diagnosis can be made by detection of larvae in the feces or eggs in respiratory secretions. Anthelmintic administration is usually effective in keeping parasite burdens low or nonexistent (see Chapter 7).

Technician Note

The importance of viruses in respiratory disease in food animals primarily resides in their ability to act synergistically to facilitate bacterial invasion.

CARDIOVASCULAR DISEASE

Heart disease, in general, is uncommon in food animals. Endocarditis is an often undiagnosed cause of cardiac disease in food animals. It is usually caused by bacteria that gain entrance through damaged valvular surfaces by hematogenous spread. Common infectious causes in cattle include *Arcanobacterium pyogenes* and alpha-hemolytic *Streptococcus.* In sheep and pigs, the common causative organisms are *Erysipelothrix rhusiopathiae, Streptococcus* spp., and *Escherichia coli.* In cattle, the tricuspid valve is most commonly affected, although multiple valves can be involved.

A systolic cardiac murmur is the most specific physical examination finding in food animals with this condition. However, affected animals may show nonspecific signs, such as constant or intermittent fever, anorexia, respiratory signs, weight loss, exercise intolerance, diarrhea, or sudden death. Dairy cows may have decreased milk production. There may be evidence of heart failure if the condition is severe or long-standing (peripheral edema, severe dyspnea, jugular pulses, distension). Isolation of pathogens on blood culture, auscultation of a murmur, and echocardiographic evidence of a vegetative lesion on a cardiac valve are highly suggestive of bacterial endocarditis.

Technician Note

Signs of congestive heart failure in food animals include submandibular edema, jugular distention and pulsation, dyspnea, and ascites.

Treatment of bacterial endocarditis involves long-term administration of antimicrobials (4 to 6 weeks); penicillin is often chosen. Adjunctive treatments include furosemide (diuretic) and oxygen therapy if there is evidence of congestive heart failure or pulmonary compromise, respectively. The prognosis is poor to guarded with posttreatment relapses common because of the inability of the antimicrobials to reach the site of infection and thrombogenic properties of the exposed heart valve leaflet. If an animal has evidence of congestive heart failure on initial evaluation, treatment response is often poor; consequently, treatment may not be economically justifiable.

Traumatic reticulopericarditis *(hardware disease)* resulting from penetration of the pericardium by ingested foreign objects, such as a wire or nail, is a common cause of pericarditis in cattle. Nontraumatic pericarditis in cattle may be caused by *Pasteurella* spp., *Clostridium* spp., and *Haemophilus* spp. In sheep and pigs, *Pasteurella* spp. and *Mycoplasma* spp. are common causes of pericarditis. *Staphylococcus aureus* and *Streptococcus* spp. are other causes in sheep and pigs, respectively. In all species, inflammation of the pericardium causes hyperemia and deposition of fibrinous exudate, followed by effusion. The animal may show nonspecific signs, such as fever, anorexia, depression, or weight loss. More specific signs may include tachycardia, friction rubs, muffled heart sounds, and absent lung sounds in the ventral thorax on thoracic auscultation. Splashing sounds are heard frequently during thoracic auscultation because of accumulation of gas and liquid in the pericardium *(washing machine murmur).* If congestive heart failure develops, the animal may develop peripheral edema, jugular venous distention and pulsation, and dyspnea (Figure 31-9). Cattle with traumatic reticulopericarditis may exhibit cranial abdominal pain (see discussion of gastrointestinal problems).

Echocardiography can be used to confirm the diagnosis of pericarditis at a referral institution. There will be evidence of an echo-free space between the two pericardial layers that is suggestive of fluid accumulation. Electrocardiograms and thoracic radiographs may be helpful, although often they are not. Treatment often is unrewarding and usually is directed toward salvage or short-term survival. Pericardial drainage with lavage and culturing may be used both diagnostically and therapeutically. Broad-spectrum antimicrobial and antiinflammatory agents are important for systemic use. Surgical removal of the foreign body in cattle with traumatic reticulopericarditis through a rumenotomy site or release of the effusion through pericardiectomy has been attempted with varying success. A common long-term sequela of pericarditis is the formation of pericardial adhesions, causing complete attachment of the pericardium to the epicardium. As a result of restriction of cardiac movement, congestive heart failure develops.

Pulmonary hypertension *(brisket disease)* can develop in susceptible cattle with prolonged exposure to high altitudes (more than 1800 m [6000 ft] above sea level). Goats and sheep are reported to be susceptible but less so than cattle. Pigs, llamas, and alpacas are resistant. The low oxygen tension at these altitudes causes hypoxic vasoconstriction of the pulmonary arteries, leading to increased pulmonary vascular resistance and hypertension. Pressure overload of the right ventricle results in cardiac hypertrophy, dilation, and failure. The disease is reversible in the early stages by moving the animal to a lower altitude.

The most common presenting clinical sign is subcutaneous edema of the brisket, ventral thorax, or submandibular area. Cattle often show dyspnea, tachypnea, chronic cough, or weight loss. A cardiac murmur may be auscultated,

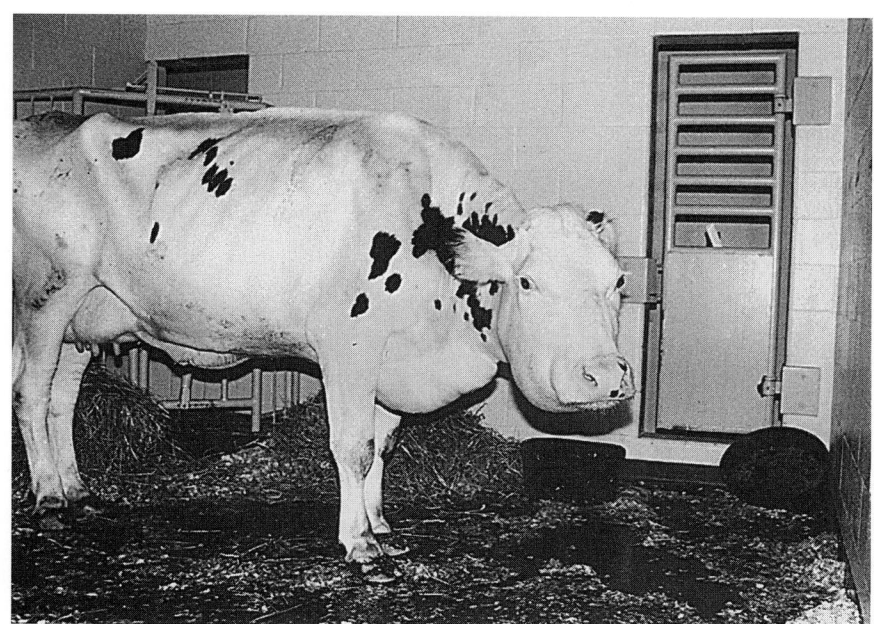

FIGURE 31-9. Cow with congestive heart failure, showing rough hair coat and edema of the ventrum and brisket.

caused by either tricuspid valve insufficiency or pulmonic valve compromise. Genetic predispositions are seen in some herds. Ingestion of locoweed can also predispose cattle to right-sided heart failure at high altitudes by causing toxic myocardial damage. Other factors, such as myocardial dystrophy, anemia, cold, pulmonary disease, or hypoproteinemia, may exacerbate the primary cardiac dysfunction.

Diagnostic tests that aid in the diagnosis of pulmonary hypertension and cardiomegaly include measurement of pulmonary arterial pressures and echocardiography. Mean pulmonary arterial pressures of more than 35 mm Hg are suggestive of high altitude disease. Echocardiography may reveal right-sided heart enlargement or valvular problems. The disease can be controlled by removing susceptible animals from the high altitude and preventing locoweed ingestion. Lung disease may need to be treated with oxygen therapy. Heart failure responds poorly to treatment; however, it may be controlled with digoxin and diuretics, such as furosemide.

Congenital heart defects occur uncommonly in all food animal species; the prevalence is highest in cattle. In some defects, heredity appears to play a role. Defects can occur alone or in combination. The most commonly reported heart defect in cattle and sheep is a ventricular septal defect (VSD). In pigs, dysplasia of the tricuspid valve and atrial septal defects are more common than VSDs. Congenital cardiac defects allow the mixing of oxygenated and reduced oxygenated blood through aberrant circuits between the pulmonary and systemic circulations. Clinical signs include heart murmur, exercise intolerance, cyanosis at rest or with exertion, lethargy, poor growth, weakness, or acute death. Often, the defect produces signs at birth and causes severe illness or death within the first few weeks of life. If adequate compensation occurs, signs may appear later in life and manifest as stunted growth as a result of reduced cardiac output, congestive heart failure, systemic infections caused by cardiac dysfunction, or sudden death from severe cardiac arrhythmias. Diagnosis is best achieved by auscultation of a characteristic heart murmur and direct

visualization of the defect and blood flow pattern with M-mode echocardiography and Doppler ultrasonography performed at a referral institution. Treatment is generally nonrewarding.

Atrial fibrillation is the most common arrhythmia of food animals. Cattle with atrial fibrillation often are asymptomatic at rest or have signs referable to the source of the arrhythmia. Gastrointestinal disease, hypocalcemia, foot rot, and pneumonia can lead to atrial fibrillation in cattle; anorexia and decreased milk production may occur as a result. Auscultation reveals an irregularly irregular heartbeat. The heart rate may be slow, normal, or rapid. The diagnosis can be confirmed with an electrocardiogram. Therapy is directed at correcting the underlying problem. Usually, the arrhythmia will resolve on its own within 5 days of treatment of the underlying problem. Quinidine can be used to convert atrial fibrillation to normal sinus rhythm in ruminants; it must be given slowly in intravenous fluids in cattle with constant monitoring. Diarrhea and depression are common side effects. If arrhythmias develop, the infusion should be discontinued. Therapy should be discontinued after the infusion, regardless of whether conversion has occurred. It should also be stopped as soon as conversion occurs.

GASTROINTESTINAL DISEASES

General Mechanisms of Disease

Ruminants use foregut microbial fermentation to extract nutrients from plant material. Regurgitation and repeated chewing are used to break down fibrous material and expose nutrients to the rumen bacteria and protozoa. Products of fermentation include organic acids and gas. The organic acids, which make rumen fluid acidic, are absorbed through the gastric or intestinal wall and are used by the animal for energy, whereas gas is released by eructation. Accumulation of either of these products in the rumen can be detrimental to the animal. Organized ruminoreticular contraction cycles, which are important for normal digestion, also prevent accumulation of acids and gas by stimulating outflow of ingesta, enhancing absorption of acids, and expelling gas. Camelids have similar gastrointestinal function, although the morphology of the gastric compartments is different. On the other hand, pigs are monogastric but have a well-developed cecum for fermentation in the caudal gastrointestinal tract.

Proper ruminoreticular (foregut) function depends on the physiologic well-being of the ruminant, as well as the continuous intake of appropriate feed. In that regard, auscultation for motility and palpation of the fill and consistency of the rumen are valuable tools in assessing the health of the ruminant. In addition, because the rumen is the biggest contributor to abdominal volume in the non-pregnant ruminant, size changes of the rumen often are mirrored by the abdominal contour.

Dysfunction of the rumen can be classified as hypomotility, shrinkage, gas distention, or fluid distention. Shrinkage is due to decreased feed or water intake and is not a primary disease. Ruminal hypomotility or stasis can be caused by lack of feed intake, rumen overdistention, gastric hyperacidity, systemic disease, and emotional stress. Hypomotility often is accompanied by a decreased fluid content in the rumen, which inappropriately is referred to as *rumen impaction*. Hypomotility is best addressed through treatment for the primary disease. Oral electrolyte fluids, liquefied feed, or gastric fluid from a healthy cow (transfaunation) may be beneficial in increasing the function of a static rumen, but mineral oil and laxatives seldom are helpful.

A thorough physical examination is necessary to determine the cause and importance of abdominal distention. Gas accumulation typically results in dorsal distention and can cause a hyperresonant area or *ping* detectable by simultaneous auscultation and percussion (Figure 31-10). Fluid accumulation typically causes ventral distention and can cause a "splashy" area detectable by simultaneous auscultation and ballottement. Transrectal palpation for distended abdominal viscera may aid in identification of the disorder. Distention of the rumen is most visible on the left side of the abdomen. A large, fluid-filled rumen is L shaped, with bilateral ventral distention and left-sided dorsal distention. Enlargement of the abomasum, cecum, or multiple loops of small intestine leads to distention of the right flank and possibly secondary rumen stasis, fluid accumulation, and left flank distention. Problems in the urogenital system also may lead to ventral abdominal distention.

Technician Note

Simultaneous ballottement and percussion of the abdomen *(pinging)* of a ruminant can help localize sites of fluid and gas accumulation.

Distention of the rumen with gas *(bloat)* can occur as a result of stasis, failure to eruct, overproduction of gas, or production of gas trapped in a stable foam. Gas distention of the rumen is important because it inhibits normal motility and prevents expansion of the lungs (Figure 31-11). Gas produced by fermentation usually is free but may be trapped in foam *(frothy bloat)* if a proteinaceous feedstuff, particularly a legume hay, is being fed. If respiration is unaffected and the skin over the rumen is not tightly stretched, emergency treatment is not necessary. An orogastric tube may be passed to release free gas, and the animal should be observed for progression of signs. If frothy bloat is suspected, a detergent (poloxalene) or mineral oil

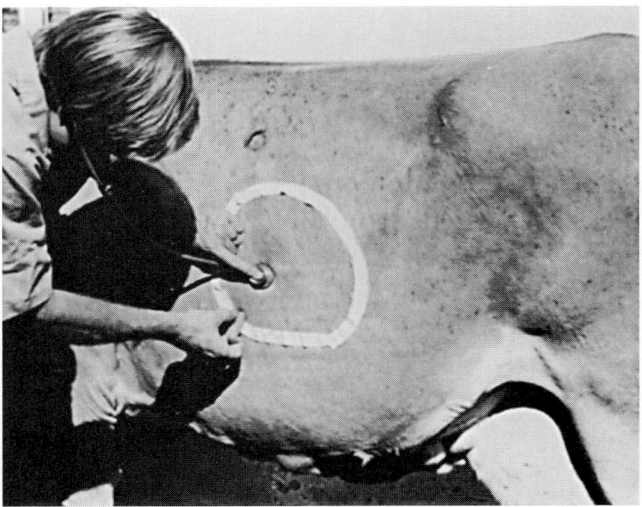

FIGURE 31-10. Auscultation and percussion of the left flank. The tape outlines the area of resonance associated with left abomasal displacement.

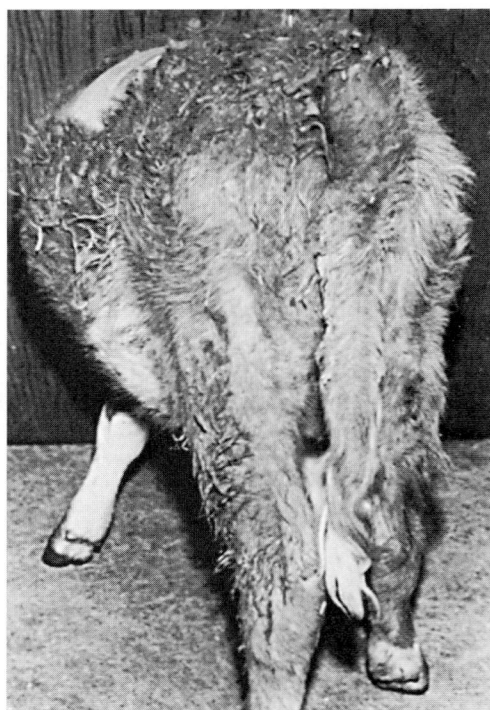

FIGURE 31-11. Ruminal gas distention (bloat) in the dorsal left paralumbar fossa of a cow.

should be given orally to destabilize the foam. If the distention is impairing the animal's ability to breathe, an aggressive attempt should be made to relieve the distention: a larger-bore stomach tube may be passed, or a fistula may be made through the dorsal left paralumbar fossa into the rumen. A temporary fistula can be made with a large-gauge hypodermic needle or trocar, but a surgical fistula will decrease abdominal contamination and provide longer relief.

Fluid distention of abdominal viscera occurs as a result of regurgitation from a distal site *(internal vomiting)*, physical or functional outflow obstruction, or fluid shifts secondary to the accumulation of osmotic particles. Thus fluid distention can occur as a primary problem or secondary to another disorder. Excess ruminal fluid inhibits eructation by causing the lower esophageal sphincter to spasm, leading to secondary gas distention. Unlike gas distention, fluid distention rarely is correctable by passage of an orogastric tube.

Specific Gastrointestinal Diseases

Overingestion of rapidly fermentable feed (carbohydrate engorgement, grain overload) results in the production of large quantities of gas and osmotically active organic acids in the rumen. Body water follows the osmotic gradient into the rumen, resulting in a "splashy," ventrally distended rumen and decreased circulatory volume. Gas accumulation leads to dorsal ruminal distention. Circulatory shock and absorption of acid into the systemic circulation lead to systemic acidosis and depression.

Treatment goals include relieving the gas and fluid distention of the rumen, reducing production and absorption of acid, and correcting systemic fluid and acid-base derangements. These goals can be accomplished through orogastric intubation with a large-bore (Kingman) stomach tube, ruminal lavage with cold water, rumenotomy to remove feed material, oral alkalinizing agents (magnesium oxide, sulfate, or hydroxide), oral mineral oil to promote gastrointestinal transit, and systemic alkalinizing fluid treatment. Secondary metabolic and infectious diseases may occur and are best treated prophylactically with thiamine and penicillin. Not all treatments are required for all animals.

Perforation of the reticulum by a metallic foreign body (hardware disease) can lead to peritonitis with possible extension into the pleural and pericardial cavities. Pain and secondary infection lead to anorexia, a drop in milk production, and cranial abdominal pain. The cow may resist ventroflexion when manual pressure is applied to the thoracic spine or may grunt when pressure is applied to the xiphoid region. Cattle with chronic hardware disease may develop weight loss, recurrent fever, and rumen distention. Retrieval of the foreign body through a rumenotomy may be beneficial if the lesion is recent. With more long-standing lesions, medical treatment with a rumen magnet and systemic antibiotics gives similar results to surgery. Because of the possibility of diffuse peritonitis and pericarditis, the prognosis for hardware disease is guarded to poor.

The abomasum of ruminants is similar to the acid-secreting stomach of monogastrics, and the lower intestinal tract is also very similar to that of other mammals. The greater curvature of the bovine abomasum has a loose omental attachment, making this organ very mobile. When filled with gas, the abomasum may displace dorsally on either side of the abdomen. Left or right abomasal displacement is most common in dairy cows and leads to anorexia, decreased milk production, and distinctive pings on abdominal auscultation and percussion. *Ketosis* (excess ketone production) is a frequent sequela to abomasal displacement because the milk production of the cow does not drop as quickly as energy intake. *Volvulus* (twisting of the bowel) of a displaced abomasum can lead to compromise of the blood supply, regurgitation of hydrochloric acid–rich fluid into the rumen, and a rapid decline in clinical condition. Surgical correction of right abomasal displacement or volvulus can be done through a right

paralumbar or paramedian incision. Left abomasal displacement can also be corrected surgically through a left paralumbar incision or percutaneously through the right paramedian area. Percutaneous fixation is not recommended for right abomasal displacements because of the inability to determine whether volvulus of the organ has occurred.

A variety of other surgical gastrointestinal lesions can occur, including intraluminal obstruction, intussusception, volvulus, and entrapment. Intraluminal obstruction is most common in pet pigs, which are prone to ingest foreign bodies, and in camelids. Clinical pathology data as well as good physical and rectal examinations are helpful in identifying these lesions. Abdominal ultrasonographic and radiographic examinations may be useful in animals too small for rectal examination. Depression, abdominal distention, colic, tenesmus, and failure to defecate may be seen. Ruminants and camelids may sequester a large volume of fluid in the forestomach (internal vomiting), making the obstruction less apparent, whereas pigs often vomit with obstruction. Disease signs and metabolic compromise are related to the location, nature, and duration of the lesion. The more cranial and complete the obstruction, the more likely gastric fluid is to be refluxed, with concomitant development of systemic dehydration and hypochloremic metabolic alkalosis. This can also develop with time with complete distal obstructions.

These metabolic abnormalities result in dehydration (dry mucous membranes, prolonged tenting of skin), forestomach distention, and depression. Strangulating lesions tend to cause a rapid decline in clinical condition, whereas nonstrangulating lesions often have a slower onset of signs. With slower onset, greater metabolic derangement can occur. Intestinal distention places pressure on mesenteric stretch receptors, causing colic; this does not occur with most gastric lesions. Exploratory laparotomy is necessary to accurately identify and correct most obstructive lesions.

Technician Note

Proximal gastrointestinal obstruction is associated with metabolic derangements without colic signs, whereas distal obstruction causes few metabolic derangements but frequent colic signs.

Paralumbar Laparotomy

A cow is best restrained while standing in a chute, although surgery can be performed with head restraint only. Small ruminants, pigs, and camelids are best restrained in lateral recumbency. The area bordered cranially by the last rib space, dorsally by midline, and caudally by the tuber coxae should be clipped and cleaned with antiseptic solutions (Figure 31-12). The ventral border of the prepared site varies but is usually one half to two thirds of the way down the lateral abdominal wall. Regional (proximal or distal paravertebral block) or local (line or inverted L block) anesthesia is used. General anesthesia or a combination of physical restraint, sedation, and local anesthesia may be used for animals in lateral recumbency. The left flank is used for rumenotomy, cesarean delivery, and repair of left abomasal displacement, especially when it is suspected that the abomasum may be adhering to the left abdominal wall. The right flank is used for most abomasal or intestinal disorders and some cesarean deliveries (Figure 31-13).

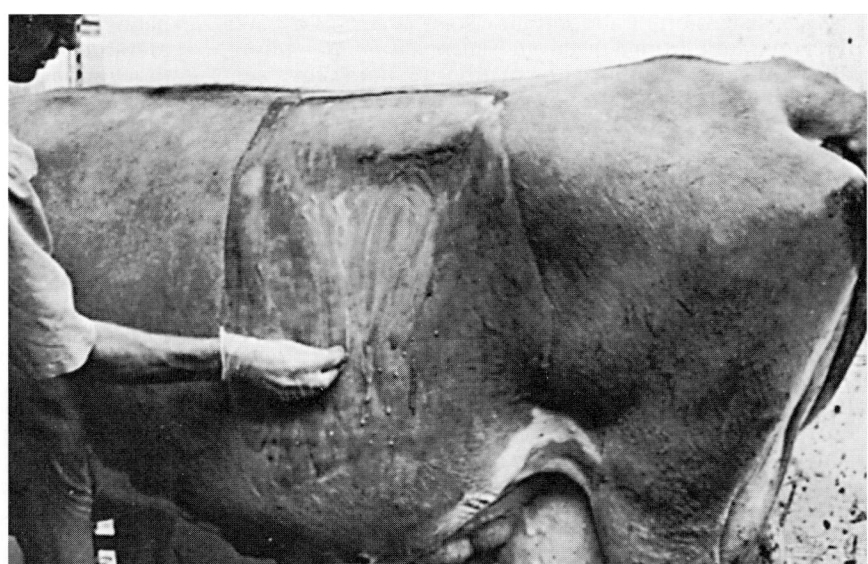

FIGURE 31-12. Preparation of the flank of a cow for aseptic surgery. The area has been clipped.

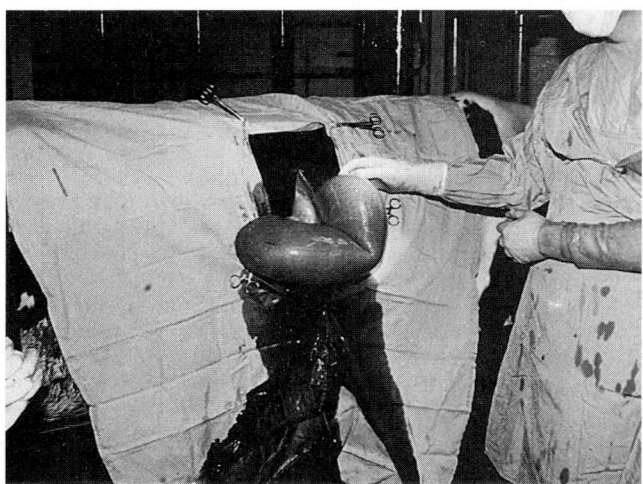

FIGURE 31-13. Dilated cecum exteriorized from the abdomen of a cow during standing right paralumbar laparotomy. The cow is restrained in a metal chute.

Ventral Paramedian or Midline Laparotomy

The cow must be restrained in dorsal recumbency. Although certain chutes are adaptable to this task, most practitioners will use hobbles to extend the legs forward and backward and a halter for head restraint. Sedation often is necessary, and a casting rope may be used to make a cow recumbent (see Chapter 1). The area between the ribs cranially and the lateral abdominal *(milk)* veins should be clipped and cleaned with antiseptics. General or local anesthesia may be used. The umbilicus is the caudal extent of the incision for cranial abdominal surgery, and the udder is the caudal extent for caudal abdominal surgery. A right paramedian incision (8 cm to the right of midline and from 10 to 20 cm caudal to the sternum) is used for abomasal problems, whereas a midline or paramedian incision between the udder and umbilicus may be

used for cesarean deliveries. Large-diameter chromic gut or absorbable synthetic suture material should be used to close the body wall. Subcutaneous tissue should be apposed carefully because fluid accumulates easily in dead space around ventral incisions. The skin is closed with large-diameter suture material. Although nonabsorbable suture is desired for skin closure, subsequent removal may not be possible in all management settings.

Diarrhea in Juveniles and Adults

Diarrhea in juvenile and adult ruminants and pigs can be caused by a variety of digestive disorders resulting from the passage of osmotically active, undigested feed into the lower gastrointestinal tract and altered intestinal motility. Cattle often have very loose feces, whereas species that normally pass pelleted feces have softer, less-formed stool. In contrast to neonatal diarrhea, most diarrhea in juveniles and adults is not accompanied by systemic signs, is self-limiting, and does not require treatment. However, diarrhea may result in reduced milk production or growth, and because severe acute infectious enterocolitis can be life threatening at any age, animals displaying diarrhea with signs of systemic disease should be examined and treated. Morbidity occurs because of fluid and electrolyte loss, bowel inflammation, systemic toxemia, and possibly viremia or bacteremia.

Several viruses cause fever and acute ulcerative enteritis and range in severity from the relatively benign winter dysentery to the more severe blue tongue, BVD, and MCF. Abortion and birth defects may also be seen. Careful examination of the mucosal surfaces of the mouth, eye, and nose for characteristic erosive lesions plus an evaluation of fecal, tissue, and blood samples by a veterinary diagnostic laboratory may aid in identification of the etiologic agent in herd outbreaks. Supportive treatment consisting of replacement fluids, antiinflammatory agents, and prophylactic antibiotic drugs may be useful in individual animals.

Acute bacterial enteritis is uncommon, except in neonates and pigs. Epizootics of severe hemorrhagic diarrhea often are attributable to *Salmonella* spp., which may be

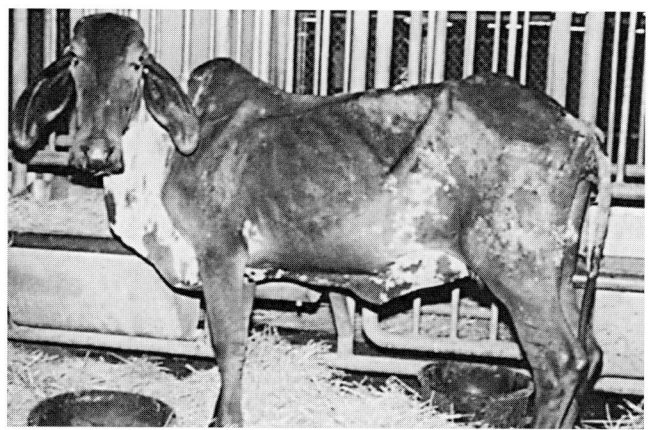

FIGURE 31-14.   Severe emaciation in a Brahman cow with Johne's disease.

introduced by rodents, contaminated feed, or asymptomatic carrier animals. Juvenile small ruminants and calves are susceptible to enterotoxemia (caused by *Clostridium perfringens*), which may be fatal before diarrhea is apparent because of gut wall necrosis and toxemia. Weanling and feeder pigs are very susceptible to hemorrhagic enteritis caused by *Serpulina (Treponema) hyodysenteria*. Secondary bacterial infection in juvenile swine with proliferative ileitis, which is caused by an unidentified organism, also may result in severe hemorrhagic or necrotizing enteritis. Individual animals are managed best with fluids, antibiotics, and antiinflammatory agents, whereas medicated water or feed may be used for large groups of animals. Specific vaccines and antitoxins are available to prevent or treat some of these disorders. With herd outbreaks, identification of the etiologic agent and management changes to prevent new cases are recommended.

Coccidiosis is the most common cause of diarrhea in juvenile ruminants. Although the diarrhea often is hemorrhagic, the affected animals usually are bright unless dehydration becomes severe. Tenesmus and neurologic disease also may be seen with coccidiosis. Fecal examination for oocysts usually is diagnostic. Effective control consists of management changes to decrease fecal contamination of feed and water plus treatment of all contact animals with a coccidiostatic or coccidiocidal drug (see Chapter 7).

Gastrointestinal parasitism may be a significant problem in ruminants on grass (strongyles) and pigs on dirt (ascarids). Bloodsucking abomasal worms in ruminants can cause poor weight gain or weight loss, diarrhea, anemia, hypoproteinemia, and death. Migrating ascarids in pigs can cause poor weight gain, diarrhea, and liver condemnation at slaughter. Fecal examination for ova may be diagnostic but also may be negative, because many of the clinical symptoms are caused by immature worms. Although worm burden may be controlled in part with anthelmintic drugs, pasture or pen sanitation and rotation also can be effective.

Chronic diarrhea often is impossible to treat because of permanent changes in the bowel wall. Johne's disease is a granulomatous disease of the ileocecal region of cattle and, rarely, other ruminants or camelids caused by *Mycobacterium* (*avium* subspecies) *paratuberculosis*; it leads to a protein-losing enteropathy. Animals are thought to become infected with the organism when young but often show clinical signs in early adulthood.

In addition to chronic diarrhea, affected animals often display weight loss, hypoproteinemia, and submandibular or brisket edema (Figure 31-14). A similar wasting syndrome may be seen in swine with the chronic form of proliferative ileitis. Removal of young from their dams, sanitation, and pasteurization of colostrum are recommended to prevent the spread of Johne's disease. These diseases must be differentiated from noninfectious causes of chronic diarrhea, including parasitism, inflammatory bowel disease, and copper deficiency, which are treatable and have a different herd significance.

LOCOMOTOR DISORDERS

Lameness in food animals is one of the most common complaints requiring veterinary attention. Bovine veterinarians or producers who deal with a high volume of lameness disorders will find it worthwhile to invest in a hydraulic table to place the cow in lateral recumbency for examination and treatment. The table allows superior restraint of the animal and the simultaneous examination of all four feet. If this option is unavailable, the head of the cow should be restrained adequately, and the affected leg should be elevated with straw bales or rope for examination. Sheep can be tipped up on their rear, whereas goats tend to struggle with this means of restraint. Llamas can be trained to allow foot handling, whereas pet pigs can be suspended in a sling to gain access to their feet. If necessary, tranquilizers may be used in all species to facilitate inspection of the affected leg.

The foot is the most common site of lameness. The normal ruminant or porcine foot consists of two digits, each of which ends in a horny hoof (Figure 31-15). A white line is found on the cranial, axial, and abaxial aspects of the bottom of each digit, where the sections of horn formed by the coriums of the sole and wall meet. The caudal portion of the weight-bearing surface is the heel bulb, which is separated by a line of demarcation from the horn of the sole. The heel bulb is covered by softer horn than the sole and is more prominent in pigs than in ruminants. Front claws bear more weight and usually have a greater solar surface area, being more ovoid than the thinner hindclaws. The angle between the dorsal wall and coronary band should be approximately 135 degrees. Weight should be borne on the abaxial wall. The camelid foot is unique; the weight-bearing bottom of the middle phalanx is covered by a keratinized digital pad. The horny claw extends from the cranial surface of the pad and normally is not weight bearing.

Because most food animals are not broken to lead, lameness examination involves careful observation of the stance and gait of the animal. Animals will shift their weight to spare sore feet or digits. Lameness is most common in the lateral digit of the hindfoot and may cause the animal to stand with a base-wide stance. Hindlimb lameness may cause the animal to shift its weight forward, lowering the head and giving the elbows an abducted appearance. The medial digit often is affected in forelimb lameness and may cause the animal to stand with a base-narrow stance or, in severe cases, the animal may stand with forelegs crossed or walk on its carpi (Figure 31-16). Forelimb lameness may cause the animal to shift its weight backward, raising the head and giving the hocks an adducted appearance. Occasionally, the medial digit of the hindleg or lateral digit of the foreleg is involved.

Horn Lesions

Lameness may be attributable simply to excessive horn growth. In some cases of chronic lameness, overgrowth of a

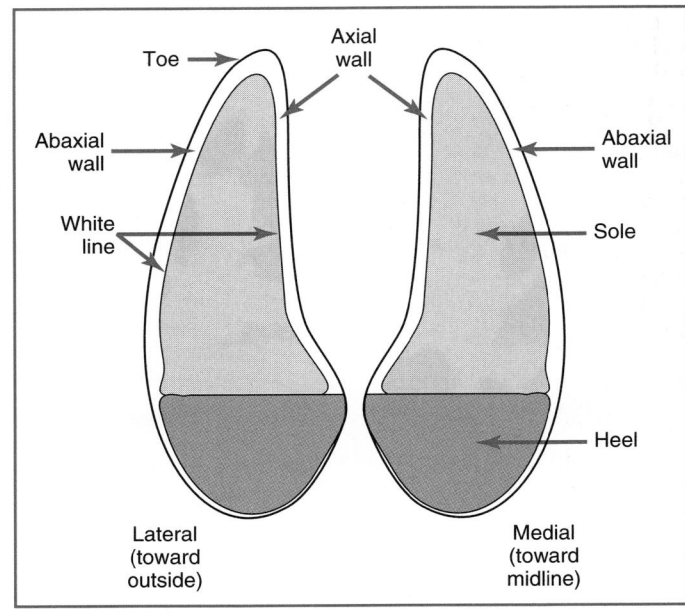

FIGURE 31-15. Cross section of bovine foot showing common anatomy.

specific region may reflect decreased wear, as the animal adapts its gait to spare a painful region. Overgrowth of horn is seen most commonly as elongated toes, excessive abaxial wall, or thickening of the heel. Overgrowth of the toes will increase the angle between the dorsal wall and coronary band and may cause the animal to bear weight on the soft tissue of the heel. Overgrowth of the abaxial walls may cause splaying of the digits and trauma to the interdigital space. Hard flooring (concrete) will exacerbate the effects of hoof overgrowth by forcing the digits into an abnormal position.

Laminitis (pododermatitis aseptica diffusa) in cattle rarely receives the attention that the disease does in horses, in part because acute clinical laminitis is rare. In contrast, subclinical laminitis is a common and important contributor to several of the hoof abnormalities of bovine lameness. Inflammation or engorgement of the horn-forming corium leads to a form of compartmental syndrome, in which the swollen corium is compressed between the pedal bone and hoof wall. Resultant damage to the corium leads to the production of abnormal, discolored horn.

The primary lesion of laminitis is not visible, but the consequences are easily seen. Partial rotation and sinking of the pedal bone can contribute to white line or toe lesions and sole hemorrhage or ulcers, respectively. Complete cessation of sole formation, followed by resumption, can lead to the formation of a double sole. Abnormal horn production by the corium of the wall can lead to horizontal fissures or laminitic rings *(hardship grooves)*. By measuring the distance from the coronary band to the laminitic ring, the timing of the laminitic event can be estimated (normal wall growth is about 0.5 cm/month). Laminitic lesions of the sole commonly become apparent 2 to 3 months after the insult, which often occurs in the early postparturient period. Bacterial invasion along the laminae may lead to heel horn erosion.

Predisposing factors to laminitis are thought to include heel conformation, high-energy diets (acidosis), disease (histamine, endotoxin), lack of exercise, high protein or

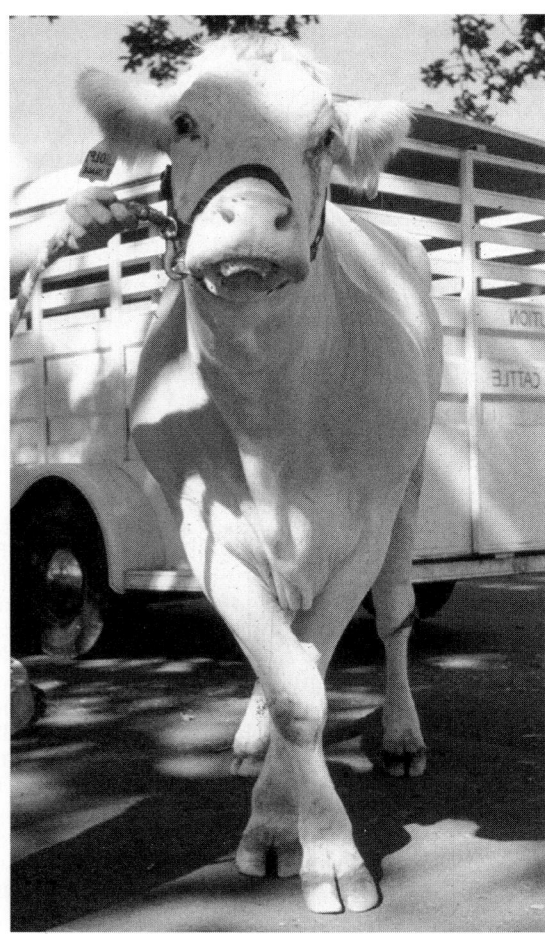

FIGURE 31-16. Cow with painful front feet. Crossing of the front feet is common when both medial claws are painful.

barley diets, concrete flooring, calving, and poorly bedded stalls (increased time standing). Gradual acclimation of an animal to a new ration or housing facility may decrease the incidence of laminitic events.

Pododermatitis circumscripta (*sole* or *Rusterholz ulcer*) is the result of damage to the corium at the sole-heel junction and may be a local form of laminitis. Hemorrhage causes discoloration of the horn as well as separation of the horn from the laminae. This weakened area ulcerates with wear and subsequently fills with granulation tissue. Secondary infection can occur, and deeper structures (most importantly, the deep flexor tendon and navicular bursa) can be affected.

Pododermatitis septica is infection and abscess formation within the horn or between the sole or wall horn and the corium. If ventral drainage is impaired, these infections often track dorsally to break out at the coronary band or heel. Laminitis predisposes to development of pododermatitis septica by allowing for soft horn formation, cracks, and white line separation. Trauma also may cause separation of the sole from the wall and deep inoculation of bacteria. These lesions are very painful and often can be localized with hoof testers. Although found in all species of hoof stock, pododermatitis septica is the most common horn lesion associated with lameness in pigs *(porcine foot rot)*.

Vertical and horizontal wall cracks are common findings and occasionally associated with lameness. Cracks form when abnormal (postlaminitis) or excessively dry horn is subjected to pressure. Overgrown toes contribute by increasing leverage on the weakened area. Lameness is uncommon unless the crack becomes full thickness through the horn or reaches the coronary band. In cases of severe lameness, secondary infection of the underlying soft tissue is likely. Vertical cracks that reach the coronary band may lead to abnormal *(corkscrew)* hoof growth.

When lameness involves the horn, corrective trimming should be performed. Excessive and separated horn should be removed. Large nippers or grinders may be used to remove large sections of horn, and knives and sanders may be used to prepare the final surface. The abaxial wall should be weight bearing, with the sole, heel, and axial wall trimmed to form a concave surface.

Dissecting tracts into the hoof should be excavated and flushed with antiseptic solutions. Subsolar lesions should be opened to allow drainage, and excessive granulation tissue should be trimmed. Partial hoof wall resections may increase drainage from lesions that track along the wall. Deep cracks may be excavated with a rotary grinding tool, and vertical cracks may be held together with wire to prevent extension of the lesion. Wall growth is slower in bulls and older animals, and bulls have proportionally less foot surface area for their weight, so care must be taken to avoid removing excessive horn from these animals. In many cases, a growing period of new hoof together with one or more trimmings is necessary to obtain a normal hoof.

If lameness can be localized to one digit, increased comfort and soundness of the animal can be achieved by supporting the sound digit of that hoof. This is done by trimming and grooving the horn of the sound digit and attaching an appropriately sized wooden, rubber, or plastic block or slipper to the sole with a cement. These usually come off or wear down after several weeks and rarely need to be removed. Open wounds may be protected with a bandage, which protects the wound, absorbs exudates, prevents drying of tissue, holds medications, and aids in hemostasis. In a clean environment, some lesions heal faster without a bandage.

Bacterial infection of horn lesions may extend into deeper tissue structures; these include joints, bones, tendons, and bursae. Rupture of the deep flexor tendon causes the toe to point up, whereas damage to other structures often results in severe lameness, swelling of the digit, and lack of response to conservative treatment. Such animals require radical debridement of lesions as well as antibiotic and antiinflammatory treatment.

Minor surgical procedures (debridement, digit amputation) are facilitated through the use of local or regional anesthesia. Local anesthesia involves infiltration of the soft tissue around the lesion. Regional anesthesia of the entire foot is achieved by the injection of 20 ml of lidocaine into a superficial vein (Figure 31-17). A tourniquet should be placed, and the skin around the vein should be clipped and disinfected before the intravenous block is attempted (see Chapter 21). Tourniquets also are useful in minimizing hemorrhage during surgical procedures.

Soft Tissue Lesions

Digital dermatitis often causes only mild lameness, especially of the hindlimb, which may be unnoticeable if bilateral. The etiology appears to be multifactorial, with poor hygiene and infectious agents (especially spirochetes) implicated, and is most common in heifers entering the milking herd. The lesion is circumscribed and partially or completely alopecic and begins as an erosion or ulcer. With time, the ulcer fills with granulation tissue *(strawberry-like)* or proliferative projections *(papillomas or warts)*. Lesions most commonly occur at the plantar or dorsal commissure but also occur at the skin-horn junction of the heel and other sites. Some lesions regress spontaneously.

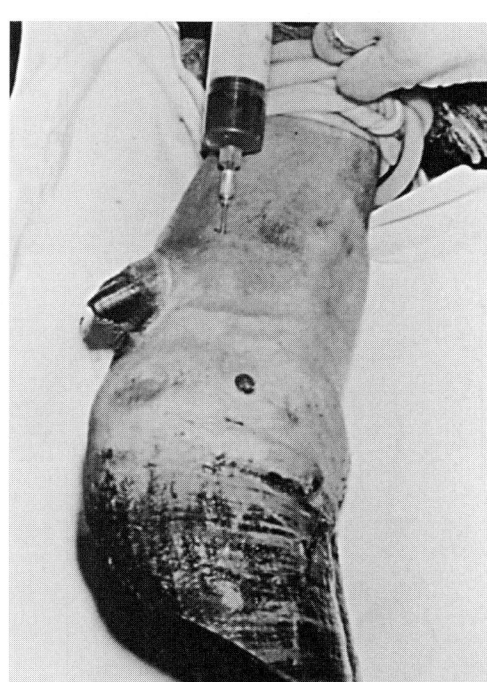

FIGURE 31-17. Local intravenous anesthesia of the bovine foot. The tourniquet, which is placed proximal to the injection site, aids in palpation of the vein and distribution of the anesthetic agent.

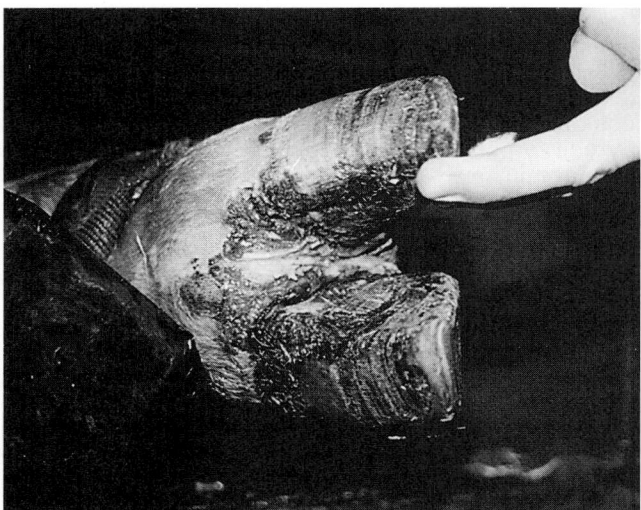

FIGURE 31-18. Interdigital dermatitis on the foot of a cow.

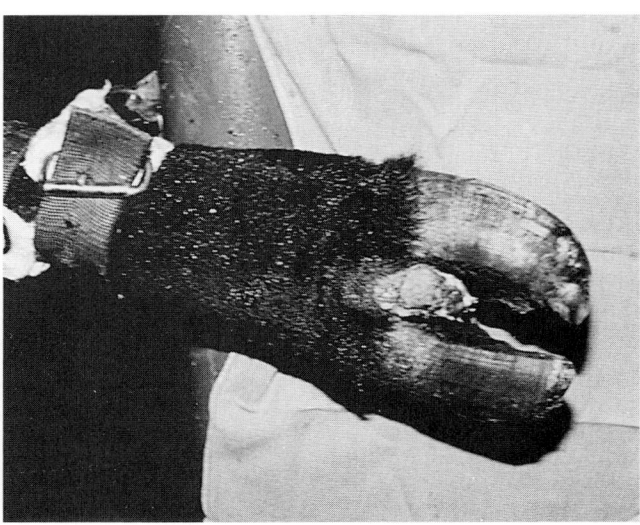

FIGURE 31-19. Interdigital hyperplasia (fibroma) on the foot of a cow.

Interdigital dermatitis *(contagious foot rot, ovine foot rot)* is the most common cause of lameness in sheep; it also occurs in other hoof-stock species. *Dichelobacter* (formerly *Bacteroides*) *nodosus* is the contagious, causative agent, whereas *Fusobacterium necrophorum* can coinvade, causing necrosis. These same organisms are thought to cause digital pad ulcers and lameness in llamas. Spirochetes also may play a role, suggesting a relationship between this disease and digital dermatitis. The lesion usually starts on the interdigital skin, and animals may be sensitive to interdigital palpation, even if no lesion is visible (Figure 31-18). With progression, a malodorous, necrotic break in the skin is formed, and deeper tissues may become infected. If the coronary band (either axial or abaxial) is affected, wall or heel separation can follow. A vaccine against *Dichelobacter* exists in some countries.

Interdigital hyperplasia (corn, fibroma) is a proliferation of fibrous tissue that protrudes into the interdigital space (Figure 31-19). Long-term irritation of the region secondary to interdigital dermatitis, hoof conformation (excessive axial sole), and housing surface probably contributes. Laxity of the distal interphalangeal (cruciate) ligaments also may allow excessive splaying of the digits and increase the risk of trauma to the interdigital space. Pain appears to increase with the size and degree of ulceration or infection of the mass.

Interdigital phlegmon *(bovine foot rot)* occurs when *F. necrophorum* and *Porphyromonas asaccharolytica* (formerly *Bacteroides melaninogenicus*) act synergistically to penetrate the epidermis and cause cellulitis. Although *Dichelobacter* is more important with interdigital dermatitis, the pathogenicity of *Fusobacterium* may dictate the severity of interdigital phlegmon. The lesion starts as a generalized soft tissue swelling in the interdigital space or heel bulb. Subsequent necrosis can lead to a splitting of the epidermis and an appearance similar to interdigital dermatitis. Deeper structures can be affected, and lameness can be severe. Because both interdigital dermatitis and phlegmon can be contagious, separation of diseased animals may be helpful.

The treatment of soft tissue lesions follows a general course: the foot should be cleaned thoroughly. Necrotic or proliferative (fibroma, proliferative dermatitis) soft tissue lesions should be debrided or resected. Granulation tissue must be debrided with care near the dorsal coronary band, because of the proximity of the joint capsule. Open soft tissue wounds may be treated with foot baths (10% zinc sulfate, 10% copper sulfate, or 5% formalin), topical disinfectants, or antibiotics, whereas systemic antibiotic therapy should be used if there is evidence of deep infection. Because most bacteria (except spirochetes) that affect the foot are anaerobic, penicillin-class antibiotics usually are effective.

Bandages may be used for open wounds, and the digits should be bandaged together if the lesion is in the interdigital space. If excessive laxity and splaying of the digits are contributing to trauma to the interdigital space, the toes may be wired together. Hoof lesions that may have contributed to soft tissue damage should be addressed through corrective hoof trimming and balancing. Management practices that promote soft tissue trauma or prolonged contact between the foot and manure or mud should be addressed, whereas routine foot baths are useful in decreasing the incidence and severity of interdigital infections. Because the disinfectants in foot baths are toxic, animals should not be allowed to drink the solutions.

 Technician Note

The source of most lameness in food animals is the foot.

Ischemic Lesions

Ischemic *(decreased blood supply)* lesions of the foot can occur as a result of *fescue foot*, ergotism, or frostbite. With ergotism, *Claviceps* spp. fungi invade the seeds of cereal and pasture grasses and produce ergot alkaloids. After ingestion, these cause arteriolar vascular spasms, which lead to ischemia. Nervous signs and agalactia also can be caused by the same or different toxins produced by the fungus. Fescue foot is a similar disease associated with tall fescue grass in cool seasons. A toxic agent produced by a fungus (not *Claviceps*) is the most likely cause. Signs with both syndromes occur days to weeks after exposure and are seen in the extremities (legs, ear tips, tail, nose), with hindlegs being the most common site. Lameness and pain are noted, with swelling and erythema from the fetlock to the coronary band. If the ischemia is severe and prolonged, a line of demarcation may be seen between healthy and affected tissues. Both syndromes are exacerbated by cold weather. Treatment consists of removing the source of toxin, avoiding cold, and enhancing circulation (hydrotherapy, hot packs). Protective salves and bandages may be helpful if the skin sloughs.

Frostbite also affects the extremities, especially of young animals. Such animals frequently have another disease condition that limits their activity. The upper hindleg is not tucked under the body in sternal recumbency and thus is the most common limb affected. Teat ends of dairy animals also can be affected, if sanitizing liquids are not dried off before exposure to cold. Clinical signs and treatment of frostbite resemble those of ergotism.

Skeletal Lesions

Septic arthritis, physitis, and osteomyelitis can be the result of direct inoculation through a wound, hematogenous seeding, or extension of infection from adjacent tissues. The larger joints are most commonly affected in septic arthritis, whereas osteomyelitis often affects long bones or vertebrae. Hematogenous origin of infection is most common in the young and often results in multiple sites being affected. Common clinical signs include lameness, joint distention, soft tissue swelling, pain on palpation, and warmth. Vertebral body osteomyelitis may lead to compression of spinal nerves or the spinal cord and can cause neurologic deficits.

Radiographs are useful in localizing and determining the extent of the lesion. Radiographic lesions include an increase or a decrease in the joint space, subchondral or medullary bone lysis, and periosteal bone reaction. Synovial fluid from infected joints contains high concentrations of protein and inflammatory cells.

Treatment consists of systemic antibiotics, nonsteroidal antiinflammatory agents, and removal of any septic focus (umbilicus). Joints may be lavaged with several liters of sterile isotonic fluids through an arthroscope or multiple large-bore hypodermic needles introduced into the affected joint space. If there are large fibrin deposits or proliferative synovium, an arthrotomy may be performed to establish drainage. Osteomyelitis or physitis may be treated with long courses of antibiotics with good bone penetration, but if there is a sequestrum or severe bone involvement, local curettage and infiltration of antibiotics may be necessary. A culture of synovial fluid or affected bone is useful in determining the appropriate antibiotic.

Digit Amputation

If the structures within the hoof are severely damaged, especially with digital osteoarthritis, amputation of the affected digit may provide the fastest and most satisfactory resolution of clinical signs. The hair should be clipped to the fetlock, and the region should be surgically prepared. After local or regional anesthesia is achieved, an incision is made through the skin from the interdigital space axially to the level of the proximal interphalangeal joint of the affected digit abaxially. Instead of completing the skin incision, the abaxial skin may be dissected off the digit before amputation and used to close the wound, but this is not recommended if infected structures are left on the

proximal stump. A wire saw is then used to excise the affected digit, using the skin incision as a guide. Care must be taken to remain below the fetlock joint. After amputation, the support structures of the remaining digit on that foot often break down because of increased weight load, although this may not occur for 1 year or longer.

Arthritis and Fractures

Viral arthropathies are very common in adult sheep and goats from flocks harboring the ovine progressive pneumonia (maedi) or caprine arthritis-encephalitis viruses, respectively. Affected adults typically have enlarged joints; they may also display long-term weight loss and respiratory disease. Lambs and kids may display weakness at birth or neurologic signs that develop over the first few months of life, with high mortality. Treatment of the individual animal is symptomatic and palliative. More important are management changes that can be made to prevent further spread of the viruses; these include serologic testing of all animals, with isolation or culling of seropositive stock or contact animals (sires). Colostrum is thought to be the major source of infection, so neonates should be separated from dams at birth and fed colostrum from seronegative dams or colostrum that has been pasteurized.

Fractures are managed as in other species, except that a poor prognosis must be given for upper limb lesions in larger animals. Economic constraints often restrict the use of internal fixation, leading to extensive use of casts, splints, and transfixation pins. Food animal species usually tolerate casts well, form exuberant callus, and are able to spend large amounts of time recumbent, contributing to the success of external fixation techniques. A block placed on the sole of the sound claw greatly increases soundness if the fracture is below the fetlock. Adequate footing and confinement are essential during the healing process.

Peripheral Neuropathies

The radial nerve is necessary to extend the elbow, and the femoral nerve is used to extend the stifle. Both may be damaged by excessive traction on the calf during a difficult birth (*obstetric paralysis of the calf*) and result in an inability to support weight on the affected leg. The sciatic and obturator nerves are most commonly damaged in the dam during birth because both course through the pelvic canal (*obstetric paralysis of the dam*). The obturator nerve is necessary for adduction of the hindlimb, especially if the animal is on poor footing, whereas the sciatic nerve is important for extension of the hip and flexion of the stifle and affects the lower hindleg through two major branches: the peroneal nerve (extension of the foot) and the tibial nerve (flexion of the foot). The peroneal branch is most commonly affected during birthing. The sciatic and tibial nerves can also be damaged by intramuscular injections given in the gluteal muscle region and on the craniolateral border of the semitendinosus muscle, respectively. Numerous nerves, including the radial, peroneal, and tibial, may also be damaged by pressure during extended periods of recumbency.

Drug treatment for peripheral nerve trauma includes corticosteroids in the acute stage, nonsteroidal antiinflammatory agents, and dimethyl sulfoxide (DMSO). Of equal or greater importance is supportive care, including making food and water easily accessible, slinging or hoisting the animal, good footing, and frequent rolling of the animal to prevent additional pressure damage to nerves and muscles. Smaller animals may benefit from physical therapy in a flotation tank, an option that is also available for cattle.

Myopathy

Any cause of excessive recumbency can lead to *downer syndrome*. This is a combination of nerve and muscle damage that tends to perpetuate the recumbency. The most common causes of recumbency are peripheral neuropathy, hypocalcemia, and severe musculoskeletal lesions. Myoglobinuria occurs with excessive muscle necrosis and can lead to renal damage; therefore adequate hydration of down animals is very important. Otherwise, treatment is similar to that recommended for peripheral neuropathy.

Tick paralysis is a myopathy that mimics peripheral neuropathy in that muscles are flaccid and neurologic reflexes are absent. The paralysis usually starts with hindlimb ataxia but progresses craniad. Death can result from respiratory paralysis or aspiration pneumonia. Geographic and seasonal factors are important in judging the likelihood of tick paralysis. Although affected animals frequently are covered with ticks, one engorged female tick can secrete sufficient toxin to affect a large animal. Therefore, in addition to downer animal care and topical or systemic acaricidal drugs, an earnest effort must be made to remove all ticks. Most animals will recover within 24 hours of removal of the tick.

Nutritional muscular dystrophy *(white muscle disease)* is a polysystemic disease caused by a deficiency in vitamin E or selenium. The disease is seen most commonly in juveniles born of dams fed deficient diets. Because these two compounds are important antioxidants, their deficiency leads to the greatest problems in metabolically active tissues, such as skeletal or cardiac muscle, and often follows periods of increased muscular exertion. In severe cases, myocardial damage leads to dyspnea or sudden death; this is the most common form in swine. The more common syndrome in ruminants is that of swollen, painful muscles; stiffness; and weakness caused by skeletal muscle involvement. Characteristic necropsy lesions include pale skeletal muscle and pale myocardial foci, although in pigs with sudden death, focal hemorrhage is seen in the cardiac muscle. Laboratory analyses for vitamin E and selenium status aid in the diagnosis. Treatment of clinical animals with injectable vitamin E and selenium compounds may be successful, although ultimately ration analysis and dietary modification are necessary.

A variety of anaerobic clostridial organisms can cause myonecrosis and cellulitis *(blackleg, malignant edema)*, especially in muscle damaged by rough handling, injections, or other trauma. The organisms may reach the site either hematogenously or through a wound. Clostridial myositis causes lameness with swollen, hot, painful muscles; fever; systemic toxemia; and sudden death. Although subcutaneous emphysema around the lesion is a hallmark sign in cattle, this is a less common finding in other species. A foul-smelling, serous fluid or gas is found when the lesion is opened or aspirated. Because of the extensive damage and toxemia, the prognosis is poor. Affected muscles can be treated by opening and cleansing the area to disrupt the anaerobic environment. Systemic penicillin and supportive care also may be beneficial. The diseases are endemic in some areas. Although information on efficacy is lacking, improved hygiene, vaccines, and management changes to avoid muscle damage may be useful in preventing these diseases.

Clostridial Neurotoxicities

Tetanus is caused by a central nervous system toxin elaborated by *Clostridium tetani* and results in generalized or localized hypertonia of skeletal muscles. Cattle are less susceptible than small ruminants. The source of infection is often the uterus for adult cattle (occurring as sequelae to metritis and retained fetal membranes) or a wound for small ruminants and pigs (caused by castration, disbudding, tail docking). Clinical signs of tetanus include stiff gait, prolapse of the third eyelid, hyperesthesia, bloat, trismus *(lockjaw)*, dysphagia, and death from asphyxiation (Figure 31-20). Diagnosis is often made on the basis of clinical signs and positive culture of an infected uterus or wound.

Treatment consists of high doses of parenteral and local procaine penicillin, tetanus antitoxin, and nursing care, which includes housing animals in dark, quiet, well-bedded stalls and provision of adequate nutrition and fluids. Prognosis is usually good for cattle and more

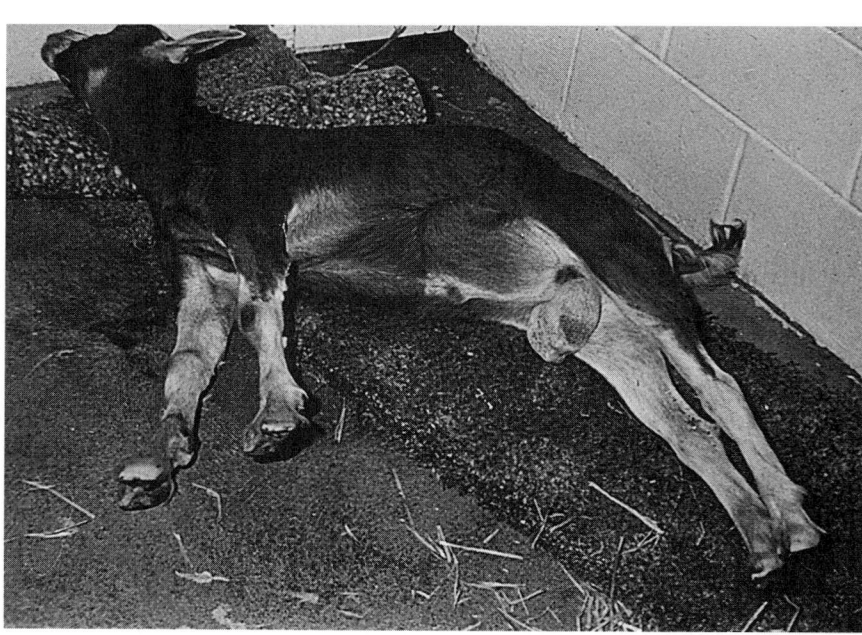

FIGURE 31-20. Goat with extensor rigidity caused by tetanus.

guarded for small ruminants. Prevention is best achieved by vaccination and improving management practices. Sheep and goats are regularly vaccinated, whereas cattle rarely need to be.

Botulism is a fatal, progressive disease of voluntary muscles resulting in flaccid paralysis. Ruminants are more susceptible than pigs. The neurotoxin acts peripherally at nerve endings and is elaborated by *Clostridium botulinum.* The source of the toxin for animals is usually a dead animal or decaying plant material. Clinical signs include reduced tongue tone, dysphagia, ataxia, ptosis, flaccid paralysis, and death. Diagnosis is often presumptive because it is difficult to grow the organism or isolate the toxin from gut contents of the animal or the feed source. Treatment is symptomatic and includes efforts to eliminate the toxin from the gut via ruminal lavage and purgatives and procaine penicillin. Polyvalent serum containing antibotulinum toxin antibodies is available and may be useful in subacute cases before the toxin is bound to nerve endings. Control measures consist mainly of good husbandry and disposal of carcasses.

BLOOD-BORNE DISEASES

Anaplasmosis occurs in cattle, sheep, and goats. It is a subclinical disease in sheep and goats. In cattle, however, it causes severe debilitation, anemia, and jaundice or abortion in adult cattle and neonatal weakness. The disease is caused by rickettsial bacteria, *Anaplasma marginale, A. centrale,* or *A. caudatam* in cattle and wild ruminants and *A. ovis* in sheep and goats. The organisms are blood borne. Mechanical transmission occurs via insect vectors, particularly ticks, or contaminated blood products. Morbidity is high during outbreaks, but mortality varies widely and increases with the age of the affected animal. Bison are naturally resistant to infection. Once infected, the food animal remains a carrier for many years. Clinical findings in cattle include fever, hemolytic anemia, jaundice, abortion, severe dyspnea, and death. Goats may occasionally succumb to a similar anemic syndrome. Diagnosis depends on serologic testing and the presence of insect vectors. Treatment consists of antibiotic administration and supportive care, including blood transfusions. Vaccines are available and are thought to be effective.

Eperythrozoonosis occurs in pigs, cattle, sheep, and llamas. The causative agent is *Eperythrozoon* spp., a rickettsia that parasitizes red blood cells. Disease is particularly important in pigs and immunocompromised llamas. Latent infections can occur in deer, elk, and goats. In swine, *Eperythrozoon suis* causes acute hemolytic anemia in stressed feeder pigs. Reproductive failure, weakness, and poor weight gain also may be seen in pigs of other ages. In cattle and sheep, *Eperythrozoon wenyoni* and *Eperythrozoon ovis* infections, respectively, often are subclinical but may cause ill-thrift, reproductive problems, and edema. Transmission is thought to occur through insect vectors or blood products. Diagnosis can be made by evaluation of a blood smear and positive identification of the organism on the periphery of red blood cell membranes or serologic testing. Treatment consists of antibiotics and blood transfusions if necessary.

URINARY DISORDERS

Urinary tract obstruction is the most common ailment of the urinary system in ruminants and potbellied pigs, as well as the most common cause of colic in many ruminant species. Castrated males are especially susceptible, although the condition also occurs in intact males and, rarely, females. Early clinical signs include colic, dysuria, and stranguria. Later signs may include anorexia, depression, death, or subcutaneous or abdominal swelling subsequent to a urethral or bladder rupture *(water belly).* Sites of obstruction, in order of occurrence, include the urethral process (small ruminants only), distal sigmoid flexure, pelvic urethra, and trigone (neck) of the bladder (Figure 31-21). Struvite calculi are most common in animals fed high-grain diets (feedlots), whereas carbonate calculi are most common overall. Silicate calculi may be seen in range animals in certain geographic areas. In most cases, multiple stones occlude the urethra, and still more are found in the bladder.

Technician Note
Urethral obstruction is the major cause of colic in many food animal species.

Optimal treatment often is dictated by the intended use of the animal. For feedlot animals, incising the ventral skin over a subcutaneous rupture site or dissecting out the sigmoid flexure and incising the urethra proximal to the obstruction will lead to resolution of the uremia and enable marketing of the animal. Amputation of the urethral process may lead to resolution of the obstruction in small ruminants, although this often is temporary. Attempts to clear the obstruction through retrograde catheterization rarely are successful because of the urethral diverticulum, and reobstruction is common.

Surgical options available for long-term correction of the obstruction include cystotomy, perineal urethrostomy, or both. Perineal urethrostomy may be performed with the animal under general, local, or regional (epidural) anesthesia and thus can be performed on animals of any size. Postoperative urethral strictures or reobstructions are common, especially in small ruminants or pigs. Preservation of breeding ability in males also precludes permanent perineal urethrostomy.

Perineal Urethrostomy
Perineal urethrostomy may be done with the animal standing or in lateral recumbency, with use of one of the above forms of anesthesia. The area behind the scrotum or scrotal

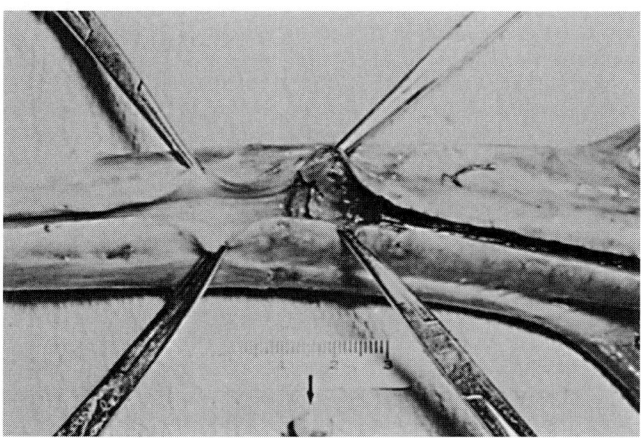
FIGURE 31-21. Obstruction of the urethra by a calculus in a steer with a corresponding mucosal lesion.

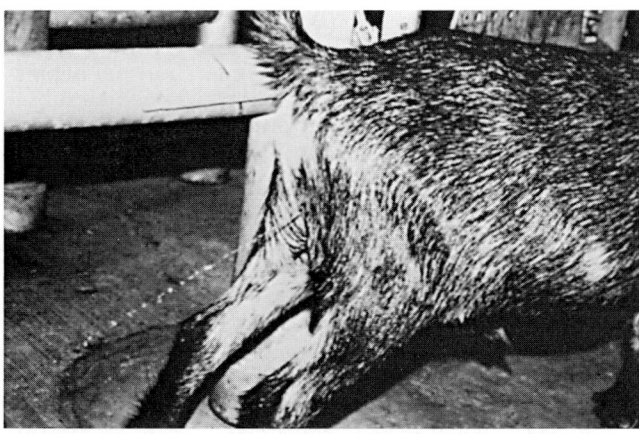

FIGURE 31-22. Healed perineal urethrostomy in a male goat. The goat is able to direct urine caudad.

remnant is clipped and surgically prepared. A midline incision is made over the distal sigmoid flexure, which then is dissected free of subcutaneous tissues, transected, and exteriorized. Care must be taken to transect the penis proximal to the attachment of the retractor muscles, or, alternatively, the distal stump should be amputated. The skin is closed around the protruding proximal penile stump, which is directed caudad, and the visible urethra is split longitudinally (Figure 31-22). Urine scald of the medial thigh is common after this procedure. Possible preservation of breeding ability may be achieved by performing a urethrotomy and removing any visible stones without anchoring or transecting the penis. In this case, the wound is left to close spontaneously once distal flow of urine is achieved.

Cystotomy

Cystotomy requires general anesthesia and is accomplished through a caudal ventral midline incision (see midline laparotomy section). The bladder is identified and exteriorized. A 2- to 4-cm incision is made into the bladder. Cystotomy allows for removal of all calculi from the bladder and normograde catheterization (passing the catheter from the bladder out to the end of the urethra) of the urethra to test patency. Distal obstruction or urethral spasms may prevent catheterization and are potential indications for performance of a perineal urethrostomy. The bladder incision is closed in two inverting layers, and the abdomen is closed routinely.

Combining cystotomy with perineal urethrostomy has given the best results in small ruminants, which rapidly reobstruct with urethrostomy alone. Conversely, recent evidence suggests that longer survival is attained by performing a tube cystotomy without urethrostomy in small ruminants, even if the distal urethra is left obstructed. This involves placing a bulb tip catheter through the body wall into the bladder during laparotomy. Temporary diversion of urine flow allows the urethra to relax and stones to pass. The catheter is removed after patency of the distal urethra is established, which may take several weeks. By performing this procedure without urethrostomy, postoperative urethral stricture is uncommon.

Medical management of other contact animals is recommended if there is a herd problem of urinary tract obstruction. Increasing dietary salt to 4% of the ration will increase water intake and urine volume, flushing small stones out of the bladder. Dietary ammonium salts acidify the urine and decrease formation of phosphate and carbonate stones. Ultimately, dietary modification is recommended to decrease formation of the specific type of stone.

Although cystitis and pyelonephritis (inflammation of the kidney) occur sporadically in ruminants, these diseases are common in pigs, especially those kept in confinement. The two most common bacterial isolates are *Eubacterium* (formerly *Corynebacterium*) *suis* and *Escherichia coli*, although many bacteria and the kidney worm *Stephanurus dentatus* also cause a similar disease. Clinical signs include repeat breeding, anorexia, pyuria or hematuria, fever, weight loss, and death. Although ascending infection after heavy fecal contamination of the perineum is blamed for the high incidence of this disorder in housed pigs, venereal transmission of *E. suis* from carrier males also can occur. Gross appearance of the urine often is sufficient to make a diagnosis, although bacteriologic culture of urine is useful in confirming the etiologic agent if there is a herd problem. Penicillin and ampicillin have good efficacy against *Eubacterium*, but a different antibiotic should be used if the infection is caused by a gram-negative organism.

REPRODUCTIVE DISORDERS

The major causes of dystocia are fetal/maternal size mismatch and fetal malpresentation. In animals with multiple fetuses (commonly pigs, sheep, and goats), malpresentation can be complicated by simultaneous entry of more than one fetus into the birth canal.

Early intervention is the key to successful resolution of dystocia. Multiparous animals should be able to deliver a fetus within 30 minutes of the onset of abdominal contractions, whereas in primiparous animals this should occur within 1 hour. If possible, examination of the animal with dystocia should begin with transrectal palpation for uterine torsion and presentation of the fetus or fetuses. If uterine torsion is not present, the dam's tail should be tied, the external vulva cleaned with surgical scrub, and vaginal examination performed. Epidural anesthesia may help reduce maternal straining during the vaginal examination or correction of a malpresentation, but this will also reduce maternal effort when the fetus is being delivered (Figure 31-23).

The fetus should be positioned so both hindlegs or the forelegs with the head are within the birth canal. To correct a flexed leg, the hoof should be directed caudomedially while the carpus or hock is directed craniolaterally until the leg can be extended. Adequate lubrication and traction should be used to deliver the fetus. If there is inadequate space in the birth canal to deliver the fetus, cesarean delivery or fetotomy should be performed. Neonates delivered after dystocia require more care than do those delivered normally.

Endometritis and retained fetal membranes are common problems in cattle, especially after induced or difficult parturition. Although such cattle typically have a fetid uterine discharge, they often are not clinically ill. Many treatments have been recommended for such cattle; however, it is generally accepted that intrauterine therapy is unnecessary, if not detrimental. Intramuscular prostaglandin injections may speed resolution of the condition, although this also is controversial. Oxytocin may be beneficial immediately postpartum but has decreasing efficacy after the first 24 hours. Cattle that demonstrate clinical signs, including fever, depression, and anorexia, should be treated aggressively because deeper layers of the uterus may be infected and fatal bacteremia or toxemia can occur.

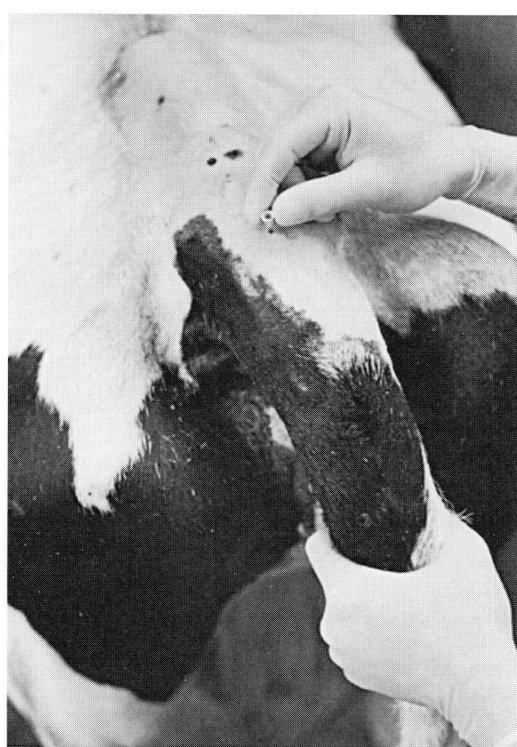

FIGURE 31-23. Epidural anesthesia in a cow. A 1.5-inch needle is placed into the epidural space between the first two coccygeal vertebrae.

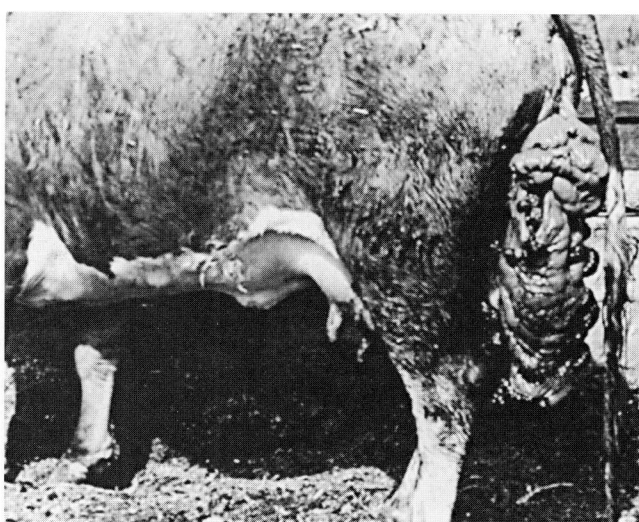

FIGURE 31-24. Complete uterine prolapse in a cow after calving, showing caruncles on the uterine wall.

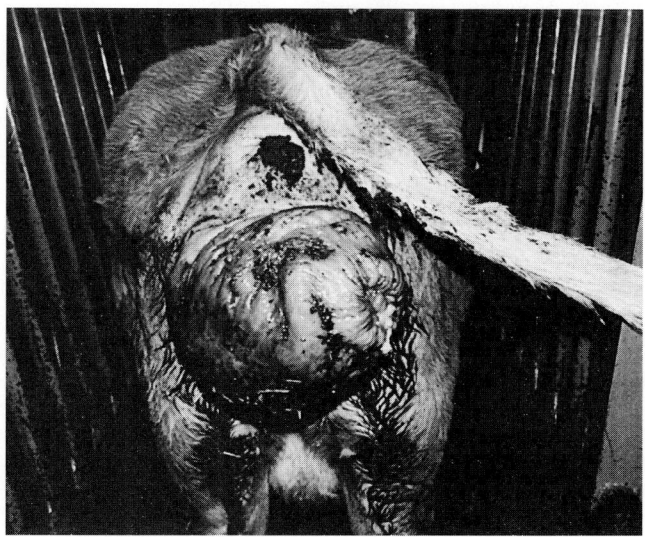

FIGURE 31-25. Cow with vaginal prolapse. The cow is restrained in a metal chute.

Systemic antibiotic treatment and lavage of the uterus with fluids to remove inflammatory debris may be beneficial for animals with systemic disease signs. Attempts to manually remove the placenta usually are not warranted. Small ruminants, pigs, and camelids are more susceptible to developing systemic disease signs with retained fetal membranes and therefore should be treated aggressively with antibiotics and oxytocin.

Postpartum straining and uterine inertia may allow prolapse of the uterus. This condition is easily recognized in ruminants by the presence of the caruncles on the inverted uterine tissue (Figure 31-24). Dystocia and hypocalcemia are important risk factors. To replace the uterus, epidural anesthesia should be administered and the prolapsed tissue should be cleaned. The cow may be left standing or restrained in dorsal recumbency with the hindlegs extended caudad *(frog legged)*. When possible, the cow should be positioned with the hindquarters higher than the forequarters, so gravity aids in replacement of the uterus. Elevation of the prolapsed uterus on a board or towel also will aid in replacement. Using firm pressure with the flat of the hands, the uterus must be worked back into the vagina. Once replaced, the horns should be palpated to ensure they are fully everted. A purse-string suture of umbilical tape may be placed in the subcutaneous tissue of the vulva to prevent recurrence of the prolapse.

Technician Note

Tetanus prophylaxis should be considered when treating uterine infections in small ruminants.

In contrast, prolapse of the vagina usually occurs in pregnant animals in which increased abdominal pressure and increased recumbency contribute (Figure 31-25). Short tail docking, hereditary factors, respiratory disease, estrogen-containing feeds, and obesity also contribute to prolapse. Vaginal prolapse usually is progressive during gestation and often will occur in that animal during subsequent pregnancies. Because of the progressive and possibly hereditary nature of this disorder, removal of the animal and its offspring from the breeding program should be considered. To treat, the prolapsed tissue should be cleaned and gently replaced with the animal under epidural anesthesia. Vaginal prolapse is very prone to recurrence despite the use of a vulvar purse-string suture or specialized retaining paddle. Epidural anesthesia with alcohol can be used to decrease straining for a longer period but should be reserved for animals that will be culled.

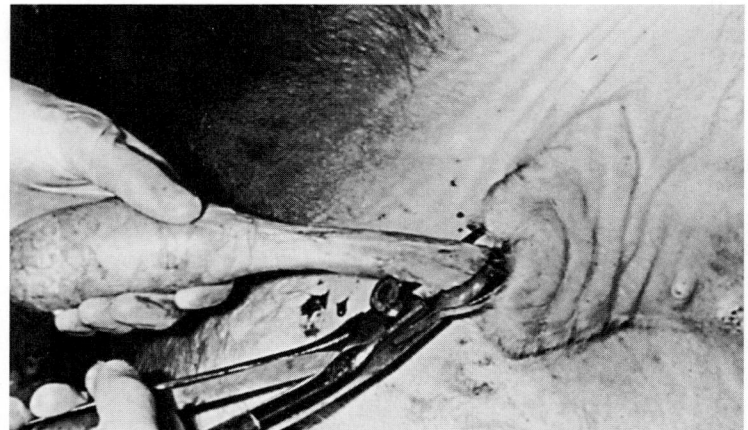

FIGURE 31-26. Open castration with an emasculator. The bottom of the scrotum has been removed with a scalpel blade.

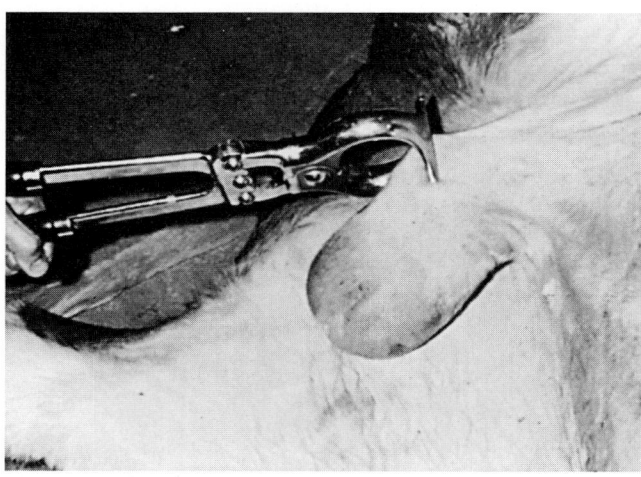

FIGURE 31-27. Closed castration with an emasculator. The two sides of the scrotum are crushed individually, with care taken to incorporate the spermatic cord in each crush.

Castration

Male ruminants have a pendulous scrotum, which allows easy access and good drainage. Castration usually can be performed without anesthesia if the animal is restrained adequately. To perform a surgical castration, the bottom third of the scrotal skin is removed. Each testicle is pulled out, a crushing clamp or emasculator is applied as high on the cord as possible, and the testicle is removed (Figure 31-26). The duration of the crush depends on the size of the animal. Because field castration is not a sterile procedure, the scrotal incision should be left open to drain, and antibiotic treatment may be indicated.

During fly season, nonsurgical castration may be preferred. This can be performed adequately on young ruminants with an Elastrator band (up to 2 weeks of age) or a Burdizzo clamp (up to 2 months of age), taking care that both testicles are completely below the level of the crush (Figure 31-27). Prophylactic vaccination against clostridial diseases, including tetanus, is recommended. Other procedures, such as dehorning and tail docking, may be performed at the same time.

Pigs and camelids do not have a pendulous scrotum but may be treated with surgical castration similar to ruminants and horses. Owners of pet pigs or camelids may prefer general anesthesia and a closed wound for castration. In those cases, the testicles should be removed using sterile technique through a prescrotal incision (similar to a canine castration), which then is closed.

DISEASES OF THE UDDER

Mastitis is the leading cause of lost income among dairy herds through treatment costs, decreased production, discard of affected milk, and premature culling of affected animals. Mastitis also is important in nondairy animals because maternal discomfort or decreased milk production may adversely affect the growth or health of nursing young. In rare cases, mastitis can be directly life threatening to the cow.

Several specialized tests are used to diagnosis mastitis. Strip-cup examination involves spraying some milk from each quarter individually onto a black surface to look for aggregations of cells *(clots or garget)*, one sign of clinical mastitis. The California Mastitis Test (CMT) involves mixing a small amount of milk from each quarter with a detergent. Detergent lysis of cell membranes allows aggregation of nucleic acids, causing a gel to form in the mixture. This test is useful for diagnosing subclinical mastitis or specific forms of mastitis in which clot formation is uncommon. A milk sample may be collected in a sterile tube for bacteriologic culture after the teat end has been cleaned with alcohol.

> **Technician Note**
>
> Because most mastitis is subclinical, prevention rather than treatment is the primary concern of dairy producers.

Staphylococcus aureus, Streptococcus agalactiae, and *Mycoplasma* spp. are commonly referred to as contagious organisms of mastitis because the main reservoir for infection is the infected gland of one cow, and the organism is spread to other cows during milking. Other streptococcal organisms (collectively referred to as *S. nonagalactiae*) are common environmental contaminants and cause mastitis after successful penetration of the teat cistern. Although invasion may occur in a contaminated environment, especially if the cow spends excessive time recumbent (seen with periparturient paresis, lameness, and inadequate stalls), these organisms usually contaminate the skin and gain access to the gland during milking.

Mastitis from gram-positive organisms is caused by bacterial attachment, invasion, and exotoxin release and the resultant inflammatory response. Often, cattle will have repeated bouts of clinical mastitis punctuating times of apparent normalcy. Subclinical mastitis results in decreased production and quality of milk and may only be detectable through CMT examination. Clinical mastitis results in visible milk clot formation and possibly reddening, warmth, and pain in the affected quarter. Systemic signs usually are absent, although the cow may display mild fever and an awkward gait. Rarely, peracute gangrenous mastitis can be caused by *S. aureus*.

There are many intramammary antibiotic preparations for the treatment of mastitis caused by gram-positive bacteria. In fact, systemic antibiotics probably are more efficacious, and many animals will clear the infection without treatment. Stripping of affected glands to remove debris and bacteria may be beneficial and is facilitated by the use of oxytocin. Proper hygiene during milking and separation of affected animals will reduce the incidence of all types of mastitis. Identification and segregation of animals with mastitis, antibiotic treatment of dry animals, and culling of persistently infected animals will help reduce herd incidence. In cases of chronic, nonresponsive mastitis, chemical destruction of the gland by injection through the teat end of formalin or chlorhexidine solution may be the best treatment option.

Mastitis caused by coliform organisms is potentially life threatening. The organisms are found in the environment and gain access to the gland in a similar fashion to *S. nonagalactiae*. Once in the gland, coliform organisms multiply rapidly and invoke a strong cellular immune response. Unlike gram-positive organisms, coliform bacteria release endotoxin during periods of rapid growth or destruction. Endotoxin triggers a cascade of endogenous inflammatory mediator release, which increases local blood flow, vascular permeability, and immune cell activity. Locally, the udder often is warm and erythematous, and the milk is replaced by a characteristic watery secretion. Clots are not always seen with coliform mastitis, but the secretion usually yields a very positive result on CMT because of the large numbers of bacteria and neutrophils.

Severe coliform mastitis resembles other diseases characterized by systemic endotoxemia or generalized weakness, making examination of the udder essential in such cows. Characteristically, there is tachycardia, tachypnea, anorexia, ruminal atony, and evidence of dehydration. Fever is an inconsistent finding. Treatment of coliform mastitis involves decreasing the effects of endotoxin. Frequent stripping out of the affected quarter will remove endotoxin and bacteria from the gland, whereas nonsteroidal antiinflammatory agents and oral or intravenous fluids will help combat the endotoxemia. Intramammary antibiotics are of limited value and should not be used in place of stripping. Systemic antibiotics may be of value in animals with severe, protracted disease. Vaccination with a gram-negative mutant bacterin appears to decrease the clinical signs of coliform mastitis.

Trauma to the teat end may allow invasion by *Arcanobacterium pyogenes* and lead to abscess formation in the gland. The characteristic secretion from the gland is thick and foul smelling. Similar to basic abscess management, adequate drainage, in this case through amputation of the distal teat end, may be necessary to resolve the infection. The affected quarter is highly unlikely to return to normal production, so chemical destruction of the gland also may be indicated to speed resolution of the infection.

Technician Note

Because of concerns about the presence of drugs and chemicals in our food supply, food animal veterinarians and producers must carefully adhere to guidelines concerning withdrawal times and extralabel use of drugs.

Teat lacerations potentially threaten the future production of a milking animal through mastitis or loss of the quarter. Trauma may also predispose the quarter to destruction by *A. pyogenes*. Surgical repair of lacerations is only necessary if the wound extends into the streak canal. In such a case, fine suture should be used to close the mucosa, submucosa, and skin in separate layers. A cannula or piece of tubing may be sutured into the streak canal to prevent stricture formation and allow milk to drain past the wound. Machine milking is less traumatic than hand milking and should be used during the recovery period. If possible, the injury should be repaired during the nonlactation period.

METABOLIC DISEASE

Hypocalcemia (*milk fever, parturient paresis*) is the most common of all metabolic diseases of dairy cattle and also occurs in sheep, goats, and pigs. It occurs when homeostatic mechanisms to mobilize calcium from bone or absorption from the gut fail to replace calcium lost from the plasma into milk at the onset of lactation or into the fetus during late gestation. Lactational hypocalcemia is most common in older dairy cows, particularly Channel Island breeds, and dairy goats. Ewes and pigs more frequently develop the problem during late gestation. Pigs fed a heavy concentrate ration with insufficient calcium supplementation can also develop clinical hypocalcemia.

Clinical signs vary depending on the severity of hypocalcemia. Signs often occur within 96 hours of delivery or within the last couple of weeks of gestation, although 7% of cases occur at other times associated with disease-induced anorexia. Signs range from mild excitement, tetany, and hyperesthesia to flaccid paralysis, loss of consciousness, and death. Sheep, goats, and pigs more frequently exhibit tetany than flaccid paralysis. If chronic calcium deficiency occurs, growing pigs may develop osteodystrophia fibrosa, whereas sows develop slipped femoral heads. Sheep often display dental maldevelopment. Other nonspecific signs of chronic calcium deficiency in food animals include poor growth, inappetence, stiffness, pathologic fractures, loss of condition, reduced milk production, and reduced fertility.

Treatment of acute hypocalcemia consists of slow intravenous or subcutaneous administration of calcium gluconate. Although subcutaneous administration is safer, intravenous administration often is necessary in severely affected animals. Products containing phosphorus also may be beneficial in hypocalcemic ruminants because many often have concurrent hypophosphatemia. Response to treatment often is rapid. Good footing and nursing care also are important to prevent recumbency-induced muscular and neurologic damage. Preventive measures in dairy cows include efforts to increase calcium mobilization during the dry period through dietary manipulation, including the feeding of high anionic salts during the dry period or reducing calcium in the diet in the last 2 weeks of gestation. Injections of vitamin D_3 at specific times during gestation also are reported to be beneficial.

> ### Technician Note
> Diagnosis of hypocalcemia is based on clinical signs and rapid response to treatment. Blood analysis can confirm the diagnosis only retrospectively.

Hypomagnesemia *(grass tetany, grass staggers, transport tetany)* occurs most commonly in lactating beef cows but can occur in dairy cows, pigs, sheep, and goats under certain management conditions. It occurs commonly in ruminants on rapidly growing grass pastures, winter wheat, or other cereal crops. Cattle and sheep that are transported long distances or ruminants or recently weaned pigs fed marginally low magnesium diets are susceptible to hypomagnesemia. Affected ruminants often are hypocalcemic as well as hypomagnesemic. Clinical signs relate to the role of magnesium in neuromuscular conduction. Ruminants frequently exhibit tetany, muscle fasciculations, excitability, aggression, seizures, and convulsions. Signs of hypocalcemia also may be present. Pigs may show weakness of the pasterns, particularly in the forelegs, causing backward bowing of the legs, sickled hocks, hyperirritability, arched back, reluctance to stand, and tetany. Death ensues if treatment is not given.

Treatment consists of subcutaneous administration of magnesium sulfate or mixtures of calcium, magnesium, phosphorus, and potassium, followed by oral magnesium oxide. Clinical signs often resolve quickly with treatment. Prevention consists of feeding magnesium supplements to animals maintained on pastures low in magnesium or concentrates low in magnesium and minimizing contact with lush, green, young pastures.

Ketosis, hepatic lipidosis, and fatty liver are all conditions associated with negative energy balance in ruminants. Ruminants typically exist in a state of low glucose availability. They have adapted to use lipids for energy, but with severe or prolonged negative energy balance, there can be clinical complications associated with the mobilization of peripheral fat stores in the form of fatty acids for energy. Some fat is incompletely oxidized by the liver to ketone bodies. These can be utilized for energy, but excessive ketones spill into the urine and milk.

Causes of negative energy balance include late pregnancy, heavy lactation, anorexia, and concurrent disease. Clinical ketosis *(acetonemia)* occurs typically in early lactation cows and often is accompanied by persistent hypoglycemia. Spontaneous recovery may occur as cows reduce their milk production to match energy intake. Hepatic lipidosis *(fatty liver)* occurs when the transport of fat to the liver overwhelms the ability of the liver to export or metabolize fat.

Pregnancy toxemia shares many metabolic similarities with ketosis. It occurs in sheep, goats, and cows with multiple fetuses or in advanced pregnancy. Unlike postpartum ketosis and fatty liver, pregnancy toxemia is irreversible without aggressive treatment because of the inability of the affected ruminant to decrease energy flow to the fetus. It also can result in hepatic lipidosis. Mortality is associated with severe dehydration and acidosis. Camelids may develop hyperlipemia and ketonuria in late gestation in response to inadequate energy intake. When faced with severe metabolic stress, camelids convert excess fatty acids to triglycerides and incorporate them in lipoproteins that are poorly cleared by peripheral tissues.

Clinical signs of clinical ketosis, pregnancy toxemia, and fatty liver are indistinguishable and include depression, lethargy, decreased milk production, and anorexia. Rabies-like neurologic signs, such as excessive salivation, excitement, blindness, and head pressing, may be seen (nervous ketosis). Diagnosis may be aided by measurement of serum glucose concentration and urine or milk dipstick for ketone bodies.

The major goal of therapy for these metabolic diseases is to reestablish normal appetite and energy balance and interrupt the destructive feedback loop of fuel utilization. Elective abortion, cesarean delivery, or induced parturition can be considered for pregnancy toxemia and hyperlipemia in camelids. Restoration of normal energy metabolism involves restoring normal blood glucose and ketone body levels. Therapeutics include intravenous fluids supplemented with glucose, oral glucose precursors such as propylene glycol and glycerol, glucocorticoids, insulin, and niacin. Often, ruminants with severe clinical ketosis and hyperlipemia are refractory to treatment.

Polioencephalomalacia *(polio)* is a noninfectious disease of ruminants characterized by cerebrocortical necrosis. Clinical signs are referable to the central nervous system and include blindness, depression, incoordination, recumbency, convulsions, and death. Polio has been associated with improper diets, such as certain milk replacers, high carbohydrates (leading to rumen acidosis), selenium toxicosis and deficiency, poisonous plants, mycotoxins, cobalt deficiency, and sulfate toxicity. Regardless of the cause, the disease is responsive to thiamine treatment during the early stages. Although thiamine deficiency has been postulated as the cause of this disease, this has not been demonstrated. Thiamine is important in cerebral energy metabolism, and the responsiveness of the syndrome to thiamine treatment suggests that the common pathogenesis involves impaired cerebral energy metabolism.

Definitive diagnosis of polio is based on postmortem evidence of cerebrocortical necrosis. Presumptive diagnosis can be achieved by measurement of erythrocyte or tissue thiamine levels, ruminal thiaminase activity, or erythrocyte transketolase activity. Responsiveness to thiamine supplementation is supportive but not conclusive of the diagnosis. Treatment consists of parenteral thiamine supplementation, dietary modification, and possibly rumen transfaunation.

NEONATAL PROBLEMS

Young stock are an important commodity for many ruminant producers. Lambs, piglets, crias, kids, and calves represent the marketable commercial product for their respective producers, as well as the genetic stock for future generations. Care and treatment of the neonate can be divided into several topics: management in the immediate postpartum period, colostral considerations, differentials for the weak neonate, general treatment approach for neonates, and other specific problems, such as diarrhea, sepsis, and congenital defects.

During parturition, the newborn experiences severe stress, temperature changes, and oxygen deprivation. These stresses trigger elevations in catecholamine and cortisol levels that stimulate the newborn to adapt to extrauterine life. Adaptation to extrauterine life is a dynamic process. Fetal organs must adjust to autonomous function in an aerobic environment. Some adaptive changes must be made immediately, such as adjusting to air breathing, whereas others are more gradual, such as development of a competent immune system.

Management of the neonate immediately postpartum

consists of facilitating the many physiologic changes occurring at that time. At birth, physical stimulation and oxygen debt encourage the newborn to develop rhythmic, productive respirations. Surfactant is produced in the lungs under the influence of cortisol and helps reduce alveolar surface tension. Fetal lung fluid is gradually absorbed, and alveoli are cleared to enable oxygen absorption. The producer or technician can facilitate adaptation of the respiratory system of the neonate by manually rubbing and stimulating the newborn, clearing fluid from the nasal and oral cavities manually or with suction, positioning the animal in sternal recumbency, and providing intranasal oxygen if necessary. With the first few respiratory efforts, the pulmonary vascular resistance in the neonate declines and the systemic vascular resistance increases comparatively. As a result, the cardiovascular system switches from fetal circulation, which is centered on the umbilicus, to the adult system of circulation, which is centered on the lungs. Cardiovascular fetal shunts, such as the foramen ovale and ductus arteriosus, close gradually. The producer and technician can facilitate these cardiovascular changes by providing oxygen as necessary and encouraging the neonate to move around and breathe well.

At birth, the neonate leaves a temperature-controlled environment (the uterus) and enters an environment with a wide range of temperature extremes. Immediately, the neonate starts to lose body heat. The neonate attempts to compensate for heat loss by nonshivering and shivering thermogenesis. Physical activity increases thermogenesis and can be encouraged by the producer and technician. Provision of external heat via blankets, hot water bottles, or heat lamps can enable the neonate to maintain body heat without as much energy and effort on its part. Glycogen is the major energy source for thermogenesis and is depleted quickly. The producer and technician can replace depleted glucose by quickly providing the neonate with high-quality, warm colostrum.

Technician Note

Basic neonatal care includes cauterization of umbilical remnants, application of suction or manual clearance of air passages, and vigorous rubbing to warm, dry, and stimulate the neonate.

The neonatal food animal is exposed to infectious agents at birth but has limited endogenous immune capabilities. Unlike carnivores, which receive maternal antibodies in utero, the neonatal artiodactylid relies on colostral ingestion to receive maternal immunoglobulins (*passive transfer*). Ability of the neonate to absorb colostral antibodies decreases with time; therefore it is important that appropriate amounts of high-quality colostrum be offered postnatally to the newborn in a timely fashion. The quality of the colostrum depends on the age and breed of the dam from which it is obtained (older animals are better), postpartum time during which it is collected (early postpartum is best), storage (stable when frozen), and source (same farm is better than from elsewhere). Ideally, the neonate should receive at least 10% of its body weight of high-quality colostrum within the first 12 hours of birth. Frequent, small feedings are best (every 2 hours if possible). The best absorption occurs if the neonate suckles the dam; however, the amount consumed cannot be regulated. Bottle feeding is better than orogastric administration via an esophageal feeder, but the latter ensures that the entire quantity reaches the gut for absorption.

Colostrum can be qualitatively assessed by use of a colostrometer, which provides a crude estimation of the specific gravity of the liquid (excellent, specific gravity of more than 1.047). Good-quality colostrum is only one part of the procedure to ensure adequate immune protection of the neonate; the other part is the absorptive capacity of the neonate, which can be reduced by hypoxemia. Techniques for assessment of neonatal immunoglobulin absorption vary in cost, ease of use, availability, and quantity measured. They include refractometry for total plasma solids, precipitation and coagulation tests (zinc sulfate, sodium sulfite, glutaraldehyde), latex agglutination, and radial immunodiffusion. Not all these tests measure the same serum component, and they must be interpreted in light of their limitations. To determine the success of passive transfer, one of these tests should be performed at approximately 24 hours of age to allow maximal time for colostral ingestion and absorption. Determination of passive transfer of immunoglobulin status of the neonate by any of these methods provides only a rough assessment of disease resistance.

There are several important problems or differentials to consider when evaluating a weak, unthrifty neonate. One of the most common is hypoxemia or perinatal asphyxia. Dystocia or prematurity contributes to these problems. An important sequela of hypoxemia and asphyxia is widespread organ damage or malfunction. The neonate usually shows neurologic signs, including the inability to maintain sternal recumbency or to stand, poor suckle reflex, hyperventilation followed by reduced respiratory efforts, and dull demeanor.

Hypoxemia can be diagnosed definitively by arterial blood gas analysis. Suspected hypoxemia should be treated by efforts to improve aeration of the lungs. Intranasal oxygen may be sufficient to correct this problem, but in some cases intubation and use of an Ambu bag or a ventilator may be required if poor ventilation is suspected. Fluid support may help correct lactic acidosis caused by tissue hypoxia. The use of epinephrine during ventilatory support may be beneficial.

Two other common differentials to consider for a weak neonate are hypoglycemia and hypothermia. These two problems are common if the food animal is born in the field during cold or damp weather and does not get dry or nurse quickly. Septicemia also can cause hypoglycemia in the later, advanced stages of the disease. Hypoglycemia and hypothermia can be diagnosed by a rectal body temperature reading for the latter and measurement of blood glucose concentrations for the former. Treatment for hypothermia consists of using towels or a hair dryer to help dry the neonate; provision of blankets, hot water bottles, or a heat lamp; provision of shelter away from adverse weather conditions; and the administration of warm isotonic fluids parenterally or warm colostrum orally. Treatment of hypoglycemia consists of fluids with glucose added and provision of warm colostrum orally.

Prenatal or postnatal infections may result in a weak neonate. The neonatal food animal may not show signs of disease for several days to weeks. Signs may be localized to a particular organ system, such as the lungs, gastrointestinal tract, umbilicus, or joints, or manifest as more widespread and generalized disease, such as diffuse septicemia. The umbilicus may serve as a wick to draw infection from the environment; therefore cauterization of the umbilical remnants at birth with iodine solutions may decrease infection entering the neonate through that route.

The major predisposing factor for the development of neonatal septicemia is failure of the neonate to acquire adequate passive immunity from colostrum. Causative organisms are those residing in the environment of the neonate and frequently include gram-negative bacteria. Clinical signs of septicemia are nonspecific and include weakness, depression, and reluctance or inability to stand and suckle; neurologic dysfunction; and ophthalmologic abnormalities. Fever and diarrhea are inconsistently observed. Confirmation of septicemia depends on isolation of the causative bacterial organism from the blood. Because blood culture results are unavailable for several days, diagnosis often is based on clinical signs and ruling out other causes of the weak neonate.

Treatment for localized infection depends on the site but consists of antibiotics, antiinflammatory agents, and possibly local wound management. Therapeutic aims for generalized septicemia are directed toward decreasing bacterial numbers, decreasing the effects of endotoxemia, improving the immune status of the neonate, and supportive care. Specific treatment includes antibiotics selected on the basis of bacterial identification and susceptibility patterns, antiinflammatory agents, intravenous fluids, and species-specific plasma or whole blood.

Another common cause of a weak neonate is infectious diarrhea. Morbidity and mortality result from dehydration and acidosis caused by fluid and electrolyte losses rather than gut damage itself. Diarrhea in neonatal food animals results from a complex interaction among etiologic, immunologic, and husbandry factors. Diarrheal disease often occurs under conditions of overcrowding and poor sanitation. Common etiologies in calves, pigs, goats, and sheep include *E. coli*; rotavirus and coronavirus; coccidia such as *Cryptosporidium* spp., *Isospora*, or *Eimeria*; and *Clostridium perfringens*. Pigs and calves also may have diarrhea caused by *Enterococcus durans*. Uncommonly, *Salmonella* spp. can cause diarrhea in neonates but often causes septicemia because of absorption of the organism into the bloodstream through the damaged gut.

The enteric viruses and *Cryptosporidium* spp. infect the cells lining the intestinal tract and thereby interfere with digestion and absorption of milk. One unique feature of the life cycle of *Cryptosporidium* is its potential for autoinfection as a result of recycling merozoites or sporozoites within the gut (see Chapter 6). Thus relapses after apparent cure are common. *E. coli* causes diarrhea by secreting a toxin that causes hypersecretion of water and electrolytes by the intestinal lining cells. Septicemic colibacillosis may occur if the bacteria enter the bloodstream through the damaged gut. These bacteria, as well as *Salmonella* spp. and *Cryptosporidium* spp., have zoonotic potential. Enterotoxemia caused by *C. perfringens* causes high mortality because of vascular effects of the exotoxin elaborated. Bovine virus diarrhea (BVD) is an uncommon cause of diarrhea in neonatal calves. Congenital defects are another manifestation of BVD infection. Historically, older cows on the farm may also have diarrhea.

All these causes of infectious diarrhea result in dehydration, depression, gastrointestinal atony, and weakness in addition to diarrhea in the neonatal food animal. Sometimes, the animal dies before diarrhea is observed, because of *C. perfringens* or *Salmonella*. In such cases, bloat, fever, colic, and anorexia may be the only clinical signs. Treatment for neonatal diarrhea involves replacement of fluid and electrolyte losses. Oral fluids may suffice if the neonate is still suckling. However, intravenous administration is required if the animal is poorly responsive or inappetent. Physical examination, blood gas, and serum biochemical panel can aid in evaluation of the calf and direct appropriate bicarbonate, electrolyte, and fluid supplementation.

Replacement fluids should consist of a balanced electrolyte mixture with amounts estimated based on percentage dehydration, with the average calf requiring 2 to 6 L. If bicarbonate deficits exceed the amounts provided in the polyionic fluids, supplemental sodium bicarbonate should be provided (Bicarbonate (mEq) = Body weight (kg) × 0.6 × Base deficit). If used, systemic administration of antibiotics is vastly superior to oral administration. Antibiotics may protect against secondary bacterial infections and septicemia, although their efficacy against the enteric pathogens per se is questionable. The neonate should be kept in a clean, warm, dry environment and be provided good nutritional support (continued milk feeding).

> **Technician Note**
>
> With undifferentiated neonatal scours, maintenance of fluid and electrolyte balance is the major goal of treatment.

Prematurity or congenital defects may be responsible for weakness in food animals. Premature food animals adapt to extrauterine life more slowly than do full-term animals. Problems may include poor suckle reflex, hypoxemia and impaired ventilatory effort, inability to stand or thermoregulate, or abnormal mentation. Some problems resolve over time with supportive therapy. Because poor colostral absorption is a common sequela to prematurity, the premature neonate should be frequently offered good-quality colostrum or provided with plasma if necessary. Congenital defects can include any number of derangements that impair normal neonatal behavior and function. Depending on the severity of the problem, directed treatment or supportive care may be warranted.

A minimum data base may help to accurately evaluate a weak, unthrifty neonate and distinguish between problems. These tests include the following:

- A measurement of serum immunoglobulin to determine passive transfer of maternal antibodies
- Complete blood count and plasma fibrinogen measurement to identify focal or widespread inflammation or infection
- Arterial blood gas analysis to diagnose respiratory impairment
- Aerobic and anaerobic blood cultures to identify causative organisms and direct antibiotic therapy
- Serum chemistry panel to identify metabolic or organ dysfunction

If the ruminant has signs specific to the gastrointestinal system (colic, abdominal distension, absence of feces), abdominal radiographs may be important. Methods for collecting samples to run these tests are described in Chapter 3.

Other tests may be appropriate for identifying focal disease processes; these include thoracic radiographs for pneumonia, fecal culture (float or smear) or viral isolation for infectious causes of diarrhea, abdominal radiographs for gastrointestinal obstructions or congenital gastrointestinal defects, joint tap for cytology and culture if joint distention is present, and ultrasound of the umbilical remnants if umbilical swelling, heat, or pain is present.

Even in the field without access to a clinical pathology laboratory, some of these tests can be performed to differentiate causes of weakness; these include a good physical examination with rectal temperature and auscultation of the chest, glucose dipstick using whole blood, and a field test for immunoglobulin estimation.

NEOPLASIA

Lymphoma

The bovine leukemia virus (BLV) is an oncogenic retrovirus spread through transmission of infected lymphocytes between animals. Hypodermic needles, rectal sleeves, dehorning and tatooing instruments, and semen may transmit the virus from one animal to another, making the veterinarian and technician important potential vectors. Although most new infections occur in calves, disease signs often take years to develop. Most infected cattle do not develop clinical disease, although many develop high peripheral blood lymphocyte counts. A small percentage of infected adult cattle develop multicentric lymphoma, with the lymph nodes, heart, uterus, abomasal wall, kidneys, and retrobulbar space being common sites of tumor formation. Clinical signs are variable, depending on the location of the masses, but include mass lesions, weight loss, melena, fever, and exophthalmia. Treatment usually is not economically feasible, and the disease is rapidly fatal. Although cattle are the primary host for BLV, other species may develop lymphoma after being infected with bovine blood products. Serologic tests can be used to identify infected animals, which may be culled from the herd. Thymic, cutaneous, and multicentric lymphomas also occur sporadically in juvenile cattle and camelids, swine, and small ruminants of all ages, but these neoplasms are not thought to have a contagious cause.

Technician Note

Although serologic testing is useful for identifying retrovirus-infected animals, only a small portion of these animals will develop clinical disease.

Squamous Cell Carcinoma

Ocular squamous cell carcinoma is the most common malignancy in cattle in many parts of the world. Ultraviolet radiation (altitude) and unpigmented ocular membranes increase risk. Growths start as pale pink plaques, usually on the limbus, eyelid margin, or third eyelid, but can become large and papillomatous (Figure 31-28). Early lesions may be treated with topical liquid nitrogen sprays or hyperthermia, whereas larger lesions or those that threaten to invade deep periorbital tissues should be removed by exenteration (ocular removal). Metastasis of tumor to local lymph nodes is rare but can occur with long-standing lesions. Gastrointestinal and urinary tract squamous cell carcinomas also occur in ruminants and camelids and are thought to have a toxic etiology.

Exenteration (Enucleation)

The skin around the eye is clipped and aseptically prepared. Regional anesthesia is achieved by infiltrating the retrobulbar space with a local anesthetic agent and blocking the auriculopalpebral nerve at the lateral canthus of the eye (Figure 31-29). The lids may be sutured or clamped together. An elliptic incision 1 cm from the lid margins is made around the eye. Subcutaneous and periorbital tissues are separated from the orbit by a combination of blunt and sharp dissection until the tissue behind the globe can be transected. All tumor tissue should be removed. The eye is removed, and the incision is closed with simple interrupted or cruciate sutures.

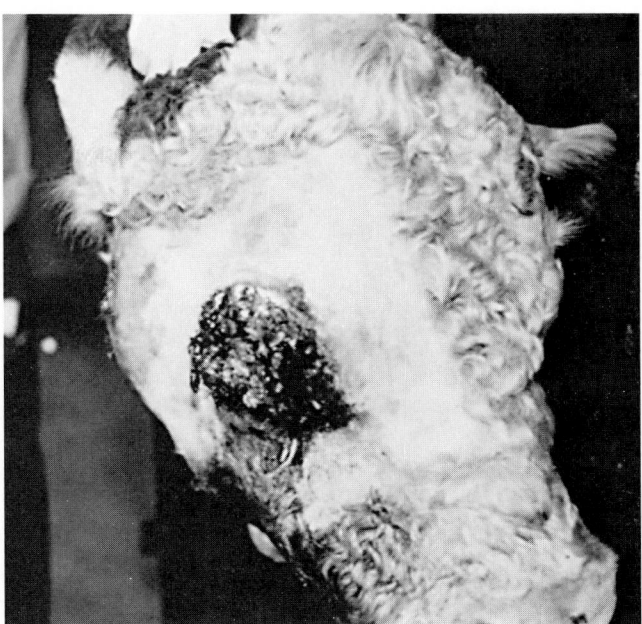

FIGURE 31-28. Advanced ocular squamous cell carcinoma (cancer eye) in Hereford bull.

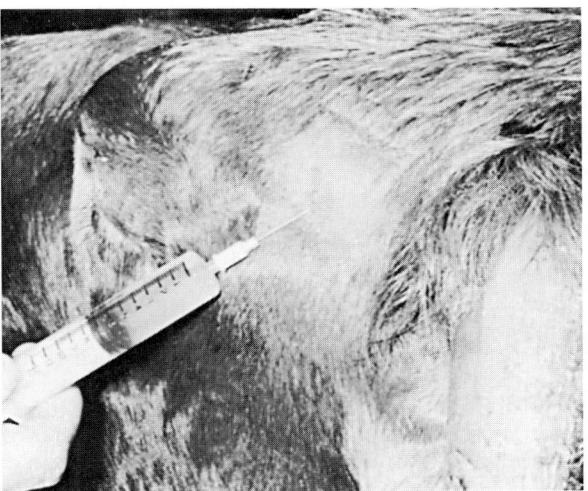

FIGURE 31-29. Corneal nerve block on a cow. The anesthetic agent is deposited subcutaneously, midway between the lateral canthus of the eye and the base of the horn.

RECOMMENDED READING

Howard JL: *Current veterinary therapy: food animal practice,* 4, Philadelphia, 1998, Lea & Febiger.

Noordsy JL: *Food animal surgery,* ed 3, Trenton, NJ, 1994, Veterinary Learning Systems.

Radostits OM, Blood DC, Gay CC: *Veterinary medicine: a textbook of the diseases of cattle, sheep, pigs and horses,* ed 8, Philadelphia, 1994, Bailliere Tindall.

Smith BP: *Large animal internal medicine,* ed 2, St Louis, 1996, Mosby.

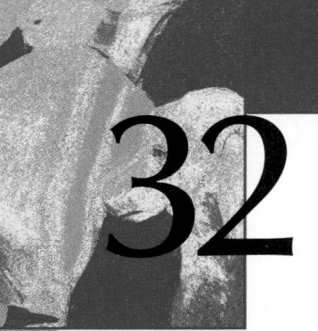

32

Veterinary Practice Management

Roger L. Lukens • Dennis M. McCurnin

Each veterinary practice is a professional business that offers medical care to animals with their owners' consent. Only willing owners consent to pay a fee for professional services provided by the veterinary team. The total cost of operating a medical business for providing these services is paid by the gross income of the practice. Therefore marketing efforts must effectively attract (and retain) sufficient clients to each practice or it will go bankrupt. No professional veterinary business will survive if it is not profitable.

The highest quality of care possible for the animals must be offered to their owners in a cost-effective (not cost-cutting) manner; this is extremely important to both patients and their owners. A high-quality practice requires keeping up with the latest medical knowledge and technologies. It also requires the most effective and caring communication possible with owners by the entire veterinary team. Quality communication is absolutely necessary to inform, educate, and obtain owner compliance for the veterinarian's recommendations to benefit the animal.

The profitability of the practice and the care of the client's animal are at risk if the veterinary team fails to deliver quality medical care for the animal coupled with caring effective communication with the owner. The services of the veterinary team are not successful unless the patient is helped and the client understands the service; the client is pleased with the caring attitude of the team; the client tells others of his or her enthusiasm for that practice; and the client wants to return for future veterinary care of pets. Veterinary technicians are very important to the success of the veterinary team in accomplishing these goals.

Effective management of the veterinary practice as a business is also necessary because of increased competition, growing malpractice threats, new technology, free Internet information, shifting client expectations, and continuing inflation of medical equipment, supply, and personnel costs. All these risks and challenges must be well managed to enhance both productivity and quality of patient care.

It has been said, "What is good business may be bad medicine, and what is good medicine may be bad business." Veterinary practice represents the *art* of balancing both business and medicine to meet the needs of patients, clients, and the veterinary team.

VETERINARY PRACTICE MANAGEMENT AREAS

Veterinary students are naturally interested in managing nursing care of patients. They must realize the necessity of effective client communication to benefit the patient and begin to understand the business side of medicine. This develops only after gaining significant experience in a veterinary practice. Managing equipment, facility, staff, and marketing is not of much interest until the student has experienced problems or limitations in these areas that have a negative impact on patient care (or technician salary).

Each of these management areas (Box 32-1) must be coordinated with the other areas to meet the veterinary team's goals for the operation (mission statement and strategic plan). A successfully managed practice enjoys success and accomplishment with people, both internally and externally. Failure to properly manage patients, people, and the business ultimately leads to a reduction in the quality of service rendered, staff dissatisfaction, staff turnover, a disorganized practice, dissatisfied clients, and decreasing business.

Veterinary Facilities

The type of practice facility will vary greatly according to the needs of the clients and the species of animals served by the practice staff. *Facility design* must accommodate the needs of the patients, the number of clients served, the interests of the veterinarians, the level of care to be provided, and the financing available for investing in the

---

BOX 32-1   MANAGEMENT AREAS

Facility design	Building
Patient care	Equipment
Client communications	Medical records
Human resources	Inventory control
Finance	Computerization
Marketing	

BOX 32-2   VETERINARY FACILITY NOMENCLATURE

Office—Room where limited or consultative type of practice is conducted

Mobile facility—A vehicle for making house or farm calls *or* a vehicle equipped with special medical and/or surgical facilities; both must have a permanent base of operations (published address and telephone number)

Clinic—Outpatient practice facility *not* offering overnight patient confinement

Hospital—Inpatient practice facility offering overnight hospitalization of patients

Emergency facility—Emergency practice facility that focuses primarily on treating and monitoring emergencies with veterinarian and staff who are always available (during specified hours of operation) and equipped to provide timely and appropriate level of emergency care

On-call emergency service—Veterinarians and staff are not on premises all the time but are available via on-call basis to handle emergency calls

Referral center—Staffed with board-certified specialist veterinarians who receive referrals from the primary care practitioners of the above facilities; sometimes called secondary care facility

Animal medical center—A large facility (veterinary teaching hospitals, large corporate practices) offering consultative, clinical, and hospital services to referred clients and their local veterinarian; also performs significant research on animal health problems and conducts advanced professional education programs; sometimes called tertiary care facility

---

facility. Many facilities are simply expanded and remodeled. Occasionally the existing facility is totally replaced with one redesigned to meet the above goals.

The practice may limit veterinary service to a single species (feline, equine, swine, cattle), to small animals (dogs, cats, exotic pets), to large animals (any livestock, horses), to exotic animals, or to a mixed practice (all species). Each type of practice has unique requirements for a facility that is designed to accommodate their patients and clients. Large animal and mixed practices may provide all veterinary services on the owner's premises, have haul-in facilities for these species, or provide both options as a convenience to the client.

The majority of practicing veterinarians are general practitioners who offer *primary care* level of services. They increasingly refer problem cases to specialists at referral practices (*secondary care* providers) or veterinary schools (*tertiary care* providers). These specialists are board-certified in one of the following: surgery, internal medicine, dermatology, ophthalmology, or other areas. Once treatment by the specialists is finished, the patient and client are transferred back to the primary care provider. Primary care providers are also able to use the skills of consultant specialists to read x-rays and ultrasound images as well as electrocardiograms (ECGs) or consult with specialists by telephone or the Internet without referring the case.

Many diseases are not fully understood because diagnostic methods are unavailable, clinical treatments are inadequate, and prevention is not yet possible. Therefore this network of referring practitioners not only is providing the best quality of care possible, but also is the foundation of supporting clinical research at the tertiary care centers at the veterinary schools. Both clinical and basic science research is absolutely necessary to discover the pathogenesis of unsolved diseases, new and effective diagnostics, effective treatments, and ultimately, the preventative steps necessary to avoid patient death and client despair.

Facility Nomenclature

Numerous terms are applied to veterinary facilities. The American Veterinary Medical Association (AVMA) has developed guidelines (Box 32-2) for consistency in naming veterinary facilities to avoid confusion by the general public. In addition, many state practice acts and regulations not only have been updated to specify standards of practice and professional competency for both veterinarians and technicians but also have adopted facility and equipment requirements and hired inspectors to ensure that these standards are being met. The American Animal Hospital Association (AAHA) also has extensive standards of excellence that cover most of the management areas listed in Box 32-1. These must be met to have the hospital accredited by AAHA.

Management of Hospital Areas

The small animal hospital (see Box 32-2) is the most complete facility for primary care practice for small animals. It provides the best model for discussing location, function, and management of each of the facility areas in this chapter. Good management of hospital areas is the foundation to understanding the principles of improving the efficiency of any practice. Conversely, lack of attention to facility area management ultimately leads to inefficiencies, disorder of the practice, staff frustration, loss of income, and decrease of the quality of client service and patient care.

Small animal hospital facilities are designed to provide overnight hospitalization, complete surgical facilities, and sufficient examination rooms to provide outpatient services. They also must have ancillary support areas to provide reception, laboratory, pharmacy, imaging, diagnostic procedures, treatment, and inpatient ward space. The appropriate size and location of each area in the hospital are related to the number of veterinarians and support staff in the practice and the number of clients and patients served.

Patient management and possibly client management are obviously the most interesting and necessary management topics for entry-level veterinary technicians. It often takes more experience and a desire for advancement before veterinary technicians become very interested in the other areas of practice management (see Box 32-1). Students need to develop a working knowledge of the principles of management of hospital areas in order to be effective technicians and to prepare for future advancement in the veterinary technology profession. This understanding is also critical for assessing practice differences when

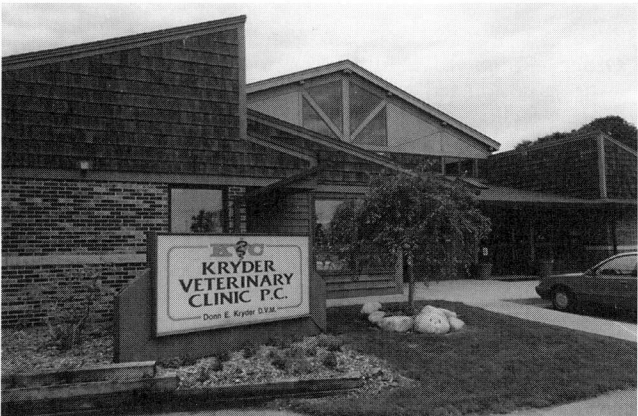

FIGURE 32-1. Hospital signs should be professional and clearly visible from the street.

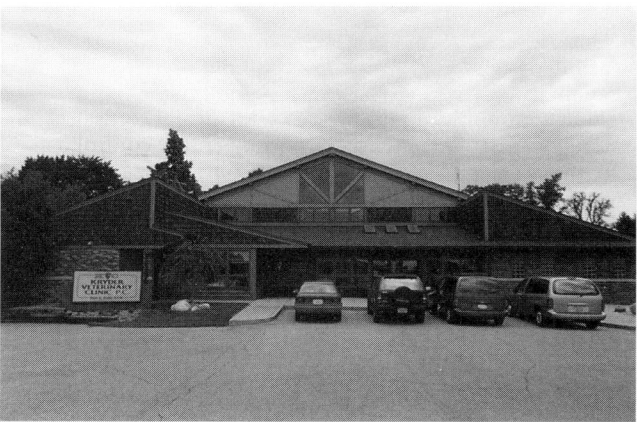

FIGURE 32-2. Client parking lot should be clearly designated and clean.

searching for the best employment opportunity (see self-marketing section at end of this chapter).

Outside Areas

Location is the primary factor (other than referrals from satisfied clients) in attracting new clients. Location will often dictate slow or rapid practice growth. Location provides visibility for potential clients and allows existing clients to easily find the practice. Prime locations within shopping centers and on main streets are expensive during the initial investment period but will repay the investment by increasing practice growth. Location of the facility should also be considered by veterinary technicians when selecting a practice for employment.

Further, the *practice sign* must be evaluated for visibility and professional appearance. The optimum would be a well-placed, neat professional sign that allows the client clear visibility and direction (Figure 32-1). The sign becomes even more important during an emergency. Some form of lighting will allow clients to identify the building entrance after dark.

Attention must be given to the *parking lot area*. Litter must be picked up, and plants and grass must be tended. The parking lot entrance and exit should be clearly marked by signs. Parking spaces should be reserved for clients only, with employee parking behind the building or in a remote area away from the building entrance (Figure 32-2).

The entrance to the veterinary facility should be in full view and well marked to allow easy access by clients. If more than one entrance is available (i.e., small animal and large animal or canine and feline), each entrance should be well marked. To prevent client congestion, the entrance and exit should be separate. Practice employees should not use the public entrance of the building. Further, routine deliveries and service activities should enter and exit the building away from client contact when possible.

Professional activities within a veterinary hospital can be grouped into four areas: outpatient, inpatient, surgical, and support. Depending on the practice size and type, the veterinarian, technician, or both may work in all four areas or focus on one or more areas. Effective management of each of these areas is needed to improve service and patient care.

Technician Note

The four professional areas of activity within a hospital are outpatient, inpatient, surgical, and support service.

Outpatient Area

The first area to be discussed is the outpatient area. This area is composed of the *reception area, examination rooms, laboratory, pharmacy,* and *public restrooms.* Most commonly, clients will only have access to this area of the hospital. Special attention must be paid to maintain the outpatient area in a clean, organized, quiet, and odor-free condition. Because the client's first contact is with the outpatient area, lasting impressions are made that may raise or lower the overall client confidence in the quality of caring. A disorganized, dirty, smelly, noisy area will be remembered just that way. Veterinarians, technicians, and other staff must be well groomed, clean, and professionally attired. A professional appearance is mandatory for a professional image. All personnel in the outpatient area should also refrain from smoking, eating, and drinking when clients are present.

The *reception area* should always be considered by all hospital employees as a reception or client greeting area and not as a waiting room. The reception area should be comfortable and project a feeling of warmth, not a sterile feeling. Plants will help to create this warm feeling, but they must be well cared for. Dead or dying plants in the reception area will not send a positive message to the client. Warm colors will also help to brighten the area. Reading material, if present, should be complete and not torn or half missing. A well-maintained fish aquarium and attractive wall hangings or paintings will help relax clients (Figure 32-3).

The clients should spend only a short period of time in the reception room before being escorted to one of the *examination rooms.* This requires effective appointment scheduling and dedication to timely service. As a general rule, two examination rooms should be available in the outpatient area for each veterinarian. The examination areas should be decorated in warm tones, as should the reception area. Medications, examination equipment, records, and so forth should be secured or out of sight so that neither clients nor their children will be tempted. It is extremely important that the examination room be clean and in excellent repair because the client will spend the greatest amount of time there (Figure 32-4). A soiled floor or wall covering, dirty sink, and marred door will be noted and remembered by the client.

The *laboratory* and *pharmacy* should be well organized and clean. Clients will only occasionally visit these areas and should always be accompanied by a hospital employee. In some practices, the laboratory and pharmacy

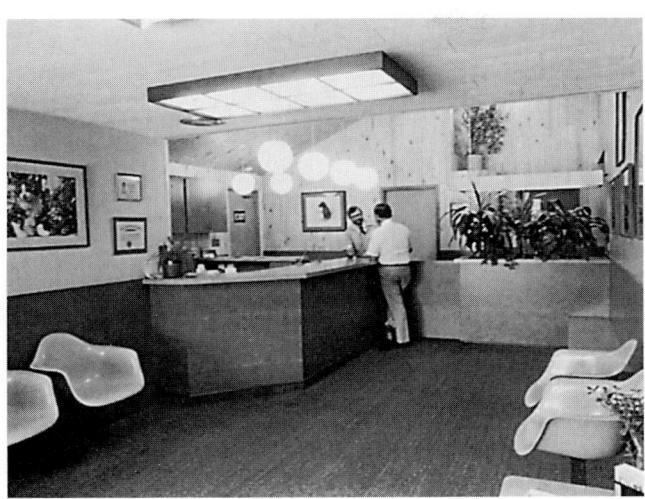

FIGURE 32-3. Reception area should give a warm, comfortable feeling to clients and staff.

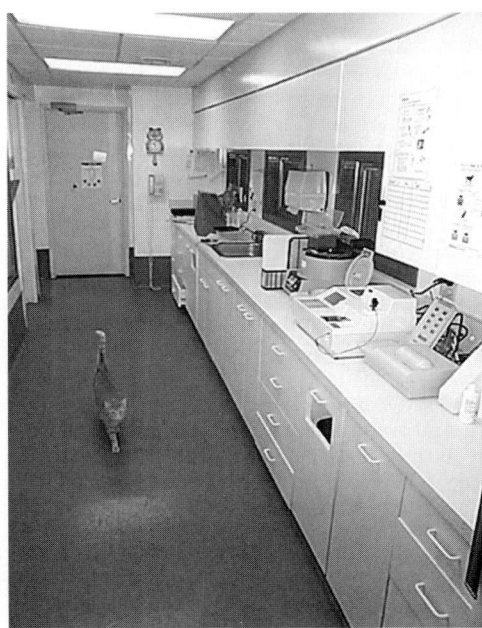

FIGURE 32-5. Clinic cat is checking out the laboratory located just beyond three examination rooms.

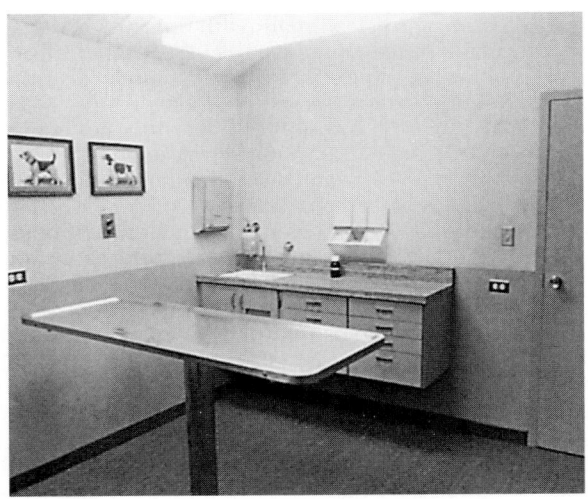

FIGURE 32-4. Examination rooms should be warmly decorated, clean, and in excellent condition.

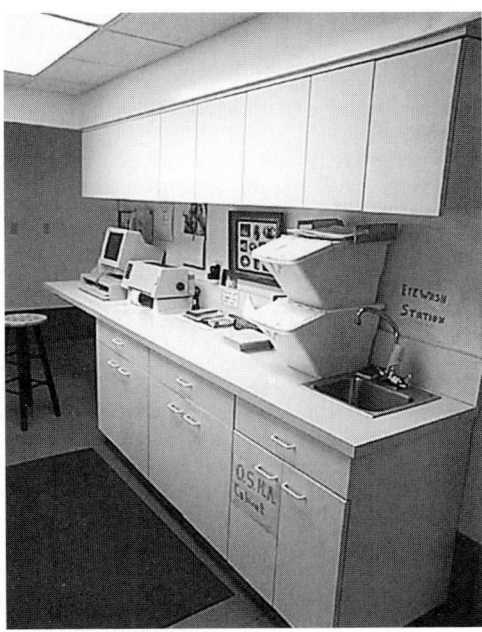

FIGURE 32-6. Pharmacy is located between examination rooms and in-patient treatment area. Note computer for printing labels and inventory control.

will be combined for more efficient use of floor space. They are usually located behind the examination rooms and accessible to the inpatient treatment areas (Figure 32-5). The pharmacy may also have Occupational Safety and Health Administration (OSHA) required material safety data sheet (MSDS) files and an eye wash station (Figure 32-6). The *public restrooms* should be cleaned and inspected regularly and should be conveniently located for client use.

Inpatient Area

The second work area is the inpatient area, consisting of a *treatment area, patient wards* and/or *large animal stalls, isolation area, exercise area,* an area in which *necropsy* is performed, a *kitchen,* and a *bathing* and *grooming* area. The client has much less contact with this area than with the outpatient area, but constant attention must be given to maintain a clean, odor-free environment to prevent nosocomial infections of patients (Box 32-3).

Box 32-3	NOSOCOMIAL INFECTIONS

Definition—New infections acquired by patients in the veterinary facility

Examples of nosocomial infection sources

Staff—Unwashed hands; contaminated equipment, including dirty needles, clothing, and boots; inadequate cleaning and disinfecting protocols; breaks in aseptic technique

Other patients—Direct contact, airborne droplets, hair, excrement, blood

Environment—Cages, feed or water pans, dust, bedding

Staff prevention

Always wash hands between patients

Always wear clean clothing and boots

Always follow established cleaning, disinfecting, sterilizing, and aseptic protocols

Train all staff in preventive protocols

NOTE: Recent studies indicate that human hospital workers wash their hands less than one half of the time before touching human patients; one factor in the recent increase of nosocomial infections in human patients!

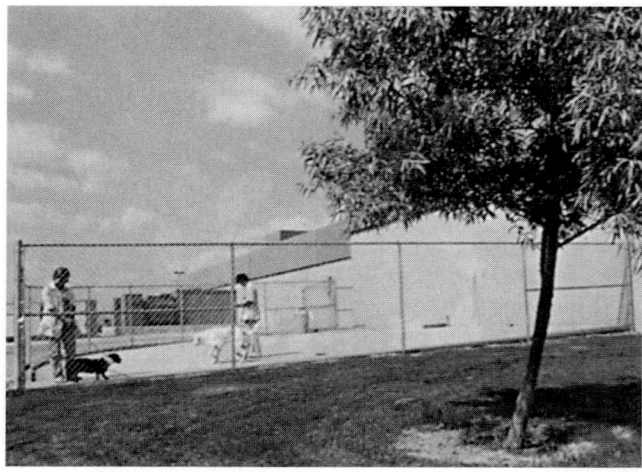

FIGURE 32-7. For security, fenced enclosures should always be used for outside exercise.

Kennels, runs, and stalls must be cleaned several times during the day. Hospitalized patients must have closer attention than animals who are just boarding. Sick animals often cannot control urination and defecation; therefore more frequent attention to these areas will be required. Some pets are not used to eliminating indoors and will be reluctant to urinate and defecate unless they are in an exercise run. To maintain a quiet environment in public areas of the hospital, patient wards must be well insulated to reduce noise.

If large animals are hospitalized, adequate holding stalls will be necessary, with regular attention given to cleaning the stall and grooming and exercising the patient. When exercising either a large animal or a small animal patient, absolute security must be maintained at all times to prevent escape. Fenced areas should always be used to ensure that in the event of escape, the animal will still be contained (Figure 32-7). The veterinarian, hospital, or both assume all liability for an animal entrusted to them. Few experiences will match the helpless feeling of watching an escaped dog, cat, horse, or cow run off into the distance (especially if close to a busy street or highway).

Because of the security problem, the ward or stall area of the hospital should be adjacent to the *exercise area,* with an escape-proof fence or walls connecting the two. Exercise areas for small animals ideally should be located within a well-insulated area of the hospital in which the temperature and humidity can be maintained at a constant level. Most city zoning laws will allow a small animal hospital to be located in proximity to residential areas because modern construction techniques use totally enclosed, attractive, and well-insulated designs.

Technician Note

Animal security within the hospital must always be a high priority. Animals that escape are the legal responsibility of the hospital.

Large animal or mixed hospitals (caring for both large and small animals) will usually be required to locate in a less developed area of a city to allow exercise areas and

odors to be properly addressed. Fewer veterinary hospitals now board animals on a regular basis. When boarding is offered, it should be explained to the client as "veterinary-supervised boarding." The recent trend has been away from construction of large boarding facilities as part of an animal hospital. Because of both the cost of construction and the cost of hospitalization, most veterinary practices work on an outpatient basis whenever possible. Construction and labor costs have made long-term hospitalization a financial burden to both client and veterinarian.

In certain instances, animals with infectious diseases must be hospitalized. Adequate *isolation facilities* must be available before a patient with an infectious disease in admitted. The isolation area should have only one entrance and exit, with proper disinfectant and clothing protection available. The air-handling system for the isolation area must be separate from the remainder of the building to prevent aerosol transmission of contagious disease organisms. In the event that adequate isolation facilities are not available on the premises, the case should be referred to a veterinarian who has the proper facility. All treatments and handling of the infectious patient should be done by one or two persons only. The patient should be treated within the isolation facility and should not be taken to the main treatment room. Staff must be trained to follow stringent isolation protocols to prevent nosocomial infections (see Box 32-3).

The *treatment area* should be the central hub of the hospital (Figure 32-8). Patients from both the wards (inpatients) and examination rooms (outpatients) will be moved to this area for diagnostic procedures, medication administration, and recheck procedures (cast, bandage, or splint changes or removal). Certified veterinary technicians are increasingly performing the prescribed medical treatment and other nursing procedures while the veterinarian is performing surgery or seeing outpatients. One of the technical staff should have the primary responsibility for organization and cleanliness of the treatment room.

On occasion, clients may accompany the patient to the treatment area to assist with a bandage change or other minor procedure. The area therefore must be presentable at all times. In addition to the routine treatment functions carried out in the treatment room, many hospitals also use

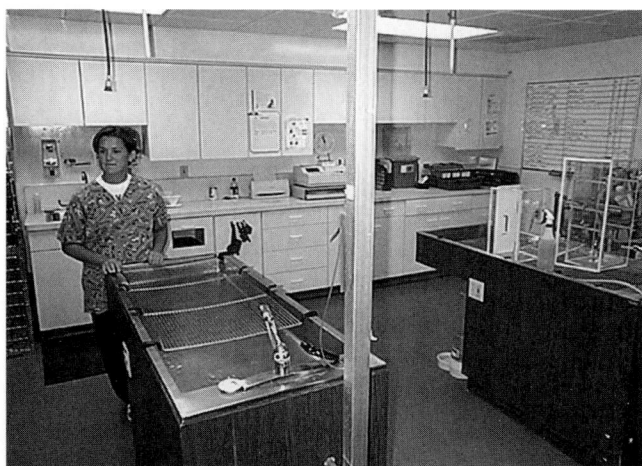

FIGURE 32-8.   Centralized treatment area accommodates both outpatient and inpatient treatment.

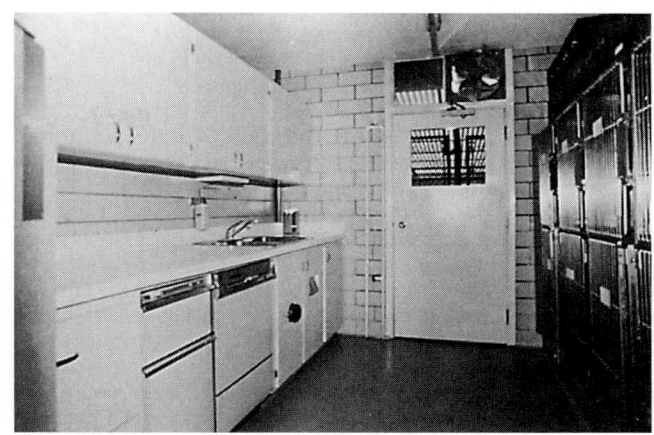

FIGURE 32-9.   Hospital kitchen should contain diet materials, dishwasher, counter space, and refrigerator.

this room for preparation of the surgical patient. In the smaller practice, the treatment room may also contain x-ray facilities, laboratory equipment, or both. Because of the high traffic volume in the treatment area, hair and other debris will build up rapidly and should be removed with a vacuum cleaner on a regular basis to prevent nosocomial infections.

The *kitchen* in a small animal hospital should be an area in which animal food is stored and prepared. Usually, both canned and dry foods are available, and it should be stored in dry, rodent-proof containers. An automatic dishwasher is of great value if any quantity of dirty pans must be cleaned on a daily basis. It will also sanitize the pans with very hot water and remove soap and significant residues that cause digestive problems in sensitive patients. Hot and cold running water, a sink, counter top space, and a refrigerator should be available in the kitchen (Figure 32-9). Human food and drinks must not be stored in this refrigerator (OSHA regulations).

In the large animal hospital, the *feed room* will usually contain several grain mixtures and ration supplements. All materials must be stored in dry, rodent-proof containers. Grass hay, alfalfa, and bedding straw should be stored in a dry area protected from the weather to prevent mold and mildew. Moldy hay or alfalfa should never be fed to an animal because of possible toxicity and allergies.

The *bathing-grooming* area in the small animal hospital will usually consist of a raised bathroom tub (elevated about 60 to 90 cm [Figure 32-10]), a combing table, and a dryer cage. It is critically important that all patients dismissed from the hospital be clean and dry. Grooming services within the hospital may not be offered, but attention to daily grooming of all patients by all employees is necessary. Attention to grooming is also important for the equine patient and is usually done in the stall on a daily basis.

The final area to be discussed within the inpatient work area of the hospital is the *necropsy area.* The veterinary technician is able to perform a prosection (initial dissection) for the veterinarian to quickly inspect all organs for lesions and decide what specimens should be collected. The technician will collect, properly prepare, and ship the designated specimens to a diagnostic laboratory with the history (see Chapter 3). The necropsy area should be located in an isolated place in the building and be well

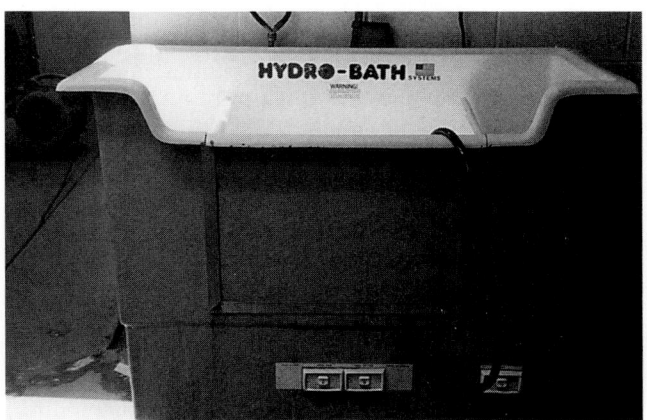

FIGURE 32-10.   Custom pet bathing tub designed to aid in controlling animal during bath. Note dryer positioned in front of run for drying previously bathed dog.

lighted and well ventilated. Hot and cold running water and a drain should also be present. Necropsy tables or racks are used for small animals, whereas the necropsy floors usually are used for dissecting large animals. Gloves, boots, and aprons should be available in addition to specific necropsy instruments and specimen bottles. The availability of a 35-mm camera, digital camera, or video camera is helpful to record specific lesions.

Acceptable carcass disposal, preferably cremation, must be offered to owners. The body may also be released to the owner for owner burial.

In conclusion, the hospital inpatient area is the most labor-intensive section because of patient contact. Most hospitals expend the greatest amount of effort in maintaining this area. Most employees spend their greatest amount of time in this area performing direct animal care, diagnostic procedures, and nursing treatments. The outcome of most cases will also be determined here.

Surgical Area

The third work area in the hospital is the *surgical area,* which consists of the *preparation room, operating rooms, radiology section,* and *recovery room.* All four areas in the surgical section must be in close proximity to one another. Frequently the surgeon may need to obtain a postoperative radiograph of a fracture reduction to determine bone alignment or implant placement. When neurosurgery is to be performed, the surgeon may request a myelogram just before surgery; this requires that the patient be moved from the preparation room to the radiology area, back to the preparation room, and then into surgery.

As stated earlier, the *preparation room* may also be the treatment room. All presurgical preparation of the patient, surgeon, and technician should take place outside the operating room. Instrument preparation and sterilization usually will be completed in the preparation room. Clipping and scrubbing the patient and hand scrubbing of the surgeon and technician should be done before entering the operating room. A vacuum cleaner should be available in the preparation room to remove all loose hair from patient, table, and floor.

The *operating room* itself should be a "dead end" room with only one entrance-exit (Figure 32-11). Dust-carrying bacteria are easily stirred into the air when people walk through the room and will settle into the open surgical incision. No one should enter the operating room without proper clothing, shoes, cap, and mask. The operating room should be used only for surgical procedures and must not double as a treatment or examination room. Storage cabinets should be kept to a minimum and should contain only items that are used in surgery. Items used elsewhere in the hospital should not be stored in the operating room. Counter tops should be kept to a minimum because flat surfaces collect dust and must be wiped down daily. Some flat surface is desirable to allow opening of packs and layout of instruments.

> ### Technician Note
> The operating room (OR) must be used only for surgery and cannot be used as an examination or treatment room.

Wall-mounted radiographic viewers should be present to allow several views of a body part to be observed at once. Surgery lights, oxygen outlets, and patient monitors should be ceiling- or wall-mounted when possible. Floors, walls, and ceiling should be washable, smooth, and seam free to allow complete and easy cleaning. Cleaning under the surgery table base, the top of surgical lights, the floor, and flat surfaces (window ledges, counter top, etc.) should be performed daily. The air-handling system for the operating room should be separate and should create a slight positive pressure to prevent dust and other debris from entering the room from other rooms when the door is opened.

All cleaning materials and utensils used in the operating room should be restricted to use in this room. Mops and sponges that are used elsewhere in the building and are then used in the operating room will bring additional contamination into the room. The cleanliness of the operating room should be everyone's concern to prevent nosocomial infection of the surgical patient.

The *radiology area* should be located near the operating room, the preparation room, and the treatment area (for diagnostic work-ups). The radiology section should not be visited by clients during film exposure because of potential radiation exposure. Protective aprons, gloves, and film exposure badges should always be worn by all personnel in radiology. The technician will usually be responsible for

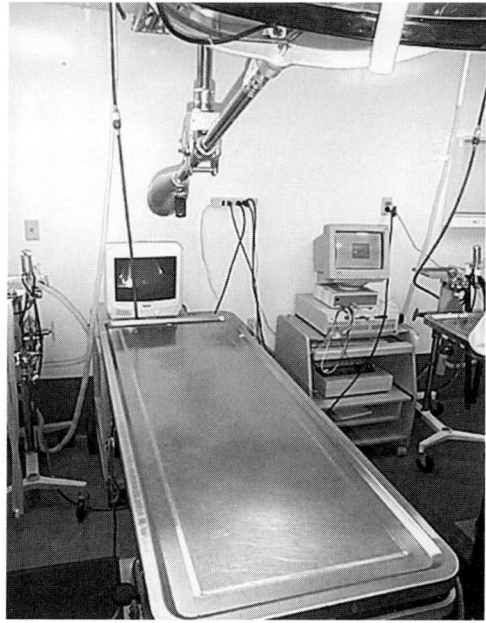

FIGURE 32-11. Surgical room with one door for both entrance and exit, ceiling-mounted lights, and minimal countertops.

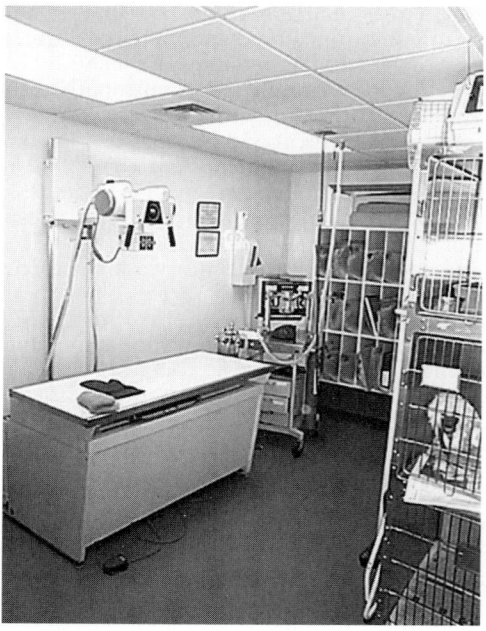

FIGURE 32-12. Radiology room with x-ray machine, x-ray storage, and holding cage. The automatic film processor is not visible.

equipment maintenance, exposure, developing, and filing radiographs (Figure 32-12). In most surgical orthopedic cases, the radiology area will be visited after surgery to evaluate bone alignment or metal implant placement or both before placing the patient in the recovery room.

The surgical recovery area should be monitored at all times by a technician until the endotracheal tube has been removed. The recovery area may be in a room adjacent to the treatment room or behind a glass partition in the treatment room, or the recovery process may occur on a blanket on the treatment room floor. Whenever surgical recovery occurs, the patient should be closely monitored by the technical staff. *Under no circumstances* should any patient recovering from anesthesia be left unattended in the ward, in a stall, or elsewhere with an endotracheal tube in place.

In review, the surgical work area is a very technical and equipment-oriented area. Clients will not be permitted in this areas except in unusual circumstances. The skill level of technical support in this area must be very high, requiring familiarization with anesthesia (induction and administration), emergency procedures, radiology, surgical assisting, medical-surgical nursing, use of fiberoptic equipment, sterile technique, sterilization, monitoring equipment hook-up, electrosurgical equipment, and necropsy techniques.

Support Area

The fourth work area of the hospital is the hospital support area. This area contains, somewhat by default, some of the "leftovers," but it also contains the planning and management areas of the hospital. The support area contains the *professional offices, business management office, library, employee lounge,* and *storage-inventory* areas.

> ### Technician Note
>
> The support area of the hospital contains the professional offices, business management office, library, employee lounge, and storage areas.

In smaller practices, the *professional office, business management office,* and *library* will be in one room. In some multiperson practices, each veterinarian may have an office or large desk area in addition to the hospital manager's office. Larger practices may also have a library and conference room combination in which weekly staff meetings and conferences can be held.

The role of the hospital manager will vary according to practice size and management philosophy, but his or her office will usually be in proximity to the admissions-discharge functions of the hospital. Credit policy, accounts receivable, inventory control, purchasing, receiving orders, accounts payable, computer information management, management reports, personnel activities, and so forth will usually be handled by the hospital manager. In many practices, some of these functions are divided among the staff, and the veterinarian or veterinarians will assume the overall management role. For most veterinary technicians, some management skills will be required for advancement. Hospital management is now developing into a specialty area of veterinary medicine for nonveterinarians.

The *professional office* of the veterinarian functions as a client consultation area, a medical management area for discussing new products with drug company salespeople, and a professional management area for writing medical records, contacting clients, and discussing difficult or interesting cases with other veterinarians or staff. Many office hours are spent by the practicing veterinarian in studying and reading textbooks, journals, and reference materials and evaluating computer information. Veterinary technicians must also keep up with the latest advances in animal nursing, imaging, and laboratory procedures. Most states also require a minimal number of hours of approved continuing education for both certified veterinary technicians and licensed veterinarians.

The last portion of the support area is *storage.* From the management viewpoint, hospital storage space is the most expensive floor space in the building because this space produces the least income. Therefore the storage areas must be given close attention so that this valuable space will function as efficiently as possible. Supplies and equipment that are no longer used or usable should be removed to make room for the essential items. Inventory control (avoiding overstocking or understocking) and space organization will ensure maximal utilization. Items that can be hung on the wall or ceiling should be removed from the floor. Metal or wooden shelving will organize space for bulk drugs, food, and cleaning supplies. Flammable or toxic materials should be safely marked and stored away from foods or drugs.

In summary, the four major hospital work areas (outpatient, inpatient, surgery, support) are somewhat separate in function but are related in patient care and support. The smaller the practice, the less distinct will the areas be. Further, the smaller the practice, the fewer the number of technical staff and assistants, resulting in less opportunity for the veterinary technician to focus on one work area. This is not to imply that the smaller practice is less desirable. Sometimes, to the contrary, the small practice can provide more personal satisfaction because of closer contact with the entire operation and a diversification of job roles. Each technician and each veterinarian need to choose the type of practice with staffing utilization patterns that provide the greatest personal and professional satisfaction.

Traffic Flow

The four work areas that have been discussed are important from both client-patient and hospital organization viewpoints. The client wants personalized and professional service that is efficient, thorough, and cost effective. If each employee fully understands and enjoys his or her work area, the client and patient will usually experience satisfaction if all communicate effectively. However, the veterinary team must be efficient at handling the necessary number of patients to provide the needed cash flow required to stay in business. An efficient traffic flow (i.e., the movement of the client and patient from admission to dismissal) becomes very important to accommodate the required number of clients each day.

LARGE ANIMAL FACILITIES

Whereas about 75% of veterinarians practice in small animal facilities, about 4% of the practices in the United States are equine and 10% are primarily food animal (swine, dairy, and/or beef) practices. A decreasing number (less than 10%) are mixed practices in which veterinarians see both large animal and small animal patients. If the livestock population is high in an area, a group practice may have several large animal veterinarians each focusing on a specific species for providing diagnostic, treatment, and surgical services as well as preventive medicine consultation.

Large Animal Mobile Units

Veterinary diagnostic and preventive medicine services for a herd of animals require the veterinarian to visit the owner's facility on the farm or in the stable. The large animal practice often makes use of a mobile facility (Figure 32-13) for conducting these farm visits. These visits require

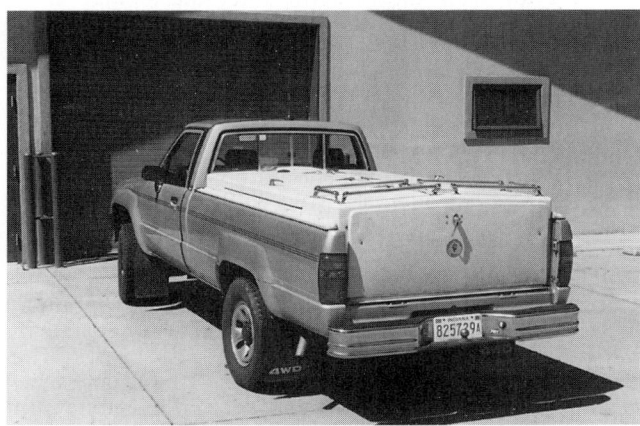

FIGURE 32-13.   A veterinary mobile unit is equipped with hot water, a refrigerator, and many compartments for equipment and supplies.

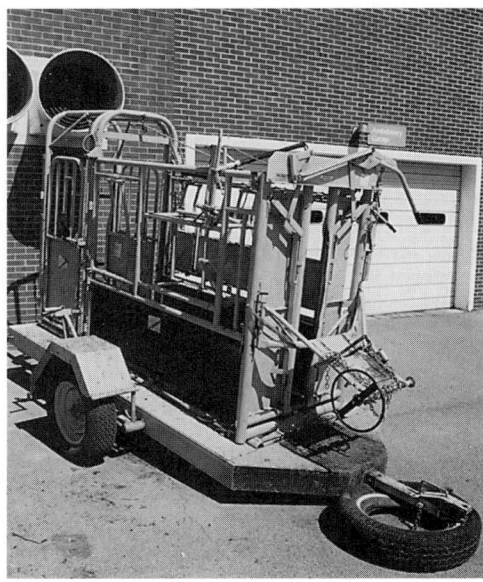

FIGURE 32-14.   A portable cattle chute on wheels is pulled behind the ambulatory truck to the farm. It has a head table on front for head work and a palpation cage on back for reproductive examinations.

stringent sanitary precautions to prevent transmitting disease among animal facilities. Washing hands, changing to clean coveralls, chemical disinfecting of boots, and cleaning of equipment between farm calls are paramount to prevent disease transmission among farms and to gain and keep the confidence of the livestock owner.

Mobile facilities used to serve large animal patients and clients may vary from a car with a few portable "grips" in the trunk, to a van with a set of drawers and containers, to a specially designed mobile truck unit. The truck units are usually fully equipped with refrigeration for biologicals plus hot water and a supply of disinfectants, drugs, vaccines, medical supplies, restraints, diagnostic and treatment equipment, and sometimes even mobile x-ray units. Everything needed for a series of planned visits plus unexpected emergencies must be on board! The water supply and disinfectants are used to clean and disinfect hands, boots, and equipment after every farm call. A portable cattle chute may be also pulled behind the mobile unit to the farm to process herds of cattle (Figure 32-14).

A veterinary technician may be responsible for stocking, organizing, and maintaining the large animal mobile unit. The mobile unit inventory will vary depending on the nature of the practice, the preferences of the veterinarian, and the species served. Preparing inventory lists and organizational charts for this daily activity ensures that the veterinarian will have what is needed on every call. Obviously, there is a wide range of specific supplies necessary for the routine practice of large animal veterinary medicine. This inventory must be replenished frequently, organized for easy and quick access, and cleaned and disinfected on a daily basis as well as after every farm call. Many technicians desire to assist veterinarians on farm calls and become efficient at maintaining and organizing the mobile unit.

Large Animal Haul-in Facilities

Some veterinarians with mixed and large practices provide haul-in facilities for individual patients to be trucked or

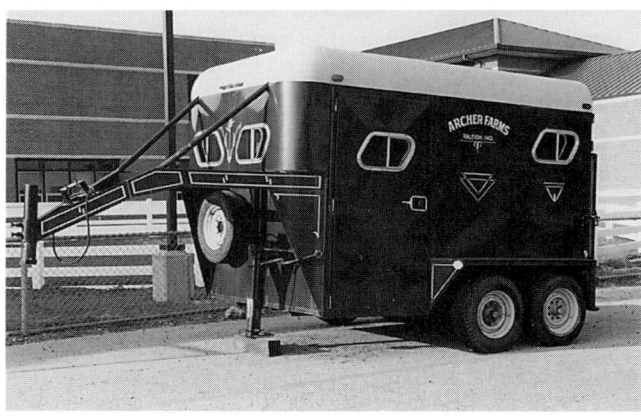

FIGURE 32-15.   A stock trailer is used by animal owners to transport farm animals to the large hospital for treatment.

brought by trailer into the practice (Figure 32-15). Unloading chutes and gates for cattle trucks and stock trailers are provided at the large animal outpatient entrance. A few even provide holding corrals and squeeze chutes for processing a truckload of cattle or sheep. Unloading chutes for cattle, sheep, and swine must adjust to different heights to accommodate the trucks, pick-ups, and trailers used for transporting the animals. It is paramount that fencing and panel arrangements be constructed to prevent escape from the premises if the animal escapes from the head-catch, alleyway, or when unloading.

When haul-in facilities for large animals are provided, each of the areas previously discussed for a small animal facility will be present for serving large animal patients. They may be in separate or combined rooms. In larger facilities they will often be separate from the small animal areas. Frequently, some areas will be used for both small animal and large animal service (e.g., the reception area,

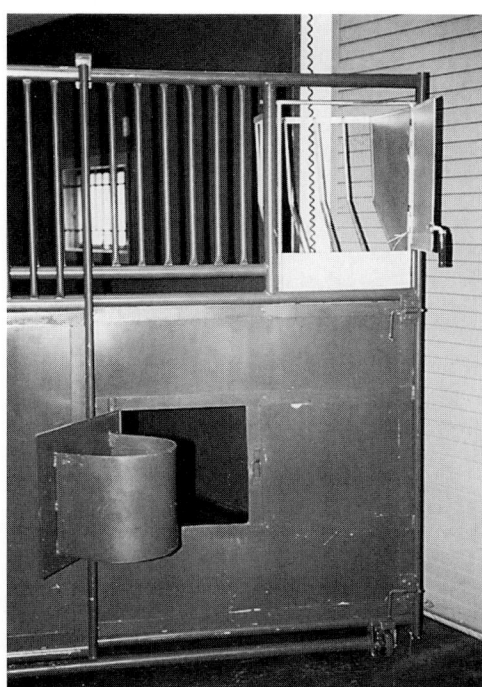

FIGURE 32-16. Large animal stall door has mini-doors to feed and water large animal patients without having to enter the stall.

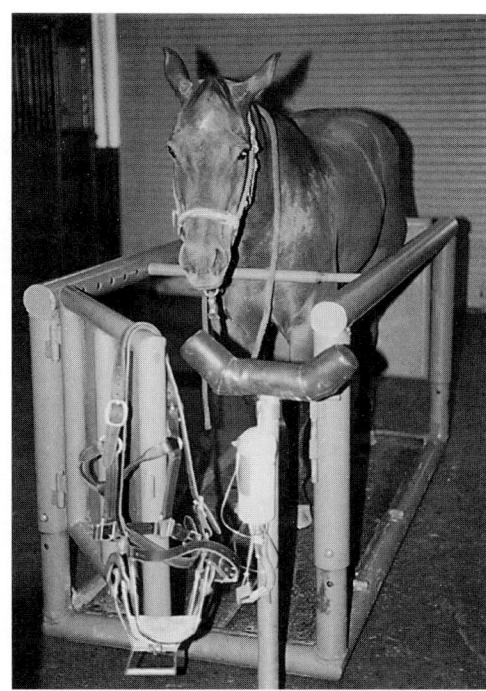

FIGURE 32-17. Horse in stocks with bar in front of chest to keep horse back against rear door. Mouth speculum is used to perform equine dental procedures.

laboratory, conference rooms, pharmacy, public restrooms). Large mixed hospitals often have a separate pharmacy for large animal supplies, separate public restrooms, and possibly a separate reception area. The nature of the large animal facilities of each practice is quite variable depending on the needs of the livestock population and owners served by the practice.

The *large animal inpatient treatment area* may be the same as the outpatient examination area for large animal patients. An alleyway with a head-catch or squeeze chute is used for bovine patients, a stock is used for equine patients, and pigs or sheep may be treated in their stall. When haul-in facilities are available for large animals, patient wards with a few stalls (Figure 32-16) are usually provided. These will often be indoors to protect the patients from bad weather, although outdoor pens may be used in good weather. Also, isolation areas in a different barn are sometimes necessary.

Examination rooms are always separate because large animal examinations require stocks for horses (Figure 32-17), a squeeze chute and head-catch for cattle, and large special examination tables for restraining cattle on their side for hoof work or minor surgery. Cattle chutes (see Figure 32-14) are manual or hydraulic squeeze chutes located at the end of an alleyway. A head-catch on the front of an alleyway will suffice for some cattle examinations and procedures. The alleyways leading to the chutes are sometimes arranged in a circular manner to facilitate easier cattle movement to the examination area. Because of the size of these species, staff should be well trained in restraint and safety procedures for protecting both large animal patients, owners, and staff. A variety of restraint procedures are used (see Chapter 1).

Most food animal practices also use the treatment area as a minor, nonsterile surgical room. Because of the large

patient size and the extensive amount of hair and excrement large animals bring to these areas, high-pressure hoses and disinfectant systems are necessary, along with removable floor drain traps. Most mixed practices use the same support areas for the small and large animal clients and patients with the exception of storage of cleaning equipment, lawn mowers, large animal hoof equipment, general supplies, and bulk pharmacy.

The *surgical room* in the equine practice facility is organized to provide the same stringent asepsis as provided in a small animal surgery. However, because the patient is much larger, mechanical or hydraulic equipment designed to lift the horse is provided. Larger equine practices have an induction room (may also be the treatment and minor surgery area), an operating room with a large animal radiology machine, and a padded recovery room. The surgical area is equipped with a surgical table on which the horse is placed after being induced with general anesthesia (Figure 32-18). Anesthesia is maintained with an equine gas anesthesia machine (Figure 32-19).

An area where a *necropsy* can be appropriately performed must also be available (see Chapter 5). Necropsies are more frequently performed when a *large* animal dies than for a small animal. Because of the economic value of large herds or flocks, necropsies of dead animals are often done to determine if the rest of the herd or flock is threatened. Confirmation of the diagnosis will often require submission of specimens to a state or university diagnostic laboratory for testing and review by a board-certified pathologist. Sometimes necropsy of several animals may be done (more common in sheep, pigs, and poultry) in order to determine which of several concurrent diseases is the probable cause of death.

Necropsies are valuable as a preventive measure to stop the spread of a disease and prevent it in the future. They are

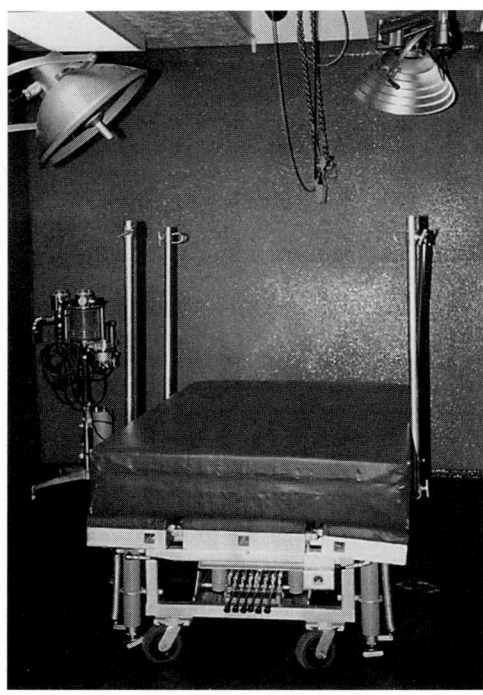

FIGURE 32-18. Large animal surgery table with anesthesia machine and padded walls of recovery room for recovering anesthetized horses.

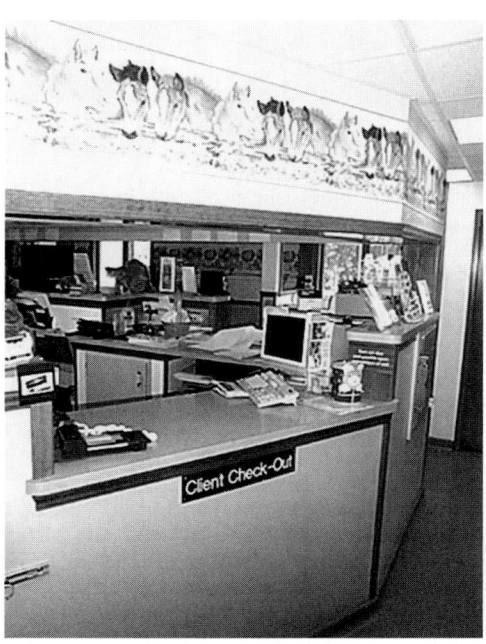

FIGURE 32-20. Common checkout desk used by both small and large animal owners in a mixed practice.

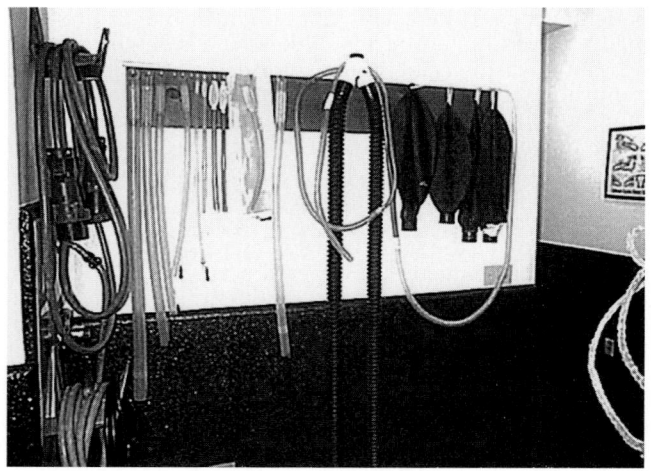

FIGURE 32-19. Large animal endotracheal tubes, rebreathing bags, and related anesthesia equipment stored on a rack for quick access.

also a great learning tool for the veterinary staff to become better prepared to recognize similar cases in the future.

Traffic flow patterns in large animal and mixed practices vary greatly. Facilities that primarily serve small animal patients with a moderately used large animal facility attached have some mixing of traffic from both groups (Figure 32-20). In some facilities, a practice that has many large animal patients may be organized with more separation to reduce crossover of traffic patterns of the small and large animal clients. Obviously if it is an exclusive large animal facility

(e.g., an equine practice), these areas are similar to a small animal practice in name, but the arrangement and size will depend on the type of horses routinely presented for treatment.

BUILDING MAINTENANCE

The building, land, and equipment in a veterinary hospital require a very large capital investment. Maintenance of this investment requires significant management attention to maximize its effective utilization for client service and to provide a good financial return on the investment. It is easy to ignore routine maintenance because the team gets busy with clients and patients and used to the working environment. Therefore routine maintenance must be assigned to someone so that a regular schedule of preventive maintenance will be followed.

Clients often initially evaluate the level of patient care by the appearance of the building and grounds. This requires professional landscaping and proper parking lot surfacing. Continual maintenance of building and grounds through regular painting and repair is *very* important. Care of the exterior of the building along with meticulous care of the lawn, shrubs, trees, and flowers often conveys an initial impression of a well-organized and caring feeling to the clients.

General Maintenance

General maintenance within the building is an ongoing challenge. Floors, flat surfaces, walls, cages, runs, and stalls must be kept sparkling clean and odor free. Counters, magazine racks, and pictures need to be organized and dusted frequently. The reception room, examination rooms, and public bathrooms must be inspected and cleaned regularly throughout each day.

Some of this general maintenance needs to be scheduled on a regular basis. However, to reach the "cleanliness is next to godliness" goal, *everyone* in the practice must assume some of the cleaning responsibility. An old adage for new graduates is that "veterinary medicine is 90% cleanup and 10% medical practice." No one should look for someone else to clean up a fresh urine or fecal deposit. It is usually quicker and easier to clean it up yourself.

One of the reasons cleanup in a veterinary practice is so challenging is the larger quantity of hair shed by animals than humans. Hair is such a major problem that a vacuum system needs to be available and used before general mopping; otherwise, there is a buildup of hair that is simply moved around the facility. Some practices have been built with a central vacuum system to improve the efficiency of hair reduction from the floors.

Clients notice hospital cleanliness. The lack of it can result in complaints or nosocomial infections. When one client actually complains, there are probably many other clients quietly forming a negative impression of the practice! If the veterinary hospital is to be considered a modern and progressive medical facility, all personnel must rigidly monitor odors and sanitation. Whenever a pet soils an area or cage it must be cleaned quickly and thoroughly. Appropriate disinfectants need to be used to avoid odor buildup. Deodorizers may be of benefit to help clean the area but should not be used to cover up a sanitation problem. The ventilation system should be capable of exhausting all air within the building within 15 to 20 minutes to facilitate odor control. In addition to exhaust fans in the wards, fans can also be useful in the examination rooms and laboratory areas.

Managing Equipment Maintenance

Equipment and cleaning must be an ongoing activity. Each major piece of equipment should be assigned to a specified member of the hospital team to keep it well maintained. It is recommended that the person most familiar with each piece of equipment be assigned to maintain it. If this is done, all equipment will last longer and always be ready for use when needed for quality patient care. Nonmedical equipment, such as typewriters, calculators, computers, air conditioning and heating units, lawn mowers, and related general maintenance equipment, should also have maintenance responsibility assigned to those who are most responsible for its use.

Major equipment items should have a specific documented maintenance schedule to ensure proper servicing (e.g., anesthetic machines, endoscopes, ultrasound machines, x-ray developer solutions, automatic processors, autoclaves, microscopes, clinical pathology laboratory analyzers, computer terminals, central vacuum systems, furnaces, hot water heaters, air conditioners). Computer software is available to organize these efforts for equipment, facility areas, and vehicles.

Managing Electrical Equipment

Supervisors should take the time to teach staff about electrical safety and how to check equipment to ensure it is in proper working order with nonfrayed electrical cords (see Chapter 35). This can prevent tragic electrocution accidents to both patient and staff.

Veterinary technicians, animal handlers, and veterinarians should be aware of some easy-to-follow rules to minimize macroshock hazards (Box 32-4). Too often people become careless when working around electricity on a continuous basis from either habit or being in a hurry.

A file of warranties, service, and repair representatives for

---

Box 32-4 Electrical Equipment Safety Rules

THE PATIENT
- Avoid touching the animal and any conductive metal surface of an electrical instrument at the same time.
- Be sure all electrical equipment in the vicinity of or attached to the animal is effectively grounded with three-wire power cords, and do not allow any equipment with two-prong plugs in the animal's vicinity.
- When two or more electrical instruments are used near a patient, connect them to the same wall outlet. Also, remove all unnecessary electrical equipment from the animal's environment.
- Always plug electrical equipment into the wall outlet with the equipment power switch off.

POWER CORDS
- Avoid using extension cords with any patient instrumentation, and never use a two-prong to three-prong cheater adapter on two-wire outlets.
- Keep electrical cords out of well-traveled pathways, and do not step on or roll equipment over electrical cables.
- Plug and unplug the power cord of the equipment by holding onto the plug firmly and straight.
- Before power cords and their connectors are used, carefully check for intermittent or loose connections, frayed wires, cracked connectors, and overall quality.

APPLIANCES
- Check all electrical appliances (especially motorized devices) periodically for current leakage and ground wire continuity.
- If performance of an instrument is unsatisfactory or a tingling sensation is felt from it, remove it from use and have it checked.
- Keep fluids, chemicals, spillable products, and heat away from electrical equipment and cables.

GENERAL
- Know the location of circuit breakers for each wall outlet serving clinical areas.
- Remember, body moisture or perspiration lowers electrical resistance and permits greater current to flow.
- Use common sense when working with electrical equipment.
- Remember that the patient is in the electrical environment and could become part of an unsuspected circuit.

Modified from Swift C, Carithers, R: Electrical safety for the veterinarian: macroshock hazards, *JAVMA* 172:903, 1978.

---

each item of major equipment should be maintained. The file should also include the instruction manuals that must be read to chart the needed schedule of required maintenance. This scheduled maintenance chart should be initialed when each maintenance is performed. Failure to do required maintenance often violates warranties and results in a shorter life of this costly equipment. Many items need to be cleaned or serviced after each use. These include electric clippers, surgical instruments, endoscopes, otoscopes, ophthalmoscopes, instrument trays, and oxygen tanks (gas levels).

To be efficient, all team members must learn to complete the last step of the action cycle (Figure 32-21) immediately after every event in the hospital. Otherwise, records are not up to date and the area or equipment is not ready when needed for the next patient! Unfinished paperwork, lack of needed cleanup, and forgotten follow-up on

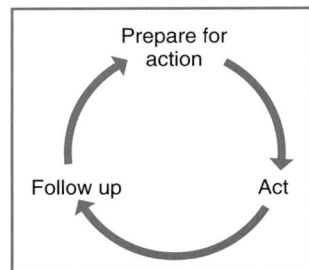

FIGURE 32-21.   Action cycle.

cases stack up and require part of the evening to finish or are forgotten. Encourage staff to be list makers and checkers to complete all the action cycles during a busy day. Tasks will be forgotten when staff members are interrupted before finishing all the follow-up tasks. Much of the disarray of a busy practice often comes from frequent lack of completion of the action cycle by one or more members of the staff team.

VETERINARY HEALTH CARE TEAM

Whereas the majority of veterinary practices were one-person practices in the twentieth century, a major shift has been occurring recently toward larger groups of veterinarians and support staff working in the same facility. This shift to increase the size of veterinary teams is being driven by an explosion of veterinary information, a demand for more and better pet health care by pet owners, and the need for a more economic delivery of veterinary services.

The team approach to veterinary practice allows different members of the team to focus on the areas of responsibility for which they have been trained and should leverage an increase of the veterinarians' effectiveness and productivity. It has also increased the demand for certified veterinary technicians. Therefore, although each of the members of the veterinary health care team has a different role, members must be hired and organized to work together efficiently as an effective team rather than as competing or isolated individuals.

Veterinarians: Owners and Associate Veterinarians

There are approximately 45,000 veterinarians practicing in about 22,000 veterinary practices in the United states. The average number of veterinarians per practice is about two, with the average range from 2.8 veterinarians per large animal practice to 1.9 for each small animal practice. Seventy percent of these veterinarians are in small animal practice with the remaining veterinarians in some form of mixed, large animal, or equine practice.

A recent development has been the increase of referral practices with board-certified specialists (e.g., veterinary radiologists, surgeons, dermatologists, ophthalmologists, internal medicine diplomates) who are receiving referral cases in their area of specialty from primary care veterinary practitioners. Also, the number of emergency clinics is increasing to handle after-hour emergencies and to provide 24-hour care for critically ill patients. Both the above practice types augment the service of primary care practices. The client returns to his or her original veterinarian after the referral or emergency service is provided. This health care network provides special or advance service to

clients when their animals need more than primary care treatment.

Each veterinary practice is usually owned by one or more of the veterinarians (business partners) in the practice. Sometimes the practice is owned by a large corporation that owns other practices. Both usually employ additional salaried veterinarians and hire their own support staff.

The veterinarians will focus the majority of their responsibilities on diagnosing illness, prescribing treatment plans, and performing surgery. These medical duties of the doctor require 4 intensive years of veterinary medical school preceded by 2 to 4 years of preveterinary college studies. Some independently minded veterinarians want to "do it all" and also perform the technician, reception, animal care, and management duties; this is not very cost effective. Every state requires all veterinarians in private practice to be licensed in that state (and follow the legal and ethical rules for veterinary practice).

Veterinary Practice Manager (VPM)

Veterinarians also managed their practices through most of the last century when one-person practices predominated. An increasing number of veterinarians (especially in group practices) are delegating the business management responsibilities to a practice manager. Medium-sized practices may divide these duties between several members of their veterinary team. In large practices a full-time, bachelor of science (B.S.) trained individual may serve as the practice manager.

Because veterinary practices are small businesses, the practice manager's role is to facilitate an efficiently operated and profitable medical business. The duties of the manager usually include hiring, supervising, and terminating personnel; managing inventory; handling client financial issues; facilitating accounting procedures needed for case control; analyzing progress toward goal; and developing and initiating new protocols for areas of hospital operation.

The owners, in concert with the hospital manager and other team members, must develop the mission statement and strategic plan for growth or change. The practice manager is delegated the responsibility for making day-to-day management decisions to meet theses goals for the business. The practice manager must also unite the team of veterinarians and support staff to work well together to meet the practice goals. Another management challenge necessary for business is the development of a marketing plan for the practice (discussed at the end of this chapter).

Veterinary Technician

A state-certified veterinary technician (VT) has had a college education in communications, science, math, animal husbandry, and other courses followed by education and training in medical and surgical nursing, anesthesia, radiography, and laboratory testing as well as client education and professional ethics. The technician's educational investment at an AVMA-accredited program totals 2 to 3 years according to the AVMA. Graduate veterinary technicians are credentialed by most states in which they practice as certified, licensed, or registered veterinary technicians after passing the Veterinary Technician National Exam (VTNE).

AVMA-accredited educational programs (85 at the beginning of the twenty-first century) focus on teaching a higher order of cognitive skills (to develop understanding of what, why, and how) than veterinarians give assistants with on-the-job training or in the few veterinary assistant programs of shorter duration. Veterinary technician students learn to understand the scientific basis of nursing. This begins with a foundation in biology, microbiology, chemistry, anatomy, and physiology and is followed by principles of hematology, radiology, anesthesia, and so forth.

Therefore graduate technicians should not only know how to perform nursing procedures, but also understand why and when they are done and be able to assess the strengths and weaknesses of procedure variations, problem solve, and recommend needed changes to the supervising veterinarian. They are also educated to anticipate early signs of changes in the clinical condition of patients. They are very adaptable and quickly learn new technologies and procedures that are available through continuing education and additional training.

There have been about 30,000 graduates of veterinary technician programs since this relatively new profession began in 1961. Only about 15,000 registered veterinary technicians were active in the profession at the start of the twenty-first century because many left for better opportunities before the profession recently began to improve technician utilization. Eighty-five AVMA-accredited programs in the United States graduated fewer than 2000 veterinary technicians and 27 veterinary schools graduated 2200 veterinarians at the beginning of the twenty-first century. This ratio of new graduates appears to be close to the need for a 1:1 ratio of technicians and veterinarians on the veterinary team but does nothing to make up the huge demand deficit that already exists. About 15,000 more technicians are needed to reach a 1:1 ratio!

The veterinary technician should be used to perform the technical procedures that veterinarians previously performed. This will provide veterinarians more time for seeing more patients, making more diagnoses and therapeutic decisions, and performing more surgery. The veterinary technician will also improve the level of patient care since veterinarians are so busy with additional clients and patients and need someone competent to handle recovery and intensive care of surgical and medical patients. The demand for technicians will definitely increase as more veterinarians delegate nursing and technical duties to certified veterinary technicians.

Veterinary Technologist

Veterinary technologists (VTG) are veterinary technicians who have invested in 4 years of education to earn a baccalaureate degree in veterinary technology. This extra education should prepare them to assume more management, supervision, or specialized technologist responsibilities in their career after gaining technician experience. Larger practices and institutions need nurse administrators to lead area teams or perform management tasks such as staff supervision, equipment management, and teaching in their area of activity (e.g., clinical laboratory, surgery room, radiology). The baccalaureate education should provide the foundation for future upward mobility. In human nursing the comparable individual is a registered nurse (R.N.) with a B.S. degree who becomes the nurse administrator or head nurse of an area. The technologist may also specialize in behavior counseling, emergency and critical care, anesthesia, or other areas.

Veterinary Technician Specialties

Emerging veterinary technician specialties are a new development in the profession. The use of the words *veterinary technician specialist* is reserved for those who pass an advanced examination (the same is true of specialties for veterinarians). The examination is administered by a na-

---

Box 32-5 | SOCIETIES WITH OR DEVELOPING SPECIALTY CERTIFICATION PROGRAMS

Veterinary Emergency and Critical Care Society (VECCS) Academy of Veterinary Emergency and Critical Care Technicians (AVECCT)
16729 San Pedro
San Antonio, TX 78232
AVECCT members can be certified as veterinary technician specialists-emergency and critical care *and will use* VTS (Emergency/Critical Care) after their name and state certification (i.e., Jane Doe, RVT, VTS (Emergency/Critical Care).

American Society of Veterinary Dental Technicians (ASVDT)
P.O. Box 1636
Venice, FL 34284-1636

Veterinary Technicians Anesthetist Society (VTAS) Academy of Veterinary Technician Nurse-Anesthetists (AVTNA)—proposed
c/o Charles Hoffman
Scott-Ritchey Research Center
Auburn University College of Veterinary Medicine
Auburn, AL 36849

Veterinary Hospital Managers Association, Inc. (VHMA)
48 Howard Street
Albany, NY 12207
To be certified, a VHMA member must be actively employed as a veterinary practice manager (not necessarily a technician or DVM), achieve 18 college credit hours in business management, pass VHMA written and oral examinations, and participate in 6 days of management continuing education every 2 years. The designation of certified veterinary practice manager (CVPM) is conveyed to successful applicants (i.e., Jane Doe, CVPM; if a registered technician, Jane Doe, RVT, CVPM).

---

tionally approved specialty society for each group (Box 32-5). It is misleading to the public to call anyone a specialist (even though one's knowledge and expertise may be advanced) until that person is accredited by a specialty organization that meets national standards. The North American Veterinary Technician Association is recognized by the AVMA as the accrediting body for veterinary technician specialties.

It is important to note that each of these specialties has a society (an organization of individuals interested in a particular area of veterinary technology) that is open to any interested veterinary technician. The society serves to provide advanced educational materials to its members, some of whom are certified and some of whom are interested in learning the specialty information without sitting for the examinations. Some societies are broader in scope, such as the Veterinary Hospital Managers Association, Inc., which is open to anyone (including nontechnicians) involved in veterinary practice management. Those who are certified become members of the respective academy.

Veterinary Assistant

Veterinary assistants (VA) are trained on the job (or in shorter courses than technician programs) with a focus on preparing for assisting both veterinarians and veterinary technicians. The veterinary assistant may have a number of different titles using one of the adjectives *animal, veterinary, technician, ward,* or *hospital,* combined with one of these nouns: *attendant, caretaker, orderly,* or *assistant.* Veterinary assistants are individuals with some training and skills that are less than the education and training required for certification as a veterinary technician. The basic tasks performed by assistants may include, but are not totally limited to, feeding, watering, bathing, restraining, transporting, and exercising animals. They may also perform cleaning, clerical office duties, and other similar-level activities. Sometimes they are also trained to do some of the basic technical procedures technicians perform.

Veterinary assistants should also be called *technician assistants.* Veterinary technicians cannot be efficiently utilized by veterinarians for performing the billable nursing and laboratory tasks of treatments, anesthesia, testing, and x-ray procedures without the help of a veterinary assistant, aide, or orderly. Also, it does not make economic sense for a veterinary technician to frequently restrain animals for the veterinarian (or perform other assistant duties) if a lower-salaried veterinary assistant is available.

Many veterinarians and technicians began their career gaining experience working or volunteering as a veterinary assistant. This does not shorten the education needed to become a technician or veterinarian but provides real world experience that motivates the student to go on with his or her education. Unfortunately, it also helps perpetuate the repetition of poor technician utilization patterns when the veterinarian graduates, especially if he or she initially worked for a veterinarian who did all the technical work without delegation to veterinary technicians.

Ward Staff

Ward staff members are individuals trained on the job to follow specific protocols for the cleaning and sanitation required to prevent nosocomial infections. They perform the basic husbandry required for keeping patients clean, groomed, fed, watered, and exercised with the safety and comfort of each patient taken into consideration. Ward staff must observe and record patient appetites, attitudes, bowel movements, and urinary output and alert the staff about observed abnormal behavior. They also move patients from the wards to the treatment area, to the reception for discharge, or to surgery. They may also be assigned basic janitorial duties in the rest of the hospital. Ward staff can also double as veterinary assistants.

Receptionists

Receptionists facilitate client service, communicate a sense of friendliness and helpfulness, and organize appointments so clients do not have to wait an unreasonable amount of time. The receptionist is a key position in any hospital operation. The "life blood" of the practice (clients) must filter through the receptionist via the telephone and one-on-one contact in the reception area. The old adages that "you don't have a second chance to make a first impression" and "the receptionist will make or break the practice" are key issues for selecting receptionists.

Receptionists have the critical role of handling the fee payments, billings, and daily cash records. These duties must be performed effectively to keep the business running smoothly, the clients happy, and the rest of the veterinary team aware of what is happening with clients and their pets. Receptionists are often the last person communicating with the client at checkout and can assess the general client satisfaction level when clients leave the premises. The business needs satisfied clients who will return as continuing clients and refer their friends and associates.

The receptionist's effectiveness is key to practice growth and happy clients!

Personnel Management

Personnel management is important because the greatest percentage of overhead is in personnel. All personnel must work as a team to ensure productivity. Working *with* someone is always better than working *for* someone. All practice employees (including veterinarians) must be as productive as possible to provide a profitable and pleasant working environment. Veterinarians and technicians are usually not professionally trained to be managers. Both must work together to have a successfully managed practice, which will result in greater career satisfaction, not just a job.

Regardless of the size of the practice and how it is managed, each position within the practice should have a backup person who is cross-trained in that area to take over when sickness, vacation, and emergencies arise. Without a cross-training plan, the practice may become crippled when one person is gone. This is especially true in smaller practices.

In most practices, the staff duties can be divided into the following job areas: (1) *reception,* (2) *examination room or outpatient duties,* (3) *inpatient duties,* and (4) *building, kennel, and barn maintenance.* The reception area is staffed and operated by one or more receptionists.

They must be friendly and caring people. The entire mood of the practice and, to a great extend, the attitude of the client will be determined by the communication skills and judgment of the receptionist. For example, the receptionist should screen patients and schedule undiagnosed medical problems or cases requiring radiography earlier in the day so that the client will have a diagnosis before the day's end. Emergencies obviously need immediate attention. The receptionist greets clients, starts the medical record by obtaining some history, answers questions by telephone, makes appointments, handles the records for patient dismissal, answers general medical questions, quotes certain fees, maintains a schedule of all veterinarians, handles money and bank deposits, and manages accounts receivable and other duties as assigned. In short, an effective receptionist in most practices is a super person.

A veterinary technician is usually assigned to *examination room* duties. In some practices, the receptionist and examination room duties will be performed by one person. The role of this individual may include backup or fill-in for the receptionist in addition to assisting in the examination rooms; obtaining medical histories; filling prescriptions; restraining patients; administering medications; demonstrating treatment techniques to clients; obtaining blood samples; performing laboratory work; escorting patients to the wards; dismissing patients; maintaining the examination, laboratory, and pharmacy areas in a clean and orderly manner; and other duties that are necessary for smooth patient flow in the public areas of the hospital. Efficiency is enhanced with multiple examination rooms and an assistant or orderly assigned to assist both technician and veterinarian. Every patient must be examined by a veterinarian to make the diagnosis to ensure that existing problems are not overlooked (e.g., hernias, retained testicles, external parasites). Patients should not be admitted unless a veterinarian has had contact with the patient and client to establish a legal client-patient-veterinarian relationship.

The duties in the *inpatient area* are more isolated, and there is usually less client contact. Most of these duties are performed by a team of technicians and assistants. These duties include administering or monitoring anesthesia or both; preparing patients for surgery; monitoring postsurgical patients; surgical assisting; collecting laboratory samples; performing dental cleanings; administering and monitoring treatments; exposing and developing radiographs; performing laboratory tests; maintaining medical records; maintaining surgical and anesthesia logs; providing direct medical and surgical nursing care; and maintaining the surgery, treatment, and radiology areas.

Maintaining *building*, *barn*, and *wards* in a clean and orderly manner and other duties that are necessary for hospitalized patients to be well cared for are usually delegated to assistants and caretakers and supervised by a veterinary technician. Animal caretakers and ward staff clean, bed, and feed patients, allowing the veterinary technician to perform additional technical support functions. The role of the technician is determined by the staffing and delegation patterns as well as the size and type of practice.

A veterinary technician must be able to work in all areas of the hospital. The most common technical support utilization in veterinary practices involves the generalist type of veterinary technician. For a technician to function effectively as a generalist, a broad base of information and techniques must be mastered and maintained with cross-training in all technical areas. Being a high-quality generalist is not an easy task.

Large private and institutional teaching hospital practices have the case load to allow the technical staff to become very skilled in one area. Examples of these areas would be surgery, intensive care, anesthesiology, cardiology, internal medicine, ophthalmology, dermatology, radiology, clinical pathology, and office management. Specialty societies and certifications for veterinary technicians are now available in critical care, dentistry, anesthesia, and management (see Box 32-5).

Delegation Principles

Personnel costs may be reduced by hiring the correct personnel for the job and delegating properly. Too many practices are still trying to hire a new veterinarian to perform veterinary technician duties. Many also hire veterinary technicians to perform non–income-producing duties of assistants and caretakers. Consequently, the practice spends more money than necessary on personnel and frustrates a new veterinarian or technician in the process as well as limiting income produced.

Both veterinarians and veterinary technicians should be paid according to gross income produced; therefore aides and assistants hired at near minimum wage levels should be relied on as much as possible to perform most non–income-producing tasks, such as restraint, general cleaning, and animal husbandry. Veterinarians should focus on making diagnoses, prescribing treatments, and performing surgery while delegating billable treatments, such as anesthesia, dental prophylaxes, imaging, and laboratory procedures, to certified veterinary technicians.

Job Descriptions

Regardless of position in the hospital setting, all personnel should have a detailed job description. A job description will allow both employee and management to maintain a clear understanding of current and new areas of responsibility. Job descriptions are also very useful when hiring new employees or replacing employees.

Through the use of the job descriptions (expectations) and periodic performance evaluations, employees can be rewarded according to their performance, poor workers can be guided and encouraged to improve, and chronically poor workers can be discharged. One of the most common mistakes in personnel management is to put off regular employee evaluations. Personnel problems resulting from poor work performance do not just go away, they only become worse. Therefore a job evaluation system that is applied equally and fairly to all employees needs to be maintained. Employees cannot improve performance unless they are given an opportunity to identify shortcomings. If improvement is not observed within a reasonable period of time, both the practice and employee will probably be better off with employee dismissal.

Hiring Procedures

When hiring a new employee, it is important that all employees have input into the decision if teamwork is to be expected. This is a very important decision. The cost of selection, training, and adaptation can equal 1 year's salary. A bad choice means disruption, turnover, and a loss of thousands of dollars to the practice.

A simple method of candidate evaluation that will satisfy most employees is to have two or three employees interview each candidate first and then make recommendations to the veterinarian. The screening committee should establish some specific questions for each interviewer to ask each candidate using the job description prepared for that specific job. The recommendations made to the veterinarian should include job suitability, personality, professionalism, knowledge, experience, dress, and other interview assessments. The veterinarian should have the final word on hiring and firing unless a practice manager has been hired for personnel management.

The major steps in the hiring process are as follows:

1. Analyze personnel requirements.
2. Develop a specific job description.
3. Develop a set of interview questions.
4. Announce and advertise the position.
5. Review the applications and resumes.
6. Rank the candidates for interview.
7. Check references.
8. Interview the top-ranked two to four candidates.
9. Make a final selection.
10. Offer the job to the best candidate.
11. Establish a starting date.

The analysis of personnel requirements will be done by the veterinarian or office manager based on the needs of the practice or business. Once the general need for the position or positions has been established (or replacement approved), a detailed job description must be prepared or the previous job description updated. The job description is usually developed on one page and consists of four or five job functions outlined in one or two sentences each. Each job function is then assigned a percentage of time. Once the job description is developed or updated, it can be used to write the advertisement to search for a specific individual. To prepare for the interview, a set of interview questions needs to be developed.

Some interview questions are unlawful or discriminatory and must not be asked (e.g., questions on race, religion, national origin, gender, handicaps, marital status). Questions should always be open ended (Box 32-6) and allow the candidates to express themselves. The following requests and questions could be considered when preparing interview questions:

1. Please review your previous position.
2. Describe your best boss.

Box 32-6   **COMMUNICATION TECHNIQUES FOR INTERVIEWING CLIENT**

OPEN-ENDED (OR PROBING) QUESTIONS   *vs.*   *LEADING (YES/NO) QUESTIONS*
Who?   Did?
How?   Was it?
What?
When?
Where?
Answers will be detailed descriptions.   Answers will be yes or no even if client is not sure!

ONE-WORD ACKNOWLEDGMENT   **PARAPHRASING**
Use one word (e.g., oh, OK, yes) with eye contact and voice   Restate client statements (in your own words) to check with
  inflection that imply you understand and want him or her   the client whether you understand what the client is trying
  to continue talking. This can be done with eye contact,   to say before going on in the interview. Use paraphrasing
  nonverbal signs of active listening, and verbal silence with periodically in each segment of the interview to give the
  some clients.   client an opportunity to clarify or confirm your under-
                                                               standing.

ACCENT QUESTIONS   **SUMMARIZING**
Restate one or two words used by the client in a questioning Restate main points at the end (or at end of major segments)
  tone, which serves to request the client to elaborate on the to emphasize key points and inform the client about what
  description of events or signs.   is going to happen next.

---

3.   Describe your worst boss.
4.   What did you like best about your last position?
5.   What did you like least about your last position?
6.   What specific skills and abilities do you have that apply to this particular position?
7.   What are your short-range and long-term employment goals?
8.   What accomplishments have made you most proud?
9.   What type of working relationships do you want to cultivate?
10. How do you feel about constructive criticism and formal performance evaluation?
11. How do you feel about being on call several times per month?
12. Do you have any questions you would like to ask?

During the interview, the evaluator should ask each candidate the same questions so the responses can be objectively compared. The interview period is the time to evaluate motivation, personal appearance, and personal hygiene. The job description, salary, and benefits should be reviewed. Each interviewer or interview team should limit their part of the interview to 30 minutes.

After the interview, personal references should be checked and past supervisors contacted. When all the above material has been collected and weighed, the individual who is the best person (and match) for the position should be offered the job.

When the final selection has been made, the most common initial contact will be by telephone. During the telephone call, the job description should be reviewed, salary and benefits discussed, and starting date established. When the above steps are followed, the best candidate should be more easily identified and successfully hired. Other candidates should be notified that the position has been filled with the applicant who best matched the position.

A potential problem in personnel management is inadequate internal communication. To avoid internal disputes, weekly (or monthly) staff meetings should be held to update all employees on various aspects of hospital operation. Often, notes on a blackboard just do not do the job! These meetings can also be used to develop teamwork via group problem-solving techniques.

 Technician Note

Practice staff meetings should be held at least once per month to ensure open communication.

Role of Veterinary Technicians and Veterinarians in Management

Technicians have an ever-increasing role in practice management. In most practice situations, technicians will be involved in management of the patient, client, equipment, and inventory. They may also be involved in staff, facility, and business management. To develop management skills, one must be willing to assume increasing levels of responsibility. As the practice changes in staffing, number of cases, facility, type of clients, new technologies, and so forth, the veterinary technician must adapt his or her management skills to these changes.

The role of the veterinary technician in management will vary depending on the type of practice and the previous experiences of the technician and the veterinarian. The technician who can (1) conceptualize the vision and goals set by the veterinarian for the practice, (2) efficiently organize each area in which he or she is given responsibility, (3) become a productive team player and a good communicator, and (4) develop the ability to solve problems constructively to enhance both patient care and the veterinary team will usually be given a greater role in practice management.

To be effective, the veterinarian-owner must act as overall hospital chief executive officer (CEO) and delegate appropriate areas of responsibility to the veterinary technician as well as to other members of the team. Effective delegation of responsibility to the technician must include billable (income producing) technical procedures of medical and surgical nursing. Ideally, veterinarians diagnose, prescribe, and perform surgery; and technicians perform venipunctures, laboratory tests, and prescribed treatments; expose and develop radiographs; and anesthetize, prepare, and manage recovery of surgical patients. The veterinary technician should also delegate most non–income-producing tasks to lesser paid aides, assistants, or animal caretakers. Clinic aides restrain, move, feed, and exercise the animals and assist both technicians and veterinarians when needed. Receptionists handle scheduling, receiving, discharging, billing, and related front office duties. There should be a direct relationship between the salary level paid and the income produced (productivity) for each veterinary technician and veterinarian in a practice if effective delegation is occurring.

Technician Note

The veterinary technician should delegate most non–income-producing tasks to assistants or aides.

Practice management efforts are necessary in all types of practice. To be effective the veterinarian and veterinary technician must be human resources managers. This requires both excellent communication skills and a policy and procedures manual for the practice team. It involves hiring, training, and scheduling performance appraisals and discharge of staff. The veterinarian and technician must work together with the rest of the staff as both a management team and a medical team.

Unfortunately, most colleges provide little training in hospital or people management for either technicians or veterinarians because it takes students so much time and effort to gain the medical expertise, technical skills, and confidence necessary to succeed medically. However, there are many new resources available to meet this need for management training after graduation, including continuing education short courses, books, journals, organizations, and consultants.

Technician Note

Never argue with a dissatisfied client.

Patient Management

Patient management and client management go hand in hand. Both should be handled together, but for the sake of this discussion they are treated separately.

Patient management can best be described by outlining the typical case as it moves through the hospital. The first contact is with the receptionist. The receptionist should move the patient and client as quickly as possible into an examination room. A patient presented as an emergency should receive priority. An emergency case is always any case that the *owner* feels is an emergency. Most of these cases are not emergencies, but each should be managed as if it were to ensure client satisfaction with quality of service.

In many practices, the patient will be escorted into the examination room by a veterinary technician. The technician will continue to develop the medical record by obtaining the temperature, pulse, respiration, and weight of the patient. Additional informational questions are asked to establish a preliminary history, and a brief physical examination may also be helpful to the veterinarian (see Box 32-6).

Once the veterinarian enters the examination room, the patient and owner should be introduced to the veterinarian by the technician. Name tags should be worn by all personnel to help clients remember whom they have met and who is the veterinarian. A veterinary assistant or technician should assist the veterinarian in the physical examination by restraining the patient as necessary. If blood, urine, or skin specimens are needed, the technician should usually take the patient to the treatment room and conduct these procedures away from the client with the help of an assistant while the veterinarian is seeing another client and patient. Once a diagnosis has been made by the veterinarian, the patient will either be treated and released or be hospitalized.

If the patient is to be treated and released, the technician will often give the treatment and will prepare prescriptions as needed. The technician will explain (or demonstrate) how to administer home medications or treatments and will then escort the client to the receptionist for dismissal and fee payment.

When the patient is to be hospitalized, the assistant or technician will escort the patient to the ward and ensure that the necessary items are present to make the patient comfortable. The veterinarian will establish each treatment regimen and evaluate its success. During hospitalization, the technician will maintain and manage most routine treatments, therapy, laboratory tests, and medical records while delegating exercise, feeding, restraint, and grooming to assistants or animal caretakers. Often the daily phone contact with the client will be through the technician. A blackboard or bulletin board in the treatment room can be used to remind personnel of the diagnostic, treatment, and surgery schedules for hospitalized patients. All patients should be evaluated several times each day, and these evaluations should be documented with appropriate entries into the medical record. Walking though ward rounds can be very helpful to all personnel to keep everyone updated on each case.

The dismissal of a hospitalized patient is similar to that of the outpatient except that dispensed medications and patient cleanup must be completed before the owner's arrival. When dismissing a hospitalized patient, the following points should be considered:

- An itemized fee statement should be ready at the time the owner is called to pick up the animal.
- All medications should be prepared in child-proof containers with proper labels.
- The veterinarian should be available for consultation with the client.
- The technician should be available to demonstrate treatment and home care techniques with handout instructions for home reference.
- Fee collection should take place.
- The next appointment or recheck should be scheduled.
- The patient should be presented dry, clean, and odor free.

Some conditions dictate that the patient be presented before fee collection and the scheduling of the next appointment. When this occurs, someone should be available to hold or control the animal until the client has completed the dismissal process.

The technician can be extremely valuable during the dismissal process by explaining to the client what to do if specific possible events occur (through reinforcement of directions given by the veterinarian). Clients will often ask technicians questions that they forgot or were afraid to ask the veterinarian.

Most clients will judge the care an animal has received by the condition and appearance of the animal at dismissal. The patient should always be as clean or cleaner than when admitted. If an animal soils itself just before dismissal, always clean or bathe the animal before sending it home even if the client has to wait a few minutes longer. The client should be informed that the animal has accidentally soiled itself and that you are cleaning it up: "We certainly do not want him to leave dirty." When dismissing surgical patients, in addition to the animal itself being clean, the surgical incision, bandages, splint, or cast must be clean and dry. The surgery technique will often be judged by the neatness of hair removal at the surgical site and the appearance of the incision.

Technician Note

Never send home a patient that has soiled itself or has an unpleasant odor.

INVENTORY MANAGEMENT

The purpose of inventory management and control is to always have every drug, vaccine, or supply item available when needed for use (or sale) yet not waste money acquiring and storing extra supplies that are not needed in the near future. This is a delicate balance because the amount and trends of use of drugs and supplies can change rapidly. Close attention to inventory levels of surgical supplies, pet food, pharmaceuticals, vaccines, x-ray film, and other items will ensure that an adequate stock is maintained without oversupply if an effective inventory control system is being used to reorder and replenish items before they are gone.

If too much stock is on hand, extra money and storage space are committed and the stock will be paid for long before the last of it is used. If too little is kept on hand, needed items will sometimes not be available to provide the preferred treatment for the patient or an opportunity for profiting from the sale of a product will be missed. If the right amount is on hand, the doctors and staff always have what is needed, large amounts do not have to be ordered and stored, and much of it is used before the payment to the supplier is due creating the needed cash flow to pay the supplier.

Inventory is the second largest expense area of operating a veterinary practice. Drugs should be used and be replaced about every 45 to 60 days (a turnover rate of six to eight times per year). The formula that is used for computing turnover rate is listed in Box 32-7. Turnover can be computed for every item in the inventory, averaged for the total inventory, or focused on the 20% of the items that account for the majority (80%) of uses (Pareto's law). Some inventory items will naturally turn over every 2 to 3 weeks (12 to 18 times per year), such as pet food, and often much or all of the item will be sold, generating income before the supplier requires payment.

Practice managers, sometimes veterinary technicians or a veterinarian, and occasionally reception staff or an assistant will be assigned responsibility for inventory control. Sometimes the responsibilities are divided among several staff members. One person should be the primary person placing orders, making sure that what is received is what was ordered and/or billed, and authorizing payment for the shipments. It is also important to set up an inventory master list of all items in stock in the hospital; keep a pharmacy library of all company product inserts, catalogs, and ordering procedures; and keep a file of material safety data sheets (MSDSs) for all products as required by OSHA.

Considerable money is involved in inventory purchases. Much can be lost through inadequate inventory control procedures. This loss may occur because the business was billed for materials that were never shipped or never received at the practice, or the business was double-billed for one shipment, billed for damaged goods, or billed for more or different items than were received. Back orders that are not canceled when the product is reordered elsewhere double the inventory! Losses also occur because of ordering too many months' supply of perishable vaccines, biologicals, antibiotics, and reagents that deteriorate beyond the printed expiration date on the container and are no longer effective or legally safe to use. Oversupply also crowds the shelf and storage space and leads to more misplacement and overordering or loss from not rotating new items to the back and oldest products forward to be used first. The best stock rotation system is "first in, first out" (FIFO).

The sales representative's responsibility is to sell their product and "deals" that may provide more product than can be used in 1 or 2 months. It makes little sense to buy and store a year's supply of an item, no matter how much the price has been reduced. On the other hand, during a seasonal increase of use of a product, it will make sense to buy a large supply instead of the normal 1-month supply, particularly if the price has been cut significantly.

There are many computerized and manual inventory systems available for upgrading a current practice's procedures on inventory control. Because computerized systems require the input of everything that is sold and used in order to be accurate, they are only moderately successful in providing all the inventory control information needed. Manual procedures, such as identifying minimum stock reorder points on the shelf, posting want lists or reorder bins for all staff to use, and taking frequent inventory count of all supplies, can go a long way to help the computerized inventory control process be a success.

An effective inventory control system should be easy to use, ensure that all medications and supplies are available when needed, and reduce expenses by achieving a turnover

---

Box 32-7	**INVENTORY MANAGEMENT FORMULAS**

$$\text{Turnover rate* of an item} = \frac{\text{Yearly inventory expense for item}}{\text{Average cost of item on hand at any one time}}$$

$$\text{Average cost of inventory on hand at one time} = \frac{\text{Inventory at midyear} + \text{Inventory at year's end}}{2}$$

*Pareto's law, or the 80/20 rule, states that 20% of the items account for 80% of the annual inventory expenses; this suggests that the above formulas should be used to evaluate and adjust the turnover rate of the biggest expense items to attain the "ideal turnover rate."

Modified from *Lukens & Landon's effective inventory control,* West Chester, Pa, 1993, Smith Kline Beecham (Pfizer).

rate of 8 to 12 times per year. It should provide a signal when each item needs to be reordered, track seasonal variations, track past usage rates, and provide purchase cost information to keep the pricing and supply of products current. It should ensure that ordered items are actually received and back-ordered items are tracked so that overordering does not occur. It should also be easy to account for when and where items are used so cost can be allocated to various profit centers within the clinic. It should ensure proper monitoring and handling of Drug Enforcement Agency (DEA) controlled substances, provide a procedure for checking invoices to make sure they are accurate for amounts ordered and prices quoted, and periodically assess the value of the inventory. It should also reduce the cost of ordering the supplies by taking advantage of minimum orders for prepaid shipments and discounts for early payments when available. The inventory control system should also allow the practice to obtain the best prices available, identify expired or outdated items for prompt removal and return to suppliers for credit if provided, and enable the manager to detect staff pilferage if it occurs (modified from *A Guide to Inventory Management for Veterinary Practices/Effective Inventory Control*, 1993, SmithKline Beecham).

All these desirable results of managing inventory will not occur if someone is not put in charge of inventory control and given adequate time and support by all members of the veterinary team to accomplish the assignment!

CLIENT MANAGEMENT

The most important person in any practice is each client. The practice of veterinary medicine is truly a *people business*. Everyone in the practice must enjoy working with and problem solving for the clients served by the practice. Veterinarians and technicians who do not like working with clients and their animal problems should not be employed in practice because they are ineffective with client communication. Many other professional careers are now available for individuals who desire less public contact.

Technician Note

The most important person in any practice is each client!

Value of the Client
The availability of veterinary services in the United States appears to be at an all-time high. New schools of veterinary medicine and expanded enrollment at existing schools have resulted in this increased availability of graduate veterinarians. The net result of the increasing supply of veterinary practitioners is increased competition for clients among established and new practices.

The practices that will financially survive must offer expanded services that are competitive. Practices can become more cost effective by using both technicians and assistants effectively to leverage the veterinarians' productivity while expanding service.

How valuable is each client? The practice will collapse unless old clients are retained and new clients are continually entering the practice. Clients are the lifeblood of the practice. Everyone in the practice works for the client. Some practices would like to think that they control their clients, but client loyalty is seldom mandated. Loyalty is won with hard work and dedicated caring service to each client.

The only unique product that a veterinary practice has to offer is service. If everyone in the practice understands that his or her primary role is to provide the finest quality medical care possible to the patient with the end result being a pleased and informed client, the practice will grow. If the staff attitude becomes one of negative feelings toward clients (e.g., not another one of these!), the practice clientele will dwindle. A practice's facilities, equipment, and techniques may be the finest available, but they will remain unused until enough clients willingly authorize or request that practice's services.

Client Selection of a Veterinarian
How does a client select a veterinarian? Most clients with small animals will select a veterinarian because the practice location is convenient. Following closely after practice location, recommendations from friends are ranked next. Once a practice is selected, the individual veterinarian will be evaluated in the following areas: friendly and caring personality, gentleness in handling the animal, communication skills, and professional knowledge. In the selection process it becomes readily apparent that practice location, facility appearance, and recommendations from satisfied clients are extremely important to practice growth.

Once the client enters the hospital the ability of the veterinarian and staff to project a concerned, caring personality, the expertise used in carefully handling the animal, and the clarity of the communication are the most important determining factors. It is interesting to note that professional knowledge falls to the bottom of the list. The general public has a limited informational basis by which to judge the professional knowledge of a physician, dentist, attorney, or veterinarian.

Technician Note

Practice location and personal referrals are the two most common methods by which new clients find a veterinarian.

When does the veterinary technician have an impact on the client selection process? Clients always view the hospital staff as an extension of the veterinarian. Therefore a friendly personality, patient-handling techniques, and caring communication skills become critically important in this whole process.

Clients with large animals usually select a veterinarian based on recommendations from others. Once the veterinarian arrives at the farm or ranch the retention and satisfaction issues are the same as the ones used by small animal owners, with the addition of economic return. In food animal practice, the veterinarian must become an economic asset to the overall farm profitability or the client cannot afford to seek veterinary services. Companion animal practice (i.e., small animal, horse) has some economic limits, but the sentimental and emotional attachment (human-animal bond) of the client to the animal is relied on to extend that economic limit, which the food animal client may not do.

Evaluation of the Client
The technician's attitude toward himself or herself will be reflected in how clients are handled. People who are happy and positive about themselves and what they are doing will find that this attitude dominates client relations. One of the most contagious attitudes is enthusiasm. Enthusiastic people turn other people on! Enthusiasm is caught, not

taught. The client must be handled effectively so that staff members do not cause a positive client to become negative. Conversely, veterinary personnel should deal with a negative client in a friendly and positive manner, identifying his or her concerns and needs and trying to help find a solution.

Generally, after working with a client for a short period of time, a staff member will get enough feedback to make some judgments about the client's expectations. These expectations are in the form of client-pet relationships, client-hospital relationships, and one-on-one personal relationships. One should not judge clients by their outward appearances only. Clients who appear to have nothing materially may value their animal highly and spend their resources to support veterinary care. In contrast, clients who drive up in a luxury car and have expensive clothes may not have the animal's best interests in mind and may be financially overextended. You cannot judge a book by its cover, and you cannot judge people by their appearance.

Technician Note

Do not judge the client's ability to pay by his or her appearance.

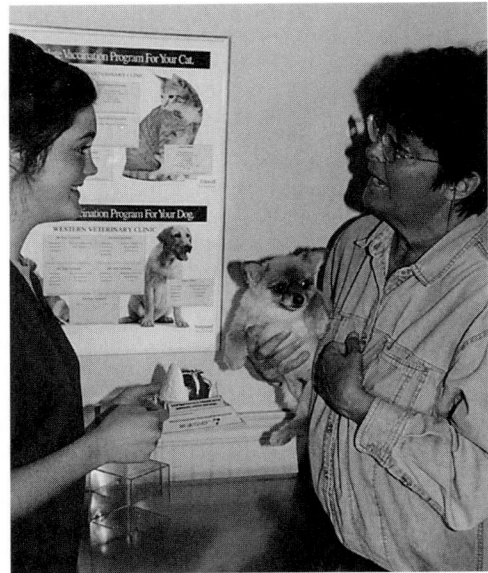

FIGURE 32-22. Veterinary technician uses a heartworm model to enhance client understanding of the impact of heartworm disease.

In most instances the technician and veterinarian will have to discuss the perceived pet's value with the client and give the client the opportunity to express himself or herself. One of the most important roles in client communication is to establish the value of the animal in that client-pet relationship. Some clients will be difficult to really figure out, and veterinary personnel may never feel they understand the client's intent or interest level.

Client Traffic Flow Patterns

When the client first enters the reception area the admission process begins. The receptionist initiates the proper business and medical records for each case. The client is escorted into one of the examination rooms. A preliminary history and examination (including temperature, pulse, and respiration [TPR]) may be taken by the technician before the veterinarian arrives. After examination and consultation with the veterinarian, either the client will leave the animal (hospitalization for further diagnostic tests, treatment, surgery, or observation) or the patient will be treated and, if necessary, medication will be dispensed before the patient returns to the receptionist for dismissal. In the event the patient is dismissed (outpatient), the client settles the account and is scheduled to return for a reexamination or to call with a follow-up report. During the routine outpatient visit, the client usually only contacts the outpatient work area. The client traffic pattern for an outpatient visit is reception→admission→examination→ (pharmacy) (laboratory)→dismissal.

If the patient is hospitalized, the client may have some contact with the inpatient area in addition to the outpatient area. A typical client traffic pattern in the hospitalized case would be reception→admission→examination→ treatment area or surgical area→hospitalization→admission (discussion of dismissal and payment-credit policy). The client would leave the hospital and return to the reception area on the day of dismissal.

On dismissal of hospitalized cases, the client enters the reception area and usually receives patient information from the receptionist or technician. The client then pro-

ceeds to the examination room for a brief consultation with the veterinarian followed by home care instructions and demonstrations from the technician (Figure 32-22). To reduce confusion at dismissal, it is advisable for the client to return to the dismissal area and settle the account before the patient is presented. Once the patient has been returned to the client, communication may be difficult during the reunion process.

In addition to the routine and outpatient client traffic pattern, a third type of contact exists when the client visits a hospitalized patient. In this event, the client usually makes an appointment with the receptionist to visit the animal at a specific time that is convenient to both client and the hospital operation. When the client arrives, he or she will proceed directly to the examination or treatment room. Visiting patients in the ward is usually discouraged because other patients in the ward are disturbed. During the visit with the animal, a technician (or veterinarian) should be present to answer questions concerning care and progress made by the patient. The client should always visit with the veterinarian at some point in the examination room or the treatment room or in the veterinarian's private office.

Client visits are often beneficial for both the hospitalized patient and the client. The mental attitudes of client and patient can be strengthened, and communication can be improved between veterinarian and client. Client visits should be encouraged rather than discouraged.

Office Procedures

General office procedure knowledge is required of all staff in a veterinary practice. Staff (veterinarians, technicians, assistants, office managers) all need to have a working knowledge of how appointments are made, personnel staffed, fees developed and collected, inventory ordered and controlled, and pet insurance utilized. Most practices have a limited number of staff positions, and therefore everyone must have the ability to perform basic office procedures. The ability to perform other jobs is obtained through *cross training.*

The additional information needed to perform the work of others is acquired by being cross trained through working in different jobs while being trained in one's new job. This allows most jobs to be temporally performed by different people when a person is out sick or on vacation. In small businesses this ability to fill in with other staff is essential to maintain a smooth running business.

Appointments

Companion animal practices can operate either through the use of an appointment or a walk-in system. Each system has advantages and disadvantages, but the appointment system is preferred by most veterinarians. Appointments allow the practice to control the flow of clients and patients into specific time periods that will improve the efficiency of the work schedule. When more clients are scheduled, most staff can be made available during the busier periods, and on the other hand, when no appointments are scheduled, staff numbers can be reduced.

The appointment system usually functions around the scheduling of consultation times (office visits) in 15-, 20-, or 30-minute blocks. When 15-minute blocks are used, then four appointments per hour can be scheduled. Companion animal practices usually schedule 3 or 4 hours of appointment times in the morning and afternoon. A typical appointment period might be from 8:00 AM to 12:00 noon and 3:00 PM to 6:30 PM. Between noon and 3:00 PM, case work-ups, treatments, and surgery are performed.

Because of clients' work schedules, practices are now scheduling consultations in the evening to help meet the needs of the working family. Several evenings may be scheduled from 6:00 PM to 8:00 PM. Saturdays are also becoming more important to many clients, because Monday through Friday are filled with work and family activity. In many practices, Saturday is becoming the busiest day of the week.

The walk-in practice is the other method of scheduling. When using this work schedule, clients simply come in whenever they want and wait to be seen. The advantages to the client are not having to make an appointment and being able to drop in at the practice when it is convenient. The disadvantages are the length of wait time and the congestion when several clients come in at the same time. For the practice, the major disadvantage is not being able to plan and somewhat control and spread the workload to prevent several people coming at the same time.

To change from a walk-in practice to an appointment schedule requires planning and client communication. The first step is to set up 1 hour for appointments in the morning and 1 hour for appointments in the afternoon. Then as clients come into the practice for service or call the practice, explain that for the convenience of the client the practice has changed to an appointment schedule. Each client should be encouraged to use the appointment system the next time. As more and more clients are educated about the use and convenience of the appointment system the 1-hour periods are expanded. Eventually, only 30 minutes of unscheduled time is left in the morning and afternoon for walk-ins and semi-emergencies.

Emergency cases are accepted at any time and are given priority over all appointments. However, if an appointment and a walk-in client come into the practice at the same time, the appointment is always given preference. Walk-in clients are always serviced, but they should not be given priority over an appointment unless it is a true emergency. Walk-in clients should never be turned away just because they do not have an appointment.

Practice Scheduling

More and more people are now employed outside the home, so clients often have difficulty in visiting the practice between 8 AM and 5 PM, Monday through Friday. To help solve this problem, many practices now are expanding their consultation hours in the evening and on Saturdays. Some practices also offer early drop-off or late pick-up service. This requires the veterinarian to communicate directly with the owner before the pick-up or drop-off time.

The technician will also need to be able to discuss the case with the owner when he or she arrives at the practice during these extended hours, since the veterinarian may not always be available.

In addition to extending the hours, the staff must be scheduled to provide coverage during all practice hours. If the practice is open 6 days per week and operates 10 hours per day, support staff must be limited to a work schedule of 40 hours per week, so that overtime can be kept at a minimum. Veterinarians who are nonowners are usually scheduled between 38 and 48 hours per week.

The larger the number of employees in the practice, the more scheduling flexibility is available. Early morning, late evening, and Saturday periods are usually rotated so that everyone shares in these hours. If part-time employees are used, they could be scheduled into these extended hours and relieve full-time staff. The use of part-time employees greatly increases the flexibility to cover the expanded hours necessary to meet clients' needs. Part-time employees are more available now for both professional and support staff and can be readily used for coverage of extended hours.

Professional Fees

The only money available for funding a veterinary practice is collected from the clients as professional fees for professional medical services and products purchased. Loans from a bank will have to be obtained to cover deficits when there are more expenses than income. Therefore the veterinary business is vulnerable to failure if sufficient income is not received from enough clients to pay the operating costs of the business.

There are no government subsidies, few if any donations, and small amounts of money from pet insurance companies paid to veterinary practices. Therefore all employees must understand that their salary level is directly related to the health of the business and their productivity in generating income from billable tasks and product sales. Health care teams must be effectively organized with this principle in mind or the business will deteriorate.

Each veterinary practice should set fees based on what it costs to deliver services. However, the methods used for determining fees vary from practice to practice just like the cost of land and staffing of the facilities will vary. Methods used to set fees vary from accounting methods for establishing fees based on the cost of offering the service, to a competitive guess of trying to match or undercut the price that other practices charge, to just estimating what each client can afford. Only the accounting method is an acceptable business procedure.

Many veterinarians try to discount fees to a level they think the client can afford. However, it is impossible to accurately judge what a client can afford and is willing to spend. Only the client can freely decide what the animal means to him or her and what he or she is willing to pay. Discounting fees will eventually lead to reducing the quality of medical service, and that is unfair to the patient.

It may also expose the team to charges of negligence and legal liabilities if the quality of care is below the accepted standard of care offered in similar practices in the area.

The practice manager or accountant must be able to identify the indirect costs and direct costs of operating the business via the financial reports to set or adjust the fees. Several steps are required to arrive at the appropriate fee for each procedure based on the cost of providing that service or product. First, direct costs are identified for each procedure related to the expendables used (drugs, bandages, film, etc.). Amortization of equipment costs over the equipment's expected useful life is also computed. For example, depreciating an x-ray machine over 7 years of useful life requires determining the number of x-rays taken per year from the radiology records. This will allow one to calculate the amount that must be included in the radiology fee for each x-ray taken. The machine will be paid for in the 7 years if the projected number of x-rays is taken (i.e., if the projected number of radiograph exposures is accurate).

The indirect costs (overhead) of operating a business must be computed. These include purchase or rental of the land, construction or rental of the building, the monthly cost of the utilities, facility upkeep, as well as taxes and interest on the debt. A new furnace, remodeling costs, and additions to the facility are included as either an annual cost or spread over several years. This cost of operation is added to each fee assessed as a percentage of overhead expense. It is spread over the number of expected client transactions in each fee to recover the indirect costs of overhead.

The biggest cost of running a professional business is the payroll for the staff. Veterinarians' salaries, whether they are owners or employees, and the salaries of the rest of the veterinary team must all be prorated to each fee. The accountant does this for each procedure based on time input for each of the team members. Therefore an estimate of the normal time the receptionist, the veterinarian, the veterinary technician, and the veterinary assistant spend to support each service must be computed. Time is valued per minute using each salary level and adding the payroll overhead costs (often 30% or more of salary). This is multiplied by the average time each person spends on the procedure and added to that fee. Once computed, all fees should be reviewed semiannually and adjusted as cost increases occur because of inflation. Obviously, fees must be refigured if anything major changes with staff time, the length of the procedure, or the purchase of new equipment.

The goal is to charge fair and equitable fees to cover the practice's cost of providing each service to clients. The fees should support using modern equipment, paying appropriate salaries to keep an effective team employed, and providing a fair return on the investment to the owners for taking business risks.

Fees fall into two groups: *shopped fees* or *nonshopped fees*. The shopped fees (examination fee, vaccination fee, and elective surgery fees: neuter, spay, declaw, etc.) should be competitive with other area practices. The level of shopped fees should be controlled by the going rate of other practices in the immediate practice area. Clients will judge the level of all practice fees by how competitive the shopped fees seem to them when they call and shop your practice.

The other group of fees are the nonshopped fees (clients do not call and shop these services), which include all other services in the practice. Examples of nonshopped fees are treatment for diarrhea or vomiting, fracture repair, chest x-ray, complete blood count, general anesthesia, cystotomy, angiogram, and cataract surgery. Most fees in practice are nonshopped. Therefore the practice can assess a fair fee for any of these services without concern about what other local practices are charging. The only fees that must be competitive are the shopped fees.

Technician Note

The only fees that must be competitive are the shopped fees.

The nonshopped fees should be increased by the inflation rate on at least an annual basis. If the annual inflation rate reaches 6%, then the nonshopped fees should be adjusted on a quarterly or monthly basis. Smaller, regular increases are not noticed by the client as much as one large annual increase. The major fees that attract client attention are the shopped fees, and these are only adjusted when local area practices adjust theirs. Computerization allows fee adjustments to be made easily and quickly even when done on a monthly basis.

Practice computerization (see Chapter 34) has allowed practices to have a much more detailed listing of fees for services and products. Fee codes can easily run into the thousands but are carefully adjusted and accounted for by the computer. This allows the client to receive a very detailed invoice at the conclusion of the practice visit. Computer software can also provide the client with a detailed fee estimate before service. This allows the client to make an informed decision about the level of service desired before the service is actually provided. This level of client communication is necessary to control collections and monthly billing.

Practice managers, owners, and the accountants that set up the accounting system of the practice will use monthly and yearly statistical summaries of incomes and expenses for evaluating changing trends for different procedures in all areas of the hospital, including profit centers. Trends of change from month to month and year to year are easy to track and recognize. The productivity of each veterinarian and veterinary technician can also be tracked with computerization software and salaries adjusted up or down based on productivity. In general the software should provide the business reports containing necessary information to make management decisions on what fees should be raised or lowered. This system enhances and rewards motivation and helps manage change. In summary, the accounting procedure for setting professional fees provides the basis for managing an effective business that will change as costs and demand for services change. The fees should be evaluated and adjusted twice yearly as appropriate to keep the fees in line with the costs and practice goals.

Collections and Billings

Most practices have a standard payment policy of "payment in full at the time service is provided." Cash payment is always the best method of payment. However, some services can be very expensive, and payment in full may not be possible at the time the service is rendered. Therefore alternative payment plans are usually required if the service is to be provided.

Alternative payment plans include the use of bank credit cards (Master Card, Visa, Discover, American Express, etc.), medical credit cards (Care Credit), and local bank credit and practice credit accounts. After all the above payment plans are discussed, the practice credit account should be used as the last option. When internal credit is provided, specific controls must be in place. The usual controls for practice credit include approval of a credit application, a 50% deposit at the time the estimate is given, the balance to be paid in three or four monthly payments, 1.5% per month interest charge on the unpaid balance, and payment of a monthly billing fee (usually $3 to $8). The monthly billing fee covers the cost of billing each client (computer time, personnel time, stationery, envelopes, postage).

The collection of a 50% deposit based on the fee estimate at the time of admission is the standard way of determining how the client will pay the account. All hospitalized cases should have a written fee estimate prepared before service. Routine outpatient services usually do not receive a written fee estimate. True emergency cases are an exception. When a written fee estimate is prepared on a hospitalized case, the client will be informed by the business manager, technician, or veterinarian that it is hospital policy to collect a 50% deposit before performing the requested services and that the balance of the account will be payable at dismissal. This allows the client and the practice the opportunity to discuss the case finances before the service.

If the client determines the estimated services are too costly, then the veterinarian will have an opportunity to recommend another possible treatment or method that is less costly or discuss credit options. By making routine use of fee estimates and deposits the level of practice credit can be carefully controlled. The level of accounts receivable (practice credit) in a practice should not exceed 25% of the average of 1 month's gross income. As an example, the level of accounts receivable should not exceed $25,000 in a practice grossing $100,000 per month ($1,200,000 annual gross income). If the level of accounts receivable goes beyond 25%, a more strict credit policy needs to be put in place or enforced.

Collections and Billings

Effective communications related to collecting the fee from the client begin with confident receptionists, technicians, and veterinarians who understand how the fee is computed and are confident that it is deserved and fair and truly represents the quality of service provided. An educated staff is more confident, positive, and informed in discussing fees with clients, whether at the time of fee estimates or at the time of payment or billing.

Billings charged by clients for future payments are called *account receivables*. The more account receivables grow, the less cash is available to pay ongoing expenses that includes the payroll of the practice. Therefore the goal must be to collect (not charge) a fee according to a defined practice policy in a business manner that does not offend or alienate clients.

Most companion animal veterinarians attempt to collect all fees and not allow clients to charge. Increased credit card availability has allowed most clients to delay actual payments by transferring the charges to a credit card. This provides almost immediate payment to the business by the credit card company and prevents the practice from losing a significant amount of money from clients who will not or cannot pay their bills in the future. Credit card payment allows money to be immediately available to pay inventory purchases, apply to payroll, or pay other bills.

If credit is to be provided, the practice manager should be involved before the services are provided to approve the client's credit application, establish down payment amounts, and develop a repayment schedule. Charging

fees and sending monthly billings by mail are more common with large animal practices. Established clients with excellent credit who have a large number of animals may negotiate a monthly payment instead of payment for each service rendered.

Cash Control

Cash control is best accomplished using some form of fee slips in triplicate that are numbered serially. One copy is kept in the examination room, one stays with the daybook ledger of income received, and one is given to the client. With this method, if someone's payment is unintentionally (or intentionally) omitted from being recorded in the daybook ledger, the numbered fee slip can be traced back to determine who that client was and what happened. This system allows errors to be corrected, prevents embezzlement, and provides a way to track clients who may have forgotten to check out and pay for a service. Computerized systems should also have these and other cash control features.

Petty cash is often needed by staff to purchase stamps and incidental supplies from local businesses. A procedure must be set up to track petty cash to prevent embezzlement and meet U.S. Internal Revenue Service (IRS) business deductibility rules. Generally, a cash box accessible to approved staff for petty cash is set up with a set amount of cash, for example, $100. The petty cash box must always contain $100 made up of the total value of signed and dated purchase receipts, cash, and temporary IOUs made out by the person as he or she removes petty cash to get supplies. When the person returns, his or her receipt plus change must equal the IOU, which is removed and replaced by the change and signed receipt. When petty cash gets low, the receipts are taken out of the box, totaled, and entered into business records as petty cash expenses. A check for expenses is made out for that amount and cashed, and that amount of cash is returned to the petty cash box. This prevents suspicion of embezzlement if every person follows this procedure, preferably overseen by the practice manager. It also makes sure all expenses are accounted for when monthly and annual reporting is due.

All staff and veterinarians should record all supplies and products taken from the practice for personal use even when these are provided free as a staff benefit. This prevents embezzlement and pilferage, accounts for the level of benefit actually provided, and keeps everyone honest and above suspicion by management, coworkers, and the IRS. It encourages honesty, avoids destructive suspicions, and promotes trust if followed by all employees, including practice owners. Consulting accountants, owners, and the practice manager have resources to set up standard business procedures for the receptionist and staff to follow to develop a smooth operating veterinary business.

BUSINESS MANAGEMENT

Professionals as a whole would often like to abstain from the business side of practice and concentrate exclusively on professional (medical) activities. In reality, without the business side of any profession, there would be few opportunities to practice that profession. The business management aspects of practice can become as challenging as patient management. Lack of available time, lack of interest, and minimal experience are limiting factors.

Clinical signs of poor business management are lax credit policies, increasing accounts receivable (total dollars clients owe), reduced operating capital, lowered gross income, lowered net income, increasing personnel costs, increasing overhead, reduced client numbers, and reduced average transaction fee per patient. Tests used to identify problems of poor business management include complete review of monthly business information to establish trends, comparison of this month's data to the same month 1 year ago, review of the fee schedule, review of the credit policy, review and comparison of inventory levels, and turnover rates.

Prognosis is generally good once the diagnosis of poor business management has been supported by a review of the diagnostic tests. Treatment will usually need to continue for the life of the practice. Some recommended treatments for the poor business management syndrome follow: Establish a firm written credit policy. Make use of a written fee estimate sheet to itemize all patient charges. Before admission, have the owner sign and retain one copy of the estimate sheet. The credit policy should be clearly stated on the fee estimate sheet (see Chapter 33 for an example of a fee estimate form). Make use of appointment systems to schedule clients for the most efficient use of time.

The practice fee schedule should be reviewed and updated at least every 3 to 6 months, and a current printed fee schedule should be available near each telephone. Accounts receivable need to be monitored monthly, with legally appropriate follow-up telephone calls and letters to stimulate payment in a timely manner.

Accounts payable should be handled in a way to obtain discounts for prompt payment. Accounts that do not provide discounts should be paid near the due date to conserve working capital. No account should be allowed to become past due. A poor credit image for the practice is difficult to remove.

One tool for analyzing and correcting poor business management is the office computer. The office computer can provide on-line storage and have information readily available at the push of a button. The computer can provide income analysis, accounts receivable information, inventory control, client information analysis, patient diagnosis analysis, and so forth. Computerization is becoming increasingly cost effective, and well-designed programs are now available through several vendors. Additional information about computers in veterinary medicine is found in Chapter 34.

If these treatments are properly applied, the outcome from "poor business management syndrome" should be complete recovery. The result of improved management is a sound and stable veterinary practice that pays dividends to clients, patients, and employees.

Pet Insurance

Health insurance has had a significant role in funding the costs of human medicine for several decades as a third-party payer insulating patients from most of the medical and surgical costs. Dental insurance also impacts dentistry practice. Pet insurance was introduced into veterinary medicine about 1985. Most pet insurance policies will cover specified services, have limits, copayment levels, and deductibles, similar to human medicine policies.

Recently, more companies have been encouraged to offer pet insurance because more pet owners value their pet as a member of the family and want some protection against catastrophic costs from unexpected accidents and disease. If these policies increase in number, they may help the business of veterinary practice. More patients will have major unexpected costs covered, wellness programs will be supported for saving money by preventing some costly

treatments, and fewer owners will choose unnecessary euthanasia of their animals. Thus everyone benefits including the animal.

Client Communication

Excellent interpersonal communication skills can serve to develop and expand veterinary service markets. Improved communication between client and veterinarian results in more personalized professional care. Reduction in spendable income of clients may reduce demand for elective procedures, but this can be offset by providing a more comprehensive preventive medicine program through improved communication skills. Clients are unable to make service selections until they fully understand all options.

Common courtesy and genuine concern affect all professions and businesses. It has been said: "I don't care how much you know until I know how much you care!" The world as a whole is becoming more depersonalized. When a veterinary practice loses sight of the individual client the personal service feeling is lost to both the client and the patient. Courtesy begins with acknowledging clients as soon as they enter the reception room, carefully explaining why an appointment is helpful, calling clients by name, asking about the clients' families—in short, treating clients as important guests in your hospital.

Courtesy also extends to telephone manners. All calls should be answered by the third ring; the caller should be greeted by "Good morning, this is ABC Animal Hospital, this is Kathy speaking. How may I help you?" The caller immediately knows that he or she has reached the correct hospital and that Kathy is there to help. Telephone courtesy is just as important as personal courtesy because most clients have their first contact with the hospital by telephone.

Technician Note

All telephone calls should be answered by the third ring, although callers prefer the telephone to be answered on the first ring.

If the veterinary staff of a hospital treat each caller and each client with common courtesy, the impression that the client will receive is genuine concern. A lack of concern for people and their pets' problems is a common complaint voiced by clients of many veterinary hospitals. If veterinary personnel treat each client as they would like to be treated when selecting or securing service, the result will be more happy clients who experience courtesy and concern.

Closely accompanying the issue of courtesy and concern is effective communication. The majority of complaints against veterinarians are the result of ineffective or misunderstood communication between veterinarian or staff and client. To communicate completely, staff members must have concern for *both* animal and client. In addition, they must learn to *listen* to the client and then communicate a caring attitude as well as information that is understandable and effective. Most people *hear* other people talking, but few people have developed the ability to *listen* effectively to what is communicated. The successful veterinary team must develop this ability.

To ensure effective communication consider these four rules:

1. Use terminology that the client will understand; scientific terms can be confusing to the client.

2. Do not rush through the information just because you are hurried or because it appears to be "common knowledge" to you, or the client will feel "brushed off."

3. Do not assume a superior manner or tone to the extent that the client feels "put down."

4. Use effective communication techniques for obtaining a history (see Box 32-6).

In short, show concern and respect. Attempt to treat each client with respect, honesty, and as a very special person even if you do not agree with him or her. If the communication is open, honest, and caring, it will be effective and most problems can be prevented. One of the most common reasons for veterinarians to refer clients to other veterinarians is because of the failure to communicate effectively with the client.

Technician Note

About 40% of all communication is verbal; 60% is body language and environmental factors.

Listening is an extremely important communication skill. The skill of listening must be practiced on a regular basis to become effective. Many people would rather talk than listen. Often, the client will assist in the diagnosis by providing important clues in the history if only someone will listen. Active listening involves listening to clients and then verbally rephrasing their messages back to them for verification. This technique ensures that the client was heard correctly and the technician or veterinarian received the entire message.

Listening requires understanding both the *music* and the *words*. The correct *words* must be sent and received. In addition, the nonverbal *music* (facial expressions, hand gestures, body stance, etc.) must also be observed and understood to allow complete communication.

Client Expectations

Most clients expect the following five things during a consultation with a veterinarian: examination of the animal, diagnosis (cause if possible), prognosis (predicted outcome), treatment plan, and fee estimate. Communication of prognosis, treatment plan, and fee estimate is difficult for most veterinarians. Clients feel unprepared to make judgments without this information and often complain if complications occur. Malpractice (professional negligence) concerns can be virtually eliminated if these areas are effectively handled with the client. Again, the veterinary technician should be part of the communication team in these areas. Clear, effective communication is a team effort and absolutely necessary for client compliance and quality patient care.

Common Complaints From Clients

When dealing with a cross section of the public, as most practices do, the goal of complete satisfaction for all clients can never be obtained. However, when clients do have complaints, careful attention must be given to them. To reduce the number of complaints from clients, several potential problem areas will be addressed. The more common areas of client complaints are fees, courtesy and concern, communication, appointment schedule, sanitation and quality of patient care.

Every client deserves a complete explanation and breakdown of all anticipated costs of each service to be performed. Whenever communication is incomplete, client complaints will result. One of the most sensitive issues practitioners deal with is financial estimates. Quoted fees must be written down and honored unless revised with full consent of the owner. The most common client complaint will concern fees. The use of a fee estimate sheet and up-front, open communication will eliminate most fee complaints.

Another common client complaint area centers on the quality of care offered to the patient and the client. Often, animal owners are hesitant to accept one veterinarian's opinion. As in human medicine, seeking multiple opinions on a case has become routine. Specialists have become more common in veterinary practice, and veterinary clients are requesting second and third opinions. Multiple opinions have been good for both the patient and the client, but they require veterinarians to be thorough and up to date with their information and techniques.

The Difficult Client

Some clients remain difficult to deal with regardless of the best efforts of everyone in the practice. Some of these difficult people actually enjoy being difficult. The attitude of the difficult client toward the technical and reception staff may be different from the attitude toward the veterinarian. A very difficult, demanding person can suddenly become quite reasonable when the veterinarian enters the room. When this happens, the technician should not feel that he or she has failed but rather should work a little harder to understand and win the client's trust.

In dealing with someone who is politely complaining, listen to their perceptions and feelings and attempt to convey that you understand the problem (you will appear to be agreeing; this will help to reduce the level of the confrontation). A good example would be the common complaint that fees are too high, which can be answered by, "Yes, fees are high. Everything is high these days!"

In situations in which the client appears to be unreasonable about the complaint, establish the specific problem (i.e., fees, unsatisfactory treatment result, poor communication) and then indicate to the client that you would like for him or her to speak to the veterinarian. Once the unreasonable client has been identified, escort the client out of the reception room and into an examination room away from other clients; then the veterinarian can handle the problem as quickly as possible.

The most difficult people to reason with are people who have been drinking or are on drugs. Be careful how you handle these people. Do not argue or confront them because they could become violent and uncontrollable. In situations in which drugs or alcohol has been consumed to excess, law enforcement officials should be contacted to handle the situation.

Never argue with a dissatisfied client. The client is "always right, even when wrong." In other words, clients have a real concern that must be acknowledged and understood. If a client leaves angry, 10 other people are told how terrible you, your veterinarian, and your hospital are. When the client leaves the practice enthusiastically, he or she will only tell three other people. We cannot have clients leaving angry. Sometimes we must all "eat a little crow" to keep the client's good will. In the long run, this will benefit all concerned.

Professional Marketing

Some professionals feel uncomfortable with the idea of marketing because the scope of marketing activity has been poorly understood. Often, the connotation of marketing is advertising. However, advertising is only a small portion of the total marketing picture for a professional business.

Professional marketing has numerous definitions, but the one that will be used here is "the communication of professional services and goods offered to existing and potential clients." The veterinary technician must understand marketing principles to be an effective communicator of professional services and goods offered by the practice.

Definition

Professional marketing consists of all activities that increase client awareness of professional services and goods. Marketing occurs through effective client relations; professional appearance of the hospital, clinic, or ambulatory vehicle; listening to owners' opinions; a convenient practice location; a polite support staff; offering full-service care; sending clients service reminders; being neat and clean; using business cards; sending clients educational newsletters; providing nutritional counseling and dietary management; providing emergency service; offering pet and livestock supplies; giving career talks at high schools; leading 4-H, FFA, or scouting groups; attending dog/cat/ horse shows; having producer or client educational nights; being involved in a community service club; setting up a website on the Internet; advertising in the yellow pages of the telephone book; providing handout material to clients; having an attractive and well-located building sign; sending thank-you and sympathy cards to appropriate clients; appearing as a guest on radio and television shows; writing a newspaper animal column; using attractive letterhead stationery; becoming active in professional associations; and group advertising in the newspaper about the annual rabies vaccination clinic.

Animals are totally dependent on owner awareness of health care needs. Professional marketing should be designed to help more animals by informing and serving more clients. If successful, it will result in increased practice income through increasing client numbers or the amount of each client transaction. It requires balancing improved animal health and public health with the needs and goals of the practice. One of the most critical questions a veterinarian should ask is "What business am I in?" To be able to conduct a successful professional business, one must be clear about specific business objectives. Some practitioners believe as long as high-quality medical and surgical skill is delivered, the client will continue to use their service based on the quality of service alone. Fortunately, clients today are usually well-informed consumers and are looking for both quality *and* value. The average client lacks the professional background to accurately judge the quality of medical or surgical services performed. However, clients do have the ability to judge the quality of caring communication that *they* received personally, which influences their perception of the value of the service received. Therefore clients' perceived value of services is their reality of the practice's quality.

Veterinary medicine is in the *people service* business. The profession cares for animals but provides professional service to their owners. Patients cannot come to the practice without the owners! If each staff member understands that she or he is in the people service business, a completely different orientation will take place. When clients call on the telephone, for example, they are not interrupting the veterinarian's or technician's time in the examination room or surgery room; they are the reason for the existence of the examination room and surgery room. Veterinary practices do provide high-quality professional service to animals but only after the agreement and support of the owner. Also, only satisfied clients return and refer others.

The professional success of most veterinarians and technicians is the result of *interpersonal skills* rather than strictly clinical skills. The ability to relate well to people and their problems will allow the practice the opportunity to provide high-quality veterinary medicine (Figure 32-23).

Once the practice is viewed as a people service business, marketing of those services becomes possible. The product to be marketed is *high-quality, people-oriented professional veterinary medical service.*

Marketing techniques must benefit the profession as a whole to achieve maximal success. The overall program must promote the *benefits* of veterinary services rather than the specific service.

If one were to compare the benefits of a program of immunization with one that sold a vaccination, the long-term effects are evident. A program that details the benefits of immunization can build a preventive medicine program through a physical examination, dental care, nutritional management, and so forth on an annual basis. The approach of selling a vaccination is just that—promoting a vaccine.

The program of promoting the benefits of a high-quality, people-oriented professional veterinary medical service must be the end goal.

Marketing techniques will not overcome the effects of poor client relations within a practice. Unless effective client communication and client orientation are practiced on a client-by-client basis, marketing will be unsuccessful.

Practice Marketing

The first step in a marketing plan is to determine client needs. One must listen closely to services being requested by each client. Determine what service trends are going on within the practice in response to economic growth of the community. As an example, both spouses usually work today. This results in some people being unable to seek

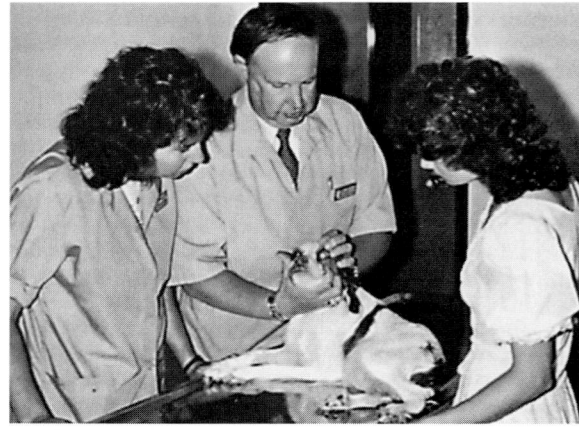

FIGURE 32-23. Technician, veterinarian, and client communicating as a team about patient care.

veterinary care during the traditional 8 AM to 5 PM period. The typical client also has less free time to devote to shopping around at several stores for items when all items could be purchased at one convenient location. By listening to clients and observing service needs, the practitioner may opt to extend the practice hours two evenings per week and open later in the mornings on those days. The practice may also expand services to include veterinary-supervised boarding and offer selected nonprofessional supplies, such as grooming aids.

The practice owner must determine the direction of the marketing plan by listening to client needs and gathering additional facts concerning community trends. The marketing process will then be guided by current facts and psychodemographic information.

Specific Marketing Techniques

Professional marketing can be divided into *internal* and *external* marketing. Internal marketing techniques are the day-to-day activities that occur within each practice, whereas external marketing involves techniques used outside the practice. The purpose of both internal and external techniques is to enlarge the number and size of the client transaction.

INTERNAL MARKETING.   Internal marketing is aimed primarily at the existing client base. Internal marketing techniques attempt to educate and inform current clients about the various veterinary services and service programs available. They also should generate client enthusiasm for the practice. The following methods are meant to serve as an idea base and not as a complete listing of techniques for internal marketing.

Client Relationships.   The most important technique to use in any marketing program is personalized, sincere client care. Most clients require as much attention and care as the patient. Clients today want both high technology and high touch. Personalized service that emphasizes each individual client will allow the opportunity for excellent communication to be established. Both veterinarian and technician must be skilled communicators as well as technically skilled professionals. All staff must support these efforts.

Practice Appearance.   The visual appearance of the clinic, hospital, or ambulatory vehicle is the first outward signal to the client concerning the potential quality of service. One must consider the appearance of the building (repair, paint, cleanliness) and the grounds (Figure 32-24). Plants and grass must be neat and trimmed and the parking lot clean and well signed for parking. The interior of the building must also be clean, well cared for, and odor free. Silent marketing messages are sent to clients through the appearance of the facility.

A practice facility does not have to be new or have the latest equipment to project a positive image. The older facility that has been given proper care and maintenance will exhibit a strong marketing message of "we care" to people passing by each day.

Support Staff Utilization.   Most internal marketing carried on within a practice will be through the veterinary team members. Support staff activities will augment the efforts of the veterinarian in client relations and personal appearance. Primarily, veterinary technicians and receptionists will be responsible for recommending services or goods and following up on hospital programs that require appointments or individual client contact. These team members are regarded as an extension of the veterinarian and must have a professional approach to client management.

Technical staff will usually deliver the majority of client education with the assistance of receptionists. Handout materials, visual aids, and video presentations will help the staff in their educational efforts. The staff will need detailed information concerning the various preventive health programs from the veterinarian. To be able to promote the product, everyone needs to be clear about the product. Therefore the veterinarian and the support staff must work together as a service team, all delivering the same high-quality service.

Professional sales point displays can add another level of service for clients. These displays need continuous monitoring by support staff to provide "on the spot" professional information. Areas in which support staff should have in-depth knowledge include nutrition, parasite control (internal and external), grooming aids, dental care, immunization programs, obedience training, and rearing orphan animals. In addition, support staff must be on the constant lookout for new clients and additional services. Staff members who are active in dog clubs have continual access to new potential clients. New clients may not be aware of services offered, and so all staff members must be willing to provide program information at any time. When certain key support staff members are given a small percentage of income from all new services and new clients they provide the practice as an incentive, a new wave of enthusiasm may develop in everyone.

Full Service Care.   Listening to client needs will verify that clients want full-service care when possible. People are exposed to 1-hour photo processing, 1-hour eyeglasses, 7-Eleven, fast food restaurants, K-Mart, Wal-Mart, drive-through banking, and so forth. Convenient, fast, economic, one-stop shopping is the rule for single-parent families and families in which both husband and wife work. People are now asking for this same type of convenient service in their veterinary care. In small animal practice, full-service care would include prepurchase counseling concerning pets, human-animal bond and behavioral problem counseling, pediatric care, preventive medicine, nutritional counseling, nutritional management, veterinary-supervised boarding, geriatric care, dentistry, bereavement counseling, cremation service, and full routine veterinary care. The service would extend from birth to death.

In a full-service practice, various programs can be packaged for marketing. The goal of marketing is to sell a

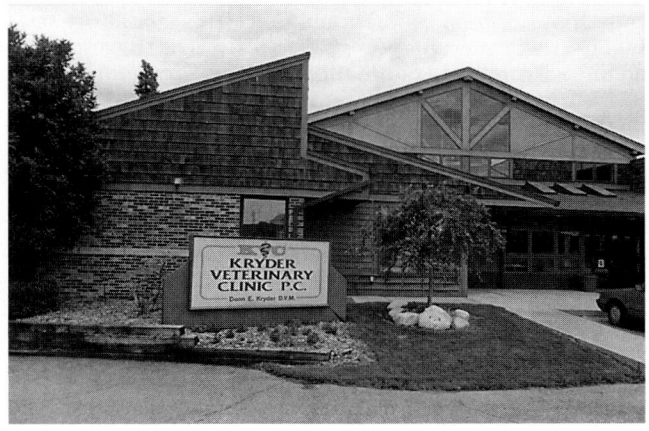

FIGURE 32-24.   Exterior appearance of the hospital should provide a positive image.

program, not an individual service. The emphasis of a quality practice is to provide preventive health care, not just disease treatment. A small animal practice must develop a complete health maintenance (wellness) program for new puppies and kittens as well as puppy training classes. This program carries into adulthood and on into the geriatric period. The wellness program could include annual physicals, nutritional counseling, dental care, and immunizations. Nutritional counseling would include pediatric, adult, and geriatric care as the patient matures. As clients continue their regular contact with the practice to purchase foods, the practice has a regular opportunity to market other health preventive care services.

Client Reminders.   One of the more successful early attempts at practice marketing was through the use of a vaccination reminder system for small animals. During the early discussions on the use of a recall system, many practitioners felt it was unprofessional to send a reminder card to clients because it was advertising. No one was considering the service provided to the client and animal. Most veterinarians thought only of how it would appear to other veterinarians.

Charles, Charles and Associates discovered that sending vaccination reminders was even more important to clients than having boarding facilities or an attractive building. Clients want to be reminded when specific services are to be done. However, clients prefer to receive reminders by mail rather than by telephone.

Technician Note

Clients now expect the practice to send annual service reminders.

A reminder system is a major marketing feature of most practice management computer software packages. A system that has the capacity to generate only one reminder is not nearly as valuable as a system that will produce a second and third reminder if the client does not respond. Using a system that will generate an additional second or third notice to be sent will greatly increase the service return rate.

Most practices now accept the use of a reminder system as a valuable marketing tool for routine immunizations. The reminder system must be expanded to include other routine services for the clients. Additional use in the small animal practice could be in the areas of dental hygiene (routine cleaning), annual physical examination, geriatric care, hip-dysplasia evaluations, follow-up laboratory testing, heartworm evaluation, and so forth. The suggestion of an annual physical examination may appear on the surface to be a poor recommendation in light of physicians now recommending fewer annual physicals. However, considering that the dog and cat age seven to nine times as rapidly as humans and that the diligent veterinarian and technician are able to find a potential problem on almost every physical examination, many clients will take advantage of the service when offered. When performing the examination, the veterinarian and technician must explain and demonstrate the findings to the client (i.e., potential problems with ears, eyes, teeth, anal sac, hair coat, obesity, etc.) (Figure 32-25).

Small animal geriatric care is another relatively untapped market area. When patients reach a specific age (i.e., 7 to 8 years of age), a reminder letter could be sent to the client providing information on specific conditions to be monitored. The letter could approach the client in the following way: "Congratulations, Blacky has just become a

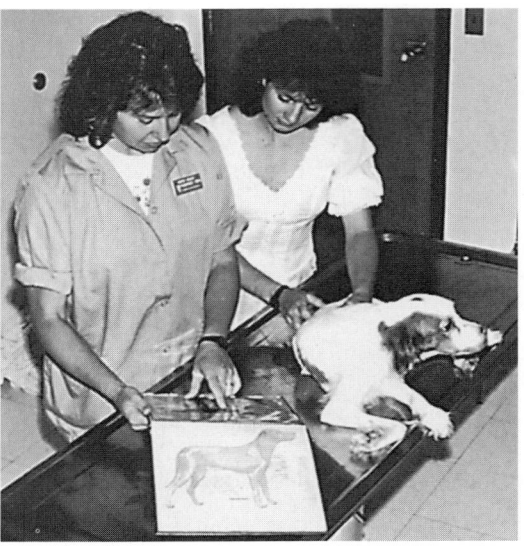

FIGURE 32-25.   Technician explaining a diagnosis to client using visual aid.

senior canine citizen. When dogs reach about 8 years of age, the care necessary to prevent and monitor disease changes. We would like to provide the following information to allow Blacky to enjoy his new senior status: . . ." This letter could be developed and recalled by the computer at a specific age.

Another area in which a reminder system could be used is to recall young animals that have been previously vaccinated but not yet neutered. The recall of unneutered animals is an opportunity to market ovariohysterectomy and castration services. This reminder may attract some clients who would otherwise go to a low-cost spay and neuter clinic. A personalized letter could detail the specific features of the service, which is not possible from the spay and neuter clinics.

The use of a recall system allows the market to be segmented (targeted). An example of market segmentation would be to send all feline owners a reminder about leukemia vaccination.

Personal Appearance.   The personal appearance and hygiene of each staff member reflect the quality of the practice. Many clients relate personal appearance to the sanitation and level of quality of the practice. If someone does not care enough to change a dirty smock, coveralls, or boots, why should he or she care enough to provide the highest-quality service? Not only should hand washing occur between all patients, but also it should be practiced in front of the client. This enhances client awareness of disease prevention efforts. Personal appearance marketing works just as building appearance—an outward signal of internal quality (Figure 32-26). A professional image is perceived by the client when all hospital members have a professional appearance. Staff uniforms, shirt and tie, dress, and smocks for doctors are recommended.

Technician Note

Personal appearance is a direct reflection of practice quality.

Handout Materials.   Marketing with handout materials has been used for a number of years. The quantity and

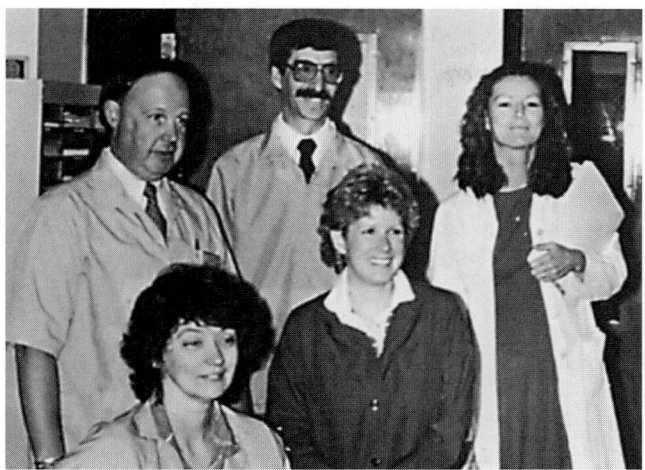

FIGURE 32-26. A professional appearance is a marketing tool.

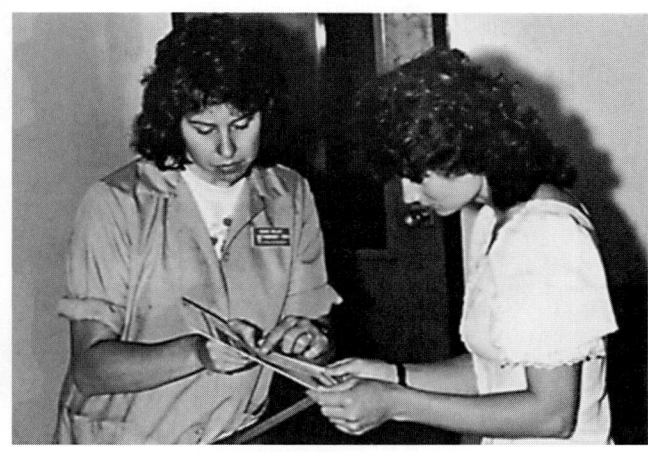

FIGURE 32-27. Technician explaining and providing a handout to client.

quality of commercially available handouts are excellent. Most commercial companies realize the value of client-oriented professional literature. These pieces should be carefully reviewed by the practice so only acceptable material is made available to clients. Once the material has been reviewed and useful pieces selected, all staff must be made familiar with how and when they should be used. A professional rubber stamp can be purchased with the practice name, location, and telephone number on it and used to personalize all commercial handout materials. Handout material must be handed directly to the client by the veterinarian or technician to be most effective (Figure 32-27). Handout materials displayed in the reception room for clients to pick up are often not well utilized. Clients will pick up material from a display rack and take it home, but few will ever read it.

In addition to commercial handouts, materials may be purchased from veterinary organizations. AVMA, the American Association of Equine Practitioners, and AAHA, among others, provide useful client handout materials.

Practices may also produce their own informational material. Quality handouts on whelping, ovarian hysterectomy, cystic calculi, colic, mastitis, and so forth can be easily prepared by the computer. Discharge instruction handouts are very effective because clients often forget verbal explanations and instructions. Practice information brochures can also be produced to more fully explain practice hours, services, equipment, facilities, and staff function (Figure 32-28). Other forms of handout materials used on a regular basis are business cards and letterhead stationery. They are effective forms of marketing. Business cards should be made available to clients from *both* veterinarians and key support staff, especially certified veterinary technicians.

Sympathy and Thank-you Communications. A very personal marketing approach is to appropriately use sympathy and thank-you types of communication. One may choose to use commercially prepared cards or develop a letter format on the computer that can be personalized. Regardless of the format used, the use of personal messages to specific clients for specific purposes has an everlasting positive effect. In the case of clients newly referred by

current clients, a note or card to both the referring clients (thanking them for the referral) and the new clients (welcoming them to the practice) is appropriate. As the use of the Internet becomes more common, e-mail notes could also be used

The sympathy card or personal note is helpful when a pet dies to demonstrate open concern for the feelings of the client during his or her emotional loss. The expression helps the client deal with the loss and allows the client to understand the "I care" attitude of the practice for both the client and pet.

Newsletter. The use of newsletters will increase client activity through improved understanding and education about veterinary services. Educational goals for newsletters should be to inform animal owners of the signs of illness, to make seasonal animal health care recommendations (i.e., heat stroke in summer), to review health care programs, and to introduce key staff members. Many clients do not understand how to tell whether an animal is ill or in serious condition. This lack of knowledge is especially true for cat and horse owners.

Newsletters will allow the client to be exposed to specific pieces of information that will help owners to know when to call a veterinarian for help. Total health care plans can also be explained to allow the owner to be aware of full-service health care that extends beyond vaccinations. The newsletter should help market the benefits of healthy animals.

Newsletters can be sent to specific segments of clients in the practice computer base; however, they can also be provided through a hand-generated list or passed out to all clients as they enter the practice. Most veterinarians do not have the experience or time to compose a complete newsletter three or four times per year. The practice manager, veterinary technicians, and receptionists may develop articles for a practice newsletter, or consideration can be given to purchasing a professionally edited newsletter service.

Each newsletter should be personalized by the practice to allow the reader easy access to the practice's location and telephone number. Another advantage newsletters have in overall marketing is the ability to reach the nonuser. If the

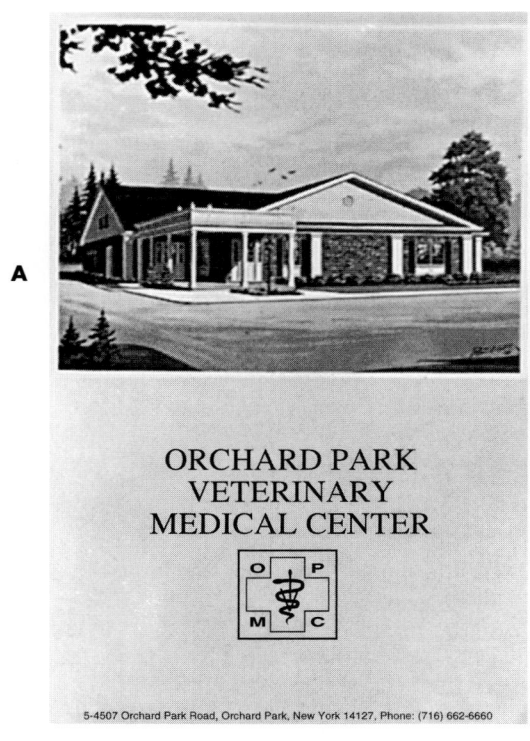

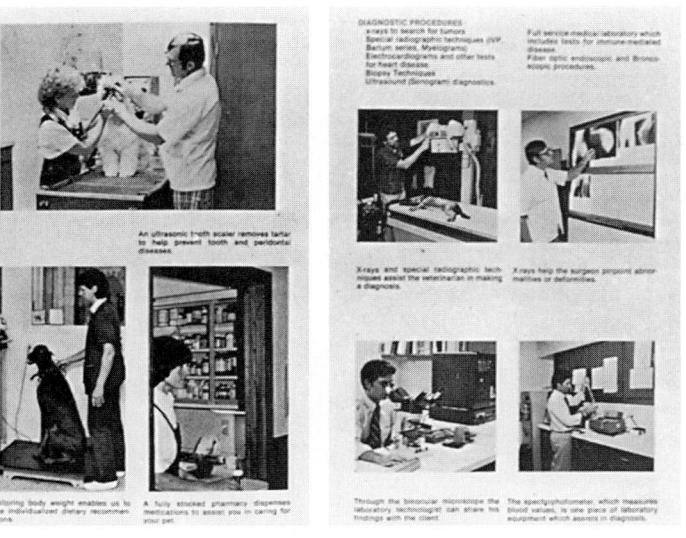

A

B

5-4507 Orchard Park Road, Orchard Park, New York 14127, Phone: (716) 662-6660

FIGURE 32-28. Practice information pamphlet. **A,** Cover. **B,** Inner page. (Courtesy Orchard Park Veterinary Medical Center, Orchard Park, NY.)

client receiving the newsletter passes it on to a nonclient friend, the nonclient has an opportunity to be exposed to various veterinary services offered by the practice.

A spinoff use of the newsletter could be through the use of news notes or Internet letters. News notes are postcard-sized updates mailed to the client three or four times per year. As more clients become connected to the Internet, short e-mail letters can be used in place of newsletters sent by regular mail.

Special Services. Practices can either expand existing services or add new services to increase their market share. In a small animal practice, market expansion might be in the areas of birds and exotic service, bereavement counseling, prepurchase evaluation of pets to determine suitability for family, behavior counseling, nutritional counseling (i.e., puppy, adult, senior), dental care (i.e., endodontics, periodontics, orthodontics), geriatric care, cremation service (Figure 32-29), emergency care, and intensive care unit. Because most small animal clinics cater to dogs, many cat owners do not feel welcome or comfortable in an environment with dog pictures on the walls and barking dogs in the reception area. Practices that want to increase feline clients might be well rewarded by considering the needs of cats and cat owners when remodeling. Having a separate reception area for cats and keeping cats in a separate ward should be a starting point. Previous lack of recognition of these needs may be the primary reason for serving fewer cat owners than dog owners with professional veterinary care.

Sales Point Displays. When displays are being considered as an internal marketing technique, several important points must be contemplated if they are to be successful. First, the practice must define the clients' needs. The specific products must be carefully selected and priced. An appropriate location or locations must be established in the clinic or hospital that may be monitored at all times by the technical staff (Figure 32-30). The products must be attractively arranged and kept neat and clean. Prices must be clearly marked on all products.

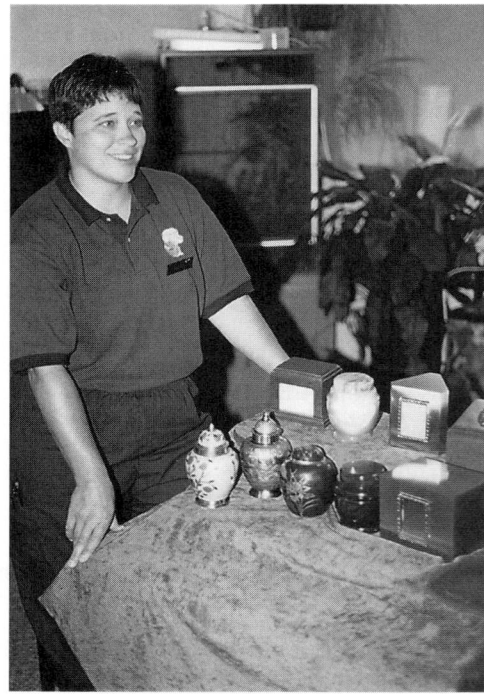

FIGURE 32-29. Veterinary technician shows a variety of urns for ashes of cremated patient. These services and compassion for the family's grief are greatly appreciated by clients.

The most important difference between a hospital or clinic display and a retail store display is the *professional* advice that is provided with each item sold. Professional counseling is not available at the feed store, grocery store, department store, or mail order outlet. The technical staff

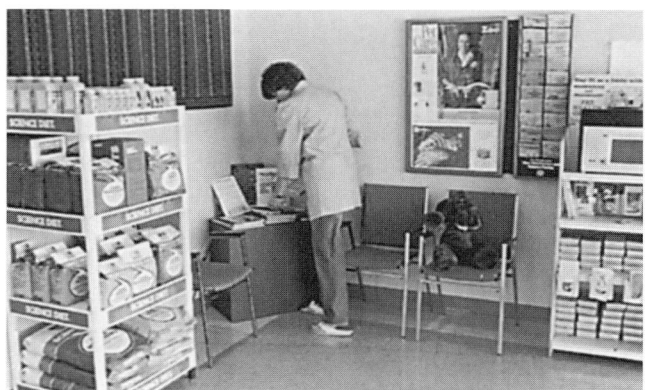

FIGURE 32-30. Professional display in reception area being organized and restocked by staff.

will pay a key role in providing product information for the client.

Professional displays may include limited product lines confined to an examination room, a specific area of the reception room, or a special room adjacent to the reception room.

Animal Care Talks. Veterinary technicians and veterinarians can both become involved in providing veterinary medical care talks to grade school and high school students as well as to adult clients. The most effective and unique visual aid is a live animal. These presentations can provide information on routine animal health care, first aid activities, signs to look for when an animal is ill, and general information on educational requirements of veterinarians and technicians. These presentations also help to change the established norms about animal care.

When a presentation has become polished, service clubs in the community make excellent audiences. Talks to service clubs are helpful to enhance awareness of quality medical care provided by the individual practice and the profession. A slide or computer presentation that features both veterinarian and technician in their team roles is very effective.

The veterinary technician could present information on care of the new puppy or kitten, exotic pets and birds, first aid, feeding the pet, whelping and queening, hip dysplasia, parasite control, pet obedience training, and pet selection. Client education programs should be given on a regular basis and offered at convenient times. Attendees should be provided with handout material to take home for future reference.

Technician Note

Technicians can present client education programs to expand professional services for preventive medicine.

When the education program is held at the practice, a complete tour of the facilities should be planned. Clients are interested in seeing hospital equipment and understanding more about hospital care. An annual hospital open house is an excellent image builder to clients. Having a "behind the scenes" tour is something most clients have not had an opportunity to experience. Many will be "amazed" to see x-ray, anesthesia, surgery, and laboratory equipment "just like in a human hospital." Children are especially impressed with "show and tell" demonstrations using live animals.

By providing client education opportunities, the client becomes more bonded to the practice. When veterinary problems arise, the client is more apt to contact the practice that has provided an inside look and veterinary medical information.

EXTERNAL MARKETING. Most external marketing activities are aimed at expanding current client activity and identifying new nonclient activity. External marketing can be carried out by an individual practice, group practice, organized veterinary medicine, and commercial companies.

Some types of external marketing are currently being used in many practices. The use of an Internet website, newsletters (direct mail to nonclients), telephone yellow page advertising, building signs, client education nights, community service activities, and AVMA's National Pet Week materials expands the image of the practice to clients and nonclients. When a practice wants to penetrate into the nonclient base, one must make use of selected forms of advertising.

Professional Advertising. Professional advertising includes hospital signs, telephone book listings, practice newsletters, vaccination reminders, and professional business cards. However, the focus on advertising in this discussion will center more on the more hard-core forms of advertising: yellow pages of the telephone book, newspapers, magazines, radio, direct mail, and telephone. Attitudes concerning advertising differ between the professional and the consumer. A great majority of professionals (physicians, dentists, attorneys, veterinarians) are against advertising for a variety of reasons: it seems to be unprofessional and unethical, and it lowers status, credibility, and sense of dignity. Just as professionals feel strongly negative toward advertising, consumers feel strongly positive. Consumers generally believe advertising by a professional would not compromise that professional's credibility, status, image, or dignity as long as it is honest and not misleading. In fact, most consumers believe advertising by professionals would help them make a more intelligent choice.

Telephone Yellow Pages. When a yellow page advertisement is deemed appropriate for external marketing purposes, several guidelines should be followed. First, the advertisement should not be larger than one-fourth page; advertisements larger than one-fourth page are perceived as being more unprofessional by the consumer. Second, the advertisement should be set in one color (preferably black). The use of multiple colors (e.g., red, green) is again perceived by the consumer as being less professional. Finally, the advertisement should provide as much information as possible about the practice and its services.

Internet Web Page. Web pages are the newest form of marketing for veterinary practices and organizations. Many practices are using their own web site to provide public access to information about the practice, its staff, pet care, and services provided, and they include pictures for a virtual tour of the medical facility and procedures. A web page may also provide the practice clientele with the ability to make an appointment on-line, as well as provide quality information about pet selection, training, feeding, and selected medical conditions. The practice web page can be updated frequently and may replace the need for practice newsletters and maybe practice brochures. Other quality sources for veterinary-related information on the Internet can be reviewed and approved and set up as a link to the practice web page (see www.avma.org for initial links to the Virtual Library, PetVet, Care for Pets, and the ElectronicZoo on the Internet).

Newspapers. Newspaper advertising, like telephone yellow page advertising, is useful for initial impact when opening or expanding a practice. Many professionals will have a newspaper listing when opening a new practice, when relocating an existing practice, or when adding new associates to an existing practice. The continual use of newspaper advertising for veterinarians has been largely prohibited by cost.

Probably the best form of newspaper advertising for veterinarians is the "animal care information" format. Weekly animal care information columns are a public service, and newspapers are always seeking educational material. Pet columns have become popular reading as the public begins to acknowledge and understand the human-animal bond. To address the need for weekly newspaper columns, several private column services have sprung up that will provide the practitioner with 52 professionally written articles on animal care each year. This service can be purchased by individual veterinarians or through associations.

Radio and Television. Veterinary associations can obtain air time essentially free by participating in talk shows. The subject of animals, animal care, and animal behavior is a fascinating subject to most listening and viewing audiences. A number of the larger radio and television markets have regularly scheduled talk shows (some hosted by veterinarians) that have a question-and-answer format devoted to animal care. The talk show format is an excellent opportunity for associations that have articulate and knowledgeable veterinarians and technicians to sell veterinary medicine for the profession as a whole.

Recently, popular television programs, such as Animal Planet and Emergency Vets, have had a large impact on marketing the veterinary profession. Likewise, the earlier James Herriot books and televised Public Broadcasting System (PBS) series attracted many animal lovers to the profession. All these media events help public awareness of the high level of medical care provided by the veterinary profession.

Community Activities. Veterinary practices that engage in community activities have a much wider client base.

Veterinarians and technicians should become involved in community service through Girl Scouts, Boy Scouts, 4-H Veterinary Science Leader, school boards, humane societies, country clubs, Rotary, Lions, and church activities. Potential client contacts are made in the course of being involved and contributing to these organizations. In addition, one becomes more knowledgeable about the species, breed, and show circuit problems when participating in animal breed clubs.

One should not join a community activity only to make client contacts. Practice is too time consuming for both veterinarian and technician to become involved in too many activities or activities that are not personally rewarding. However, a reasonable involvement in some of these activities is an important marketing tool in addition to being necessary for supporting the community.

Graduate Technician Self-Marketing

Veterinary technicians must learn to choose employment in practices in which veterinarians will delegate sufficient billable technical tasks to allow the technician to also generate income. This must be sufficient for adequate leveraging of the veterinarian's productivity to provide the technician an adequate salary sufficient to stay in the veterinary technology profession. The IAMS publication "How to Market Yourself—A Veterinary Technician Placement Program" is an excellent resource to plan this critical choice. Also see Recommended Reading at the end of this chapter.

Technician Note

Leveraging the veterinarian's productivity through delegation of billable tasks to the technician should provide adequate salary support for the technician.

The second phase of technician marketing occurs after the initial adjustment period of employment. Once a technician is a productive and trusted part of the veterinary team, strategies must be undertaken to improve and enhance the technician's productive role on the veterinary team. "I can do that" spoken at appropriate times is one of many ways to encourage greater delegation. Keeping a log of technical duties performed by the veterinarian and preparing an analysis of potential time (and money) that could be saved through delegation can also be effective. The same process can be applied to tasks performed by the technician that could be economically done by a minimum-wage assistant.

Obviously, there must be some role delineation between technicians and assistants and between veterinarians and technicians while maintaining the most productive teamwork possible. In general, tasks should be delegated to the lowest paid person who can perform them correctly, especially when other income-producing tasks are available.

SUMMARY

In conclusion, practices that will flourish in the twenty-first century will be those that integrate well-trained technicians with responsible client communication, deliver high-quality medicine and surgery, maintain excellent client-patient and personnel-business management, practice in attractive facilities aided by a good location, and practice preventive maintenance on the facility, equipment, and grounds. These flourishing practices will be exciting and rewarding for clients, patients, and staff.

RECOMMENDED READING

American Veterinary Medical Association (AVMA): *Your professional image*, Schaumburg, Ill, 2000, The Association.

Finch L: *Telephone courtesy and client service*, Schaumburg, Ill, 1991, American Veterinary Medical Association.

Gerson RF: *Beyond customer service: keeping clients for life*, Schaumburg, Ill, 1993, American Veterinary Medical Association.

Haberer JB, Webb MW: *Teamwork: 50 ways to make it work in your practice*, Schaumburg, Ill, 1996, American Veterinary Medical Association.

Lukens RI, Landon RM: *Effective inventory control*, West Chester, Pa, 1993, SmithKline Beecham (Pfizer).

McCarthy JB: *Basic guide to veterinary hospital management*, ed 2, Lakewood, Colo, 1995, American Animal Hospital Association.

McCurnin DM, editor: *Veterinary practice management*, Philadelphia, 1988, Lippincott.

Petit TH: *Hospital administration for veterinary staff*, Goleta, Calif., 1994, American Veterinary Publications.

Scott D: *Client satisfaction: the other half of your job*, Schaumburg, Ill, 1991, American Veterinary Medical Association.

Wise JK: *US pet ownership and demographics sourcebook,* Schaumburg, Ill, 2000, American Veterinary Medical Association.

MANUALS AND DIRECTORIES

AAHA hospital standards and accreditation manual, Denver, 2000, American Animal Hospital Association.

2000 AVMA membership directory and resource manual, ed 11, Schaumburg, Ill, 2000, American Veterinary Medical Association.

How to market yourself: a veterinary technician placement program, Dayton, 2000, The IAMS Co.

Waltham veterinary hospital management, ed 3, Vernon, Calif, 1998, Waltham.

JOURNALS

DVM: The Newsmagazine of Veterinary Medicine, Cleveland, Advantstar Communications, monthly.

Trends, Denver, American Animal Hospital Association, monthly.

Veterinary Economics, Lenexa, Kan, Veterinary Medicine Publishing Group, monthly.

Veterinary Practice News, Mission Viejo, Calif, monthly.

MANAGEMENT SHORT COURSES

Veterinary Management Development School, Denver. Contact AAHA for details.

Veterinary Management Institute at Purdue University. Contact AAHA for details.

INTERNET SITES

http://www.avma.org (information on veterinary medicine and links to pet care sites)

http://www.avma.org/navta/ (veterinary technology profession information)

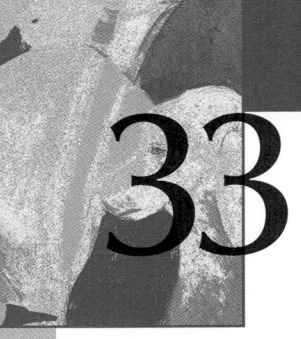

33

Medical Records

Sharee A. Chavis • Judith L. Hutton • Joanna M. Bassert

Veterinary medical records include a wide range of forms and logs that document the treatment and care of animal patients. The results of physical examinations, laboratory tests, and diagnostic procedures, such as radiographic imaging, ultrasound, electrocardiograms, and endoscopy, are examples of information that is included in the record. In addition, medical records document treatment protocols, such as the administration of medication and intravenous fluids, surgery, wound care, and radiation or physical therapy. Medical records also describe the progress of patients, list daily observations, and chart vital signs and other monitoring data. Finally, medical records document euthanasia and postmortem examinations and include important authorization and consent forms.

The number and types of forms and logs that comprise medical records vary from practice to practice. Large teaching hospitals, for example, such as those associated with schools of veterinary medicine, tend to have more extensive medical records than those used by small private practices. Many companion animal hospitals combine information into a concise chart or folder that is easy to store and interpret, whereas large teaching hospitals (or referral centers) tend to employ a separate form for each department, procedure, or study. This chapter emphasizes understanding the comprehensive medical record and the many forms that comprise it.

PATIENT RECORD

The patient record forms the core of medical records and is therefore simply called *the medical record*. It comprises pertinent facts about the patient's life and health history. It describes past and present illnesses and treatments ordered by the clinician. In addition, it serves as a guide for planning the animal's care and provides continuity in evaluating its condition and treatment. The history provided by the animal's owner or agent, the clinician's observations, and the results of any laboratory tests help to determine a diagnosis and course of treatment in each case.

Patient records are usually stored in a central area. In private practices, this area is usually located behind the receptionist's desk for convenience and easy access. On the other hand, in large university animal hospitals, medical records may be housed in a separate room located on a different floor of the hospital.

The patient record must be compiled in a timely manner. Important medical details may be overlooked if they are not recorded quickly. The record should contain sufficient data to identify the animal, support the diagnosis, justify the treatment, and have accurate documented results. Pertinent and correct information helps the health professional diagnose and treat the animal's condition.

The process of ensuring that the medical record is complete and useful is an important task. It includes a thorough knowledge of the medical record and its contents and requires knowledge of its purpose, ownership, value, and uses. It is important that the entire veterinary health care team participates in the maintenance of the record and the accurate entry of daily information.

A complete record should contain the owner's name, address, place of employment, and telephone numbers at work and at home (Figure 33-1). It should also include animal identification, such as the case number, name, and signalment (age, gender, breed, species). All treatment sheets, laboratory results and electrodiagnostic strips should be stamped with the animal's identifying information to avoid loss of important data from the record. When the forms are not identifiable because of lack of information, they must be discarded and important data are therefore lost.

Technician Note

Remember to stamp or write the patient's identifying information on each page of the record.

Some veterinary practices use paperless medical records. This means that the patient record is stored entirely on a computer. Today many veterinary hospitals are outfitted with a computer network that includes multiple computer workstations located throughout the veterinary facility. This enables the veterinary health care team to enter medical, billing, and boarding information about each

DATE _____   CASE NUMBER _____

COMPANION ANIMAL CLIENT/PATIENT INFORMATION FORM

Please provide the following information for our records: **PLEASE PRINT!**

OWNER INFORMATION

OWNER'S NAME	SOCIAL SECURITY NUMBER

STREET ADDRESS

CITY STATE	ZIP CODE	PARISH OR COUNTY

TELEPHONE NUMBER(S) (Area Code, if long distance) →	HOME	BUSINESS

DRIVER'S LICENSE NUMBER	PLACE OF EMPLOYMENT	HOW LONG?

ANIMAL INFORMATION

ANIMAL SPECIES (Dog, Cat, Other)	BREED

ANIMAL'S NAME	SEX	HAS ANIMAL BEEN SEXUALLY ALTERED? ☐ Yes ☐ No

COLOR	BIRTHDATE (Month/year, or approximate)	The undersigned owner or agent certifies that the herein described animal has a maximum value of approximately **$**

REFERRAL INFORMATION

WERE YOU REFERRED BY A VETERINARIAN? ☐ Yes ☐ No	IF YOU WERE REFERRED BY A VETERINARIAN, PLEASE COMPLETE THE FOLLOWING:

VETERINARIAN'S NAME	PHONE

STREET ADDRESS

CITY/STATE	ZIP CODE

You will be advised of estimated cost and anticipated procedures. Please feel free to discuss the proposed treatment and its cost with the veterinarian. A minimum deposit of 50% of the initial estimated charges will be required for hospitalization of an animal patient.

STATEMENT OF OWNERSHIP AND CONSENT: I am the owner of the above described animal, or have authorization from the owner to consent to its treatment.

I hereby authorize the performance of professionally accepted diagnostic, therapeutic, anesthetic, and surgical procedures necessary for its treatment.

I accept financial responsibility for these services.

I have read the above consent and understand why the above procedures may be necessary. I also have been told of the possible complications and alternatives to the listed procedures.

PAYMENT CHOICE: ☐ Cash   ☐ Check   ☐ Bank Card

SIGNATURE (Owner/Agent)	DATE

FIGURE 33-1.   Client/patient information form.

animal on an ongoing basis. The records are then "backed up" on floppy or zip disks or on CD/ROM.

A comprehensive patient record includes, but is not limited to, the following sections:

- Patient's history
- Physical examination
- Symptoms
- Diagnosis
- Prognosis
- Biopsy or necropsy findings (if applicable)
- Vaccination status
- Client education about patient's aftercare
- Client's authorization for patient's treatment
- Discharge summary
- Fee estimate (on all hospitalized cases)
- Financial information (mode of fee payment), such as credit card, cash, or check

HERD RECORDS

It is impractical for food animal veterinarians, who are responsible for the health of entire herds of livestock, to maintain an individual record for every animal treated. In this situation, records are kept on the herd as a whole. Immunizations and reproductive histories are maintained for the group, although individual records may be generated for animals that have undergone special surgical or treatment procedures.

OWNERSHIP OF MEDICAL RECORDS

The original medical record, along with radiographic films, electrodiagnostic tests, and laboratory reports, is the property of the hospital or hospital owner. Although the client purchased the veterinary services that generated the medical information, the client is *not*, by law, the owner of the medical record. However, the owner may request a copy of the record at any time. In fact, it is customary for clients to request copies of their pet's medical record when they are moving and changing veterinary practices. This facilitates continued care of the patient and prevents repetition of immunizations or diagnostic tests. It is recommended that copies of medical records be mailed to the successive veterinarian and not hand delivered by the owner who may be apt to misinterpret the status of his or her animal's health. A cover letter should be included with the copy of the record so that the original veterinary hospital and veterinarian can be easily contacted if necessary. A flat fee for copying the record may be charged, or the practice may levy a fee on a per-page basis.

RELEASE OF MEDICAL INFORMATION

A signed authorization form (Figure 33-2) or a written letter of request for record copies should be obtained from the animal's owner before any information is released to him or her, another veterinarian, or an insurance company. The practice owner should be the only person to authorize release of information contained in the record. However, there is an exception to this rule. Local, state, and federal agencies require the reporting of certain diseases that may be dangerous to the public or to the widespread health of animals. These are called *reportable diseases* and include rabies, brucellosis, and equine encephalitis. Additional regulations regarding reportable diseases can be found in the Animal Movement Quarantine Regulations Manual that is published by the U.S. Department of

Agriculture (USDA). In addition, physicians, animal control agencies, and the regional department of health may inquire about the rabies immunization status of an animal that had bitten a human.

Technician Note

The medical record is a legal document and can be subpoenaed by a court of law.

MEDICAL AND LEGAL REQUIREMENTS

It is important to keep in mind that the medical record is a legal document and could be used in a court of law. It is generated not only to ensure consistent and accurate veterinary care, but also to protect the veterinarian against potential malpractice litigation. Any written data contained in the medical record must therefore be complete, accurate, and legible. Entries should either be typed or written in black ink. Errors should *not* be scratched out, erased, or blotted out. Instead, a single line should be drawn through the mistake and initialed. The correct information should then be written in and initialed next to the mistake. Any erasure or blotting out may suggest tampering of the record and could render the document inadmissible in a court of law. Otherwise, the medical record is considered legal evidence of services and procedures performed by the veterinary health care team. In the event of litigation, such as during a malpractice or insurance suit, the record could be subpoenaed and admitted as evidence.

Legal guidelines for medical records vary from state to state and may dictate the type of information that should be included, how long the record should be kept, and restrictions on the release of medical information. It is recommended that all members of the veterinary health care team be familiar with the laws of the state in which they work.

Technician Note

Do not white out or scribble through mistakes in records. It is a legal document! Draw a line through the mistake once and write "void," plus your initials next to the mistake. Example:

void DM
~~blood~~

ORGANIZATION OF THE MEDICAL RECORD

Because many different types of forms are contained within the medical record, organization and completion of the record can be challenging. However, good organization is of critical importance and enables health professionals to efficiently locate needed information. Different colored tabs or dividers may be added to the patient's record to assist with the location of information. In addition, different types of forms may be printed on paper of different colors so that staff may quickly locate, for example, the blue consent form or the yellow history form.

The order of the record can be different for outpatients and inpatients. Outpatient records may be organized so the outpatient physical examination and client consult sheet

CONSENT TO DISCLOSURE OF MEDICAL RECORD

WAIVER OF CONFIDENTIALITY

BY AUTHORIZED PATIENT REPRESENTATIVE

I, _____ am the _____

of _____ a _____

I understand that the information contained in_____'s

medical record is confidential. However, I specifically give my consent for _____

_____

to release the following specific information concerning

_____ to _____

_____

_____

_____

The above-listed information is to be disclosed for the specific purpose of _____

_____

_____

It is further understood that the information released is for professional purposes only and may not be provided in whole or part to any other person than that stated above.

_____

Signature of
Authorized Representative

_____

Date

FIGURE 33-2.   Authorization form.

are placed on top and in immediate view, whereas inpatient records may place the most recently completed progress sheets on top. In both the inpatient and the outpatient records, the master problem list is an important and easily located document. Although every veterinary clinic and hospital tend to establish their own procedure for the order of records, most veterinary practices employ *reverse chronologic order*. In this organizational plan, the most recent data are positioned on the top so that they are readily available to the clinician. This saves time for the health care team, who would otherwise have to dig through volumes of paperwork to find the most recent information.

During the patient's hospitalization, the progress notes, current laboratory results, and description of treatments performed need to be readily available and are placed in an order so that they are accessible. However, after patient dismissal, the diagnosis and billing information may become more pressing issues and the forms providing this information are preferentially positioned. After all transactions with the patient and client are completed, the record is subsequently organized into its permanent order. Regardless of the system used, the organization of medical records must be *uniform* and *consistent* to ensure efficient retrieval of client and patient information by the veterinarian and hospital staff.

Missing information should be readily noted and added to the chart as soon as it becomes available. For example, the results of laboratory tests, such as tissue biopsies, which are submitted to outside laboratories for analysis, must be added to the medical record as they are received.

MEDICAL RECORD FORMATS

Two formats are generally used in medical records: *conventional* and *problem oriented.*

The conventional method is source oriented. Information is entered into the record as it occurs chronologically. The record therefore ends with the most recent entry. The conventional method is easy to learn and requires less time than the problem-oriented format. It is therefore commonly employed in very busy private practices in which time is limited. In addition, the conventional format lends itself to less voluminous medical records and can be applied to a wide range of record styles (e.g., folder, card, pocket files). The greatest disadvantage of the conventional method, however, is that it lacks detail and includes fewer documents to protect against potential litigation.

The problem-oriented veterinary medical record (POVMR) was adapted from the field of human medicine. It provides an organized and detailed record for each patient. It has also proven to be a valuable teaching and research tool and is therefore commonly employed in most university and teaching veterinary hospitals. Problem-oriented veterinary medical records offer improved professional communication by providing a complete compilation of the patient's problem along with any treatments or procedures that may have been performed on the patient. Although the time to compile this type of record is lengthier, it makes available more historical data and other information to support case planning and provide protection in case of a legal claim.

MASTER PROBLEM LIST

An important part of the POVMR is a master problem list. A problem is defined as anything that requires veterinary medical attention or care. It may be a symptom that the animal's owner noticed or an abnormal finding from a physical examination or laboratory report. The master problem list serves as a mini history for the medical record. It lists immunizations, fecal analyses, and heartworm tests according to the dates on which they were performed, along with problems that the animal has encountered healthwise. The sheet also includes a place where the owner and the animal's identification can be placed (Figure 33-3).

LABORATORY DIAGNOSTIC FLOW SHEET

The laboratory diagnostic flow sheet is a compilation of laboratory data collected from an individual animal. It can be used for outpatients or inpatients. It shows at a glance the different laboratory values for the tests that have been performed on the patient. Specific values can be compared on the different dates for blood counts, chemistry panels, blood gases, urinalyses, and coagulation rates (Figure 33-4). This sheet is of particular value when evaluating patients with diabetes, anemia, chronic renal failure, hepatic failure, Addison's disease, and Cushing's disease. Two spaces at the bottom of the left column are reserved for additional laboratory data that are not already listed in the grid.

DATA BASE

The history, physical examination, chief complaint, and laboratory tests and radiographs if needed are considered the core data base of the medical record. Each hospital may have its own required minimal data base. Animals admitted for either a routine visit or a hospital stay may have, for example, a complete blood count, urinalysis, and fecal analysis. In this way, the data base can vary depending on the needs of the patient. This portion of the record will expand with the addition of data from future visits. The tests done on the first visit will be considered the original data base, and any subsequent visits should provide data for the current problems.

In many emergency and critical care units the data base is considered to include five or six important elements (PCV, total solids, potassium [K^+], Azo, Sticks [checks blood urea nitrogen levels], dextrose, urinalysis). These data can be acquired quickly with a small amount of blood, countertop analyzers, and dipsticks.

COMPREHENSIVE HISTORY FORM

A comprehensive history is acquired with every new patient and those that have not been seen in longer than 1 year. The comprehensive history form contains information on ownership, habitat, diet, environment, and a preventive medical program. It also should include a brief systems review area, along with space for the date seen, time of appointment, and clinician examining the animal (Figure 33-5).

PHYSICAL EXAMINATION FORM

The physical examination is one of the most important diagnostic tools for the clinician. The efficiency of the examination can be maximized with the aid of a well-organized physical examination form. Each of the 11 systems examined is listed clearly so that none is overlooked. In addition, ample space is given to record abnormal findings (Figure 33-6).

WORKING PROBLEM LIST

The working problem list is used in the inpatient file. It provides a comprehensive overview of the pet's problems during a particular hospitalization period. The working problem list provides a quick review of previous problems without the entire record having to be read through (Figure 33-7).

PROGRESS NOTES (SOAP)

SOAP is an acronym formed by the initials of the divisions of the progress notes: S = subjective, O = objective, A = assessment, and P = procedure.

While an animal is hospitalized, clinical notes are kept daily. In the POVMR system, each of the problems is said to be "SOAPed." Any incoming information from a referring veterinarian or an animal's owner during a current hospital stay or on a subsequent visit should also be placed in the progress notes section in chronologic order. Verbal agreements made with the owner either in person or by telephone (including progress reports on the animal) should be recorded in the progress notes (Figure 33-8); each problem is "SOAPed" separately.

Many forms compose the total record, and these can be of various sizes. What is essential for the record to be considered complete is consistency of format. This consistency will ensure that anyone taking care of the animal on a professional or paraprofessional level will readily have available all the information on the patient. When client communication occurs in person, notes are taken and

Text continued on p. 826

JONATHAN HART DVM
2441 TREASURE HILL BLVD
HOUSTON, TEXAS 78550

BERNARD DAVIS   66444
1087 TARA BLVD
BATON ROUGE, LA 70825

CAN LAB F/S
BO BLK 11/30/87

210 389 4726

IMMUNIZATION PREVENTATIVE RECORD

DATE	5/10/98	6/14/99								
RABIES	X	X								
DA2PL	X	X								
PARVO	X	X								
FVRCP										
FELV VACC.										
FELV/FIV										
FECAL	neg.	neg.								
HEARTWORM	neg.	neg.								

	PROBLEM LIST	DATE ENTERED	DATE RESOLVED
1.	Elective Ovariohysterectomy	8/10/90	8/10/90
2.	Malassezia-otitis externa	8/10/90	8/17/90
3.	Dental prophylaxis	11/3/93	11/3/93
4.	Gastroenteritis — small bowel diarrhea	3/15/94	3/18/94
5.	Uncomplicated UTI	2/3/00	2/16/00
6.	Recurrent UTI — E. coli	3/14/00	3/28/00
7.	Recurrent UTI	6/10/00	6/20/00
8.	Right renomegaly; Cystic kidney mass	6/20/00	
9.	Right unilateral nephrectomy	6/23/00	6/23/00
10.	Renal carcinoma	6/24/00	
11.	Lethary, anorexia	7/2/00	7/5/00
12.			
13.			

BREED=   SEX=

FIGURE 33-3.   Master problem list.

Hospital Name _____

Address _____

City _____ **State** _____ **Zip Code** _____

SIGNALMENT

LABORATORY DIAGNOSTICS FLOW SHEET

CHEMISTRY PANEL	DATES					HEMOGRAM	DATES				
GLUCOSE mg/dL						WBC ($\times 10^3$)/μL					
AST U/L						RBC ($\times 10^6$)/μL					
ALT U/L						HGB g/dL					
ALP U/L						HCT %					
CK U/L						MCV fl					
T. BILIRUBIN mg/dL						MCH pg					
T. PROTEIN g/dL						MCHC g/dL					
ALBUMIN g/dL						PLT ($\times 10^3$)/μL					
GLOBULIN mg/dL						PCV/TS %					
CHOLESTEROL mg/dL						SEGS ($\times 10^3$)/μL					
UREA NITROGEN mg/dL						BANDS ($\times 10^3$)/μL					
CREATININE mg/dL						LYMPHS ($\times 10^3$)/μL					
CALCIUM mg/dL						MONO ($\times 10^3$)/μL					
PHOSPHORUS mg/dL						EOS ($\times 10^3$)/μL					
SODIUM mmol/L						BASOS ($\times 10^3$)/μL					
POTASSIUM mmol/L						nRBC					
CHLORIDE mmol/L						RETIC %					
TCO$_2$ mmol/L						**URINALYSIS**					
ANION GAP mmol/L						COLOR					
BLOOD GAS						TURBIDITY					
pH						SPECIFIC GRAVITY					
PCO$_2$ mm Hg						pH					
PO$_2$ mm Hg						PROTEIN mg/dL					
HCO$_3$ mmol/L						GLUCOSE mg/dL					
TCO$_2$ mmol/L						KETONES					
BASE EXCESS						BILIRUBIN					
COAGULATION						HEMOGLOBIN					
ACT sec						VOLUME					
PT sec PATIENT / CONTROL						CASTS (+/−)					
PTT sec PATIENT / CONTROL						WBC					
FDP μg/mL						RBC					
BMBT (Sec)						EPITH CELLS (+/−)					
						CRYSTALS (+/−)					
						BACTERIA (+/−)					

FIGURE 33-4.   Laboratory flow sheet with reference ranges.

Continued

CLINICAL PATHOLOGY REFERENCE RANGES

	units	CANINE	FELINE	EQUINE	BOVINE
Total leukocytes	(x10³/μL)	6–17	5.5–19.5	5.5–12.5	4–12
Neutrophils	(x10³/μL)	3–11.5	2.5–12.5	2.7–6.7	0.6–4
Bands	(x10³/μL)	0–0.3	0–0.3	0–0.1	0–0.1
Eosinophils	(x10³/μL)	0.1–1.2	0–1.5	0–0.9	0–2.4
Basophils	(x10³/μL)	rare	rare	0–0.2	0–0.2
Monocytes	(x10³/μL)	0.1–1.4	0–0.8	0–0.8	0–0.8
Lymphocytes	(x10³/μL)	1–4.8	1.5–7	1.5–5.5	2.5–7.5
Erythrocytes	(x10⁶/μL)	5–8.5	5–10	6.5–12.5	5–10
Hemoglobin	(g/dL)	12–18	9–16	11–19	8–15
Hematocrit	(%)	35–55	28–45	32–52	24–46
MCV	(fl)	60–77	39–55	34–58	40–60
MCH	(pg)	21–27	13–17	10–18	11–18
MCHC	(g/dL)	32–36	30–36	30–35	30–36
Platelets	(x10³/μL)	200–700	200–700	100–600	100-800
Plasma Protein	(g/dL)	6–7.8	6–7.5	5.2–7.8	6–8
Fibrinogen (HPP)	(mg/dL)	–	–	100–500	100–700
Glucose	(mg/dL)	75–115	85–115	70–100	60–100
ALT	(IU/L)	<100	<90	–	–
AST	(IU/L)	<60	<40	<350	<150
CK	(IU/L)	<285	<300	<300	<300
ALP	(IU/L)	<135	<45	<300	<140
GGT	(IU/L)	–	–	<45	<45
T. Bilirubin	(mg/dL)	<0.4	<0.2	<2.0	<0.5
T. Protein	(g/dL)	5.7–7.4	6.0–8.1	6.0–8.0	6.4–8.2
Globulins	(g/dL)	2.1–4.1	2.8–4.9	2.0–4.4	2.7–4.5
Albumin	(g/dL)	2.9–4.0	2.9–3.5	3.0–4.1	3.1–4.0
BUN	(mg/dL)	6–22	15–30	14–27	10–24
Creatinine	(mg/dL)	0.4–1.5	0.6–2.2	1.2–2.5	0.7–1.8
Calcium	(mg/dL)	8.6–11.2	8.9–11.0	10–13	8.5–11.1
Phosphorus	(mg/dL)	2.5–5.5	3.1–5.8	1.9–4.7	4.0–7.2
Cholesterol	(mg/dL)	130–240	90–160	–	–
Magnesium	(mmol/L)	–	–	0.60–0.95	0.70–1.10
Amylase	(IU/L)	<900	<900	<20	–
Lipase	(IU/L)	<600	<400	<20	<50
Bile Acids, fasting	(μmol/L)	<5	<2	–	–
Bile Acids, post	(μmol/L)	<20	<20	–	–
Ammonia, fasting	(μmol/L)	<32	–	<55	–
SDH	(IU/L)	–	–	<7	<15
Sodium	(mmol/L)	140–155	140–155	130–145	135–150
Potassium	(mmol/L)	3.5–5.5	3.0–5.5	3.0–5.0	3.5–5.0
Chloride	(mmol/L)	105–120	110–125	95–110	95–110
Total CO₂	(mmol/L)	20–28	20–28	24–30	21–31
Anion Gap	(mmol/L)	8–20	8–20	6–15	6–15
pH		7.31–7.50	7.24–7.40	7.30–7.43	7.35–7.50
PCO₂	(mm Hg)	29–42	29–42	36–50	35–44
HCO₃	(mmol/L)	17–24	17–24	21–30	20–30
TCO₂	(mmol/L)	18–25	18–25	22–31	21–31

FIGURE 33-4, CONT'D.   For legend see opposite page.

TEACHING HOSPITAL AND CLINICS

School of Veterinary Medicine
Louisiana State University
Baton Rouge, Louisiana 70803

LSU

| SMALL ANIMAL | | NUMBER |

NAME BERNARD DAVIS   66444
          1087 TARA BLVD   CASE NO.
STREET BATON ROUGE, LA 70825
CITY, STATE, ZIP
PHONE CAN LAB F/S   HOME
          BO BLK 11/30/87
          SPECIES   BREED   SEX

ANIMAL'S NAME   DATE OF BIRTH

COLOR—IDENTIFYING MARKS

CHIEF COMPLAINT: *Frequent UTI*

REFERRING VETERINARIAN:

JONATHAN HART DVM
2441 TREASURE HILL BLVD
HOUSTON, TEXAS 78550

210 389 4726

Date: *6/20/00*

Appt. Time:

Admitting Clinician: *Ryan*

ENVIRONMENTAL HISTORY:
Length of time owned:

12 1/2 years

Kept In:
☒ Louisiana
☐ Other _____

Obtained From: Bred ☐   Breeder ☐   Friend ☒
Pet Shop ☐   Humane Society ☐   Stray ☐   Other ☐

Environment:		Confined to:		Other Pets:		Diet:			
Urban House	☒	Home , *(yard)*	☒	Yes	☒	Commercial Dry	☒	Frequency	*1 x /day*
Apartment	☐	Outdoor pen/chain	☐	No	☐	Semimoist	☐	Amount:	
Suburban	☐	Roams	☐	*5 cats*		Canned	☐		*3 cups*
Rural	☐	Other	☐	*2 dogs*		Table Scraps	☐		
						Other	☐		

PREVENTATIVE MEDICINE PROGRAM:

YES		DATE	NO	YES		DATE	NO
☒	Distemper-Hepatitis	*6/99*	☐	☐ Fecal Check			☒
☐	Feline Panleukopenia		☐	☒ Heartworm Check		*6/99*	☐
☐	FVR-Calci-Panleukopenia		☐	☒ Heartworm Preventative	*(Heartguard) monthly*		☐
☒	Distemper-Hep-Parainfluenza	*6/99*	☐	☐ Flea Control			☒
☒	Rabies	*6/99*	☐	☐ Tick Control			☒

MEDICAL HISTORY:
Past Medical History—prior illness, surgery, drug reactions, etc.
Current Medical History—signs, chronological course, prior therapy, system review.

System Review
Attitude ✓
Exercise
Tolerance
Ocular or
Nasal
Discharge
Sneezing ✓
Coughing ✓
Appetite ✓
Vomiting ✓
Diarrhea ✓
P/D - P/U ✓
Pruritus
Incoordination
Paresis
Seizures
Estrus

Normal attitude, appetite, activity level.
No cough, sneeze, vomit, or diarrhea, discharge
water intake increased (subjectively)
No neurologic signs.

Primary complaint: ① *Urinates in house*
② *Drinking more; urinating more frequently*
③ *Straining to urinate*
    No hematuria; increased urgency
④ *Not apparently painful*
⑤ *Two similar episodes in past 6 months*

COMPREHENSIVE HISTORY   **MEDICAL RECORDS**   V-1

FIGURE 33-5. Example of a comprehensive history form.

TEACHING HOSPITAL AND CLINICS
School of Veterinary Medicine
Louisiana State University
Baton Rouge, Louisiana 70803

LSU

Date: 6/20/00

SMALL ANIMAL | NUMBER

NAME
BERNARD DAVIS
1087 TARA BLVD
BATON ROUGE, LA 70825
STREET
CITY, STATE, ZIP
PHONE BUS. HOME
CASE NO. 66444

CAN LAB F/S
BO BLK 11/30/87
SPECIES BREED SEX
ANIMAL'S NAME DATE OF BIRTH
COLOR—IDENTIFYING MARKS

Temp 102.5 °F Attitude BAR
Fem. Pulse 100 Charac. normal Resp. 24
Memb. Color pink Cap. Refill Time < 1.5 sc
Hydration normal Body Weight 70 #
Color & Consistency of feces on Therm. normal
Body Condition — Underweight ☐ Overweight ☒ Normal ☐

SYSTEM REVIEW

1. Integumentary ☐ Normal ☑ Abnormal	2. Otic ☐ Normal ☑ Abnormal	3. Ophthalmic ☑ Normal ☐ Abnormal	4. Musculoskeletal ☑ Normal ☐ Abnormal
5. Nervous ☑ Normal ☐ Abnormal	6. Cardiovascular ☑ Normal ☐ Abnormal	7. Respiratory ☑ Normal ☐ Abnormal	8. Digestive ☑ Normal ☐ Abnormal
9. Lymphatic ☑ Normal ☐ Abnormal	10. Reproductive ☑ Normal ☐ Abnormal	11. Urinary ☑ Normal ☐ Abnormal	

DESCRIBE ABNORMAL:

1) multiple dermal, epidermal, and subcutaneous masses
—(R) lateral stifle, (R) cranial shoulder, (L) muzzle, (L) distal cranial antebrachium

2) Moderate otitis externa — erythema, waxy exudate, bilateral

EXAMINER K. Ryan DVM

PHYSICAL EXAMINATION MEDICAL RECORDS V-1

FIGURE 33-6. Example of a physical examination form.

**VETERINARY TEACHING HOSPITAL
LOUISIANA STATE UNIVERSITY**

WORKING PROBLEM LIST

BERNARD DAVIS   66444
1087 TARA BLVD
BATON ROUGE LA 70825

CAN LAB F/S
BO BLK 11/30/87

PROBLEM NUMBER	ACTIVE DATE	PROBLEM	DATE RESOLVED
①	6/20/00	Recurrent lower urinary tract signs (stranguria, pollakiuria)	6/24/00
②	6/20/00	Polyuria/Polydipsia	
③	6/20/00	Right Renomegally; Cystic Kidney mass	6/24/00
④	6/24/00	Renal Carcinoma	

MEDICAL RECORD

Figure 33-7. Working problem list.

VETERINARY TEACHING HOSPITAL AND CLINICS
LOUISIANA STATE UNIVERSITY

Progress Notes must be recorded at least once every
24 hours. All entries must be in the SOAP format.

Page __1__ of __3__

BERNARD DAVIS   66444
1087 TARA BLVD
BATON ROUGE, LA 70825

CAN LAB F/S
BO BLK 11/30/87

DATE	TEMP:	100.4	
6/20/00	PULSE:	120	
	RESP:	30	
	APPETITE:	good	
	BOWELS:	normal x 1	

(S) Bo is a 13 year old female spayed Labrador retriever who presented for evaluation of a recurrent lower urinary tract infection. She appears bright, alert, and responsive with no obvious signs of sytemic illness.

(O) wt = 70 #

vital signs recorded – see margin

multiple cutaneous masses, moderate ear debris (both ears)

Normal abdominal palpation; normal thoracic ausc.

(A) Problem List:

(1) Cutaneous masses — these masses have a benign appearance, and seem unrelated to current presenting complaint. Differential diagnoses include: 1. Neoplasia (benign or malignant) (i.e., mast cell tumor, lipoma, sebaceous adenoma, etc.)

(2) Inflamed ear canals with debris — This is classic for otitis externa. Differentials include yeast and bacterial infection. However, otitis is also a common manifestation of allergic skin disease (i.e., atopy, food allergy, etc.). Less likely causes include ear mites and foreign bodies and neoplasia.

(3) Recurrent Stranguria and Pollakiuria
These signs suggest recurrent lower urinary tract infection (UTI). Causes of recurrent UTI include neoplasia, urinary calculi, polyps, anatomic defects (strictures, diverticuli, etc.), and decreased immune response; the most common bacteria include E. coli, proteus, and staph. Other causes of stranguria and pollakiuria include noninfectious inflammatory disease, neoplasia,

KR   V-5

FIGURE 33-8.   Progress notes.

Continued

**VETERINARY TEACHING HOSPITAL AND CLINICS
LOUISIANA STATE UNIVERSITY**

Progress Notes must be recorded at least once every
24 hours. All entries must be in the SOAP format.

Page __2__ of __3__

BERNARD DAVIS   66444
1087 TARA BLVD
BATON ROUGE, LA 70825

CAN LAB F/S
BO BLK 11/30/87

DATE	TEMP:	(A) Continued
6/20/00	PULSE:	and urinary calculi. Top differentials include neoplasia or
	RESP:	calculi.
	APPETITE:	(P)(1) Cutaneous masses should be identified via fine needle aspirate
	BOWELS:	cytology. Excisional biopsy is recommended if the mass in question
		is a malignancy, or is irritating to owner or pet.
		(2) Otitis externa should be evaluated via otoscopic exam to rule
		out ear canal masses or foreign bodies. Swab cytology can identify
		infectious agents (difQuick, gram stain) associated with current
		problem. This information will help dictate topical and systemic
		medication. Underlying causes such as atopy should be further
		evaluated via historical questioning. If present, atopy should be
		managed medically with consultation with a dermatologist as
		needed.
		(3) The recurrent lower urinary tract signs in this dog are the
		most important problem. The age of this dog and the number of
		previous episodes indicate a thorough evaluation for an underlying
		cause. Tests should include:
		1.) Urinalysis and urine culture
		— to document infection, assess urine
		concentration, and examine urine sediment
		2.) Chemistry panel — to assess general
		health especially kidney function
		3.) Complete blood count — to assess systemic
		inflammatory component (if present)

KR   V-5

FIGURE 33-8, CONT'D. For legend see p. 823.

Continued

VETERINARY TEACHING HOSPITAL AND CLINICS
LOUISIANA STATE UNIVERSITY

Progress Notes must be recorded at least once every
24 hours. All entries must be in the SOAP format.

Page ___3___ of ___3___

BERNARD DAVIS   66444
1087 TARA BLVD
BATON ROUGE, LA 70825

CAN LAB F/S
BO BLK 11/30/87

DATE	TEMP:	(P) Continued
6/20/00	PULSE:	4.) Abdominal radiographs — to rule out radio opaque
	RESP:	calculi and search for supportive evidence of neoplasia
	APPETITE:	or renal disease
	BOWELS:	5.) Abdominal ultrasound will likely be needed to assess
		bladder wall and rule out intraluminal neoplasia. Renal
		architecture can be seen
		6.) Vaginal and rectal exam (under sedation) to search
		for neoplasia or inflammation in these areas
		Treatment with antibiotics based on culture results may occur
		while work up is proceeding. Amoxicillin would be a good choice
		empirically.
		K. Ryan V-5

FIGURE 33-8, CONT'D.   For legend see p. 823.

included with the progress (SOAP) sheets in chronologic order, with the most recent data on top (see Figure 33-8). If client communication occurs by telephone, a telephone report form should be filled out (Figure 33-9). This form should be placed within the progress notes if the patient is in the hospital or on top of the most recent visit if the patient has gone home.

> **Technician Note**
>
> When writing in charts, use only approved abbreviations. Do not abbreviate the final diagnosis.

CARD FILE

To conserve space and costs, some veterinary practices use a card file system instead of maintaining medical record files on each patient. The size of the card most often used is 5 × 8 inches, with a plastic pocket attached in which to store laboratory data, radiology reports, or electrocardiogram strips. This card can be stored in a file drawer (Figure 33-10).

Another card system involves the use of a 10- × 16-inch card, which accommodates more information on the patient. It can be folded in half and stored in a file drawer. Information contained on this type of record is brief; it must contain owner and patient information along with sufficient data to allow the proper and adequate care of the animal (Figure 33-11). As society has become more litigious, fewer veterinary practices are using the card system. The limited amount of available writing space precludes recording what may prove to be important details. Many practices therefore use files rather than cards and often employ the conventional medical format.

> **Technician Note**
>
> When using the file folder format for the chart, keep all information related to each visit stapled together.

COLOR-CODING SYSTEMS

Two types of color-coding systems are used in medical records: *alphabetic* and *numeric*. In alphabetic color coding, a different color is assigned to each letter of the alphabet, and all names that fall within that letter group are filed behind that color in alphabetic order. Additional colors may be added, depending on the desired extent of the color-coding system.

In numeric color coding, one color is assigned to each digit from 0 to 9, and the colors on the record vary according to the record number. This system is invaluable in preventing chart misfiles and as a signaling device in the search for a specific record.

Color coding may also be used to signal files to be purged or files for dead animals, bad debts, or return visits, and it can be used to mark when vaccinations are due so the client can be notified.

This system can be simple or complex, depending on the size of the practice and the personnel available to keep the system running smoothly. It is important, regardless of the size of the practice, that the coding system be maintained and updated regularly.

FILE PURGING

Each practice or hospital will set its own rules for purging files. Generally, active records covering a 3-year period are kept in the medical records area, including files of animals that have a new veterinarian because the owner has moved. The charts of animals that have died within this period are also kept so the clinician will have them available for review or research purposes. Any inactive record that is 4 years old or older is placed in a separate storage area.

Files should be purged on a yearly basis to allow easier filing and make room available for new records. Color coding can be a big help in signaling inactive records so the entire file will not have to be checked. Recording the date of the client's last visit on the front of the file folder will allow inactive files to be easily identified and purged.

The inactive file should be in a convenient place that is easily accessible and safe, so the record can be quickly reactivated if necessary. In general, records 8 years old or older can be purged from the inactive file. They should be destroyed by shredding or burning.

LOST RECORDS

The risk of losing records in both a small and a large hospital is problematic. They can be lost through misfiling, incorrect spelling of names, or misplacement. At times, even after an exhaustive search, the record continues to be missing. Sometimes the loss is not discovered until the animal comes back to the practice for a return visit.

It is best, in this case, to explain to the client that the record has been misplaced. A new record should be started and information requested from the client and veterinarian. In addition, copies of laboratory data, pathology reports, and radiologic information should be obtained and added to reestablish the file.

Although the problem of lost records is embarrassing to the practice and inconvenient to the client, it happens with even the most elaborate record system; however, every effort possible should be made to quickly and accurately file each record after each visit. Clients feel more at ease and welcomed if the record is complete and easily accessible.

LOGS

Logs are maintained in a veterinary facility for the purpose of recording procedures and tests performed, radiology studies, mortality and euthanasia rates, quality and inventory control, and data collection for quick retrieval and to compare or justify procedures. They also contain brief owner and pet identifying information should the need arise to look up data in this matter. Logs are kept in binders or bound composition books within the area of the hospital that provides that service.

Biopsy Log

The biopsy log is kept in the pathology or laboratory department. Each biopsy performed through the pathology department is recorded in the log book. It serves as a retrospective study of disease frequencies within a region, such as cancer or other diseases, and provides a review of treatment of these diseases and the outcome.

Necropsy Log

The necropsy log is a compilation of data regarding animal deaths, including their cause and type of necropsy

TELEPHONE REPORT

Date: _____ Case Number: _____

Name: _____
Species: _____ Breed: _____
Sex: _____ Animal's Name: _____
Phone #: _____ DOB: _____

Client History: _____

_____

_____

_____

Instructions to Client: _____

_____

_____

_____

_____

_____

_____

_____

_____

Prescription: _____

_____

_____

_____

_____

_____

_____

Signature: _____

FIGURE 33-9.   Telephone report.

Client Name ________ Address ________ Zip Code ________ Phone ________

Employment ________ Phone ________ Referred by ________

Animal's Name ________ Color ________ Species ________ Breed ________ Age ____ Sex ____

Vaccination History	Date		

Allergies ________

Fecal Exams ________

Date	Chief Complaint	Exam	Treatment/Surgery	Doctor

FIGURE 33-10. Veterinary medical record card (5 × 8 inches).

Client Name ________ Address ________ Phone ________

Employment ________ Phone ________ Referred by ________

Animal's Name ________ Case No. ________ Color ________ Species ________

Breed ________ Age ____ Sex ____ Altered ____ Date ________

Vaccination History

Date Vaccination Revaccinate

Fecal Exams

Date Results

Dental Care

Allergies

Date	Examination/Treatment	Dr.	Charge	Pd.	Balance

FIGURE 33-11. Veterinary medical record card (10 × 16 inches).

performed. The log contains the owner's name, case number, species, date, veterinarian performing the evaluation, histopathology, or special tissue submitted. It is kept in the necropsy area (Figure 33-12).

Radiology Log

The radiology log is completed by a technician who is designated within the department to post information. The log contains date of examination, type of examination performed, owner's name, case number, animal's species and breed, exposure settings, and veterinarian's name (Figure 33-13). This log is very useful when improved exposure technique is desired or repeat films are requested.

Anesthesia Log

Every patient that undergoes anesthesia has a preliminary physical examination. Laboratory studies are also completed to evaluate the patient's ability to recover from anesthesia. The result of these findings are included in the "anesthesia request and data form" (Figure 33-14). In addition, a record is made before, during, and after surgery that notes the process of induction, maintenance of anesthesia, and recovery from anesthesia. This document carries particularly important legal data began some patients die during the surgical and perisurgical period (Figure 33-15).

Finally, after an animal is moved to the recovery room,

NECROPSY LOG

DATE	PATH #	VTH&C #	DIAG LAB #	SPECIES	CLINICIAN	OWNER	PATH	GRAD.	DATE REC TYPE	DATE TYPED	DATE CORR.	DATE MAILED
16 June	0507	70048	33791	Ovine	Quinn	Douglas	Smith	Toole	17 June	18 June	19 June	19 June
16 June	0508	63378	27590	Equine	Brown	Breaux	Homes	——	17 June	18 June	19 June	19 June
17 June	0509	52215	20079	Avian	Lucky	McCasey	Baer	——	18 June	19 June	19 June	19 June
21 June	0510	40021	13386	Feline	Grant	Sprickett	Cadd	Black	22 June	23 June	24 June	24 June
2 July	0511	57740	25005	Canine	O'Connor	Page	Dicks	——	3 July	6 July	6 July	6 July
8 July	0512	60020	30059	Antelope	Pine	Brumfield	Cones	——	9 July	10 July	10 July	11 July
	0513											
	0514											
	0515											
	0516											
	0517											
	0518											
	0519											
	0520											
	0521											
	0522											
	0523											
	0524											
	0525											
	0526											
	0527											
	0528											
	0529											

Sample of Necropsy Log

FIGURE 33-12. Example of a necropsy log.

the animal continues to be monitored. Vital signs, analgesic drugs given, and other notes are recorded on a form such as the one in Figure 33-16.

Surgery Log

The surgery log contains information on the procedure performed (major or minor), animal's name, case number, owner's name, date on which surgery was performed, anesthesia used, surgeon's name, duration of the surgical or anesthesia procedure, and fee. Through this log, retrospective studies are made of costs, procedures, and surgical complications (Figure 33-17).

THE FAX CONNECTION

The facsimile (fax) machine plays a major role in the field of health care communication. The rapid transmission of information is important, especially when handling emergency cases.

This method of data transmittal is also used for, but not limited to, record transfer when the animal's owner has moved to another area, information transmittal to a veterinary specialist from a referring veterinarian, or information transmittal from the specialist back to the referring veterinarian.

Although this has proved to be a convenient way to send data, confidentiality must be maintained so the integrity of the medical record is not compromised. Procedures for sending information by fax should be established and explained to the office personnel who will carry out the transmittal procedure.

It is suggested that fax communication be used only if the mail will not serve the purpose or in the event of an emergency. For information to be sent, a properly completed and authorized release of information should be obtained, to be used for that one time only. A hard copy (original form) should also be mailed to the veterinary practice to be kept as a permanent part of the record. The faxed copy is kept as a part of the record until the original is received. In an emergency, the release form may not be obtainable before treatment. A policy should be developed within each practice regarding the emergency request of information. It is also recommended that fax data be sent only when used in a patient care encounter and not for routine use. When data are sent via fax, a cover letter with the sender's and receiver's names, addresses, date, telephone numbers, and fax identifications should be included (Figure 33-18). It should be established beforehand whether the copies should be destroyed after having been transmitted or returned to the medical record department for their disposition. A fax copy is as admissible in court as an original copy in the event of legal proceedings. Therefore fax copies must also be legible and complete so the validity of the medical record is not questioned. In all cases, the original copy of the cover letter should be placed in the medical record for future reference. Regular mail or messenger service should cover the routine release of information by the practice. A nominal fee per page is charged for the transmission and transfer of the medical record. This fee helps defray costs of telephone line use, paper, and time.

Text continued on p. 835

RADIOLOGY LOG

DATE	CASE NUMBER	OWNER	BREED	DOCTOR	EXAMINATION
1/28	12167	Jones	K-9	Woods	STC
1/28	12257	Kaiser	K-9	Little	PO2
1/29	12257	Pearson	K-9	Green	AS
1/29	12287	White	K-9	Drennon	AS
1/29	12215	Major	K-9	Davis	AS
1/29	8527	Golden	K-9	Gomez	AS
1/29	12297	Jenks	K-9	Gomez	RUC X 2
1/29	307630	Ryan	EQ	Meyers	TRANQ + TL X 2
1/30					
1/30					
1/30					
1/30					
2/1					
2/1					
2/1					
2/1					
2/1					
2/1					
2/1					
2/2					
2/2					
2/2					
2/2					
2/3					

FIGURE 33-13. Example of a radiology log.

TEACHING HOSPITAL AND CLINICS
School of Veterinary Medicine
Louisiana State University
Baton Rouge, Louisiana 70803
ANESTHESIA REQUEST AND DATA FORM

IDENTIFICATION

Total Fee: _____

Charge to: ☐ Client
            ☐ Research
            ☐ Grant # _____

Date request submitted: Date of surgery:

Preferred surgery time: Estimated surgery length:

Surgeon:

Surgery Student:

Patient position   ☐ LL   ☐ RL   ☐ D   ☐ S

CAGE/STALL #   DATE: /   /

WEIGHT: _____ lb. _____ kg.   Temperament: _____

EMERGENCY   ☐ yes   ☐ no

Previous anesthetics used _____ when? _____

Other medications (last 24 hours): _____

Procedure(s):

1. _____

2. _____

3. _____

Recent treatment for ecto- or endoparasites (within last 6 weeks)?   ☐ yes   ☐ no

If yes, what agent? _____

Known allergies?   ☐ yes   ☐ no _____   Known drug rxns?   ☐ yes   ☐ no _____

History (of current problem): _____

_____

Abnormal Physical exam findings: _____

_____

Laboratory Data: (if unavailable, has it been submitted?   ☐ yes   ☐ no)

CBC	Panel	Blood gases a or v
WBC _____/ul	glucose _____mg/dl	pH _____
Neut _____/ul	BUN _____mg/dl	pCO$_2$_____mm Hg
Lymp _____/ul	creatinine _____mg/dl	pO$_2$_____mm Hg
Mono _____/ul	albumin _____gm/dl	HCO$_3$_____mEq/L
Eos_____/ul	calcium _____mg/dl	TCO$_2$_____mEq/L
Baso_____/dl	phosphorus _____mg/dl	BE _____mEq/L
PCV _____%	T. Bili _____mg/dl	
Hgb _____gm/dl	SAST (LA) _____U/L	Electrolytes
TP _____gm/dl	SALT (SA) _____U/L	Na _____mEq/L
Fib _____gm/dl	SGGT _____U/L	K _____mEq/L
Other _____	SALP _____U/L	Cl _____mEq/L
_____	CPK _____U/L	AG _____mEq/L
_____		

Preanesthetic considerations: _____

_____

Postanesthetic considerations _____

_____

Preoperative examination: Temp:_____ HR:_____ RR:_____ membrane color_____ CRT:_____sec.

Physical status: _____1 _____2 _____3 _____4 _____5

Preanesthetic agents: _____

Induction agents: _____

Maintenance: _____

Fluids: type:_____   rate:_____   ml/lb/hr x_____lbs=_____ml/hr_____

FIGURE 33-14.   Identification log for anesthesia.

TEACHING HOSPITAL AND CLINICS
School of Veterinary Medicine
Louisiana State University

ANESTHESIA RECORD

IDENTIFICATION

DATE: / /

Case No.

Premedications

Drug	Dose	Route	Time

Induction Agents

Drug	Dose	Route	Time

Physical Status 1 2 3 4 5 E

Preop: Temp:________ HR:________ RR:________ Weight:________

Time	15	30	45	15	30	45	15	30	45	15	30	45	15	30	45
Oxygen Flow															
N20 Flow															
Vaporizer Setting															

SYMBOLS

Symbol		Scale
		200
Anes	A	180
Oper	x	160
End O	ⓧ	140
End A	Ⓐ	120
BP Mean	—	100
Syst	V	80
Diast	Λ	
		60
Pulse	●	
Resp	○	40
		35
		30
		25
		20
		15
		10
Temp	▲	8
		6
		4
		2

CODE NO:

FLUIDS

Time to standing:____________ EXTUBATION:________ ET tube used:_____ mm i.d.__________ Total fluids:________

Postoperative Exam: Time______________ Temp______________ HR______________ RR______________

Complications: ____

Student signature ______________________ Clinician signature ______________________

FIGURE 33-15. Anesthesia record.

DATE _____

TEACHING HOSPITAL AND CLINICS
SCHOOL OF VETERINARY MEDICINE

SURGERY/PROCEDURE: _____

_____

CLINICIAN _____

ANESTHESIA STUDENT _____

STUDENT _____

SMALL ANIMAL RECOVERY ROOM

BODY WT. _____

❏ WILL BITE   ❏ WILL NOT BITE

POST OPERATIVE ANALGESIA

Drug	Time	Amount Drug mg	Route	Initials

PATIENT VITAL SIGNS

Time	Temp	Pulse Rate	Resp. Rate	MM Color		Treatments/ Medications/Observations	Initials

INSTRUCTIONS: Patient vital signs should be monitored and recorded every 30 minutes until T°=99.0°F or more and/or patient is ambulatory. IV catheters should remain in place until patient is completely recovered and is ready to return to the wards.

SPECIAL INSTRUCTIONS: _____

_____

PRE-OPERATIVE ANESTHETICS: _____

ANESTHETICS/INTRA-OP MEDS: _____

RETURN TO WARDS? _____ WARD/CAGE NO. _____ REMOVE CATHETER POST-RECOVERY? _____

FIGURE 33-16. Recovery record.

SURGERY LOG

CASE NUMBER	CLIENT	SURGEON	ANESTHESIA	PROCEDURE	MAJOR	MINOR	TIME	FEE

FIGURE 33-17.   Example of a surgery log.

FIGURE 33-18.   Facsimile cover sheet.

Hospital Name _____
Address _____
City _____ State _____ Zip Code _____

TELEFACSIMILE COVER SHEET

DATE: _____

TO: _____

DEPT. / ADDRESS: _____

_____

FAX NUMBER: _____
          Country Code   City Code   Area Code   Phone Number

FROM: _____

MESSAGE: _____

_____

_____

_____

_____

_____

_____

_____

TOTAL PAGES TO BE TRANSMITTED, INCLUDING COVER: _____

MORBIDITY – MORTALITY REPORT FOR _____ (MONTH)

CASE NUMBER:	CASE NUMBER:
CLINICIAN:	CLINICIAN:
SURGERY: YES NO	SURGERY: YES NO
DIED: EUTHANIZED:	DIED: EUTHANIZED:
DIAGNOSIS:	DIAGNOSIS:
CASE NUMBER:	CASE NUMBER:
CLINICIAN:	CLINICIAN:
SURGERY: YES NO	SURGERY: YES NO
DIED: EUTHANIZED:	DIED: EUTHANIZED:
DIAGNOSIS:	DIAGNOSIS:
CASE NUMBER:	CASE NUMBER:
CLINICIAN:	CLINICIAN:
SURGERY: YES NO	SURGERY: YES NO
DIED: EUTHANIZED:	DIED: EUTHANIZED:
DIAGNOSIS:	DIAGNOSIS:

FIGURE 33-19. Example of a morbidity-mortality log.

Technician Note

Copying and faxing of medical records should be done only by authorized personnel.

MORBIDITY-MORTALITY REPORT

The morbidity-mortality record includes the patient case number, clinician in charge of the case, whether surgery was performed, whether the animal was euthanized or died of natural causes, and diagnosis at time of death. Information is entered daily or monthly, making this record a convenient source for compilation of statistics (Figure 33-19).

AUTHORIZATIONS

Authorizations are not a legal requirement. Their purpose is to protect the veterinarian and to ensure each client understands all treatments, surgical procedures, fee estimates, euthanasia approval, necropsy approval, and release of responsibility.

Several different forms may be needed to accommodate each situation. All authorizations should contain owner and animal information and become part of the permanent medical record.

The fee estimate sheet is an important form provided to the client for approval before service. This form provides an estimate for all services the animal may need during diagnosis and treatment. A total fee estimate may be difficult to establish on admission to the hospital but must be attempted to avoid financial misunderstandings with the client. If the estimate changes during the treatment period, the client should be informed. Both the owner and veterinarian should sign the fee estimate form, and a

duplicate copy should become a part of the medical record (Figure 33-20). The euthanasia/donation authorization is critical at the time the owner is agreeing to donate or euthanize an animal. Occasionally, an owner may wish to change his or her instructions or cancel a euthanasia. When this occurs, the completed and signed consent form is the only legal document in the medical record that authorizes such activity (Figure 33-21).

COMPUTERS

The computer is an invaluable tool in the field of veterinary medicine. Most veterinary practices today use computer resources. The compilation of regular reports by the computer can provide financial statistics, caseload by species, type of diagnoses and treatments, procedures performed, management reports, and herd health data. Computer-generated management information can help in planning for future practice expansion or in the retrospective evaluation of case management. Pharmacy and medical supply inventory can also be maintained through computerization. Some practices are using computerized (paperless) medical records. Computerized medical records are legally useful when the record program has been protected by security levels. If the software of the program has been secured through the transaction file, then all changes, additions, and deletions will be recorded and can be audited at any time. Computerized medical records have become easy to use and are efficient. Additional information concerning the use of computers in practice can be found in Chapter 34.

VETERINARY MEDICAL DATA BASE

The Veterinary Medical Data Base (VMDB) is a national data bank located at Purdue University. It contains computerized veterinary medical data supplied by 24 veterinary schools in the United States and Canada. Each institution submits data for the VMDB on a quarterly basis to a central processing center. The data consist of abstracted data from each clinical case seen at each teaching hospital. The national data base allows studies of national trends in various animal diseases. It provides patient chart number, institution code, date of visit, length of stay, clinician code, gender, species, breed, discharge status, age, weight, diagnosis, and procedures for each animal. The VMDB is available for use in retrospective studies and in the evaluation of national and regional disease patterns.

AMERICAN ANIMAL HOSPITAL ASSOCIATION

The American Animal Hospital Association (AAHA) is geared to small animal hospitals and small animal practitioners. Member hospitals are certified if they meet certain standards required by the organization. Hospital evaluations are carried out every 2, 3, or 4 years to ensure that the practice and veterinarians are complying with approved standards. A complete medical record is part of these standards. AAHA publishes a *Medical Records Manual* that contains the regulations for medical records, along with samples of forms that can help to develop or improve a medical record system within each practice.

It is of utmost importance to maintain a retrievable, complete, and legible medical record at all times and to make it available to anyone in the practice. A high-quality record can be developed by use of computer

HOSPITAL NAME _____			FEE ESTIMATE		

HOSPITAL NAME _____
ADDRESS _____
CITY _____ STATE ____ ZIP CODE _____

FEE ESTIMATE

NAME _____ CASE NO. _____
STREET _____
CITY, STATE, ZIP _____
PHONE BUS. _____ HOME _____

DATE:	**TIME:**	SPECIES BREED SEX

CLINICIAN:

ANIMAL'S NAME   DATE OF BIRTH

COLOR—IDENTIFYING MARKS

INITIAL EXAM	Routine Visit	Referral		Emergency	$
HOSPITALIZATION NO. OF DAYS	Standard	ADDITIONAL FEES FOR : Isolation		ICU	
LABORATORY Data base	Clin Path Microbiology Parasitology	LASMDL Endocrinology Histopathology		Cytology Immunology Other	
RADIOLOGY Survey Exams	Ultrasound	Other			
DIAGNOSTIC **PROCEDURES** Consultations	ECG EEG EMG ERG	CSF Tap Endoscopy Skin Test Biopsy		Aspirate/Washes Ultrasound Special Exams Other	
ANESTHESIA Sedation	Local	General		Other	
SURGERY O.R. Fee	Materials Supplies	Professional Service		Implants Other	
THERAPEUTICS Vaccinations Medicated Bath/Dip	In–Hosp.Trmt Fluids Transfusions	Oxygen Therapy Physical Therapy		Deworming Dentistry Other	
PHARMACY Hospital Meds	Bandage Materials	Discharge Meds		Special Diets	
OTHER	Contingencies/Comments:				

You have been advised of estimated costs and procedures. Please feel free to discuss the proposed treatment and its cost with the veterinarian. A minimum deposit of 50% of the initial charges will be required for hospitalization of an animal patient.

Amt. of Deposit $ _____ Receipt # _____ TOTAL ESTIMATE $ _____

<u>STATEMENT OF OWNERSHIP AND CONSENT:</u> I am the owner of the above described animal, or have authorization from the owner to consent to its treatment.

I hereby authorize the performance of professionally accepted diagnostic, therapeutic, anesthetic, and surgical procedures necessary for its treatment.

I accept financial responsibility for these services.

I have read the above consent and understand why the above procedures may be necessary. I also have been told of the possible complications and alternatives to the listed procedures.

I will not hold _____ or its agents liable in any manner regarding the care, treatment, or safekeeping of the animal described above.

I understand that if further services are required for this animal (even if for treatment of the same condition), additional expenses will occur. Do not allow the total bill to exceed $ _____ without my authorization.

I have read and understand the above statement and have received a copy of this estimate.

_____   _____
Signature (Owner or agent)   Date

White: Client   Canary: Discharge Office   Pink: Medical records

FIGURE 33-20.   Fee-estimation form.

HOSPITAL NAME _____

ADDRESS _____

CITY _____ STATE _____ ZIP CODE _____

NAME _____ CASE NO. _____

STREET _____

CITY, STATE, ZIP _____

PHONE BUS. _____ HOME _____

SPECIES   BREED   SEX

ANIMAL'S NAME   DATE OF BIRTH

COLOR—IDENTIFYING MARKS

EUTHANASIA – UNRESTRICTED DONATION RELEASE

Animal's Name _____   Brand, Tattoo, or ID Chip _____

Owner's Driver License #_____   Owner's Vehicle License # _____
                             STATE   NUMBER   STATE   NUMBER

The insurance company has been notified on _____ and has forwarded permission.

I, the undersigned, certify that I am the owner, or authorized agent of the owner of the above described animal. I hereby unconditionally release the above animal

☐   1.   To euthanatize and dispose of the animal.

☐   2.   To euthanatize and return the animal.

☐   3.   Unrestricted donation.

Special Instructions: _____

_____

_____

_____

Date: _____

Owner or Agent: _____

Witness: _____

_____   _____
Clinician ordering euthanasia   Date

Euthanasia was performed with _____
                                                          Drug & Amount

on _____ at _____ a.m./p.m.
          Date   Time

_____   _____
Person performing euthanasia   Date

FIGURE 33-21.   Euthanasia-unrestricted donation release form.

support along with individual record forms. This record is the only legal and tangible evidence that the veterinarian maintains.

RECOMMENDED READING

American Animal Hospital Association: *Hospital standards and accreditation manual*, Denver, 2000, The Association.

Hannah HW: Practice and the law. In McCurnin DM, editor: *Veterinary practice management*, Philadelphia, 1988, Lippincott.

Huffman EK: *Medical record management*, Berwyn, Ill, 1994, Physician's Record Co.

Terry GR, Stallard JJ: *Office management and control*, Homewood, Ill, 1980, Richard D. Irwin, Inc.

34

Computer Applications in Veterinary Medicine

E. David Stearns

Veterinary practices have been computerizing their business for more than 20 years. Computers have offered and continue to offer increasing efficiency and provide outcomes often unmanageable or unable to be done by the human mind. The application of the system is literally left to the imagination of the user. Computers are the greatest inventions of modern times because they have completely revolutionized many occupations and industries. This chapter looks at computer applications in veterinary practice and ways in which they can enhance veterinary medicine.

The most logical reason for using computers in this profession, or any other profession or industry, is that the instruments do some aspects of the job that humans are incapable of doing or that they can accomplish certain functions better than humans. With an ever-changing society, technology has played an important role in evolving social and personal conditions as well as business. Advances in technology occur very rapidly. The observation made in 1965 by Gordon Moore, founder of Intel, that the number of transistors per square inch on integrated circuits will double every 12 to 18 months since the integrated circuit was invented has held true and is expected to continue for the next 2 decades. Computers are most efficient at handling large volumes of data and handling complex or repetitive tasks. Obviously, veterinarians have practiced successfully for several hundred years without computers; however, it is difficult to deny that computers are capable of doing many tasks better, faster, more accurately, and more conveniently than humans. The ultimate decision to computerize must be based on whether the instruments improve service to the animal-owning public and provide an adequate return on investments of time and money. We are convinced that computers can fulfill both of these criteria—provided veterinarians and staff understand their opportunity and that they are utilized efficiently.

Much of this chapter is devoted to describing how computers can be used to the greatest advantage in the practice of veterinary medicine. Its aim is to provide the reader with insights into routine and innovative uses of computers in veterinary medicine. Because of space limitations, the discussion is limited to applications in private practice. However, the same principles can be applied to public, industrial, corporate, and academic veterinary medicine.

Before entering into discussions of applications in the profession, a brief introduction to the terminology of computers is warranted. A detailed list of computer terms is provided for the convenience of the reader in the Glossary at the end of the chapter.

COMPUTER HARDWARE

Hardware used in computerization of a veterinary medical practice includes any digital or analog device used to develop or process an electronic signal. Hardware includes the *central processing unit* or *units (CPUs)*, or the "server," and peripheral devices, such as monitors, printers, scanners, modems, disk drives, tape drives, speakers, terminals, and pointing devices (mice). Hardware is the "machinery" over which a computer system runs. Often, practice information management systems (PIMSs) vendors consider the operating system part of the hardware. However, technically the operating system is a software component; therefore it will be discussed in the computer software section. Hardware systems come in as many varieties as there are manufacturers. As is the case with other applications, veterinary PIMSs can usually be run on a variety of computers and hardware. With the steady increase in computing power and decreasing cost of computers, the decision regarding which hardware to purchase is based on the level of technology desired. When introduced to the marketplace, the newest, state-of-the-art technology may be considered "leading edge" and more expensive than currently available components. Remember Moore's Law: when purchasing hardware for a veterinary practice: the type of hardware purchased should be primarily dictated by the type of software (and its vendor) selected.

The intended use of the application software and system is of primary importance when considering the type and configuration of computer hardware. Some considerations that must be made before committing to a particular brand, model, or configuration of computer include the number of users that will have simultaneous access to the software, the number and location of the data entry stations, and the performance requirements of the application software (e.g., color and graphic display requirements, data size, laptop synchronization, bar coding). Another primary consideration in the selection of hardware is the availability of rapid and reliable service. Rapid service generally equates with a company that guarantees overnight or next business day replacement of malfunctioning hardware. Such service is offered by both local and remote companies. Some PIMS vendors may offer next day loaner service. Having one service vendor to contact for hardware, software, and operating system needs is very advantageous because often an error is reported by the software but is actually an operating system, networking, or hardware malfunction.

COMPUTER SOFTWARE

Software for computerization of a veterinary practice is by far the most important consideration. Software consists of the operating system, the application program, and, with some PIMS programs, the networking system. As mentioned previously, the operating system is often considered by many PIMS vendors as part of the hardware when it comes to system support and troubleshooting. However, the *operating system* is a software platform that enables the computer to operate the application program. It is considered the most important program that runs on a computer.

Every general-purpose computer must have an operating system to run other programs. Operating systems perform basic tasks, such as recognizing input from the keyboard, sending output to the display screen, keeping track of files and directories on the disk, and controlling peripheral devices, such as disk drives and printers (Figure 34-1). Operating systems provide a software platform on top of which other programs, called *application programs*, can run. The application programs must be written (developed) specifically to run on top of a particular operating system. The choice of operating system therefore determines to a great extent the applications that can run. For personal computers (PCs), the most popular operating systems are DOS (disk operating system) and Windows, but others are available, such as Macintosh, OS/2, UNIX, and LINUX. Some of the most commonly used operating systems in veterinary medicine today are DOS; Windows, which provides a graphic user interface; Macintosh, another graphic user interface; and UNIX.

The DOS system is the operating platform that was specifically developed for IBM personal computers. The DOS platform has the disadvantage of being able to only run character-based applications, and also it can only run as a single-user, single-application system, meaning that only one user is allowed to use the application program and only one application program can be operated at one time. It has the advantage of being fairly simple to use and of having been in use for many years. Very few, if any, PIMS programs are developed today specifically for DOS.

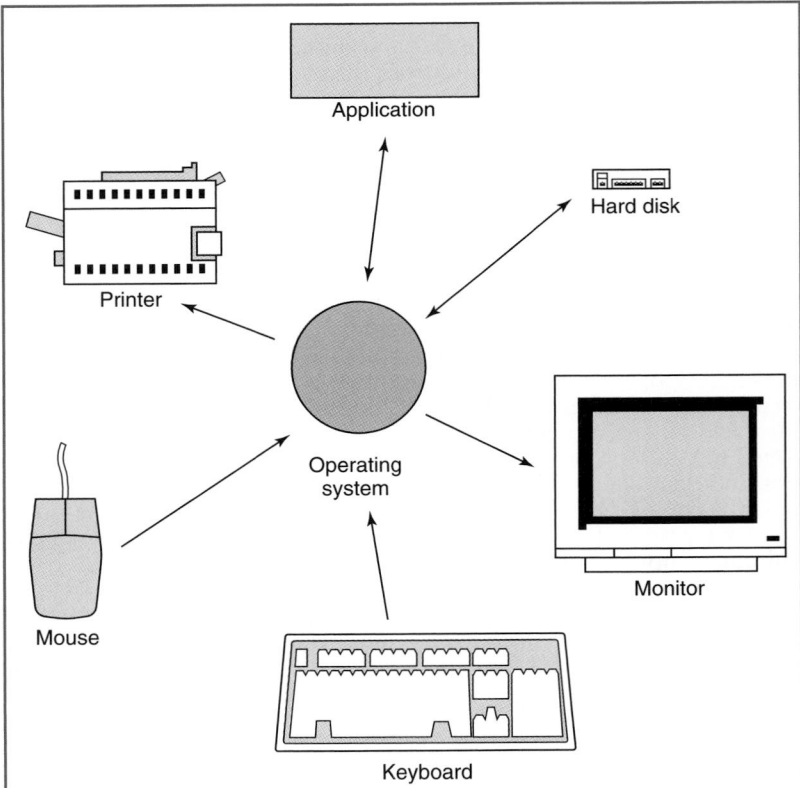

FIGURE 34-1. This diagram depicts the function of the operating system and the flow of information (direction) by and among peripheral devices.

Microsoft Windows provides a family of operating systems for personal computers. Windows dominates the personal computer world, running, by some estimates, on 90% of all personal computers. The remaining 10% are mostly Macintosh computers. Like the Macintosh operating environment, Windows provides a *graphic user interface (GUI)*, virtual memory management, multitasking, and support for many peripheral devices. In addition to Windows 3.x , Windows 95/98, Windows 2000, and Windows ME (Millenium), which run on Intel-based machines, Microsoft also sells Windows NT, a more advanced operating system that runs on a variety of hardware platforms and provides advanced networking capabilities.

Another GUI operating system used to run veterinary practice management applications is the Macintosh system. Although less popular than DOS or Windows, the Macintosh system has die-hard proponents who are partial to a GUI and are adept at the use of a mouse. The PowerPC, developed jointly by Apple Computers, Motorola, and IBM, make it possible for other operating systems to run on that PC, including Windows NT. Macintosh-based PIMSs are not as widely used in the veterinary marketplace as DOS or Windows systems.

The UNIX operating system (and its XENIX-type counterparts) is a multitasking, multiuser system developed by Bell Labs in the 1970s. Today it is still one of the most widely used operating systems in the veterinary industry and in many other business applications. UNIX was one of the first operating systems to be written in a high-level programming language, namely, C. This meant that it could be installed on virtually any computer for which a C compiler existed. This natural portability combined with its low price made it a popular choice among many businesses and universities. Disadvantages of this operating system are lack of standardization among versions, third-party application integration, and increased skill and knowledge required to operate and maintain the system.

The *networking platform* is software that enables CPUs (or workstations) to communicate with one another and with the server (the main CPU that runs the operating system and networking and application software); dumb terminals to communicate with the CPU; and CPUs to communicate with remote peripheral devices, such as printers, modems, and disk drives. Commonly used networking platforms in veterinary practice include Novell, Lantastic, Windows and Windows NT, UNIX, and XENIX. The use of a networking platform is generally dictated by the application software vendor because the vendor's proprietary software is usually developed to run in a specific networking environment. Networking capabilities are also directed by the "traffic" on the network; in other words, how many users and how many transactions are being driven through the system. Networking capabilities are particularly important when two or more practices (sites) are linked together and want to share data.

The importance of the application software (PIMS) warrants an in-depth discussion, which will be presented later. However, the section on application software is preceded by uses of computers in a veterinary practice. Currently used applications are discussed, and an attempt is made to predict future uses as technology develops.

USES OF COMPUTERS IN A CLINICAL PRACTICE

Uses of computers in veterinary practices are limited only by the imagination of the software developers and the users, and the only justifications for use of computers are that tasks will be performed faster, more efficiently, or

more reliably and that there will be a fair return on the investment. With the above statements in mind, computer uses will be discussed. Computers in veterinary practices are commonly used for medical records management, inventory management, appointment scheduling, client communication, accounting (billing, accounts receivable [A/R]), employee time clocks, general hospital or practice management and evaluation, laboratory results, and other practice-related programs. In addition, increased use of the World Wide Web and the Internet allows more access to both medical and business information, which enables veterinary practices to practice better medicine and better business.

Accounting

The creation and recording of transactions, commonly called *invoices*, in veterinary practices probably constitute one of the most commonly used computer applications. They are the nucleus around which most, if not all, PIMS software was designed. Newer software technology from some vendors now allows transactions to be created from the medical record, making them "medical record driven." This function is discussed under Medical Records. A completely integrated accounting package that provides income from receipts, accounts receivable, and accounts payable and incorporates them all into a general ledger is not commonly supplied by most PIMS vendors. Many PIMS vendors are, however, providing integration from their PIMS into popular general ledger programs, such as QuickBooks and Peachtree Accounting. Many practices use the computer solely to maintain the accounts receivable or the amounts owed to the practice. If this is the case, one could easily create a custom application using one of several commercially available spreadsheets or database programs. Maintaining only accounts receivable records on a computer is not recommended. PIMS software today offers much more to veterinary practices.

There are several advantages to using the accounting features of PIMS. Among these advantages are automated client billing, credit management (alerts staff to clients who have more than the allowable balance or who are bad credit risks), business management reports (daily, weekly, monthly, annual), and maintenance of tax records. The advantage of automated client billing with professional itemized invoices and automated recording of service entries is sufficient to warrant a comprehensive computer system. This automation of the invoice helps practices not only to charge for services and supplies rendered but also to standardize fees. One of the most common justifications for computerizing a veterinary practice, even today, is missed fees or undercharges.

Appointment Scheduling

Appointment scheduling is one of the most valuable features of veterinary PIMSs and should be utilized to its maximum. Proper use of the scheduling features can balance workloads among days; can fill in appointment gaps with vaccinations, heartworm checks, and routine dental maintenance; and can minimize the number of clients who become angry because of long waits in the reception area. Electronic appointment scheduling is far more efficient than paper appointment books and can make the practice proactive rather than reactive. When a client calls the veterinary practice to schedule an appointment, most receptionists or technician-receptionists will typically check for the next available appointment. Appointment schedulers in many PIMSs can provide automatic alerts, such as overdue reminders for all animals, previous failed appointments, or clients that have bad credit, all of which make the practice more efficient and may increase revenues. In addition, with an electronic appointment book, the medical record of each patient, the account history, and the doctor's schedule are one button away for review, all while the client is on the phone. Another advantage of a computerized appointment scheduler is the ability to allow clients to make their own appointment through the use of the practice's web site.

Many appointment scheduler modules of PIMSs work in the same fashion. Most are aligned with a grid much like a spreadsheet with time slots along one side and types of appointments titled in columns along the top (Figure 34-2). When in the market for a scheduling module seek one that has the following attributes: effortless shuttling from the scheduling module to all other functions within the practice management program, ability to schedule appointments of variable lengths of time, and ability to graphically display daily and weekly schedules of all providers of veterinary services. Additional features that are desirable in a scheduling program are the ability to time multiple simultaneous events and to set multiple alarms and the ability to display "intelligent" colors for appoint-

ment slots depicting the type or classification of appointment (Figure 34-2).

Inventory Management

Drug and supply inventories are important functions of PIMSs that are, without a doubt, best done by computers. Management of drug and supply inventories so that the practice does not run out of an item, does not have to pay high costs for overnight shipment, or does not become overstocked or have outdated products can result in considerable savings over a 1-year period. The ability to determine with a few keystrokes the amount of any drug or item on hand, its cost, and retail value and automatic notification when inventory numbers reach predetermined levels are highly desirable. However, the reader is cautioned that a significant initial investment is necessary to establish the inventories and a moderate amount of time and effort is required to maintain inventory accuracy. Most veterinary practices spend 15% to 20% of their annual gross income on drugs and supplies. Therefore, for example, a practice that annually grosses $500,000 could spend $100,000 on drug and supply inventory. A 5% increase in efficiency would make it worthwhile to use the PIMS to manage inventory.

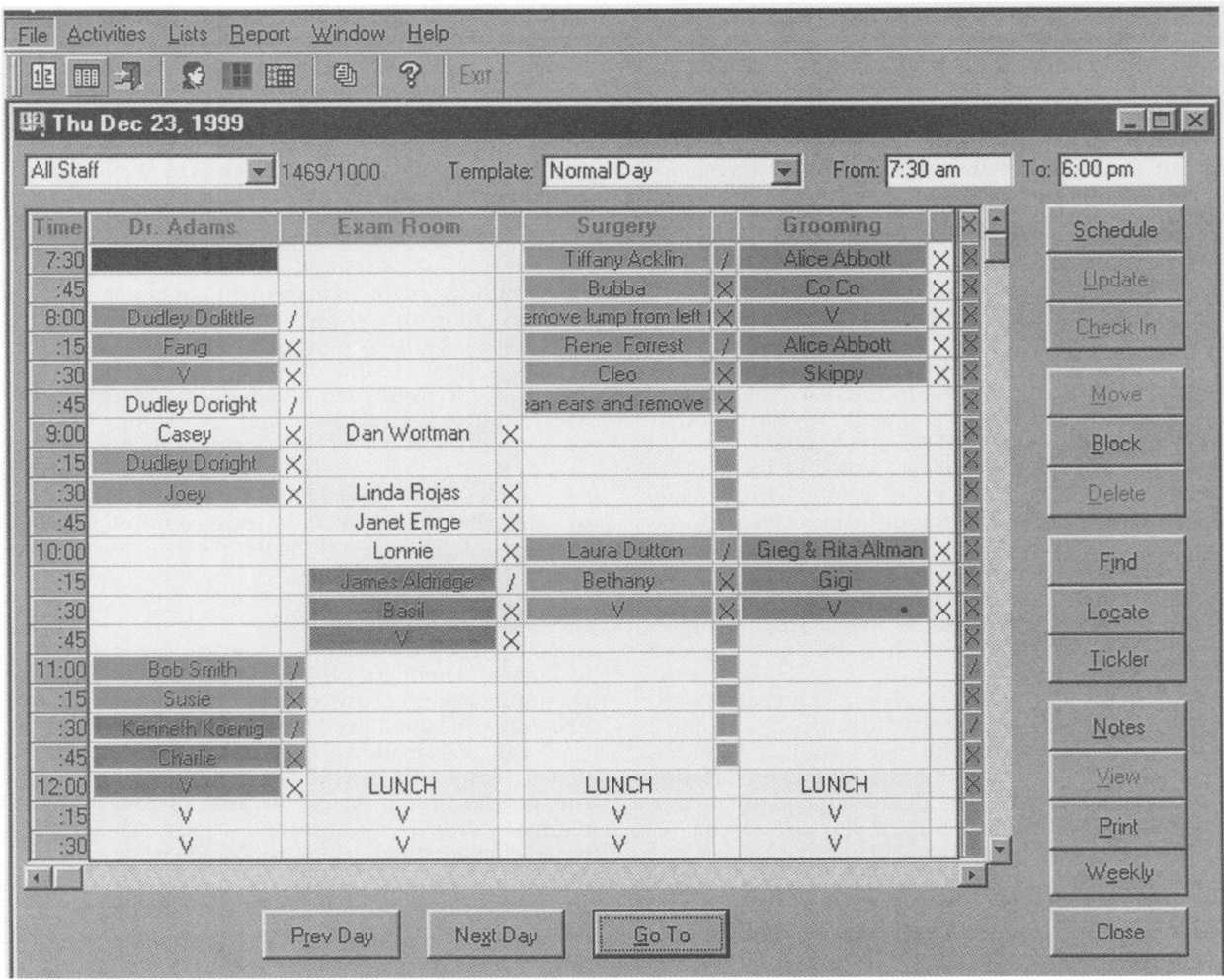

FIGURE 34-2.   Electronic appointment schedule showing a grid of appointment time slots and columns of types of appointments. Intelligent color can be used to see appointment types at a glance.

In addition to drug inventory, many practice management programs have desirable features associated with the pharmacy program, either as part of the overall package or as add-on modules. Features frequently included in the pharmacy package are automatic reordering including customized order forms, a data base of drug and supply vendors, automatic prescription label printing with intelligent signalment, and a drug formulary. With increased use of the Internet, many drug and supply vendors make on-line ordering available. Integration of automated on-line ordering into PIMSs based on clinic use and stocking levels is in the future of PIMSs.

Medical Records

Maintenance of good medical records on every patient is imperative in the practice of quality veterinary medicine and has strong legal implications. The medical record, as used in the context of this discussion, is the chronologic record of all physical observations, electronic measurements, imagery, and laboratory data collected on a patient and all therapy administered. Medical records may be as extensive as problem-oriented medical records (POMRs) or as simple as small cryptic notes on observations and therapy. In POMRs, each problem observed in an animal or reported by the client is recorded and "SOAPed." The acronym *SOAP* is used to describe four steps in dealing with each problem: subjective observations, objective data, assessment, and procedures performed. Additional information on medical records is given in Chapter 33.

Medical records on patients must be kept if acceptable veterinary medicine is to be practiced and, from a legal standpoint, a client-veterinarian-patient relationship is to be documented. Whether to keep records in hard copy or electronically is a decision to be made by the owner or administrator of the practice. Approximately 5% of practices have paperless, or electronic, medical records. After this decision is made, decisions on operational procedures must be made and accurately communicated to all members of the practice team. Who is allowed or required to make entries into the medical record? What is the level of security for medical records? When and where are these entries made? If medical records are maintained electronically, who has access to the information and when?

Complete and detailed medical records are imperative to the practice of sound, modern veterinary medicine. No matter how good one's memory is, it is unlikely that anyone can maintain knowledge of even the common signalments of temperature, pulse, and respiration from day to day. To think that one can mentally maintain the entire medical history of even a few patients is foolhardy. Further, consider the scenario of different veterinarians seeing the same patient on different office visits. There is no better means of communication among veterinarians in the same practice than through good records. This same argument holds true for communication among the veterinarian and the veterinary technician, the referring veterinarian, and the diagnostic laboratory.

Maintenance of complete and accurate medical records has profound legal implications. Following a problem that developed involving over-the-counter dispensing of prescription drugs by veterinarians and their staff, it was determined by the local court that the simple dispensing of a drug was a violation of state practice acts. The court ruled that veterinarians may dispense prescription drugs only to clients with whom there is a valid client-veterinarian-patient relationship. This is usually interpreted as that relationship in which the client's animal was recently physically observed by the prescribing veterinarian. The best proof of such a relationship is an accurate medical record. Aside from proof of the client-veterinarian relationship, medical records are the best evidence that a veterinarian can have in court when accused of malpractice. False malpractice suits, although not anticipated by anyone, are filed even by the best of clients because of some misunderstanding between client and veterinarian or because of financial problems experienced by the client. Electronic medical records are legal, and, just as with hard copy records, they must be maintained for several years, depending on local and state laws.

Practice Management

Practice management, as used in this discussion, involves analyses of all areas of the practice of veterinary medicine with the ultimate goals of improving the efficiency of service, lowering the cost of that service, and improving the income generated by a clinical practice. Computerized systems for operation of clinical practices provide the ultimate tool for true practice management. The information from these systems is critical for practicing better medicine and better business management. A majority of the commercially available PIMSs have the ability to automatically analyze the practice and to provide daily, weekly, monthly, and yearly reports. Reports built into the various software packages vary greatly, but most provide analyses of multiple levels of income categories. Other analyses that are helpful to the owner or administrator of a veterinary hospital include analyses of time, services, and personnel. Analyses of the average time spent with each appointment should be the basis for scheduling appointments and the cost of an office visit. Analyses of time required for various medical and surgical procedures should also be the basis of fees assessed. Analysis of services provides the administrator with knowledge of income generated by each service of the practice and which service warrants additional personnel or is overstaffed.

Practice management capabilities of many PIMSs include the ability to determine the revenue generated by each of the veterinarians and, from some PIMSs, by each "provider" in the practice. The income analysis of each veterinarian can also be used to establish salary bonus plans (see Chapter 32). If one has an accurate analysis of the various services in a veterinary hospital, it is possible to make fairly reliable inferences as to the productivity of providers for a particular service.

Electronic Mail

Although most PIMSs do not include electronic mail capabilities, the network and operating systems may provide this function. As a general rule, practices with multiple locations or staff that work multiple shifts value this feature more than smaller practices. E-mail is an excellent means of communication in a practice provided everyone agrees or is required to use the feature.

E-mail has gained importance and popularity in recent times among veterinarians in private practice as a result of access to the Internet and commercial network services. Use of e-mail through the available networks enables veterinarians to communicate with colleagues, veterinary specialists, emergency clinics, diagnostic laboratories, university faculty, drug and pharmaceutical companies, and government regulatory agencies without having to play telephone tag. Some practices are beginning to communicate with clients through the use of e-mail newsletters.

Word Processing

Although word processing is available as a stand-alone software program, most PIMSs integrate a word processing program into the overall system. Such an arrangement lets the word processing program merge with many files within the PIMS, allowing customization of the reminders, follow-up letters, correspondence to referring practices, and many other client communications.

The word processing portion of the PIMS is one of the primary means of communication between the practice and the public that it serves. For this reason, when using the word processor to communicate, practice staff must be careful to put their best foot forward. Stated from another viewpoint, it is important not to portray the practice or the profession negatively. An error in subject-verb agreement or syntax made in a telephone conversation with a client may be quickly forgotten, but a glaring error of tense or spelling in a document makes a lasting impression on most people. Any document, whether a fee statement or a newsletter, that is forwarded from a veterinary practice should be and *look* professional. The document should be on professional statement forms or letterhead with an appropriate logo. Documents should be free of typographic, grammatic, and spelling errors and should be printed by a letter-quality printer, preferably of the laser variety, on quality bond paper.

Aside from merely being a mode of communication, the word processing software can be a very effective practice-building tool. Consider the effectiveness of a well-timed letter of sympathy to a client who is grieving the loss of a loved pet. The letter need not be original but should be sincere and should reflect the caring nature of the veterinarian and the practice staff. It is not recommended that the same sympathy letter be sent to all clients or that an original letter be composed for the death of every animal that dies in a practice. Sympathy letters and other types of correspondence that are used routinely could be created as basic templates in the word processing program and customized for individual purposes.

Many modern word processing programs can also function as a desktop publishing program. Although most veterinary practices today choose to have their newsletters printed professionally, some practices may choose to create and publish their own newsletters. Other uses of word processing programs integrated with the PIMS could include correspondence to referring hospitals (specialty practices) and welcome and thank-you letters. The mail-merge function of word processors from data within the PIMS makes this type of correspondence very customized by client and very efficient to create and print in bulk.

On-Line Services

Network and Internet services available to veterinarians and veterinary technicians within the last several years are unprecedented and very exciting. Veterinarians and technicians have access to several networks devoted specifically to veterinary medicine. One popular network dedicated to veterinarians is the Veterinary Information Network (VIN), a privately owned network accessed through America On-line and other networks. Another popular network developed for the veterinary profession is the Network of Animal Health (NOAH), created by the American Veterinary Medical Association (AVMA).

VetConnect.com has recently become available to the veterinary community and offers specialized services to practices, such as website hosting, laboratory results on-line, on-line ordering, and access to specialists. Other services available through veterinary networks include special interest bulletin boards or messaging services, e-mail, real-time chat capabilities, electronic medical literature retrieval systems, online consultation with specialists, continuing education, and access to veterinary medical

data bases. One new and exciting area available through specialized networks and the Internet is transmission of digitized images (x-rays, ultrasound, other digital pictures) to specialists for interpretation and consultation (telemedicine).

Access to the Internet by the practicing veterinarian and the practice staff is important today and will continue to grow in the future because, in addition to providing access to information from throughout the world, it provides an electronic link to academic and regulatory medicine. Internet access provides veterinarians with e-mail access to faculty at veterinary schools and other specialists throughout the world, to diagnostic laboratories, and to regulatory agencies such as the Food and Drug Administration (FDA), U.S. Department of Agriculture (USDA/Animal and Plant Health Inspection Service [APHIS]), the Drug Enforcement Administration (DEA), the Occupational Safety and Health Administration (OSHA), and state boards. Another growing area in the use of the Internet is distance learning, which is becoming popular at some AVMA-accredited technician education programs and veterinary medical colleges.

Another cutting-edge technology that is being introduced into the veterinary marketplace today is application service providers (ASPs). This model allows software applications to reside on a remote server. Thus PIMS software could be on a server across the United States from the local veterinary practice, and the local practice would have simple desktop computers or terminals at the practice to access data and run the system through the Internet. As Internet access speeds increase with increasing bandwidth and security over the Internet is increased, the ASP model will become more and more popular.

Utility and Miscellaneous Applications

Computer systems in veterinary practices are seldom used exclusively to execute practice management programs. Many people who are familiar with computers are partial to certain software programs and cannot function without them. These types of programs include but are not limited to spreadsheets, data base search programs, programs for managing herd health, inventory management, tax computations, human resource packages (employee scheduling, data base, time clock), and vehicle logs. PIMS software is not usually purchased for these programs, but they do constitute significant added value to some practices. It is unlikely that any PIMS will have all the features desired by all users. Fortunately, users with unique requirements can execute their favorite programs on the same computer that is used for the PIMS. This section discusses some programs that can be used to supplement or even enhance the practice software. The purpose of the section is to suggest useful programs and not to endorse any specific application or program. The reader should not consider this a complete listing of useful utility programs. In addition, users should consult their PIMS vendors before purchasing or installing any third-party software on the PIMS.

Among the most useful software programs are the general utility programs, which assist users in such tasks as recovery of deleted files, recovery of a crashed hard disk, optimization of hard disk functions, and routine file management including backup of data files. A convenient and reliable method of backing up data from the PIMS, whether provided in the program or as a stand-alone utility, is absolutely essential. Without a good daily backup, a simple power failure or the inadvertent flip of a switch could cost the practice thousands of dollars and the loss of patient and client records. Most PIMS vendors will recommend their preferred method. Although many media types are available to write data to, streaming tape drives continue to be very popular and reliable.

Another important group of programs for users of PIMS is antivirus computer software. The software will stop application programs in progress and alert the user when a virus is introduced into the memory. Antivirus software can also destroy the virus and usually restore files to their original form. Antivirus software is important, particularly if files or programs are introduced from home, the Internet, or other external sources.

If users are to access remote computers and networks, a communication package is needed in addition to a modem. The communication programs facilitate and, in most cases, automate the communication between computers. These programs facilitate communication between servers whether they are networked together or linked via telephone lines and modems. Some PIMS vendors require their users to purchase modems and communication programs because this allows vendors to dial into the practice and service and correct problems remotely.

The professional staff of veterinary hospitals is frequently called on to make presentations to student groups, civic clubs, and professional organizations. Such presentations are best received when supplemented with quality visual aids with vivid text and graphics. Presentation software can allow users to import files, photographs, and digital images to provide a very enhanced presentation from a desktop or laptop computer through a video projector.

Another type of software program that is used by many veterinary practices is a spreadsheet program. Spreadsheets allow data to be formatted with mathematic formulas, providing users unique analysis of clinic data. Some PIMSs are open database compliant (ODBC), which allows the user to save data from the PIMS and import the data into a spreadsheet for further analysis and manipulation. Spreadsheets can be used for graphic analysis, comparative analysis of practice revenues and provider revenues, and budgeting.

COMPUTER CONFIGURATION TYPES IN A VETERINARY PRACTICE

In determining the type of computer configuration to employ in a veterinary practice, it is important to first determine the uses for the computer system, the flow of traffic within the practice, and, finally, which staff will be responsible for entering data into the system. An in-depth needs analysis of the requirements and functionality of the software is recommended before purchasing a PIMS. Once these questions have been answered, the software can be selected. Most PIMS vendors will assist (if not provide) the practice in recommending a proper configuration of computer hardware.

The simplest configuration of computer hardware in veterinary practices is the single personal computer operating in the DOS or Windows operating system (Figure 34-3, *A*). Because this system has one workstation for data entry, this important task is often entrusted to the receptionist at the front desk. The receptionist obtains input information, usually in written form, such as a "circle" or "travel" sheet that lists services, or directly from the patient record (chart). This written form of communication is entered into the PIMS and is an efficient arrangement with minimal chance of error.

Another configuration seen frequently in veterinary practices, particularly those in which several veterinarians are employed, is a server with several personal computers attached to it through a network (see Figure 34-3, *B*). In this system, workstations (PCs) are located in service areas where data entry may occur, such as the treatment room, reception desk, pharmacy, laboratory, doctor's office, and sometimes examination rooms. The server in this type of system may be dedicated or nondedicated. A nondedicated server is one in which the user may input data into the PIMS through the server. A dedicated server is used only to drive the rest of the networked computers, and users do not typically use the server to input data (see Figure 34-3, *C*). The amount of traffic (both transactions and the number of workstations in use) on the network will influence the decision of a dedicated versus nondedicated server. Most PIMS vendors will recommend a configuration that maximizes performance of the system.

A third system that has been popular for many years is a single central processing unit (CPU) with attached "dumb" terminals (see Figure 34-3, *D*). This configuration is used by the UNIX operating system and considered very fast and efficient. Practices with multiple locations and the need to share a common database with real-time updates may prefer this configuration.

FACTORS IN THE SUCCESS OR FAILURE OF THE COMPUTER SYSTEM

Of primary importance in the success of a computer system is the selection of the proper PIMS. There are at least two dozen PIMS vendors with programs commercially available that are designed specifically for veterinarians. Some of these programs are marketed and intended to be used just as they are installed "out of the box." Other vendors offer a foundation package with additional modules that offer added functionality and allow veterinarians to purchase only the desired modules. Before purchase, there should be a clear understanding between the purchaser and the vendor as to the desired function and use of the application. Many vendors will provide consultation and demonstration at the veterinary practice so staff can get an in-depth review of the PIMS's functionality.

Most PIMSs are designed to accomplish the same basic tasks but often do so in different fashions. In addition, the kinds and numbers of utility and special programs included in the packages differ greatly. Therefore, before selection of software, the type of veterinary practice and the long-term goals of the practice should be considered. After matching the software to the type of practice, a number of considerations need to be made before the final decision to purchase takes place. There must be a well-understood agreement between the vendor and the purchaser as to whether both hardware and software are provided, type and cost of hardware and software support (maintenance contracts), technical manuals, training provided, frequency and cost of software updates, and cost of supplies (labels, invoice paper, reminder cards) required by the software.

A prime consideration in the selection of PIMS is the availability and quality of technical support for both the software and, if purchased from the PIMS vendor, the hardware. It is extremely important that the contract to purchase a PIMS package include specifications as to the type and amount of training the vendor will provide to the veterinary staff. The contract should also specify the amount of technical support the purchaser is entitled to, the cost per unit of time, and the hours that technical support is available. Response time by the vendor should also be specified. Software support, even for the most experienced users, is necessary because problems, such as

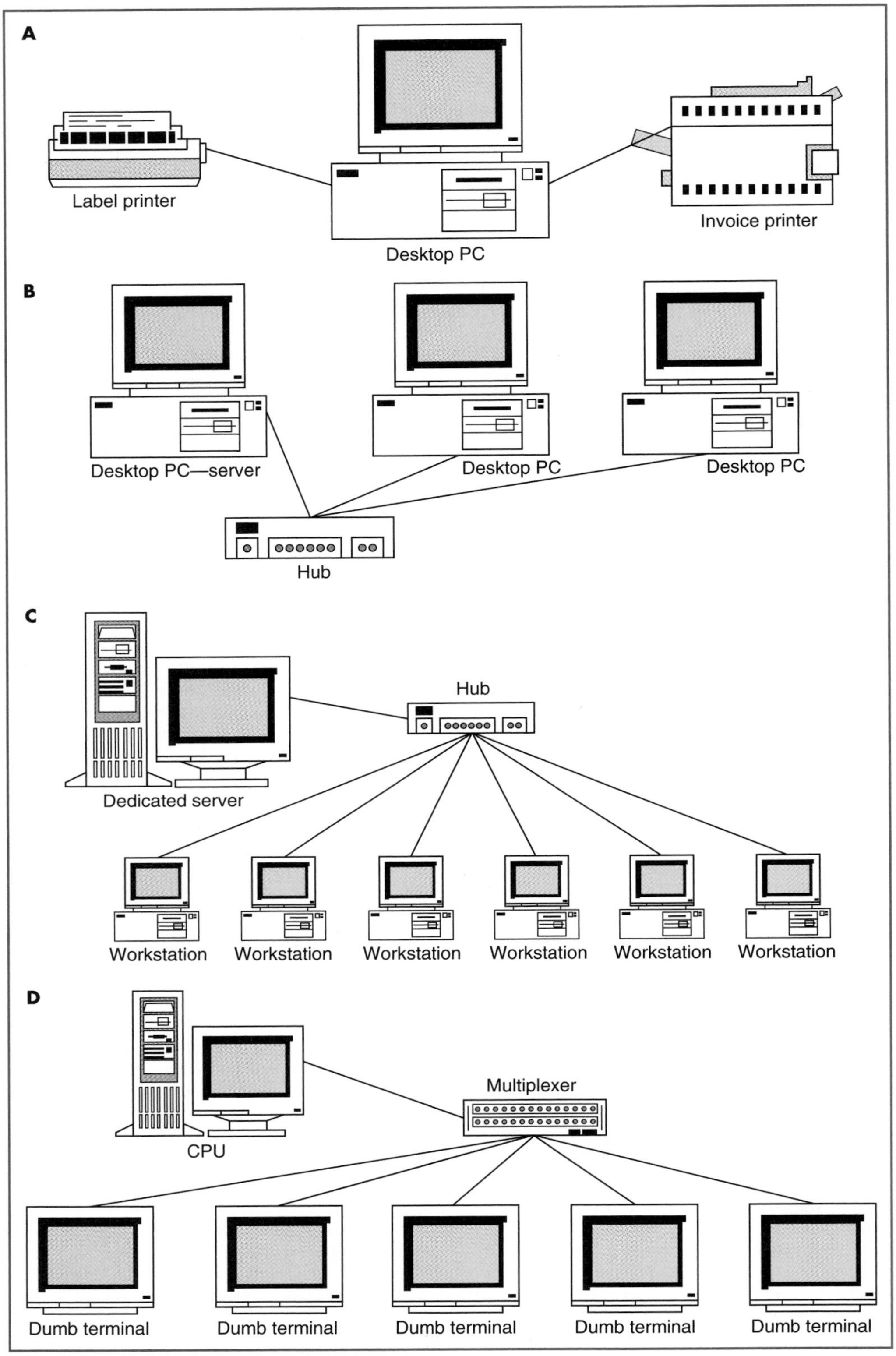

FIGURE 34-3.   **A,** Single station system. **B,** Multistation system with nondedicated server. **C,** Multistation system with dedicated server. **D,** A configuration by the UNIX operating system with one central processing unit (CPU) and "dumb" terminals attached. *PC,* Personal computer.

file corruption, invariably occur. The time to negotiate these services needs is at the time of purchase, not when a problem develops.

Technical support for computer hardware is as important as that needed for the software. Whether the hardware is purchased separately or from the software vendor as a total package, a service contract should be negotiated at the time of purchase. Response time of the vendor, minimal service fees, and initial warranties should be included in the contract. In addition, specifications for the vendor to provide comparable hardware on loan while nonfunctional equipment is being repaired is highly recommended.

Of all the factors involved in the success or failure of a computerized veterinary practice system, the personnel of the practice are the most important. The owner of the practice may be a genius with a doctorate in computer science, but if the staff of the practice are improperly trained or unmotivated, the PIMS is destined for failure. It does not really matter whether the owner, the receptionist, or the kennel staff enter charges for an office visit; it is imperative that someone be charged with the responsibility and that he or she discharge it. Income is lost daily in many veterinary practices because someone forgets to enter charges for services rendered or drugs dispensed. This reason alone is still the best economic justification today for computerizing a veterinary practice or moving to a PIMS that can best enhance this process.

In computerized practices, it is important that the management delegate the responsibilities for all aspects of the system. There should be no question as to who has the responsibility to enter charges from the various services, who has authority to grant credit and discounts, who can initiate or delete a record, and, most important, who is responsible for backup and other technical service of the system. Once decisions have been made as to the duties of the hospital staff, it is the responsibility of management to provide training in operation of the system.

Computerization of an established practice is highly recommended but is not without a degree of stress to all involved. Good change management is required for smooth transitions to computerized systems. Staff are asked to convert to a system that requires a change in their normal process, may be difficult for some to comprehend, and often requires extra hours or effort during the conversion process. They are asked to endure all this on the good faith that their jobs will be made easier by the computer. It must be pointed out that the degree to which the staff's jobs are made easier depends on the investment of the staff in learning the finer points of the software *and its application to their practice*. It is safe to say that the more features of the program that are used, the easier the duties of the hospital staff become. There is truth to the old adage, "the duration of the assigned tasks usually fills the time allowed." Therefore the greatest advantage of proper use of the practice's computer system is the marked increase in efficiency.

A discussion of computer use in a veterinary practice would be lacking without a brief discussion of do's and don'ts. This discussion starts with the don'ts. When a veterinary practice is computerized, there is the risk, or at least it is the perception of some clients, that the business is being "dehumanized." Many people have experienced the frustration of trying to correct an error in billing from a large department store or credit card company. The person one usually speaks to seems to be a lifeless individual who is not ashamed to be subservient to "the computer." These individuals seem reluctant or incapable of making even the most trivial decisions on their own. Veterinary medicine must not become dehumanized.

Receptionists should greet clients with eye contact and a warm personal smile. Computer monitors should not be positioned so that they will interfere with the receptionist's view of the clients or vice versa. Receptionists should not hide behind the monitor. It is necessary to view the monitor when entering data on a client's record or when totaling a bill, but questions should not be asked of clients without providing periodic eye contact. A good study on proper ergonomics is recommended, and consultations in this regard may be available from the PIMS vendor. Finally, when a client points out an error on the invoice, do not blame the error on the computer. In today's society, in which most people have some degree of computer literacy, blaming human mistakes on a computer is no longer acceptable. Further, it may aggravate most people.

Now for the do's of computer use in a veterinary practice. For reasons previously mentioned, it is recommended that the veterinary technician take the initiative in learning the practice management system. Reading the manual for the PIMS may be effective for some users, however time consuming. Training provided by the vendor is usually the most cost effective. Some vendors may have computer-based training (CBT) available on CD/ROM. This interactive method is also a very efficient way of learning the system. The more one knows about the computer system, the more efficient it will make the user. It is equally important to take the time to learn aspects of the system that are assigned to fellow workers and to train someone else to handle your responsibilities (cross training). This ensures continuity in the veterinary practice when someone leaves the practice, is sick, or is on vacation. Another do that is worthy of mention is to maintain the security of the system and the confidentiality of patient records. This entails scrupulous care to maintain the confidentiality of passwords. Patient-veterinarian confidentiality is regulated by state law and professional ethics. Veterinary medical records must be treated as confidential materials.

IMPLICATIONS FOR THE FUTURE

There are PIMS packages available to veterinary practices that offer many new and innovative features. However, these are only hints at what will be available in the near future. With the few exceptions where multiple clinics are linked by a network, PIMSs are largely stand-alone packages. Most have modems in the system that are primarily used by the vendor for technical support. Software of the future will emphasize communication external to the practice. The ASP model previously discussed will become more prevalent in the veterinary industry. Such communication will be rapid, have worldwide access, and be transparent to the user. As technology advances, veterinary practices will be "live" on the Internet from all workstations linked through a router. The communication of the future will have more graphic and voice capabilities and will offer many conveniences that are unheard of today.

Even today, some PIMS vendors are beginning to bring these technologic advances to the veterinary practice. Communication to outside consultants via telemedicine, the downloading of reference laboratory results and in-clinic testing instruments into a patient record, and connection to pharmaceutical companies and product distributors are now becoming a reality. In addition, interfaces between the veterinary client and the PIMS will become more popular. This could allow clients to tap into the PIMS (at the practice's discretion) and view appointment availability, check fees, or even review their animal's medical record.

Veterinary practices of the future will have access to computer-assisted laboratory and clinical diagnostic programs, many of which will be based on artificial intelligence. This will enable veterinarians and veterinary technicians to be more accurate in their diagnoses and will reduce the amount of information that must be memorized. In addition, continuing education will be more accessible to veterinarians and the entire practice team. Individuals, within the confines and comfort of their offices or workstations, will have access to a wide variety of quality continuing education programs that are interactive and feature text, sight, and sound. The practice of veterinary medicine in the future will be made more exciting and productive through the use of computer technology.

PRACTICAL APPLICATIONS OF PRACTICE COMPUTERIZATION

Nearly every aspect of veterinary medicine has been computerized from rabies tag tracking to diagnostic programs. The veterinary practice team (owner, professional staff, receptionists) must determine what tasks are done in the practice and then decide which tasks they want done by a computer, which tasks are best done by people, and which tasks are best done by people with the assistance of a computer. Computers are good at storing and processing large volumes of data and doing repetitive tasks but poor at decision making and thought processes. People, on the other hand, are relatively inefficient at remembering large volumes of data or doing repetitive tasks but are better at decision makingespecially with subjective or emotional issues. The computer has no morals; it is brutally cold when it comes to sending bills and has no regard for the person's ability to pay, employment status, and so forth. Every practice is faced with certain moral or ethical decisions that the computer is incapable of making. Therefore, in spite of the great strides in computerization and technology, the functions of the daily practice must be tempered with human judgment.

PIMSs are designed and developed to manage information by storing data, assembling facts, and performing calculations. As a part of managing data, the computer provides an excellent means of communicating the information. The term *practice management* is something of a misnomer because the program does not manage the practice; the practice team manages the practice. Therefore the term practice *information management system* (PIMS) is most appropriate. The computer system just collects and assembles information in a format that is useful to the various members of the practice team.

Because no two practices are alike, the tasks in which the veterinarians, technicians, and receptionists are involved must be itemized and the advantages and disadvantages of computerizing discussed. Only after these items are resolved can the computer software be selected. The benefits may not be readily identified and may be somewhat intangible and must be balanced against the cost of receiving those benefits. Some tasks that should be considered are shown in Box 34-1.

Box 34-1   COMPUTER APPLICATIONS IN VETERINARY PRACTICE

Demographic data collection
   Name, address, phone number of the client
   Name, age, gender, species, breed, color of the animal
Scheduling time use
   Client appointments by doctor
   Boarding reservations
   Vacation scheduling
   Conference scheduling
Billing
   Accounts receivable
   Accounts payable
Mass mailings
   Monthly statements
   Newsletters and client information
   Reminders
      Vaccinations, fecal or dental examinations, heartworm tests
      Rechecks and follow-ups
Inventory management
   Drugs, controlled substances
   Supplies
Financial
   Cash drawer reconciliation
   Deposit slips automatically generated
   Payment records—cash, check, credit card receipts
   Payroll calculations
   Profit and loss reports
   Productivity reports—which areas are making or losing money
   Fee code entry to keep track of clients' and patients' bill status
   Income analysis
   Practice profile and analysis

Medical records
   Patient's history
   Daily progress reports and treatment records
   Laboratory data storage and retrieval
   Surgical procedures
   Diagnostic codes—storage and retrieval
   Physical examination results
   Fee code entry to keep track of treatments done and prescriptions
   Certificates and forms
      Vaccinations, rabies tag number tracking
      Spay/neuter
      Euthanasia
      Release forms—surgery
Communication
   Patient's medical and financial records available to all staff at any time
   Security—who can and cannot access certain data
Diagnostic aids
   Diagnostic programs
   Drug formulary
Remote modem communications
   Home to hospital
   Ranch or farm to hospital
   Satellite clinic to hospital
   Meeting or conference to hospital
   Cellular phone to hospital

Demographic Data Collection

At the heart of any system, be it by hand or computer, is demographic data collection (Figure 34-4). In essence, there is no option: name, address, and other pertinent data must be collected for each client. Having demographic data computerized has many advantages. Looking up names and addresses is much faster and easier than searching a paper record system. The data are accessible from any computer in the practice and even from home through a modem. One is not limited by the physical restraints of a paper record system. Paper records can be in only one place at a time, whereas electronic data are accessible to any staff member at any terminal or computer.

Traditionally, PIMSs have been developed around client and patient demographics and accounting functions, mostly on the receivables side. This has occurred because the demographics are easy to program, and numerous accounting software packages are already developed and can be integrated into the PIMS. Therefore one of the prime uses for PIMSs has been tracking demographic information and accounting.

Appointment Scheduling

Appointment scheduling can be one of the most beneficial and revenue-generating functions of the PIMS, but its usefulness will be dictated, to a large degree, by the software vendor. The convenience of using the scheduling function and its integration with the rest of the system will determine its use. If the receptionist has to work his or her way through multiple menus to get from one function to another or just to enter basic demographic data, the scheduling program will probably not be used. Assuming the appointment scheduler is used, it can offer some significant advantages. The electronic appointment scheduler can make the practice proactive rather than reactive. In most veterinary practices when clients call for an appointment, the receptionist marks a convenient time to see the patient, depending on the medical need. Rarely do staff members review the medical record for all the needs of the patient or for other animals owned by the same client. An efficient appointment scheduler will flag reminders for all animals, alert the client's accounts receivable status, and give the user immediate access to the entire medical record and account history.

Some PIMS appointment schedulers use "intelligent color" on the screen to indicate appointment type, past due reminders, and past due balances (Figure 34-5). In addition, the paper appointment book is usually located at the front reception desk where, in a busy practice, congestion can occur during busy times. An electronic appointment scheduler can be viewed and appointments made from any workstation in the practice, or it can be viewed from home or remote sites through modem connectivity. Most PIMS appointment schedulers allow flexibility in time

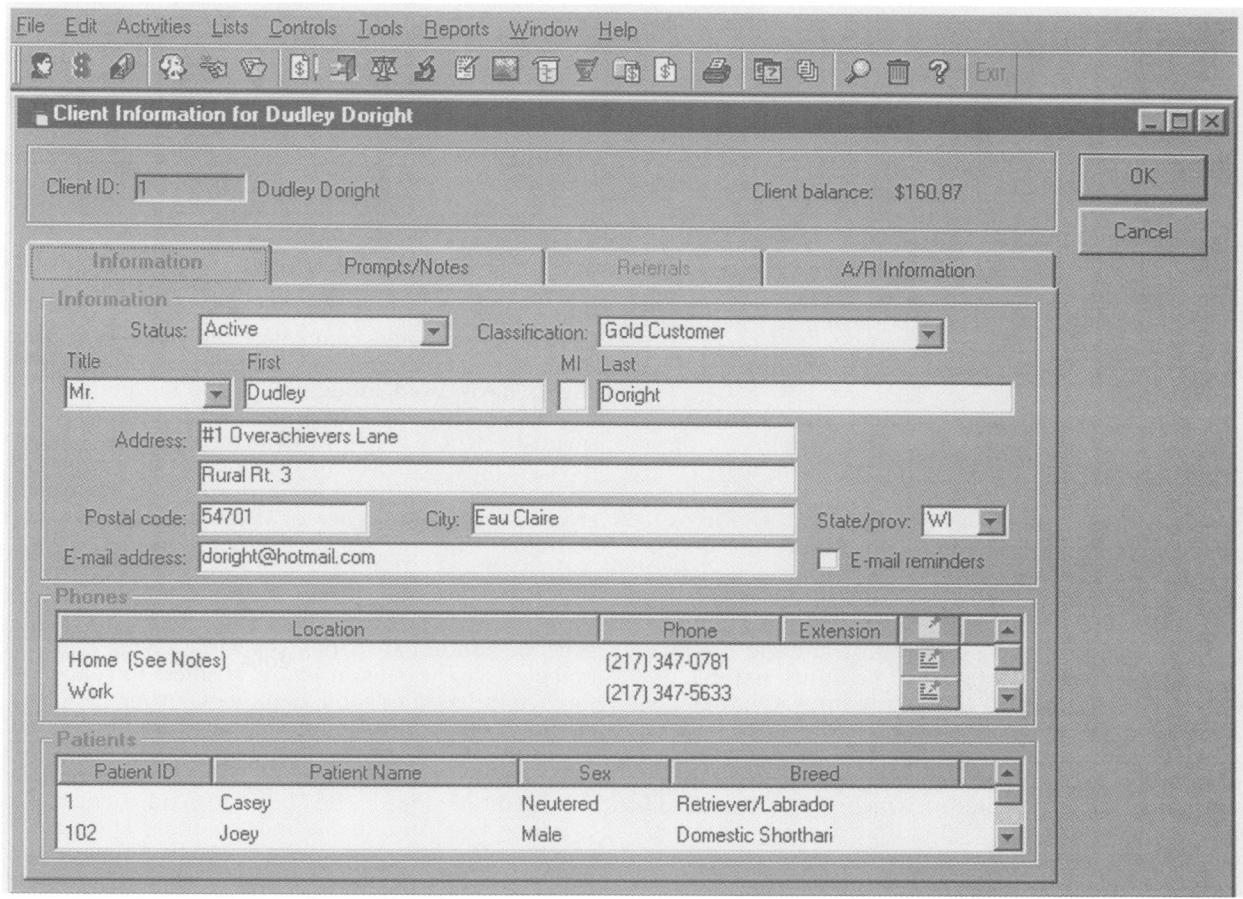

FIGURE 34-4. Example of a screen that captures most client demographics, such as name, address, and phone number, along with balance due, accounts receivable (A/R) information, and e-mail address.

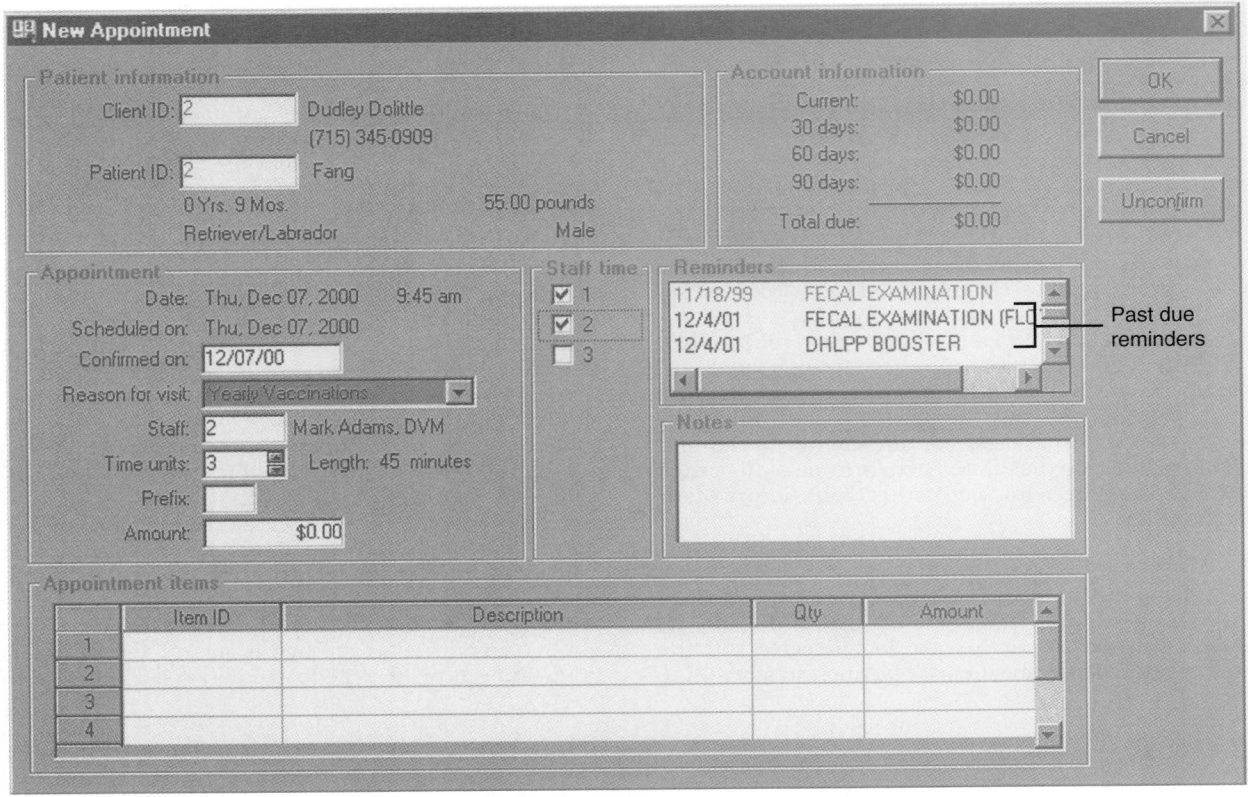

FIGURE 34-5.   Appointment screen showing intelligent color to visualize past due reminders, along with being able to view balance due.

increments as well as scheduling by provider, room, or activity. Scheduling should be considered in the following areas:

- Routine appointments
- Surgery
- Boarding
- Grooming
- Vaccinations
- Conferences
- Dentistry
- Geriatric workups
- Radiology
- Consultations (specialists, colleagues, vendors)

Billing

One of the most desirable features of the PIMS is the ability to keep track of billing—both daily invoicing and the ability to send statements at the end of each month. Accounts receivable and invoicing are the features that are at the heart of most software programs and are used as integral sections of all programs. Accounts payable is usually interfaced through a third-party software program.

Adding new charges to a patient's record does several things. First, the fee codes become part of the medical record of that patient and give a history of what was done to that patient and the date on which it was provided. Second, in hospitalized or complicated cases, the fees entered give a running total of expenses incurred to date and allow estimates to be provided for clients. Third, if there are financial limitations on the treatment regimen, the fee totals keep everyone informed of the status. Finally,

the time saved at the end of the month to send statements is greatly reduced. Most software packages let the practice define the dates of the billing cycle, and the computer does the rest.

On the other end of the billing spectrum are those bills for which payment is overdue. When charges are entered into the computer, an internal date timer is set. It keeps track of when charges were made and when payments were made. On a command, the computer will calculate which clients have owed money for a specific period of time. Clients who have an account balance of more than 30 days might be sent a nicely worded reminder. For those who have account balances of over 60 or 90 days, the letter might be more stern and pointed. If desired, the system can calculate and add service or interest charges for overdue accounts.

Client Communication and Mass Mailings

Mass mailings provide service information to clients and generate additional client visits while saving time. Private practices rely heavily on return business to survive; therefore reminders are a good method of encouraging periodic, routine health care. Traditionally, vaccination; dental, fecal, and heartworm examinations; and routine health examination reminders are used whether or not the practice is computerized. The ability to send client reminders has long been one of the most popular enticements for purchasing a computer system. PIMS programs have a feature that allows linkage of a fee code entry with a trigger to automatically generate a reminder letter or postcard; or, because the Internet is becoming more popular in the

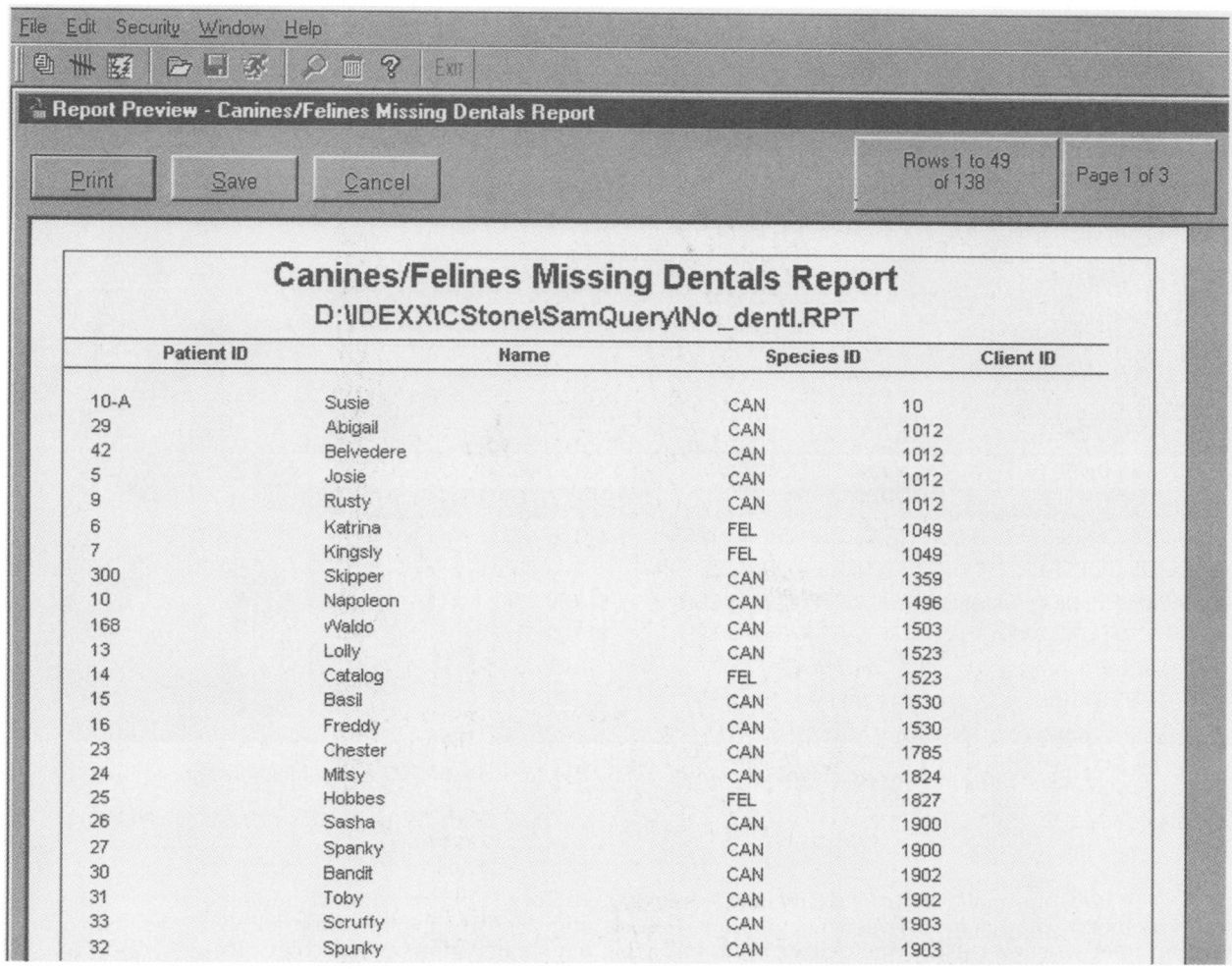

FIGURE 34-6. A report showing a query on all pets that have not had a dental examination. This type of report can be merged into a word processing document to create a letter to be sent to all clients with these pets.

general public, the capability of sending reminders via e-mail is becoming available from some PIMS vendors. For instance, when a rabies vaccine (or any other service) is charged to a patient, five steps are immediately completed by the computer:

1. The service automatically becomes part of the patient's medical record.
2. The inventory quantity of dispensed product is updated.
3. A rabies certificate is generated.
4. A reminder is generated and stored in the system for sending at the proper time.
5. The fee is entered on the client's account for billing purposes.

Internally, the computer keeps track of when a vaccination was given and then calculates when the next visit needs to be scheduled. This information, which is stored in the computer for automatic reminder generation, is also readily available for display on the computer screen if a client should inquire about his or her animal's vaccination status.

Other reminders can be developed and are usually lumped under a category of "word processing" or "mail merges." Reminders, newsletters, or other types of marketing correspondence can be directed to specific clients if the demographics and history meet the criteria input by the practice staff. For example, if the practice wishes to target all dogs and cats that have not had a dental examination, a letter indicating the importance of teeth cleaning can be sent to all canine- and feline-owning clients with pets that have not had a dental examination (Figure 34-6). General client information, such as the addition of a new staff member, a change in operating hours, or other items of widespread interest, can be easily disseminated to all clients or to specific types of client (e.g., all clients who own animals over 10 years of age).

Inventory Management: Drugs and Supplies

Inventory management is an application that will take serious planning before implementation. Much information can be generated from inventory management, and it is believed to be an effective tool to manage the practice; however, much time can be spent maintaining inventory. Therefore proper planning and assessment of the need will help the practice become more efficient with inventory management. Inventory items used on the patient must be entered into the system in order to generate charges for the

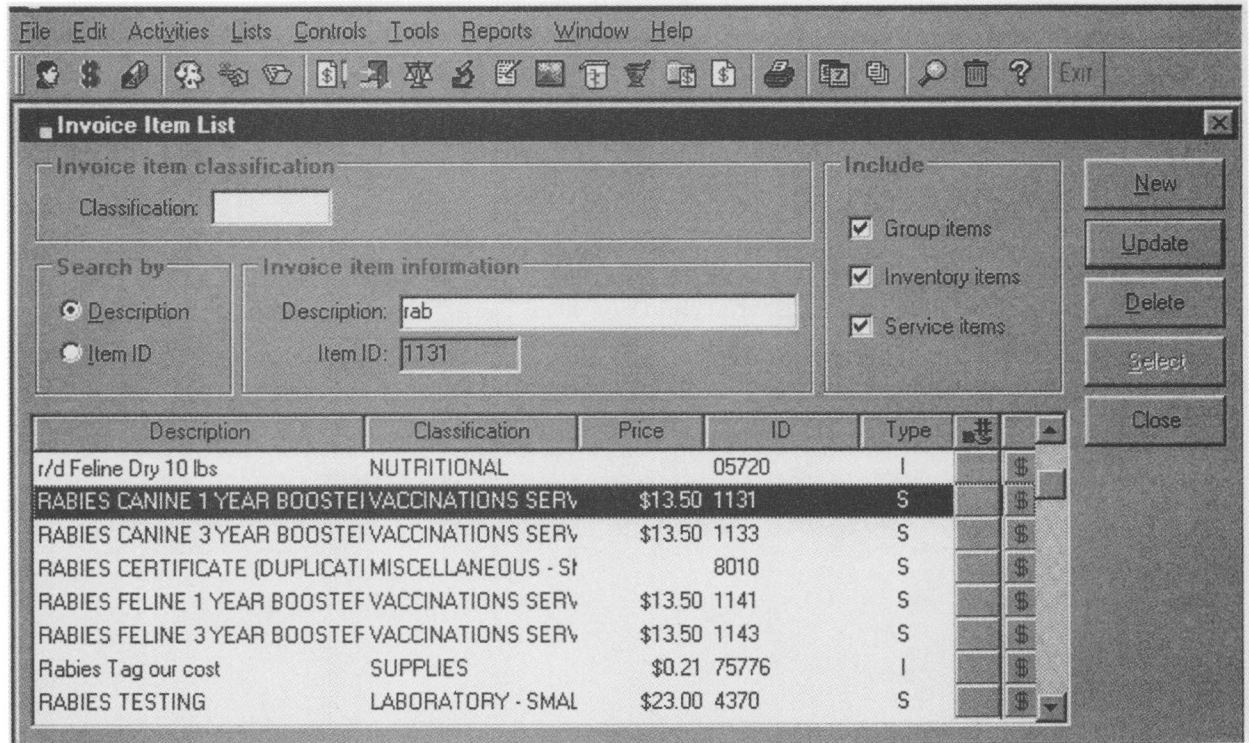

FIGURE 34-7. A screen showing inventory items listed by description along with classifications, price, and identification number or code.

client. This is the minimal level of activity needed for inventory management (Figure 34-7). The computer will subtract an item whenever it is dispensed or used, but a person must be in charge of entering quantities into the computer when shipments arrive. Entering the orders received may become time consuming but may be outweighed by the efficiencies gained in inventory control and management. In a relatively small practice that does not keep a large inventory, implementing all the features of inventory management may not be needed. Multisite practices or practices with a large inventory may wish to take advantage of all inventory features, including purchase orders, controlled substance control, and seasonal stocking levels. If inventory management and control are a high priority, bar coding systems might be considered. Each drug or product is given a bar code number (Universal Product Code [UPC]) that is linked to the individual drug information. The system then becomes similar to a grocery line checkout. When a product is dispensed, the bar code scanner is run over the bar code label and the quantity of product is entered. As with the rest of the inventory program, there is a cost/benefit ratio. It should be noted that all veterinary products today do not include UPC codes on the labels. Often, the PIMS inventory system must also generate the bar code label.

Financial Applications

Cash drawer verification, automatic deposit slips, and payment method itemization are features that are usually most helpful to the reception and accounting staff. During the daily transactions, the computer keeps a record of what charges were paid and by what method: cash (amount tendered and change given), check, or credit card. At the

end of the day or at the beginning of the next day, reports and deposit slips are automatically generated so that the day's transactions can be reconciled.

A profile of the practice with demographic comparisons along with the income analysis have often been touted as one of the main reasons to purchase a computer system. These types of reports are generated daily, monthly, yearly, or for any period desired (Figure 34-8). They are usually tied to the daily fee entries and give an overall analysis of the activities of a practice. As professional marketing becomes more sophisticated, more data are needed to make management decisions. Can the practice justify additional staff? Will the volume of a certain laboratory procedure justify buying an instrument for that procedure? Are the fees for radiographs at a level to support all costs of the equipment and film? Where do clients live? Who has referred clients to the practice? Can the practice afford a salary increase for all staff?

Usually, when statements are done, month-to-date and year-to-date statistics are generated. Which doctor did which procedures? How many of each type of procedure were done? How much income was collected? These data can provide valuable information when making management decisions.

When all charges for a patient are entered into the PIMS, a monthly billing becomes a relatively painless chore. The ability of various staff members to access a client's bill status can be an important part of the program. One of the main things that both the client and the practice have in common is the status of charges for a patient. It is easy to let charges get out of hand, especially on a hospitalized case. It is in the best interest of both parties that an accurate record of charges be kept.

Daily Summary Report
Wednesday, January 05, 2000 10:25 am

Description	Today	Month to Date	Year to Date
New Clients:	0	0	102
Patient Visits:	2	0	329
No. Of Invoices:	2	0	280
Gross Sales:	$104.50	$0.00	$28,577.95
Avg. Gross per Invoice:	$52.25	$0.00	$102.06
Minus: Manual Discount:	$0.00	$0.00	$0.00
Minus: Preset Discount:	($5.50)	$0.00	($583.00)
Net Sales:	$99.00	$0.00	$27,994.95
Avg. Net per Invoice:	$49.50	$0.00	$99.98
Taxes:	$1.10	$0.00	$1,152.99
Total Potential Collections:	$100.10	$0.00	$29,147.94
Net Service Revenues:	$99.00	$0.00	$5,504.03
Net Inventory Revenues:	$0.00	$0.00	$856.40
Total Net Revenue:	$99.00	$0.00	$6,360.43
New Receivables:	$100.10	$0.00	$14,976.16
Old Receivables Paid:	$0.00	$0.00	($6,041.64)
Net Change:	$100.10	$0.00	$8,934.52
Total Payments:	$0.00	$0.00	$21,012.60

A

FIGURE 34-8. A, A sample daily report showing income and demographic analysis.   *Continued*

Medical Records

The ability to enter medical histories and treatments for a patient is a feature that has become much more efficient in modern PIMSs. Entering medical data on a patient can be one of the most useful tools in a computer system. Some of the larger PIMS vendors have a part of the program where data such as the problem list for the patient, the current and past histories, vital signs data, laboratory data, daily progress notes, and diagnostic codes can be entered. In addition, the information gathered in the veterinarian's routine examination can be easily communicated to the client (Figure 34-9). Instead of entering all this information on paper, which is useful only to the person who possesses the medical record, the information in the computer is accessible to anyone at any terminal or workstation.

Many PIMSs have the ability to create customized data entry templates to enter medical records information. For example, a form could be developed that would allow the examination, using SOAP notes, to be recorded, and the program would guide the technician through the form, section by section, for data input (Figure 34-10). A template could be developed to record vital signs and enter physical examination and laboratory data (Figure 34-11). These data then become part of an individual animal's history. Customized patient forms are an area where the staff must make some real decisions on how much, if any, patient data they want on the computer. Generally, this feature is a plus because it gives everyone easy access to those data. The legality of computerized medical records versus paper records has always been in question. In general, if adequate backups of the hard disk are made and there is a reasonable amount of security in the system, electronic medical records have had equal legal status with paper records. Laws may vary among states; therefore it is advised that the practice obtain legal advice before implementing electronic medical records.

PROCESS OF SOFTWARE EVALUATION

In the evaluation of PIMSs, not only the veterinarian but also the technician and receptionist staff should have significant input into the selection process. Computerization is an area in which all members of the team must be happy for the entire system to succeed. This is not a process, for example, whereby a surgical instrument is evaluated only by the veterinarian because he or she will be the only one using that instrument. In fact, one of the main objectives of installing or switching a computer system should be to make communication better for everyone—

Net Inventory Revenues:	$0.00	$0.00	$856.40
Total Net Revenue:	$99.00	$0.00	$6,360.43
New Receivables:	$100.10	$0.00	$14,976.16
Old Receivables Paid:	$0.00	$0.00	($6,041.64)
Net Change:	$100.10	$0.00	$8,934.52
Total Payments:	$0.00	$0.00	$21,012.60
Cash Refunds	$0.00	$0.00	$0.00
Total Deposits:	$0.00	$0.00	$21,012.60
Returned Checks:	$0.00	$0.00	$321.89
Service Charges:	$0.00	$0.00	$75.00
Adjustments	$0.00	$0.00	$1,922.65
Write Offs:	$0.00	$0.00	$0.00

B

| Top 10 Invoice Item Classifications | LABORATORY - SMALL
VACCINATIONS SERVICE
PROFESSIONAL SERVICES - S | | PROFESSIONAL SERVICES - S
VACCINATIONS SERVICE
Pharmaceuticals
LABORATORY - SMALL
SURGERY - SMALL
ANESTHESIA - SMALL
PROFESSIONAL SERVICES - L
NUTRITIONAL
SKIN CARE
DENTAL - SMALL |

Figure 34-8, cont'd.   B, Additional daily report showing end of day financial summaries.

this is not just a tool for the veterinarian. Although this discussion is about the initial decision to computerize a veterinary practice, the same rationale and process can be used in evaluating, changing, or upgrading a PIMS.

The first task in deciding to computerize is for the management staff to decide what they want the computer system to do for them. Initially, do not even consider what computer or configuration to use; consider only the functions and tasks to be done. The next step is to contact several PIMS vendors for a demonstration or to visit exhibits at one of the national or state meetings (e.g., AVMA, American Animal Hospital Association [AAHA], Western Veterinary Conference, North American Veterinary Conference, Central Veterinary Conference). During the demonstration, veterinary staff will probably be overwhelmed by all the functions available. The veterinary management staff should have their list of requirements prepared to help focus and direct the demonstration. Many PIMS programs that have been around for a long time offer the basic functions: invoicing, reminders, inventory management, and appointment scheduling. Primary consideration should be given to ease of use, staff support, and training.

How does one decide which PIMS vendors to evaluate? Periodically, different veterinary publications publish a list of current practice management software. AAHA's *Trends* magazine lists multiple vendors in the marketplace. These articles generally provide a brief synopsis of the state of

veterinary practice management computing and then publish a list of vendors and the main features of their programs. These are excellent articles since they usually provide information such as the length of time the company has been in business, number of employees, number of installations, hardware and software platforms, and main features. Remember that PIMS should not be considered a commodity, but rather an investment in the future of the practice.

Several items should be considered when choosing a software vendor. How long has the company been in business, how many programs have they sold, and how many programs are in operation? Is the company's user base generally happy? The veterinary staff should ask for references of users who are in the same type of practice or have the same type of needs as their practice does. In the early days of the veterinary computer revolution (1970s), some hospital systems were programmed by individual practitioners who had an interest in computers and programming. The practitioner used the program in his or her own practice, and if someone else liked it, the program would be disseminated. Some of them developed into larger systems if there was enough financial backing, but for the most part they were unsuccessful. The competition in the veterinary software market is narrowing and still somewhat fierce, and the roads are lined with skulls of the small vendors who cannot continue to develop and support their product in today's market. Programs need to be

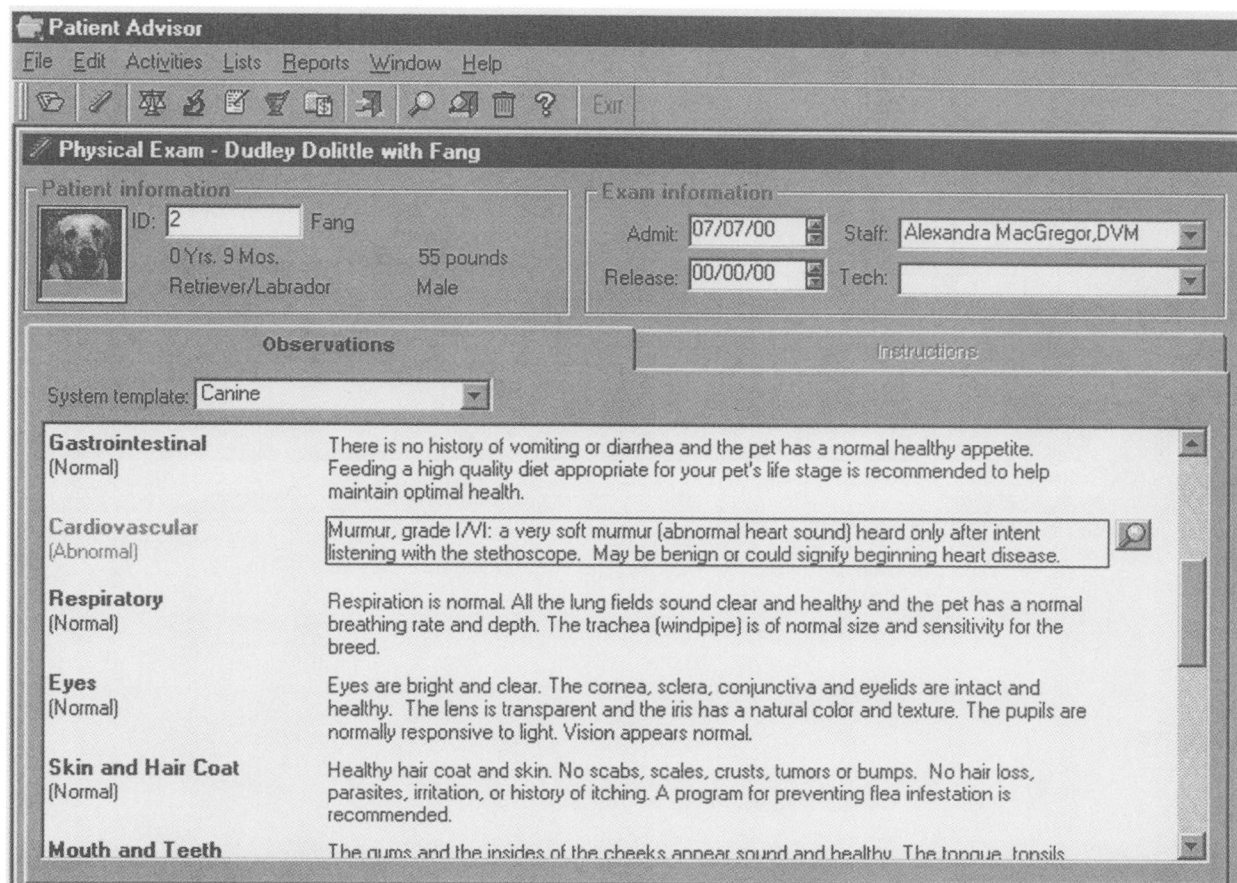

FIGURE 34-9.   A patient health report indicating normal or abnormal values from a routine examination. This report can be reviewed with the client to increase compliance and communicate examination findings.

purchased from survivors; they probably have a reliable product and service. Therefore look for longevity, number of installations, and a quality support staff and record.

A vital element to look for is support for both hardware and software. This is a feature that is not given enough attention but is of extreme importance. Most companies concern themselves primarily with software and provide the hardware as a service to the customer. What kind of software support do they provide, and during what hours of the day do they provide it? Is support available 24 hours per day, 7 days per week in case of an emergency? What is the cost? The vendor should know his or her program inside and out; there are often features or shortcuts that are not documented in the instructions. Even people who think they know what they are doing with computers have to rely heavily on software support because of the proprietary nature of the systems. Without easily reached, competent support, the system will never survive. A monthly support fee will usually provide telephone support and upgrades when new programs are developed. The number of true system upgrades (not just feature fixes) and the regularity with which upgrades are issued are other indicators of the stability of the program and the company. A progressive company will consistently be improving its product.

Probably the last feature to evaluate is hardware. There is an idiom in the computer world that states that one should always select the software first; there will always be a computer to make it run. It is always best to go on the PIMS vendor's advice and if possible, choose a vendor that sells and supports the full system, not just the software. Networking and computers have changed considerably since the early 1970s. Computer hardware has become so inexpensive and powerful that it is much less a concern than in years past. The prices of powerful computers have come down drastically in the last few years, and there are wide selections of computers and operating systems that offer excellent benefits.

As state above, it is advised to purchase the entire system from a reputable vendor. Most practice personnel do not have enough knowledge or time to buy and install their own computers and networks. Prices at local computer stores may look slightly better than those of the software vendor, but the local vendor or technician is probably not knowledgeable about the particular PIMS package to be of real support. Software vendors have tried and developed the software on a particular type of computer or network on which they know it will work. They probably will not provide hardware support, and possibly not even software support, if the veterinary practice does not comply with their hardware specifications.

The larger and most reputable software companies will usually provide an on-site demonstration by a trained representative. This is a highly desirable time to get a good overview of the software and to ask questions and consult an expert on the needs of the practice. It is a good time to

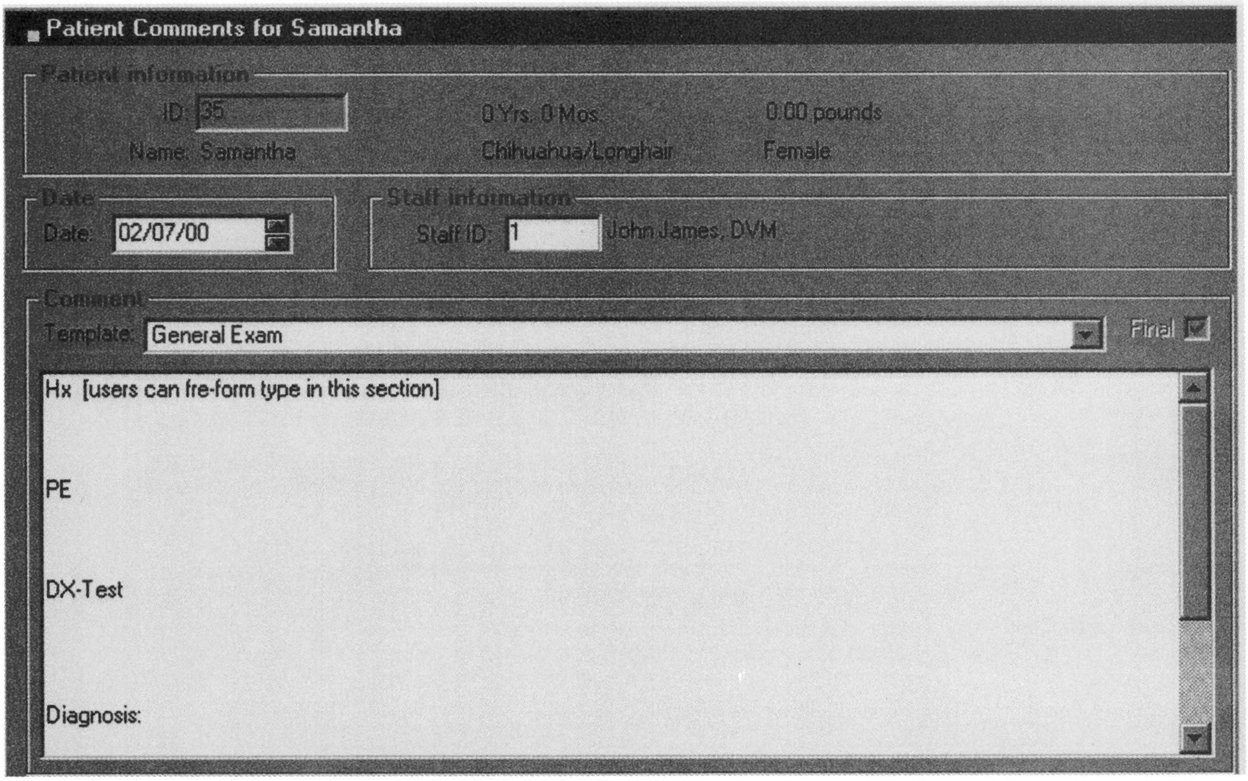

FIGURE 34-10. A patient template allowing user to type notes into sections.

let the staff review the features and see how easily the software will do everyday functions. Smaller companies may not have the resources to send a representative but will allow on-site evaluation of the system for some period. Evaluation of systems at meetings is an alternative, but usually the itinerary at veterinary meetings is too hectic to allow participants to be able to do a good evaluation.

It is during the demonstration or the evaluation period that a decision should be made regarding what portions of the program are needed. Most programs offer built-in modules that can be added to the basic system. A small animal boarding and grooming package would be of no use to an equine practice. An equine trainer list would be of no use to a small animal practice. A good way to hold down prices is by purchasing just what the practice can use.

THE DECISION TO BUY: WHAT HAPPENS NEXT?

After the decision to buy is made, what happens next? Depending on the agreement with the vendor, the delivered computer system will be set up either by the practice or the vendor. If a single-user computer system has been purchased and the software is already loaded into the computer, setup will be minimal. It is worth the extra expense to have the vendor set up a networked system. Network operating systems are complex and require trained personnel for installation and management. Exten-

sive network maintenance is far beyond the capabilities of most practices.

If the purchase is a conversion to a new system, much consideration should be given to maintaining the integrity of the practice data. The current practice data are vital for client lists, accounts receivable, medical records, reminders, and so forth. The PIMS vendor should provide the practice with a specific list of data fields that can be converted along with data that cannot be converted. Veterinary practices are cautioned to choose a vendor who has extensive experience with conversions of the existing PIMS.

After installation is complete, the next step is training on the actual system. Most of the large vendors provide on-site training by one of their own education specialists, usually for 2 to 5 days. During the training period, a reduced appointment schedule is recommended because it becomes too hectic to handle a normal business load and learn the computer system. This is the time when all staff members need to be deeply involved in the new system. The more attention the practice can devote to the training, the better the system will be utilized in the practice. The practice staff must take responsibility for learning and implementing the PIMS.

No matter how easy the program is to use and no matter how intelligent the staff, the initial stages of computerization can be hectic. Most programs are well organized and intuitive so that everyday functions become second nature in a matter of days.

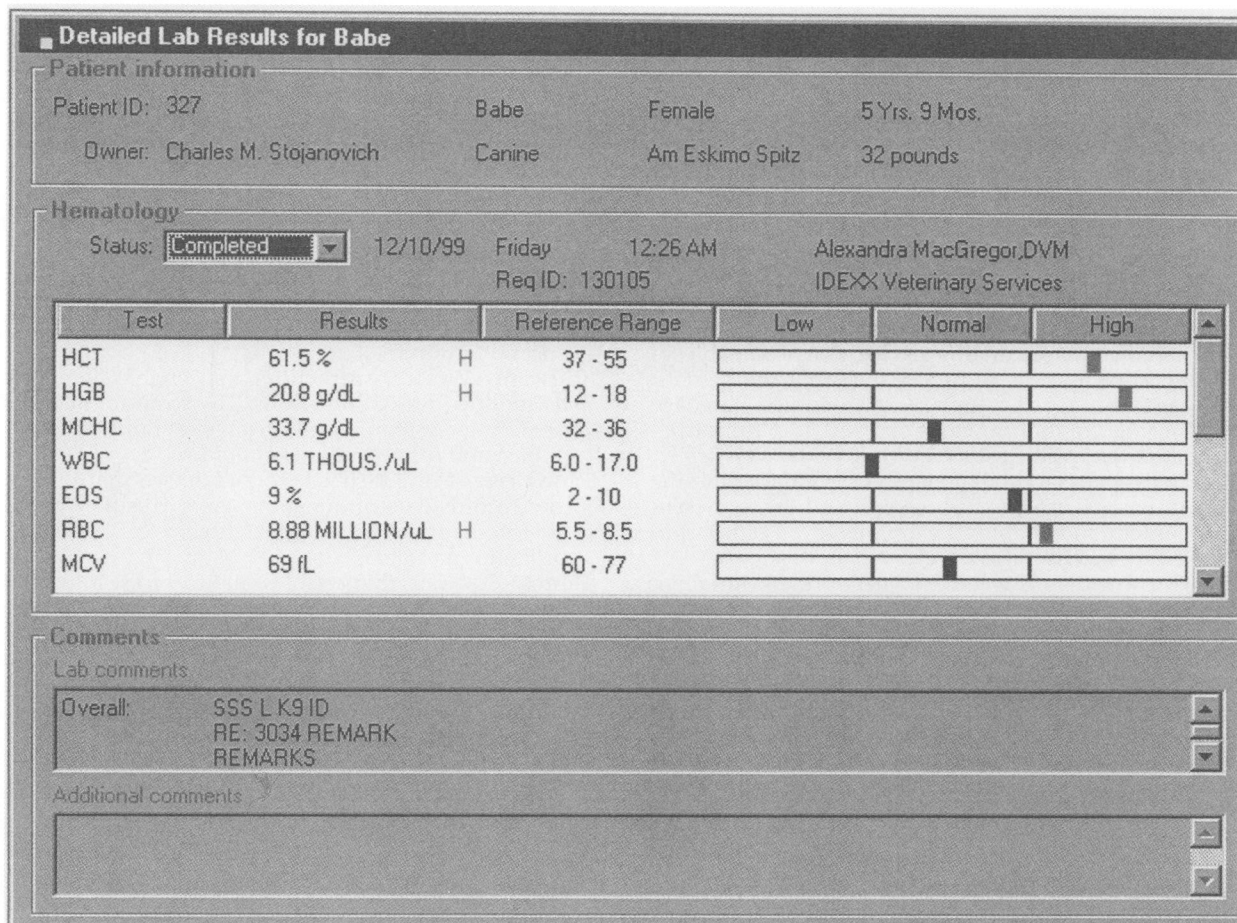

FIGURE 34-11.   A patient record showing laboratory results embedded within the medical record.

GLOSSARY

ASCII—American Standard Code for Information Interchange. A standard format for representing characters. This format is used in text files and is useful when files are shared between programs.

AUTOEXEC.BAT file—A file containing disk operating system (DOS) commands written in ASCII text form, which is automatically executed when the computer is turned on or booted.

Batch file—An executable file with DOS commands written in ASCII text, which is used for automating frequently used commands.

BIOS—Basic input/output system. This is part of the read-only memory (ROM) of the central processing unit (CPU), which is installed in the form of a chip and which controls how the CPU interacts with the screen, keyboard, printer, and other peripheral devices.

Bit—Unit of data in binary form; the smallest storage unit for data in a computer.

Byte—A fixed number of bits that represents a character. The most common byte size is eight bits.

CD/ROM—Compact disk read-only memory. A data storage system based on conversion of data from digital to analog and storage of the analog data on optical disks.

CPU—Central processing unit. That part of a computer or computer system responsible for the actual computations.

CRT—Cathode ray tube. This is the electronic tube making up the visual display of the terminal or the computer.

Database—A collection of interrelated data stored together with a minimum of redundancy to serve multiple applications.

DOS—Disk operating system. This is software that controls movement of information in a computer and allows the CPU to use peripheral devices, such as printers, diskette drives, and fixed disk drives.

Driver—A set of commands that are used to run a peripheral device, such as a printer.

EGA—Enhanced graphics adapter. This acronym refers to the ability of a computer to display graphic images in color.

E-mail—Electronic mail. An electronic method of communication between network users.

Expanded memory—The RAM of a computer in excess of 640 kilobytes and less than 1 megabyte.

Extended memory—The random access memory (RAM) of a computer in excess of 1 megabyte.

Facsimile—A device for transmission of graphic files from one location to another; also called *fax*. The graphic image is converted to digital signals by the sending device, and the receiving device converts the digital signals to a graphic image. Facsimile machines act as remote copying machines.

File—A collection of one or more records.

Fixed disk—A high-volume magnetic storage device that is usually built into the computer.

Floppy disk—Small, portable, magnetic storage device for storage of computer programs and data.

Font—A specific typeface, including its point size and weight.

FTP—File transfer protocol. A protocol for remote transfer of files from one CPU to another.

Gopher—A program that facilitates access and retrieval of textual (ASCII) information on servers connected to the Internet. Gopher is also referred to as a text browser.

Graphics display—A CRT or monitor that is capable of displaying graphic images.

Hardware—A digital or analog device that is capable of detecting, transmitting, or processing electronic signals.

Home page—A specific hypertext markup language (HTML) program that provides text and graph information that is retrievable from a World Wide Web server.

HTML—Hypertext markup language. A system for marking up documents that instructs browsers on how to present the document and enables documents (even remote) to be linked by specific tags.

Internet—A worldwide electronic network of interconnected computers operating in Transmission Control Protocol/Internet Control Protocol (TCP/ICP).

LAN—Local area network. An electronic network permitting communication between the CPUs or CPUs and peripheral devices, such as terminals, printers, and plotters.

Language—A computer language is a particular format in which programs are written, such as BASIC, FORTRAN, COBOL, and MUMPS.

MB—Megabyte. One million bytes; refers to amount of memory available or used. To be more specific, it is 1024 kilobytes or 1,048,576 bytes.

Modem—A device that accepts a digital signal and converts it into an analog signal and accepts an analog signal and converts it to a digital signal.

Operating system—Software that enables the computer to run the application software programs.

Optical scanner—A device that converts printed text or graphic images to digital files.

Printer, daisywheel—An impact printer that functions by a device striking a wheel containing the alphabet and the numbers 1 to 10.

Printer, dot matrix—An impact printer that functions by pins striking the inked ribbon to form the letters, numbers, and graphic forms. Dot matrix printers have 9 to 32 pins. The more pins in the print head, the better the quality of print.

Printer, ink jet—A relatively inexpensive, letter-quality printer that operates by fluid ink being forced through nozzles and transferred to the paper by resistive heaters.

Printer, laser—A printer that produces high-resolution images utilizing the same process as photocopy machines.

RAM—Random access memory. Memory that is used to store application programs and data while the program is in use. All data in RAM will be lost when the computer is turned off.

ROM—Read-only memory. That part of a computer memory that contains prewritten instructions. These instructions cannot be erased or rewritten by application programs.

Server—A computer that provides digital programs and information that can be accessed by networked computers and terminals.

Software—Written instructions that enable the computer to conduct desired functions. The software includes the operating system, application programs, utility programs, and other types of programs.

Tape drive—A high-speed storage device that reads from and records data on magnetic tape. This type of storage device is often used for archiving or "backing up" programs and data.

Telnet—Software that enables one to access and manipulate a computer from a remote CPU.

Terminal—An input/output device with a visual display and keyboard that is utilized to send and receive data from the CPU. Terminals are referred to as "dumb" terminals because they are incapable of processing information.

VGA—Video graphics adapter. A board installed in a computer that allows one to view graphic images in color.

WAN—Wide area network. This is usually a network linking two to several LANs.

Web browser—A program that facilitates access and retrieval of graphic data and HTML documents from World Wide Web servers connected to the Internet.

Windows—An operating system with a graphic interface that allows two applications to be active at the same time and the transfer of information between applications.

World Wide Web—A network of computers interconnected via the Internet that provides access to graphic data and HTML documents.

WYSIWYG—"What you see is what you get." This acronym refers to programs that print exactly what is seen on the display screen.

RECOMMENDED READING

Bohlender E: 2000 reader's choice software survey, *Trends* 16(3):17, 2000.

35

Occupational Health and Safety in Veterinary Hospitals*

Diane McKelvey

By the very nature of their work, veterinary technicians are frequently exposed to potential safety hazards, including bite wounds and other animal-related injuries, laboratory accidents, x-ray radiation, waste anesthetic gas, noise, and toxic chemicals. This chapter surveys these and other potential dangers and the means by which injury or disease can be prevented. Zoonotic diseases are covered in Chapter 18.

There are many published surveys of injury and disease in veterinary hospital workers. A study of 773 insurance claims made by injured American veterinarians between 1967 and 1969 (Thigpen, Dorn, 1973) found that most injuries occurred on a farm or ranch. The authors state:

While in the process of treating, restraining, castrating or examining animals, the veterinarians were bitten, kicked, gored, pawed, knocked down, trampled, run over, and even fallen upon by these animals. While treating resisting farm animals, veterinarians cut themselves, fell, stumbled, or slipped on wet ground or ice in attempts to avoid injuries. These veterinarians jumped off fences, twisting ankles or landing on nails, stepped on pitchforks, and were injured with chutes, speculums, lariats, nose tongs, halters, broken syringes, and an array of practice equipment. They were knocked over and through fences, squeezed against fences, and caught between bulls fighting. They were fallen on by horses while working cattle or else they twisted an ankle while getting off the horse.

Things did not improve much when the veterinarians returned to the hospital:

In the clinics they were bitten, scratched, and knocked down by the animals. They were burned when steam valves burst, and slipped while reaching in a cage for an animal. They injured their backs picking up dogs and bumped their heads and legs on clinic equipment. They cut themselves during surgery and ran pinning equipment into their fingers and wrists.

Obviously, there is ample opportunity for injury within a veterinary environment. Basic safety precautions are listed in Box 35-1.

If a technician or other hospital employee is injured on the job, there are many unfortunate sequelae. The injury itself may result in pain, disability, and lost workdays for the affected person. In addition, both the employee and the hospital may be affected financially, or there may be legal and regulatory issues to face. Hospital morale may also suffer if staff members are convinced that the hospital is not a safe work environment. Employees may be required to take on additional duties if a co-worker is absent because of an injury or disease acquired at work. It is therefore in everyone's interest to learn about the hazards that are present in a veterinary environment and to take all reasonable steps to protect the hospital staff, patients, and clientele from injury and illness.

In all jurisdictions within the United States and Canada, the employer has the primary responsibility for hospital safety. The employer's duties include the following:

- To ensure that all employees are adequately trained to protect themselves from injury

Box 35-1   BASIC SAFETY PRECAUTIONS FOR VETERINARY EMPLOYEES

MACHINERY AND EQUIPMENT

- Do not attempt to operate a machine unless you are familiar with its use.
- Tie long hair back to prevent it from getting caught in equipment. For the same reason, avoid loose-fitting clothing.
- Vent all autoclaves before opening, and keep hands and face away from steam. Avoid handling autoclaved materials until they have cooled.
- Use the insulated handle when picking up cautery or branding devices.
- When using a centrifuge, ensure that the centrifuge is balanced with equal numbers of tubes and that the lid is securely bolted on. No attempt should be made to stop the centrifuge arm or remove samples until the arm has come to a complete stop.

FLOORS

- Wear slip-proof shoes and avoid running.
- Use nonslip mats or strips in areas that are frequently wet.

HOUSEKEEPING

- Clean up spills as soon as possible.
- Return equipment and chemicals to the proper storage area immediately after use.
- Avoid clutter in drawers or counters.
- Hallways, exits, and stairs should be free of obstructions. Equipment or chemicals should not be stored in these locations.
- Store chemicals and heavy equipment on lower shelves to avoid injury or exposure to chemicals in case the container falls off the shelf.
- Replace lids tightly on all containers.
- Use a ladder or step stool to reach high places.
- Follow a checklist for regular facility maintenance, including daily, weekly, monthly, semiannual, and annual procedures.

HYGIENE

- Food and beverages should not be stored with chemicals, drugs, vaccines, or patient samples. Human food can be stored with animal food.
- Prepare and consume foods only in designated eating areas, away from chemicals, work surfaces, and patient handling areas.
- Wash hands with a surgical soap after treating every patient, before and after using the bathroom, and before eating.

LABORATORY

- Wear a laboratory coat or uniform when working with chemicals or diagnostic specimens in a laboratory. In some circumstances, the use of additional protective equipment (gloves, face mask, face shield, biologic containment cabinet) may be advisable.
- All persons should wash their hands after completing laboratory activities and should remove protective clothing before leaving the workplace.
- Persons should not remove or insert contact lenses when working in a laboratory.

- Work surfaces should be cleaned with a disinfectant at the end of the day and after any spill. Useful disinfectants include chlorhexidine, 70% isopropyl alcohol, and a 1:10 dilution of 5% bleach. Bleach is especially suitable for cleaning up blood spills but is corrosive and will damage metal surfaces with prolonged use. If samples contain *Mycobacterium* or if the surface to be cleaned is metallic, glutaraldehyde is the recommended disinfectant. Gloves should be worn when using glutaraldehyde, and care should be taken to avoid inhalation of glutaraldehyde vapors.

CHEMICALS
Storage

- Corrosive chemicals should not be stored above shoulder height, because accidental dislodgment of the container could result in chemical splashing onto a person below. Storage in a closed cupboard at floor level is preferred.
- Hazardous chemicals should not be stored in passageways, aisles, or hallways or next to emergency exits.
- Separate storage areas should be used for each group of hazardous chemicals, including strong oxidizers (peroxides), flammable liquids, acids, alkalis, and compressed gases.
- Flammable materials (ether, acetone) and compressed gases should not be stored where there is a possibility of exposure to heat, sunlight, or a source of combustion, including cigarettes. A fireproof cabinet is ideal.
- For any hazardous chemical, it is advisable to purchase the smallest quantity that is needed, because there will be less material to spill or catch fire.
- Storage areas should be tidy, with good access to all materials without climbing over bottles or reaching over boxes.
- Some type of absorbing agent, such as kitty litter, should be kept in the storage area for use in cleaning up spills. If a spill occurs, it should be cleaned up immediately.
- All containers should have purchase and expiration dates written on the label or box, and stocks should be reviewed at least annually. Expired or deteriorated chemicals should be discarded.

Use

- Caps should be replaced on chemical bottles immediately after use.
- Wear gloves, a laboratory coat or waterproof apron, and protective goggles when mixing or diluting chemicals.
- Chemicals should not be mixed together unless the label or material safety data sheet (MSDS) states that the chemicals are compatible. One example of incompatible chemicals is bleach and ammonia-containing disinfectants. Mixtures of these two compounds may release clouds of extremely toxic chlorine gas.
- If a material is to be diluted with water, start with the water and gradually add the chemical to it. That way, if the solution is spilled or reacts, it is the water or diluted chemical that is splashed, rather than the chemical in concentrated form.

Continued

Box 35-1   BASIC SAFETY PRECAUTIONS FOR VETERINARY EMPLOYEES—CONT'D

CHEMICALS—cont'd

Disposal

- Many chemicals cannot be safely (or legally) discarded with regular garbage. The MSDS should be consulted to determine correct disposal options for any particular chemical. Municipalities often have regulations that govern disposal of chemicals and should be consulted for further information.
- Waste materials, including solvents, oils, grease, paints, and other flammable substances, should be placed in covered metal containers before disposal.
- Broken glass must be clearly identified and placed in a puncture-proof container.
- Although small amounts of some liquid chemicals may be discarded into the sewer system and flushed with copious amounts of water, this is not a good option for chemicals that can damage sewer pipes or chemicals that are an environmental hazard.

ELECTRICITY

- Do not remove light switch or electrical outlet covers.
- Keep circuit breaker boxes closed.
- When using electrical equipment in wet areas (e.g., a portable dryer), it must be properly grounded and only plugged into a ground-fault circuit interruption outlet.
- Extension cords must never be run across aisles or floors or through a window or door.
- Appliances with defective plugs should not be used until repaired. Never alter or remove the ground terminals on plugs.

ERGONOMICS

- When lifting a heavy object, whether an animal, equipment, or container, keep the back straight and use the leg muscles—not the back muscles—to lift. Bend at the knees, rather than at the waist.
- Do not attempt to lift an object weighing more than 50 lb without assistance. Pregnant persons should not lift any heavy object.
- Use portable or fixed steps for moving large dogs onto examination tables or into a bathing area. Some dogs can be readily led up the steps rather than being lifted.
- Use a walk-on weigh scale rather than lifting an animal to be weighed.
- When restraining an animal or working with a microscope or computer, avoid a fixed, static posture. Occasional stretching or movement is helpful in preventing fatigue.
- When using a computer, adjust the monitor position, brightness, and contrast to the most comfortable level. To

avoid glare, locate the monitor at right angles to windows and other light sources. Windows should have blinds or drapes to minimize glare. Characters on the screen should not have a visible flicker or waver.
- Computer keyboards should be thin and detached from the screen, allowing the user to adjust the keyboard position.
- A foam support placed under the wrist may help avoid strain during prolonged keyboard use.
- Office chairs should be stable, with an adjustable seat height and angle and an adjustable backrest. The front edge of the seat should be contoured. The backrest should provide firm support to the lumbar region of the back and should extend up almost to the lower end of the shoulder blade. A woven fabric covering is more comfortable than plastic or wood.
- Petite persons and pregnant women should use a footrest, especially if the table height is fixed.
- Ensure adequate lighting in all workplaces.

NOISE

- Occupational Safety and Health Administration (OSHA) standards require a hearing conservation program if employees are exposed to noise levels above 85 decibels (dB) based on an 8-hour time-weighted average. This level may be exceeded in areas where dogs are housed. The noise level from a single barking dog may be 80 to 90 dB, and if several dogs are housed in one area, noise levels may be as high as 115 dB. At 115 dB, an employee can only work approximately 15 minutes in the area without hearing protection before the daily limit is exceeded.
- The employer must identify a noise hazard area by means of signs placed at all entrances to the room, indicating that a noise hazard exists and hearing protection is required for prolonged exposure.
- Noise levels can be reduced by acoustical tiles or sound-absorbing panels hung from the ceiling. Commercial panels are available for this purpose, or homemade baffles can be constructed.
- If sound-absorbing panels cannot be installed, personal hearing protection is an alternative means of reducing exposure to noise. Several varieties of earphones or earplugs are available, but the protection method chosen must reduce noise by at least 20 dB. Personal hearing protection is not necessary for persons who enter and leave the room immediately.
- Some attempt may be made to reduce barking noise through the use of citronella collars and by closing doors to the kennel area.

- To provide employees with the facilities and protective equipment necessary to do their jobs safely
- To establish emergency procedures in case of accident or fire and to ensure that employees are familiar with these procedures
- To collect and make available mandatory forms and posters, including material safety data sheets (MSDSs) for chemicals
- To notify employees of impending inspections and special hazards
- To report accidents that result in serious injury
- To maintain a log of occupational illnesses and injuries (in the United States, this applies to businesses with 11 or more employees)

- To post warning signs at emergency exits, radiation areas, and areas in which hearing protection is required (in the United States)

Technician Note

In all jurisdictions within the United States and Canada, the employer has the primary responsibility for hospital safety.

The responsibilities of the employee are to learn the safety hazards and approved procedures for avoiding injury in the workplace, to wear the protective equipment

BOX 35-2   REFERENCES FOR OCCUPATIONAL SAFETY AND HEALTH ADMINISTRATION (OSHA) REQUIREMENTS

The Complete Veterinary Practice Regulatory Compliance Manual
Philip Seibert
RR 1 Box 313
Calhoun, TN 37309
(423) 336-1925

AVMA Guide to Hazard Communication
American Veterinary Medical Association
1931 N. Meacham Road, Suite 100
Schaumburg, IL 601734360
1-800-248-2862

Hazard Communication Compliance Kit and *OSHA Compliance Guide for the Veterinary Practice*
American Animal Hospital Association
PO Box 150899
Denver, CO 80215-0899
1-800-252-2242

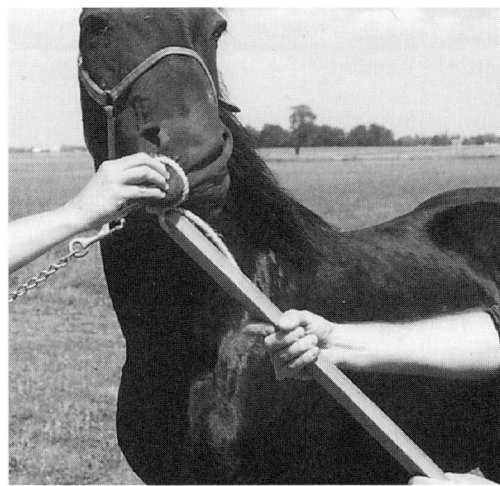

FIGURE 35-1. Horses are a common source of animal-related injury.

provided, and to report incidents or conditions that could result in injury.

In the United States, the Occupational Safety and Health Administration (OSHA) has been established under the Department of Labor to ensure that health and safety standards are maintained in every workplace. Many states have developed their own OSHA plans, which may vary in some details from the federal standards. In Canada, workplace safety is a provincial responsibility. Regardless of the jurisdiction, safety regulations are enforced by means of inspections by government personnel, and noncompliance is subject to stiff penalties (in the United States, up to $70,000 for each infraction). Any hospital is subject to an unannounced inspection, although most visits arise from employee complaints or workers' compensation claims. During the visit, the compliance officer checks for unsafe conditions and procedures and inspects the hospital's written documentation regarding hospital safety hazards, emergency procedures, safe work procedures, and staff training. The inspector also ensures that required notices, such as the OSHA Workplace Safety and Health Protection poster or the provincial Occupational Health and Safety Act, are displayed in the workplace. Inspectors ensure that all necessary personal protection equipment is available and in good repair. Persons seeking more information on regulatory requirements are advised to contact their local state or provincial veterinary association or consult the references listed in Box 35-2.

ANIMAL-RELATED INJURY

Veterinary technicians are constantly exposed to sick or fractious animals and their blood, urine, and feces, and the potential for animal-related injury or disease is always present. The most important animal-related hazards in the veterinary environment are as follows:

- Animal kicks, bite wounds, scratches, squeeze injuries, and other physical trauma
- Parasites and zoonotic diseases (see Chapters 7 and 18)

- Allergy to animal dander or fleas
- Exposure to feces, urine, blood, and tissues that contain pathogenic microorganisms, such as *Salmonella* and *Listeria*
- Handling contaminated needles, bacterial cultures, and other biomedical wastes.

Trauma

Animals are capable of inflicting serious injury to people that handle them. Dogs primarily defend themselves with their teeth, cats scratch as well as bite, rabbits can inflict deep scratches with the nails of their powerful hind legs, budgerigars can nip with their beaks, and larger birds can bite or scratch with their claws. Persons working with cattle are at risk of being kicked, squeezed, or trampled, and those working with horses can be bitten, struck by the front hooves, squeezed, or kicked by the rear hooves (Figure 35-1). Persons working with ratites, exotic pets, or captive wildlife, such as deer or elk, may also sustain an injury when handling or treating these patients. In fact, animals are the most common source of injury to veterinarians and their staff (see Figure 35-1). Restraint and handling of animals are discussed in Chapter 1.

Surveys undertaken to investigate the incidence of animal-related trauma have shown the animal species most commonly associated with injury to veterinarians are cattle, cats, horses, and dogs. The most common injuries are lacerations and puncture wounds, followed by fractures (including facial fractures and dislodged teeth) and sprains and torn ligaments.

Technician Note

Newer studies show that dog and cat bites are the most common source of injury to veterinarians.

Basic guidelines for avoiding animal-related injury are given in Box 35-3.

Bite Wounds

Veterinary technicians, veterinarians, and other hospital employees are frequently bitten by dogs, cats, and other animals. The most common location of canine bite wounds is the radius or ulna, and the most common location for feline bite wounds is the hand.

Bite wounds are potentially more serious than other puncture wounds because of the amount of bruising and tissue injury that occurs. This is not surprising, given that the jaws of a large dog can produce 150 to 450 psi of pressure, which is enough to bend steel bars and penetrate stainless steel feeding bowls.

Technician Note

Bite wounds are potentially more serious than other puncture wounds because of the amount of bruising and tissue injury that occurs.

Bite wounds not only traumatize tissue but may also become infected. The risk of infection is estimated to be 2% to 5% for a dog bite and 30% to 50% for a cat bite. Usually, wounds are contaminated with the bacteria that reside in the dog's or cat's mouth, although occasionally human skin bacteria may invade the wound. Of the more than 64 species of bacteria that are found in the canine and feline mouth, the one most commonly associated with wound infections is *Pasteurella multocida*. This small gram-negative coccobacillus is present in 50% of canine mouths and 80% of feline mouths. Other bacteria, including *Capnocytophaga*, *Streptococcus*, *Staphylococcus*, *Klebsiella*, *Enterobacter*, and anaerobic bacteria, may also cause bite wound infections.

Typically, *P. multocida* infection causes rapid development of local swelling, erythema (redness), and pain, usually within a few hours of the bite. Shortly after the bite occurs, the wound may start to exude a blood-tinged fluid. After 24 to 48 hours, local swelling may resolve, or the bacteria may spread into other tissues, causing swelling and pain some distance away from the wound. In some cases, systemic signs, such as swollen lymph nodes, and flulike symptoms, such as fever, chills, and muscle pain, may be present. Occasionally, even more severe complications may develop, including osteomyelitis, septic arthritis, tendon and joint infections, meningitis, brain abscess, and septicemia, as well as scar formation and disfigurement. Persons with underlying diseases or immune system dysfunction are at particularly high risk of serious wound complications. Victims of bite wounds may also develop diseases transmitted by animal bites, including rabies and cat-scratch disease.

Capnocytophaga has recently been recognized as the causative agent of a distinctive illness that follows a scratch or bite. The incubation time is 3 to 6 days, followed by symptoms resembling influenza. These symptoms may be present even if there is no significant lesion at the site of trauma. As with other bacteria that invade bite wounds, *Capnocytophaga* infections are potentially most dangerous in persons who are immunocompromised or who have undergone a splenectomy.

The risk of complications from bite or scratch wounds can be substantially reduced by prompt first aid following a bite wound (Box 35-4).

Allergies

Allergies to animal dander, fur, urine, and saliva are common among persons working in veterinary hospitals. Cats are frequently the allergen source, although allergies to dogs, horses, cows, and laboratory species (rabbits, rats, mice, hamsters, gerbils, guinea pigs) are also commonly reported. The route of exposure to animal allergens is usually airborne, with common clinical signs including itchy and runny nose and eyes, conjunctivitis, or urticaria (raised, red, itchy lesions). More serious symptoms include coughing, wheezing, and shortness of breath. Symptoms usually peak within 1 hour of exposure to the allergen, although delayed asthmatic reactions may be seen up to 12 hours after contact. Allergic symptoms may occur following a lick, scratch, or bite, but this is relatively rare.

Affected persons usually have a positive skin test to allergens from one or more animal species. Desensitization using repeated injection of allergen extracts is sometimes successful in reducing the severity of the allergic response. An experimental vaccine against feline allergies is currently being developed.

Allergic persons are advised to avoid contact with the offending animal species and to consult an allergist regarding the use of antihistamines and other drugs to prevent or treat symptoms. If contact with the animal species cannot be avoided, use of gloves and a surgical mask is effective in reducing exposure to most allergens.

Vaccine Self-Inoculation

Veterinary hospital employees occasionally accidentally inject themselves with vaccines intended for use in animals. Adverse reactions, including anaphylaxis and delayed hypersensitivity, have been reported and are thought to be induced by the adjuvants (mineral oils, aluminum

---

BOX 35-4   TREATMENT OF CANINE OR FELINE BITE WOUNDS

1. Wash the wound thoroughly with a surgical preparation solution such as chlorhexidine or povidone-iodine. Surgical preparation solutions are preferred to soaps, which may contain detergents that cause pain and delay wound healing. A sterile gauze may be used to gently clean the wound, but vigorous scrubbing should be avoided. After washing, an open wound should be irrigated with up to 1 L of normal saline using an 18-gauge blunted needle on a 35-ml syringe. The saline should be applied with maximal pressure in order to flush out bacteria, devitalized tissue, and other materials.

2. If the wound is severe, seek medical attention within 24 hours. The infection potential of a bite wound is reduced if it is treated promptly with deep irrigation and debridement, which should only be administered by a physician. Some physicians advocate suturing, but many do not unless the wound is on the face or is deep and hemorrhagic. If signs of infection are present, the physician will likely culture the wound and prescribe antibiotics.

3. Use of prophylactic antibiotics in persons with fresh, clean wounds is controversial. Studies show that the incidence of canine bite wound infections is not reduced when antibiotics are given prophylactically. Feline bite wounds have a higher risk of infection, and most physicians routinely prescribe antibiotics for persons with deep cat bites. In the case of a bite wound that is already visibly infected, it is generally agreed that antibiotics should be administered. There is no single antibiotic that is effective against all the aerobic and anaerobic bacteria that cause wound infections, and therefore culture and sensitivity testing are commonly required. Antibiotics should only be used if prescribed by a physician.

4. Soaking the affected region in hot water (or applying a hot, damp cloth) may give temporary pain relief. If purulent material accumulates, it may require drainage by a physician.

5. Tetanus is a potential (although uncommon) complication of any bite wound. There are two ways to prevent tetanus: use of tetanus toxoid (which causes the formation of antibodies and confers long-term immunity) and use of human tetanus immune globulin (injection of preformed antibody, which gives short-term protection only). It is advisable that all persons working in veterinary hospitals be vaccinated with tetanus toxoid every 5 years to develop active immunity to this disease. Tetanus toxoid must be administered before a bite wound occurs, to allow time for an immune response to develop. Persons who have not been previously immunized with tetanus toxoid should be given tetanus immune globulin immediately after a bite wound occurs.

6. If the biting animal is potentially rabid, the local health department and the victim's physician should be contacted, because rabies prophylaxis may be necessary.

---

hydroxide) contained in the vaccines. Anaphylactic reactions occur shortly after inoculation and are characterized by difficult breathing, skin eruptions, and shaking. Immediate administration of epinephrine is an effective treatment but should be undertaken under the supervision of a physician.

Some vaccines, including brucellosis (strain 19), *Mycobacterium paratuberculosis* (Johne's disease), and *Aeromonas salmonicida* (salmon furunculosis) are associated with a particularly high incidence of reactions following accidental self-inoculation. Delayed hypersensitivity reactions to these vaccines usually occur hours to days after inoculation, with clinical signs of swelling, redness, and pain at the injection site. Granuloma formation may also occur.

If self-inoculation occurs with any vaccine, the site should be immediately washed with soap and water. Bleeding should be encouraged to help drain injected material from the wound. Medical treatment should be sought at once. Tetanus prophylaxis is recommended following self-inoculation if the victim does not have a current tetanus toxoid immunization. Treatment with warm packs and immobilization of the area is helpful in reducing local pain and irritation.

Technician Note

If self-inoculation occurs with any vaccine, the site should be immediately washed with soap and water.

Laboratory Hazards

Most technicians and other hospital employees are well aware of the potential for catching a zoonotic disease from a living patient (e.g., a dog with rabies). Equally serious but less obvious hazards are associated with handling diagnostic samples, including bacterial or fungal cultures, blood, feces, urine, and tissue specimens, which may contain the same viruses, bacteria, protozoa, or parasites that cause zoonotic diseases.

Infections are usually acquired by one of three routes: ingestion, direct contact, or inhalation.

Ingestion of contaminated materials may occur by eating or drinking, smoking, biting nails, chewing on pens, or otherwise placing articles in the mouth after handling contaminated specimens. Frequent, thorough hand washing is the best way to prevent ingestion of infective substances. It is also a good idea to avoid touching the face or eyes with the hands when doing laboratory work.

Ingestion may also occur when pipetting liquids by mouth. Mouth pipetting should *never* be employed when working with urine, blood, serum, or other specimens from a veterinary patient.

Infections may also be acquired through *direct skin* or *mucous membrane contact* with contaminated materials. A few infectious agents are able to penetrate intact skin, and many can cross intact mucous membranes in the mouth, nose, and conjunctiva. Almost all agents can invade if there are cuts or abrasions present in the skin. Again, hand washing is the single best way to prevent infection by this route. In some circumstances the use of protective equipment, such as gloves, goggles, a face shield, or biologic safety cabinet, may be advisable.

Infection by *inhalation* of microorganisms may occur whenever aerosols are produced, such as when performing a dental prophylaxis using an ultrasonic scaler. Infective aerosols may also be inhaled when examining a fungal or bacterial culture that is producing spores or when flaming an inoculating loop or needle that has been used to culture bacteria. The risk of inhaling microorganisms is greatly reduced if a surgical mask is worn. Goggles are also recommended in some cases, particularly dental procedures.

Spills may occur when working with a diagnostic sample, such as urine or blood, or when handling a broth or other liquid culture. Because of the potential for disease transmission, it is a good practice to treat all spills with disinfectant such as chlorhexidine or a 1:10 dilution of 5% bleach, followed by application of an absorbent material, such as cat litter, to absorb all liquid. Gloves should be worn for spill cleanup if a zoonotic agent is present or if a strong disinfectant, such as bleach or glutaraldehyde, is used. If spills are likely to occur, it may be helpful to place a paper towel on the work surface before starting.

Universal Precautions

Health care workers who treat human patients are very aware of the risks of disease transmission when working with human blood and other body fluids. This caution is justified because of the risk of acquiring the human immunodeficiency virus (HIV) or hepatitis B or C viruses from human specimens. The most common route of exposure to these agents in a health care setting is a needle-stick injury, although infection may also occur after direct skin or mucous membrane contact with infected blood.

In response to this problem, the human health care professions have adopted universal precautions when handling blood, saliva, and other body fluids. Universal precautions specify that gloves should be worn when touching blood and body fluids, mucous membranes, or nonintact skin on all human patients. Gloves are also worn when handling items or surfaces soiled with blood or body fluids and for performing venipuncture. Hands and other skin surfaces are washed immediately and thoroughly after contact with blood or other body fluids. Because it is impossible to reliably identify all patients infected with HIV or hepatitis viruses, precautions are used when handling blood and body fluid from *all* patients (hence the term *universal*).

Although universal precautions are not routinely applied when working with veterinary patients or their body fluids and excretions, a few agents may be transmitted from animal blood and fluids to humans (either directly or by inhalation of aerosols) and universal precautions should be applied when working with samples containing these agents. Samples from patients diagnosed with anthrax, brucellosis, tularemia, *Erysipelothrix* infection, rabies, equine encephalitis, viral disease in monkeys, plague, Q fever, chlamydiosis, *Hantavirus* infection, and other readily transmissible zoonotic diseases should be handled only with universal precautions. Pregnant women should also use universal precautions when handling specimens that may contain toxoplasmosis oocysts or *Listeria* organisms.

Sharps

Caution is needed when handling sharps (needles, scalpel blades), particularly those that have been used for necropsy or surgical procedures. Not only are these materials often coated with infectious materials but also they can cause a skin wound that will inoculate the infectious material into the wound site, vastly increasing the probability of infection. Exposure to infectious material may also occur if syringe contents leak or are sprayed on skin, eyes, or mucous membranes.

All scalpel blades, needles, and other sharp disposable objects should be capped or discarded in a puncture-proof, sturdy container immediately after use. Needles and other sharps should never be thrown into regular trash containers, even if capped. Once filled, sharps containers should not be opened and the contents should not be transferred to another container.

Technician Note

All scalpel blades, needles, and other sharp disposable objects should be capped or discarded in a puncture-proof, sturdy container immediately after use.

To prevent needle-stick injuries, needles should not be purposely bent or broken or otherwise manipulated by hand. It is safer to dispose of a syringe and needle together rather than to attempt to remove the needle and to reuse the syringe. Recapping needles is a common cause of needle-stick injury, and capping is not advised before disposal. If capping is necessary, the "one-handed" method should be used (the cap is placed on a flat surface, and the needle is threaded onto the syringe using only one hand).

RADIATION SAFETY

Persons working in veterinary hospitals may be exposed to electromagnetic radiation produced by x-ray machines, fluoroscopes, lasers, radioisotopes, and ultraviolet lamps. Electromagnetic radiation consists of photons of energy traveling at the speed of light. Photons are identical, no matter what type of electromagnetic radiation is involved; however, different forms of radiation have different wavelengths.

Some forms of electromagnetic radiation, including x-rays, have a potential to damage cells even in relatively small doses. One factor that determines the risk associated with a given type of radiation is whether it is an *ionizing* or a *nonionizing* form of radiation. Ionizing radiation (e.g., x-rays) causes the formation of ions and free radicals as it passes through tissues. These ions may cause chromosomal damage and have other deleterious effects. The tissues most sensitive to radiation are the skin, ovaries or testes, intestine, and bone marrow. Nonionizing radiation either does not penetrate very well through tissues (e.g., visible light), or it may penetrate tissues and pass through them with minimal harmful effects (e.g., radio waves). High doses of nonionizing radiation can damage tissue (e.g., too much infrared or ultraviolet radiation can cause a burn), but the potential for chromosomal damage is less than for ionizing radiation.

X-rays and other forms of ionizing radiation cannot be detected by human senses, and a person may be bombarded with even a fatal dose of x-rays yet feel no unusual sensation. X-rays are able to penetrate human tissue in the same way that they penetrate through the chest or leg of an animal being radiographed and can therefore cause damage not only to the skin but also to underlying organs. This also means that if the abdomen of a pregnant woman is irradiated with x-rays, the fetus is exposed.

An individual's exposure to x-rays can come from a variety of sources: environmental, medical, and occupational. *Environmental sources* include cosmic rays produced by the sun and building materials, such as concrete, soil, and brick (which contain minute amounts of radioactive materials such as uranium and radon). In North America, the average environmental exposure is approximately 2 mSv (millisievert) per year.* *Medical exposure* results from x-rays ordered by a physician or dentist, including dental x-rays, chest or abdominal x-rays, and mammograms. The average dose of medical and dental x-rays has been calculated to be 0.5 to 0.7 mSv per person per year in the United States (DHHS, 1988). *Occupational exposure* refers to the radiation that is received when a person takes x-rays as part of his or her job. Veterinary hospital personnel have a potential occupational exposure whenever they are in a room where a radiograph is being taken, unless they are standing behind a lead screen. The extent of occupational exposure depends on many factors, including the number of x-rays taken, the use of shielding devices such as lead aprons and gloves, and the person's proximity to the x-ray beam. For any person who operates an x-ray machine in the United States, the maximal permissible whole-body dose is 50 mSv (5 rem) per year. In Canada, the maximal permissible dose is 20 mSv (2 rem) per year. Veterinary personnel using appropriate precautions are rarely exposed to more than a fraction of this. One survey of veterinarians reported a maximal exposure equivalent to 14.4 mSv (1.44 rem) per year.

The 50-mSv yearly limit applies only to nonpregnant adults who are required to take x-rays as part of their job. For persons under 18 years old (including student trainees) the allowable whole-body exposure is only 5 mSv (0.5 rem) in the United States and 1 mSv (0.1 rem) in Canada. Canadian regulations also specify that the maximal permissible occupational exposure to a pregnant woman's abdomen during the 9 months of pregnancy is 2 mSv (0.2 rem). The U.S. National Council on Radiation Protection and Measurements recommends that fetal radiation not exceed 5 mSv during pregnancy.

Effect of Radiation on Adults

It has been well established that the risk of health problems rises as the amount of radiation exposure increases. In the case of a low-dosage exposure, cellular damage may result but is usually repaired and no permanent harm is likely. Higher levels of radiation can cause permanent damage to chromosomes and may injure the skin, gonads, bone marrow, and other tissues. Chromosomal damage may also lead to increased risk of cancer, particularly of the thyroid gland, bone, and lymphatic and hematopoietic systems. There is also some potential for development of lens cataracts following long-term exposure of the eyes to low levels of radiation.

Technician Note

It has been well established that the risk of health problems rises as the amount of radiation exposure increases.

---

*A sievert (Sv) is a metric unit that indicates the amount of biologic damage that can occur from radiation. One sievert is equal to 100 rem, which is equal to the biologic effect of 100 rad of x-rays being absorbed by the body. The higher the Sv, the higher the exposure to x-rays and the more potential for tissue damage. It is most common for low doses to be expressed in millisieverts (mSv), one of which is equal to one thousandth of a sievert. 1 Sv = 1000 mSv = 100 rem. Similarly, 1 mSv = 0.1 rem = 100 mrem.

Veterinary staff using appropriate safety precautions are at very low risk for these problems provided their exposure is under the occupational limit, 50 mSv per year (Wiggins et al, 1989; Schenker et al, 1990).

Effect of Radiation on the Fetus

Pregnant woman who receive high doses of radiation are at increased risk of spontaneous abortion or congenital defects in the fetus. The effect on the fetus depends on the amount of radiation received and the time during gestation that it occurs. If a woman is exposed to a large dose of radiation in the period *immediately before* pregnancy begins, there is an increased incidence of leukemia and Down's syndrome in the children conceived after exposure. Presumably these children are affected because the egg cell from which they arose was damaged by the radiation. If a woman is extensively exposed to radiation during the *first 2 weeks after conception*, there is no higher incidence of fetal malformations, but a very high incidence of embryo death is observed. If extensive radiation exposure is received *between 3 and 11 weeks after conception*, severe abnormalities may result, including brain abnormalities (epilepsy, retardation, microcephaly) and ocular, genital, and skeletal defects. If high doses of radiation are received *between 11 and 16 weeks after conception*, abnormalities such as stunted growth, mental retardation, and microcephaly are seen but are generally less severe than for fetuses affected in the 3- to 11-week period. Fetuses who receive high doses of radiation *after 16 weeks* have a lower incidence of defects, and the defects reported are generally minor (including hair loss and skin lesions).

Given the potential for fetal loss or damage, many women hesitate to undertake radiographic duties when pregnant. However, it is generally accepted that there is no increased risk of obvious birth defects or embryonic death for the children of mothers who are exposed to less than 50 mSv of x-ray radiation during pregnancy. Some investigators believe there is a possibility that lower doses of x-rays may have subtle effects on the fetus, including increased risk of leukemia and nervous system changes. There is some evidence of a slightly increased risk of spontaneous abortion among veterinarians and veterinary assistants who take more than four radiographs per week during pregnancy, even though the 5-mSv exposure limit is not exceeded (Schenker et al, 1990). A pregnant employee should discuss this issue with her physician to determine the course of action with which she is most comfortable. If an employee continues to perform radiography duties while pregnant, she must wear a dosimeter and good-quality protective equipment (apron, gloves) and use care to avoid unnecessary exposure to x-rays (in particular, exposure to the primary x-ray beam).

Technician Note

If an employee continues to perform radiographic duties while pregnant, she must wear a dosimeter and good-quality protective equipment (apron, gloves) and use care to avoid unnecessary exposure to x-rays (in particular, exposure to the primary x-ray beam).

Protecting Yourself from X-Ray Radiation

The basic principle of protection from x-ray radiation is simply to avoid unnecessary exposure to x-rays. The level of exposure should be ALARA (*as low as reasonably achievable*). This can be done in three ways:

- *Time:* decreasing the time one is exposed to x-rays
- *Distance:* increasing the distance from the source
- *Shielding:* use of protective clothing containing lead

Exposure to x-rays may occur in two ways. The first (and by far the most serious) is contact with the primary beam, which is the stream of x-rays that flows from the machine and passes through the animal, the photographic film, and the hands of any personnel who are "in the way" of the beam. It is a basic principle of veterinary radiography safety that no human hands or other body parts should be placed in the primary beam, even if lead gloves are worn. The other form of exposure, more common but less intense, is the x-rays that are bounced off (scattered) after contacting the x-ray table and the animal.

To prevent unnecessary exposure to x-rays, the following precautions should be taken:

1. *Do not take any more x-rays than necessary.* Some practices rotate x-ray duties among staff members so that no one employee receives the entire exposure to x-rays. It also makes sense to use the best technique possible to limit the number of retakes. Careful measurement of the animal, adequate sedation, proper positioning, use of a technique chart, and optimal film processing all help to reduce the frequency of retakes.

2. *When exposing a film, use the least amount of radiation possible.* Fast screens and film should be used to reduce the amount of radiation required to produce an image. Use of higher-kilovoltage techniques allows the milliampere-seconds (mAs) setting to be reduced, which in turn decreases the dose of x-rays received by the animal and hospital employees. Obviously, only persons who are thoroughly familiar with the operation of the x-ray machine should adjust machine controls.

3. *Stay as far from the x-ray beam as possible when the radiograph is being taken.* The closer a person stands to an x-ray beam, the greater the amount of scattered radiation that strikes him or her. In the case of the primary beam, the strength of x-rays falls off as the square of the distance from the source. Thus a person who is in the path of the primary beam, 2 feet away from the source of the beam, will receive only one fourth the amount of radiation received by the person who is 1 foot away from the source of the beam. The ideal solution is to be out of the room or behind a lead screen when the radiograph is taken, and in some states this is a legal requirement. Restraint of the animal can be achieved through the use of anesthetics or passive restraint devices, such as sandbags and foam wedges. Walls composed of concrete block or double-thick dry wall provide some protection, and by leaving the room one increases the distance from the primary beam such that very little radiation exposure occurs anyway. If a person stays in the room to press the button, he or she can be effectively protected by a lead-lined screen placed between the control panel and the x-ray table. If no lead screen is available, protective equipment must be worn.

4. *Any person restraining an animal for radiography must keep the hands out of the primary beam.* Exposure to high doses of radiation occurs whenever hands are exposed to the primary beam, whether or not lead-lined gloves are worn. Gloves are not designed to protect the hands

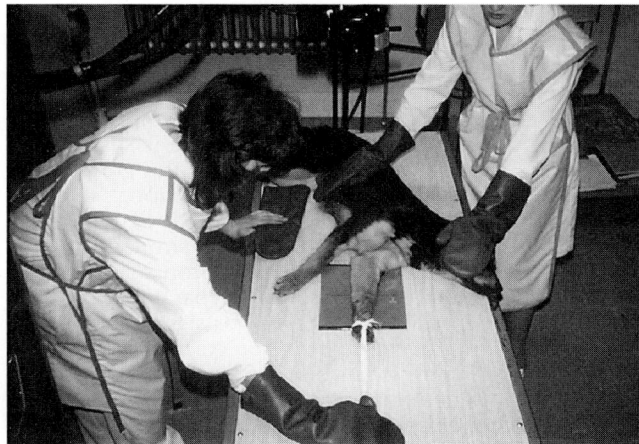

FIGURE 35-2.   Use of gauze ties to restrain animals. The hands are kept well away from the direct x-ray beam.

from these levels of radiation. If the outline of fingers or gloves appears on the developed image, the hands were exposed to the primary beam. This type of exposure usually arises when handling very small patients, such as a bird, or when photographing extremities. Small patients can be taped to the cassette, and rope or gauze can be used to hold a leg that is being radiographed (Figure 35-2).

It is much easier to avoid exposure to the primary beam if it is collimated down to the bare minimum. Ideally, there should be a clear (nonexposed) border of 12 inches around the outside of the exposed film, which indicates that the beam size was reduced to cover less than the area of the photographic plate.

If it is necessary to restrain animals for radiographic procedures, it is a good idea to stand as upright as possible. Persons who sit on or lean over the x-ray table are exposed to much greater amounts of scattered radiation.

5. All persons in the room where an x-ray is being taken must wear protective clothing, including lead-lined gloves and an apron, unless standing behind a lead barrier or control booth.

   a. *Gloves.* Bulky, full-hand gloves offer good protection from x-ray exposure. Seamless lead-vinyl gloves are available that are lighter and more flexible than conventional gloves yet offer comparable protection. One-sided gloves (hand shields) are commercially available and have the advantage of allowing greater dexterity. However, one-sided gloves may not adequately protect the hands from scatter radiation and are not legal for use in some jurisdictions in the United States. Whatever type of glove is used, there should be enough gloves for every person in the room (usually a minimum of two pairs per practice).

   b. *Aprons.* Aprons used for x-ray voltages up to 150 kVp must contain 0.5 mm of lead sheet. The thickness of lead contained in an apron must be permanently marked on the outside of the apron. At 70 kVp, this amount of shielding reduces exposure by a factor of 800.

In addition to mandatory gloves and aprons, other protective equipment is available and its use is recommended. Thyroid collars protect the thyroid gland, which is a potential site of x-ray-induced cancer. Lead glasses protect the eyes from radiation and thus help to prevent the development of cataracts.

All equipment must be in good repair and tested yearly for leaks (more often if damage is suspected). This testing can be done by placing the glove on a cassette and taking a radiograph using enough kilovolt peak and milliampere-seconds to slightly penetrate the lead.* Aprons can be examined in a similar manner, using masking tape to divide the apron into sections and radiographing each section separately. The test radiographs should be checked for signs of exposure (black), which indicate tears or cracks in the lead. Gloves and aprons can also be tested using fluoroscopic equipment if available.

X-ray aprons and gloves should not be folded for storage, because creases may cause permanent weak lines and cracks. It is acceptable to leave the apron on the x-ray table between uses, or it may be hung over a round surface. Gloves should be stored in a vertical position to allow air circulation inside the glove. Equipment containing lead should never be machine washed but can be safely wiped with hospital disinfectants.

X-ray safety equipment is expensive and easily damaged and should never be used to restrain or capture fractious animals. A single bite can damage the lead and make the glove virtually useless.

6. *If a portable x-ray unit is used, special precautions must be taken to prevent exposure.* Persons in the vicinity should be warned that x-rays are about to be taken and cautioned to put adequate distance between themselves and the x-ray beam. Persons near the x-ray source must wear protective gloves and aprons. No person should stand in the direct path of the beam, even at a distance. X-ray cassettes should never be held by hand, since any person who holds or stands behind the cassette when a radiograph is taken receives direct exposure to the primary beam. In addition, the portable x-ray machine should never be held by hand when the exposure is being made.

7. *Monitor x-ray exposure using a dosimeter (also called a monitor or film badge).* A dosimeter is a small piece of thermoluminescent material or radiosensitive film that should be worn by each person taking radiographs. Badges used in veterinary radiography are usually worn on the outside collar of the apron, at the level of the thyroid gland, although wrist badges and waist-level monitors are also available. The dosimeter records the amount and type of radiation received by that person. After a period of use (1 to 3 months), the thermoluminescent plaque from the dosimeter is returned to the dosimeter service so that the exposure to x-rays can be measured. Exposure results are returned to the employer and must be made available to all employees.

Every person who is occupationally exposed to ionizing radiation (in other words, in the room when a radiograph is taken or assisting in a procedure using a portable x-ray machine) is required to wear a dosime-

ter. Staff members who assist in radiography should have their own dosimeters clearly marked with their names.

Dosimeters provide several types of useful information. They verify that the legal dose limit has not been exceeded, and they give each employee an exact measure of occupational exposure. Comparison of dosimeter readings also allows the veterinarian or employee to detect changes in exposure levels, which may be the result of poor technique, increased workload, or equipment problems. Dosimeters are sensitive to dosages as small as 0.2 mSv (20 mrem). Exposures smaller than this are indicated on the report as a dash (—).

8. Persons under 18 years of age should not be in the room when a radiograph is taken.

> ### Technician Note
> Persons under 18 years of age should not be in the room when a radiograph is taken.

Developing X-Ray Films

Poor darkroom procedures can lead to excessive exposure to x-rays. If incorrect developing times or temperatures are used, it will be necessary to retake numerous films, increasing employee exposure to radiation. A common problem is the use of developer that is over 1 month old or that has not been mixed or replenished according to the manufacturer's recommendations. Another common mistake is failure to agitate the chemicals in hand tanks before use. Failure to use good darkroom technique may lead to underdevelopment of the films (films appear too light). In order to compensate, the x-ray machine operator may increase exposure settings, causing unnecessary exposure to radiation. When the developing problem is corrected, the radiographs often appear very dark, an indication that the settings on the x-ray machine have been set artificially high to overcome the poor developing performance.

Chemicals used to develop and fix x-ray film are corrosive. The chief hazards associated with exposure to these chemicals are as follows:

- Severe eye irritation, including the potential for permanent corneal damage if the liquid is splashed in the eye
- Respiratory tract irritation and burning if concentrated vapors are inhaled
- Skin irritation if there is direct contact with unprotected skin; allergic dermatitis has also been reported after long-term exposure to these chemicals

Federal regulations in the United States and Canada require that hazard labels be present on or adjacent to developing tanks. Staff must be trained in safe handling techniques for pouring, mixing, or transporting chemicals. Protective equipment, such as gloves and goggles, must be provided for persons who hand develop x-rays using tanks. Hands should be washed after hand developing films, even if gloves are worn. The darkroom should be equipped with an eyewash fountain in case of eye exposure.

Ventilation of the darkroom by means of an exhaust fan or similar device is usually necessary to prevent the accumulation of toxic vapors. Tanks should be kept covered when not in use.

The use of automatic processors greatly reduces the potential exposure to developing chemicals. There is some risk of chemical exposure when cleaning or replenishing the automatic processor, and employees should use appro-

---

*The following are approximate settings that can be used to check protective clothing for leaks: aprons and thyroid shields: 90 kVp and 5 to 10 mAs; gloves: 90 kVp and 10 to 20 mAs. At the correct exposure, a gray image should result.

BOX 35-5   SOURCES OF WASTE ANESTHETIC GAS

- Anesthetic machines in use
- Expired air from anesthetized patients (leaking around endotracheal tubes or masks)
- Expired air from recovering patients
- Anesthetic chambers
- Liquid anesthetic spills
- Anesthetic machine components, such as rubber reservoir bags and rubber hoses (absorb anesthetic gases and release them into the air of the room in which they are stored)

TABLE 35-1   HALOTHANE CONCENTRATIONS WITHIN VETERINARY HOSPITALS

Location	ppm
Personnel breathing zone	
With scavenging	1.45
No scavenging	2.00
Air around unscavenged anesthetic chamber	>10
Nose and mouth of anesthetized patient	
Intubated, cuff inflated	3.25
Intubated, cuff not inflated	6.10
Air outside recovery cage door	1.07
Nose of patient in recovery cage	5.43

Modified from Short CE, Harvey RC: Anesthetic waste gases in veterinary medicine, *Cornell Vet* 73:363, 1983.

---

priate protective clothing and equipment (gloves, protective eye wear, waterproof apron) for these procedures.

Developing chemicals may react dangerously with other chemicals, including liquid drain cleaners, and should never be poured into a sink or drain in which other chemicals may be present. Environmental regulations in many areas prohibit disposal of fixer solutions into sinks or drains. Silver recovery units are a responsible alternative method of disposal.

HAZARDS ASSOCIATED WITH ANESTHESIA

In recent years, concerns have been raised about the safety of operating room personnel exposed to high levels of waste anesthetic gas in human and veterinary hospitals. The term *waste anesthetic gas* refers to vapors of nitrous oxide, halothane, isoflurane, or methoxyflurane that are present in the room air of a veterinary hospital. Exposure to these agents can occur in several ways (Box 35-5).

Surveys of veterinary hospitals reveal a wide range in waste anesthetic gas levels, depending on the location within the clinic and the anesthetic equipment and techniques used. The highest levels of contamination are associated with spills of anesthetic liquids. Liquid anesthetic rapidly evaporates when it is poured or spilled, producing a large amount of anesthetic vapor that rapidly mixes with room air. Accidental spillage of only 1 ml of liquid halothane, for example, will evaporate to form 200 ml of gas with a concentration of 1 million parts per million (ppm).* Liquid anesthetic can also penetrate intact skin and be absorbed into the circulation.

Even without a spill, considerable amounts of waste gas may be generated within the average veterinary hospital (Table 35-1). This is a silent danger, often undetected by the staff or veterinarian. It is sometimes erroneously believed that if the odor of anesthetic gas is not present, the room air is safe. Unfortunately, the human nose can only detect halothane if the concentration is at least 30 ppm. This level is already 15 times higher than the maximal recommended level.

Significant levels of waste gas are commonly found in areas where anesthetic machines are in use, including surgery suites, surgical preparation rooms, and treatment rooms where dentistry or minor surgery is performed.

Recovery rooms may also be contaminated by waste gas as it is exhaled by animals awakening from anesthesia.

During the anesthetic period itself, the level of waste gas is highest immediately adjacent to the anesthetic machine and the patient's mouth. The actual level depends on several factors, including the duration of anesthesia (the longer the machine is in use, the higher the waste gas concentration in the room air), the flow rate of the carrier gas (higher flow rates may lead to more waste gas pollution), and whether an effective scavenging system is used. If no scavenging system is present, anesthetic gas mixed with oxygen is vented through an open pop-off valve at a rate approximately equal to the oxygen flow rate (usually 500 ml to 3 L/min). If a nonrebreathing system, such as a Bain circuit, is in use, the gas exits through the relief valve or reservoir bag outlet. Either way, all the waste gas enters the room air when no scavenger is present.

Surveys of veterinary hospitals indicate that levels of waste anesthetic gas in *unscavenged* veterinary surgeries range from 1 to 34 ppm for halothane, 1 to 62 ppm for methoxyflurane, and 6 to 270 ppm for nitrous oxide. Levels for *scavenged* surgery rooms are usually between 0 and 10 ppm depending on the sampling location (see Table 35-1).

Room ventilation also affects the waste gas level, and rooms with a ceiling fan, wall fan, or other ventilating device generally have lower levels of waste gas. It is advised that all rooms in which anesthetic gases are released have at least 15 air changes per hour.

Effects of Waste Anesthetic Gas

Since the first study of waste anesthetic gas was published in 1967, many investigators have attempted to determine the toxicity of isoflurane, halothane, methoxyflurane, nitrous oxide, and other anesthetic agents used for medical and veterinary anesthesia. Although much of the evidence is contradictory, it is generally accepted that exposure to waste anesthetic gas is associated with a higher than normal incidence of both acute and chronic health problems. These problems appear to be dose dependent (i.e., the greater the exposure, the greater the risk).

Short-term problems, such as those that occur during or immediately after exposure to waste anesthetic gas, include drowsiness, headache, fatigue, nausea, pruritus, depression, and irritability. These symptoms usually resolve spontaneously when the affected person leaves the area, but their frequent occurrence indicates that excessive levels of waste gas are present and a potential for long-term toxicity exists.

---

*The term *parts per million* is a measure of concentration. An atmosphere that is 100% composed of a certain gas has 1 million ppm of that gas. If the concentration of a gas is 1% in room air, this is equivalent to 10,000 ppm. Patients connected to an anesthetic machine delivering 1% halothane in oxygen are therefore breathing 10,000 ppm of halothane and 990,000 ppm of oxygen.

Long-term effects of anesthetic gas may include any of the following: reproductive disorders (including increased risk of spontaneous abortion and increased incidence of congenital defects), liver or kidney damage, and nervous system dysfunction (muscle weakness, tingling sensations, numbness). It is thought that these effects are due to the action of metabolites produced by the breakdown of anesthetic agents within the body. These toxic metabolites include inorganic fluoride or bromide ions, oxalic acid, free radicals, and other substances known to have harmful effects on animal tissues. If this theory is correct, anesthetics that are retained by the body and metabolized (e.g., methoxyflurane, halothane) have greater potential for long-term toxicity than those that are rapidly eliminated through the lungs (e.g., isoflurane). Significant amounts of methoxyflurane or halothane may linger in the liver, kidney, and body fat stores for long periods. For example, anesthetists have been shown to have traces of halothane in their breath as long as 64 hours after administering this gas to a patient.

All hospital staff (and in particular, pregnant women) should avoid exposure to high levels of waste anesthetic gas, particularly nitrous oxide, during pregnancy. Controls should be introduced to reduce waste gas levels to 2 ppm in room air. When volatile anesthetics are used with nitrous oxide, the maximal advisable concentration is 0.5 ppm for isoflurane, methoxyflurane, and halothane and 25 ppm for nitrous oxide (8-hour time-weighted average). It is generally accepted that provided these limits are not exceeded, exposure to waste anesthetic gas is associated with minimal risk, even to pregnant women.

Minimizing Exposure to Waste Gas

There are five important ways in which exposure to waste gas can be reduced to a minimum:

- Install an effective scavenging system.
- Test the anesthetic machine for gas leaks before it is used each day.
- Utilize anesthetic techniques that reduce waste gas release.
- Use and maintain anesthetic equipment as advised by the manufacturer.
- Use protective equipment when exposure is unavoidable (e.g., when cleaning up liquid anesthetic spills) (Figure 35-3).

Scavenging Systems

A scavenger (more properly termed a *gas-scavenging system*) is an apparatus that collects waste gas from the pop-off valve of an anesthetic machine and conducts it to a disposal point outside the building. The installation and use of an effective scavenger constitute the single most important step in reducing the exposure of hospital employees to waste anesthetic gas. One survey of veterinary hospitals showed that scavengers reduced waste halothane concentrations by up to 94%.

Technician Note

The installation and use of an effective scavenger constitute the single most important step in reducing the exposure of hospital employees to waste anesthetic gas.

Many types of scavengers are available, but all of them have the same basic design. Waste gas from the anesthetic machine is conveyed to a disposal point by a tube or hose

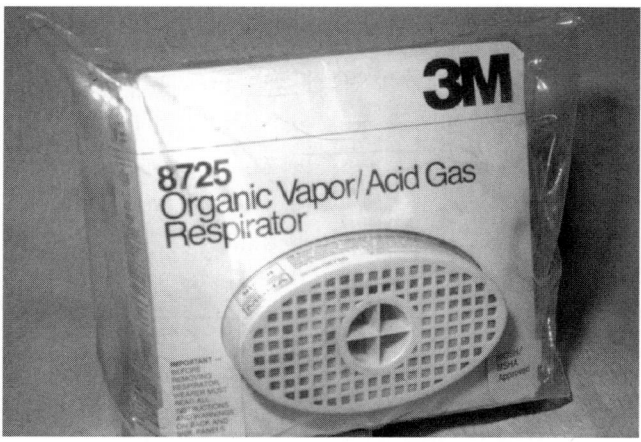

FIGURE 35-3. A cartridge respirator suitable for cleaning up spills of anesthetic liquids and other organic chemicals.

connected to the pop-off valve of the anesthetic machine. In some systems (passive scavenging systems) the tube simply carries the waste gas to an open window or exhaust vent in the wall. The gas flows by gravity and because it is pushed by the pressure of gas in the anesthetic machine. Another type of system (active scavenging system) uses a vacuum pump or fan to draw the gas away from the anesthetic machine and discharges it through a vent to the outdoors. The vacuum system can be part of the hospital's central vacuum system, or (preferably) it can be an independent system. Both active and passive scavenging systems are effective, provided they are correctly installed.

Modern anesthetic machines are equipped with pop-off valves that are designed to allow easy connection to scavenging systems. Adapters for use with older equipment are also available from anesthetic equipment suppliers. It is important to choose the type of pop-off connection that matches the type of scavenging system used, whether high vacuum, low vacuum, or passive. Nonrebreathing systems (e.g., a Bain circuit or Ayre's T-piece) should also be connected to a scavenger or other exhaust system. This can be achieved by connecting the scavenger hose to the outlet of the reservoir bag or the circuit. "Bag tail valves" and other adapters can be obtained from suppliers of anesthetic equipment.

No matter which type of scavenging system is chosen, the guidelines given in Box 35-6 should be followed.

Every anesthetic machine or anesthetic chamber in the hospital must be connected to a scavenger when in use. If it is not practical to install scavenging equipment in a specialized room (e.g., the radiography room), it is advised that either anesthesia be maintained with an injectable agent or that an anesthetic machine with an activated charcoal cartridge be used. These cartridges, available from safety supply firms, can effectively absorb isoflurane, halothane, and methoxyflurane vapors (not nitrous oxide) but must be replaced after 12 hours of use.

Leak Testing

Leakage of gas from anesthetic machines is a significant source of operating room pollution. Contamination from this source is not reduced by a scavenging system, because the gas escapes before it can reach the scavenger. In some cases, the presence of a leak is obvious—there may be an audible hiss, the odor of anesthetic, or a jet of air coming from the rebreathing bag or hose. Unfortunately, small

Box 35-6	GUIDELINES FOR THE USE OF WASTE GAS SCAVENGING SYSTEMS

- The anesthetic gas should be confined within the hose from the pop-off valve to the outlet, without passing through open air gaps.
- Air from the scavenging system must be discharged outside the building, away from doors, windows, and air intakes. Scavengers that discharge gas onto the floor of the surgery room, into the attic or basement of the clinic, or into a recirculating central vacuum system will contaminate all building rooms with waste gas.
- If a passive system is used, the hose should be as short as possible (maximum 10 feet in length) and should travel a downward course toward the exhaust. If possible, the hose should not travel on the floor, where it may be stepped on or trapped under equipment and occluded.
- Scavenging systems may become blocked, leading to accumulation of gas in the anesthetic circuit. The obvious indication that this is occurring is an overdistended reservoir bag. Such a blockage must be immediately resolved (if necessary, by disconnecting the scavenger), or it may lead to circulatory problems or lung damage in the patient. Some anesthetic machines are equipped with pressure-releasing valves that minimize this hazard.
- If an active system is used, the vacuum should not be so strong that it draws too much air from the anesthetic machine. The reservoir bag should always contain a sufficient amount of air to allow the patient to breathe comfortably. Anesthetic machines equipped with negative pressure-releasing valves will allow room air to enter the circuit if a vacuum inadvertently develops within the circuit.
- Scavenging systems with exhaust fans should be explosion proof and designed to handle waste gases that contain oxygen.

Box 35-7	LEAK TESTING PROCEDURES

1. Assemble the anesthetic machine together with all hoses and connections.
2. Close the pop-off valve, and place a hand or stopper over the Y-piece, closing off all avenues of gas escape from the machine.
3. Turn on the oxygen tank, and adjust the flowmeter to supply at least 2 L of oxygen per minute.
4. The reservoir bag is allowed to gradually fill with oxygen. The anesthetist should be able to squeeze the inflated bag with significant pressure without causing escape of air from the bag. Alternatively, the anesthetist can adjust the oxygen flow such that a circuit pressure of 30 cm H_2O is maintained for 30 seconds (this is indicated on the manometer). If the oxygen flow required to maintain this pressure is over 200 ml/min, there is significant leakage from the machine.
5. If nitrous oxide is used, a high-pressure test should also be performed. The nitrous oxide cylinder is turned on, and the tank pressure gauge reading is noted. The cylinder is then turned off. With the flowmeter set to zero, the pressure should be maintained in the system such that the tank pressure gauge reading is unchanged after 1 hour.

leaks are often inaudible and the odor is undetectable and can only be found by leak testing the machine. Leak-testing procedures should be performed at least daily, following a procedure similar to that outlined in Box 35-7. In addition, periodic inspection of the anesthetic machine (including leak testing) should be undertaken by a qualified medical equipment repair technician.

Once it has been determined that a leak is present, its location can sometimes be found by listening carefully for the source, or it may be located using a solution of liquid soap (e.g., dish-washing detergent) mixed with water. This solution is gently squirted on all potential leakage points, and each location is observed for bubble formation, indicating the escape of gas. Common locations for gas leaks include the tank connection to the machine, carbon dioxide absorbers, unidirectional valves, and reservoir bags. Once the source of the leak is identified, it can often be fixed by tightening a connection or replacing a part. If the leak cannot be fixed, the machine should not be used until it is serviced by qualified personnel.

Anesthetic Techniques
The anesthetist, by his or her choice of anesthetic techniques, can considerably reduce the amount of waste gas released into the room air. The procedures outlined Box 35-8 help to minimize waste gas release.

Equipment Concerns
Hoses, reservoir bags, masks, endotracheal tubes, and other rubber components of the anesthetic circuit should be washed with soap and water and air dried after each procedure. Washing not only removes absorbed waste gas but also reduces the transfer of microorganisms between patients.

Anesthetic vaporizers should be filled or drained only in a well-ventilated area. When pouring liquid anesthetic into the machine it is a good idea to use a filling device (supplied by most anesthetic manufacturers). Care should be taken to avoid overfilling the vaporizer or spilling the anesthetic.

Technician Note

Waste gas concentrations around the patient's head can be reduced by 50% if an endotracheal tube is used instead of a mask.

Because of the risk of exposure to significant levels of waste gas when emptying or filling anesthetic vaporizers, pregnant personnel should not be assigned to these tasks.

Empty anesthetic bottles should be capped before being discarded, because residual anesthetic may evaporate into the room air. Likewise, filling devices should be stored between uses in a sealed plastic bag.

If a bottle of anesthetic is accidentally broken or a spill occurs, the area should be immediately evacuated and cleanup procedures initiated as discussed under chemical spills.

Technician Note

Because of the risk of exposure to significant levels of waste gas when emptying or filling anesthetic vaporizers, pregnant personnel should not be assigned to these tasks.

Box 35-8   ANESTHESIA PROCEDURES AND PRECAUTIONS

- Avoid the use of anesthetic chambers as much as possible. Unless a scavenging system is connected to the chamber, large amounts of waste gas are released when the chamber is opened. In addition, the fur of the patient is saturated with anesthetic during the induction and gives off significant waste gas vapor when the animal is removed from the chamber. If a chamber must be used, it should be connected to a scavenging device and the chamber should be washed with soap and water immediately after each use to remove residual anesthetic. Chambers should only be used where ventilation is excellent, and the use of an exhaust fan or other means of evacuating room air to the outside is recommended.

- Avoid the use of face masks to maintain anesthesia. Waste gas concentrations around the patient's head can be reduced by 50% if an endotracheal tube is used instead of a mask. The high contamination level associated with masks is probably due to the escape of anesthetic gas around the mask, particularly if it is not fitted tightly over the animal's face. If face mask inductions are required, the animal should be intubated as soon as it reaches an appropriate depth.

- Cuffed endotracheal tubes significantly reduce the escape of waste gas into room air, compared with uncuffed tubes. To be effective, however, the tube must be of adequate size and the cuff must be inflated and in good repair.

- The vaporizer or nitrous oxide flowmeter should not be turned on until the anesthetic machine is connected to the endotracheal tube and the cuff is inflated. It is inadvisable to fill the reservoir bag with anesthetic gas before connecting the machine to the patient, because the gas is released directly into the room air. Once the procedure is under way, the patient should not be disconnected from the breathing circuit unless the vaporizer has first been turned to zero.

- The contents of the reservoir bag should not be released into the room air. Rather, the bag should be squeezed gently while still attached to the machine, to allow the scavenger to retrieve the waste gas.

- If possible, maintain the connection between the animal and the machine, with the animal breathing pure oxygen, for several minutes after the vaporizer is turned off. This allows expired anesthetic from the animal's lungs to enter the scavenging system rather than the room air. Obviously this is not always possible, for example, if the animal is awakening from anesthesia and is chewing on the endotracheal tube.

- Whenever possible, avoid being closer than 3 feet to the nose of a recovering or anesthetized animal.

Measurement of Waste Gas Levels in a Veterinary Hospital

A hospital can periodically monitor waste anesthetic gas levels to ensure that the 2-ppm limit is not exceeded in several ways. One method is to hire a professional monitoring service to visit the hospital to evaluate ventilation and scavenging techniques and to collect air samples to be analyzed for waste gas concentration. These monitoring services may be available through the companies that install and maintain anesthetic gas machines, or they may be listed under "Safety," "Industrial Hygiene," or "Air Sampling" in the yellow pages of the telephone book. It is also possible for clinic employees to monitor waste gas levels using detector tubes or dosimeter badges (similar to radiation badges) obtained from safety supply companies and monitoring services such as Assay Technology (800-833-1258). Some badges detect only one chemical, such as halothane or nitrous oxide, whereas others are sensitive to all organic vapors, including methoxyflurane, isoflurane, and halothane. The badges are worn for a timed period in a location where anesthetic gases are being used and then returned to the supplier for analysis. Results are given as time-weighted average in parts per million.

Compressed Gas Cylinders

Oxygen and nitrous oxide are purchased as compressed gases in metal cylinders. Several potential safety hazards associated with compressed gas cylinders are listed in Box 35-9.

CHEMICAL HAZARDS

Veterinary technicians frequently treat animals that have been poisoned or burned by chemicals such as pesticides, pharmaceuticals, and cleaning agents. These same chemicals are handled by veterinary hospital employees on a daily basis and may be as harmful to humans as they are to animals. Fortunately, it is possible to reduce the hazards significantly by taking commonsense safety precautions when storing, using, or disposing of chemicals (see Box 35-2).

How Chemicals Enter the Body

No matter how a chemical enters the body, it can cause two types of problems: acute and chronic. Acute effects are those experienced after a single large dose or exposure (e.g., pesticide splashing into the eyes) and often result in a trip to a hospital emergency room. Chronic effects are more insidious, since they usually result from repeated small doses absorbed over a long period. Chronic effects may not be apparent for years after the chemical exposure and are therefore difficult to trace back to any particular chemical or other cause. Both the acute and chronic effects of any given chemical are listed on its MSDS.

Chemicals normally enter the body by one of three routes: *inhalation, mucous membrane* or *skin exposure,* and *ingestion.*

Inhalation

Hazardous vapors are given off by many substances used in veterinary hospitals, including ethylene oxide, some pesticides, film-developing chemicals, and formaldehyde. Harmful vapors may also be given off by items that seem innocuous, including correction fluid, marker pens, and photocopy machine toner.

Hazardous vapors and dusts affect the body in several ways. Vapors such as formaldehyde may cause direct irritation of the eyes and respiratory tract. Vapors from chemicals such as ethylene oxide or ether may be absorbed from the lungs, enter the bloodstream, and affect internal organs. A few gases (e.g., pure nitrous oxide) can cause asphyxiation if oxygen is unable to reach and bind to hemoglobin in the red blood cells.

There are two important ways to prevent inhalation of injurious gases, vapors, and dusts: increase ventilation and wear protective equipment.

VENTILATION. There is less likelihood of injury from chemical vapors if the vapor is immediately diluted with

Box 35-9   SAFETY PRECAUTIONS FOR COMPRESSED GAS CYLINDERS

- Although oxygen and nitrous oxide are not flammable, they support combustion and should not be used in a room with an open flame. It is recommended that no sources of ignition (matches, Bunsen burners, etc.) be present in any room in which oxygen or nitrous oxide cylinders are stored or used and that smoking be prohibited in these areas. Cylinders should be stored in a dry, cool place, away from furnaces, water heaters, and direct sunlight. The storage area should be identified by a sign indicating that compressed gases are present and that smoking is prohibited. Gas cylinders should be stored away from emergency exits or areas with heavy traffic.
- Oxygen and nitrous oxide must not be stored or used near flammable chemicals such as ether, acetone, or gasoline.
- Care should be taken to avoid dropping cylinders containing compressed air. Pressurized gas may be suddenly released if a cylinder is damaged or knocked over and the regulator (pressure-reducing valve) becomes detached from the tank. The force of the gas escaping from the tank may cause the tank to move like a rocket through walls and other objects. To prevent this occurrence, large cylinders should be chained or belted to a wall and should always be stored in an upright position. Transportation carts and floor-mounting collars are also acceptable means of securing compressed gas cylinders. Valve caps should be used on all large cylinders that are not connected to gas lines.
- If a cylinder must be moved to another location, a handcart should be used, rather than rolling the cylinder.
- Full tanks should be kept separate from empty tanks and should be labeled for quick identification. Cylinders should be used in the order in which they are received (first in, first out).
- Supply tanks should be turned off when not in use. Supply lines from central gas supply systems should be identified with the gas they contain. All staff should know the location of the emergency shutoff valve for the central gas supply.
- Impact-resistant protective goggles should be worn when connecting or disconnecting tanks, because air escaping from the tanks can potentially cause severe eye damage. Similarly, high-pressure leaks can cause severe injury to skin and underlying tissues and one should never attempt to stop such leaks by using hand pressure.

fresh air. Open doors or windows, or exhaust fans that direct exhaust outside the room may be used to increase ventilation in critical areas, such as a surgical preparation room where patients are masked with anesthetic gases, a bathing area where pesticides are in use, or a darkroom where tanks are used to develop x-rays. More sophisticated ventilation devices, such as biologic containment cabinets, fume hoods, and ventilation systems, are available for special purposes, including preparation of cytotoxic drugs and sterilization using ethylene oxide.

PROTECTIVE EQUIPMENT.   If dangerous fumes or dusts are present and ventilation is not adequate, it is necessary to use protective equipment. Three types of equipment are commonly used: surgical masks, disposable respirators, and cartridge respirators. *Surgical masks* are an effective barrier against some dusts and bacterial spores. They are most useful when working with potentially harmful bacteria or fungal cultures and when performing a dental prophylaxis. *Disposable respirators* are similar to surgical masks but are designed to screen out dust, nuisance odors, hot air, and hazardous mists. *Cartridge respirators* fit over the nose and mouth area so that the wearer breathes only air that has passed through the respirator filters. The most common use of cartridge respirators in veterinary clinics is for persons handling liquid anesthetics (e.g., when filling vaporizers) and for cleaning up spills of toxic liquids, such as x-ray fluids and ethylene oxide. Respirators can be obtained at a reasonable cost through safety supply catalogs, safety supply outlets, and some hardware stores. Use of respirators is only permitted where prevention or elimination of a hazardous condition is not reasonably practicable or where the exposure results from temporary or emergency conditions only. Any person who uses a respirator must be given instruction on its proper use and its limitations.

 Technician Note

To prevent accidental ingestion of chemicals, food and drink should not be stored in proximity to chemicals or in a refrigerator that is used for chemical storage.

Ingestion

It is unlikely that a veterinary clinic employee would knowingly eat or drink a hazardous chemical, but there is a potential to ingest these materials by smoking, eating, or drinking while handling chemicals.* Ingestion of harmful materials not only irritates the gastrointestinal tract but also may lead to absorption of the material and resultant spread throughout the body. Nursing mothers who are exposed to toxic chemicals, such as pesticides, may excrete them in breast milk.

To prevent accidental ingestion of chemicals, food and drink should not be stored in proximity to chemicals or in a refrigerator that is used for chemical storage. Food or other items that are suspected to have been contaminated by a chemical spill or splash should be discarded.

Hands should be washed immediately after handling chemicals, and both the hands and face should be washed again before eating. After handling toxic chemicals on the job, it is a good idea to shower and change clothes after arriving home from work.

Absorption Through Direct Contact

Absorption of chemicals such as pesticides through the eyes, mucous membranes, or skin is very common. Some chemicals may be absorbed through intact skin, or (more commonly) they can enter through a rash, skin puncture, or wound. One obvious effect of chemical absorption is local irritation and tissue damage. The eyes are particularly sensitive to chemicals, as is evident to anyone who has splashed formalin or x-ray fixer into the eyes. The skin, although less sensitive than the eyes, may also be irritated by chemicals, and the use of concentrated disinfectant solutions and other chemicals may lead to skin rashes and even allergic dermatitis.

---

*Smoking not only creates the risk of chemical ingestion but also may lead to fire or explosion. Smoking should not be permitted in areas where oxygen, nitrous oxide, flammable liquids, pesticides, ethylene oxide, and other chemicals are stored or used.

Chemicals that are absorbed through the skin or mucous membranes may enter the blood and be distributed throughout the body. This phenomenon is familiar to anyone who has applied dimethyl sulfoxide (DMSO) without wearing gloves and has shortly after perceived a garlic taste in the mouth. Once present in the tissues, chemicals may affect almost any organ, including the brain, heart, liver, kidney, reproductive tract, immune system, and bone marrow. Some chemicals are teratogenic (cause birth defects), carcinogenic (cause cancer), or mutagenic (cause chromosomal mutations, leading to increased risk of birth defects in future offspring and increased risk of cancer).* Some chemicals used in veterinary hospitals, including ethylene oxide, formaldehyde, and cytotoxic drugs, have the potential to cause multiple adverse effects, including local inflammation, internal organ damage, chromosomal changes, increased risk of miscarriage, and cancer.

Use of Protective Equipment

To minimize exposure to hazardous chemicals, it is necessary to wear protective equipment when working with these substances. The employer must provide all personal protective equipment (including equipment used for handling chemicals and laboratory samples, preventing exposure to x-rays, and restraining animals), and the employee must wear it as required by the employer. Protective equipment is readily accessible through safety supply companies and hardware stores. The employer must ensure that protective equipment is properly cleaned and maintained and that sufficient equipment is available to fit each employee correctly.

Technician Note

To minimize exposure to hazardous chemicals, it is necessary to wear protective equipment when working with these substances.

OSHA regulations require that staff members be trained to recognize when use of the equipment is necessary, the type of equipment to use in each situation, how to wear and adjust the equipment, the limitations of the equipment, and the proper care of the equipment. In the United States, the employer must certify in writing that each employee has completed this training before working with the hazard.

Wherever possible, engineering controls are preferred over protective equipment. For example, it is better to install an exhaust fan in the darkroom than to require employees to wear a respirator when developing x-rays.

The type of protective equipment worn should reflect the hazards that are present. Simply wearing a laboratory coat or uniform over street clothes may be sufficient when working with chemicals that have low toxicity (e.g., diluted hospital disinfectants). Long-sleeved shirts and pants offer more protection than shorts or a skirt. Similarly, conventional shoes offer more protection than open-toed shoes and sandals. If significant exposure is expected (e.g., when

cleaning up a chemical spill), rubber boots, coveralls, and a rubber or plastic apron should be worn.

Gloves

It is sometimes advisable to wear hand protection when using chemicals. This is particularly true when working with concentrated solutions, because they have more potential for harm than diluted solutions. Gloves should be worn when handling formalin and formaldehyde, carbon dioxide absorber (soda lime or barium hydroxide lime), concentrated pesticides and disinfectants, chemicals used to fix and develop x-ray films, and cytotoxic drugs.

Unfortunately, gloves do not always provide full protection, since some chemicals (particularly acids and solvents) can penetrate gloves or may be splashed onto skin and clothing beyond the glove margins. Hands should always be washed after removing the gloves. Protective creams can be worn under gloves or on their own and are helpful in preventing skin contact with irritating substances.

Eye Protection

Almost all chemicals are harmful if splashed or sprayed into the eyes, and in situations where an eye splash may occur it is advisable to wear safety glasses, goggles, or a face shield. Protective eye wear should be worn when pouring or handling concentrated pesticides and disinfectants, corrosive or toxic chemicals (including chemicals used to develop x-rays), and cytotoxic drugs. Protective eye wear should also be worn when connecting or disconnecting compressed gas cylinders and when performing dentistry with ultrasonic equipment.

Technician Note

Every practice must have at least one eyewash station available in case of accidental eye splash with a toxic chemical.

Every practice must have at least one eyewash available in case of accidental eye splash with a toxic chemical. Faucet-mounted eyewash devices are relatively inexpensive and provide copious amounts of fresh water, unlike hand-held eyewash bottles. Hand-held devices are used to remove foreign bodies but are not suitable for chemical splash injuries. Eyewash devices must be available within 100 feet (or 10 seconds) of any area where chemicals are used. Persons working with chemicals must know the location of the eyewash and be able to safely reach the eyewash in the event of eye exposure, even if they cannot see (as would be the case after a corrosive chemical was splashed into the eye).

Contact lenses may increase the damage caused by any chemical that is splashed into the eye by trapping the material next to the cornea. Contact lenses should be removed immediately after a chemical is splashed into the eye. Persons who wear contact lenses should notify their co-workers of this fact, so a co-worker giving first aid will know to remove the contact lens if the eye is injured. Once removed, contact lenses should not be replaced until a physician is consulted.

Regulatory Requirements

In the United States, employers must conduct a formal hazard assessment to determine the safety hazards present in the workplace, including chemicals. A complete list of hazardous chemicals used in the hospital must be pre-

---

*Obviously, birth defects and cancer may arise from many causes other than exposure to chemicals. Birth defects most commonly occur if a teratogen is ingested between 25 and 35 days after conception, although some risk is present throughout the entire period from 21 days to 90 days of pregnancy. The most common teratogenic effects include low birth weight, mental retardation, and functional deficits.

pared, and a written plan must list the protective equipment and procedures that are to be used when handling each chemical. This information is usually obtained by conducting a systematic inventory of all chemicals in the hospital, and by consulting the MSDS for each chemical. Details on preparation of the hazardous chemical list and other OSHA requirements are given in the references listed in Box 35-2. Generally, any chemical that has a label or MSDS warning that it is toxic, carcinogenic, an irritant or sensitizer, flammable or combustible, unstable, reactive, or corrosive is considered to be hazardous. Most veterinary practices have more than 100 materials (injectable drugs, cleaning products, laboratory chemicals) in use at any given time that are considered to be hazardous by OSHA. Foods, drugs, or cosmetics intended for personal consumption by employees are exempt from listing and training requirements, as are many common consumer products when purchased and used in small quantities (e.g., laundry detergent). Pills or tablets are also exempt from these requirements.

In addition, OSHA regulations require that employees know specific details on what chemicals they are handling, the type of dangers associated with the material, and how to protect themselves from injury. In the United States, a written plan must be prepared giving details on the safety training program for staff members and the person responsible for ensuring that all training is received.

Labels

In order to work safely with a chemical, it is necessary that the container be clearly labeled with the identity of the substance and the potential hazards associated with it. If the chemical is unfamiliar, the employee should consult the label for information on protective equipment that should be worn. It is a wise practice to routinely double check the label before using a chemical, in the same way that persons handling pharmaceuticals double check the label before dispensing a drug. Labels should be replaced when they start to peel off or become illegible. If a container is difficult to label (e.g., a shampoo container) a color-coded system can be used instead of an adhesive label, provided all persons using that material are familiar with the identification system used.

Any chemical received by the practice should already have a supplier label when it is delivered. This label is produced by the manufacturer and gives the name of the chemical and a brief description of the risks associated with handling it. Some labeling requirements are waived for common consumer chemicals, such as those purchased in small quantities from retail outlets and small quantities of laboratory chemicals.

When a chemical is diluted or transferred to another container (e.g., when transferring isopropyl alcohol from a large bottle to a dispensing bottle) the new container must be identified by a new label. This is particularly important if the new container is to be used by several people or over several days. If the chemical is hazardous, the label must also outline brief hazard warnings and handling precautions. These labels, called workplace labels or secondary labels, can be prepared by the practice or purchased from safety suppliers.

Material Safety Data Sheets

Every company that supplies chemicals to a veterinary practice must provide material safety data sheets (MSDSs) for all hazardous chemicals. These sheets are valid for 3 years, after which time the supplier should send a new MSDS with the next shipment. The MSDS has detailed information on the chemical, including the following:

- A list of hazardous ingredients
- Information on normal use of the chemical
- Physical data, such as the boiling point and vapor pressure
- Warning of fire or explosion hazard and how to extinguish fires
- List of incompatible materials and decomposition products
- Toxicologic properties, including effects of short-term and long-term exposure, carcinogenicity, and teratogenicity
- First-aid measures in case of exposure
- Preventive measures when handling the product, including personal protective equipment that should be used
- Disposal options

The MSDS is only useful as a reference if every person in the hospital has easy access to it. Regulations therefore require that the MSDSs for all hazardous chemicals used by the hospital staff be gathered together and kept in a place that is readily accessible to all staff.

Technician Note

Every company that supplies chemicals to a veterinary practice must provide material data safety sheets (MSDSs) for all hazardous chemicals.

HAZARDOUS CHEMICALS USED IN VETERINARY HOSPITALS

Pesticides

Any chemical used to control pests can be described as a "pesticide." Most pesticides fall into one of five classes: rodenticides, fungicides, herbicides, fumigants, and insecticides. Insecticides are the class most commonly used by veterinary hospital staff, in the form of flea and tick sprays and repellents, collars, shampoos, dips, foams, tablets, and similar products. These products may contain organophosphates, carbamates, chlorinated hydrocarbons, pyrethrins and other botanicals, insect growth regulators, amitraz, or DEET (diethyltoluamide). Human exposure may occur when handling or diluting insecticides or when applying them to animals.

Technician Note

Of all the insecticides used in veterinary hospitals, the organophosphates and carbamates are most frequently associated with human toxicity.

Of all the insecticides used in veterinary hospitals, the organophosphates and carbamates are most frequently associated with human toxicity. These agents inhibit acetylcholinesterase, the enzyme that degrades the neurotransmitter acetylcholine. Persons experiencing acute organophosphate or carbamate poisoning may show a multitude of clinical signs that reflect overstimulation of the central nervous system, skeletal muscles, and parasympathetic nervous system. Clinical signs include salivation, lacrimation, nausea, cramps, diarrhea, sweating, muscle weakness, twitching, blurred vision, restlessness, headache, dizziness,

---

BOX 35-10   SAFE USE OF PESTICIDES

- All staff who handle or dispense pesticides must be familiar with the chemicals contained in the preparations used in the hospital and the class of insecticide to which each chemical belongs (organophosphate, pyrethrin, insect growth regulator, etc.). Consult the MSDS (material safety data sheet) for information on hazards and protective equipment that should be worn for a particular pesticide.
- When treating an animal it is wise to use the least toxic chemical that is effective, for both human and animal safety. Follow the label directions, and avoid "extra label" use unless it is backed by an expert opinion. Agricultural insecticides and preparations intended for use in cattle should not be used on pets, since excessive exposure to both humans and animals may result. When dispensing a pesticide to an animal owner, advise him or her to read the label carefully before using the product and to follow all label directions.
- All pesticide containers must be clearly labeled with the name of the pesticide and brief hazard warnings.
- Many pesticides (pyrethrins, carbamates, any pour-on product) can be readily absorbed through intact skin. Skin exposure to pesticides can be avoided by wearing gloves. An apron or waterproof coveralls should also be worn when bathing an animal with insecticidal shampoos or dips. Gloves and coveralls must also be worn when applying insecticidal dips and spray to livestock. Protective gloves should not be reused indefinitely, be-cause pesticides are absorbed into the rubber and will eventually penetrate through them. Laboratory coats, coveralls, and other protective clothing should be laundered between uses.
- Protective eye wear should be worn when pouring or mixing concentrated pesticide solutions or when working around pesticide mists and sprays. Eyewashes should be available in case of accidental exposure.
- All pesticides (even shampoos) should be used only in areas with good ventilation. If the odor of insecticidal chemicals is strong in the area in which they are used, ventilation is inadequate. If this is the case, doors and windows should be opened or portable fans used to increase air flow. Use of a pesticide filter mask or respirator may be necessary in some situations (e.g., when spraying a barn). The MSDS lists the respiratory protection required when working with specific chemicals.
- Open containers of food, beverages, cigarettes, and similar articles should not be left on the counter of a room in which insecticides are being used. Obviously, it is inadvisable to eat, drink, or smoke when using insecticides.
- If possible, insecticide administration should not be assigned to only one person on the staff. Administration of baths and dips should be assigned to several staff members on a rotating basis. Pregnant employees may want to minimize exposure to pesticides, since some authorities suggest that human fetuses and infants are particularly sensitive to the effects of pesticides.

---

confusion, and slurred speech. One survey of large animal veterinarians who used pour-on organophosphates to treat cattle grubs reported that many veterinarians experienced headache, nausea, dizziness, and irritation of the nose and throat, particularly when these products were used in a poorly ventilated location (Beat, Morgan, 1977). Treatment of affected persons includes washing the skin with mild soap and water in cases of skin exposure, removal of contaminated clothing, and administration of atropine and pralidoxime chloride (2-PAM).

Attention has been focused on possible chronic toxicity of organophosphates and carbamates. Long-term exposure to organophosphates may cause subtle behavioral effects for weeks to months after exposure, including decreased mental alertness and intellectual functioning; poor neuromuscular control; sleep disorders; memory loss; and psychotic, schizoid, and paranoid reactions. As with waste anesthetic gases, it is probably wise to minimize exposure to organophosphates as much as possible.

Pyrethrins and other botanicals, such as limonene, pennyroyal, oil of citronella, *Melaleuca* oil ("tea tree"), and rotenone, are derived from natural sources, such as plant oils and flowers. The most commonly reported adverse effect associated with botanical agents is dermatitis as a result of a contact allergy. Rotenone is reported to cause reproductive problems in pregnant laboratory animals, including increased incidence of babies born dead and reduced maternal and fetal weight gains.

Amitraz (Mitaban), a chemical used in the treatment of demodectic mange in dogs, can be absorbed through intact skin and may cause dizziness and fatigue in persons who bathe dogs without wearing gloves and other protective equipment. It is essential to use gloves and an apron when mixing amitraz with water or when treating dogs. Hands and arms should be washed with soap and water after treatment. There is also some danger of toxicity if amitraz vapors are inhaled, and the drug should only be applied in areas where ventilation is excellent. Because of the toxicity associated with inhalation of vapors or skin absorption of amitraz residues, it is a good idea to avoid close contact with dogs bathed with amitraz within the past 24 hours.

Insect growth regulators (e.g., lufenuron) appear to have very low toxicity for humans but are often combined with more toxic insecticides for quick kill of adult insects. For example, one commonly used insecticide contains chlorpyrifos (an organophosphate) as well as methoprene.

Despite this list of potential hazards, pesticides can be safely used in veterinary hospitals provided a few commonsense rules are observed (Box 35-10). Although it is unlikely that a person will show signs of illness after giving a single flea bath, the risk of toxicity increases with exposure. Many signs of pesticide exposure are subtle and nonspecific (nausea, dizziness, headache, fatigue), and it is often difficult to know if a staff member is being exposed to toxic levels of these drugs. Any person who experiences symptoms suggestive of pesticide toxicity or observes these symptoms in others should immediately contact medical personnel or a poison control center for advice.

Disinfectants

Most disinfectants used in veterinary hospitals are relatively nontoxic, particularly when diluted with water. The most common health problem arising from the prolonged use of disinfectants is skin irritation. Disinfectants remove protective lipids and protein from the skin and after prolonged use may cause dehydration and death of superficial cells. Affected skin has a red, peeling, dry, and cracked appearance and may be itchy. Dermatitis can be prevented by wearing gloves when handling disinfectants.

> **Technician Note**
>
> The most common health problem arising from the prolonged use of disinfectants is skin irritation.

If persons with skin irritation continue to have contact with the offending disinfectant, they may develop an allergy to that disinfectant. Symptoms of a contact allergy to disinfectants (allergic contact dermatitis) are more severe than for simple irritation and include blistering of the skin and extreme itchiness following contact with the offending substance. Fortunately, allergic dermatitis can usually be successfully treated by applying corticosteroid ointments and avoiding future skin contact with the offending agent.

Concentrated disinfectant solutions may be irritating to the hands, eyes, and respiratory tract. Gloves should be used when handling concentrated solutions, and safety goggles should be used if there is a possibility of splashing. Repeated exposure to vapors from concentrated bleach solutions may cause coughing, runny nose, wheezing, and other respiratory problems, and persons should ensure adequate ventilation when using these agents. Bleach should never be mixed with any disinfectant containing ammonia (e.g., quaternary ammonium compounds) because the combination of bleach and ammonia produces chlorine gas, which is extremely toxic.

Glutaraldehyde is somewhat toxic, particularly if used as a concentrated solution. Glutaraldehyde vapors may cause lung irritation, cough, and headaches. Glutaraldehyde is also known to be mutagenic and toxic to fetuses. For these reasons, it is wise to avoid breathing vapors from concentrated solutions, to wear goggles if there is any possibility of eye splash, to wear protective clothing including gloves when handling this agent, and to wash skin that has been exposed to this agent.

Latex Allergies

Persons who routinely wear latex gloves may eventually develop a contact allergy to latex. Reactions to latex gloves include dermatitis (similar to a contact allergy to a pesticide or disinfectant); nasal congestion and sneezing; conjunctivitis; and swelling of the lips, eyelids, and throat. Severe reactions may involve the respiratory tract and include asthma, coughing, and dyspnea.

Persons with an allergy to latex should use plastic, vinyl, or nitrile gloves, or glove liners inside latex gloves. Barrier creams may also help reduce contact with latex. Hypoallergenic latex gloves are available but may cause allergic reactions in some individuals.

Formalin and Formaldehyde

Formaldehyde and its derivatives (including formalin, which is a 37% solution of formaldehyde in methanol and water) are used in hospital disinfectants, in some diagnostic test kits, and for preservation of tissue samples being sent to a laboratory for histopathologic study. Both liquid formaldehyde and formaldehyde vapors are toxic. *Liquid formaldehyde* is intensely irritating to eyes and skin, causing burning, tearing, and, in severe cases, corneal damage. *Formaldehyde vapors* are irritating to the nose, throat, and respiratory tract. The eyes are particularly sensitive to formaldehyde vapors, and lacrimation (watery eyes) may occur even at low concentrations (0.1 to 3 ppm in room air). Long-term exposure to formaldehyde is known to cause cancer in hamsters and rats, and formaldehyde is considered to be a potential human carcinogen.

OSHA has established a short-term formaldehyde exposure limit of 2 ppm and an 8-hour time-weighted average limit of 8 ppm. If there is a chance that employees will be exposed to higher concentrations, the hospital must develop a written plan for safe storage and handling of formaldehyde and emergency procedures in case of spills. Exposure levels can be monitored using dosimeter badges.

To minimize the concentration of formaldehyde vapors in room air, formaldehyde and formalin should only be used in areas with excellent ventilation. Gloves should be worn when working with formaldehyde or tissues preserved in formalin. Goggles and an emergency eyewash station are recommended if there is a danger of splashing formaldehyde into the eyes. Formalin should be ordered in small, prediluted containers to minimize handling of this agent.

> **Technician Note**
>
> To minimize the concentration of formaldehyde vapors in room air, formaldehyde and formalin should only be used in areas with excellent ventilation.

Ethylene Oxide

Ethylene oxide is a gas sterilization agent, most commonly used in veterinary clinics for sterilizing materials that cannot withstand conventional autoclaving. Ethylene oxide for veterinary hospital use is usually purchased as a liquid in ampules.

Many concerns have been raised regarding the safety of this agent. Several hazards are associated with ethylene oxide use:

- Ethylene oxide is flammable and potentially explosive.
- Liquid ethylene oxide can cause severe burns if it is accidentally splashed onto the skin or eyes.
- Exposure to ethylene oxide vapors may irritate the eyes and respiratory system.
- Long-term exposure to moderate levels of ethylene oxide (10 ppm) has been shown to cause chromosomal abnormalities in male and female laboratory animals and may cause similar problems in humans. It is therefore considered to be a "mutagenic" agent and has been classified as a potential human carcinogen.

Given the potential adverse health problems associated with ethylene oxide, OSHA has set an exposure limit of 1 ppm (8-hour time-weighted average), with a maximal level of 5 ppm (time-weighted average) for any 15-minute period. OSHA requires hospitals using ethylene oxide to prepare a detailed written plan for safe handling, storage, and use of ethylene oxide if there is a chance that workers may be exposed to concentrations above this level. Persons handling this agent should complete the certified key operator training course offered free of charge by the manufacturer (Andersen Products, 800-523-1276).

Cytotoxic Drugs

Probably the most hazardous pharmaceuticals the veterinary technician is likely to handle are the cytotoxic drugs used in cancer chemotherapy (also called antineoplastic, chemotherapeutic, or anticancer agents). The agents most commonly used in veterinary medicine include cyclophosphamide (Cytoxan), vincristine (Oncovin), cisplatin (Platinol), azathioprine (Imuran), and doxorubicin (Adriamycin). If technicians and other hospital personnel are assigned to handle or administer cancer chemotherapeutic agents or to dispose of materials contaminated with these drugs, they must receive special training in the toxicity of these agents and the techniques required for safe handling. Staff must also be familiar with spill cleanup procedures and first aid after acute exposure to these agents.

There is ample evidence that cytotoxic drugs can induce cancers in laboratory animals. Many anticancer agents can induce birth defects and miscarriage. Cytotoxic drugs are also extremely irritating to eyes, skin, and tissues, even in very low doses. A single needle prick to a finger with a syringe containing the cytotoxic drug mitomycin C has caused the eventual loss of function of that hand.

Nurses working in cancer wards have shown a higher than expected incidence of liver damage, nausea, dizziness and lightheadedness, chronic headaches, hair loss, dermatitis (particularly after exposure to cisplatin, methotrexate, and vincristine), menstrual cycle irregularities, and miscarriage. Many side effects observed in nurses were the same as those noted by patients receiving antineoplastic drugs. Exposure was thought to arise from accidental contact through routine handling of the drug preparations.

It is suspected that inhalation of drug aerosols and skin absorption of powders and liquids are the chief routes by which cytotoxic drugs gain entry into the body. Skin exposure may occur when crushing or dividing a tablet or when handling urine or stool from an animal that has been treated with antineoplastic drugs. Inhalation of aerosols may occur when breaking an ampule, when withdrawing a syringe from a vial, when adjusting the amount of drug in a syringe, when expelling air from a partly filled syringe, or when liquid containing the drug leaks from tubing or a syringe.

The minimal necessary protective equipment when handling or administering cytotoxic drug tablets is a long-sleeved laboratory coat and disposable latex gloves. Whether intact or broken, cytotoxic drug capsules and tablets should never be manipulated with bare hands. Hands should be washed thoroughly after removing gloves. For procedures involving liquid cytotoxic drugs, it is recommended that personnel handling the drugs wear a disposable surgical gown (or other long-sleeved, back-closure, disposable protective garment with tight-fitting cuffs and neck) and disposable latex gloves. Special techniques are required to avoid generating aerosols when opening ampules, removing liquid from an ampule, reconstituting powders, and administering these agents to a patient.

Technician Note

Persons who are pregnant, breast-feeding, or attempting to conceive are advised not to handle cytotoxic drugs.

Cytotoxic wastes (syringes, intravenous sets, gauzes, gloves) should be placed in a sealable plastic bag and disposed by incineration or held for biomedical waste pickup. Latex gloves should be worn when handling urine, feces, vomitus, and other body fluids from an animal that has received cytotoxic drugs within the previous 48 hours. Patient waste may be disposed of through the sewage system.

Persons who are pregnant, breast-feeding, or attempting to conceive are advised not to handle cytotoxic drugs.

If a veterinary hospital regularly prepares and administers injectable cytotoxic drugs, consideration should be given to the purchase of a glove box, biologic safety cabinet, or a vertical laminar flow hood. This equipment has been shown to significantly reduce exposure to aerosols of cytotoxic drugs. Alternatively, preparation of cytotoxic agents may be contracted to a local pharmacy or hospital.

FIRST AID AND EMERGENCY RESPONSE

Despite the best of precautions, accidental exposure to chemicals may occur. Basic guidelines for handling chemical spills are given in Box 35-11, and guidelines for treatment of eye and skin exposure to chemicals are given in Boxes 35-12 and 35-13. A written cleanup procedure for chemical spills should be posted in the clinic, giving details of cleanup procedures and protective equipment required. If an employee is unfamiliar with the procedure for clean-

---

Box 35-11   EMERGENCY PROCEDURES FOR CHEMICAL SPILLS

- All veterinary hospitals should have a chemical spill kit prepared in advance and stored in an easily accessible location. The spill kit should contain an absorbent material such as cat litter, gloves, a dustpan and brush, and a plastic bag. Commercial spill kits can be purchased for cleanup of mercury, acids, and flammable solvents.
- **If the spill involves a relatively nontoxic liquid or solid** (e.g., overturning a bottle of laboratory stain), the technician should immediately place a towel, newspaper, kitty litter, or other absorbent material on top of the spill. When the liquid is completely absorbed, the absorbent material should be swept up (or picked up using gloved hands) and placed in an airtight, sealed plastic bag for disposal outside the hospital.
- **If the spilled material gives off potentially hazardous vapors** (formalin, anesthetic liquid, ethylene oxide, bleach), all adjacent doors and windows should be opened to increase ventilation. If a large amount of material is present and toxic fumes are being produced (e.g., a whole bottle of halothane is dropped and broken, or a vial of ethylene oxide is opened and exposed to the room air), all personnel should leave the area at once. A person who is trained in the use of a respirator and wearing protective clothing (apron, gloves) should reenter the room and clean up the mess by first increasing ventilation and then using cat litter or other absorbent as described above. If a respirator is not available or if staff members are not trained in its use, the fire department should be contacted.

Box 35-12   TREATMENT OF CHEMICAL SPLASH TO THE EYES

If a corrosive chemical is splashed into the eyes, the affected person should first call for help. Contact lenses, if worn, should be removed. Then both eyes must be continuously washed for 15 minutes with lukewarm or cold water, using an eyewash fountain or bottle. It is necessary to hold the eyelids open during the washing period; otherwise, the natural inclination is to close the eyes, which keeps water away from the cornea. The affected person should not rub or touch the eyes, because this is likely to introduce more chemical. After 15 minutes of continuous washing, the person should seek medical attention. Take the MSDS (material safety data sheet) from the chemical, or the labeled bottle, to the hospital with the injured person.

ing up the spilled chemical, the MSDS should be consulted before cleaning up.

All veterinary hospitals should have a fire safety plan that includes specifics on safe storage of chemicals and garbage, a list of fire hazards and potential ignition sources, precautions when using portable heaters, location and type of fire extinguishers available, and identification of emergency exits and alarm systems. Hospitals with more than 10 employees must prepare written plans, but smaller hospitals may communicate the plan orally.

Emergency exits must be kept free from obstructions, and at least two exits must be available for use so that persons within the building can escape without using a key.

Box 35-13   TREATMENT AFTER SKIN CONTACT WITH CHEMICALS

In case of splashing or other skin contact with a corrosive or toxic substance, all contaminated clothing should be removed and placed in a plastic bag. If the chemical is a powder or other dry material, brush away as much of the chemical as possible using gloved hands. The affected area should then be rinsed with water. For liquid chemicals, immediate water rinse is advisable. If the chemical is not corrosive (e.g., isopropyl alcohol) it is probably adequate to wash the exposed area with soap and water. If the chemical is toxic or corrosive (e.g., concentrated bleach or formaldehyde) the exposed skin should be flushed with cold water and soap for 15 minutes. If the exposure is extensive or the material is very toxic (e.g., ethylene oxide liquid), the person should be transported to medical attention immediately after the 15-minute flushing period. During transport, the affected area should be covered with a loose clean cloth. Cold packs or ice can be used as necessary to relieve pain.

Box 35-14   FIRE RESPONSE

1. The first person to detect the fire calls for help immediately. Notify the fire department by calling 911 (or other applicable phone number for your area). Stay on the line, and follow the dispatcher's instructions.
2. Alert all staff and clients that a fire has occurred. The veterinarian will report immediately to the site of the fire and decide if evacuation is necessary. If the fire is not contained, instruct all clients and staff not involved in fighting the fire to leave the hospital. All persons should meet in a preassigned location outside the building to determine if everyone has been evacuated. No person is to reenter the building unless directed to do so.
3. If possible to do so without endangering human safety:
   a. Close windows and doors.
   b. Turn off oxygen tanks and natural gas lines.
   c. Turn off fans.
   d. Use a fire extinguisher if the fire is small and the employee knows how to handle the fire extinguishing equipment. Do not attempt to fight a fire if it is spreading beyond the immediate area where it started or if it could spread to block the escape route.
   e. Evacuate animals.

Fire prevention also includes designation of duties in case of a fire and a fire response plan (Box 35-14). This plan should be posted at a central location within the clinic.

Technician Note

All laboratories and veterinary clinics should be equipped with one or more fire extinguishers of a size easily manipulated by the employees.

All laboratories and veterinary clinics should be equipped with one or more fire extinguishers of a size easily manipulated by the employees. Different classes of fire extinguishers are designed to extinguish different types of fires (flammable solvents, paper, electrical). A veterinary hospital should have an extinguisher that is effective against a wide range of materials: a dry chemical (ABC) type is often recommended. Hospitals with computer equipment may prefer to use a carbon dioxide extinguisher, which has less potential for harming electrical equipment. Fire extinguishers should be placed no less than 75 feet apart. They should be inspected monthly by a hospital employee to ensure that they are properly charged, and a qualified person should inspect each fire extinguisher annually. Hospitals, like homes, should be equipped with smoke detectors on each floor, including the basement.

REFERENCES
Beat VB, Morgan DP: Evaluation of hazards involved in treating cattle with pour-on organophosphate insecticides, *J Am Vet Med Assoc* 170:812, 1977.

DHHS (U.S. Department of Health and Human Services): *Guidelines for protecting the safety and health of health care workers.* National Institute for Occupational Safety and Health (NIOSH), Washington, DC, 1988, US Government Printing Office.

Schenker MB et al: Adverse reproductive outcomes among female veterinarians, *Am J Epidemiol* 132:96, 1990.

Thigpen CK, Dorn RC: Nonfatal accidents involving insured veterinarians in the United States 1967-1969, *J Am Vet Med Assoc* 163:369, 1973.

Wiggins P et al: Prevalence of hazardous exposures in veterinary practice, *Am J Ind Med* 16:55, 1989.

RECOMMENDED READING
GENERAL
Faris R et al: *Health hazards in veterinary practice,* ed 3, Schaumburg, Ill, 1995, American Veterinary Medical Association.

Langley RL: *Occupational medicine state of the art reviews: animal handlers,* vol 14, no. 2, Philadelphia, 1999, Hanley and Belfus.

McKelvey D: *Safety handbook for veterinary hospital staff,* Lakewood, Col, 1999, American Animal Hospital Association.

Seibert PJ: *Safety issues for the veterinary hospital staff,* 1996 (self-published).

Wilkins JR, Steele JJ: Occupational factors and reproductive outcome among a cohort of female veterinarians, *J Am Vet Med Assoc* 213:61, 1998.

ANIMAL-RELATED INJURY
Barber JL, Ford RB: Animal bite wounds in humans, *Anim Health Tech* 3:277, 1982.

Underman AE: Bite wounds inflicted by dogs and cats, *Vet Clin North Am Small Anim Pract* 17(1):195, 1987.

RADIATION

Moore RM, Davis YM, Kaczmarek RG: An overview of occupational hazards among veterinarians, with particular reference to pregnant women, *Am Ind Hyg Assoc J* 54:113, 1993.

Oppenheim BE, Griem ML, Meier P: The effects of diagnostic x-ray exposure on the human fetus: an examination of the evidence, *Radiology* 114:529, 1975.

Rendano VT, Ryan G: Technical assistance in radiology. II. Basic considerations and radiation safety, *Vet Technician* 9:547, 1988.

Seibert PJ: Radiation issue, *Vet Safety Health Digest*, vol 9, March-April 1995.

WASTE ANESTHETIC GAS

Ad Hoc Committee of the American Society of Anesthesiologists: Occupational disease among O.R. personnel: a study, *Anesthesiology* 41:321, 1974.

Gross ME, Branson KR: Reducing exposure to waste anesthetic gas, *Vet Tech* 14:175, 1993.

McKelvey D, Hollingshead KW: *Small animal anesthesia*, ed 2, St Louis, 1999, Mosby.

Potts DL, Craft BF: Occupational exposure of veterinarians to waste anesthetic gases, *Appl Ind Hyg* 3:132, 1988.

Shenkar MB et al: Adverse reproductive outcomes among female veterinarians, *Am J Epidemiol* 132:96, 1990.

Short CE, Harvey RC: Anesthetic waste gases in veterinary medicine, *Cornell Vet* 73:363, 1983.

PESTICIDES

Wiggins P et al: Prevalence of hazardous exposures in veterinary practice, *Am J Ind Med* 16:55, 1989.

DISINFECTANTS

Vainio H: Inhalation anesthetics, anticancer drugs and sterilizants as chemical hazards in hospitals, *Scand J Work Environ Health* 8:94, 1982.

ETHYLENE OXIDE

National Institute of Occupational Safety and Health: *Ethylene oxide sterilizers in health care facilities. Current Intelligence Bulletin 52*, Cincinnati, 1989, US Department of Health and Human Services.

Seibert PJ: *Vet Safety Health Digest*, vol 11, July-August 1995.

Vainio H: Inhalation anesthetics, anticancer drugs and sterilizants as chemical hazards in hospitals, *Scand J Work Environ Health* 8:94, 1982.

CYTOTOXIC DRUGS

Bacovsky R: Guidelines for handling and disposal of hazardous pharmaceuticals, *Can Soc Hosp Pharmacists* 416:979, 1991.

Dickinson KL, Ogilvie GK: Safe handling and administration of chemotherapeutic agents in veterinary medicine. In Kirk RW, editor: *Current veterinary therapy 12*, Philadelphia, 1995, WB Saunders.

Hahn KA, Morrison WB: Safety guidelines for handling chemotherapeutic drugs, *Vet Med*, Nov 1991, pp 1094-1099.

Holt L: Cytotoxic drugs, *Vet Tech* 16:675, 1995.

Morrison W: *Cytotoxic drug safety* (video), distributed by the American Animal Hospital Association, PO Box 150899, Denver, CO 80215-0899.

Swanson LV: Potential hazards associated with low-dose exposure to antineoplastic agents. I. Evidence for concern, *Compend Contin Educ Small Anim Pract* 10:290, 1988.

Swanson LV: Potential hazards associated with low-dose exposure to antineoplastic agents. II. Recommendations for minimizing exposure, *Compend Contin Educ Small Anim Pract* 10:615, 1988.

Vainio H: Inhalation anesthetics, anticancer drugs and sterilizants as chemical hazards in hospitals, *Scand J Work Environ Health* 8:94, 1982.

Yodaiken RE, Bennett D: OSHA work-practice guidelines for personnel dealing with cytotoxic (antineoplastic) drugs, *Am J Hosp Pharmacists* 43:1193, 1986.

36

Personal Leadership*

Ray L. Russell

Study and application of the principles in this chapter will help the veterinary technician develop the skills of *personal leadership (PL)* (Russell, 1996a). The most important business in life is the business of leading yourself to be all you can possibly be through the process of PL.

In a time of rapidly changing technology, when there is so much new information to learn, it is easy to overlook the importance of continuing to learn some of the so-called soft skills, such as communication, leadership, and interpersonal relations. For a veterinary practice to reach its potential, it is important to maintain a balance between critical technical skills and leadership skills. The veterinary technician who is willing to develop PL skills will become an even better technician and a greater asset to a practice.

The importance of learning these skills is pointed out in a study by the American Management Association that revealed two of three workers in the United States believe their supervisors are incompetent. This is a shocking indictment of the failure of management to learn and practice PL.

Technician Note

Two out of three workers believe their leaders are incompetent.
—American Management Association

There will always be a demand for position or public leadership; however, today's changing world will necessitate greater emphasis on PL than on organizational leadership.

Technician Note

A major shift is occurring today from organizational to personal leadership.

Humanity's quest should be to find better methods of leading, managing, learning, teaching, motivating, and interacting with others. Acquiring new competencies will be necessary to effectively compete and adapt to the challenges of society, which are different than anything previously experienced.

Competent technicians and front office staff are absolutely essential to the operation of a successful practice. In managing my clinical practice, I often said, "I would rather replace a veterinarian than a technician or receptionist." I have had many outstanding technicians; however, one technician who was also a behavioral consultant opened up a new dimension in our practice with her knowledge of animal behavior. Kay Bickford added to her value as a technician because she had answers and training techniques for clients with pet behavioral problems.

Kay's interest and knowledge of animal behavior started when she was a young child. She trained her dogs to do unusual things; her German shepherd rode bareback with her on her horse. Kay said, "My best friends were my dogs." She developed a reputation in show circles by training and showing her golden retrievers. Her proficiency in working with canine behavior is attested to by the fact that she trained five of the number 1 obedience dogs in the United States.

Kay's advice to new veterinary technicians is as follows:

- Love animals; be firm with them so they will not make a mistake that could harm them.
- Go through the best technician program available, and become certified.
- Talk to veterinarians, and find out what they want in a technician.
- Get all the experience you can by doing the dirtiest jobs and working your way up. Do not worry about the pay. If you are good, the pay will follow.
- Treat people like they are long-lost relatives.
- Enjoy what you do.

Kay is an outstanding example of a personal leader who has developed master skills that have complemented her technical training.

OTHER ROLES

A person's role as a veterinary technician may often expand beyond the work done as a technician into the management of the practice. In this role, one needs to be sure the practice is in compliance with U.S. Occupational Health and Safety Administration (OSHA) controlled substances and environmental standards. In addition, many technicians need to learn how to do the following:

- Order drugs and supplies.
- Hire staff, negotiate contracts, and review performance.
- Operate computers, faxes, and other business equipment.
- Supervise, train, and provide leadership to the practice staff.
- Handle payables, receivables, and deposits; and balance the checkbook.

If some of these roles are new to the veterinary technician, he or she may have to obtain the information and training to learn these skills in addition to keeping current with advances in technology. Lifelong learning is essential to contributing to a successful practice as well as having a good quality of life.

WHAT IS LEADERSHIP?

Everyone has his or her own definition of *leadership*, and most use the word without a clear understanding of what it really means. This is understandable because there are more than 350 definitions according to leadership authorities.

My favorite definition of a *leader* is someone who knows where he or she is going and can convince others to go along.

Technician Note

Leaders know where they are going and can convince others to go with them.

President Harry Truman said, "Leadership is the ability to get other people to do what they don't want to do and like it! "The management and leadership guru Peter Drucker taught, "The essence of leadership is performance. The ultimate task of leadership is to create human energies and human vision. Lifting vision, raising performance, and building personality is the very essence of leadership."

Regardless of the definition, one thing is certain: there is a huge leadership gap in the world at a time when leadership is needed the most.

BOTTOM-UP PERSONAL LEADERSHIP

In conversing with a student employed by a major hotel, he said, "I think I could do a better job of managing than the manager of the hotel. Eight of our student employees are turned off by how they are treated by management—their attitude is terrible and morale is low."

This student decided this was the wrong attitude to have, so he arranged a meeting with his department and they all agreed to put the customer first. They decided to do everything in their power to help each hotel guest feel glad he or she stayed at the hotel.

Instead of being a "hostile takeover" by the employees, it became an employee "makeover." Their department completely changed, and it is now the very best and most motivated department in the hotel. He told me, "Everyone works harder and we enjoy our work so much more—we take pride in giving our very best to every customer."

The employee responsible for this turnaround acted on his own without any direction or authority from management. His personal action changed the attitude of every employee and energized his department. His motivation and attitude of quality customer service had a positive impact on all the other employees. This demonstrates the power of one person who exercises PL.

Bottom-up PL was very effective in changing attitudes and creating positive results for the entire organization. Top-down leadership may not have been effective.

As a veterinary technician, one's own PL can have a positive influence on the entire practice. Let's discover how the technician can build these skills so that, in addition to technical skills, he or she can have a major impact on the staff and clients in a practice.

A NEW LEADERSHIP MODEL

PL is a new leadership model that radiates life, spirit, and energy to all who come within the leader's energy field. It enables and empowers individuals to visualize and achieve the pictures they paint.

How can PL be defined?

Technician Note

Personal leadership is the ability to create a vision, develop a strategy, and generate the energy and empowerment necessary to accomplish personal objectives.

—Ray Russell

Study Figure 36-1, and observe the visual relationships of the five elements of PL. The model shows an interrelationship among the parts. The two-way arrows illustrate a dynamic synergism in leadership. If any part of the model is neglected or eliminated, the energy and empowerment components are weakened.

The PL model is very direct and straightforward. Learning to do these five things well will start the veterinary technician on the way to being a successful personal leader.

Five Principles of Personal Leadership

- Paint a picture.
- Develop a personal strategy.
- Energize self.
- Become personally empowered.
- Set an example.

The veterinary technician who understands and applies these five principles will become a proactive personal leader. While reading about each of these principles, ask the following questions:

- Do I have a clear mental picture of what I want to achieve for the rest of my life?
- Have I written a strategy for accomplishing my vision?
- How much energy am I willing to put into accomplishing my strategy?
- Do I have the personal empowerment to make my vision come true?
- Am I setting a quality example for my family, friends, and co-workers?

Painting a Picture

It is said that pictures are worth a thousand words. Some people have the natural ability to visualize and dream,

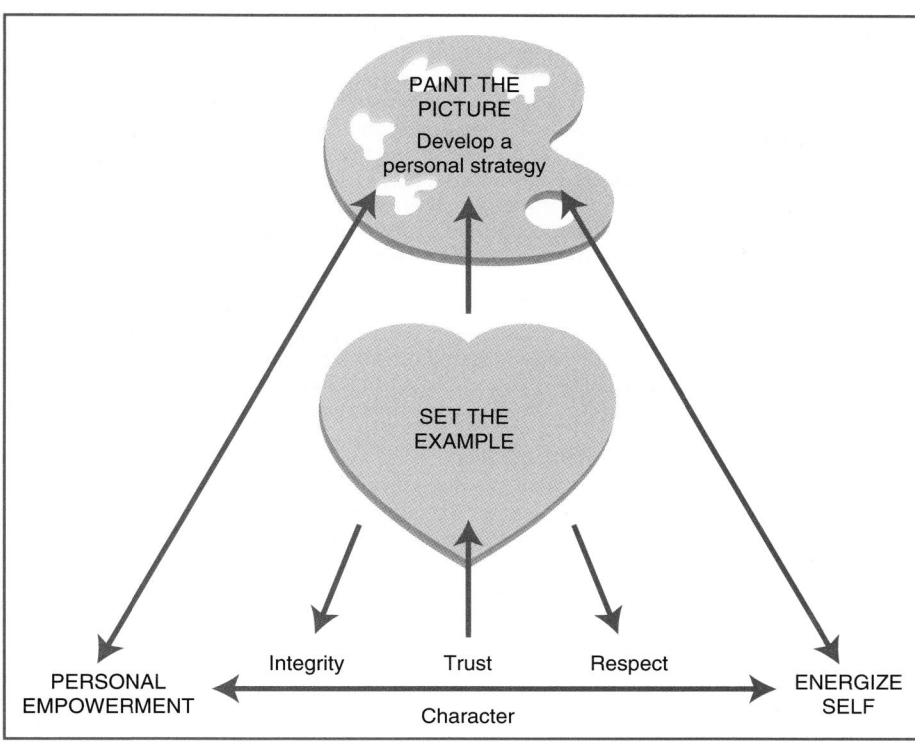

FIGURE 36-1. Personal leadership model.

whereas others have to work at developing this skill. Seeing clear, living pictures painted in color inside one's mind is an important quality to develop. Leaders can visualize what the finished product will look like and have the ability to see things as they will be in the future. *Vision* is a constant source of internal drive and motivation; it keeps individuals focused on their purpose in life.

Technician Note

Successful people have developed the habit of doing what failures don't like to do. They don't like to do them either, but their dislike is subordinated to their strength of purpose.

—E.N. Gray

Power of Purpose

Having a purpose in life and work generates an energy that propels a person forward to achieve objectives. My *purpose statement* was about 50 words long when I first wrote it. Each year I have refined and shortened it. After years of experimenting and refining my statement, I have arrived at an eight-word purpose statement: Raise people and organizations to their highest value.

Technician Note

Raise people and organizations to their highest value.
—Ray Russell

Purpose is often referred to in business as a *vision* or *mission statement*. Technically, there is a difference between vision and mission; however, for our purposes, I use painting a picture, mission, and purpose interchangeably.

Without a clearly identified mission, a person is likely to wander—not focusing on what is most important. Many business owners struggle and even go bankrupt because they have lost sight of their mission. If businesses fail, it is reasonable that each of us also may wander and lose focus without a clearly identified purpose or mission. Consider the following mission or purpose statements:

- Quality without compromise . . . because we care (James S. Reid, V.M.D., Vienna, Va.)
- Serve others each day by some small act of service (Loe Pierce, Sandy, Utah)
- Because we care . . . we treat them like family (Terry Sippel, D.V.M., Wichita, Kan.)

Gita the philosopher said, "You are what you believe in . . . and [you will] become what you believe you can become."

I have met several people who have achieved extraordinary results in their lives. When I asked them how they were able to accomplish seemingly impossible projects, they frequently told me their project was constantly before them in their mind's eye.

The ability to clearly see and paint vivid pictures of how things will appear when they are finished is an important talent for people to develop. Two people who exemplify what could be accomplished when they painted a picture in their mind are Dr. Otto Shill and his wife, Betty.

Otto enrolled in college with aspirations of becoming a veterinarian. He was accepted into the College of Veterinary Medicine at Kansas State University and 4 years later graduated second in his class.

Betty's parents were divorced when she was 16 months old. Her mother died when she was 8 years old, so she lived with various relatives during her childhood. She became a registered nurse, worked for 1 year as a school nurse, and then returned to college for further study.

Otto and Betty were married during Otto's first year in veterinary college. She worked for a pediatrician to support them while he finished school. Before Otto graduated, Betty contracted poliomyelitis and was hospitalized for 4 months; for one of those months she lived in an iron lung. After the acute illness, she began the long process of rehabilitation to overcome extensive paralysis.

On graduation, Otto became an associate in a veterinary practice in El Paso, Texas, while awaiting his call into the Air Force. During this time, he was exposed to rabies and had to take the Pasteur treatment. He reacted to the treatment, developed transverse myelitis, and for 3 weeks was unable to move from the waist down. He was told if he ever had to take the treatment again, he would die.

Otto recovered to the point where he was able to enter the Air Force and spend the next 5 years doing public health and radiation research. He resigned from the Air Force to return to medical school. At graduation, he received the Wintrobe Award as the outstanding student of his class. After his internship, he moved to Houston, where he completed a 4-year residency in otolaryngology at Baylor University College of Medicine.

Otto and Betty have five children—three by birth and two by adoption. Betty miraculously was able to raise her three sons and two daughters, even though some observers may have wondered how she could manage with her physical challenge and paralysis. The Shills' experiences have given them a deep appreciation for life. They also know the heartache of losing a 25-year-old son to death.

If you feel you are not able to lead your life through education, find the right practice, or take care of your family (even if you are a single parent), practice painting a picture in your mind and you will be amazed at the results you may obtain.

Developing a Strategy

The Small Business Administration reports lack of planning as one of the principal reasons businesses fail. Similarly, one of the primary reasons people do not achieve as much as they could is because they fail to make personal plans. A person who fails to plan is operating by *chance* instead of by *choice*.

Technician Note

Failing to plan means operating by *chance* instead of by *choice*.

Pictures painted in the mind's eye will become reality when clear and vivid personal strategies are developed and acted on.

While serving as a member of the American Animal Hospital Association (AAHA) board of directors, I learned an important lesson about the power of a written strategy. The board had a strong desire to move the national headquarters to a city more centrally located and near a major airport. It was interesting to observe the excitement among the board members; however, after a period of time, the energy died. The headquarters were never moved because the board failed to develop a written moving strategy.

As fate would have it, several years later I became the executive director of AAHA. I moved my family from sunny Arizona to Indiana so we could live close to the association headquarters. After my first year, it became apparent that we were limiting our growth by remaining in this location.

Even though the board had wanted to move several years previously, it had given up hope because of the expense and difficulty involved in moving the computer system. Interest was revived when a clear, written moving strategy was presented to the board, which they quickly approved. As the strategy was implemented, Denver was selected over eight other cities.

Following this written strategy made the move easier than expected. The move and eventual construction of a new headquarters injected a new enthusiasm into the membership. The many dedicated volunteers, staff, and members have earned AAHA the reputation of being one of the finest nonprofit associations in North America. Many people and organizations never reach their potential because they do not take the time to develop a *written strategy* that has the power to turn dreams into reality.

Energizing Self

Many people have developed habits that rob them of natural energy. To stay energized, avoid the following *enemies of energy*, or *energy drains*.

Common Enemies of Energy

- Low self-esteem
- Inaction
- Worry
- Fear
- Criticism
- Anger
- Negative thinking
- Jealousy
- Dictatorial leadership style
- Poor physical and mental conditioning

Avoid these energy robbers. They are contagious and extremely destructive to high energy.

In addition to avoiding things that drain energy, there are numerous ways to *build energy*.

To Develop Greater Personal Energy:

- Take charge of your life, and "just do it."
- Keep in top physical and mental condition.
- Learn something new every day.
- Communicate effectively.
- Act enthusiastically.
- Associate with high-energy people.
- Lose yourself in serving others.
- Build up other people.
- Set a powerful example.
- Listen; give others your full attention.
- Express sincere interest and concern for others.
- Look on the bright side of life.
- Relax; take time for recreation *(re-creation)*.
- Build your self-confidence, commitment, and control.
- Develop a "light touch"; have a playful attitude.

Life is energy! Death is when all the energy leaves the body. Energy is the fuel of PL. The person who loses zest for living may die at 20 years old, even though he or she may not be buried until 80 years old.

Technician Note

Life is exciting and interesting to interesting and exciting people. It is only dull and boring to dull and boring people.

The quality of life will largely depend on the degree to which people keep their lives active and involved.

The First Seeing Eye Dog

One of the most energized persons I have ever known was Dr. Mark L. Morris, who is well known in the veterinary profession because of his contribution to nutrition and organized veterinary medicine.

Mark once told me about his experience in researching and developing Science Diet Prescription Diet k/d in the clinical laboratory and in his kitchen at his Raritan Hospital for Animals. One of his clients was a blind man, Morris Frank, whose dog, Buddy, was the first Seeing Eye dog. Buddy had kidney failure, and Mark and his wife, Louise, were preparing food for Buddy in the hospital kitchen. Mr. Frank persuaded Mark to put the k/d in a can so he could take this special diet on the road to feed Buddy while he was traveling around the country raising money for the Seeing Eye Foundation during its formative stage.

Dr. Morris has left a lasting legacy as a dynamic visionary personal leader, pioneering small animal practice, nutrition, organized veterinary medicine, and companion animal research. Pets throughout the world have benefited from his research and innovative contributions to animal nutrition.

Personal Empowerment

Empowerment has been a much overused buzzword in recent years. Some authorities say an individual cannot empower a person, just like he or she cannot motivate a person. Motivation is internal; it is something people do to themselves.

Anything that causes an increase in performance or improves your ability to lead yourself to accomplish your purpose is empowerment. People are empowered if they have the ability to get things done and can achieve their objectives.

The word *power* comes from the Latin word *potere*, which means "able." *Roget's II New Thesaurus* defines power as "the capacity to exert an influence or force."

Think of empowerment in terms of having personal power or the ability to act and take ownership for actions. The person who fails to act loses personal empowerment.

H.B. Karp wrote, "Power is strictly an interpersonal phenomenon and is measured in terms of obtained objectives. . . . You cannot empower or disempower anyone else and nobody else can do this for or to you either. . . . Power resides with the individual, authority resides with the organization."

Dan McCormick is a very successful businessperson who exemplifies this. His burning desire, consistency, and work ethics have carried him to the top of his businesses. I asked him what his secret was in earning $1.5 million in his first 4 years in business. He said, "Life is a marathon—not a 100-meter dash." His formula is as follows:

- Do not let other people steal your dreams.
- Be teachable; read motivational books, and listen to tapes.
- Find a mentor you respect, and model his or her behavior.
- Be consistent.
- Develop a burning desire.
- Paint clear vivid pictures in your mind of what you want to achieve.

Rudy Lavik, a university professor, took control of his life by running several miles each day. He continued to run nearly every day well into his 80s. Rudy said, "We are soft—we need to run an extra mile each day and read an extra book each week."

Technician Note

We need to run an extra mile each day and read an extra book each week.

　　　　　　　　　　　　　　　　　　　—Rudy Lavik

The personal discipline exemplified by Rudy is an essential characteristic for proponents of PL to develop. Discipline builds character and will help a person become a great technician.

There is a big difference between being interested in something and being committed. The person who is interested will do something when it is convenient. The person who is committed will do something no matter what it takes and will find a way to accomplish objectives with no excuses.

The two essential empowering skills technicians must learn are *people skills* and *performance skills*. A person can be a very competent technician, but without these skills, he or she will not be as effective as possible.

Interpersonal Skills

Business and professional people are learning to understand the vital importance of developing interpersonal skills. Recent research reveals that 70% of all litigation with physicians is the result of poor attitude, relationships, or communication skills. More than 200 practice owners told me that it was difficult to find employees who have the ability to communicate with and relate to clients (Russell, 1994).

The technician's role may require supervision of other staff members. In this role, many managers have tried to manage people like inventory, which will not work. A person manages things and leads people. Both management and leadership are necessary to a successful practice, but most people do not possess both skills.

Technician Note

People are underled and overmanaged.

　　　　　　　　　　　　　　　　　　　—Warren Bennis

Trust and respect form the foundation on which all human relationships are built. You can respect a person without agreeing with him or her. The secret is to learn to disagree agreeably. Relationships grow stronger when every encounter is a win-win situation. Even when it is necessary to discipline or terminate employees, veterinary personnel can preserve the person's dignity by treating him or her with respect.

Research demonstrates that the more one understands other people and oneself, the more effective that person will be in working relationships. Sensitivity to these differences will strengthen relationships.

While observing others, try to recognize their primary behavioral style. With practice, a person can read other people and predict their style by the way they walk, talk, sit, and gesture. People are quite predictable in their behavior, so the ability to read people will assist an individual to more effectively interact with others. While focusing on the other person, one's own interpersonal relationships will usually improve.

Thus it does not matter what style a person employs. There is no need to change style unless a certain behavior is affecting the success of work, marriage, or relationships. A person can learn to blend his or her style when this would improve a job or relationships with others. For several years, I have used computerized behavioral reports (*Managing for Success*, 1991) as a tool to build strong practices and businesses. These reports are simple and accurate. They are useful in helping staff members understand themselves, their clients, and other staff members. After a person completes a 24-question instrument, a computer prints a 14- to 20-page report about his or her unique behavior, with startling accuracy. This report is used by many executives, supervisors, and other business and professional leaders.

These computerized reports are a valuable tool in helping students, technicians, and practitioners develop skills in leadership, team building, client service, staff supervision, and mentoring. This technology combined with training has produced significant improvements in productivity and helping people work together. It is the operations manual for working with people.

The computer report describes the following aspects:

- General characteristics
- Value to the organization
- Checklist for communication
- Cautions on communication
- Ideal environment
- Perceptions
- Natural and adapted style
- Motivated style
- Keys to motivating
- Keys to managing
- Areas for improvement
- Action plan

I have observed significant improvements in productivity, service/quality, teamwork, and profitability as a direct result of using these reports (Russell, 1996b). They are a particularly effective tool for improving communication within organizations.

Developing Rapport

People tend to be attracted to similar people. This attraction or relationship is referred to as being in rapport with others. *Rapport* is defined as a harmonious, empathetic, or sympathetic relation with mutual trust of another person.

Rapport is essential for successful communication; it is the glue that holds together relationships. Exceptional client service depends on developing and maintaining harmonious relationships.

Many business and professional owners have said their greatest need is to find employees who can relate to their customers. It is relatively easy to find people who have good technical skills but more difficult to locate employees who can relate to and communicate effectively with clients.

A technology known as *neurolinguistic programming (NLP)* was developed by Dr. John Grinder and Richard Bandler. Dr. Michael Brooks, an industrial psychologist, presents this technology in his books *Instant Rapport* (Brooks, 1989) and *The Power of Business Rapport* (Brooks, 1990). He describes how people experience the world through one of three senses: *sight, sound,* or *feelings*.

The veterinary technician who can diagnose whether clients or associates are visual, auditory, or kinesthetic has a better chance of establishing rapport with them. Until rapport is established, there will be no openness and trust, which are needed to communicate and relate effectively.

Observe clients closely, and become sincerely interested in them. Listen carefully, noting their voice, rate of speech, and tone. Pay attention to their eyes and position of their pupils. Match and mirror their rate and tone of speech and body language. This will assist the technician in quickly developing rapport.

Communication

Most people are completely unaware of their communication habits. They may say one thing yet convey a different message because of their nonverbal language. If this happens to you, analyze your speaking and listening habits.

The ability to clearly communicate a message through written and spoken language is important for accomplishing objectives.

When you communicate, do you speak rapidly? Slowly? Talk too much? Or not enough? Is your verbal message saying one thing and your body language something else? Do you have credibility? Are people influenced by your message?

Most people think they are good communicators; however, after a review, they frequently find weaknesses that can be corrected with identification and coaching.

Listening Is Essential to Effective Communication

The inability to communicate effectively with others is often the reason for a breakdown in relationships. After working with many different organizations over the years, it has been my observation that the majority of problems originate because of a failure to communicate. Much of this problem is specifically related to listening skills.

Even when people think they listen, they commonly retain less than 25% of what they hear. The ability to be a good listener is one of the rarest yet most important of the interpersonal skills. A person really feels important when someone listens to him or her, really listens, with both ears and heart.

There are many reasons why people do not listen. Frequently, they are busy talking or preoccupied with what they will say next. Being aware of your listening barriers will improve your ability to listen.

Here are some tips for becoming a better listener:

- Have a desire to listen.
- Maintain eye contact, and concentrate on the other person.
- Listen with your heart, ears, and eyes.
- Take notes.
- Build rapport by pacing the speaker (match and mirror gestures, voice patterns, and expressions).
- Tell someone else what you have learned.
- Do not jump to conclusions.
- Control distractions.
- Expect to be a good listener.

Be aware of what kind of listener you are. Work at it, and you will build stronger relationships. Other people will like you more, and you will have a greater capacity to contribute to the practice.

Make Others Feel Important

One of the most effective listeners I have known is the late Dr. Jacob Mosier, former president of the American Veterinary Medical Association (AVMA) and former head of clinics at Kansas State University. He seldom talked about himself. His eyes focused on the speaker while he asked questions to draw out comments. His complete attention and interest made the speaker feel very important! Emulating his example in speaking to clients and other staff members will greatly increase the technician's effectiveness.

Develop a Light Touch

Life would be a lot happier and more interesting if more people had a sense of humor. I was recently in a practice in which a technician was a great example of a person with a light touch. This technician intently listens to clients with her heart and eyes. Her keen sense of humor erases any communication barriers and instantly draws people to her. She makes a client feel important because of her sincere interest and sense of humor.

Practical Ideas to Build Rapport and Develop Relationships

Try the following simple practical suggestions to improve interpersonal relations with clients:

- Greet clients with a warm salutation.
- Look them in the eye, smile, and call them by name.
- Develop rapport.
- Become genuinely interested; find out about them.
- Ask more questions, talk less, and listen more.
- Welcome criticism, and avoid being defensive.
- Make every person you meet feel important.

There is a saying in business, "If you don't succeed with people—you don't succeed in business." Interactive skills are synonymous with being a successful technician.

Setting an Example

At the center of the leadership model is the heart of a leader. This represents the role model that is the most important part of leadership.

A person's character is the building block of PL because every person must be able to look in the mirror with respect; otherwise, energy and confidence are diminished. Each individual must know what John Gray meant when he said, "Success lies in doing not what others consider to be great, but what you consider to be right."

Technician Note

Success lies in doing not what others consider to be great, but what you consider to be right.

—John Gray

The heart of PL is example. Values, character, trust, respect, and integrity are the core of one's example. It has been said that "the way one wins shows much of his or her character, and the way he or she loses shows all of it."

Dr. Albert Schweitzer, the French theologian and jungle physician, said, "Example is not the main thing in influencing others. It is the only thing." He taught, "There are only three ways to teach. . . one is by example, two is by example, and three is by example!"

Dr. Hugh Nibley said, ". . . leadership is an escape from mediocrity . . . the leader being simply the one who sets the highest example."

It is important to feel good about yourself and recognize your worth. The feeling that you are a person of value is closely related to developing as a personal leader. Your ability to set a good example is also closely linked to self-esteem.

The Journey of Jim and Naomi Rhode

A good example of two inspirational role models is provided by Jim and Naomi Rhode. They founded Smart/

Practice, one of the most successful medical marketing companies in the world. They supply practices throughout the world with more than 14,000 products, ranging from consumable and disposable infection-control products to "soft paws" for the veterinary profession, which keep cats from scratching the furniture.

Naomi Rhode, CSP, CPAE and James Rhode, CSP, are motivational speakers who are in great demand. They both have served as president of the National Speakers Association.

Despite busy schedules, Jim and Naomi have been able to maintain a balance in their business, family, and church. I asked them, "What has been your greatest internal motivation for accomplishing so much?" They answered, "Our involvement and love for the spiritual part of life are what light the fire within us." Naomi added, "Our family, faith in God, and dedication to living life abundantly are most important to us. Through the years, we have come to know the value of little things. Our lives have been happy and fulfilled as we have been able to serve others."

Technician Note

Our energy comes from the love of the spiritual part of life.

—Naomi Rhode

BEING A LIFELONG LEARNER

Knowledge is power! Keeping current requires the processing of a huge amount of information. Jeanne Bosson, a veterinary technician, says, "Take every seminar you can; study during your free time." Vicky Kasel echoes this advice. She says, "After 30 years' experience as a veterinary technician, the most important thing I can say is don't become stagnant; keep learning." Unless a person is truly motivated to lifelong learning, he or she will fall hopelessly behind.

Harvard Psychology Professor B.F. Skinner writes, "Education is what survives when what has been learned has been forgotten."

Technician Note

Education is what survives when what has been learned has been forgotten.

—B.F. Skinner

Formal education is a place to start, but it will not fulfill all one's learning requirements throughout life. Workshops, seminars, training sessions, coaching, videos, audiocassettes, interactive computer programs, and visits to other practices are other excellent sources of new information. Also, there is no substitute for reading and studying books and periodicals.

The veterinary technician with a desire to get a formal education but who feels he or she cannot afford it should consider the story of Dr. Gabor Vajda. Looking back on his childhood, he remembers the bombings, deaths, and destruction in his neighborhood in Bolatonszemes, Hungary; his family lived on a small farm in this village of about 1000 people during the dark days of World War II. His father was away fighting in the war, and the Vajda family had to fend for themselves, surviving on only the crops they could grow.

When conditions improved after the war, Gabor accompanied a German country veterinarian on his farm calls to neighboring farms. His love for animals grew, and his boyhood dream of preventing suffering and diseases among animals became dominant in his mind. He prepared to become a veterinarian and was studying veterinary science at the University of Budapest when the Communists again took over the country in the Hungarian Revolution. Gabor protested the presence of tanks and destruction of thousands of lives. His family's farm and business were taken over by the Communists, and Gabor and his younger brother fled the country. They were successful in getting to Salzburg, where they obtained sponsorship to immigrate to America.

Gabor spent 3 months learning to speak English and was accepted into the Iowa State University College of Veterinary Medicine. Four years later, he graduated with a doctoral degree in veterinary medicine. He paid his way through school by milking cows, making doughnuts, caring for a research colony of beagles, and working as a janitor.

Gabor obtained his first position with Dr. Bella Marriassy, who had also escaped from Hungary after the war. Through hard work and sacrifice, Gabor eventually was able to lease his own small animal clinic. In the next few years, he worked 7 days each week, concentrating on delivering quality medicine and exceptional client service. His efforts earned him the respect of his clients and colleagues, as attested to by being selected Arizona's Veterinarian of the Year and later being elected the national president of the American Animal Hospital Association.

How was Gabor able to overcome the obstacles that hold back most people? He told me that he was able to achieve his dream despite a lack of money and family support because he had confidence that he could achieve his goals. He said, "I have never known failure—I believed I could accomplish anything through hard work and by giving other people their money's worth."

Technician Note

I have never known failure—I believed I could accomplish anything through hard work and by giving other people their money's worth.

—Gabor Vajda

Gabor gives the following advice to others who would like to be stronger personal leaders:

- Love people; put people first.
- Always be sincere, appreciative, and grateful.
- Treat others with respect.
- Be willing to work as hard as necessary to achieve your goals.
- Be honest and open, and count your blessings.

Gabor Vajda lives by the philosophy of George Bernard Shaw, which (paraphrased) is, "Life is like a burning torch; live it to its fullest and pass the torch along to others."

OVERCOMING OBSTACLES

It is easy to look at other people with envy, not realizing the obstacles they have had to overcome to achieve success.

A good example is Emmett Smith. He was diagnosed with a fatal brain tumor and given no hope of living. A decision was made to have experimental surgery that had been performed only four times. Two of the patients had died on the operating table, and the other two were in a vegetative state for the rest of their lives.

After Emmett's surgery, he was partially paralyzed and confined to a wheelchair. His inner balance system had been destroyed. To complicate matters, infection set in, and he again was given no hope of survival. However, after 14 days of a temperature of 104° F, he miraculously began to respond and slowly recovered.

Most people would have resigned themselves to remain in a wheelchair for the remainder of their lives, but not Emmett! He challenged himself to not only walk again but also run 20 miles just 1 year from the day of his operation. As impossible as it seemed, Emmett had the faith and determination needed to accomplish this goal.

Emmett literally forced himself to get out of the wheelchair and start walking. He struggled because he could not maintain his balance and would fall. He eventually conquered this problem and threw away his canes. Soon he was able to jog slowly. At exactly 1 year after his surgery—through sheer determination, practice, and persistence—he accomplished his goal of running 20 miles. Emmett believes, "It is how you handle the difficulties in your life that determines your success." Experience taught him that true happiness is achieving victory over self.

Technician Note

It is how you handle the difficulties in your life that determines your success. True happiness is victory over self.

—Emmett Smith

Emmett demonstrated that the human spirit cannot be held down if there is a will to fight back and succeed. In his speeches, he challenges others to find success and happiness in life by doing the following:

- Meeting trouble as a friend
- Realizing that all great human endeavor results from doing common things in an uncommon way
- Taking chances; the fear of failure holds people back
- Daring to meet luck halfway
- Daring to be honest
- Setting an example; being a role model

Regardless of circumstances, problems, or challenges, an individual can achieve personal objectives if he or she believes in a goal and is committed to overcome all obstacles to achieve that goal.

ALL THINGS ARE POSSIBLE

Ryan Zinn, the son of a Tiffin, Ohio, veterinarian, is a 100- and 200-meter sprinter. He was voted the most valuable member of his Sycamore Mohawk High School track team and elected captain of the 4 × 100 relay team, which set a new school record.

You may wonder what is so unusual about this. The remarkable thing is that he accomplished this with someone else's heart. Yes, Ryan is proud of the fact that he is alive today and has earned two degrees in mechanical engineering from The Ohio State University. The heart of a 21-year-old college ROTC and honor student was transplanted into Ryan's chest cavity when Ryan was only 15 years old.

I wondered how Ryan was able to keep going, without slowing down, in the face of death. Ryan said, "I focused on what I could do—not on what I couldn't do."

> ### Technician Note
> I focused on what I could do—not on what I couldn't do.
> —Ryan Zinn

How was Ryan so successful in recovering from this life-threatening event? He has been successful in leading himself through a stroke and transplant surgery by learning to do the following:

- Follow and learn from the example and values of parents.
- Be goal oriented.
- Manage time effectively.
- Relate well to other people.
- Never give up.
- Recognize that no matter how tough it may seem, it always gets better.

THE PRECIOUS FAMILY-PET BOND

Dr. Martin Becker has dedicated his life to promoting "the celebration and protection of the family-pet bond" on a global basis.

A highly motivated and skilled communicator, Martin's goal is to educate and enlighten practice staffs on everything they need to delight clients and nurture and protect animals. He believes, "To be a successful technician, you should treat every animal as if [his or her] owner was watching."

His parents taught him the following ideas to help him craft emotional wealth and financial success:

- The harder you work, the luckier you'll get.
- Don't look for opportunities. Create them!
- If you want your ship to come in, you've got to send some out.
- ROA: Be responsible for (your) own actions.

"Every day when I leave my house, I pause to look at our family mission statement, which is at eye level on the door: Remember yesterday; live for today; plan for tomorrow; no regrets!"

> ### Technician Note
> Remember yesterday.
> Live for today.
> Plan for tomorrow.
> No regrets!

This is good advice for technicians or any personal leader who wants a better quality of life. To accelerate personal growth, follow Martin's example and do not wait for success to fall into your lap. Make your mark on society by having a purpose, developing a strategy, taking action, evaluating your progress, and living a life of self-improvement. Dr. Becker truly believes, "You won't get to the top of the mountain by falling there!"

APPLICATION OF PERSONAL LEADERSHIP

PL will lift vision to higher sights, raise performance to higher standards, and build personality beyond its normal limitations. The person who faithfully follows the PL formula and applies these five principles will be amazed at the results in his or her professional as well as personal life. Do not be discouraged by failure. Just remember, no one succeeds 100% of the time. Keep in mind that losing is the first step to winning. Failing should not be thought of as a failure, but as a valuable learning experience.

> ### Technician Note
> Losing is the first step to winning.

Why are there are so many half-read books, uncleaned garages, and diets and exercise programs that have been started and stopped? We have failed to lead ourselves to accomplish our objectives. It could result from not having a specific plan, a weak commitment, or failure to follow the five principles of PL.

My challenge to the reader is to read and reread this chapter and then apply this information after making a commitment to be all you can be. Reading this chapter will be beneficial, but real power will not come from reading but from the application of PL.

REFERENCES

Brooks M: *The power of business rapport,* New York, 1990, Harper-Collins.

Brooks M: *Instant rapport,* New York, 1989, Warner Books.

Managing for success software: employee manager version, Scottsdale, Ariz, 1991, TTI Software, Ltd.

Russell RL: *The miracle of personal leadership,* Dubuque, Iowa, 1996a, Kendall/Hunt.

Russell RL: People: the keys to profitability, *Semin Vet Med Surg (Small Anim),* vol 11, 1996b.

Russell RL: Preparing veterinary students with the interactive skills to effectively work with clients and staff, *J Vet Med Educ* 21:40, 1994.

RECOMMENDED READING

Laborde GZ: *Influencing with integrity,* Palo Alto, Calif, 1983, Syntony.

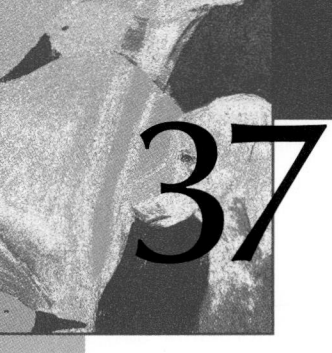

37

Stress and Its Management

Sandra S. Brackenridge

During the last 25 years, information from the medical community regarding stress and its deleterious effect on human beings has been abundant. According to current research, stress is responsible for physical illness, mental illness, and even death more often than any other factor. Further, stressful living has become accepted, even considered unavoidable, in our technologically modern, fast-paced society. In choosing to work in veterinary medicine, especially if responsibilities entail direct service to clients, one chooses a work environment with a high potential for daily stress. However, stress can be managed, controlled, and sometimes alleviated through personal and professional awareness, understanding, monitoring, and revision of lifestyle. This chapter provides a basic understanding of stress, identification of some of the stressors in life and those specific to veterinary medicine, suggestions for management and coping, and awareness of burnout signals.

 Technician Note

In choosing to work in veterinary medicine, one chooses a work environment with a high potential for daily stress.

A DEFINITION OF STRESS

Stress can be defined as the state produced when the body responds to any demand for adaptation or adjustment. The infinite demands that produce this response state are called *stressors*. These stressors may be external (e.g., time schedules, workload), environmental (e.g., heat, cold, noise), or internal (e.g., emotions, sensitivities). The nature of stress is nonspecific in that certain biochemical reactions are common with exposure to all types of stressors. However, stress is not always negative. Stress responses can be pleasurable and even beneficial in certain situations.

GOOD STRESS/BAD STRESS

Stressors can mobilize a person into being energized to meet specific challenges and take action. As action is taken, the body's stress management system functions in exactly the way it was intended, and with "good" stress, the person experiences a feeling of satisfaction, relief, or exhilaration. Stressors can also be excessive in number or intensity, prolonged, and unavoidable. When a person experiences stressors of this nature, the stress reaction of the body works overtime. The body mobilizes, attempts to adjust to an ongoing drain of energy, and eventually becomes overwhelmed and exhausted. Three factors determine whether stress is negative or positive: *choice, control,* and *consequences.*

 Technician Note

Stress may be negative or positive depending on choice, control, and consequences.

Choice

When a person responds to a stressor that is perceived as self-chosen, the response itself is viewed more positively. Generally speaking, if individuals are attracted to veterinary medicine, pursue training, and obtain their desired employment, they will be more likely to perceive stressors encountered at work without excessive negativity or resentment. However, if employment in veterinary medicine is perceived as necessary simply to make ends meet financially, or if the person feels his or her true career choice is an impossibility, stressors common to veterinary medicine may be less tolerable. For example, an aggressive animal may be perceived as a challenging stimulation by one who has chosen this career, whereas the same animal would be perceived as a burden or an obstacle by one who truly wishes to be in a different position of employment.

Control

Good or bad stress is also determined by whether the stressor is perceived as within the person's control. In veterinary practice, clients control the schedule, patients provide emergencies and unpredictability, and employers control much of the working environment. When staff are consulted as to scheduling and offered control over certain areas of the working environment, the stressful effect of these factors can be minimized. Again, an aggressive animal provides a good example. Such a situation can seem

TABLE 37-1	EXAMPLES OF GOOD AND BAD STRESS	
	Good Stress	**Bad Stress**
Personal	You exert yourself and win a game of tennis.	Your car breaks down, and you must walk 3 miles for help.
Professional	You are asked to speak at the next professional conference.	A co-worker fails to show up for work, and you must work doubly hard.
Personal	You throw a party for 150 people.	Your house is burglarized.
Professional	You perform euthanasia on an elderly animal, and the family thanks you.	A young animal unexpectedly dies while boarding.
Personal	You reenter higher education.	Your spouse is laid off.
Professional	The practice expands, you work harder, but your income increases.	A type A co-worker constantly competes with you.

intolerable when the client insists on being present during treatment, and the employer refuses to muzzle the animal. However, when the client responds in the desired way, and when the employer considers others' opinions, the staff feel that the treatment of the animal and the aggression is within their control. Although the aggressive animal continues to be a stressor during the working day, perceived control of the stressor alleviates much of its negative impact.

Consequences

Stressors are more likely to be perceived as positive stimulation when consequences can be anticipated. In veterinary medicine, the death of a patient is always a source of stress. However, when the animal is properly diagnosed and death is expected or euthanasia is performed, stress in the situation is manageable. On the other hand, when an apparently healthy animal unexpectedly dies during surgery, treatment, or boarding, resulting stress can feel acutely negative and overwhelming. Because the stressor could not have been anticipated, the stress response has become "bad" stress.

Therefore each stressful situation provides an opportunity for choice, a feeling of control, and anticipation of consequences. Table 37-1 provides further examples of good and bad stress within veterinary medicine. Because stress is unavoidable, knowledge of these three factors can help one to transform adverse stressors into tolerable stressors.

STRESS AND THE BODY

Stress, whether good or bad, is a response of the body. An understanding of how and where stress originates within the body, its pathway, and the physical toll it can extract is necessary to manage stress and maintain good health.

Flight or Fight

Humans are equipped, as are all mammals, with a physical system to assist them in handling threatening situations. This system has been necessary for survival as a species. Historically, this physical system enabled humans to flee or to fight when externally threatened. In the primitive state, enemies included wild animals, other primitive peoples, and natural occurrences. Today, this physical system shifts into gear when anything or anyone is perceived as threatening, externally or internally. In fact, perceived threats are pervasive. We drive defensively and cope with pollution of all sorts, and crime has become a realistic cause for concern. Internally, we fear bad news, losses, rejection, and failure; we are threatened by financial crises, in consider-

ation by others, illness, and aging. The list of internal stressors is unique to every person, depending on background, temperament, and aspirations. The stress response is nonspecific and is mobilized when one is faced with any of these threats, perceived or real.

The Pathway of Stress

Dr. Hans Selye, who is often called the father of stress research, termed the body's response to stress the *general adaptation syndrome (GAS)*. On a person's exposure to any threat or stressor, the first phase of GAS, the alarm reaction, is elicited. After this phase, the person enters a stage of adaptation or resistance. If the stressor continues to threaten, the person enters a third phase, which Dr. Selye called the stage of exhaustion. Unless interrupted, and if the stressor is severe enough and present long enough, the third stage results in physical illness, burnout, or even death.

Technician Note

The general adaptation syndrome (GAS) is the body's response to stress.

During the alarm phase, the body's physical system designed for fight or flight is mobilized. The human body is "supercharged" for action with all muscles and organs in a state of readiness. Many changes are happening internally. The real or perceived stressor signals the hypothalamus to produce hormones, such as endorphins. These hormones stimulate the autonomic nervous system as well as the pituitary gland. The autonomic nervous system affects the digestive system and other vital organs. The stimulation of the pituitary gland increases blood flow, discharging more hormones into the bloodstream. This action stimulates the adrenal glands, which affect breathing, cortisone production, muscle tension, perspiration, and blood sugar levels. Figure 37-1 charts the pathway of the stress response through the body.

The stimulation of the adrenal glands is responsible for many stress-related illnesses. Increased epinephrine production causes increased respiration and heart rate. Rapid breathing causes the injection of additional oxygen into the bloodstream, which alters the amount of carbon monoxide in the bloodstream and causes dry mouth, irritated nasal passages, and chest contractions. A prolonged increase in heart rate can cause hypertension, leading to cardiovascular problems. The pituitary and adrenal glands influence cortisone levels, which are responsible for the body's immune responsiveness. Prolonged muscular

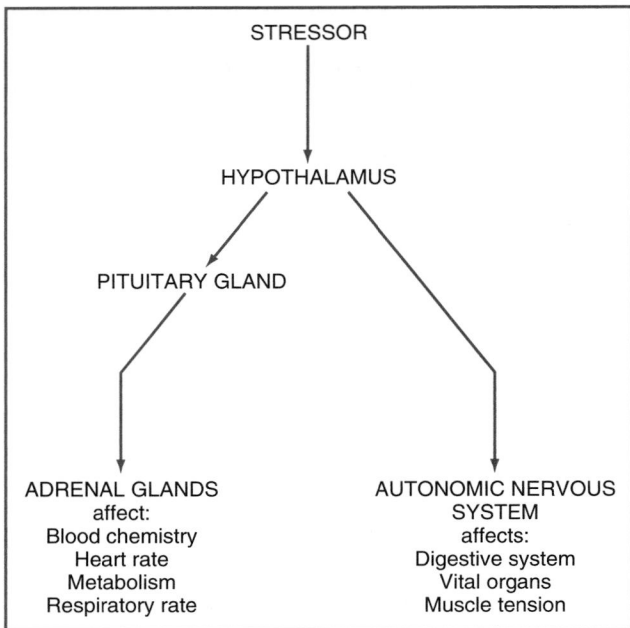

FIGURE 37-1. Pathway of the stress response through the body.

Box 37-1	PHYSICAL PROBLEMS TRIGGERED BY STRESS
Insomnia	Chest pains
Headaches	Hypertension
Allergies	Heart attacks
Temporomandibular joint (TMJ) disorder	Sexual dysfunction
	Chronic fatigue
Nausea	Depression
Indigestion	Dizziness
Heartburn	Anxiety
Backaches	Alcoholism
Ulcers	Muscle aches
Colitis	Dry mouth
Problems swallowing	Facial tics
Hyperventilation	Erratic breathing
Asthma	Upper respiratory illnesses
Rheumatoid arthritis	Nosebleeds
Dermatitis	Perspiration

tension, caused by the adrenal glands and by stimulation of the autonomic nervous system, results in various aches and pains, as well as digestive disorders. Stress-induced digestive disorders are exacerbated by the fluctuation in blood sugar levels, resulting in poor eating habits, ulcers, nausea, or constipation. Prolonged stress can result in ongoing endocrine disorders. Box 37-1 shows the various physical disorders that can be considered stress-related disorders.

All the mentioned physical changes originally occur during the alarm phase of GAS. However, when the stressor or stressors continue, the adaptation phase ensues, in which the body attempts to adjust to its new level of activity. When exposure to the stressor continues, any level of adaptation that the body has acquired may be lost, depending on factors unique to each person. Exhaustion may appear physically, or it may be demonstrated psycho-

logically. Burnout can be defined as psychologic, and sometimes physical, exhaustion prompted by prolonged subjection to a stressor without adaptation or interruption.

Although all humans will respond to stressors through activation of the above described physical syndrome, not all will proceed through all three phases of GAS. Whether a person can adapt to stress, what stressors are felt most acutely, and which physical or psychologic manifestations of stress will appear depend on various factors, including personality.

PERSONALITY FACTORS

Certain personality variables predispose individuals to susceptibility to stress or to resistance to stress. These variables may be inherent in the personality, or they may be learned behaviors and attitudes. Science has not yet determined how much of the personality is genetic and how much is learned, but personalities can be grouped into types. Personality type is a reliable indicator of predisposition to stress-related disorders.

 Technician Note

Personality factors predispose individuals to be resistant or susceptible to stress.

The Stress-Prone Individual

The term *type A personality* was first used by Dr. Meyer Friedman and Dr. Ray Rosenman in their book *Type A Behavior and Your Heart.* One study concluded that type A personalities were three times as likely to have coronary artery disease, and personality type was found to be the most reliable predictor of heart attack. Type A people are competitive, impatient, perfectionist, often angry, suffering from "hurry sickness," and insecure.

 Technician Note

Type A people are susceptible to coronary artery disease.

Overt and covert feelings of competition with others represent a characteristic of type A personalities. These feelings may be motivated by an ambition to win or succeed, or they may stem from a fear of defeat or failure. Specific areas for competition may be chosen, such as within the workplace, or the type A person may compete in every activity, even in driving, recreation, and social groups.

Type A personalities are impatient, and they find it trying to stand in line or to wait. They would rather be late to appointments than be left waiting; thus type A personalities can be chronically late. They are impatient with receptionists, waiters and waitresses, car mechanics, and, frankly, almost anyone on whom they depend for service. They are also impatient with employers and sometimes with their families. This behavior may be motivated by the need to be in control of situations, or it may be motivated by the desire to avoid anxiety-provoking thinking time.

Perfectionism is a characteristic included in identification of many personality types, and it is also a sign of type A personality. The need for approval and the desire to avoid criticism are paramount in the minds of type A people. Combined with their competitive behavior, perfectionism accounts for the priority type A individuals seem

TABLE 37-2 TYPE A OR TYPE B?		Type A	Type B
1.	I become impatient when events move slowly.	Often	Rarely
2.	I bring work home from the job.	Often	Rarely
3.	I set deadlines and schedules for myself.	Often	Rarely
4.	I feel guilty when I relax and "do nothing."	Often	Rarely
5.	I speak, eat, and move at a quick pace.	Often	Rarely
6.	I am achievement oriented.	Very	Slightly
7.	I have a strong need for success.	Yes	No
8.	I hurry through or do not finish sentences.	Often	Rarely
9.	I try to do two or more things at once.	Often	Rarely
10.	I like to count my achievements and possessions.	Yes	No
11.	I have angry or hostile feelings toward competitive people.	Often	Rarely
12.	I am generally observant of my surroundings.	Yes	No

to place on performance. They have difficulty delegating and appear critical of others to whom they do delegate. Type A people wage a true inner struggle between the need to share responsibility and fear that delegation will backfire on them.

Hostile and *aggressive* are terms often used by co-workers to describe a type A personality. Because the type A personality is competitive and impatient, he or she will expect the same from others. Type A individuals then defend themselves against what they perceive as other people's aggression and hostility. As a self-fulfilling prophecy, they often find themselves working with others who are also type A. Their sense of humor is often directed toward others' inferiority, and they have difficulty believing that anyone likes them for themselves rather than for their performance. As a result, type A people can be difficult as employers and as fellow employees. Ironically, they usually get rave reviews from their own supervisors or mentors.

The type A individual experiences what Friedman and Rosenman called "hurry sickness" or polyphasic behavior. This is the easiest behavior to identify, because type A persons constantly seem to juggle more than one activity at a time. They talk on the telephone at the same time that they write in charts and eat lunch. Type A secretaries are able to simultaneously answer the telephone, file charts, and schedule appointments. A type A technician might be found attending to a patient, setting up for surgery, and taking a telephone call from a client at the same time. Type A personalities impose so many deadlines on themselves. In short, they deprive themselves of opportunities to relax, while thinking that efficiency is another word for speediness in all activities.

Often, type A individuals appear judgmental of others; however, they are usually most judgmental about themselves. They have high standards and high expectations for themselves and for others. This behavior stems from insecurity about their own worth, and they are constantly trying to prove their worth through performance, production, and status. Type A people are often truly compassionate individuals, empathic to the pain and sensitivities of others.

Although type A behaviors place these individuals at risk in regard to stress, many of the same behaviors are responsible for the success that they experience in their chosen field. In veterinary medicine, as in many other professions, there is a higher proportion of type A individuals at the top of the profession. Veterinarians often exemplify type A behavior, and thus technicians frequently work for type A

individuals. Because of the fact that type A individuals often approve of behavior similar to their own, these same veterinarians enjoy employing type A technicians.

An alternative to the type A personality is termed the *type B personality*. To determine whether you are a type A or type B personality, answer and score the questionnaire provided in Table 37-2. No one is a perfect type A or type B, but the more that type B fits one's personality, the lower the incidence of stress-related illness.

The Stress-Hardy Individual

Research has focused on personality types who are stress prone as well as on the characteristics of individuals who are more resistant to stress. Friedman and Rosenman described type B individuals as more resistant to stress-related illness. Other studies use the term *hardiness* to stress and outline certain components of the personality that appear to protect against stress.

 Technician Note

Type B people are more resistant to stress.

Type B individuals have realistic expectations and are not worried about failure. They have an appreciable acceptance of themselves that is not based on status or production. Type B people have a good sense of security and self-esteem, and they are comfortable delegating responsibilities to others without fear of backfire. Deadlines are based on an appraisal of what the type B person can do, not on a misperception of what others believe he or she should do. Type B individuals enjoy time off for recreation and quiet time. They can be as ambitious and successful as type A individuals and sometimes more so. In fact, because they do not experience the same sense of urgency as type A personalities, type B personalities can avoid mistakes and therefore be more efficient. They have good relationships in their world because they are not hostile, guarded, or judgmental.

Other qualities of personality that help individuals in their resistance to stress have been identified and grouped under the term *stress hardy*. These individuals have in common three notable attitudes toward living that appear to make a difference in their response to stress:

- *Control.* Hardy individuals approach experiences with the attitude and belief that they are in control of their own life, responses, and destiny. They believe that they can influence events and do not have a "victim" attitude. They take responsibility for what happens to them and for the situations in which they are placed.

- *Commitment.* Hardiness also indicates an attitude of curiosity and involvement in situations that are faced. They do not withdraw from situations; instead, they attempt to understand the people and activities in their life.
- *Challenge.* The belief that change and adjustment are exciting and conducive to personal growth is important to hardy individuals. They see life as an opportunity to learn and develop as people, and experiences of all kinds help them to do so.

Hardy individuals ride out stress or cope with it better. In addition, they are often people who have deeply spiritual connections. This spirituality is not necessarily dependent on affiliation with any religious institution, yet it is important to hardy individuals in their private moments, their belief systems, and their approach to life.

Thus personality can be an advantage or disadvantage in regard to stress management. Certain qualities of behavior and of attitude may buffer a person against stress, and awareness of these personal risk factors is the first step in managing stress. Identifying specific stressors is the next step.

IDENTIFYING STRESSORS

A veterinary technician's stressor load includes general stressors and those that are unique to veterinary medicine. There are life event stressors, environmental stressors, personal stressors, client stressors, and career stressors common to many technicians.

Technician Note

Technicians are often subjected to stress from the environment, workplace, clients, and personal issues.

Life Event Stressors

Many events encountered within a lifetime are stressful, regardless of the perception of the event as positive or negative. Thomas Holmes and Richard Rahe created a scale to measure the impact of 43 life events (Table 37-3). An individual who accrues more than 300 life change units within 1 year is at risk for stress-related illness. If the total is 150 to 299, the risk is reduced by 30%. Only a slight risk is posed if the total is under 150 life change units. The scale is only an indicator, however, and some people are simply more susceptible to stress than others. Total stressor load must be analyzed to determine true risk for stress-related illness and the need to alleviate stress load.

Environmental Stressors

General environmental stressors include climate and weather, pollution, where one lives and works, crime, and traffic. Other environmental stressors include the people with whom one spends time; for example, a mother-in-law who has come for a 1-month visit may be a stressor for some individuals. Government concerns, such as the threat of war or U.S. Internal Revenue Service (IRS) auditing, may be an environmental stressor. Many environmental stressors can affect individuals in their personal and professional lives. Identification of general environmental stressors can help in determining stressor load and need for revision of lifestyle.

TABLE 37-3 SOCIAL READJUSTMENT RATING SCALE	
Life Event	Number of Life Change Units
Death of a spouse	100
Divorce	73
Marital separation	65
Jail term	63
Death of close family member	63
Personal injury or illness	53
Marriage	50
Fired at work	47
Marital reconciliation	45
Retirement	45
Change in family member's health	44
Pregnancy	40
Sex difficulties	39
Gain of new family member	39
Business readjustment	39
Change in financial state	38
Death of close friend	37
Change to different line of work	36
Change in number of arguments with spouse	35
Mortgage of $100,000	31
Foreclosure of mortgage or loan	30
Change in work responsibilities	29
Son or daughter leaving home	29
Trouble with in-laws	29
Outstanding personal achievement	28
Spouse begins or stops work	26
Begin or end school	26
Change in living conditions	25
Revision of personal habits	24
Trouble with boss	23
Change in work hours or conditions	20
Change in residence	20
Change in schools	20
Change in recreation	19
Change in church activities	19
Change in social activities	18
Mortgage or loan less than $100,000	17
Change in sleeping habits	16
Change in number of family get-togethers	15
Change in eating habits	15
Vacation	13
Christmas	12
Minor violations of the law	11

Modified from Holmes TH, Rahe R: *J Psychosom Res* 11:213, 1967; with permission.

Veterinary environmental stressors, which are more pertinent for the purposes of this chapter, may also be numerous and greatly affect an individual's stress level. Environments will differ for those who work in a small animal clinic and for those who work in large animal or mixed animal practices.

Environmental stressors in a veterinary practice may include noise level, space limitations, equipment and supply factors, orderliness, record-keeping factors, scheduling demands, geographic area, co-workers, and population served. Noise in a clinic is often constant because of vocalization of animals, telephones ringing, and conversation. Most people who work in a clinic accustom themselves to the noise level and are able to tune it out.

However, if the stimulation becomes irritating, more frequent breaks may be required to combat this stressor.

Space limitations are also a stressor in most veterinary practices. Clientele and staff frequently become larger in number before additional space is discussed or affordable. Crowding is stressful for humans, and each person in a practice needs his or her own personal space, even if it is just a locker or desktop. Attention should also be paid to arrangement, design, colors, lighting, temperature, and flow of traffic, all of which have been shown to affect stress levels. Clinic arrangement should make work easier and not more difficult. Equipment and supplies should be available and accessible to avoid unnecessary stress, and this is true in all practices, whether stationary or mobile. Inadequate equipment is a stressor and should be discarded. Regular maintenance of equipment avoids the stress of breakdowns and burdensome catch-up maintenance. Orderliness in storage is important, as is storage near the working area. Orderliness and efficiency are necessary to avoid stress in record keeping. Computers have become a huge asset in record keeping, but training must be thorough and provided to all staff so that software is an asset, not an additional stressor. Most software companies offer support in sales contracts, and companies should be required to provide training. In addition, forms should be customized, whether on computer or manually, to the needs of the practice so as to assist in speed, accuracy, and efficiency without stress.

Scheduling can be one of the most formidable veterinary environmental stressors. Despite best efforts, schedules frequently go awry because of emergencies, a verbose client, or an unexpected lengthy surgery or treatment. In a small animal clinic, scheduling is frequently interrupted by an emergency, such as an animal hit by a car or a resident case in cardiac arrest. In an equine practice, a case of colic can disrupt scheduling for several days. All staff members must work together to ensure that scheduling is as stress free as possible, allowing breaks while maintaining a good level of productivity. Type A employers may need to be approached about the problem of overscheduling. Walk-ins or emergencies on a slower day may be manageable, but the same case during a busy day may be stress producing. Encourage the development of policy regarding walk-ins and emergencies, making certain that all opinions are heard.

Geographic location is important, especially in large animal or mixed practices. Traffic, distance, and travel time to and from appointments may require special flexibility in scheduling. Emergencies and unexpected situations occur frequently and can be stressful if one is compulsively attached to schedule. The stressors of population served and co-workers will be discussed later under Career Stressors.

Personal Stressors

Each person brings to employment certain qualities that make him or her either resistant to the stressors in veterinary medicine or sensitive to those stressors. Amount of experience is a factor in that all initial employment in a chosen field is stressful. Moreover, each person's temperament is unique and may or may not be suited to the various duties of being a veterinary technician. Some people are naturally more sensitive to stimulation and environmental stressors. Some people are more comfortable with animals than with clients, finding professional contact with clients stressful; yet in most practices, technicians will be expected to deal with both animals and people. Flexibility is a quality of temperament necessary to manage stress in veterinary medicine. Each person also

brings the baggage of individual personal problems and backgrounds. These make the person vulnerable to certain types of people, certain situations, and certain animals that are reminders of similar personal experiences. Further, coping with various stressors in one's personal life (e.g., relationships, family) makes one more vulnerable to stressors within the workplace.

Self-confidence and self-esteem are important in the workplace and in all areas of life. Without those two qualities, almost every situation is stressful. With successful experience and acceptance and support by co-workers and employers, both qualities will develop to their fullest positive extent in a healthy person. If an individual struggles constantly with confidence and self-esteem, counseling can help in management of stress and avoidance of further deterioration in these areas.

Some professionals believe that people who work with animals are empathetic by nature. After all, they learn to recognize pain and contentment in patients who cannot use words. Empathy can be defined as the vicarious experience of another person's emotions. Further, empathy has been said to be the foundation of compassion. However, empathy may be stressful in a veterinary environment, where patients are often in pain and treated without being able to inform or to object. Empathy also is stressful in situations of patient death and euthanasia when the experience of another person's grief is painful. It cannot be avoided, but it can be useful in every work situation. Technicians must learn to distinguish between their own empathy and another person's emotions to manage stress.

Client Stressors

All clients may be stressors for the person who would rather spend time with animals than with humans. However, certain types of clients are always stress producing. The elderly client, angry client, independent client, and grieving client are mentioned most often as the most difficult to deal with and therefore the most stressful.

Technician Note

The angry and demanding client always produces stress for the technician.

The *elderly client* is often attached to a pet. In fact, the animal can even be important to the quality of life of an elderly person who is widowed and living alone. Because of the health problems of the elderly population, their decreasing mobility, their ever-fluctuating memory, and sometimes their loneliness, more time can be expended with these clients than with all others combined. Instructions are given and are not always understood, or they must be repeated several times. When in the clinic, elderly clients would like to talk not only about the animal being treated but also about all the animals they have owned and even their children's animals. When an animal desperately needs conscientious treatment, treatment is not always followed by the elderly client, who cannot bear to leave the animal for treatment at the clinic. One can manage the stress of elderly clients by scheduling them for slower times of the day, allowing time to talk, returning their telephone calls when extra time can be allotted, and talking to their loved ones when painful decisions must be made. When an elderly person is your client, take a mental step backward, take a deep breath, and be patient.

The *angry client* can disrupt a perfectly good day. If the technician's confidence is not functioning well, the angry client can quickly find and mangle all of his or her sensitivities. No matter what the provocation, angry clients feel that they (or their animals) have been neglected, abused, or taken advantage of in some way. Assuming a defensive position is counterproductive with angry clients. Listening to their complaints, even making notes, reporting what they have said, and following up with them and their complaints can salvage positive feelings. Even when an angry client's accusations are correct, listening is the best response. Making excuses or defending actions will not alleviate the anger. These clients need the feeling that they, and their animals, are cared for, paid attention to, and important. Contact with angry clients, even when remediation has been successful, produces stress, and support from other staff members is essential to relieve stress.

The *independent client* consults a veterinarian but continues to treat his or her animal in a predetermined fashion. Such clients hear only what they decide makes sense in regard to instructions. They may have attempted every old-fashioned remedy before the animal is seen for treatment. They may be uneducated clients, or they may be clients who have obtained higher education, even within another area of medicine. In short, they act as if they know more than the professionals do about treating the animal. These clients unwittingly provoke anger and frustration among the veterinary team. To resist stress in dealing with independent clients, hear them out and tell them that you agree with some of their points. Explain, in terms that they can understand, your opinion as to diagnosis, justification for the diagnosis, and treatment. Treat them importantly, and make them feel as though they are a part of the treatment team and as though their opinions are carefully considered.

The *grieving client* is a stressor because of the emotionality of the situation. As mentioned, an empathetic response is helpful to clients yet stressful for the veterinary professional. Death of a patient is always stressful in veterinary practice. Not only do technicians frequently witness death and participate in causing death, but also they face the grief of clients, and sometimes they must even deal with their own grief for the patient. Management of this stressor involves several activities. First, technicians must separate their own feelings of grief (and/or failure and guilt) from the client's feelings. Second, they must deal with their own philosophy and feelings about death, including their feelings about their own and their loved ones' deaths. Third, technicians can become more comfortable with functioning during times of client bereavement. Literature and seminars are available that allow veterinary professionals to learn how to deal with bereavement. Chapter 20 gives assistance in this situation. An understanding of the stages of grief and what the technician may do to help clients during each stage is necessary to make the technician more comfortable in dealing with bereavement. Grief is an emotional process that cannot be avoided and must be experienced. Nothing can transform bad news into good news, but certain behaviors can allow an individual to confidently support others through bereavement.

Career Stressors

In choosing a career as a veterinary technician, individuals open themselves to various stressors. Veterinary technicians frequently must cope with long hours and demanding work responsibilities in return for minimal financial compensation. As in many careers, they must also cope with stressors provided by participating in a medical team.

Daily vulnerability to stress is much more justifiable when monetary compensation is on a par with the level of risk. Unfortunately, the salaries of veterinary technicians (and many veterinarians) do not reflect the long hours and demands of their careers. Technicians must at some point decide whether they can cope with this reality on a long-term basis. Only a conscious decision to accept a financial ceiling to remain in this rewarding career can prevent resentment because of terms of financial compensation.

Finances today are a stressor for most Americans. Budgets, consumer counseling services, and cutting back on credit can help. Veterinary technicians must accustom themselves to this stressor as ongoing, and they must use management techniques to cope.

The long hours of sometimes intense physical work to which veterinary technicians expose themselves are another stressor. Fatigue is an enemy that must be guarded against if one is to successfully manage stress. Becoming overtired, missing breaks, and working too many hours per week should be infrequent occurrences if longevity on the job and good health are desirable.

Work responsibilities for most veterinary technicians are demanding and stressful. Often, the veterinary technician spends more time caring for the animals and the clients than does the veterinarian. High-pressure cases, full schedules, emergencies, demanding clients, and monotonous tasks are stressors that can take their toll.

Finally, working as part of a medical team has advantages and disadvantages. When relationships within a medical team are amicable, compatible, and supportive, each person is better able to tolerate stressors. However, when there is even one conflicting relationship within the team, all members are vulnerable to the stress of this conflict. Communication, fairness, and trust within the team are necessary to meet the demands of the career. All team members should work conscientiously to ensure that the team functions as a buffer against stress rather than having the opposite effect.

Evaluation

After identifying all stressors in an individual's life, the total stressor load should be analyzed. Which stressors can be alleviated? Which ones can be prevented? In the workplace, team effort is usually required to alleviate many of the stressors mentioned in this chapter. If other people must be involved in lowering the stressor load, are they willing to cooperate to do so? Now, take a look at how much of the stress is ongoing and unavoidable. The following section discusses techniques for coping with stress and building stressor resistance.

COPING WITH STRESS

Resistance to stress can be developed by instituting new habits within the lifestyle, increasing mental health and awareness, developing support systems, and performing relaxation activities that are known to miraculously protect against stress within the body and psyche. Some of these techniques may require more extensive explanation than this chapter can provide, and the reader is encouraged to consult Recommended Reading for more information. Table 37-4 outlines some common solutions for stressors found in the environment, career, and personal life.

 Technician Note

A slightly altered lifestyle along with certain mental and physical requirements can combat the effects of stress.

TABLE 37-4	ALLEVIATION OF STRESS	
Stressor Type	**Stressor**	**Solution**
Environment	Noise	More frequent breaks
	Space	Redesign of clinic
	Equipment	Maintenance, discard faulty equipment
	Orderliness	Organization with routine staff maintenance
	Records	Customization of forms, computerization with consultation and training
Career	Scheduling	Team scheduling with attention to breaks, avoid overscheduling
	Geography	Avoid compulsivity in scheduling, make schedules flexible, maintenance of transportation, communication links
	Co-worker conflicts	Team meetings, mediation
	Client population	Training of staff in communication
	Finances	Budgetary counseling
	Long hours	Vacations, shift work
Personal	Personal/home/family	Counseling, peer support

Stress Resister Habits

Individuals can become more resistant to stress if they incorporate specific healthy habits into their daily lives. Attention to certain mental and physical requirements and the institution of a slightly altered lifestyle can combat the effects of stress. Aspects of nutrition, sleep, exercise, and mental recreation are relevant in the management of stress.

Nutrition is important in coping with stress. Regular healthy eating habits are the best protection against stress. However, during more stressful periods or if one is living a highly stressful daily life, the body's requirements are somewhat altered. Protein is important in counteracting the impact of stress on the body, and attention should be paid to the consumption of adequate protein while under stress. Vitamin C is helpful in combating the lowered immune response that stress produces and in avoiding stress-related illness. Vitamin D, calcium, iron, and the B-complex vitamins are thought to be important in reducing the impact of stress on the body and the psyche as well, especially in women. Because the amount of sugar within the bloodstream is altered during the body's response to stress, many people have a tendency to overeat or to eat too many sugars, fats, and carbohydrates during stressful periods. This tendency should be avoided because it is directly counterproductive in alleviating stress. Finally, good nutrition includes moderation in negative habits, such as the use of alcohol, caffeine, tobacco, and sodium.

Sleep is often neglected by veterinary professionals. More and more information from researchers is becoming available involving sleep, the need for it, and the type and duration of sleep needed. Every person has a unique requirement for duration of sleep, and one must examine this habit over a period of time to determine how much sleep makes him or her feel best, work best, and enjoy rising in the morning. An optimal amount of nighttime sleep is important in coping with stress, as is the type of sleep. The phase of sleeping called *rapid eye movement (REM) sleep* is when dreams occur. This phase does not occur normally in those who use drugs or alcohol or in those who are constantly tired and sleep deprived. In addition, it is known that this phase is abnormal in many people with mental illness. Good sleep habits particular to each individual provide the rest that both the body and mind need to be strong in response to stress.

Exercise is one of the best antidotes to stress. Its benefits include release from tension, restoration of normal chemical balance, resistance to the physiologic reaction to stress and resultant cardiovascular diseases, and relief from depression. To achieve these benefits, an exercise program should be convenient and inexpensive, be rhythmic and part of a daily routine, and require some exertion and concentration. Because aerobic exercises can be performed free indoors or outdoors, are rhythmic, and require focus, they are well suited for incorporation into a program of stress management.

Mental recreation describes the activity of pleasantly refocusing the mind away from stress-producing thoughts. So many stressors involve mental and emotional components that no coping program is effective unless there is attention to strengthening and relaxing the mind. Humor is important because laughter produces endorphins and combats illness. It is helpful if habits are developed so that some time is spent amusing ourselves, even laughing, each day. Television is sometimes, but not always, helpful. Other sources of humor include various forms of literature and art. The best source of humor is oneself, and learning to laugh at oneself is an irreplaceable gift.

Various other forms of mental recreation exist. Music, reading, and conversation are pleasing and interrupt the stress response. Hobbies that are enjoyable and require concentration are also effective. Contact with animals, coincidentally, has been found to lower blood pressure, respiration rate, and pulse rate. Animals are certainly available to veterinary technicians, but some time each day could be spent enjoying them rather than working on them. Spirituality and prayer are also effective in refocusing mental activity. Some form of mental recreation should be built into the weekly routine for each individual.

Mental Health and Awareness

Mental health is the best predictor of physical health. When an individual's stressor load includes a higher proportion of personal stressors from his or her present and past personal backgrounds, a more concentrated effort toward mental health may be recommended. Fears of rejection, inadequacy, or abandonment and problems with self-esteem, relationships, depression, or anger may render a person more vulnerable to stress.

Awareness, not only of one's own state of mental health but also of what personal stressors are and how one reacts to stressors, can make management of stress more effective. Which parts of the body are the first to react or are more sensitive to stress? How does the person respond to stress emotionally? In terms of behavior, where and with whom is stress released, and are those behaviors inappropriate or hurtful to others? Individuals may need professional help

Box 37-2	BENEFITS OF THE RELAXATION RESPONSE

- Oxygen consumption is lowered to a degree commonly reached only after 6 or 7 hr of sleep.
- Heart and respiration rates are decreased.
- Blood flow and skin temperature increase (circulation eases).
- Electrical resistance of the skin increases markedly, suggesting decreased anxiety.
- An electroencephalogram (EEG) shows high alpha and occasional theta, beta, and delta waves, suggesting a fluid level of consciousness comprising both wakefulness and deep sleep.
- A person becomes desensitized regarding disturbing thoughts or stimuli.
- A person feels enlivened after relaxation, with a fresher view of the world.
- The workload of the cerebral hemispheres becomes more equalized.
- Alertness is sharpened, stress-related illnesses improve, and productivity increases.
- Depression, self-blame, and irritability decrease.

Box 37-3	PROGRESSIVE MUSCULAR RELAXATION

1. Frown hard, count to 10, let go. Repeat. Repeat again.
2. Squeeze eyes shut, count to 10, let go. Repeat. Repeat again.
3. Wrinkle nose while counting to 10. Let go. Repeat twice.
4. Press lips together, count to 10. Let go. Repeat twice.
5. Tighten neck, pushing back. Count to 10. Let go. Repeat.
6. Lift left shoulder up, tighten, relax. Again.
7. Lift right shoulder up, tighten, relax. Repeat.
8. Press arms back against imaginary wall. Tighten. Relax. Repeat.
9. Clench fists, count to 10. Let go. Repeat.
10. Slump over, let head fall forward, and up. Repeat.
11. Tighten buttock muscles, count to 10, relax. Repeat.
12. Tighten leg muscles, count to 10. Relax. Repeat.
13. Flex feet, count to 10, relax. Repeat.
14. Repeat whichever spots were tense, at least once.

to answer these questions and to change their external and internal lives. Counselors can be of help in this area. In choosing a counselor, make sure that the professional is licensed in your state. Interview the counselor, and ascertain that his or her style and philosophy are compatible with those of the person to be treated. Finally, choose a counselor who appears knowledgeable about stress and the medical field and who is goal oriented.

Support

One of the more essential coping techniques concerns human relationships. Friendships, support, and ventilation of feelings are vital for human mental health in general but are also necessary for stress resistance. Veterinary technicians may need to work at developing healthy support networks at work and outside of work. Spouses cannot be the only resource for support because the system then becomes out of balance and the marriage begins to take pressure. Staff meetings and socials can help to develop rapport among co-workers. Employers should be required to offer support to their employees in many ways. Association meetings and conferences are another way to develop professional friendships and widen support networks. As mentioned, the veterinary medical profession, at all levels, is stressful, and the stressors within employment are common to many individuals. The feeling of commonality with others, even in stress, can be helpful in managing stress. Creative solutions for common stressors can be shared within office relationships, and some stressors can even be alleviated.

Relaxation Techniques

Dr. Herbert Benson wrote a book in 1975 called *The Relaxation Response* in which he popularized the response of the body to self-induced relaxation techniques. Meditation, self-hypnosis, and power naps all have the same function in eliciting the relaxation response. The benefits of these techniques are extensive and are listed in Box 37-2. This chapter cannot teach all these valuable techniques; however, two of them, progressive muscular relaxation and autohypnosis, are described in Boxes 37-3 and 37-4.

Box 37-4	AUTOHYPNOSIS

1. Put your feet flat on the floor, and support your hands on your lap. Sit up straight but comfortably. Roll your head to loosen your neck.
2. Pick a focal point for your eyes.
3. Breathe in deeply through your nose, out through your mouth, using your abdomen to breathe. Repeat twice.
4. Begin saying the word *relax* silently as you breathe normally, and let your eyes close.
5. Repeat the word *relax* in rhythm with your breathing.
6. Let your thoughts come, note them, and let them go. Then return your attention to the word *relax*.
7. Just let yourself relax, feel peaceful, and feel safe as you repeat the word *relax*. You may stay in this space for 10 minutes.
8. Now take a slow, deep breath, hold it, and breathe out. Begin to open your eyes as you take another breath, and breathe out. Stretch, and move about slowly.

When All Else Fails: Burnout

Burnout is psychologic, and sometimes physical, exhaustion caused by prolonged, uninterrupted exposure to a stressor or stressors. Many individuals in the veterinary profession experience burnout; veterinarians may burn out within 15 years and veterinary technicians within a shorter period of time. Physical symptoms of burnout include any of the illnesses noted earlier in the chapter, such as ulcers, gastroenteritis, cardiac arrhythmia, and even heartburn, backache, or nausea. Early behavioral symptoms of burnout include withdrawal, overeating, increase in alcoholic intake, constant fatigue, agitation, distraction, aggressive behaviors, facial tics and spasms, and increased spending. Georgia Witkin-Lanoil, Ph.D., wrote about the psychologic warning signs, which she characterizes as the "six D's": defensiveness, depression, disorganization, defiance, dependency, and decision-making difficulties.

Technician Note

When stress becomes overwhelming, burnout occurs.

When burnout has occurred, the professional hates to get up and go to work, has lost passion and enthusiasm for the once-loved career, and feels lost internally. Good counseling may help in reversing the burnout, but many times professionals consider and make a career change. To recover from burnout, one may need counseling and support. Reconnection with the initial enthusiasm is important; once desire to remain in the career has been established, reorganization of lifestyle and business regimen may be necessary.

However, the individual who is burned out is often the last to know. Loved ones and co-workers may recognize the syndrome much earlier than does the individual in question. As with many emotional problems, when the defense mechanism of denial is in place, the individual will only move to awareness when ready and able to cope. Working (or living) with this individual can be frustrating and difficult. Offer support, gentle confrontation and observations, readings, and personal experiences, and, most importantly, LISTEN. Encourage vacations, start an office exercise program, be creative. Suggest counseling only if the relationship is a close one and if the individual would not be alienated by the suggestion.

SUMMARY

Stress is a fact of life today, and it is a problem within the field of veterinary medicine that can cause mental and physical problems and even disrupt this rewarding career. However, it can be prevented, alleviated, and managed to the extent that its ramifications are not severe. The changes made, originally intended for management of stress, can also enrich lives and provide untold secondary rewards.

RECOMMENDED READING

Almeida DM, Kessler RC: Everyday stressors and gender differences in daily stress, *J Pers Soc Psych*, vol 75, 1998.

Benson H: *The relaxation response*, New York, 1975, Wm. Morrow & Co.

Boryshenko J: *Mending the body, mending the mind*, New York, 1988, Bantam Books.

Brackenridge S, Elkins D: *Stress management for the veterinary practice team*, Santa Barbara, Calif, 1996, Veterinary Practice Publishing.

Elkins AD: Burnout: is it a problem for the veterinary practice team? *Vet Pract Staff* 2:1, 1990.

Friedman M, Rosenman RH: *Type A behavior and your heart*, Greenwich, Conn, 1974, Fawcett Publications.

George JM et al: *Stress management for the dental team*, Philadelphia, 1986, Lea & Febiger.

Selye H: *Stress without distress*, Philadelphia, 1974, Lippincott.

Witkin G: *The female stress syndrome survival guide*, New York, 2000, Newmarket Press.

Witkin-Lanoil G: *The male stress syndrome*, New York, 1988, The Berkley Publishing Group.

APPENDIX

Common Abbreviations Used in Veterinary Medicine

a	Artery
aa	Of each
AA	Amino acid
AAHA	American Animal Hospital Association
Ab	Antibody; antibiotics
ABG	Arterial blood gas
ac	Before meals
ACD	Acid-citrate-dextrose
ACE	Angiotensin-converting enzyme
ACTH	Adrenocorticotropic hormone
AD	Right ear
ADH	Antidiuretic hormone
ad lib	Freely, as wanted
ADR	Active defense reflex; adverse drug reaction
A Fib	Atrial fibrillation
Ag	Antigen
A:G	Albumin-globulin ratio
AGID	Agar gel immunodiffusion
AL	Left ear
ALB	Albumin
ALK PHOS	Alkaline phosphatase
ALP	Alkaline phosphatase
ALT	Alanine aminotransferase
AM	Antemortem
AMA	Against medical advice; American Medical Association
AMI	Acute myocardial infarction
amp	Ampule
ANA	Antinuclear antibody
ANS	Autonomic nervous system
AP	Anterior-posterior; arterial pressure
APC	Atrial premature contraction
APTT	Activated partial thromboplastin time
ARF	Acute renal failure
ARR	Arrhythmia
AS	Aortic stenosis; left ear
ASAP	As soon as possible
ASD	Atrial septal defect
ASIF	Association for the Study of Internal Fixation
AST	Aspartate aminotransferase
AU	Each ear
AV	Atrioventricular
AV block	Atrioventricular as in first-, second-, third-degree AV block
BAR	Bright, alert, and responsive
BAER	Brain stem auditory-evoked response
BBB	Blood-brain barrier
BE	Barium enema colon only
BER	Basal energy requirement
bid	Twice daily
BLD	Blood
BLV	Bovine leukosis virus
BM	Bowel movement
BMR	Basal metabolic rate
BOL	Large pill (hora)
BP	Blood pressure
BRD	Bovine respiratory disease

BRSV	Bovine respiratory syncytial virus
BSA	Body surface area
BSP	Bromsulphalein
BT	Blue tongue
BUN	Blood urea nitrogen
BUTE	Phenylbutazone
BV	Bronchovesicular
BVD	Bovine virus diarrhea
BW	Body weight
$\bar{c}$	With
C & S	Culture and sensitivity
C-S	Coughing-sneezing
C-spine	Cervical spine
Ca	Calcium
CA	Carcinoma; coronary artery; cardiac arrest
CAE	Caprine arthritis-encephalitis
caps	Capsules
CAV-1	Canine adenovirus type 1
CBC	Complete blood count
cc	Cubic centimeter
CC	Chief complaint
CCM	Congestive cardiomyopathy
CD	Canine distemper
CEA	Canine erythrocyte antigen
CEM	Contagious equine metritis
CFJ	Coxofemoral joint
CGP	Circulating granulocyte pool
CHD	Canine hip dysplasia; coronary heart disease
CHF	Congestive heart failure
CHOL	Cholesterol
CHV	Canine hepatitis virus
CI	Cardiac insufficiency
CID	Combined immunodeficiency
CIN	Chronic interstitial nephritis
CITE	Concentration immunoassay technology
Cl	Chloride
CM	Cardiomyopathy
CMS	Cervical stenotic myelopathy
CMT	California mastitis test
CNE	Canine distemper encephalitis
CNS	Central nervous system
COB	Care of body
CODE E	Used in emergency for cardiac arrest
CPA	Cardiopulmonary arrest
CPD	Citrate-phosphate-dextrose
CPK	Serum creatine phosphokinase
CPR	Cardiopulmonary resuscitation
CPU	Central processing unit
Creat	Creatinine
CRF	Chronic renal failure; corticotropin-releasing factor
CRT	Capillary refill time; cathode-ray tube
CSF	Cerebrospinal fluid; colony-stimulating factor
CTZ	Chemoreceptor trigger zone
CVA	Cardiovascular accident; cerebrovascular accident

CVP	Central venous pressure	GUI	Graphical-user interface
CVS	Cardiovascular system	h	Hour
cwt	Hundredweight	Hb	Hemoglobin
CXR	Chest x-ray	HBC	Hit by car
D BILI	Direct bilirubin	HBs	Harsh bronchial sounds
D/S	Dextrose in saline	HC	Health certificate
D₅W	5% dextrose in water	HCT	Hematocrit
Ddx	Differential diagnosis	HIS	Hospital information systems
DEC	Decrease; diethylcarbamazine	HR	Heart rate
DES	Diethylstilbestrol	hs	At bedtime (hora somni)
DHL	Canine distemper-hepatitis-leptosirosis vaccine	HSA	Hemangiosarcoma
		Hx	History
DIC	Disseminated intravascular coagulation	I BILI	Indirect bilirubin
DJD	Degenerative joint disease	IBK	Infectious bovine keratoconjunctivitis
DLH	Domestic longhair	IBR	Infectious bovine rhinotracheitis
DM	Diabetes mellitus	IC	Intracardiac
DMSO	Dimethyl sulfoxide	ICF	Intracellular fluid
DOA	Dead on arrival	ICH	Infectious canine hepatitis
DOS	Disk operating system	ICU	Intensive care unit
DRG	Diagnosis-related group	ID	Intradermal
DS	Dose or days not acceptable	IM	Intramuscular
DSH	Domestic shorthair	IN	Intranasal
DTM	Dermatophyte test medium	IOP	Intraocular pressure
DV	Dorsal ventral	IP	Intraperitoneal
Dx	Diagnosis	ISE	Ion-selective electrode
EAE	Enzootic abortion of ewes	IT	Intratracheal
ECF	Extracellular fluid	IU	International unit
ECG or EKG	Electrocardiogram	IV	Intravenous
ECHO	Echocardiogram	IVD	Intervertebral disk disease
EDTA	Ethylenediaminetetraacetic acid	IVP	Intravenous pyelogram
EEE	Eastern equine encephalomyelitis	K	Potassium
EEG	Electroencephalogram	K-9	Canine
EENT	Eyes, ears, nose, throat	Kcal	Kilocalorie
EFA	Essential fatty acids	KCS	Keratoconjunctivitis sicca
EHV	Equine herpesvirus	kg	Kilogram
EIA	Equine infectious anemia	L or LT	Left
ELISA	Enzyme-linked immunosorbent assay	LBBB	Left bundle branch block
EM	Electron microscopy	LDA	Left displaced abomasum
EMD	Electromechanical dissociation	LDH	Lactate dehydrogenase
EMG	Electromyogram	LN	Lymph node
ER	Emergency room	LRS	Lactated Ringer's solution
ERG	Electroretinogram	LSA	Lymphosarcoma
ESR	Erythrocyte sedimentation rate	m²	Meter squared
F-A	Fecal analysis	MAC	Minimum alveolar concentration
FA	Fluorescent antibody; fatty acids	MAOI	Monoamine oxidase inhibitor
FB	Foreign body	MAP	Mean arterial pressure
FD	Feline distemper	μg	Microgram
FeLV	Feline leukemia virus	μl	Microliter
FeSV	Feline sarcoma virus	mcg	Microgram
FIP	Feline infectious peritonitis	MCH	Mean corpuscular hemoglobin
FIV	Feline immunodeficiency virus	MCHC	Mean corpuscular hemoglobin concentration
FPV	Feline panleukopenia virus		
FSH	Follicle-stimulating hormone	MCT	Mast cell tumor
FUO	Fever of unknown origin	MCV	Mean corpuscular volume
FUS	Feline urologic syndrome	MEA	Mean electrical axis
FVR	Feline viral rhinotracheitis	mEq	Milliequivalents
Fx	Fracture	MER	Maintenance energy requirements
g	Gram	Mg	Magnesium
gal	Gallon	MGP	Marginated granulocyte pool
GAS	General adaptation syndrome	MI	Mitral insufficiency or myocardial insufficiency; myocardial infarction
GDV	Gastric dilation volvulus		
GFR	Glomerular filtration rate	MIC	Minimal inhibitory concentration
GGT	Gamma-glutamyltransferase	MIP	Mare's immunological pregnancy test
GI	Gastrointestinal	ml	Milliliter
gm	Gram	MLV	Modified live virus
GnRH	Gonadotropin-releasing hormone	MM	Mucous membrane
gtt	Drops (guttae)	MRI	Magnetic resonance imaging
GU	Genitourinary	Na	Sodium

NC	No change	q	Every
NCC	Nucleated cell count	q2h	Every 2 hours
NMR	Nuclear magnetic resonance	q6h	Every 6 hours
non rep	Do not repeat	QBC	Quantitative buffy coat
NPL	No palpable lesions	qd	Every day
NPO	Nothing per os (nothing by mouth)	qh	Every hour
NR	Not remarkable	qid	Four times a day
NRBC	Nucleated red blood cell	qns	Quantity not sufficient
NRC	National Research Council	qod	Every other day
NS	Normal saline	qs	Quantity sufficient
NSF	No significant findings	R or RT	Right
NSR	Normal sinus rhythm	RACL	Ruptured anterior cruciate ligament
NVL	No visible lesions	RADs	Radiographs
OB	Obstetrics	RAM	Random access memory
OCD	Osteochondritis dissecans	RAS	Reticular activating system
OD	Right eye (oculus dexter)	RBBB	Right bundle branch block
OFA	Orthopedic Foundation for Animals	RBC	Red blood cell
OHE	Ovariohysterectomy (spray)	RDA	Right displaced abomasum
OL	Left eye	RER	Resting energy requirement
OPP	Ovine progressive pneumonia	Retic	Reticulocyte
OS	Left eye (oculus sinister)	RHF	Right heart failure
OSA	Osteosarcoma	RID	Radical immunodiffusion
OTC	Over the counter	R/O	Rule out
OU	Both eyes	RTG	Ready to go
P	Phosphorus	RV	Rabies vaccination; residual volume
P3	Third phalanx or coffin bone	Rx	Take (prescription)
PAC	Premature atrial contraction	s̄	Without (sine)
PAT	Paroxysmal atrial tachycardia	SC or SQ	Subcutaneous
pc	After meals	SCC	Squamous cell carcinoma
PCV	Packed cell volume	SDH	Sorbitol dehydrogenase
PDA	Patent ductus arteriosus	SGOT	Serum glutamic-oxaloacetic
PDQ	Pretty darned quick		transaminase
PDR	Passive defense reflex	SGPT	Serum glutamic-pyruvate transaminase
PE	Pulmonary edema; physical	Sig	Label (prescription)
	examination	SIM	Sulfide-indole-motility (medium)
PEA	Phenylethyl alcohol	SMEDI	Stillbirths, mummified fetuses, embry-
PEG	Percutaneous endoscopic gastrostomy		onic death, and infertility
per os	Orally, by mouth	SNS	Sympathetic nervous system
PG	Prostaglandin	SOAP	Subjective, objective, assessment, plan
PGA	Polyglycolic acid	SOB	Shortness of breath
PI3	Parainfluenza-3	S/P	Status post
PK	Pigmentary keratitis	sp.	Species
PM	Postmortem	sp. gr.	Specific gravity
PMSG	Pregnant mare serum gonadotropin	SR	Suture removal
PNS	Parasympathetic nervous system	ss	One half
PO	Postoperative, per os	stat	Statum (immediately)
POVMR	Problem-oriented veterinary medicine	Sx	Signs, symptoms
	record	T BILI	Total bilirubin
PPH	Pertinent past history	tab	Tablet
ppm	Parts per million	TAT	Tetanus antitoxin
PPM	Persistent pupillary membrane	TBW	Total body water
PPN	Partial parenteral nutrition	TDN	Total digestible nutrients
PPV	Porcine parvovirus	TEME	Thromboembolic meningoencephalitis
PRA	Progressive retinal atrophy	TGC	Time gain compensation
PRAA	Persistent right aortic arch	TGE	Transmissible gastroenteritis
prn	As necessary	TGEV	Transmissible gastroenteritis virus
PRRS	Porcine reproductive and respiratory	TI	Tricuspid insufficiency
	syndrome	tid	Thrice daily
PRV	Pseudorabies virus	T-L	Thoracolumbar vertebra
PS	Pulmonic stenosis	TLC	Tender loving care
PSS	Physiologic saline	TP	Total protein
PTA	Prior to admission	TPN	Total parenteral nutrition
PTH	Parathyroid hormone	TPP	Total plasma protein
PTS	Put to sleep	TPR	Temperature, pulse, respiration
PTT	Partial thromboplastin time	TR	Trace
PU	Penile urethrostomy	TRF	Thyrotropin-releasing factor
PVC	Premature ventricular contraction	TRH	Thyrotropin-releasing hormone
PWD	Powder	TRIG	Triglycerides

TS-FIPV	Temperature-sensitive feline infectious peritonitis virus
TSH	Thyroid-stimulating hormone
TSI	Triple sugar iron
TT	Tetanus toxoid
Tx	Treatment
U	Unit
UA	Urinalysis
UG	Urogenital
UGI	Upper gastrointestinal tract (includes esophagus, stomach, and duodenum)
ung	Ointment
UO	Urinary obstruction
URI	Upper respiratory infection
US	Ultrasound
USG	Urine specific gravity
UT DICT	As directed (ut dictum)
UTI	Urinary tract infection
v.	Vein

V TACH	Ventricular tachycardia
vc	Vital capacity
VD	Ventral dorsal
V-D	Vomiting and diarrhea
VECCS	Veterinary Emergency and Critical Care Society
VEE	Venezuelan equine encephalomyelitis
VER	Visual evoked response
VES	Ventricular extrasystole
VMDB	Veterinary medical data base
VPC	Ventricular premature contraction
VS	Vital signs
VSD	Ventricular septal defect
VSV	Vesicular stomatitis virus
WBC	White blood cell
WEE	Western equine encephalomyelitis
WNL	Within normal limits
XRT	Radiation therapy

INDEX

f denotes figure; *t* denotes table.